THE COMPLETE
RESOURCE GUIDE FOR
PEOPLE WITH
DISABILITIES

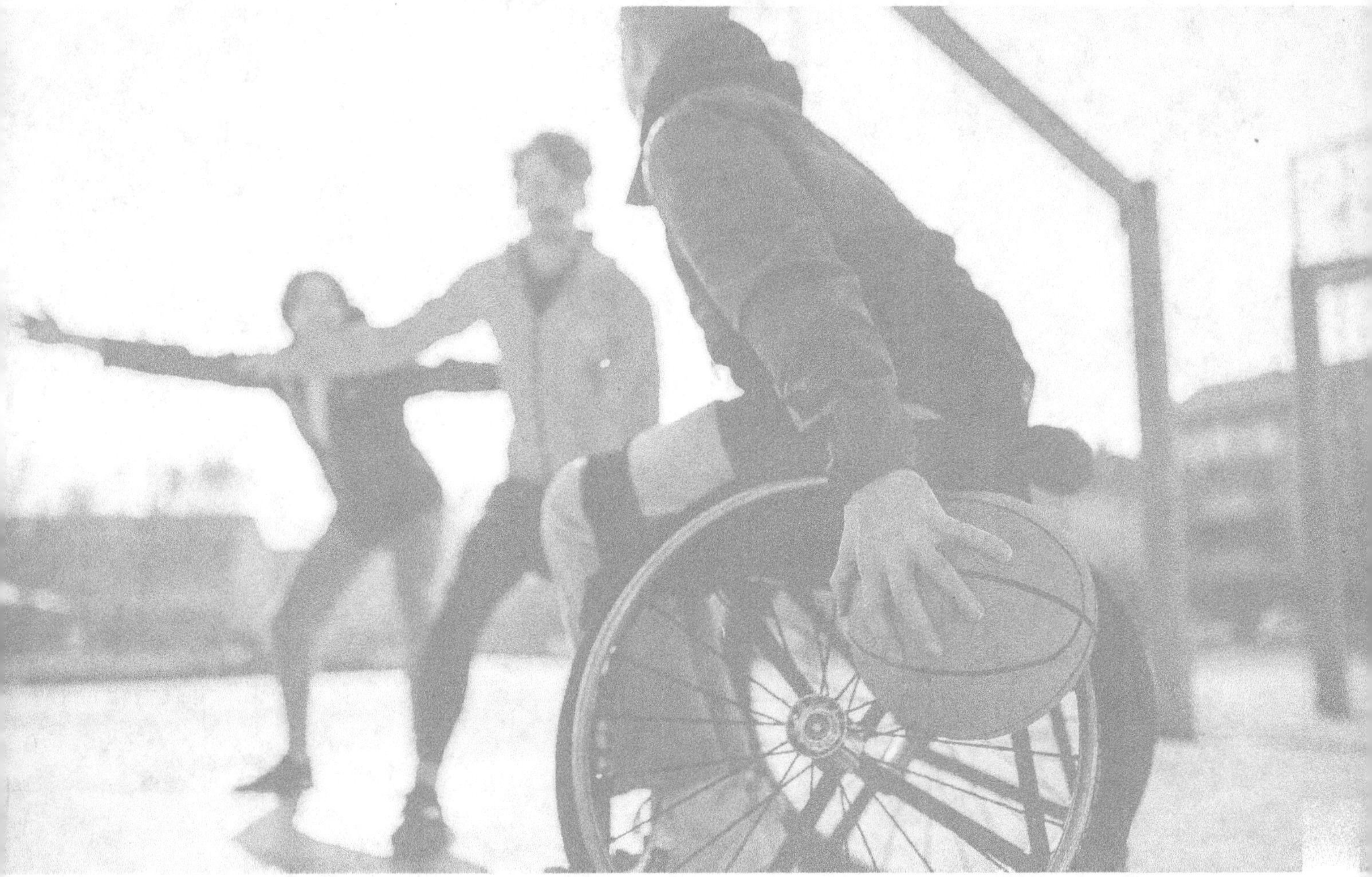

2023
THIRTY-FIRST
EDITION

THE COMPLETE RESOURCE GUIDE FOR
PEOPLE WITH DISABILITIES

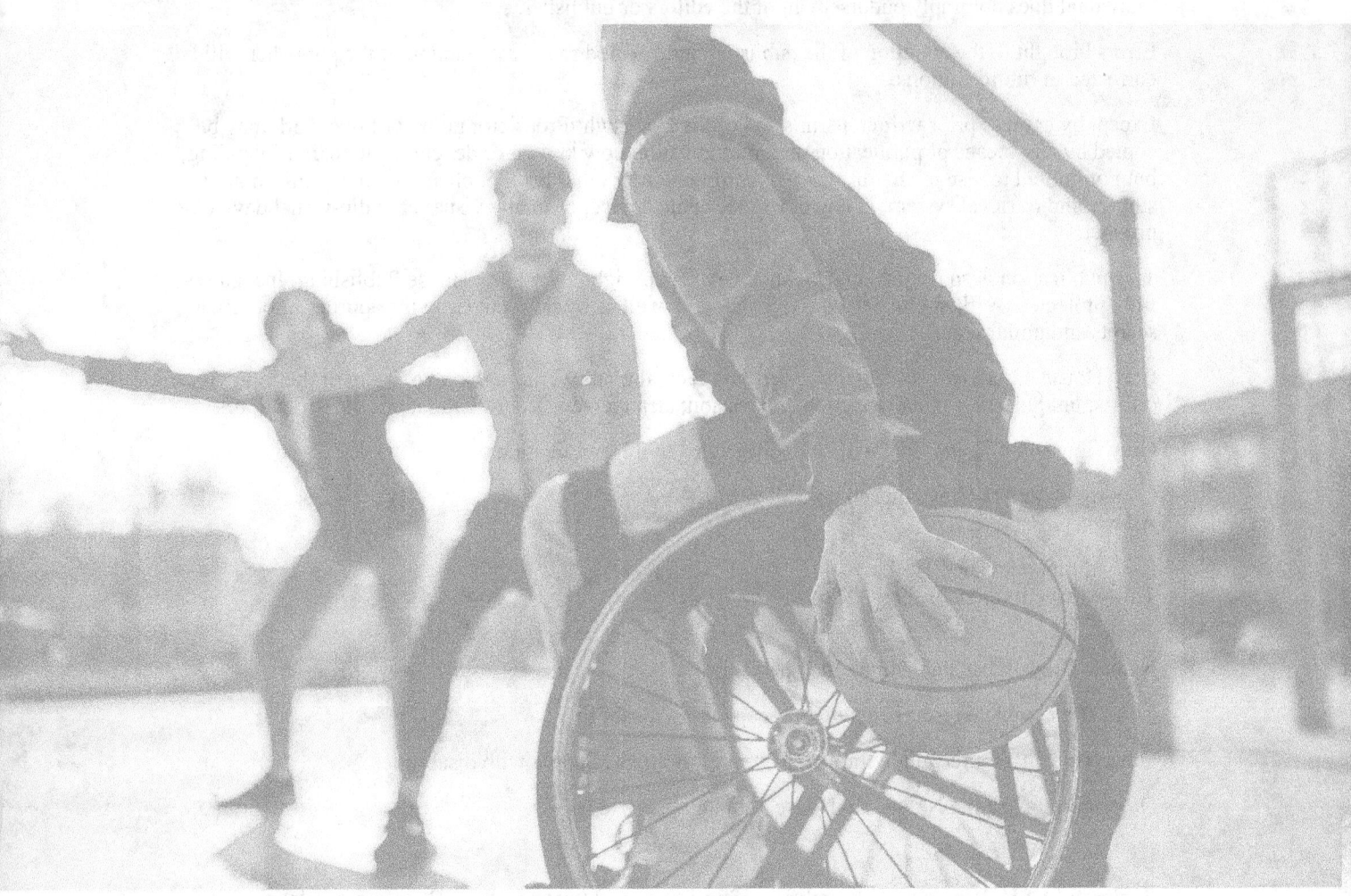

GREY HOUSE PUBLISHING

PUBLISHER: Leslie Mackenzie
EDITORIAL DIRECTOR: Stuart Paterson
STATISTICS: David Garoogian
MARKETING DIRECTOR: Jessica Moody

Grey House Publishing, Inc.
4919 Route 22
Amenia, NY 12501
518.789.8700
Fax: 845.373.6390
www.greyhouse.com
books@greyhouse.com

First edition published 1991
Thirty-first edition published 2022

Names: Grey House Publishing, Inc., publisher.

Title: The complete resource guide for people with disabilities.

Other Titles: Resource guide for people with disabilities | People with disabilities

Description: Amenia, NY : Grey House Publishing, 2018-

Identifiers: ISSN 2643-234X

Subjects: LCSH: People with disabilities—Services for—United States—Directories. | People with disabilities—Services for—United States—Periodicals. | People with disabilities—Services for—United States—Bibliography—Periodicals.

Classification: LCC HV1553 .C58 | DDC 362.4—dc23

Printed in Canada
ISBN 13: 978-1-63700-151-6 Softcover

Table of Contents

Arts & Entertainment

Assistive Devices

Associations

Camps

Clothing

Computers

Table of Contents

Introduction

This 31st edition of the award-winning *Complete Resource Guide for People with Disabilities* is invaluable for all those living with a disability, their personal and professional community, and all those committed to empowering these individuals. It offers thousands of ways for people with disabilities to succeed at work, in school, and in their community.

Careful research and compilation of the best data available maintains the reputation of *The Complete Resource Guide for People with Disabilities* among educators, librarians and the disability community. This resource is a repeat recipient of the **National Mature Media Award** and the **National Health Information Award**.

This comprehensive resource opens with the following valuable front matter:
- An in-depth report on the impact of the COVID-19 pandemic on people living with disabilities, including the following sections: Healthcare; Congregate Care Facilities; The Direct Care Workforce; Education; Employment; Effective Communication; Mental Health and Suicide
- User Guide and Key
- Glossary of Disability-Related Terms

Coverage continues with subject-specific listing sections (i.e. Arts, Assistive Devices, Camps, Vocational Programs), Rehabilitation Facilities, and disability-specific sections (i.e. Aging, Cognitive, Mobility, Speech). Each disability section includes a range of resources from Associations to Support Groups. The comprehensive Table of Contents guides you through the 33 chapters and more than 100 subchapters contained in this rich resource.

Following the listing chapters is a 2020 Annual Disability Statistics Compendium: a robust section of easy-to-read tables featuring the latest available data. The first part of the compendium features numbers of disabled individuals by both state and disability—hearing, vision, cognitive, ambulatory, and self-care and independent-living disabilities—and the second part features individuals who are employed, broken down by the categories listed above.

Sure to save hours of Internet research time, *The Complete Resource Guide for People with Disabilities* provides comprehensive, critical and immediate information in one source that can be accessed quickly and easily. This edition provides 9,192 descriptive listings, 23,365 key contacts, 7,219 fax numbers, 5,804 email addresses, and 8,193 web sites.

Indexes

Three indexes provide quick, easy access to the data.
- **Subject Index** alphabetically organizes directory listings by relevant topics, i.e. autism, language disorders.
- **Geographic Index** organizes listings alphabetically by state.
- **Entry & Publisher Index** lists all directory listings alphabetically.

In addition to the print work, The Complete Resource Guide for People with Disabilities is available by subscription on G.O.L.D., Grey House OnLine Databases. This gives you immediate access to the most valuable disability community contacts in the United States, plus offers easy-to-use keyword searches, organization type and subject searches, hotlinks to web sites and emails, and so much more. Call 800-562-2139 for a free trial or visit http://gold.greyhouse.com for more information.

Praise for previous editions:

> *"This comprehensive directory is an excellent starting point...a very useful resource for public, hospital, and consumer-health libraries as well as social-service agencies and nonprofits serving the disabled."*

—Booklist

> *"The strength of this source is in the information referral portion for each entry: the wide range of resources and organizations presented that can assist with additional information and support."*

—ARBA

> *"...thousands of resources...covering a diverse range of services...separate section for specific disabilities...from aging to mobility and from the blind and deaf to speech and language disorders. Libraries...will want to consider..."*

—Against the Grain

We welcome your comments, and look forward to another year of serving the disability community.

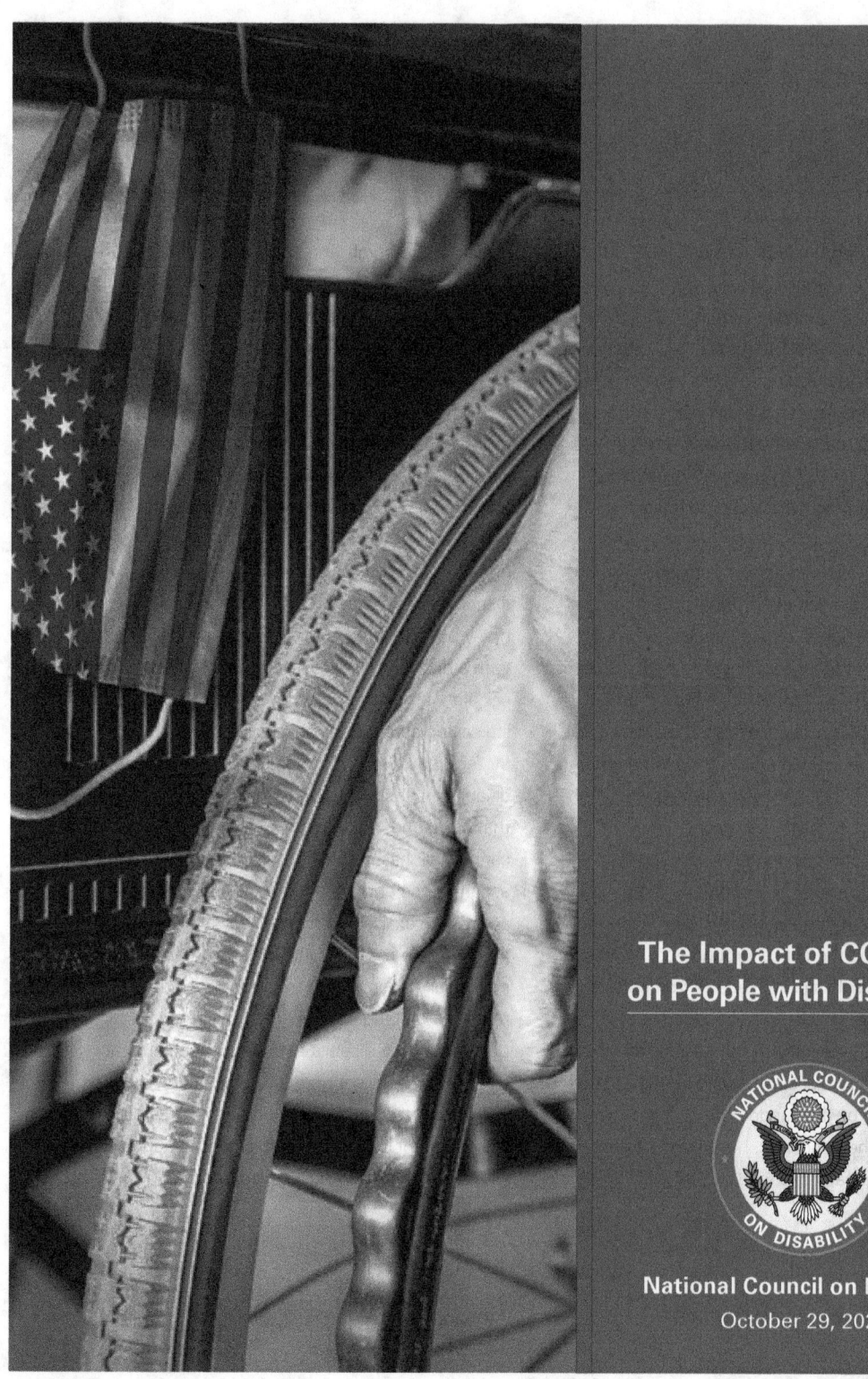

The Impact of COVID-19
on People with Disabilities

National Council on Disability
October 29, 2021

Introduction

When the first case of COVID-19 in the United States was officially confirmed in January 2020, people with disabilities were living their lives: attending schools, working, raising families, enjoying their communities, and planning for the future. The pandemic caused by the novel coronavirus upended the lives of people with disabilities just as it disrupted the lives of nondisabled persons, but this statement does not reveal the full story. By 2020, people with disabilities had spent decades fighting for equal opportunity and their civil rights. Key federal laws such as Section 504 of the Rehabilitation Act of 1973,[1] the Individuals with Disabilities Education Act (IDEA),[2] and the Americans with Disabilities Act[3] had helped people with disabilities integrate into their communities, receive improved educational services, and increase their presence in the workforce, but many barriers remained before the pandemic struck. The impact of the pandemic on people with disabilities cannot be understood without laying the critical groundwork of what living with disabilities looked like immediately before the pandemic. This introduction provides context for the report using brief topical "snapshots" of disability discrimination that were exacerbated by the pandemic.

Prior to the pandemic, health and healthcare disparities already exposed people with disabilities to heightened risk for poor health outcomes.[4] Moreover, despite the fact that people with disabilities are a population subject to healthcare disparities, many healthcare professionals continue to see the poor health outcomes of people with disabilities as an inevitable function of disability rather than an avoidable consequence of accessibility barriers, lack of needed modifications in policies and procedures, and explicit and implicit bias among providers.[5] In 2019, NCD reported that the disability bias of healthcare providers leads many providers to "critically undervalue life with a disability,"[6] representing a real threat to people with disabilities who may be denied life-saving care due to physicians relying on stereotypes about the lives of people with disabilities, including the common assumption that someone who cannot walk or who cannot talk has no quality of life. In addition to assumptions and attitudinal barriers, the lack of accessible examination and medical equipment in medical care means that people with disabilities, specifically people with mobility disabilities, receive substandard primary care compared to people without disabilities.[7] When people with disabilities require a period of acute care, they can encounter denials of their personal care attendants or support persons, even though they benefit greatly from having their regular assistants in the hospital. Prior to the pandemic, hospital policies on support persons were opaque and varied greatly among institutions and among providers, leading to harmful medical results.[8] As a result of these factors, people with disabilities entered the pandemic in a far worse position than people without disabilities. They found themselves in need of intensive care or life-sustaining services and devices, and being treated by emergency room physicians who typically had little or no extended contact with patients who go through their daily lives with chronic disabilities,[9] and who were quick to deem them expendable in a situation where medical resources were becoming scarce. Notably, those physicians who acknowledged ableist medical rationing policies that occurred during the pandemic tended to be specialists who work regularly with people with disabilities.[10]

The pandemic brought renewed attention to the medical, social, and economic vulnerability of those living in CCFs or institutions. The history of people with physical, mental, or developmental disabilities is illustrated by involuntary institutionalization in terrible conditions, even where a facility's origins may have been benign.[11] CCFs are usually justified on the basis that people with significant disabilities could not otherwise survive or stay well, yet recent research across states has found that those states where residents have higher measures of implicit disability prejudice also institutionalize more people, even controlling for state size, and these same states tend to spend more on institutional funding, controlling for both state size and wealth.[12] These facts

[P]eople with disabilities entered the pandemic in a far worse position than people without disabilities.

indicate that disability prejudice has more to do with the assumption that people with disabilities need to be cared for in nursing homes than the objective health needs of people with disabilities. The disability community has long fought to avoid the overuse and misuse of institutions, and this battle was brought to a head in the U.S. Supreme Court decision *Olmstead v. L.C.* in 1999.[13] The Court held that people with disabilities must receive community-based care in the least restrictive environment possible if they are qualified. Unfortunately, many remain confined in institutions because community-based services and supports are lacking. Medicaid, the largest single payer of home- and community-based services (HCBS) has a historic "institutional bias" because federal law requires states to cover institutional care in nursing homes but makes Medicaid coverage of community living through HCBS optional for Medicaid enrollees,[14] even though services in the community are less expensive than institutional care. The reliance on CCFs for lower-income people with disabilities is worsened when housing expenses rise. For example, the approximately 4.8 million people with disabilities who rely on SSI cannot afford to live in their own home, even where home-based care might be available.[15] When natural disasters and public emergencies occurred prior to the pandemic, people with disabilities were often relegated to institutions in contravention of federal law that prohibits institutionalization.[16] When people without disabilities lose their jobs, their income, their housing, their health coverage, or their personal support network, they are not confronted with the specter of institutionalization as are people with disabilities, and especially people with disabilities who have long-term services and supports (LTSS) needs. People with significant disabilities must have access to equally effective healthcare and needed services and supports in their communities, or they are at risk of losing functional capacity and being subject to institutionalization.

The well-being of people with disabilities who have LTSS needs has always been closely intertwined with the well-being of the direct care workforce, including personal care attendants, home health aides, and nursing assistants, who can be employed in institutional, agency, and individual-pay community contexts. Due to the low rates of pay and difficulty with obtaining full-time positions, direct care workers can be holding multiple jobs at the same time,[17] though doing so can inhibit close relationships with individual clients that are of mutual benefit.[18] If people with disabilities are to realize their rights under *Olmstead* and avoid institutionalization, they must have access to a reliable HCBS workforce that is stable in all respects—pay, benefits, job satisfaction, working conditions, and availability. The availability of HCBS permitting persons with disabilities to live in the community is the alternative to living in CCFs, and Medicaid, which issues HCBS waivers to transition people out of institutions to the community, or to keep a person at risk of institutionalization in their home with proper supports,[19] is subject to all kinds of restrictions and policy disagreements among federal and state lawmakers. Well before the pandemic, the direct care workforce was already subject to frequent turnover and a shortage of providers who could supply personal care services throughout the country, particularly as an aging U.S. population added to the demand. Direct care workers are often in short supply due to low wages, the difficulty of maintaining full-time work, and the lack of health insurance for many.[20] In 2019, one in six direct care workers lived below the federal poverty level.[21] The direct care workforce before 2020 was inconsistent because workers had the option of leaving their positions for better paying jobs; thus, people with disabilities have long been struggling to find and maintain direct care workers necessary for their continued health and, for many, even their independence.

Education and employment opportunities are among the many opportunities that are lost when

When people without disabilities lose their jobs, their income, their housing, their health coverage, or their personal support network, they are not confronted with the specter of institutionalization as are people with disabilities . . .

If people with disabilities are to realize their rights under Olmstead *and avoid institutionalization, they must have access to a reliable HCBS workforce that is stable in all respects—pay, benefits, job satisfaction, working conditions, and availability.*

a person is living in a CCF or community with insufficient HCBS to maintain health and critical function. When students with disabilities don't receive educational services that are guaranteed under law, it can affect their social, physical, and emotional well-being and their greatest chances for economic self-sufficiency for the rest of their lives, as well as the lives of the family members who may have to act as unpaid caregivers for extended periods. NCD reported in 2018 that the longstanding federal underfunding of the Individuals with Disabilities Education Act was already adversely affecting the ability of students with disabilities to receive Free and Appropriate Public Education (FAPE), placing many students with disabilities at a disadvantage.[22] There was also a national shortage of special education providers, and qualified staff for in-home education can be wholly unavailable.[23] Coronavirus and the public health emergency have only exacerbated these existing disadvantages.

For years, people with disabilities have been chronically unemployed and underemployed despite the ADA prohibitions on discrimination in employment.[24] Though the ADA prompted a national increase in employment for people with disabilities when it was passed in 1990, there are still significant numbers of people with disabilities "persistently locked out of employment," many of whom rely on federal public assistance programs.[25] For working-age people with disabilities prior to COVID-19, almost "two-thirds of working-age Americans [were] left out of the labor market all together."[26] Despite the many opportunities for employment that an increasingly digital world may provide job-hunters with disabilities, the fastest-growing and most dynamic technology-based industries have the poorest representation of people with disabilities.[27] Looking at employment in the context of education and healthcare for people with disabilities is instructive. The failure to fund the IDEA, discussed above, means that young people with disabilities entering the workforce are twice as likely as their peers without disabilities to have no high school diploma, leaving them unqualified for many jobs.[28] Young people with disabilities (ages 20–24) were nearly 30 percent less likely to be employed than their peers without disabilities. Further, a certain portion of people with disabilities who are counted as employed are working for less than the minimum wage in sheltered workshops, as a consequence of the Fair Labor Standards Act section 14(c).[29] For people with disabilities with significant chronic care needs, and especially for those with personal care assistance needs,

> *Direct care workers are often in short supply due to low wages, the difficulty of maintaining full-time work, and the lack of health insurance for many. In 2019, one in six direct care workers lived below the federal poverty level.*

> *When students with disabilities don't receive educational services that are guaranteed under law, it can affect their social, physical, and emotional well-being and their greatest chances for economic self-sufficiency for the rest of their lives . . .*

Medicaid provides critical services and supports that cannot be easily replicated or afforded. However, the income limits on both Medicaid and the Social Security programs that are a gateway to Medicaid enrollment can also act as a reverse disincentive to employment and income. People with disabilities who get a job and earn too much or get too many hours can fall off the "Medicaid cliff" and find themselves losing the very healthcare services that enable them to work and thrive in their communities while still not earning enough to pay out of pocket for the HCBS that private insurance rarely covers. While federal Medicaid buy-in and work incentive programs can alleviate some of the problems raised by the Medicaid cliff, the programs are administratively challenging to understand and follow and usually offer limited employment supports.[30]

People with sensory disabilities were met with barriers in communication during emergencies well before the COVID-19 pandemic. In 2014, in the wake of several devastating hurricanes, NCD reported that the communications needs of people with disabilities were not being met in emergency settings by either federal or local agencies.[31] The failures of effective communication included, but were not limited to, a lack of American Sign Language (ASL) interpreters in televised announcements, web sites with emergency information not accessible to screen readers, inaccessible emergency notification systems, and inaccessible shelter locations.[32] Even outside of an emergency context, complaints and lawsuits continue to be brought as education,[33] state,[34] and private business entities[35] ignore basic effective communications for thousands of people with disabilities, failing to provide sign language in complex legal matters and only sending benefit eligibility and coverage information to blind persons in print letters. All too often, covered entities seek an easy way out of providing effective communication and place an ongoing burden on the person with a disability to "make do" and adjust to the situation, rather than follow the dictates of federal law. For example, the National Association of the Deaf advises that qualified sign language interpreters are still often the best option in medical settings and that the use of Video Remote Interpreting (VRI) should be reserved for emergencies, reporting with concern that overreliance on VRI has detrimentally impacted Deaf and Hard-of-Hearing healthcare consumers.[36] Failures of communication continued to be unsurprisingly pervasive during the pandemic,[37] placing people with disabilities at an increased likelihood of danger, from the highest levels of public briefings from the White House when the pandemic began (see chapter 6, section E on Government Activities) all the way through to vaccination, a process that began almost a year into the public emergency.[38]

> *Failures of communication continued to be unsurprisingly pervasive during the pandemic, placing people with disabilities at an increased likelihood of danger, from the highest levels of public briefings from the White House when the pandemic began . . . all the way through to vaccination, a process that began almost a year into the public emergency.*

People with a range of disabilities were already at higher risk of experiencing depression and suicidality before the pandemic, due in part to social isolation, abuse, and increased likelihood of living in poverty.[39] These facts were made worse by the lack of accessible mental healthcare for people with disabilities,[40] particularly for people with physical disabilities who found most counselors' offices in inaccessible buildings and tele-mental health services unavailable. Though the Affordable Care Act (ACA) made progress toward expanding mental healthcare for Medicaid coverage, millions of Medicaid-eligible Americans continued to lack access to behavioral health services.[41] Medicaid services reimburse behavioral healthcare providers at lower rates, which contributes to a lack of mental healthcare providers serving people with disabilities who rely on Medicaid.[42] Those with employment or private insurance face cost-control and other embedded gatekeeping barriers to obtaining the mental and behavioral health services they need to maintain well-being and functional capacity in their lives.[43] Stigma, ableism in society, and a lack of coordinated expertise in the medical field also exacerbated mental health problems for people with disabilities. People with co-occurring mental or behavioral health and other disabilities encountered a lack of experience and fragmented communication among their providers, leading to undiagnosed or untreated mental health symptoms.[44]

One final thing to note in the 17 months since COVID-19 first appeared is the growing awareness in the United States and globally of systemic racism and implicit bias against people of color, and how Black, Brown, and Indigenous persons have been subjected to authoritarian violence. In light of increasingly documented links between disability and race/ethnicity,[45] this report tries to note where and when compounded disparities of treatment and outcome occurred during the pandemic; for example, in the educational opportunities of Indigenous children with disabilities or in the application of crisis standards of care to significantly disabled Black persons.

The phrase "a rising tide lifts all boats" is generally used to explain how changes in circumstance or policy that directly benefit some segments in society will nonetheless benefit all in society. Similarly, a pandemic is a great equalizer because the coronavirus's inherent capacity to infect, hospitalize, or kill does not change with a given individual's personal characteristics. Such truisms disregard the extent to which people with disabilities, as with other identifiable groups such as Black and Brown persons or low-income female employees, have endured particular and avoidable harms during the pandemic that are rooted in longstanding physical and programmatic barriers as well as implicit bias and systemic discrimination. When an emergency hits, people with disabilities typically have fewer reserves to draw upon, their options for housing and healthcare are more limited, and it can be harder for them to recover once the immediate emergency has

> *When an emergency hits, people with disabilities typically have fewer reserves to draw upon, their options for housing and healthcare are more limited, and it can be harder for them to recover once the immediate emergency has passed.*

passed. The pandemic has also revealed how much employees with disabilities are among those first to be let go and last to be rehired in an economic crisis. If we focus on the harms that have been universally imposed on all people, we pay insufficient attention to the loss of disability-specific programs and activities that were still needed to ensure effective and equal opportunities for people with disabilities. A rising tide might float all boats, but some of the boats were deep in the sea already, on top of schools of fish, while others were barely clear of sandbars or caught in shoals, far from economic opportunity and freedom from want. In a world where personal characteristics historically determine where one's boat is located in a sea of unequal opportunity, some will be no closer to recovery and well-being post-pandemic.

The pandemic has also revealed how much people with disabilities are among those "first to be let go and last to be rehired" in an economic crisis.

This report will provide data on major life areas where people with disabilities of all ages experienced fallout from the pandemic. We focus specifically on healthcare, congregate care facilities, the direct care workforce, mental health and suicide policy, education, employment, effective communication, and elements of transportation. Beyond data, which is not always available, we try to describe what people with disabilities have been living through as the coronavirus raced through the country. It is the story of disability communities forced to cope with historic systemic failures that continued to have implications for their economic, social, and educational well-being and recommends action to avoid leaving this population behind in a future pandemic or public health emergency.

Chapter 1: Healthcare

Context of COVID-19 and Disability Discrimination in Healthcare

The story of COVID-19[46] in the world and in the United States is one of loss: lost opportunities to prepare for the pandemic, lost time to institute contract tracing and testing, lost chances to rally behind population protocols that would lessen infection, and, ultimately, a terrible loss of physical, mental, emotional, and financial health and life. The global pandemic has raised a multitude of urgent national systemic issues involving the economy, education, employment, business, politics, culture, and race, but more than 17 months and 34 million cases later, the pandemic remains at its core a healthcare crisis. It is no surprise, then, that for people with disabilities who have long endured healthcare discrimination and barriers to equally effective healthcare, COVID-19 was not only a healthcare crisis but an extended test of the nation's recognition of their human and civil rights.

Early press reports on coronavirus cases and deaths in the United States stressed the virus'

When reports of rapid infection and high death rates exploded across the country and within LTCFs, the primary discussion was about the impact of age and rarely acknowledged that more than 14 percent of the residents in those facilities are people with disabilities younger than 65 years.

outsize impact on older persons and people with preexisting conditions, giving the false reassurance that healthy younger people had little to fear. Practically, this approach placed pressure on people with disabilities to withdraw from society while simultaneously lulling the wider public into a false sense of security about relying on hand washing, social distancing, mask wearing, and other behaviors that would reduce community infection rates of a virus that is transmitted through the air. It was an approach that cast people with disabilities and older persons as intrinsically distinct from the rest of society and portrayed them as inevitable victims of a new virus that the rest of us could just "shrug off" like a cold.[47] When reports of rapid infection and high death rates exploded across the country and within LTCFs, the primary discussion was about the impact of age and rarely acknowledged that more than 14 percent of the residents in those facilities are people with disabilities younger than 65 years.[48] The idea that COVID-19 death rates could be diminished by rapidly diverting and deinstitutionalizing people with disabilities from nursing homes was not widely considered, seriously embraced, or explicitly included or funded in federal and state emergency measures. New York, New Jersey, Pennsylvania, and Michigan adopted the reverse policy, ordering nursing homes in the state to admit residents even if they were COVID-19 positive and irrespective of insufficient coronavirus testing, PPE, and infection control procedures in care facilities.[49]

There is no question that the pandemic made it harder for many people with disabilities to be in the world, and equally no doubt that the pandemic exacerbated existing discrimination and inequities experienced by people with disabilities when they sought or received healthcare, as described in this report's introduction. This point was strongly noted in each stakeholder convening that we held. Stereotypes about people with disabilities, inaccessible diagnostic and treatment equipment, and systemic difficulties in obtaining needed accommodations have been documented for years, and led to healthcare disparities for everyone, from women with developmental disabilities seeking gynecological services to Deaf persons needing surgical interventions.[50] The dissemination and use of CSC by states and hospital facilities during the pandemic, which would allow delay or denial of care based on a person's disability or age, was a high-stakes example of long-standing disability stereotypes and implicit bias among healthcare systems and providers.

It is important to point out the fact that civil rights laws protecting people with disabilities apply broadly to the healthcare industry. Federal and state disability nondiscrimination laws have included healthcare entities for decades. Virtually every hospital or healthcare facility is subject to disability rights law because they receive federal financial assistance through, for example, treating Medicaid or Medicare patients,[51] they are part of the programs or activities of a state or local government,[52] or because they are a private healthcare entity that is subject to Title III of the ADA.[53] Health insurers that offer insurance products, including managed care plans, on a federal or state health insurance exchange are subject to Section 1557 of the ACA, which incorporates the disability nondiscrimination protections of Section 504.[54] At this point, healthcare entities have no excuse for failing to recognize that they have nondiscrimination obligations that include requirements for physical accessibility, effective communication, and the obligation to make reasonable modifications in policies, practices, or procedures[55] for people with disabilities.

Key Healthcare Discrimination Issues During the COVID-19 Pandemic

Five aspects of COVID-19 affected the health and well-being of people with disabilities during the pandemic. In one sense, people with disabilities contended with the same challenges of avoiding infection, finding effective treatment in the event of infection, and obtaining vaccination once available that any nondisabled individual faced. But this view discounts how the U.S. healthcare system was rife with physical, communication, programmatic, and attitudinal barriers to healthcare for people with disabilities. People with disabilities were simply not at the same starting line in healthcare when the pandemic hit. The public health emergency led to a few possibly temporary healthcare delivery changes that may benefit some people with disabilities, such as broader coverage and availability of telehealth.[56] For the most part, however, COVID-19 worsened existing barriers.

People with disabilities experienced multiple overlapping layers of healthcare discrimination during the pandemic in the following specific areas: access to personal protective equipment, COVID-19 testing, and the capacity to shelter in place and isolate; medical rationing, CSC, and DNR orders; visitation policies and other healthcare policy modifications and accommodations; and accessible vaccination and vaccination prioritization. Data collection on infection, hospitalization, treatment, and death rates of people with disabilities in the healthcare and public health context is also addressed, as a decades-long dearth in the collection of detailed disability and functional status information has left people with disabilities facing not only the burden of being overlooked, but also bearing the burden, as a group and sometimes individually, of trying to prove their capacity to respond to treatment or their higher susceptibility to COVID-19 before full treatment and vaccination prioritization would be extended to them.

At its worst, these and additional barriers during the pandemic led to people with disabilities losing their lives. Approximately one-third of reported COVID-19 deaths in the United States throughout the pandemic occurred in LTCFs, among a group that makes up only 1 percent to 3 percent of the nation's population depending on what is included in the LTCF category beyond nursing homes.[57] We still do not know if these statistics tell the true number of deaths in these facilities or for those living outside facilities. While nursing home residents are generally thought of primarily as seniors, they are also people with disabilities and include residents aged 31 to 64 years who make up 14 percent of the nursing home population.[58]

Long-term care statistics are likely undercounted for various reasons, including the fact that federal data requirements do not apply to the skilled nursing facilities where hundreds of thousands of people with disabilities live and the complete lack of standardized or historical gathering of death rates among LCTFs.[59] Unfortunately, even though data on the impact of the coronavirus in LTCFs is both incomplete and unreliable, it is among the only data that is available on COVID-19 infection, hospitalization, and death rates of people with disabilities during the pandemic. That is largely because disability status is not a recognized component of mortality data in this country.

People with disabilities were simply not at the same starting line in health care when the pandemic hit . . . For the most part, . . . COVID-19 worsened existing barriers.

The U.S. Standard Certificate of Death contains fields for a limited degree of personal information that the funeral director is responsible for filling in with information derived from an "informant" (usually a relative).[60] These fields include age/date of birth, sex, race, length of residence in a county/state, whether someone has served in the armed forces, marital status and occupation at time of death, names of spouse and/or parents, level of educational attainment, and the informant's name. There is no space for recording disability status as a demographic characteristic of a deceased person. The middle "cause of death" section on the certificate must be filled out by the person who pronounces or certifies death, usually a medical examiner or coroner.[61] This section requires an "underlying cause of death" and has room for "conditions, if any, leading to" the primary cause of death, as well as "other significant conditions contributing to death but not resulting in the underlying cause." There are also a few questions concerning tobacco use, current or past pregnancy, and the manner of death that have public health value to the NCHS, which eventually receives and compiles death certificate information.

When organizations such as the Kaiser Family Foundation sounded the early alarm on how Black, Hispanic, and American Indian and Alaska Native populations were bearing a disproportionate burden of COVID-19 cases, hospitalization, and deaths,[62] the analysis was grounded in state data on provisional death counts made available by the NCHS, as well as race/ethnicity population distribution information from surveys such as the American Community Survey.[63] Because disability status as a demographic fact is not required or asked on death certificates, it is extremely difficult to establish even the bare fact of how many people with disabilities died from COVID-19, and we know even less about the personal characteristics or health of those who have died. As a result, more time-consuming and original analytical research has to be conducted. The elevated risks of coronavirus infection and death among nonelderly people with disabilities who receive Medicaid HCBS, for example, was established

Because disability status as a demographic fact is not required or asked on death certificates, it is extremely difficult to establish . . . how many people with disabilities died from COVID-19 . . .

using source data from published private insurance data claims, Medicaid data, National Health Interview Survey data, and a gradually growing stream of medical research on specific "high-risk" health conditions and disabilities.[64] It is still not, however, an actual count of the numbers of COVID-19 infections or deaths of people with disabilities who have died directly as a result of contracting COVID-19, or indirectly as a consequence of being unable to gain access to needed care or losing necessary services and supports during the pandemic.[65] CDC has reported, with regard to medical care, that:

Avoidance of both urgent or emergency and routine medical care because of COVID-19 concerns was highly prevalent among unpaid caregivers for adults, respondents with two or more underlying medical conditions, and persons with disabilities. For caregivers who reported caring for adults at increased risk for severe COVID-19, concern about exposure of care recipients might contribute to care avoidance. Persons with underlying medical conditions that increase their risk for severe COVID-19 are more likely to require care to monitor and treat these conditions, potentially contributing to their more frequent report of avoidance. (Internal citations omitted)[66]

For people with disabilities, the fact that they vanish as a demographic population when COVID-19 deaths are reported except in so far as they overlap with the population of institutionalized persons raises an overarching discrimination issue that has persisted throughout the public health emergency. The Supreme Court's 1999 decision in *Olmstead v. L.C.*[67] established that people with disabilities have the right to receive state or another public entity's services in the most integrated setting. Yet, as the next two chapters on CCFs and the direct care workforce document, persistent systemic, economic, and legal barriers hinder the capacity of people with disabilities to live independently in the communities of their choice with appropriate supports and services. The "institutional bias" in Medicaid means public funding of institutional long-term care is mandatory, although states have the option of providing HCBS.[68] At the same time, the direct care workforce's decades of poor pay and a lack of worker protections for physically and emotionally demanding work have contributed to a worsening shortage of the direct care workforce on which people with disabilities rely.[69] During the pandemic, the long-standing insufficiency of emergency direct service back-up systems for those living in the community also threatened people with disabilities as their usual personal care assistants became ill or had to take care of ill family members or supervise children when schools and daycares were closed.

The public health emergency starkly revealed how institutionalized people with disabilities are at risk of extreme isolation from family and community and subject to infection and loss of life. Yet a number of states at the height of COVID-19 adopted policies that *required nursing homes to readmit COVID-19 positive residents from hospitals*, placing all residents and staff at heightened risk, rather than provide residents with safer community placements and HCBS using innovative practices such as those discussed in the following chapter. This disregard for the safety of people with disabilities is yet another example of the degree to which people with disabilities were discounted in the pandemic—left off of basic data gathering on death certificates, left out of emergency planning and distribution of supplies, and subject to ongoing stereotypes and assumptions about their health and quality of life by healthcare providers, which led to further deadly consequences for people with disabilities who needed urgent intensive care at the height of the pandemic. Although the federal government funded programs in May 2020 to address some emergency preparedness issues related to the needs of people with disabilities, the results of that work could not be realized quickly enough to change the unnecessary deaths and general treatment of people with disabilities during this pandemic.[70]

The life of a person with disabilities is neither more nor less valuable than the life of a person without disabilities. But when people with disabilities lost their lives because they were unnecessarily housed in CCFs where infectious diseases cannot be controlled, or COVID-19

> *[A] number of states at the height of COVID-19 adopted policies that required nursing homes to readmit COVID-19 positive residents from hospitals, placing all residents and staff at heightened risk, rather than provide residents with safer community placements and HCBS . . .*

treatment was denied because of discriminatory medical rationing, or because states failed to recognize that people with significant disability need priority for vaccination because they are subject to higher risks of infection and death, these were not only "pandemic losses." These lives were lost due to the devaluation of the lives of people with disabilities, a devaluation that is rooted in the medical establishment and that continues to pervade our educational, economic, cultural, and social systems.

Individuals with disabilities who could not drive or carry packages on their own, or shop or assess their PPE needs independently, and who did not have internet access or funds to spare on unbudgeted expenses, found it extremely difficult to find and maintain a PPE supply.

Access to Personal Protective Equipment, COVID-19 Testing, Capacity to Shelter in Place and Isolate

Once the highly infectious nature of the coronavirus became widely known, federal agencies and infectious disease experts recommended key strategies for staying safe that included the consistent use of personal protective equipment, regular testing for COVID-19, and isolating in place as much as possible, including self-quarantine in the event of a positive COVID-19 test. People with a range of disabilities encountered numerous barriers to achieving these strategies.

The public demand for PPE such as fitted masks, gloves, and gowns, as well as hand sanitizer and wipes, quickly overwhelmed the U.S. supply, which was simultaneously subject to a worldwide shortage.[71] Some individual market abuses and instances of PPE price gouging became almost legendary.[72] Letting purchasing

and distribution responsibilities for PPE float freely in an overheated free market environment pitted states against the federal government and individual consumers against workplaces and healthcare facilities. Those individuals with the time and resources to readily monitor for, drive to, and quickly snap up supplies were instantly at an advantage. Individuals with disabilities who could not drive or carry packages on their own, or shop or assess their PPE needs independently, and who did not have internet access or funds to spare on unbudgeted expenses, found it extremely difficult to find and maintain a PPE supply. People with long-term care needs were especially vulnerable to coronavirus infection because the direct care workers who came to their homes to provide care were often the last in line to have access to PPE, as is documented in chapter 3.

Another shortage that left people with disabilities at a disadvantage was the inaccessibility of many COVID-19 testing sites, including the procedures for making testing appointments. The Federal Emergency Management Agency (FEMA) noted that people with disabilities nationwide encountered "[l]imited access to effective communication, facilities, transportation, and programs that allow for improved access to COVID-19 treatment, testing sites, and Alternate Care Sites. . . ." Drive-through testing sites became common in many parts of the country because they allowed for

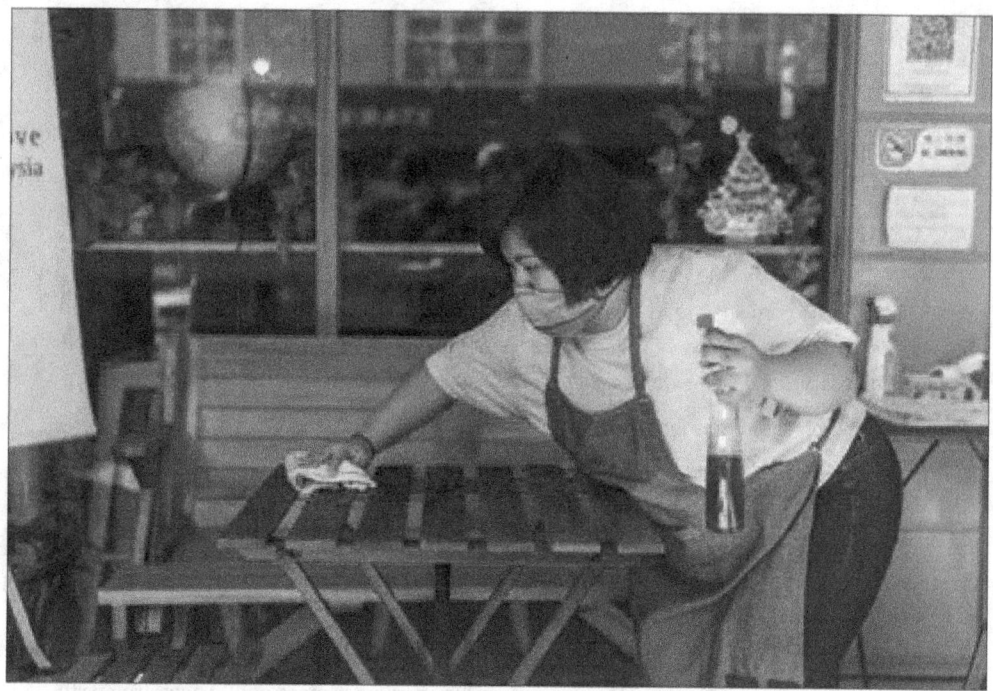

greater social distancing between those seeking and those administering tests, but FEMA further warned that "[p]eople with disabilities may not be able to access COVID-19 testing sites which include, but are not limited to, community-based drive-through testing sites. Drive-through testing is especially inaccessible in urban areas, where fewer people have access to cars."[73]

Additional testing barriers included physical inaccessibility and procedural barriers such as long lines, inaccessible online portals for making test appointments, and a lack of sign language or other interpreters on-site given that anyone who has not taken a test could be shocked by the physical invasiveness of the procedure if an explanation for how the procedure works is not effectively communicated.[74]

Though test manufacturer shortages, unclear information about the accuracy and interpretation of different types of tests, and delays in getting results affected every person who sought testing, the problems had a disproportionate impact on persons with disabilities who relied on personal care assistants. Given the low minimum wages common to direct care workforce jobs, as well as the fact that individuals with disabilities may typically need less than 40 hours per week of personal care attendance, many direct care workers work for more than one client or in both institutional and community settings. When PPE and timely testing are not consistently available in any one of those situations, it left the direct care worker with an elevated coronavirus infection risk and constant uncertainty about their COVID-19 status. In turn, those negatively affected individuals with significant disabilities who received direct care assistance because they faced additional risks of death upon infection from the way their disabilities could interact with the virus *and* the risk that they could be prioritized lower to receive treatment for COVID-19.

Barriers to Goods and Services

Multiple factors combined to turn "shelter in place" orders for persons with disabilities into an extended period of isolation with little access to needed COVID-19 resources or other needed goods and services. People with specific disabilities experienced the following barriers:

- The common use of opaque face masks diminished communication for Hard-of-Hearing and Deaf persons trying to meet their daily needs and get healthcare.

- Transit systems that stopped completely or cut routes and hours made it difficult for people with mobility, vision, and other disabilities to get beyond their immediate neighborhoods, not only because routes themselves were cut but because it was difficult to get timely, accurate, and fully accessible information about changed routes and times.[75]

- Reduced accessibility to transportation in conjunction with lower income levels[76] and having high-risk conditions such as a compromised immune system or other chronic health conditions left some individuals with disabilities unable to get essentials such as groceries and medicines.[77] Food insecurity among U.S. households grew overall during the pandemic but "[a]dults who have a disability—in particular adults who have a disability and are not in the work force—also experience more than two times the rate of food insecurity as adults who do not have a disability."[78] Some food banks began distributing food using a drive-through model, but not all food banks adapted to provide home delivery to people with disabilities who did not independently drive or lift groceries. In rural areas, grocery and food delivery options were already limited and were further limited by store policies that did not allow people with Supplemental Nutritional Assistance Program (SNAP) or food stamps to use those benefits for home delivery of groceries.[79]

- Individuals at high risk of death from contracting COVID-19 had to risk exposure to receive necessary healthcare such as infusions or therapy, or forego the services and therapies that allowed them to maintain function and good health; some healthcare providers stopped certain treatments altogether.

- Individuals who needed assistance with activities of daily living and became infected with the virus faced being unable to keep or find new personal care assistants for their most basic needs, given the heightened risk of infection.

In short, people with disabilities who lived in the community were confronted daily with choosing between life necessities such as food and healthcare and high risks of infection with COVID-19, which led to the risk of forgoing personal assistance from a direct care worker who might not be able to access PPE or of losing assistants who became ill or stopped working because they were afraid of bringing the virus home to their families.

News media quickly covered the "perfect storm" of medically and/or cognitively vulnerable and often older residents living in facilities with well-documented infection control problems and tragic state policies that encouraged keeping or even returning infectious residents at some facilities, but similar attention has not been given to the situation of people with disabilities living in the community, for whom there is a dearth of detailed demographic data. Without this data and analyses, it is extremely hard to get a full picture of how much emergency Medicaid and other measures developed as a response to the pandemic benefitted people with disabilities in the community at large, and even more difficult to try and see, for example, if subpopulations within the disability community, such as Black or Brown persons, face discernible compound discrimination.

> [T]esting barriers included physical inaccessibility and procedural barriers such as long lines, inaccessible online portals for making test appointments, and a lack of sign language or other interpreters on-site given that anyone who has not taken a test could be shocked by the physical invasiveness of the procedure if an explanation for how the procedure works is not effectively communicated.

One study that tried to determine if COVID-19 had a disparate impact among people with disabilities who are subject to sociogeographic disadvantage analyzed county-level data on confirmed COVID-19 cases from Johns Hopkins with a number of disability variables from the 2018 American Community Survey. What may be the first study published in the United States to look at disability from an explicit intersectional lens during the pandemic found that:

> Greater COVID-19 incidence rate is significantly associated with: (1) higher percentages of PwDs [people with disabilities] who are Black, Asian, Hispanic, Native American, below poverty, under 18 years of age, and female; and (2) lower percentages of PwDs who are non-Hispanic White, above poverty, aged 65 or more years, and male, after controlling for spatial clustering. . . . Socio-demographically disadvantaged PwDs are significantly overrepresented in counties with higher COVID-19 incidence compared to other PwDs.[80]

This study helps demonstrates the need for much better data collection on people with disabilities and their experiences during COVID-19 in ways that will allow for a nuanced look at how

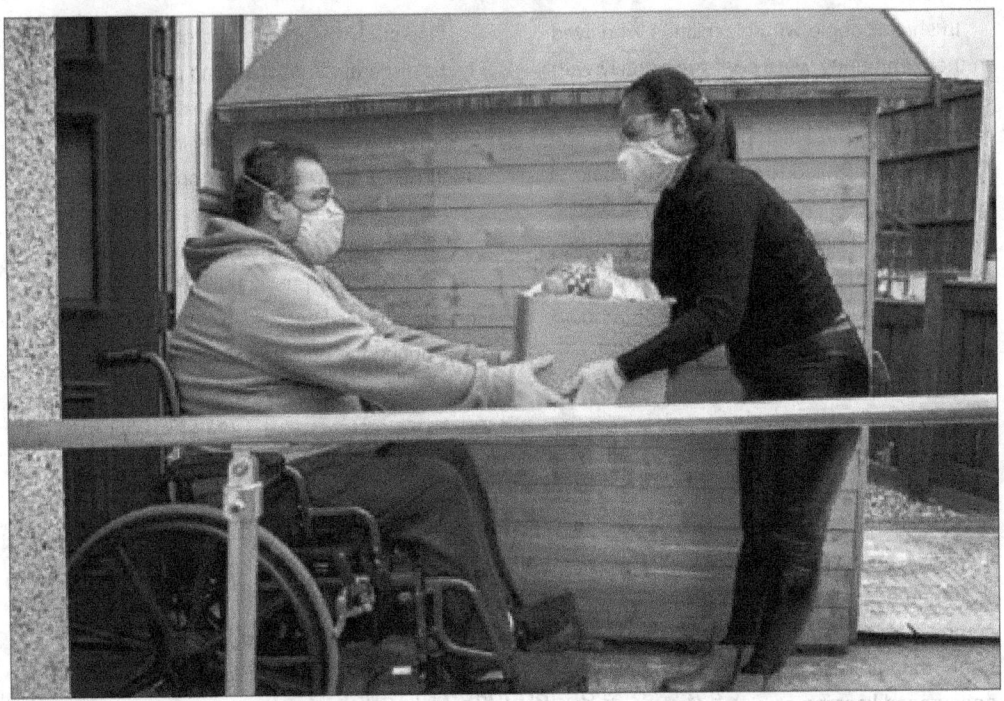

Findings from Study of Disability from an Intersectional Lenses

Greater COVID-19 incidence rate is significantly associated with: (1) higher percentages of PwDs [people with disabilities] who are Black, Asian, Hispanic, Native American, below poverty, under 18 years of age, and female; and (2) lower percentages of PwDs who are non-Hispanic White, above poverty, aged 65 or more years, and male, after controlling for spatial clustering. . . .Socio-demographically disadvantaged PwDs are significantly overrepresented in counties with higher COVID-19 incidence compared to other PwDs.

disability, for example, makes a further difference to the health disparities that Black persons and people of color already face because of race.

Medical Rationing, Crisis Standards of Care, and Do Not Resuscitate Orders

The issue of medical rationing and how intensive care beds, treatment, equipment, and personnel would be made available during a period of widespread simultaneous virus infection emerged early during the pandemic. Stories of overwhelmed health systems and providers in Italy were soon followed by surge circumstances closer to home in places such as New York City. A medical surge occurs when the number of patients needing care is greater than a hospital or health system's capacity to serve those patients. When a surge threatens, some facilities have policies to guide doctors and staff on the standards of care that should be applied when there are not enough beds, medical supplies or equipment, or trained staff to provide a normal level of care (i.e., doing everything possible to save every life) to every current or imminently expected patient. In response, some states revived or put out CSC guidelines in spring 2020.

The application of CSC guidelines during the pandemic profoundly affected people with disabilities, family members, disability advocates, and even many members of the public who were surprised that they could be denied medical care at the moment in which it was most needed. Why did a different set of rules evolve, and how could those rules apply when so few had provided input or even knew what the rules were?

What might be termed the "modern era" of CSC guidelines in the United States can be traced to the terrorist attacks of September 11, 2001, and subsequent fears of anthrax attacks. As the federal Agency for Healthcare Research and Quality (AHRQ) started to work on national plans to respond to bioterrorism and public health emergencies, it came to recognize that an event with mass casualties could at least temporarily overwhelm local or regional health systems and prevent the application of normal standards of medical care. AHRQ convened

The application of CSC guidelines during the pandemic profoundly affected people with disabilities, family members, disability advocates, and even many members of the public who were surprised that they could be denied medical care at the moment in which it was most needed.

experts in "the fields of bioethics, emergency medicine, emergency management, health administration, health law and policy, and public health" in August 2004, and eventually published "Altered Standards of Care in Mass Casualty Events."[81] The document states explicitly that the overall goal of altering standards of care in a mass casualty event is "to save as many lives as possible."[82] The Institute of Medicine subsequently held a series of workshops and published a 2009 letter report on developing CSC guidelines for disaster situations.[83] The letter report concluded that:

"[i]n an important ethical sense, entering a crisis standards of care mode is not optional—it is a forced choice, based on the emerging situation. Under such circumstances, failing to make substantive adjustments to care operations—i.e., not to adopt crisis standards of care—is very likely to result in greater death, injury, or illness." The committee also concluded that there is an urgent and clear need for a single national guidance for states with crisis standards of care that can be generalized to all crisis events and is not specific to a certain event.[84]

This short background on CSC reveals that when CSC guidelines are triggered and how they apply are thought of as matters for medical and policy experts. The Institute of Medicine letter report was written in response to a request by the HHS Office of the Assistant Secretary for Preparedness and Response. Subsequent publications by both AHRQ and the Institute of Medicine addressing CSC criteria similarly involved convenings of experts. It is unclear whether any of the federal or academic entities that worked on these CSC reports prioritized participation or engagement with members of the public who would be directly affected by CSC guidelines, though AHRQ describes "issues related to populations with special needs" as an "important nonmedical" issue. The tendency toward "expert delegation" is highlighted in a recent paper that analyzes how state and hospital CSC guidance changed over the course of the pandemic in response to the assertion of disability rights and nondiscrimination.[85]

CSC guidelines varied considerably among states, with some several years old and designed for an indeterminate public health emergency or a generic "flu" epidemic/pandemic, and others updated or developed specifically for the highly infectious novel coronavirus. As COVID-19 cases and hospitalizations spiked in several states in the spring of 2020, the disability community became increasingly aware of the impact that CSC guidelines could have on individuals with disabilities who sought medical treatment upon infection with the coronavirus. People with disabilities and disability advocates recognized how CSC language approved by medical and policy experts discriminated, both explicitly and implicitly, on the basis of disability in the following ways:

Methods of Discrimination in CSC Guidelines

1. *Categorical exclusion on the basis of specific diagnosis or categories of disability*: One example of a categorical exclusion is found in Florida's 2011 CSC guideline that barred from hospital admission individuals with "complex disorders with significant neurological component and prognosis for imminent expected lifelong assistance with most basic activities of living (i.e., toileting, dressing, feeding, respiration)."[86] Another example is found in Colorado's CSC guideline that lists "cystic fibrosis with post-bronchodilator FEV1 <30% or baseline Pa02 <55 mm Hg" as criteria for excluding an individual from admission or transfer to critical care.[87] The origins of the cystic fibrosis exclusion can be traced to a 2004 CSC guideline developed in Ontario, Canada, that based this diagnostic exclusion on a study published in 1992 that used cohort data derived between 1977 and 1989. In short, the categorical exclusion of people with cystic fibrosis who meet certain clinical criteria was based on 40-year-old mortality data.[88] There is no reason to think that other states

Methods of Discrimination in CSC Guidelines: *continued*

and hospital systems were or are using the most current or even more current medical research when developing criteria for deprioritizing individuals with certain disabilities or health conditions, especially where CSC guidelines were developed in the midst of an ongoing emergency situation. Individuals with intellectual or developmental disabilities and their families in Washington and Alabama raised strong allegations that those states' CSC guidelines discriminate against people with cognitive disabilities by deprioritizing their access to ventilators. Alabama's CSC guideline from early 2020 stated that "persons with severe mental retardation, advanced dementia or severe traumatic brain injury may be poor candidates for ventilator support" and "persons with severe or profound mental retardation, moderate to severe dementia, or catastrophic neurological complications such as persistent vegetative state are unlikely candidates for ventilator support."[89] The state's CSC guideline was revised in April 2020 after disability rights groups filed a formal discrimination complaint with HHS OCR.[90]

2. *Application of medical rationing or triage criteria that allow or encourage physicians to import their subjective assumptions about a patient's length or quality of life:* An example of this can be found in Washington State's CSC guideline that states that individuals can be considered for removal to out-patient or palliative care on the basis of "[b]aseline functional status (consider loss of reserves in energy, physical ability, cognition and general health)."[91] Given that hospital physicians will be unfamiliar with the energy levels, physical ability, cognition levels, or general health of virtually every patient brought to the hospital with COVID-19, this appears to be an open invitation for physicians to make admission and treatment decisions that rest on how a physician interprets the current "functional status" of a person with disabilities.

3. *Relying on physician assessments of years of remaining life in the long or medium term, despite the notorious and established inaccuracy of such assessments:* Some CSC guidelines prioritize the goal of saving "life years" rather than saving lives. Pennsylvania, for example, considers a patient's "prognosis for long-term survival," assessing a patient's comorbid conditions with the goal to "save the most life-years."[92] (See Pennsylvania Department of Health.) A goal of maximizing life years not only shortchanges the value of both people with disabilities and older persons, it invites physicians to make predictions about life expectancy even though they are notoriously bad at doing so.[93] It also penalizes people with disabilities with conditions that appear to have shorter life spans, regardless of whether that information reflects unequal medical treatment, physician stereotypes

(continued)

Methods of Discrimination in CSC Guidelines: *continued*

about a disability, or a dearth of medical research into a particular condition, or is simply outdated.[94]

4. *Failing to recognize or make any kind of adjustment for the impact of disability on the clinical measures that were applied to determine patient priority for COVID-19 treatment:* Many CSC guidelines elevated the use of medical assessment tools such as the Sequential Organ Failure Assessment (SOFA), developed as a way to measure how likely patients' with sepsis were to survive in the near term, as a way to objectively assign a clinical priority score to individual patients for COVID-19 treatment. However, these tools commonly use variables that fail to take disability into account when they should. For example, the SOFA includes the Glasgow Coma Score as a component that measures a patient's consciousness level partly through their ability to articulate intelligible words. People with developmental, speech, hearing, or other disabilities may not be able to articulate intelligible words but that would not signal anything about their conscious functioning. As another example, clinicians should use clinical judgment to adjust SOFA scores downward (the higher the score the lower the chances of survival) as appropriate to account for chronic baseline levels of physiological functional impairment that are not caused by COVID-19, such as low oxygenation ratios for individuals with post-polio or complex neuromuscular conditions who use ventilation to support the muscles around the lungs rather than because of any functional incapacity in the lungs themselves. It is discriminatory to not adjust the application of SOFA or other tools so that they do not automatically and unjustly equate long-term functional impairments with lower survivability.[95]

5. *Refusing to allow individuals to use their personal ventilators during hospitalization and maintaining the possibility of redistributing private ventilators:* People with a range of disabilities use personal ventilators to assist their breathing for some or all of their day. This equipment is personally calibrated to the individual user and medically necessary for maintaining that individual's life and function. Other persons with disabilities may use personal ventilators on a more intermittent "as needed" basis. Personal ventilator users became concerned that some CSC guidelines would allow hospitals to reallocate personal ventilators for the use of patients deemed to have a better chance of benefitting from COVID-19 treatment; some community members became fearful that not only would they be denied treatment if they arrived at a hospital with COVID-19, they risked active harm and death if their ventilator were taken from them.[96] Disability rights advocates in Kansas and in New York raised concerns about personal ventilator reallocation with the

Methods of Discrimination in CSC Guidelines: *continued*

HHS Office for Civil Rights last spring,[97] though the concern has been raised in New York since 2009.[98] New York's Governor Cuomo issued an executive order in April 2020, calling upon nonhospital facilities to give up their ventilators as much as possible so they could be used in intensive care units (ICUs) for COVID-19 treatment.[99] Nursing homes were not captured in the executive order, but a nursing home in Long Island voluntarily lent 11 of its 16 ventilators out to a hospital when asked to do so.[100] This specific concern of personal ventilator allocation resonates strongly within the disability community and raised the specter of medical experts making decisions that would lead directly to the death of people with disabilities. Some of these experts have pointed out that "taking away someone's PV [personal ventilator] is a direct assault on their bodily and social integrity, that PVs should not be part of reallocation pools, and that triage protocols should be immediately clarified and explicitly state that PVs will be protected in all cases."[101]

We cannot know whether the above practices found in CSC guidelines were developed with discriminatory intent, but the practices, if acted upon, would deny life-saving care based on a preexisting disability. The presence or absence of individual or even systemic malice is neither relevant nor a defense. As disability rights advocates pointed out:

Congress intended disability nondiscrimination protections to reach not only discrimination that is the result of "invidious animus," but also of "thoughtlessness," "indifference," and "benign neglect." The implementing regulations make clear that illegal discrimination includes providing "an aid, benefit, or service that is not as effective in affording equal opportunity to obtain the same result, to gain the same benefit, or to reach the same level of achievement" as that provided to people without disabilities; and also "eligibility criteria that screen out or tend to screen out an individual with a disability or any class of individuals with disabilities from fully and equally enjoying any service, program, or activity." No provision in the ADA, Section 504, or Section 1557 of the ACA nor in any other federal law authorizes the waiver of these requirements during a public health emergency. [Internal citations omitted][102]

The CSC guidelines . . . and others like them are discriminatory when their application tends to automatically place people with disabilities in a lower priority category for receiving COVID-19 treatment.

The CSC guidelines highlighted above and others like them are discriminatory when their application tends to automatically place people with disabilities in a lower priority category for receiving COVID-19 treatment. The guidelines establish this priority if they do not require an individualized assessment of whether an individual with disabilities could benefit from the treatment, without consideration for whether a particular disability requires modification of the guideline's application to have an equal opportunity for treatment, and absent any examination of whether and how implicit disability bias influences physicians' clinical perceptions and policymakers' understanding of efficient and fair decision-making. This last point has implications beyond the immediate topic of CSC guidance.

Implicit disability bias was the common factor in prepandemic healthcare discrimination to early pandemic CSC guidelines that devalued the lives of people with disabilities to later vaccine prioritizations that ignored how people with disabilities receiving HCBS and their caregivers were at high risk from the coronavirus. CSC guidelines were developed by experts from many fields who are subject to many kinds of disability bias. Many CSC guidelines recommend a triage panel to make treatment prioritization decisions with a required bioethicist on the panel to provide ethical counterweight to utilitarian concerns, but many bioethicists have utilitarian beliefs as well—that disabled lives are less valuable and, as such, it is ethical to devalue or even deny care when resources become scarce. Bioethicists are not immune from holding implicit biases of their own.

An examination of CSC guidelines developed or repurposed for the coronavirus pandemic makes clear that CSC drafters failed to understand the lived experience and goals of people with disabilities, especially those living in the community using HCBS; failed to understand the value and quality of life of people with disabilities; failed to acknowledge the myriad barriers and failures to accommodate that people with disabilities commonly encounter in the healthcare setting; and assumed that medical providers will do what is best for people with disabilities even when there is a growing body of research confirming that healthcare professions are rife with false assumptions about living with disability and uncomfortable with treating people with chronic conditions who cannot be "cured" or "fixed."[103]

A recent study of physician attitudes toward people with disabilities, released in early 2021, captured the prepandemic views of more than 700 U.S. physicians in active practice across the country.[104] More than 80 percent self-reported

> *Implicit disability bias was the common factor in prepandemic health care discrimination to early pandemic CSC guidelines that devalued the lives of people with disabilities to later vaccine prioritizations that ignored how people with disabilities receiving HCBS and their caregivers were at high risk from the coronavirus.*

> *More than 80 percent [of over 700 U.S. physicians] self-reported the belief that people with significant disabilities have a worse quality of life than nondisabled people.*

the belief that people with significant disabilities have a worse quality of life than nondisabled people. As the study's authors point out, it would be difficult to imagine four out of five physicians freely stating that Black people have a worse quality of life than white people, though some might indicate that Black people face significant challenges in their life from things such as police violence or systemic racism in housing, employment, and other major areas. However, only about 18 percent of this same group "strongly agreed that the healthcare system often treats [disabled] patients unfairly."[105] Taken together, these two findings indicate that physicians base the perceived lack of quality of life for people with disabilities on the fact of the disability, not in how people with disabilities are treated when they seek healthcare. At the same time, "only 40.7% of physicians were very confident about their ability to provide the same quality of care to patients with disability" and "just 56.5% strongly agreed that they welcomed patients with disability into their practices."[106] Interpreting these two figures together, it is clear that a minority of physicians do not feel fully confident in their ability to provide quality care to people with disabilities, and a small majority agree that they welcome patients with disabilities. This leaves about 16 percent of surveyed doctors who welcome patients with disabilities even though they are not very confident that they can provide those patients with the same quality of care that they give to nondisabled patients. This

"[O]nly 40.7% of physicians were very confident about their ability to provide the same quality of care to patients with disability" and "just 56.5% strongly agreed that they welcomed patients with disability into their practices."

discrepancy leads again to the inference that at least some physicians attribute the challenge of providing quality care to people with disabilities to the fact of disability, not seeing it as a problem that is sourced in doctors or that physicians should address by improving their abilities to provide quality healthcare individually or as a group.

CSC guidelines, whether issued by states, health systems, or hospitals, all make the physician a key decision maker and, sometimes, the sole decisionmaker. Findings such as those described in the physicians' attitudes study mean that people with disabilities are particularly disadvantaged by CSC guidelines that give physicians discretion for using and determining "severity" of condition, "quality of life," and "healthy remaining years of life" to assess a patient's treatment prioritization. These same problematic attitudes can be seen in how doctors talk about Do Not Resuscitate (DNR) orders with patients with disabilities and their families.

When approaching, or in, surge situations, some state CSC guidelines encourage doctors to ask their patients about DNR orders with the laudable goal of obtaining and honoring a patient's informed choice to forgo ventilation or other means of invasive care under certain circumstances. In England, stories emerged of hospitals unilaterally placing DNR orders in the files of patients with intellectual disabilities.[107] In the United States, there have also been media reports about physicians pressuring patients and families to adopt DNR orders or rescind an existing POLST form that can express a patient's wish for full resuscitation attempts.

For example, when Sarah McSweeney, a 45-year-old woman with disabilities who lived in a group home in Oregon developed a high fever in April 2020, her support team and guardian brought her to the hospital and submitted her POLST form on her behalf.[108] Tests showed that McSweeney did not have COVID-19, but she developed life-threatening aspiration pneumonia during her stay. At one point, two members of her support team were discussing the use of a ventilator with the lead doctor as the logical next treatment step when he surprised them and "pushed to rewrite McSweeney's care document. He wanted a new order that would say the disabled woman should not be resuscitated or intubated. That would be an order to deny McSweeney the ventilator the doctor had just said she needed." The nurse manager at her group home, Kimberly Conger, recalled that the lead doctor "said intubating her was a matter of risk versus quality of life . . . I was like, 'But she has quality of life.' And he looked at me and goes, 'Oh, she can walk? And talk?'"[109] The doctor accompanied his words by scissoring his index and middle fingers in a simulation of walking. When the medical team looked at McSweeney, they saw a significantly disabled nonverbal woman who used a feeding tube and needed assistance with multiple activities of daily living. Her guardians and friends saw a lively young woman who loved country music, "girly" activities, making her friends laugh, and was actively taking steps to get a part-time job. This difference in views especially clashed around the issue of DNR; the hospital viewed intubation as an extraordinary measure that could do more harm than good, but McSweeney had been intubated before and spent time with good friends who used ventilators 24 hours a day and had tracheostomies. In the end, McSweeney died of aspiration pneumonia after her third week in the hospital. During her nearly three weeks in the hospital, "doctors and social workers had questioned why this disabled woman had medical instructions for full care, instead of a Do Not Resuscitate order. McSweeney's advocates had pushed back. Says Conger of McSweeney's care at the hospital: 'I don't feel like they—and this is my personal opinion—I feel like they didn't feel like she was worth that.'"[110]

McSweeney and her guardians experienced explicit pressure to formally adopt a DNR. In the case of Michael Hickson, a 46-year-old Black man with quadriplegia and other disabilities who was hospitalized in Austin, Texas, in the summer of 2020 with COVID-19, the hospital did not have to press for a DNR because the court-appointed

> *When the medical team looked at McSweeney, they saw a significantly disabled nonverbal woman who used a feeding tube and needed assistance with multiple activities of daily living. Her guardians and friends saw a lively young woman who loved country music, "girly" activities, making her friends laugh, and was actively taking steps to get a part-time job. This difference in views especially clashed around the issue of DNR . . .*

guardian agreed to the treating doctor's request to transfer Hickson from the ICU to palliative care. The treating doctor spoke to Mr. Hickson's wife in a disturbing conversation that she recorded. He evoked Hickson's quality of life, the fact that he did not walk or talk like others who had recovered after being placed on ventilators in the ICU, and the desire to make a "humane" decision for Mr. Hickson, but because Melissa Hickson was not her husband's legal guardian, her objections did not prevent the hospital's planned transfer of Mr. Hickson, who died after care and treatment were withdrawn.[111]

McSweeney and Hickson had family or support persons present. The pandemic context moves even further away from that situation as a norm as pointed out by Arthur Caplan, New York University's chief ethicist.[112] Typically, people go to hospitals for help and see doctors as an advocate for their care. People with disabilities, however, have met with implicit bias in the provision of urgent care that links the potential withdrawal/withholding of medical treatment as "futile" to questions on the quality of the life led by a person who is disabled.[113] Even accepting the premise that under surge conditions normal standards of care must be adjusted, this does not automatically lead to the further step of burdening individuals with disabilities with not only fighting for their lives should COVID-19 or another health emergency arise during the pandemic, but with simultaneously having to fight for medical treatment and to prove to one's own physicians that one's existence is "worth living."

According to Arthur Caplan, NYU's chief medical ethicist:

We're trying to go into not just who's coming in the door and triaging, but what

will we do if we can't resuscitate. Do I care what your living will says in a pandemic? I probably don't. I probably won't even read it. I probably don't even know where it is. Remember, many people are isolated in these units. Their loved ones may or may not be around to communicate something. It's not business as usual. Rarely do we find living wills that get read to guide treatment in normal times. It's usually your friends or family, your partner who speaks up and says, you know, they wanted everything or they didn't. But if they're in the hall far away and we don't want them in the intensive care unit, or surrounded by coronavirus patients, that isn't even going to happen.[114]

While most media coverage over the last year was on the development and actual use of state CSC guidelines, the situation where hospital administrators and staff know that they are rapidly approaching capacity but *before* a CSC policy is formally triggered and individual physicians are still in primary charge of their patients' care options is equally fraught. In this situation of "contingency capacity" where the hospital's resources are stretched but there is still some possibility of maintaining normal standards of care, disability implicit bias and stereotypes about disability are highly likely to influence care decisions as well as the advice providers give to patients and their families. The hospital that treated Michael Hickson did not have a triggered CSC even though he was admitted for COVID-19, leaving his doctor(s) free to decide whether to steer him toward a DNR order or hospice care instead of aggressive ICU treatment.[115] In a convening held in furtherance of researching this report that included a range of adult and pediatric primary care and specialty providers, both physicians and nurses, participants agreed that there is systemic ableism within the healthcare system. Bias is baked into the curriculum in medical school where quality of life is a major focus and disabilities are viewed purely as "medical conditions" that decrease quality of life. The entire group, which included family members of people with disabilities as well as bioethicists, strongly endorsed the need for implicit bias training in the healthcare context that especially focuses on disability.[116]

Understanding and addressing disability discrimination in healthcare as a systemic issue will require investing in sustained action throughout the entire healthcare education, delivery, and funding system. A 2021 equity report and strategic plan by the American Medical Association appears to acknowledge this. The report focuses primarily on race and ethnicity, but also explicitly includes women, LGBTQ+ persons, and people with disabilities as groups that have "experienced a history of harm and discrimination in medical settings."[117] Within the report, there is a page that focuses on structural violence and people with disabilities that mentions state sterilization laws, federal civil rights laws, and key court cases for the disability community such as *Holland v. Sacramento*[118] and *Olmstead v. L.C.*[119] There is also the statement that an equity model that simply treats everyone the same "fails individual patients and communities. For example, high-quality and safe care for a person with a disability

does not translate to 'equal' care. A person with low vision receiving the 'same' care might receive documents that are illegible, depriving them of the ability to safely consent to and participate in their own treatment."[120] The American Medical Association's report does not have cutting edge examples of ableism and, as a strategic plan, has been criticized for lacking bold commitments to inclusive changes in such specific areas as its prestigious research journals and boards, for example,[121] but the clear inclusion of people with disabilities as a group that experiences redressable health and healthcare disparities signals an opening for change.

Physicians and other healthcare providers enter their fields presumably because they want to provide care, not triage it. But healthcare providers cannot develop nondiscriminatory CSC guidelines and administer them fairly unless they are supported in their ability to make nonbiased and nonableist treatment prioritizations when surge or contingency capacity is reached. Such support can run the gamut from encouraging ongoing professional education on what federal disability rights laws require in the healthcare context, a topic on which considerable ignorance appears to remain,[122] to the active identification and dissemination of research that will inform clinical diagnosis and treatment of persons with disabilities during an emergency like the COVID-19 pandemic.[123] Without interventions, such as training in disability cultural competency,

Without interventions, such as training in disability cultural competency, health care providers will fall back on their own assumptions about the likely length and quality of life of people with disabilities, especially in conjunction with other factors such as age or race and income level.

healthcare providers will fall back on their own assumptions about the likely length and quality of life of people with disabilities, especially in conjunction with other factors such as age or race and income level. As one qualitative study of close to 100 physicians found, "[w]hile most clinicians did not feel that they had been in the position of having to ration scarce resources, some nevertheless described practices, such as selection by age or comorbidity, that may be subject to implicit biases and may not be supported by societal priorities for fairness in resource allocation." [Internal citations omitted.][124] This gap between physicians feeling like they are not engaged in medical rationing even as they engage in triage may be particularly relevant with emergency room specialists, who are expected to make rapid diagnostic and urgent care decisions, and who rarely have longer-term experience working with people who have disabilities and chronic conditions.

At the end of May 2021, the coronavirus appeared to be in retreat in the United States, and most signs indicated that both cases and death rates would continue to go down.[125] The subjects of medical rationing and CSC guidelines seemed less urgent than they had been a few short months before, but the disability community and the nation must retain an ongoing concern on this topic. The underlying biases that made medical rationing and triage so dangerous for people with disabilities during the

The underlying biases that made medical rationing and triage so dangerous for people with disabilities during the pandemic, and the potential for CSC polices to be applied in the future, will exist in any emergency whether caused by natural disasters, terrorist attack, or failings of critical infrastructure.

pandemic, and the potential for CSC polices to be applied in the future, will exist in any emergency whether caused by natural disasters, terrorist attack, or failings of critical infrastructure. Within the relatively short time period of the pandemic, there was an evolution of the language used in state CSC guidelines. Comparative research conducted on CSC guidelines across 35 states found that "CSC plans revised later in the pandemic were more likely to align with disability rights priorities than those revised early in the pandemic or never revised. This pattern is consistent with growth over time in both the familiarity of state policymakers with disability rights concerns and the capacity of disability activists to influence public policy on a topic that quickly moved from obscurity to prominence."[126] Medical and legal authors are writing journal pieces that openly acknowledge the need for CSC guidelines to be assessed for compliance with antidiscrimination laws as well as broader goals of social justice.[127] Advocates must be prepared to maintain momentum and repeat effective strategies for fighting discriminatory CSC guidelines now while also strategizing on what still needs to be done on a longer-term basis.

One helpful strategy pursued by state and national advocates was the coordinated effort to challenge discriminatory CSC guidelines by bringing administrative complaints with HHS OCR. HHS OCR was receptive to these complaints and early in 2020 bolstered disability advocacy efforts by issuing nondiscrimination CSC guidance for healthcare entities in a civil rights bulletin,[128] and working with individual states that had some of the most egregious CSC policies.[129] HHS' early resolutions with Alabama, Pennsylvania, Tennessee, and Utah,[130] plus the ongoing work of disability advocates and community members to develop CSC principles, have prompted a number of states to incorporate explicit baseline protections for patients with disabilities who use personalized ventilators and/or require accommodations, and establish a framework of due process for medical rationing decisions. HHS OCR also worked with the state of North Carolina, the North Texas Mass Critical Care Guidelines Task Force, the Southwest Texas Regional Advisory Council, and the Indian Health Service to ensure that each entity's CSC guidelines contain best practices for serving individuals with disabilities and older persons.[131] In addition, some physicians, researchers, and bioethicists began to speak out and bolster the need for alternative best practices by questioning the accuracy and ethical assumptions behind common mortality prediction scores in existing CSC guidelines.[132] Mainstream media support also pointed out the ethical and equitable shortcomings in medical triage approaches that, in practice, pushed people with disabilities and people from vulnerable populations to the back of the COVID-19 treatment line.[133]

While some of the worst and older state CSC guidelines are using much improved language that eliminates discriminatory references to categorical disability exclusions from ICU care and a requirement for a prognosis of long-term

The allocation of health care resources needs to be based on living with a disability, not dying with a disability.

survival, disability advocates continue to meet continued resistance on CSC guidelines. Some states and many private healthcare entities fail to make their CSC guidance readily available to the public, and if the CSC guideline or policy is not known, it cannot be protested or potentially changed through advocacy. Not every CSC guideline includes a strong explicit commitment to nondiscrimination; nor does every guideline come with a clear set of due process instructions that would allow individuals and/or their families to question their prioritization for care or appeal the denial of care. The states and healthcare entities that work on CSCs need to proceed with less deference to "expertise" and more inclusion of people with disabilities in developing updated CSC guidelines for any situation where surge conditions might arise. And critically, all stakeholders need to find ways to effectively implement and enforce nondiscriminatory CSC guidelines in the urgent situations where people with disabilities face irreparable harm. For patients with disabilities who face the imminent potential for being taken off a ventilator or having their ICU admission delayed indefinitely, there are few or no viable options for immediate assistance, or at least, assistance to appeal or delay implementation of what could be a fatal decision. Finally, as a society we need a much greater understanding of how implicit biases are compounded in the case of specific individuals such as Michael Hickson who was both Black and disabled. Disability advocates, the federal government (e.g., HHS OCR), and ethicists who support the value of every life, must continue this work because even when CSC guidelines are not triggered, their principles clearly influence the decisions that are made in "pre-surge" conditions, and the roots of medical rationing decisions lie in the same implicit bias that affected healthcare for people with disabilities long before the coronavirus came into existence.

Even if all states make their CSC guidelines nondiscriminatory, that may be only the substantial first step in protecting people with disabilities from medical rationing. State CSC guidelines are generally regarded as only guidelines. Individual hospitals and health systems may fail to formally adopt any CSC policy, and individuals with disabilities may make find themselves subject to policies that are not publicly available even if they exist, and that look very different from those developed in their state. In addition, public health and other state agencies that typically have authority over hospitals and health systems may lack the experience, legislative mandate, sufficient personnel, or the will to enforce disability and other civil rights laws in the arena of CSC, instead, treating medical rationing and triage decisions as purely medical decisions to be made by healthcare professionals. For the sake of every stakeholder, from patients with disabilities to doctors, from family members to medical educators, we must find ways to work together on developing nondiscriminatory standards of care, and to do so before we are actually in the midst of the next crises or emergency shortage. The allocation of healthcare resources needs to be based on living with a disability, not dying with a disability.

Throughout the pandemic, many health care facilities and plans seemed unclear on the critical point that civil rights laws apply during a public health emergency . . .

Visitation Policies and Other Healthcare Policy Modifications and Accommodations

People with a range of disabilities often develop a close and trusted relationship with their support person(s), who gain specific expertise in their employer, client, or family member's physical, communicative, social, and emotional needs. The no-visitor policies adopted by hospitals, healthcare facilities, and ambulatory clinics/offices since the pandemic began have been challenging for primarily adult people with disabilities[134] (most hospitals recognize an exception for minors that allows them to be accompanied by at least one adult for both inpatient and outpatient hospital procedures). Some professional provider associations such as the American Academy of Developmental Medicine and Dentistry also recognized the need and the capacity for no visitor policies to be modified.[135] The American Academy of Developmental Medicine and Dentistry statement "recommended that hospitals provide reasonable accommodations in accord with the Americans with Disabilities Act in their visitor policies for persons who need support from known and acknowledged support persons" and recognized that "policies should permit a caregiver to be present to the greatest extent possible," while also recognizing the hospital's responsibility to develop appropriate infection control protocols for the presence of support persons.[136]

Throughout the pandemic, many healthcare facilities and plans seemed unclear on the critical point that civil rights laws apply during a public health emergency. As explained earlier in this chapter, healthcare entities have been subject to federal and state disability civil rights for decades. With the declaration of a public health emergency, however, many hospitals and urgent care systems seemed to assume that they could adopt blanket policies that would apply throughout the pandemic. Moreover, some hospitals did not publicly acknowledge any obligation to make individualized assessments of the needs of people with disabilities or to consider disability-related policy modifications or exceptions in care for people who contracted the virus. HHS OCR identified "[a]voiding separating people from their sources of support, such as service animals, durable medical equipment, caregivers, medication and supplies" as a practice needed to help ensure that people with disabilities have equal access to emergency services,[137] and emphasized that "government officials, healthcare providers, and covered entities should not overlook their obligations under federal civil rights laws to help ensure all segments of the community are served."[138] As the following examples show, covered healthcare entities around the county have been slow to publicly acknowledge disability-based accommodations to their no-visitor policies, and even where policies exist, frontline hospital staff may not know or understand them or may implement them in overly narrow ways.

HHS OCR was directly involved in this issue after receiving several distinct complaints about hospital facilities denying the support persons needed by patients with disabilities. In May 2020, Disability Rights Connecticut and other disability rights groups filed a complaint with HHS OCR against a Connecticut hospital that refused to modify its no-visitor policy to allow the support person of a 73-year-old generally nonverbal patient with aphasia and severe short-term memory loss; the complainant's support person provided assistance with communication and comprehension.[139] Connecticut state was also included in the complaint because the state's visitation guidance only recognized a narrow exception to no-visitation policies, limiting support person modifications to those "individuals with disabilities receiving certain services from the state Department of Developmental Services."[140] Individuals with very similar functional limitations to those with developmental disabilities were arbitrarily denied their support persons merely because their disabilities first manifested in adulthood or were the result of an accident, and therefore fell outside eligibility criteria under the state's Department of Developmental Services funding stream.

Later in 2020, HHS OCR received three distinct complaints about MedStar Heath's denial of a disability-related exemption to its no-visitor policy. MedStar Health operated health facilities that operated in more than 100 locations throughout Maryland, Virginia, and Washington, D.C., including hospitals and urgent care centers. The three complainants had sought surgical or emergency care unrelated to COVID-19 but were confronted with the no-visitor policies that MedStar Health hospital facilities had adopted because of the coronavirus. Each of the complainants had physical disabilities and either cognitive or memory impairments, and two complainants also had hearing or vision loss. The complainants alleged that MedStar Health's visitation policy denied them effective communication with their treating providers, denied them the ability to provide informed consent, and subjected them to physical and pharmacological restraints that would have been unnecessary if their support persons had been allowed.[141]

A close look at the complaint brought by Disability Rights D.C. and other disability organizations in September 2020 on behalf of William King[142] shows numerous common discriminatory elements in the hospital visitation policies brought to HHS OCR's attention:

These common elements of visitation policies that are not in compliance with disability civil rights obligations can be found in the Connecticut complaint and also in other visitation policies that were the subject of complaints brought from around the county.[143] In a series of complaints filed with the California Department of Public Health (CDPH) in August 2020 against five separate hospitals across the state, encompassing four different health systems,[144] family members and support persons detailed a trail of ignorance

Discrimination in Hospital Visitation Policies

- Narrowly or exclusively defining a subgroup of persons with disabilities (e.g., people with developmental disabilities or specific diagnoses) as patients who can receive an exception to the no-visitor policy;

- Narrowly or exclusively defining who the hospital will accept as a support person (e.g., someone with legal decision-making authority over the patient, or a paid disability service provider) and limiting the disability-related functions that will be recognized as tasks that a support person undertakes (e.g., direct interpretation is recognized but recognizing and alleviating anxiety so effective communication can take place is not recognized), and/or limiting when and how a support person can be present;

- Little emphasis on communicating policies and policy changes to frontline hospital staff, ultimately leaving discretion for the admittance of support persons in the hands of untrained staff who might not know exceptions to no-visitation even exist;

- No clear obligation on the part of hospitals and urgent care facilities to make their policies *and the disability-related exceptions to those policies* publicly available on websites, physically displayed at entrances, or handed out upon hospital admission;

- State departments of public healthcare that provided only advisory rather than mandatory guidance, did not mention civil rights or nondiscrimination obligations, and gave individual hospitals unfettered discretion to create individualized visitation policies without any consideration for elevating or appealing frontline decisions.

concerning the needs and rights of people with disabilities.[145] One 68-year-old person with a disability was hospitalized for a week and her support person, her daughter, was excluded every night for 12 hours.[146] As the complaints show, many hospitals disregarded CDPH's statement that "'recommends that one support person be allowed to be present with the patient when medically necessary,"[147] or would interpret "medically necessary" in the narrowest possible way; frontline hospital staff were unfamiliar with and disregarded even their own hospital's policy exceptions to a no-visitation rule.

When a needed support person is denied, the health and well-being of the person with a disability can quickly deteriorate, and the initial failure to accommodate will be compounded by an extended stay and a resulting increased risk of being subject to medical rationing if crisis standards of care are triggered or close to being triggered. Even when a support person is not a requested accommodation, people with various disabilities can need modifications in policy: someone with quadriplegia may need extra assistance during meals or frequent visits for repositioning because of existing pressure sores, someone who is developmentally disabled may require additional checks to ensure that intravenous and monitoring connections stay in place, and someone with limited vision may need initial assistance using unfamiliar technology

When a needed support person is denied, the health and well-being of the person with a disability can quickly deteriorate, and the initial failure to accommodate will be compounded by an extended stay and a resulting increased risk of being subject to medical rationing if crisis standards of care are triggered . . .

for online visitation. A person with mobility disabilities needs an accessible toilet and may need assistance with any needed transfers. A failure to meet these needs is not only likely to result in unequal care, it can lead over time to complications and worsening health that then also raise the threat of medical rationing during surge or near-surge conditions. This is why a common lack of accommodations, policy modifications, and individualized care assistance related to disability needs can lead directly to patient concerns about staying in a hospital. As one well-known disability researcher and doctor who is a person with disabilities herself has noted:

Each of us makes choices about the care that is confronting us, and especially at the height of the COVID crisis, it would have been rational for a person with disabilities to decide to remain at home and receive care at home—even if it ultimately resulted in their death. We didn't understand the virus well back then.[148]

Policymaking that did not consider the need for disability modification of pandemic-motivated policies or individualized assessment of the healthcare needs of individuals with disabilities led to discriminatory CSC, and also prompted hospitals to adopt strict "no-visitor" policies as an infection control measure without considering the need for exceptions. A central part of the problem is that there was already a preexisting assumption by many physicians and the general public that when a person with a disability goes to the hospital, hospital staff will be equipped to meet all of their healthcare–related needs. During the pandemic, this assumption shortchanged both support persons' expertise and hospital staff, who during the best of times may not have the training or capacity to meet the assistance needs of multiple significantly disabled adults, much less during a pandemic. A majority of healthcare providers working in hospitals, and especially those in emergency rooms and intensive care units, focus on urgent care. They are not necessarily trained to recognize how people with intellectual or developmental disabilities may not give straightforward answers to questions about their pain levels, or how people who use personal ventilators will deteriorate mentally and physically without their ventilators, or how preexisting disabilities or conditions, including mental health medications, may require additional assistance during a hospital stay. One professor of nursing has agreed that visitation has become an ethical dilemma for nurses, who "are often disadvantaged, forced to act as 'gatekeepers' without sufficient direction or training on disability-related exceptions to general policy, and expected to deal with additional care requirements when someone with significant disabilities is admitted without the experienced support person who would willingly perform many of these care functions." By refusing to admit support persons or provide other needed policy modifications during a pandemic or similar health crisis, hospitals hurt people with disabilities as well as the very staff who would benefit most from having support persons on site.

It is difficult to conceive of any public health emergency, natural disaster, hostile act, or infrastructure failing that would not place a significant strain on the health system in the affected geographic area. Once that occurs, it is entirely foreseeable that healthcare providers and administrators will deny needed policy modifications and accommodations because they will assume that emergency conditions dictate common rules for every patient, without exception. But disability-based policy modifications are required in healthcare under federal and many state laws. Those laws are not neutralized or diminished in an emergency, as this chapter has repeatedly stressed.

Accessible Vaccination and Vaccination Prioritization

The first Emergency Use Authorization (EUA) for a coronavirus vaccine in the United States was granted for individuals aged 16 years and older on December 11, 2020.[149] The second EUA followed one week later for individuals aged 18 years and older.[150] The third vaccine, which required only a single shot rather than two spaced weeks apart and did not need storage at ultra-cold temperatures, was approved at the end of February 2021, again for individuals aged 18 years and older.[151] And on May 10, 2021, the EUA granted for the first vaccine was expanded to include persons aged 12 to 15 years old,[152] while both the first and second EUA grantees applied May 7 and June 1, respectively, for full use authorization and not just EUA status.[153] Even though the full authorization process is likely to take months, the applications showed the developers' confidence in their product. Full authorization allows each developer to market its vaccine directly to consumers and reassure those with vaccine hesitancy because of concerns that the vaccines were insufficiently tested in a rushed process.

Vaccination was described by federal administration and state governors as the light at the end of COVID-19's long dark tunnel. Vaccination helped the nation reach a crucial turning point of both falling case and death rates[154] and economic recovery,[155] though not all of these positive changes happened evenly across all states.[156] Vaccination itself can be a divisive subject, but monthly polling showed that even though the percentages of the public who said they will definitely not get the vaccine or will only get vaccinated if required to do so stayed consistent for months at approximately 13 percent and 7 percent respectively, the percentage of the public who received shots steadily increased, reaching 62 percent in May 2021 with only 4 percent indicating they had not yet been vaccinated but would like to be as soon as possible.[157] The proportion of people who said they would "wait and see" if they would get vaccinated steadily dropped from 22 percent in January 2021 to 12 percent in May 2021.[158] By August 2021, about 52 percent of U.S. residents were fully vaccinated.[159] Nonetheless, the vaccine success story should not obscure the fact that the *same* preexisting foundational problems that made PPE and COVID-19 testing so hard to get for those needing or providing HCBS, made medical rationing fearful, and made the denial of needed policy modifications so common for people with disabilities, also plagued the equitable and accessible inclusion of people with disabilities in COVID-19 vaccine distribution across the country.

Generally speaking, the groundwork for vaccination can be placed into three overlapping categories of work that had to be done before any shot was given: outreach, prioritization of population groups (assuming at least some period[s] during which demand outstrips supply) and establishing the mechanics of eligibility sign-up and delivery. The needs of people with disabilities must be considered in all these categories or many will be left out. Equitable outreach and education efforts focused on race and ethnicity, as is appropriate, but they also had to consider effective communication requirements and the need to reach and reassure groups, such as Deaf persons, who may be experiencing vaccine hesitancy because breaking public health news is full of technical jargon and often only available through error-prone automatic captioning,[160] or they are reluctant to place themselves in situations where they are unsure that full communication access will be provided.[161] In Rochester, New York, which has one of the largest per capita communities of Deaf persons in the world, the full communication access provided to refugees who are Deaf and seeking vaccination exemplified how effective communication was integral to both equitable vaccination and achieving public health goals.[162] Vaccine information and outreach written in plain language benefits Limited English–speaking populations, persons with intellectual or developmental disabilities, and people with lower literacy levels.

In the category of vaccine sign-up and delivery, there were numerous reports across the country of inaccessible online registration forms, physically inaccessible vaccination sites, lack of ASL interpreters and alternative formats, and the failure of vaccine personnel to recognize direct care workers and unpaid support persons as frontline healthcare workers.[163] Both HHS OCR and ACL made attempts to address some of these barriers by developing legal guidance on how vaccine providers needed to ensure that people with disabilities had equal access to vaccine processes[164] and on best practices and strategies for providing that access on the ground.[165] Another key accessibility factor was having sufficiently reliable internet access to reach vaccination sites. Analysis of 2019 American Community Survey data established that people with disabilities, older persons, and people of color had lacked internet access in higher proportions.[166]

The two categories of outreach and vaccine delivery also affected other populations that include and/or directly intersect with the well-being of people with disabilities. For example, states were not equally effective in early efforts to proactively target outreach and vaccination to low-income counties with racial and ethnic groups that had multiple social vulnerability indicators; Arizona and Montana were notably successful, while California ran into problems of misuse when special vaccination codes intended for communities of color circulated among wealthier nonresidents.[167] A majority of direct care workers are low-income women of color, as explained in chapter three, and vaccine hesitancy deeply influenced uptake of the COVID-19 vaccines among healthcare workers—those who put off the vaccine comprised at least 40% of healthcare workers at some historical points and was most prevalent among lesser-paid healthcare workers of color.[168] Some states, such as Virginia and Missouri appeared to have reached Latino populations effectively, but nationally "a dearth of transportation options, an inability to take off from work to get a vaccine,

and concerns about documentation and privacy dampened uptake among Hispanics, according to experts."[169] These same accessibility barriers concerned organizations such as the National Medical Association and other Black healthcare professionals, who emphasized that "the fear of Covid-19, which is this invisible looming foe, that fear does not always outweigh the very clear and well-documented danger of going to a system that has proven itself to be as deadly as disease," and pointed to "the forced sterilization of poor, disabled, and Black women through much of the 20th century as just one of many examples."[170] People with disabilities were therefore disadvantaged by vaccination barriers they encountered themselves, as well as barriers that lowered vaccination rates among current and potential direct care workers who provide necessary personal assistance.

As problematic as vaccine outreach and delivery have been for people with disabilities, however, the most revealing systemic difficulties occurred in the category of vaccine prioritization. Given multiple reports emerging in 2020 on the unequal impact of the coronavirus on racial and ethnic population groups in particular, the federal government took steps to address the potential inequalities in how COVID-19 vaccines would be distributed once approved. In the late summer of 2020, the National Institutes of Health and CDC asked the National Academies of Science, Engineering, and Medicine (NASEM) to form a committee of experts who would create a consensus statement on how to equitably allocate COVID-19 vaccines. Vaccine supply would almost certainly be less than demand, both domestically and globally, for a period likely to be months or even years for some poorer countries. The committee, largely made up of individuals with medical, scientific, bioethics, or legal expertise, was asked to:

> consider what criteria should be used to set priorities for equitable distribution among groups of potential vaccine recipients, considering factors such as population health disparities; individuals at higher risk because of health status, occupation, or living conditions; and geographic distribution of active virus spread. In addition, the committee will consider how communities of color can be assured access to COVID-19 vaccines in the U.S. and recommend strategies to mitigate vaccine hesitancy among the American public.[171]

The NASEM committee's equitable framework for vaccination gave limited recognition to disability as a factor in prioritization, and *it failed to recognize people with disabilities* as a group subject to identifiable risks of coronavirus infection and severe COVID-19 illness. Instead, the committee paid almost exclusive attention to age and medical factors and failed to grapple with multiple high-risk factors that affect people with disabilities, such as reliance on HCBS, living in smaller CCFs such as group homes whatever one's age, the historical and ongoing impact of being a health disparity population, and the existence of discriminatory CSC that would ration people with various significant disabilities out of COVID-19 treatment in surge conditions.[172] People with disabilities were not specifically consulted or asked about the unavoidable risks of infection and severe consequences from COVID-19 that they live with because of disability-related needs. The final framework noted the risks of infection experienced by people with disabilities who could not forego or socially distance from their direct care workers, but the committee's prioritization recommendation pointed only to CDC's then-current listing of comorbid conditions associated with increased risk of severe illness or death from COVID-19: cancer, chronic kidney disease, chronic obstructive pulmonary disease, immunocompromised state from solid organ transplant, obesity (body mass index ≥30), serious heart conditions (e.g., heart failure, coronary artery disease, cardiomyopathies), sickle cell disease, and type 2 diabetes mellitus. Recognizing the limited initial vaccine supply, Phase 1c proposed setting a priority on individuals with two or more of these conditions, recognizing that these priorities could be refined as better evidence emerges.[173]

CDC's list of conditions, not intended to be used as a way to distinguish between people with disabilities who were or were not at high risk from COVID-19, was not a particularly timely or efficient way of keeping up with emerging evidence about comorbid conditions.[174] At the simplest, comorbid conditions are two or more conditions or diseases that exist at the same time in a person. Scientists researched comorbid conditions in those individuals who were infected with the coronavirus or who were hospitalized or died most often from COVID-19. Researchers could then make reasoned conclusions about whether people with certain health conditions were at higher risk of becoming seriously ill or dying from COVID-19 if they were exposed to the coronavirus.[175] The idea that national or state guidance on vaccinations would equitably include people with disabilities by consistently and constantly incorporating the very latest scientific investigations into what constitutes a comorbid condition, in the middle of a pandemic, was flawed to begin with. Medical researchers gravitated toward more common conditions among the general population such as type 2 diabetes or chronic obstructive pulmonary disease, tended to focus on specific diagnostic conditions rather than the functional impairments that reveal more about disability status and healthcare needs, and relied on death certificate information that incompletely captures a deceased person's health conditions. Scientists and institutions conducting research also tended to overlook persons with rarer health conditions because it is harder to find enough subjects to make statistically significant findings.[176]

Nonetheless, as NCD highlighted in its February 2021 letter to the National Governors' Association, the NASEM equitable vaccination framework as well as the federal Advisory Committee for Immunization Practices (ACIP) Updated Interim Recommendations for Allocation of COVID-19 Vaccine[177] explicitly included at least some people with disabilities in their recommendations and did not impose additional arbitrary age divisions on those with high-risk medical conditions. Each recommendation "proposed persons of all ages with comorbid and underlying conditions that put them at significantly higher risk be included in Phase 1b or Phase 1c."[178] But the NASEM framework was purely a model. Even ACIP's recommendations to CDC on who should get vaccinated and when

> *The idea that national or state guidance on vaccinations would equitably include people with disabilities by consistently and constantly incorporating the very latest scientific investigations into what constitutes a comorbid condition, in the middle of a pandemic, was flawed to begin with.*

only served as "guidance" for states. Most states adopted ACIP's 1a prioritization of healthcare personnel and residents of LTCFs, but as time progressed, states increasingly established their own prioritizations with varying degrees of specificity.

The degree of specificity in a state's vaccine priorities can and did become a barrier in and of itself. Washington, D.C., and Ohio indicated by January 11, 2021, that inpatient psychiatric patients should be included in phase 1a as residents of LTCFs,[179] but in states that were unclear on this point, psychiatric patients could be completely overlooked or only included in the event that some advocate at the facility had connections with a state or federal vaccine provider. On the other hand, some states were narrowly specific in ways that could result in prioritized individuals being turned away. For example:

- Massachusetts included "home-based healthcare workers, including: Personal Care Attendants (PCAs) and Home-Based Respite and Individual/Family Support staff (DDS and DDS Self Directed)" among its 1a category of healthcare workers, but Illinois stated that "those providing "Home Health" or serving as a "Home Aide/Caregiver" for a relative with a disability include those who care for people with any of . . . : Cerebral Palsy, Down Syndrome, Epilepsy, Specialized healthcare needs, including dependence upon ventilators, oxygen, and other technology."[180] Even though the Illinois priority list indicated its list of stated conditions was not exhaustive, a list makes it that much harder for caregivers of individuals with disabilities that are not specified on the list to establish their prioritization.

- Maryland and Ohio included people with developmental disabilities in its phase 1b, a deliberate and explicit inclusion that necessarily excludes people with other disabilities from vaccination unless they happen to be institutionalized or over 75 years old and fit into the age prioritization.[181]

- Florida appeared to broadly include people deemed to be "extremely vulnerable to COVID-19" in phase 1a but the determination had to be made by a hospital physician using a specific form.[182]

> ... [T]he first months of 2021 reveals that vaccine prioritization was the "Wild West" of COVID-19.

- Pennsylvania was one of the few states to explicitly and early mention people receiving HCBS and include them in phase 1b.[183]

Once Phase 1a was underway, some states such as California, Colorado, Kentucky, Montana, New Hampshire, New Jersey, New Mexico, and Ohio quickly pivoted in early January to an age-based framework that included age limits as young as 50 years in phase 1c. However, only some of these same states, such as Montana, New Hampshire, New Mexico, and Oklahoma *also* included people 16 years and older with high-risk medical conditions in phase 1b. Montana went so far in phase 1c as to include people 16 years and older with medical conditions that were not included in phase 1b. Even among these four states, however, one state required people to have two or more underlying health conditions while the other three states explicitly or implicitly required only one condition. States also changed their own prioritizations over time, especially in the first weeks of 2021. New Jersey, for example, did not include people with high-risk medical conditions on January 11 but by January 19 included persons 16–64 years with high-risk medical conditions in phase 1b.[184] By March 9, the situation had reshuffled with at least thirty-seven states including at least some residents with high-risk conditions in their vaccine prioritization, but "the health issues granted higher priority differ from state to state, and even county to county."[185] In marked contrast, California moved to a primarily age-based framework in January, placing people aged 65–74 years in phase 1b and those aged 50–64 in phase 1c. Phase 1b also included essential workers, defined in terms of agriculture/food services, education/childcare, and emergency services.[186]

The above review of vaccination among states through the first months of 2021 reveals that vaccine prioritization was the "Wild West" of COVID-19. States talked about equity and tried to achieve speed, but a great deal of vaccination procedures on the ground were determined by local public health authorities and vaccine providers who seemed to have default discretion to interpret state rules that could change weekly. The needs of people with disabilities and older individuals, especially those who could not leave their homes for vaccination, were partially met if there happened to be a strong local advocate, a healthcare decision maker, or even just a single provider who saw the need,[187] but heroic individual efforts should not have been required and cannot redeem systemic failures. The degree of seemingly arbitrary variance in how people with disabilities as a population group were treated when it came to COVID-19 vaccination cannot be overstated. Such treatment, coming after people with disabilities were seemingly left to die in nursing homes and subject to discrimination under some CSCs, left members of the disability community fearful that governments and public health authorities simply didn't care if some of them died during the pandemic.[188] It is foreseeable that in a free-for-all environment, people with disabilities will get pushed to the back of the line virtually every time, with their rights obscured and forced to be dependent upon charity.

California is a case study in how people with disabilities and high-risk conditions had to battle to be included in the state's vaccine prioritization, irrespective of a public commitment to equity in the vaccination process. The state had established a "Community Vaccination Advisory Committee" (CVAC) in November 2020 with nearly 80 advocates and representatives from racial, ethnic, and underserved communities, with the state goal of ensuring that COVID-19 vaccines would be distributed equitably, and the hope of avoiding exacerbation of existing health and healthcare disparities.[189] The CVAC met frequently and tried to achieve consensus results on the population groups that would be prioritized once vaccination began. However, demand far outweighed supply for many weeks and as reports of a slow vaccination pace and unused spoiled doses spread across the state,

California moved away from nuanced attempts to balance exposure, infection, and death risks among California communities. The state instead adopted age as a prioritization factor that is logistically easy to administer and widely acknowledged as a strong risk factor for dying from COVID-19.[190] A few CVAC members worked together bringing original data verifying how younger Medicaid-enrolled people who require HCBS usually have a range of health conditions and are at high risk of infection, hospitalization, and death from COVID-19.[191] These members also circulated breaking studies and information to the CVAC on how COVID-19 placed people with various disabilities at higher risk, such as those with intellectual and developmental disabilities,[192] people with schizophrenia,[193] and those for whom other countries gathered data.[194] Mainstream state and national media also played a useful role by reporting on rates of coronavirus infection and death from COVID-19 among people with specific disabilities[195] and providing a forum for younger people with disabilities to express their personal concerns on vaccination and the impact of COVID.[196]

In the end, younger people with high-risk disabilities or conditions were not included in phase 1b or 1c until February 12, 2021, at which time CDPH issued a bulletin to vaccine providers advising them that people with high-risk conditions or disabilities would be eligible for vaccination as of March 15.[197] High-risk conditions were defined primarily through CDC's finite list of health conditions, but high-risk disability encompassed circumstances in which:

- an individual is likely to develop severe life-threatening illness or death from COVID-19 infection;

- acquiring COVID-19 limits the individual's ability to receive ongoing care or services vital to their well-being and survival; or

- providing adequate and timely COVID-19 care will be particularly challenging as a result of the individual's disability.[198]

The more open-ended nature of high-risk disability was a victory for California's disability community.[199] California was experiencing near-surge conditions at the end of 2020 through the first few months of 2021, making this period a particularly anxious time, and once people with high-risk conditions and disabilities were included within California's vaccine priority populations, state representatives and disability advocates had to consider how vaccine providers could confirm that individuals belonged within this group. If the verification process called for "a doctor's note," people with disabilities and advocates were concerned that the requirement would become yet another barrier to low-income people of color who were disproportionately less likely to have a regular healthcare provider who could write such a note, and primary care doctors did not always know when their patients received HCBS or understand its significance for coronavirus infection.[200] In the end, CPHD agreed that people with high-risk medical conditions and disabilities could self-attest to that fact to establish their vaccination priority.[201]

Now that the United States has reached a point where supply seems to match or even outstrip remaining demand in at least some parts of the country, it is easy to look back and characterize the inaccessibility and uneven treatment of people with disabilities in vaccination as just one of many flawed government responses during an emergency. But vaccine problems persisted for some people with disabilities as states reopened and vaccination totals are celebrated. Individuals with disabilities who had difficulty leaving their homes remained unvaccinated months after they were first eligible because of their age or having a high-risk condition/disability.[202] There was a sharp contrast between states like Ohio, New York, and Colorado initiating vaccination lotteries with large cash prizes to incentivize vaccination among those who remain hesitant[203] even as unvaccinated people filled COVID-19 wards in Cleveland, New York City, and Denver, including people who were unable to get vaccinated because "[c]ities and states have slowly been rolling out programs to reach some of the nation's estimated 4 million homebound Americans, but the programs tend to have modest goals and target only a fraction of the people who likely need outreach."[204]

When states, local governments, and public health authorities made decisions in or after May to use narrow definitions of "homebound" to gatekeep the house call vaccination process and consequently missed people with disabilities who face multiple barriers to leaving their homes,[205] they were not deciding something in the heat of an emergency. They were making deliberate decisions about where to expend resources and who is worthy of those resources. Even as states fully reopened their economies and modified social distance and mask rules, persons with disabilities of all ages who still could not get vaccinated were left to weather a profound social isolation that is even longer than the period of isolation that nursing home and congregate residents had to endure when they quarantined in their own rooms. Ironically, institutional residents were told that they could not be placed into alternative housing because they would be lonely, while nursing home residents and their families were told they had to endure loneliness to remain healthy. But as poignantly observed by the adult daughter of a memory care facility resident, "Is physical health so important that we deny social isolation as potentially furthering illness and death?"[206] Six months after the first vaccine was authorized, we had unvaccinated people with disabilities who fought to remain in the community who had to continue curtailing visitors, maintaining social distance, and enduring anxiety when they received personal support services or other medical services in their homes. Their deprioritization for COVID-19 vaccination was also a choice of sorts, but one that was imposed upon them rather than a decision they got to make.

The cycle of insufficient data, inadequate accommodations and modifications, untrained frontline responders, and implicit bias cannot be left to trap people with disabilities in an endless loop of actions that come "too little, too late."

The common thread that ran from inadequate PPE to discriminatory medical rationing of COVID-19 treatment to failing to be accounted for in vaccination schemes is rooted in how many levels of public health and emergency decision makers fail to recognize the lives of people with disabilities, and particularly those with significant disabilities living in the community. The failure to collect relevant health data on those lives—where people with disabilities live, where they get healthcare, how they are or are not accommodated, the health and healthcare disparities that they experience, the intersection of disability characteristics with racial, ethnic, LGBTQ+ and other personal characteristics—constitutes ignorance that was systemic, and at this point in history, willful. This idea will be addressed more fully in the following section.

Even though several states were approaching 70 percent vaccination rates of adults 16 and over, vaccination-related issues continued to be relevant for some time for a number of reasons. These reasons include the fact that experts could not pin down exactly when herd immunity will be achieved in the United States, vaccination rates remained uneven across states and identifiable population groups, COVID-19 variants continued to evolve and spread across the globe, vaccine use was not yet granted for children 12 years and under, and there was still much discussion and uncertainty around how proof of vaccination would play out in such contexts as employment, travel, and attendance at mass events held in music or sports venues. So many of the problems outlined throughout this chapter occurred because governments, public health entities, and healthcare providers failed to take account of the disparate needs of *all* persons when planning and executing pandemic and emergency response measures. The cycle of insufficient data, inadequate accommodations and modifications, untrained frontline responders, and implicit bias cannot be left to trap people with disabilities in an endless loop of actions that come "too little, too late."

COVID-19 Data Collection—Infection, Hospitalization, Treatment, and Death Rates of People with Disabilities, Collected in Conjunction with Race, Ethnicity, Age, and Other Demographic Characteristics

The dearth of disability-specific COVID-19 information has left the nation uncertain of such basic figures as how many COVID-19–related deaths of people with disabilities occurred in the United States and where they occurred; the number of people with disabilities younger than 65 who died in long-term care and other congregate settings; the functional disabilities among those who have been infected with the coronavirus and those who received treatment in hospitals; and how many people with disabilities were vaccinated to date.

Without this data, it is challenging to make tailored legal and policy recommendations to reduce disparities in COVID-19 testing, receipt of treatment, and vaccination among people with disabilities because it is difficult to even establish that disparities exist. It is also almost impossible to make a cross-analysis of how disability intersects with age, race, ethnicity, income levels, LGBTQ+ status, and other personal characteristics.

When disability advocates and communities sought vaccination prioritization for younger people with disabilities, they were confronting a complex application of disability rights. People with disabilities can clearly evoke disability rights laws when they face physically or programmatically inaccessible vaccination locations, for example, or if they are explicitly excluded from vaccination because they are disabled. In such cases, they face targeted barriers that prevent their equal access to vaccines to which they would otherwise have the same right as everyone else. It is a less straightforward argument to say that people with disabilities are being discriminated against when a state establishes vaccination priorities that give higher priority to groups of individuals on the basis of a characteristic other than disability, for example age. Infection and death rates have established that the coronavirus is having a greatly disproportionate impact on older individuals. If people with disabilities who also fit the age criteria are being vaccinated, it is difficult to establish that younger people with disabilities are actively discriminated against just because disability in and of itself is not being prioritized above age. Similarly, a state's prioritization of other equity or social factors such as emphasizing frontline healthcare workers or essential workers is difficult to impugn as inherently discriminatory. Arguably, a governing entity is free to prioritize saving older lives that are disproportionately at risk or people working in occupations that are particularly needed for maintaining population health and infrastructure. If advocates could establish similarly high rates of risk of infection, severe illness, and death from the coronavirus for younger people with disabilities to those cited for older persons, but the state nonetheless refused to prioritize on the basis of disability, then the presence of discrimination becomes more probable.

Ultimately, the country must achieve finely detailed or "granular" collection of health data on people with disabilities because it cannot achieve equitable well-being in healthcare and public health for people with disabilities without it. The U.S. government must recognize the need for the data, information collection must be mandated, and a variety of health entities must agree to develop and use validated methods for collecting data both at the point at which a service such as hospitalization or vaccination is administered and through the use of national surveys such as the American Community Survey or the Behavioral Risk Factor Surveillance System (BRFSS). Though the surveys are national some are administered by and through states. The BRFSS, for example, has "a standardized core questionnaire, optional modules, and state-added questions" and is administered by state health departments through telephone surveys using random digit dialing to landlines and cell phones; the BRFSS is administered throughout the year and is particularly important for detecting trends that can point to emerging illnesses such as COVID-19.[207] The ACS, on the other hand, is conducted directly by the U.S. Census Bureau through paper or online surveys sent out randomly every month to addresses in any of the 50 states, the District of Columbia, and Puerto Rico in five-year cycles, and "provides information about the social and economic needs of your community every year."[208] It is particularly important in helping all levels of government to plan spending and infrastructure for educational, housing, healthcare, transportation, and other needs in American communities.

Disability data collection efforts and standardization in healthcare and in programs and activities conducted or sponsored by federal HHS were not broadly required until Section 4302 of the ACA was enacted in 2010.[209] An interagency committee had developed a six-item set of functional disability questions that had undergone extensive cognitive and field testing and was being used in the ACS and some other major national surveys, but it had not been officially adopted as a minimum standard or uniformly required by HHS;[210] but the Section 4302 mandate

covers only national population-based surveys and does not extend to "administrative data (such as data captured at the time of enrollment in a program or data collected from a medical record), clinical data (collected as part of clinical care), and research data (collected from participants in research studies)" that would allow analysis of disparities in the public health inclusion of people with disabilities.[211] The adequacy of inclusion of people with disabilities in state health surveillance, public health, and emergency measures is also not captured. There has not been any attempt to extend Section 4302's minimum data standards to private entities, even to entities that receive federal financial assistance through their participation in federal and state insurance exchanges, for example.

For the most part, private health providers and insurers treat diagnostic information as disability information. This tends to obscure functional disability status because someone with a diagnosis of multiple sclerosis, for example, can have a range of symptoms from nonvisible fatigue to loss of mobility requiring use of a wheelchair; a diagnosis in itself fails to reveal a patient's accommodation needs or their likelihood of experiencing disability-related healthcare disparities. Nonetheless, private health insurance claims data helped to establish how persons with certain health conditions were at high risk of severe consequences after contracting COVID-19[212] and could be even more helpful if claims data included demographic data from the ACS disability set.

Given the current limited state of granular disability health data collection, it is useful to trace how granular data on race, ethnicity, and language (REL) has come to be widely embraced as an important component for measuring health and healthcare disparities in the United States.

The information we now have on health and healthcare disparities experienced by racial and ethnic groups is due to government policies that date back decades. Starting with "the landmark 1985 Secretary's Task Force on Black and Minority Health," HHS reports came to recognize how timely and reliable data could be used to identify racial and ethnic health disparities and the factors that cause and accompany disparities and to monitor progress in reducing disparities.[213] In 1997, HHS finally adopted a "Data Inclusion policy that "required the collection of uniform standard data on race and ethnicity in all HHS-sponsored data collection activities."[214] Years later, the Institute of Medicine issued its seminal report in 2003, *Unequal Treatment: Confronting Racial and Ethnic Disparities in Healthcare*, that acknowledged how racial and ethnic disparities are "significant predictors" for of the quality of care that a person of color receives even after accounting for other socioeconomic differences.[215]

Almost 20 years of advocacy later, we see far greater awareness among experts and the general public of health and healthcare disparities related to race, ethnicity, and language (REL). During the pandemic, all levels of government openly accepted that systemic racial/ethnic discrimination and implicit bias contributed to COVID-19 infection, treatment, and vaccination disparities among people of color, particularly Black, Hispanic, and Indigenous persons, a response that was likely heightened by cultural and social changes in the wake of George Floyd's death in 2020. Media sources established regularly updated dashboards that showed disproportionate infection and death rates among people of color and the racial and ethnic demographic characteristics of vaccinated individuals.[216] CDC providing national rates of vaccination by race and ethnicity, stated that "[i]mproving COVID-19 vaccination coverage in communities with high proportions of racial/ethnic minority groups and persons who are economically and socially marginalized is critical because these populations have been disproportionately affected by COVID-19–related morbidity and mortality."[217] The great majority of states are also reporting state vaccination rates by race and ethnicity.[218]

Even with far greater awareness and intentionality, though, state-level collection of race and ethnicity data remains highly imperfect. Some states' existing Immunization Information Systems still lack capacity to track REL data, and adding that capacity could take months, while other states have the capacity to record race and ethnicity data but the fields are not required during data entry.[219] Moreover, those states that track race and ethnicity have not uniformly adopted the clearly defined racial and ethnic categories used in federal census data or committed to a minimum set of data collection standards.[220] Inconsistencies and gaps can also compound across states and further impede any attempt to get a clear national picture of vaccine equity; for example, South Carolina "lumps together Asians, Native Americans, and Pacific Islanders in one category,"[221] while "data gaps and separate reporting of data for vaccinations administered through the Indian Health Service [further] limit the ability to analyze vaccinations among American Indian and Alaska Native and Native Hawaiian and Other Pacific Islander people."[222] With race and ethnicity information known for only 53 percent of those vaccinated as of March 29, 2021, numbers still consistently showed that Black and Hispanic populations across states received proportionately less vaccine than their percentage share of cases, of deaths, and of the state's total population.[223] As pointed out by one population health expert, incomplete and inconsistent data makes it "harder for us to hold ourselves accountable to our own work and to stand up and say to the public 'Here's the evidence that we are trying and we're making progress.'"[224] Not all states agreed that improving data collection and transparency was crucial to accountability for achieving greater equity in the pandemic's impact. "Only about half of US states still provide daily updates on key Covid-19 metrics—such as new cases, deaths, hospitalizations and vaccinations—a trend that worries some public health experts."[225]

Lessons Learned on Data Collection

The ways in which race and ethnicity data collection was elevated, carried out, and reported during the pandemic provide valuable lessons for disability advocates.

- **Persistence Paid Off:** REL communities and advocates developed evidence for decades on the existence of health and healthcare disparities across multiple delivery contexts and argued that without granular REL data and uniform collection standards, there was no way to effectively hold providers accountable and encourage measurable quality improvement for delivering equitable healthcare. During the pandemic, most government and healthcare entities took steps to track race and ethnicity data that confirmed the inequitable impact of COVID-19 and showed that states fell far short of achieving vaccination equity.

- **National Leadership is Critical:** Federal standards facilitate regional and national data analysis and information technology interoperability. The Office of Management and Budget (developed a federal government-wide standard for REL data collection in 1997 after holding a wide-ranging public process of engagement and field testing. This early standard grounds the REL minimum data collection standard under Section 4302 of the ACA and paved the way for further work by federal agencies such as the AHRQ when it suggests ways for REL data collection to take place.[226]

- **The Pandemic Exposed Data Gaps:** Many experts agree that the pandemic "has shined a light on racial data problems that have persisted in U.S. public health for far too long. . . . [the hope] is that our lessons from COVID really cause all of us to think about the infrastructure we need within out state and nationally to make sure we are prepared next time. Data is our friend."[227]

- **Data Collection Needs Will Continue:** pandemic data collection cannot end prematurely, particularly while disparities in vaccination rates persist among specific populations and herd immunity has not been achieved in the country. Moreover, the public health reporting systems that states have built or improved since the pandemic started do *not* have to be limited to use with COVID-19. "States have spent 15 to 18 months building up this infrastructure . . . By winding down, the question is what will happen to this new infrastructure and skill set. By putting this genie back in the bottle, we lose the capacity to take advantage of them."[228]

The disability community has made significant strides in establishing itself as a population group that is subject to health and healthcare disparities,[229] but it clearly has not reached the point where health and government entities will put out disability-specific statistics related to coronavirus infection, treatment, deaths, and vaccination or search for ways to do so. Even at the height of CDC and state reporting of COVID-19 cases and deaths, there was no attempt to capture the full extent of the virus's toll on people across a range of disabilities, except for people with disabilities who happened to intersect with characteristics that were already tracked, such as age. Even when the pandemic eased, some people with disabilities, including those who are immunocompromised, adults with disabilities who have difficulty leaving their homes, or young children with disabilities who are not yet eligible for vaccination, could be harmed by the decision to cut back on vaccination reporting as "[d]aily data reporting provides critical "backup" information to help people and public officials alike make decisions about the safety of engaging in various social activities,"[230] and especially until the nation reaches herd immunity.

The fragmented nature of healthcare delivery and insurance coverage in the United States makes it particularly difficult to compile complete data on where, how, and under what circumstances COVID-19 circulated among and killed people with disabilities. Without common ways to identify people with functional disabilities, common standards for data collection, and a common mandate to collect this information across states and healthcare systems, people with disabilities will remain shut out of policymakers' increased commitment to emergency interventions that account for disparities and to equitable healthcare overall. As one prominent healthcare research organization observed, the "wide variety in state reporting makes it difficult to compare between states or have a complete understanding of how people with disabilities have been affected by the pandemic."[231]

The best tools we have for baseline granular identification of people with disabilities, the six-disability question set in the ACS and the Washington Short Set on Functioning[232] are not in broad use, and this shortcoming makes it difficult to even begin thinking about how those tools can be further refined to better capture people with communication disabilities, mental health or behavioral health disabilities, and people with HCBS needs. All these factors proved to be relevant to the high risk borne by people with disabilities during the pandemic, but potential users of disability identification tools have little current incentive to find effective ways to obtain additional information.

> *Without common ways to identify people with functional disabilities, common standards for data collection, and a common mandate to collect this information across states and health care systems, people with disabilities will remain shut out of policymakers' increased commitment to emergency interventions that account for disparities and to equitable health care overall.*

Surveillance tools such as the BRFSS offer another opportunity to gather vaccination information, albeit some time after vaccination. The BRFSS's focus on noninstitutionalized adults will leave out some people with disabilities residing in CCFs, but that is a population for which additional demographic information on functional disability, race, ethnicity, and other characteristics can and should be obtained in any event. CDC requested approval on March 12, 2021, to add an optional module on COVID-19 vaccination to BRFSS that would be available by mid-2021. The proposed questions include when the respondent received their vaccination shot(s) and "what kind of place" the shot(s) were received.[233] By early June, Alaska, Illinois, Missouri, New Jersey, and North Carolina had reported their intention to administer the optional COVID-19 vaccine-related module, and North Carolina intended to include an additional question: "What is the MAIN reason you have NOT received a COVID19 vaccination?"[234] These questions have great potential for providing important information about the vaccine barriers that people with disabilities encountered and the set will be coupled with the six-question disability set used in national surveys. The downside is that the vaccine module is optional, and any given state that chooses to include it may have insufficient sample sizes of people with specific functional limitations to provide reliable and meaningful analysis. If all states administered the vaccine module or went so far as to include

[A]ttempts to establish the overall impact of the coronavirus on people with disabilities are continually stymied by the failure to collect functional disability as a demographic characteristic and not just an individual medical need or a patient diagnosis.

vetted disability-specific data questions, it might be possible to combine disability samples across states or within a geographic region that included a number of states.

Another data collection option is the administration of independent, state-specific polls or surveys that could be tailored and achieve results quite quickly when offered by such entities as state or local public health departments, health policy groups, university research entities, and media, or even large healthcare systems such as a managed care entity, but such surveys can be costly, which in turn tends to limit sample size.[235] And again, the lack of mandated disability inclusion in state surveillance means that disability is easily excluded from data gathering. Even with REL data, none of the many public and private players in healthcare "has the capability by itself to gather data on race, ethnicity, and language for the entire population of patients."[236] Some individuals, including people with disabilities, may have sporadic contact with the healthcare system for various reasons, such as the lack of a regular source of healthcare or being homeless, making the gathering of standardized data for quality improvement across all health and healthcare entities even more important.

The evidence that people with disabilities comprise a population group that experiences health and healthcare disparities continues to grow. The pandemic has established higher rates of coronavirus infection, and serious illness and death upon infection, for at least some persons with specific disabilities. But attempts to establish the overall impact of the coronavirus on people with disabilities are continually stymied by the failure to collect functional disability as a demographic characteristic and not just an individual medical need or a patient diagnosis. Health information technology interoperability rules provide yet another potential way for patients with disabilities to disclose functional disability information, but neither version 1 of the U.S. Core Data Set for Interoperability put forth by the U.S. Office of the National Coordinator for Health Information Technology, nor version 2 which is in draft form, asks for disability-related demographic information.[237] A category called "functioning" is included in the health record and includes questions relating to mental function, mobility, and self-care among other elements, but its placement in the electronic health record among purely medical questions indicates that it is likely not a field that could be used to help identify or verify people with disabilities as a group subject to health disparities. The "missed policy opportunity to advance health equity" through the inclusion of more granular race, ethnicity, disability, and gender identity demographic information was noted when the Core Data Set was first being adopted: "CMS declined to adopt disability status or sexual orientation and gender identity because of the lack of consensus on definitions, lack of agreed-upon standards, data collection and reporting challenges, and disagreement over where and how to collect this information in an [electronic health record]."[238]

At some point, the fact that federal and state governments continually overlook the need for functional disability data begins to cross the line from simply being overlooked in prioritization to

negligence. It is virtually impossible to provide real-time accurate data about the impact of COVID-19 on people with disabilities or the healthcare disparities they experienced during the pandemic if state, public health, health plan, and provider databases fail to identify someone as a person with a disability. This simple fact has become increasingly clear over the past couple of decades as the U.S. healthcare system has come to gradually recognize REL-related health and healthcare disparities, and concentrated effort has been put into transitioning to electronic health records. The fundamental failure of healthcare data collection to recognize people with disabilities must be decisively changed on multiple levels, or policymakers, researchers, and the public will never know whether people with disabilities are disproportionately dying in the next pandemic or emergency, and they will assume that any disproportionate impact is purely attributable to the presence of disability or a health condition rather than a matter of systemic or implicit bias.

Summary of Findings

- Needed PPE was widely unavailable to both those providing and receiving long-term services and supports, placing people with disabilities, both those living in congregate care situations and those living in the community, at higher risk of infection, severe illness, and death during the pandemic.

- Implicit bias about living with a significant disability is widely prevalent among healthcare providers, hospital administrators, bioethicists, and healthcare decision makers and likely influenced denials of treatment and inappropriate referrals to hospice care of people with disabilities, including people of color with disabilities who are also subject to intersecting stereotypes and systemic racism.

- There is some awareness among healthcare providers and professional associations of how people with disabilities have suffered historic harm, structural discrimination, and unequal care in the delivery of healthcare, but this awareness has not yet translated into concrete commitments to changing healthcare education, professional accreditation, and academic research policies.

- Many of the CSC policies established or used by states and hospitals during periods when medical beds, equipment, and personnel were first strained by high levels of coronavirus infection and hospitalization discriminated explicitly and implicitly against people with disabilities.

- Longstanding failures of healthcare providers and administrators to know and follow federal and state disability nondiscrimination laws resulted in patients with disabilities being denied critical policy modifications and accommodations during the pandemic.

- Basic physical and programmatic inaccessibility was widespread in many public health responses to the emergency, from the establishment of drive-in testing sites to procedures for making vaccine appointments and providing vaccination.

- Policymakers have limited data or understanding about people with disabilities who live in the community and receive HCBS, some of whom cannot maintain access to the necessities of life while sheltering in place and practicing strict social distancing.

- Current restrictions on how SNAP benefits can be used exacerbated the food shortages experienced by people with disabilities who need assistance with Complex Activities of Daily Living or who live in remote rural areas, particularly when public transportation is also restricted or unavailable.

- The rollout of COVID-19 vaccines in the United States raised competing priorities for achieving equitable distribution and achieving speedy and efficient vaccination, which left out people with disabilities who were at high-risk from COVID-19 but who did not have health conditions already established as medically high-risk or who needed logistically complex accommodations, such as vaccination in their homes.

- Federal and state healthcare data collection practices failed to capture baseline information about the functional disability status of patients and the public, leaving people with disabilities uncounted during and after public health emergencies, and healthcare workers and policymakers unaccountable for both failing to include people with disabilities during crises and improving quality and inclusion for people with disabilities in the aftermath of crises.

- Private health insurance claims information contains valuable data on health and healthcare disparities experienced by people with disabilities, but this information cannot be fully accessed or effectively analyzed unless these insurers collect demographic functional disability information in addition to standard information about medical diagnoses and health conditions.

Recommendations

To ensure the United States is prepared to swiftly recognize healthcare discrimination and appropriately monitor and enforce disability civil rights laws on behalf of people with disabilities in a future pandemic or similar national health crisis, NCD recommends the following actions based on our findings about the impact of COVID-19 on people with disabilities:

Recommendations for Congress

Congress should:

- Include functional disability status among any bills that propose improved demographic data collection relating to testing, infection, injuries, hospitalizations, and fatalities that are related to pandemics, natural disasters, climate change–related emergencies, or any other public health emergencies, both within every type of congregate care setting (e.g. psychiatric facilities, facilities for people with intellectual and developmental disabilities, board and care homes, group homes, and so forth) as well as community settings.

- In any legislation that addresses shortfalls in the nation's supply of healthcare providers (physicians, nurses, therapists, and so forth) through changes to training programs, inclusive recruitment for a diverse healthcare workforce, loan forgiveness that encourages healthcare providers to work with underserved populations, or other innovative targeted incentive measures, include healthcare providers who are familiar with the needs of disability communities such as Deaf and Hard-of-Hearing people, people with complex rehabilitative needs, people with intellectual and developmental disabilities, people with serious mental illness, and so forth.

- Require state collection of healthcare demographic data relating to functional disability and HCBS use for all Medicaid enrollees, including better data collection across the full range of long-term care, group homes, and congregate settings licensed, certified, or approved by the state.

Recommendations for Federal Agencies

HHS should:

- Require all hospitals, hospital systems, and managed care plans that receive federal financial assistance to increase public transparency of, and nondiscrimination and due

Recommendations for Federal Agencies: *continued*

process within, CSC guidelines and medical rationing policies adopted during public health emergencies and emergency surge situations. These guidelines and policies should be clearly posted on all the entity's websites and hospital and appropriate provider network websites.

- Conduct a national convening of experts, including disability advocates and people with disabilities to review how discriminatory CSC and medical rationing policies developed and may continue to influence healthcare decision making in future public health emergencies, and to make further recommendations for alleviating the impact of CSCs and medical rationing on people with disabilities, people of color, older persons, and other groups that experience health and healthcare disparities.

- Include functional disability status among the demographic data that must be collected by the Secretary of HHS and posted on Nursing Home Compare on COVID-19 cases and deaths under the COVID-19 Nursing Home Protection Act (S.333) or other bills introduced to improve demographic data collection on nursing home infections, illnesses, deaths, or resident transfers to hospitals

- Expand on the data collection standards and requirements laid out in Section 4302 of the ACA to require any healthcare or public health program, activity, or survey (including population surveys conducted by the Bureau of the Census) that is federally conducted or that receives federal financial assistance to collect and report data on functional disability status for applicants, recipients, or participants (though the provision of such information from individual applicants, recipients, and participants should always be voluntary).

- ***HHS OCR and DOJ*** should work with state civil rights counterparts to issue early general guidance clarifying that there is nothing in federal or state law that automatically relieves covered entities from their preexisting disability nondiscrimination obligations, including the obligation to provide reasonable modifications and accommodations to people with disabilities, in the event of an epidemic, pandemic, natural disaster, climate change disaster, or other public health emergency.

- ***HHS OCR*** should:

  - Develop a Patient Bill of Rights for People with Disabilities, written in plain language, and including information on the following rights that pertain to healthcare: effective communication, policy modifications, treatment without discrimination, access to personal support persons, use of personal medical equipment, physical accessibility,

(continued)

Recommendations for Federal Agencies: *continued*

choice of less invasive reasonable treatment or health maintenance alternatives; having an advance directive, POLST, or DNR orders without undue influence, information on and assistance for returning to the community from hospital or institutional care, and freedom from assumptions about one's quality of life and capacity to benefit from treatment or survive treatment because of the presence of a disability or particular condition.

- Initiate an ongoing process for reviewing crisis standards of care and medical rationing policies of states, healthcare systems, and hospitals in anticipation of other public health emergencies that will strain local, regional, or national resources, and provide technical assistance for compliance with disability nondiscrimination in the formulation of CSC and rationing policies.

- *HHS and FEMA* should require disability expertise and representation on federal pandemic planning committees, and ensure true inclusivity in all local, state and federal emergency responses for a wide range of disabilities and co-occurring conditions, including lesser known or nonvisible disabilities such as multiple chemical sensitivity, and disability-specific concerns such as including personal care assistants and direct support professionals in federal emergency measures for strengthening Medicaid and frontline healthcare workers during an emergency (e.g., authorization of overtime hours or hazard payment if providing assistance to a person with disabilities who is sick or has other direct care workers who are sick, distribution of virus tests and PPE, and so forth).

- *HHS, U.S. Census Bureau, FEMA*—Interagency Cooperation: Federal agencies including CDC, CMS, FEMA, and the U.S. Census Bureau, should collaborate and form a broader interagency work group to identify methods to efficiently collect functional disability information during public health and other emergencies in order to identify how many people with disabilities are affected (e.g., infection, illness, injury, hospitalization, death), whether they live in a type of congregate care facility or in the community or transition between them during the emergency, and whether they have HCBS needs. They should also develop methods to identify how HCBS workers are affected by public health or other emergencies (e.g., infection, illness, injury, hospitalization, death) to inform policies and actions that will be needed to maintain necessary HCBS during and after these emergencies. Data should be published on regularly updated publicly available websites.

- *HHS* should assume primary responsibility for implementing, monitoring, and enforcing the data collection requirements in Section 4302 of the ACA. Data should be collected at

Recommendations for Federal Agencies: *continued*

the smallest geographic level such as state, county, zip code, or institutional levels, using disability data collection tools such as current population survey questions included in the ACS, those recommended by the Washington Group on Disability Statistics, or other equivalent data collection measures developed through interagency cooperation. Disability data collection tools should also be further developed to better capture people with intellectual and developmental disabilities, communication disabilities, and other diagnostic or functional limitations that may be currently excluded from or undercounted by the ACS or Washington Group survey questions. The U.S. Census Bureau, the HHS, CMS, and the CDC should aggregate the data on a common website for use by researchers and the public.

- *HHS, working through the Health Resources and Services Administration* should assume primary responsibility for implementing and appropriately funding Section 5307 of the ACA,[239] including establishing and developing criteria for grants, contracts, or cooperative agreements for developing and evaluating research, demonstration projects, and model curricula in cultural competency, prevention, public health proficiency, reducing health disparities, and aptitude for working with individuals with disabilities. HHS should identify effective best practices and model curricula identified through projects initiated under Section 5307 and mandate their use in health professions schools and continuing education programs to address systemic and implicit disability bias in the health professions.

- *NCHS* should work with state vital statistics offices to initiate revisions in the U.S. Standard Certificate of Death to include functional disability and HCBS consumer information in the demographic section of death certificates and obtain the approval of completed revisions from the HHS Secretary.

- *HHS/ACL, HHS/OCR, and DOJ* should work together to establish and fund a national healthcare technical assistance center to inform a range of healthcare providers on civil rights issues regarding patients with disabilities. The Center would provide healthcare providers, medical educators, professional associations, and public health authorities with information and trainings on implicit disability bias, the importance of policy modifications and reasonable accommodations to providing effective healthcare, and the critical role that support persons play in maintaining the health and functional capacity of people with disabilities. ACL could play a central coordinating role over the Center, either as an

(continued)

Recommendations for Federal Agencies: *continued*

independent entity or as an adjunct component of existing entities that provide disability expertise such as the regional ADA Centers, while both HHS OCR and DOJ can provide technical and legal expertise, given their overlapping regulatory authority over the gamut of healthcare entities and providers.

- **Department of Agriculture** should monitor and enforce physical, website, and procedural accessibility to ensure that people with disabilities are able to enroll in SNAP and fully use their SNAP benefits, including modifications needed by people with disabilities who may require grocery delivery and assistance during pandemics and public health emergencies. In addition, rather than require all persons with disabilities to meet the strict asset tests imposed on Supplemental Security Income and Social Security Disability Insurance payments, recognize persons with disabilities through broad-based categories for eligibility, for example, HCBS consumers as they are likely to have higher disability-related household expenses that make it harder to meet food expenses.

Recommendations for States

States should:

- Specify and adequately fund a designated state agency or entity that will take individual complaints, provide real-time technical assistance, and initiate investigations on allegations of discrimination and accessibility barriers by healthcare entities during public health emergencies, including communication accessibility, access to support persons and needed policy modifications and accommodations, and nondiscrimination in medical rationing and crisis standards of care.[240]

- Require hospitals, managed care entities, and healthcare systems operating in the state, including university teaching hospitals and systems, that are licensed, regulated, or certified in the state or that receive any state funding or that serve any Medicaid enrollees to include people with disabilities or disability advocates on their medical ethics committees and in the development, adoption, or revision of crisis standard of care or medical rationing policies.

Recommendations for States: *continued*

- State Departments of Public Health must strengthen ties with disability and community-based organizations such as independent living centers and aging and disability networks to build capacity to reach people with disabilities through trusted messengers if outreach is needed on newly developed or repurposed medications or treatments, and to strengthen the department's capacity to ensure full accessibility, including threshold languages, in its own outreach, emergency guidance, and logistical operations.[241]

Recommendations For Additional Entities

- *Association of State Governors:* Develop a set of strategies, best practices, and data collection standards (including privacy concerns and addressing interoperability needs) for collecting functional disability information on residents across the full range of congregate living facilities that are licensed, certified, or otherwise recognized or funded by a state (e.g., psychiatric facilities, intermediate care facilities, board and care homes, group homes, and so forth).

- *American Medical Association:* Develop and disseminate mandated requirements and standards relating to disability rights and implicit bias training for physicians and related healthcare professions involved in setting public health emergency procedures, medical rationing, and standard setting. Such training should be a required component of continuing professional education. The American Medical Association should also encourage reporting and academic investigation that reveals health and healthcare disparities experienced by people with disabilities, including people of color with disabilities.

- *National Association of Insurance Commissioners:* Develop model disability data collections standards and best practices that state departments of insurance could enact as part of Market Conduct Annual Statement reporting requirements on healthcare insurers licensed or practicing in the state.

Chapter 2: Impact of COVID-19 on People with Disabilities in Congregate Care Facilities

COVID-19 Had a Devastating Impact on People with Disabilities in Congregate Care Facilities

No demographic in the United States experienced COVID-19 more dramatically than people living in CCFs. The way people in congregate settings live and receive care made the pandemic especially difficult to contain and, as a result, greatly increased the risk of exposure for residents and staff.

CCFs include LTCFs like nursing homes and assisted living facilities, and other congregate settings such as state psychiatric hospitals, intermediate care facilities for individuals with intellectual and developmental disabilities, board and care homes, and group homes. On the front lines of a fast-changing pandemic, CCFs reported staff shortages, inadequate PPE, inconsistent and slow testing, and limited space for resident isolation and quarantine. Residents of CCFs also experienced extreme isolation due to COVID-related restrictions on visitors, and many died alone.

Most significantly, due to the difficulty of ensuring physical distancing, isolation, and quarantine in CCFs, rates of transmission and death from COVID-19 in these facilities were extraordinary. As of March 2021—a year into the pandemic—over one-third of all COVID-19 deaths in the United States occurred in LTCFs, including nursing homes and assisted living facilities. One hundred and eighty-one thousand individuals in LTCFs died from COVID-19, accounting for more than one-third of all COVID-19 deaths in the United States, from a group of individuals constituting less than 3 percent of the nation's population.[242] Almost 1.5 million cases of COVID-19 occurred in LTCFs, with nearly 35,000 facilities reporting known cases.[243]

> *As of March 2021—a year into the pandemic—over one-third of all COVID-19 deaths in the United States occurred in LTCFs, including nursing homes and assisted living facilities. One hundred and eighty-one thousand individuals in LTCFs died from COVID-19, accounting for more than one-third of all COVID-19 deaths in the United States, from a group of individuals constituting less than 3 percent of the nation's population.*

However, these numbers do not account for cases and deaths in other types of CCFs for people with disabilities, like state psychiatric hospitals, intermediate care facilities for individuals with intellectual and developmental disabilities, board and care homes, and group homes.

Data from these other types of CCFs is less available, but what data exists indicates that residents and staff who lived and worked in other types of CCFs also had a heightened risk of contracting COVID-19 and of dying from the virus. One would expect the data in these facilities to be comparable to that in LTCFs, given the similarities in how they operate.

Living in a CCF exposes people with disabilities to the many individuals who enter the facility on a regular basis—including caregivers, other residents, and staff. A study of Connecticut nursing homes found that those with "more residents at the beginning of the pandemic and with greater shares of beds filled had significantly more cases and deaths per licensed bed than facilities operating at lower capacity . . . speak[ing] to the importance of density and intrafacility spread."[244] Moreover, nursing homes with higher staffing rates and a lower staff-to-resident ratio had fewer COVID-19 incidences and deaths.[245] The risk of transmission based on density and traffic in and out is similar in all types of CCFs.

The high frequency with which residents and staff interact and the difficulty of practicing physical distancing within these facilities contribute to transmission.[246] Consistent with these observations, a July 2020 report found that people with intellectual disabilities residing in group homes were four times more likely to contact COVID-19, twice as likely to die than people with intellectual disabilities receiving care in noncongregate settings, and eight times more likely to die than the general population.[247] Further, a recent study found that individuals admitted to a psychiatric inpatient setting faced an increased risk for infection and death compared with similarly situated individuals in the community.[248]

These risks may be heightened where residents have certain types of impairments that make them particularly vulnerable. For example, studies have shown higher rates of COVID-19 and death in people with intellectual disabilities, including a recent study showing that people with intellectual disabilities are 2.5 times as likely as others to be diagnosed with COVID-19 and 5.9 times as likely to die from it.[249] Similarly, a recent study published in the *Journal of the American Medical Association* found that individuals with a diagnosis of schizophrenia were 2.7 times as likely to die from COVID-19 as individuals without psychiatric diagnoses, controlling for demographic factors such as age, race, and sex and for known medical risk factors.[250]

Staffing shortages further exacerbated the vulnerabilities of CCF residents and staff. As one state human services official explained, "Pre-COVID, we have had staffing shortages in [congregate care and group home] settings across Minnesota, but what we're experiencing right now is something different . . . as staff test positive for COVID-19, they're having to

> *[P]eople with intellectual disabilities are 2.5 times as likely as others to be diagnosed with COVID-19 and 5.9 times as likely to die from it.*

quarantine, which leaves care facilities in a precarious position."[251]

All types of CCFs reported experiencing the same unprecedented staff shortages due to COVID-19. A state-run psychiatric hospital in Pennsylvania was so short-staffed that even after closing a patient ward on weekends and some weekdays, the hospital still could not meet a 1:4 aide to patient ratio, the professional recommendation.[252] Some states looked to staffing agencies to recruit emergency workers, others called in the National Guard as a last resort.[253]

Where visitation restrictions combined with staff shortages, facilities altered the provision of care, including fewer therapies and greater restrictions on the mobility of residents within facilities. As a result, CCF residents experienced increased rates of isolation, depression, and physical deterioration.[254] In Connecticut, "despite differences in methods and frequency of visitations, nearly all family members reported the physical and emotional health of residents declined significantly without frequent, in-person interactions with the family members and caregivers who had provided critical support for activities of daily living."[255]

Limited access to testing and PPE worsened the already dire situation in CCFs. A fall 2020 investigative report from Senator Elizabeth Warren (D-MA) found that none of the 10 large behavioral health treatment program operators surveyed "conduct[ed] routine daily or weekly testing of staff or patients at all their facilities" and "experienc[ed] turnaround times of a week or more for test results."[256] These facilities were "generally not able to perform routine testing of asymptomatic individuals" in line with CDC recommendations for CCFs. Only two of the 10

providers reported testing new patients upon admission. One provider attributed limited testing to the "difficulty of obtaining testing supplies" and reliance on "local health departments."[257] Another provider shared that "as a sub-acute provider, our company facilities and staff seemed to be near the bottom of the list to receive both assistance with emergency supplies or financial assistance," so they had to rely on "their own supply chains for PPE, without the assistance of local health or emergency response officials."[258] The report also found that "most providers reported shifting care into telehealth formats and using technology to arrange virtual visits and group meetings," yet difficulties "obtaining reimbursement from commercial insurers for services provided by telehealth" remained a large barrier to care."[259]

In sum, the COVID-19 pandemic exposed anew many vulnerabilities of our congregate care systems, including that congregate settings placed people with disabilities at a high risk of infection, serious illness, and death. While vaccinations greatly reduced the death tolls in CCFs across the country, the unpredictability of the virus, difficulties of getting vaccines to some facilities, and high rates of vaccine hesitancy among many facility staff led to outbreaks at dozens of facilities even after vaccinations occurred at the facilities.[260]

People with Disabilities were Stuck as Diversions and Transitions from CCFs Slowed to a Near Halt

While the dangers imposed by the pandemic in CCFs created an urgency to transition residents to their own homes or other noncongregate community settings to keep people safe and to allow for distancing within facilities, the opposite happened. Due to the pandemic's impact on community service providers like direct support professionals, assertive community treatment team staff, case managers, employment services providers, and peer support workers, transitions and diversions in most places ground to a halt, even as unprecedented efforts were made to reduce the census of many jails and prisons due to COVID-19 transmission risks.[261] The National Governors Association observed that while at least some states continued facilitating discharges from state psychiatric hospitals, others "halted or slowed discharges."[262]

Among other things, community service providers were unable to enter CCFs to engage and assist residents with transitions to the community, and in many cases had fewer staff available due to staff illness, quarantining after exposure to the virus, or family or childcare issues. While Centers for Medicare & Medicaid Services (CMS) guidance allowed essential workers into nursing homes and other LTCFs, many states did not designate community service providers and individuals conducting "in-reach" to engage people with disabilities in institutions and assist them with transition as essential workers. In North Carolina, in-reach workers helping people with psychiatric disabilities transition out of adult care homes were designated as essential workers able to enter the facilities as a result of advocacy by the court monitor in an *Olmstead* settlement, but that designation took four months to accomplish.[263]

> *[A]dvocates filed lawsuits seeking to quickly move people out of state psychiatric hospitals in the District of Columbia, California, Connecticut, and Massachusetts where high rates of COVID-19 transmission and deaths were occurring.*

Complicating the situation, many nursing homes and group homes for people with IDD/DD could not safely readmit people who needed to be temporarily hospitalized during the pandemic. In New York, for example, the "OPWDD [Office for People with Developmental Disabilities] issued guidance instructing providers to accept individuals only if they could safely accommodate them in the group home" such that "people who could not be safely accommodated either remained at the hospital or were served in one of the over 100 temporary sites established for COVID-19 recovery efforts."[264]

While telehealth was used to facilitate communication between community providers and individuals in many CCFs, CCFs often lacked reliable internet access, tablets and other devices were often difficult for individuals to use, and residents were often not trained in how to use them. This lack of technology and training impaired provider access to residents, and isolated residents from communication with loved ones and other forms of social interaction. Moreover, many activities essential for community transition that could have been conducted virtually were often not—for example, in-reach activities, assessments and service planning by community providers, and tours of community housing.[265]

In response to deaths in CCFs from COVID-19, advocates filed lawsuits seeking to quickly move people out of state psychiatric hospitals in the District of Columbia, California, Connecticut, and Massachusetts where high rates of COVID-19 transmission and deaths were occurring.[266] A mental health expert in one of these cases observed:

> State psychiatric wards are typically designed to hold between twenty to forty patients per unit. Having that many people living in rooms with two or more other patients and interacting in a confined area with a large number of staff is obviously not consistent with "social distancing." . . . Even if congregate care facilities could be rendered safe by observance of CDC guidelines, it would not happen. There is no effective way to enforce social distancing in a psychiatric ward. . . . Psychiatric units are designed to facilitate staff and patient interaction. Patients are encouraged with a variety of incentives to attend group treatment, eat, socialize, and watch television together in an open area, attend community meetings, and exercise as a group. Avoiding the isolation that is compelled by the virus is so ingrained in treatment protocols that licensing standards typically prohibit staff from requiring patients to stay in their room unless they are an imminent danger to themselves or others."[267]

Some of this litigation resulted in better infection control practices in the hospitals. It did not, however, succeed in securing facility census reductions, in part because vaccination efforts and decreases in COVID-19 outbreaks made this relief more difficult to secure.[268]

These cases demonstrate the difficulty that disability advocates have experienced in trying to secure relief that would increase the pace of discharges from institutional settings, even where deaths from COVID-19 in institutions reached alarming rates.

COVID-19 Exacerbated Existing Civil Rights Violations Involving Needless Institutionalization and Segregation

The disability community and disability advocates have long fought to reduce the use of congregate settings for people with disabilities. Individuals with disabilities overwhelmingly thrive in the community when they are provided HCBS. The ADA and its integration mandate require that public entities administer services to people with disabilities in the most integrated setting appropriate, unless doing so would fundamentally change their service systems.[269] HCBS provides people with an opportunity to live full lives in the communities where they and their support systems are located, and, as we learned during COVID-19, serving people at home rather than in a CCF, along with other safety precautions, such as PPE, helps to control the spread of the virus.

[S]erving people at home rather than in a CCF, along with other safety precautions, such as PPE, helps to control the spread of the virus.

In 1999, the U.S. Supreme Court affirmed that people with disabilities have a legal right to community-based care. The Court found that needless institutionalization "perpetuates unwarranted assumptions that persons so isolated are incapable or unworthy of participating in community life."[270] In addition, "confinement in an institution severely diminishes the everyday life activities of individuals, including family relations, social contacts, work options, economic independence, educational advancement, and cultural enrichment."[271] As such, the needless segregation of people with disabilities in institutional settings is a form of disability-based discrimination. *Olmstead* established that people with disabilities have the right to receive a public entity's services in the most integrated setting.

The impact of COVID-19 on CCFs meant that people with disabilities not only experienced needless segregation on a widespread basis, but now that segregation also came with serious risks of infection and death from COVID-19. Moreover, the pandemic's impact in slowing down discharges and diversions from CCFs and hampering the community service system meant that people with disabilities had little chance of achieving their right to community integration and were stuck in CCFs that in many cases had become dangerous.

Even for individuals who were class members in *Olmstead* settlement agreements that afforded them specific rights to transition out of CCFs, enforcing those rights became an enormous challenge as states fell far behind on the obligations in these settlements and were unable to conduct certain activities required by the settlements due to the pandemic, including activities that required face-to-face contact or that could not be conducted through telehealth because of poor internet access, lack of equipment, the inability to train individuals in how to use the equipment, or other issues.

In one state, community providers advocated for the state to halt diversion and transitions under two *Olmstead* settlements because they said they could not maintain adequate staffing and considered all individuals transitioning out of these institutions as "high-risk" for community living in light of the providers' capacity concerns. Providers also expressed concerns about the impact of loneliness on individuals living in the community if providers were not spending as much time with them, even though isolation was even more dramatic in CCFs, particularly with staff reductions during the pandemic, and some facilities prohibited residents from even going outside.[272] Despite budget increases to support diversion and transition, including the hiring of additional staff and allowing telehealth for services, and despite the fact that hundreds of individuals died of COVID-19 in the nursing homes at issue in one of these settlements, transitions under the settlements were largely halted. During 2020, the rate of transitions of individuals from these institutions was the lowest since the settlements had begun more than 10 years earlier.[273]

The Biden Administration DOJ is reinvigorating the federal government's *Olmstead* enforcement efforts. In June 2021, it entered an *Olmstead* settlement with Maine's Department of Health and Human Services requiring an "exceptions process" allowing individuals to show that modifying Maine's caps on HCBS Medicaid waiver costs and/or service amounts is necessary to ensure that people with intellectual disabilities or autism spectrum disorders can receive adequate and appropriate services in the most integrated setting appropriate to their needs. The settlement resolved a complaint by a man with intellectual disabilities who, as a result of the state's waiver caps, was at risk of having to move to a congregate setting to access needed services.[274] One month earlier, it issued a findings letter detailing *Olmstead* violations by Alameda County, California, in placing people with psychiatric disabilities at risk of institutionalization and incarceration by failing to provide needed community-based services.[275]

More Could Have Been Done to Discharge and Divert People with Disabilities from CCFs during the Pandemic

While the pandemic created real challenges for transitioning and diverting individuals from CCFs, in most instances many steps could be taken to work around these challenges. For example, North Carolina, to promote compliance with an *Olmstead* settlement, developed protocols for local management entities in order to quickly transition people out of state psychiatric hospitals, including challenging providers to report barriers to the state for remediation. As a result, the state successfully diverted 40 percent of people from entering board and care facilities called "adult care homes."[276] Though transitions out of these facilities did not reach prepandemic levels, they continued despite barriers and obstacles with visitation and transportation. The state transitioned and diverted 331 individuals into supported housing between March 1 and December 31, 2020, and the number of people who stayed in the community after exiting adult care homes remained steady.

In addition, a number of individual Centers for Independent Living led efforts to transition individuals out of CCFs. These centers took advantage of funds directed to independent living centers through the Coronavirus Aid, Relief, and Economic Security Act of 2021 (CARES) as well as other emergency resources to quickly set up temporary housing and transition people out of congregate settings. These innovative partnerships provided potential solutions to long-standing problems with transition and diversion, and investments should continue beyond the pandemic.

In Denver, Atlantis Community, Inc., an independent living center, launched a pilot program called "the Emergency Relocation of People with Disabilities out of Congregate Settings" to transition people out of CCFs including acute care hospitals, assisted living facilities, nursing homes, congregate shelters for people experiencing homelessness, hospitals, and physical rehabilitative hospitals. The program "started with the basic idea of gathering a group of 9 people and moving them into a hotel for a minimum 14 day quarantine period while services, supports, and housing are set up with the individuals for more permanent housing in the community."[277] Using a combination of funds from CARES Act, Medicaid, state housing vouchers, and private foundations and donors, Atlantis also hired and trained (and housed) people experiencing homelessness as caregivers for the individuals transitioning. Every person who participates in the pilot program is set up with a state housing voucher and supported in finding long-term, sustainable housing. Roads to Freedom independent living center in Pennsylvania used a similar model of moving people from nursing homes to hotels and

> *[North Carolina] transitioned and diverted 331 individuals into supported housing between March 1 and December 31, 2020, and the number of people who stayed in the community after exiting adult care homes remained steady.*

then to more permanent housing, using CARES Act, FEMA funds, grants, and other funding. Both of these programs found that once individuals were transferred to a hotel, they were able to secure permanent housing of the person's choice within approximately a month or one and a half months.[278] In the Denver program, state rental subsidies paid for community housing. The Pennsylvania program used federal subsidies, including Section 8 Housing Choice Vouchers, Section 811 supportive housing for people with disabilities, and public housing. In both programs, Medicaid paid for supportive services.

Experts in one of the cases seeking to reduce the census of institutions during the pandemic stated: "Based on our years of experience managing psychiatric hospitals and other facilities, planning for the successful transition of individuals with serious mental illness from state psychiatric hospitals can be accomplished, even under these circumstances, through individualized planning and using all available resources, including natural supports."[279] Experts in these cases recommended that discharge determinations be made using a different standard than in ordinary times, ensuring that individuals' basic needs will be met in the community; that facilities explore whether residents have family or friends who could house them if provided with appropriate supports; that available capacity in community programs be used to permit discharges; that temporary housing in hotels be used if more permanent housing options are not immediately available; that community providers be included in the process of assessing discharge potential and planning for transition; and that additional funding to enhance community services be considered.[280]

Concerns about isolation and loneliness in the community should not be used as an excuse to keep people institutionalized; similar concerns exist in institutional settings, particularly during a pandemic.[281] Providing individuals with technology to more easily communicate can reduce isolation and can also help with telehealth services and virtual transition efforts.[282] For example, the California Foundation for Independent Living Centers purchased and distributed laptops to people with disabilities living in the community and agreed to pay internet costs for several months.[283] These tablets "allow[ed] people to take cooking classes, peer classes, and even attend a disability athletics fair."[284] Similarly, many peer support providers have transitioned efforts to Zoom to continue engagement during the pandemic. In North Carolina, community providers used Zoom to communicate with psychiatric facility social workers to facilitate quick discharges of individuals to the community.[285] One North Carolina community service provider employed robots to assist individuals in the community with medication and case management during the pandemic.[286]

Unfortunately, efforts to move people into the community remained sparse because little was done on a state level to facilitate discharges and diversions from CCFs, and most people in congregate settings at the start of the pandemic remained there.

> *Concerns about isolation and loneliness in the community should not be used as an excuse to keep people institutionalized; similar concerns exist in institutional settings, particularly during a pandemic.*

Limited Federal Guidance for CCFs Hindered Responses During Early Days of COVID-19

As the federal government wrestled with the COVID-19 pandemic in its early days, the CDC issued general guidance instructing how nursing homes and healthcare settings should control infection and ensure equitable delivery of care but not for other CCFs, like group homes. CDC reports issuing general guidance for nursing homes and healthcare settings as early as January 2020 and on March 1, 2020.[287] CMS issued a memo on March 13, 2020, and a toolkit on April 4, 2020, with best practices for nursing homes, and, together, CMS and CDC issued recommendations on April 2, 2020, concerning COVID-19 transmission in nursing homes.[288] A March 30, 2020, CMS guidance concerning intermediate care facilities for people with intellectual disabilities and psychiatric residential treatment facilities addressed infection control and prevention practices to prevent the transmission of COVID-19 in these facilities.[289] These guidance documents focused mainly on infection control, including recommendations for visitor restrictions, and emphasized the importance of social distancing.[290] In many facilities, compliance with this distancing guidance would require the facilities to discharge and divert people, but CDC did not specifically discuss the need to increase discharges and diversions to community settings.

CDC also published guidance to administrators of assisted living facilities on April 16, 2020.[291] This guidance, again, focused almost exclusively on basic infection control within facilities—including recommendations that facilities mandate residents wear cloth face masks, regularly disinfect, cancel group activities, implement social distancing, "restrict . . . all non-essential personnel," and "ask residents not to leave the facility except for medically necessary purposes." The guidance also instructed facilities to isolate suspected positive individuals in their rooms or, where facilities could not provide adequate care, to transfer individuals to another location (e.g., alternate care setting, hospital) that was equipped to adhere to recommended infection prevention and control practices.[292]

Despite the widespread deaths of individuals with disabilities in CCFs during the first weeks of the pandemic—by April 23, 2020, more than 10,000 deaths had been reported in LTCFs in the 23 states that publicly reported death data for these facilities[293]—it was not until May 28, 2020, that CDC released targeted guidance for community-based congregate settings. In CDC's "Guidance for Group Homes for Individuals with Disabilities" and, later, its "Guidance for Shared or Congregate Housing," CDC acknowledged that some individuals with disabilities may be unable to socially distance or wear face masks and recommended that facilities consult with local "Departments of Behavioral Health and Developmental Disabilities" for "information on and resources for behavioral techniques." The guidance recommended that facilities "plan for essential outings," but focused only on resident use of public transportation to continue working

> *By April 23, 2020, more than 10,000 deaths had been reported in LTCFs in the 23 states that publicly reported death data for these facilities.*

or attending medically necessary medical appointments, not to partake in diversion or transition efforts. CDC also recommended that CCF residents "continue to receive medical care for underlying conditions and evaluation or new symptoms or illnesses," including by investigating where "providers . . . have new ways to be contacted or new ways of providing appointments," like telehealth.

Though CDC revised its prior recommendations to fully restrict the mobility of CCF residents, it continued to recommend that CCFs only allow "essential" visitors, which contributed to limited access for necessary direct support workers and community service providers.[294] The dividing line between essential and nonessential visitors proved murky, and, in practice, was often a difficult one for facilities to manage.[295] While facility staff and personal care attendants were considered essential and therefore allowed into facilities to provide necessary care to residents, community transition support workers were not always considered essential, which slowed transitions out of CCFs. CDC also said facilities should "avoid transferring residents with disabilities to alternate settings, whenever possible, as a solution to staffing issues," which contributed to the hampering of moving individuals into lesser density community-based settings.[296]

Similarly, states offered little guidance for CCFs beyond infection control procedures within the facilities. For example, New York issued guidance for congregate residential settings, but the guidance focused on policies for group environments, social distancing, infection control, visitation, and testing.[297] Pennsylvania

issued guidance for individuals in personal care homes, assisted living residences, and private intermediate care facilities.[298] The guidance mostly provided guidance for infection control, but also detailed the allowance of compassionate care visitation if a resident has a "significant change" in condition.[299]

Until the early months of 2021, under the Biden Administration, there was little public recognition that without efforts to move people out of crowded institutional or congregate settings, infection control efforts that relied primarily on social distancing would continue to leave CCF residents and staff at risk.

Initial federal guidance for emergency use vaccines also failed to prioritize all residents of CCFs equitably. The National Academies of Science, Engineering, and Medicine's "Framework for Equitable Allocation of COVID-19 Vaccination" tiered groups for vaccine distribution in priority order, including as key populations "people who live and/or work in congregate settings," "older adults living in senior facilities," and "long-term care facility residents."[300] Phase 1a, making vaccination available to the highest priority group, included "high-risk health workers" that "are involved in direct patient care."[301] Phase 1b, the next phase, "focuse[d] attention on two groups that [we]re particularly vulnerable to severe morbidity and mortality due to COVID-19: (1) people of all ages with comorbid and underlying conditions that put them at significantly higher risk and (2) older adults living in congregate or overcrowded settings."[302] However, even though the guidance recognized the risk in congregate settings, the guidance left until Phase 2 "group homes . . . for people with disabilities, including serious mental illness, developmental and intellectual disabilities, and physical disabilities or in recovery, and staff who work in such settings" despite similarities in transmission rates and population risks across these congregate settings.[303] Moreover, the guidance did not detail whether staff or residents should be prioritized first, how residents with different disabilities in different types of CCFs should be prioritized based on underlying risk, or how facilities could ensure the continued availability of vaccines for new residents. In response, many states vaccinated CCF staff much earlier than residents, similarly to the manner in which some states made COVID-19 testing available more frequently to CCF staff than residents.[304]

The Biden Administration Brought New Focus to People with Disabilities in CCFs, Though Many Steps Came Late and Others Remain Undone

President Biden issued a National Strategy for the COVID-19 Response and Pandemic Preparedness immediately upon assuming office. Among other things, it included a commitment to make "significant investments in home and community based services," and, through HHS, CMS, and ACL, identify "opportunities and funding mechanisms to provide greater support for individuals receiving home and community based services, with particular attention to people with disabilities and the home care workforce crisis."[305]

On January 21, 2021, President Biden issued an Executive Order directing the federal government to take a more active role in providing assistance to CCFs.[306] The Executive Order requires the Secretaries of Defense, HHS, and Veterans Affairs to "provide targeted surge assistance to critical care and LTCFs, including nursing homes and skilled nursing facilities, assisted living facilities, intermediate care facilities for individuals with disabilities, and residential treatment centers in their efforts to combat the spread of COVID-19."[307] Since then, CDC has updated its guidance for LTCFs to include procedures for handling PPE, visitation, and physical distancing with "a description of quarantine recommendations including resident placement, recommended PPE, and duration of quarantine,"[308] and updated its guidance for individuals with disabilities in group homes,[309] but neither recommends facilitating transitions out of these facilities or describes strategies to do so.

HHS's Office for Civil Rights issued a guidance prohibiting discrimination in COVID-19 vaccination programs on April 13, 2021,[310] and around the same time, the Administration for Community Living issued strategies for improving equitable vaccine access for older adults and people with disabilities.[311] These guidance documents were helpful but did not specifically address individuals in CCFs.

The Biden Administration engaged in significant interagency coordination to identify ways to pair services and housing resources to promote transitions and diversions of people with disabilities and older adults from institutions, particularly in light of the virus transmission that occurred and could recur in the future.

The federal government first addressed legal requirements to transition individuals from CCFs during COVID-19 almost a year into the pandemic. On December 17, 2020, CMS issued guidance stating that community service providers "should have direct access to service recipients prior to discharge;" that facilities should use telehealth strategies to engage outside providers in transition planning, developing relationships, and facilitating transition if visitation restrictions are in place for these providers; and that institutional settings should work together with community providers to ensure that individuals who no longer need or want facility-based care can transition to the community, including through the use of virtual technology for team meetings, client engagement, service planning, and apartment walk-throughs.[312] On February 10, 2021, CMS issued guidance noting that federal disability rights laws *may* require facilities to permit entry of support staff to facilitate an individual's transition from an institutional setting to the community.[313] The guidance, later updated on June 3, 2021, says that under federal law, "facilities may be required to permit entry of a designated support person to meet an individual's disability-related needs, including, as may be appropriate in some cases, supporting an individual's transition from an institutional setting into the community, and offering strategies as well for allowing safe outdoor visitation."[314] Despite CMS's acknowledgment that visitation restrictions should not impede community providers from entering facilities to provide transition support, the guidance could be clearer that these providers

> *Despite CMS's acknowledgment . . ., the guidance could be clearer that these providers should be considered "essential care providers."*

should be considered "essential care providers." The guidance also could have clarified what newly available funding sources could help fund transition-related costs.

On April 2, 2021, DOJ issued a statement recommending "services in home- and community-based settings instead of in long-term care facilities" and requiring "governments" to "comply with the ADA and Section 504."[315] Moreover, the guidance acknowledged that these HCBS services "can satisfy the ADA integration mandate by preventing unnecessary institutionalization . . . [and] also reduce COVID-19 risk."[316]

Though the spring 2021 guidance documents from CMS and DOJ were necessary, they came too late; the worst of the pandemic had already occurred and had taken the lives of thousands of CCF residents during the previous year. Furthermore, by the time they were released, the United States had made vaccines widely available to this population. An earlier investment in infrastructure and guidance to move people out of these high-density settings and requiring compliance with *Olmstead* during the pandemic could have prevented mass casualties and infection.

> *[T]he federal government has not fully addressed the need for federal guidance to facilitate transitions and diversions from CCFs.*

Moreover, the federal government has not fully addressed the need for federal guidance to facilitate transitions and diversions from CCFs. While rates of COVID-19 transmission in CCFs have dramatically decreased, such guidance is important for the future. No federal guidance has detailed with specificity how HCBS could facilitate transitions and diversions of individuals from CCFs during a pandemic, nor how states could reduce census within facilities by enhancing HCBS, despite similar CDC guidance recommending release of individuals from correctional and detention facilities to prevent intrafacility transmission.[317] Guidance could have detailed how providers could use telehealth for transition services and could highlight temporary discharge options like motels or other housing.

For example, to speed up transitions amid staff and provider shortages, CMS guidance could have identified strategies for discharging individuals with disabilities from CCFs to temporary housing—possibly with a lower but critical level of support initially, affording additional time to secure permanent housing and full supportive services. Guidance could have considered subsidies or financial stipends for friends and family of persons in CCFs to provide short-term housing and care while permanent supports were found. It could also have given states a framework for innovative ways to use emergency funds and existing resources to fund other short-term, emergency housing like hotel stays, so people could be safely moved from CCFs while providers were given a window to find stable housing.

The full extent of vaccinations among CCF residents is not known due to inadequate data collection for facilities other than LTCFs. Around 3 million people in LTCFs were fully vaccinated, but, even so, the federal program bringing vaccines to nursing homes missed around half of the staff working within those facilities, according to a March 2021 report.[318] More data is needed to understand where and how vaccines should have been prioritized differently.

On May 13, 2021, CMS issued an interim final rule requiring intermediate care facilities for individuals with intellectual and developmental disabilities, along with LTCFs, to offer residents and staff vaccinations and to collect and report data on these vaccinations to CDC.[319] CMS solicited public comment on whether it would be feasible to impose similar requirements on other facilities including psychiatric hospitals, psychiatric residential treatment facilities, forensic hospitals, adult foster care homes, group homes, assisted living facilities, supervised apartments, and inpatient hospice facilities. NCD believes that all of these facilities should be required to comply with these rules.

During future pandemics and national emergencies, guidance is needed at every step of the way for *all* types of CCFs, not just nursing homes and LTCFs. The guidance must detail how facilities can accelerate discharges and ensure diversion and how states can pay for those efforts—both by increasing the availability of funds and detailing ways in which

> *During future pandemics and national emergencies, guidance is needed at every step of the way for all types of CCFs, not just nursing homes and LTCFs. The guidance must detail how facilities can accelerate discharges and ensure diversion . . .*

those funds can be used most efficiently to provide equitable care.

Financing Community Services and Housing to Enable Transitions from CCFs

Understanding the key funding sources available to expand community services and housing is critical to accelerating discharges and diversions from CCFs. Medicaid is the primary payer of HCBS for people with disabilities. Key Medicaid authorities for financing these services include HCBS waiver services, the Medicaid rehabilitation option (which covers assertive community treatment, peer support services, mobile crisis, and other crisis services), personal care services, home health services, intensive case management, transition services, tenancy support services, and supported employment. The Medicaid "Money Follows the Person" program also funds HCBS for people with disabilities who have been institutionalized for at least 90 days, but states have had difficulty relying on it due to short reauthorization periods,[320] and features of the program have made it largely unavailable to people with psychiatric disabilities.

HCBS services were already in short supply before the pandemic. For example, most states' HCBS wait lists averaged around three years,[321] and community mental health services were in similarly short supply. Additionally, the Trump Administration weakened its enforcement of the Medicaid HCBS "Settings Rule," which is designed to ensure that scarce resources designated for HCBS are provided in integrated community settings, and not in segregated settings that isolate people.[322] The Settings Rule has been important in expanding opportunities for individuals with disabilities to live, work, and receive services in integrated settings and thus in reducing some COVID-19 risks. CMS's enforcement in recent years has been less assertive, however, and its new policies have weakened the impact of the rule. In 2017, CMS extended the deadline for states to come into full compliance with the rule by three years, from March 2019 to March 2022,[323] and in 2020 CMS extended the timeline by another year due to COVID-related issues.[324] In 2019, CMS issued guidance making a number of changes allowing states to avoid federal scrutiny of whether federal HCBS funds are appropriately used for settings that are presumptively institutional in nature but for which states seek HCBS funding.[325] Had the Settings Rule been in full effect during the pandemic, persons with disabilities may have had more opportunities to secure community-based services to transition from or avoid placement in a CCF. The Trump guidance should be reversed, and CMS should take a more active role in scrutinizing which settings meet the requirements of the rule.

As described above, the pandemic's impact on community service providers made HCBS services even more difficult to access. In addition to these services, housing subsidies are critical to ensure that people with disabilities can transition or be diverted from CCFs. A lack of housing is often the biggest barrier to

> *Medicaid is the primary payer of HCBS for people with disabilities. . . . [A]s of July 2021, there are more than 850,000 people with IDD/DD on waiting lists for HCBS services.*

transition. Many states have programs providing state rental subsidies as part of supported housing. In addition, federal housing funding streams are often used, including HUD's Housing Choice Vouchers (formerly known as "Section 8" housing), "Section 811" supportive housing vouchers for people with disabilities, "Mainstream vouchers" for nonelderly people with disabilities, and Continuum of Care subsidies to house homeless individuals. The availability of both federal and state rental subsidies falls far short of the need. As a result, there are nearly 400,000 people with disabilities living on the streets, in shelters, and another 200,000–300,000 people with disabilities in institutional settings.[326] Further, as of July 2021, there are more than 850,000 people with IDD/DD on waiting lists for HCBS services.[327] According to one report, "federal rental subsidy programs administered by the U.S. Department of Housing and Urban Development (HUD) currently reach only 35 of every 100 extremely low-income (ELI) households. . . . This shortfall translates into long waiting lists at Public Housing Agencies (PHAs) and affordable housing developments, and a critical shortage of permanent supportive housing (PSH) opportunities for people with significant disabilities who have SSI-level incomes."[328]

Congress has made available new funding available for HCBS and housing in its COVID-19 relief legislation, most significantly in the American Rescue Plan Act (ARPA).[329] However, it is incumbent upon state and local governments to take advantage of these funds to expand their ability to transition and divert people with

> *A lack of housing is often the biggest barrier to transition [to the community].*

disabilities from CCFs. States also have the ability to use certain Medicaid flexibilities during an emergency to cover services that would otherwise not be reimbursable—including "Appendix K" waivers for Medicaid HCBS waivers as well as waivers permitted under Section 1135 of the Social Security Act.

Enhanced Medicaid Funding for HCBS

Increased funding for HCBS is critical to speed up the rate of transitions out of congregate settings for people with disabilities. HCBS are health services "designed to enable people to stay in their homes, rather than moving to a facility for care."[330] For community providers who were hit hard by the pandemic including with staff shortages, expenses of acquiring PPE, telehealth equipment, vehicle shields, and other necessary supplies, additional funding that could be used to provide HCBS and cover such supplies and extra staffing was key to shore up their ability to function and to expand. ARPA provided $12.7 billion to states for HCBS—including home healthcare, personal care, habilitation services, supported employment, and rehabilitative services, among other services. Congress provided a 10 percent increase in federal Medicaid reimbursement for these services for one year, from April 2021 through March 2022. If states choose to use this newly available funding, they must use it to supplement current HCBS spending.[331] This ensures that states do not reduce their financial investments in HCBS as they receive an influx of federal funds; the funds must be used to add to the state's existing investments. The Act also provided enhanced federal Medicaid reimbursement for mobile crisis services for a three-year period beginning in April 2022.

Congress also extended the Money Follows the Person program for three years in the Consolidated Appropriations Act in December 2020.[332] Money Follows the Person "provides states with enhanced federal matching funds for services and supports to help . . . people with disabilities move from institutions to the community" and "was designed to . . . increase the use of home and community-based, rather than institutional, long-term care services."[333]

Using Medicaid "Appendix K" and Section 1135 Waivers to Cover Family Caregiver Support

Many states have used "Appendix K" waivers, which may be used to modify Medicaid HCBS waivers during an emergency, to cover services that they ordinarily would not cover. Appendix K waivers, which must be approved by HHS, enable states to "pay legally responsible relatives to provide care that is 'extraordinary'" and that is "necessary in order to prevent the beneficiary from being institutionalized."[334] For example, states could expand eligibility for community services by increasing flexibility for payment to family caregivers and by temporarily modifying minimum provider qualifications. States could also use these waivers to increase the amount they currently pay home caregivers and to provide them with PPE. As of April 19, 2021, 39 states were using Appendix K waivers to pay family caregivers.[335] The use of Appendix K has helped to prevent the transmission of COVID-19.

As of April 19, 2021, 39 states were using Appendix K waivers to pay family caregivers.

Likewise, "Section 1135" waivers can be used during emergencies to temporarily halt certain requirements for providers of home healthcare. As of April 19, 2021, 14 states were using Section 1135 waivers to pay for personal care provided by legally responsible family caregivers.[336] By keeping family members together and out of congregate settings, the use of Section 1135 to pay for family caregivers, like Appendix K, has helped to prevent transmission of COVID-19.

One flexibility that CMS commonly granted in Section 1135 waivers is a waiver of preadmission screening (PASRR) requirements to ensure that individuals with psychiatric and intellectual disabilities are not inappropriately admitted to nursing homes. As it is, these requirements have had limited effectiveness in stopping nursing home admissions of individuals who could live in more integrated settings, and waiving them only increases needless institutionalization and exposes more people with disabilities to risks of coronavirus transmission.

FEMA Reimbursement for Emergency Housing

The Federal Emergency Management Agency (FEMA) quickly became a leading source of funding for housing assistance grants. The main source of FEMA funding for housing relief is Category B Public Assistance under the Stafford Act.[337] The CARES Act added supplementary funding to Category B Public Assistance and enhanced Emergency Food and Shelter Program grants. By an Executive Order dated February 2, 2021, President Biden increased the federal match to 100 percent of approved expenses (up from the usual 75 percent rate) for work through September 30, 2021.[338] FEMA Category B grants can be made to states, territories, tribes, and local governments if the area is under a public health order that recommends noncongregate housing to address COVID-19 in a target population. According to FEMA, target populations may include, for example, people who test positive for COVID-19 but do not require hospitalization, people who have been exposed to COVID-19, and individuals who are high-risk and require physical distancing as a precautionary measure.[339] Localities may then use Category B funds to reimburse the cost of renting hotels, motels, and "other forms of non-congregate sheltering" to house individuals at risk of homelessness.[340]

At least four states—California, Pennsylvania, Connecticut, and North Carolina—received approval for FEMA Category B funds to provide noncongregate housing to a target population during the pandemic, which could include, "those who test positive for COVID-19 who do not require hospitalization but need isolation (including those exiting from hospitals); those who have been exposed to COVID-19 who do not require hospitalization; and asymptomatic high-risk individuals needing social distancing as a precautionary measure, such as people over 65 or with certain underlying health conditions (respiratory, compromised immunities, chronic disease)."[341] California and Pennsylvania applied for and were granted funds for noncongregate sheltering for the groups outlined in FEMA's target populations.[342] North Carolina expanded the target population to also include "those whose living situation makes them unable to adhere to social distancing guidance."[343] Finally, Connecticut's approved application broadly extended to cover noncongregate housing for individuals currently living in "at-risk facilities such as group homes, nursing homes, long-term care sites, and alternative care facilities" and "homeless individuals in congregate shelters."[344]

In the fall of 2020, independent living centers reported that FEMA funds were difficult to access during the pandemic, sometimes because they were allocated to other entities early on and also because independent living centers would have to contract with a local agency or a county than directly with a state, to access Category B funds covering the areas in which they worked.[345] As an example, Roads to Freedom, the Center for Independent Living of North Central Pennsylvania, entered into an agreement with the county to receive FEMA Category B funds to transition people with disabilities from congregate settings. FEMA acknowledged that these funds could be used to transition people with disabilities from congregate settings to noncongregate settings about seven months later.

While Category B funds offer an important temporary solution for moving people out

> *Category B funds offer an important temporary solution for moving people out of CCFs and into supported housing quickly while more permanent housing is found, but recipients cannot use the funds for the wrap-around services that individuals in temporary housing need.*

of CCFs and into supported housing quickly while more permanent housing is found, but recipients cannot use the funds for the wrap-around services that individuals in temporary housing need. For example, FEMA explicitly disallows subsidies for case management and mental health counseling, and states must apply separately for sheltering subsidies and crisis counseling funds. Additionally, Category B funds provide only for *temporary* housing. Other federal subsidies are needed to ensure permanent, supportive housing for individuals with disabilities.

The CARES Act also provided $200 million to FEMA's Emergency Food and Shelter Program (EFSG), which is not contingent on a local disaster declaration.[346] Emergency Food and Shelter Program grants reimbursed 30-day stays in noncongregate housing and sheltering transportation costs.

The only housing funding targeted directly for people with disabilities in the COVID-19 relief legislation to date has been $15 million for Section 811 supportive housing and $65 million for the Housing Opportunities for Persons with AIDS (HOPWA) program. . . .

New Funding for Housing

Congress also appropriated significant new funding for federal housing programs in its COVID-19 relief packages. Most of these funds are targeted to individuals who are homeless or at risk of homelessness, but some may be used for people with disabilities being discharged or diverted from CCFs to the extent that they meet the criteria for the funds.

For example, ARPA included $5 billion for emergency vouchers that can be used by people who are homeless or at risk of homelessness, recently homeless, or fleeing domestic violence. These vouchers should be able to be used by people with disabilities discharged from CCFs who do not have access to stable housing.

CARES Act provided nearly $4 billion in new funding for HUD Emergency Solutions Grants (ESG).[347] These grants, authorized by the McKinney-Vento Homeless Assistance Act, provide funding to cities, counties, states, and territories to provide services to individuals at risk of homelessness (typically through subgrants to nonprofit organizations).[348] They can be used for individuals exiting an institution who meet certain qualifications—having income below 30 percent of the median family income and having spent 90 days or less in an institution and lived in an emergency shelter or were homeless prior to entering the facility.[349] Upon discharge, qualifying individuals leaving institutions are eligible for short-term rental assistance as well as housing relocation and stabilization. Funds can only be spent "to the extent that the assistance is necessary to help the program participant regain stability in [their] current permanent housing or move into other permanent housing and achieve stability in that housing."[350]

The only housing funding targeted directly for people with disabilities in the COVID-19 relief legislation to date has been $15 million for Section 811 supportive housing and $65 million for the Housing Opportunities for Persons with AIDS (HOPWA) program, both included in the CARES Act. However, Section 811 funds did not include any requirement to provide new housing units, but only to ensure maintenance of operations of existing Section 811 units during the pandemic. The HOPWA funds can be used to maintain existing housing assistance or to respond to COVID-19, including isolation and relocation expenses to protect people living with HIV/AIDS,[351] but most HOPWA funds tend to serve individuals who are not coming out of CCFs.

Since the vast majority of funding that can be used for new housing subsidies is targeted at people who are homeless or at risk of homelessness, guidance indicating that these funds can be used for purposes of transitioning eligible individuals with disabilities out of CCFs is important to ensure that some of this funding is directed to that purpose. Likewise, in any future health crisis, legislation establishing emergency funding should make clear that funds may be used for transition purposes.

> [T]he Better Care Better Jobs Act . . . would make states eligible for a 10 percent increase in federal Medicaid reimbursement for HCBS services if they take certain steps to expand HCBS services, strengthen the HCBS workforce . . . , and demonstrating improved availability of services and competitive wages for workers.

> CMS routinely collects data on nursing homes and therefore had built-in channels to begin requiring nursing homes to track and report on incidences of COVID-19 in their facilities; but neither CMS, the CDC, nor any other federal agency required reporting of this data in other types of CCFs, including CDC's COVID-19 Data Tracker.

Forthcoming Infrastructure Investments

On March 31, 2021, the Biden Administration released its $2.3 trillion infrastructure plan, the American Jobs Plan.[352] Among the plan's provisions are a proposal to spend $400 billion to shore up the HCBS workforce and expand HCBS services for people with disabilities and older adults, as well as a proposal to further extend the Money Follows the Person program. Congressional enactment of new funding for HCBS would be an opportunity to extend the American Rescue Plan's important incentive for expansion of HCBS into the future. On June 24, 2021, the Better Care Better Jobs Act was introduced in the House and Senate.[353] This legislation would make states eligible for a 10 percent increase in federal Medicaid reimbursement for HCBS services if they take certain steps to expand HCBS services, strengthen the HCBS workforce including by raising HCBS payment rates and ensuring that rate increases are passed through to direct care workers, and demonstrating improved availability of services and competitive wages for workers. The legislation would also make the Money Follows the Person program permanent.

Better Collection and Analysis of the Impact of COVID-19 on People Living and Working in Congregate Care Facilities

Data capturing the spread and transmission of COVID-19 in CCFs outside of LTCFs (and, especially, nursing homes) is sparse. CMS routinely collects data on nursing homes and therefore had built-in channels to begin requiring nursing homes to track and report on incidences of COVID-19 in their facilities; but neither CMS, the CDC, nor any other federal agency required reporting of this data in other types of CCFs, including CDC's COVID-19 Data Tracker.[354] This left gaps in critical information and an unclear picture of the impact on people with disabilities living in other CCF's, such as group homes and assisted living facilities.

To track the spread of the pandemic in CCFs, advocates had to piece together data from news reports on specific facilities, state databases and reports (where they existed), narratives from providers and caregivers, and private insurance data. The lack of federal data collection efforts stymied efforts to monitor compliance with federal disability protections and intensified civil rights concerns. Motivated by these grave consequences, in every Congressional negotiation on COVID-related packages, advocates pushed for federal collection of data to track the impact of COVID-19 on residents and staff of CCFs and to compare it to the impact on similarly situated individuals living at home. Such data requests included, for example:

Data Requests in Federal COVID Legislation

- Numbers of tests and rates of testing for COVID-19 of people with disabilities and staff in nursing homes, psychiatric facilities, facilities for people with intellectual and developmental disabilities, board and care homes, group homes, and other congregate facilities for people with disabilities in supported housing and other community settings.

- Numbers of people with disabilities and staff testing positive for COVID-19 and rates of positive tests in each of these settings.

- Numbers of COVID-19–related hospitalizations of people with disabilities and staff in each of these settings.

- Numbers of COVID-19–related deaths and death rates among people with disabilities and staff in each of these settings.

- Numbers of people who have recovered from COVID-19 and recovery rates among people with disabilities and staff in each of these settings.

- Numbers of people who have been transferred from community settings to institutional settings as a result of COVID-19.

- Numbers of people with disabilities who have been discharged from institutions as a result of COVID-19.

- Analysis of the data to identify trends and factors such as facility type, disability type, location or geographical area, or other factors that correlate with rates of testing, positive cases, or outcomes."[355]

Though the House-passed Health and Economic Recovery Omnibus Emergency Solutions (HEROES) Act included a provision requiring the Secretary to work with covered agencies to support the modernization of data collection to increase data related to "health inequities, such as racial, ethnic, socioeconomic, sex, gender, and disability disparities," the bill did not ultimately become law.[356]

The primary provision in the various pieces of COVID-19 relief legislation that could be used to require expanded data collection and analysis concerning people with disabilities is in the Paycheck Protection and Healthcare Enhancement Act. This Act included a provision requiring HHS to report incidences of COVID-19 diagnoses, hospitalizations, and deaths, broken down by several factors including race, ethnicity, age, sex, region, and "other relevant factors," but did not specifically require reporting by disability.[357] HHS should issue guidance indicating the "other relevant factors" provision includes disability, and data should be separated by housing status, including community care. Data is needed on community care to compare the difference in outcomes for people who experienced the pandemic in congregate settings and those that were able to receive care at home.

ARPA included provisions calling for the Secretary, acting through the Director of CDC, to provide funds to be used for data related to vaccine distribution and vaccinations, and funds for activities to support data collection systems. While the provisions are not currently disability-specific, these provisions might be a tool to track vaccination data for people with disabilities in and out of CCFs.[358] Further, as noted above, CMS issued an interim final rule requiring nursing facilities and intermediate care facilities

for people with intellectual and developmental disabilities to collect and report vaccination data for residents and staff.[359]

In January 2021, President Biden released the "National Strategy for the COVID-19 Response and Pandemic Preparedness," which included a call for increased data collection.[360] The strategy recognized that "the fragmented and limited availability of data by race, ethnicity, geography, disability and other demographic variables delays recognition of risk and a targeted response," and called upon HHS to "optimize data collection from public and private entities to increase the availability of data by . . . disability . . . and other demographic variables, as feasible," and established that CMS "will work to report Medicare and Medicaid data on COVID-19 testing, cases, vaccinations, hospitalizations, therapeutic utilization, and deaths by . . . disability and other sociodemographic factors.'[361] Additionally, President Biden issued an Executive Order directing federal agencies to "expand their data infrastructure to increase collection and reporting of health data for high risk populations."[362]

Summary of Findings

- COVID-19 exposed many of the worst vulnerabilities of congregate care systems and emphasized the weaknesses in existing efforts to move individuals out of these settings. In the face of the century's worst public health crisis, states had dramatically less capacity to fund and implement legally required diversion and transition initiatives. As a result, people with disabilities residing in congregate settings experienced disproportionate rates of severe illness and death due to COVID-19.

- Without adequate data to track the rates of transmission, testing, morbidity, mortality, and vaccination in each category of CCF, it is hard to say whether the federal government's prioritization of older adults and disabled persons, facility adherence to visitation restrictions, and provider hesitancy to move people out of congregate settings had a positive net effect on controlling the spread of COVID-19 in congregate settings (as claimed), despite the negative impact on transitions and diversion and the isolation that people experienced in these facilities. More information is needed to understand the full experiences that people with disabilities had during the pandemic. Moreover, CDC and CMS must build systems and capacities to track future public health emergencies in CCFs.

- Two positive gains from the pandemic include added investments in HCBS and housing for people with disabilities—including enhanced Medicaid reimbursement for HCBS, Medicaid flexibilities to reimburse family caregivers, a three-year extension of the Money Follows the Person demonstration project, and FEMA funding for emergency housing. Yet, it is not clear how fully states used these new funding streams, and if they did not, whether such oversight was intentional or a result of limited guidance and/or a lack of awareness of potential uses. Even with these positive steps, more investments are needed to expand Medicaid HCBS services, make permanent the Money Follows the Person program, strengthen enforcement and interpretations of the HCBS Settings Rule, and to expand the availability and affordability of housing units.

Recommendations

To ensure that diversions and transitions from CCFs continue prior to a future health crisis or pandemic, and to ensure quality standards of care for those who prefer or need to reside in CCFs, NCD recommends:

Recommendations for Federal Agencies

CMS, ACL, SAMHSA, HUD, FEMA, and DOJ should:

- Develop a multi-agency national strategy to mitigate the risks of COVID-19 transmission in CCFs and address the civil rights concerns that continue to impact the lives of people with disabilities in CCFs. The agencies should clarify how community services can be paired with housing resources to ensure that people with disabilities have the opportunity to receive services in the most integrated setting and avoid needless risk of infection and death. They should also issue guidance identifying strategies and resources available to state and local governments to facilitate transitions and diversions from CCFs, flexibilities

Recommendations for Federal Agencies: *continued*

that may be used, and how these resources factor into public entities' *Olmstead* obligations in future crises; for example:

- **CMS** should issue guidance explaining how states can combine HCBS funding with housing resources to facilitate transitions and diversions from CCFs; and ensure that temporary funds are available in future emergency settings with an explicit directive to transition people with disabilities out of CCFs.

- **CMS** should encourage states to use Appendix K and Section 1135 waivers to support family caregivers.

- **CMS** should rescind Trump-era guidance that weakens the interpretation of the HCBS Settings Rule and ensure that HCBS funding is used to fund services in integrated community settings.

- **CMS** should rescind its approval of PASRR waivers and HHS should prohibit their use in any future health emergency except under very limited circumstances.

- **HUD** should issue guidance clarifying that federal housing funds made available through ARPA and the CARES Act, as well as Emergency Solutions Grant funding more generally, may be used for individuals with disabilities transitioning or being diverted from CCFs.

- **HUD** should increase the availability of additional housing vouchers so states can curtail lengthy waiting lists, increase housing options—including accessible units—and speed up the process of transitioning people with disabilities into the community.

- **FEMA** should issue guidance clarifying that Category B funds and the Individuals and Households Program may be used for individuals with disabilities transitioning out of CCFs.

- **DOJ** should issue guidance concerning public entities' *Olmstead* obligations and how those entities should take advantage of specific federal resources to facilitate transition and diversion from CCFs, including emergency resources. The guidance should clarify that *Olmstead* and the ADA's integration mandate require that transitions and diversion from CCFs continue even during pandemics and other emergencies and offering strategies and examples of how that can be accomplished.

- ***CDC and CMS*** should work together to emphasize census reduction in all CCFs as an infection control strategy. Accordingly,

  - ***CDC*** should expand its guidance beyond LTCFs to include all CCFs and emphasize that reducing the census of CCFs through accelerating discharges and diversions as a

(continued)

Recommendations for Federal Agencies: *continued*

critical strategy to ensure that the physical distancing required for infection control can be effectively done in CCFs. CMS guidance should explain ways to reduce the level of services required for discharge when needed to speed up transitions amid staff and provider shortages during an emergency. In many cases, minimally necessary services and supports could, in an emergency setting, simply include medication and case management.

- **HHS** should improve disability data collection: The Paycheck Protection and Healthcare Enhancement Act required HHS to report incidences of COVID-19 diagnoses, hospitalizations, and deaths, broken down by several factors including "other relevant factors," but not specifically disability.[363] For data collection purposes, the Secretary of HHS should define "other relevant factors" to include data points that capture people with disabilities in CCFs. Future legislation should also require the collection of this data for each type of congregate care setting as well as for individuals with disabilities living in their own homes (specific data recommendations for Congress are addressed in the recommendations in chapter 1). Further, the CDC's COVID-19 Data Tracker should release COVID-19 data separated by housing status—for each type of CCF and for individuals who live independently in the community.[364]

- **CMS** should prioritize all CCFs to receive equipment such as test kits and proper PPE from federal, state, and local governments that is necessary to follow CDC guidelines in any similar health emergency. CMS should recognize and clarify that community providers conducting in-reach transition support to facility residents are "essential care providers," not "visitors," and should not be restricted from entering facilities during future pandemics or crises. All CCFs should receive priority designation for vaccine allocation. Federal and state investments to expand telehealth infrastructure to ensure continuity of care are likewise needed.

- **FEMA** should issue guidance to regional administrators reiterating their ability to approve broader eligibility definitions for sheltering-related Public Assistance reimbursements and to state governments explaining how they can access upfront FEMA Public Assistance payments in line with President Biden's January 21 executive order. It should:

  - Expand Reimbursement to Cover Expenses for Supportive Services and Personal Assistance Services (PAS) To Ensure Accessibility: Supportive services can be necessary to ensure that people experiencing homelessness, residents of CCFs, and other individuals with disabilities have access to noncongregate sheltering. To ensure greater

Recommendations for Federal Agencies: *continued*

access to the Public Assistance program, FEMA should expand the types of expenses eligible for reimbursement to include supportive services and encourage states and localities to provide supportive services alongside noncongregate shelter.

- Allow Independent Living Centers and Homeless Service Organizations to Apply for and Receive Direct Public Assistance Reimbursements: Currently, FEMA allows Public Assistance program reimbursements to be applied for and received by PNPs. The standing definition of PNPs, however, often exclude facilities such as independent living centers, homeless service centers, and similar nonprofits that operate in an open and public manner to ensure that certain populations have the services they need to survive. FEMA must issue guidance expanding the definition of PNP to include these organizations, ensuring they can continue operating after a disaster—including the current pandemic.

Recommendations for States

- *State Medicaid agencies* should expand Medicaid HCBS services including through taking advantage of new HCBS funding made available through ARPA and use Appendix K and Section 1135 waivers to support family caregivers.

- *State housing authorities and disability services agencies* should support the expansion of available housing to enable people with disabilities, including by increasing requests for federal housing assistance through HUD programs and targeting housing resources to people with disabilities, as well as expanding the use of state housing subsidy programs to support people with disabilities.

- *States*
  - Should ensure that requests for FEMA emergency housing assistance include the needs of people with disabilities to move from congregate settings from CCFs.
  - Should collect and make public, data concerning the numbers and rates of infections, hospitalizations, and deaths from COVID-19 or other viruses among residents and staff of all CCFs.

Chapter 3: The Direct Care Workforce

Overview of Direct Care Workforce

The direct care workforce, including personal care assistants, home health aides, and nursing assistants, is critical to the independence and well-being of any person with long-term care needs. Similarly, unpaid family caregivers assist family and friends who have chronic or other health conditions, functional limitations, or disabilities, allowing them to remain living at home and, for some, avoid institutionalization in nursing homes. As the coronavirus pandemic spread across the United States, direct care workers, primarily women and people of color, continued to shoulder responsibility for providing essential care and assistance for people with disabilities and older people. Yet they often received little or no training on the risks of COVID-19 and were not provided with adequate coronavirus testing or PPE and supplies that could shield them from infection and death.[365] Moreover, for these workers, the pandemic laid bare other long-standing inequities, including low wages, lack of comprehensive employee benefits such as paid family and medical leave, adequate unemployment insurance benefits, and hazard pay, and limited training and advancement opportunities.

Family caregivers met unforeseen challenges arising from COVID-19, including uncertainty about the likely impact of the disease on themselves and their families, the impact of shelter-at-home restrictions, lack of access to routine medical care, school, childcare, adult day program closures, potential job loss, income insecurity, and restricted access to prescriptions and home care supplies. The pandemic caused hardship and loss, yet it brought the essential and undervalued role of direct care workers into the national conversation. It also shined a light on urgently needed reforms, including improvements in compensation, career development, care team integration, training, and improved employee benefits. Similarly, the pandemic heightened public awareness of the invaluable role family caregivers play in maintaining people with disabilities and older adults at home[366] and focused on reforms that would support and enable unpaid workers to continue in these critical roles.[367]

> *The pandemic caused hardship and loss, yet it brought the essential and undervalued role of direct care workers into the national conversation.*

Direct Care Workforce and Family Caregiver Characteristics

An estimated 4.6 million individuals make up the direct care workforce in the United States, with a subset of more than 2.4 million who provide home care for people with disabilities and older individuals. An estimated 1 million home care workers are employed directly by people with disabilities and older people who receive services through publicly funded, consumer-directed programs. Other workers are hired privately in the "gray market," however, workforce data is not available for this group.[368] The direct care workforce assists an estimated 17 million people with disabilities and older people living in the community who require help with daily activities. It also assists an additional 1.5 million people living in nursing homes and 1 million people living in residential care facilities such as assisted living facilities and group homes.[369]

DC workers include personal care assistants, home health aides, and nursing assistants. People who work with individuals with intellectual and developmental disabilities are referred to as direct support professionals. Personal care assistants typically assist people with disabilities living in community settings and homes of their own with Activities of Daily Living (ADLs) such as bathing, dressing, eating, and toileting, and Instrumental Activities of Daily Living (IADLs) such as shopping, preparing meals, housekeeping, and handling finances. Home health aides and nursing assistants who work in institutional and community settings are

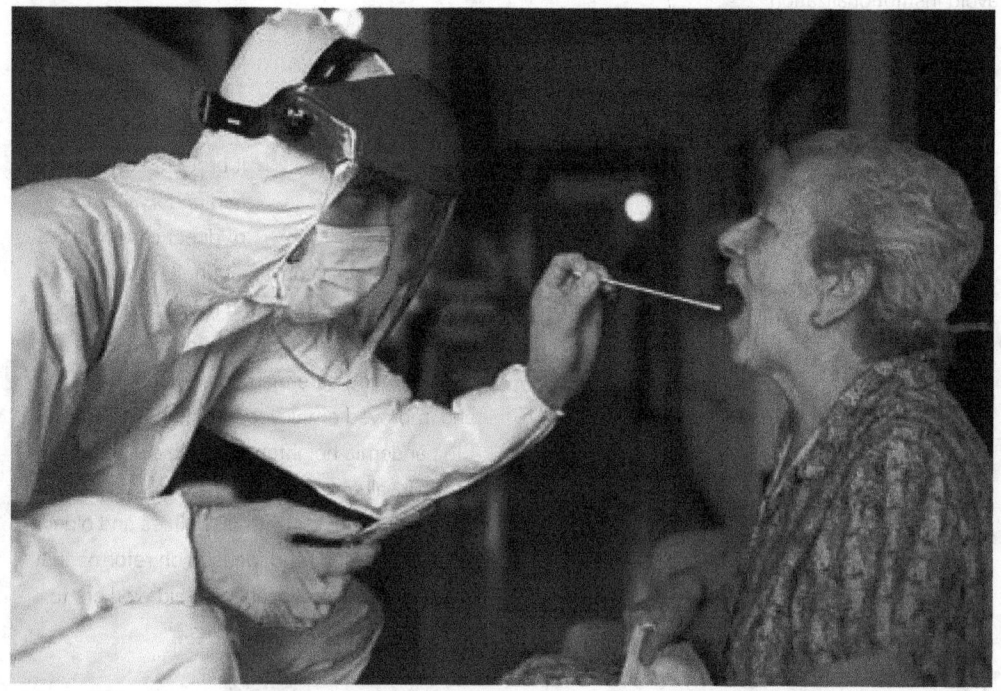

allowed to perform some clinical tasks, such as medication management, that some personal care assistants may not be allowed to carry out. An estimated 53 percent of direct care workers come into close, frequent contact with the individuals they assist, which placed them and the people with whom they worked at risk of contracting COVID-19 during the pandemic.[370]

The direct care workforce is comprised mostly of women (87 percent) and people of color (59 percent). Immigrants—noncitizens living in the United States, including lawful permanent residents, "nonimmigrants,"—such as visitors, students, and temporary workers, and undocumented immigrants—make up about 27 percent of the direct care workforce. The median age of the workforce is 45 years of age.[371] The direct care workforce in the United States, especially home health and personal care assistants, is projected to grow 34 percent from 2019 to 2029, according to the Bureau of Labor Statistics, as the baby boom generation ages and demand for home health and personal care assistance increases.[372] Even as millions of people with disabilities and older people rely on the care they provide, these undervalued and undercompensated workers were affected by structural racism, gender inequality, and anti-immigrant sentiments in the United States.[373]

Before the coronavirus pandemic, the workforce as a whole was subject to consistently low wages, challenging work conditions, and limited workplace protections and employee benefits.[374] Because they earned a median hourly wage of only $11.57, nearly 20 percent of direct care workers lived in poverty, and more than 40 percent depended on public assistance, including Medicaid and the Children's Health

Insurance Program (CHIP).[375] Sixteen percent did not have any form of health insurance.[376] These factors also contributed to high job turnover.[377] During the height of the pandemic, one study revealed that home care workers felt invisible and forgotten when it came to hazard pay, health insurance, paid leave, and lack of child care when schools were closed. Moreover, many direct care workers who lived in multigenerational households where most adults continued to work, often as essential employees, expressed fear of bringing the coronavirus home to their families.[378] Other studies revealed that direct care workers in nursing homes and assisted living communities were statistically more likely than home care workers to report COVID-19–related workplace challenges including increased workload demands and understaffing. Thirty-seven percent of nursing home direct care workers and 33 percent of assisted living workers reported understaffing as a challenge, compared to 13 percent of workers in agencies that provide HCBS including home healthcare agencies.[379] Staffing shortages placed additional pressure on already overburdened workers.

As the coronavirus spread, direct care workers continued to shoulder responsibility for providing essential care and assistance for people with disabilities and older people. Moreover, in light of the disproportionate impact of the virus on communities of color, direct care workers who were members of racial, ethnic, and immigrant groups also faced more significant health and economic risks during the pandemic.[380] Long-standing healthcare inequities left them more likely to experience severe COVID-19 illness if they become infected. Yet they often received little or no training beyond narrowly focused COVID-19 safety measures and were not provided with adequate coronavirus testing or PPE and supplies that could shield them from infection and death. Moreover, they lacked employee benefits that could help them avoid a financial crisis if they contracted the virus, lost their jobs, chose to isolate to protect themselves or their families, or left jobs to care for their own family members.[381] While we lacked accurate COVID-19 death rates for all direct care workers, high rates of nursing home staff and resident infection and death had been reported and are referenced in chapter 2 of this report.[382]

DC workers were acutely affected by the inadequacy of the federal response during the early days of the pandemic. COVID-19 precipitated an extraordinary and widespread human rights and public health crisis in nursing facilities, but direct care workers caring for people with disabilities and older adults living in home- and community-based care settings also experienced threats to their jobs and difficulty protecting themselves and their clients from the danger of coronavirus infection and death. The most effective methods to avoid contracting the coronavirus—social distancing and working remotely from home—were not options for direct care workers whose jobs in nursing facilities and community-based settings required close and sometimes intimate contact with clients. Lack of PPE and training on its use, worker and client fear of infection, and personal, economic, and family demands and stress led to an estimated loss of 232,000 homecare jobs during just the first three months of the pandemic in 2020.[383] However, the fragmented systems that pay for and facilitate HCBS also could not generate a coordinated response as the pandemic swept across the country. And notably, the lack of accurate data on the prevalence of COVID-19 illness and death among home care workers and the people they cared for also made it impossible to understand with any accuracy the true scope of the national COVID-19 disaster. Even as some data was available on the devastating effects of COVID-19 on people with intellectual and developmental disabilities, and states and the CDC reported nursing home infections, illness, and deaths for staff and residents, age-adjusted data was not available on COVID-19 infections, illness, and death based on disability status alone or the combined characteristics of race, ethnicity, and disability status.[384] Lack of this critical information meant that policy advocates had to base recommendations mostly on anecdotes and early qualitative research. A dearth of accurate occupational data on the direct care workforce also obscured a full understanding of COVID-19's impact on these workers. Existing data did not consider the varied roles, job duties, work environments, and titles of direct care workers, which led to undercounting certain workers and excluding others entirely.[385]

A direct care workforce that makes a living wage, has access to comprehensive healthcare, appropriate employment protections, benefits, job security, and career track opportunities is a matter of racial, ethnic, and gender equity.

> *[D]irect care workers caring for people with disabilities and older adults living in home- and community-based care settings also experienced threats to their jobs and difficulty protecting themselves and their clients from the danger of coronavirus infection and death.*

These employment rights also ensure that the disability community has consistent access to services and supports needed to maintain health and live full, independent lives. The pandemic created new and distinct employment and health threats and challenges for direct care workers in addition to those they were already experiencing. While these threats eased somewhat, especially for residents and staff of nursing facilities, as vaccinations and PPE became more readily available, longstanding inequities remained. Direct care workers and home care agencies providing HCBS still reported PPE shortages and barriers to being vaccinated. For the foreseeable future policymakers must continue to recognize that the direct care workforce is made up of essential workers who are eligible for free coronavirus testing and vaccinations, who must have sufficient PPE and training in PPE use and infection control. They must also recognize that these workers are entitled to living wages and employment benefits that incentivize continued employment in the field, especially in light of threats posed by COVID-19.

In addition to the paid direct care workforce, research suggested that more than 50 million caregivers are currently providing unpaid help for adults or children with disabilities in the United States.[386] A family caregiver is generally defined as an adult family member or another individual who has a significant relationship with a person who has a chronic or other health condition, a functional limitation, or a disability. These caregivers represent all ages, racial and ethnic groups, and socioeconomic backgrounds. They assist with ADLs, IADLs, medication management, and emotional and other support for family members or close friends. Among people caring for adults, almost 90 percent care for an adult relative, while about 10 percent care for a friend or neighbor. As the U.S. population

lives longer with more chronic and complex functional limitations and medical conditions, the prevalence of unpaid caregiving will increase.

Family caregivers provide care for people with long-term physical conditions and emotional, mental health, or memory problems, including dementia or Alzheimer's. Recent studies suggested that not only are more people in the United States taking on unpaid caregiver roles; they also are caring for people who have increasingly complicated support requirements or medical needs. Even before COVID-19, some family caregivers reported experiencing emotional stress and short- and long-term financial consequences to devoting significant time to caregiving, and a decline in self-reported health status.[387] Furthermore, studies reported that over 50 percent of family caregivers had jobs that pay hourly wages, including some direct care workers, suggesting that taking unpaid time off threatened their economic stability.[388]

The coronavirus pandemic added additional stress and uncertainty for family caregivers, many of whom experienced new and unforeseen challenges arising from COVID-19. After the pandemic began, millions of family caregivers were forced to shelter in place, and some had to take a leave from their jobs to care for family members. Many had little or no paid leave while they struggled to fill caregiving gaps for their family members with disabilities when scheduled workers contracted COVID-19 themselves or choose to stay home to avoid either contracting the virus or passing it on to clients and their families. Caregivers also encountered difficulties coordinating care for family members living in nursing homes and other facilities that closed to visitors.[389] COVID-19 hit communities of color especially hard, and reports indicated that 16 percent of Latino and 13 percent of Black adults left their jobs to care for family members during the pandemic.[390] Many of these individuals held low-paying jobs and lacked paid leave even as they needed to shelter in place to avoid contracting the virus or to care for a person with a disability or an older adult.[391] Refining the focus even more to women of color, 28 percent of Latina women and 27 percent of Black women indicate that they have taken days off without pay or quit a job to care for either a child or an elderly relative, compared to 12 percent of white women and men of all ethnicities.[392]

Federal and State COVID-19 Responses to Direct Care Workers

After the pandemic began, Congress and state legislatures enacted significant COVID-19 relief measures and approved specific short-term solutions for the most pressing threats and problems brought on by the pandemic. These legislative and policy

16 percent of Latino and 13 percent of Black adults left their jobs to care for family members during the pandemic.

actions rolled out during 2020 and 2021 as advocates, researchers, the media, and those directly affected reported the COVID-19 landscape and associated workforce challenges. Even as federal COVID-19 relief bills did not seek to reform the long-standing structural problems that direct care workers experienced, they afforded a glimpse into what was possible and practicable.

PPE and COVID-19 Testing

Lack of timely coronavirus testing and PPE, including gowns, masks, gloves, and face shields, placed many direct care workers in increased danger of becoming infected and spreading the virus to clients and family members. COVID-19 testing was limited in the early days of the pandemic, and people who were able to be tested had long waits for test results. Provisions of the Paycheck Protection Program and Healthcare Enhancement Act,[393] signed into law on March 18, 2020, allocated funds to scale up coronavirus surveillance and testing capabilities. However, the direct care workforce, especially those serving people with disabilities and older people living at home or in other community-based settings and at high risk for infection, found testing challenging: limited availability of testing during the early months of the pandemic and other barriers such as lack of transportation, difficulty taking time off from work, concerns over the cost of testing, and fear of revealing their immigration status to authorities were common barriers to testing. A survey of states conducted by Health Management Associates and the Kaiser Family Foundation for fiscal years 2020–2021 confirmed these problems. The survey found that nearly three-quarters of states indicated concerns about access to COVID-19 tests for direct care workers, and almost all states reported that access to PPE for direct care workers was a serious concern. Several states reported the length of COVID-19 test processing times as a particular challenge. A small number of states reported limited testing due to lack of transportation to testing sites, which remained problems for rural areas.[394]

Confusion over who was responsible for payment of testing also persisted for months during 2020. Two federal COVID-19 relief bills, the Families First Coronavirus Response Act (FFCRA)[395] and the CARES Act,[396] signed into law during the onset of the pandemic, in March 2020, required most private health plans, Medicare, and Medicaid to pay for the COVID-19 testing procedure, the test itself, and other related costs, with no cost sharing required.

Some resources were also made available to finance free testing for uninsured people. However, the CARES Act limited access to free testing for immigrants and temporary workers, although states could provide testing for these groups through Medicaid programs. The CARES Act provided $1 billion for free coronavirus testing and treatment at federally supported community health centers where many immigrants sought care, regardless of citizenship status or insurance coverage. Immigrants who would have been eligible in some states to enroll in Medicaid during the pandemic and thus eligible for free testing were reluctant to do so, due to the Trump Administration's "public charge" rule that would make immigrants who applied for public assistance ineligible to pursue legal residency status or citizenship.[397] The rule discouraged immigrants from applying for Medicaid and the CHIP by interpreting "public charge" to include immigrants who either had previously received or who might rely on some types of public assistance in the future.

On March 14, 2020, the U.S. Citizenship and Immigration Services (USCIS) announced that it would not count the use of free COVID-19 testing services when determining if immigrants would potentially rely on public benefits in the future. However, likely many immigrants, including those who were direct care workers, chose not to take advantage of available testing, either because they were unaware of the March 14 clarification or because they were uncertain that USCIS would implement it.[398] Responding to advocates' concerns about the devastating impact of the public charge rule on immigrant communities during the pandemic, the Biden Administration, on Tuesday, March 10, 2021, halted implementation of the policy following the reinstatement of a federal court order blocking it. The Department of Homeland Security would no longer consider receipt of Medicaid (except for Medicaid-supported institutionalization), public housing, or SNAP benefits as disqualifying factors in a public charge determination. The Department of Homeland Security also stated that it would not consider vaccination for the coronavirus or COVID-19 treatment in public charge determinations.[399]

Even though FFCRA and the CARES Act explicitly required that COVID-19 testing be free in most cases, the laws also required that testing be medically necessary. Guidance from CMS said that free testing was required "when medically appropriate for the individual, as determined by the individual's attending healthcare provider in accordance with accepted standards of current medical practice."[400] Relying on this guidance, some health insurance plans applied cost sharing or denied COVID-19 testing claims for members who were asymptomatic when they were tested unless they knew or suspected they had been exposed to someone who was positive for the coronavirus.[401] Where testing was offered, this interpretation placed the payment burden on the individual, undoubtedly making it difficult for even those direct care workers who had insurance to navigate the cost obstacles.[402] Federal guidance issued by the Biden Administration early in 2021 clarified that health insurers must cover testing without any cost to the individual being tested except when testing was a requirement in employee return-to-work programs.[403]

Reports in 2021 indicated that testing demand had dropped off even as testing availability was widespread in most areas. This suggested that testing barriers related to cost and availability had eased, making it somewhat easier for direct care workers to be tested later in the pandemic.[404] Even so, the structural barriers related to testing and treatment for COVID-19 that some direct care workers encountered reveal the complex effects of historical racism.[405]

PPE, including gowns, masks, and gloves, was scarce for many months during 2020. direct care workers interviewed for a study in New York reported receiving conflicting information on COVID-19 safety protocols and varied amounts of PPE from their home care agencies. They also reported relying on nonagency sources for news, PPE, and other supplies.[406] DC workers, along with other health workers, reported being forced to use trash bags as gowns, reuse face masks for weeks, and sometimes go totally without gloves.[407] The CARES Act appropriated considerable federal funding to hospitals and other healthcare entities, which they could use for PPE. Still, the law did not allocate such funding to nursing homes and other LTCFs.[408] The Health Management Associates–Kaiser Family Foundation study confirmed that in a few states, making PPE available for workers in institutional settings was a high priority, thus leaving community-based workers with fewer options for obtaining these supplies.[409] The CARES Act also expressly provided funds for PPE to protect home health workers providing care for veterans from contracting or spreading the coronavirus.[410]

A year and several months into the pandemic, most hospitals had access to PPE in bulk. Specific items, such as surgical masks, could be relatively easily purchased in stores. However, a few reports suggested that PPE supplies were still not readily and consistently available to small entities such as healthcare clinics, homeless shelters, home health agencies, and individual direct care workers. Even some nursing homes were still experiencing occasional shortages: One in 10 nursing homes reported not having a week's PPE supply on hand during the four weeks ending March 7, 2021.[411] This disparity in access to PPE was still evident as COVID-19 infections increased in some states during the spring of 2021.[412]

DC workers, along with other health workers, reported being forced to use trash bags as gowns, reuse face masks for weeks, and sometimes go totally without gloves.

COVID-19 Vaccination

As word that COVID-19 vaccinations would likely be available in early 2021, people with disabilities, older people, home care workers (direct care workers providing care for people in their homes and community settings), and family caregivers worried that they might not be included in federal and state vaccine allocation policies. Disproportionate rates of COVID-19 infection and death among nursing home residents and staff were well known, and CDC and state and local public health leaders responded by identifying nursing home workers and residents as top priority populations for vaccination. However, home care workers who worked for multiple clients faced a risk of COVID-19 infection similar to nursing home staff, yet federal and state officials did not include these direct care workers in recommended early vaccination eligibility. Public health officials based these decisions on the need to set priority populations because vaccine availability was limited, and public health data showing populations at greatest risk of COVID-19 infection should receive the first available shots. Little data was available about COVID-19 infection, illness, and death among home care workers, family caregivers, people with disabilities, and older people living in community settings. Therefore, these vulnerable groups were unnoticed and ignored by public health officials in many states' early vaccine allocation protocols, as further detailed in chapter 1.

Also emerging as a concern was how structural racism, especially in healthcare, would affect how Black, Indigenous, and other communities of color, including direct care workers who were members of these communities, would gain access to the vaccine and be interested in being vaccinated. Researchers have noted that the long-standing effects of historical racism underpin inequalities in the processes for vaccine distribution. Disparities in access to computers and other digital technologies, for example, made it difficult or impossible for some people to access the array of vaccine scheduling websites. While internet websites were intended to make access to vaccine appointments equitable, relying on them had the effect of widening access disparities for some marginalized communities. The long history of racism in science and healthcare also caused some people from communities of color to express a wait-and-see

attitude about the safety and efficacy of the COVID-19 vaccines.[413]

In December 2020, the same month that the U.S. Food and Drug Administration (FDA) approved two COVID-19 vaccinations for emergency use, the CDC's Advisory Committee on Immunization Practices (ACIP) recommended priorities for demographic populations who would receive the vaccine first in light of limited supply. The CDC placed healthcare personnel and residents of long-term care facilities (LTCF) in Phase 1(a), the highest priority tier to receive the vaccine based on their risk of exposure to the virus and the high rate of COVID-19 deaths in nursing homes.[414] The CDC included home healthcare workers and people who deliver services for older people and people with disabilities, among many healthcare job classifications, in Phase 1(a) based on a comprehensive list of essential workers initially created by the US Department of Homeland Security.[415] However, ACIP's December 3 advisory defines essential healthcare workers for purposes of inclusion in Phase 1(a) at that time as, ". . . all paid and unpaid persons serving in *healthcare settings* who have the potential for direct or indirect exposure to patients or infectious materials." ACIP also explicitly noted that residents of LTCFs required personal care, thus DC workers who provided such services in these facilities were considered eligible healthcare personnel and included in Phase 1(a). Although the CDC was aware of the diverse workforce employed in the healthcare field, ACIP's early vaccination guidance was expressly aimed at healthcare personnel who worked in settings where healthcare was delivered.[416] The strong emphasis on vaccinating these workers first led many states to craft vaccine allocation policies that excluded DC workers who delivered personal care services in the homes of people with disabilities or in other community settings rather than healthcare settings. Moreover, people with disabilities under age 65 living in the community who required DC worker assistance to live independently were not specifically ranked within any of the four primary phases even though many were at high risk of coronavirus infection, serious COVID-19 illness, and even death. Disability advocates recommended that younger people with disabilities in the community be included in a high priority category, but most states did not mention disability in their initial vaccine allocation plans.[417]

The Advisory Committee on Immunization Practices' Updated Interim Recommendation for Allocation of COVID-19 Vaccine—United States December 2020[418]

Phase	Groups Recommended to Receive COVID-19 Vaccine
1a	Healthcare personnel
	Long-term care facility residents
1b	Frontline essential workers
	Persons aged ≥75 years
1c	Persons aged 65–74 years
	Persons aged 16–64 years with high-risk medical conditions
	Essential workers not recommended for vaccination in Phase 1b
2	All persons aged ≥16 years not previously recommended for vaccination

Some states and locales modified the federal vaccine guidance to include direct care workers who provide home care in a higher Phase 1 tier. For example, California initially placed home care workers in Phase 1b, Tier 2. Vaccination of these workers began in some counties in February 2021. However, this did little to protect people with disabilities in HCBS since it was unclear at the time whether vaccination precluded the capacity to infect others.[419]

Massachusetts planned to start vaccinating all home care workers in February 2021. The state defined home care worker as "a clinical or non-clinical healthcare or home care worker doing in-person consumer or patient-facing care when the work is performed in the home of the patient/healthcare consumer." Personal care attendants, home health, hospice, home care agency staff performing visits in the home, and an array of others who might have contact with an individual in their home were included.[422] Even as some states included home care workers in their earliest vaccine phases, others did not, such as Louisiana. Moreover, officials in some locales were confused about direct care worker eligibility for the vaccine. For instance, some Florida vaccination sites initially turned away home care workers, thinking they were not yet eligible for the shots.[423] Widespread media reports revealed that multiple vaccination websites were overwhelmed and hard to navigate, and the few available appointment slots were often filled. Rural direct care workers reported minimal availability, and they often had to travel long distances to get to a vaccine distribution site. Workers with limited English proficiency did not necessarily have access to technology or linguistically appropriate information about making a vaccine appointment

Guidelines to California's Health Departments Allocation of COVID-19 Vaccine During Phase 1[420]

PHASE 1a	▪ Persons at risk of exposure to SARS-CoV-2 through their work in any role in direct healthcare or long-term care settings. • This population includes persons at direct risk of exposure in their nonclinical roles, such as, but not limited to, environmental services, patient transport, or interpretation. ▪ Residents of skilled nursing facilities, assisted living facilities, and similar long-term care settings for older or medically vulnerable individuals.
1b **Tier 1**	▪ Acute care, psychiatric, and correctional facility hospitals ▪ Skilled nursing facilities, assisted living facilities, and similar settings for older or medically vulnerable individuals • Also, in concordance with ACIP, residents in these settings ▪ Paramedics, EMTs, and others providing emergency medical services ▪ Dialysis centers
Tier 2	▪ Intermediate care facilities for persons who need noncontinuous nursing supervision and supportive care ▪ *Home healthcare and in-home supportive services* ▪ Community health workers, including promotoras[421] ▪ Public health field staff ▪ Primary Care clinics, including Federally Qualified Health Centers, Rural Health Centers, correctional facility clinics, and urgent care clinics
Tier 3	▪ Specialty clinics ▪ Laboratory workers ▪ Dental and other oral health clinics

or navigating the multiple complex vaccine websites. Often, alternative methods to make an appointment, such as a telephone line, were overwhelmed with long wait times, could not record messages, or were not working. Other direct care workers were concerned about the cost of the vaccine and the possible need to reveal their immigration status in order to receive shots, problems similar to those they faced being tested for the coronavirus. Even if they could make an appointment and surmount other hurdles, some workers simply could not take time off from work to travel to a vaccination site.[424]

As vaccine eligibility eased and availability of vaccines increased, CDC stated that everyone 16 years of age and older was eligible to get a COVID-19 vaccine as of April 19, 2021. On

May 10, 2021, the FDA approved emergency use authorization for the Pfizer-BioNTech COVID-19 vaccine for adolescents age 12 through 15 years.[425] Even with increased vaccine availability, communities of color hit hardest by the pandemic were not always receiving an equitable share. Federal vaccination data indicated that communities with the highest level of disadvantage and health vulnerabilities, based on the Social Vulnerability Index,[426] were being vaccinated at a lower rate than communities with fewer disadvantages and vulnerabilities.[427] Moreover, decades of research confirmed that race and ethnicity status are factors that predict unequal access to healthcare and health disparities outcomes. The cumulative effect of these multiple, generational inequities disproportionally affected Black, Indigenous, and other communities of color, including direct care workers who are members of these communities. Such systemic inequities inevitably contributed to poor healthcare experiences and distrust of medical professionals, establishing the basis for concern about the COVID-19 vaccine's safety and effectiveness.[428] These influences were reflected in vaccination figures: By early March 2021, only about a quarter of home care workers had been vaccinated, compared with approximately two-thirds of hospital workers and half of nursing home workers.[429]

> *Even with increased vaccine availability, communities of color hit hardest by the pandemic were not always receiving an equitable share.*

> *By early March 2021, only about a quarter of home care workers had been vaccinated, compared with approximately two-thirds of hospital workers and half of nursing home workers.*

Enhanced Employment Wages and Benefits

Federal COVID-19 relief legislation contained provisions that very likely benefitted many direct care workers, their families, and family caregivers, while other provisions specifically worked against direct care workers. The FFCRA,[430] the first of the COVID-19 relief packages, signed into law on March 18, 2020, included assistance to states for payment of unemployment insurance claims. Emergency paid sick leave was also included, but nursing homes and home health agencies were among various health providers and educational organizations that could exempt their direct care workers from eligibility if they chose to do so. Tax credits for paid sick and paid family and medical leave were also made available for employers of a specific size, including home care agencies and nursing facilities. Congress intended these credits to encourage employers to pay sick, family, and medical leave.[431] While FFCRA provided sick leave and paid family and medical leave, gaps in the legislation excluded some direct care workers from eligibility for the enhanced benefit. For instance, FFCRA excluded independent contractors from eligibility for emergency family medical leave. Therefore, home care workers employed as independent contractors were ineligible for this temporary benefit. FFCRA also exempted businesses with fewer than 50 employees from providing emergency family medical leave, thus limiting eligibility for home care workers employed by some smaller home healthcare agencies.[432]

Some states responded to these gaps. For instance, California sought federal approval under FFCRA to increase sick leave for Medicaid home care workers. This request enabled workers in California's In-Home Supportive Services (IHSS) program who were employed by people with disabilities and who met specific eligibility requirements to receive the new federal COVID-19 sick leave. IHSS provides in-home assistance to eligible people with disabilities to enable them to live in the community.[433] Because FFCRA expired at the end of 2020, California passed a measure in March 2021 that provided for supplemental paid sick leave for specified IHSS and other personal care service providers who were unable to work or telework due to certain reasons related to COVID-19. The measure made sick leave available retroactively to January 1, 2021.[434]

Many direct care workers and family caregivers who lost or left their jobs during the pandemic depended on income support provided by unemployment insurance. The CARES Act included a 6.2 percent increase in federal Medicaid matching funds available to states to ensure continued insurance coverage for beneficiaries. It also focused on expanding unemployment insurance by providing an additional, federally financed $600 benefit, referred to as Federal Pandemic Unemployment Compensation, that supplemented weekly unemployment insurance benefits, expanded benefit eligibility, and provided weeks of additional federally financed benefits.[435] Later in the year, on December 27, 2020, Congress passed the Consolidated Appropriations Act extending Federal Pandemic Unemployment Compensation through March 2021.[436] The Act added a $300 additional benefit to all recipients, extended benefits for people who had been unemployed long-term and for low-wage and self-employed workers who were not eligible for regular unemployment.[437] Another new law, the Coronavirus Response and Relief Supplemental Appropriations Act[438] re-instituted some enhanced unemployment insurance benefits, covering January 1, 2021, through March 14, 2021. However, the law did not extend COVID-19–related paid sick leave or increase funding for Medicaid, long-term services and supports, and home and community-based services.[439]

The CARES Act also provided a recovery rebate for the 2020 tax year of $1,200 for an individual return ($2,400 for a joint return) with an additional $500 per qualified dependent child. Income limited eligibility for these rebates, but they nonetheless likely benefitted direct care workers and some family caregivers.

During the spring of 2020, Congressional interest was building to provide federal funding for hazard pay for the nation's essential workers, including the direct care workforce. However, that interest never culminated in legislation, so individual employers had to decide whether they would provide this form of compensation for their workers. Research suggested that most chose not to do so. However, some states took advantage of CARES Act funding to allocate temporary hazard pay for some public and private sector essential workers, including direct care workers in some cases. For instance, Pennsylvania established a grant program that afforded about 40,000 workers who earned less than $20 per hour a $3 per hour raise for 10 weeks. The program only helped a fraction of those who qualified. So, with equity in mind, the state emphasized assisting those with the greatest financial need. Direct care workers, including home health aides, personal care aides, and nursing home workers, benefitted most from the program. With $120 million from the CARES Act, Michigan temporarily paid Medicaid-funded direct care workers an additional $2 per hour.[440] Virginia made $1,500 one-time payments to over 43,500 home healthcare workers who provided support for Medicaid beneficiaries.[441] Comprehensive data is lacking on how many direct care workers received COVID-19 wage compensation; however, one study reported that 70 percent of direct support professionals who work with people with intellectual and developmental disabilities did not receive COVID-19 wage augmentation or bonus pay, suggesting that many other direct care workers were likely left out of these benefits.[442]

70 percent of direct support professionals who work with people with intellectual and developmental disabilities did not receive COVID-19 wage augmentation or bonus pay, suggesting that many other direct care workers were likely left out of these benefits.

In September 2020, CMS announced the availability of up to $165 million in supplemental funding for 33 states that had been operating Money Follows the Person demonstration programs. Money Follows the Person, officially slated to end in 2018, had been extended several times temporarily. Its funding helped people with disabilities move from nursing homes to their own homes or other community settings. Among many options, states could use the new funding for direct care worker recruitment, education, training, technical assistance, and quality improvement activities. States could also elect to include training people with disabilities to become direct service workers. Eligible states could submit supplemental budget requests under this funding opportunity on a rolling basis through June 30, 2021.[443]

Congress enacted the American Rescue Plan Act of 2021 (ARPA),[444] a $1.9 trillion response to the pandemic, on March 11, 2021. ARPA included $350 billion for state and local governments and $12.7 billion to allow more low-income people with disabilities and older people to receive care at home instead of nursing homes. It included a one-year, 10 percentage point boost in the federal contribution for Medicaid HCBS to states.

According to CMS, funds could be used for a variety of purposes, provided they supplemented and did not supplant existing state funds used for HCBS. Of importance to the direct care workforce, funds could support caregiver training and education and create financial incentives to expand the number, retention rates, and skills of the direct care workforce. States could provide hazard pay, overtime pay, and shift differential pay for home health workers and direct support professionals, including those who worked with people with intellectual and developmental disabilities. Funds could also be used to increase rates for home health and other HCBS agencies or individuals who employed direct support professionals, with the expectation that they would increase pay rates for workers.[445]

California unveiled a preliminary ARPA HCBS spending plan in early May 2021.[446] Following a short public comment period and additional discussion with lawmakers, HHS submitted a final, revised plan to CMS on July 12, 2021. The plan included expanding existing IHSS worker training to support people with complex care needs and supporting and incentivizing career pathways.[447]

ARPA also provided several other types of assistance for direct care workers, e.g., tax cuts and immediate cash relief for low- and middle-income families, renter assistance, help for homeowners to avoid foreclosure, extended unemployment benefits, and an additional $300 per week federal increase in unemployment benefits. This provision prevented direct care workers and family caregivers who left their jobs to care for family members or who were laid off, or who contracted COVID-19, from losing their unemployment insurance benefits.[448] ARPA also allocated $145 million for the National Family Caregiver Support Program, which provided grants to states and territories to fund various supports that helped family and informal caregivers care for older adults in their homes for as long as possible.[449]

Medicaid and Medicare

As the pandemic spread, states soon recognized its effect on people with disabilities and older people who required Medicaid-funded HCBS, direct care workers, family caregivers, and others who provided these services. As infection engulfed congregate care settings, affecting residents and workers alike, some direct care workers and family caregivers fell ill or stayed home to care for family members or avoid becoming ill themselves. Others continued working in homes, community settings, and nursing homes for the usual low wages and without hazard pay, even at the risk of becoming ill, especially when PPE was scarce. Recognizing the emergency, some states and the federal government used various Medicaid emergency waiver authorizations to respond to participant and workforce challenges, including severe staff shortages, historically low direct care worker wages, and inadequate benefits, that had been brought to the forefront by the pandemic.

CMS approved 34 states to pay spouses and parents of minor children as Medicaid providers through various waivers, and 33 states gained permission to add family members as eligible providers for adults with disabilities.

For instance, CMS approved various state requests for Medicaid "Appendix K" and Section 1135 emergency waivers, including raising direct care workforce wages and increasing benefits. CMS approved 34 states to pay spouses and parents of minor children as Medicaid providers through various waivers, and 33 states gained permission to add family members as eligible providers for adults with disabilities.[450] CMS approved these waivers as mitigation strategies to limit exposure to COVID-19 in the family home and to provide support for individuals who returned from congregate settings to family homes to avoid the risk of transmission. They also responded to the existing direct care workforce and family caregiver challenges that had been intensified by COVID-19.[451]

Thirty-three states also received CMS approval to modify Medicaid HCBS provider payment rates. For instance, Michigan and Wisconsin received Medicaid Section 1115 waivers allowing them to pay higher pay rates for direct care workers providing HCBS to maintain worker capacity. Delaware, Hawaii, Massachusetts, North Carolina, Rhode Island, and Washington were granted Section 1115 waivers to enable retainer payments to certain habilitation and direct care workers to maintain capacity during the COVID-19 emergency. In California, an approved 1915(c) waiver extended emergency paid sick leave for direct care workers unable to work during COVID-19. California allocated money to hire social workers and pay overtime when clients and Medicaid-funded direct care workers needed their services.[452]

Recent changes to the Medicare program, including some that responded to the pandemic, also affected older people with disabilities and their family caregivers. The CARES Act permitted nonphysicians such as nurses and physician assistants to approve Medicare home healthcare services, streamlining the approval process and reducing the burden on family caregivers who often had to coordinate skilled long-term care services through a physician.

The 2018 Chronic Care Act, contained in the Bipartisan Budget Act of 2018, another federal law that benefited family caregivers and people with disabilities during the pandemic, expanded Medicare supplemental benefits and allowed health plans to provide services that were not primarily health-related.[453] For instance, supplemental services could include medical transportation for nonemergencies, caregiver support including respite and in-home services, and bathroom safety devices. By 2021, 95 plans offered support for caregivers of enrollees.[454] While the availability of these benefits varied widely regionally and by health insurance plan, some family caregivers and Medicare beneficiaries nevertheless likely benefited during the pandemic.[455]

ARPA and other pandemic relief laws partially responded to the economic and other hardships the direct care workforce experienced before and during the pandemic. States' actions to achieve flexibility within the complex Medicaid program, the main source of funding for HCBS, also foretold a possible future when direct care workers could gain recognition, wages, and benefits commensurate with their critical roles. Changes in Medicare before and during the pandemic also provided some modest help to family caregivers and increased access to a few new services for beneficiaries in specific geographic health insurance markets.

These stopgap measures provided some short-term help for a struggling direct care workforce and family caregivers. However, because they were a temporary response to a public health crisis, they did not establish a permanent pathway to reversing the inequities that direct care workers and family caregivers experienced every day. Even so, these measures spurred an overdue conversation about the critical, yet undervalued and underrecognized role direct care workers and family caregivers played

> *Thirty-three states also received CMS approval to modify Medicaid HCBS provider payment rates.*

in the lives of people with disabilities and older people. This heightened awareness, driven by a worldwide public health emergency, presented advocates and policymakers with a unique opportunity to create permanent reforms built on state and federal emergency Covid-19 policies.

Federal Policy Proposals

Two federal policy proposals, the Better Care Better Jobs Act, as initially outlined in the American Jobs Plan,[456] and the HCBS Access Act[457] aimed to increase funding and reduce waiting lists for Medicaid HCBS services and invest in the nation's caregiving infrastructure. These proposals represented decades of advocacy by people with disabilities and older people, allies, organizations of home care workers, unions, researchers, and policy leaders.[458] They were brought to the forefront because the coronavirus pandemic revealed deficiencies in HCBS and deep inequities in the treatment and status of direct care workers and family caregivers. If these proposals are enacted, people with disabilities and older adults would have greater access to Medicaid HCBS and direct care workers could experience improvement in wages, benefits, and collective bargaining opportunities. Family caregivers could also gain access to additional assistance and supports.

Building on the $12.7 billion short-term funding included in the American Rescue Plan, the Biden Administration sought an additional $400 billion investment in the nation's caregiving infrastructure. The Better Care Better Jobs Act,[459] introduced in the Senate on June 24,

[T]he coronavirus pandemic revealed deficiencies in HCBS and deep inequities in the treatment and status of direct care workers and family caregivers.

2021, if enacted, would strengthen and expand access to Medicaid HCBS, promote adequate wages and benefits for direct care workers, and ensure opportunities to organize or join a union. The Better Care Better Jobs Act would support quality and accountability and would facilitate state planning. It would also help states build innovative workforce programs and connect workers with people with disabilities and older people. The proposed legislation would permanently authorize protections against impoverishment for people whose spouses receive Medicaid HCBS and make permanent the Money Follows the Person program.[460]

The HCBS Access Act,[461] a federal legislative discussion draft introduced in March 2021, would amend Title XIX of the Social Security Act to make coverage of HCBS mandatory rather than optional under the Medicaid program. This proposal advances a long-standing recommendation from disability advocates to reverse the institutional bias in the Medicaid program in favor of HCBS.

Another Biden Administration proposal, the American Families Plan, directly addressed issues that affect direct care workers throughout the country and emphasized reforms that responded to the effects of the pandemic. If enacted, the American Families Plan would extend key tax cuts and child tax credits in the American Rescue Plan, create a national paid family and medical leave program, and reform unemployment. It would also improve healthcare affordability, ensure that childcare is affordable, and provide two years of free community college.

The U.S. Citizenship Act of 2021,[462] another Biden Administration proposal, would provide an earned pathway to citizenship for the U.S. undocumented population. The bill was introduced on February 18, 2021. While it is beyond the scope of this chapter to report fully on immigration proposals, the U.S. Citizenship Act, if enacted, would directly bear on some immigrant members of the direct care workforce and provide remedies to some of the starkest problems they faced before and during the pandemic. Immigrants make up a substantial part of the direct care workforce and fill a crucial role in meeting the growing national need for direct care workers. Barriers to legal residency and citizenship have forced some of these workers into the shadows, even as they provide critical services that enable people with disabilities and older people to remain in their homes and community-based settings. Expediting immediate routes to lawful immigrant status would help expand the direct care workforce to meet the growing need, provide important long-term economic benefits, and create career advancement opportunities for these workers.[463]

Social Insurance

The National Academy of Social Insurance (NASI) has proposed Universal Family Care (UFC), a social insurance program model that states could consider for early childcare and education (ECCE), paid family and medical leave (PFML), and long-term services and supports (LTSS). NASI argues that large-scale social forces inspire the need for social insurance that would respond to race, ethnicity, gender, and disability inequalities that social institutions have created over decades. The UFC model envisions that all workers would contribute to a single care insurance fund that would pay out ECCE, PFML, and LTSS benefits when these needs arise. The fund would provide these benefits through a single, integrated access point for families. Program designs would be based on state priorities, such as funding sources, eligibility requirements, who is covered, and adequacy of benefits. Federal programs, including Social Security and state programs including for LTSS and PFML, have successfully used this social insurance model and serve as examples of how programs can be successfully structured.[464]

The impact of the coronavirus pandemic on direct care workers illustrates the appeal of social insurance by revealing structural inequalities that have affected direct care workers disproportionately and pointing out the inadequacies of the current social safety net in times of crisis. The pandemic has brought to the forefront the urgency of increasing wages for the direct care workforce as a means of acknowledging the critical work they do, retaining them in the workforce, attracting people to the field, and meeting their basic economic needs. At the same time, policy advocates have expressed concern that providing direct care workers with a living wage over the long term will be difficult

> *The pandemic has brought to the forefront the urgency of increasing wages for the direct care workforce as a means of acknowledging the critical work they do, retaining them in the workforce, attracting people to the field, and meeting their basic economic needs.*

if the primary funding source is Medicaid, which must compete with other public programs for general tax revenue.

Over many years, federal policymakers proposed public insurance plans in response to the need to find ways to pay for the nation's growing demand for LTSS/HCBS. The Community Living Assistance Services and Supports (CLASS) program was passed as part of the Affordable Care Act,[465] but later was repealed, in 2013, because it was considered financially unstable.[466] Since then, at least four states—California, Maine, Michigan, and Minnesota—have explored models for making LTSS available beyond Medicaid.[467] Washington has passed legislation establishing a Long-Term Care Trust that would provide a daily benefit of $100 beginning in 2025, after a 10-year vesting period. The lifetime benefit was capped at $36,500 and would be available to individuals who require help with three or more ADLs. Revenue came from a small tax (.58 percent) on each person's earnings.[468] Hawaii enacted the Kūpuna Care Program in 2008, making limited LTSS available to non-Medicaid-eligible residents 60 or older so they can continue living at home or in the community.[469]

These state policies mark a trend that recognizes the current system of support for people with disabilities and older people is unsustainable, leaving gaps in service for people who do not meet income eligibility requirements for Medicaid. Moreover, it does not provide adequate pathways to achieve pay equity, provide a living wage, or expand career opportunities for direct care workers. The social insurance model offers an alternative to Medicaid-funded LTSS/HCBS that could bolster and stabilize wages for the direct care workforce, spur improvements in training and job performance, and foster economic stability.

Summary of Findings

- Improvements in wages and employment benefits, including healthcare insurance, have long been identified as fundamental reforms required to reduce direct care worker shortages, boost job opportunity and satisfaction, and increase financial security for this diverse and underrecognized workforce. In addition to low wages and limited benefits, few career development and advancement opportunities spurred high job turnover in a workforce made up disproportionately of women and people of color. Moreover, some direct care workers faced additional insecurities based on their immigration status. The coronavirus pandemic laid bare these deficiencies.

- DC workers who are members of racial, ethnic, and immigrant groups faced disproportionate health and economic risks during the pandemic. Long-standing health and healthcare inequities left them more likely to experience severe COVID-19 illness if they become infected. Yet, they often were overlooked and were not provided with adequate coronavirus testing or PPE and supplies. Such systemic inequities contributed to distrust of medical professionals and established the basis for concern about the COVID-19 vaccine's safety and effectiveness. Moreover, the direct care workforce lacked employee benefits such as paid medical and family leave that could help them avoid a financial crisis if they contracted the virus, lost their jobs, chose to isolate to protect themselves or their families, or left their jobs to care for their own family members.

- Lack of accurate data on the prevalence of COVID-19 illness and death among home care workers and the people they cared for made it impossible to understand with any accuracy the true scope of the national COVID-19 disaster. Occupational data on the direct care workforce was incomplete and did not consider the varied roles and titles of direct care workers, which led to undercounting certain workers and excluding others entirely, thus obscuring a full understanding of COVID-19's impact. Without accurate data, policy advocates had to base recommendations mostly on anecdotes and early qualitative research.

- In addition to the paid direct care workforce, millions of caregivers provided unpaid help for adults or children with disabilities in the United States. Even before the pandemic, family caregivers experienced emotional stress, short- and long-term financial consequences to devoting significant time to caregiving, and a decline in self-reported health status. During the pandemic, millions of family caregivers were forced to shelter in place, and some had to take a leave from their jobs to care for family members. Many had little or no paid leave while they struggled to fill gaps in caregiving services for their family members.

- As the pandemic in the United States moved into its second year, direct care workers still reported shortages of PPE. Federal legislation increased production and distribution of PPE during the first year of the pandemic; however, regional and local distribution channels were uneven, and smaller home care agencies and other HCBS service providers reported unequal access to these essential supplies. If policymakers do not address the reasons for these lingering deficiencies now, they will carry forward to future public health emergencies.

- Federal COVID-19 relief legislation, emergency Medicaid authorizations, changes to Medicare, and actions by some states provided limited, partial relief for some of the most severe economic and health challenges direct care workers and unpaid family caregivers experienced during the pandemic. These short-term actions did not resolve the long-standing deficiencies reported in this chapter; however they served as a road map that could guide long-term, permanent transformations.

- Building on the lessons of the COVID-19 pandemic, the Biden Administration developed several legislative proposals intended to spur long-term reforms affecting direct care workers and family caregivers. One proposal would increase direct care worker pay and benefits, encourage opportunities to organize or join a union, build state HCBS infrastructures, and extend key tax cuts and child tax credits. Another would increase support to family caregivers and make Medicaid HCBS mandatory rather than optional, thus increasing the need for direct care workers. Still others would create a national paid family and medical leave program, reform unemployment, and provide an earned pathway to citizenship that would open opportunities for undocumented direct care workers. If enacted, these legislative proposals would support family caregivers and fully acknowledge the value and worth of direct care workers by reducing some of the most pervasive barriers to their recruitment, retention, and promotion.

- Even as the Biden Administration proposals held promise for improving wages, benefits, and employment opportunities for direct care workers, policy advocates worried that providing direct care workers with a living wage and benefits over the long term would be difficult if the primary funding source was Medicaid. Social insurance program models

that include HCBS, such as Universal Family Care, offered payment alternatives and responded to race, ethnicity, gender, and disability inequalities that social institutions had created over decades.

Recommendations

To ensure the United States will have the necessary DC workforce that will be needed to support people with disabilities safely in the community in the event of a future pandemic or similar national health crisis or emergency, NCD recommends the following actions.

Recommendations for Congress

Congress should:

- Enact the Better Care Better Jobs Act, the American Families Plan, the U.S. Citizenship Act of 2021, and the HCBS Access Act. Enact federal legislation based on the principle of Universal Family Care, a social insurance program model for early childcare and education, paid family and medical leave, and long-term services and supports as envisioned by the National Academy of Social Insurance. Built on the models of Social Security and Medicare, Universal Family Care is an integrated approach to care policy that recognizes long-standing social inequities based on race, ethnicity, and disability. Ensure that future and proposed legislation, such as the Better Care Better Jobs Act, which builds on the ARPA's expanded funding for Medicaid home and community-based services, includes funding to improve direct service workforce wages and benefits and increase recruitment and retention. This funding should include a mechanism to ensure that workers' wages and benefits are adequate for the present and adjusted as necessary in the future to ensure a stable workforce that is paid a living wage. It should also require as a condition of receiving such funding that states either provide directly or require that home healthcare agencies, CCFs, and other service providers provide paid family and medical leave for their direct care workers. States should also be required to ensure that direct care workers have access to adequate, affordable healthcare insurance either as an employer or union-sponsored benefit, through the Health Insurance Marketplace, or by other means.

(continued)

Recommendations for Congress: *continued*

Provide federal tax credits for employers offering a minimum number of weeks of paid leave to family caregivers as an incentive to make such leave available. Tax credits should also be offered to offset out-of-pocket expenses related to caregiving, such as housing costs, home modifications, respite, medical costs and other expenses incurred from providing care.

Recommendations for Federal Agencies

- *HHS and CMS* should require State Medicaid waiver requests to include assurances that the direct care workforce will receive fair and living wages and benefits, including paid family and medical leave, if waiver funds are used for direct care workforce compensation.

- *HHS, DOL, and BLS* should collaborate to update the occupational codes assigned to direct care workers to reflect more accurately the wide range of jobs they perform and to better include those workers who do not fit squarely into current classifications.

- *FEMA, HHS, and ACL* should collaborate to develop specific distribution networks with state and local departments of public health and community-based organizations that are in direct contact with direct care workers and family caregivers (e.g., Aging and Disability Resource Centers, Independent Living Centers, grantees of the National Family Caregiver Support Program [NFCSP], veterans' organizations) that can assist with distribution of PPE and other resources and supplies during natural or public health emergencies, with an emphasis on reaching individual home care workers who do not work for a home health agency, in nursing homes, or other residential facilities and therefore do not have ready access to resources or collective purchasing power.

Recommendations for States and State Medicaid Agencies

- *States and State Medicaid agencies* should implement permanent policies that encourage and facilitate paid family caregiving and invest in support services for such caregivers.

Chapter 4: Education and COVID-19

Students with Disabilities Before and After the Pandemic

Under ordinary circumstances, students with disabilities—about 14 percent of students from kindergarten to 12th grade, and more than 7 million children—face multiple and substantial barriers to education. In 2018, NCD reported that the longstanding federal underfunding of the Individuals with Disabilities Education Act (IDEA) was adversely affecting the ability of students with disabilities to receive Free and Appropriate Public Education (FAPE), causing delays and denials of services, and triggering unfair social resentment and discrimination.[470] NCD also found a nationwide shortage of qualified special education teachers and related service providers.[471]

In this funding context, districts often fail to comply fully with the IDEA, and instead make decisions that ration and deny services and supports to meet the unique needs of students with disabilities.[472] Students with disabilities then suffer the consequences. Students with disabilities have lower test scores and are less likely to graduate high school.[473] Just over 67 percent of students with disabilities graduate

Just over 67 percent of students with disabilities graduate high school, compared to about 85 percent of all students.

high school, compared to about 85 percent of all students.[474] Students with disabilities are more likely to be chronically absent.[475] The "academic achievement gap" between students with and without disabilities has remained roughly unchanged over the last decade.[476]

Students with disabilities also have higher rates of discipline, including suspensions and referrals to law enforcement. Students with disabilities represent 12 percent of students enrolled, but are 26 percent of students receiving an out-of-school suspension, and 25 percent of students referred to law enforcement.[477] Students with disabilities are much more likely than students without disabilities to be restrained and secluded at school,[478] a dangerous and ineffective practice that has caused serious injuries and deaths.[479] Rates of discipline and handcuffings at school are even higher and more disproportionate for Black students with disabilities.[480]

Discipline often causes exclusion from the classroom and lost instruction[481] and can advance the "school to prison pipeline."[482] Up to 85 percent of youth in juvenile detention facilities have disabilities that make them eligible for special education services, and a disproportionate number of percentages of these detained youth are youth of color.[483]

Many students with disabilities are multiply marginalized, which creates additional barriers to equal educational opportunity. Students with disabilities are more likely to be low-income.[484] They are disproportionately Black.[485] They may be in the foster care system, or juvenile justice systems, or both. About 32 percent of children in foster care are children with disabilities,[486] and, as noted, up to 85 percent of children in juvenile detention have disabilities. Children with disabilities may be homeless;[487] they may be English language learners.[488] Many experience intersectional discrimination based on multiple statuses, such as disability, sex, race, ethnicity, sexual orientation, gender identity, and size. These additional statuses and traumas exacerbate the vulnerabilities of those who are already struggling with academics, behavior, planning, speech, motor skills, and other areas essential to long-term success.

The COVID-19 pandemic worsened the educational experience for many students with disabilities.[489] The shift from an in-person model of learning to fully remote education as the sole option for education exacerbated the exclusion of students with disabilities.[490] Barriers to education were worse for students with disabilities in low-income households who did not have access to reliable high-speed internet and appropriate computers, or to adults with expertise in this technology.[491]

> *Many students with disabilities are multiply marginalized, which creates additional barriers to equal educational opportunity. Students with disabilities are more likely to be low-income. They are disproportionately Black.*

During the pandemic, families with students with disabilities experienced the failure of school districts to provide notices, meetings, assessments, plans, and services, and to comply with the procedural and substantive requirements of the IDEA and Section 504 of the Rehabilitation Act. A GAO study that interviewed researchers, representatives from national organizations, and officials from four school districts, and reviewed the learning plans from 15 school districts, supported much of the anecdotal evidence of the pandemic's impacts on education for students with disabilities. It found that some students with disabilities did not receive all of the services and supports contained in their IEPs or Section 504 plans during shelter in place,[492] and many school districts shortened their school day for all students, making it difficult to find time to provide the specialized instruction and related services detailed in students' IEPs.[493]

The onset of the pandemic and remote learning for K-12 students triggered the abrupt cessation, often for months, of essential services and supports that are typically provided to students with disabilities in person or on school campuses, such as occupational therapy, speech and language therapy, behavioral and mental health supports, small group instruction, and one-on-one aides.[494] Students with disabilities no longer had access to Braille or tactile learning tools. Officials from the school districts studied by the GAO reported that it was particularly difficult to deliver these "related services" that would ordinarily include hands-on instruction or equipment not available in families' homes.[495] While some school districts implemented small in-person cohorts for children with disabilities or provided an in-person (at-home) aide for students who could not access a free and appropriate public education (FAPE) without in-person services, many school districts refused to do so.[496] Even students with disabilities who were provided with an in-person setting on school campuses were often still receiving their instruction through a computer screen. In-person staff wore masks and maintained distance, making any communication difficult for many students with disabilities, particularly those with hearing loss. Many K-12 students with disabilities were denied FAPE for months and even more than one year (the length of the pandemic). Many students with disabilities who rely upon in-person supports experienced substantial regression in their behaviors and educational goals.[497]

Many students with disabilities, including not only K-12 students but also students with disabilities at colleges and universities, struggled to engage and participate in their education once all learning moved to a virtual environment.[498]

The onset of the pandemic and remote learning for K-12 students triggered the abrupt cessation, often for months, of essential services and supports that are typically provided to students with disabilities in person or on school campuses, such as occupational therapy, speech and language therapy, behavioral and mental health supports, small group instruction, and one-on-one aides.

A survey of more than 30,000 students at nine universities found that college students with disabilities were less likely during the pandemic to feel that they "belonged" at their schools, or that their institution supported them, compared to students without disabilities.

Some schools failed to ensure that their remote educational programs and materials were accessible to students with disabilities, including students who are Deaf or Hard of Hearing, students who have low vision or are blind, students with learning or attention disabilities, and students with psychiatric disabilities.[499] A survey of more than 30,000 students at nine universities found that college students with disabilities were less likely during the pandemic to feel that they "belonged" at their schools, or that their institution supported them, compared to students without disabilities.[500] These students with disabilities were also more likely to be experiencing food and housing insecurity.[501] As the pandemic continued, disability resource professionals—staff who ensure access and reasonable accommodations at colleges and universities—faced budget cuts, in some cases triggering layoffs.[502]

Some students with disabilities flourished in the remote classroom or experienced unexpected benefits. Some students with disabilities that affect their social and emotional functioning experienced decreased social anxiety in the virtual learning environment and were able to participate more freely.[503] Some students with disabilities had fewer challenging behaviors while learning from home because they faced fewer transitions in location and activity. Remote education also benefited some students with disabilities who rely on attendants, because it made it easier for these individuals to go off-camera when they needed to engage in personal care.

As a result of the pandemic and the gaps in the federal response to COVID, many K-12 students with disabilities experienced an extended exclusion from FAPE, and now need compensatory education to recover and regain skills they have lost. Students with disabilities at all levels including K-12 and postsecondary experienced barriers in remote educational programs and activities, including discrimination and denials of effective communication and reasonable accommodations.

The Heavy Impact of the Pandemic on Low-Income Families with Children with Disabilities

Children with disabilities disproportionately live in low-income households.[504] These children, often children of color with disabilities, experienced particularly severe barriers to education during the pandemic. Many low-income parents lost their jobs or had work hours decreased after COVID-19 hit, and they struggled to feed their families.[505] Among low-income families, families of Black, Hispanic/Latino, and Native American children were more likely to experience income loss and food insecurity.[506] Parents who retained employment often had to work in person,[507] preventing them from providing their children

with at-home supports for remote learning. Many low-income families did not have reliable internet, appropriate computers, or an area free of distraction for distance learning.[508]

A survey of 1,000 low-income families in Tulsa, Oklahoma, found that opportunities for learning shrank dramatically with the shift to remote instruction, especially for children with disabilities.[509] Low-income parents of children with disabilities were more likely than other low-income parents to report problems with distance learning (83 percent versus 63 percent).[510] And almost half of low-income parents of children with and without disabilities reported that their children experienced increased emotional and behavioral problems during the pandemic.[511]

Broadband Technology, Computer Equipment, and Related Supports

When the pandemic hit, many students with disabilities were unable to access remote education due to technology barriers, including poor internet connections, outdated equipment, and difficulties with accessing and navigating online platforms.[512] Some parents of students with and without disabilities were reported to child welfare agencies when their children did not participate in remote education and were found truant, even though in many cases the absences were related to technology, disabilities, lack of supports, the competing demands of the pandemic, or combinations of these factors.[513]

Many students with disabilities, including children with learning, attention, and behavioral disabilities, struggled to focus and learn through a computer screen.[514] The consequences for students with disabilities, and particularly

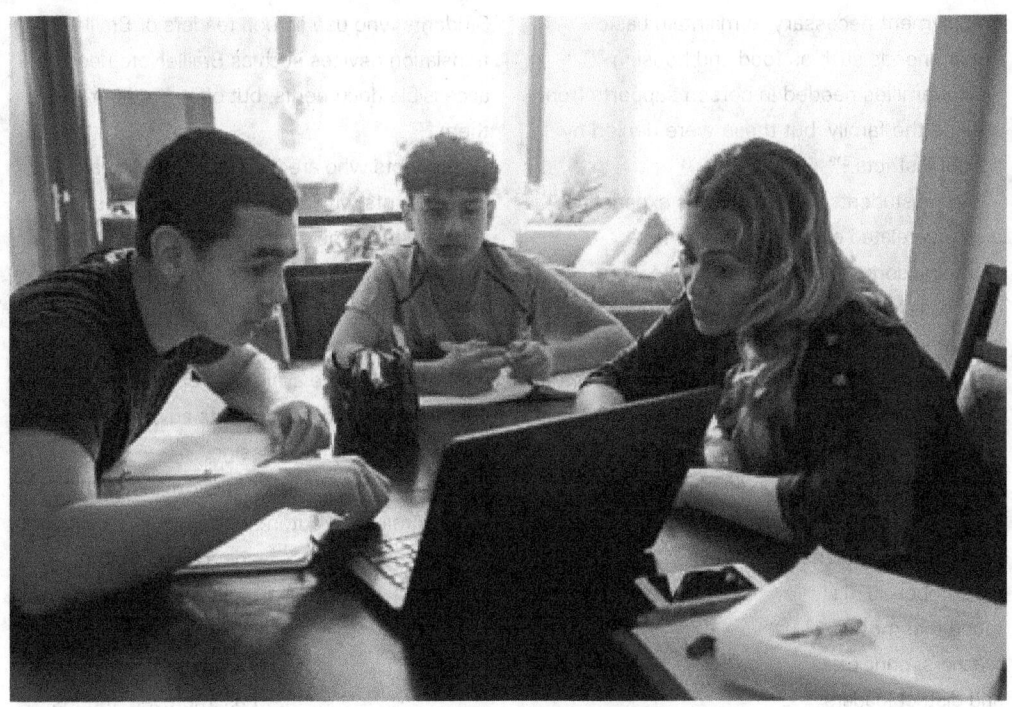

students of color with disabilities, were at times dire. Grace, a 15-year-old Black girl in Michigan with Attention Deficit Hyperactivity Disorder (ADHD), spent 78 days in juvenile detention when her probation was revoked for her not completing her online work.[515] She reported feeling unmotivated and overwhelmed by online learning and got easily distracted without live instruction or structure.

Access to equipment and connectivity slowly improved as the pandemic continued, but barriers persisted.[516] And the primary response to the "digital divide" was for school districts to distribute tablets and hotspots. While this was an essential intervention, it did not represent a permanent solution. Tablets do not have the same level of functionality as laptops, and

hotspots—which can be slow and unreliable—are not a substitute for high-speed connection to the internet.[517]

Reasonable Accommodations, Supports, and Accessibility in Remote Education

Many students with disabilities have disability-related barriers to learning in a remote environment. During the pandemic, some K-12 students with disabilities needed in-person supports such as one-on-one aides to prompt and sustain their attention to on-screen lessons. While in some cases this was the student's parent or family member, some families were unable to perform this role for a variety of reasons, including competing employment necessary to maintain basic human needs such as food and housing.[518] Some families needed in-person supports from outside the family, but these were denied by school districts.[519]

Some students with disabilities experienced disability-related conduct during remote sessions; sometimes these students were removed from the digital "room" without appropriate procedures or documentation for the removal.[520] Some students with disabilities could not participate with their camera turned on, including because of disruptive anxiety or other disability-related conditions, or due to aspects of their home environments. Despite such equity concerns, an October 2020 survey found that most K-12 teachers, principals, and district leaders required cameras to be turned on during remote sessions, and imposed consequences—including losing points and being marked absent—if students turned them off.[521] And as described above, some students with disabilities were reported as "truant" when they did not log in to class, including when this occurred because of disability-related barriers in accessing the virtual classroom.

Students with disabilities faced barriers when education moved online, because the digital platforms and related digital documents were not accessible. Students who are blind need audio description, sound options for verification, adjustments to increase font size, type, and color, magnification that does not destroy the integrity of the text or page, and compatibility with assistive technology such as screen readers.[522]

Students with disabilities faced barriers when education moved online, because the digital platforms and related digital documents were not accessible.

Students who use screen readers or Braille translation devices such as BrailleNote need accessible documents, but often did not receive them.[523]

Students who are Deaf or Hard of Hearing, and students with other disabilities, need accurate real-time captioning. Students with disabilities often need transcripts of remote sessions, including transcripts that can be converted into other formats such as large print or Braille. The availability of captions and transcripts for all students advances the principles of universal design.[524]

During the pandemic, many colleges and schools relied on automatic captioning to convert speech into text for students who need captions in class.[525] While automatic captioning has improved, it does not offer many functions critical to the classroom setting such as proper grammar and punctuation markers, identification of multiple speakers and changes in speakers, and accurate captioning of technical vocabulary, jargon, and proper nouns. Automatic captioning does not allow for clarification or corrections.[526] In many educational settings, students needed a professional captioner.

Students who are Deaf and who communicate using sign language need sign language interpreters integrated into the video platform. To see and understand the interpreter, Deaf students need to be able to view the speaker and the interpreter on the computer screen in larger boxes, and to reduce the size of the other video participants. These features were not available during much of the pandemic.[527]

Students with various disabilities may have needed other adjustments to remote educational platforms. Examples include having participants speak one at a time, ensuring that participants not speaking are on "mute," and having instructors on video, with proper lighting and their faces clearly visible in the frame, to facilitate lip reading or perception of other visual cues.[528]

In-Person Services and Supports

During the pandemic, K-12 students with disabilities were particularly harmed by the cessation of virtually all services and supports that are typically provided to students with disabilities in person. Many students went months without essential services and supports such as occupational therapy, speech and language therapy, behavioral and mental health supports, small group instruction, and one-on-one aides. A review by GAO of the COVID-19 distance learning plans of 15 school districts found that none included details on how the specialized instruction or related services specified in students' IEPs would be provided.[529]

For some students with disabilities, access to a free and appropriate public education and to equal employment opportunity thereafter is only possible with in-person instruction and/ or supports. Many school districts across the country established and maintained in-person instruction for small cohorts of students with disabilities who could not learn in a remote environment. Some provided at-home aides for students with disabilities who needed support. However, other school districts refused to provide any in-person instruction or supports for months or for as long as one year during the pandemic.[530] Many parents did not have the specialized training, or the time, to fill these roles. The result for many students with disabilities was substantial regression.[531]

Children with disabilities also experienced mental health crises during shelter in place, exacerbated by the lack of in-person mental health and behavioral health services. According to the CMS, between March and May 2020, children on Medicaid received 44 percent fewer outpatient mental health services—including therapy and in-home support—compared to the same time period in 2019.[532] It is challenging to provide effective therapy in the remote environment to children with mental health disabilities. Many children do not have a private space with appropriate technology (including broadband internet) to speak confidentially with a therapist. Children with mental health disabilities may struggle with attention, behavioral regulation, and dissociation, making it more difficult for clinicians to therapeutically engage through a video screen.[533] Children with disabilities experienced significantly more mental health problems such as fear and anxiety than other children.[534]

With fewer effective outpatient options, children with disabilities increasingly ended up in emergency rooms, psychiatric hospitals, and residential treatment, and even jail.[535] Across

A review by GAO of the COVID-19 distance learning plans of 15 school districts found that none included details on how the specialized instruction or related services specified in students' IEPs would be provided.

the country, journalists profiled the devastating impact of the pandemic on families of children with significant disabilities who needed in-person supports. For example, in Philadelphia, Aaron and Syrita Powers parent three children with disabilities, a 12-year-old girl with autism, a 10-year-old nonverbal girl with intellectual disability, and an eight-year-old nonverbal girl with autism. Before the pandemic, the three children attended school every day, and were supported in their educational goals by therapies, tutoring, and paraprofessionals. The oldest child attended an afterschool program.[536] That all changed abruptly when schools closed in March 2020. Because of a lack of technology available to students, online teacher-led instruction did not begin until May 2020. Even when online school began, it was not effective for the two younger children due to their disabilities. Some therapies were offered by the district, but only remotely, which did not work for the younger children. And the oldest child was distracted from her online education by the needs of her siblings. With the demands of parenting during the pandemic, Aaron and Syrita skipped doctors' appointments for their own disabilities (kidney disease and fibromyalgia).[537]

All three children regressed substantially during the pandemic, when they did not attend in-person school for more than one year. The two younger children lost their toilet training, and their educational goals—holding a pencil, writing some words, sitting down, and following instructions—deteriorated. The oldest child lost ground in math and social skills and began carrying and speaking with a stuffed animal. Even after one month of in-person instruction beginning in April 2021, there was no change in the youngest child's regression.[538]

Outside of Atlanta, 17-year-old Lindsay who has autism experienced a mental health crisis when schools closed. Without the routine of in-person school and the support of in-person therapies, Lindsay began walking out of the house and wandering several times a week. Her mother, a nurse, would try to call the mental health crisis line to seek a crisis team, but would often be put on hold for 40 or 50 minutes. After an incident in which Lindsay walked into a Family Dollar retail store in a t-shirt and underwear to get Doritos, she ended up tackled and handcuffed by police, and spent most of a night in jail until her mother was able to post bail.[539]

In Los Angeles, Luis Martinez, an 11-year-old nonverbal fifth grader with autism, rarely missed a day of school before the pandemic, and enjoyed seeing his friends and teachers. But after ten months of remote education, Luis stopped looking at his tablet or making any attempt to interact with his peers online. He began acting out nearly every day, scratching and biting himself and members of his family out of frustration.[540]

In Whittier, California, six-year-old Mateo has Phelan-McDermid syndrome, a rare genetic condition causing developmental delays and limited fine motor skills. He has difficulty walking and is nonverbal, and usually uses a device to communicate. During the in-person portion of the school year, he made progress working with his teacher and speech, occupational, and physical

With fewer effective outpatient options, children with disabilities increasingly ended up in emergency rooms, psychiatric hospitals, and residential treatment, and even jail.

therapists. After the pandemic hit, his progress stalled. His speech therapy, which was previously three times a week for half an hour each time, was cut to once a week for about 15 minutes. He stopped learning new vocabulary, tasks, or modes of communication.[541]

On May 6, 2021, a parent testified about his experiences during the pandemic with his nine-year-old son with autism and ADHD, and his nine-year-old daughter with cerebral palsy and intellectual disability, before the U.S. House of Representatives Subcommittee on Early Childhood, Elementary, and Secondary Education.[542] He described how his children regressed and deteriorated with no in-person services, and his son ended up suicidal and hospitalized. Because his daughter cannot engage in learning over an iPad, his wife had to quit her job to stay home to provide schooling. When schools opened part-time in March 2021, his son was a whole year behind in reading. So far, the school has only offered this child 30 minutes of extra support per week.

These are just a handful of accounts of the experiences of thousands of families of children with disabilities. These stories and others attest to how the effects of the pandemic will be long lasting for families of children with disabilities who need in-person education and supports to learn and thrive in the community.

Sustained access to compensatory education will be critical for students with disabilities who needed in-person supports and services, but who did not get them during the pandemic.

The Pandemic's Impact on Native American Students with Disabilities

Native American students with disabilities served through the Bureau of Indian Education (BIE) received few educational services during the pandemic, effectively losing more than one year of education. Throughout the pandemic, BIE failed to issue comprehensive distance learning guidance to BIE schools, despite a need for such guidance.[543] Instead, in August 2020, BIE issued a reopening guide for the 2020–2021 school year focused on in-person school, even though COVID-19 infection rates were high in rural Native communities, and nearly all schools were closing or planning for distance learning for the fall of 2020.[544]

The BIE and other Interior offices provided over 7,000 hotspots to students to improve home internet access, but they did not order laptops for most students until September 2020. Most BIE schools received laptops from late October 2020 to early January 2021, and some laptops still had not been delivered as of late March 2021. Once laptops were delivered, schools faced challenges configuring them, leading to further delays in distributing them to students. By the end of December 2020, more than 80 percent of the laptops had not been delivered by schools to students. As a result, most BIE students who received laptops did not get them until several months after the school year began.[545]

While these failures in pandemic response affected all students, BIE students with disabilities also did not receive the services and supports required by IDEA. The National Indian Education Association (NIEA) found that 21 percent of BIE schools closed during COVID-19 and did not provide any services to their students, including students with disabilities. Thirty-four percent of BIE schools sent home learning packets for their students to work on during school closures, and 30 percent sent students technology devices to use at home.[546]

The relatively high percentage of BIE schools using learning packets correlates to the substantially lower level of connectivity in Native American communities. According to a survey by the NIEA, 40 percent of students who attended BIE schools reported that they had no access to internet services during school closures. Another 34 percent reported that they used a cell phone for their internet service. Only about 21 percent of BIE students had access to broadband internet.[547] The American Community Survey also found that fewer than half of households in many BIE school communities had access to broadband internet prior to the pandemic, and that connectivity is particularly limited on the Navajo Nation Reservation, the site of more than one-third of BIE schools.[548] Internet access was higher for Native American students who were in public school, but still much lower than for non-Native students, with 16 percent reporting no access to the internet during school closures and 22 percent accessing the internet through a cell phone.[549]

During the pandemic, Native American households had fewer resources to pay for internet or cell phone data during the pandemic. Families were struggling to secure food, as sources of revenue were closed, and children were not eating any meals at school.[550] Moreover, providing hotspots and laptops could not resolve barriers to connectivity. Native American families in remote tribal areas may not have electric service at all and must depend on generators to power all appliances that require electricity, including laptops and hotspots.[551] Moreover, hotspots do not function in rural areas without cell coverage.[552]

Educators who attempted to serve Native students with disabilities in these challenging environments reported using a variety of approaches. Some examples included: sending text messages to family members with ideas for gross and fine motor activities that could be done at home; having the speech pathologist, occupational therapist, and physical therapist provide consultation to the family through phone calls, and then sending parents hard copies of suggested activities to do at home with their children; sending special education and general education packets to the student's home, or delivering these packets by school bus; making materials available for pickup or delivering equipment such as walkers, communication devices, and assistive technology; and conducting

> *21 percent of [Bureau of Indian Education] schools closed during COVID-19 and did not provide any services to their students, including students with disabilities. Thirty-four percent of BIE schools sent home learning packets for their students to work on during school closures, and 30 percent sent students technology devices to use at home.*

> *During the pandemic, Native American households had fewer resources to pay for internet or cell phone data during the pandemic. Families were struggling to secure food, as sources of revenue were closed, and children were not eating any meals at school.*

IEPs by phone. Where families and children had connectivity, special education teachers and related service providers conducted short classes or sessions online, and IEPs could be conducted by videoconference. In some cases, parents declined special educational services or requested that teachers and service providers stop calling them, which may have been due to concerns about increased use of the family's cell phone minutes.[553]

The efforts of some dedicated educators did not change the fact that for over a year many Native American students with disabilities received none of the services in their IEPs. Moreover, the failure of BIE to provide or ensure necessary IDEA services and supports predates the pandemic. In an analysis of BIE school documentation from late 2017 and early 2018, the GAO found that the BIE either did not provide or did not document 38 percent of special education and related service time for students with disabilities.[554] The agency also failed to comply with an obligation to verify that IDEA services were provided at all BIE schools each year, and instead only checked services at one-third of schools.[555] The BIE failed to provide required technical assistance to 14 schools that were determined to be at high risk of not complying with IDEA, and provided required monitoring reports late.[556] The BIE acknowledged that its field staff were not qualified to support schools on their IDEA obligations.[557]

Summary of Findings

- The federal, state, and local response to COVID-19 left behind many K-12 and postsecondary students with disabilities.
- During the shelter-in-place period, many K-12 students with disabilities did not receive

FAPE over an extended period of time and went months without essential services and supports that are usually provided in person. Many students with disabilities did not learn and experienced regression in their behavioral and educational goals.

- Children with disabilities in low-income households, and particularly children of color with disabilities in low-income households, experienced particularly severe barriers to remote education during the pandemic.
- Many students with disabilities were unable to access remote education due to technology barriers, including lack of access to broadband internet and appropriate equipment.
- While some students with disabilities flourished in the remote learning environment, many students with disabilities struggled to focus and learn through a computer screen. Punitive responses to students with disabilities who did not attend or engage in remote education were counterproductive and had particularly dire consequences for students of color with disabilities.
- At all levels including K-12 and postsecondary, students who are Deaf, Hard of Hearing, blind, or with other disabilities faced access barriers in digital platforms and related digital documents.
- Without access to effective mental health supports, including in-person supports, some children with disabilities experienced mental health crises during the COVID-19 pandemic, ending up in emergency rooms, psychiatric hospitals, residential treatment, and even jail.

- Native American students with disabilities served through the BIE received few educational services during the pandemic, effectively losing more than one year of education.

- Many students with disabilities now require compensatory education to allow them to recover and regain skills lost during the COVID-19 pandemic, or to learn them for the first time.

Without better guidance, planning, and investment before the next national public health crisis or other emergency, students with disabilities will again experience the denial of FAPE and equal education opportunity.

Recommendations

To ensure the United States is prepared to continue providing special education services and supports needed by students with disabilities to maintain educational benefit during a future pandemic or similar national health crisis, NCD recommends the following actions:

Recommendations for Congress

Congress should:

- Ensure that new or amended legislative proposals.

- Include funds dedicated to compensatory education for students with disabilities who were denied necessary educational services and supports during the pandemic and who have experienced disruption and regression in their behavioral and educational goals. Priority should be given to compensatory education for children with disabilities living in low-income families, children with disabilities who needed—but did not receive—in-person instruction and supports, and Native American children with disabilities.

- Include funds dedicated to making high-speed broadband internet available to and affordable for everyone, and particularly for low-income families, homeless families, and families in rural and other areas where high-speed internet access is not consistently available. Federal recovery efforts must continue to expand connectivity in Native American communities, with a focus on BIE school communities and American Indian reservations. Funds should be allocated soon to ensure that every student has an appropriate laptop or tablet for remote education so that education is not interrupted by another emergency.

- Include funds dedicated to the U.S. Departments of Education and Justice, and to state departments of education, for prompt and effective complaint processing, including free voluntary mediation, for complaints of denial of FAPE and disability discrimination in education during the COVID-19 pandemic.

Recommendations for Federal Agencies

U.S. Department of Education (ED) should:

- Direct school districts to provide compensatory education to students with disabilities to allow them to recover and regain skills. The right to and need for compensatory education should be presumed for children with disabilities who did not receive necessary instruction and supports during the COVID-19 pandemic. Given the extended crisis and national emergency caused by the pandemic, the extent and duration of gaps in educational services, and the known impacts on children with disabilities, families should have a right to "opt in" to compensatory education without any requirement of an extensive individualized factual showing. Sustained access to compensatory education will be critical for many students with disabilities because they were virtually excluded from all education for more than one year.

- Direct school districts to structure compensatory education to provide families with the option to receive additional educational services over several years following the pandemic. Such services should extend past age 22 if the student needs them to make up for the education lost.

- Direct school districts to assess and support access to computer technology for students with disabilities as part of the IEP or Section 504 plan, and should clarify that computer equipment, broadband internet, and computer training are appropriate IEP services.

- Direct school districts to provide in-person services and supports as necessary for students with disabilities to access FAPE and to prevent regression, mental health crises, institutionalization, and family separation, even during a pandemic or public health emergency.

- Affirm that removals from a digital classroom are subject to the same procedures and documentation requirements that apply to removals from a regular classroom. ED should direct schools not to remove students with disabilities from remote sessions for purported misconduct without considering reasonable accommodations and supports. These principles should be established and made known to parents in the event of a future public health emergency.

- Prioritize resolution of complaints of denial of FAPE and disability discrimination that occurred during the COVID-19 pandemic, including through the use of free voluntary mediation.

(continued)

Recommendations for Federal Agencies: *continued*

ED and DOJ should:

- Issue joint guidance to school districts and child welfare agencies directing them to intervene in a problem-solving rather than punitive manner to address student truancy from remote education caused by disabilities, lack of technology, or lack of supports.

- Issue a joint guidance document outlining the elements of accessible remote education for students with disabilities. The guidance should review accessibility requirements for digital platforms and digital documents and emphasize the necessity of designing remote education to be fully accessible to students who are Deaf, Hard of Hearing, and/or blind, or who have other disabilities. The guidance should review necessary auxiliary aids and services such as real-time captioning, accessible transcripts, sign language interpreting, and alternative formats. The guidance should specify the educational contexts in which automatic captioning is not appropriate and detail the features necessary to properly integrate sign language interpreters into a video platform.

Federal Communications Commission (FCC) should:

- Take affirmative steps to make high-speed broadband internet available to and affordable for everyone, including Native Americans and people with disabilities living in rural areas. The FCC's Lifeline program should be expanded to provide high-speed broadband internet to low-income households for $10.00 a month.

Congress should task GAO with:

- Continuing to audit the performance of the BIE during and after the pandemic, including for children with disabilities.

ED and U.S. Department of the Interior should:

- Cooperatively develop, and have the BIE implement, a plan for bringing BIE schools into compliance with the IDEA and Section 504 and delivering compensatory education for Native American children with disabilities who were impacted by the pandemic.

Recommendations for States and State Agencies

State Education Agencies should:

- Direct school districts to provide compensatory education to students with disabilities to allow them to recover and regain skills. The right to and need for compensatory education should be presumed for children with disabilities who did not receive necessary instruction and supports during the COVID-19 pandemic. School districts should offer flexible options for receiving compensatory education over several years following the pandemic.

- Direct school districts to provide in-person services and supports necessary for students with disabilities who require them to receive FAPE and to prevent regression, mental health crises, institutionalization, and family separation, even during a pandemic or public health emergency.

- Direct school districts that student removals from a digital classroom are subject to the same procedures and documentation requirements that apply to removals from an in-person classroom.

- Prioritize resolution of complaints of denial of FAPE and disability discrimination that occurred during the COVID-19 pandemic, including through the use of free voluntary mediation.

- Work with appropriate federal and state agencies to develop and implement plans for ensuring timely and effective delivery of special education services to Native American children in geographic areas where those children can attend public schools or BIE schools.

Chapter 5: Employment and COVID-19

Employment of People with Disabilities Before and After the Pandemic

The passage of the ADA more than 30 years ago advanced a vision for people with disabilities that included among its core principles economic self-sufficiency and full participation in the mainstream economy. The ADA instituted new requirements for how employers were required to evaluate the capabilities of people with disabilities, and spurred the development of accommodations, services, and supports for individuals with significant support needs to succeed in many work environments. Since its enactment, barriers to employment have been lifted for millions, and many individuals with disabilities have been able to secure employment.[558]

At the same time, a large proportion of people with disabilities remain "persistently locked out of employment,"[559] and people with disabilities disproportionately live in poverty.[560] Prior to the COVID-19 pandemic, nearly two-thirds of working-age Americans with disabilities were left out of the labor market altogether.[561]

Fewer than one-third of working-age people with disabilities had a job, compared to nearly three quarters of working-age people without disabilities.[562] This employment gap of 40 or more points has remained steady for years.[563] Federal investments in vocational services, and tax credits for employers that hire and retain people with disabilities,[564] have not been adequate to significantly alter employment and labor participation rates for people with disabilities.

Many people with disabilities excluded from the labor market are in a "poverty trap"; they rely on federal public assistance programs, and cannot work without losing essential healthcare.[565] For example, people with disabilities who need Medicaid to pay for necessary services like personal care attendants face an abrupt loss of this life-sustaining coverage should their earnings exceed certain modest caps.[566] Congressional efforts to reduce the barriers to work imposed by the SSA programs have resulted in complex exemptions that have achieved only very small positive effects.[567] Individuals with disabilities who rely upon SSI receive a benefit amount below the federal

> *Many people with disabilities excluded from the labor market are in a "poverty trap"; they rely on federal public assistance programs, and cannot work without losing essential healthcare.*

poverty level, and more than two-fifths of SSI beneficiaries live below the poverty line.[568]

The unemployment rate for persons with a disability, at 12.6 percent in 2020, increased by 5.3 percentage points from 2019. Their jobless rate continued to be much higher than the rate for those without a disability. (Unemployed persons are those who did not have a job, were available for work, and were actively looking for a job in the four weeks preceding the survey.)[569] The 2019 unemployment rate for persons without a disability increased by 4.4 percentage points to 7.9 percent in 2020. In 2020, 17.9 percent of persons with a disability were employed, down from 19.3 percent in 2019.[570] In contrast, 61.8 percent of people without a disability were employed in 2020, down from 66.3 percent in the prior year. In 2020, persons with a disability were more likely to work in service occupations than those with no disability (18.0 percent, compared with 15.4 percent). Workers with a disability were also more likely than those with no disability to work in production, transportation, and material moving occupations (14.9 percent, compared with 12.2 percent). Persons with a disability were less likely to work in management, professional, and related occupations than those without a disability (36.1 percent, compared with 43.3 percent),[571] a fact that closely related to their ability to telework—as the ability to telework was far greater in these occupations.

These significant problems of exclusion and unemployment for people with disabilities have persisted throughout a time period that has otherwise been characterized by a rapid pace of innovation and disruptive changes in the American workplace—including greater flexibilities, technology, and diversity—and the recovery from the Great Recession to the lowest overall unemployment rate in decades.[572] Emerging employment opportunities in an increasingly digital world have not translated into more jobs for people with disabilities. The fastest growing and most dynamic technology-based industries have the poorest representation of people with disabilities.[573]

The sustained failure to fund and implement the IDEA exacerbates and contributes to the employment gap experienced by people with disabilities. Young people with disabilities are twice as likely as their peers without disabilities to have no high school diploma, leaving them unqualified for many jobs.[574] Only 16.1 percent of people with disabilities earn a bachelor's degree or more, compared to 39.2 percent of people without disabilities.[575]

These failures in education translate into exclusion from employment for young adults with disabilities. In 2019, before the onset of the pandemic, 40.2 percent of young people with disabilities ages 20–24 years were employed, as compared to 73.4 percent of their peers without disabilities.[576] One year out of school, only 17 percent of youth with intellectual and developmental disabilities and 12 percent of youth with multiple disabilities were employed.[577] Many of these youth are made to participate in school transition programs where they are trained to perform manual tasks. These youth are often referred to sheltered workshops directly from school, where they earn far less than the minimum wage under section 14(c) of the Fair Labor Standards Act.[578]

> *The fastest growing and most dynamic technology-based industries have the poorest representation of people with disabilities.*

The onset of the COVID-19 pandemic triggered a massive decline in employment, and the initial hit had a disproportionate impact on people with disabilities. By the end of April 2020, nearly 1 million people with disabilities lost their jobs, representing about 20 percent of working people with disabilities. By comparison, 14 percent of people without disabilities lost their jobs.[579]

School closures forced by the pandemic also had a disproportionate impact on young people with disabilities, who were depending upon transition and other IDEA services to prepare to leave school and enter the workforce. These services are typically provided in person to students with disabilities. With school days shortened and instruction moved to remote platforms, school districts struggled to deliver required IDEA services.[580] Many states and districts failed to plan for or provide postsecondary preemployment transition services during the COVID-19 pandemic.[581] Although the U.S. Department of Education stated that state departments of rehabilitation must continue to make "good faith and reasonable efforts" during the pandemic to provide preemployment transition services to students with disabilities,[582] deadlines were extended and in practice such services were interrupted and delayed.[583]

> By the end of April 2020, nearly 1 million people with disabilities lost their jobs, representing about 20 percent of working people with disabilities. By comparison, 14 percent of people without disabilities lost their jobs.

> School closures forced by the pandemic also had a disproportionate impact on young people with disabilities, who were depending upon transition and other IDEA services to prepare to leave school and enter the workforce.

Against this backdrop of historic barriers, and the disproportionate impact of the pandemic, individual people with disabilities worked, teleworked, looked for work, lost their jobs, and navigated unemployment benefits. Many workers with disabilities have medical statuses putting them at risk for severe outcomes from COVID-19 infection and struggled to balance their own safety with their need to go to work and earn a wage. Households including people with disabilities faced the multiple challenges of managing COVID-19 safety protocols, employment, job loss, caregiving, and remote K-12 learning.

"Reasonable accommodations" under the ADA helped some workers but not others. Gaps in civil rights protections became apparent. Some workers at sheltered workshops were denied unemployment benefits. And the extended duration of the pandemic pushed some workers with disabilities—and particularly older workers with disabilities—out of the labor market altogether.

Unemployment and Other Income and Job Supports

As discussed above, people with disabilities who rely upon SSI and/or SSDI frequently cannot work because their earnings would threaten their access to the essential healthcare coverage that is provided through these assistance programs—a "poverty trap." The COVID-19 relief packages have included three economic incentive payments totaling a maximum of $3,200 per individual. These incentive payments were available to beneficiaries of SSI and SSDI without the need for complicated paperwork and without jeopardizing their benefits. For individuals receiving the maximum federal SSI benefit of $783 per month, the three economic incentive payments raised their income by nearly 35 percent and posed no threat to their healthcare coverage. The simplicity of this approach should be the standard for a reimagining of the "working while disabled" programs of the SSA, which are complex and have had only very small positive effects of bringing people with disabilities into employment.[584]

For people with disabilities facing unemployment during the pandemic, federal relief has been necessary but inadequate. The Paycheck Protection Program helped employers keep some people employed, particularly in the service industries in which many people with disabilities work. But many businesses closed and could not retain employees. It is difficult to know how many jobs were saved,[585] and there is no way to know how many were held by people with disabilities.

People with disabilities who lost their jobs due to the pandemic could apply for unemployment, and people who quit because they have medical conditions making them vulnerable to severe effects from COVID-19, or because of a household member with such

[The] incentive payments were available to beneficiaries of SSI and SSDI without the need for complicated paperwork and without jeopardizing their benefits. . . . The simplicity of this approach should be the standard for a reimagining of the "working while disabled" programs of the SSA . . .

a medical condition, were generally able to access unemployment benefits.[586] Many people with disabilities have medical conditions that made them more vulnerable to severe or life-threatening outcomes from COVID-19.[587] Access to unemployment benefits for people with disabilities vulnerable to COVID-19, and for their household members, was critical to the safety and economic stability of people with disabilities.

In response to the overall loss of employment due to the pandemic, the federal government, which ordinarily pays a share of state unemployment benefits, boosted the weekly amounts available to many beneficiaries, by $600 for about four months, and by $300 for longer, but provided no supplement at all during a gap in the fall and winter of 2020. Without the federal supplements, the unemployment benefit amounts varied greatly from state to state, and at best were modest (one-third to half of the individuals' earnings, with a cap). This was particularly true for people with disabilities because the amount of unemployment benefits is based upon the amount of the person's prior earnings, which is generally lower for people with disabilities.[588] Federal pandemic support also included access to unemployment benefits for self-employed, gig, freelance, and part-time workers. This was critical to many workers with disabilities, who are more likely than workers without disabilities to work for themselves or to work part-time.[589]

In many states, there were huge backlogs before people received unemployment benefits.

Some people waited weeks to get their application processed. The waits were even longer for people who had to appeal the denial of benefits. It was virtually impossible for claimants to reach a benefits worker by phone to resolve issues such as delayed payments or website problems.[590] Many people were deterred from filing or pursuing these claims due to these problems.[591] While there are no formal studies yet, it is likely that those deterred from accessing the benefits owed to them included large numbers of people with disabilities, including people with cognitive, intellectual, developmental, and attention disabilities, who faced disability-related barriers in accessing state unemployment benefit systems.[592]

Technology, Telework, and Remote Work

The pandemic created an unprecedented expansion in telework in certain sectors.[593] Up to half of American workers teleworked during the pandemic, and remote workdays doubled.[594] The expansion of telework had disparate effectiveness, positive and negative, on employees with disabilities.

The ability of employees with and without disabilities to telework was closely related to education level, which had a disproportionate impact on people with disabilities. Very few people with no education beyond high school were able to telework during the pandemic.[595] Those who switched to telework reported higher income and education and better health than those who did not change their typical in-person work.[596] Data shows that people with disabilities are less likely than people without disabilities to graduate from high school[597] or to achieve a bachelor's degree.[598]

The switch to telework was of great benefit to many people with disabilities who, prior to the pandemic, had advocated for more telework.[599] Telework offered workers with disabilities more flexibility, and improved the ability to avoid barriers to working such as inadequate accessible public transportation.[600] Many people with disabilities flourished in a digital environment, in some cases more so than in person. Among people with and without disabilities, more than half of those telecommuting during the pandemic said that, given a choice, they would want to keep working from home even after the pandemic.[601] Many said that telework provided greater flexibility, and made it easier to balance work and family responsibilities.[602]

Expanded telework and remote work also offer the hope of increased job opportunity for the disproportionate number of people with disabilities who live in rural areas.[603] Rates of employment are lower in rural areas for both people with and without disabilities, but the differences are more pronounced for people with disabilities.[604] Computers and

> *Telework offered workers with disabilities more flexibility, and improved the ability to avoid barriers to working such as inadequate accessible public transportation.*

> *Among people with and without disabilities, more than half of those telecommuting during the pandemic said that, given a choice, they would want to keep working from home even after the pandemic.*

high-speed internet must be viewed as necessary utilities for people with disabilities, particularly in rural areas.[605] While the large majority of working-age people with disabilities have broadband internet, a computer, and a smart phone,[606] people with disabilities experience a "digital divide" and are less likely than people without disabilities to have these technologies.[607]

Some employees with disabilities were not able to telework, including those with jobs that are not well suited for telework, those who are not allowed by their employers to telework, those for whom telework is not accessible, and those who have been laid off or whose jobs have been eliminated.[608] Some supports, such as job coaching for people with intellectual disabilities, moved to digital platforms, which worked for some but not all people with disabilities in supported employment.[609]

Some employees with disabilities faced barriers to participating in employment-related meetings on Zoom or other digital platforms. These include some workers with medical conditions such as migraines who experience triggered or worsening symptoms when they look at a computer for too long or when they use digital meeting platforms,[610] or employees with sensory disabilities, such as people who are Deaf, Hard of Hearing, blind, or low vision, who experienced barriers in using digital platforms. In many cases, accessibility can be feasibly provided in the platform by employers.[611]

In 2018, the federal government employed about 269,000 people with disabilities.[612] About 40,000 of them had "Targeted Disabilities," defined as severe disabilities that are associated with high rates of unemployment and underemployment.[613] Most federal workers who telecommuted during the pandemic, and who responded to an anonymous online survey, said that their productivity either increased or stayed the same since the pandemic began.[614] Most said that they think that their agencies will have greater support for remote work even after the pandemic is over.[615] On June 10, 2021, the U.S. Office of Personnel Management together with the General Services Administration issued a guidance document to federal agencies on personnel policies for reentry that includes guidance on telework.[616] The document states that the federal government's nationwide operating status remains at "open with maximum telework flexibilities" for workers eligible for telework,[617] and emphasizes the value of tools such as telework, remote work, and flexible work schedules to advance federal agency goals effectively and efficiently:

OPM/GSA Guidance on Telework

Agency leaders can leverage issues such as telework, remote work, and flexible work schedules as tools in their broader strategies for talent recruitment and retention, and for advancing diversity, equity, inclusion, and accessibility in the Federal workforce. . . . As shown during the pandemic, agencies can, where appropriate, deploy personnel policies such as telework, remote work, and flexible work schedules effectively and efficiently as strategic management tools for attracting, retaining, and engaging talent to advance agency missions, including in the context of changes in workplaces nationwide as a result of the pandemic and in response to long-term workforce trends.[618]

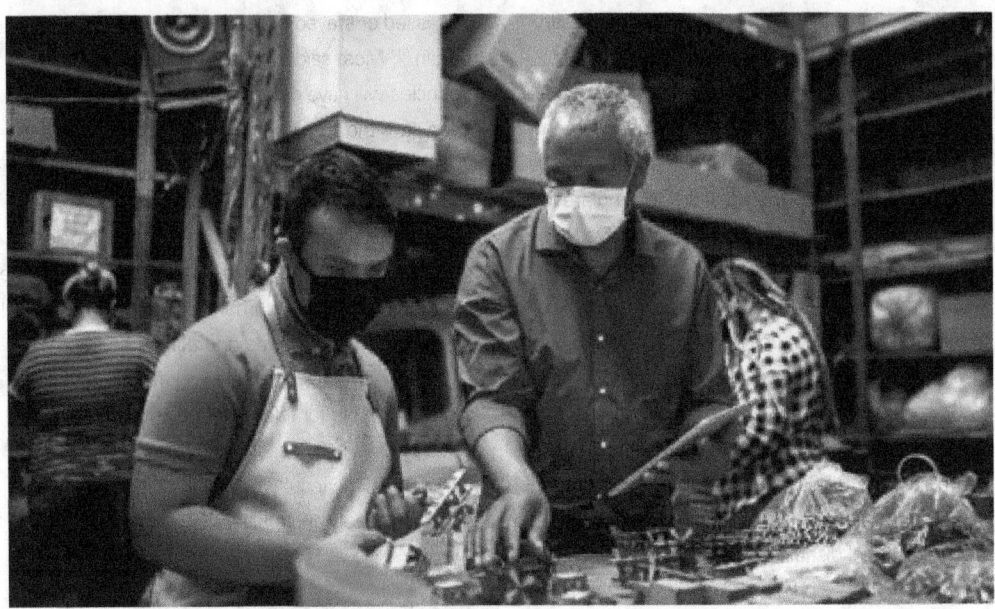

The document urges all agencies "to consider telework as part of overall strategic workforce planning," and "to think of remote work as another option in their overall strategic workforce planning to assist them in competing for top talent."[619] The document states that decisions about telework should be based on job functions and other mission-related priorities, "rather than mere managerial preference."[620] Workers with disabilities have a greater opportunity to succeed when the flexibility of telework is incorporated into the ordinary policies and practices of the employer, which may now be the case for the federal government.

Reasonable Accommodations and Leaves of Absence

Telework

Prior to the COVID-19 pandemic, telework was used by relatively few employees—about 7 percent of private sector workers and 4 percent of state and local workers.[621] But when the pandemic hit, many employers had no choice but to switch to a largely remote work environment for all workers, with and without disabilities.[622] Over the months of the pandemic, working from home became the "new normal" for many workers, with up to half of the workforce telecommuting.[623] As a result of this experience, there is renewed interest in and acceptance of teleworking, which offers cost savings and a recruitment edge for employers and flexibility for workers, including individuals with disabilities.[624] Employees with disabilities may benefit from the expansion of telework, which has resulted from economically common needs and experiences during the pandemic.[625]

EEOC has long recognized telework as a form of reasonable accommodation under the Americans with Disabilities Act.[626] A qualified employee with a disability may be entitled to telework as an accommodation when they need the arrangement to perform the essential functions of the job and/or to enjoy equal employment opportunity.[627] Telework can help remove a range of disability-related work barriers, including difficulties commuting to and from work, accessibility barriers or environmental issues at the worksite, and the need for regular access to private spaces or the bathroom to attend to disability treatment or symptoms.[628] During the pandemic, telework was an essential reasonable accommodation for workers with disabilities who were at increased risk for severe illness or death from acquiring COVID-19. These disabilities included diabetes, HIV, cancer, stroke, Down syndrome, lung, heart, and liver diseases, and additional disabilities.[629]

At the same time, telework was not always easily granted by all employees everywhere. Disability Rights Texas, in testimony submitted to an April 2021 EEOC hearing, reported that it received dozens of employment-related intakes in Texas during the pandemic.[630] More than 60 percent involved an employer rejecting a telework accommodation. In some cases, the workers were permitted partial telework, but were refused a full-time remote assignment.[631] Most of the intakes were from employees with a high-risk health condition or disability, but in some cases telework was needed by individuals who had a mental health condition that was exacerbated by the pandemic.[632]

These telework cases reflected a broad range of jobs. The most common setting was in the school context, both public and private, including teachers, professors, coaches, administrators, counselors, instructional aides, and support personnel. But many other parts of

the economy were also represented, including real property management, real estate, state and local employees, mental health and addiction counselors, social workers, call center employees, and technical writers.[633] Some employers required a certain date by which the person with a disability would stop teleworking and start working on site. But before vaccine appointments became widely available, there was no way to provide such a date.[634]

Where telework was refused as a reasonable accommodation during the pandemic, the employee with a disability was left with bad choices: requesting unpaid leave, quitting, or returning to work and risking acquiring the virus. Workers with disabilities who went on unpaid leave lost their usual income, and were more likely to lose their jobs altogether, particularly as the pandemic went on. There is also indication that women with disabilities and particularly women of color with disabilities were hit particularly hard by employers' refusal to grant telework. Many women with "high-risk" disabilities were insufficiently accommodated in entry-level jobs and also had greater caregiving responsibilities. Now these workers must explain a significant gap in their employment history as they seek new employment.[635] During fiscal year 2020, which included seven months of the pandemic, the EEOC saw a small uptick in the frequency of claims of disability discrimination (from 24,238 to 24,324), while a number of other types of claims decreased.[636]

In 2020, the District Court for Massachusetts granted a preliminary injunction to allow the plaintiff, an assistance manager for a mental health provider, to continue to telework. The plaintiff had moderate asthma that imposed a greater risk of serious illness if they contracted COVID-19. The employee tried to return to the office but was not given PPE and was exposed to other people not wearing masks. The plaintiff returned to teleworking without the accommodation being approved and understood that they would be fired as a result; the lawsuit followed.[637] After the court granted the injunction, the case settled.[638] Many employees with disabilities do not have a lawyer to represent them in court.[639]

Some employers who allowed telework during the pandemic ended the practice once vaccines became available and directed employees to return to the workplace.[640] But some workers with disabilities still needed telework as a reasonable accommodation, either because of the continued effects of the pandemic, or for other disability-related reasons. The EEOC has stated that the fact that an employer has permitted telecommuting for a period of time during the pandemic does not mean that it is a required reasonable accommodation.[641]

If, because of the experience during the pandemic, more employers offer flexible hours, remote work, and telework into the future, this could greatly expand employment opportunities for workers with disabilities.[642] Telework can allow individuals with disabilities to work even if they have disability-based limitations to travel such as not driving due to disability, and despite ongoing access barriers in the transportation system.[643] Increased availability of remote work could also improve job opportunity for the disproportionate number of people with disabilities who live in rural areas and who experience lower rates of unemployment.[644] The success of the federal government in maintaining its efficiency and productivity during the 18 months that most federal employees teleworked should guide public policy with respect to telework.

Leaves of Absence

For people with disabilities who were vulnerable to severe outcomes from COVID-19 infection, accessing sufficient job-protected unpaid leave during the pandemic was difficult. While the Family and Medical Leave Act was helpful, it grants only 12 weeks of job-protected leave and is available only to a small portion of the workforce—those employees who work for large employers and who have one year's tenure and sufficient hours.

The ADA may provide additional job-protected leave, but the case law is mixed. While some ADA case law is protective, other ADA cases hold that indefinite or lengthy leaves are not required as reasonable accommodations. For example, in *Hwang v. Kansas State University*, a professor with cancer requested an extension of leave beyond six months because there was a flu epidemic on campus and her immune system was compromised. She was fired. In 2014, the court of appeals for the Tenth Circuit ruled that her termination was not disability discrimination.[645] During the pandemic, leaves of absence sufficient to reach the end of the pandemic or the rollout of vaccines were typically both indefinite and lengthy.

Accommodations for People with COVID-19–Vulnerable Household Members

The pandemic revealed a substantial gap in civil rights protections: Many employees needed reasonable accommodations such as telework, not because of their own vulnerability, but because they were household members and caregivers of people with disabilities who were vulnerable to severe effects from COVID-19 infection. There is no civil rights law that adequately protects this group of workers. According to EEOC guidance, employees without disabilities are not entitled to reasonable accommodations needed to protect a vulnerable household member or care recipient.[646]

Some of these household members and caretakers took unpaid leave. Some went to work and took the risk that they would spread the virus to the vulnerable person. Some quit. For those who took unpaid leave, leave was often not guaranteed or job-protected. As noted above, most employees are not covered by the Family and Medical Leave Act, and even those who are covered are only entitled to up to 12 weeks of unpaid leave.

Many employees needed reasonable accommodations such as telework, not because of their own vulnerability, but because they were household members and caregivers of people with disabilities who were vulnerable to severe effects from COVID-19 infection. There is no civil rights law that adequately protects this group of workers.

Masks and Other COVID-19 Safety Protocols at Work

CDC recommended l cloth masks or other face coverings and social distancing for individuals older than two years during the pandemic, including people who were not medically at risk.[647] During the pandemic, as a matter of basic workplace safety for all employees, employers should have monitored and enforced compliance with COVID-19 protocols such as masks and social distancing.

In addition, compliance with COVID-19 protocols was a form of reasonable accommodation that was needed by some employees with disabilities during the pandemic. These included people who had conditions that made them vulnerable to severe effects from COVID-19 such that they could not safely work without masks and social distancing in place, as well as people who had anxiety disabilities or other conditions that made them extremely fearful of the coronavirus. Where requested by an employee with a disability as a reasonable accommodation, employers should have enforced safety protocols such as masks and social distancing.

Unfortunately, COVID-19 protocols including masks were resisted in some workplaces, sometimes because they have been harmfully politicized. In these environments, employees with disabilities had difficulties resolving their accommodation needs without facing harassment and hostility.[648]

At the same time, employers must also provide reasonable accommodations to employees who cannot wear masks or cannot wear them consistently or for long periods of time, due to their disabilities. Examples may include individuals with developmental or intellectual disabilities, including autistic people, who cannot tolerate masks, and people with mobility impairments who cannot independently put on or take off a mask. During a pandemic, under the ADA, employers must provide reasonable accommodations to all employees with disabilities, including employees with disabilities who have needs that appear to conflict (such as an employee with a disability who needed safety protocols in place due to their preexisting condition that made them vulnerable to severe effects from COVID-19, and a fellow employee with a disability who was not able to consistently wear a mask due to their developmental disability). This requires creativity and flexibility to reach safe and inclusive outcomes.[649]

Older Workers with Disabilities

Older workers with disabilities who have lost their jobs due to the pandemic face a high risk that they will never rejoin the workforce.[650] Many of these workers have been or will be forced into early retirement, with the serious financial and other losses that accompany this change in status.[651]

During and after the Great Recession, it took older workers longer to find work.[652] Older workers are more likely to suffer long-lasting negative consequences due to recessions, including job loss, pay cuts, loss of healthcare, poverty, and decreased longevity or life expectancy.[653] The COVID-19 pandemic and resulting recession hit older people, especially older women, even harder than past recessions.[654] Workers over age 55 experienced higher unemployment from the pandemic than midcareer workers and returned to work more slowly.[655] Older workers who are Black, female, or lack a college degree experienced even higher rates of job loss.[656]

Workers over age 55 experienced higher unemployment from the pandemic than midcareer workers and returned to work more slowly. Older workers who are Black, female, or lack a college degree experienced even higher rates of job loss.

Even if a prior workplace reopens after being closed due to the pandemic, older employees with disabilities may not be called back to work with the others.[657] This kind of discrimination is extremely difficult to demonstrate or remedy. Research shows that age discrimination in hiring increases during recessions, contributing to longer periods of unemployment for older workers.[658] Age discrimination is also a significant barrier for older workers who look for temporary jobs to delay retirement.[659]

Some older workers with disabilities may have worked somewhere for a very long time before the pandemic, with reasonable accommodations and job supports in place (whether formal or informal).[660] Once these tailored positions were lost due to the pandemic, they were extremely hard to recreate later. These workers may not be very knowledgeable about how to go about getting a job in the current reality. They may not be proficient at using computers and application portals to apply for jobs.

Older people also experience more severe aftereffects of COVID-19 infection. New or more severe disabilities are primary reasons that older workers with disabilities leave the labor force.[661] Workers with new disabilities may have less ability to successfully advocate for reasonable accommodations at work, compared to individuals with long-standing, chronic disabilities who may better understand their rights.[662] Robust and explicit accommodation programs can help keep older workers with disabilities on the job.[663]

People with Disabilities Earning Subminimum Wage at Sheltered Workshops

Since 1938, Section 14(c) has allowed employees with disabilities to be paid less than the minimum wage under special certificates used to operate sheltered workshops. Some employees with disabilities earn as little as cents per hour.[664] Section 14(c) creates a federally sanctioned segregated jobs system for people with disabilities, and is contrary to the civil rights principles of the ADA and its integration mandate.[665] NCD has long recommended that Congress phase out Section 14(c) of the Fair Labor Standards Act as a policy relic from the 1930s, when discrimination was inevitable because service systems were based on a charity model, rather than empowerment and self-determination.[666] NCD favors instead investment into training programs and competitive, integrated employment, including supported employment. The U.S. Commission on Civil Rights recently made the same recommendation.[667] The Transformation to Competitive Integrated Employment Act (H.R. 2373) would provide states and employers with resources to transition workers with disabilities into fully integrated and competitive jobs while phasing out the subminimum wage for individuals with disabilities.[668]

The onset of the pandemic caused many sheltered workshops to close. These congregate workplaces posed substantial health risks to workers with intellectual and developmental disabilities, who are at increased risk of severe illness and death from COVID-19.[669] Many people with disabilities who worked in sheltered workshops under Section 14(c) of the Fair Labor Standards Act found that they were not eligible for unemployment when their work stopped due to the pandemic. This was because they were classified as "trainees" or recipients of services rather than as employees, and their employer-provider did not pay into the state unemployment system.[670] These workers found themselves overlooked and disregarded while nondisabled workers were able to access unemployment benefits.

Many of these segregated programs have reopened or are slowly reopening.[671] The ongoing recovery effort provides an opportunity for a substantial federal investment into developing integrated employment opportunities as alternatives to sheltered workshops.

> *Many people with disabilities who worked in sheltered workshops under Section 14(c) of the Fair Labor Standards Act found that they were not eligible for unemployment when their work stopped due to the pandemic.*

Summary of Findings

- Before the onset of the COVID-19 pandemic, nearly two-thirds of working-age Americans with disabilities were left out of the labor market altogether, caught in a "poverty trap" created by federal public assistance programs. People with disabilities who were working or looking for work experienced an unemployment rate more than twice that of people without disabilities.

- The onset of the COVID-19 pandemic triggered a massive decline in employment, and the initial losses were borne disproportionately by people with disabilities, with nearly 1 million people with disabilities—about one in five—losing their jobs.

- Young people with disabilities, who were already disproportionately excluded from the workforce, did not receive mandated IDEA services during the COVID-19 pandemic, including preemployment transition services.

- The expansion of telework during the pandemic was of great benefit to many people with disabilities. It offered workers with disabilities more flexibility, and reduced barriers to working such as those associated with transportation.

- While in many cases accessibility can be feasibly provided by employers in digital platforms such as Zoom, some employees with disabilities faced barriers to participating in remote employment–related meetings.

- Some employees with disabilities were not able to telework during the pandemic, including those with jobs that were not well suited for telework, those who were not allowed by their employers to telework, those for whom telework is not accessible, and those who have been laid off or whose jobs have been eliminated.

- Telework has long been recognized by the EEOC as a reasonable accommodation under the ADA. Telework can help remove disability-related work barriers, including difficulties commuting, accessibility barriers at the worksite, and the need for regular access to private spaces to attend to disability treatment or symptoms.

- During the pandemic, telework was an essential reasonable accommodation for workers with disabilities who were at increased risk for severe illness or death from acquiring COVID-19. When telework was refused as a reasonable accommodation, these employees with disabilities were left with bad choices: quit, request unpaid leave, or return to work and risk acquiring the virus.

- For people with disabilities who were vulnerable to severe outcomes from coronavirus infection, accessing sufficient job-protected unpaid leave during the pandemic was difficult because the leaves needed were long and often indefinite.

- The pandemic revealed a substantial gap in civil rights protections: no federal civil rights law protected employees who needed a reasonable accommodation such as telework, not because of their own disability, but because they were household members and caregivers of people with disabilities who were vulnerable to severe effects from acquiring COVID-19.

- The availability of benefits from the COVID-19 relief packages was critically important to the safety and economic stability of people with disabilities. These benefits included three EIPs that were made available to beneficiaries of SSI and SSDI without jeopardizing their benefits. These benefits included extended unemployment insurance, including for self-employed and part-time workers, with federal supplements of $300 or $600 during most weeks of the pandemic. The unemployment benefits were valuable to people with disabilities, who are more likely to have lower earnings, meaning that their unemployment benefit amounts were lower, and who are more likely to work for themselves or to work part-time.

- State unemployment insurance claims systems experienced huge backlogs, and it is likely that those deterred from accessing the benefits owed to them included large numbers of people with disabilities.

- The federal government maintained its efficiency and productivity during the 18 months that most federal employees teleworked. If implemented, the June 2021 guidance issued by the U.S. Office of Personnel Management and the General Services Administration will afford workers with disabilities a greater opportunity to succeed by incorporating the flexibility of telework into the ordinary employment policies and practices of the federal government.

- If, because of experiences during the pandemic, more employers offer flexible hours, remote work, and telework into the future, this could greatly expand employment opportunities for workers with disabilities. Telework can allow individuals with disabilities to work even if they have barriers to commuting, such as not driving due to disability, or inaccessible public transportation. Increased availability of remote work could also improve job opportunity for the disproportionate number of people with disabilities who live in rural areas and who experience lower rates of unemployment.

- Section 14(c) to the Fair Labor Standards Act creates a federally sanctioned segregated jobs system for people with disabilities and is contrary to the civil rights principles of the ADA and its integration mandate. The onset of the pandemic caused many sheltered workshops to close. These congregate workplaces posed substantial health risks to workers with intellectual and developmental disabilities, who are at increased risk of severe illness and death from COVID-19.

- Many people with disabilities who worked in sheltered workshops under Section 14(c) of the Fair Labor Standards Act found that they were not eligible for unemployment when their work stopped due to the pandemic.

- Many of these segregated programs have reopened or are slowly reopening. The ongoing recovery effort provides an opportunity for a substantial federal investment into developing integrated employment opportunities as alternatives to sheltered workshops.

- Older workers with disabilities who have lost their jobs due to the pandemic face a high risk that they will never rejoin the workforce. Many of these workers have been or will be forced into early retirement, with the serious financial and other losses that accompany this change in status.

Recommendations

To ensure the United States is prepared for a future pandemic or similar national health crisis, NCD recommends the following actions based on our findings about the impact of COVID-19 on workers with disabilities and working-aged people with disabilities:

Recommendations for Congress

Congress should:

- Task GAO with examining the gaps in employment protections that occurred during the COVID-19 pandemic, including for people with disabilities who were vulnerable to severe outcomes from COVID-19, and for people who have COVID-19–vulnerable household members, or who are caregivers to COVID-19–vulnerable individuals. This examination should consider whether existing laws and federal policies will provide adequate protections to these workers during future pandemics, or whether new laws or federal policies are needed.

- Pass legislation to decouple eligibility for Medicaid and Medicare from eligibility for cash benefits. The legislation should allow people with disabilities covered by Medicaid and/or Medicare through the SSI and SSDI programs to work and to retain their existing healthcare coverage permanently, without cost to the individual and without any complex paperwork.

- Pass legislation to allow people with disabilities receiving Social Security Administration benefits to work without fear of losing necessary income and supports, such as the Work Without Worry Act (S. 2108) which would allow adults with disabilities who receive the Disabled Adult Child benefit to work without jeopardizing their benefits. Congress should also raise the benefit amount for SSI to above the federal poverty line.

- In the event of a future national disaster or public health emergency, pass legislation immediately to provide dedicated unemployment and relief funds to stabilize households, including those of part-time workers, self-employed individuals, and gig workers, who are disproportionately people with disabilities, working families with children with disabilities, individuals with caregiving obligations, and people with disabilities receiving SSI and SSDI benefits.

- Enact the Transformation to Competitive Integrated Employment Act (TCIEA), which would phase out and repeal 14(c) from the Fair Labor Standards Act and would invest in alternative service models prioritizing competitive integrated employment.

- Adequately fund vocational rehabilitation by increasing authorization for preemployment transition services, training programs, and integrated competitive employment, including supported employment, for individuals with disabilities.

- Enhance tax credits for employers who hire and retain employees with disabilities by enacting the Disability Employment Incentive Act.

(continued)

Recommendations for Congress: *continued*

- Authorize and fund a federal exchange for state unemployment benefits, to be overseen by the U.S. Department of Labor, that is accessible to and usable by everyone eligible for unemployment benefits, including people with disabilities. Require states that are unable to provide an accessible and usable system for state unemployment benefits to join the federal exchange.

Recommendations for Federal Agencies

EEOC should:

- Work to strengthen legal protections for workers with disabilities who seek telework, leaves of absence, and safety policy modifications as reasonable accommodations. EEOC should offer guidance to employers in accommodating employees with needs that appear to conflict.

- Consider amending Section 501 regulations to include a sub-goal for older people with disabilities, and/or to require reporting on older workers with disabilities.

EEOC and DOL should:

- Prioritize enforcement of the Americans with Disabilities Act and Sections 501 and 503 of the Rehabilitation Act to ensure that workers with disabilities receive reasonable accommodations needed to secure or maintain employment, including accommodations needed due to the pandemic.

Office of Personnel Management (OPM) should:

- Maintain maximum telework flexibility for all federal agencies on a permanent basis and ensure that federal employees with disabilities receive necessary, reasonable accommodations in their technology while working remotely and retain flexibility to work from their designated federal office as needed or desired.

DOL and OPM should:

- Issue joint guidance on effective telework tools and highlight the benefit of telework for many people with disabilities. The guidance should describe the need for accessibility in remote work platforms and allow agencies to use the platforms that are most accessible based on employee needs.

Recommendations for Federal Agencies: *continued*

Federal Communications Commission (FCC) should:

- Take affirmative steps now to ensure that high-speed broadband internet is available to and affordable for everyone. The FCC's Lifeline program should be expanded to provide high-speed broadband internet to low-income households for $10.00 a month.

Department of Labor should:

- Audit state systems of unemployment benefits, and issue notices of correction to agencies that failed to maintain functional and accessible systems for applying for and maintaining benefits during the COVID-19 crisis, so that such agencies will be better prepared for any similar public emergency. The Department should require states to join a federal exchange if they cannot offer eligible workers such a system.

Office of Federal Contract Compliance Programs (OFCCP) should:

- Consider amending Section 503 regulations to include a sub-goal for older people with disabilities, and/or to require reporting on older workers with disabilities.

Recommendations for States and State Agencies

Fair Employment Practices (FEP) Agencies should:

- Review any gaps in state employment law protections that occurred during the COVID-19 pandemic, including for people with disabilities who were vulnerable to severe outcomes from COVID-19, and for people who have COVID-19–vulnerable household members, or who are caregivers to COVID-19–vulnerable individuals. State FEP agencies should report on their findings to state legislatures.

Chapter 6: Effective Communication

Overview of Effective Communication Before and During the Pandemic

The COVID-19 pandemic has uniquely impacted Deaf and Hard of Hearing communities, people who are blind, and people who cannot rely on speech to be heard and understood. Today, there are over 37.5 million people with difficulty hearing, and an additional 5 million people who cannot rely on speech to communicate, in the United States.[672] Prior to the pandemic, they faced communication barriers across healthcare, education, employment, and government contexts. The provision of disability-related accommodations and proper auxiliary aids and services by public entities, employers, and public accommodations—as required by the ADA,[673] Section 504 of the Rehabilitation Act,[674] and Section 1557 of the Affordable Care Act[675]—was inconsistent and often a barrier to equal access.

With the pandemic, disparities in effective communication deepened. Widespread mask use and social distancing protocol, as well as increased reliance on virtual forums of communication, among other pandemic-era policies, created new challenges for people with hearing, vision, speech, and/or intellectual or developmental disabilities to interact with their communities and equally access healthcare, education, and employment. These new communication barriers also hindered the dissemination of public health information critical to slowing the spread of COVID-19 and exacerbated the difficulties that people with disabilities already faced in accessing essential services. When, as during the pandemic, written and oral communications related to the provision of medical care and public health precautions are of the utmost importance, it is critical that public entities, employers, and places of public accommodation ensure that their

> *Widespread mask use and social distancing protocol, as well as increased reliance on virtual forums of communication, among other pandemic-era policies, created new challenges for people with hearing, vision, speech, and/or intellectual or developmental disabilities to interact with their communities and equally access health care, education, and employment.*

communications are fully accessible to people with disabilities.

Healthcare Setting

The failure to provide proper accommodations to people with communication disabilities in healthcare settings can have life-threatening consequences. During the COVID-19 pandemic, which disproportionately caused serious illness and death among people with disabilities,[676] it was crucial for patients and family members with disabilities to have the auxiliary aids and services that they need to be able to effectively communicate in healthcare settings. The failure of a hospital, doctor's office, or medical provider to provide accurate, real-time communication in accessible formats can lead to a misunderstanding of a patient's symptoms, inappropriate diagnosis, and/or delayed or improper medical treatment.[677] While the entire country feared contracting COVID-19, millions of people with disabilities experienced the additional anxiety of being unable to learn about, communicate, and express decisions regarding their medical circumstances.[678]

Face Masks and Physical Distancing

COVID-19 is transmitted is through exposure to respiratory fluids carrying infectious virus. Exposure occurs in three principal ways: (1) inhalation of very fine respiratory droplets and aerosol particles, (2) deposition of respiratory droplets and particles on exposed mucous membranes in the mouth, nose, or eye by direct splashes and sprays, and (3) touching mucous membranes with hands that have been soiled either directly by virus-containing respiratory fluids or indirectly by touching surfaces with virus on them. To prevent infection and spread of the virus, including those were disabled and those medically at risk, the CDC recommended maintaining a physical distance of at least six feet from other individuals, practicing hand hygiene and environmental cleaning, By April 3, 2020, CDC recommended the universal use of face coverings.[679] Following this guidance, healthcare entities, as well as many government entities, businesses, and employers, mandated the use of face masks. These measures have been a double-edged sword for disability communities. These requirements are important to protecting high-risk individuals from contracting COVID-19, such as people with lung disease, asthma, heart conditions, diabetes, kidney disease, or conditions that deem a person immunocompromised.[680] At the same time, however, the common use of opaque masks created new challenges for people who are Deaf and others with disabilities that impact their hearing or speech.

People who are Deaf and Hard of Hearing have varying degrees of hearing loss and rely on a variety of auxiliary aids and services in the healthcare setting, such as sign language interpreters, assistive technologies, and/or amplification of sound. Everyone has different needs and preferences, but auditory cues and visual cues such as mouth and lip movements and facial expressions can play an important role in effective communication for many of these individuals.[681]

The use of face masks can muffle sound, making it more difficult for people with hearing loss to understand speech and higher pitched voices.[682] It can also take away an individual's ability to lip read and contextualize communications through the observation of facial expressions.[683] People with hearing loss have reported "widespread difficulty" in understanding healthcare providers who are wearing face masks during the COVID-19 pandemic.[684] For example, one participant in a recent study, who had significant but not complete hearing loss, reported that they "attended a clinic appointment . . . [and] struggle[d] to understand what was said [] by the consultant wearing [a] facemask."[685] Others report having to ask healthcare workers to repeat themselves and speak more loudly because of the barriers created by the face mask.[686]

Physical distancing can also create heightened communication challenges. Distance causes speech to sound quieter and makes it more difficult to see visual cues, especially when an individual also has vision loss.[687] It can also be more difficult for individuals to focus their attention on a speaker from a distance, because other sounds and movements in the environment can distract or overshadow the communication.[688] The change in nature of face-to-face interactions caused by the pandemic "hinder[ed] speech understanding" among people with hearing loss and/or intellectual or developmental disabilities.[689]

Several solutions were suggested to lessen the communication difficulties created by face mask use and social distancing in the healthcare setting. First, the use of adaptable, clear masks has been widely endorsed as an alternative that accommodates people who lip read.[690] In one study, the sentiment that key healthcare workers should be supplied with a transparent face mask was "widely shared."[691] However, while some clear masks were approved by the FDA, they were not N95-rated and therefore were inappropriate in certain healthcare settings, such as when a provider is interacting with COVID-19 patients.[692] Additionally, they do not alleviate communication barriers created by muffled sound and certainly cannot be a substitute for an ASL interpreter, when that is the patient's primary language.

Alternative accommodations must also be considered. Depending on the needs and preferences of the individual, the use of a sign language interpreter; assistive technology such as video-remote interpreting (VRI), transcription services, Communication Access Realtime Translation (CART), and assistive listening devices; low-tech solutions such as communication boards; or moving an appointment to an accessible telemedicine forum may be appropriate. While each of these accommodations have their own complications related to the COVID-19 pandemic (as further discussed in the following subsections), it is essential that healthcare providers and administrators continue to listen to the needs of people with communication disabilities and devise effective solutions to ensure that they can learn and communicate about their health conditions.

In addition to the challenges that face mask mandates create in the *receipt* of information from healthcare professionals, they also can create barriers for people with disabilities

> *In addition to the challenges that face mask mandates create in the receipt of information from health care professionals, they also can create barriers for people with disabilities to provide information to their health care providers.*

to *provide* information to their healthcare providers. There are individuals who, by virtue of their disability, cannot wear a mask either at all or for an extended period of time.[693] Examples include individuals with developmental or intellectual disabilities who cannot tolerate masks, people with mobility impairments who cannot independently put on or take off a mask, people who use ventilators to support breathing, people with seizure disorders who may be in danger if they experience a seizure while wearing a mask, people with lung diseases or breathing difficulties, and people who experience panic attacks while wearing masks.[694]

In-Person Interpretation

Prior to the COVID-19 pandemic, in-person interpretation in the hospital setting was the highest standard of care for people who communicate through sign language. Healthcare experiences can be fast-paced and dynamic. Especially in emergency situations, there are often multiple healthcare providers (doctors, nurses, technicians, etc.) in a room at once, performing several tasks, and attempting to communicate multiple pieces of information, all while the patient is potentially in a supine or prone position and in pain. In such situations, it is critical that the auxiliary aids or services provided to an individual with a communication disability be built for this dynamic environment. Digital interpretation services,

To protect all parties involved, while still providing the in-person interpretation services that are necessary in many critical healthcare circumstances, interpreters need adequate safety gear. Likewise, healthcare entities must be provided the resources they need . . ., including funding to ensure the availability of qualified interpreters and other augmentative communication tools.

such as VRI, have limited effectiveness in crisis care situations and are inferior to an in-person interpreter, who can observe the whole scene and move around the room as needed to facilitate communication.

However, at the onset of the pandemic, sign language interpreters expressed concern for their lives and safety, given the increased chance of contracting COVID-19 in the hospital setting.[695] Likewise, patients expressed concern that interpreters could spread COVID-19 to the people who use their services, other patients in the facility, and hospital staff. These safety concerns were amplified by nationwide shortages in PPE.[696] The economic crisis caused by the pandemic also significantly reduced the number of sign language interpreters available to provide services to people with disabilities.[697] Many interpreters lost their jobs as funding for interpreter services decreased and public and private health insurers failed to cover interpretation and disability accommodation services.[698]

In order to balance the competing need for in-person interpretation services in hospital settings with the safety concerns of potential COVID-19 exposure from the use of such a service, interpreters must have access to PPE. Just like any other individual who is working in a hospital, a sign language interpreter is essential staff. To protect all parties involved, while still providing the in-person interpretation services that are necessary in many critical healthcare circumstances, interpreters need adequate safety gear. Likewise, healthcare entities must be provided the resources they need to effectively communicate with patients or family members with a communication disability, including funding to ensure the availability of qualified interpreters and other augmentative communication tools.

Assistive Technology

As an alternative to in-person interpretation, healthcare entities increased reliance on assistive technologies such as VRI, transcription services, or Communication Access Realtime Translation (CART), and communication boards during the COVID-19 pandemic. These communication tools have the advantage of bypassing the need for another individual—a potential vector for COVID-19—to be in the room. However, as explained in the previous section, the use of remote interpretation and other auxiliary aids is not always appropriate, especially in critical care settings. In situations where an in-person interpreter is not required, however, they can provide an effective tool to facilitate effective communication—when used properly and when certain technological performance standards are met.

For example, VRI is a videoconferencing technology for accessing an offsite interpreter to provide real-time sign language or oral interpretation services for conversations between hearing people and the Deaf or Hard of Hearing.[699] To be effective, VRI must be used over a dedicated high-speed, wide-bandwidth internet connection; the screen must be large enough to display the interpreter's entire upper body; the audio must be clear; and facility staff must be trained in its set-up and proper operation.[700] Provided that the situation does not require an in-person interpreter and the individual with hearing loss prefers VRI over an in-person interpreter, then properly used VRI can be an effective solution to communication in healthcare settings, while also reducing potential exposure to the COVID-19 virus.[701]

Alternatively, some people with hearing loss may prefer to use remote real-time transcription services like CART to communicate with their healthcare providers,[702] or low-tech communication methods, such as supplemental communication boards.[703]

Telemedicine

In an effort to slow the spread of the COVID-19 virus, healthcare entities have rapidly adopted telephone and video visits (collectively "telemedicine") as an alternative to traditional in-person care. Prior to the pandemic, telemedicine was widely unavailable due to a preference for seeing patients in person and potential Health Insurance Portability and Accountability Act of 1996 (HIPAA) concerns related to the perceived lack of security of telecommunications. Where available, if a person with a disability faced barriers accessing the platform or communicating with healthcare providers, then they could revert to in-person care. For this reason, some argue that the focus of communication access has concentrated almost exclusively on how to adapt the in-person healthcare environment to accommodate the needs of people with disabilities; while telemedicine, up until the pandemic, was largely an afterthought.[704] COVID-19 has swiftly changed that.

For some people with disabilities, particularly those who are immunocompromised and/or have mobility disabilities, telemedicine was a welcome addition to healthcare systems. It created a safer and more affordable method of receiving healthcare when physical presence is not necessary—reducing potential exposure to communicable diseases like COVID-19, lowering transportation costs and hardships, and lowering the cost of care.[705] On the other hand, however, it has created a host of new communication barriers for people with hearing loss, vision loss, and/or intellectual or developmental disabilities.[706]

Most HIPAA-compliant telemedicine platforms do not have built-in accessibility features to facilitate communications with patients with disabilities.[707] Features such as live captioning and three-way video visits (which allow an interpreter to join the meeting and facilitate communication) are not yet commonplace.[708] This means that telemedicine visits can be useless to the Deaf or Hard of Hearing, who may be able to see but not communicate with their healthcare providers. While a telephone visit—when coupled with a relay service operator such as Text Telephone (TTY)—may be a more viable option, quality of care is questionable when the only means of communication is through text, especially when visits are further constrained by time limits.

Most HIPAA-compliant telemedicine platforms do not have built-in accessibility features to facilitate communications with patients with disabilities.

[D]ue to the inflexibility, lack of exemptions, . . . regarding these [no visitor] policies, they also had the unintended consequence of blocking people with disabilities from accessing the direct care workers/direct support professionals and family members they needed . . . to effectively communicate . . . to health care providers, . . . and make informed medical decisions.

Likewise, telemedicine platforms and the patient education materials posted on them are often not accessible to people with vision loss.[709] Websites, software programs, and electronic documents are often not designed and formatted to be accessible with a screen reader. Compliance with World Wide Web Consortium's (W3C) Web Content Accessibility Guidelines (WCAG) is not widespread.[710]

To remedy the communication barriers in telemedicine, the digital interfaces must be customized to accommodate the needs of people with disabilities. This includes ensuring that three-way video visits are supported by the platform and the interface is visually accessible.

No-Visitor Policies

During the course of the COVID-19 pandemic, some hospitals have enacted no-visitor policies.[711] These policies were aimed at decreasing the number of people in hospital settings, thus curbing the spread of COVID-19 among patients and hospital staff alike. However, due to the inflexibility, lack of exemptions, and lack of forethought regarding these policies, they also had the unintended consequence of blocking people with disabilities from accessing the direct care workers/direct support professionals and family members they needed by their side in order to effectively communicate their symptoms and needs to healthcare providers, accurately understand information provided by those staff members, and make informed medical decisions.[712]

A person with a disability's daily direct care workers and family members know the individual, their conditions, and their needs better than anyone else. Blocking a support person from accompanying an individual during a hospital visit can decrease the quality of their care and put their lives at risk. As an example, consider the experience of Cindy (name changed for privacy reasons) and her adult son, who has an intellectual disability that impacts his ability to perform self-care. In Fall 2020, Cindy's son experienced a medical emergency and needed to be transported to the hospital. Cindy, as the support person for her son, accompanied him to the emergency room. Cindy has the greatest perspective on and knowledge of her son's needs. She knows, for example, when he needs respiratory suction and how to properly administer it. She also knows how to communicate with her son better than anyone else. When she visited the hospital in Fall 2020, the staff members refused to allow her to be by her son's side. Despite bringing supporting documentation with her to the emergency room and citing relevant laws and State policy, the hospital refused to let her attend to her son for an hour and a half. Cindy feared for her son's life the entire time.

Situations like what Cindy and her son experienced are unacceptable. Many people with disabilities rely on direct care workers or family members in order to effectively communicate with their providers. Exceptions to no-visitor policies must be made when it is necessary to effectuate the communication rights of people with disabilities. HHS OCR agrees with this position.[713] As discussed in detail in Chapter 1, HHS OCR asserted in a series of resolutions with healthcare entities that no-visitor policies that fail to make exemptions for support persons of people with disabilities violate the ADA, Section 504 of the Rehabilitation Act, and Section 1557 of the Affordable Care Act, and can result in a denial of effective communication within the meaning of those laws.[714]

While the law is clear, federal and state entities must remind hospitals and healthcare facilities of their obligations to provide reasonable accommodation and policy modifications when needed by people with disabilities, including providing exceptions to general "no-visitor" policies during the pandemic when a patient needs a support person for disability-related reasons such as effective communication. These reminders must be clear that effective communication needs are one of the disability-related reasons that a support person may be needed, and for which an exception must be granted.

Congregate Care Settings

The COVID-19 pandemic also impacted the communication methods of people with disabilities who are in CCFs. By virtue of the danger of the COVID-19 virus spreading quickly through CCFs, in-person communication with individuals outside of the facility was sharply curtailed. Outside of staff members, very few individuals were able to connect with residents. This includes close family members, whose physical presence could place their loved one and other residents at risk of contracting COVID-19.

As a replacement for in-person interaction, CCFs increasingly relied on technology to provide residents with social interaction and healthcare. Technologies such as smartphones and tablets, which allow for video conferencing and telemedicine, became commonplace. Such technologies also created opportunities for social workers and other providers to assist residents in touring potential housing, assessing site accessibility and safety, picking out furniture, and engaging in other activities that ease transitions out of the CCF.

With the increased use of communication technologies, however, also came new barriers for some people with disabilities. An individual may not have the capacity to communicate via video screen if, for example, screen use triggers migraines; instead they may need telephone or in-person communication. Likewise, the communication platform being used may not be accessible for people with hearing or vision loss, as was discussed in greater detail in the previous section.

As in the healthcare context, in order to improve communication in CCFs, accessibility in virtual communication technologies must be prioritized. WCAG 2.1 standards should be adopted, and individuals living in CCFs should be given the assistance they need in learning and using new communication technologies.

Education Setting

Students with disabilities, as well as their parents and educators, were intimately affected by the social distancing policies enacted during the COVID-19 pandemic. While constantly evolving, the K-12 education system has incorporated remote learning modalities in a way never envisioned prior to the pandemic.

Remote Learning

At the beginning of the COVID-19 pandemic, many K-12 schools shifted from an in-person model of learning to a fully remote education system. Many still remained remote in 2021. The rise of remote education was a double-edged sword for the communication needs of students with disabilities: It has benefitted some students, but it has severely disadvantaged others.

For some disabled students, the remote learning modality allowed them to interact with their teachers and fellow students in a manner not previously possible. For example, the use of video conferencing provided them with greater exposure to the world and connectivity with their classmates as they could, quite literally, see into each other's homes. An act as simple as sharing one's pets with each other over a video platform can provide a valuable social interaction to some students with disabilities who may not otherwise be able to experience such close interaction with other students. Learning from home can also benefit some disabled students who have attendants, because remote learning makes it easier for these individuals to go off-camera when they need to engage in personal care. This can reduce stigma associated with the presence of the attendant and decrease any generalized classroom disruption. Further, particularly

> *As a replacement for in-person interaction, CCFs increasingly relied on technology to provide residents with social interaction and healthcare.*

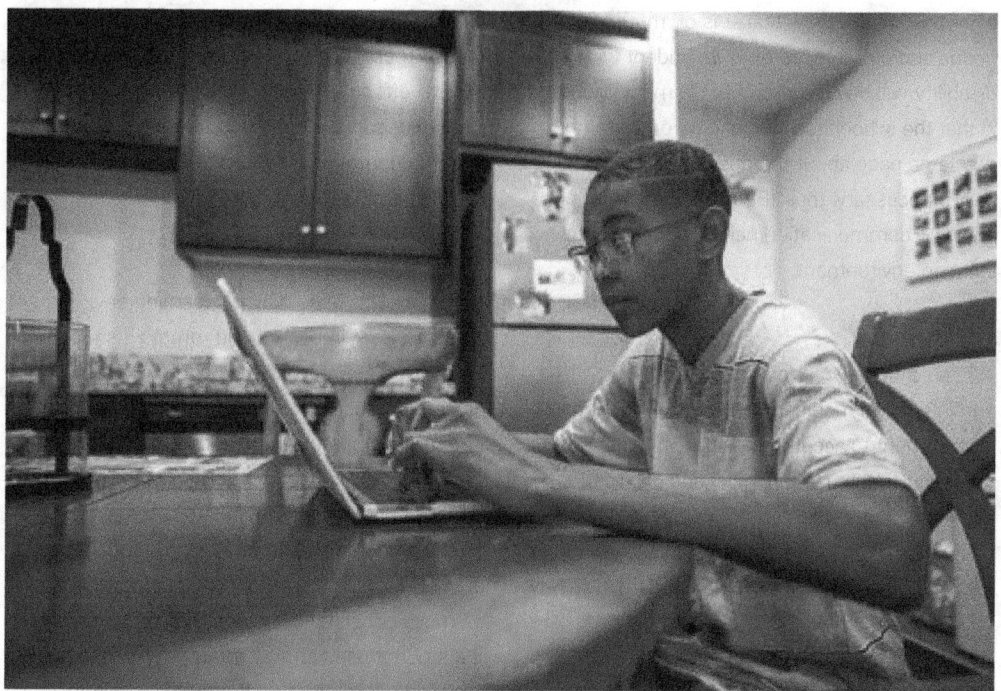

for students with disabilities that affect their social and emotional functioning, the degree of separation created by the virtual learning environment can decrease their social anxiety and actually encourage greater communication in the classroom.[715]

For other students with disabilities, however, the COVID-19 pandemic had a devastating impact on classroom communications.[716] For many students, remote learning cut off access to education attendants, physical therapists, occupational therapists, and speech therapists. Parents do not have the specialized training, or, often, the time, to fill these roles. Many disabled students no longer had access to Braille or tactile learning tools that they may have relied on in the physical classroom. These problems were only amplified by the lack of proper accessibility in

remote learning platforms. Video platforms are not always compatible with assistive technology, and sign language is difficult through video. Technological inadequacies can severely hinder educational accommodations.

Because of these concerns, it is critical that schools and teachers using remote learning make assistive technologies and services available for students, including real-time captioning of video lectures, video interpreter services, and other assistive technologies that a student who is Deaf or Hard of Hearing may need.[717] Teachers should also ensure that they are on video, with proper lighting and their faces clearly visible in the frame, to facilitate lip reading and perception of other visual cues. If a student has a disability that affects their concentration or they easily become overstimulated, then teachers should ensure that everyone except the speaker is on mute.[718] The needs and preferences of each student with a disability will be different. What is most important is that the school, teacher, and parents are on the same page about the needs of the students and, if necessary, their IEP is updated to reflect any new communication needs in the remote learning environment.

Modified In-Person Instruction

When schools reopened, teachers and administrators modified the physical learning environment to account for safety precautions. In particular, the use of masks and physical distancing changed the nature of in-person instruction and affected students with hearing loss and other disabilities that cause them to rely on visual cues to effectively communicate.

Masks can muffle sound, hide lip movements, and hide facial expressions; while increased physical distance from the teacher decreases the volume of communications. These new challenges made in-person learning even more difficult for students with communication disabilities. Depending on the needs of the student, measures such as wearing clear masks, amplifying the teacher's voice, and following communication best practices (such as directly facing a student while talking, speaking slower and louder, and providing extra written resources that bolster verbal instruction) are helpful.[719] All students who are commonly

Masks can muffle sound, hide lip movements, and hide facial expressions; while increased physical distance from the teacher decreases the volume of communications. These new challenges made in-person learning even more difficult for students with communication disabilities.

expected to participate in classroom discussions should receive some basic instructions on how to effectively communicate with all their classmates in a modified in-person, hybrid learning context, or simulcast context. IEPs should also be updated, as needed.

Hybrid Learning Models

Some schools used a hybrid learning environment involving both in-person and remote instruction. This mixed approach can be confusing and anxiety-producing for students, especially for students with intellectual or developmental disabilities or with learning disabilities, who benefit from regular routines.

If a student is a part of a hybrid model, then it is important for the school and parents to foster as much consistency as possible. For example, if a student uses an ASL interpreter in person, then that interpreter should also be available to help with remote instruction as well.[720] It is also important that the student have regular check-ins to determine whether the new way of learning is working for them and how it can be modified to better meet their needs. Like all learning models, IEPs should be modified as needed.

Government Activities

The most important aspect of slowing the spread of COVID-19 was to empower people with accurate information about the virus, its transmission, and vaccines.[721] If facts about mask

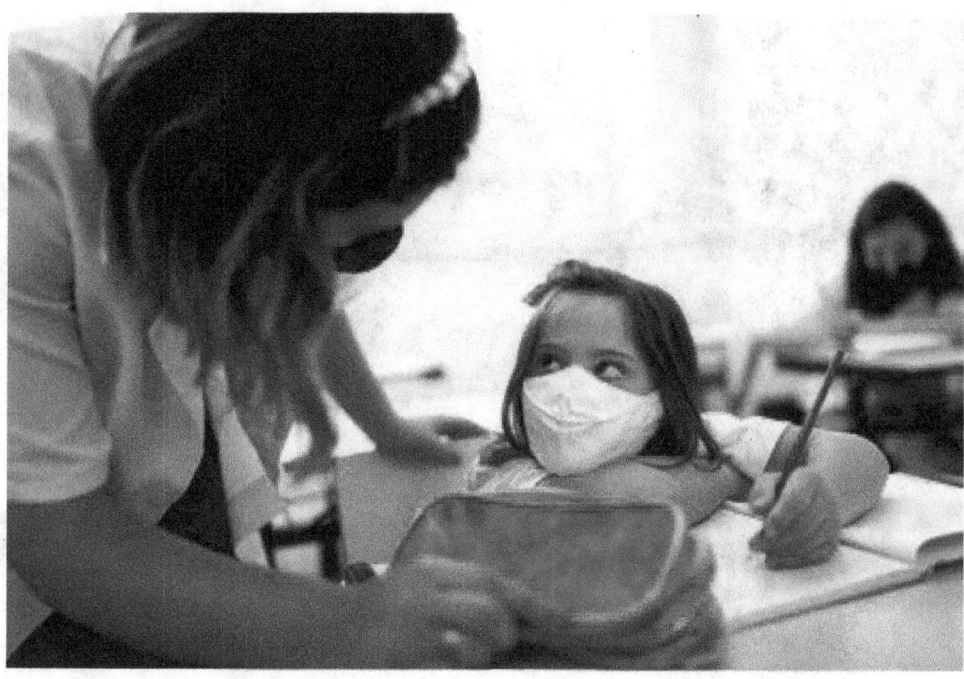

use, physical distancing, and other protective practices were not available to everyone then we could not expect to slow the spread of the virus or decrease infection rates and the development of dangerous variants.[722] Likewise, if accurate information about the efficacy and side effects of vaccines, or the availability of economic stimulus support related to COVID-19, was not made accessible to all individuals, then we could not expect equity in vaccination and economic support.

Traditionally, the role of disseminating public health information has been tasked to federal, state, and local governments. All federal programs and agencies, and all entities receiving federal financial assistance, are subject to disability rights laws that require information to be made available in alternative formats such as large print, electronic format, and Braille.[723] Likewise, all federal websites and the content posted on them must be fully accessible.[724] This includes all documents, videos, charts, graphs, or infographics that are made public.[725]

Despite clear legal requirements, people with disabilities were overlooked on multiple governmental levels during the COVID-19 pandemic. Not only did state public health departments and local municipalities fail to make critical information accessible to people with communication disabilities,[726] but so too did the federal government. For example, while the pandemic was still in its infancy—arguably at its most critical stage in relation to stopping or at least slowing the spread of the deadly COVID-19 virus—the Trump administration's White House consistently failed to provide sign language

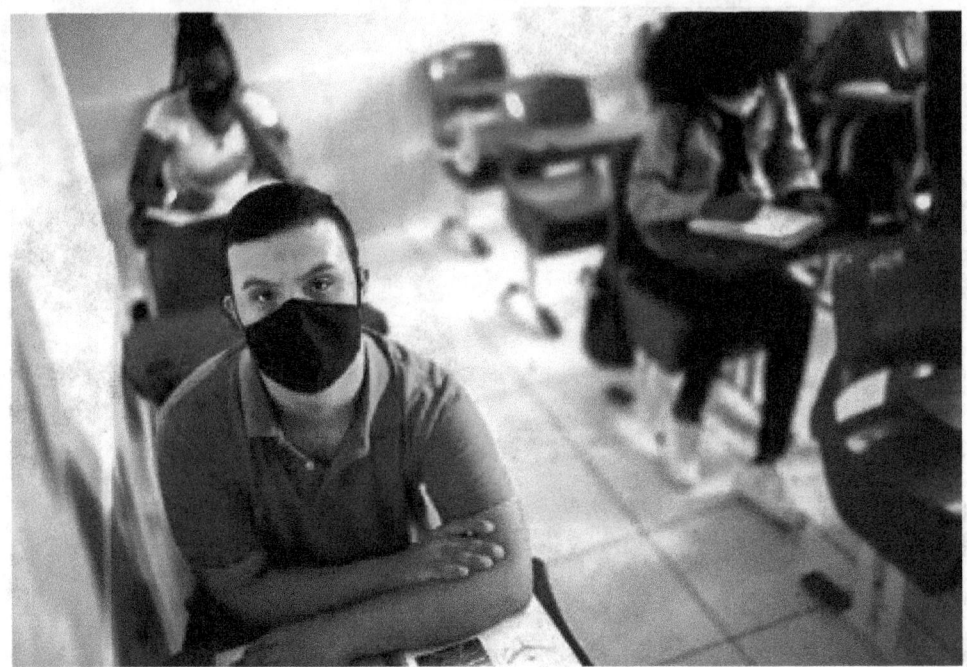

interpreters during its COVID-19 briefings.[727] This left millions of U.S. residents who communicate using ASL, a language distinct from English,[728] without access to critical, up-to-date information related to the pandemic.[729] It took a lawsuit from the National Association of the Deaf in order to change this injustice. In September 2020, six months into the known pandemic, a federal court ordered the White House to provide live ASL interpreters for all COVID-19–related briefings.[730] The decision made clear: "With their lives at risk due to the pandemic, it is important to provide the information in ASL so that Deaf and Hard of Hearing people have access to this information."[731]

Federal, state, and local governments must ensure that their programs and activities during the pandemic, and communications related to the pandemic, are fully accessible for people with disabilities. In the middle of this national crisis, it is essential that people with disabilities have access to the same information that any other individual does.[732]

All information shared by governmental entities must be accessible to people with disabilities, and this includes persons who may have limited English proficiency and require information in another language. Video briefings from the federal government must provide sign language interpretation and live captions, to ensure that individuals with hearing loss can have equal access. All written materials must be provided in formats accessible to people with visual impairments, including the availability of large print, Braille, and electronic copies of documents. All forms related to COVID-19 care and vaccination must be accessible and fillable. Additionally, all information disseminated on federal websites must be accessible for people with vision and/or hearing impairments. The failure to ensure accessibility in these contexts is not only a violation of the law but puts the lives of a population that is already particularly vulnerable to COVID-19 at even more risk.

Summary of Findings

- The widespread use of opaque face masks served as a communication barrier to people with disabilities who rely on lip-reading and facial cues for effective communication.

- There was a months-long nationwide shortage of PPE, and sign language interpreters in healthcare settings did not have sufficient access to it, hindering the safe use of their services.

- Telemedicine platforms were initially inaccessible to people with communications disabilities, with many platforms not supporting three-way video visits with interpreters or screen-reader accessibility.

- Hospital protocols, such as mask mandates and no-visitor policies, failed to account for the needs of people with communication disabilities at the onset of the pandemic.

- Remote and hybrid learning modalities failed to provide proper communication accommodations to students with disabilities at the beginning of the pandemic, rendering the school environment inaccessible for many children with disabilities.

- Local, state, and federal government entities did not disseminate information related to the COVID-19 pandemic, its transmission, and vaccines in fully accessible formats.

Recommendations

To ensure that the United States is prepared to support effective communication for people with disabilities as fully as possible in a future pandemic or similar national health crisis, NCD recommends the following actions based on our findings about the impact of COVID-19 on people with disabilities:

Recommendations for Congress

- Congress should increase funding to healthcare entities and providers during public health emergencies specifically aimed at ensuring effective communication services and PPE for in-person interpreters.

Recommendations for Federal Agencies

- **HHS OCR and DOJ** should direct hospitals and other healthcare entities to include in their nondiscrimination notices and staff training the recognition of policy modifications as part of a patient's right to effective communication, in addition to the provision of auxiliary aids and services when needed by patients with disabilities to receive effective care. Concrete examples should be provided, such as giving exceptions to face mask mandates when an individual cannot wear a mask by reason of their disability and to general "no-visitor" policies when needed for disability-related communication needs.

- **HHS** should release guidance outlining appropriate exemptions to face mask mandates and encouraging the use of adaptable face masks.

- **HHS OCR** should enforce the WCAG 2.1 standards in the telemedicine.

- **ED** should direct schools to assess and provide necessary reasonable accommodations and supports, including auxiliary aids and services such as captioning, sign language interpreting, and audio description, to students with disabilities during in-person, remote, and hybrid learning.

- **All federal entities involved in public health, emergency management, and the provision of public announcements or briefings of broad public importance:** Disseminate information related to any pandemic or public health emergency in accessible formats, including information about the nature of the emergency, mitigating actions that individuals should take, available federal and state assistance and support, and available medical treatments, This includes providing sign language interpretation and/or captions during live and pre-recorded video briefings; making all written materials available in alternative formats; and making all online materials accessible.

Recommendations for Other Entities

- **State Hospital Associations:** Work with state departments of public health and disability advocacy groups to develop guidance and best practices for ensuring effective communication in hospitals and associated urgent care clinics during public emergencies, including:

  - The provision of clear, adaptable masks to hospital staff, to be used when an N-95 mask is not required;

  - The provision of qualified in-person interpretation when a person with a disability requests it, with PPE made readily available to interpreters;

  - Fully accessible telemedicine platforms to ensure effective communication for people with communication disabilities, including ensuring that their interface supports three-way video visits with interpreters and that the platform and its content are screen-reader accessible, consistent with the WCAG 2.1 standards.

Chapter 7: Addressing the Impact of COVID-19 on Mental Health and Suicide

Introduction

The pandemic has had a tremendous adverse impact on the nation's mental health. The economic impact of job losses resulting from the pandemic, the social isolation caused by remote work, closed businesses, stay-at-home orders, and physical distancing, the burnout experienced by healthcare workers, and the difficulty of obtaining needed accommodations in school and at work all contribute to increased rates of mental health disabilities, substance use disorders, and suicide. Rates of anxiety and depression have risen significantly, particularly for healthcare workers and other essential workers. Crisis hotlines have experienced high call volumes and surveys show rising rates of individuals contemplating suicide, particularly people of color, unpaid caregivers, and essential workers.

At the same time, the pandemic has created severe limitations on the availability of mental health services. Behavioral health services in public systems were already strained before COVID-19, and the pandemic has tremendously hampered service delivery due to the impact on provider staffing and the need to shift service delivery mechanisms and find new flexibilities. The pandemic has presented opportunities for service improvements, however, including changes to policies to facilitate telehealth services that may enable greater numbers of people to access services. Moreover, the pandemic presents opportunities to revisit our approach to suicide prevention, which is ineffective and focuses primarily on hospitalization, placing people at risk of COVID-19 transmission.

> *The social isolation caused by protective measures to combat COVID-19—including physical distancing, quarantining, and a dramatic reduction in social activities—has resulted in isolation, loneliness, and depression.*

The Pandemic Has Had a Dramatic Effect on the Nation's Mental Health

The pandemic's impact on the mental health of adults and children across the United States has been well documented. The social isolation caused by protective measures to combat COVID-19—including physical distancing, quarantining, and a dramatic reduction in social activities—has resulted in isolation, loneliness, and depression. Literature and studies showing that these results of the pandemic have negatively affected the mental health of adults and children abound.[733] Surveys consistently show high percentages of adults and children experiencing anxiety and depression as a result of this situation, as well as an increase in suicidal thoughts.[734] Surveys conducted in June 2020 found that symptoms of anxiety disorder and depression increased considerably in the United States during April through June compared with the same period in 2019, with anxiety symptoms three times as high and depression symptoms four times as high.[735] About twice as many people reported serious consideration of suicide within the previous 30 days than did adults in the United States during 2018.[736]

These trends have continued throughout the pandemic. In January 2021, CDC's National Health Interview Survey and Census Bureau Household Pulse data showed that 41 percent of adults reported symptoms of anxiety and/or depressive disorder that month—a figure that had changed little since the spring of 2020—compared to 11 percent between January and June of 2019.[737]

The negative impact on mental health has not only amplified the impact of preexisting mental health disabilities but also resulted in individuals developing mental health disabilities that they did not have before the pandemic. Indeed, many people with psychiatric disabilities had already experienced loneliness and social isolation prior to the pandemic, and that isolation was further magnified as a result of the pandemic's public

In January 2021, CDC's . . . data showed that 41 percent of adults reported symptoms of anxiety and/or depressive disorder that month—a figure that had changed little since the spring of 2020—compared to 11 percent between January and June of 2019.

health measures.[738] For people with chronic illness, already high rates of concurrent mental health disabilities may have been heightened further because of their vulnerability to severe effects of COVID-19.[739] Older adults are also at particular risk, as many "have experienced an acute, severe sense of social isolation and loneliness with potentially serious mental and physical health consequences."[740] Further, having COVID-19 itself may have led to mental health disabilities for some people; one study found that 18 percent of people with and without a past psychiatric diagnosis were later diagnosed with a mental health disability after having been diagnosed with COVID-19.[741]

The pandemic's mental health impact has been felt with particular force in communities of color, which have experienced disproportionately high rates of COVID-19 cases and deaths. Black and Latinx adults have more commonly reported symptoms of anxiety and/or depressive disorder during the pandemic than White adults. Further, Black and Latinx adults were less likely to receive needed mental health services than others prior to the pandemic.[742]

In addition, the impact of the pandemic on veterans' mental health is significant. Veterans already face isolation and a sense of social disconnectedness due to the challenges of explaining past traumatic experiences to those who have not served in the military. Ordinarily, between 17 and 18 veterans die by suicide each day in the United States.[743] According to the Wounded Warriors Project, a national veteran services organization, "lack of social connection (loneliness) along with co-occurring mental health conditions (PTSD, depression, suicidal ideation) exacerbates and magnifies the burden warriors experience during adverse events like COVID-19."[744] The Project reported that at the time of its 2020 survey, "60% of warriors were experiencing moderate to severe depression symptoms, 56% were experiencing PTSD symptoms, 66% reported loneliness, and 30% reported recent suicidal ideations."[745]

The mental health impact on children from prolonged periods of time outside of school, without physical interaction with peers, remains to be seen; but grave concerns have been raised about the impact of this situation in the short and long term. As one stakeholder convening participant observed, "this pandemic is a perfect storm of those suicide risk factors, including social stressors, . . . loss, adverse life events, life transition, physical illness, feeling trapped and isolated," and COVID-19 increases the presence as well as the severity of all of these risk factors.[746]

Mental Health Impact on Healthcare Workers and Other Essential Workers

Frontline healthcare workers and other essential workers have been particularly impacted by the pandemic. Essential workers had the highest rates of adverse mental health outcomes compared to all other employment groups surveyed by CDC.[747] Research has shown that frontline healthcare workers are generally at higher risk of negative mental health outcomes

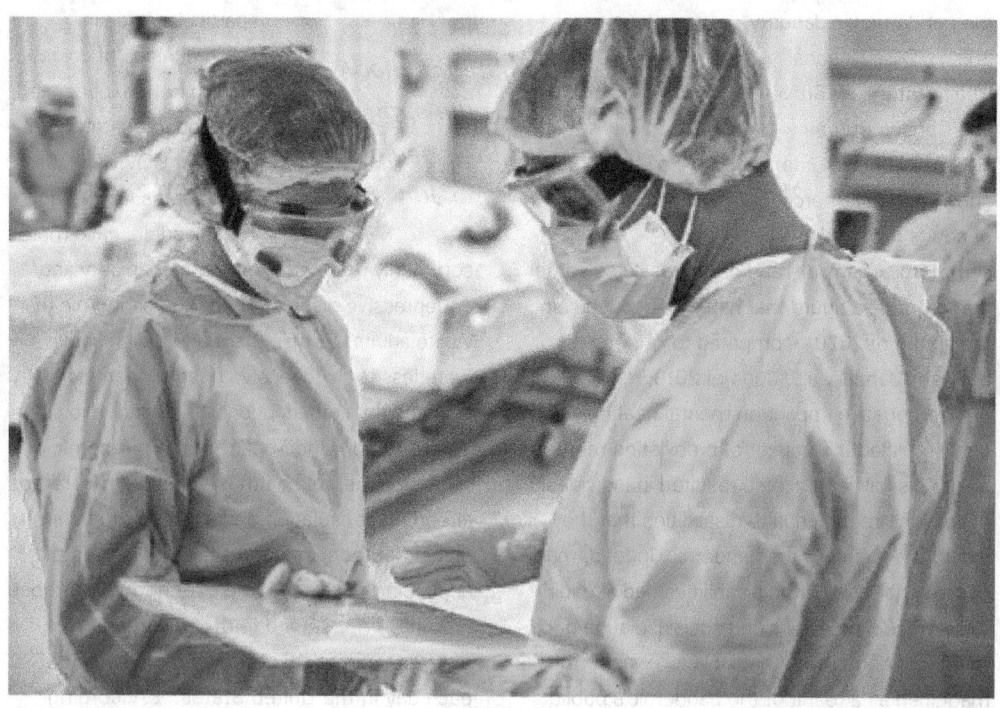

during pandemics.[748] During the COVID-19 pandemic, caregivers working in LTCFs and those providing unpaid care to family members or other loved ones have faced particular mental health risks due to the stressors of high coronavirus infection risks and burnout.[749] Staffing challenges due to COVID-related illness, exposure, or childcare or other family responsibilities during the pandemic have also exacerbated stresses on healthcare workers.

Approximately one third of U.S. adults reported being essential workers required to work outside their homes during the pandemic.[750] These workers are disproportionately Black and low-income.[751] Women of color are particularly overrepresented.[752] More than 90 percent of workers in the bottom 25th income percentile cannot work from home.[753] In the healthcare industry, more than 6.5 million healthcare support workers earn less than the U.S. median wage, and many do not receive basic benefits such as paid sick leave or personal leave.[754]

A significant proportion (30 percent) of adult workers reported symptoms of anxiety or depression in a June 2020 survey, but essential workers reported such symptoms at even higher rates (42 percent). Twenty-two percent of essential workers also reported suicidal thoughts, compared with 8 percent of nonessential workers.[755] Nearly three in ten essential workers said that their mental health has worsened, and 75 percent said they could have used more emotional support than they received.[756] Thirty-one percent of unpaid caregivers for adults "seriously considered suicide" during the past 30 days.[757] Moreover,

multiple studies have found that frontline healthcare workers with preexisting mental health conditions "were more likely to exhibit severe mental health outcomes during outbreaks."[758]

This level of distress suggests that many of these workers experience psychiatric disabilities, whether or not they had such disabilities before the pandemic. Indeed, 25 percent of essential workers reported being diagnosed with a mental health disorder since the start of the pandemic.[759] Essential workers were more than twice as likely as those who are not to have received treatment from a mental health professional (34 percent vs. 12 percent) and to have been diagnosed with a mental health disorder since the coronavirus pandemic started (25 percent vs. 9 percent).[760]

. . . 25 percent of essential workers reported being diagnosed with a mental health disorder since the start of the pandemic.

The mental health impact on healthcare workers in particular has manifested itself not only in the anxiety, depression, and loneliness that many have experienced during the pandemic, but also in trauma-related disorders. Frontline healthcare workers have experienced sickness and death on a daily basis during the pandemic, and have repeatedly been placed at risk for infection, often without adequate staffing and resources.[761] Thirty-five percent of healthcare workers have experienced trauma-related symptoms.[762] These symptoms were particularly common in women, nurses, frontline workers, and workers who experienced physical symptoms of COVID-19.[763]

Recommendations to address these issues have included both clinical approaches, such as expanding the mental health workforce to expand the availability of services, and nonclinical approaches including making available peer support services (provided by individuals with lived experience with psychiatric disability to help individuals develop skills in managing illness and recovery, in self-advocacy, and in identifying and using natural supports) and workplace supports such as employee assistance programs.[764] Peer support is a highly effective intervention that has been used for many decades and recognized by the CMS as an evidence-based service.[765] It has also been a widely used and successful intervention for veterans with mental health disabilities including PTSD.[766]

Other recommendations have included employers providing flexibility and support to essential workers, including making reasonable accommodations, removing nonessential tasks, ensuring essential workers have access to PPE and to needed transportation, recognizing the phenomenon of burnout, and helping employees prioritize critical tasks.[767] Diversifying the mental health workforce has also been recommended, given the disproportionate representation of Black Americans and other people of color among the essential workers impacted by the pandemic.[768]

Mental Health Impact Resulting from Remote Work and from Increased Job Loss and Unemployment

The isolation and stress of remote work also seem to have had a significant impact on individuals' mental health. The closure of many schools, daycares, and public spaces has meant that many people who have been able to work from home during the pandemic are facing new stresses, additional responsibilities at home, and diminished work-life balance.[769] Surveys found that nearly half of adults working from home during the pandemic experienced stress, anxiety, or depression; for many, these experiences began or worsened after they started working from home.[770]

Further, the increased job loss and unemployment associated with the COVID-19 pandemic has contributed to the development of mental health and substance use disabilities.[771] During April 2020, the U.S. unemployment rate peaked at 14.8 percent, the highest since data collection began in 1948.[772] Unemployment rates have been higher for workers without a college degree and for racial and ethnic minorities during the pandemic.[773] People of color have historically experienced higher unemployment rates than white people in the United States, but the disparities in unemployment rates spiked during April 2020 and unemployment rates for people of color remained high through the end of 2020, even though the overall unemployment rate fell.[774] Estimates of how many Americans lost employment due to the pandemic range from 13 million to 36 million, depending on the methodology used.[775]

Half or more of those who became unemployed during the COVID-19 pandemic have developed behavioral health conditions.[776] Research has consistently found that rises in unemployment are directly associated with increases in suicide.[777] The Meadows Mental Health Policy Institute estimated that a COVID recession on par with the 2007–2009 recession, which brought a 5 percent increase in unemployment, would result in the loss of approximately 4,000 additional Americans to

> *Half or more of those who became unemployed during the COVID-19 pandemic have developed behavioral health conditions.*

suicide.[778] Individuals who are most at risk of having adverse mental health impacts are those for whom unemployment is an immediate threat to their survival.[779]

Moreover, during and after a major recession, individuals who have developed behavioral health conditions have an especially difficult time becoming re-employed.[780] In addition, research has shown that people with behavioral health conditions are disproportionately likely to contract COVID-19 and die from it. Thus, as one set of prominent mental health experts observed, "COVID-10 infection and behavioral health conditions influence each other in a bidirectional relationship."[781]

It is no surprise that the job loss and unemployment caused by the pandemic have had such a significant adverse effect on mental health. Not only is unemployment associated with negative mental health effects, but conversely, work is associated with improved mental health outcomes. Work is not only a means to economic security: "[E]mployment is itself an effective behavioral health intervention" and "part of the [mental health] recovery process itself."[782]

Accordingly, one key measure that has been recommended as a strategy to address the mental health effects of the pandemic is making evidence-based supported employment services available to individuals who have developed behavioral health conditions as a result of the pandemic. The experts recommending this strategy pointed out that the rate at which the Individual Placement and Support model of supported employment for people with psychiatric disabilities succeeded in getting people competitively employed during the fourth quarter of 2020, when the pandemic was at its height, was 42 percent—just as high as it has averaged over the past decade.[783]

The success of these services even during the pandemic reflects that individual placement and support (IPS) teams continued to provide services remotely throughout the pandemic and developed expertise in providing all phases of supported employment with minimal face-to-face contact.[784] Since the behavioral health disabilities developed by individuals unemployed due to the pandemic are less severe than those experienced by individuals who have traditionally received IPS, these unemployed individuals may be helped with lower levels of service than IPS usually requires.[785]

Mental Health Impact on Children and Youth

The pandemic has particularly affected the mental health of children and youth due to the isolation, stresses, and difficulties associated with remote learning. A November 2020 report from CDC showed a dramatic increase in mental health emergencies among children and youth.[786] Beginning in March 2020 and continuing through the end of the reporting period in October 2020, the proportion of mental health–related emergency department visits increased sharply, with increases of 24 percent among children aged 5–11 years and 31 percent among adolescents aged 12–17 years compared with the same period in 2019.[787] While CDC cautions that this data has limitations, including that the percentage of children's mental health emergency department visits may appear proportionally inflated due to the sharp declines in emergency department use for other issues such as asthma and musculoskeletal injuries in 2020, it is still troubling.[788] Most emergency departments do not have adequate capacity to treat pediatric mental health concerns.[789]

In addition to the loneliness and social isolation experienced by children and youth who spent months isolated from their peers and school communities, one cause of increased mental health concerns may be the reduced access to the mental health services that many children receive through their school or in their communities, leading to increased reliance on emergency department services for routine treatment as well as crisis services.[790] Between March and May 2020, children on Medicaid received 44 percent fewer outpatient mental health services, such as therapy and in-home support, compared to the same time period in 2019.[791]

Story of Student Mental Health Crisis

Crisis services were impacted. One story of a 17-year-old girl with autism who experienced mental health crises when her school closed is particularly poignant. The girl continued to get up early and wait for the school bus and began wandering when the bus did not show up. Her mother began calling a mental health crisis line and was routinely put on hold for 40 or 50 minutes. Out of frustration, the mother called the police for help. When the police showed up the girl became agitated and hit her mother in the back, leading police to arrest her and take her to jail. The mother pleaded with the police instead to drive the girl home so that she could take her medication, but the police indicated that they were unable to do that and the only places they could transport her were the jail or the hospital. The girl spent most of the night in jail until her mother posted bail.[792]

Additionally, with many children having been away from school and disconnected from adults who might ordinarily identify signs of abuse or neglect, the potential for children to be exposed to trauma as abuse or neglect goes unaddressed is high.[793] Such adverse childhood experiences are strongly correlated with the development of mental health disabilities.[794]

A survey of college students conducted by Active Minds, a mental health organization with chapters on hundreds of college campuses, found that 80 percent of college students reported that COVID-19 has negatively affected their mental health, and one in five reported that their mental health has significantly worsened during the pandemic.[795] Another survey found that college students' mental health needs had changed during the pandemic, and many did not feel supported by their schools.[796]

Barriers to conducting mental health counseling and other services through telehealth have generally been removed, although some challenges may impede the effectiveness of telehealth to deliver these services, including the availability of adequate technology and the ability to ensure that students and staff can use that technology.[797] For example, the above-referenced 44 percent decrease in outpatient mental health services for children on Medicaid between March and May 2020 occurred despite the increased use of telehealth services.[798] In addition, for some students, telehealth visits simply may not substitute for in-person interactions, and academic-focused mental health services may be more challenging to deliver through telehealth technology.

At the same time, the use of telehealth actually presented an opportunity to expand availability of mental health services to a greater number of children and youth who could benefit from them, given the reductions in time needed for providers or clients to travel to in-person appointments. Hybrid in-person and virtual approaches, where providers serve some children through virtual appointments and others in person, could be an important part of that expansion and may help reach children who need additional support or do not have regular access to the internet.[799]

The Pandemic Has Limited Access to Mental Health Services at a Time When They Are Most Needed

While the COVID-19 pandemic created greater need for mental health services, at the same time it has significantly impaired the availability of mental health services. The National Governors Association reported that capacity and operations of the behavioral health system are increasingly strained due to the negative impact of illness and job loss on the direct care workforce.[800] Most behavioral health community service

providers suspended site-based services early in the pandemic. Providers struggled with staffing challenges, including for assertive community treatment (ACT), in-home services, and other services.[801] Some agencies enhanced rates and other incentives to maintain staffing. Ensuring access to PPE was also a challenge.[802]

As noted above, state and federal rules restricting billing for behavioral health telehealth services were largely lifted during the pandemic. Nonetheless, use of telehealth by behavioral health providers remained limited due to lack of staff training, internet connectivity issues, and insufficient funds for technology, as well as concerns about clinical efficacy and privacy concerns.[803] In addition, some services require face to face interaction.[804]

Federal and state efforts to address these issues made some difference, though more remains to be done, particularly in light of the challenges that mental health service systems faced even before the pandemic. Some of the strategies that were used include:

Strategies to Address the Need for Mental Health Services

- Utilizing Medicaid flexibilities permitted due to the public health emergency.[805] Florida, for example, waived prior authorization and limits on the frequency and duration of behavioral health services. North Carolina waived prior authorizations, limits on length of services, certain staff training requirements, supervision requirements, and face-to-face requirements for certain behavioral health services.[806] Connecticut used an Appendix K waiver (these are discussed in the CCF chapter) to increase staff providing services for individuals with psychiatric disabilities coming out of nursing facilities.[807] By November 17, 2020, 36 states temporarily increased provider payment rates and 39 were temporarily using retainer payments to address emergency issues through Appendix K.[808]

- Using Medicaid State Plan Amendments or other administrative actions to increase reimbursement rates for providers more permanently.[809]

> **Strategies to Address the Need for Mental Health Services:** *continued*
>
> - Taking advantage of CMS guidance allowing states to request authority for advance payments to providers. States and Medicaid managed care organizations used prospective payments and advanced cash flow to help providers during the pandemic. New Hampshire, for example, asked its managed care plans to reallocate 1.5 percent of the capitation dollars for provider rate enhancements for certain providers, and Washington has worked with its managed care organizations to direct advance payments, capitated contracts, and other funding strategies toward providers at the highest risk of closing.[810]
>
> - Using state resources and providing guidance and training to support community-based provider needs related to the pandemic. For example, Washington paid for Zoom licenses for providers to ensure access to telehealth services.[811]
>
> - Taking advantage of new federal resources available through the COVID-19 relief legislation. These resources include a 10 percent increase in federal Medicaid reimbursement for HCBS, including a wide array of community mental health services, available through the American Rescue Plan (available for one year beginning April 1, 2021), an 85 percent federal match rate for mobile crisis services available through the American Rescue Plan (available for three years beginning April 1, 2022), new funding for Certified Community Behavioral Health Clinics available through the American Rescue Plan and prior COVID-19 relief legislation, and increased mental health and substance use disorder block grant funding through the various COVID relief packages.[812]

As the National Governors Association observed, additional support for technical assistance, training, and general capacity building by community behavioral health providers is needed given that these providers were already under-resourced for years prior to the pandemic.[813]

More Effective Suicide Prevention Strategies are Needed

As noted above, during the pandemic, the United States has seen significant increases in the percentage of individuals considering suicide. Participants in an NCD stakeholder convening concerning the pandemic's impact on mental health and suicide universally identified problems with the way that suicide has been understood and the strategies being discussed to address and prevent suicide during the pandemic.

Participants noted that it was unsurprising that the pandemic had caused an increase in suicides, given all of the associated losses that it has caused, including loss of friends, family members and others, adverse life events, loss of jobs and housing, physical illness, a sense of feeling trapped and isolated, and life transitions.[814] One participant mentioned that the first suicide that her organization saw during the pandemic was that of a transgender woman stuck in a hotel who took her life within hours after unsuccessfully asking someone for help with housing. That participant described how both the COVID-19 pandemic and the individuals' past experiences with coercive mental health treatment led to a sense of loss of power and control that, consistent with research findings, increases the likelihood of suicidal thoughts.[815] One survey found that for individuals who had been involuntarily confined in a psychiatric facility in the past or subjected to coercive mental health services, more than twice as many reported increased suicidal thoughts during the pandemic compared to individuals who had not been involuntarily hospitalized or subjected to force.[816]

Participants observed that suicide should not be understood as a "mental health problem," and suicides during the pandemic have not been limited to individuals with preexisting mental health disabilities or individuals with newly developed mental health disabilities. They highlighted that efforts to focus on suicide itself as the problem to be stopped miss the root causes of suicide—the underlying stressors and problems that individuals who attempt suicide are trying to "solve" or escape.[817] Rather than focusing on clinical approaches that target suicide itself, participants urged a public health approach that focuses on the systemic needs and inequalities that cause people to be in distress—for example, measures that focus on ensuring a living wage and measures that focus on preventing evictions.[818]

Participants pointed out that the common strategies discussed for addressing suicide during the pandemic are problematic or ineffective and that suicide prevention efforts should focus on alternative strategies. First, a great deal of attention has been given to screening and identifying individuals who may be suicidal, including particularly through the use of crisis or suicide hotlines.[819] For example, the recommendation to call suicide or crisis hotlines features prominently in documents published by CDC, the National Institute of Mental Health, and the National Governors Association concerning strategies to address the mental health impact of the pandemic.[820] Due to the passage of legislation designating a national "988" crisis line that will use the National Suicide Prevention Line for calls relating to both suicide and mental health crises generally, 988 has featured prominently in discussions of how to address mental health crises as we emerge from the pandemic.[821]

Convening participants noted, however, that little attention has been paid to what happens when individuals call these hotlines.[822] Many individuals have come to avoid using these hotlines for assistance because of concerns about the requirement that hotlines contact law enforcement in certain circumstances and calls that have led to the frequent outcome of

Many individuals have come to avoid using these hotlines for assistance because of concerns about the requirement that hotlines contact law enforcement in certain circumstances and calls that have led to the frequent outcome of involuntary hospitalization.

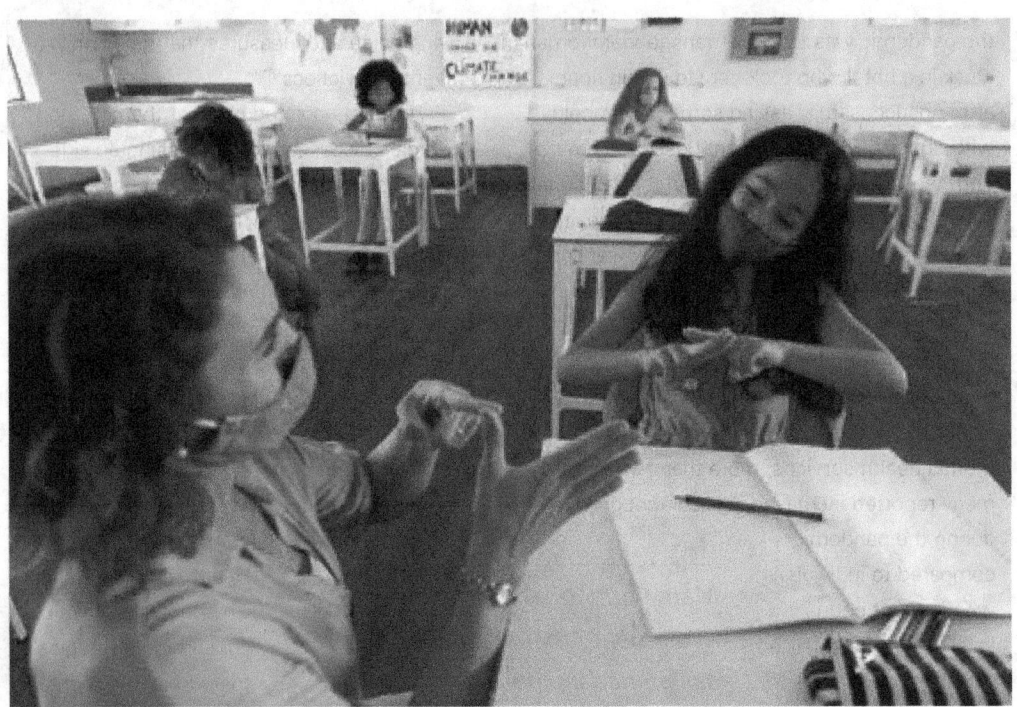

involuntary hospitalization.[823] A recent article chronicling the experiences of individuals who experienced unwanted police encounters and involuntary hospitalization as a result of calls to the National Suicide Prevention Line observed:

> Driving much of this is growing awareness that calling 911 for issues of emotional distress can lead to deadly police interventions. Yet under-reported and under-investigated is the fact that calls to the National Suicide Prevention Lifeline (NSPL)—which prominently advertises itself as "confidential"—are often covertly traced. Callers get subjected to police interventions and forced psychiatric hospitalizations. Police shootings occur. Many callers describe their experiences

as terrifying and traumatizing and say the betrayal has made them feel more isolated than ever.[824]

Among the examples described in the article are:

- A veteran who called the NSPL during his lunch break at work when he was "feeling pretty down" but not actively suicidal. The man hung up after 10 minutes to return to work, and 20 minutes later police arrived, took his access badge, and escorted him to an ambulance that brought him to a veterans' hospital. The man relayed that it was embarrassing and traumatizing because "[a]ll my coworkers and my lead and supervisor, they saw me get taken away." The man, who is Black, was particularly intimidated by the police encounter because growing up he was frequently subjected to random stop-and-frisks by police. He was detained in the hospital until a family member came to pick him up several hours later. He was required to get clearance from a doctor in order to return to work, and subsequently received an ambulance bill for $1,000. He wonders whether the incident played a role in his being laid off several months later while individuals with less seniority were kept on.

■ A student who called the NSPL because she had no health insurance, could not afford therapy, and "was just depressed and kind of wishing that I might just die" and "wanted to talk to another person and maybe be reassured a little." When the call attendant urged her to go to a psychiatric hospital immediately and the student explained she had a class that was about to start, the call attendant threatened to send police and the student hung up. Fifteen minutes later, the police and an ambulance showed up, strapped the student to a stretcher, and took her to a hospital where she was forced to strip and sit in an empty room for 12 hours without explanation. When her 72-hour involuntary detention period expired, the student consented to a voluntary admission out of fear that going through a court proceeding for involuntary commitment could threaten her ability to obtain a law license. The student received a $50,000 hospital bill at the end of her two-week stay.[825]

According to the NSPL, its call centers dispatch emergency services in only 2 percent of calls. But if its projection of up to 40 million annual 988 calls by 2027 is accurate, a 2 percent rate of dispatching police and ambulances could affect up to 800,000 callers each year.[826] Thus, while crisis or suicide hotlines may help many people, they may create other problems including expanding law enforcement involvement with people with psychiatric disabilities.

Moreover, suicide hotlines rely on screening tools that research has consistently demonstrated have little effectiveness in predicting suicide. The lead author of a widely read meta-analysis of the past 50 years of research on assessing suicide risk stated:

> Our analyses showed that science could only predict future suicidal thoughts and behaviors about as well as random guessing. In other words, a suicide expert who conducted an in-depth assessment of risk factors would predict a patient's future suicidal thoughts and behaviors with the same degree of accuracy as someone with no knowledge of the patient who predicted based on a coin flip. This was extremely humbling—after decades of research, science had produced no meaningful advances in suicide prediction.[827]

Convening participants noted that little has changed in the interventions that we offer once someone has been identified as at risk of suicide; the primary intervention continues to be hospitalization, despite research demonstrating that hospitalization does not result in lower rates of suicide and despite the dangers to which institutionalized people are exposed during the COVID-19 pandemic.[828]

Participants urged a demedicalized approach to suicide prevention that addresses the root causes of suicidality such as loss of jobs and housing, the need for culturally competent services to understand the different expressions of suicidality across cultures, expanded public and private coverage of suicidality treatments that focus on the underlying problems that are causing distress, including Collaborative Assessment and Management of Suicidality and Dialectical Behavioral Therapy for suicidality, and efforts to remove lethal means from individuals' environments.[829] They also urged the expansion of peer-run peer support services and approaches such as the "Alternatives to Suicide" groups conducted by the Western Massachusetts Recovery Learning Community, which are run by suicide attempt survivors and prohibit calls to law enforcement.[830]

Participants noted the challenges in expanding peer support, including extremely low wages in many areas, the general limitation of private insurance coverage to services provided by licensed professionals, and the strictures of Medicaid reimbursement for peer support services, which requires peer support workers to be supervised by clinical professionals. Participants also discussed the challenges of clinician involvement because clinicians may face potential liability connected with licensure obligations if they do not warn others or act if a person may be at risk of suicide.[831] These concerns make it difficult for many individuals to speak freely to professionals about their distress, limiting the

effectiveness of treatment. One participant referenced a survey concerning "Alternatives to Suicide" groups in which over 90 percent of respondents indicated that the most useful thing about these groups is being able to talk openly to someone without the prospect of being subjected to force.[832]

Many of these recommendations have been echoed by the American Foundation for Suicide Prevention. Its chief medical officer has developed priorities for addressing suicide that include involving individuals with lived experience (including COVID-19-related lived experience) in decision-making related to policy, clinical practice, and research; expanding the use of peer specialists and peer educators; expanding access to evidence-based suicide risk-reducing treatments such as Cognitive Behavioral Therapy, Dialectical Behavioral Therapy, and Collaborative Assessment and Management of Suicidality; and reducing access to lethal means.[833]

Summary of Findings

The COVID-19 pandemic had a devastating impact on the mental health of Americans. Due to the social isolation caused by remote work, job loss, closed schools, stay-at-home orders, shuttered businesses, and physical distancing, many adults and children experienced new mental health disabilities or exacerbations of existing ones. The adverse mental health effects of the pandemic hit certain groups particularly hard, including frontline and other essential workers, children and youth, veterans, and those who lost jobs. Women and people of color also experienced high rates of mental health disabilities due to their disproportionate representation among essential workers. Rates of anxiety and depression rose significantly, crisis hotlines saw high call volumes, and more people experienced suicidal thoughts.

At the same time that the pandemic caused increased mental health needs, it hamstrung the ability of mental health service systems to address those needs. Service providers experienced staffing shortages due to illness, exposure, and family or childcare responsibilities during the pandemic. Providers dramatically expanded their use of telehealth, but not everyone could access the technology needed for telehealth and not every service could be delivered remotely.

Expanded access to mental health services in public and private insurance is important to address the lasting impact of the pandemic even as it recedes. Peer support services and supported employment are particularly critical.

Policymakers should also take this opportunity to rethink suicide prevention strategies and expand approaches that focus on the root causes of suicide such as job loss and housing unaffordability, as well as expanding insurance coverage of clinical strategies that address these root causes rather than relying so heavily on hospitalization.

Recommendations

To address the dramatic impact of the pandemic on the mental health of adults and children in the United States, expanding access to mental health services is urgent. The services needed include clinical services but also nonclinical approaches, including expansion of peer support services, services and accommodations that support individuals with mental health disabilities in the workplace, and housing supports.

Recommendations for Congress

Congress should:

- Permanently authorize telehealth flexibilities that enable tele-mental health services while also ensuring that in-person services and hybrid in-person and virtual services are available options for those who need and want them. (This recommendation also applies to state lawmakers, as well as to private insurance regulators).[834]

- Promote effective suicide prevention efforts. Rather than promoting screening and identification of individuals who may be suicidal and involuntarily hospitalizing them, Congress should promote suicide prevention efforts focusing on approaches that address the underlying problems that cause people to consider suicide. These should include helping individuals secure housing, preventing evictions, and helping individuals secure and maintain employment. They should also include peer-run support services for individuals who are experiencing suicidal thoughts. (This recommendation also applies to state lawmakers, as well as to private insurance regulators).

Recommendations for Federal Agencies

- **SAMHSA and state mental health agencies** should robustly promote effective suicide prevention efforts focusing on approaches that address the underlying problems that cause people to consider suicide. These should include helping individuals connect with housing services and referring individuals to vocational rehabilitation or other employment programs for people with disabilities.

- **CMS** should:

  - Revisit Medicaid rules requiring that peer support services be delivered under the supervision of clinicians. While clinical input and consultation may be beneficial, it should not be a requirement for reimbursement of all peer support services.

Recommendations for States

States should:

- Take steps to expand the mental health workforce, and particularly the peer support workforce, including through using new HCBS dollars and mobile crisis dollars available through the American Rescue Plan and new block grant and Certified Community Behavioral Health Center (CCBHC) funds. States should ensure that their service systems include robust peer support services.

- Provide guidance, training and supplies to support community-based mental health provider needs related to new and increased operational needs raised during the pandemic, including paying for Zoom licenses to ensure access to tele-mental health services.

- Invest in peer-run services including peer crisis respite centers, peer "bridger" services that help individuals transitioning from institutional to community settings, and peer-run services for individuals experiencing suicidal thoughts.

- Expand supported employment services using the Individual Placement and Support (IPS) model. Peer specialists should be part of the IPS teams.

- Make efforts to diversify the mental health workforce so that it reflects the racial, ethnic, cultural, sexual orientation, and gender identity diversity of the communities it serves.

(continued)

Recommendations for States: *continued*

Peer support workers should not only have lived experience with mental health disabilities but also reflect the lived experiences of communities of color and particularly Black communities.

- Take advantage of federal Medicaid flexibilities permitted due to the public health emergency to suspend premiums and other cost sharing, suspend the need for prior authorizations for community mental health services, make advanced or supplemental payments to community mental health providers, increase payment rates for these services, allow early or extended refills of medication without prior authorization, and add benefits including peer support, supported employment, and housing-related services.

- Take advantage of CMS guidance allowing states to request authority for advance payments to providers in order to support community mental health providers at risk of closure.

- Reconcile the important suicide prevention measure of removing lethal means from individuals' environments with privacy and equity concerns. Removal efforts most commonly take the form of "extreme risk protection orders" that allow the removal of guns from individuals' homes when those individuals have engaged in conduct that indicates that continuing to possess a gun would be dangerous. Such laws should identify individuals based on conduct and not based on a disability diagnosis, treatment, or history.

- Review evidence on effective suicide prevention efforts. Rather than focusing on trying to screen and identify individuals who may be suicidal and involuntarily hospitalizing them, suicide prevention efforts should focus on approaches that address the underlying problems that cause people to consider suicide. These should include helping individuals secure housing, preventing evictions, and helping individuals secure and maintain employment. They should also include peer-run support services for individuals who are experiencing suicidal thoughts.

User Guide

Descriptive listings in *The Complete Resource Guide for People with Disabilities* are organized into 31 chapters, by either resource type or disability category type. You will find the following types of listings throughout the book:

- National Agencies & Associations
- State Agencies & Associations
- Camps & Exchanges Programs
- Manufacturers of Assistive Devices, Clothing, Computer Equipment & Supplies
- Print & Electronic Media
- Living Centers & Facilities
- Libraries & Research Centers
- Conferences & Trade Shows

Below is a sample listing illustrating the kind of information that is or might be included in an Association entry. Each numbered item of information is described in the paragraphs on the following page.

---

1 ➤ 1234
2 ➤ **Advocacy Center for Seniors with Disabilities**
3 ➤ 1762 South Major Drive
New Orleans, LA 98087

4 ➤ **800-000-0000**

5 ➤ **058-884-0709**

6 ➤ **Fax: 058-884-0568**

7 ➤ **TDD: 800-000-0001**

8 ➤ **email: info@sadvoc.com**

9 ➤ **www.sadvoc.com**

10 ➤ Barbara Pierce, Executive Director
Diane Watkins, Marketing Director
Robert Goldfarb, Administrative Assistant

11 ➤ The mission of the Center is to advance the dignity, equality, self-determination and choices of senior citizens with disabilities. It provides referrals, publishes information, including a monthly newsletter, offers workshops and consultation on legal, social, travel, and medical issues. The Center works with various local organizations to help seniors with disabilities stay active in their community.

12 ➤ Founded 1964

13 ➤ 18 pages

14 ➤ Monthly

User Key

1 ➤ **Record Number**: Entries are listed alphabetically within each category and numbered sequentially. The entry numbers, rather than page numbers, are used in the indexes to refer to listings.

2 ➤ **Organization Name**: Formal name of company or organization. Where organization names are completely capitalized, the listing will appear at the beginning of the alphabetized section. In the case of publications, the title of the publication will appear first, followed by the publisher.

3 ➤ **Address**: Location or permanent address of the organization.

4 ➤ **Toll Free Number**: This is listed when provided by the organization.

5 ➤ **Phone Number**: The listed phone number is usually for the main office of the organization, but may also be for the sales, marketing, or public relations office as provided by the organization.

6 ➤ **Fax Number**: This is listed when provided by the organization.

7 ➤ **TDD Number**: This is listed when provided. It refers to Telephone Device for the Deaf.

8 ➤ **E-Mail**: This is listed when provided by the organization and is generally the main office e-mail.

9 ➤ **Web Site**: This is also referred to as an URL address. These web sites are accessed through the Internet by typing *http://* before the URL address.

10 ➤ **Key Personnel**: Name and titles of department heads of the organization.

11 ➤ **Organization Description**: This paragraph contains a brief description of the organization and their services.

12 ➤ **Year Founded**: The year in which the organization was established or founded. If the organization has changed its name, the founding date is usually for the earliest name under which it was known.

13 ➤ **Number of Pages**: Number of pages if the listing is a publication.

14 ➤ **Frequency:** The frequency of the listing if it is a publication.

Glossary of Disability-Related Terms

Accessible: In the case of a facility, readily usable by a particular individual; in the case of a program or activity, presented or provided in such a way that a particular individual can participate, with or without auxiliary aids(s); in the case of electronic resources, accessible with or without the use of adaptive computer technology.

Access barrier: Any obstruction that prevents people with disabilities from using standard facilities, equipment and resources.

Accessible Web design: Creating World Wide Web pages according to universal design principles to eliminate or reduce barriers, including those that affect people with disabilities.

Accommodation: An adjustment to make a workstation, job, program, facility, or resource accessible to a person with a disability.

Adaptive technology: Hardware or software products that provide access to a computer that is otherwise inaccessible to an individual with a disability.

ALT attribute: HTML code that works in combination with graphical tags to provide alternative text for graphical elements.

Americans with Disabilities Act of 1990 (ADA): A comprehensive Federal law that prohibits discrimination on the basis of disability in employment, telecommunications, public services, public accommodations and services.

American Standard Code for Information Interchange (ASCII): Standard for unformatted text which enables transfer of data between platforms and computer systems.

Assistive technology: Technology used to assist a person with a disability (e.g., a handsplint or computer-related equipment).

Auxiliary aids and services: May include qualified interpreters or other effective methods of making aurally delivered materials available to individuals with hearing impairments; qualified readers, taped texts, or other effective methods of making visually delivered materials available to individuals with visual impairments; acquisition or modification of equipment or devices; and other similar services and actions.

Braille: A system of embossed characters formed by using a Braille cell, a combination of six dots consisting of two vertical columns of three dots each. Each simple Braille character is formed by one or more of these dots and occupies a full cell or space.

Browser: A program that runs on an Internet-connected computer and provides access to the World Wide Web. Web browsers may be text-only, such as Lynx, or graphical, such as Internet Explorer and Netscape Navigator.

Captioned film or videos: Transcription of the verbal portion of films or videos is displayed to make them accessible to people who have hearing impairments.

Closed Circuit TV Magnifier (CCTV): A camera used to magnify books or other materials on a monitor.

Cooperative education: Programs that work with students, faculty, staff, and employers to help students clarify career and academic goals, and expand classroom study by allowing students to participate in paid, practical work experiences.

Compensatory tools: Adaptive computing systems that allow people with disabilities to use computers to complete tasks that would be difficult without a computer (e.g., reading, writing, communicating, accessing information).

Disability: A physical or mental impairment that substantially limits one or more major life activities; a record of such an impairment; or being regarded as having such an impairment (Americans with Disabilities Act of 1990).

Discrimination: The act of treating a person differently in a negative manner based on factors other than individual merit.

Dymo Labeller: A device used to create raised print or Braille labels.

Electronic information: Any digital data for use with computers or computer networks, including disks, CD-ROMs, and World Wide Web resources.

Essential job functions: Those functions of a job or task which must be completed with or without an accommodation.

Facility: All or any portion of a physical complex, including buildings, structures, equipment, grounds, roads, and parking lots.

FM sound amplification system: An electronic amplification system consisting of three components: a microphone/transmitter, monaural FM receiver and a combination charger/carrying case. It provides wireless FM broadcasts from a speaker to a listener who has a hearing impairment.

Frame tags: A means of displaying Web pages. The browser reads the frame tags and produces an output that subdivides output within a browser into discrete windows.

Graphical user interface (GUI): Program interface that presents digital information and software programs in an image-based format as compared to a character-based format.

Hardware: Physical equipment related to computers.

Hearing impairment: Complete or partial loss of the ability to hear, caused by a variety of injuries or diseases, including congenital causes. Limitations, including difficulties in understanding language or other auditory messages and/or in production of understandable speech, are possible.

Independent study: A student works one-on-one with individual faculty members to develop projects for credit.

Informational interview: An activity where students meet with people working in careers to ask questions about their jobs and companies, allowing students to gain personal perspectives on career interests.

Input: Any method by which information is entered into a computer.

Internet: Computer network connecting governmental, educational, commercial, other organizations, and individual computer systems.

Internship: A time-limited, intensive learning experience outside of the typical classroom.

Interpreter: Professional person who assists a person who is deaf in communicating with hearing people.

Job shadowing: A short work-based learning experience where students visit businesses to observe one or more specific jobs to provide them with a realistic view of occupations in a variety of settings.

Keyboard emulation: Uses hardware and/or software in place of a standard keyboard.

Kinesthetic: Refers to touch-based feedback.

Large-print: Most ordinary print is six to ten points in height (about 1/16 to 1/8 of an inch). Large-print type is fourteen to eighteen points (about 1/8 to 1/4 of an inch) and sometimes larger.

Link: a connection between two electronic files or data items.

Lynx: A text-based World Wide Web browser.

Macro: A mini-program that, when run within an application, executes a series of predetermined keystrokes and commands to accomplish a specific task. Macros can automate tedious and often-repeated tasks or create special menus to speed data entry.

Mainstreaming: The inclusion of people with disabilities, with or without special accommodations, in programs, activities, and facilities with non-disabled people.

Major life activities: Functions such as caring for oneself, performing manual tasks, walking, seeing, hearing, speaking, breathing, learning, working, and participating in community activities (Americans with Disabilities Act of 1990).

Multimedia: A computer-based method of presenting information by using more than one medium of communication, such as text, graphics, and sound.

Optical Character Recognition (OCR): Machine recognition of printed or typed text. Using OCR software with a scanner, a printed page can be scanned and the characters converted into text in an electronic format.

Output: Any method of displaying or presenting electronic information to the user through a computer monitor or other device (e.g., speech synthesizer).

Glossary of Disability-Related Terms

Portable Document Format (PDF): The file format for representing documents in a manner that is independent of the original application software, hardware and operating system used to create the documents.

Physical or mental impairment: Any physiological disorder or condition, cosmetic disfigurement, or anatomical loss affecting one or more, but not necessarily limited to, the following body systems: neurological; musculoskeletal; special sense organs; respiratory, including speech organs; cardiovascular; reproductive; digestive; genitourinary; hemic and lymphatic; skin and endocrine; or any mental or psychological disorder, such as mental retardation, organic brain syndrome, emotional or mental illness, and specific learning disabilities (Americans with Disabilities Act of 1990).

Plug-ins: Programs that work within a browser to alter, enhance, or extend the browser,s operation. They are often used for viewing video, animation or listening to audio files.

Proprietary software: Privately owned software based on trade secrets, privately developed technology, or specifications that the owner refuses to divulge, thus preventing others from duplicating a product or program unless an explicit license is purchased. The opposite of proprietary is open (publicly published and available for emulation by others).

Qualified individual with a disability: An individual with a disability who, with or without reasonable modification to rules, policies or practices, the removal of architectural, communication, or transportation barriers, or the provision of auxiliary aids and services, meets the essential eligibility requirements for the receipt of services or participation in programs or activities provided by a public entity (Americans with Disabilities Act of 1990).

Reader: Volunteer or employee of a blind or partially sighted individual who reads printed material in person or records to audiotape.

Relay service: A third-party service (usually free) that allows a hearing person without a TTY/TDD device to communicate over the telephone with a person who has a hearing impairment. The system also allows a person with a hearing impairment who has a TTY/TDD to communicate in voice through a third party, with a hearing person or business.

Screen reader: A text-to-speech system intended for use by computer users who are blind or have low vision that speaks the text content of a computer display using a speech synthesizer.

Service learning: A structured, volunteer work experience where students provide community service in non-paid, volunteer positions to give them opportunities to apply knowledge and skills learned in school while making a contribution to local communities.

Sign language: Manual communication commonly used by people who are deaf. Sign language is not universal; deaf people from different countries speak different sign languages. The gestures or symbols in sign language are organized in a linguistic way. Each individual gesture is called a sign. Each sign has three distinct parts: the hand shape, the position of the hands, and the movement of the hands. American Sign Language (ASL) is the most commonly used sign language in the United States.

Specific learning disability (SLD): A disorder of one or more of the basic psychological processes involved in understanding or in using language, spoken or written, which may manifest itself in difficulties listening, thinking, speaking, reading, writing, spelling, or doing mathematical calculations. Limitations may include hyperactivity, distractibility, emotional instability, visual and/or auditory perception difficulties and/or motor limitations, depending on the type(s) of learning disability.

Speech output system: A system that provides the user with a voice alternative to the text presented on the computer screen.

Speech impairment: A problem in communication and related areas, such as oral motor function, ranging from simple sound substitutions to the inability to understand or use language or use the oral-motor mechanism for functional speech and feeding. Some causes of speech and language disorders include hearing loss; neurological disorders; brain injury; mental retardation; drug abuse; physical impairments, such as cleft lip or palate; and vocal abuse or misuse.

Speech input system: A computer-based system that allows the operator to control the system using his/her voice.

Sticky keys: Enables a computer user to do multiple key combinations on a keyboard using only one finger at a time. The sticky keys function is usually used with the Ctrl, Alt, and Shift keys. Simultaneous keystrokes can be entered sequentially.

Telecommunications Device for the Deaf (TDD) or Teletypewriter (TTY): A device which enables someone who has a speech or hearing impairment to use a telephone when communicating with someone else who has a TDD/TTY. TDD/TTYs can be used with any telephone, and one needs only a basic typing ability to use them.

Trackball: A pointing device consisting of a ball housed in a socket containing sensors to detect the rotation of the ball " like an upside down mouse. The user rolls the ball with his thumb or the palm of his hand to move the pointer.

Traumatic Brain Injury (TBI): An open or closed head injury resulting in impairments in one or more areas, such as cognition; language; memory; attention; reasoning; abstract thinking; judgment; problem-solving; sensory, perceptual, and motor abilities; psychosocial behavior; physical functions; information processing; and speech. The term does not apply to brain injuries that are congenital or degenerative, or brain injuries induced by birth trauma.

Undue hardship: An action that requires significant difficulty or expense in relation to the size of the employer, the resources available, and the nature of the operation (Americans with Disabilities Act of 1990).

Universal design: Designing programs, services, tools, and facilities so that they are usable, without additional modification, by the widest range of users possible, taking into account a variety of abilities and disabilities.

Vocational Rehabilitation Act of 1973: An act prohibiting discrimination on the basis of disability which applies to any program that receives federal financial assistance. Section 504 of the act is aimed at making educational programs and facilities accessible to all people with disabilities. Section 508 of the act requires that electronic office equipment purchased through federal procurement meets disability access guidelines.

Voice input system: A computer-based system that allows the operator to control the system using his/her voice.

Vision impairments: A complete or partial loss of the ability to see, caused by a variety of injuries or diseases including congenital causes. Legal blindness is defined as visual acuity of 20/200 or less in the better eye with correcting lenses, on the widest diameter of the visual field subtending an angular distance no greater than 20 degrees.

World Wide Web (WWW, W3, or Web): Hypertext and multimedia gateway to the Internet.

DO-IT
University of Washington
Box 354842
Seattle, WA 98195-4842
doit@uw.edu
http://www.washington.edu/doit/
206-685-DOIT (3648) (voice/TTY)
888-972-DOIT (3648) (toll free voice/TTY)
206-221-4171 (FAX)
509-328-9331 (voice/TTY) Spokane

Director: Sheryl Burgstahler, Ph.D.

Arts & Entertainment

Resources for the Disabled

1 AbleArts
P.O. Box 831
Bear, DE 19701   302-368-7477

AbleArts is a nonprofit, community based performing arts organization composed of people with and without disabilities. Their mission is to entertain and inform the public of the abilities and talents possessed by individuals with disabilities. Performances include dance, poetry, comedy skits, and satire.

2 American Art Therapy Association (AATA)
4875 Eisenhower Ave.
Suite 240
Alexandria, VA 22304   703-548-5860
                                        888-290-0878
                                   Fax: 703-783-8468
                                   info@arttherapy.org
                                        arttherapy.org
Cynthia Woodruff, Executive Director
Barbara Florence, Director, Events & Education
Kat Michel, Senior Manager, Member Services
Not-for-profit organization dedicated to advancing the art therapy profession.

3 American Council of the Blind
1703 N Beauregard St
Suite 420
Alexandria, VA 22311   202-467-5081
                                        800-424-8666
                                   Fax: 703-465-5085
                                        info@acb.org
                                        www.acb.org
Eric Bridges, Executive Director
Sharon Lovering, Editor
Tony Stephens, Director, Advocacy and Governmental Affairs
The American Council of the Blind (ACB) is an association working to increase the independence, security, and opportunity for all blind or visually impaired individuals. The Council primarily focuses on developing and maintaining policies to implement the services needed for the blind or visually impaired.

4 American Dance Therapy Association (ADTA)
230 Washington Ave.
Suite 101
Albany, NY 12203-3539   518-704-3636
                                   Fax: 518-463-8656
                                        info@adta.org
                                        www.adta.org
Michelle Lavoy, Manager, Operations
Lora Wilson, Continuing Education Administrator
Lauren Hoyt, Office Administrator
Supports the dance and movement therapy profession by promoting education, training, practice and research.

5 American Music Therapy Association (AMTA)
8455 Colesville Rd.
Suite 1000
Silver Spring, MD 20910   301-589-3300
                                   Fax: 301-589-5175
                                   info@musictherapy.org
                                        www.musictherapy.org
Adonia Calhoun Coates, Chief Executive Officer
Jane P. Creagan, Director, Professional Programs
Angie K. Elkins, Director, Membership Services & Information Systems
AMTA's purpose is the progressive development of the therapeutic use of music in rehabilitation, special education and community settings. Predecessors to the American Music Therapy Association included the National Association for Music Therapy founded in 1950 and the American Association for Music Therapy founded in 1971. AMTA supports the music therapy profession through the advancement of education, training, professional standards, credentialing, and research.

6 Arena Stage
The Mead Center for American Theater
1101 Sixth St. SW
Washington, DC 20024   202-554-9066
                                   Fax: 202-488-4056
                                   TTY: 202-484-0247
                                   info@arenastage.org
                                        arenastage.org
Edgar Dobie, Executive Director
Molly Smith, Artistic Director
Joseph Berardelli, CFO
Arena Stage has played a pioneering role in providing access to all productions for people with disabilities. Access services and programs include wheelchair accessible seating; infrared assistive listening devices; Braille, large print, audio description and sign interpretation at designated performances.

7 Art Therapy SourceBook
McGraw-Hill Company
2 Penn Plaza
New York, NY 10121-101   212-904-2000
                                   www.mhhe.com/hper/physed
Cathy Malchiodi, Author
An overview of the uses of art as a mentally therapeutic tool.
$18.00
272 pages
ISBN 1-565658-84-1

8 Art and Disabilities
Brookline Books
8 Trumbull Rd
Suite B-001
Northampton, MA 01060   413-584-0184
                                        800-666-2665
                                   Fax: 413-584-6184
                                   brbooks@yahoo.com
                                   www.brooklinebooks.com
Florence Ludins-Katz, Author
A step-by-step guide to establishing creative arts centers for people with disabilities. Includes philosophy and making creative arts centers happen.

9 Art and Healing: Using Expressive Art to Heal Your Body, Mind, and Soul
Three Rivers Press/Crown Publishing-Random House
1745 Broadway
New York, NY 10019   212-782-9000
                              crownpublicity@randomhouse.com
                         www.randomhouse.com/crown/trp.html
Barbara Ganim, Author
Markus Dohle, Chairman & CEO
Melanie Fallon-Houska, Dir., Corporate Contributions
The author believes creating a visual image through any medium can produce physical and emotional benefits for both the creator as well as those who view it. *$17.00*
256 pages
ISBN 0-609803-16-6

10 Art for All the Children: Approaches to Art Therapy for Children with Disabilities
Charles C. Thomas
2600 S First St
Springfield, IL 62704-4730   217-789-8980
                                        800-258-8980
                                   Fax: 217-789-9130
                                   books@ccthomas.com
                                        www.ccthomas.com
Frances E Anderson, Author
Sharon Moorman, Editorial Assistant
This second edition is for art therapists in training and for in-service professionals in art therapy, art education and special education who have children with disabilities as a part of their case/class load. *$56.95*
398 pages Paperback
ISBN 0-398060-07-7

1

11   Arts Unbound
542/544 Freeman Street
Orange, NJ 07050   973-675-2787
                                     Fax: 973-678-4408
                                     www.artsunbound.org
Margaret Mikkelsen, Executive Director
Catherine Lazen, Founder and Board Chair
Alan Hirsh, Executive Vice President
Arts Unbound is a nonprofit organization dedicated to the artistic achievement of youth, adults, and senior citizens with disabilities.

**12   Association of Mouth and Foot Painting Artists
       (AMPFA)**
2070 Peachtree Court
Suite 101
Atlanta, GA 30341   770-986-7764
                                          877-637- 872
                                     Fax: 770-986-8563
                                     mfpausa@bellsouth.net
                                     www.mfpausa.com
Erich Stegmann, Founder
The AMPF is an international, for-profit association wholly owned and run by disabled artists to help them meet their financial needs. Members paint with brushes held in their mouths or feet as a result of a disability sustained at birth or through an accident or illness that prohibits them from using their hands.

13   Awakenings Project, The
PO Box 177
Wheaton, IL 60187   www.awakeningsproject.org
Robert Lundin, Co-Director
Irene O'Neill, President and Co-Director
Mary Lou Lowry, Secretary
The Awakenings Project is an organization whose mission is to assist those artists with psychiatric illnesses in developing their talent and finding an outlet for their creative abilities through art in all forms.

14   Brookline Books
8 Trumbull Rd
Suite B-001
Northampton, MA 01060   413-584-0184
                                          800-666-2665
                                     Fax: 413-584-6184
                                     brbooks@yahoo.com
                                     www.brooklinebooks.com
Brookline Books has been publishing reader-friendly and informative education literature for more than 20 years, with a mission to reach both a specialized and non-specialized audience. They have a strong list of books for people with disabilities, including general information on advocacy, assistive technology, parent involvement, professional resources, early childhood intervention, as well as on specific disabilities.

**15   Clinical Applications of Music Therapy in
       Developmental Disability, Pediatrics and Neurolog**
Taylor & Francis
400 Market Street
Suite 400
Philadelphia, PA 19106-4738   215-922-1161
                                         866-416-1078
                                    Fax: 215-922-1474
                                    hello.usa@jkp.com
                                    www.jkp.com
Tony Wigram, Editor
Jessica Kingsley, Chairman, Managing Director
Jemima Kingsley, Director
More and more, music therapy is being practiced as an intervention in medical and special educational settings. This book describes and explains the planning and evaluation of music therapy intervention and how it can be used for assessing complex organic and emotional disabilities. *$34.95*
312 pages
ISBN 1-853027-34-0

16   Contemporary Art Therapy with Adolescents
Taylor & Francis
400 Market Street
Suite 400
Philadelphia, PA 19106-4738   215-922-1161
                                         866-416-1078
                                    Fax: 215-922-1474
                                    hello.usa@jkp.com
                                    www.jkp.com
Shirley Riley, Author
Jessica Kingsley, Chairman, Managing Director
Jemima Kingsley, Director
Reviews contemporary theories on adolescent development and therapy and offers solutions to the treatment of young people. *$ 26.95*
285 pages
ISBN 1-853026-37-9

17   Creative Arts Resources Catalog
MMB Music
9051 Watson Road
Ste 161
St. Louis, MO 63126   314-531-9635
                                     Fax: 314-531-8384
                                     info@mmbmusic.com
                                     www.mmbmusic.com
Norm Goldberg, Founder & Chair
Publisher and distributor of creative arts therapy materials in the areas of music, dance, art, drama, and poetry. Free catalog contains hundreds of books, recordings, and videos.

18   Creative Growth Art Center
355 - 24th St
Oakland, CA 94612   510-836-2340
                                     Fax: 510-836-0769
                                     info@creativegrowth.org
                                     www.creativegrowth.org
Becki Couch-Alvarado, Executive Director
Tom Di Maria, Director
Jennifer Strate O'Neal, Partnerships & Communications Manager
Creative Growth Art Center serves adult artists with developmental, mental and physical disabilities, providing a professional studio environment for artistic development, gallery exhibition and representation and a social atmosphere among peers.

19   Creativity Explored
3245 16th St.
San Francisco, CA 94103   415-863-2108
                                     Fax: 415-863-1655
                                     info@creativityexplored.org
                                     www.creativityexplored.org
Linda Johnson, Executive Director
Creativity Explored is a nonprofit visual arts center giving artists with developmental disabilities the means to create and share their work with the community, celebrating the power of art to change lives.

20   Dancing from the Inside Out
Fanlight Productions
c/o Icarus Films
32 Court Street, 21st Floor
Brooklyn, NY 11201   718-488-8900
                                          800-876-1710
                                     Fax: 718-488-8642
                                     info@fanlight.com
                                     www.fanlight.com
Ben Achtenberg, Founder
This eloquent video looks at the lives and work of three talented dancers who dance professionally with the acclaimed AXIS Dance Troupe, which includes both disabled and non-disabled dancers. They discuss the process they went through in adapting to their disability and how they came to re-discover physical expression through dance.

21   Deaf West Theatre
5114 Lankershim Blvd.
Los Angeles, CA 91601   818-762-2998
                                      Fax: 818-762-2981
                                      info@deafwest.org
                                          deafwest.org

Ed Waterstreet, Founding Artistic Director
David Kurs, Artistic Director
Mark Freund, President
Deaf West Theatre, Inc., was founded in 1991 to directly improve and enrich the cultural lives of the 1.2 million deaf and hard-of-hearing individuals who live in the Los Angeles area. DWT provides exposure and access to professional theatre, filling a void for deaf artists and audiences.

22   Disability and Social Performance: Using Drama to Achieve Successful Acts
Brookline Books
8 Trumbull Rd
Suite B-001
Northampton, MA 01060   413-584-0184
                                          800-666-2665
                                      Fax: 413-584-6184
                                      brbooks@yahoo.com
                                   www.brooklinebooks.com

Bernie Warren, Author
This book makes a major contribution to the understanding of disability, people with disabilities and the creative power they possess which can be unleashed through performance. The books name is Disability and Social Performance: Using Drama to Achieve Successful Acts of Being. *$17.95*

23   Expressive Arts for the Very Disabled and Handicapped of All Ages
Charles C. Thomas
2600 S First St
Springfield, IL 62704-4730   217-789-8980
                                          800-258-8980
                                      Fax: 217-789-9130
                                    books@ccthomas.com
                                      www.ccthomas.com

Marilyn Wannamaker, Co-Author
Jane G. Cohen, Co-Author
The ideas presented are not only designed to hold the interest of the children and adults, but to meet the needs of professionals and volunteers working with the disabled artists. All crafts are rated on a sliding scale, are of a low difficulty rating, use inexpensive and safe materials, and include explicit instructions. *$ 49.95*
236 pages Spiral-Paper 1996
ISBN 0-398067-04-5

24   Fanlight Productions
c/o Icarus Films
32 Court Street, 21st Floor
Brooklyn, NY 11201   718-488-8900
                                          800-876-1710
                                      Fax: 718-488-8642
                                      info@fanlight.com
                                      www.fanlight.com

Ben Achtenberg, Founder
Fanlight Productions is a leading distributor of innovative film and video works on the social issues of our time, with a special focus on healthcare, mental health, professional ethics, aging and gerontology, disabilities, the workplace, and gender and family issues. Select titles include Acting Blind, Autism: A World Apart, Dancing from the Inside Out, and Able to Laugh.

25   Fountain House Gallery
702 Ninth Ave at 48th St
New York, NY 10019   212-262-2756
                                   fountaingallerynyc.com

Ariel Wilmott, Director
Camille Tibaldeo, Communications Director
Fountain House Gallery provides an environment for artists living and working with mental illness to pursue their personal visions and to challenge the stigma that surrounds mental illness.

26   Friends In Art (FIA)
4317 Vermont Court
Columbia, MO 65203   573-445-5564
                                      www.friendsinart.com

Peter Altschul, President
Lynn Hedl, Vice President
Don Horn, Corresponding Secretary
Friends in Art is a national organization for blind, visually impaired, and deaf-blind artists, musicians and writers, and art enthusiasts. The organization is dedicated to enhancing the skills and broadening the opportunities of the individuals involved with the organization.

27   Future Horizons
721 West Abram Street
Arlington, TX 76013-6995   817-277-0727
                                          800-489-0727
                                      Fax: 817-277-2270
                                      www.fhautism.com

R. Wayne Gilpin, President
Jennifer Gilpin, VP, Foreign Translations
Kelly Gilpin, Editorial Dir.
Founded in 1996, Future Horizons is devoted to supporting and fostering works and programs for those who live and work with autism and asperger's syndrome.

28   Guide to the Selection of Musical Instruments
MMB Music
9051 Watson Road
Ste 161
St. Louis, MO 63126   314-531-9635
                                          800-543-3771
                                      Fax: 314-531-8384
                                      info@mmbmusic.com
                                      www.mmbmusic.com

Norm Goldberg, Founder & Chair
A marvelous resource book to aid therapists teaching those who are disabled to play musical instruments. *$7.75*

29   In-Definite Arts Society
8038 Fairmount Drive SE
Calgary, AB T2H0Y   403-253-3174
                                      Fax: 403-255-2234
                                      www.indefinitearts.com

Darlene Murphy, Executive Director
Dijana Andric, Client Services Manager
Peter Kelsch, Accountant
Promotes opportunities for people with developmental disabilities to express themselves and to grow and develop through their involvement in art.

30   Infinity Dance Theater
220 W 93rd St
New York, NY 10025   212-877-3490
                                      info@infinitydance.com
                                      infinitydance.com

Kitty Lunn, RDE, Founder/Artistic Director
Michael A. Fitch, Executive Director
Infinity Dance Theater is a non-traditional dance company committed to expanding the boundaries of dance by featuring dancers with and without disabilities. The company aims to inspire people with and without disabilities, encourage their artistic and other professional aspirations, and empower them through the organization's educational and performance programs.

31   Instrumental Music for Dyslexics: A Teaching Handbook
Wiley & Sons
111 River Street
Hoboken, NJ 07030-5774   201-748-6000
                                      Fax: 201-748-6088
                                      info@wiley.com
                                      www.wiley.com

Sheila Oglethorpe, Author
Stephen M. Smith, President and CEO
Ellis E. Cousens, Executive Vice President, Chief Operations Officer
Describes dyslexia in layman's terms and explains how the various problems that a dyslexic may have can affect all aspects of learning to play a musical instrument. It alerts the music teacher with a problem pupil to the possibilities of that pupil having some form of dyslexia. It offers suggestions as to how to teach dyslex-

ics, with particular reference to piano teaching, and it suggests ways in which the music teacher may contribute to the welfare of a dyslexic pupil. *$ 34.95*
200 pages
ISBN 1-861562-91-8

32   Interact Center for the Visual and Performing Arts
Interact Center
1860 Minnehaha Ave W
St. Paul, MN 55401   651-209-3575
                                              Fax: 651-209-3579
                                      info@interactcenter.com
                                            interactcenter.com
Jeanne Calvit, Artistic & Executive Director
Shannon Forney, Managing Director
Beth Bowman, Director, Advancement
Creates art in a spirit of radical inclusion; Inspires artists and audiences to explore the full spectrum of human potential; Transforms lives by expanding ideas of what is possible.

33   Kaleidoscope: Exploring the Experience of Disability through Literature & the Fine Arts
United Disability Services
701 South Main St
Akron, OH 44311-1019   330-762-9755
                                              Fax: 330-762-0912
                                      kaleidoscope@udsakron.org
                               www.udsakron.org/services/kaleidoscope
Howard Taylor, President & CEO
Lisa Armstrong, Director of Community Relations & Managing Editor
Gail Willmott, Editor in Chief
Kaleidoscope is a magazine published by United Disability Services. Kaleidoscope challenges and transcends stereotypical, patronizing and sentimental attitudes about disability, looking at the experience of actually living with a disability from a more personal/individual perspective rather than a clinical, sociological or rehabilitative point of view. Included are a variety of articles, fiction, art and poetry relating to issues of disability, literature and the fine arts. *$10.00*
64 pages BiAnnually

34   Keshet Dance and Center for the Arts
4121 Cutler Ave NE
Albuquerque, NM 87110   505-224-9808
                                          info@keshetarts.org
                                              keshetarts.org
Shira Greenberg, Artistic Director
Adrian Moore Trask, Director of Business Advancement
Emily Dunkin, Events Director
Keshet offers youth and adult classes and workshops for individuals with varying levels of physical disabilities and dance experience. Within the Adaptive Dance programming, Keshet pairs dancers with disabilities with able-bodied dancers, which often include siblings, parents, and peers, to create professional-quality dance works.

35   Learning Disabilities Sourcebook, 3rd Ed.
Omnigraphics
615 Griswold Street
Suite 520
Detroit, MI 48226   610-461-3548
                                                    800-234-1340
                                              Fax: 800-875-1340
                                      contact@omnigraphics.com
                                            www.omnigraphics.com
Peter Ruffner, Co-Founder
Fred Ruffner, Co-Founder
Learning Disabilities Sourcebook, Third Edition provides updated information about specific learning disabilities and other conditions that make learning difficult. These include dyscalculia, dysgraphia, dyslexia, auditory and visual processing, communication disorders, autism spectrum disorders, attention deficit and hyperactivity disorder, hearing and visual impairments, and brain injury. *$84.00*
600 pages Hard cover
ISBN 0-780810-39-6

36   Manual of Sequential Art Activities for Classified Children and Adolescents
Charles C. Thomas
2600 S First St
Springfield, IL 62704-4730   217-789-8980
                                                    800-258-8980
                                              Fax: 217-789-9130
                                          books@ccthomas.com
                                              www.ccthomas.com
Rocco A L Fugaro, Author
Offers information to the special education professional on art therapy and management. *$41.95*
246 pages Softcover
ISBN 0-39805 -85-6

37   Mozart Effect: Tapping the Power of Music to Heal the Body, Strengthen the Mind
Harper Collins Publishers
10 E 53rd St
New York, NY 10022-5244   212-207-7000
                                              www.harpercollins.com
Don Campbell, Author
Brian Murray, President and CEO
Michael Morrison, President and Publisher, U.S. General Books and Canada
Offers dramatic accounts of how doctors, shamans, musicians, and others use music to deal with everything from anxiety, cancer, and chronic pain, to dyslexia and mental illness. *$14.95*
352 pages
ISBN 0-060937-20-3

38   Music Therapy
Future Horizons, Inc.
721 West Abram St
Arlington, TX 76013-6995   817-277-0727
                                                    800-489-0727
                                              Fax: 817-277-2270
                                              www.fhautism.com
Betsey King Brunk, Author
R. Wayne Gilpin, President
Jennifer Gilpin, VP, Foreign Translations
Music therapy is the use of music to address non-musical goals. Parents and professionals are finding that music can break down barriers for children with autism in areas such as cognition, socialization, and communication. *$19.95*
123 pages
ISBN 1-885477-53-8

39   Music Therapy and Leisure for Persons with Disabilities
Sagamore Publishing
1807 N Federal Drive
Urbana, IL 61801   217-359-5940
                                                    800-327-5557
                                              Fax: 217-359-5975
                                      books@sagamorepub.com
                                            www.sagamorepub.com
Alicia L. Barksdale, Author
Joseph J. Bannon, Sr., Ph.D., Publisher & CEO
Peter L. Bannon, MBA, President
Explores the use of musical therapy in order to enhance the development of independent leisure skills with a variety of special populations. Suggestions are provided for alternative avenues through musical experiences enabling individuals to achieve their greatest potential for independence and a high quality of life. *$19.95*
ISBN 1-571675-11-6

40   Music Therapy for the Developmentally Disabled
Sage Publications
2455 Teller Road
Thousand Oaks, CA 91320   805-499-9774
                                                    800-818-7243
                                              Fax: 800-583-2665
                                          info@sagepub.com
                                              www.sagepub.com
S. Venkatesan, Author
Included are practical guidelines, case samples and step-by-step instructions that enable a music therapist to bring about dramatic

improvements in developmentally disabled adults and children.
$40.00
269 pages Hardcover
ISBN 0-890791-90-2

41   Music Therapy in Dementia Care
Jessica Kingsley Publishers
400 Market Street
Suite 400
Philadelphia, PA 19106-4738
215-922-1161
866-416-1078
Fax: 215-922-1474
hello.usa@jkp.com
www.jkp.com

David Aldridge, Editor
Jessica Kingsley, Chairman, Managing Director
Jemima Kingsley, Director
A comprehensive look at music therapy as a means of improving memory, health, and identity in those suffering from dementia, particularly Alzheimer's. For music therapists and those involved in psychogeriatry. *$29.95*
256 pages
ISBN 1-853027-76-6

42   Music Therapy, Sensory Integration and the Autistic Child
Jessica Kingsley Publishers
400 Market Street
Suite 400
Philadelphia, PA 19106-4738
215-922-1161
866-416-1078
Fax: 215-922-1474
hello.usa@jkp.com
www.jkp.com

Dorita S. Berger, Author
Jessica Kingsley, Chairman, Managing Director
Jemima Kingsley, Director
Examines the human physiologic function, the brain, information processing, functional adaption, and how that might be affected by music interventions in persons with sensory integration difficulties. *$23.95*
256 pages
ISBN 1-843107-00-7

43   Music and Dyslexia: A Positive Approach
Wiley & Sons
111 River Street
Hoboken, NJ 07030-5774
201-748-6000
Fax: 201-748-6088
info@wiley.com
www.wiley.com

John Westcombe, Editor
Stephen M. Smith, President and CEO
Ellis E. Cousens, Executive Vice President, Chief Operations Officer
This book shows how some people who have Dyslexia can be gifted musicians. The main point this books makes is that Dyslexic musicians can succeed provided only that they are given sufficient encouragement and understanding. *$34.95*
200 pages
ISBN 1-861562-05-5

44   Music for the Hearing Impaired
MMB Music
9051 Watson Road
Ste 161
St. Louis, MO 63126
314-531-9635
800-543-3771
Fax: 314-531-8384
info@mmbmusic.com
www.mmbmusic.com

Norm Goldberg, Founder & Chair
A resource manual and curriculum guide. It is the product of a four-year developmental music program, placing emphasis on the needs of those with severe and profound losses. *$29.95*

45   Music: Physician for Times to Come
Quest Books
P.O.Box 270
Wheaton, IL 60187-270
630-665-0130
800-669-9425
Fax: 630-665-8791
submissions@questbooks.net
www.questbooks.net

Don Campbell, Author
A resource guide for various types of music and their therapeutic outcome.
365 pages
ISBN 0-835607-88-7

46   NIAD Art Center (Nurturing Independence through Artistic Development)
551 23rd St.
Richmond, CA 94804-1626
510-620-0290
Fax: 510-620-0326
admin@niadart.org
www.niadart.org

Deborah Dyer, Executive Director
NIAD Art Center) promotes creativity, independence, dignity, and community integration for people with developmental and other disabilities. The visual arts studio supports artists with disabilities by providing materials, space to make art and facilitators to teach skills in drawing, painting, ceramics, printmaking, fiber arts and mixed media. The work that they make is exhibited in the Richmond gallery as well as in other galleries, on-line and other exhibition spaces.

47   National Arts and Disability Center (NADC)
Tarjan Center at UCLA
760 Westwood Plaza
Los Angeles, CA 90095-1759
310-825-5054
Fax: 310-794-1143
bstoffmacher@mednet.ucla.edu
www.semel.ucla.edu/nadc

Olivia Raynor, Director
Beth Stoffmacher, Center Coordinator
NADC has a database and website advocating for access to and participation in the arts by people with disabilities.

48   National Association for Drama Therapy
1450 Western Avenue
Suite 101
Albany, NY 12203
571-223-6440
888-416-7167
Fax: 518-463-8656
office@nadta.org
www.nadt.org

Nadya Trytan, MA, RDT/BCT, President
Jeremy Segall, MA, RDT, LCAT, Vice President
Jason Butler, RDT/BCT, LCAT, President-Elect
The National Association for Drama Therapy (NADT) was incorporated in 1979 to establish and uphold rigorous standards of professional competence for drama therapists. The NADT promotes drama therapy through information and advocacy.

49   National Endowment for the Arts: Office for AccessAbility
1100 Pennsylvania Ave NW
Washington, DC 20506-0001
202-682-5034
Fax: 202-682-5666
TTY: 202-682-5496
webmgr@arts.gov
www.arts.gov/

Jane Chu, Chairman
Beth Bienvenu, Accessibility Director
Wendy Clark, Director of Museums, Visual Arts, and Indemnity
The National Endowment for the Arts Office for AccessAbility is the advocacy-technical assistance arm of the Arts Endowment to make the arts accessible for people with disabilities, older adults, veterans, and people living in institutions.

50 National Library Service for the Blind and Physically Handicapped (NLS)
1291 Taylor St NW
Washington, DC 20011   202-707-5100
800-424-8567
Fax: 202-707-0712
nls@loc.gov
www.loc.gov/nls
Administers a national library service that provides Braille and recorded books and magazines on free loan to anyone who cannot read standard print because of visual or physical disabilities.
Annual

51 National Theatre Workshop of the Handicapped (NTWH)
535 Greenwich Street
New York, NY 10013-1004   212-206-7789
Fax: 212-206-0200
www.ntwh.org
Jason Matthews, Director of Admissions
Rick Curry, President & CEO
John Spalla, General Manager
A non-profit organization that provides individuals within the disabled community with the communication skills and the artistic discipline necessary to pursue a life in professional theatre.

52 National Theatre of the Deaf
139 N Main St
West Hartford, CT 06107-1264   860-236-4193
Fax: 860-574-9107
Info@NTD.org
www.ntd.org
Betty Beekman, Executive Director
William C. Martin, Marketing/PR Director
George Ghista, Accountant
The mission of the National Theatre of the Deaf is to produce theatrically challenging work of the highest quality, drawing from as wide a range of the world's literature as possible and to perform these original works in a style that links American Sign Language with the spoken word.

53 New Music Therapist's Handbook, 2nd Ed. Berklee School of Music
Berklee Press Publications
1140 Boylston Street
Boston, MA 02215   617-747-2146
866-237-5533
www.berkleepress.com
Suzanne B. Hanser, Author
Dr. Hanser's well-respected Music Therapist's Handbook has been revised and thoroughly updated to reflect the latest developments in the field of music therapy. *$29.95*
256 pages
ISBN 0-634006-45-2

54 No Limits
9801 Washington Blvd
2nd Fl
Culver City, CA 90232   310-280-0878
Fax: 310-280-0872
michelle@nolimitsfordeafchildren.org
nolimitsfordeafchildren.org
Michelle Christie, Founder & Executive Director
Juliana Scott, Director, Operations & Development
The mission of No Limits is to meet the auditory, speech and language needs of deaf children and enhance their confidence through the theatrical arts and individual therapy as well as provide family support and community awareness on the needs and talents of deaf children who are learning to speak.

55 Non-Traditional Casting Project
Ste 1600
1560 Broadway
New York, NY 10036-1518   212-730-4750
Fax: 212-730-4820
TTY: 212-730-4913
www.ntcp.org/
Nancy Kim, Manager
The Non-Traditional Casting Project (NTCP) is a not-for-profit advocacy organization whose purpose is to address and seek solutions to the problems of racism and exclusion in theatre, film and television. NTCP's principal concerns are those of artists of color, female artists, Deaf and hard of hearing artists, and artists with disabilities.

56 Nuvisions For Disabled Artists, Inc.
C/O Rose Marcus
1319 Magee Street
Philadelphia, PA 19111
Kaye E Schonbach, Executive Director
Nuvisions was established to enable physically challenged artists to pursue professional and semi-professional artistic opportunities. Nuvisions supports these artists by sponsoring accessible exhibitions, special projects and educational opportunities in Southeastern Pennsylvania and Southern New Jersey.

57 Open Circle Theatre
102-500 King Farm Blvd
Rockville, MD 20850   240-683-8934
info@opencircletheatre.org
opencircletheatre.org
Suzanne Richard, Artistic Director
Ian Armstrong, Executive Producer
Open Circle Theatre is a professional theatre dedicated to producing productions that integrate the considerable talents of artists with disabilities. OCT was formed by a group of people with and without disabilities, who possess professional theater experience, love of the theater, and a commitment to full access for all persons in every opportunity our community has to offer.

58 Pied Piper: Musical Activities to Develop Basic Skills
Jessica Kingsley Publishers
400 Market Street
Suite 400
Philadelphia, PA 19106-4738   215-922-1161
866-416-1078
Fax: 215-922-1474
hello.usa@jkp.com
www.jkp.com
John Bean, Author
Jessica Kingsley, Chairman, Managing Director
Jemima Kingsley, Director
Describes 78 enjoyable music activities for groups of children or adults who may have learning difficulties. The emphasis is on using music, rather than learning songs or rhythms, so group members do not need any special skills to be able to participate. Full details are given about any equipment required for the games, as well as suggestions for variations or modifications. *$21.95*
96 pages
ISBN 1-853029-94-

59 Project Onward Gallery
Bridgeport Art Center
1200 W. 35th St
4th Fl
Chicago, IL 60609   773-940-2992
info@projectonward.org
projectonward.org
Project Onward is dedicated to supporting the career development of artists with mental and developmental disabilities. Operating as both a studio and gallery, Project Onward supports the work of visual artists who have exceptional talents but face challenges ranging from autism to mental illness.

60 Pure Vision Arts
The Shield Institute
114 W 17th St
3rd Fl
New York, NY 10011   212-366-4263
Fax: 718-269-2059
progers@shield.org
purevisionarts.org
Pamala Rogers, Director
Pure Vision Arts mission is to provide people with autism and developmental disabilities opportunities for artistic expression and to build public awareness of their important creative contributions.

61 **Reaching the Child with Autism Through Art**
Future Horizons, Inc.
721 W Abram St
Arlington, TX 76013-6995   817-277-0727
                                        800-489-0727
                                        Fax: 817-277-2270
                                        www.fhautism.com
Toni Flowers, Author
R. Wayne Gilpin, President
Jennifer Gilpin Yacio, Vice President and Editorial Director
This book uncovers how art encourages communication, positive self-image, concept development, spatial relationships, fine-motor skills, and many more facets of health child development. *$19.95*
130 pages

62 **Survivors Art Foundation**
PO Box 383
Westhampton, NY 11977   www.survivorsartfoundation.org
Michael Herships, Ph.D, Project Leader & Board President
Candyce Brokaw, Art Director
Candyce M. Brokaw, Executive Director
Dedicated to encourage healing through the arts, committed to empowering Trauma-Survivors with Effective Expressive Outlets via Internet Art Gallery, Outreach Programs, National Exhibitions, Publications and Development of Employment Skills.

63 **Teaching Asperger's Students Social Skills Through Acting**
Future Horizons, Inc.
721 W Abram St
Arlington, TX 76013-6995   817-277-0727
                                        800-489-0727
                                        Fax: 817-277-2270
                                        www.fhautism.com
Amelia Davies, Author
R. Wayne Gilpin, President
Jennifer Gilpin Yacio, Vice President and Editorial Director
This book provides the theories and activities needed for setting up acting classes that double as social skills groups for individuals with Asperger's or high-functioning autism. Using these skills, students will be able to develop social understanding through repetition and generalization. *$19.95*
211 pages

64 **Teaching Basic Guitar Skills to Special Learners**
MMB Music
9051 Watson Road
Ste 161
St. Louis, MO 63126   314-531-9635
                                        800-543-3771
                                        Fax: 314-531-8384
                                        info@mmbmusic.com
                                        www.mmbmusic.com
Norm Goldberg, Founder & Chair
The first-of-its-kind guitar book for use with persons who have difficulty learning to play via traditional methods. *$16.00*

65 **The Arts of Life**
2010 W. Carroll Ave
Chicago, IL 60612   312-829-2787
                                        info@artsoflife.org
                                        artsoflife.org
Denise Fisher, Co-Founder & Executive Director
Sara Bemer, Development Coordinator
An organization comprised of people with and without disabilities seeking to promote artistic expression, community building, self-respect, and independence.

66 **Theatre Without Limits**
P.O.Box 4002
Portland, ME 04101   207-607-4016
                                        Fax: 207-761-4740
                                        www.vsartsmaine.org
Kippy Rudy, Executive Director
VSA Maine is a 501(c)(3) non-profit organization providing educational, arts, and cultural opportunities to children and adults with disabilities in Maine.

67 **VSA - The International Organization on Arts and Disability**
2700 F Street, NW
Washington, DC 20566   202-467-4600
                                        800-444-1324
                                        Fax: 202-429-0868
                                        TTY: 202-737-0645
                                        www.kennedy-center.org/education/vsa/
Ambassador J Kennedy Smith, Founder
David M. Rubenstein, Chair
Michael M. Kaiser, President
VSA offers a large selection of guides, publications, and other resources dealing with a wide variety of subject matter in education, arts, and disabilities.

68 **VSA arts**
2700 F Street, NW
Washington, DC 20566   202-467-4600
                                        800-444-1324
                                        Fax: 202-429-0868
                                        TTY: 202-737-0645
                                        www.kennedy-center.org/education/vsa/
Ambassador J Kennedy Smith, Founder
David M. Rubenstein, Chair
Michael M. Kaiser, President
VSA arts is an international, nonprofit organization founded in 1974 by Ambassador Jean Kennedy Smith whose mission is to create a society where all people with disabilities learn through, participate in, and enjoy the arts. Most states offer local programs, such as Arts in Action, that showcases the accomplishments of artists with disabilities and promotes increased access to the arts for people with disabilities.

69 **We Are PHAMALY**
Fanlight Productions
c/o Icarus Films
32 Court Street, 21st Floor
Brooklyn, NY 11201   718-488-8900
                                        800-876-1710
                                        Fax: 718-488-8642
                                        info@fanlight.com
                                        www.fanlight.com
Ben Achtenberg, Owner
Stands for Physically Handicapped Musical Actors League. This dynamic troupe doesn't cut any corners or make any compromises. The musicals they perform are chosen for their appeal to the audience, not because they are easy for the performers, who have a variety of sensory and mobility handicaps. *$199.00*
ISBN 1-572954-08-6

Assistive Devices

Automobile

70 AUT Secondary Control
Ace Mobility, LLC
9850 E 30th St.
Indianapolis, IN 46229
317-241-2444
877-223-5301
info@acemobility.us
www.acemobility.us

Doron Mishor, President & CEO
Zvika Amir, Vice President, Marketing & Sales
Controls up to 35 secondary functions.

71 AUTone
Ace Mobility, LLC
9850 E 30th St.
Indianapolis, IN 46229
317-241-2444
877-223-5301
info@acemobility.us
www.acemobility.us

Doron Mishor, President & CEO
Zvika Amir, Vice President, Marketing & Sales
Sound-activated signal device that allows drivers to momentarily activate a secondary function by pressing a button, which will play one to eight tones.

72 Ability Center
4797 Ruffner St.
San Diego, CA 92111
858-541-0552
833-919-2581
Fax: 858-541-1941
www.abilitycenter.com

Terry Barton, General Manager
Specializes in accessible vehicles and mobility products; the company has more than 100 employees in 14 locations across the western U.S.
1994

73 Accelerator Shield
Handicaps, Inc.
4335 S Santa Fe Dr.
Englewood, CO 80110-5417
303-781-2062
800-782-4335
info@handicapsinc.com
www.handicapsinc.com
Designed to help prevent vehicles from accelerating during leg spasms.

74 Accelerator/Brake Foot Control
Ace Mobility, LLC
9850 E 30th St.
Indianapolis, IN 46229
317-241-2444
877-223-5301
info@acemobility.us
www.acemobility.us

Doron Mishor, President & CEO
Zvika Amir, Vice President, Marketing & Sales
Electronic foot pedals designed for drivers with adaptive driving needs. The pedals can be mounted at any height, spacing, and angle.

75 Accelerator/Brake Hand Control
Ace Mobility, LLC
9850 E 30th St.
Indianapolis, IN 46229
317-241-2444
877-223-5301
info@acemobility.us
www.acemobility.us

Doron Mishor, President & CEO
Zvika Amir, Vice President, Marketing & Sales
Hand control device that controls the vehicle's acceleration and brakes. The device can be modified to the needs of the client through the push and pull functions.

76 Automobile Lifts for Scooters, Wheelchairs and Powerchairs
Bruno Independent Living Aids, Inc.
1780 Executive Dr.
PO Box 84
Oconomowoc, WI 53066
262-567-4990
800-454-4355
Fax: 262-953-5501
www.bruno.com

Michael R. Bruno, II, President & CEO
Offers automobile lifts for scooters, wheelchairs and powerchairs for nearly any car, van, truck or sport utility vehicle that can raise scooters or wheelchairs under 200 pounds and power chairs up to 300 pounds.

77 BraunAbility
645 W Carmel Dr.
Carmel, IN 46032
800-488-0359
888-365-9417
questions@braunability.com
www.braunability.com

Staci Kroon, President & CEO
Manufactures wheelchair lifts and lowered floor minivans as well as many other mobility products.

78 COM Hand Control
Ace Mobility, LLC
9850 E 30th St.
Indianapolis, IN 46229
317-241-2444
877-223-5301
info@acemobility.us
www.acemobility.us

Doron Mishor, President & CEO
Zvika Amir, Vice President, Marketing & Sales
A hand control device that integrates Ace Mobility's Hand Control and JoySpinner devices.

79 Car Cane with Transfer Swivel Cushion
Maxi Aids
42 Executive Blvd.
Farmingdale, NY 11735-4710
631-752-0521
800-522-6294
Fax: 631-752-0689
TTY: 631-752-0738
sales@maxiaids.com
www.maxiaids.com

Elliot Zaretsky, Founder, President & CEO
This device is designed for those who have trouble getting in and out of a car. The portable handle slides into any car door and can be easily stored in the door or glove box. *$64.90*

80 DW Auto & Home Mobility
1208 N Garth Ave.
Columbia, MO 65203-4056
573-449-3859
800-568-2271
contactus@dwauto.com
www.dwauto.com

Shawn Bright, Owner
DW manufactures paratransit conversions and personalized conversions for the physically challenged. Products include home elevators and lifts, scooters, and wheelchairs.
1967

81 Digital Shifter
Ace Mobility, LLC
9850 E 30th St.
Indianapolis, IN 46229
317-241-2444
877-223-5301
info@acemobility.us
www.acemobility.us

Doron Mishor, President & CEO
Zvika Amir, Vice President, Marketing & Sales
Enables drivers with limited arm strength and range of motion to use buttons to switch between the vehicle's gears. The switch console can be placed at any location to suit the needs of the driver.

82   Drive Master Company
37 Daniel Rd. W
Fairfield, NJ 07004-2521   973-808-9709
Fax: 973-808-9713
info@drivemastermobility.com
www.drivemastermobility.com
Peter B. Ruprecht, President
The Drive Master Company offers a full service mobility center, raised tops/doors, drop floors, custom driving equipment. Distributor of name brand devices and systems for full sized and mini vans.

83   Driving Systems Inc.
16139 Runnymede St.
Van Nuys, CA 91406-2913   818-782-6793
www.drivingsystems.com
DSI is the manufacturer of the Scott Driving System for disabled drivers. DSI manufactures the 'Wave Grip' grab rails and bathroom accessories for the disabled and elderly. DSI is also the importer of the Carospeed Menox Hand Controls, Left Foot Pedals and other disability driving aids.

84   Dual Brake Control
Kroepke Kontrols
104 Hawkins St.
Bronx, NY 10464   718-885-1100

This product includes one lever fingertip brake controls and precision steel machines. Does not take up lots of legroom. *$105.00*

85   Entervan
BraunAbility
645 W Carmel Dr.
Carmel, IN 46032   800-488-0359
888-365-9417
questions@braunability.com
www.braunability.com
Staci Kroon, President & CEO
The Entervan's accessible features include a power sliding door, ramp, and auto-kneel system, allowing for easier entry and exit for wheelchair and scooter users.

86   Foot Steering Systems
Drive Master Company
37 Daniel Rd. W
Fairfield, NJ 07004-2521   973-808-9709
Fax: 973-808-9713
info@drivemastermobility.com
www.drivemastermobility.com
Peter B. Ruprecht, President
Custom installed foot steering systems for drivers without the use of their arms.

87   Four Way Switches
Gresham Driving Aids
30800 S Wixom Rd.
Wixom, MI 48393-2418   248-624-1533
800-521-8930
Fax: 248-624-6358
www.greshamdrivingaids.com
David Ohrt, General Manager
Craig Wigginton, Sales Consultant
Joyce Martell, Customer Service
Multi-function switches for hand controls. Up to four functions can be added, including left turn signal, right turn signal, horn and dimmer.

88   Freedom Motors USA, Inc.
740 Watkins Rd.
Battle Creek, MI 49015   269-244-3497
866-581-7463
Fax: 269-580-8291
www.freedommotors.com
Sieto van Dillen, Chief Executive Officer
Freedom Motors offers van conversions with equipment that is easily installed and accessible for the physically challenged.

89   Gas and Brake Pedal Guard
Gresham Driving Aids
30800 S Wixom Rd.
Wixom, MI 48393-2418   248-624-1533
800-521-8930
Fax: 248-624-6358
www.greshamdrivingaids.com
David Ohrt, General Manager
Craig Wigginton, Sales Consultant
Joyce Martell, Customer Service
Designed for drivers who use hand controls, this device guards gas and brake pedals so they do not get accidentally pushed.

90   Gear Shift Adaptor
Handicaps, Inc.
4335 S Santa Fe Dr.
Englewood, CO 80110-5417   303-781-2062
800-782-4335
info@handicapsinc.com
www.handicapsinc.com
This device allows column mounted gear shift to be used with the left hand.

91   Gear Shift Extension
Gresham Driving Aids
30800 S Wixom Rd.
Wixom, MI 48393-2418   248-624-1533
800-521-8930
Fax: 248-624-6358
www.greshamdrivingaids.com
David Ohrt, General Manager
Craig Wigginton, Sales Consultant
Joyce Martell, Customer Service
Allows for easier gear shift operation.

92   Gresham Driving Aids
30800 S Wixom Rd.
Wixom, MI 48393-2418   248-624-1533
800-521-8930
Fax: 248-624-6358
www.greshamdrivingaids.com
David Ohrt, General Manager
Craig Wigginton, Sales Consultant
Joyce Martell, Customer Service
Gresham Driving Aids offers mobility solutions to physically challenged individuals including lowered floors, raised roofs and doors and high-quad driver control systems. Dealer for Braun, Ricon, Crow River and Bruno wheelchair lifts.

93   Hand Brake Control Only
Kroepke Kontrols
104 Hawkins St.
Bronx, NY 10464   718-885-2100

These devices include one-lever, fingertip-operated brake controls that are custom designed to fit each car, are completely adjustable, and offer positioning operation at your fingertips. *$130.00*

94   Hand Control Multi-Function Buttons
Gresham Driving Aids
30800 S Wixom Rd.
Wixom, MI 48393-2418   248-624-1533
800-521-8930
Fax: 248-624-6358
www.greshamdrivingaids.com
David Ohrt, General Manager
Craig Wigginton, Sales Consultant
Joyce Martell, Customer Service
Enables the driver to operate multiple vehicle controls using only one hand.

95   Hand Gas & Brake Control
Kroepke Kontrols
104 Hawkins St.
Bronx, NY 10464   718-885-2100

Driving controls that are attached by a control level right on to the gas and brake pedals for easy maneuvering and convenience. *$220.00*

9

96 Hand Parking Brake
Kroepke Kontrols
104 Hawkins St.
Bronx, NY 10464   718-885-2100

These devices include one lever, fingertip-operated brake controls that are custom designed to fit each car. *$25.00*

97 HandBrake
Ace Mobility, LLC
9850 E 30th St.
Indianapolis, IN 46229   317-241-2444
                                    877-223-5301
                                    info@acemobility.us
                                    www.acemobility.us
Doron Mishor, President & CEO
Zvika Amir, Vice President, Marketing & Sales
Electrical power parking brake aid device for drivers with limited arm or hand strength.

98 Handicaps, Inc.
4335 S Santa Fe Dr.
Englewood, CO 80110-5417   303-781-2062
                                    800-782-4335
                                    info@handicapsinc.com
                                    www.handicapsinc.com
Handicaps, Inc. is a manufacturer of 'SuperArm' wheelchair lifts, hand driving controls, and left foot gas pedals for vans and motor homes.

99 Headlight Dimmer Switch
Kroepke Kontrols
104 Hawkins St.
Bronx, NY 10464   718-885-2100

This device is a one lever, fingertip controls for disabled drivers. *$23.00*

100 Horizontal Steering Systems
Drive Master Company
37 Daniel Rd. W
Fairfield, NJ 07004-2521   973-808-9709
                                    Fax: 973-808-9713
                                    info@drivemastermobility.com
                                    www.drivemastermobility.com
Peter B. Ruprecht, President
The Horizontal Steering System is designed to meet the needs of drivers with spinal cord injuries and other individuals with limited arm strength and range of motion.

101 Horn Control Switch
Kroepke Kontrols
104 Hawkins St.
Bronx, NY 10464   718-885-2100

This device is one lever, fingertip control for disabled drivers that does not interfere with the regular operation of the vehicle. *$23.00*

102 JoySpinner
Ace Mobility, LLC
9850 E 30th St.
Indianapolis, IN 46229   317-241-2444
                                    877-223-5301
                                    info@acemobility.us
                                    www.acemobility.us
Doron Mishor, President & CEO
Zvika Amir, Vice President, Marketing & Sales
An ergonomic built-in remote-control joystick for secondary driving operations, including turn signals, beams, wipers, and hazard signals.

103 Kersey Mobility
6015 160th Ave. E
Sumner, WA 98390   253-863-4744
                                    www.kerseymobility.com
Mike Kersey, Owner
Kersey Mobility is a wheelchair van dealer serving the Pacific Northwest. Also offers a line of mobility products and accessories, including lifts, wheelchair restraints, vehicle transfer seating, and adaptive driving aids.

104 Kessler Institute for Rehabilitation
1199 Pleasant Valley Way
West Orange, NJ 07052   973-731-3600
                                    877-322-2580
                                    Fax: 973-243-6819
                                    www.kessler-rehab.com
Sue Kida, President
Driver evaluation training for the physically/mentally challenged. Offers state certified driving instructors. Door-to-door pickup at home, work or rehab centers are available.

105 Left Foot Gas Pedal
Kroepke Kontrols
104 Hawkins St.
Bronx, NY 10464   718-885-2100

This device is one lever, fingertip control for disabled drivers that does not interfere with the regular operation of the vehicle. *$90.00*

106 Left Foot Gas Pedal, The
Handicaps, Inc.
4335 S Santa Fe Dr.
Englewood, CO 80110-5417   303-781-2062
                                    800-782-4335
                                    info@handicapsinc.com
                                    www.handicapsinc.com
Designed for drivers with limited use of the right foot.

107 MobilityWorks
4199 Kinross Lakes Pkwy.
Suite 300
Richfield, OH 44286   877-275-4907
                                    www.mobilityworks.com
Bryan Everett, Chief Executive Officer
Offers a selection of wheelchair accessible vehicles, mobility equipment, adaptive systems, and seating solutions.

108 Multi-Function Spinner Knobs
Gresham Driving Aids
30800 S Wixom Rd.
Wixom, MI 48393-2418   248-624-1533
                                    800-521-8930
                                    Fax: 248-624-6358
                                    www.greshamdrivingaids.com
David Ohrt, General Manager
Craig Wigginton, Sales Consultant
Joyce Martell, Customer Service
Spinner knobs that can include up to six vehicle accessory controls.

109 Park Brake Extension
Handicaps, Inc.
4335 S Santa Fe Dr.
Englewood, CO 80110-5417   303-781-2062
                                    800-782-4335
                                    info@handicapsinc.com
                                    www.handicapsinc.com
This is designed for cars with foot operated parking brake, to operate with hand.

110 Parking Brake Extension
Gresham Driving Aids
30800 S Wixom Rd.
Wixom, MI 48393-2418   248-624-1533
                                    800-521-8930
                                    Fax: 248-624-6358
                                    www.greshamdrivingaids.com
David Ohrt, General Manager
Craig Wigginton, Sales Consultant
Joyce Martell, Customer Service
Enables drivers to operate the foot parking/emergency brake by hand.

111 Portable Hand Controls by Handicaps, Inc.
Handicaps, Inc.
4335 S Santa Fe Dr.
Englewood, CO 80110-5417   303-781-2062
                                    800-782-4335
                                    info@handicapsinc.com
                                    www.handicapsinc.com

To be used on a temporary basis only. Must be used on vehicles with automatic transmission, power brakes, and power steering. Unimpaired hand use is required.

112 Power Transfer Seat Base (6-Way)
Ricon
1135 Aviation Pl.
San Fernando, CA 91340   818-267-3000
                                        800-322-2884
                                        Fax: 800-962-1201
                                        ricinsales@wabtec.com
                                        www.riconcorp.com
Facilitates a driver's self-transfer from a wheelchair to the driving seat and allows optimal driving positioning.

113 Push Pull Hand Controls
Gresham Driving Aids
30800 S Wixom Rd.
Wixom, MI 48393-2418   248-624-1533
                                        800-521-8930
                                        Fax: 248-624-6358
                                        www.greshamdrivingaids.com
David Ohrt, General Manager
Craig Wigginton, Sales Consultant
Joyce Martell, Customer Service
These controls are operated by pushing for brake and pulling back for acceleration.

114 Push Rock Hand Controls
Gresham Driving Aids
30800 S Wixom Rd.
Wixom, MI 48393-2418   248-624-1533
                                        800-521-8930
                                        Fax: 248-624-6358
                                        www.greshamdrivingaids.com
David Ohrt, General Manager
Craig Wigginton, Sales Consultant
Joyce Martell, Customer Service
These controls allow the driver to apply the accelerator and brakes by hand.

115 Rampvan
BraunAbility
645 W Carmel Dr.
Carmel, IN 46032   800-488-0359
                                        888-365-9417
                                        questions@braunability.com
                                        www.braunability.com
Staci Kroon, President & CEO
Fully accessible minivan conversions with automatic doors and ramps.

116 Reduced Effort Steering
Drive Master Company
37 Daniel Rd. W
Fairfield, NJ 07004-2521   973-808-9709
                                        Fax: 973-808-9713
                                        info@drivemastermobility.com
                                        www.drivemastermobility.com
Peter B. Ruprecht, President
Reduced effort steering modifications available for nearly all vehicles. Additional products are pedal extensions which are 1 inch to 4 inch clamp-on aluminum blocks and 6 inch to 12 inch adjustable fold-down pedals.

117 Right Angle Hand Controls
Gresham Driving Aids
30800 S Wixom Rd.
Wixom, MI 48393-2418   248-624-1533
                                        800-521-8930
                                        Fax: 248-624-6358
                                        www.greshamdrivingaids.com
David Ohrt, General Manager
Craig Wigginton, Sales Consultant
Joyce Martell, Customer Service
These controls apply the gas and accelerator at a right angle to the brake.

118 Right Hand Gas and Brake Control
Gresham Driving Aids
30800 S Wixom Rd.
Wixom, MI 48393-2418   248-624-1533
                                        800-521-8930
                                        Fax: 248-624-6358
                                        www.greshamdrivingaids.com
David Ohrt, General Manager
Craig Wigginton, Sales Consultant
Joyce Martell, Customer Service
Floor-mounted hand control that allows drivers to accelerate and brake using their right hand.

119 SWAB Steering Wheel
Ace Mobility, LLC
9850 E 30th St.
Indianapolis, IN 46229   317-241-2444
                                        877-223-5301
                                        info@acemobility.us
                                        www.acemobility.us
Doron Mishor, President & CEO
Zvika Amir, Vice President, Marketing & Sales
The SWAB (Steering Wheel Accelerator-Brake) allows drivers to steer the vehicle and control gas and brake functions with low effort.

120 Spider Network Systems
Ace Mobility, LLC
9850 E 30th St.
Indianapolis, IN 46229   317-241-2444
                                        877-223-5301
                                        info@acemobility.us
                                        www.acemobility.us
Doron Mishor, President & CEO
Zvika Amir, Vice President, Marketing & Sales
Modular control network system that allows drivers with disabilities to activate secondary driving functions, including gear-shift, hand-brake, signaling, lights, and more. Also available in touch screen format.

121 Spinner Knobs
Ace Mobility, LLC
9850 E 30th St.
Indianapolis, IN 46229   317-241-2444
                                        877-223-5301
                                        info@acemobility.us
                                        www.acemobility.us
Doron Mishor, President & CEO
Zvika Amir, Vice President, Marketing & Sales
Knobs designed to maximize the comfort of drivers with disabilities who have difficulty turning the steering wheel.

122 Steering Device
Handicaps, Inc.
4335 S Santa Fe Dr.
Englewood, CO 80110-5417   303-781-2062
                                        800-782-4335
                                        info@handicapsinc.com
                                        www.handicapsinc.com
Mounts to one side of steering wheel. Allows for easier steering using only one hand.

123 Steering Wheel Devices
Drive Master Company
37 Daniel Rd. W
Fairfield, NJ 07004-2521   973-808-9709
                                        Fax: 973-808-9713
                                        info@drivemastermobility.com
                                        www.drivemastermobility.com
Peter B. Ruprecht, President
Steering devices for disabled drivers, including steering knobs, steering cuffs, amputee rings, tri-pins, and grips.

124 Super Grade IV Hand Controls
Handicaps, Inc.
4335 S Santa Fe Dr.
Englewood, CO 80110-5417   303-781-2062
                                        800-782-4335
                                        info@handicapsinc.com
                                        www.handicapsinc.com

Hand controls the operation of accelerator and brakes. VA tested. Right angle style.

125 TapGear
Ace Mobility, LLC
9850 E 30th St.
Indianapolis, IN 46229   317-241-2444
                                877-223-5301
                                info@acemobility.us
                                www.acemobility.us
Doron Mishor, President & CEO
Zvika Amir, Vice President, Marketing & Sales
Electronic device that allows the driver to control gear positions.

126 Tim's Trim
25 Bermar Park
Rochester, NY 14624-1542   585-429-6270
                                888-468-6784
                                info@timstrim.com
                                www.timstrim.com
Tim Miller, Owner
Offers vehicle modifications, drop floors, raised tops/doors, driving equipment, touch pads and lifts.

127 Transportation Equipment for People with Disabilities
Gresham Driving Aids
30800 S Wixom Rd.
Wixom, MI 48393-2418   248-624-1533
                                800-521-8930
                                Fax: 248-624-6358
                                www.greshamdrivingaids.com
David Ohrt, General Manager
Craig Wigginton, Sales Consultant
Joyce Martell, Customer Service
Wheelchair lifts and ramps, hand and foot controls, steering and braking modifications, complete van conversions, home modifications, wheelchairs and scooters and wheelchair accessible van rentals.

128 Turn Signal Cross-Over
Gresham Driving Aids
30800 S Wixom Rd.
Wixom, MI 48393-2418   248-624-1533
                                800-521-8930
                                Fax: 248-624-6358
                                www.greshamdrivingaids.com
David Ohrt, General Manager
Craig Wigginton, Sales Consultant
Joyce Martell, Customer Service
This device enables the driver to operate the turn signal lever using the right hand.

129 United Access
9389 Natural Bridge Rd.
St. Louis, MO 63134   877-578-1962
                                www.unitedaccess.com
John Beering, President
Various automobile control systems that use hand, foot and steering aids for the disabled, including complete vehicle modifications.

130 Vantage Mobility International
5202 S 28th Pl.
Phoenix, AZ 85040   855-864-8267
                                www.vantagemobility.com
Mark Shaughnessy, Chief Executive Officer
Manufacturer and distributor of accessible vehicles and mobility products.

131 Vehicle Access Remote Control
Ace Mobility, LLC
9850 E 30th St.
Indianapolis, IN 46229   317-241-2444
                                877-223-5301
                                info@acemobility.us
                                www.acemobility.us
Doron Mishor, President & CEO
Zvika Amir, Vice President, Marketing & Sales
Universal remote control that opens and closes vehicle doors, raises and lowers hoist and chair elevators, and includes full lift control.

132 Wheelers Accessible Van Rentals
6614 W Sweetwater Ave.
Glendale, AZ 85304   623-776-8830
                               800-456-1371
                               Fax: 623-900-2708
                               corporate@wheelersavr.com
                               www.wheelersvanrentals.com
Offers daily, weekly and monthly rentals to accommodate various disabilities at locations across the U.S.
1987

Bath

133 Adjustable Raised Toilet Seat & Guard
Invacare
1 Invacare Way
Elyria, OH 44035-4190   800-333-6900
                               www.invacare.com
Matthew E. Monaghan, Chairman of the Board & Chief Executive Officer
Rick A. Cassiday, Senior Vice President & Chief Human Resources Officer
Kathleen P. Leneghan, Senior Vice President & Chief Financial Officer
The seat features an exclusive pivot locking system so it won't slip or tip and the adjustable guard rail fits all toilets.

134 ArjoHuntleigh
ArjoHuntleigh
2349 W Lake St.
Suite 250
Addison, IL 60101   800-323-1245
                               us.cc@arjohuntleigh.com
                               www.arjohuntleigh.us
Joacim Lindoff, President & CEO
Daniel F,,ldt, Chief Financial Officer
ARJO offers a complete line of patient bathing, showering and lift/transport systems, bariatric solutions, and accompanying skin care products for long-term and acute care facilities.

135 Bath Fixtures
Fiat Products
41 Cairns Rd.
Mansfield, OH 44904   833-549-2887
                               Fax: 816-763-9244
                               www.fiatproducts.com
Manufacturers plumbing fixtures for the disabled. Products include toilets, lavatories, showers and tub/shower units.

136 Bath Products
R82, Inc.
13137 Bleinheim Lane
Matthews, NC 28105   844-876-6245
                               Fax: 704-882-0751
                               sales.us@etac.com
                               www.etac.com
Michael Wirzberger, Chief Executive Officer
Johan Nylander, Chief Financial Officer
Kim Ankj'r, Vie President, Quality Assurance & Regulatory Affairs
Offers a wide range of products to meet the transportation, mobility, seating and bath aid needs for people of all ages. From car seats and standers for children with special needs to versatile wheelchairs that offer adults customized options and the freedom to go anywhere with confidence.

137 Bath Shower & Commode Chair
Clarke Health Care Products
7830 Steubenville Pike
Oakdale, PA 15071-9226   724-695-2122
                               888-347-4537
                               Fax: 724-695-2922
                               info@clarkehealthcare.com
                               www.clarkehealthcare.com
Aquatic Stainless steel shower/commode chairs and powered bathlifts. Mobeli portable grab bars, Dolomite rollators, Arco bed rails, Care bags for hygiene collection, DecPac portable ramps, Ableware eating, hygiene and dressing aids.

138   Bath and Shower Bench 3301B
Mada Medical Products
625 Washington Ave.
Carlstadt, NJ 07072-2901   201-460-0454
                                           800-526-6370
                                   Fax: 201-460-3509
                        saragannon@madamedical.com
                               www.madamedical.com
The bath and shower bench is corrosion-resistant, has a cross
brace design and angled legs to prevent tipping, and seat height
adjustments.

139   Bathroom Transfer Systems
Inspired By Drive
11724 Willake St.
Santa Fe Springs, CA 90670-5032   800-454-6612
                              info@inspiredbydrive.com
                              www.inspiredbydrive.com
Michael Gipson, Senior Director
Offers a complete line of bathroom transfer systems, bath lifts, reclining bath chairs, bath/shower/commode chairs, wrap-around
bath supports, toilet supports, positioning commodes, premium
air, foam and gel seat cushions, giant trainers and positioning restraint car seats that accommodate individuals from 20-130
pounds.

140   Bathtub Safety Rail
AliMed, Inc.
297 High Street
Dedham, MA 02026-2852   781-329-2900
                                           800-437-2966
                                   Fax: 781-437-2966
                       customerservice@alimed.com
                                    www.alimed.com
Adam S. Epstein, Chief Executive Officer
Made of stainless steel, this safety rail fits in any size bathtub and
offers safety and independence at bathing time. *$55.00*

141   Can-Do Products Catalog
Independent Living Aids
137 Rano Rd.
Buffalo, NY 14207   716-332-2970
                                           800-537-2118
                                   Fax: 877-498-1482
                        can-do@independentliving.com
                             www.independentliving.com
Can-Do Products Catalogue provides aids and products for the
blind and visually impairments.
84 pages Quarterly

142   Clarke Healthcare Products, Inc.
7830 Steubenville Pike
Oakdale, PA 15071-9226   724-695-2122
                                           888-347-4537
                                   Fax: 724-695-2922
                          info@clarkehealthcare.com
                               www.clarkehealthcare.com
Aquatic Stainless steel shower/commode chairs and powered
bathlifts. Mobeli portable grab bars, Dolomite rollators, Arco bed
rails, Care bags for hygiene collection, DecPac portable ramps,
clarke aluminum ramps.

143   Commode
Maxi Aids
42 Executive Blvd.
Farmingdale, NY 11735-4710   631-752-0521
                                           800-522-6294
                                   Fax: 631-752-0689
                                   TTY: 631-752-0738
                               sales@maxiaids.com
                                    www.maxiaids.com
Elliot Zaretsky, Founder, President & CEO
Adjustable seat height for patient comfort. Easily assembled, alu-
minum frame.

144   Deluxe Bath Bench with Adjustable Legs
Maxi Aids
42 Executive Blvd.
Farmingdale, NY 11735-4710   631-752-0521
                                           800-522-6294
                                   Fax: 631-752-0689
                                   TTY: 631-752-0738
                               sales@maxiaids.com
                                    www.maxiaids.com
Elliot Zaretsky, Founder, President & CEO
Bath bench with back support and adjustable legs. *$ 69.95*

145   Electric Leg Bag Emptier
RD Equipment, Inc.
230 Percival Dr.
West Barnstable, MA 02668-1244   508-362-7498
                                   Fax: 508-362-1458
                               r_dag@hotmail.com
                                    www.rdequipment.com
Richard Dagostino, Owner and Founder
Designed for independence, this small, lightweight, battery-operated valve attaches to the bottom of the leg bag. A simple flip of
the switch empties the leg bag, allowing the user to take in unlimited amounts of fluids. *$550.00*

146   Freedom Bath
ArjoHuntleigh
2349 W Lake St.
Suite 250
Addison, IL 60101   800-323-1245
                               us.cc@arjohuntleigh.com
                                    www.arjohuntleigh.us
Joacim Lindoff, President & CEO
Daniel F,,ldt, Chief Financial Officer
Residents can relax on a semi-reclining seat and enjoy the sooth-
ing deluxe whirlpool system. Freedom Bath offers a revolution-
ary solution with its unique Roll-Door. Includes head cushion and
safety belt.

147   Heavy-Duty Bath and Shower Seat
AliMed, Inc.
297 High Street
Dedham, MA 02026-2852   781-329-2900
                                           800-437-2966
                                   Fax: 781-437-2966
                       customerservice@alimed.com
                                    www.alimed.com
Adam S. Epstein, Chief Executive Officer
Bath and shower seat that fits easily in any tub or shower. In-
cludes easy-to-grip handles for safety and convenience. *$ 59.25*

148   Long Handled Bath Sponges
Therapro, Inc.
225 Arlington St
Framingham, MA 01702-8723   508-872-9494
                                           800-257-5376
                                   Fax: 508-268-6624
                               info@therapro.com
                                    www.therapro.com
Karen Conrad Weihrauch, President & Owner
Plastic-handled, 18-inch bath sponge. Handle may be heated and
bent for easy reach. *$2.50*

149   Modular Wall Grab Bars
Invacare
1 Invacare Way
Elyria, OH 44035-4190   800-333-6900
                                    www.invacare.com
*Matthew E. Monaghan, Chairman of the Board & Chief Executive
Officer*
*Rick A. Cassiday, Senior Vice President & Chief Human Resources
Officer*
*Kathleen P. Leneghan, Senior Vice President & Chief Financial
Officer*
Engineered for strength and beauty, these bars can be assembled
in various combinations to fit any bath or shower.

150 P.T. Rail
Maxi Aids
42 Executive Blvd.
Farmingdale, NY 11735-4710   631-752-0521
800-522-6294
Fax: 631-752-0689
TTY: 631-752-0738
sales@maxiaids.com
www.maxiaids.com

Elliot Zaretsky, Founder, President & CEO
Wall-mounted support rail for safer transfer to and from the toilet.
Left side and right side rails available.

151 Portable Shampoo Bowl
JK Designs
4500 Williams Dr.
Suite 212-140
Georgetown, TX 78633- 1332   206-999-8226
info@portableshampoobowl.com
www.portableshampoobowl.com
A bowl designed to allow a person who is in a wheelchair or sitting on a regular chair to shampoo hair; useful for assisted living environments.

152 Prelude
ArjoHuntleigh
2349 W Lake St.
Suite 250
Addison, IL 60101   800-323-1245
us.cc@arjohuntleigh.com
www.arjohuntleigh.us

Joacim Lindoff, President & CEO
Daniel F,,ldt, Chief Financial Officer
Prelude shower cabinet allows patients to be showered in comfort and privacy, at the same time as protecting staff from excessive splashing.

153 Shower Bathtub Mat
Maxi Aids
42 Executive Blvd.
Farmingdale, NY 11735-4710   631-752-0521
800-522-6294
Fax: 631-752-0689
TTY: 631-752-0738
sales@maxiaids.com
www.maxiaids.com

Elliot Zaretsky, Founder, President & CEO
Tub mat provides security against falls in the bath and shower.
$22.95

154 Superior Clear Voice Talking Scale
Independent Living Aids
137 Rano Rd.
Buffalo, NY 14207   716-332-2970
800-537-2118
Fax: 877-498-1482
can-do@independentliving.com
www.independentliving.com
Speaks in a clear voice. Automatically calibrates when stepped on and turns off once weight is announced. Maximum weight of 550 lbs. *$69.95*

155 Suregrip Bathtub Rail
Invacare
1 Invacare Way
Elyria, OH 44035-4190   800-333-6900
www.invacare.com

Matthew E. Monaghan, Chairman of the Board & Chief Executive Officer
Rick A. Cassiday, Senior Vice President & Chief Human Resources Officer
Kathleen P. Leneghan, Senior Vice President & Chief Financial Officer
Compact and versatile, the bars have a soft-touch, contoured, white vinyl gripping area for added safety.

156 Transfer Tub Bench
Arista Surgical Supply Company/AliMed
297 High Street
Dedham, MA 02026-2852   781-329-2900
800-437-2966
Fax: 781-437-2966
customerservice@alimed.com
www.alimed.com

Adam S. Epstein, Chief Executive Officer
Curved padded backrest for comfortable support. Backrest also assists patient during lateral transfer. *$64.00*

157 Tri-Grip Bathtub Rail
Maxi Aids
42 Executive Blvd.
Farmingdale, NY 11735-4710   631-752-0521
800-522-6294
Fax: 631-752-0689
TTY: 631-752-0738
sales@maxiaids.com
www.maxiaids.com

Elliot Zaretsky, Founder, President & CEO
Two gripping heights for easy bathtub entrance or exit. *$54.95*

Bed

158 ASSISTECH Special Needs
42 Executive Blvd.
Farmingdale, NY 11735   631-752-0521
800-522-6294
Fax: 631-752-0689
TTY: 800-281-3555
www.assistech.com
ASSISTECH is a division of Maxi-Aids that sells hearing, visual, and mobility aid devices.

159 Bye-Bye Decubiti Air Mattress Overlay
Rand-Scot, Inc.
209 Christman Drive
Fort Collins, CO 80524   970-484-7967
800-467-7967
Fax: 970-484-3800
info@randscot.com
www.randscot.com

Joel Lerich, Co-Founder
Barbara Lerich, Co-Founder
Originally designed for hospital beds, the overlay converts any bed into a therapeutic flotation unit when used between the conventional mattress and pad. The complete overlay is comprised of five individually inflatable, 100 percent natural rubber, ventilated sections enclosed within separate pockets of a soft fleece cover. Conforms to any configuration of electric or manual beds. The overlay comes in a kit that includes an overlay cover, overlay sections, air pump, and patch kit. *$1588.00*

160 Dual Security Bed Rail
Maxi Aids
42 Executive Blvd.
Farmingdale, NY 11735-4710   631-752-0521
800-522-6294
Fax: 631-752-0689
TTY: 631-752-0738
sales@maxiaids.com
www.maxiaids.com

Elliot Zaretsky, Founder, President & CEO
Bed safety rails for the injured or elderly to help getting in and out of bed, and to prevent falling out of bed. The rails are made of steel with a powder coat. *$150.00*

161 Foam Decubitus Bed Pads
Profex Medical Products
P.O. Box 140188
Memphis, TN 38114   800-325-0196
Fax: 901-454-9850
customercare@ProfexMed.com
www.profexmed.com

Robert Gates Watel, Founder
Convoluted foam provides extra back support and comfort for wheelchair users.

162   **Hard Manufacturing Company**
230 Grider Street
Buffalo, NY 14215   800-873-4273
                                            www.hardmfg.com
Manufacturer of pediatric cribs and age-appropriate youth beds.

163   **Hausmann Industries**
130 Union Street
Northvale, NJ 07647   201-767-0255
                                               888-428-7626
                                          info@hausmann.com
                                              hausmann.com
David Hausmann, Chief Executive Officer
Lori Picano, Sales & Marketing Administrator
Wheelchair accessible exam tables, treatment tables and mat platforms. Hausmann Industries has been in the healthcare sector for over 60 years.

164   **Home Bed Side Helper**
Maxi Aids
42 Executive Blvd.
Farmingdale, NY 11735-4710   631-752-0521
                                               800-522-6294
                                          Fax: 631-752-0689
                                          TTY: 631-752-0738
                                         sales@maxiaids.com
                                            www.maxiaids.com
Elliot Zaretsky, Founder, President & CEO
The rail attaches to home bed frames and provides support for those who require assistance getting in and out of bed. *$149.95*

165   **SleepSafe Beds**
3629 Reed Creek Drive
Bassett, VA 24055   276-627-0088
                                               866-852-2337
                                          Fax: 276-627-0234
                              SleepSafeBed@SleepSafeBed.com
                                         www.sleepsafebed.com
Gregg Weinschreider, President
Edward Hettig, Marketing Director
Rachel Markwood, Marketing Director
Perfect for adult home or home care use. SleepSafe offers twin or full size bed frames in classic style. The beds offer an attractive alternative to a hospital bed. SleepSafe beds keeps the user safe during rest and electrically adjusts smoothly for user comfort and caregiver ease of use.

166   **Sonic Alert Alarm Clock with Bed Shaker**
ASSISTECH
42 Executive Blvd.
Farmingdale, NY 11735   631-752-0521
                                               800-522-6294
                                          Fax: 631-752-0689
                                          TTY: 800-281-3555
                                            www.assistech.com
A vibrator that is put under the pillow or between the mattress and box spring that helps to wake heavy sleepers or individuals who are hard of hearing and/or have hearing impairments. The Sonic Alert Alarm Clock features a large and easy-to-read display. *$47.95*

167   **iLuv SmartShaker 2**
ASSISTECH
42 Executive Blvd.
Farmingdale, NY 11735   631-752-0521
                                               800-522-6294
                                          Fax: 631-752-0689
                                          TTY: 800-281-3555
                                            www.assistech.com
The iLuv SmartShaker 2 is a smartphone-controlled bed shaker for individuals with hearing loss. The alarm comes with three vibration settings and works with a variety of smartphones. *$29.99*

Communication

168   **Accent 1400**
Prentke Romich Company
1022 Heyl Road
Wooster, OH 44691   330-262-1984
                                               800-262-1984
                                          Fax: 330-263-4829
                                        info@prc-saltillo.com
                                            www.prentrom.com
Dave Hershberger, President & CEO
Barry Romich, Co-Founder
A portable electronic communication device that uses Minspeak so that symbols are used to represent words, sentences, or phrases. Accent 1400 can be accessed by touching the screen or optical/head tracking. Other versions of the Accent are also available. *$7595.00*

169   **Access Control Systems: NHX Nurse Call System**
Aiphone Corporation
6670 185th Ave NE
Redmond, WA 98052   425-455-0510
                                               800-692-0200
                                          Fax: 800-525-3372
                                           info@aiphone.com
                                            www.aiphone.com
Toshiki Yamazaki, President/CEO
AIPHONE manufactures audio and video intercom systems for home or business to help the physically disabled answer doors and communicate through physical barriers; also ADA-compliant emergency call intercom stations for use in public facilities and an Environmental Control System for persons with limited mobility. NHX Nurse Call System provides staff alert in nursing homes, assisted-living facilities, clinics, wards, and hospitals.

170   **Adaptek Systems**
14224 Plank Street
Fort Wayne, IN 46818   260-637-8660
                                          Fax: 260-637-8597
                                      sales@adapteksystems.com
                                         www.adapteksystems.com
Developers of a voice output module designed to work with the Kurzweil voice-recognition system. The device provides voice output of what the computer hears for persons with visual impairments.

171   **Amplified Handsets**
HARC Mercantile
5413 S Westnedge Ave.
Suite A
Portage, MI 49002   800-445-9968
                                          TTY: 269-324-1615
                                              info@harc.com
                                               www.harc.com
Michael Martinson, Owner
Amplified handsets are phones for individuals who are hard of hearing. The phones are louder than other headsets, and can also include extra loud ringers, larger press keypads, and designated speed dial buttons.

172   **Amplified Phones**
HARC Mercantile
5413 S Westnedge Ave.
Suite A
Portage, MI 49002   800-445-9968
                                          TTY: 269-324-1615
                                              info@harc.com
                                               www.harc.com
Michael Martinson, Owner
Amplified phones are phones for individuals who are hard of hearing. Amplified phones enhance and/or amplify sound, and can have a low frequency ringer, an indicator light, and lighted easy-to-read dial pads.

173 Amplified Portable Phone
HARC Mercantile
5413 S Westnedge Ave.
Suite A
Portage, MI 49002   800-445-9968
                                    TTY: 269-324-1615
                                       info@harc.com
                                        www.harc.com

Michael Martinson, Owner
Cordless phones with amplified or enhanced sound for individuals with hearing loss.

174 Assistive Technology
Tobii Dynavox
2100 Wharton Street
Suite 400
Pittsburgh, PA 15203   800-344-1778
                                    Fax: 866-804-1267
                                         www.tobii.com

Anand Srivatsa, Chief Executive Officer
Magdalena Rodell Andersson, Chief Financial Officer & Vice President
Ann Emilson, Executive Vice President, Sales & Marketing
A premiere developer of innovative touch and eye-tracking technology solutions for people with physical and learning disabilities. Breakthrough products enable people of all ages and abilities to live and learn independently. Supportive material for teachers, clinicians, and those with disabilities.

175 Big Red Switch
AbleNet, Inc.
2625 Patton Road
Roseville, MN 55113-1137   651-294-2200
                                          800-322-0956
                          customerservice@ablenetinc.com
                                     www.ablenetinc.com

Jennifer Thalhuber, President & CEO
Paul Sugden, CFO & Trustee
Five inches across the top and activates no matter where on its surface it is touched. It is made of shatterproof plastic and contains a cord storage compartment. The Big Red Switch provides auditory, visual, and tactile feedback. Also available in green, yellow, and blue.

176 Closed Caption Decoder
HARC Mercantile
5413 S Westnedge Ave.
Suite A
Portage, MI 49002   800-445-9968
                                    TTY: 269-324-1615
                                       info@harc.com
                                        www.harc.com

Michael Martinson, Owner
Provides closed captions for TV programs, with text displayed as white letters on a black background. *$50.00*

177 Cornell Communications
7915 North 81st Street
Milwaukee, WI 53223   414-351-4660
                                          800-558-8957
                                    Fax: 414-351-4657
                                        www.cornell.com

Cornell's Rescue Assistance Systems allow personnel to request emergency assistance. Applications include handicapped evacuations, parking garages, and elevators. Voice, intercom, and visual only signaling systems are available.

178 Harc Mercantile, Ltd.
HARC Mercantile
5413 S Westnedge Ave.
Suite A
Portage, MI 49002   800-445-9968
                                    TTY: 269-324-1615
                                       info@harc.com
                                        www.harc.com

Michael Martinson, Owner
HARC sells assistive devices for the hard of hearing and deaf, such as amplified telephones, personal amplifiers, personal and large area fm systems, induction hearing loops, signaling systems for wake-up, smoke/fire door and telephone, and hearing aid batteries and supplies.

179 InfoLoop Induction Receiver
HARC Mercantile
5413 S Westnedge Ave.
Suite A
Portage, MI 49002   800-445-9968
                                    TTY: 269-324-1615
                                       info@harc.com
                                        www.harc.com

Michael Martinson, Owner
Sound-induction receiver to be used with any loop system (a length of wire around the perimeter of a room and connected to an amplifier). *$99.00*

180 Large Button Speaker Phone
HARC Mercantile
5413 S Westnedge Ave.
Suite A
Portage, MI 49002   800-445-9968
                                    TTY: 269-324-1615
                                       info@harc.com
                                        www.harc.com

Michael Martinson, Owner
HARC Mercantile amplified phones have large, easy-to-read buttons for individuals who have visual impairments. Most phones also have a speakerphone option.

181 Metropolitan Washington Ear
12061 Tech Rd.
Silver Spring, MD 20904   301-681-6636
                                    Fax: 301-625-1986
                         information@washear.org
                                       www.washear.org

Terry Pacheco, President
Amir Rahimi, Secretary
John F. Anderschat, Treasurer
Multi-media reading service for the blind and visually impaired. Offering 24-hour audio radio reading, dial-in newspapers and webcasting, as well as audio description at theaters, museums and films.

182 Microloop III Basic
HARC Mercantile
5413 S Westnedge Ave.
Suite A
Portage, MI 49002   800-445-9968
                                    TTY: 269-324-1615
                                       info@harc.com
                                        www.harc.com

Michael Martinson, Owner
Home induction loop amplifier for use with hearing aids equipped with T-Coil. Small and compact, the Microloop is also suitable for use in a vehicle. *$198.00*

183 MyAlert Body Worn Multifunction Receiver
HARC Mercantile
5413 S Westnedge Ave.
Suite A
Portage, MI 49002   800-445-9968
                                    TTY: 269-324-1615
                                       info@harc.com
                                        www.harc.com

Michael Martinson, Owner
Composed of a small wireless personal device that receives coded signals and a group of transmitters that send them. Transmitters can send alert signals for telephone, smartphone, door, and window. *$39.00*

184 PLA240 Room Loop System
HARC Mercantile
5413 S Westnedge Ave.
Suite A
Portage, MI 49002   800-445-9968
                                    TTY: 269-324-1615
                                       info@harc.com
                                        www.harc.com

Michael Martinson, Owner
Helps hearing aid users listen to TV or audio equipment via the "T" or "Loop" programs of their hearing aids. *$325.00*

185 Personal FM Systems
HARC Mercantile
5413 S Westnedge Ave.
Suite A
Portage, MI 49002

800-445-9968
TTY: 269-324-1615
info@harc.com
www.harc.com

Michael Martinson, Owner
Wireless FM systems transmit sound via a radio carrier wave.

186 Phone Ringers
HARC Mercantile
5413 S Westnedge Ave.
Suite A
Portage, MI 49002

800-445-9968
TTY: 269-324-1615
info@harc.com
www.harc.com

Michael Martinson, Owner
Uses loud ringers and/or bright flashers to signal phone rings and messages.

187 Phone Strobe Flasher
Independent Living Aids
137 Rano Rd.
Buffalo, NY 14207

716-332-2970
800-537-2118
Fax: 877-498-1482
can-do@independentliving.com
www.independentliving.com

Once the phone is plugged into the Phone Strobe Flasher, the light will flash with each ring, alerting individials that there is a phone call. *$23.95*

188 Pocketalker Personal Amplifier
HARC Mercantile
5413 S Westnedge Ave.
Suite A
Portage, MI 49002

800-445-9968
TTY: 269-324-1615
info@harc.com
www.harc.com

Michael Martinson, Owner
Amplifies sounds and voices for better understanding.

189 Prentke Romich Company
1022 Heyl Road
Wooster, OH 44691

330-262-1984
800-262-1984
Fax: 330-263-4829
info@prentrom.com
www.prentrom.com

Dave Hershberger, President & CEO
Barry Romich, Co-Founder
The Prentke Romich Company is a full-service company offering easy yet powerful communication aids. The company believes in supporting customers before and after the sale by providing funding assistance, distance learning training, extended warranty, service assistance, etc.

190 Silent Call Communications
5095 Williams Lake Rd.
Waterford, MI 48329

800-572-5227
TTY: 800-572-5227
customerservice@silentcall.com
www.silentcall.com

George J. Elwell, President
Diana Elwell, President
Lisa DeLeuil, Director of Sales & Marketing
Alerting devices such as paging systems and smoke detectors for deaf and deaf-blind people.

191 Sonic Alert
Harris Communications
15155 Technology Dr
Eden Prairie, MN 55344

800-825-6758
Fax: 952-906-1099
TTY: 952-388-2152
info@harriscomm.com
www.harriscomm.com

Ray Harris, CEO
Offers visual alerting devices that provide safety and convenience by turning vital sound into flashing light: telephone ring signalers, doorbell signalers, baby cry signalers, and wake up alarms. Free catalog available.

192 Speech Adjust-A-Tone Basic
Maxi Aids
42 Executive Blvd.
Farmingdale, NY 11735-4710

631-752-0521
800-522-6294
Fax: 631-752-0689
TTY: 631-752-0738
sales@maxiaids.com
www.maxiaids.com

Elliot Zaretsky, Founder, President & CEO
Speech Adjust-A-Tone improves speech amplification for use with telephone, TV, radio, tape recorder, or computer sound card. *$155.00*

193 Step-by-Step Communicator
AbleNet, Inc.
2625 Patton Road
Roseville, MN 55113-1137

651-294-2200
800-322-0956
Fax: 651-294-2259
customerservice@ablenetinc.com
www.ablenetinc.com

Jennifer Thalhuber, President & CEO
Paul Sugden, CFO & Trustee
Allows individuals to record a series of messages for later communication. It has a 2 1/2 inches diameter switch surface and is 3 inches at its tallest point. The Step-by-Step Communicator includes 2 minutes of record time, and comes in yellow, green, blue, or red.

194 TTYs: Telephone Device for the Deaf
HARC Mercantile
5413 S Westnedge Ave.
Suite A
Portage, MI 49002

800-445-9968
TTY: 269-324-1615
info@harc.com
www.harc.com

Michael Martinson, Owner
A telecommunications device for individuals who are deaf. The device is a teleprinter that creates text communication over a telephone line. *$239.00*

195 TalkTrac Wearable Communicator
AbleNet, Inc.
2625 Patton Road
Roseville, MN 55113-1137

651-294-2200
800-322-0956
Fax: 651-294-2259
customerservice@ablenetinc.com
www.ablenetinc.com

Jennifer Thalhuber, President & CEO
Paul Sugden, CFO & Trustee
The TalkTrac Wearable Communicator is a personal, portable communication aid that is wearable on the wrist. TalkTrac features simple to use, 80 seconds of recording time, as well as four message locations, rechargeable battery, water resistant coating, and adjustable band. *$145.00*

196 Talking Calculators
ASSISTECH
42 Executive Blvd.
Farmingdale, NY 11735

631-752-0521
800-522-6294
Fax: 631-752-0689
TTY: 800-281-3555
www.assistech.com

17

Calculators for blind and low vision users that announce numbers and calculation results.

197 Talking Watches
Maxi Aids
42 Executive Blvd.
Farmingdale, NY 11735-4710

631-752-0521
800-522-6294
Fax: 631-752-0689
TTY: 631-752-0738
sales@maxiaids.com
www.maxiaids.com

Elliot Zaretsky, Founder, President & CEO
Digital display watches that announce the time at the touch of a button.

198 Unity Language System
Prentke Romich Company
1022 Heyl Road
Wooster, OH 44691

330-262-1984
800-262-1984
Fax: 330-263-4829
info@prentrom.com
www.prentrom.com

Dave Hershberger, President & CEO
Barry Romich, Co-Founder
A Minspeak application program designed for adolescent and adult individuals with developmental disabilities and associated learning difficulties. The software is used with Prentke Romich Company augmentative communication devices.

199 Voice Amplified Handsets
HARC Mercantile
5413 S Westnedge Ave.
Suite A
Portage, MI 49002

800-445-9968
TTY: 269-324-1615
info@harc.com
www.harc.com

Michael Martinson, Owner
Designed for the person who has a weak speaking voice. Control increases the level of the user's voice and can increase as much as 30%.

Chairs

200 Adjustable Chair
Bailey Manufacturing Company
P.O. Box 130
Lodi, OH 44254-0130

330-948-1080
800-321-8372
Fax: 330-948-4439
baileymfg@baileymfg.com
www.baileymfg.com

The seat and footboard of this versatile chair can be adjusted to accommodate children of various sizes. A classroom-suitable variation of this model is also available.

201 Adjustable Clear Acrylic Tray
Bailey Manufacturing Company
P.O. Box 130
Lodi, OH 44254-0130

330-948-1080
800-321-8372
Fax: 330-948-4439
baileymfg@baileymfg.com
www.baileymfg.com

An clear tray that adjusts for heigh and depth, and is equipped with a spill rim for easy to clean edges.

202 Adjustable Tee Stool
Bailey Manufacturing Company
P.O. Box 130
Lodi, OH 44254-0130

330-948-1080
800-321-8372
Fax: 330-948-4439
baileymfg@baileymfg.com
www.baileymfg.com

May be used to encourage balance as well as develop integrative and perceptual motor skills. The stool has five adjustable height ranges.

203 BackSaver
BackSaver Products Company
3000 East Imperial Highway
Lynwood, CA 90262

310-661-3044
800-251-2225
www.backsaver.com

A recliner desinged to relieve the pressure on the spine and reduce muscle tension. The recliner aids in expanding lung capacity, increasing circulation, and increasing blood oxygen levels.
$1999.00

204 Carendo
Arjo Inc
2349 West Lake Street
Suite 250
Addison, IL 60101

800-323-1245
888-594-2756
www.arjo.com

Joacim Lindoff, President & CEO
The Carendo hygiene chair has been designed for caregivers. The chair is battery powered, and allows for easy access to most parts of the body for sensitive hygiene tasks. Its innovative, ergonomic design makes for better grooming and hygiene routines.

205 Century Bath System
Arjo Inc
2349 West Lake Street
Suite 250
Addison, IL 60101

800-323-1245
888-594-2756
www.arjo.com

Joacim Lindoff, President & CEO
This bathing system is used with a hygiene lift chair and has a built-in cleaning/disinfectant injection system with adjustable flowmeter. The incorporation of an automatic hot water alarm/shut-off system, and digital temperature monitors, helps to assure resident safety and comfort.

206 Convert-Able Table
REAL Design
187 S. Main St.
Dolgeville, NY 13329

315-429-3071
800-696-7041
rdesign@twcny.rr.com
www.realdesigninc.com

Sam Camardello, Owner
Kris Wohnsen, Vice President
This table has push button height adjustment and interchangeable tops so it can become a desk, art easel, or a sensory stimulation bowl.

207 Drive DeVilbiss Healthcare
99 Seaview Boulevard
Port Washington, NY 11050

877-224-0946
Fax: 516-998-4601
customerSupport@drivemedical.com
www.drivemedical.com

Derek Lampbert, Chief Executive Officer
Jeffrey Schwartz, Executive Vice President, Commerical Operations
Nora Coleman, Executive Vice President, General Counsel
Supplies durable medical equipment, including those dealing with mobility, wheelchairs, beds and sleeping surfaces, personal care products, and electrotherapy devices. Company's goals are to promote independence and improve people's quality of life.

208 Evac + Chair Emergency Evacuation Chair
Evac + Chair North America LLC
3000 Marcus Ave.
Suite 3E6
Lake Success, NY 11042-1012

516-502-4240
Fax: 516-327-8220
sales@evac-chair.com
www.evac-chair.com

David Egen, Founder
Gravity-driven evaluation chair allows one nondisabled person to smoothly glide a seated passenger down fire stairs and across landings to exit on a combination of wheels and track belts. Pivots

in own width for tight landing turns. Features include ability to compactly store on wall mount, a maximum capacity of 400 pounds, and braking features. No installation needed and works on all fire exit stairs.

209 Golden Technologies
401 Bridge Street
Old Forge, PA 18518   570-451-7477
                                               800-624-6374
                                           Fax: 800-628-5165
                                           www.goldentech.com

Richard Golden, CEO
Robert Golden, Chair
Fred Kiwak, Vice President, Research & Development
The largest facility in the world dedicated to the manufacture of lift chairs, scooters, and power chairs.

210 High-Low Chair
REAL Design
187 S. Main St.
Dolgeville, NY 13329   315-429-3071
                                               800-696-7041
                                           rdesign@twcny.rr.com
                                           www.realdesigninc.com

Sam Camardello, Owner
Kris Wohnsen, Vice President
A high chair and mobile floor sitter in one. The High-Low Chair comes with colorful upholstered wipe clean seat and height adjustable tray. The chair has a single lever adjustment to change the seat height. Lateral and head supports are available as options. *$ 1720.00*

211 Ladybug Corner Chair
REAL Design
187 S. Main St.
Dolgeville, NY 13329   315-429-3071
                                               800-696-7041
                                           rdesign@twcny.rr.com
                                           www.realdesigninc.com

Sam Camardello, Owner
Kris Wohnsen, Vice President
For children 0-3 years. This chair is adjustable for long leg or conventional sitting positions. The back can also be removed for independent sitting. The Ladybug Chair is upholstered in padded vinyl, and includes an H-strap harness, hip belt, abductor, and removable tray.

212 Lumex Recliner
Graham-Field Health Products
One Graham-Field Way
Atlanta, GA 30340-4700   770-368-4700
                                           Fax: 770-368-4932
                                           cs@grahamfield.com
                                           www.grahamfield.com

Kenneth Spett, President & CEO
Cherie Antoniazzi, Senior Vice President, Quality, Regulatory & Risk Management
Marc Bernstein, Senior Vice President, Consumer Sales
A recliner designed to improve the mobility of residents in extended care facilities. This chair combines therapeutic benefits of position change with attractive appearance.

213 Prime Engineering
Prime Engineering
4202 W Sierra Madre Ave.
Fresno, CA 93722   559-276-0991
                                               800-827-8263
                                           Fax: 800-800-3355
                                           info@primeengineering.com
                                           www.primeengineering.com

Bruce Boegel, CFO
Mary Boegel, President
Mark Allen, Vice President
Prime Engineering is a leading manufacturer of adult and pediatric standing devices and patient transfer equipment. Products include Superstand HLT, Granstand III MSS Standing System, Kidstand III MSS Standing System, Superstand Standing System, Symmetry Youth Standing Systen, UpRite Standing System, and the Symmetry Standing System.

214 Rifton Equipment
P.O. Box 260
Rifton, NY 12471-0260   845-658-7750
                                               800-571-8198
                                           Fax: 845-658-7751
                                           sales@rifton.com
                                           www.rifton.com

A leader in manufacturing furniture and equipment for children with special needs.

215 Roll Chair
Bailey Manufacturing Company
P.O. Box 130
Lodi, OH 44254-0130   330-948-1080
                                               800-321-8372
                                           Fax: 330-948-4439
                                           baileymfg@baileymfg.com
                                           www.baileymfg.com

A chair with a padded roll seat that helps maintain proper hip abduction and prevents scissoring of the legs.

216 Safari Tilt
Convaid
2830 California Street
Torrance, CA 90503   888-266-8243
                                           Fax: 310-618-2166
                                           convaidsales.us@etac.com
                                           www.convaid.com

Chris Braun, President
A semi-contour seat provides positioning with 5-45 degree tilt adjustment. One step design folds compactly into a lightweight chair.

217 Transfer Bench with Back
Invacare
1 Invacare Way
Elyria, OH 44035-4190   800-333-6900
                                           www.invacare.com

Matthew E. Monaghan, Chairman of the Board & Chief Executive Officer
Rick A. Cassiday, Senior Vice President & Chief Human Resources Officer
Kathleen P. Leneghan, Senior Vice President & Chief Financial Officer
A shower bench with back rest designed to help individuals get in and out of the bathtub. Features a textured seat with drain holes, built-in soap dish, and hand-held shower holder. *$268.84*

Cushions & Wedges

218 Action Products
954 Sweeney Dr.
Hagerstown, MD 21740   301-797-1414
                                               800-228-7763
                                           service@actionproducts.com
                                           www.actionproducts.com

Mistie Witt, President
Janet Kaplan, Marketing Director
Wheelchair pads, mattress pads, positioning cushions, and insoles that aid in the prevention and cure of pressure sores by reducing pressure. All products are made of Akton viscoelastic polymer that does not leak, flow, or bottom out. Manufacturer of the Xact line of positioning cushions for patients with high risk of skin breakdown.

219 Adjustable Wedge
Bailey Manufacturing Company
P.O. Box 130
Lodi, OH 44254-0130   330-948-1080
                                               800-321-8372
                                           Fax: 330-948-4439
                                           baileymfg@baileymfg.com
                                           www.baileymfg.com

Orthopedically and neurologically disabled children can freely move arms and hands while lying on this adjustable wedge.

220 Back-Huggar Pillow
Bodyline Comfort Systems
3730 Kori Rd.
Jacksonville, FL 32257   904-262-4068
                               800-874-7715
                          Fax: 800-323-2225
                          info@bodyline.com
                          www.bodyline.com

Dr. John W. Fiore, Owner
Exclusive design makes almost any seat more comfortable by exerting soothing pressure against back muscles and discs. *$32.95*

221 Bye-Bye Decubiti (BBD)
Rand-Scot, Inc.
209 Christman Drive
Fort Collins, CO 80524   970-484-7967
                                800-467-7967
                           Fax: 970-484-3800
                           info@randscot.com
                           www.randscot.com

Joel Lerich, Co-Founder
Barbara Lerich, Co-Founder
The BBD therapeutic wheelchair cushions have been market-proven since 1951 in the prevention and cure of pressure sores (decubiti). These natural rubber inflatable products have recently been expanded to include pediatric, sports, and double-valve models.

222 Dynamic Systems, Inc.
Dynamic Systems, Inc.
104 Morrow Branch Road
Leicester, NC 28748   828-683-3523
                             855-786-6283
                        Fax: 844-270-6478
                        dsi@sunmatecushions.com
                        www.sunmatecushions.com

Mardi Norman, President & CEO
Dynamic Systems, Inc. manufactures high-performance, medical-grade, orthopedic cushion materials for applications where pressure relief, body support, and skin health are critical. Molding seat inserts.

223 Geo-Matt for High Risk Patients
Span-America Medical Systems
70 Commerce Ctr
Greenville, SC 29615   864-288-8877
                              800-888-6752
                         Fax: 864-288-8692
                         www.spanamerica.com

James Ferguson, President & CEO
Provides a line of healthcare products concerned with pressure management and patient positioning, including therapeutic mattress systems, overlay and seat cushions, wound-care seating, and skincare. Helps prevent pressure sores in high-risk patients.

224 Inflatable Back Pillow
Corflex Inc.
669 East Industrial Park Dr
Manchester, NH 03109-5625   603-623-3344
                                   800-426-7353
                              Fax: 603-623-4111
                              sales@corflex.com
                              www.corflex.com

Paul Lorenzetti, President & CEO
Corflex specializes in orthopedic rehabilitation products. ReFolds flat to fit into its own carrying case, this inflatable back pillow ensures comfort while at home or traveling.

225 Jobri
Jobri
510 Fountain Pkwy
Grand Prairie, TX 75050   972-641-9680
                          Sales@AlexOrthopedic.com
                          www.jobri.com

Brian Gourley, CEO
Jobri manufactures ergonomic back supports, ergonomic chairs, orthopedic soft goods and sleep products.

226 Lumbar Cushions
Graham-Field Health Products
One Graham-Field Way
Atlanta, GA 30340-3140   770-368-4700
                           Fax: 770-368-4932
                           cs@grahamfield.com
                           www.grahamfield.com

Kenneth Spett, President & CEO
Cherie Antoniazzi, Senior Vice President, Quality, Regulatory & Risk Management
Marc Bernstein, Senior Vice President, Consumer Sales
Line of cushions and pillows give comfort and independence to the physically challenged.

227 Medpro Static Air Chair Cushion
Medpro
1950 Rutgers Blvd
Lakewood, NJ 08701-4537   732-905-9001
                                 800-257-5145
                            Fax: 732-905-9899

Jody Gorran, President
Provides a protective layer of air beneath the patient helping prevent and treat pressure ulcers. *$94.95*

228 Medpro Static Air Mattress Overlay
Medpro
1950 Rutgers Blvd
Lakewood, NJ 08701-4537   732-905-9001
                                 800-257-5145
                            Fax: 732-905-9899

Jody Gorran, President
Supports the patient on a cushioned network of air designed to redistribute the patient's weight reducing tissue interface pressure. Medpro's design incorporates a series of 65 air-breather vents that maintain air circulation. Medpro effectively reduces pressure and helps prevent and treat pressure ulcers. *$164.95*

229 Silicone Padding
Spenco Medical Group
P.O.Box 2501
Waco, TX 76702-2501   254-772-6000
                             800-877-3626
                        spenco@spenco.com
                        www.spenco.com

For the management of pressure sores, this padding provides a special support system which allows even distribution of pressure and cool, comfortable, well-ventilated support.

230 Spenco Medical Group
Spenco Medical Group
P.O.Box 2501
Waco, TX 76702-2501   254-772-6000
                             800-877-3626
                        spenco@spenco.com
                        www.spenco.com

Wheelchair cushions, silicone mattress pads, wound dressings, second skin blister and burn pads, polysorb insoles, elbow, knee and wrist supports and walking shoes.

231 Stryker
2825 Airview Boulevard
Kalamazoo, MI 49002   269-385-2600
                        Fax: 269-385-1062
                        www.stryker.com/us/en/about.html
Kevin A. Lobo, Chair & CEO
Yin C. Becker, Vice President & Chief Corporate Affairs Officer
William E. Berry Jr., Vice President & Chief Accounting Officer
Leader in medical technology companies, with the drive to improve healthcare. Provides services and products in Orthopaedics, Medical and Surgical, and Neurotechnology and Spine.

232 Sun-Mate Seat Cushions
Dynamic Systems, Inc.
104 Morrow Branch Road
Leicester, NC 28748   828-683-3523
                             855-786-6283
                        Fax: 844-270-6478
                        dsi@sunmatecushions.com
                        www.sunmatecushions.com

Mardi Norman, President & CEO

Line of cushions, pads and accessory items for personal comfort of the disabled. SunMate Orthopedic foam cushions and sheets that contours slowly to give uniform pressure distribution and soft spring back. Liquid SunMate for Foam-in-Place Seating (FIPS) to make custom molded seat inserts.

Dressing Aids

233   Button Aid
Maxi Aids
42 Executive Blvd.
Farmingdale, NY 11735-4710

631-752-0521
800-522-6294
Fax: 631-752-0689
TTY: 631-752-0738
sales@maxiaids.com
www.maxiaids.com

Elliot Zaretsky, Founder, President & CEO
Makes buttoning possible with the use of only one hand. *$10.95*

234   Dressing Stick
Maxi Aids
42 Executive Blvd.
Farmingdale, NY 11735-4710

631-752-0521
800-522-6294
Fax: 631-752-0689
TTY: 631-752-0738
sales@maxiaids.com
www.maxiaids.com

Elliot Zaretsky, Founder, President & CEO
Helps put on coats, sweaters and garments even when arm and shoulder movement is limited. *$16.95*

235   Elastic Shoelaces
Therapro, Inc.
225 Arlington St
Framingham, MA 01702-8723

508-872-9494
800-257-5376
Fax: 508-268-6624
info@therapro.com
www.therapro.com

Karen Conrad Weihrauch, President & Owner
The elastic laces allow the wearer to slip tied shoes on and off. *$8.75*

236   Mirror Go Lightly
AbleNet, Inc.
2625 Patton Road
Roseville, MN 55113-1137

651-294-2200
800-322-0956
Fax: 651-294-2259
customerservice@ablenetinc.com
www.ablenetinc.com

Jennifer Thalhuber, President & CEO
Paul Sugden, CFO & Trustee
Framed in plastic, the mirror can be tilted to provide either a normal or magnified image or to direct its lights at, or away from, the user. *$22.00*

237   Molded Sock and Stocking Aid
Therapro, Inc.
225 Arlington St
Framingham, MA 01702-8723

508-872-9494
800-257-5376
Fax: 508-268-6624
info@therapro.com
www.therapro.com

Karen Conrad Weihrauch, President & Owner
Sock or stocking is pulled over the molded plastic and then can be put on more easily. *$13.00*

238   Say What Clothing Identifier
Maxi Aids
42 Executive Blvd.
Farmingdale, NY 11735-4710

631-752-0521
800-522-6294
Fax: 631-752-0689
TTY: 631-752-0738
sales@maxiaids.com
www.maxiaids.com

Elliot Zaretsky, Founder, President & CEO
Braille the tag with information that the wearer wants on the tag and place the tag on a hanger. The custom-identification program makes it easier for the user to remember and identify the right clothes. *$4.95*

239   Shoe Horn and Sock Remover
Maxi Aids
42 Executive Blvd.
Farmingdale, NY 11735-4710

631-752-0521
800-522-6294
Fax: 631-752-0689
TTY: 631-752-0738
sales@maxiaids.com
www.maxiaids.com

Elliot Zaretsky, Founder, President & CEO
Helps with the removal of socks and shoes. Designed for those with arthritic or weak hands. Easily assembled and taken apart. The handle is 28" (13.75" when disassembled). *$11.95*

Health Aids

240   AMI
Aqua Massage International
P.O.Box 808
Groton, CT 06340-0808

860-536-3735
800-248-4031
Fax: 860-536-4362
sales@aquamassage.com
www.aquamassage.com

The Aqua PT provides the major benefits of Hydrotherapy, Massage Therapy and Dry Heat Therapy. 36 water jets provide continuous full body or localized massage while the user remains clothed and dry. Adjustable water pressure, temperature and pulsation frequency can massage in either a two direction travel mode for musculoskeletal pain management or a one direction mode, flowing water from head to foot for a contrast massage-relax therapy.

241   American Medical Industries
EZ Healthcare
19550 N. 10th Street
Covington, LA 70433

504-717-4884
www.ezhealthcare.com

Rick Martin, CEO
Software solutions that allow for healthcare providers to cut back on operational expenses through the automation of office procedures. Tailored to physicians in managing office practices and procedures.

242   BIPAP S/T Ventilatory Support System
Respironics
1010 Murry Ridge Ln
Murrysville, PA 15668-8517

724-733-0200
www.respironics.com

John L. Miclot, CEO
Gerald McGinnis, Chair
Daniel Bevevino, Vice President & CFO
Respironics, a recognized resource in the medical device market, provides innovative products and unique designs to the health care provider while helping them to grow and manage their business efficiently. As a global leader in the sleep and respiratory fields, Respironics provides innovative products that deal with sleep apnea management, oxygen therapy, noninvasive ventilation, and respiratory drug delivery.

243   Coast to Coast Home Medical
Coast to Coast Home Medical
100 Waldron Rd.
Fall River, MA 02720   774-888-1000
                                             c2cmed.com

Keri Suess, Owner
Home-delivered medical supplies for diabetes, respiratory, arthritis and impotence.

244   Compass Health
6753 Engle Road
Middleburg Heights, OH 44130   440-572-1962
                                          800-376-7263
                                      Fax: 440-572-4261
                    corporate@compasshealthbrands.com
                               www.roscoemedical.com
For over 20 years, Compass Health Brands has been offering Pain Management, Respiratory and Home Medical Equipment. Delivers products of high quality in addition to unparalleled personal service.

245   Drew Karol Industries
Drew Karol Industries
633 Highway 1 North
P.O.box 1066
Greenville, MS 38702- 1066   662-378-2188
                                      Fax: 601-378-3188

Andrew K. Hoszowski, Owner
Orally operated toothbrush and dental care system for persons with limited or complete loss of hand or arm use - wheelchair accessible. *$600.00*

246   Duraline Medical Products Inc.
Duraline Medical Products Inc.
P.O.Box 67
324 Werner Street
Leipsic, OH 45856-1039   419-943-2044
                                          800-654-3376
                                      Fax: 419-943-3637
                                  duraline@fairpoint.net
                                     www.dmponline.com
An assortment of quality incontinence products for adults and children.

247   Duro-Med Industries
Duro-Med Industries
128 Rockingham Road
Suite 1
Windham, NH 03087   800-563-0433
                                      Fax: 603-898-9348
                                         hello@hpms.com
            www.hpms.com/Duro-Med-Industries-s/184.htm
Mike Mazza, President
Tony D'Antonio, Senior Vice President of Sales
Alan Yefsky, Exec Vice President, Sales & Marketing
Manufacturers of a complete line of home health care products. Featured products are patient gowns, back and seat cushions, pillows and a complete line of aids for daily living.

248   Ekso Bionics
1414 Harbour Way S.
Suite 1201
Richmond, CA 94804   510-984-1761
                                  hello@eksobionics.com
                                         eksobionics.com

Steven Sherman, Chairman & CEO
Scott Davis, President & COO
Jack CFO, CFO
Develops and manufactures exoskeleton solutions to enhance the mobility of users with paralysis. Provides research for the U.S. defense capabilities.

249   Electronic Amplified Stethoscopes
HARC Mercantile
5413 S Westnedge Ave.
Suite A
Portage, MI 49002   800-445-9968
                                     TTY: 269-324-1615
                                          info@harc.com
                                         www.harc.com

Michael Martinson, Owner

A stethoscope designed for hearing aid users. Amplifies heart, breath, and Korotkoff sounds. *$335.00*

250   Healing Dressing for Pressure Sores
Baxter Healthcare Corporation
1 Baxter Pkwy
Deerfield, IL 60015-4625   224-948-1812
                                          800-422-9837
                                        media@baxter.com
                                         www.baxter.com
Jos, E. Almeida, Chairman, President & CEO
A dressing specifically designed to promote healing of pressure sores and other dermal ulcers.

251   Invacare Corporation
Invacare
1 Invacare Way
Elyria, OH 44035-4190   800-333-6900
                                        www.invacare.com
Matthew E. Monaghan, Chairman of the Board & Chief Executive Officer
Rick A. Cassiday, Senior Vice President & Chief Human Resources Officer
Kathleen P. Leneghan, Senior Vice President & Chief Financial Officer
The world's leading manufacturer and distributor of innovative home and long-term care medical products which promote recovery and active lifestyles.

252   MedDev Corporation
MedDev Corporation
730 N Pastoria Ave
Sunnyvale, CA 94085-3522   408-730-9702
                                          800-543-2789
                                      Fax: 408-730-9732
                                  info@meddev-corp.com
                                   www.meddev-corp.com
Aids to rehabilitate hands following injury or illness, including patented complementary FingerHelper, ThumbHelper and Iso HandHelper models. MedDev also manufactures Soft Touch foam exercisers and the FiddlLink exerciser for digital dexterity. The Ultimate Hand Helper, an ergonomically designed hand exerciser, is curved to conform to the shape of the hand.

253   Osborn Medical Corporation
Osborn Medical Corporation
9800 E. Easter Ave.
Suite 130
Centennial, CO 80112   303-223-1800
                                          800-535-5865
                                      Fax: 507-932-5044
                                   www.rookeproducts.com
Bill Davis, President & CEO
Keith Walli-Ware, Vice President, Sales & Marketing
Strider allows the user to exercise in most chairs found in at home. No more small, uncomfortable bicycle seats to sit on while exercising. A hands-free exercising experience.

254   Talking Digital Cooking Thermometer
Maxi Aids
42 Executive Blvd.
Farmingdale, NY 11735-4710   631-752-0521
                                          800-522-6294
                                      Fax: 631-752-0689
                                     TTY: 631-752-0738
                                     sales@maxiaids.com
                                       www.maxiaids.com
Elliot Zaretsky, Founder, President & CEO
Clearly announces temperature in Fahrenheit or Celsius. *$24.95*

255   Talking Digital Thermometer
Maxi Aids
42 Executive Blvd.
Farmingdale, NY 11735-4710   631-752-0521
                                          800-522-6294
                                      Fax: 631-752-0689
                                     TTY: 631-752-0738
                                     sales@maxiaids.com
                                       www.maxiaids.com

Elliot Zaretsky, Founder, President & CEO

Talking and large print thermometer. Announces and displays temperature in Fahrenheit or Celsius. *$16.95*

256   Thinklabs One Stethoscope
HARC Mercantile
5413 S Westnedge Ave.
Suite A
Portage, MI 49002   800-445-9968
                                  TTY: 269-324-1615
                                      info@harc.com
                                       www.harc.com

Michael Martinson, Owner
Stethoscope that amplifies sounds by more than 100x. Works with any headphones or hearing aid streamer.

Hearing Aids

257   Auditech: Personal PA Value Pack System
Auditech
P.O.Box 510476
St. Louis, MO 63151   314-416-1050
                                      800-669-9065
                               auditecinfo@auditec.com
                                    www.auditec.com

Reliable hearing assistance. This wireless FM system broadcasts to listeners with a hearing assistance system, helping them overcome background noise at a distance from the sound source. *$899.00*

258   Battery Device Adapter
AbleNet, Inc.
2625 Patton Road
Roseville, MN 55113-1137   651-294-2200
                                      800-322-0956
                                  Fax: 651-294-2259
                        customerservice@ablenetinc.com
                                  www.ablenetinc.com

Jennifer Thalhuber, President & CEO
Paul Sugden, CFO & Trustee
A cable which connects to and adapts battery-operated devices for external switch control. Two sizes are available to adapt devices with either AA or C and D size batteries. *$8.00*

259   Cochlear
10350 Park Meadows Drive
Lone Tree, CO 80124   303-790-9010
                                      800-523-5798
                                  Fax: 303-790-1157
                            www.cochlear.com/us/en/home

Dig Howitt, President & CEO
Stuart Sayers, Chief Financial Officer
Jan Janssen, Chief Technology Officer
For over three decades, Cochlear has been delivering hearing implant innovation worldwide. Cochlear helps with the communication of implant recipients.

260   Custom Earmolds
Lloyd Hearing Aid Corporation
P.O.Box 1645
4435 Manchester Drive
Rockford, IL 61109   815-964-4191
                                      800-323-4212
                                  Fax: 815-964-8378
                              info@lloydhearingaid.com
                               www.lloydhearingaid.com

Andrew Palmquist, President
Hearing aid molds, custom built to the exact fit of the customer. *$29.95*

261   Digital Hearing Aids
Lloyd Hearing Aid Corporation
P.O.Box 1645
4435 Manchester Drive
Rockford, IL 61109   815-964-4191
                                      800-323-4212
                                  Fax: 815-964-8378
                              info@lloydhearingaid.com
                               www.lloydhearingaid.com

Andrew Palmquist, President

Latest hearing technology. *$7.50*

262   Duracell & Rayovac Hearing Aid Batteries
Lloyd Hearing Aid Corporation
P.O.Box 1645
4435 Manchester Drive
Rockford, IL 61109   815-964-4191
                                      800-323-4212
                                  Fax: 815-964-8378
                              info@lloydhearingaid.com
                               www.lloydhearingaid.com

Andrew Palmquist, President
Reliable and long-lasting, these batteries power the user's hearing aid. Easy to insert into hearing aid.

263   Harris Communications
Harris Communications
15155 Technology Dr
Eden Prairie, MN 55344   800-825-6758
                                  Fax: 952-906-1099
                                  TTY: 952-388-2152
                                 info@harriscomm.com
                                  www.harriscomm.com

Ray Harris, CEO
A national distributor of assistive devices for the deaf and hard-of-hearing with many manufacturers represented. Catalog includes a wide range of assistive devices as well as a variety of books and video tapes related to deaf and hard-of-hearing issues. Products available for children, teachers, hearing professionals, interpreters and anyone interested in deaf culture, hearing loss and sign language.
180 pages Yearly

264   Hearing Aid Batteries
HARC Mercantile
5413 S Westnedge Ave.
Suite A
Portage, MI 49002   800-445-9968
                                  TTY: 269-324-1615
                                      info@harc.com
                                       www.harc.com

Michael Martinson, Owner
Hearing aid batteries in all popular sizes in mercury, zinc air, silver as well as Nicad and Varta and batteries for electrolarynx and infrared systems.

265   Hearing Aid Battery Testers
HARC Mercantile
5413 S Westnedge Ave.
Suite A
Portage, MI 49002   800-445-9968
                                  TTY: 269-324-1615
                                      info@harc.com
                                       www.harc.com

Michael Martinson, Owner
From pocket size to professional type battery testers which test mercury, zinc air, silver, specialty and general usage batteries. *$7.00*

266   Hearing Aid Care Kit
HARC Mercantile
5413 S Westnedge Ave.
Suite A
Portage, MI 49002   800-445-9968
                                  TTY: 269-324-1615
                                      info@harc.com
                                       www.harc.com

Michael Martinson, Owner
Includes a hearing aid dehumidifer, stethoset, and cleaning tools. *$40.00*

267   MED-EL Corporation, USA
2645 Meridian Parkway
Suite 100
Durham, NC 27713   919-572-2222
                                      888-633-3524
                                  Fax: 919-484-9229
                                    www.medel.com/us

Ingeborg Hochmair, CEO

MED-EL is the leader in implantable hearing solutions. In 2017, the company launched the RONDO 2, a revolutionary cochlear implant powered by wireless charging technology.

268   Micro Audiometrics Corporation
Micro Audiometrics
1901 Mason Ave
Suite 104
Daytona Beach, FL 32117

386-888-7878
866-327-7226
Fax: 866-683-4447
sales@microaud.com
www.microaud.com

Jason Keller, President
Manufacturer and distributor of hearing testing instruments, including the complete line of Earscan.

269   Mushroom Inserts
Lloyd Hearing Aid Corporation
P.O.Box 1645
4435 Manchester Drive
Rockford, IL 61109

815-964-4191
800-323-4212
Fax: 815-964-8378
info@lloydhearingaid.com
www.lloydhearingaid.com

Andrew Palmquist, President
A universal earplug useful in wearing behind the ear type hearing instruments. *$2.50*

270   Oval Window Audio
33 Wildflower Ct
Nederland, CO 80466

303-447-3607
Fax: 303-447-3607
TTY: 303-447-3607
info@ovalwindowaudio.com
www.ovalwindowaudio.com

Norman Lederman, Director of Research & Development
Paula Hendricks, Educational Director
Manufacturer of induction loop hearing assistance technologies compatible with telecoil-equipped hearing aids used by many hard of hearing people. The company also makes multisensory sound systems for use in speech and music therapy and science classes.

271   Sonova USA Inc.
Phonak
4520 Weaver Parkway
Warrenville, IL 60555-3927

800-679-4871
Info@Phonak.com
www.sonova.com/usa/en-us

Provides innovative technology and solutions to every form of hearing loss. Hearing aid brands Sonova carries aside from Phonak are Unitron, Advanced Bionics, and Connect Hearing.

272   Starkey Hearing Foundation
P.O. Box 41514
Minneapolis, MN 55441

866-354-3254
info@starkeyfoundation.org
www.starkeyhearingfoundation.org

Richard S. Brown, President
Brady Forseth, Executive Director
Keith Becker, Senior Director of Operations
The Starkey Hearing Foundation works to assist those with hearing impairments by offering hearing aids and aftercare services.
Quarterly

273   Ultratec
450 Science Dr
Madison, WI 53711

800-482-2424
Fax: 608-204-6167
TTY: 800-482-2424
service@ultratec.com
www.ultratec.com

Jackie Morgan, Marketing Director
Ultratec works to make telephone access more convenient and reliable for people with hearing loss by providing assistive devices such as amplified phones and text phones.

274   Widex USA, Inc.
185 Commerce Drive
Hauppauge, NY 11788

800-221-0188
www.widex.com/en-us

Provider and producer of hearing aids, Widex's design combines technology with functionality and aesthetics.

Kitchen & Eating Aids

275   Bagel Holder
Maxi Aids
42 Executive Blvd.
Farmingdale, NY 11735-4710

631-752-0521
800-522-6294
Fax: 631-752-0689
TTY: 631-752-0738
sales@maxiaids.com
www.maxiaids.com

Elliot Zaretsky, Founder, President & CEO
Holds bagels in place for easy slicing. *$4.95*

276   Big and Bold Low Vision Timer
Maxi Aids
42 Executive Blvd.
Farmingdale, NY 11735-4710

631-752-0521
800-522-6294
Fax: 631-752-0689
TTY: 631-752-0738
sales@maxiaids.com
www.maxiaids.com

Elliot Zaretsky, Founder, President & CEO
Sixty-minute mechanical timer with large, easy-to-read numbers for the visually impaired. *$14.75*

277   Big-Grip Cutlery
Therapro, Inc.
225 Arlington St
Framingham, MA 01702-8723

508-872-9494
800-257-5376
Fax: 508-268-6624
info@therapro.com
www.therapro.com

Karen Conrad Weihrauch, President & Owner
Stainless steel utensils have a special twist built into the metal to facilitate bending of a spoon or fork at any angle for right or left handed people. *$11.95*

278   Box Top Opener
Performance Health
28100 Torch Parkway
Suite 700
Warrenville, IL 60555-3938

630-393-6000
800-323-5547
Fax: 630-547-4333
customersupport@performancehealth.com
www.performancehealth.com

Francis Dirksmeier, Chief Executive Officer
Greg Nulty, Chief Financial Officer
Jim Plewa, Chief Sales Officer
This handy device exerts the pressure on those hard-to-open boxes of laundry/dishwasher soap, rice and prepared dinners. *$2.95*

279   Braille Timer
Maxi Aids
42 Executive Blvd.
Farmingdale, NY 11735-4710

631-752-0521
800-522-6294
Fax: 631-752-0689
TTY: 631-752-0738
sales@maxiaids.com
www.maxiaids.com

Elliot Zaretsky, Founder, President & CEO
Three raised dots at 15, 30 and 45, two raised dots at 0, and one raised dot on all other numbers.

280 Cordless Receiver
AbleNet, Inc.
2625 Patton Road
Roseville, MN 55113-1137   651-294-2200
800-322-0956
Fax: 651-294-2259
customerservice@ablenetinc.com
www.ablenetinc.com
Jennifer Thalhuber, President & CEO
Paul Sugden, CFO & Trustee
The Cordless Receiver in conjunction with the Cordless Big Red Switch, can be used anywhere a switch is currently used to control battery or electrically-operated toys, games or appliances; augmentative communication systems; and computers (through a computer switch interface). *$79.00*

281 Deluxe Roller Knife
Performance Health
28100 Torch Parkway
Suite 700
Warrenville, IL 60555-3938   630-393-6000
Fax: 630-393-7600
customersupport@performancehealth.com
www.performancehealth.com
Francis Dirksmeier, Chief Executive Officer
Greg Nulty, Chief Financial Officer
Jim Plewa, Chief Sales Officer
Stainless steel blade rolls smoothly, cutting food cleanly. *$10.95*

282 Dual Brush with Suction Base
Performance Health
28100 Torch Parkway
Suite 700
Warrenville, IL 60555-3938   630-393-6000
Fax: 630-393-7600
customersupport@performancehealth.com
www.performancehealth.com
Francis Dirksmeier, Chief Executive Officer
Greg Nulty, Chief Financial Officer
Jim Plewa, Chief Sales Officer
Two brushes clean the inside and outside of bottles and glasses at the same time using just one hand. *$14.50*

283 Etac Relieve Angled Table Knife
R82, Inc.
13137 Bleinheim Lane
Matthews, NC 28105   844-876-6245
Fax: 704-882-0751
sales.us@etac.com
www.r82.com
The design of these knives allows a better working posture and makes optimal use of strength in the arms and hands.

284 Folding Pot Stabilizer
Maxi Aids
42 Executive Blvd.
Farmingdale, NY 11735-4710   631-752-0521
800-522-6294
Fax: 631-752-0689
TTY: 631-752-0738
sales@maxiaids.com
www.maxiaids.com
Elliot Zaretsky, Founder, President & CEO
This device holds onto the pot handle and secures the pot in place, allowing for easier use for those with physical challenges. *$35.95*

285 H.E.L.P. Knife
Maxi Aids
42 Executive Blvd.
Farmingdale, NY 11735-4710   631-752-0521
800-522-6294
Fax: 631-752-0689
TTY: 631-752-0738
sales@maxiaids.com
www.maxiaids.com
Elliot Zaretsky, Founder, President & CEO
Adjustable food slicing system guides the knife for even, uniform slices while protecting the user. *$22.95*

286 Innerlip Plates
Therapro, Inc.
225 Arlington St
Framingham, MA 01702-8723   508-872-9494
800-257-5376
Fax: 508-268-6624
info@therapro.com
www.therapro.com
Karen Conrad Weihrauch, President & Owner
Food may be pushed to the side of the plate, then scooped up with a fork and spoon. Available in beige or blue. *$8.50*

287 Long Oven Mitts
Performance Health
28100 Torch Parkway
Suite 700
Warrenville, IL 60555-3938   630-393-6000
Fax: 630-393-7600
customersupport@performancehealth.com
www.performancehealth.com
Francis Dirksmeier, Chief Executive Officer
Greg Nulty, Chief Financial Officer
Jim Plewa, Chief Sales Officer
Protect hands and forearms from heat, flames and oven grates with these practical mitts that allow a longer reach and less bending. *$8.95*

288 Nosey Cup
Therapro, Inc.
225 Arlington St
Framingham, MA 01702-8723   508-872-9494
800-257-5376
Fax: 508-268-6624
info@therapro.com
www.therapro.com
Karen Conrad Weihrauch, President & Owner
For those with a stiff neck or persons who can't tip their head back while drinking. *$5.95*

289 Performance Health
Performance Health
28100 Torch Parkway
Suite 700
Warrenville, IL 60555-3938   630-393-6000
Fax: 630-393-7600
customersupport@performancehealth.com
www.performancehealth.com
Francis Dirksmeier, Chief Executive Officer
Greg Nulty, Chief Financial Officer
Jim Plewa, Chief Sales Officer
Performance Health is a leading provider of rehabilitation and assistive devices to help those with disabilities meet daily physical challenges and achieve their greatest level of independence. With one of the industry's largest catalogs, Sammons Preston Rolyan offers a wide range of products available.
Annually

290 PowerLink 4 Control Unit
AbleNet, Inc.
2625 Patton Road
Roseville, MN 55113-1137   651-294-2200
800-322-0956
Fax: 651-294-2259
customerservice@ablenetinc.com
www.ablenetinc.com
Jennifer Thalhuber, President & CEO
Paul Sugden, CFO & Trustee
The PowerLink 4 Control Unit allows switch operation of electrical appliances. It can be used to activate 1 or 2 appliances (up to 1700 watts combined). If 2 appliances are used, they will activate simultaneously. There are four modes of control on the PowerLink 2; direct mode, timed (seconds) mode, timed (minutes) mode and latch mode. Meets safety standards from Underwriters Laboratory (UL) and Canadian Standards Association (CSA) for electrical appliances. *$330.00*

291 Steel Food Bumper
Maxi Aids
42 Executive Blvd.
Farmingdale, NY 11735-4710   631-752-0521
                                    800-522-6294
                               Fax: 631-752-0689
                               TTY: 631-752-0738
                               sales@maxiaids.com
                               www.maxiaids.com

Elliot Zaretsky, Founder, President & CEO
Provides stable area to push against while eating. *$ 16.95*

292 Stove Knob Turner
Maxi Aids
42 Executive Blvd.
Farmingdale, NY 11735-4710   631-752-0521
                                    800-522-6294
                               Fax: 631-752-0689
                               TTY: 631-752-0738
                               sales@maxiaids.com
                               www.maxiaids.com

Elliot Zaretsky, Founder, President & CEO
Lightweight aluminum rod for turning stove knobs. Designed for wheelchair users. *$34.95*

293 Talking Food Cans
Maxi Aids
42 Executive Blvd.
Farmingdale, NY 11735-4710   631-752-0521
                                    800-522-6294
                               Fax: 631-752-0689
                               TTY: 631-752-0738
                               sales@maxiaids.com
                               www.maxiaids.com

Elliot Zaretsky, Founder, President & CEO
Voice recording device for recording descriptions of hard to identify objects, such as food cans, bottles and storage containers. *$25.95*

294 Undercounter Lid Opener
Performance Health
28100 Torch Parkway
Suite 700
Warrenville, IL 60555-3938   630-393-6000
                               Fax: 630-393-7600
                               customersupport@performancehealth.com
                               www.performancehealth.com

Francis Dirksmeier, Chief Executive Officer
Greg Nulty, Chief Financial Officer
Jim Plewa, Chief Sales Officer
The gripper of this unit which installs under the counter can help unscrew any cap. *$5.75*

295 Uni-Turner
Performance Health
28100 Torch Parkway
Suite 700
Warrenville, IL 60555-3938   630-393-6000
                               Fax: 630-393-7600
                               customersupport@performancehealth.com
                               www.performancehealth.com

Francis Dirksmeier, Chief Executive Officer
Greg Nulty, Chief Financial Officer
Jim Plewa, Chief Sales Officer
Odd-shaped handles can be turned easily with one-handed, L-shaped Uni-Turner. *$16.50*

296 Universal Hand Cuff
Therapro, Inc.
225 Arlington St
Framingham, MA 01702-8723   508-872-9494
                                    800-257-5376
                               Fax: 508-268-6624
                               info@therapro.com
                               www.therapro.com

Karen Conrad Weihrauch, President & Owner
·Comfortable cuff with Velcro strap holds utensils, toothbrushes, etc. Washable and adjustable to the user's condition and hand size. *$8.50*

Lifts, Ramps & Elevators

297 Accessibility Lift
Inclinator Company of America
601 Gibson Blvd
Harrisburg, PA 17104   800-343-9007
                               info@inclinator.com
                               www.inclinator.com

Cliff Warner, President & CEO
Mark Crispen, Director of Marketing, Corporate Secretary & Board Member
Marcia Cleland, Human Resource Manager/Accounting
An economical lift for restricted usage that provides barrier-free access that can be used by churches, schools, lodging halls and meeting halls to meet compliance requirements, with the dignified convenience and freedom they deserve.

298 Adjustable Incline Board
Bailey Manufacturing Company
P.O. Box 130
Lodi, OH 44254-0130   330-948-1080
                                    800-321-8372
                               Fax: 330-948-4439
                               baileymfg@baileymfg.com
                               www.baileymfg.com

Incline board for the physically challenged with a foot board with non-slip tread.

299 AlumiRamp
AlumiRamp, Inc.
855 East Chicago Road
Quincy, MI 49082-9450   517-639-8777
                                    800-800-3864
                               Fax: 517-639-4314
                               sales@alumiramp.com
                               www.alumiramp.com

Doug Cannon, Sales & Customer Service
Complete line of modular, aluminum and portable ramps for both home and vehicle use. Welded construction and non-skid extruded surfaces are featured on all our ramps.

300 Area Access
Area Access
7131 Gateway Court
Manassas, VA 20109-1015   703-396-4949
                               www.areaaccess.com

Serving the entire Mid-Atlantic with scooters, stairway lifts and elevators. Large inventory and fully stocked showrooms.

301 Back-Saver
Bruno Independent Living Aids, Inc.
1780 Executive Dr.
PO Box 84
Oconomowoc, WI 53066   262-567-4990
                                    800-454-4355
                               Fax: 262-953-5501
                               webinfo@bruno.com
                               www.bruno.com

Michael R. Bruno, II, President & CEO
Exterior platform lift for transporting manual folding wheelchairs. 100 lb lift capacity.

302 Basement Motorhome Lift
Handicaps, Inc.
4335 S Santa Fe Dr.
Englewood, CO 80110-5417   303-781-2062
                                    800-782-4335
                               info@handicapsinc.com
                               www.handicapsinc.com

Wheelchair lifts made for vans and motor homes. Lift is made without a platform so no doorways are blocked.

303 Big Lifter
Bruno Independent Living Aids, Inc.
1780 Executive Dr.
PO Box 84
Oconomowoc, WI 53066   262-567-4990
                                     800-454-4355
                               Fax: 262-953-5501
                               webinfo@bruno.com
                                   www.bruno.com
Michael R. Bruno, II, President & CEO
Hoist-style lift for scooters and power chairs. Can be manually
rotated; 400 lb lift capacity.

304 BraunAbility
645 W Carmel Dr.
Carmel, IN 46032   800-488-0359
                                     888-365-9417
                          questions@braunability.com
                               www.braunability.com
Staci Kroon, President & CEO
Manufactures wheelchair and mobility scooter lifts and ramps for
vehicles.

305 Bruno Independent Living Aids
Bruno Independent Living Aids, Inc.
1780 Executive Dr.
PO Box 84
Oconomowoc, WI 53066   262-567-4990
                                     800-454-4355
                               Fax: 262-953-5501
                               webinfo@bruno.com
                                   www.bruno.com
Michael R. Bruno, II, President & CEO
An ISO 9001 Certified Manufacturer of automotive lifts for
scooter, wheelchairs, powerchairs, three and four wheel scooters,
and straight and custom curve stairlifts.

306 Butlers Wheelchair Lifts
Butler Mobility Products
571 Industrial Drive
Lewisberry, PA 17339   717-938-4253
                                     888-847-0804
                               Fax: 717-938-4238
                               www.butlermobility.com
Wheelchair lift can be equipped with a ramp and guard. Automatically retractable, it locks firmly into place when the lift is in operation.

307 Chariot
Bruno Independent Living Aids, Inc.
1780 Executive Dr.
PO Box 84
Oconomowoc, WI 53066   262-567-4990
                                     800-454-4355
                               Fax: 262-953-5501
                               webinfo@bruno.com
                                   www.bruno.com
Michael R. Bruno, II, President & CEO
Exterior lift for transporting scooters and power chairs. The lift
includes 360-degree spinning wheels and has a 350 lb lift capac-
ity.

308 Clearway
Ricon
1135 Aviation Pl.
San Fernando, CA 91340   818-267-3000
                                     800-322-2884
                               Fax: 800-962-1201
                               ricinsales@wabtec.com
                                   www.riconcorp.com
Wheelchair lift featuring an automatic split platform that allows
for clear access to the vehicle.

309 Columbus McKinnon Corporation
Columbus Mckinnon Corporation
205 Crosspoint Parkway
Getzville, NY 14068   716-689-5400
                                     800-888-0985
                                   www.cmworks.com
David J. Wilson, President & CEO

Supplies various lift and transfer systems for independent or attended applications including ceiling mounted or freestanding
overhead track lifts and mobile floorbase units for homes,
schools and healthcare facilities. Lift Systems for transferring
between bed, chair, commode or bath are available with a variety
of slings, scales and accessories.

310 Curb-Sider
Bruno Independent Living Aids, Inc.
1780 Executive Dr.
PO Box 84
Oconomowoc, WI 53066   262-567-4990
                                     800-454-4355
                               Fax: 262-953-5501
                               webinfo@bruno.com
                                   www.bruno.com
Michael R. Bruno, II, President & CEO
A hoist lift that stores fully or partially assembled scooters or
power chairs weighing up to 450 pounds in the rear of a van,
minivan, SUV, pickup truck, or some station wagon applications.

311 Custom Lift Residential Elevators
Waupaca Elevator Company
1726 N. Ballard Road
Suite 1
Appleton, WI 54911-2404   800-238-8739
                          info@waupacaelevator.com
                                   waupacaelevator.com
Bill Mc Michael, Owner
Waupaca Elevator residential elevators and dumbwaiters add
value, convenience and reliability to today's homes.

312 Deluxe Convertible Exercise Staircase
Performance Health
28100 Torch Parkway
Suite 700
Warrenville, IL 60555-3938   630-393-6000
                               Fax: 630-393-7600
                  customersupport@performancehealth.com
                               www.performancehealth.com
Francis Dirksmeier, Chief Executive Officer
Greg Nulty, Chief Financial Officer
Jim Plewa, Chief Sales Officer
An exercise staircase to fit any department configuration. Just re-
position a few nuts and bolts to change from a straight to a corner
type staircase.

313 Digital Wheelchair Ramp Scale
Graham-Field Health Products
One Graham-Field Way
Atlanta, GA 30340-3140   770-368-4700
                               Fax: 770-368-4932
                               cs@grahamfield.com
                                   www.grahamfield.com
Kenneth Spett, President & CEO
*Cherie Antoniazzi, Senior Vice President, Quality, Regulatory &
Risk Management*
Marc Bernstein, Senior Vice President, Consumer Sales
Weight capacity of 1,000 lbs; 270 patient memory; platform with
wheels for mobility.

314 Easy Pivot Transfer Machine
Rand-Scot, Inc.
209 Christman Drive
Fort Collins, CO 80524   970-484-7967
                                     800-467-7967
                               Fax: 970-484-3800
                               info@randscot.com
                                   www.randscot.com
Joel Lerich, Co-Founder
Barbara Lerich, Co-Founder
The Easy Pivot Patient Lifting System allows for strain-free,
one-caregiver transfers of the disabled individual.

315   Easy Stand
Altimate Medical
262 W. 1st St.
Morton, MN 56270-180   507-697-6393
                                     800-342-8968
                                Fax: 507-697-6900
                                info@easystand.com
                                www.easystand.com
Designed to make standing fast and simple. The easy-to-operate,
hydraulic lift system provides controlled lifting and lowering.
With the convenience of simply transferring to the chair and
reaching a standing position in seconds with no straps to struggle
with.

316   Elan Stair Lift
Bruno Independent Living Aids, Inc.
1780 Executive Dr.
PO Box 84
Oconomowoc, WI 53066   262-567-4990
                                     800-454-4355
                                Fax: 262-953-5501
                                webinfo@bruno.com
                                www.bruno.com
Michael R. Bruno, II, President & CEO
Indoor stairlift; vertical rail design; 300 lb lift capacity.

317   Elite Curved Stair Lift
Bruno Independent Living Aids, Inc.
1780 Executive Dr.
PO Box 84
Oconomowoc, WI 53066   262-567-4990
                                     800-454-4355
                                Fax: 262-953-5501
                                webinfo@bruno.com
                                www.bruno.com
Michael R. Bruno, II, President & CEO
Curved stairlift with 400 lb lift capacity; indoor and outdoor
stairlifts available.

318   Elite Stair Lift
Bruno Independent Living Aids, Inc.
1780 Executive Dr.
PO Box 84
Oconomowoc, WI 53066   262-567-4990
                                     800-454-4355
                                Fax: 262-953-5501
                                webinfo@bruno.com
                                www.bruno.com
Michael R. Bruno, II, President & CEO
Stairlift with 400 lb lift capacity; indoor and outdoor stairlifts
available.

319   Freedom Wheels
Freedom Wheels
580 TC Jester Blvd
Houston, TX 77007   713-864-1460
                                Fax: 713-864-1469
                                info@freedomwheels.com
                                www.freedomwheels.com
Carlos Saez, Owner
Assistive technology and mobility-equipment provider commit-
ted to people with disabilities and personal transportation options
for an independent lifestyle.

320   Handi Lift
Handi-Lift
730 Garden St
Carlstadt, NJ 07072   201-933-0111
                                     800-432-5438
                                sales@handi-lift.com
                                www.handi-lift.com
Douglas Boydston, Founder
Accessibility with Dignity. Solutions that enable users with mo-
bility impairments to live freely with products like wheelchair
lifts and home elevators.

321   Handi Prolift
Handi-Lift
730 Garden St
Carlstadt, NJ 07072   201-933-0111
                                     800-432-5438
                                sales@handi-lift.com
                                www.handi-lift.com
Douglas Boydston, Founder
Provides dependable vertical transportation for multi-level
buildings.

322   Handi-Ramp
Handi-Ramp
5600 99th Ave
Unit A1
Kenosha, WI 53144   847-876-7267
                                info@handiramp.com
                                www.handiramp.com
Thomas Disch, President & CEO
Provides a complete line of economic, ADA-compliant access
ramping products. Line includes van attachable and wheelchair
tie-downs; aluminum or expanded metal folding portables; aluminum channels; portable, sectional ramp systems; semi-perma-
nent ramps, platforms and systems. All ramp series are available
in varied lengths and widths combined with platforms, optional
hand railing, and single or double bar construction with return
ends. Special Order ramps and ramp systems.

323   Home Elevators
Handi-Lift
730 Garden St
Carlstadt, NJ 07072   201-933-0111
                                     800-432-5438
                                sales@handi-lift.com
                                www.handi-lift.com
Douglas Boydston, Founder
Home Elevators answers access problems in churches, schools
and small offices.

324   Homewaiter
Inclinator Company of America
601 Gibson Blvd
Harrisburg, PA 17104   800-343-9007
                                info@inclinator.com
                                www.inclinator.com
Cliff Warner, President & CEO
Mark Crispen, Director of Marketing, Corporate Secretary &
Board Member
Marcia Cleland, Human Resource Manager/Accounting
Easy to install and highly adaptable to existing conditions. Can
travel up to 35 feet, opening on any or all three sides at different
stations, whether at counter level or floor level.

325   Horcher Lifting Systems
Horcher Medical Systems
324 Cypress Rd
Ocala, FL 34472-3102   352-687-8020
                                     800-582-8732
                                Fax: 866-378-3318
                                info@horcherlifts.com
                                www.horcherlifts.com
Barrier Free Lifts by Horcher leads the industry for excellence in
patient transfers and technology for over 18 years. They offer
state of the art ceiling track systems, floor base lifts and bathing
systems such as the Unilift, PC-2, Diana, Lexa, and Raisa to
achieve greater mobility.

326   Inclinette
Inclinator Company of America
601 Gibson Blvd
Harrisburg, PA 17104   800-343-9007
                                info@inclinator.com
                                www.inclinator.com
Cliff Warner, President & CEO
Mark Crispen, Director of Marketing, Corporate Secretary &
Board Member
Marcia Cleland, Human Resource Manager/Accounting
Inclinette provides comfort and convenience in providing
multi-floor access to persons who have difficulty climbing stairs.

327 Independent Driving Systems
Independent Driving Systems
580 T.C. Jester
Houston, TX 77007
713-864-1460
info@independentdrivingsystems.com
www.independentdrivingsystems.com
Chad Donnelly, Owner
Provides adaptive driving systems for individuals with disabilities with more severe higher levels of injury that require more sophisticated types of assistive technology to enable them to drive safely.

328 Joey Interior Platform Lift
Bruno Independent Living Aids, Inc.
1780 Executive Dr.
PO Box 84
Oconomowoc, WI 53066
262-567-4990
800-454-4355
Fax: 262-953-5501
webinfo@bruno.com
www.bruno.com
Michael R. Bruno, II, President & CEO
Lifts and stores unoccupied scooters or powerchairs in the back of a minivan at the touch of a button.

329 KlearVue
Ricon
1135 Aviation Pl.
San Fernando, CA 91340
818-267-3000
800-322-2884
Fax: 800-962-1201
riconsales@wabtec.com
www.riconcorp.com
Wheelchair lift and folding platform with an unobstructed view from inside the vehicle.

330 Lift-All
Amigo Mobility International
6693 Dixie Highway
Bridgeport, MI 48722
989-777-0910
service@myamigo.com
www.myamigo.com
Al Thieme, Chair & Founder
Beth Thieme, President & CEO
Leading manufacturer of electric mobility; Amigo's Lift-All transports your wheelchair easily into the trunk of an automobile and neatly stores it for easy access. *$965.00*

331 Lifter
Bruno Independent Living Aids, Inc.
1780 Executive Dr.
PO Box 84
Oconomowoc, WI 53066
262-567-4990
800-454-4355
Fax: 262-953-5501
webinfo@bruno.com
www.bruno.com
Michael R. Bruno, II, President & CEO
Raises and stows folding manual wheelchairs, travel scooters, and travel power chairs. 200 lb lift capacity.

332 Lifts for Swimming Pools and Spas
Aquatic Access
1921 Production Dr
Louisville, KY 40299-2110
502-425-5817
800-325-5438
Fax: 502-425-9607
info@AquaticAccess.com
www.aquaticaccess.com
Linda Nolan, President
David Nolan, Vice President & CEO
Aquatic Access manufacturers and sells water-powered lifts providing access to in-ground and above-ground swimming pools, spas, boats and docks. *$2310.00*

333 Mac's Lift Gate
Mac's Lift Gate, Inc.
2801 South Street
Long Beach, CA 90805
800-795-6227
Fax: 562-529-3466
sales@macsliftgate.com
www.macsliftgate.com
Rick Pearce, Contact
Paul Hemmingway, Contact
Sales and service of van and truck lifts. Sales and service of wheel chair lifts for vans and automobiles. Sales, installation and service of vertical home lifts, scooter lifts and pool lifts. Sales of scooters.

334 Mecalift Sling Lifter
Arjo Inc
2349 West Lake Street
Suite 250
Addison, IL 60101
800-323-1245
888-594-2756
www.arjo.com
Joacim Lindoff, President & CEO
Tailored to the mobility level and needs of the resident and patient for the purpose of lifting manoeuvers.

335 Motorhome Lift
Handicaps, Inc.
4335 S Santa Fe Dr.
Englewood, CO 80110-5417
303-781-2062
800-782-4335
info@handicapsinc.com
www.handicapsinc.com
Wheelchair lifts made for vans and motor homes. Lift is made without a platform so no doorways are blocked.

336 Out-Sider III
Bruno Independent Living Aids, Inc.
1780 Executive Dr.
PO Box 84
Oconomowoc, WI 53066
262-567-4990
800-454-4355
Fax: 262-953-5501
webinfo@bruno.com
www.bruno.com
Michael R. Bruno, II, President & CEO
Exterior platform lift. Maintains seating and cargo space. Designed specifically for rear-view visibility. Platform folds automatically when not being used. 350 lb lift capacity.

337 Parker Bath
Arjo Inc
2349 West Lake Street
Suite 250
Addison, IL 60101
800-323-1245
888-594-2756
www.arjo.com
Joacim Lindoff, President & CEO
This product involves no manual lifting, strain or stress for the caregiver.

338 Patient Lifting & Injury Prevention
Arjo Inc
2349 West Lake Street
Suite 250
Addison, IL 60101
800-323-1245
888-594-2756
www.arjo.com
Joacim Lindoff, President & CEO
Aids in patient lifting while protecting the caregiver from the risk of backstrain.

339 Platform Lifts
Handi-Lift
730 Garden St
Carlstadt, NJ 07072
201-933-0111
800-432-5438
sales@handi-lift.com
www.handi-lift.com
Douglas Boydston, Founder
Designed to provide access over stairs that impede movement.

340   Portable Wheelchair Ramp
Maxi Aids
42 Executive Blvd.
Farmingdale, NY 11735-4710
631-752-0521
800-522-6294
Fax: 631-752-0689
TTY: 631-752-0738
sales@maxiaids.com
www.maxiaids.com
Elliot Zaretsky, Founder, President & CEO
Single-fold ramp designed to help wheelchair or scooter users easily transition from one surface level to another.

341   Rickshaw Exerciser
Access to Recreation
8 Sandra Ct
Newbury Park, CA 91320-4302
805-498-7535
800-634-4351
Fax: 805-498-8186
customerservice@accesstr.com
www.accesstr.com
Don Krebs, President & Founder
This Exerciser develops the muscle used most by those in wheelchairs. It develops the strength you need to lift yourself for pressure relief, doing transfers and pushing your wheelchair.

342   Ricon Classic
Ricon
1135 Aviation Pl.
San Fernando, CA 91340
818-267-3000
800-322-2884
Fax: 800-962-1201
ricinsales@wabtec.com
www.riconcorp.com
Wheelchair lift featuring Ricon Safety Zone, an occupant restraint belt system, as well as Sto-Loc, a design that prevents lift drift.

343   Ricon Corporation
1135 Aviation Pl.
San Fernando, CA 91340
818-267-3000
800-322-2884
Fax: 800-962-1201
ricinsales@wabtec.com
www.riconcorp.com
Ricon Corporation is a manufacturer of lifts and other mobility products for people with disabilities. It is a subsidiary of Wabtec Corporation and Faiveley Transport.

344   Smart Leg
Invacare
1 Invacare Way
Elyria, OH 44035-4190
800-333-6900
www.invacare.com
Matthew E. Monaghan, Chairman of the Board & Chief Executive Officer
Rick A. Cassiday, Senior Vice President & Chief Human Resources Officer
Kathleen P. Leneghan, Senior Vice President & Chief Financial Officer
An elevating leg rest that automatically extends to correctly fit every outstretched leg.

345   Smooth Mover
Dixie EMS
300 Liberty Ave
Brooklyn, NY 11207
718-257-6400
800-347-3494
Fax: 718-257-6401
info@dixieems.com
www.dixieems.com
Eva Silverstein, President
Patient mover is a board designed to transfer patients from bed to stretcher or table with one or two people. Being radio-translucent makes it suitable for x-ray procedures. *$199.95*

346   SpectraLift
Inclinator Company of America
601 Gibson Blvd
Harrisburg, PA 17104
800-343-9007
info@inclinator.com
www.inclinator.com
Cliff Warner, President & CEO
Mark Crispen, Director of Marketing, Corporate Secretary & Board Member
Marcia Cleland, Human Resource Manager/Accounting
A newly designed hydraulic wheelchair lift made of fiberglass construction suitable for commercial and residential use.

347   Spectrum Products
Spectrum Aquatics
7100 Spectrum Lane
Missoula, MT 59808
800-791-8056
www.spectrumproducts.com
Manufacturers of swimming pool disabled access products such as lifts, ramps, railings, ladders, and stainless steel hydrotherapy tanks for the swimming pool and medical therapy markets.

348   Spectrum Products Catalog
Spectrum Aquatics
7100 Spectrum Lane
Missoula, MT 59808
800-791-8056
www.spectrumproducts.com
Manufacturers of swimming pool disabled access products such as lifts, ramps, railings, ladders, and stainless steel hydrotherapy tanks for the swimming pool and medical therapy markets.

349   StairLIFT SC & SL
Inclinator Company of America
601 Gibson Blvd
Harrisburg, PA 17104
800-343-9007
info@inclinator.com
www.inclinator.com
Cliff Warner, President & CEO
Mark Crispen, Director of Marketing, Corporate Secretary & Board Member
Marcia Cleland, Human Resource Manager/Accounting
Simple, self-contained and efficient stair units.

350   Superarm Lift for Vans
Handicaps, Inc.
4335 S Santa Fe Dr.
Englewood, CO 80110-5417
303-781-2062
800-782-4335
info@handicapsinc.com
www.handicapsinc.com
Wheelchair lifts made for vans and motor homes. Lift is made without a platform so no doorways are blocked.

351   SureHands Lift & Care Systems
982 County Route 1
Pine Island, NY 10969-1205
800-724-5305
info@surehands.com
www.surehands.com
Thomas Herceg, President
SureHands specializes in lift & care systems for both homecare and professional settings where safety is most important, to assist an individual in overcoming physical and architectural barriers. Some of their products include lifting and body support systems, handi-slides, accessories and bathing equipment.

352   Vangater, Vangater II, Mini-Vangater
BraunAbility
645 W Carmel Dr.
Carmel, IN 46032
800-488-0359
888-365-9417
questions@braunability.com
www.braunability.com
Staci Kroon, President & CEO
Tri-fold and fold-in-half lifts for adapted van transportation.

353   Versatrainer
Pro-Max/ Division Of Bow-Flex Of America
800-605-3369
customerservice@bowflex.com
www.bowflex.com

One exercise system for the disabled person that does everything. Incorporates full-body strength, muscle development, and cardiovascular conditioning, giving full muscle movement and balanced muscle development.

354 Vestibular Board
Bailey Manufacturing Company
P.O. Box 130
Lodi, OH 44254-0130

330-948-1080
800-321-8372
Fax: 330-948-4439
baileymfg@baileymfg.com
www.baileymfg.com

Creates tilting in a rolling motion for reclining patients who need help developing balance.

355 Wheelchair Carrier
Wheelchair Carrier
5254 Jackman Road
Unit B
Toledo, OH 43613

800-541-3213
admin@WheelChairCarrier.com
wheelchaircarrier.com

David Makulinsky, President
Wheelchair, scooter and powerchair carriers for hitch mount on vehicles, both manual and electric, making it easy and simple to transport the user's mobility device.

356 Williams Lift Company
24 S Ave.
Fanwood, NJ 07023

908-325-3648
Fax: 308-322-8020
contact@williamslifts.com
www.williamslifts.com

Barry Williams, Owner
A division of Williams Surgical, Williams Lift Company offers stairlifts, wheelchair ramps, and power lift recliners. Services include installation, repairs, and rentals.

Major Catalogs

357 Access to Recreation
Access to Recreation
8 Sandra Ct
Newbury Park, CA 91320-4302

805-498-7535
800-634-4351
Fax: 805-498-8186
customerservice@accesstr.com
www.accesstr.com

Don Krebs, President & Founder
The Access to Recreation catalog is full of recreation and exercise equipment. One can find items such as electric fishing reels and other fishing and hunting equipment for the disabled sportsman. There are also adapted golf clubs, swimming pool lifts, wheelchair gloves and cuffs and bowling equipment. There are devices to help with embroidery, knitting and card playing, videos, books and practical aides such as wheelchair ramps and book.
64 pages Bi-Annually

358 Adaptive Technology Catalog
Synapse Adaptive
14 Lynn Ct
San Rafael, CA 94901-5114

415-455-9700
800-317-9611
Fax: 415-455-9801
info@synapse-ada.com
www.synapseadaptive.com

Martin Tibor, President
Adaptive technology for individuals with disabilities, ADA compliant workstations, and ergonomic furniture. Products accommodate blindness, low vision, mobility impairments or learning differences.

359 AliMed
Alimed, Inc.
297 High Street
Dedham, MA 02026

781-329-2900
800-437-2966
Fax: 781-437-2966
customerservice@alimed.com
www.alimed.com

Adam S. Epstein, Chief Executive Officer
AliMed is a leading provider of medical and healthcare products serving all segments of the healthcare market, including hospitals and clinics, nursing homes and care facilities, private medical practices, therapists and more.

360 Apria Healthcare
Apria Healthcare Group, Inc.
1975 Wehrle Dr
Buffalo, NY 14221

716-631-8726

Lifts, chairs, bathroom aids, bedroom aids, eating utensils and independent living aids for the physically challenged.

361 Armstrong Medical
American Medical Industries, Inc.
575 Knightsbridge Parkway
P.O. Box 700
Lincolnshire, IL 60069-0700

847-913-0101
800-323-4220
Fax: 847-913-0138
csr@armstrongmedical.com
www.armstrongmedical.com

John Armstrong, Founder
Jim Armstrong, Vice President
Training aids, anatomical models, medical equipment, pediatrics equipment and rehabilitation equipment.

362 Assistive Technology Journal
Technologists, Inc.
3120 Fairview Park Drive
Suite 610
Falls Church, VA 22042

202-681-3851
email@technologistsinc.com
www.technologistsinc.com

Sayed "Aziz" Azimi, President & CEO
Integrates technical and management in difficult environments. Various disciplines include architecture, engineering, construction management, etc. *$32.50*
Bi-Annually

363 Bailey
Bailey Manufacturing Company
P.O. Box 130
Lodi, OH 44254-0130

330-948-1080
800-321-8372
Fax: 330-948-4439
baileymfg@baileymfg.com
www.baileymfg.com

Ambulation aids, balance aids, benches, chairs, exercise devices, tables, stools, rehabilitation and physical therapy equipment for the physically challenged.
70 pages

364 Cambridge Career Products Catalog
Cambridge Educational
132 West 31st Street
16th Floor
New York, NY 10001

800-322-8755
Fax: 800-678-3633
custserv@films.com
cambridge.films.com

A full-color catalog featuring hundreds of products designed to aid people in career exploration, selecting specific occupations and obtaining these jobs through resume and interview preparation.
64 pages BiAnnual

365 Carex Health Brands
Carex Health Brands

800-526-8051
carex.com

Duane Wagner, CEO

The Carex brand provides a full line of home healthCare mobility, bath safety and personal care products that improve quality of life and increase independence. Consistently provides innovative, high-quality, safe and reliable products that exceed customer expectations.

366   Carolyn's Low Vision Products
3938 S. Tamiami Trail
Sarasota, FL 34231-3622   941-373-9100
                               800-648-2266
                               info@carolynscatalog.com
                               www.carolynscatalog.com

John Colton, Owner

A trusted leader in low-vision products. Free national mail-order catalog of items for visually impaired and blind people. Well versed in a variety of eye diseases that damage vision and have an expertise in helping customers making product purchasing decisions for their needs.

367   Connect Hearing
Hearing Center
750 N Commons Dr
Suite 200
Aurora, IL 60504   630-303-5380
                              info@connecthearing.com
                              www.connecthearing.com

Marcello J. Celentano, President & CEO

Specializes in products for the hard of hearing and deaf as required under ADA including visual alerting products for fire, phone, door, wake up, phone amplification, TTY, FM and infrared listening systems. Provides expertise on diagnosing hearing loss.

368   Danmar Products
221 Jackson Industrial Dr
Ann Arbor, MI 48103   800-783-1998
                              Fax: 734-761-8977
                              sales@danmarproducts.com
                              www.danmarproducts.com

Dan Russo, President & COO

Manufactures adaptive equipment for persons with physical and mental disabilities. Products include seating and positioning equipment, flotation devices, toileting aids, and hard and soft shell helmets.

369   Disabilities Sourcebook
Omnigraphics
132 West 31st Street
16th Floor
New York, NY 10001   800-322-8755
                             Fax: 800-678-3633
                             contact@omnigraphics.com
                             www.omnigraphics.com

Peter Ruffner, Co-Founder
Fred Ruffner, Co-Founder

For people with disabilities and caregivers, this product gives general information concerning birth defects, loss in hearing and vision, speech disorders, learning disorders, intellectual and cognitive disabilities, and other impairments due to illness, injury, and trauma. *$78.00*
616 pages
ISBN 0-780803-89-2

370   Enrichments Catalog
Performance Health
28100 Torch Parkway
Suite 700
Warrenville, IL 60555-3938   630-393-6000
                             Fax: 630-393-7600
                             customersupport@performancehealth.com
                             www.performancehealth.com

Francis Dirksmeier, Chief Executive Officer
Greg Nulty, Chief Financial Officer
Jim Plewa, Chief Sales Officer

Provides people with physical challenges with the products they need to help live their lives to the fullest. Includes items for everyday tasks and personal care; assistive products for home use; toileting and bathing aids; grooming and dressing devices; kitchen and dining aids. Also items for range of motion, mobility and exercise such as weights, therapy putty and exercise equipment; ergonomic gloves and supports; canes, crutches, walkers and wheelchair accessories. 36-page catalog.

371   Equipment Shop
34 Hartford Street
P.O. Box 33
Bedford, MA 01730   781-275-7681
                             800-525-7681
                             Fax: 781-275-4094
                             sales@equipmentshop.com
                             www.equipmentshop.com

Ken Larson, President
Carrie Larson, Manager

Specializing in oral motor therapy equipment, including Flexi Cut Cups, Maroon Spoons, Chewy Tubes, ARK grabbers and z-vibes. Also tricycle foot peal attachments and trike back supports as well as fat wheels.

372   Essential Medical Supply, Inc.
6420 Hazeltine National Drive
Orlando, FL 32822   407-770-0710
                             essentialmedicalsupply.com

John Hoepner, President
Carol Ann Hoepner, Secretary & Treasurer
Michael J. Hoepner, Vice President & COO

A broad based supplier of home medical and health related products designed with the needs of the user in mind.

373   Express Medical Supply
218 Seebold Spur
Fenton, MO 63026   800-633-2139
                             customerservice@exmed.net
                             www.exmed.net

William Nahm, President

Offers a full line of high quality medical and ostomy supplies to individuals, clinics, and medical institutions.

374   FlagHouse, Inc.
601 Flaghouse Drive
Hasbrouck Heights, NJ 07604-3116   201-288-7600
                                   800-793-7900
                                   Fax: 800-793-7922
                                   sales@flaghouse.com
                                   www.flaghouse.com

George Carmel, President

Global supplier of products for physical activity, recreation, education and special needs with the mantra of improving the lives of everyone.
Bi-Annually

375   Freedom Rider
Freedom Rider
5225 Tudor Court
Naples, FL 34112   603-540-0933
                             888-253-8811
                             Fax: 866-522-4708
                             info@freedomrider.com
                             www.freedomrider.com

Victoria Surr, President

A catalog of equipment for people with disabilities who ride and drive horses which includes instructional aids, vaulting equipment, and lots of hard to find items. Provides safety in their prod for riders, horses, instructors, and trainers.

376   Graham Field
One Graham-Field Way
Atlanta, GA 30340-4700   770-368-4700
                             Fax: 770-368-4932
                             cs@grahamfield.com
                             www.grahamfield.com

Kenneth Spett, President & CEO
Cherie Antoniazzi, Senior Vice President, Quality, Regulatory & Risk Management
Marc Bernstein, Senior Vice President, Consumer Sales

Manufactures more than 200 items for persons with physical disabilities, including wheelchairs, seat cushions, shower chairs, grab bars and more.

377 Health and Rehabilitation Products
Luminaud, Inc.
8688 Tyler Blvd
Mentor, OH 44060
440-255-9082
800-255-3408
Fax: 440-255-2250
info@luminaud.com
www.luminaud.com
Thomas M. Lennox, President
Dorothy Lennox, Vice President
Switches for limited capability, stoma and trach covers, shower protectors and thermo-stim oral motor stimulator. Personal voice amplifiers for people with weak voices. Artificial larynges for people with no voices. Small electronic communication boards. Books for laryngectomies and speech pathologists.

378 Huntleigh Healthcare
2349 W. Lake Street
Suite 250
Addison, IL 60101
800-323-1245
Fax: 888-594-2756
www.huntleigh-healthcare.us
Offers quality products including support surfaces, seating surfaces, fetal monitoring, vascular Assessment and treatment, and intermittent pneumatic compression devices.

379 Invacare Corporation
1 Invacare Way
Elyria, OH 44035-4190
800-333-6900
invacare.com
Matthew E. Monaghan, Chairman of the Board & Chief Executive Officer
Rick A. Cassiday, Senior Vice President & Chief Human Resources Officer
Kathleen P. Leneghan, Senior Vice President & Chief Financial Officer
A global leader in the manufacture and distribution of innovative home and long-term care medical products that promote recovery and active lifestyles.

380 Kleinert's
433 Newton St
Elba, AL 36323
800-498-7051
Fax: 305-937-0825
customercare@kleinerts.com
www.kleinerts.com
Michael Brier, President
Offers a complete line of sweat and odor protection products, incontinence products, and skin care products consisting of disposable and reusable panties for women and pants for men. Also disposable liners, diapers, underpads, antiperspirant wipes, deodorants, bedding, underpads, and cleaning solutions.

381 LS&S
145 River Rock Drive
Buffalo, NY 14207
716-348-3500
800-468-4789
Fax: 877-498-1482
LSSInfo@LSSproducts.com
www.LSSproducts.com
Melissa Balbach, President
John K. Bace, Executive Vice President
Specializes in products for the blind, visually impaired, hearing impaired, and deaf. A variety of hearing helpers, daily living aids, and vision aids. LS&S aids in the adjustment of alterations in life.

382 Lighthouse Low Vision Products
Lighthouse Guild
250 West 64th Street
New York, NY 10023
800-284-4422
www.lighthouseguild.org
Calvin W. Roberts, President & CEO
James M. Dubin, Chairman
Lawrence E. Goldschmidt, Vice Chairman & Treasurer
This organization provides health care services related to vision loss; Career and academic services for people with vision loss; Music instruction and pre K curriculum for visually impaired students.

383 Luminaud, Inc.
8688 Tyler Blvd
Mentor, OH 44060
440-255-9082
800-255-3408
Fax: 440-255-2250
info@luminaud.com
www.luminaud.com
Thomas M. Lennox, President
Dorothy Lennox, Vice President
Offers a line of artificial larynx, personal voice amplifiers, special switches, stoma covers and other communication, health and safety items.

384 MOMS Catalog
Home Delivery Incontinent Supplies
9385 Dielman Ind Dr
Saint Louis, MO 63132
800-269-4663
custcare@hdis.com
www.hdis.com
Bruce Grench, President
MOMS catalog features high quality, incontinence supplies, mobility products, bath safety products urological products, aids for daily living products, ostomy supplies and many other adaptive items. MOMS offers low prices, excellent customer service and convenient home delivery to your doorstep.
52 pages

385 Maddak Inc.
661 Route 23 South
Wayne, NJ 07470
973-628-7600
Fax: 973-305-0841
custservice@maddak.com
maddak.com
Brian Larkin, President & CEO
Maddak is proud to be a leading manufacturer of home healthcare products for seniors, people with disabilities and people recovering from injuries and illnesses. Marketed under the Ableware brand name, our products make daily living activities easier enabling you to remain active and independent.

386 Maxi Aids
Maxi Aids
42 Executive Blvd.
Farmingdale, NY 11735-4710
631-752-0521
800-522-6294
Fax: 631-752-0689
TTY: 631-752-0738
sales@maxiaids.com
www.maxiaids.com
Elliot Zaretsky, Founder, President & CEO
Products specially designed for blind, low vision, visually impaired, deaf, deaf-blind, hard of hearing, arthritic, diabetic, and disabled persons.

387 Memory Tips for Making Life Easier
Attainment Company
504 Commerce Parkway
P.O. Box 930160
Verona, WI 53593- 160
608-845-7880
800-327-4269
Fax: 800-942-3865
info@attainmentcompany.com
www.attainmentcompany.com
Autumn Garza, President
Don Bastian, CEO
Offers more than 100 resources specially designed or easy-on/easy-off clothing for men, women, children and wheelchair users. An invaluable resource for older adults on mild impairments or advanced memory loss. *$25.00*
167 pages 2006
ISBN 1-578615-72-0

388 Performance Health
28100 Torch Parkway
Suite 700
Warrenville, IL 60555-3938
630-393-6000
800-323-5547
Fax: 630-393-7600
customersupport@performancehealth.com
www.performancehealth.com
Francis Dirksmeier, Chief Executive Officer
Greg Nulty, Chief Financial Officer
Jim Plewa, Chief Sales Officer
Performance Health is a global provider of rehabilitation, assistive, and splinting products, working with occupational therapists, physical therapists, long-term care facilities, and clinics.

389 Performance Health Enrichments Catalog
Performance Health
28100 Torch Parkway
Suite 700
Warrenville, IL 60555-3938
630-393-6000
Fax: 630-393-7600
customersupport@performancehealth.com
www.performancehealth.com
Francis Dirksmeier, Chief Executive Officer
Greg Nulty, Chief Financial Officer
Jim Plewa, Chief Sales Officer
Performance Health Enrichments Catalog offers products that make the tasks and challenges of living at home - bathing, getting dressed, getting around - a little easier. Choose from personal care items to kitchen and dining aids, household helpers to mobility devices, plus a complete selection of pain-reducing products, exercise items, health monitoring equipment and more.
40 pages Yearly

390 Prentke Romich Company Product Catalog
1022 Heyl Road
Wooster, OH 44691
330-262-1984
800-262-1984
Fax: 330-263-4829
info@prentrom.com
www.prentrom.com
Dave Hershberger, President & CEO
Barry Romich, Co-Founder
A full-line product catalog containing information on speech-output communication devices, environmental controls and computer access products.

391 Products for People with Disabilities
LS&S
145 River Rock Drive
Buffalo, NY 14207
716-348-3500
800-468-4789
Fax: 877-498-1482
LSSInfo@LSSproducts.com
www.LSSproducts.com
Melissa Balbach, President
John K. Bace, Executive Vice President
LS&S, LLC has a free catalog of products for the blind, deaf, visually and hearing impaired including: TTYs, computer adaptive devices, CCTVs, talking blood pressure, blood glucose and talking scales.

392 Rehabilitation Engineering and AssistiveTechnology Society of North America (RESNA)
2001 K Street NW
3rd Floor North
Washington, DC 20006
202-367-1121
Fax: 202-367-2121
info@resna.org
www.resna.org
Maureen Linden, President
Andrea Van Hook, Interim Executive Director
RESNA improves the potential of people with disabilities to achieve their goals through technology. RESNA promotes research, development, education, advocacy and provision of technology.

393 SafePath Products
SafePath Products
530-893-1596
800-497-2003
info@safepathproducts.com
www.safepathproducts.com
Tim Vander Heiden, Owner
As a ramp manufacturer, Safe Path solves vertical rises with a variety of product solutions. One of the largest online ADA Compliance Catalogs available. Offers everything from innovative barrier removal products to survey equipment, to unique specialty products.

394 Sportaid
78 Bay Creek Rd
Loganville, GA 30052
770-554-5033
800-743-7203
Fax: 770-554-5944
stuff@sportaid.com
www.sportaid.com
Stacy Green, Co-Owner
Jimmy Green, Co-Owner
Offers an assortment of wheelchairs (everyday and racing), wheelchair sports equipment, replacement tires, hubs, spokes, pushrims, cushions and more.
68 pages Yearly

395 Store @ HDSC Product Catalog
Hearing, Speech & Deafness Center (HDSC)
1625 19th Ave.
Seattle, WA 98122
206-323-5770
888-222-5036
Fax: 206-328-6871
TTY: 800-761-2821
clinics@hsdc.org
www.hsdc.org
Lindsay Klarman, Executive Director
Hearing, Speech & Deaf Center (HSDC) is a nonprofit for clients who are deaf, hard of hearing, or who face other communication barriers such as speech challenges. Their mission is to foster inclusive and accessible communities through communication, advocacy, and education.
32 pages Yearly

396 Walgreens Home Medical Center
200 Wilmot Rd.
MS #2002
Deerfield, IL 60015
800-925-4733
www.walgreens.com
John Standley, Executive Vice President, WBA & President
Hospital supplies and home medical equipment with nationwide direct mail delivery.

397 Weitbrecht Communications, Inc. (WCI)
310-656-4924
800-233-9130
Fax: 310-450-9918
www.weitbrecht.com
Robert Weitbrecht, Co-Founder
James C. Marsters, Co-Founder
This catalog offers a variety of products for the deaf and hard of hearing, such as wake-up devices, alarm clocks, alerting systems, assistive listening devices, signalers, smoke detectors, TTY, captioned telephones and telephone amplifiers. Novelties and educational books and videos are also available.
24 pages

Miscellaneous

398 Access-USA
242 James St.
P.O. Box 160
Clayton, NY 13624-160
800-263-2750
Fax: 800-563-1687
info@access-usa.com
www.access-usa.com
Deborah Webster, Manager
Produces Braille business Cards. Access-USA also provides Alternate Format transcription services for documentation, i.e., re-

ports, schedules, menus, statements, brochures, and more. submissions accepted via email or hard copy. AF formats include Braille, Large Print, Accessible Audio as well as Captioning Audio Description. Accessible products are also available for custom projects.

399   Access-USA: Transcription Services
242 James St.
P.O. Box 160
Clayton, NY 13624-160
800-263-2750
Fax: 800-563-1687
info@access-usa.com
www.access-usa.com

Deborah Webster, Manager
Access-USA produces Braille business cards as well as offering alternate format services and products to enhance accessibility. Braille, large print, captioning, audio-descriptive forms are available.

400   BeOK Key Lever
Performance Health
28100 Torch Parkway
Suite 700
Warrenville, IL 60555-3938
630-393-6000
Fax: 630-393-7600
customersupport@performancehealth.com
www.performancehealth.com

Francis Dirksmeier, Chief Executive Officer
Greg Nulty, Chief Financial Officer
Jim Plewa, Chief Sales Officer
Handy accessory helps position key to provide maximum leverage enabling the user to work the most stubborn lock. *$11.50*

401   Big Lamp Switch
Maxi Aids
42 Executive Blvd.
Farmingdale, NY 11735-4710
631-752-0521
800-522-6294
Fax: 631-752-0689
TTY: 631-752-0738
sales@maxiaids.com
www.maxiaids.com

Elliot Zaretsky, Founder, President & CEO
This three-spoked knob replaces small rotating knobs which are a problem for those with arthritis or other limitations of the fingers. *$10.95*

402   Bookholder: Roberts
Therapro, Inc.
225 Arlington St
Framingham, MA 01702-8723
508-872-9494
800-257-5376
Fax: 508-268-6624
info@therapro.com
www.therapro.com

Karen Conrad Weihrauch, President & Owner
Gray plastic, ideal for hands-free reading, adjusts to all sizes of books and prevents pages from flipping for the physically challenged. *$32.90*

403   Brandt Industries
4461 Bronx Blvd.
Bronx, NY 10470-1496
718-994-0800
800-221-8031
Fax: 718-325-7995
brandtequip@yahoo.com
www.brandtind.com

Shaun Semple, President
Family-owned, Brandt Industries is a provider of Wholesale Medical Equipment desgined for maintaining and operating healthcare facilities. Carries and manufactures medical equipment widely used across the medical industry.

404   Child Convertible Balance Beam Set
Bailey Manufacturing Company
P.O. Box 130
Lodi, OH 44254-0130
330-948-1080
800-321-8372
Fax: 330-948-4439
baileymfg@baileymfg.com
www.baileymfg.com

This convertible set is used to develop balance in two stages.

405   Child Variable Balance Beam
Bailey Manufacturing Company
P.O. Box 130
Lodi, OH 44254-0130
330-948-1080
800-321-8372
Fax: 330-948-4439
baileymfg@baileymfg.com
www.baileymfg.com

The four walking beams can be arranged in several different ways for variable balance training.

406   Child's Mobility Crawler
Bailey Manufacturing Company
P.O. Box 130
Lodi, OH 44254-0130
330-948-1080
800-321-8372
Fax: 330-948-4439
baileymfg@baileymfg.com
www.baileymfg.com

Neurologically delayed or orthopedically impaired small children can perform crawling and coordination exercises while being comfortably supported by the crawler.

407   Dazor Lighting Technology
2360 Chaffee Drive
St. Louis, MO 63146
314-652-2400
800-345-9103
info@dazor.com
www.dazor.com

Dazor is a U.S. manufacturer of quality task lighting. Products include fluorescent, incandescent and halogen lighting fixtures. Illuminated magnifiers combine light and magnification to greatly enhance activities such as reading and make hobbies more enjoyable. All lamps come in various mounting options, including desk bases, floor stands and wall tracks.

408   Digi-Flex
Therapro, Inc.
225 Arlington St
Framingham, MA 01702-8723
508-872-9494
800-257-5376
Fax: 508-268-6624
info@therapro.com
www.therapro.com

Karen Conrad Weihrauch, President & Owner
This is a unique hand and finger exercise unit. Recommended for use of individuation of fingers, web space and general strengthening of work hands. Available in a variety of resistances. *$20.00*

409   Digital Talking Compass
Maxi Aids
42 Executive Blvd.
Farmingdale, NY 11735-4710
631-752-0521
800-522-6294
Fax: 631-752-0689
TTY: 631-752-0738
sales@maxiaids.com
www.maxiaids.com

Elliot Zaretsky, Founder, President & CEO
Compass that speaks the direction it is pointed to. Includes eight points for noisy conditions for hard of hearing users. *$89.95*

410   Door Knock Signaler
HARC Mercantile
5413 S Westnedge Ave.
Suite A
Portage, MI 49002
800-445-9968
TTY: 269-324-1615
info@harc.com
www.harc.com

Michael Martinson, Owner
Flashes light to signal a knock on the door. *$31.00*

411 Doorbell Signalers
HARC Mercantile
5413 S Westnedge Ave.
Suite A
Portage, MI 49002
800-445-9968
TTY: 269-324-1615
info@harc.com
www.harc.com

Michael Martinson, Owner
Doorbell signalers to alert with either louder chime or flashing light.

412 Dormakaba USA Inc.
1 DORMA Drive, AC Drawer
Reamstown, PA 17567
717-336-3881
866-401-6063
Fax: 717-336-2106
archdw@dorma-usa.com
www.dormakaba.com/en

Riet Cadonau, CEO
Bernd Brinker, CFO
Alwin Berninger, COO Access Solutions DACH
DORMA provides a complete line of door controls, including barrier-free units that comply with the Americans with Disabilities Act. A wide variety of surface-applied and concealed closers, low-energy operators, exit devices and electronic access control systems are available to address this equipment.

413 Dual Switch Latch and Timer
AbleNet, Inc.
2625 Patton Road
Roseville, MN 55113-1137
651-294-2200
800-322-0956
Fax: 651-294-2259
customerservice@ablenetinc.com
www.ablenetinc.com

Jennifer Thalhuber, President & CEO
Paul Sugden, CFO & Trustee
A Dual Switch Latch and Timer allows two users to activate two devices at a time in the latch. Timed seconds or timed minutes mode of control. *$235.00*

414 Enabling Devices
50 Broadway
Hawthorne, NY 10532
914-747-3070
800-832-8697
Fax: 914-747-3480
sales@enablingdevices.com
www.enablingdevices.com

Seth Kanor, President & CEO
For more than 25 years, Enabling Devices has been dedicated to providing affordable learning and assistive devices for the physically challenged. Products include augmentative communicators, adapted toys, capability switches, training and sensory devices and activity centers.

415 Foot Inversion Tread
Bailey Manufacturing Company
P.O. Box 130
Lodi, OH 44254-0130
330-948-1080
800-321-8372
Fax: 330-948-4439
baileymfg@baileymfg.com
www.baileymfg.com

Effective for correcting flat feet. These angled boards require the patient to walk on the outside of the foot instead of the arch.

416 Foot Placement Ladder
Bailey Manufacturing Company
P.O. Box 130
Lodi, OH 44254-0130
330-948-1080
800-321-8372
Fax: 330-948-4439
baileymfg@baileymfg.com
www.baileymfg.com

Adjustable cross bars for different length steps. Reinforced metal crosses for easier climbing for the physically disabled.

417 HealthCraft SuperPole
Maxi Aids
42 Executive Blvd.
Farmingdale, NY 11735-4710
631-752-0521
800-522-6294
Fax: 631-752-0689
TTY: 631-752-0738
sales@maxiaids.com
www.maxiaids.com

Elliot Zaretsky, Founder, President & CEO
A floor-to-ceiling grab bar designed for those who require assistance with standing, transferring, or moving. Can be used beside a bed, bath, toilet or chair.

418 Hocoma AG
77 Accord Park Drive
Suite D-1
Norwell, MA 02061
877-944-220
Fax: 781-792-0104
service.usa@hocoma.com
www.hocoma.com

Dr. Gery Colombo, President & CEO
Mark Faris, CFO
Leader in developing, manufacturing and marketing robotic and sensor-based products for functional movement therapy on a global level.

419 Home Alerting Systems
HARC Mercantile
5413 S Westnedge Ave.
Suite A
Portage, MI 49002
800-445-9968
TTY: 269-324-1615
info@harc.com
www.harc.com

Michael Martinson, Owner
Alerting systems featuring bright flasher, loud speaker, and/or bedshaker signals.

420 Hospital Environmental Control System
Prentke Romich Company
1022 Heyl Road
Wooster, OH 44691
330-262-1984
800-262-1984
Fax: 330-263-4829
info@prentrom.com
www.prentrom.com

Dave Hershberger, President & CEO
Barry Romich, Co-Founder
Permits the non-ambulatory patient to operate a variety of electrical items in a single room. A large liquid crystal display is mounted in front of the user and they scan through the menu of operations and make a selection using a sip-puff switch. Options include nurse call, standard telephone functions, electric bed control, hospital television operation and electrical appliance on and off. *$3860.00*

421 Identity Group
10 Burton Hills Blvd
Suite 101
Nashville, TN 37215
800-237-9447
help@identitygroup.com
www.identitygroup.com

Sam Richardson, President & CEO
Bob Tate, CFO
Manufacturer of signs and visual decor for office and personal use.

422 Leg Elevation Board
Bailey Manufacturing Company
P.O. Box 130
Lodi, OH 44254-0130
330-948-1080
800-321-8372
Fax: 330-948-4439
baileymfg@baileymfg.com
www.baileymfg.com

Includes seven positions to a 30 degree incline, three pillows with Velcro, easy carry hand slot and a natural finish.

423 Leveron Door Lever
Lindustries
440 E. Southern Ave.
Tempe, AZ 85282   877-794-9511
customer.service@trademarkia.com
www.trademarkia.com/leveron-73486756.ht ml
Dave Lind, Jr., President & CEO
Leveron is a doorknob lever handle for ease of operation. Leveron converts standard doorknobs to lever action without removing existing hardware. No gripping, twisting or pinching when hands are wet, arthritic or arms are full. Leveron provides convenience. ADA access requirements in public and private places. *$16.95*

424 Loop Scissors
Therapro, Inc.
225 Arlington St
Framingham, MA 01702-8723   508-872-9494
800-257-5376
Fax: 508-268-6624
info@therapro.com
www.therapro.com
Karen Conrad Weihrauch, President & Owner
Pliable, plastic handles that allow for easy and controlled cutting. Extra finger room provides better control when cutting. *$17.95*

425 Pacific Rehab, Inc.
36805 N Never Mind Tr.
P.O. Box 5406
Carefree, AZ 85377-5406   888-222-9040
Fax: 480-575-7907
information@pacificrehabinc.com
pacificrehabinc.com

426 Pet Partners
Delta Society National Service Dog Center
345 118th Ave SE
Suite 100
Bellevue, WA 98005   425-679-5550
Fax: 425-379-5539
www.petpartners.org
C. Annie Peters, President & CEO
Jenn Gilbertson, Chief Marketing & Technology Officer
Linda Dicus, Executive Assistant
Pet Partners, formerly Delta Society, is a non-profit organization that helps people live healthier and happier lives by incorporating therapy, service and companion animals into their lives.

427 Plastic Card Holder
Therapro, Inc.
225 Arlington St
Framingham, MA 01702-8723   508-872-9494
800-257-5376
Fax: 508-268-6624
info@therapro.com
www.therapro.com
Karen Conrad Weihraucher, President & Owner
For those with reduced finger control. Front extension for pencils and coins.

428 ProtectaCap, ProtectaCap+PLUS, ProtectaChin Guard and ProtectaHip
Plum Enterprises
800-321-7586
info@plument.com
www.plument.com
Janice Carrington, Founder & CEO
Plum Enterprises award winning, exquisite, ergonomic protective wear keeps you safe from the dangers of falls. ProtectCap+Plus and ProtectHips are engineered for superior shock-absorption and designed for exquisite simplicity and amazing lightweight comfort.

429 Real Design Inc.
187 S. Main Street
Dolgeville, NY 13329   800-696-7041
Fax: 315-429-3071
rdesign@twcny.rr.com
sites.google.com/site/realdesign95/

Real Design inc. (Rehab and Educational Aids for Living) specializes in rehabilitation products for children with disabilities. To understand the needs of child with disabilities, the company deals with therapists, parents, and caregivers.

430 Rex Bionics, Ltd.
50 Milk Street
Floor 16
Boston, MA 02109   info@rexbionics.com
www.rexbionics.com
Rex Bionics develops and manufactures exoskeletons, capable of performing exercises in multiple positions: upright, backward, sideways, lunge, or squat. REX exoskeletons. Permits both at home or gym exercises and stretches for the upper and lower body, accessing different groups of muscles.

431 Rocker Balance Square
Bailey Manufacturing Company
P.O. Box 130
Lodi, OH 44254-0130   330-948-1080
800-321-8372
Fax: 330-948-4439
baileymfg@baileymfg.com
www.baileymfg.com
The rocker is used in developing activity, balance control and coordination.

432 Room Valet Visual-Tactile Alerting System
HARC Mercantile
5413 S Westnedge Ave.
Suite A
Portage, MI 49002   800-445-9968
TTY: 269-324-1615
info@harc.com
www.harc.com
Michael Martinson, Owner
ADA compliant built-in visual-tactile alerting system. The Room Valet is fully supervised and has power failure back up. Alerts to in-room smoke, building alarm, door, phone, and alarm clock. Designed for permanent installation.

433 Series Adapter
AbleNet, Inc.
2625 Patton Road
Roseville, MN 55113-1137   651-294-2200
800-322-0956
Fax: 651-294-2259
customerservice@ablenetinc.com
www.ablenetinc.com
Jennifer Thalhuber, President & CEO
Paul Sugden, CFO & Trustee
Allows two-switch operation of any battery-operated device or electrical devices. *$20.00*

434 Signaling Wake-Up Devices
HARC Mercantile
5413 S Westnedge Ave.
Suite A
Portage, MI 49002   800-445-9968
TTY: 269-324-1615
info@harc.com
www.harc.com
Michael Martinson, Owner
Wake up devices. Vibrating alarm clocks, available with flashing lights, louder alarm noises and more.

435 Smoke Detector with Strobe
HARC Mercantile
5413 S Westnedge Ave.
Suite A
Portage, MI 49002   800-445-9968
TTY: 269-324-1615
info@harc.com
www.harc.com
Michael Martinson, Owner
Detects smoke within a radius of 100' and flashes a strobe as a signal.

436 Spinal Network: The Total Wheelchair Resource Book
No Limits Communications & New Mobility
120-34 Queens Blvd.
Suite 330
Kew Gardens, NY 11415   800-404-2898
www.newmobility.com

Jean Dobbs, Publisher & Editorial Director
Josie Byzek, Executive Editor
Ian Ruder, Editor
Nearly 600 pages of profiles, articles and resources on every topic of interest to wheelchair users. Subjects include health, coping, relationships, sexuality, parenthood, computers, sports, recreation, travel, personal assistance services, legal rights, financial strategies, employment, and media images. *$34.95*
400 pages

437 SteeleVest
Steele
P.O. Box 7304
Kingston, WA 98346   888-783-3538
Fax: 360-297-2816
steelevest@gmail.com
www.steelevest.com

Lynn Steele, Owner
Vest developed by NASA provides an external cooling system. Cooling Vests are tailored to industrial workers while operating in warm environments to keep cool and safe.

438 Strobe Light Signalers
HARC Mercantile
5413 S Westnedge Ave.
Suite A
Portage, MI 49002   800-445-9968
TTY: 269-324-1615
info@harc.com
www.harc.com

Michael Martinson, Owner
Strobe alerts that plug into receivers for signaling systems. A strobe light on the device will flash to alert for calls, visitors, and home alarms.

439 Tactile Braille Signs
Maxi Aids
42 Executive Blvd.
Farmingdale, NY 11735-4710   631-752-0521
800-522-6294
Fax: 631-752-0689
TTY: 631-752-0738
sales@maxiaids.com
www.maxiaids.com

Elliot Zaretsky, Founder, President & CEO
Contains raised text and pictograms, Grade 2 braille, and contrasting colors. Stairs, No Smoking, and various Restroom signs available. *$19.95*

440 Tactile Thermostat
ASB
919 Walnut Street
Philadelphia, PA 19107-5237   215-627-0600
Fax: 215-922-0692
asbinfo@asb.org
www.asb.org

Karla S. McCaney, President & CEO
Beth Deering, Chief Program Officer
Sylvia Purnell, Director of Learning & Development
Large embossed numbers on cover ring and raised temperature setting knob. *$31.50*

441 Therapy Putty
Therapro, Inc.
225 Arlington St
Framingham, MA 01702-8723   508-872-9494
800-257-5376
Fax: 508-268-6624
info@therapro.com
www.therapro.com

Karen Conrad Weihrauch, President & Owner
Designed to exercise and strengthen hands, ranging from soft to firm, for developing a stronger grasp. Available in two, four and six-ounce sizes. Three-ounce putty in a clear fist-shaped container.

442 Window-Ease
A-Solution
1331 Wind Ridge Dr NW
Albuquerque, NM 87120   505-856-6632
Fax: 505-856-6652
www.windowease.com
Device adapts horizontally and vertically sliding windows to ANSI A117.1 standards. 10:1 mechanical advantage at the crank arm opens a 50lb window with 5lbs force.

Office Devices & Workstations

443 BAT Personal Keyboard
Infogrip
Ventura, CA 93001   503-828-1221
866-606-8551
support@infogrip.com
www.infogrip.com

Liza Jacobs, President
Aaron Gaston, Vice President
Infogrip has creative computer access solutions for people with all types of disabilities. Alternative keyboards and mice, switches, screen readers, magnifiers and educational software. *$200.00*

444 Computer Workstation and Activity Table
Maxi Aids
42 Executive Blvd.
Farmingdale, NY 11735-4710   631-752-0521
800-522-6294
Fax: 631-752-0689
TTY: 631-752-0738
sales@maxiaids.com
www.maxiaids.com

Elliot Zaretsky, Founder, President & CEO
Height-adjustable wheelchair accessible table. Adjusts with a hand crank. ADA compliant. *$989.00*

445 Desk-Top Talking Calculator
Maxi Aids
42 Executive Blvd.
Farmingdale, NY 11735-4710   631-752-0521
800-522-6294
Fax: 631-752-0689
TTY: 631-752-0738
sales@maxiaids.com
www.maxiaids.com

Elliot Zaretsky, Founder, President & CEO
Full-function calculator that announces results in a clear voice. Also features a large 8-digit display. *$13.85*

446 Don Johnston
26799 West Commerce Drive
Volo, IL 60073   847-740-0749
800-999-4660
Fax: 847-740-7326
info@donjohnston.com
www.donjohnston.com

Don Johnston, Founder
Ruth Ziolkowski, President
Kevin Johnston, Director of Product Design
A provider of quality products and services that enable people with special needs to discover their potential and experience success. Products are developed for the areas of Physical Access, Augmentative Communication and for those who struggle with reading and writing.

447 Freedom Ryder Handcycles
Brike International
20589 SW Elk Horn Ct
Tualatin, OR 97062-9518   503-692-1029
michaelslofgren@gmail.com
www.freedomryder.com

The finest handcycle in the world. The cycles incorporate body, lean steering and the finest bicycle components to make this a three-wheeled vehicle without equal. Suitable for both recreation and competition. *$1995.00*

448 Golf Xpress
Emotorsports
4400 West M-61
Standish, MI 48658
989-846-6255
mitch@golfxpress.com
www.golfxpress.com
Patented single-rider adaptive golf cart allows users to play golf, seated or supported. Hit woods, irons, and putt from the car. Drives onto tees and greens and into traps without damaging the course.

449 Pencil/Pen Weighted Holders
Therapro, Inc.
225 Arlington St
Framingham, MA 01702-8723
508-872-9494
800-257-5376
Fax: 508-268-6624
info@therapro.com
www.therapro.com
Karen Conrad Weihrauch, President & Owner
Securely hold any pencil or pen. These weighted holders allow for more control along with proprioceptive feedback to encourage better writing skills.

450 Perkins Electric Brailler
Maxi Aids
42 Executive Blvd.
Farmingdale, NY 11735-4710
631-752-0521
800-522-6294
Fax: 631-752-0689
TTY: 631-752-0738
sales@maxiaids.com
www.maxiaids.com
Elliot Zaretsky, Founder, President & CEO
Can emboss 25 lines with 42 cells on an 11 x 11 1/2 sheet. *$1035.00*

451 Raised Line Drawing Kit
Maxi Aids
42 Executive Blvd.
Farmingdale, NY 11735-4710
631-752-0521
800-522-6294
Fax: 631-752-0689
TTY: 631-752-0738
sales@maxiaids.com
www.maxiaids.com
Elliot Zaretsky, Founder, President & CEO
For writing script or drawing graphs by the use of special plastic paper. *$34.95*

452 Reizen RL-350 Braille Labeler
Maxi Aids
42 Executive Blvd.
Farmingdale, NY 11735-4710
631-752-0521
800-522-6294
Fax: 631-752-0689
TTY: 631-752-0738
sales@maxiaids.com
www.maxiaids.com
Elliot Zaretsky, Founder, President & CEO
For labeling in braille with 3/8 or 1/2 wide labeling tape. *$32.87*

453 SciPlus 3200 Low Vision Scientific Vision
Independent Living Aids
137 Rano Rd.
Buffalo, NY 14207
716-332-2970
800-537-2118
Fax: 877-498-1482
can-do@independentliving.com
www.independentliving.com
Large scientific calculator with large illuminated numbers, full color display, and large buttons/display for visually impaired users. *$405.00*

454 Steady Write
Maxi Aids
42 Executive Blvd.
Farmingdale, NY 11735-4710
631-752-0521
800-522-6294
Fax: 631-752-0689
TTY: 631-752-0738
sales@maxiaids.com
www.maxiaids.com
Elliot Zaretsky, Founder, President & CEO
Furnishes the writer with increased holding capacity and stabilizes the hand. *$8.95*

455 Television Remote Controls with Large Numbers
Independent Living Aids
137 Rano Rd.
Buffalo, NY 14207
716-332-2970
800-537-2118
Fax: 877-498-1482
can-do@independentliving.com
www.independentliving.com
Television remote control with large, easy-to-see, and color-coded buttons. *$49.95*

456 Touch-Dots
Maxi Aids
42 Executive Blvd.
Farmingdale, NY 11735-4710
631-752-0521
800-522-6294
Fax: 631-752-0689
TTY: 631-752-0738
sales@maxiaids.com
www.maxiaids.com
Elliot Zaretsky, Founder, President & CEO
Adhesive-backed dots for identification. Can be used with keyboards, telephones, calculators and more. *$1.95*

Scooters

457 Ability Center
4797 Ruffner St.
San Diego, CA 92111
858-541-0552
833-919-2581
Fax: 858-541-1941
www.abilitycenter.com
Terry Barton, General Manager
Specializes in accessible vehicles and mobility products; the company has more than 100 employees in 14 locations across the western U.S.
1994

458 Aerospace Compadre
Aerospace America, Inc.
900 Parkway Drive
Bay City, MI 48706
989-684-2121
800-237-6414
sales@aerospaceamerica.com
www.aerospaceamerica.com
Mike Alley, President
Fully customized golf-cart type vehicle for the physically impaired person. Fully equipped with hand controls, wheelchair rack, storage racks, head and tail lights and full safety belts. *$2500.00*

459 Alante
Golden Technologies
401 Bridge Street
Old Forge, PA 18518
570-451-7477
800-624-6374
Fax: 800-628-5165
www.goldentech.com
Richard Golden, CEO
Robert Golden, Chair
Fred Kiwak, Vice President, Research & Development
Rear-wheel-drive vehicle that represents the best in powered mobility.

460 **Amigo Mobility International**
Amigo Mobility International
6693 Dixie Highway
Bridgeport, MI 48722   989-777-0910
service@myamigo.com
www.myamigo.com

Al Thieme, Chair & Founder
Beth Thieme, President & CEO
An industry leader in power operated vehicles and scooters, Amigo provides innovative, durable, and customized mobility solutions for the disabled, injured, and seniors worldwide. Other services include healthcare, travel and transportation services. *$1295.00*

461 **Amigo Mobility International Inc.**
6693 Dixie Highway
Bridgeport, MI 48722   989-777-0910
service@myamigo.com
www.myamigo.com

Al Thieme, Chair & Founder
Beth Thieme, President & CEO
Amigo Mobility designs and manufactures a complete line of power operated vehicles/mobility scooters and accessories.

462 **Cruiser Bus Buggy 4MB**
Convaid
2830 California Street
Torrance, CA 90503   888-266-8243
Fax: 310-618-2166
convaidsales.us@etac.com
www.convaid.com

Chris Braun, President
In sizes from infant through young adult, this positioning buggy is crash-tested.

463 **E-Wheels Electric Senior Mobility Scooter**
Maxi Aids
42 Executive Blvd.
Farmingdale, NY 11735-4710   631-752-0521
800-522-6294
Fax: 631-752-0689
TTY: 631-752-0738
sales@maxiaids.com
www.maxiaids.com

Elliot Zaretsky, Founder, President & CEO
Three-wheel, high-powered scooter for seniors. Travels up to 45 miles on a single charge.

464 **EMS 2000 - Analog Muscle Stimulator**
BioMedical Life Systems
1954 Kellogg Avenue
Calsbad, CA 92008-6581   760-579-0801
800-726-8367
Fax: 760-929-9953
information@bmls.com
www.bmls.com

This three-mode device has four adjustable modulations and is powered by one 9-volt battery.

465 **Electric Power Scooter**
Electro Kinetic Technologies
W194 N11301 McCormick Drive
Germantown, WI 53022   262-250-7740
800-824-1068
Fax: 262-250-7741
info@ek-tech.com
www.ek-tech.com

Designed to increase your mobility indoors. Features up to 20 hours of continuous operation between charges. Weight capacity: 750 lbs.

466 **Espree Atlas**
PaceSaver
1800 Merriam Lane
Kansas City, KS 66106   913-722-5658
Fax: 913-722-2614
leisure-lift@leisure-lift.com
www.pacesaver.com

Bill Burke, Founder
This easily maneuverable scooter boasts the industry's best incline stability rating. Weight capacity: 500 lbs. *$2695.00*

467 **Invacare Fulfillment Center**
Invacare
1 Invacare Way
Elyria, OH 44035-4190   800-333-6900
www.invacare.com

Matthew E. Monaghan, Chairman of the Board & Chief Executive Officer
Rick A. Cassiday, Senior Vice President & Chief Human Resources Officer
Kathleen P. Leneghan, Senior Vice President & Chief Financial Officer
Invacare Corporation is a leading manufacturer and distributor of non-acute medical products which promote recovery and active lifestyles for people requiring home and other non-acute health care.

468 **Outdoor Independence**
Palmer Industries
71 Cyrpress St
Warwick, RI 02888
Electric, outdoor scotter. Includes bench seat, push button control panel, headlight and stop light, horn, on-off key, rear basket, moped/motorcycle tires, and stainless steel foot platform.

469 **PaceSaver Power Scooter**
PaceSaver
1800 Merriam Lane
Kansas City, KS 66106   913-722-5658
Fax: 913-722-2614
leisure-lift@leisure-lift.com
www.pacesaver.com

Bill Burke, Founder
The scooter combines outdoor ruggedness with indoor maneuverability at a low price.

470 **Polaris Trail Blazer**
Polaris Industries
2100 Highway 55
Medina, MN 55340-9770   763-542-0500
888-704-5290
Fax: 763-542-0599
www.polarisindustries.com

Michael T. Speetzen, CEO
Michael F. Donoughe, SVP, Chief Technical Officer & Head of Electrification
Lucy Clark Dougherty, SVP, General Counsel & Corporate Secretary
A four-wheeler that has many engineered innovations, features such as: full floorboards for full comfort, single lever breaking with auxiliary foot brake, electronic throttle control, parking brake and adjustable handlebars.

471 **Quickie LXI/LX**
Sunrise Medical
2842 Business Park Avenue
Fresno, CA 93727   800-333-4000
Fax: 800-300-7502
www.sunrisemedical.com

Thomas Babacan, President & CEO
Roxane Cromwell, Chief Operating Officer
Adrian Platt, Chief Financial Officer
This custom, ultralight, folding, everyday wheelchair offers portability and performance.

472 **Rascal Scooter**
Mobility Parts and Service
1501 Grandview Avenue
Suite 400
West Deptford, NJ 08066   800-257-7955
info@mobilitypartsandservice.com
mobilitypartsandservice.com

An electric vehicle that serves as both a compact mobile chair and a rugged outdoor scooter. Usable in both indoors and outdoor environments. Also available with joystick controls.

473 **Regent**
Golden Technologies
401 Bridge Street
Old Forge, PA 18518   570-451-7477
                                         800-624-6374
                                    Fax: 800-628-5165
                                    info@goldentech.com
                                    www.goldentech.com
Richard Golden, CEO
Robert Golden, Chair
Fred Kiwak, Vice President, Research & Development
Top-rated performance scooter, with extra features and economically priced.

474 **Scoota Bug**
Golden Technologies
401 Bridge Street
Old Forge, PA 18518   570-451-7477
                                         800-624-6374
                                    Fax: 800-628-5165
                                    www.goldentech.com
Richard Golden, CEO
Robert Golden, Chair
Fred Kiwak, Vice President, Research & Development
A lightweight, completely modular scooter that disassembles and fits into most auto trunks.

475 **SoloRider Industries**
Regal Research & Manufacturing Company
1200 East Plano Parkway
Plano, TX 75074   800-898-3353
                                    info@solorider.com
                                    www.solorider.com
Roger Pretekin, Founder
Manufacturer and distributor of the Solorider Golf Cart. This revolutionary single rider adaptive cart is specifically designed to meet the needs of individuals with mobility impairments.

476 **Terra-Jet: Utility Vehicle**
TERRA-JET USA
P.O. Box 918
Innis, LA 70747   225-492-2249
                                         800-864-5000
                                    Fax: 225-492-2226
                                    Terrajet@Yahoo.com
                                    www.terra-jet.com
Larry Rabalais, President & CEO
TERRA-JET utility vehicles are unique in their ability to traverse many different types of terrain in remote areas otherwise inaccessible. It has a multitude of uses for industry, sportsmen or the whole family. Uniquely designed, industrial duty construction of low-maintenance and low-fuel consumption.

477 **Terrier Tricycle**
TRIAID
P.O. Box 1364
Cumberland, MD 21501   301-759-3525
                                    Fax: 301-759-3525
                                    sales@triaid.com
                                    www.triaid.com
Provides fun therapy and actively encourages participation, awareness and the building of self-confidence. Designed for children from about five years, it features ATB styling, 16-inch wheels, an adjustable steering stop and a supportive saddle. Handlebar and seat adjustments combine with a broad wheelbase to ensure the rider is in the optimum position to pedal, and the tricycle gives good stability and confident handling.

478 **Tracer Tricycle**
TRIAID
P.O. Box 1364
Cumberland, MD 21501   301-759-3525
                                    Fax: 301-759-3525
                                    sales@triaid.com
                                    www.triaid.com
These tricycles provide fun therapy for teenagers and adults. Highly recommended by therapists for users whose use of the lower limbs is restricted. *$740.00*

Stationery

479 **Access-USA**
242 James St.
P.O. Box 160
Clayton, NY 13624-160   800-263-2750
                                    Fax: 800-563-1687
                                    www.access-usa.com
Deborah Webster, Manager
Access-USA provides one-stop alternate format transcription services for almost any type of document-reports, schedules, menus, monthly statements, brochures, reports, etc. Items may be submitted on computer disk, hard copy or email. Alternate formats include Braille, large print, Braille and print, audio recordings, adapted disks as well as video services-open/closed captioning and video descriptions. Accessible products also include Braille Business Cards and ADA signage.

480 **Address Book**
ASB
919 Walnut Street
Philadelphia, PA 19107-5237   215-627-0600
                                    Fax: 215-922-0692
                                    asbinfo@asb.org
                                    www.asb.org
Karla S. McCaney, President & CEO
Beth Deering, Chief Program Officer
Sylvia Purnell, Director of Learning & Development
The big print address book is the first personal book to provide enlarged writing spaces, making it easier to write down and retrieve information. *$12.50*

481 **Bold Line Paper**
ASB
919 Walnut Street
Philadelphia, PA 19107-5237   215-627-0600
                                    Fax: 215-922-0692
                                    asbinfo@asb.org
                                    www.asb.org
Karla S. McCaney, President & CEO
Beth Deering, Chief Program Officer
Sylvia Purnell, Director of Learning & Development
This pad consists of 100 sheets of paper with bold lines to help guide the writing of an individual with limited vision. *$2.50*

482 **Braille Calendar**
Maxi Aids
42 Executive Blvd.
Farmingdale, NY 11735-4710   631-752-0521
                                         800-522-6294
                                    Fax: 631-752-0689
                                    TTY: 631-752-0738
                                    sales@maxiaids.com
                                    www.maxiaids.com
Elliot Zaretsky, Founder, President & CEO
Calendar with braille markings for touch reading. *$14.99*

483 **Braille Notebook**
Maxi Aids
42 Executive Blvd.
Farmingdale, NY 11735-4710   631-752-0521
                                         800-522-6294
                                    Fax: 631-752-0689
                                    TTY: 631-752-0738
                                    sales@maxiaids.com
                                    www.maxiaids.com
Elliot Zaretsky, Founder, President & CEO
Made of heavy-duty board, covered with waterproof plastic and contains three rings for binding. *$18.95*

484 **Braille: Greeting Cards**
ASB
919 Walnut Street
Philadelphia, PA 19107-5237   215-627-0600
                                    Fax: 215-922-0692
                                    asbinfo@asb.org
                                    www.asb.org
Karla S. McCaney, President & CEO
Beth Deering, Chief Program Officer
Sylvia Purnell, Director of Learning & Development

Birthday, anniversary, get well, sympathy and Christmas cards offering Braille print for the blind. *$.95*

485   Clip Board Notebook
ASB
919 Walnut Street
Philadelphia, PA 19107-5237   215-627-0600
Fax: 215-922-0692
asbinfo@asb.org
www.asb.org

Karla S. McCaney, President & CEO
Beth Deering, Chief Program Officer
Sylvia Purnell, Director of Learning & Development
Kit includes a pack of Bold Line paper and black ink pen. *$5.95*

486   Deluxe Signature Guide
Maxi Aids
42 Executive Blvd.
Farmingdale, NY 11735-4710   631-752-0521
800-522-6294
Fax: 631-752-0689
TTY: 631-752-0738
sales@maxiaids.com
www.maxiaids.com

Elliot Zaretsky, Founder, President & CEO
Consisting of rods supported by two rubber blocks, this device helps to facilitate writing. *$1.95*

487   Giant Print Address Book
Maxi Aids
42 Executive Blvd.
Farmingdale, NY 11735-4710   631-752-0521
800-522-6294
Fax: 631-752-0689
TTY: 631-752-0738
sales@maxiaids.com
www.maxiaids.com

Elliot Zaretsky, Founder, President & CEO
Large print address book for storing up to 360 names. Three-ring hardcover binder with removable pages. *$16.95*

488   Letter Writing Guide
Independent Living Aids
137 Rano Rd.
Buffalo, NY 14207   716-332-2970
800-537-2118
Fax: 877-498-1482
can-do@independentliving.com
www.independentliving.com

Sturdy plastic sheet with 13 apertures corresponding to standard line spacing. *$3.95*

489   Ottobock
11501 Alterra Parkway
Suite 600
Austin, TX 78758   800-328-4058
supportUS@OttoBock.com
www.ottobockus.com

Provides prosthetic devices to people with amputations. Assists users in maintaining and gaining their freedom of movement.

490   Writing Guide Value Kit
Independent Living Aids
137 Rano Rd.
Buffalo, NY 14207   716-332-2970
800-537-2118
855-746-7452
Fax: 516-937-3906
can-do@independentliving.com
www.independentliving.com

Included in this useful pack are four durable plastic lettering and number guides for tracing letters when the individual is unable to write letters unassisted. *$9.95*

Visual Aids

491   Adjustable Folding Support Cane for the Blind
Maxi Aids
42 Executive Blvd.
Farmingdale, NY 11735-4710   631-752-0521
800-522-6294
Fax: 631-752-0689
TTY: 631-752-0738
sales@maxiaids.com
www.maxiaids.com

Elliot Zaretsky, Founder, President & CEO
Adjustable canes for the visually impaired. *$21.95*

492   All Terrain Cane
Maxi Aids
42 Executive Blvd.
Farmingdale, NY 11735-4710   631-752-0521
800-522-6294
Fax: 631-752-0689
TTY: 631-752-0738
sales@maxiaids.com
www.maxiaids.com

Elliot Zaretsky, Founder, President & CEO
A rigid aluminum cane with a curved nylon tip and golf grip with hook handle. Designed to help blind and visually impaired persons navigate unpaved areas. *$49.95*

493   Audio Book Contractors
P.O. Box 96
Riverdale, MD 20738-0096   301-439-5830
audiobookcontractors@verizon.net
www.audiobookcontractors.com

Flo Gibson, Founder
Over 950 titles of unabridged classic books in a variety of genres on audio cassettes in sturdy vinyl covers with picture and spine windows. Discounted prices for disabled patrons.

494   Beyond Sight, Inc.
5650 S Windermere St
Littleton, CO 80120   303-795-6455
www.beyondsight.com

Products for the blind and visually impaired, including talking clocks, watches and calculators. Beyond Sight, Inc. also carries a large selection of Braille products, magnifiers, reading machines and computer equipment.
Site is under construction.

495   Big Button Talking Calculator with Function Replay
Independent Living Aids
137 Rano Rd.
Buffalo, NY 14207   716-332-2970
800-537-2118
Fax: 877-498-1482
can-do@independentliving.com
www.independentliving.com

Big Button Talking Calculator features color-coded buttons ideal for hard of hearing and low vision users. New repeat function lets you listen to the most recent entry. *$15.95*

496   Braille Elevator Plates
Maxi Aids
42 Executive Blvd.
Farmingdale, NY 11735-4710   631-752-0521
800-522-6294
Fax: 631-752-0689
TTY: 631-752-0738
sales@maxiaids.com
www.maxiaids.com

Elliot Zaretsky, Founder, President & CEO
The plates have curing type pressure sensitive material applied for metal to metal bonding. *$49.95*

497 Braille Touch-Time Watches
Independent Living Aids
137 Rano Rd.
Buffalo, NY 14207   716-332-2970
                                800-537-2118
                         Fax: 877-498-1482
          can-do@independentliving.com
              www.independentliving.com
White dial with black numerals and hands makes telling time possible quickly and easily for the visually impaired. *$44.95*

498 Circline Illuminated Magnifier
Dazor Lighting Technology
2360 Chaffee Drive
St. Louis, MO 63146   314-652-2400
                                800-345-9103
                           info@dazor.com
                           www.dazor.com
Provides even, shadow-free light under the magnifying lens with a 22-watt circline fluorescent. The magnifier is mounted on a floating arm that allows you to position the light source and lens with the touch of a finger.

499 Large Display Alarm Clock
HARC Mercantile
5413 S Westnedge Ave.
Suite A
Portage, MI 49002   800-445-9968
                          TTY: 269-324-1615
                            info@harc.com
                            www.harc.com

Michael Martinson, Owner
Features a large, easy-to-read display, as well as an extra-loud alarm and bedshaker. *$54.00*

500 Low Vision Watches & Clocks
Maxi Aids
42 Executive Blvd.
Farmingdale, NY 11735-4710   631-752-0521
                                800-522-6294
                          Fax: 631-752-0689
                          TTY: 631-752-0738
                        sales@maxiaids.com
                          www.maxiaids.com

Elliot Zaretsky, Founder, President & CEO
Offers a wide range of watches and clocks, including braille watches, talking watches, and large display clocks.

501 Magni-Cam & Primer
Innoventions

Magni-Cam and Primer are hand-held, light weight, inexpensive auto-focus electronic magnification systems designed to meet the reading and writing needs of those with low vision. The systems present the image in black and white or in color with three different view modes. Connects to any TV monitor in minutes. Systems read any surface with no distortion. A battery powered system is available, providing total portability and flexibility. *$25.00*

502 Magnifier Paperweight
Levenger
420 S Congress Ave
Delray Beach, FL 33445-4693   800-544-0880
                          Fax: 800-544-6910
                       Cservice@levenger.com
                         www.levenger.com

Margaret Moraskie, CEO
The Magnifier Paperweight features an optical quality magnifier and is long enough to enlarge the entire width of most book pages while holding the pages open. *$25.00*

503 Man's Low-Vision Quartz Watches
Independent Living Aids
137 Rano Rd.
Buffalo, NY 14207   716-332-2970
                                800-537-2118
                         Fax: 877-498-1482
          can-do@independentliving.com
              www.independentliving.com
An inexpensive, easy-to-read watch with chrome case. *$27.95*

504 MonoMouse Electronic Magnifiers
Maxi Aids
42 Executive Blvd.
Farmingdale, NY 11735-4710   631-752-0521
                                800-522-6294
                          Fax: 631-752-0689
                          TTY: 631-752-0738
                        sales@maxiaids.com
                          www.maxiaids.com

Elliot Zaretsky, Founder, President & CEO
Portable magnifier for people with low vision. Just about the size of a standard computer mouse. Compatible with any desktop or notebook PC. Variable magnification from 3x to 100x.

505 Stretch-View Wide-View Rectangular Illuminated Magnifier
Dazor Lighting Technology
2360 Chaffee Drive
St. Louis, MO 63146   314-652-2400
                                800-345-9103
                           info@dazor.com
                           www.dazor.com
Provides even, shadow-free light under the magnifying lens with a 22-watt circline fluorescent. The magnifier is mounted on a floating arm that allows you to position the light source and lens with the touch of a finger.

506 Unisex Low Vision Watch
Independent Living Aids
137 Rano Rd.
Buffalo, NY 14207   716-332-2970
                                800-537-2118
                         Fax: 877-498-1482
          can-do@independentliving.com
              www.independentliving.com
Unisex watch with large numbers and wide hands. Gold-toned case with either expansion or leather band. *$31.95*

Walking Aids: Canes, Crutches & Walkers

507 Aluminum Kiddie Canes
Maxi Aids
42 Executive Blvd.
Farmingdale, NY 11735-4710   631-752-0521
                                800-522-6294
                          Fax: 631-752-0689
                          TTY: 631-752-0738
                        sales@maxiaids.com
                          www.maxiaids.com

Elliot Zaretsky, Founder, President & CEO
Rigid and folding canes for children.

508 Aluminum Walking Canes
Maxi Aids
42 Executive Blvd.
Farmingdale, NY 11735-4710   631-752-0521
                                800-522-6294
                          Fax: 631-752-0689
                          TTY: 631-752-0738
                        sales@maxiaids.com
                          www.maxiaids.com

Elliot Zaretsky, Founder, President & CEO
Lightweight walking canes made of a heavy gauge aluminum tube with safety locknuts and heavy-duty rubber tips.

509 Axillary Crutches
Arista Surgical Supply Company
297 High Street
Dedham, MA 02026-2852   781-329-2900
                                800-437-2966
                          Fax: 781-437-2966
                customerservice@alimed.com
                          www.alimed.com

Adam S. Epstein, Chief Executive Officer
Lightweight crutches with wood underarms and handgrips. Adjusts to custom fit any user. *$43.25*

510   Days Hemi Walker
Performance Health
28100 Torch Parkway
Suite 700
Warrenville, IL 60555-3938   630-393-6000
                                    Fax: 630-393-7600
CustomerSupport@performancehealth.com
www.performancehealth.com
Francis Dirksmeier, Chief Executive Officer
Greg Nulty, Chief Financial Officer
Jim Plewa, Chief Sales Officer
For upper extremity trauma. An alternative to crutches that allows safe, stable ambulation for elderly or disabled individuals with the use of only one arm. *$74.50*

511   Deluxe Nova Wheeled Walker & Avant Wheeled Walker
Performance Health
28100 Torch Parkway
Suite 700
Warrenville, IL 60555-3938   630-393-6000
                                    Fax: 630-393-7600
CustomerSupport@performancehealth.com
www.performancehealth.com
Francis Dirksmeier, Chief Executive Officer
Greg Nulty, Chief Financial Officer
Jim Plewa, Chief Sales Officer
Lightweight and simple to handle with an easy-to-operate braking system. *$425.40*

512   Equalizer 6000 Single Stack Gym
Access To Recreation
8 Sandra Ct
Newbury Park, CA 91320-4302   805-498-7535
                                         800-634-4351
                                    Fax: 805-498-8186
customerservice@accesstr.com
www.accesstr.com
Don Krebs, President & Founder
Provides dynamic leg motion for individuals who are unable to stand upright or walk on their own.

513   Europa Superior Folding Cane
Maxi Aids
42 Executive Blvd.
Farmingdale, NY 11735-4710   631-752-0521
                                         800-522-6294
                                    Fax: 631-752-0689
TTY: 631-752-0738
sales@maxiaids.com
www.maxiaids.com
Elliot Zaretsky, Founder, President & CEO
Aluminum folding cane with tapered joints, golf grip with wrist loop, and screw-on glide tip. *$23.95*

514   Foot Harness
Consumer Care Products, LLC
W282 N7109 Main Street
Merton, WI 53056   262-820-2300
info@consumercarellc.com
www.consumercarellc.com
This sandle-like Foot Harness is designed for wheelchair plates and pedals. Available in small, medium, and large sizes.

515   Mobility Aid Trike
Consumer Care Products, LLC
W282 N7109 Main Street
Merton, WI 53056   262-820-2300
info@consumercarellc.com
www.consumercarellc.com
This mobility aid promotes postural alignment, balance, exercise and coordination.

516   Rand-Scot
Rand-Scot, Inc.
209 Christman Drive
Fort Collins, CO 80524   970-484-7967
                                         800-467-7967
                                    Fax: 970-484-3800
info@randscot.com
www.randscot.com
Joel Lerich, Co-Founder
Barbara Lerich, Co-Founder
Manufactures the Easy Pivot patient lift, the BBD wheelchair cushion line and Saratoga Exercise products for the disabled. Offers a line of patient lifts and standers for the disabled. Rand-scot products are designed to help the disabled achieve independence, comfort, and stamina.

517   Rollators
Maxi Aids
42 Executive Blvd.
Farmingdale, NY 11735-4710   631-752-0521
                                         800-522-6294
                                    Fax: 631-752-0689
TTY: 631-752-0738
sales@maxiaids.com
www.maxiaids.com
Elliot Zaretsky, Founder, President & CEO
Offers a wide range of rolling walkers.

518   Stable Base Quad Cane
Arista Surgical Supply Company/AliMed
297 High Street
Dedham, MA 02026-2852   781-329-2900
                                         800-437-2966
                                    Fax: 781-437-2966
info@alimed.com
www.alimed.com
Adam S. Epstein, Chief Executive Officer
A reliable walking cane offering independence to the physically challenged user. *$29.75*

519   T-Handle Cane
Arista Surgical Supply Company/AliMed
297 High Street
Dedham, MA 02026-2852   781-329-2900
                                         800-437-2966
                                    Fax: 781-437-2966
info@alimed.com
www.alimed.com
Adam S. Epstein, Chief Executive Officer
A standard old-fashioned wooden cane for the physically challenged. Ideal for those with arthritis. *$33.00*

520   TIDI Products, LLC
570 Enterprise Drive
Neenaha, WI 54956   920-751-4300
                                         800-521-1314
                                    Fax: 920-751-4370
excellence@tidiproducts.com
www.tidiproducts.com
Kevin McNamara, President & CEO
Jeff Hebbard, Vice President & COO
Jennifer Jones, Vice President, Marketing
TIDI Products meets the needs of caregivers for job optimization and providing solutions to other healthcare professionals. Supplies Brand name medical equipment and devices including: POSEY patient safety devices, TIDISHIELD eyewear and devices, C-AMOR drapes, STERILE-Z drapes, GRIP-LOK securement items, and ZERO-GRAVITY radiation protection.

521   U-Step Walking Stabilizer: Walker
Maxi Aids
42 Executive Blvd.
Farmingdale, NY 11735-4710   631-752-0521
                                         800-522-6294
                                    Fax: 631-752-0689
TTY: 631-752-0738
sales@maxiaids.com
www.maxiaids.com
Elliot Zaretsky, Founder, President & CEO

Stabilizing walker with braking system, seat and basket. Easily foldable. Weight capacity is 375 lbs. Suitable for users 5'1 to 6'1 tall. *$539.95*

522   Ventura Enterprises
4431 S. Eastern Avenue
Las Vegas, NV 89119   702-457-7676
                                    info@venturaenterprises.com
                                    www.venturaenterprises.com

Sam Ventura, President & CEO
Ron Ventura, Vice President of Development
Galit Rozen, Vice President of Acquisitions
Manufacturer of everyday living mobility aids. Products include carrying aids for walkers and wheelchairs and also wheelchair cushions.

523   WCIB Heavy-Duty Folding Cane
Maxi Aids
42 Executive Blvd.
Farmingdale, NY 11735-4710   631-752-0521
                                    800-522-6294
                                Fax: 631-752-0689
                                TTY: 631-752-0738
                                    sales@maxiaids.com
                                    www.maxiaids.com

Elliot Zaretsky, Founder, President & CEO
A four section aluminum folding cane with a golf-type grip handle and flexible wrist loop. *$27.95*

Wheelchairs: Accessories

524   Advantage Wheelchair & Walker Bags
Advantage Bag Company

                                    310-540-8197
                                advantagebag@verizon.net
                                    www.advantagebag.com
Wheelchairs with and without push handles. Pac slips over back of almost any wheelchair.

525   Automatic Wheelchair Rollback Lock
Alzheimer's Store
3197 Trout Place Rd
Cumming, GA 30041-8260   678-947-4001
                                    800-752-3238
                                Fax: 678-947-8411
                                    contact@alzstore.com
                                    www.alzstore.com

Ellen Warner, President & Co-Founder
Mark Warner, Co-Founder
Automatic anti-rollback safety device automatically locks the wheels whenever the user stands or sits.

526   Battery Operated Cushion
DA Schulman
3827 Creekside Lane
Holmen, WI 54636   608-782-0031
                                    866-782-9658
                                Fax: 608-782-0488
                                    aquila@aquilacorp.com
                                    www.aquilacorp.com

Steve Kohlman, Owner & President
Justine Kohlman, Vice President
Battery-operated, dynamic cushion for wheelchairs. The Airpulse PK wheelchair cushion system is Aquila Corporation's most dynamic cushion system. It was designed to be the most advanced solution to help prevent and heal pressure ulcers.

527   Dual-Mode Charger
Lester Electrical
625 West A Street
Lincoln, NE 68522-1794   402-477-8988
                                    sales@lesterelectrical.com
                                    www.lesterelectrical.com

Spencer Stock, President & CEO
Fully automatic battery charger.

528   Equalizer 1000 Series
Helm Distributing
Deer Park P.O.
PO Box 25105
Red Deer, Alberta, Canada, T4R-2M2   403-309-5551
                                Fax: 403-342-5509
                                    james@equalizerexercise.com
                                    www.equalizerexercise.com
Weight training equipment designed for wheelchair users. Features 7 stations targeting different major muscle parts: Vertical Bench Press, Seated Military Press, High/Low Pulleys, Lat Pull Down, Vertical Butterfly, Leg Curl and Extension, Lateral Deltoid, and Seated Leg Press/Calf Extension, in addition to a variety of accessories. *$ 7050.00*

529   Equalizer 6000 Series
Helm Distributing
Deer Park P.O.
PO Box 25105
Red Deer, Alberta, Canada, T4R-2M2   403-309-5551
                                Fax: 403-342-5509
                                    james@equalizerexercise.com
                                    www.equalizerexercise.com
Weight training equipment designed for wheelchair users. Includes Vertical Bench Press, Rowing/Long Pull, Lat Pull Down, Vertical Butterfly, Low Pulley/Prchr. Bench, Gripless Bicep Curl, Gripless Tricep Extension, Mid Pulley, and Removable Rolling Stool. *$4250.00*

530   Featherspring Shoe Inserts
Luxis International, Inc.
1292 South 7th St.
DeKalb, IL 60115   815-981-3793
                                    800-628-4693
                                Fax: 800-261-1164
                                    www.luxis.com
Foot supports for wheelchair users to prevent and treat cold feet, sore heels, swollen feet and weak ankles. *$199.95*

531   Gem Wheelchair & Scooter Service: Mobility & Homecare
176-39 Union Turnpike
Flushing, NY 11366   718-969-8600
                                    800-943-3578
                                    help@gemwheelchairservice.com
                                    www.gemwheelchairservice.com
GEM sells, repairs and rents all models of manual and motorized wheelchairs, power scooters, ramps, stairway lifts, and homecare products including diapers, chux, and bathroom safety equipment.

532   MAT Factory, Inc.
6726 North Figueroa Street
Los Angeles, CA 90042   800-628-7626
                                    888-266-7590
                                Fax: 888-266-9555
                                    sales@matfactoryinc.com
                                    www.matfactoryinc.com
Wheelchair access mats for pathways, walkways, trails and playgrounds.

533   Permobil
300 Duke Dr
Lebanon, TN 37090   800-736-0925
                                    www.permobilus.com

Bengt Thorsson, President & CEO
Charlotta Nyberg, Chief Financial Officer
Jonas Cederhage, Executive Vice President, Group Supply Chain
Develops and manufactures wheelchairs, communication systems, and seating and positioning systems for users with disabilities. Offers a full line of standing wheelchairs for manual operation. *$ 7000.00*

534   Safety Deck II
MAT Factory, Inc.
6726 North Figueroa Street
Los Angeles, CA 90042   800-628-7626
                                    888-266-7590
                                Fax: 888-266-9555
                                    sales@matfactoryinc.com
                                    www.matfactoryinc.com

The Safety Deck II is an interlocking grid system made from recycled rubber tires and recycled PVC. The tiles are set directly on top of the ground and permit grass to grow through the holes and cover the surface. The system provides safe, non-barrier access for wheelchairs over grass. Once the grass has covered the tiles the only maintenance required is watering and mowing. Safety Deck II also allows for beach and sand access. *$7.80*

535   Scooter & Wheelchair Battery Fuel Gauges and Motor Speed Controllers
Curtis Instruments, Inc.
200 Kisco Ave.
Mount Kisco, NY 10549   914-666-2971
                                            www.curtisinst.com
Provides a readable, accurate indication of battery in easy to read type of display. Innovative, efficient motor speed controllers for single or dual PM motor vehicles.

536   Softfoot Ergomatta
MAT Factory, Inc.
6726 North Figueroa Street
Los Angeles, CA 90042   800-628-7626
                                              888-266-7590
                                         Fax: 888-266-9555
                                    sales@matfactoryinc.com
                                        www.matfactoryinc.com
Interlocking roll-up mat system with antimicrobial additive. Allows wheelchairs and walkers to move easily and safely along wet and potentially hazardous surfaces. *$9.90*

537   Wheelchair Accessories
Diestco Manufacturing Company
370 Ryan Ave.
Chico, CA 95973   800-795-2392
                                             www.diestco.com
Diestco makes innovative accessories for wheelchairs, scooters and walkers. Products include canopies, backpacks, cupholders, pouches, threshold ramps, laptrays and others.

538   Wheelchair Back Pack and Tote Bag
Med Covers
321 Route 59
Suite 147
Tallman, NY 10982   718-302-1923
                                              800-320-7140
                                         Fax: 866-522-6967
                                   info@1800wheelchair.com
                                      www.1800wheelchair.com
Accessories are specifically designed with the wheelchair user in mind. The Back Pack has a main roomy pouch for larger items and has a full length zipper with four sliders for convenient access.

539   Wheelchair Positioning Tray
Graham-Field
One Graham-Field Way
Atlanta, GA 30340-4700   770-368-4700
                                         Fax: 770-368-4932
                                      cs@grahamfield.com
                                        www.grahamfield.com
Kenneth Spett, President & CEO
Cherie Antoniazzi, Senior Vice President, Quality, Regulatory & Risk Management
Marc Bernstein, Senior Vice President, Consumer Sales
This is a heavy-duty wheelchair comfort tray which surrounds the wheelchair user and provides a large, smooth surface for dining, writing, hobbies or work. Includes washable nylon cover with zippered pockets.

540   Wheelchair Roller
Access To Recreation
8 Sandra Ct
Newbury Park, CA 91320-4302   805-498-7535
                                              800-634-4351
                                         Fax: 805-498-8186
                                  customerservice@accesstr.com
                                            www.accesstr.com
Don Krebs, President & Founder
The McClain Wheelchair Roller allows you to build strength and stamina in the comfort of your own home.

541   Wheelchair Work Table
Bailey Manufacturing Company
P.O. Box 130
Lodi, OH 44254-0130   330-948-1080
                                              800-321-8372
                                         Fax: 330-948-4439
                                      baileymfg@baileymfg.com
                                           www.baileymfg.com
An adjustable height, functional, individual cut-out work table featuring a wood-grain laminate, scratch resistant top with chrome plated steel legs.

Wheelchairs: General

542   21st Century Scientific, Inc. - Bounder Power Wheelchair
4931 N Manufacturing Way
Coeur D Alene, ID 83815-8931   208-667-8800
                                              800-448-3680
                                         Fax: 208-667-6600
                                      21st@wheelchairs.com
                                            wheelchairs.com
Ronald E. Prior, Ph.D., President & Founder
High-performance power chairs for active individuals. High-speed (11 + MPH), OFF-ROAD, and Bariatric options are available. Power seating options include tilt, recline, 13-inch seat elevator, reverse tilt, leg rests, standing, and front load (latitude). 6-drive programmable electronics standard; lights, horn, electric bag emptier and many other options available.

543   Ability Center
4797 Ruffner St.
San Diego, CA 92111   858-541-0552
                                              833-919-2581
                                         Fax: 858-541-1941
                                        www.abilitycenter.com
Terry Barton, General Manager
Specializes in accessible vehicles and mobility products; the company has more than 100 employees in 14 locations across the western U.S.
1994

544   Advantage Wheelchair
Sizewise
8601 Monrovia Street
Lenexa, KS 66215   800-814-9389
                                         info@sizewise.com
                                           www.sizewise.com
A large-frame wheelchair constructed of high-quality, stress-tested stainless steel to ensure durability and peak performance.

545   Breezy
Sunrise Medical
2842 Business Park Avenue
Fresno, CA 93727   800-333-4000
                                         Fax: 800-300-7502
                                        www.sunrisemedical.com
Thomas Babacan, President & CEO
Roxane Cromwell, Chief Operating Officer
Adrian Platt, Chief Financial Officer
This lightweight chair is durable, comfortable and flexible enough to meet the needs of a wide range of wheelchair users.

546   Breezy Elegance
Sunrise Medical
2842 Business Park Avenue
Fresno, CA 93727   800-333-4000
                                         Fax: 800-300-7502
                                        www.sunrisemedical.com
Thomas Babacan, President & CEO
Roxane Cromwell, Chief Operating Officer
Adrian Platt, Chief Financial Officer
A lightweight, portable folding wheelchair. *$750.00*

547   Champion
Kuschall of America
                                               kuschall.com

The ultra-light, compact, foldable Champion wheelchair has the feel and performance of a rigid chair.

548 Choosing a Wheelchair: A Guide for Optimal Independence
Patient-Centered Guides
1005 Gravenstein Highway North
Sebastopol, CA 95472
707-827-7000
Fax: 707-829-0104
support@oreilly.com
www.oreilly.com

Linda Lamb, Series Editor
Shawnde Paull, Marketing
Tim O'Reilly, Publisher
With the right wheelchair, quality of life increases dramatically and even people with severe disabilities can have a considerable degree of independence and activity. Choosing the wrong chair can indeed the tantamount to confinement. This book describes technology, options, and the selection process to help you identify the chair than can provide you with optimal independence.
$11.19
186 pages Paperback
ISBN 1-565924-11-8

549 Compact
Kuschall of America
kuschall.com
The Compact wheelchair is lightweight, foldable and features new, ergonomic bended knee shape for maximum convenience.

550 Convaid
2830 California Street
Torrance, CA 90503
888-266-8243
Fax: 310-618-2166
convaidsales.us@etac.com
www.convaid.com

Chris Braun, President
Five different styles of wheelchairs.

551 Etac USA
P.O. Box 1739
Matthews, NC 28106-1739
262-717-9910
800-678-3822
Fax: 262-796-4605
sales.us@etac.com
www.etac.com/en-us/us/
Offers wheelchairs designed to provide function, comfort and flexibility. Seat frame and upholstery are adjustable to fit each individual. Swing away, detachable footrests are standard. Numerous accessories are available in order to individualize each chair. Lifetime warranty on frame for original user.

552 Evacu-Trac
Garaventa Lift Canada
18920 - 36th
Surrey, BC, Canada, V3Z-0P6
604-594-0422
800-663-6556
info@garaventalift.com
www.garaventalift.com
This emergency evacuation chair is designed for safety and fast operation.

553 Gem Wheelchair & Scooter Service: Mobility & Homecare
176-39 Union Turnpike
Flushing, NY 11366
718-969-8600
800-943-3578
help@gemwheelchairservice.com
www.gemwheelchairservice.com
GEM sells, repairs and rents all models of manual and motorized wheelchairs, power scooters, ramps, stairway lifts, and homecare products including diapers, chux, and bathroom safety equipment.

554 Gendron
GF Health Products, Inc.
P.O. Box 47510
Doraville, GA 30362-0510
770-368-4700
cs@grahamfield.com
www.gendroninc.com

Katie Johnson, Director of Customer Service & Technical Support

Manufacturer of wheelchairs for a variety of other applications, specializing in bariatric mobility products.

555 K-Series
Kuschall of America
kuschall.com
Fully-adjustable wheelchair that can be modified independently from the frame.

556 Lounge Chairs
Graham-Field Health Products
One Graham-Field Way
Atlanta, GA 30340-4700
770-368-4700
Fax: 770-368-4932
cs@grahamfield.com
www.grahamfield.com

Kenneth Spett, President & CEO
Cherie Antoniazzi, Senior Vice President, Quality, Regulatory & Risk Management
Marc Bernstein, Senior Vice President, Consumer Sales
Provides all-day comfort and safe, independent mobilization with feet or hands. The ergonomically engineered seat back provides correct support.

557 Majors Medical Service
2601 W Mockingbird Ln
Suite 101
Dallas, TX 75235
214-951-9710
Fax: 214-951-9720
www.majorsmedicalservice.com

Pat Metz, Owner
Offers selection of wheelchairs and homecare medical equipment for safety and mobility needs.

558 Pride Mobility
401 York Avenue
Duryea, PA 18642
800-522-7391
info@pridemobility.com
www.pridemobility.com

Scott Meuser, Chair & CEO
Dan Meuser, Owner
Pride Mobility manufacturers a variety of electric wheelchairs, mobility scooters, and lift chairs for users of all sizes. As a global innovator, Pride Mobility is dedicated to improving the lives of users through mobility solutions.

559 Regency XL 2002
GF Health Products, Inc.
P.O. Box 47510
Doraville, GA 30362-0510
770-368-4700
cs@grahamfield.com
www.gendroninc.com

Katie Johnson, Director of Customer Service & Technical Support
Bariatric wheelchairs for users weighing up to 600 pounds.

560 Rock-King X3000 Wheel Chair Kit
Maxi Aids
42 Executive Blvd.
Farmingdale, NY 11735-4710
631-752-0521
800-522-6294
Fax: 631-752-0689
TTY: 631-752-0738
sales@maxiaids.com
www.maxiaids.com

Elliot Zaretsky, Founder, President & CEO
Wheelchair that can turn into a rocking chair with the flip of a lever. The kit includes wheels, footrests, lateral supports, black frame finish, heal-leg strap, cushion and standard head pillow.
$1995.00

561 Rolls 2000 Series
Invacare
1 Invacare Way
Elyria, OH 44035-4190
800-333-6900
www.invacare.com

Matthew E. Monaghan, Chairman of the Board & Chief Executive Officer
Rick A. Cassiday, Senior Vice President & Chief Human Resources Officer
Kathleen P. Leneghan, Senior Vice President & Chief Financial Officer

The first light-weight wheelchairs designed for rental use. Comes with optional elevating footrests.

562 Skyway
Skyway Machine
4451 Caterpillar Rd
Redding, CA 96003
530-243-5151
800-332-3357
Fax: 530-243-5104
www.skywaywheels.com

Ken Coster, Sales Department
Parrey Cremeans, Sales Department
Rein Stolz, Engineering Department
Supplies wheel combinations for wheelchairs, lawn and garden products, bicycles, and a large assortment of wheeled devices to serve the Health Care industry. Wheel sizes range from 4-inch to 24-inch diameter.

563 The KSL
Kuschall of America
kuschall.com
Ultralight wheelchair designed to improve mobility.

564 Vista Wheelchair
Arista Surgical Supply Company/AliMed
297 High Street
Dedham, MA 02026-2852
781-329-2900
800-437-2966
Fax: 781-437-2966
info@alimed.com
www.alimed.com

Adam S. Epstein, Chief Executive Officer
Vista has a rugged cold-rolled steel frame, durable vinyl upholstery and steel bearings to assure a smooth ride. *$220.00*

565 Wheelchairs and Transport Chairs
Maxi Aids
42 Executive Blvd.
Farmingdale, NY 11735-4710
631-752-0521
800-522-6294
Fax: 631-752-0689
TTY: 631-752-0738
sales@maxiaids.com
www.maxiaids.com

Elliot Zaretsky, Founder, President & CEO
Offers a wide range of wheelchairs, including lightweight transport chairs, full-reclining wheelchairs, bariatric wheelchairs, and more.

Wheelchairs: Pediatric

566 Convaid
2830 California Street
Torrance, CA 90503
888-266-8243
Fax: 310-618-2166
convaidsales.us@etac.com
www.convaid.com

Chris Braun, President
Convaid manufactures Mobile Positioning Systems for children. The Expedition, Safari Tilt, Cruiser, EZ Rider and Metro offer a non-institutional styling and are lightweight and compact-folding. The steel/aluminum structure is engineered for maximum comfort and durability. The mobile positioning lines come with more than 20 positioning features and a full range of positioning adaptations.

567 Imp Tricycle
TRIAID
P.O. Box 1364
Cumberland, MD 21501
301-759-3525
Fax: 301-759-3525
sales@triaid.com
www.triaid.com

Provides fun therapy and actively encourages participation, awareness and the building of self confidence. Designed for children from 2 1/2 years, it features ATB styling, 12 1/2 inch wheels, an adjustable steering stop and a supportive saddle. Handlebar and seat adjustments combine with a broad wheelbase to ensure

the rider is in the optimum position to pedal, and the tricycle gives good stability and confident handling. Support accessories are available. *$590.00*

568 Koala R-Net
Permobil USA
300 Duke Dr
Lebanon, TN 37090
800-736-0925
www.permobilus.com

Bengt Thorsson, President & CEO
Charlotta Nyberg, Chief Financial Officer
Jonas Cederhage, Executive Vice President, Group Supply Chain
The Koala Miniflex is a powered wheelchair designed for use by children with lower extremity, mobility, or neurological disabilities or spinal cord injury.

569 TMX Tricycle
TRIAID
P.O. Box 1364
Cumberland, MD 21501
301-759-3525
Fax: 301-759-3525
sales@triaid.com
www.triaid.com

Provides fun therapy and actively encourages participation, awareness and the building of self confidence. Designed for children from about eight years, it features ATB styling, 20-inch wheels, adjustable steering stop and a supportive saddle. Handlebar and seat adjustments combine with a broad wheelbase to ensure the rider is in the optimum position to pedal and the tricycle gives good stability and confident handling. Support accessories are available. *$795.00*

Wheelchairs: Powered

570 Bounder 450
21st Century Scientific
4931 N Manufacturing Way
Coeur D Alene, ID 83815-8931
208-667-8800
800-448-3680
Fax: 208-667-6600
21st@wheelchairs.com
wheelchairs.com

Ronald E. Prior, Ph.D., President & Founder
The Heavy Duty Bounder 450 Power Wheelchair is designed for users up to 450 lbs.

571 Bounder Power Wheelchair
21st Century Scientific
4931 N Manufacturing Way
Coeur D Alene, ID 83815-8931
208-667-8800
800-448-3680
Fax: 208-667-6600
21st@wheelchairs.com
wheelchairs.com

Ronald E. Prior, Ph.D., President & Founder
The Bounder Power Wheelchair is designed for users up to 300 lbs. *$8695.00*

572 Chief 107-ZRx
Redman Powerchair
1601 S Pantano Rd
Suite 107
Tucson, AZ 85710
800-727-6684
Info@RedmanPowerChair.com
www.redmanpowerchair.com

Don Redman, Co-Founder
Paula Redman, Co-Founder
Motorized standing chair which allows you to stand, recline, and tilt comfortably. Custom sizing is available for power chairs from 3'8 40 lbs. to 6'8 350 lbs.

573 Damaco D90 Biomedical Battery
Damaco
28381 Constellation Rd.
Valencia, CA 91355
877-528-2288
Fax: 661-775-2025
www.atbatt.com

Sealed Lead Acid battery for Damaco D90 Power Wheelchair. Nominal voltage of 12.0V/rated capacity of 26.0Ah. 2/Unit Required. *$ 2495.00*

574 Folding Lightweight Power Wheelchair
Maxi Aids
42 Executive Blvd.
Farmingdale, NY 11735-4710
631-752-0521
800-522-6294
Fax: 631-752-0689
TTY: 631-752-0738
sales@maxiaids.com
www.maxiaids.com

Elliot Zaretsky, Founder, President & CEO
Folding power wheelchair with large foot platform, foam seat design and back seat pocket for storage. Weight capacity is 400 lbs. *$2579.00*

575 Gem Wheelchair & Scooter Service: Mobility & Homecare
176-39 Union Turnpike
Flushing, NY 11366
718-969-8600
800-943-3578
help@gemwheelchairservice.com
www.gemwheelchairservice.com
GEM sells, repairs and rents all models of manual and motorized wheelchairs, power scooters, ramps, stairway lifts, and homecare products including diapers, chux, and bathroom safety equipment.

576 Permobil F3 Corpus
Permobil
800-736-0925
www.permobil.com/en-us
An easily maneuverable power wheelchair featuring the smallest footprint of the Permobil F-series.

577 Permobil M300 Corpus HD
Permobil
800-736-0925
www.permobil.com/en-us
The power wheelchair is designed for users up to 450 lbs.

578 Power Wheelchairs
LaBac Systems
8245 Quebec St
Commerce City, CO 80022
800-370-6808
Fax: 303-340-3863
www.falconrehab.net
Power tilt and recline seating systems for wheelchairs, offering more comfort and dependability for the physically challenged.

Wheelchairs: Racing

579 Eagle Sportschairs, LLC
2351 Parkwood Road
Snellville, GA 30039-4003
770-972-0763
Fax: 770-985-4885
eaglesportschairs@gmail.com
www.eaglesportschairs.com

Barry Ewing, Owner
The Eagle line of custom lightweight performance chairs includes various options to fit all racing and sports needs, including track, baseball, quad-rugby, tennis, field events and waterskiing. Also popular for daily use. Ability to customize any chair to accommodate size and disability.

580 East Penn Manufacturing Company
East Penn Manufacturing Company
102 Deka Rd.
Lyons, PA 19536
610-682-6361
Fax: 610-682-4781
contactus@eastpenn-deka.com
www.eastpennmanufacturing.com

Daniel Langdon, President & CEO
DeLight Breidegam, Co-Founder & Chair
David Byrne, Director of Finance & Accounting

Specially engineered for demanding deep-cycle applications, Gelled electrolyte Deka Dominator Batteries provide maintenance-free operation and longer battery life.

581 Invacare Top End
Invacare
1 Invacare Way
Elyria, OH 44035-4107
800-333-6900
www.invacare.com
Matthew E. Monaghan, Chairman of the Board & Chief Executive Officer
Rick A. Cassiday, Senior Vice President & Chief Human Resources Officer
Kathleen P. Leneghan, Senior Vice President & Chief Financial Officer
Manufacturers of lightweight, rigid, sport-specific wheelchairs, such as the Eliminator line of racing chairs, T-3 tennis and softball chairs, and the Terminator for quad rugby and basketball. The Excelerator, XLT three-wheel hand cycle for adults and juniors.

Associations

General Disabilities

582 A Loving Spoonful
1449 Powell St.
Vancouver, BC, Canada V5L-1G8   604-682-6325
Fax: 604-682-6327
info@alovingspoonful.org
alovingspoonful.org

Gerald Regio, President
Quinn Newcomb, Vice President
Ken Channon, Treasurer
A Loving Spoonful is a volunteer-driven, non-partisan Society that provides free, nutritious meals to people living with HIV/AIDS in Greater Vancouver. Every week volunteers deliver frozen meals and snack packs to men, women, and children who are primarily homebound with AIDS.
1989

583 ADA National Network
ADA Knowledge Translation Center
University of Washington
Seattle, WA 98382   800-949-4232
adakt@uw.edu
adata.org
The Network offers information and training on how to implement the Americans with Disabilities Act (ADA). It consists of 10 regional centers across the U.S., plus an ADA Knowledge Translation Center, and is funded by the National Institute on Disability, Independent Living, and Rehabilitation Research (NIDILRR).

584 AHF Federation
AIDS Healthcare Foundation
6255 Sunset Blvd.
21st Floor
Los Angeles, CA 90028   323-860-5200
www.aidshealth.org

Michael Weinstein, President
Peter Reis, Senior Vice President
Scott Carruthers, Chief Pharmacy Officer
A consortium of AIDS Service Organizations under the umbrella of the AIDS Healthcare Foundation.

585 AIDS Healthcare Foundation
6255 Sunset Blvd.
21st Floor
Los Angeles, CA 90028   323-860-5200
www.aidshealth.org

Michael Weinstein, President
Peter Reis, Senior Vice President
Scott Carruthers, Chief Pharmacy Officer
The Los Angeles-based AIDS Healthcare Foundation (AHF) is a global nonprofit organization providing medicine and advocacy to people all around the world. AHF is currently the largest provider of HIV/AIDS medical care in the U.S.
1987

586 AIDS Vancouver
1101 Seymour St.
4th Floor
Vancouver, BC, Canada V6B-0R1   604-893-2201
Fax: 604-893-2205
contact@aidsvancouver.org
aidsvancouver.org

Phillip Banks, Interim Executive Director
Janet Cheng, Finance Director
Adam Reibin, Director of External Relations
AIDS Vancouver strives to create a community with no new HIV infections while ensuring support for those who are affected through case management services, financial assistance, grocery and nutrition support, and confidential helplines.
1983

587 Abilities, Inc.
The Viscardi Center
201 I.U. Willets Rd.
Albertson, NY 11507   516-465-1400
info@viscardicenter.org
viscardicenter.org/services/abilities-inc
Dr. Chris Rosa, President & Chief Executive Officer
Sheryl P. Buchel, Executive Vice President & Chief Financial Officer
Michael Caprara, Chief Information Officer
The Viscardi Center is a network of nonprofit organizations that provides a lifespan of services for children and adults with disabilities. The Abilities, Inc. program prepares adolescents and adults with disabilities for entering the workforce.
1952

588 Academy of Integrative Health & Medicine (AIHM)
6919 La Jolla Blvd.
San Diego, CA 92037   info@aihm.org
aihm.org

Tabatha Parker, Executive Director
Erika Cappelluti, Fellowship Director
April Gruzinsky, Fellowship Admissions Director
The Academy of Integrative Health & Medicine unites health care professionals from family doctors to psychologists, acupuncturists to nurses, to build bridges between disciplines and offer credible educational and certification programs for licensed health care providers.
1996

589 Access & Information Network
2600 N Stemmons Fwy
Suite 151
Dallas, TX 75207   214-943-4444
Fax: 469-329-0717
info@aindallas.org
aindallas.org

Steven Pace, President & Chief Executive Officer
Joni Wysocki, Chief Operating Officer
Hosea Crowell, Compliance Coordinator
AIN is a nonprofit organization providing services for individuals with chronic health conditions and prevention programs for at-risk communities.

590 Accreditation Commission for Acupuncture & Oriental Medicine
8941 Aztec Dr.
Suite 2
Eden Prairie, MN 55347   952-212-2434
info@acaom.org
acaom.org

Mark McKenzie, Executive Director
Karl Gauby, Director, Regulatory Affairs
Jason Wright, Director, Accreditation Services
National accrediting agency of programs in acupuncture and Oriental medicine (AOM), and related institutions.

591 Accreditation Commission for Midwifery Education (ACME)
American College of Nurse Midwives
8403 Colesville Rd.
Suite 1230
Silver Spring, MD 20910   240-485-1800
Fax: 240-485-1818
membership@acnm.org
midwife.org/acme

Katrina Holland, Executive Director
Amy Kohl, Director, Advocacy & Government Affairs
Marc Rucker, Vice President, Finance & Operations
Commission of the American College of Nurse Midwives responsible for overseeing all aspects of the accreditation review process.

592   Advocacy Centre for the Elderly (ACE)
2 Carlton St.
Suite 701
Toronto, ON, Canada M5B-1J3   416-598-2656
                                               855-598-2656
                                      Fax: 416-598-7924
                          www.advocacycentreelderly.org
Graham Webb, Executive Director
Susan Bryson, Chair
Alexander Henderson, Vice Chair
The Advocacy Centre for the Elderly is a specialty community legal clinic that provides a range of legal services to low-income seniors in Ontario. Legal services include advice and representation to individual and group clients, public legal education, law reform, and community development activities.
1984

593   Advocates for Children of New York (AFC)
151 West 30th St.
5th Floor
New York, NY 10001   212-947-9779
                                      Fax: 212-947-9790
                          info@advocatesforchildren.org
                          www.advocatesforchildren.org
Kim Sweet, Executive Director
Matthew Lenaghan, Deputy Director
Ivette Greenblatt, Director, Development
AFC works on behalf of children from infancy to age 21 who are at risk for school-based discrimination and/or academic failure. These include children with disabilities, ethnic minorities, immigrants, homeless children, foster care children, English language learners, and those living in poverty.

594   Advocates for Developmental Disabilities
1301 Lincoln Ave. S.
Owatonna, MN 55060
Advocates for Developmental Disabilities is a local agency that advocates for the dissemination of information regarding developmental disabilities, the enhancement of existing services, and the development of new programs on behalf of individuals with developmental disabilities. Its goal is to develop a better understanding of developmental disabilities by families and others interested in the welfare of individuals with developmental disabilities.

595   American Academy of Audiology (AAA)
11480 Commerce Park Dr.
Suite 220
Reston, VA 20191   703-790-8466
                                      Fax: 703-790-8631
                               infoaud@audiology.org
                               www.audiology.org
Patrick E. Gallagher, Executive Director
Kathryn Werner, Vice President, Public Affairs
Amy Miedema, Vice President, Communications & Membership
The American Academy of Audiology is the world's largest professional organization for audiologists. The Academy is dedicated to providing quality hearing care services through professional development, education, research, and increased public awareness of hearing and balance disorders.

596   American Academy of Environmental Medicine (AAEM)
PO Box 195
Ashland, MO 65010   316-684-5500
                                      Fax: 888-411-1206
                               www.aaemonline.org
Dane Mosher, President
Lauren Grohs, Executive Director
William A. Ingram, Secretary
The Academy is an association of physicians and other professionals engaged in investigating and coming up with preventive strategies for medical care relating to environmentally triggered illnesses.
1965

597   American Academy of Medical Acupuncture
2512 Artesia Blvd.
Suite 200
Redondo Beach, CA 90278   310-379-8261
                          info@medicalacupuncture.org
                          www.medicalacupuncture.org
Kendra Unger, President
Donna Pittman, Vice President
Montiel Rosenthal, Secretary
Professional organization for physicians in North America who have incorporated acupuncture into their traditional medical practice.
1987

598   American Academy of Pain Medicine (AAPM)
1705 Edgewater Dr.
Suite 7778
Orlando, FL 32804   800-917-1619
                                      Fáx: 407-749-0714
                               info@painmed.org
                               painmed.org
W. Michael Hooten, President
Vitaly Gordin, Vice President, Scientific Affairs
Farshad M. Ahadian, Treasurer
AAPM is an organization created for physicians practicing the specialty of pain medicine in the United States. AAPM works to provide the most up-to-date information available on the practice of pain medicine, advocate for its members, and bring visibility and credibility to the specialty of pain medicine.
1983

599   American Academy of Pain Medicine Foundation
American Academy of Pain Medicine
1705 Edgewater Dr.
Suite 7778
Orlando, FL 32804   800-917-1619
                                      Fax: 407-749-0714
                               info@painmed.org
                          painmed.org/aapm-foundation
W. Michael Hooten, President
The Foundation supports AAPM's core purpose to optimize the health of patients in pain and eliminate the major health problem of pain by advancing the practice and the specialty of pain medicine.
1911

600   American Academy of Pediatrics (AAP)
345 Park Blvd.
Itasca, IL 60143   800-433-9016
                                      Fax: 847-434-8000
                               mcc@aap.org
                               www.aap.org
Mark Del Monte, Chief Executive Officer & Executive Vice President
Christine Bork, Chief Development Officer & Sr. Vice President, Development
Roberta Bosak, Chief Administrative Officer & Sr. Vice President, HR
An organization of pediatricians committed to attaining the best physical, mental, and social health and well-being for all infants, children, adolescents, and young adults.
1930

601   American Acupuncture Council
1100 W Town & Country Rd.
Suite 1400
Orange, CA 92868   800-838-0383
                                      Fax: 714-571-1863
                          info@acupuncturecouncil.com
                          acupuncturecouncil.com
Marilyn Allen, Contact
Provides acupuncture malpractice insurance across the country.

602 American Association of Acupuncture and Oriental Medicine (AAAOM)
PO Box 96503
Suite 44114
Washington, DC 20090-6503   admin@aaaomonline.org
                                   www.aaaomonline.org

Carlos Chapa, President
Drea Miller, Vice President
Fotios Sardelis, Treasurer
A national professional organization that is dedicated to the promotion and advancement of high ethical, educational, and professional standards in the practice of acupuncture and Oriental medicine (AOM) in the U.S.

603 American Association of People with Disabilities (AAPD)
2013 H St. NW
5th Floor
Washington, DC 20006   202-521-4316
                                  800-840-8844
                          communications@aapd.com
                                   www.aapd.com

Maria Town, President & Chief Executive Officer
Jasmin Bailey, Manager, Business Operations
Christine Liao, Programs Director
Nonprofit cross-disability member organization dedicated to ensuring economic self-sufficiency and political empowerment for Americans with disabilities. AAPD works in coalition with other disability organizations for the full implementation and enforcement of disability nondiscrimination laws, particularly the Americans With Disabilities Act (ADA) of 1990 and the Rehabilitation Act of 1973.

604 American Association on Health and Disability (AAHD)
110 N Washington St.
Suite 407
Rockville, MD 20850   301-545-6140
                             Fax: 301-545-6144
                                 contact@aahd.us
                                   www.aahd.us

Roberta Carlin, Executive Director
Karl Cooper, Director, Public Health Programs
E. Clarke Ross, Director, Public Policy
The American Association on Health and Disability is a cross-disability national nonprofit organization committed to promoting health and wellness initiatives for children and adults with disabilities.

605 American Association on Intellectual and Developmental Disabilities (AAIDD)
8403 Colesville Rd.
Suite 900
Silver Spring, MD 20910   202-387-1968
                             Fax: 202-387-2193
                                       aaidd.org
Margaret A. Nygren, Executive Director & Chief Executive Officer
Paul D. Aitken, Director, Finance & Administration
Ravita Maharaj, Director, Supports Intensity Scale Program
The organization focuses on intellectual and developmental disabilities, advocating for quality of life and rights for individuals with such disabilities.

606 American Board of Disability Analysts (ABDA)
1483 N. Mt. Juliet Rd.
Suite 175
Nashville, TN 37122   629-255-0870
                             Fax: 615-296-9980
                             office@eventsm3.com
                        www.americandisability.org
Certifies physicians, psychologists, attorneys, and counselors as specialists in disability and personal injury.

607 American Board of Medical Psychotherapists and Psychodiagnosticians
American Board of Disability Analysts
1483 N. Mt. Juliet Rd.
Suite 175
Nashville, TN 37122   629-255-0870
                             Fax: 615-296-9980
                             office@eventsm3.com
                        www.americandisability.org

Affiliated organization of the American Board of Disability Analysts (ABDA).

608 American Board of Professional Disability Consultants
American Board of Disability Analysts
1483 N. Mt. Juliet Rd.
Suite 175
Nashville, TN 37122   629-255-0870
                             Fax: 615-296-9980
                             office@eventsm3.com
                        www.americandisability.org
Affiliated organization of the American Board of Disability Analysts (ABDA).

609 American Botanical Council (ABC)
6200 Manor Rd.
Austin, TX 78723-4345   512-926-4900
                                  800-373-7105
                            Fax: 512-926-2345
                               abc@herbalgram.org
                                    herbalgram.org

Mark Blumenthal, Founder & Executive Director
Stefan Gafner, Chief Science Officer
Denise Meikel, Development Director
The American Botanical Council is an independent, nonprofit, international member-based organization providing education using science-based and traditional information to promote the responsible use of herbal medicine.
1988

610 American Camp Association (ACA)
5000 State Rd. 67 North
Martinsville, IN 46151-7902   765-342-8456
                                  800-428-2267
                            Fax: 765-342-2065
                                 www.acacamps.org
Tom Rosenberg, President & Chief Executive Officer
Lizabeth Fogel, Chair
Dayna Hardin, Vice Chair
The American Camp Association is a community of camp professionals who have joined together to share their knowledge and experience and to ensure the quality of camp programs. Children and adults have the opportunity to engage with a community, developing character building and other skills.

611 American Chiropractic Association (ACA)
1701 Clarendon Blvd.
Suite 200
Arlington, VA 22209   703-276-8800
                             Fax: 703-243-2593
                           memberinfo@acatoday.org
                                 www.acatoday.org

Michele J. Maiers, President
Karen Silberman, Executive Vice President
Kim Hodes, Vice President, Finance
The ACA is a professional organization representing chiropractors. Its mission is to preserve, protect, improve, and promote the chiropractic profession. The purpose of the ACA is to provide leadership in health care and a positive vision for the chiropractic profession and its natural approach to health and wellness.

612 American College of Advancement in Medicine (ACAM)
380 Ice Center Lane
Suite C
Bozeman, MT 59718   800-532-3688
                               members@acam.org
                                   www.acam.org

Ahvie Herskowitz, President
Allen Green, Treasurer
Neal Speight, Secretary
The American College for Advancement in Medicine is a nonprofit society dedicated to educating physicians and other health care professionals on the latest findings and emerging procedures in integrative medicine. ACAM's goals are to improve skills, knowledge, and diagnostic procedures as they relate to integrative medicine; to support research; and to develop awareness of alternative methods of medical treatment.

613 American College of Nurse Midwives (ACNM)
8403 Colesville Rd.
Suite 1230
Silver Spring, MD 20910
240-485-1800
Fax: 240-485-1818
membership@acnm.org
midwife.org

Katrina Holland, Chief Executive Officer
Marc Rucker, Vice President, Finance & Operations
Amy Kohl, Director, Advocacy & Government Affairs
The American College of Nurse-Midwives is the oldest women's health care organization in the U.S. ACNM provides research, accredits midwifery education programs, administers and promotes continuing education programs, establishes clinical practice standards, and creates liaisons with state and federal agencies and members of Congress.

614 American Counseling Association (ACA)
P.O. Box 31110
Alexandria, VA 22310-9998
800-347-6647
Fax: 800-473-2329
www.counseling.org

S. Kent Butler, President
Kimberly Frazier, President-Elect
Erik Hines, Treasurer
The American Counseling Association is a not-for-profit, professional and educational organization dedicated to advancing the counseling profession.
1952

615 American Disabled Golfers Association (ADGA)
United States Golf Teachers Federation
200 S Indian River Dr.
Suite 206
Fort Pierce, FL 34950
772-888-7483
info@usgtf.com
www.usgtf.com

Brandon Lee, President
Mark Harman, Director, Education
The American Disabled Golfers Association helps create accessibility to golf courses for disabled golfers.
1989

616 American Disabled for Attendant Programs Today (ADAPT)
4513 Tyson Ave.
Philadelphia, PA 19135
adapt.org
National organization fighting for the rights of disabled people through non-violent activism tactics and advocacy. The national body is made up of local groups and individuals.

617 American Foundation for Suicide Prevention (AFSP)
199 Water St.
11th Floor
New York, NY 10038
212-363-3500
888-333-2377
Fax: 212-363-6237
info@afsp.org
afsp.org

Robert Gebbia, Chief Executive Officer
Christine Yu Moutier, Chief Medical Officer
Stephanie Rogers, Senior Vice President, Communications & Marketing
The American Foundation for Suicide Prevention is a voluntary health organization that gives those affected by suicide a nationwide community empowered by research, education, and advocacy to take action against this disease. AFSP achieves their goal by funding scientific research, educating the public about mental health and suicide prevention, and supporting survivors of suicide loss and all those affected by suicide.

618 American Herbalists Guild (AHG)
PO Box 3076
Asheville, NC 28802-3076
617-520-4372
office@americanherbalistsguild.com
www.americanherbalistsguild.com

Denise Cusack, Chair
Mary Colvin, Vice Chair
Tenby Owens, Treasurer
A nonprofit, educational organization that represents the voices of herbalists specializing in the medicinal use of plants. Their mission is to promote a high level of professionalism and education in the study and practice of therapeutic herbalism.
1989

619 American Massage Therapy Association (AMTA)
500 Davis St.
Suite 900
Evanston, IL 60201
877-905-2700
info@amtamassage.org
www.amtamassage.org

Michaele M. Colizza, President
AMTA is a nonprofit professional organization for massage therapists. AMTA works to establish massage therapy as integral to the maintenance of good health and complementary to other therapeutic processes. AMTA aims to advance the profession through ethics and standards, certification, school accreditation, continuing education, professional publications, legislative efforts, public education, and fostering the development of members.

620 American Occupational Therapy Association (AOTA)
6116 Executive Blvd.
Suite 200
North Bethesda, MD 20852-4929
301-652-6611
800-729-2682
customerservice@aota.org
www.aota.org

Sherry Keramidas, Executive Director
Neil Harvison, Chief Officer, Knowledge Division
Matthew Clark, Chief Officer, Innovation & Engagement
A national professional association that advances the quality, availability, use, and support of occupational therapy through standard setting, advocacy, education, and research on behalf of its members.

621 American Organization for Bodywork Therapies of Asia (AOBTA)
391 Wilmington Pike
Suite 3, Box 260
Glen Mills, PA 19342
484-841-6023
office@aobta.org
www.aobta.org

Sarah Goldenberg, President
Andrea Sullivan, Vice President
Sheryl Huske, Treasurer & Secretary
The American Organization for Bodywork Therapies of Asia is a professional membership organizaton that promotes Asian Bodywork Therapy and its practitioners while honoring a diversity of disciplines. AOBTA serves its community of members by supporting appropriate credentialing; defining scope of practice and educational standards; and providing resources for training, professional development, and networking. AOBTA advocates public policy to protect its members.
1989

622 American Public Health Association (APHA)
800 I St. NW
Washington, DC 20001
202-777-2742
Fax: 202-777-2534
TTY: 202-777-2500
www.apha.org

Georges C. Benjamin, Executive Director
Kaye Bender, President
James Carbo, Chief of Staff
The association works to protect all Americans and their communities from preventable, serious health threats. APHA represents a broad array of health officials, educators, environmentalists, policy-makers, and health providers at all levels working both within and outside governmental organizations and educational institutions.
1972

623 American Red Cross
430 17th St. NW
Washington, DC 20006
800-733-2767
www.redcross.org

Bonnie McElveen-Hunter, Chair
Gail J. McGovern, President & Chief Executive Officer
Brian J. Rhoa, Chief Financial Officer
The American Red Cross is an emergency assistance organization offering services in the following areas: disaster relief and recov-

ery; blood donations; health and safety training and education; support for military and veteran families; and international relief and development programs.

624 American Society for the Alexander Technique (AmSAT)
11 W Monument Ave.
Suite 510
Dayton, OH 45402-1233   937-586-3732
800-473-0620
info@amsatonline.org
www.amsatonline.org

Matthew Dubroff, Chair
Renee Schneider, Secretary
Rick Carbaugh, Treasurer
The Alexander Technique is a self-help method for improving balance and coordination and increasing movement awareness by eliminating habitual reactions of misuse in every day activities. AmSat, a professional organization of Alexander Technique teachers, aims to define, maintain, and promote the Alexander Technique at its highest standard of professional practice and conduct.
1987

625 American Society of Clinical Hypnosis (ASCH)
180 Admiral Cochrane Drive
Suite 370
Annapolis, MD 21401   410-940-6585
Fax: 630-351-8490
info@asch.net
www.asch.net

Joe Tramontana, President
John Hall, Treasurer
David Alter, Secretary
The American Society of Clinical Hypnosis is an organization of health and mental health care professionals using clinical hypnosis. ASCH aims to further the knowledge, understanding, and application of hypnosis in health care; to promote the recognition and acceptance of hypnosis as an important tool in clinical health care; and to provide a professional community for clinicians and researchers using hypnosis.
1957

626 American Therapeutic Recreation Association
25 Century Blvd.
Suite 505
Nashville, TN 37214   703-234-4140
www.atra-online.com

Tracey Crawford, President
Cathy L. Jordan, Secretary
Laura Kelly, Treasurer
Represents the interests and needs of more than 10,000 recreational therapists.
1984

627 American Tinnitus Association (ATA)
PO Box 424049
Washington, DC 20042-4049   800-634-8978
ata.org

Torryn P. Brazell, Chief Executive Officer
David Hadley, Chair
Gordon Mountford, Vice Chair
ATA is an organization dedicated to finding cures for tinnitus and hyperacusis. ATA's research program focuses on providing seed grants for new areas of tinnitus scientific exploration.

628 Amputee Coalition
601 Pennsylvania Ave. NW
Suite 600, South Bldg.
Washington, DC 20004   888-267-5669
www.amputee-coalition.org

Mary Richards, President & Chief Executive Officer
The Amputee Coalition is a nonprofit organization dedicated to assisting and empowering people affected by limb loss through education, support groups, and vocal advocacy.
1986

629 Anxiety and Depression Association of America (ADAA)
8701 Georgia Ave.
Suite 412
Silver Spring, MD 20910   240-485-1001
Fax: 240-485-1035
information@adaa.org
adaa.org

Susan K. Gurley, Executive Director
Lise Bram, Deputy Executive Director
Vickie Spielman, Associate Director, Membership & Education
The Anxiety and Depression Association of America is an international nonprofit organization and a leader in education, training, and research for anxiety, OCD, PTSD, depression, and related disorders. ADAA encourages the advancement of scientific knowledge about the causes and treatment for mental health issues.

630 Aspies For Freedom (AFF)

www.aspiesforfreedom.com

Gwen Nelson, Co-Founder
Amy Nelson, Co-Founder
Seeks to change the discourse on autism, including negative treatment in the media. Runs an online chatroom and promotes Autistic Pride Day.

631 Assistive Technology Industry Association (ATIA)
330 N Wabash Ave.
Suite 2000
Chicago, IL 60611-4267   312-321-5172
877-687-2842
Fax: 312-673-6659
info@atia.org
www.atia.org

David Dikter, Chief Executive Officer
Caroline Van Howe, Chief Operating Officer
Emily Schmitt, Marketing Manager
Dedicated to manufacturers, sellers and providers of assistive technology, offering education and research.

632 Association for Applied Psychophysiology and Biofeedback (AAPB)
4400 College Blvd.
Suite 220
Overland Park, KS 66211   303-422-8436
800-477-8892
info@aapb.org
www.aapb.org

Fred B. Shaffer, President
Michelle Cunningham, Executive Director
Jessica Eure, Treasurer
AAPB is a nonprofit organization that aims to advance applied psychophysiology and biofeedback through scientific research, practice, and education.
1969

633 Association of Assistive Technology Act Programs (ATAP)
1440 G St. NW
Washington, DC 20005   atapadmin@ataporg.org
www.ataporg.org

Audrey Busch, Executive Director
Dave Scherer, PI & Grant Administrative Lead
Jamie Anderson, Membership & Opertions Director
The Association of Assistive Technology Act Programs (ATAP) is a national, member-based organization consisting of state Assistive Technology Act Programs funded under the Assistive Technology Act (AT Act). It promotes, represents, and coordinates the state AT Programs at a national level.

634 Association of Children's Residential Centers (ACRC)
648 N Plankinton Ave.
Suite 245
Milwaukee, WI 53203   877-332-2272
info@togetherthevoice.org
togetherthevoice.org

Kari Sisson, Executive Director
Amanda Prange, Training Coordinator
McKenzie Melchoir, Membership Services Specialist
The Association of Children's Residential Centers advocates for quality treatment and residential interventions for youth. The or-

ganization provides support, training and resources to help members better serve children and families through residential interventions.
1956

635 **Association of Educational Therapists (AET)**
7044 S 13th St.
Oak Creek, WI 53154   414-908-4949
                                    customercare@aetonline.org
                                            www.aetonline.org

Kaye Ragland, President
Susan Grama, Treasurer
Pamm Scribner, Secretary
AET is a professional association for educational therapists. Educational Therapy offers children and adults with learning disabilities and other learning challenges a wide range of intensive, individualized interventions designed to remediate learning problems.
1979

636 **Association of Independent Camps**
American Camp Association
5000 State Rd. 67 North
Martinsville, IN 46151-7902   765-342-8456
                                              800-428-2267
                                          Fax: 765-342-2065
                                            www.acacamps.org
Tom Rosenberg, President & Chief Executive Officer
The Association of Independent Camps is an affiliate of the American Camp Association. Originally founded as a committee in 1954, the AIC has served the independent camp community since 1996. They provide accreditation and public credibility, as well as camper scholarship programs.

637 **Association of Medical Professionals with Hearing Losses (AMPHL)**

                                            admin@amphl.org
                                                amphl.org
Christopher Moreland, President
Ian DeAndrea-Lazarus, Vice President
Robert Radtke, Secretary
The Association of Medical Professionals with Hearing Losses provides information, promotes advocacy and mentorship, and creates a network for individuals with hearing loss interested in or working in health care fields.
1999

638 **Association of People Supporting Employment First (APSE)**
7361 Calhoun Place
Suite 680
Rockville, MD 20855   301-279-0060
                                          Fax: 301-279-0075
                                             info@apse.org
                                             www.apse.org
Erica Belois-Pacer, Director, Professional Development
Julie Christensen, Director, Policy & Advocacy
Erynn Pawlak, Director, Operations
Through advocacy and education, this nonprofit organization advances employment and self-sufficiency for all people with disabilities.
1988

639 **Association of University Centers on Disabilities (AUCD)**
1100 Wayne Ave.
Suite 1000
Silver Spring, MD 20910   301-588-8252
                                          Fax: 301-588-2842
                                           aucdinfo@aucd.org
                                             www.aucd.org

John Tschida, Executive Director
Michele Lunsford, Director, Communications, Events & Development
Dawn Rudolph, Senior Director, Technical Assistance & Network Engagement
AUCD is a membership organization consisting of University Centers for Excellence in Developmental Disabilities (UCEDD), Leadership Education in Neurodevelopmental Disabilities (LEND) Programs, and Intellectual and Developmental Disabil-

ity Research Centers (IDDRC). AUCD supports its members through advocacy, technical assistance, information dissemination, networking, and leadership.

640 **Association on Higher Education & Disability (AHEAD)**
8015 West Kenton Circle
Suite 230
Huntersville, NC 28078   704-947-7779
                                          Fax: 704-948-7779
                                             www.ahead.org
Amanda Kraus, President
Stephan Smith, Executive Director
Oanh Huynh, Chief Financial Officer
AHEAD is a professional membership organization for individuals involved in the development of policy and in the provision of quality services to meet the needs of persons with disabilities involved in all areas of higher education, promoting full and equal participation.
4,000+ members 1977

641 **Bastyr Center for Natural Health**
3670 Stone Way N
Seattle, WA 98103   206-834-4100
                                          Fax: 206-834-4131
                                          www.bastyrcenter.org
The Bastyr Center is the teaching clinic of Bastyr University, which provides a range of programs in science-based natural medicine. Services include naturopathic medicine, acupuncture, nutrition services, ayurvedic medicine, and counseling.

642 **Beacon Tree Foundation**
9201 Arboretum Pkwy.
Suite 140
N. Chesterfield, VA 23236   800-414-6427
                                          info@beacontree.org
                                            beacontree.org
Beacon Tree Foundation is dedicated to being an advocate for the family, providing education about treatment and financial resources to help heal children and teens struggling with mental health issues and to provide hope for the future.

643 **Birth Defect Research for Children (BDRC)**
976 Lake Baldwin Lane
Suite 104
Orlando, FL 32814   407-895-0802
                                         staff@birthdefects.org
                                         www.birthdefects.org
Betty Mekdeci, Executive Director
A nonprofit organization that provides information about birth defects of all kinds to parents and professionals. Offers a library of medical books and files of information on less common categories of birth defects and is involved in research to discover possible links between environmental exposures and birth defects.
1982

644 **Bonnie Prudden Myotherapy**
4330 E Havasu Rd.
Tucson, AZ 85718   520-529-3979
                                         www.bonnieprudden.com
Enid Whittaker, Managing Director
Sandy Dirks, Treasurer
Lori Drummond, Secretary
Myotherapy is a method for relaxing muscle spasms, improving circulation, and alleviating pain. Pressure is applied using elbows, knuckles or fingers, and held for several seconds to defuse trigger points. The success of this method depends upon the use of specific corrective exercises of the freed muscles.

645 **Brain & Behavior Research Foundation**
747 Third Ave.
33rd Floor
New York, NY 10017   646-681-4888
                                              800-829-8289
                                         info@bbrfoundation.org
                                           bbrfoundation.org
Jeffrey Borenstein, President & Chief Executive Officer
Louis Innamorato, Vice President, Finance & Chief Financial Officer
Lauren Duran, Vice President, Communications, Marketing & PR

The Brain & Behavior Research Foundation is a nonprofit organization committed to alleviating the suffering caused by mental illness by awarding grants in the field of mental health research.
1987

646   Brain Injury Association of America (BIAA)
3057 Nutley St.
Suite 805
Fairfax, VA 22031-1931   703-761-0750
                                      Fax: 703-761-0755
                                      info@biausa.org
                                      www.biausa.org
Susan H. Connors, President & Chief Executive Officer
Shana De Caro, Chairwoman
Page Melton Ivie, Vice Chairwoman
The Brain Injury Association of America is a national organization serving and representing individuals, families and professionals who are touched by a traumatic brain injury (TBI). Its mission is to improve the quality of life for people affected by brain injury through the advancement of research, treatment, education and awareness.
1980

647   Burton Blatt Institute (BBI)
Syracuse University
950 Irving Ave.
Dineen Hall, Suite 446
Syracuse, NY 13244-2130   315-443-2863
                                      Fax: 315-443-9725
                                      bbi.syr.edu
Peter Blanck, Chair
Michael Morris, Senior Advisor
Jonathan Martinis, Senior Director, Law & Policy
Seeks to advance the full inclusion of people with disabilities through program development, research, and public policy guidance in economic and community participation.
1905

648   CARF International
6951 East Southpoint Rd.
Tucson, AZ 85756-9407   520-325-1044
                                      888-281-6531
                                      Fax: 520-318-1129
                                      TTY: 520-495-7077
                                      info@carf.org
                                      carf.org
Brian J. Boon, President & Chief Executive Officer
Leslie Ellis-Lang, Managing Director, Child & Youth Services
Darren M. Lehrfeld, Chief Accreditation Officer
An independent, nonprofit accreditor of human service providers in the areas of aging services, behavioral health, child and youth services, DMEPOS, employment and community services, medical rehabilitation, and opioid treatment programs.
1966

649   Cambia Health Foundation
100 SW Market St.
Suite E15B
Portland, OR 97201   503-225-4813
                                      cambiahealthfoundation.org
Peggy Maguire, President & Chair
Rob Coppedge, Chief Executive Officer
Anjie Vannoy, Vice President, Finance & Controller
Cambia Health Foundation is the corporate foundation of Cambia Health Solutions dedicated to transforming the way people experience health care to create a more person-focused and economically sustainable health care system.
1907

650   Canadian Art Therapy Association (CATA)
PO Box 658, Stn Main
Parksville, BC, Canada V9P-2G7   admin@canadianarttherapy.org
                                      canadianarttherapy.org
Amanda Gee, President
Nicole Le Bihan, Vice President
Waqas Yousafzai, Treasurer
CATA is a nonprofit organization that works in cooperation with other provincial art therapy associations to promote education

and understanding of the value of art therapy, as well as provide ongoing education and professional standards for this field.
1977

651   Canine Companions for Independence (CCI)
PO Box 446
Santa Rosa, CA 95402-0446   866-224-3647
                                      800-572-2275
                                      www.canine.org
Paige Mazzoni, Chief Executive Officer
Leslie Hennessy, Treasurer
W. Stephen Boyd, Secretary
A nonprofit organization that enhances the lives of people with disabilities by providing highly trained assistance dogs and ongoing support to ensure quality partnerships.
1975

652   Canine Helpers for the Handicapped
Canine Helpers for the Handicapped, Inc.
5699 Ridge Rd.
Lockport, NY 14094   716-433-4035
                                      chhdogs@aol.com
A nonprofit organization dedicated to training dogs in order to assist people with disabilities and promote independence.

653   Case Management Society of America (CMSA)
5034A Thoroughbred Lane
Brentwood, TN 37027   615-432-0101
                                      800-216-2672
                                      Fax: 615-523-1715
                                      cmsa@cmsa.org
                                      www.cmsa.org
Melanie Prince, President
Patricia Noonan, Treasurer
Nadine Carter, Secretary
The Case Management Society of America is an international, nonprofit organization dedicated to the support and development of the profession of case management through educational forums, networking opportunities, and legislative involvement. Case management workers play a vital role in taking care of patients' health care needs.
1990

654   Center for Creative Arts Therapy
2600 Warrenville Road
Suite 205
Downers Grove, IL 60515   847-477-8244
                                      info@c4creativeartstherapy.com
                                      c4creativeartstherapy.com
Azizi Marshall, Founder & Chief Executive Officer
Rachel Wagner-Cantine, Clinical Director
Leslie Kane, Coordinator, Marketing & Outreach
The Center for Creative Arts Therapy offers arts-based psychotherapy services to individuals and their families as a healthy, proactive way to achieve wellness and balance in their lives. Provides art therapy, music therapy, dance therapy and drama therapy, as well as professional counseling.

655   Center for Disability Resources
University of South Carolina School of Medicine
Department of Pediatrics
8301 Farrow Rd.
Columbia, SC 29208   803-935-5231
                                      Fax: 803-935-5059
                                      david.rotholz@uscmed.sc.edu
                                      uscm.med.sc.edu/cdrhome
A University Affiliated Program which develops model programs designed to serve persons with disabilities and to train students in fields related to disabilities.

656   Center for Inclusive Design and Innovation
512 Means St. NW
Suite 250
Atlanta, GA 30318   404-894-8000
                                      866-279-2964
                                      Fax: 404-894-8323
                                      cidi-support@design.gatech.edu
                                      cidi.gatech.edu
Eric Trevena, Senior Director, Operations
Carolyn Phillips, Director, Services & Learning

CIDI supports individuals with disabilities of any age within the State of Georgia and beyond through expert services, research, design and technological development, information dissemination, and educational programs.

657 Center for Mind-Body Medicine
5225 Connecticut Ave. NW
Suite 414
Washington, DC 20015   202-966-7338
Fax: 202-966-2589
www.cmbm.org
James S. Gordon, Founder & Chief Executive Officer
Rosemary L. Murrain, Executive Director
Lynda Richtsmeier, Clinical Director
The Center for Mind-Body Medicine is a nonprofit educational organization dedicated to reviving the spirit and transforming the practice of medicine. The Center is working to create a more effective, comprehensive, and compassionate model of health care and education. The Center's model combines the precision of modern science with the best of the world's healing traditions.

658 Cerebral Palsy Foundation (CPF)
3 Columbus Circle
15th Floor
New York, NY 10019   212-520-1686
info@yourcpf.org
yourcpf.org
Rachel Byrne, Executive Director
Michelle Kassner, Chairman of the Board
James P. Volcker, Vice President & Secretary
The Cerebral Palsy Foundation is dedicated to assisting and empowering people with cerebral palsy through research in both medical breakthroughs and assistive technologies.

659 Challenged Athletes Foundation (CAF)
9591 Waples St.
San Diego, CA 92121   858-866-0959
Fax: 858-866-0958
caf@challengedathletes.org
challengedathletes.org
Kristie Entwistle, Chief Executive Officer
J.D. Douglas, Chief Financial Officer
Virginia Tinley, Chief Legacy Officer
The Challenged Athletes Foundation provides opportunities and support to physically challenged persons so they can pursue active lifestyles through physical fitness and competitive athletics.
1994

660 Change, Inc.
115 Stoner Ave.
Westminster, MD 21157   410-876-2179
info@penn-mar.org
www.changeinc.cc
Gregory T. Miller, President & Chief Executive Officer
A nonprofit organization that partners with families, caregivers, and advocates to provide opportunities for children with developmental disabilities. A division of Penn-Mar Human Services.

661 Child and Parent Resource Institute (CPRI)
600 Sanatorium Rd.
London, ON, Canada N6H-3W7   519-858-2774
877-494-2774
Fax: 519-858-3913
TTY: 519-858-0257
www.cpri.ca
Provides highly specialized services to children and youth from 0-18 years of age with complex mental health and/or developmental challenges on a short term inpatient and community basis.

662 Children's Alliance
420 Capitol Ave.
Frankfort, KY 40601   502-875-3399
Fax: 502-223-4200
www.childrensallianceky.org
Michelle Sanborn, President
Melissa Muse, Director, Member Services
Kathy Adams, Director, Public Policy
An association of individuals and human services organizations committed to being a voice for at-risk children and families. Interacts with the legislative and executive branches of government and assists members in developing services that most effectively meet the needs of at-risk children and families.

663 Children's Mental Health Network (CMHN)
Chapel Hill, NC 27516   information@cmhnetwork.org
www.cmhnetwork.org
Scott Bryant-Comstock, President & Chief Executive Officer
Provides neutral, independent information on children's mental health issues, while sharing ideas on ways to improve the lives of affected children and their families.

664 Children's National Medical Center
111 Michigan Ave. NW
Washington, DC 20010   202-476-5000
888-884-2327
childrensnational.org
Kurt Newman, President & Chief Executive Officer
Donna Anthony, Vice President & Chief of Staff
Denice Cora-Bramble, Chief Diversity Officer
The Children's National Medical Center provides health care services that enhance the health and well-being of children regionally, nationally, and internationally. Through leadership and innovation, the organization will create solutions to pediatric health care problems.

665 Clay Tree Society
838 Old Victoria Rd.
Nanaimo, BC, Canada V9R-6A1   250-753-5322
Fax: 250-753-2749
info@claytree.org
www.claytree.org
Dan Dube, President
Jennifer Fowler, Executive Director
Alexandria Stuart, Secretary
A nonprofit society providing day programming, assistance and support for people with developmental disabilities.
1957

666 Coalition for Health Funding
c/o Cavarocchi Ruscio Dennis Associates, LLC
600 Maryland Ave. SW
Suite 220E
Washington, DC 20024   202-271-8963
Fax: 202-484-1244
emorton@dc-crd.com
www.publichealthfunding.org
Erin Will Morton, Executive Director
Erika Miller, Senior Vice President & Counsel
Katina Pierce, Vice President, Administration & Finance
Nonprofit alliance working to preserve and strengthen public health investments via funding for federal agencies and programs.

667 Communitas Supportive Care Society
103-2776 Bourquin Cres. W
Abbotsford, BC, Canada V2S-6A4   604-850-6608
800-622-5455
Fax: 604-850-2634
office@communitascare.com
www.communitascare.com
Kathy Doerksen, Chair
John Wiebe, Vice Chair
Jacquie Lepp, Secretary & Treasurer
Communitas Supportive Care Society is a nonprofit, faith-based organization providing care in communities across British Columbia to those living with disabilities. Services include skills-based day programs, residential care, and respite care for families.

668 Council for Exceptional Children (CEC)
3100 Clarendon Blvd.
Suite 600
Arlington, VA 22201-5332   888-232-7733
TTY: 866-915-5000
service@exceptionalchildren.org
www.exceptionalchildren.org
Chad Rummel, Executive Director
Laurie VanderPloeg, Associate Executive Director, Professional Affairs
Craig Evans, Chief Financial Officer

The Council for Exceptional Children aims to improve the educational success of individuals with disabilities and/or gifts and talents by advocating for appropriate policies, setting professional standards, and providing resources and professional development for special educators.

669 Council of Colleges of Acupuncture & Oriental Medicine
9615 E. County Line Road
Suite B-584
Centennial, CO 80112   410-464-6040
Fax: 410-464-6042
support@ccaom.org
www.ccaom.org

Kris LaPointe, President
Thomas Kouo, Vice President
Jennifer Brett, Treasurer
The Council seeks to advance the standing of acupuncture and Oriental medicine (AOM) in the U.S. by promoting educational excellence within the field by deepening the knowledge, understanding and skills of the AOM practitioner.
1982

670 Council of Parent Attorneys and Advocates (COPAA)
PO Box 6767
Towson, MD 21285   844-426-7224
www.copaa.org

Denise Stile Marshall, Executive Director
Selene A. Almazan, Legal Director
Marcie Hipple, Director, Member Services & Events
Group of attorneys, advocates, parents and related professionals working to protect the rights of students with disabilities and their families, including promoting excellence in education.

671 Council of State Administrators of Vocational Rehabilitation (CSAVR)
1 Research Ct.
Suite 450
Rockville, MD 20850   301-519-8023
info@csavr.org
www.csavr.org

Stephen A. Wooderson, Chief Executive Officer
Rita Martin, Deputy Director
Kathy West-Evans, Director, Business Relations
The Council is made up of the chief administrators of the public rehabilitation agencies that serve people with physical and mental disabilities across the U.S.

672 Department of Physical Medicine & Rehabilitation at Sinai Hospital
LifeBridge Health
2401 W Belvedere Ave.
Baltimore, MD 21215-5271   410-601-9355
www.lifebridgehealth.org
Provides health-related services to the people of the Northwest Baltimore region. LifeBridge is dedicated to advancing the health of the community through a variety of health and wellness programs and services. The Department of Physical Medicine & Rehabilitation provides care to individuals with disabling conditions such as traumatic brain injury, spinal cord injury, amputees, and more.

673 DisAbility LINK
1901 Montreal Rd.
Suite 102
Tucker, GA 30084   404-687-8890
Fax: 404-687-8298
TTY: 711
kgibson@disabilitylink.org
www.disabilitylink.org
Kim Gibson, Executive Director
Ken Mitchell, Disability Rights & Peer Support Training Advocate
Joseph Bryant, Financial Director
disABILITY LINK is an organization committed to promoting the rights of all people with disabilities in allowing them to be independent, achieve goals, have access to their community, and make decisions for themselves.

674 Disability Funders Network (DFN)
14241 Midlothian Turnpike
Suite 151
Midlothian, VA 23113-6500   703-795-9646
info@disabilityfunders.org
www.disabilityfunders.org
Kim Hutchinson, President & Chief Executive Officer
Disability Funders Network is a national membership organization dedicated to advocating for equality and rights for disabled individuals and communities.
1990

675 Disability Research and Dissemination Center
Arnold School of Public Health, USC
Discovery 1 Bldg.
915 Greene St.
Columbia, SC 29208   info@disabilityresearchcenter.com
www.disabilityresearchcenter.com
Suzanne McDermott, Research & Administration
Margaret A. Turk, Training & Evaluation
Roberta S. Carlin, Dissemination
The DRDC was formed in 2012 and is a partnership between the University of South Carolina (USC), the State University of New York Upstate Medical University (SUNY Upstate), and the American Association on Health and Disability (AAHD). Its five core areas are Administration, Research, Research Translation, Evaluation, and Dissemination & Policy.

676 Disability Rights Bar Association (DBRA)
c/o Burton Blatt Institute
950 Irving Ave.
Dineen Hall, Suite 446
Syracuse, NY 13244-2130   315-443-2863
Fax: 315-443-9725
drba-law@law.syr.edu
disabilityrights-law.org
Lydia X.Z. Brown, Co-Chair
Mehgan Sidhu, Co-Chair
Michelle Nunez, Secretary
The DRBA is an online network of attorneys who specialize in disability civil rights law.

677 Disability Rights Florida
2473 Care Dr.
Suite 200
Tallahassee, FL 32308   850-488-9071
800-342-0823
Fax: 850-488-8640
TTY: 800-346-4127
www.disabilityrightsflorida.org
Peter Sleasman, Executive Director
Ann Siegel, Legal Director
Cherie E. Hall, Director, Operations
A federally mandated Protection & Advocacy (P&A) organization working to ensure the safety, well-being and success of people with disabilities.
1977

678 Disability Rights International (DRI)
1825 K St. NW
Suite 600
Washington, DC 20006   202-296-0800
Fax: 202-697-5422
info@driadvocacy.org
www.driadvocacy.org
Laurie Ahern, President
Eric Rosenthal, Founder & Executive Director
Priscila Rodriguez, Associate Director, Advocacy
Promotes international oversight of disability rights by documenting human rights abuses and publishing reports on enforcement.

679 Disability Rights Louisiana
8325 Oak St.
New Orleans, LA 70118   800-960-7705
info@disabilityrightsla.org
disabilityrightsla.org
Ron Lospennato, Interim Executive Director & Director, Legal Services
Tory Rocca, Director, Public Policy and Community Engagement
Debra Weinberg, Director, Community Advocacy

Protects and advocates for the rights of seniors and individuals with disabilities in Louisiana.

680 Disability:IN
3000 Potomac Ave.
Alexandria, VA 22305   info@disabilityin.org
disabilityin.org
Jill Houghton, President & Chief Executive Officer
Brian Horn, Chief Operating Officer
Elizabeth Taub, Executive Vice President, Programs
Nonprofit specializing in disability inclusion in the workplace.

681 Disabled Athlete Sports Association (DASA)
1600 Mid Rivers Mall Circle
Suite 2272
St. Peters, MO 63376   dasa@dasasports.org
www.dasasports.org
Kelly Behlmann, Executive Director
Meghan Morgan, Program Director
The Disabled Athlete Sports Association is a nonprofit organization specializing in adaptive sport and fitness opportunities. DASA relies heavily upon fundraising events, grants, and individual and corporate donations to sustain its mission.
1997

682 Disabled Businesspersons Association (DBA)
6367 Alvarado Crt.
Suite 350
San Diego, CA 92120   619-594-8805

Urban Miyares, Founder
The Disabled Businesspersons Association is a nonprofit public charity and educational organization to help disabled entrepreneurs maximize their potential in the business world, and to encourage the participation and enhance the performance of disabled individuals in the work force.
1991

683 Disabled Children's Fund (DCF)

info@achildthrives.org
achildthrives.org
Bill Collins, Co-Founder
Erma Collins, Co-Founder
Disabled Children's Fund is a humanitarian organization serving oppressed children and families worldwide. It distributes braces, wheelchairs, crutches, walkers and rehabilitative services globally.
1997

684 Disabled Drummers Association (DDA)

www.disableddrummers.org
The Disabled Drummers Association is a nonprofit organization representing drummers with disabilities. The DDA seeks to raise public awareness and funds, advocate for the development of adaptive equipment, and provide resources and opportunities to members.
1996

685 Disabled In Action (DIA)
PO Box 30954
Port Authority Station
New York, NY 10011- 0109   646-504-4342
Fax: 646-504-4342
TTY: 711
treasurer@disabledinaction.org
www.disabledinaction.org
Jean Ryan, President
Phil Beder, Treasurer
A democratic, nonprofit, membership organization advancing civil rights and seeking to end discrimination for people with disabilities.

686 Disabled Peoples' International (DPI)
160 Elgin St.
Place Bell RPO, PO Box 70073
Ottawa, ON, Canada K2P-2M3   dpi.org
Rachel Kachaje, Chair
Jean Luc Simon, Secretary
Shoji Nakanishi, Treasurer

Aims to protect the rights of people with disabilities, while promoting their full and equal role in society.
1981

687 Disabled and Alone: Life Services for the Handicapped, Inc. (Act for Life Services)
1441 Broadway
23rd Floor
New York, NY 10018-2326   212-532-6740
800-995-0066
Fax: 212-532-6740
info@disabledandalone.org
www.actforlifeservices.org
Leslie D. Park, Chair
Rex L. Davidson, Vice President
Lee Alan Ackerman, Executive Director
A national nonprofit humanitarian organization whose primary concern is the well-being of disabled persons, particularly when their families can no longer care for them. The organization helps families do sensible planning for and with their disabled children; provides advocacy and oversight when the parents cannot do so; and advises families, attorneys, and financial planners about life planning for a family with a member with a disability.
1988

688 Dr. Ida Rolf Institute (DIRI)
5055 Chaparral Ct.
Suite 103
Boulder, CO 80301   303-449-5903
Fax: 303-449-5978
www.rolf.org
Christina Howe, Executive Director
Mary Contreras, Director, Admissions & Recruitment
Samantha Sherwin, Director, Financial Aid & Compliance
The Rolf Institute is a nonprofit corporation, dedicated to educating individuals on Rolfing Structural Integration. It is recognized by the US Government as a tax-exempt educational and scientific research organization.
1971

689 Early Childhood Technical Assistance Center (ETCA)
CB 8040
Chapel Hill, NC 27599-8040   919-962-2001
Fax: 919-966-7463
ectacenter@unc.edu
ectacenter.org
Christina Kasprzak, Co-Director
Meghan Vinh, Co-Director
Julie Austen, Technical Assistance Specialist
ECTA Center, funded by the Office of Special Education Programs, is a technical assistance center supporting Part C and Section 619 IDEA programs in building quality early intervention and preschool special education service systems, improving and sustaining state systems, and enhancing outcomes for children with disabilities and their families.

690 Easterseals
141 W Jackson Blvd.
Suite 1400A
Chicago, IL 60604   312-726-6200
800-221-6827
Fax: 312-726-1494
info@easterseals.com
easterseals.com
Kendra E. Davenport, President & Chief Executive Officer
Glenda Oakley, Chief Financial Officer
Marcy Traxler, Senior Vice President, Network Advancement
Easterseals provides services, education, outreach and advocacy for people with disabilities, veterans, senior citizens and their families. Programs include early intervention, workforce development, adult day care, autism services, mental health services, and more.

691 Elwyn
111 Elwyn Rd.
Media, PA 19063   610-891-2000
info@elwyn.org
elwyn.org
Charles S. McLister, President & Chief Executive Officer
Rex Carney, Chief of Staff
Len Kirby, Chief Operating Officer

A nonprofit organization developing programs for children and adults with disabilities and disadvantages.
Founded in 1852. 1952

692 Employer Assistance and Resource Network on Disability Inclusion (EARN)
Cornell University, ILR School
201 Dolgen Hall
Ithaca, NY 14853   askearn@cornell.edu
                           www.askearn.org
Susanne Bruyere, Co-Director
Wendy Strobel Gower, Co-Director
Free network for employers providing education on building inclusive workplace cultures.

693 Enable America Inc.
101 E Kennedy Blvd.
Suite 3250
Tampa, FL 33602   877-362-2533
                          Fax: 813-221-8811
                  richard.salem@enableamerica.org
                          www.enableamerica.org
Richard J. Salem, Founder & Chief Executive Officer
Enable America is a nonprofit organization that is dedicated to increasing employment among people with disabilities in the United States.

694 Esalen Institute
55000 Highway One
Big Sur, CA 93920   831-667-3000
                          888-837-2536
                          info@esalen.org
                          www.esalen.org
Gordon Wheeler, President
Camille Wright, Chief Executive Officer & Chief Financial Officer
An alternative education center devoted to East/West philosophies, experiential/didactic workshops, and a steady influx of philosophers, psychologists, artists, and religious thinkers.
1962

695 Family Resource Center on Disabilities
11 E. Adams St.
Suite 1002
Chicago, IL 60603   312-939-3513
                          info@frcd.org
                          www.frcd.org
A not-for-profit advocacy organization dedicated to improving services for all children with disabilities by providing support and services to affected families, informing parents of their rights, and helping parents become advocates for their children. Offers family support services, training, seminars, and information and referral services. Publishes a monthly newsletter.

696 Family Run Executive Director Leadership Association (FREDLA)
10632 Patuxent Pkwy.
Suite 234
Columbia, MD 21044   410-707-4547
                          info@fredla.org
                          www.fredla.org
Pat Hunt, Executive Director
Millie Sweeney, Deputy Director
Malisa Pearson, Project Coordinator
Aims to strengthen the leadership and organizational capacity of family-run organizations.

697 Family Voices
110 Hartwell Ave.
Lexington, MA 02421   781-674-7224
                          888-835-5669
                          www.familyvoices.org
Nora Wells, Executive Director
Cara Coleman, Director, Public Poicy & Advocacy
Beth Dworetzky, Associate Director, Programs
A not-for-profit organization dedicated to ensuring that children's health issues are addressed as public and private health-care systems undergo change in communities, states, and the nation. They are a national grassroots clearinghouse for information and education in ways to improve health care for children with disabilities and chronic conditions. Family Voices provides

materials including pamphlets, a newsletter, and one-page papers on important topics.

698 Favarh ARC
225 Commerce Dr.
Canton, CT 06019-2478   860-693-6662
                          Fax: 860-693-8662
                          favarh@favarh.org
                          www.favarh.org
Suzanne Sinacore, President
Ernie Mack, Vice President
Tom Smith, Treasurer
Favarh ARC provides a variety of programs and services to adults with developmental, physical, or mental disabilities and their families throughout the Farmington Valley communities of Avon, Burlington, and more. Favarh's programs are designed to enhance the personal, social, emotional, vocational, and living capabilities of persons with disabilities.
1958

699 Fedcap Rehabilitation Services
633 Third Ave.
6th Floor
New York, NY 10017   212-727-4200
                          Fax: 212-727-4374
                          TTY: 646-606-5950
                          info@fedcap.org
                          www.fedcap.org
Steve Coons, President
George Rios, Director, Operations
Amy Reisner, Director, Contract Administration
Fedcap helps people with barriers achieve economic independence through employment. Through evaluation, vocational and soft-skills training, job placement, job creation, and support programs, each year Fedcap helps thousands of Americans overcome obstacles, rebuild their lives, and find and keep meaningful employment.
1935

700 Federation for Children with Special Needs
529 Main St.
Suite 1M3
Boston, MA 02129   617-236-7210
                          800-331-0688
                          Fax: 617-241-0330
                          fcsinfo@fcsn.org
                          www.fcsn.org
Pam Nourse, Executive Director
Mary Lewis-Pierce, Director, Development
Jacqui Koelsch, Director, Finance
The Federation for Children with Special Needs provides information, support, and assistance to parents of children with disabilities, their professional partners, and their communities.
1975

701 Feingold Association of the US
10955 Windjammer Dr. S
Indianapolis, IN 46256   631-369-9340
                          help@feingold.org
                          www.feingold.org
Deborah Lehner, Executive Director
An organization of families and professionals, the Feingold Association of the United States is dedicated to helping children and adults apply proven dietary techniques for better behavior, learning, and health.
1976

702 Feldenkrais Guild of North America (FGNA)
401 Edgewater Pl.
Suite 600
Wakefield, MA 01880   781-876-8935
                          800-775-2118
                          Fax: 781-645-1322
                          www.feldenkraisguild.com
Nancy Haller, President
Maxine Sidenfaden, Vice President
Erik LaSeur, Treasurer
This organization sets the standards for and certifies all Feldenkrais practitioners in North America. In order to practice, a practitioner must be a graduate of an FGNA accredited program (a minimum of 800 instruction hours over a three to four year pe-

riod), and agree to follow both the Code of Professional Conduct and the Standards of Practice. FGNA may be contacted for further information about the Feldenkrais Method or for a list of Feldenkrais practitioners sorted by region.

703 Flying Manes Therapeutic Riding, Inc.
PO Box 508
Scarsdale, NY 10583   917-524-6648
                                    info@flyingmanes.org
                                          flyingmanes.org
Flying Manes is a therapeutic riding center located at Riverdale Stables in New York. Flying Manes aims to help individuals with emotional, cognitive, and physical disabilities in a safe and enjoyable environment.
Founded in 2009. 1909

704 Freedom from Fear
308 Seaview Ave.
Staten Island, NY 10305   718-351-1717
                                   help@freedomfromfear.org
                                       freedomfromfear.org
Mary Guardino, Founder & Executive Director
Freedom From Fear is a national nonprofit mental health advocacy organization whose goal is to better the lives of all those affected by anxiety, depressive, and related disorders through advocacy, education, research, and community support.
1984

705 Fos Feminista

                                           212-248-6400
                                    online@fosfeminista.org
                                      www.fosfeminista.org
Giselle Carino, Chief Executive Officer
Works to generate health and population policies, programs, and funding that promote and protect the rights and health of girls and women worldwide.

706 Genova Diagnostics
63 Zillicoa St.
Asheville, NC 28801   828-253-0621
                                           800-522-4762
                                             info@gdx.net
                                            www.gdx.net
Jeffrey Ledford, Chief Executive Officer
Craig Thiel, Chief Financial Officer
Jeff Ellis, Chief Commercial Officer
Genova Diagnostics specializes in nutritional, metabolic, and toxicant analyses. Genova is committed to helping health care professionals identify nutritional influences on health and disease, and laboratory procedures in nutritional and biochemical testing.
1984

707 Goodwill Industries International
15810 Indianola Dr.
Rockville, MD 20855   contactus@goodwill.org
                                         www.goodwill.org
Steven C. Preston, President & Chief Executive Officer
Goodwill strives to achieve the full participation in society of disabled persons and other individuals with special needs by expanding their opportunities and occupational capabilities through a network of autonomous, nonprofit, community-based organizations providing services throughout the world in response to local needs.

708 Grand Lodge of the International Association of Machinists and Aerospace Workers
9000 Machinists Pl.
Upper Marlboro, MD 20772   301-967-4500
                                            info@iamaw.org
                                            www.goiam.org
Robert Martinez, Jr., International President
Dora Cervantes, General Secretary-Treasurer
Mark Blondin, General Vice President, Aerospace
Offers placements, programs, and resources for persons with disabilities.

709 HEATH Resource Center at the National Youth Transitions Center
George Washington University
2134 G St. NW
Washington, DC 20052-0001   askheath@gwu.edu
                                          www.heath.gwu.edu
Joan Kester, Principal Investigator
Christopher Nace, Research Assistant
The HEALTH Resource Center is a national clearinghouse for information about education after high school for people with disabilities. Also serves as an information exchange about educational support services, policies, procedures, adaptations, and opportunities on American campuses, vocational-technical schools, adult education programs, independent living centers, and other training entities after high school.

710 Habilitation Benefits Coalition
c/o Powers Pyles Sutter & Verville PC
1501 M St. NW
7th Floor
Washington, DC 20005   habcoalition.wordpress.com
The HAB Coalition coordinates, sustains and promotes a unified voice for organizations who are independently active in their support for habilitative services and devices.

711 Haldimand-Norfolk Resource Education and Counseling
101A Nanticoke Creek Parkway
Townsend, ON, Canada N0A-1S0   519-587-2441
                                           800-265-8087
                                       Fax: 519-587-4798
                                       info@hnreach.on.ca
                                       www.hnreach.on.ca
Leo Massi, Executive Director
Wendy Carron, Director, Early Childhood Services
Deb Young, Director, Services, Moving on Mental Health
Haldimand-Norfolk REACH is a multi-service agency, providing children's mental health services, developmental services, Autism services, youth justice services, family services, a residential program for transitional-aged youth and several early learning and care services including licensed childcare, Ontario Early Years Centre(s) and Community Action Program for Children.

712 Hanger, Inc.
4534 Westgate Blvd.
Suite 114
Austin, TX 78745   512-614-4612
                                           877-442-6437
                                       Fax: 512-614-4615
                                          hangerclinic.com
Vinit K. Asar, President & Chief Executive Officer
Thomas E. Kiraly, Executive Vice President & Chief Financial Officer
C. Scott Ranson, Executive Vice President & Chief Information Officer
Hanger Clinic specializes in orthotic and prosthetic services with clinic locations across the country.

713 Health Action
5276 Hollister Ave.
Suite 257
Santa Barbara, CA 93111   805-617-3390
                                          www.healthaction.net
Roger Jahnke, Co-Founder & Chief Executive Officer
Rebecca McLean, Co-Founder
Health Action's mission is to foster innovation in health care that will increase health status, customer satisfaction, profitability, support provider efficiency, enhance clinical outcomes, and encourage consumer self-managed care.

714   Hearing Health Foundation (HHF)
575 Eighth Ave.
Suite 1201
New York, NY 10018   212-257-6140
                                            866-454-3924
                                       Fax: 212-257-6139
                                       TTY: 888-435-6104
                                            info@hhf.org
                                   hearinghealthfoundation.org
Timothy Higdon, President & Chief Executive Officer
Noemi Disla, Director, Finance, Operations & Administration
Christopher Geissler, Director, Program & Research Support
Hearing Health Foundation promotes hearing health and advocates for the prevention and cure of hearing loss and tinnitus through research.
1958

715   High Technology Foundation
1000 Galliher Dr.
Suite 1000
Fairmont, WV 26554   304-363-5482
                                            877-363-5482
                                            info@wvhtf.org
                                            www.wvhtf.org
Michael I. Green, Chairman
James L. Estep, President & Chief Executive Officer
High Technology Foundation is dedicated to maximizing economic development in West Virginia through the high-technology business sector.
1990

716   Hogg Foundation for Mental Health
3001 Lake Austin Blvd.
Austin, TX 78703   512-471-5041
                          hogg-operations@austin.utexas.edu
                                            hogg.utexas.edu
Octavio N. Martinez Jr., Executive Director
Vicky Coffee, Director, Programs
Crystal Viagran, Director, Finance & Operations
The Hogg Foundation for Mental Health is a nonprofit organization that is dedicated to the advancement of mental wellness for the people of Texas through outreach programs, conferences, seminars, research grants, and more.

717   Homeopathic Educational Services
812C Camelia St.
Berkeley, CA 94710   510-649-0294
                                            800-359-9051
                                       email@homeopathic.com
                                       www.homeopathic.com
Dana Ullman, Owner & Director
Resource center for homeopathic products and services including books, tapes, research, medicines, medicine kits, software for the general public and health professionals, and correspondence courses.
1975

718   Hope Network Neuro Rehabilitation
3075 Orchard Vista Dr. SE
PO Box 890
Grand Rapids, MI 49546   616-301-8000
                                            800-695-7273
                                       Fax: 616-301-8010
                                   www.hopenetworkrehab.org
Phil Weaver, President & Chief Executive Officer
Tim Becker, Chief Operating Officer
Andre Pierre, Chief Financial Officer
Neuro Rehabilitation is a service line of Hope Network, helping those with brain or spinal cord injuries or other neurological conditions recover through treatment techniques and person-centered care.

719   Humanity & Inclusion (HI)
8757 Georgia Ave.
Suite 420
Silver Spring, MD 20910   301-891-2138
                                       Fax: 301-891-9193
                                            info.usa@hi.org
                                            www.hi-us.org
Jeff Meer, Executive Director
Nancy A. Kelly, President
Christine Kaunch, Treasurer
International organization promoting disability rights, rehabilitation, and safety in areas of emergency and conflict.

720   Immune Deficiency Foundation
110 West Rd.
Suite 300
Towson, MD 21204   800-296-4433
                                       Fax: 410-321-9165
                                   info@primaryimmune.org
                                       primaryimmune.org
Jorey Berry, President & Chief Executive Officer
Sarah Rose, Chief Financial Officer
Katherine Antilla, Vice President, Education
The Immune Deficiency Foundation is the national patient organization dedicated to improving the diagnosis, treatment, and quality of life of persons with primary immunodeficiency diseases through advocacy, education, and research.

721   Indiana Association for Home and Hospice Care (IAHHC)
6320-G Rucker Rd.
Indianapolis, IN 46220   317-775-6675
                                       Fax: 317-775-6674
                                            evan@iahhc.org
                                            www.iahhc.org
Evan Reinhardt, Executive Director
Katie Ociepka, Director, Development
Tori Raderstorf, Director, Communications & Events
The Indiana Association for Home & Hospice Care represents home nursing services and inpatient hospice care services. The association offers education and resources, advocacy, and a career center to its members.

722   Institute for Educational Leadership (IEL)
4301 Connecticut Ave. NW
Suite 100
Washington, DC 20008   202-822-8405
                                       Fax: 202-872-4050
                                            iel@iel.org
                                            iel.org
Eddie Koen, President
Maame Appiah, Vice President, Finance & Talent
S. Kwesi Rollins, Vice Resident, Leadership & Engagement
Assists under-funded communities by preparing children, youth, adults, and families for postsecondary education and training, leading to better career options and greater community engagement.

723   International Academy of Independent Medical Evaluators
1061 E Main St.
Suite 300
East Dundee, IL 60118   847-752-5355
                                            iaime@iaime.org
                                            www.iaime.org
Fabrice Czarnecki, President
Diana Kraemer, President Elect
James Underhill, Secretary & Treasurer
IAIME is an organization serving physicians involved in disability management. Their courses and products cover disability management and evaluations for physicians, health care providers, attorneys, regulators, legislators, and others involved in the care of injured persons.

724   International Association of Yoga Therapists (IAYT)
PO Box 251563
Little Rock, AR 72225   928-541-0004
                                            www.iayt.org
Alyssa Wostrel, Executive Director
Beth Whitney-Teeple, Chief of Staff
Nancy Sinton, Manager, Certification

IAYT supports research and education in yoga and serves yoga practitioners, teachers, therapists, health care professionals, and researchers worldwide. Its mission is to establish yoga as a recognized and respected therapy in the Western world. IAYT also serves members, the media, and the general public as a comprehensive source of information about contemporary yoga education, research, and statistics.
1989

725   International Child Amputee Network
PO Box 13812
Tuscon, AZ 85732   child-amputee.net
I-CAN provides information, support and education to children with traumatic and congenital limb difference and their families.

726   International Chiropractors Association (ICA)
6400 Arlington Blvd.
Suite 650
Falls Church, VA 22042   703-528-5000
                                        Fax: 703-528-5023
                                        info@chiropractic.org
                                        www.chiropractic.org
Beth Clay, Executive Director & Chief Executive Officer
The Association strives to protect, promote and advance chiropractic throughout the world.
1926

727   International Clinic of Biological Regeneration (ICBR)
PO Box 509
Florissant, MO 63032   800-826-5366
                                        Fax: 314-921-8485
                                        icbr@aol.com
                                        www.icbr.com
Judith A. Smith, Co-Founder & Director
William Johnson, Director, Medical Services
The International Clinic of Biological Regeneration is an international cell therapy center dedicated to constantly improving therapeutic results by selecting newer, safer, and more effective treatments.
1981

728   International Expressive Arts Therapy Association (IEATA)
PO Box 40707
San Francisco, CA 94140-0707   415-489-0698
                                        info@ieata.org
                                        ieata.org
Christina Hampton, Co-Chair
Janet Rasmussen, Co-Chair
Susan Johnson, Treasurer
The International Expressive Arts Therapy Association is a nonprofit organization dedicated to supporting expressive arts therapists, artists, educators, consultants, and others using creative processes for personal growth and community development.

729   International League Against Epilepsy (ILAE)
2221 Justin Rd.
Suite 119-352
Flower Mound, TX 75028   860-586-7547
                                        Fax: 860-201-1111
                                        ilae.org
Julie Hall, Executive Director
Linda Beza, Director, Finance
Priscilla Shisler, Director, Engagement & Education
ILAE is a nonprofit organization dedicated to the advancement and dissemination of knowledge about epilepsy and to promoting research, education, and training to improve service and care for patients.
Founded in 1909. 1909

730   International Ventilator Users Network (IVUN)
50 Crestwood Executive Ctr.
Suite 440
St. Louis, MO 63126-1916   314-534-0475
                                        Fax: 314-534-5070
                                        info@ventusers.org
                                        www.ventnews.org
Mark Mallinger, President & Chairperson
Frederick M. Maynard, Vice President
Marny K. Eulberg, Secretary

To enhance the lives and independence of individuals using ventilators by promoting education, networking and advocacy. IVUN is an affiliate of Post-Polio Health International.

731   Invisible Disabilities Association (IDA)
PO Box 4067
Parker, CO 80134   invisibledisabilities.org
Wayne Connell, Founder, President & Chief Executive Officer
Jess Stainbrook, Executive Director & Vice President
The Invisible Disabilities Association (IDA) encourages, educates, and connects people and organizations touched by illness, pain, and disability around the globe.

732   JDRF
200 Vesey St.
28th Floor
New York, NY 10281   800-533-2873
                                        Fax: 212-785-9595
                                        info@jdrf.org
                                        www.jdrf.org
Timothy Doyle, President & Chief Operating Officer
Sanjoy Dutta, Chief Scientific Officer
Syndey Yovic, Chief of Staff & Head of Global Initatives
A nonprofit, nongovernmental diabetes research organization. JDRF's mission is to find a cure for diabetes and its complications through the support of research. JDRF also sponsors international workshops and conferences for biomedical researchers, and individual chapters offer support groups and other activities for families affected by diabetes. JDRF has more than 110 chapters and affiliates worldwide. They publish a quarterly newsletter.
1970

733   Job Accommodation Network (JAN)
PO Box 6080
Morgantown, WV 26506-6080   800-526-7234
                                        TTY: 877-781-9403
                                        jan@askjan.org
                                        askjan.org
JAN's mission is to facilitate the employment and retention of workers with disabilities by providing employers, employment providers, people with disabilities, their family members, and other interested parties with information on job accommodations, self-employment, and small business opportunities and related subjects.

734   Joni and Friends (JAF)
30009 Ladyface Ct.
Agoura Hills, CA 91301   818-707-5664
                                             800-736-4177
                                        Fax: 818-707-2391
                                        www.joniandfriends.org
Joni Eareckson Tada, Founder & Chief Executive Officer
John Nugent, President & Chief Operating Officer
Laura Gardner, Executive Vice President & Chief Financial Officer
A nonprofit organization seeking to accelerate Christian ministry with people affected by disabilities. JAF provides resources and training to churches to help create disability-welcoming environments, offers family retreats and mobility programs, and mentors people with disabilities to lead and provide service in their churches and communities.

735   Lambton County Developmental Services (LCDS)
339 Centre St.
Petrolia, ON, Canada N0N-1R0   519-882-0933
                                        Fax: 519-882-3386
                                        humanresources@lcds.on.ca
                                        www.lcdspetrolia.ca
Jill Cousins, President
Barb Frayne, Treasurer
John Douglas, Secretary
A network of experts and volunteers working together to provide support services and employment services for people with developmental disabilities.

736 Laurent Clerc National Deaf Education Center
800 Florida Ave. NE
Washington, DC 20002   202-651-5855
Fax: 202-651-5857
TTY: 202-250-2856
clerc.center@gallaudet.edu
www.clerccenter.gallaudet.edu
Provides resources, information, training and research on deaf
education and deaf and hard of hearing children.

737 Learning Disabilities Association of America (LDA)
4068 Mount Royal Boulevard
Suite 224B
Allison Park, PA 15101   412-341-1515
info@ldaamerica.org
www.ldaamerica.org

Cindy Cipoletti, Executive Director
Tracy Gregoire, Director, Healthy Children Project
Nina DelPrato, Administrative Manager
LDA aims to provide opportunities for success and support to individuals with learning disabilities, their parents, teachers, and
other professionals. It carries out its mission by supporting research on learning disabilities, advocating for early identification and best practice interventions, and protecting the rights of
all persons with learning disabilities.
1964

**738 Learning Disabilities Association of New York State
(LDANYS)**
300 Hylan Dr., Suite 6
PO Box 144
Rochester, NY 14623   518-608-8992
Fax: 518-608-8993
www.ldanys.org

Jeffrey Baker, President
Helene Fallon, Vice President
Kathryn Cappella, Treasurer
A nonprofit organization advocating for children and adults with
learning disabilities. LDA is a three-tiered organization comprised of a national organization, state affiliates and local chapters. They aim to support and empower individuals with learning
disabilities throughout their lives.

739 Learning Disabilities Worldwide
179 Bear Hill Rd.
Suite 104
Waltham, MA 02451   help@ldworldwide.org
www.ldworldwide.org

Teresa Allissa Citro, Chief Executive Officer
Nicholas D. Young, Chairman
Matthias Grünke, Vice Chairman
Learning Disabilities Worldwide, Inc. is an international professional organization dedicated to improving the educational, professional, and personal outcomes for individuals with learning
disabilities and other related disorders.
1965

740 LoSeCa Foundation
215-1 Carnegie Dr.
St. Albert, AB, Canada T8N-5B1   780-460-1400
Fax: 780-459-1380
chorpestad@loseca.ca
www.loseca.ca

Carmen Horpestad, Executive Director & Chief Executive Officer
Jules Lefebvre, Director, Operations
Rebecca McLeod, Manager, Human Resources
A nonprofit organization that provides support services to adults
with developmental disabilities.

741 Mainstream
300 S Rodney Parham Rd.
Suite 5
Little Rock, AR 72205   501-280-0012
800-371-9026
Fax: 501-280-9267
TTY: 501-280-9262
www.mainstreamilrc.com
A non-residential, consumer-driven independent living resource
center for persons with disabilities. Mainstream operates with the
conviction that people with disabilities have the right and responsibility to make choices, to control their lives and to participate

fully and equally in the community. Mainstream offers the following services free of charge: Advocacy, Peer Support, Training
and Education, Information and Referral, Ramp program, and
more.
1988

742 March of Dimes
1550 Crystal Dr.
Suite 1300
Arlington, VA 22202   888-663-4637
www.marchofdimes.org
Stacey D. Stewart, President & Chief Executive Officer
*Adrian P. Mollo, Senior Vice President, General Counsel & Assis-
tant Secretary*
*David C. Damond, Senior Vice President, CFO & Assistant
Treasurer*
The mission of the March of Dimes is to improve the health of ba-
bies by preventing birth defects and infant mortality.

743 McKinnon Body Therapy Center
2940 Webster St.
Oakland, CA 94609   510-465-3488
info@mckinnonbtc.com
mckinnonbtc.com
The McKinnon Body Therapy Center offers certificate programs
and courses in massage therapy. They provide continuing education for massage therapists and other health professionals seeking to expand their skills.
1973

744 Mental Health America (MHA)
500 Montgomery St.
Suite 820
Alexandria, VA 22314   703-684-7722
800-969-6642
Fax: 703-684-5968
info@mhanational.org
www.mhanational.org
Schroeder Stribling, President & Chief Executive Officer
Mary Giliberti, Chief Public Policy Officer
Jessica Kennedy, Chief of Staff & Chief Financial Officer
A nonprofit organization addressing issues related to mental
health and mental illness. MHA works to improve the mental
health of all Americans, especially individuals with mental disor-
ders, through advocacy, education, research, and service.
Founded in 1909. 1909

745 MindFreedom International (MFI)
454 Willamette, Suite 216
PO Box 11284
Eugene, OR 97440-3484   541-345-9106
877-623-7743
Fax: 480-287-8833
office@mindfreedom.org
mindfreedom.org

Celia Brown, President
Ronald Bassman, Executive Director
Sarah Smith, Office Manager
Nonprofit organization dedicated to winning human rights and
alternatives for people with psychiatric disabilities.

746 Muscular Dystrophy Association USA (MDA)
161 N Clark
Suite 3550
Chicago, IL 60601   800-572-1717
resourcecenter@mdausa.org
www.mda.org
Donald S. Wood, President & Chief Executive Officer
Kristine Welker, Chief of Staff
*Sharon Hesterlee, Executive Vice President & Chief Research
Officer*
MDA provides comprehensive medical services to people with
neuromuscular diseases at hospital-affiliated clinics across the
country. The Association's worldwide research program, which
funds over 400 individual scientific investigations annually, represents the largest single effort to advance knowledge of
neuromuscular diseases and to find cures and treatments for
them. In addition, MDA conducts far-reaching educational
programs for the public and professionals.
1950

747 National Association for Holistic Aromatherapy (NAHA)
6000 S. 5th Ave.
Pocatello, ID 83204
877-232-5255
Fax: 919-894-0271
info@naha.org
www.naha.org

Sharon Falsetto, Chief Journal Editor
Kelly Holland Azzaro, Assistant Journal Editor
The NAHA is an educational, nonprofit organization dedicated to enhancing public awareness of the benefits of true aromatherapy. It offers aromatherapy Tele-classes & membership benefits, and acts as a referral service.

748 National Association of Blind Merchants (NABM)
National Federation of the Blind
7450 Chapman Hwy.
Suite 319
Knoxville, TN 37920
888-687-6226
president@merchants-nfb.org
blindmerchants.org

Nicky Gacos, President
Harold Wilson, First Vice President
Ed Birmingham, Second Vice President
Serving as an advocacy and support group, NABM is a membership organization of blind persons employed in self-employment work or the Randolph-Sheppard Vending Program. The organization provides information on issues affecting blind merchants, including rehabilitation, social security, and tax.

749 National Association of City and County health Officials
1201 Eye St. NW
4th Floor
Washington, DC 20005
202-783-5550
Fax: 202-783-1583
info@naccho.org
naccho.org

Lori Tremmel Freeman, Chief Executive Officer
E. Oscar Alleyne, Chief, Programs & Services
Adriane Casalotti, Chief, Government & Public Affairs
Strengthens and advocates for local health departments to improve the health of communities.

750 National Association of Councils on Developmental Disabilities (NACDD)
1825 K St. NW
Suite 600
Washington, DC 20006
202-506-5813
info@nacdd.org
www.nacdd.org

Donna A. Meltzer, Chief Executive Officer
Erin Prangley, Director, Public Policy
Sheryl Matney, Director, Technical Assistance
NACDD is the national association for the 56 State and Territorial Councils on Developmental Disabilities (DD Councils) which receive federal funding to support programs that promote self-determination, integration, and inclusion for all Americans with developmental disabilities.

751 National Association of Disability Representatives (NADR)
1305 W 11th St.
Suite 222
Houston, TX 77008
202-822-2155
800-747-6131
Fax: 972-245-6701
admin@nadr.org
www.nadr.org

Michael Wener, President
Christopher Mazzulli, Vice President
Cliff Berkley, Secretary
NADR is an organization of Professional Social Security Claimants Representatives that focus on issues involving policies to protect the interest of people with disabilities. NADR conducts annual conventions open to members and non-members with educational seminars to keep practitioners up to date on Social Security rulings, regulatory changes, and practice improvements.

752 National Association of State Directors of Developmental Disabilities Services (NASDDDS)
301 N Fairfax St.
Suite 101
Alexandria, VA 22314-2633
703-683-4202
cmcgraw@nasddds.org
www.nasddds.org

Mary P. Sowers, Executive Director
Dan Berland, Director, Federal Policy
Barbara Brent, Director, State Policy
NASDDDS is the representative for the nation's agencies providing services to people with intellectual and developmental disabilities. They aim to promote the development of effective, efficient service delivery systems for individuals with disabilities.

753 National Business & Disability Council (NBDC)
The Viscardi Center
201 I.U. Willets Rd.
Albertson, NY 11507
516-465-1400
info@viscardicenter.org
viscardicenter.org/services/nbdc

Dr. Chris Rosa, President & Chief Executive Officer
Sheryl P. Buchel, Executive Vice President & Chief Financial Officer
Michael Caprara, Chief Information Officer
The NBDC is a resource for employers seeking to integrate people with disabilities into the workplace and companies seeking to reach them in the consumer marketplace.

754 National Care Planning Council
PO Box 1118
Centerville, UT 84014
801-298-8676
800-989-8137
Fax: 801-295-3776
info@longtermcarelink.net
www.longtermcarelink.net

Thomas E. Day, Director
The National Care Planning Council's mission is to help families with long term care planning for seniors. Services include training, eldercare articles, books, workshops and seminars, networking and more.

755 National Center for College Students with Disabilities (NCCSD)
8015 West Kenton Circle
Suite 230
Huntersville, NC 28078
844-730-8048
TTY: 651-583-7499
nccsd@ahead.org
www.nccsdonline.org

Wendy Harbour, Co-Principal Investigator & Center Director
Stephan Smith, Co-Principial Investigator & Project Director
Richard Allegra, Associate Director, Education & Outreach Services
A federally-funded project under the U.S. Department of Education, housed at the Association on Higher Education And Disability (AHEAD). It provides assistance and information to students, families, educators and more; collects information and conducts research; and reports to the Department of Education.
Founded in 2015. 1915

756 National Center for Education in Maternal and Child Health (NCEMCH)
Georgetown University
MCHnavigator@ncemch.org
www.ncemch.org

Rochelle Mayer, Research Professor & Director
John Richards, Executive Director
Provides information on children with special health needs, child health and development, adolescent health, nutrition, violence and injury prevention, and other issues of maternal and child health for health professionals and the public.

757   National Center for Health, Physical Activity and Disability
4000 Ridgeway Dr.
Birmingham, AL 35209   800-900-8086
                                          Fax: 205-313-7475
                                          email@nchpad.org
                                          www.nchpad.org
James Rimmer, Principal Investigator
Angela Grant, Business Manager
Jeff Underwood, Program Director
NCHPAD promotes health for people with disability through increased participation in all types of physical and social activities. These include fitness and aquatic activities, recreational and sports programs, adaptive equipment usage, and more.
1999

758   National Center on Deaf-Blindness (NCDB)
Hellen Keller National Center
141 Middle Neck Rd.
Sands Point, NY 11050   541-800-0412
                                          support@nationaldb.org
                                          www.nationaldb.org
Sam Morgan, Director
Julie Durando, Evaluation Coordinator
Peggy Malloy, Information Services & Technology Coordinator
Funded by the federal Department of Education, the Center seeks to improve quality of life for children who are deaf-blind and their families.

759   National Center on Disability and Journalism (NCDJ)
Walter Cronkite School of Journalism, AZ State U.
555 N Central Ave.
Phoenix, AZ 85004   ncdj.org
Kristin Gilger, Director
Rachel Konieczny, Graduate Assistant
Jake Geller, Inaugural Director
Supports journalists as they cover people with disabilities, concerned with accuracy, fairness and diversity in news coverage.
1998

760   National Certification Commission for Acupuncture and Oriental Medicine
2001 K St. NW
3rd Floor
Washington, DC 20036   202-381-1140
                                          888-381-1140
                                          Fax: 202-381-1141
                                          info@thenccaom.org
                                          www.nccaom.org
Mina Larson, Chief Executive Officer
Olga Cox, Chief Operations Officer
Irene Basore, Director, Administration & Governance
National organization that provides professional certification for entry-level practitioners of acupuncture and Oriental medicine (AOM), representing 98 percent of the states that regulate acupuncture.

761   National Collaborative Workforce on Disability (NCWD/Youth)
c/o Institute for Educational Leadership

Provides assistance to state and local workforce development systems to better serve youth of all types of ability.

762   National Council on Independent Living (NCIL)
P.O. Box 31260
Washington, DC 20006   202-207-0334
                                          844-778-7961
                                          Fax: 202-207-0341
                                          TTY: 202-207-0340
                                          ncil@ncil.org
                                          www.ncil.org
Darrell Lynn Jones, Interim Executive Director
Jenny Sichel, Director, Operations
Denise Law, Coordinator, Member Services
A national cross-disability grassroots organization, NCIL advances independent living and the rights of people with disabilities through consumer-driven advocacy.

763   National Disability Rights Network (NDRN)
820 1st St. NE
Suite 740
Washington, DC 20002   202-408-9514
                                          Fax: 202-408-9520
                                          TTY: 202-408-9521
                                          info@ndrn.org
                                          www.ndrn.org
Curtis Decker, Executive Director
Belinda Miller, Deputy Executive Director, Finance & Administration
David Hutt, Deputy Executive Director, Legal Services
Voluntary national membership association of protection and advocacy systems and client assistance programs. Promoting and strengthening the role and performance of its members in providing quality legally based advocacy services.

764   National Federation of Families for Children's Mental Health (NFFCMH)
15800 Crabbs Branch Way
Suite 300
Rockville, MD 20855   240-403-1901
                                          ffcmh@ffcmh.org
                                          www.ffcmh.org
Lynda Gargan, Executive Director
Michelle Covington, Project Manager
Kelsey Engelbracht, Project Manager
A national family-run organization serving to provide advocacy at the national level for the rights of children and youth with emotional, behavioral, and mental health challenges and their families. The FFCMH provides leadership and technical assistance to a nation-wide network of family run organizations, and collaborates with organizations to transform mental and substance abuse health care in the U.S.
1989

765   National Guild of Hypnotists (NGH)
PO Box 308
Merrimack, NH 03054-0308   603-429-9438
                                          Fax: 603-424-8066
                                          ngh@ngh.net
                                          www.ngh.net
Dr. Dwight Damon, President
Don Mottin, Vice President
Jereme Bachand, Executive Director
The National Guild of Hypnotists is a not-for-profit, educational corporation committed to advancing the field of hypnotism.
1950

766   National Health Council
1730 M St. NW
Suite 500
Washington, DC 20036-4561   202-785-3910
                                          Fax: 202-785-5923
                                          nationalhealthcouncil.org
Randall L. Rutta, Chief Executive Officer
Linda Beza, Senior Vice President, Finance & Administration
Susan Gaffney, Executive Vice President, Membership, Development & Events
Seeks to provide a unified voice for people living with chronic diseases and disabilities, and their caregivers.

767   National Institute on Disability, Independent Living, and Rehabilitation Research (NIDILRR)
Administration for Community Living
330 C St. SW
Washington, DC 20201   202-401-4634
                                          acl.gov
Anjali Forber-Pratt, Director
Alison Barkoff, Principal Deputy Administrator
Vicki Gottlich, Director, Center for Policy & Evaluation
NIDILRR, formerly the National Institute on Disability and Rehabilitation Research (NIDRR), aims to promote new research into the abilities of individuals with disabilities, and to use that research to allow those individuals to improve and use those skills within their community. NIDILRR also aims to maximize the full inclusion and integration of individuals with disabilities into society.

768   National Organization on Disability (NOD)
77 Water St.
13th Floor
New York, NY 10005   646-505-1191
                                   Fax: 646-505-1184
                                        info@nod.org
                                        www.nod.org
Carol Glazer, President
Moeena Das, Chief Operating Officer
Priyanka Ghosh, Director, External Affairs
The National Organization on Disability is a private, nonprofit
organization that promotes the full and equal participation of
men, women, and children with disabilities in all aspects of
American life.
1982

769   National Rehabilitation Association (NRA)
PO Box 150235
Alexandria, VA 22315   703-836-0850
                                        888-258-4295
                                   info@nationalrehab.org
                                        nationalrehab.org
Satinder Atwal, Chief Administrator Officer
James Liin, Coordinator, Membership
NRA members work to eliminate barriers and increase employ-
ment opportunities for people with disabilities. They provide op-
portunities for advocacy and increase awareness of issues
through professional development and access to current research
topics.

770   National University of Natural Medicine (NUNM)
49 South Porter St.
Portland, OR 97201   503-552-1555
                                    reception@nunm.edu
                                        nunm.edu
Melanie Henriksen, Interim President
Gerald Bores, Executive Vice President & Chief Financial Officer
Kathy Stanford, Vice President, Human Resources
NUNM is an accredited naturopathic medical university, and
leads the research on natural medicine. They offer programs in
naturopathic medicine, classical Chinese medicine, integrative
mental health, global health, massage therapy, and more.
1956

771   National Vaccine Information Center (NVIC)
21525 Ridgetop Circle
Suite 100
Sterling, VA 20166   703-938-0342
                                   Fax: 571-313-1268
                                     contactus@nvic.org
                                        www.nvic.org
Barbara Loe Fisher, Co-Founder & President
Kathi Williams, Co-Founder & Vice President
Theresa Wrangham, Executive Director
Provides resources on vaccination and health.

772   National Women's Health Network (NWHN)
1413 K St. NW
4th Floor
Washington, DC 20005   202-682-2640
                                   Fax: 202-682-2648
                                       nwhn@nwhn.org
                                        www.nwhn.org
Teri Bordenave, Interim Executive Director
Abigail Arons, Board Chair
Kimberly Robinson, Vice Chair
The National Women's Health Network seeks to improve
women's health by developing and promoting a critical analysis
of health issues in order to affect policy and support consumer decision-making. The Network aspires to a health care system that
is guided by social justice and reflects the needs of diverse
women.
1975

773   Native American Disability Law Center
905 W. Apache St.
Farmington, NM 87401   505-566-5880
                                        800-862-7271
                                   Fax: 505-566-5889
                              info@nativedisabilitylaw.org
                                 www.nativedisabilitylaw.org
Therese Yanan, Executive Director
Laura McClenny, Director, Development
The Native American Disability Law Center is a private nonprofit
organization that advocates for the legal rights of Native Americans with disabilities. Through advocacy and education, the center empowers Native people with disabilities to lead independent
lives in their own communities.

774   North Hastings Community Integration Association
2 Alice St.
PO Box 1508
Bancroft, ON, Canada K0L-1C0   613-332-2090
                                   Fax: 613-332-4762
                                 communityliving@nhcia.ca
                                        www.nhcia.ca
Sandra Phillips, Executive Director
Teena Surma, Manager, Independent Living
Bev Lloyd, Manager, Community Resources
NHCIA offers daily living supports, life planning, community access, dual diagnosis supports, respite services, assistance with
funding and resource referral information. The association works
closely with many community services, groups, schools, and
businesses to offer individualized supports to children, youth and
adults with an intellectual disability and their families.

775   Not Dead Yet
497 State St.
Rochester, NY 14608   708-420-0539
                                        notdeadyet.org
Diane Coleman, President & Chief Executive Officer
Anita Cameron, Director, Minority Outreach
Disability rights group opposing the legalization of assisted sui-
cide and euthanasia.

**776   PACER Center (Parent Advocacy Coalition for
        Educational Rights)**
8161 Normandale Blvd.
Bloomington, MN 55437   952-838-9000
                                        800-537-2237
                                   Fax: 952-838-0199
                                       pacer@pacer.org
                                        www.pacer.org
Paula F. Goldberg, Executive Director
Mission is to expand opportunities and enhance the quality of life
of children and young adults with disabilities and their families
based on the concept of parents helping parents. Offers workshops, individual assistance, and written information for children
with disabilities, their parents and families, and professionals
working with them. Computer Resource Center/Software
Lending Library available.
1977

777   PEAK Parent Center
917 East Moreno Ave.
Suite 140
Colorado Springs, CO 80903   719-531-9400
                                   Fax: 719-531-9452
                                     info@peakparent.org
                                        www.peakparent.org
Michele Williers, Executive Director
Pam Christy, Director, Parent Training & Information
PEAK Parent Center is Colorado's federally-designated Parent
Training and Information Center (PTI). As a PTI, PEAK supports
and empowers parents, providing them with information and
strategies to use when advocating for their children with disabilities. PEAK works one-on-one with families and educators helping them realize new possibilities for children with disabilities by
expanding knowledge of special education and offering new
strategies for success.
1986

778   Pacific Institute of Aromatherapy
PO Box 6723
San Rafael, CA 94903   415-479-9120
                                                   Fax: 415-479-0614
www.pacificinstituteofaromatherapy.com
Kurt Schnaubelt, Founder & Director
The Pacific Institute on Aromatherapy offers certification
courses, seminars, books, and products on aromatherapy treatments and essential oils.
1983

779   Parent Professional Advocacy League (PPAL)
77 Rumford Ave.
Waltham, MA 02453   866-815-8122
                                                   Fax: 617-542-7832
                                                       info@ppal.net
                                                       www.ppal.net

Lisa Lambert, Executive Director
Meri Viano, Associate Director
Joel Khattar, Program Manager
A statewide organization focusing on the interests of families
with children with mental health needs. PPAL advocates for improved and better access to mental health services for children
and their families.

780   Parents Helping Parents (PHP)
1400 Parkmoor Ave.
Suite 100
San Jose, CA 95126   408-727-5775
                                                        855-727-5775
                                                   Fax: 408-286-1116
                                                       info@php.com
                                                       www.php.com

Maria Daane, Executive Director
Janet Nunez, Director, Programs
Mark Fishler, Director, Development
Dedicated to assisting children with any type of special need:
mental, physical, emotional, or learning disability. Mission is to
help children with special needs receive love, hope, respect, and
services needed to achieve their full potential by strengthening
their families and the professionals who serve them. Develops
programs and produces educational and support materials, including information packets, brochures, and a newsletter.

**781   Partnership on Employment and Acessible Technology
        (PEAT)**
                                                   info@peatworks.org
                                                   www.peatworks.org
Funded by the U.S. Department of Labor's Office of Disability
Employment Policy (ODEP), PEAT fosters collaboration around
building and buying accessible technology in the workplace.

782   Partnership to Improve Patient Care
100 M St. SE
Suite 750
Washington, DC 20003   www.pipcpatients.org
Sara van Geertruyden, Executive Director
Thayer Surette Roberts, Deputy Director
Promotes a patient-centric healthcare system including compara-
tive effectiveness research, the assessment of treatment value
through shared decision-making, and alternate payment models.

783   People First of Canada
20-226 Osborne St. North
Winnipeg, MB, Canada R3C-1V4   204-784-7362
                                                   Fax: 204-784-7364
                                          info@peoplefirstofcanada.ca
                                          www.peoplefirstofcanada.ca
Shelley Fletcher, Executive Director
Catherine Rodgers, Director, Communications
People First of Canada is the national voice for people who have
been labeled with an intellectual disability. People First is a
movement of people who want all citizens to live equally in the
country.

784   Peter and Elizabeth C. Tower Foundation
2351 North Forest Rd.
Suite 106
Getzville, NY 14068-1225   716-689-0370
                                                   Fax: 716-689-3716
                                           info@thetowerfoundation.org
                                               thetowerfoundation.org
Tracy A. Sawicki, Executive Director
Donald W. Matteson, Chief Program Officer
Charles E. Colston Jr., Program Officer
The Peter and Elizabeth C. Tower Foundation supports community programming that results in children, adolescents, and young
adults affected by substance use disorders, learning disabilities,
mental illness, and intellectual disabilities achieving their full
potential.
1990

785   Post-Polio Health International
50 Crestwood Executive Ctr.
Suite 440
St. Louis, MO 63126   314-534-0475
                                                   Fax: 314-534-5070
                                                    info@post-polio.org
                                                   www.post-polio.org

Mark Mallinger, President
Frederick M. Maynard, Vice President
Brian M. Tiburzi, Executive Director
To enhance the lives and independence of polio survivors, home
ventilator users, their caregivers and families, and health profes-
sionals through education, networking, and advocacy.

786   Postpartum Support International (PSI)
6706 SW 54th Ave.
Portland, OR 97219   503-894-9453
                                                        800-944-4773
                                                   Fax: 503-894-9452
                                            support@postpartum.net
                                                       postpartum.net
Wendy N. Davis, Executive Director
Lianne Swanson, Executive Administrator
Birdie Gunyon Meyer, Certification Director
The mission of Postpartum Support International is to promote
awareness, prevention, and treatment of mental health issues re-
lated to childbearing in every country worldwide.
1987

787   Primary Care Collaborative
601 13th St. NW
Suite 430N
Washington, DC 20005   202-417-2076
                                                    spadre@pcpcc.org
                                                       www.pcpcc.org
Ann Grenier, President & Chief Executive Officer
Loren Vandegrift, Director, IT
Stephen Padre, Senior Communications Manager
Advocates for a health system built on patient-centered primary
care. Its four aims are better care, better health, lower costs, and
greater joy for clinicians and staff in delivery of care.

**788   Professional Association of Therapeutic Horsemanship
        International (PATH Intl.)**
PO Box 33150
Denver, CO 80233   303-452-1212
                                                        800-369-7433
                                                   Fax: 303-252-4610
                                                    pathintl@pathintl.org
                                                       www.pathintl.org
Kathy Alm, Chief Executive Officer
Carrie Garnett, Director, Membership & Operations
Kaye Marks, Director, Marketing & Communications
A national nonprofit equestrian organization dedicated to serving
individuals with disabilities by giving disabled individuals the
opportunity to ride horses. Establishes safety standards, provides
continuing education, and offers networking opportunities for
both its individuals and center members. Produces educational
materials including fact sheets, brochures, booklets, audio-visual
tapes, a directory, and PATH Intl. magazine Strides.

789 Raising Deaf Kids
3440 Market St.
4th Floor
Philadelphia, PA 19104   215-590-7440
                                      Fax: 215-590-1335
                                      TTY: 215-590-6817
                                 info@raisingdeafkids.org
                                      raisingdeafkids.org
Annie Steinberg, Director
This website provides parents/guardians of children with hearing impairments with information and resources. The website is run and funded by the Deafness and Family Communication Center based at the Children's Hospital of Philadelphia.

790 Rehabilitation International
866 United Nations Plaza
Office 422
New York, NY 10017   212-420-1500
                                      Fax: 212-505-0871
                                         info@riglobal.org
                                         www.riglobal.org
Teuta Rexhepi, Secretary General
Zhang Haidi, President
RI and its members develop and promote initiatives to protect the rights of people with disabilities and improve rehabilitation and other crucial services for disabled people and their families. RI also works toward increasing international collaboration and advocates for policies and legislation recognizing the rights of people with disabilities and their families, including the establishment of a UN Convention on the Rights and Dignity of Persons with Disabilities.
1922

791 RespectAbility
11333 Woodglen Dr.
Suite 102
Rockville, MD 20852   202-517-6272
                                  info@respectability.org
                                  www.respectability.org
Deborah Fisher, Interim President & Chief Executive Officer
Lauren Appelbaum, Vice President, Communications, Entertainment & News Media
Philip Kahn-Pauli, Director, Policy & Practices
Nonprofit, nonpartisan organization providing free educational tools and resources to end stigmas and advance opportunities for people with disabilities and their families.

792 Ronald McDonald House Charities (RMHC)
110 N Carpenter St.
Chicago, IL 60607   630-623-7048
                                           info@rmhc.org
                                           www.rmhc.org
Kelly Dolan, President & Chief Executive Officer
Stacey Bifero, Chief Financial Officer
Janet Burton, Chief Operating Officer
Ronald McDonald House programs for families with sick children can be found in more than 64 countries around the world. Each house is run by a local nonprofit agency comprised of members of the medical community, McDonald's owners, businesses and civic organizations, and parent volunteers.

793 Ryan White HIV/AIDS Program
Health Resources & Services Administration
5600 Fishers Lane
Rockville, MD 20857   301-443-3376
                    hab.hrsa.gov/about-ryan-white-hivaids-program
Carole Johnson, Administrator
Diana Espinosa, Deputy Administrator
Jordan Grossman, Chief of Staff
The Ryan White HIV/AIDS Program provides a comprehensive system of care that includes primary medical care and essential support services for people living with HIV who are uninsured or underinsured. The Program works with cities, states, and local community-based organizations to provide HIV care and treatment services to more than half a million people each year.

794 Shirley Ryan AbilityLab
355 East Erie
Chicago, IL 60611   312-238-1000
                                           844-355-2253
                                      Fax: 312-238-1369
                                           www.sralab.org
Peggy Kirk, Co-President & Chief Executive Officer
Nancy E. Paridy, Co-President & Chief Administrative Officer
Richard L. Lieber, Chief Scientific & Senior Vice President of Research
Shirley Ryan AbilityLab is a research hospital integrating medical and research experts together in real time, applying research and providing patient care in physical medicine and rehabilitation. The AbilityLab has five Innovation Centers, each focusing on an area of biomedical science: Brain; Nerve, Muscle & Bone; Cancer; Spinal Cord; and Pediatric.

795 Society for Post-Acute and Long-Term Care Medicine (AMDA)
10500 Little Patuxent Pkwy.
Suite 210
Columbia, MD 21044   410-740-9743
                                           800-876-2632
                                      Fax: 410-740-4572
                                           info@paltc.org
                                           paltc.org
Suzanne M. Gillespie, President
Milta Little, Vice President
Swati Gaur, Treasurer
The Society for Post-Acute and Long-Term Care Medicine is a medical society representing medical directors, physicians, nurse practitioners, physician assistants, and other professionals working in post-acute and long-term care settings. The Society's mission is to advance the development of medical practitioners in all post-acute and long-term care settings through professional development, clinical guidance, and advocacy.
1977

796 Sofia University
3333 Harbor Blvd.
Costa Mesa, CA 92626   888-820-1484
                                student_services@sofia.edu
                                           sofia.edu
Allan Cahoon, President
Chris Nguyen, Chief Financial Officer & Vice President, Administration
Sofia University is a private, WSCUC-accredited institution focusing on humanistic and transpersonal psychology.
1975

797 Spartan Stuttering Laboratory
Michigan State University
1026 Red Cedar Rd.
East Lansing, MI 48824   517-884-2406
                                           jsy@msu.edu
                                   stutteringlab.msu.edu
The Spartan Stuttering Laboratory is a nonprofit organization that provides specialized assessment and treatment for children, adolescents, and adults who stutter and their families. They also provide education, training, and support for speech-language pathologists who work with people who stutter, and conduct an active program of basic and clinical research on the nature and treatment of stuttering across age groups.

798 St. Paul Abilities Network
4637 - 45 Ave.
St. Paul, AB, Canada T0A-3A3   780-645-3441
                                           866-645-3900
                                      Fax: 780-645-1885
                                 www.stpaulabilitiesnetwork.ca
Anthony Opden Dries, Executive Director
Provides support and opportunities to encourage the development of an individual's full potential through education, advocacy, and community partnerships.
1964

799 Starbridge
1650 South Ave.
Suite 200
Rochester, NY 14620   585-546-1700
800-650-4967
Fax: 585-224-7100
www.starbridgeinc.org
Colin Garwood, President & Chief Executive Officer
Nikisha Ridgeway, Chief Operating Officer
Terry O'Hare, Chief Financial Officer
A nonprofit organization dedicated to educating, supporting, and advocating for people who have disabilities, their families, and their circles of support.

800 Student Disability Services (SDS)
Wayne State University
5155 Gullen Mall
1600 Undergraduate Library
Detroit, MI 48202   313-577-1851
Fax: 313-577-4898
TTY: 313-202-4216
studentdisability@wayne.edu
www.studentdisability.wayne.edu
Cherise Matthews Frost, Interim Director
Mission is to ensure a university experience in which individuals with disabilities have equitable access to programs and to empower students to self-advocate in order to fulfill their academic goals.

801 TASH
1101 15th St. NW
Suite 206
Washington, DC 20005   202-817-3264
Fax: 202-999-4722
info@tash.org
www.tash.org
Michael Brogioli, Executive Director
Linda Metchikoff-Hooker, Director, Special Events
Donald Taylor, Manager, Membership & Operations
Formerly The Association for Persons with Severe Handicaps, it is an international association of people with disabilities, their family members, other advocates, and professionals fighting for a society in which inclusion of all people in all aspects of society is the norm.
ther pages 1975

802 The Advocacy Centre
205 Hall Street
Nelson, BC, Canada V1L-4E9   250-352-5777
877-352-5777
Fax: 250-352-5723
advocacycentre@nelsoncares.ca
advocacycentre.org
The Advocacy Centre's mission is to advocate for the rights of women, children, and other oppressed groups. The Centre aims to provide one-on-one advocacy, change unfair legislation and policy, and support those working on issues such as poverty, violence against women, mental illness, and child abuse and neglect. The Centre serves communities in the West Kootenay region.
1988

803 The Cherab Foundation
2301 NE Savannah Rd
Suite 1771
Jensen Beach, FL 34957   772-335-5135
help@cherab.org
cherabfoundation.org
Lisa Geng, Founder & President
Jolie Abreu, Vice President
The Cherab Foundation is a world-wide nonprofit organization working to improve the communication skills and education of all children with speech and language delays and disorders. The Cherab Foundation is committed to assisting with the development of new therapeutic approaches, preventions, and cures to neurologically-based speech disorders.

804 The Davis Center
110 Wesley St.
PO Box 508
Manlius, NY 13104   862-251-4637
Fax: 862-251-4642
npdunn@thedaviscenter.com
www.thedaviscenter.com
Dorinne S. Davis, Director
Offers sound-based therapies supporting positive change in learning, development, and wellness. All ages/all disabilities. Uses The Davis Model of Sound Intervention, an alternative approach.

805 The Hanen Centre
1075 Bay St.
Suite 515
Toronto, ON, Canada M5S-2B1   416-921-1073
877-426-3655
Fax: 416-921-1225
info@hanen.org
hanen.org
Elaine Weitzman, Executive Director
The Hanen Centre's mission is to provide parents, caregivers, early childhood educators, and speech-language pathologists with the knowledge and training they need to help young children develop the best possible language, social, and literacy skills. This includes children with or at risk of language delays and those with developmental challenges such as Autism Spectrum Disorder.

806 The Obesity Medicine Association (OMA)
7173 S Havana St.
Suite 600-130
Centennial, CO 80112   303-770-2526
Fax: 303-779-4834
info@obesitymedicine.org
obesitymedicine.org
Teresa Fraker, Executive Director
Joan Hablutzel, Director, Education
Christin Eriksen, Director, Marketing & Sales
The Obesity Medicine Association is an organization of physicians, nurse practitioners, physician assistants, and other health care providers with special interest and experience in the comprehensive treatment of obesity.

807 The Steve Fund
PO Box 9070
Providence, RI 02940   401-249-0044
info@stevefund.org
stevefund.org
Tia Dole, Executive Director
Monica Ingkavet, Director, Programs & Partnerships
Anelle B. Primm, Senior Medical Director
The Steve Fund is dedicated to the mental health and emotional well-being of young people of color. It offers programs and services designed to assist both institutions of higher education and nonprofits in improving their capacity to support the mental health and emotional well-being of students of color. Programs and services include workshops, webinars, expert speakers, training, and technology innovations.

808 Therapeutic Touch International Association (TTIA)
TTIA Box 130
Delmar, NY 12054   518-325-1185
Fax: 509-693-3537
ttia@therapeutictouch.org
therapeutictouch.org
Mary Anne Hanley, President
Madonna Pence, Treasurer
Lin Bauer, Contact, Education
This international cooperative network of health care professionals is committed to excellence in healing through Therapeutic Touch. The organization serves as a resource for persons in the field of health care, laypersons, and other organizations interested in information on Therapeutic Touch, and for therapists and teachers searching for teaching and learning materials related to Therapeutic Touch.
1979

809　**Thresholds**
4101 N Ravenswood Ave.
Chicago, IL 60613　　　　　　　773-572-5500
thresholds@thresholds.org
www.thresholds.org
Mark Ishaug, Chief Executive Officer
Mark Furlong, Chief Operating Officer
Brent Peterson, Chief Development Officer
Provider of recovery services for persons with mental illnesses and substance abuse disorders in Illinois. It offers 30 programs at more than 75 locations throughout Chicago and surrounding suburbs and counties. Services include case management, housing, employment, education, psychiatry, primary care, substance use treatment, and research.

810　**United States Disabled Golf Association (USDGA)**
598 Dixie Rd.
Clinton, NC 28328　　　　　　910-214-5983
info@usdga.net
www.usdga.net
Jason Faircloth, Founder
The US Disabled Golf Association provides people with physical, sensory, and mental disabilities an opportunity to play golf at the highest level in the USA.
Founded in 2015. 1915

811　**United States Trager Association**
550M Richie Highway
Severna Park, MD 21146　　　　440-834-0308
Fax: 888-525-7645
exec@tragerus.org
www.tragerapproach.us
Offers sessions and courses on the Trager Approach, a gentle and effective approach to movement education and mind/body integration.

812　**Universal Pediatrics**
10654 Justin Dr.
Urbandale, IA 50322　　　　　800-383-0303
www.universalpediatrics.com
Tucker Anderson, Chief Executive Officer
Universal Pediatrics provides high-tech in-home medical care to children and young adults. Emphasis is placed on the provision of services in the rural areas, the ability to service high tech needs, and the promotion of primary nurse concept.
1985

813　**Upledger Institute International (UII)**
11211 Prosperity Farms Rd.
Suite D-325
Palm Beach Gardens, FL 33410　　561-622-4334
800-233-5880
Fax: 561-622-4771
upledger@upledger.com
www.upledger.com
Kathy Woll, Chief Operating Officer
Dawn Langnes Shear, Chief Development Officer
Alex Jozefyk, Chief Financial Officer
A healthcare resource center focused on comprehensive education programs, advanced treatment options, and outreach initiatives. The Institute has trained more than 125,000 healthcare professionals throughout the globe in the therapeutic approach.

814　**Viability**
60 Brookdale Dr.
Springfield, MA 01104　　　　413-781-5359
viability.org
Francis Fitzgerald, Chair
Jonathon Stephen "Steve" Dean, Vice Chair
Charlene Smolkowicz, Treasurer
Viability's mission is to help individuals with disabilities achieve their full potential. Services include day programs, employment services, and job training and placements.

815　**Volunteers of America (VOA)**
1660 Duke St.
Alexandria, VA 22314　　　　　703-341-5000
800-899-0089
info@voa.org
www.voa.org
Michael King, President & Chief Executive Officer
Joseph A. Budzynski, Executive Vice President & Chief Financial Officer
Jatrice Martel Gaiter, Executive Vice President, External Affairs
Volunteers of America is a nonprofit organization serving vulnerable groups, including veterans, at-risk youth, people with disabilities, homeless persons and families, and individuals recovering from addiction. Services include housing, behavioral and mental health services, and community outreach.

816　**WORLD**
389 30th St.
Oakland, CA 94609　　　　　　510-986-0340
Fax: 510-986-0341
mroberts@womenhiv.org
womenhiv.org
Women Organized to Respond to Life-threatening Disease supports women, girls, families and communities affected by HIV through education, wellness, advocacy, and leadership development.

817　**Waban Projects**
5 Dunaway Dr.
Sanford, ME 04073　　　　　　207-324-7955
Fax: 207-324-6050
connect@waban.org
www.waban.org
Jennifer Putnam, Executive Director
Gervaise Flynn, Deputy Director
Ashley Bjornson, Chief Financial Officer
Waban Projects is a nonprofit corporation working to create programs and services for individuals with autism and intellectual, developmental, and other disabilities.

818　**Women to Women Healthcare**
170 US Route 1
Suite 110
Falmouth, ME 04105　　　　　207-846-6163
800-540-5906
Fax: 207-846-6167
support@womentowomenhealthcarecenter.com
www.womentowomenhealthcarecente r.com
Marcelle Pick, Co-Founder & Director
Aims to combine alternative and conventional medicine in women's health. Provides integrative care for women and specializes in chronic and difficult cases.

819　**World Federation for Mental Health**
6800 Park Ten Blvd.
Suite 220-N
San Antonio, TX 78213　　　　info@wfmh.global
wfmh.global
Nasser Loza, President
Silvia Raggi, Corporate Secretary
Andrew Mohanraj, Treasurer
WFMH is an international membership organization that seeks to prevent mental and emotional disorders, advance the proper treatment and care of those with such disorders, and promote mental health.
1948

820　**World Institute on Disability (WID)**
3075 Adeline St.
Suite 155
Berkeley, CA 94703　　　　　510-225-6400
Fax: 510-225-0477
wid@wid.org
www.wid.org
Marcie Roth, Executive Director & Chief Executive Officer
Katherine Zigmont, Senior Director, Operations & Deputy Director
Reggie Johnson, Senior Director, Marketing & Communications
The mission of the World Institute on Disability (WID) is to eliminate barriers to full social integration and increase employment, economic security, and health care for persons with disabilities. WID creates innovative programs and tools; conducts research,

public education, training, and advocacy campaigns; and provides technical assistance.

821   YAI: National Institute for People with Disabilities
220 E 42nd St.
8th Floor
New York, NY 10017   212-273-6100
                                              communications@yai.org
                                                        www.yai.org

George Contos, Chief Executive Officer
Kevin Carey, Chief Financial Officer
Alek Hoyos, Chief of Staff

YAI is dedicated to enhancing the lives of people with developmental disabilities and their families. The organization works with individuals, families, government, corporate partners, donors, and foundations to ensure that people with disabilities are recognized for their abilities, achieve the goals that are important to them, and are integrated in the community.

822   Youth MOVE National
PO Box 215
Decorah, IA 52101   800-580-6199
                                                youthmovenational.org

Johanna Bergan, Executive Director
Kristin Thorp, Director, Youth Program
Victoria Eckert, Director, Operations

Aims to strengthen services and systems for issues such as mental health, juvenile justice, education, and child welfare.
Founded in 2007. 1907

823   Youth as Self Advocates (YASA)
Family Voices
110 Hartwell Ave.
Lexington, MA 02421   781-674-7224
                                                     888-835-5669
                                              bbaker@familyvoices.org
                                              www.familyvoices.org/yasa

Nora Wells, Executive Director, Family Voices

National program created by youth with disabilities for other youth, helping them to better advocate for themselves.

Camps

Alabama

824 Camp ASCCA
Alabama's Special Camp for Children and Adults
PO Box 21
5278 Camp Ascca Dr.
Jacksons Gap, AL 36861   256-825-9226
                                          Fax: 256-269-0714
                                          info@campascca.org
                                          www.campascca.org

Matt Rickman, Camp Director
John Stephenson, Administrator
Jocelyn Jones, Secretary
Camp Evoked Potential is held one week out of the year for children aged 6-18 with epilepsy at Camp ASCCA. Fully funded by The Epilepsy Foundation, persons wishing to attend the camp must apply. The camp provides a barrier free setting situated on 230 acres of wooded land at Lake Martin. The camp is staffed with medical personnel trained to care for children with all types of disabilities and provides a variety of camp activities.
1976

825 Camp Seale Harris
Southeastern Diabetes Education Services
500 Chase Park S.
Ste 104
Birmingham, AL 35244   205-402-0415
                                          Fax: 205-402-0416
                                          info@campsealeharris.org
                                          www.campsealeharris.org

Rhonda McDavid, Executive Director
John Latimer, Director, Camp & Community Programs
Shelby Harrison, Manager, Communications & Events
Offering overnight, family, day and community program camps, Camp Seale Harris is a nonprofit organization that offers residential camps for children and teens with diabetes. With multiple programs in Alabama, the volunteer camp counselors are trained adults living with diabetes, to better help the camp attendees gain independence in learning to manage their diabetes. Camp programs run all year round.
1949

826 Camp Shocco for the Deaf
216 North St. E
PO Box 602
Talladega, AL 35161   800-264-1225
Camp Shocco for the Deaf is a Christian Camp for children and teens with a hearing impairment, whose parents are deaf or are siblings of a person that are deaf. The camp runs for 1 week and offers a range of camp activities.

827 Camp Smile-A-Mile
Smile-A-Mile Place
1600 2nd Ave. S.
Birmingham, AL 35233   205-323-8427
                                          Fax: 205-323-6220
                                          info@campsam.org
                                          www.campsam.org

Bruce Hooper, Executive Director
Kellie Reece, Chief Operating Officer
Katie Langley, Special Events Director
Camp Smile-A-Mile offers 7 different educational camp opportunities for children and their families who have been affected by childhood cancer in Alabama. The programs run all year long, in a variety of formats.

828 Camp Smile-A-Mile: Jr./Sr. Camp
Smile-A-Mile Place
1600 2nd Ave. S.
Birmingham, AL 35233   205-323-8427
                                          Fax: 205-323-6220
                                          info@campsam.org
                                          www.campsam.org

Carrie Pomeroy, Program Director
Kellie Reece, Chief Operating Officer
Camp Smile-A-Mile's Jr./Sr. Camp is for high school juniors, seniors, and new high school graduates that are both on and off therapy. The weekend camp works to instill independence and responsibility in regards to their diagnosis.

829 Camp Smile-A-Mile: Off Therapy Family Camp
Smile-A-Mile Place
1600 2nd Ave. S.
Birmingham, AL 35233   205-323-8427
                                          Fax: 205-323-6220
                                          info@campsam.org
                                          www.campsam.org

Carrie Pomeroy, Program Director
Kellie Reece, Chief Operating Officer
Camp Smile-A-Mile's Off Therapy Family Camp is a specialized camp for off-therapy patients and their families. Campers up to the age of 18 who are no longer receiving therapy are eligible to attend the camp.

830 Camp Smile-A-Mile: On Therapy Family Camp
Smile-A-Mile Place
1600 2nd Ave. S.
Birmingham, AL 35233   205-323-8427
                                          Fax: 205-323-6220
                                          info@campsam.org
                                          www.campsam.org

Carrie Pomeroy, Program Director
Kellie Reece, Chief Operating Officer
A program of Camp Smile-A-Mile, On Therapy Family Camp is for patients up to 18 years of age, who are currently receiving therapy. The Family Camp is designed to give patients and their immediate families the opportunity to connect outside of an hospital environment.

831 Camp Smile-A-Mile: Sibling Camp
Smile-A-Mile Place
1600 2nd Ave. S.
Birmingham, AL 35233   205-323-8427
                                          Fax: 205-323-6220
                                          info@campsam.org
                                          www.campsam.org

Carrie Pomeroy, Program Director
Kellie Reece, Chief Operating Officer
Camp Smile-A-Mile's Sibling Camp is a specialized camp for the siblings of children and teens with cancer. Campers attending the Sibling Camp range in age from 6-18 and no patients or parents attend the camp.

832 Camp Smile-A-Mile: Teen Weeklong Camp
Smile-A-Mile Place
1600 2nd Ave. S.
Birmingham, AL 35233   205-323-8427
                                          Fax: 205-323-6220
                                          info@campsam.org
                                          www.campsam.org

Carrie Pomeroy, Program Director
Kellie Reece, Chief Operating Officer
A weeklong summer camp session for children, 13 through to the 10th grade, who have cancer. The session is open to those who are and aren't receiving therapy, with campers participating in activities such as swimming, snorkeling, and campfires.

833 Camp Smile-A-Mile: Young Adult Retreat
Smile-A-Mile Place
1600 2nd Ave. S.
Birmingham, AL 35233   205-323-8427
                                          Fax: 205-323-6220
                                          info@campsam.org
                                          www.campsam.org

Carrie Pomeroy, Program Director
Kellie Reece, Chief Operating Officer
A program of Camp Smile-A-Mile, the Young Adult Retreat is for childhood cancer survivors ages 19-30. The retreat is held over a summer weekend and offers educational and camping activities for participants. Those wanting to attend the retreat do not have to be former campers of Camp Smile-A-Mile.

834 **Camp Smile-A-Mile: Youth Weeklong Camp**
Smile-A-Mile Place
1600 2nd Ave. S.
Birmingham, AL 35233   205-323-8427
                              Fax: 205-323-6220
                              info@campsam.org
                              www.campsam.org

Carrie Pomeroy, Program Director
Kellie Reece, Chief Operating Officer
A weeklong summer camp session for children, ages 6-12, who have cancer. The session is open to those who are and aren't receiving therapy, with campers participating in activities such as arts and crafts, fishing, boating, archery, and canoeing.

835 **Camp WheezeAway**
YMCA Camp Chandler
880 South Lawrence Street
Montgomery, AL 36104   334-229-4362
                    jikner@ymcamontgomery.org
                    ymcamontgomery.org/camp/wheezeaway

Jennifer Ikner, Contact
For children ages 8-12 with moderate to severe asthma, Camp WheezeAway offers week long summer camp programs that foster confidence building skills. The camp is free and managed by medical professionals. Those with children wishing to attend must apply to the camp and complete a selection process.

836 **Easterseals Camp ASCCA**
PO Box 21
5278 Camp Ascca Dr.
Jacksons Gap, AL 36861   256-825-9226
                              Fax: 256-269-0714
                              info@campascca.org
                              www.campascca.org

Matt Rickman, Camp Director
John Stephenson, Administrator
Jocelyn Jones, Secretary
Easterseals Camp ASCCA is Alabama's Special Camp for Children and Adults, offering therapeutic recreation for children and adults with both physical and intellectual disabilities. The camp is located on 260 acres of barrier free woodland on Lake Martin and campers experience a wide variety of educational and recreational activities, including but not limited to: horseback riding, fishing, tubing, swimming, environmental education, arts, canoeing, and zip-lining. 1 week camp fees are $750.00.
1976

837 **Happy Camp**
Merrimack Hall Performing Arts Center
3320 Triana Blvd SW.
Huntsville, AL 35805   256-534-6455
                              info@merrimackhall.com
                    www.merrimackhall.com/happy-headquarters
For ages 3-12, Happy Camp is Merrimack Hall's annual half-day performing arts camp for children with special needs. Open to children with a wide range of physical or intellectual disabilities at any art level, activities include: music, theater, dance, and visual art. Happy Camp has a 1:1 staff-to-camper ratio. Camp time is from 9am - 12pm every day of the week.

838 **Rapahope Children's Retreat Foundation**
205 Lambert Ave.
Suite A
Mobile, AL 36604   251-476-9880
                              info@rapahope.org
                              www.rapahope.org

Melissa McNichol, Executive Director
Roz Dorsett, Assistant Director
Rapahope is an organization that offers a one week long summer camp for children who have, or who have had cancer. For children ages 7-17, the camp offers a wide range of summer camp activities, including but not limited to, swimming, kayaking, horseback riding, and arts. The camp is offered at no cost to campers or their families.

839 **Adam's Camp**
56 Inverness Drive East
Suite 250
Englewood, CO 80112   303-563-8290
                              contact@adamscamp.org
                              www.adamscampcolorado.org

Brian Conly, Executive Director
Paige Heydon, Director, Finance & Development
Adam's Camp is a nonprofit organization providing therapeutic programs and recreational camps for children and the families of children with special needs. Programs offered include Early Start Therapy Camp (6 months to 4 years old), Mountain Therapy Camps (ages 5 and up), and the Overnight Adventure Camps (ages 9 and up). Additional location offered in Northern Ireland.

840 **Camp Webber**
Alpine Alternatives
750 E. Fireweed Lane
Suite 101
Anchorage, AK 99507-1105   907-561-6655
                              Fax: 907-563-9232
                              admin@alpinealternatives.net
                              alpinealternatives.net
A program of Alpine Alternatives, Camp Webber is a developmental sports camp for children ages 8-19 who are blind or visually impaired. The camp provides 1-on-1 instructional education, with campers participating in physical activities such as swimming, goalball, beep baseball, tandem biking, tack and field events, rock climbing, hiking, canoeing, and archery.
1984

841 **Arizona Camp Sunrise & Sidekicks**
530 E. McDowell Road
Suite 107-295
Phoenix, AZ 85004   480-382-8564
                              info@swkcf.org
                              www.swkidscancerfoundation.org
Arizona Camp Sunrise & Sidekicks offers a variety of programs running all year long for children and their siblings who have had or currently have cancer. Arizona Camp Sunrise & Sidekicks, was the first camp in the state specifically tailored for children with cancer, and the camp is the only one in Arizona offering a camp for siblings affected by cancer through their Sidekicks program. Offered for children ages 8-18.

842 **Camp AZDA**
American Diabetes Association
2451 Crystal Drive
Suite 900
Phoenix, AZ 85014   800-342-2338
                              ampazda@diabetes.org
                              www.diabetes.org/node/1086
Camp AZDA is the Arizona summer camp program of the American Diabetes Association for children with diabetes. The camp is held at Friendly Pines in Prescott, Arizona with children participating in traditional camp activities while receiving educational information on managing their diabetes.

843 **Camp Abilities Tucson**
8987 East Tanque Verde Rd.
Suite 309-104
Tucson, AZ 85749   campabilitiestucson@gmail.com
                              www.campabilitiestucson.org

Murry Everson, Camp Director
Maria Lepore-Stevens, Camp Director
Camp Abilities is a privately funded educational sport camp for children and young adults who are blind, deaf-blind or have multiple disabilities including visual impairment. The camp offers sports instruction, with a 1:1 camper to coach ratio, tailored to fit the needs of the individual. The location of camp sessions is the Arizona School for the Deaf and Blind and costs $300.00 per person.

844 Camp Candlelight
Epilepsy Foundation Arizona
941 S Park Lane
Tempe, AZ 85281
602-282-3515
800-332-1000
AZ@EFA.org
epilepsyaz.org/events/campcandlelight
Suzanne Matsumori, Executive Director
Min Skivington, Program Manager
Camp Candlelight provides children ages 8 to 17 a unique camp experience that mixes traditional summer camp with special sessions that teach campers about their seizures and gives them resources to manage the challenges that the seizures represent. Staff inclues a neurologist, several nurses, and a school psychologist, in addition to traditional camp staff who are given specialized training in responding appropriately to the needs of kids with epilepsy.

845 Camp Civitan
Civitan Foundation, Inc.
12635 N. 42nd Street
Phoenix, AZ 85032
602-953-2944
info@campcivitan.org
www.civitanfoundationaz.com
Dawn Trapp, Executive Director
Camp Civitan offers week long summer camp programs, and weekend programs throughout the year, to children with developmental disabilities. The camp is fully wheelchair accessible, is staffed by medical professionals and there is a 2:1 ratio of campers to staff. Camp Civitan offers campers the experience of traditional camp activities including, swimming, adaptive sports, fishing, music, arts and crafts, and talent shows.
1968

846 Camp H.U.G.
Arizona Hemophilia Association
826 North 5th Ave
Phoenix, AZ 85003
602-955-3947
info@arizonahemophilia.org
www.arizonahemophilia.org/camp-programs
Leigh Goldstein, Executive Director
Vickie Parra, Programs & Conferences Manager
Jessica Jackson, Finance Manager
Camp H.U.G (Hemophilia Uniting Generations) is a weekend camp program of the Arizona Hemophilia Association. The camp is for families who have a member with hemophilia, WWD, and/or other bleeding disorders.

847 Camp Honor
Arizona Hemophilia Association
826 North 5th Ave
Phoenix, AZ 85003
602-955-3947
info@arizonahemophilia.org
www.arizonahemophilia.org/camp-programs
Leigh Goldstein, Executive Director
Vickie Parra, Programs & Conferences Manager
Jessica Jackson, Finance Manager
Camp Honor offers a week long summer camp to children affected by an inherited bleeding disorders. Camp Honor offers children the chance to partcipate in outdoor activities and educational opportunities.

848 Camp Not-A-Wheeze
2689 E Michelle Way
Gilbert, AZ 85234
602-336-6575
Fax: 602-336-6576
info@campnotawheeze.org
campnotawheeze.org
Alan Crawford, Camp Director
Week-long summer camp for children aged 7-14 with moderate to severe asthma living in Arizona. Campers attending Camp Not-A- Wheeze, participate in a wide range of activities such as, horseback riding, hiking, canoeing, and fishing as well as an asthma education class. Those wishing to attend must fill out and send in a camper application.

849 Camp Rainbow
Phoenix Childrens Hospital
1919 E Thomas Rd
Phoenix, AZ 85016
602-933-1000
888-908-5437
camprainbow@phoenixchildrens.com
www.phoenixchildrens.org
Emilie Jarboe, Camp Director
Camp Rainbow is for children aged 7-17 who have or had cancer or a chronic blood disorder. The camp is offered for one week during the summer, held at camp Friendly Pines in Prescott, Arizona. Campers must be patients of Phoenix Children's Hospital's Center for Cancer and Blood Disorders, with the camp offering participants the opportunity to experience traditional camp activities including but not limited to, horseback riding, canoeing, fishing, swimming, and archery.

850 Lions Camp Tatiyee
5283 W White Mountain Blvd
Lakeside, AZ 85929
480-380-4254
pam@camptatiyee.org
camptatiyee.org
Richard Page, President
Lions Camp Tatiyee is the only organization in Arizona providing a week long summer camp for individuals with special needs. There is no cost for the camp and all of the programs are adaptable. Some activities that campers can participate in are, go-karting, fishing, art, games, cooking, rock wall, swimming, dances and campfires.

851 Nick & Kelly Heart Camp
Nick & Kelly Children's Fund
1321 E Bayview Dr
Tempe, AZ 85283
480-838-1529
contact@nickandkellyfund.org
www.nkheartcamp.org
Nick & Kelly's Heart Camp is a free camp for children and teens ages 7-17 with congenital heart disease. The camp is held at Friendly Pines in Prescott, Arizona with campers participating in activities such as nature walks, water sports, arts and crafts, and recreational activities.

Arkansas

852 Camp Aldersgate
2000 Aldersgate Road
Little Rock, AR 72205
501-225-1444
Fax: 501-225-2019
hello@campaldersgate.net
www.campaldersgate.net
Sonya S. Murphy, Chief Executive Officer
Shelley Myers, Chief Operating Officer & Chief Financial Officer
Brooke Wilson, Director, Communications
Camp Aldersgate is a nonprofit organization, offering summer, weekend camps, and year-round social service programs to children, teens and adults with special needs. The camp promotes outdoor recreation and socialization in a completely accessible environment.

853 Camp Quality Arkansas
PO Box 7754
Little Rock, AR 72217
870-926-3324
arkansas@campqualityusa.org
www.campqualityusa.org/ar
Nick Hankins, Executive Director
Jordan Law, Assistant Director
Audrey Wilkins, Camper Coordinator
Camp Quality is an international camping program for children with cancer. The Arkansas Camp Quality is held at Camp Powderfork in Bald Knob, Arkansas and offers children and their siblings summer camps and year round camping opportunities. Volunteer doctors and nurses are at the camp 24 hours a day, and there is a 1:1 staff to camper ratio.

854 Camp Sunshine
Burn Program at Arkansas Children's
1 Children's Way
Slot 225
Little Rock, AR 72202   501-364-1635
                        wilkinsonge@archildrens.org
                www.archildrens.org/services/burn-program
Gretta Wilkinson, Camp Director
Camp Sunshine is a 4-day no-cost summer camp for children and
teens, 4-16, who have experienced burn injuries. Camp Sunshine
works to assist campers in the transformation from burn victim to
burn survivor. In order to attend the camp, campers must have survived a 10% or greater full thickness burn and/or may have significant scarring, disability or scarring to the hands or face.
1991

855 Kota Camp
Junior League Of Little Rock
401 South Scott Street
Little Rock, AR 72201   501-375-5557
                                info@jllr.org
                        www.jllr.org/community/kota-camp/
Maradyth McKenzie, President
Tabitha McNulty, President Elect
Jenna Martin, Treasurer
Kota Camp is offered to children aged 6-16 with disabilities or
medical conditions. Kota derived from a word used by the
Quapaw Native American Tribe indigenous to Arkansas, means
friend, and reflects the goals of the camp. Children with a disabil-
ity bring a sibling or friend without a disability, to create a envi-
ronment of inclusion, participate in camp activities, and promote
an understanding of those with special needs. The camp is held at
Camp Aldersgate in Little Rock.

California

856 Bearskin Meadow Camp
Diabetic Youth Families
5167 Clayton Rd
Suite F
Concord, CA 94521   925-680-4994
                                Fax: 925-680-4863
                                info@dyf.org
                                www.dyf.org
Davey Warner, Executive Director
Kaylor Glassman, Director, Programs
*Marissa Clarke-Howard, Director, Development & Communica-
tions*
Bearskin Meadow Camp, is a camp program offered by the Diabe-
tes Youth Families organization to children (7-13), teens (14-17),
and families who are affected by type 1 diabetes. The camp has
traditional camp activities as well as educational opportunities
for campers.

857 Camp Beyond The Scars
Burn Institute
8825 Aero Drive
Suite 200
San Diego, CA 92123-2269   858-541-2277
                                Fax: 858-541-7179
                        ccoppenrath@burninstitute.org
                www.burninstitute.org/camp-beyond-the-scar s
Susan Day, Executive Director
Tessa Haviland, Director, Marketing & Events
Benjamin Hemmings, Director, Operations
Camp Beyond the Scars, is a weeklong sleepaway summer camp
for children aged 8-17 who have survived a burn injury. Staffed
by adult burn survivors, healthcare professionals, and off-duty
firefighters, the camp provides an inclusive environment for burn
survivors to participate in activities including, swimming, basketball, volleyball, archery, golf, and arts and crafts. The camp is
free of charge, and is hosted at a camp facility in Romano,
California.
1987

858 Camp Bloomfield
Wayfinder Family Services
5300 Angeles Vista Blvd.
Los Angeles, CA 90043   323-295-4555
                                800-352-4555
                                Fax: 323-296-0424
                                www.wayfinderfamily.org
Miki Jordan, Chief Executive Officer
Jay Allen, President & Chief Operating Officer
Fernando Almodovar, Chief Financial Officer
Camp Bloomfield is a summer camp with week long sessions for
children and youth who are blind, visually impaired or multi-disabled. The 45 acre campground offers campers a variety of activities, specifically designed to meet the needs of the children, with
campers attending at no cost.

859 Camp Christian Berets
2508 Oakdale Rd.
Suite 10
Modesto, CA 95355   209-524-7993
                                Fax: 209-524-7979
                                www.christianberets.org
Kevin Van Donselaar, Executive Director
Mark Burns, Chairperson
Kelly Luth, Treasurer
Camp for children, students and adults with special needs.

860 Camp Conrad Chinnock
Diabetes Camping And Educational Services, Inc.
2400 E. Katella Ave.
Suite 800
Anaheim, CA 92806   844-744-2267
                                Fax: 909-752-5354
                        info@diabetescamping.org
                        www.diabetescamping.org
Rocky Wilson, Executive Director
Ryan Martz, Development & Program Director
Dale Lissy, Camp Manager
Camp Conrad Chinnock offers year round recreational, social,
and educational opportunities for children and families with type
1 diabetes.

861 Camp Grizzly
NorCal Services For Deaf & Hard Of Hearing
4044 N Freeway Blvd.
Sacramento, CA 95843   916-349-7500
                                Fax: 916-349-7578
                                TTY: 916-349-7500
                        campgrizzly@norcalcenter.org
                        www.campgrizzly.org
Molly Bowen, Program Leader
Cheryl Bella, Program Leader
A program of NorCal Services for Deaf & Hard of Hearing, Camp
Grizzly is a coed camp for children aged 7-18 who have a hearing
impairment. Camp Grizzly takes place at the Camp Lodestar
campground facilities and offers sporting activities, performing
and creative arts, hiking, swimming, playgrounds and campfires.

862 Camp Hollywood HEART
One Heartland
26001 Heinz Rd.
Willow River, MN 55795   888-216-2028
                        helpkids@oneheartland.org
                        www.oneheartland.org
Patrick Kindler, Executive Director
Katie Donlin, Operations Manager
Kadien Bartels-Merkel, Program Director
A program of One Heartland, a nonprofit organization working to
provide camping programs for children with serious illnesses or
experiencing social isolation. Camp Hollywood HEART is a
weeklong summer camp for youths, ages 15-20, who are infected
or affected by HIV/AIDS. The camp is held in Malibu, California
and is partnership camp between One Heartland and Hollywood
Heart.

863   Camp Kindle
Project Kindle
27203 Golden Willow Way
Santa Clarita, CA 91387   877-800-2267
                                     eva@projectkindle.org
                                     www.projectkindle.org
Eva Payne, Founder & Chief Executive Officer
Mandy Nickolite, Vice President
Camp Kindle provides year-round cost free recreational, educational and support services for children with special needs and life challenges.
1998

864   Camp Krem
Camping Unlimited
102 Brook Lane
Boulder Creek, CA 95006   831-338-3210
                                     campkrem@campingunlimited.org
                                     campingunlimited.org
Christina Krem DiGirolamo, Camp Director
Leon Wong, Head of Camper Services
Kristen Carter, Virtual Program Coordinator
Camp Krem - Camping Unlimited offers year-round and summer camping programs for children and adults with developmental disabilities. With a variety of different programs and many facilities on the campground such as a swimming pool, arts and crafts building, amphitheater, music pavilion, and archery range, Camp Krem provides its campers with recreation, education, and adventure opportunities.

865   Camp No Limits California
No Limits Foundation
700 S Wren Dr.
Big Bear Lake, CA 92315   207-569-6411
                                     Fax: 877-406-5106
                                     campnolimits@gmail.com
                                     www.nolimitsfoundation.org
Mary Leighton, Founder & Executive Director
Kelsey Moody, Program Operations Manager
Alix Sandler, Marketing & Development Director
Camp No Limits California, a location of Camp No Limits, is a recreational and educational camp for youth who have experienced limb loss. Camp No Limits, is a program of the nonprofit organization No Limits Foundation. The California camp is held in Big Bear where campers have access to ropes courses, zip lines, and a swimming pool.

866   Camp Okizu
Okizu Foundation
83 Hamilton Dr.
Suite 200
Novato, CA 94949-5755   415-382-9083
                                     Fax: 415-382-8384
                                     info@okizu.org
                                     www.okizu.org
Suzie Randall, Executive Director
Heather Ferrier, Director, Family Services
Sarah Uldricks, Director, Marketing & Special Events
Camp Okizu offers a variety of medically supervised, residential camp programs for families who have a child diagnosed with cancer. Programs are offered throughout the year free of charge.

867   Camp Okizu: Family Camp
Okizu Foundation
83 Hamilton Dr.
Suite 200
Novato, CA 94949-5755   415-382-9083
                                     Fax: 415-382-8384
                                     enrollment@okizu.org
                                     www.okizu.org
Suzie Randall, Executive Director
Heather Ferrier, Director, Family Services
Sarah Uldricks, Director, Marketing & Special Events
Camp Okizu's Family Camp is no-cost camp designed for the families of children, and children who have been diagnosed with cancer. The Family Camp is offered as a weekend program, running on multiple weekends from April to September.

868   Camp Okizu: Oncology Camp
Okizu Foundation
83 Hamilton Dr.
Suite 200
Novato, CA 94949-5755   415-382-9083
                                     Fax: 415-382-8384
                                     enrollment@okizu.org
                                     www.okizu.org
Suzie Randall, Executive Director
Heather Ferrier, Director, Family Services
Sarah Uldricks, Director, Marketing & Special Events
A program of Camp Okizu, the Oncology Camp is for children and teens, ages 6-17, who have or have had cancer. The camp is a residential summer camp program and is staffed by pediatric oncology departments from the participating hospitals.

869   Camp Okizu: SIBS Camp
Okizu Foundation
83 Hamilton Dr.
Suite 200
Novato, CA 94949-5755   415-382-9083
                                     Fax: 415-382-8384
                                     enrollment@okizu.org
                                     www.okizu.org
Suzie Randall, Executive Director
Heather Ferrier, Director, Family Services
Sarah Uldricks, Director, Marketing & Special Events
SIBS (Special and Important Brothers and Sisters) Camp is for the sibling or siblings, ages 6-17, of a child who has, has had, or has died from cancer. The camp is a no-charge, residential summer program, that provides campers the opportunity to learn new skills and get support from others who have experienced having a sibling with cancer.

870   Camp Okizu: Teens-N-Twenties Camp
Okizu Foundation
83 Hamilton Dr.
Suite 200
Novato, CA 94949-5755   415-382-9083
                                     Fax: 415-382-8384
                                     enrollment@okizu.org
                                     www.okizu.org
Suzie Randall, Executive Director
Heather Ferrier, Director, Family Services
Sarah Uldricks, Director, Marketing & Special Events
Camp Okizu: Teens-N- Twenties Camp is a weekend recreation and support program that is offered 4 times a year for pediatric oncology patients and their siblings ages 18-25.

871   Camp Pacifica
California Lions Camp
1836 K Street
Merced, CA 95340-4818   559-373-0961
                                     deafcamppacifica@gmail.com
                                     camp-pacifica.org
Angelica Martinez, Camp Director
John Martinez, Assistant Director
Camp Pacifica provides a summer camp experience for children, boys and girls, aged 7-15 who have a hearing impairment. The camp is located in the foothills of Sierra on 52 acres of forested woodland. Activities include, but are not limited to, archery, canoeing, ropes course, swimming, horseback riding, and riflery. The camp costs $360, plus a registration fee.
1978

872   Camp Paivika
Ability First
PO Box 3367
Crestline, CA 92325   909-338-1102
                                     Fax: 909-338-2502
                                     camppaivika@abilityfirst.org
                                     www.abilityfirst.org/camp-paivika
Kelly Kunsek, Camp Director
Lauren Wilson, Program Director
Tina Ronning-Fraynd, Coordinator, Camper Services
As a program of AbilityFirst, Camp Paivika offers overnight summer programs for children, teens and adults with developmental and physical disabilities. The camp is completely accessible and the staff is trained to provide any assistance or personal care a camper needs. Located in San Bernardino National Forest, Camp

Paivika provides a traditional summer camp experience in a safe and fun environment.
1947

873   Camp ReCreation
9272 Madison Ave.
Orangeville, CA 95662   916-988-6835
                                        camprecreation@outlook.com
                                              www.camprecreation.org
Kathi Barber, Camp Director
Camp ReCreation offers residential summer camps and year round programs for children, teens, and adults with developmental disabilities. The summer camp is held at Camp Ronald McDonald in Lassen National Forest. With a 1:1 staff to camper ratio, Camp ReCreation offers wide variety of camp activities, and campers wishing to participate must fill out a camper application.
1983

874   Camp Reach for the Sky
The Seany Foundation
3530 Camino del Rio N
Suite 101
San Diego, CA 92108   858-551-0922
                                              www.theseanyfoundation.org
Amy Robins, Co-Founder, The Seany Foundation
Paula Lutzky, Chief Financial Officer
Emily Brody, Director, Marketing & Media
Previously run by the American Cancer Society, Camp Reach for the Sky (CR4TS) is now run by The Seany Foundation and provides an opportunity for children with cancer and their siblings to attend a free summer camp. Camp Reach for the Sky offers a multiple programs, including a Resident Oncology Camp, a Sibling Camp and Day Camps.

875   Camp Ronald McDonald at Eagle Lake
2555 49th Street
Sacramento, CA 95817   916-734-4230
                                            Fax: 916-734-4238
                                              info@rmhcnc.org
                                              www.campronald.org
Catherine Ithurburn, Chief Executive Officer
Pip Pipkins, Camp Manager
Camp Ronald McDonald at Eagle Lake collaborates with other nonprofit organizations to provide week long summer camp opportunities for children with special medical needs, financial hardship and/or emotional, developmental or physical disabilities. The camp is fully accessible.

876   Camp Ronald McDonald for Good Times
4560 Fountain Avenue
Los Angeles, CA 90029   323-666-6400
                                            Fax: 626-744-9969
                                              www.campronaldmcdonald.org
Erica Mangham, Executive Director
Brian Crater, Associate Executive Director
Chad Edwards, Program Director
Free year-round residential camping for children with cancer and their families.

877   Camp Sunburst
Sunburst Projects United States Headquarters
2143 Hurley Way
Suite 240
Sacramento, CA 95825   916-440-0889
                                            Fax: 916-440-1208
                                        admin@sunburstprojects.org
                                              www.sunburstprojects.org
Jacob Bradley-Rowe, Executive Director
Camp Sunburst is a youth oriented leadership camp that promotes and creates an environment to help youth learn self confidence to change negative social patterns and break cycles of HIV/AIDS infections. Activities campers will participate in include, boating, swimming, art, dance, and sports.

878   Camp Sunshine Dreams
PO Box 28232
Fresno, CA 93729-8232   stephanie@campsunshinedreams.org
                                              www.campsunshinedreams.org
Stephanie Scharbach, Contact
Pam Aiello, Contact

Camp Sunshine Dreams provides a summer camp experience to children aged 8-15 with cancer and their siblings.

879   Camp Taylor
Camp Taylor, Inc.
8224 West Grayson Rd.
Modesto, CA 95358-9094   209-545-3853
                                        camp@kidsheartcamp.org
                                              www.kidsheartcamp.org
Kimberlie Gamino, Founder & Executive Director
With several programs, Camp Taylor provides youth, teens, and the families of children with heart disease the opportunity to go to a free medically supervised summer sleepaway camp. Campers are able to enjoy activities such as, swimming, snorkeling, horseback riding, rock-wall, skits, archery, and heart education.
Founded in 2002. 2002

880   Camp Taylor: Family Camp
Camp Taylor, Inc.
8224 West Grayson Rd.
Modesto, CA 95358-9094   209-545-3853
                                        camp@kidsheartcamp.org
                                              www.kidsheartcamp.org/familycampca
Kimberlie Gamino, Founder & Executive Director
A program of Camp Taylor, Family Camp is for children of all ages, with congenital heart disease and/or acquired heart disease, and their family including parents and siblings. The camp offers parental heart education and support programs for parents and siblings. Family Camp is geared towards children too young to attend Youth or Teen Camp, or those who are not ready to attend a residential camp.

881   Camp Taylor: Leadership Camp
Camp Taylor, Inc.
8224 West Grayson Rd.
Modesto, CA 95358-9094   209-545-3853
                                        camp@kidsheartcamp.org
                                              www.kidsheartcamp.org/leadershipcamp
Kimberlie Gamino, Founder & Executive Director
Leadership Camp is for teens and youth, ages 16-21, who have previously attended a Camp Taylor California camp program, wishing to be camp mentor for youth, teen, and family camps. Campers wishing to attend this camp should make it known to either a camp counselor or camp director.

882   Camp Taylor: Teen Camp
Camp Taylor, Inc.
8224 West Grayson Rd.
Modesto, CA 95358-9094   209-545-3853
                                        camp@kidsheartcamp.org
                                              www.kidsheartcamp.org/teencamp
Kimberlie Gamino, Founder & Executive Director
The Teen Camp program at Camp Taylor is for teens ages 13-17, with congenital heart disease and/or acquired heart disease. Campers participate in heart education and traditional camp activities. Campers wishing to attend the camp must apply, with campers being accepted on a first come basis.

883   Camp Taylor: Young Adult Program
Camp Taylor, Inc.
8224 West Grayson Rd.
Modesto, CA 95358-9094   209-545-3853
                                        camp@kidsheartcamp.org
                                              www.kidsheartcamp.org/leadershipcamp
Kimberlie Gamino, Founder & Executive Director
The Young Adult Program at Camp Taylor is designed for previous heart campers ages 18-35 with congenital heart disease. The program works to provide support, education, and the opportunities to participate in social events in order to help with the transition to adulthood.

884   Camp Taylor: Youth Camp
Camp Taylor, Inc.
8224 West Grayson Rd.
Modesto, CA 95358-9094   209-545-3853
                                        camp@kidsheartcamp.org
                                              www.kidsheartcamp.org/youthcamp
Kimberlie Gamino, Founder & Executive Director
A program of Camp Taylor, Youth Camp is designed for children, ages 7-12, with congenital heart disease and/or acquired heart disease. Campers participate in heart education and traditional

camp activities. Campers wishing to attend the camp must apply, with campers being accepted on a first come basis.

885 Camp Tuolumne Trails
22988 Ferretti Road
Groveland, CA 95321   209-962-7534
                                        info@tuolumnetrails.org
                                        www.tuolumnetrails.org
Jacqui Montero, Director of Camper Operations
Tuolumne Trails is a camp for individuals with special medical needs. With week-long summer camp options, Camp Tuolumne Trails is a completely accessible camp, with a 3:1 staff to camper ratio, that allows campers to participate in camping activities in a safe environment. Campers wishing to attend must complete the application and session assignment process.
Founded in 2002. 2002

886 Camp del Corazon
11615 Hesby St
North Hollywood, CA 91601-3620   818-754-0312
                                        Fax: 818-754-0377
                                        info@campdelcorazon.org
                                        www.campdelcorazon.org
Kevin Shannon, President & Medical Director
Chrissie Endler, Executive Director
Kristina Caberto Wallace, Director of Development & Operations
Camp del Corazon is a nonprofit corporation offering a no cost summer camp and other programs to children aged 7-17 living with heart disease. Campers or their guardians must fill out a camp application, with acceptance into the camp dependant upon a nurse review of the parent and cardiology portions of the application.
1995

887 Camp-A-Lot and Camp-A-Little
The Arc of San Diego
3030 Market Street
San Diego, CA 92102   619-685-1175
                                        Fax: 619-234-3759
                                        info@arc-sd.com
                                        www.arc-sd.com
Anthony J. DeSalis, President & Chief Executive Officer
Programs of The Arc of San Diego, Camp - A - Lot (ages 18 and up) and Camp - A - Little (ages 5-17) offer recreational summer camp opportunities for individuals with physical and developmental disabilities.

888 Coelho Epilepsy Youth Summer Camp
Epilepsy Foundation Of Northern California
909 Marina Village Pkwy
Suite 239
Alameda, CA 94501   510-922-8687
                                        800-632-3532
                                        Fax: 510-922-8659
                                        efnca@epilepsynorcal.org
                                        www.epilepsynorcal.org
Carlos Quesada, Chief Executive Officer
Miriam Swanson, Programs Manager
Kimberly Bari, Programs Ambassador
Offered to children aged 9-17, Coelho Epilepsy Youth Summer Camp provides a week-long sleepaway camp for children with epilepsy. Staffed by medical professional throughout the entire week, campers participate in traditional camp activities. Parents or guardians must fill out an application for a camper.

889 Dream Street
Dream Street Foundation
324 S. Beverly Dr.
Suite 500
Beverly Hills, CA 90212   424-333-1371
                                        Fax: 310-388-0302
                                        www.dreamstreetfoundation.org
Patty Grubman, Founder
Run by The Dream Street Foundation, Dream Street Camps provide camping programs for children (aged 4-14) and young adults (18-24) with chronic and life threatening illnesses. The kids program runs in California, with the young adults program running in Arizona. The programs are free of charge, and campers can participate in different activities such as, swimming, arts and crafts, sports, horseback riding, and archery.

890 Easterseals Camp
Easterseals Southern California
1063 McGaw Avenue
Suite 100
Irvine, CA 92614   951-264-4855
                                        amanda.showalter@essc.org
                                        www.easterseals.com/southerncal
Mark Whitley, President & Chief Executive Officer
Easterseals Camp is a week long summer camp for children and adults with disabilities. Held at Camp Oakes in the San Bernardino Mountains. Campers participate in activities including, crafts, hayrides, talent shows, dances, swimming, canoeing, archery, hiking, and rope courses. There is a 1:2 counselor to camper ratio. The cost of the camp is $1,248 per camper.

891 Easterseals Camp Harmon
16403 Highway 9
Boulder Creek, CA 95006   831-338-3383
                                        campharmon@es-cc.org
                                        www.campharmon.org
Jeff Terpstra, Chair
Robert Guerin, Vice Chair
Greg Jensen, Secretary
Camp Harmon, the Easterseals Central California camp, offers residential summer camps programs to individuals ages 8-65 with disabilities. Each session at Camp Harmon is designed for a specific age group and offers campers the opportunity to experience traditional summer camp activities. There is a 3:1 counsellor to camper ratio, with camp fees are based on $140.00 a day base.

892 Enchanted Hills Camp for the Blind
Lighthouse for the Blind
1155 Market St.
10th Floor
San Francisco, CA 94103   415-431-1481
                                        Fax: 415-863-7568
                                        info@lighthouse-sf.org
                                        www.lighthouse-sf.org
W. Brandon Cox, Chief Operating Officer
Michelle Knapik, Chief Financial Officer
Enchanted Hills Camp for the Blind is located on 311 acres of land on Mt. Veeder, offering programs for children, teens, adults, deaf-blind, seniors, and families of the blind. The camp gives campers the experience of traditional summer camp but is adapted to meet the needs of the campers.

893 Firefighters Kids Camp
Firefighters Burn Institute
3101 Stockton Blvd.
Sacramento, CA 95820   916-739-8525
                                        valorie@ffburn.org
                                        www.ffburn.org
Valorie Smart, Camp Contact
Joe Pick, Executive Director
Rachel Crowell, Assistant Director
Firefighters Kids Camp is a program run by the Firefighters Burn Institute for children ages 6-17, who are survivors of burns. With activities such as rocking climbing, bicycling, hiking, kayaking, swimming, and arts and crafts, the ratio of staff to campers is 3:1, with on site 24/7 nurse and physical therapist ensuring a safe and fun environment.

894 Lions Wilderness Camp for Deaf Children, Inc.
Lions Wilderness Camp Headquarters
PO Box 8
Roseville, CA 95661-9998   lionscampfordeaf@gmail.com
                                        www.lionswildcamp.org
David Velasquez, Camp Program Director
Lions Wilderness Camp gives deaf children aged 7-15 an outdoor camp experience helping children to learn outdoor skills and enjoy nature.

895 Little Heroes Family Burn Camp
Firefighters Burn Institute
3101 Stockton Blvd.
Sacramento, CA 95820   916-739-8525
                                        www.ffburn.org
Valorie Smart, Camp Contact
Joe Pick, Executive Director
Rachel Crowell, Assistant Director

Little Heroes Preschool Burn Camp is a burn recovery program run by the Firefighters Burn Institute. The camp is for children ages 1-6, who are survivors of burns, and their families. The program runs for 3 days, providing support and education for those attending.

896   New Horizons Summer Day Camp
YMCA of Orange County
13821 Newport Ave.
Suite 150
Tustin, CA 92780   714-508-7616
                                    newhorizons@ymcaoc.org
                                    www.ymcaoc.org/new-horizons
Jeff McBride, Chief Executive Officer
New Horizons is a program by the YMCA offering day camps for adults with developmental disabilities. Outings in the community are supervised and create an environment that fosters social interaction, skill building, and friendship.

897   Quest Camp
907 San Ramon Valley Blvd.
Suite 202
Danville, CA 94526   925-743-2900
                                    800-313-9733
                                    Fax: 925-743-1937
                                    www.questcamps.com
Robert B. Field, PhD., Founder & Executive Director
Debra Forrester-Field, MA, Administrative Director
Aprilyn Artz, MA, Clinical Director
Quest Camps are designed using the Quest Camp Therapeutic System developed specifically to help and reduce a campers psychological disability. With locations in San Francisco East Bay, California, Huntington Beach, California, and Pittsburgh, Pennsylvania, camps have a 6:1 camper to staff ratio, with campers receiving sport instruction and participate in physical activity, arts, and games.
1989

898   Special Camp For Special Kids
31641 La Novia Ave
San Juan Capistrano, CA 92675   949-661-0108
                                    Fax: 949-661-8637
                                    lindsay.eres@smes.org
                                    www.specialcamp.org
Lindsay Eres, Executive Director
Katie McCombs, Associate Program Director
Katie Schwartz, Assistant Director
For youths with disabilities, Special Camps for Special Kids, offers day camps with a 1:1 volunteer counselor to camper.

899   The Painted Turtle
1300 4th Street
Suite 300
Santa Monica, CA 90401   310-451-1353
                                    866-451-5367
                                    Fax: 310-451-1357
                                    info@thepaintedturtle.org
                                    www.thepaintedturtle.org
Page Adler, Chairman of the Board & Co-Founder
Lou Adler, Producer & Co-Founder
The Painted Turtle provides year round camp programs for children, siblings, and families with children who have chronic and life threatening illnesses. The camp is located in Lake Hughes, California.

Colorado

900   Adam's Camp: Colorado
Adam's Camp
1101 County Road 53
Granby, CO 80446   303-563-8290
                                    Fax: 303-563-8291
                                    Contact@AdamsCamp.org
                                    www.adamscampcolorado.org
Brian Conly, Executive Director
Paige Heydon, Director, Finance & Development
Adam's Camp is a nonprofit organization providing therapeutic programs and recreational camps for children and the families of children with special needs. The Colorado location of Adam's

Camp, offers both therapy and adventure camps. The adventure camp is held at the YMCA - Snow Mountain Ranch in Granby, Colorado.

901   Aspen Camp
4862 Snowmass Creek Rd.
Snowmass, CO 81654   970-315-0513
                                    TTY: 970-315-0513
                                    hi@aspencamp.org
                                    www.aspencamp.org
Karen Immerson, Vice President
Eric Kaika, Treasurer
Open to the deaf community, including family members and friends as well as those who are deaf, deaf blind, hard of hearing, and late deafened, Camp Aspen provides year round programs for youth and adults.

902   Breckenridge Outdoor Education Center
PO Box 697
Breckenridge, CO 80424   970-453-6422
                                    800-383-2632
                                    Fax: 970-453-4676
                                    boec@boec.org
                                    www.boec.org
Sonya Norris, Executive Director
Karen Skruch, Finance Director
Jeff Inouye, Ski Program Director
Breckenridge Outdoor Education Center (BOEC) provides year round educational outdoor experiences to individuals with physical and intellectual disabilities. Some programs BOEC offer include, Adaptive Ski and Ride School, Wilderness Programs and adaptive programs for individuals with brain injuries, multiple sclerosis, and Parkinson's Disease.
1976

903   Camp Rocky Mountain Village
Easterseals Colorado
393 S. Harlan St.
Suite 250
Lakewood, CO 80226   303-233-1666
                                    Fax: 303-569-3857
                                    campinfo@easterealscolorado.org
                                    www.easterseals.com/co
Roman Krafczyk, President & Chief Executive Officer
Krasimir Koev, Chief Operating Officer
Kerry Erdahl, Chief Financial Officer
A program of Easterseals Colorado, Rocky Mountain Village in Empire Colorado is a fully accessible camp, with summer camps sessions for children and adults with disabilities. Activities include but are not limited to swimming, fishing, overnight camping, outdoor cooking, arts and crafts, and a zip line.

904   Camp Wapiyapi
191 University Blvd.
PO Box 294
Denver, CO 80206   303-534-0883
                                    Fax: 303-534-0874
                                    Wapiyapi@wapiyapi.org
                                    www.campwapiyapi.org
Darla Dakin, Chief Executive Officer
Megan Blanc, Summer Camp Director
Camp Wapiyapi is a nonprofit organization that fosters friendships, fun and healing outside of the hospital for families facing childhood cancer through a camp experience. For patients ages 6-17. Full-time onsite volunteer medical staff available 24/7.

905   Challenge Aspen
PO Box 6639
Snowmass Village, CO 81615   970-923-0578
                                    Fax: 970-923-7338
                                    info@challengeaspen.org
                                    www.challengeaspen.org
Lindsay Cagley, Chief Executive Officer
Anne Adams, Chief Operating Officer
Jenni Petersen, Chief Financial Officer
Challenge Aspen provides recreational, cultural experiences and summer camps for individuals who have cognitive or physical challenges. Programs are tailored to fit a diversity of needs and interests.
1995

906   Children's Hospital Burn Camps Program
13123 E 16th Ave.
PO Box 580
Aurora, CO 80045   720-777-8295
                                                 Fax: 720-777-7270
                               learnmore@noordinarycamps.org
                                      www.noordinarycamps.org
Trudy Boulter, Camp Director
Tim Schuetz, Outreach Coordinator
The Children's Hospital Colorado Burn Camps Program provides
rehabilitation and reintegration opportunities for children, teens,
adults, and families who have been affected by burn injuries. The
Camps Program has partnerships with 7 hospitals across the
United States and offers year-round programs.

**907   Children's Hospital Burn Camps Program: England
Exchange Program Burn Camp**
13123 E 16th Ave.
PO Box 580
Aurora, CO 80045   720-777-8295
                                                 Fax: 720-777-7270
                               learnmore@noordinarycamps.org
                                      www.noordinarycamps.org
Trudy Boulter, Camp Director
Tim Schuetz, Outreach Coordinator
An international exchange program for campers, ages 13-15, be-
tween the Children's Hospital Burn Camps Program and The
Manchester Children's Hospital Burns Camp in England. Camp-
ers are able to explore a new culture, food, and climate. The camp
is located in the Lake District.

**908   Children's Hospital Burn Camps Program: Family Burn
Camp**
13123 E 16th Ave.
PO Box 580
Aurora, CO 80045   720-777-8295
                                                 Fax: 720-777-7270
                               learnmore@noordinarycamps.org
                                      www.noordinarycamps.org
Trudy Boulter, Camp Director
Tim Schuetz, Outreach Coordinator
The Family Burn Camp is for families who have been affected by
a burn injury. The camp is designed to give families the opportu-
nity to interact and connect with other families who have had a
similar experiences.

**909   Children's Hospital Burn Camps Program: Summer
Burn Camp**
13123 E 16th Ave.
PO Box 580
Aurora, CO 80045   720-777-8295
                                                 Fax: 720-777-7270
                               learnmore@noordinarycamps.org
                                      www.noordinarycamps.org
Trudy Boulter, Camp Director
Tim Schuetz, Outreach Coordinator
The Summer Burn Camp is part of the Children's Hospital Colo-
rado Burn Camps Program, and offers a weeklong summer camp
for children and teens, ages 8-18 who have been affected by burn
injuries. The camp is held in Estes Park in partnership with
Cheley Colorado Camps, and activities include, hiking, mountain
biking, challenge courses, horseback riding, mountain climbing,
fishing, archery, crafts, riflery, and swimming.

**910   Children's Hospital Burn Camps Program: Winter Burn
Camp**
13123 E 16th Ave.
PO Box 580
Aurora, CO 80045   720-777-8295
                                                 Fax: 720-777-7270
                               learnmore@noordinarycamps.org
                                      www.noordinarycamps.org
Trudy Boulter, Camp Director
Tim Schuetz, Outreach Coordinator
The Winter Burn Camp is for older campers, ages 13-18, who
have previously attended the Cheley Children's Hospital Colo-
rado Summer Burn Camp. Held in Steamboat Springs, Colorado
at the Steamboat Grand Lodge campers participate in a week of
skiing and/or snowboarding.

**911   Children's Hospital Burn Camps Program: Young Adult
Retreat**
13123 E 16th Ave.
PO Box 580
Aurora, CO 80045   720-777-8295
                                                 Fax: 720-777-7270
                               learnmore@noordinarycamps.org
                                      www.noordinarycamps.org
Trudy Boulter, Camp Director
Tim Schuetz, Outreach Coordinator
A program of the Children's Hospital Colorado Burn Camps Pro-
gram, the Young Adult Retreat is designed to address the specific
issues facing burn survivors ages 18-25. The retreat offers a variety of recreational and workshop opportunities working to address the topics of relationships, body image, and goal setting.

**912   City of Lakewood Recreation and Inclusion Services for
Everyone (R.I.S.E.)**
City Of Lakewood
480 S Allison Pkwy
Lakewood, CO 80226   303-987-4867
                                              TTY: 303-987-7057
                                            rise@lakewood.org
                                        www.lakewood.org/rise
The Recreation and Inclusion Services for Everyone (R.I.S.E.) of
Lakewood is a therapeutic recreation program for individuals
with disabilities, age 6 through senior adult. Some programs offered by R.I.S.E include field trips, social dances, sports and
camping.

913   Cochlear Implant Camp
Listen Foundation
6950 E Belleview Ave.
Suite 203
Greenwood Village, CO 80111   303-781-9440
                                   cochlearimplantcamp@gmail.com
                                www.listenfoundation.org/cicamp
Janette Cantwell, Camp Director
Held at the YMCA Rockies Estes Park Center, the camp offers a
wide range of activities for children from 3-17 years old with cochlear implants. The camp is held during the summer and also offers programs for parents and families. The cost is $800 for a
family of four.

914   Colorado Lions Camp
28541 Hwy 67 N
PO Box 9043
Woodland Park, CO 80863   719-687-2087
                                                 Fax: 719-687-7435
                                   coloradolionscamp@msn.com
                                     www.coloradolionscamp.org
Erin Newport, Camp Director
Brenna Bonnelycke, Executive Assistant
Colorado Lions Camp offers summer camp and weekend respite
programs for individuals aged 8 and up with special needs. The
camp is designed to promote independence and provide an opportunity for campers to discover their potential in a safe
environment.

915   First Descents
3827 Lafayette St.
Suite 161
Denver, CO 80205   303-945-2490
                                                 Fax: 866-592-6911
                                          info@firstdescents.org
                                        www.firstdescents.org
Brad Ludden, Founder
Debbie King-Ford, Chairperson
Michael Kantor, Treasurer
First Descents offers free outdoor adventure programs for young
adults ages 18-39 who have, or who have had cancer. Activities
include climbing, paddling and surfing, all offered in a safe
environment.

916   Roundup River Ranch
8333 Colorado River Rd.
Gypsum, CO 81637   970-524-2267
                                        Fax: 888-524-2477
                                   info@roundupriverranch.org
                                   www.roundupriverranch.org
Ruth B. Johnson, President & Chief Executive Officer
Sterling Nell Leija, Director of Operations
Kendra Perkins, Camp Director
Roundup River Ranch provides traditional camp experiences for
children and their families with chronic and serious illnesses. The
Ranch is located in Gypsum, Colorado, with all programs offered
free of charge.

Connecticut

917   Arthur C. Luf Children's Burn Camp
Connecticut Burns Care Foundation
601 Boston Post Rd.
Milford, CT 06460   203-878-6744
                                        Fax: 203-878-4044
                                   cbcf@ctburnsfoundation.org
                                   www.ctburnsfoundation.org
Armand J. Cantafio, President
Thomas Smith, Camp Director
The Arthur C. Luf Children's Burn Camp provides a free of
charge camp experience for children and teens, ages 8-18, who
have survived life altering burn injuries. Camp activities include
hiking, fishing, archery, boating, ropes course, and campfires.
The volunteer staff is composed of retired firefighters, medical
personnel, and burn survivors.
1978

918   Camp Discovery
American Academy of Dermatology
PO Box 1968
Des Plaines, IL 60017   847-240-1280
                                           866-503-7546
                                           888-462-3376
                                        Fax: 847-240-1859
                                    www.campdiscovery.org
A program of the American Academy of Dermatology, Camp Discovery is a camp held in 5 locations across the United States for
children with chronic skin conditions. Campers can participate in
activities such as fishing, swimming, archery and horseback riding. The Connecticut camp is held in Andover, Connecticut at
Channel 3 Kids Camp.
1993

919   Camp Harkness
The Arc Eastern Connecticut
125 Sachem St.
Norwich, CT 06360   860-889-4435
                                        Fax: 860-889-4662
                                        info@thearcect.org
                                   thearcect.org/camp-harkness
Kathleen Stauffer, Chief Executive Officer
A week-long summer camp program for individuals with intellec-
tual and developmental disabilities. The camp is held at Camp
Harkness in Waterford, CT.

920   Camp Horizons
127 Babcock Hill Rd.
PO Box 323
South Windham, CT 06266   860-456-1032
                                        Fax: 860-456-4721
                                        www.horizonsct.org
Adam Milne, Chair
Chris McNaboe, President & CEO
Kathleen McNaboe, Vice President
Camp Horizons offers summer camp and weekend camps for chil-
dren and adults with developmental disabilities.

921   Camp Isola Bella
410 Twin Lakes Rd.
Salisbury, CT 06079   860-824-5558
                                        Fax: 860-824-4276
                                        TTY: 860-596-0110
                                   ibdirector@asd-1817.org
                              asd-1817.org/programs/camp-isola-bella
David Guardino, Director
Owned and operated by the American School for the Deaf, Camp
Isola Bella provides summer camp opportunities for children who
are deaf or hard of hearing. Staff is able to communicate with the
campers regardless of the mode of communication, including
sign language, oral, aural, lipreading or a mix, and activities include, but are not limited to, swimming, ropes course, canoeing,
water skiing, archery, hiking, sports, and sailing.

922   Camp No Limits Connecticut
No Limits Foundation
Quinnipiac University
305 Sherman Avenue
Hamden, CT 06518   207-569-6411
                                   campnolimits@gmail.com
                                   www.nolimitsfoundation.org
Mary Leighton, Founder & Executive Director
Kelsey Moody, Program Operations Manager
Alix Sandler, Marketing & Development Director
Camp No Limits Connecticut, a location of Camp No Limits, is a
recreational and educational camp for youth who have experienced limb loss. Camp No Limits, is a program of the nonprofit
organization No Limits Foundation. The Connecticut camp is
hosted at Quinnipiac's York Hill campus and provides campers
the opportunity to participate in a variety of different sports,
including ice and sled hockey.

923   Easterseals Camp Hemlocks
Easterseals Oak Hill
120 Holcomb St.
Hartford, CT 06112   860-286-3108
                                   jillian.mccarthy@oakhillct.org
                                   www.easterseals.com/oakhill
Barry M. Simon, President & CEO
Jillian McCarthy, Camp Director
A summer camp program of Easterseals Oak Hill, Camp Hem-
locks is a completely accessible camp for youth and adults with
physical, sensory, intellectual, and developmental disabilities.
Activities include swimming, boating, fishing, arts and crafts,
and climbing tower.

924   SeriousFun Children's Network
SeriousFun Support Center Office
230 East Ave.
Suite 107
Norwalk, CT 06855   203-562-1203
                                        Fax: 203-341-8707
                                   info@seriousfunnetwork.org
                                   www.seriousfun.org
Blake Maher, Chief Executive Officer
Justin Fusaro, Chief Financial Officer
Tara Fisher, Chief Marketing Officer
The SeriousFun Children's Network is an international organiza-
tion of camps and programs for children and the families of chil-
dren with serious illnesses. The Network has 30 camps and
programs worldwide.

925   The Hole in the Wall Gang Camp
565 Ashford Center Rd.
Ashford, CT 06278   860-429-3444
                                   info@holeinthewallgang.org
                                   www.holeinthewallgang.org
James H. Canton, Chief Executive Officer
Padraig Barry, Chief Strategy Officer
Kevin Magee, Chief Financial Officer
The Hole in the Wall Gang Camp offers summer and weekend
camp experiences for children and the siblings of children with
serious illnesses. Located in Ashford, Connecticut, campers are
able to participate in traditional camp activities in a medically
safe environment.

926 The Rainbow Club
The Barton Center for Diabetes Education, Inc.
30 Ennis Rd.
PO Box 356
North Oxford, MA 01537-0356   508-987-2056
                                     Fax: 508-987-2002
                                     info@bartoncenter.org
                                     www.bartoncenter.org

Lynn Butler-Dinunno, Executive Director
Jenna Dufresne, Director, Health Services
Sarah Balko, Director, Camps & Programs
A program of The Barton Center for Diabetes Education, The Rainbow Club is a day camp held in Greenwich, Connecticut for children and teens, ages 5-15 with diabetes. Campers receive diabetes education and participate in games, crafts, and water activities. An adult program designed for parents runs in conjunction with the day camp session.

Delaware

927 Camp Manito & Camp Lenape
United Cerebral Palsy Of Delaware
700A River Rd.
Wilmington, DE 19809   302-764-2400
                              Fax: 302-764-8713
                              TTY: 302-764-8708
                              ucpde@ucpde.org
                              www.ucpde.org/summer-camps
Moni Edgar, Executive Director
Kim Evans, Director, Camp Program
Camp Manito, located in New Castle County and Camp Lenape, serving Kent and Sussex Counties, are summer camps run by United Cerebral Palsy of Delaware for children and young adults, ages 3-21, with orthopedic disabilities. Both campsites are accessible and activities include swimming, arts and crafts, music, sports, computer education, and outings.

928 Children's Beach House
100 W 10 St.
Suite 411
Wilmington, DE 19801-1674   302-655-4288
                                   Fax: 302-655-4216
                                   www.cbhinc.org
Richard T. Garrett, Executive Director
Patrice Tosi, Vice President, Advancement
Children's Beach House (CBH) is a nonprofit organization providing support and education for children with special needs. CBH offers summer and weekend programs at the Lewes facility on Delaware Bay. Activities are modified for each camper and include, but are not limited to, swimming, sailing, kayaking, arts and crafts, sports, and campfires.

District of Columbia

929 Camp Lighthouse
Columbia Lighthouse for the Blind
1825 K St. NW
Suite 1103
Washington, DC 20006   202-454-6400
                              Fax: 202-955-6401
                              info@clb.org
                              www.clb.org
Tony Cancelosi, President & CEO
Jocelyn Hunter, Senior Director, Communications
Toya Horten, Director, Administrative Operations
Camp Lighthouse is a one week day camp program run by Columbia Lighthouse for the Blind. The camp is for children ages 6-12 with visual impairments.

930 Paddy Rossbach Youth Camp
Amputee Coalition
601 Pennsylvania Ave. NW
Suite 600, South Bldg.
Washington, DC 20004   888-267-5669
                              www.amputee-coalition.org
Mary Richards, President & Chief Executive Officer

A 6-day camp for youths ages 10-17 who have limb loss or limb difference. Activities include sports, swimming, fishing, arts and crafts. Also offers a Leadership Camp for 18- and 19-year-olds transitioning from high school to college and careers.

Florida

931 Camp Amigo
Children's Burn Camp Of North Florida, Inc.
PO Box 368
Tallahassee, FL 32302   850-509-6200
                               www.campamigo.com
Rusty Roberts, President
Camp Amigo provides a one week summer camp experience for children ages 6-18 who live in Florida and have survived a burn injury.

932 Camp Boggy Creek
30500 Brantley Branch Rd.
Eustis, FL 32736   352-483-4200
                          866-462-6449
                          Fax: 352-483-0589
                          info@campboggycreek.org
                          www.boggycreek.org
June Clark, President & CEO
Lisa Hicks, Chief Development Officer
David Mann, Camp Director
Part of the SeriousFun Children's Network, Camp Boggy Creek provides year round camping opportunities for children with serious illnesses throughout Florida. The camp has week-long summer camp sessions and retreat weekends.

933 Camp No Limits Florida
No Limits Foundation
8411 25th Street East
Parrish, FL 34219   207-569-6411
                           campnolimits@gmail.com
                           www.nolimitsfoundation.org
Mary Leighton, Founder & Executive Director
Kelsey Moody, Program Operations Manager
Alix Sandler, Marketing & Development Director
Camp No Limits Florida, a location of Camp No Limits, is a recreational and educational camp for youth who have experienced limb loss. Camp No Limits is a program of the nonprofit organization No Limits Foundation. The Florida camp is hosted at the Clearwater Marine Aquarium in Clearwater, Florida.

934 Camp Thunderbird
Quest, Inc.
PO Box 531125
Orlando, FL 32853   407-218-4300
                           888-807-8378
                           Fax: 407-218-4301
                           contact@questinc.org
                           www.questinc.org/quests-camp-thunderbird
John Gill, President & Chief Executive Officer
Brooke Eakins, Chief Operating Officer
Todd Thrasher, Chief Financial Officer
A program of Quest, Inc. Camp Thunderbird provides recreational programs for children and adults with developmental disabilities. The camp has six-day overnight sessions with age specific programming. Activities include sports, games, arts and performance, and nature studies.

935 Center Academy at Pinellas Park
6710 86th Ave. N
Pinellas Park, FL 33782   727-541-5716
                                 Fax: 727-544-8186
                                 infopp@centeracademy.com
                                 www.centeracademy.com
Mack R. Hicks, Founder & Chair
Andrew P. Hicks, Chief Executive Officer & Clinical Director
Eric V. Larson, President & Chief Operating Officer
Specifically designed for the learning disabled child and other children with difficulties in concentration, strategy, social skills, impulsivity, distractibility and study strategies. Programs offered include attention training, visual-motor remediation, socialization skills training, relaxation training, and more.

936   Dr. Moises Simpser VACC Camp
Nicklaus Children's Hospital
3200 SW 62nd Ave.
Suite 203
Miami, FL 33155-4076   305-662-8222
                                      Fax: 786-268-1765
                                   bela.florentin@mch.com
                                       www.vacccamp.com

Bela Florentin, Camp Coordinator
Tania Diaz, Camp Clinical Coordinator
VACC Camp is a week-long overnight camp program for ventilation-assisted children and their families. The program includes sailing, swimming, field trips to local attractions, campsite entertainment, structured games, free play, and more. Parents have formal and informal opportunities to network among themselves.

937   Dream Oaks Camp
Foundation For Dreams, Inc.
16110 Dream Oaks Pl.
Bradenton, FL 34212   941-746-5659
                                 www.foundationfordreams.org

Elena Cassella, Executive Director
AnnaMaria Carleton, Director, Children Services
Lauralie Benge, Office Manager
Dream Oaks Camp offers weekend, summer day, summer residential, and specialty camps for children ages 7-17 with special needs and chronic illnesses. The camp is a program of the Foundation for Dreams with a 3:1 staff to camper ratio. Activities include horseback riding, nature programs, sports, games, swimming, talent shows, and arts and crafts.

938   Easterseals Camp Challenge
Easterseals Florida
31600 Camp Challenge Rd.
Sorrento, FL 32776   352-383-4711
                                   camp@fl.easterseals.com
                                   www.easterseals.com/florida

Susan Ventura, President & CEO
Maggie Denk, Camp Director
Located in Sorrento, Florida, Easterseals Camp Challenge provides camp opportunities for children and adults with cognitive and physical disabilities.

939   Florida Diabetes Camp
Florida Camp for Children & Youth with Diabetes
PO Box 14136
Gainesville, FL 32604-2136   352-334-1321
                                      Fax: 352-334-1326
                              fccydd@floridadiabetescamp.org
                                 www.floridadiabetescamp.org

Gary Cornwell, Executive Director
Chris Stakely, Assistant Director
Janet Silverstein, Medical Director
The Florida Diabetes Camp offers weekend and summer camps for children with type 1 diabetes. The camp combines traditional camp activities and diabetes related educational sessions for campers in order to provide a fun and safe environment.

940   Hand Camp
Hands to Love
3450 Hull Rd., Suite 3341
PO Box 140572
Gainesville, FL 32614-0572   352-273-7382
                                      Fax: 352-273-7388
                                     info@handstolove.org
                                       www.handstolove.org

John Hosman, President
Sean Branch, Vice President
Brian Caslow, Treasurer
A program of Hands to Love, an organization for children and the families of children with upper limb differences, Hand Camp is an annual event held in Starke, Florida at Camp Crystal Lake. Hand Camp offers camp activities, networking and support groups, and special guests.

941   Kris' Camp
Kris' Camp/Therapy Intensive Programs, Inc.
1132 Green Hill Trace
Tallahassee, FL 32317   850-445-4821
                                    kberger62@gmail.com
                                       www.kriscamp.org

Kathy Berger, Director
Kris' Camp provides programs for children with autism and special needs. The camp offers therapy programs led by art, education, music, occupational, physical, and speech therapists.

942   Sertoma Camp Endeavor
1300 Camp Endeavor Blvd.
Dundee, FL 33838   352-422-3435
                               campendeavorceo@gmail.com
                                  www.campendeavorfl.org

Maureen Tambasco, Camp CEO
Scott Botelho, Camp Assistant Director
Sertoma Camp Endeavor provides camp programs for deaf and hard of hearing youth. Programs are designed to promote social and personal growth, environmental awareness, and independence.

Georgia

943   Aerie Experiences
GA   404-285-0467
                              mdweneta@aerieexperiences.com
                                      aerieexperiences.com

Matthew Weneta, Owner & Director
Located north of Atlanta, Georgia with summer camp expeditions taking place in Georgia, North Carolina, and Tennessee, Aerie Experiences provides programs for children, families and individuals with special needs. Aerie Experiences is focused on those affected by Aspergers, High Functioning Autism, Learning Disabilities, ADHD, and Neurobiological Disorders.

944   Camp Breathe Easy
American Lung Association
2452 Spring Rd. SE
Smyrna, GA 30080
Operated by the Georgia Chapter of American Lung Association, Camp Breathe Easy is a summer camp program for children ages 6-13 with asthma. Campers are able to participate in a wide variety of camp experiences such as swimming, fishing, archery, and canoeing, with asthma education incorporated into the program. Camp Breathe Easy is held at Camp Twin Lakes in Rutledge, GA.

945   Camp Caglewood
Caglewood, Inc.
5182 Glen Forrest Dr.
Flowery Branch, GA 30542   info@caglewood.org
                                       www.caglewood.org

Paul Freeman, Co-Founder
Jessica Freeman, Co-Founder
A special needs camping program, Camp Caglewood provides active weekend programs for children and adults with developmental disabilities.

946   Camp Dream
Camp Dream Foundation
4355 Cobb Pkwy.
Suite J117
Atlanta, GA 30339   678-367-0040
                                     info@campdreamga.org
                                       www.campdreamga.org

Gary Marshall, Executive Director
Hunter Steng, Operations Director
Amy Blankenship, Medical Director
Camp Dream provides recreational camp programs, Summer Camp and Camp Out, for children and young adults with physical and developmental disabilities.

947   Camp Firefly
The Firefly Foundation
5737 Kanan Rd.
Suite 180
Agoura Hills, CA 91301   campfirefly89@gmail.com
                                       www.campfirefly.com

Camp Firefly offers a week-long camping experience for terminally and seriously ill children and their families. Camp Firefly is held in Georgia.

948   Camp Hawkins
GA Baptist Children's Homes & Family Ministries
800 Rudeseal Rd.
Mount Airy, GA 30563   770-463-3800
georgiachildren.org/camp-hawkins
Kenneth Z. Thompson, President & CEO
Camp Hawkins is a residential summer camp for youth ages 8-21 with developmental disabilities, learning disorders, traumatic brain injury or other special needs. Activities include swimming, canoeing, arts and crafts, games, and Bible study. The camp has locations in Baxley, GA and Mt. Airy, GA.

949   Camp Independence
Camp Twin Lakes
1391 Keencheefoonee Rd.
Rutledge, GA 30663   404-785-0631
campindependence@choa.org
www.choa.org/camps/camp-independence
Donna Hyland, President & CEO, Children's Healthcare of Atlanta
Camp Independence is an overnight, week-long summer camp for children and teens ages 8-18 who have kidney disease, are on dialysis, or have received an organ transplant.

950   Camp Juliena
Georgia Center of the Deaf and Hard of Hearing
2296 Henderson Mill Rd.
Suite 115
Atlanta, GA 30345   404-381-8447
888-297-9461
Fax: 404-297-9465
info@gcdhh.org
www.gcdhh.org/camp-juliena
Jimmy Peterson, Executive Director
Andrea Alston, Coordinator, Community Outreach
A week-long residential summer camp for deaf or hard of hearing youth. Activities help campers develop leadership, team-building, social, and communication skills.

951   Camp Kudzu
Camp Kudzu, Inc.
5885 Glenridge Dr.
Suite 160
Atlanta, GA 30328   833-995-8398
info@campkudzu.org
www.campkudzu.org
Robert G. Shaw, Executive Director
Danielle Holmes, Senior Development Coordinator
Carrie Claiborne, Medical Coordinator
Camp Kudzu is a nonprofit organization, offering overnight summer camp, day camp, family camps, and teen programs for individuals and the families of individuals with type 1 diabetes. Programs are held at various locations across Georgia and provide campers with traditional camp experiences and diabetes education.

952   Camp Sunshine
1850 Clairmont Rd.
Decatur, GA 30033   404-325-7979
866-786-2267
Fax: 404-325-7929
info@mycampsunshine.com
www.mycampsunshine.com
Sally Hale, Executive Director
Tenise Newberg, Program Director
Ann Baker, Program Director
Camp Sunshine provides recreational, educational, support, and camp programs for children with cancer and their families.

953   Camp Twin Lakes
1100 Spring St.
Suite 406
Atlanta, GA 30309   404-231-9887
Fax: 404-577-8854
camps@camptwinlakes.org
www.camptwinlakes.org
Jill Morrisey, Chief Executive Officer
Daniel C. Mathews, Chief Operations Officer
Cheryl Belair, Chief Development Officer
Camp Twin Lakes provides fully accessible, year round camp programs for children with serious illnesses, disabilities, and other life challenges. Camp Twin Lakes has locations in Rutledge and Winder, Georgia.

954   Camp Twin Lakes: Rutledge
1391 Keencheefoonee Rd.
Rutledge, GA 30663   706-557-9070
Fax: 706-557-9147
camps@camptwinlakes.org
www.camptwinlakes.org
Jill Morrisey, Chief Executive Officer
Daniel C. Mathews, Chief Operations Officer
Cheryl Belair, Chief Development Officer
A location of Camp Twin Lakes, which offers camp programs for children with serious illnesses, disabilities, and other life challenges. The Rutledge campus is fully accessible and includes a pool, ropes course, farm, and paddleboat activities.

955   Camp Twin Lakes: Will-A-Way
210 S Broad St.
Unit 5
Winder, GA 30680   770-867-6123
Fax: 770-867-6130
camps@camptwinlakes.org
www.camptwinlakes.org
Jill Morrisey, Chief Executive Officer
Daniel C. Mathews, Chief Operations Officer
Cheryl Belair, Chief Development Officer
A location of Camp Twin Lakes, which offers camp programs for children with serious illnesses, disabilities, and other life challenges. The Will-A-Way campus is fully accessible and includes a gymnasium, ropes course, zip line, rock wall, outdoor ampitheater, beachfront, and equestrian program.

956   Squirrel Hollow Summer Camp
The Bedford School
5665 Milam Rd.
Fairburn, GA 30213   770-774-8001
Fax: 770-774-8005
info@thebedfordschool.org
www.thebedfordschool.org
Betsy Box, Admissions Director
Jeff James, Head of School
Allison Day, Associate Head of School
A program of The Bedford School, Squirrel Hollow Summer Camp offers summer sessions for students with academic needs due to a learning disability. Students receive academic instruction in reading, writing, and math through a variety of teaching techniques, with students grouped by age and skill level. The camp also incorporates recreational activities such as swimming, games, and a challenge course.

Hawaii

957   Camp Anuenue
Honolulu, HI   808-349-7325
campanuenue@gmail.com
www.campanuenue.com
B.K. Cannon, President & Director
Alison James, Vice President & Director
Des Medeiros, Medical Director
Camp Anuenue is a nonprofit organization that offers a week long camping experience for children ages 7-18 who have or have had cancer. The camp is held at Camp Mokule'ia on the North Shore of Oahu and accepts children from Hawaii and US territories in the Pacific including Guam, Saipan, Samoa, and Marshall Islands.

958 Camp Taylor: Family Camp
Camp Taylor, Inc.
Hilton Hawaiian Village
2005 Kalia Road
Honolulu, HI 96815   209-545-3853
camp@kidsheartcamp.org
www.kidsheartcamp.org/familycamphi
Kimberlie Gamino, Founder & Executive Director
A program of Camp Taylor, Family Camp is for children of all
ages, with congenital heart disease and/or acquired heart disease,
and their family including parents and siblings. The camp offers
parental heart education and support programs for parents and
siblings. The camp is held at the Hilton Hawaiian Village and is
open to families from all of the Hawaiian Islands.

Idaho

959 Camp Hodia
Idaho Diabetes Youth Programs, Inc.
5439 W Kendall St.
Boise, ID 83706   208-891-1023
info@hodia.org
www.hodia.org
Lisa Gier, Executive Director
Morgan Coenen, Director, Programs
Ciera Miller, Director, Marketing
Camp Hodia offers a variety of educational camp programs for
children and teens with type 1 diabetes.

960 Camp No Limits Idaho
No Limits Foundation
Camp Cross Marine Rt.
Coeur d'Alene, ID 83814   207-569-6411
campnolimits@gmail.com
www.nolimitsfoundation.org
Mary Leighton, Founder & Executive Director
Kelsey Moody, Program Operations Manager
Alix Sandler, Marketing & Development Director
Camp No Limits Idaho, a location of Camp No Limits, is a recre-
ational and educational camp for youth who have experienced
limb loss. Camp No Limits, is a program of the nonprofit organi-
zation No Limits Foundation. The camp is held at Camp Cross on
Lake Coeur d'Alene. Unavailable in 2022 due to COVID-19
restrictions.

961 Camp Rainbow Gold
216 W Jefferson St.
Boise, ID 83702   208-350-6435
info@camprainbowgold.org
www.camprainbowgold.org
Elizabeth Lizberg, Executive Director
Tracy Bryan, Program Director
Christl Holzl, Development Director
Camp Rainbow Gold is a independent, nonprofit organization
providing year round camp programs, support groups, and scholarships for children, siblings, and the family of children who have
been diagnosed with cancer. All camp programs are offered free
of charge, with campers participating in activities such as fishing,
hiking, campfires, and crafts. The camp is held in the Sawtooth
National Forest.

962 Cristo Vive International: Idaho Camp
139 McLean Lane
Kooskia, ID 83539   208-507-1241
www.cristovive.net
Carol McLean, Camp Coordinator
Christian camp with programming for individuals who are
blind/deaf, physically or mentally challenged, have multiple disabilities, Down Syndrome, Autism/Asperger's, ADHD/ADD,
Cerebral Palsy, and their families and siblings.

Illinois

963 ADA Camp GranADA
American Diabetes Association
55 E Monroe St.
Suite 3420
Chicago, IL 60603   312-346-1805
illinoiscamps@diabetes.org
www.diabetes.org
Camp GranADA is an American Diabetes Association resident
camp located in Monticello, Illinois at the 4H Memorial Campground. For children with diabetes, ages 8-16.

964 ADA Teen Adventure Camp
American Diabetes Association
55 E Monroe St.
Suite 3420
Chicago, IL 60603   312-346-1805
illinoiscamps@diabetes.org
www.diabetes.org
Paula Williams, Contact
Camping for teenagers with diabetes. Coed, ages 14 to 17. Camp
dates are early in August. Located at the YMCA Camp Duncan in
Ingleside, Illinois. Featured activities include archery, boating,
roller skating, ropes course, and swimming.

965 ADA Triangle D Camp
American Diabetes Association
55 E Monroe St.
Suite 3420
Chicago, IL 60603   312-346-1805
illinoiscamps@diabetes.org
www.diabetes.org
Triangle D Camp is a resident camp program for children with diabetes. A coed camp for participants aged 9-13 years old, with
swimming, row boating, canoeing, ropes course, camp games, archery, soccer, basketball, volleyball, and diabetes education as
the camp's featured activities. The camp is held at YMCA Camp
Duncan in Ingleside, Illinois.

966 Camp "I Am Me"
Illinois Fire Safety Alliance
426 W Northwest Hwy.
Mount Prospect, IL 60056   847-390-0911
Fax: 847-390-0920
ifsa@ifsa.org
www.ifsa.org/programs/camp
Philip Zaleski, Executive Director
Riley Anderson, Program Coordinator
Jenny Tzortzos, Community Outreach Coordinator
Camp I Am Me is a one-week summer camp for children and teens
who have experienced burn injuries. The camp is held in
Ingleside, Illinois at YMCA Camp Duncan. Activities include ar-
chery, games, canoes, kayaks, sailboats, campfires, fishing, ropes
course, swimming, and specialized workshops related to burn
injuries.

967 Camp Callahan
Camp Callahan, Inc.
PO Box 5253
Quincy, IL 62305   217-883-0137
www.campcallahan.com
Peg Ratliff, Camp Director
Brandy Schlieper, Program Director
Camp Callahan is dedicated to providing a camp experience for
youth with disabilities. The camp is held at Saukenauk Scout Res-
ervation.

968 Camp Discovery
American Academy of Dermatology
PO Box 1968
Des Plaines, IL 60017   847-240-1280
866-503-7546
888-462-3376
Fax: 847-240-1859
www.campdiscovery.org
A program of the American Academy of Dermatology, Camp Discovery is a camp held in 5 locations across the United States for
children with chronic skin conditions. Campers can participate in

activities such as fishing, swimming, archery and horseback riding.
1993

969 Camp FRIENDship
Easterseals Chicagoland & Greater Rockford
1939 W 13th St.
Suite 300
Chicago, IL 60608-1226   312-491-4110
www.easterseals.com/chicago
Sara Ray Stoelinga, President & CEO
A program of Easterseals, Camp FRIENDship is a summer camp program designed to help children ages 5-14 with autism, nonverbal learning disabilities, and intellectual disabilities. The camp promotes the acquiring of social skills in a safe and fun learning environment.

970 Camp Little Giant
Touch of Nature Environmental Center
Southern Illinois University
Mail Code 6888
Carbondale, IL 62901   618-453-3950
Fax: 618-453-1188
jcave@siu.edu
www.ton.siu.edu
Jasmine Cave, Director
A program of the Southern Illinois University and held at the Touch of Nature Environmental Center, Camp Little Giant is a residential camp offering camping opportunities for people with physical, cognitive and developmental disabilities.

971 Camp New Hope
PO Box 764
Mattoon, IL 61938   217-895-2341
Fax: 217-895-3658
officemanager@campnewhopeillinois.org
campnewhopeillinois.org
Paul Semple, Office Manager
Pat Crum, Site Coordinator
Camp New Hope is a year round recreational experience for individuals 8 and up with developmental and physical disabilities. The camp offers summer, weekend respite, and bowling programs. Camp New Hope is situated on 41 acres of land on Lake Mattoon.

972 Camp One Step
Children's Oncology Services Inc.
213 W Institute Pl.
Suite 410
Chicago, IL 60610   312-924-4220
Fax: 312-878-7374
info@camponestep.org
www.camponestep.org
Jeff Infusino, President
Darryl Winston Perkins, Jr., Chief Programs Officer
Katie Weil, Vice President, Philanthropy
Camp One Step provides 11 different year round camp programs for children and teens ages 7-19 who have been diagnosed with cancer. Camp One Step is open to children and families who live in Illinois, Wisconsin, and the Midwest.

973 Camp Quality Illinois
PO Box 641
Lansing, IL 60438   708-895-8311
illinois@campqualityusa.org
www.campqualityusa.org/il
Mary Lockton, Executive Director
Dawn Winters, Treasurer
Camp Quality is an international camping program for children with cancer. The Illinois Camp Quality is held in Frankfort, Illinois at Camp Manitoqua & Retreat Center and offers children and their siblings summer camps and year round support programs. Volunteer doctors and nurses are at the camp 24 hours a day, and there is a 1:1 staff to camper ratio.

974 Camp Red Leaf
26710 W Nippersink Rd.
Ingleside, IL 60041   847-740-5010
Fax: 847-740-5014
www.campredleaf.org
Ari Strulowitz, Executive Director
Angela McNeal, Camp Director
Tyesha Smith, Business Manager
Camp Red Leaf provides camp programs for individuals ages 9 and up with developmental disabilities. Programs include youth day and overnight as well as adult overnight and travel camp sessions.

975 Illinois Wheelchair Sport Camps
University of Illinois
1207 S Oak St.
Champaign, IL 61820   217-333-1970
Fax: 217-244-0014
sportscamp@illinois.edu
www.disability.illinois.edu/camps
Illinois Wheelchair Sport Camps is hosted at the University of Illinois and offers a variety of summer resident wheelchair sport programs such as track, basketball, and individual skills camps.

976 MDA Summer Camp
Muscular Dystrophy Association National Office
161 N Clark
Suite 3550
Chicago, IL 60601   800-572-1717
resourcecenter@mdausa.org
mda.org/summer-camp
Donald S. Wood, President & Chief Executive Officer
Kristine Welker, Chief of Staff
Sharon Hesterlee, Executive Vice President & Chief Research Officer
MDA Summer Camp is a program of the Muscular Dystrophy Association providing a one-week summer camp for children with muscular dystrophy and related muscle-debilitating diseases.

977 Nothern Suburban Special Recreation Association Day Camps
3105 MacArthur Blvd.
Northbrook, IL 60062   847-509-9400
Fax: 847-509-1177
TTY: 711
info@nssra.org
www.nssra.org/programs/camps
Blair Hill, Recreation Manager, Camps
The Northern Suburban Special Recreation Association (NSSRA) offers year round day camps for children and youth with disabilities.

978 Rimland Services for Autistic Citizens
1265 Hartrey Ave.
Evanston, IL 60202   847-328-4090
Fax: 847-328-8364
TTY: 847-328-4090
www.rimland.org
Lorraine Ganz, President
Barbara Cooper, Secretary
Services include residential living, community day services, and health and wellness programs.

979 Shady Oaks Camp
16300 Parker Rd.
Homer Glen, IL 60491   708-301-0816
Fax: 708-301-5091
soc16300@sbcglobal.net
www.shadyoakscamp.org
Scott Steele, Executive Director
Katie Clark, Camp Director
Gary Schaid, Assistant Director
Shady Oaks is a summer camp for people with disabilities. The camp provides a recreational camp experience with a 1:1 camper to staff ratio.

980 Timber Pointe Outdoor Center
Easterseals Central Illinois
20 Timber Pointe Lane
Hudson, IL 61748
309-365-8021
Fax: 309-365-8934
tpoc@eastersealsci.com
www.easterseals.com/ci

Steve Thompson, President & CEO
Allen McBride, Camp Director
Timber Pointe Outdoor Center (TPOC) is a specialized outdoor recreational center for individuals with disabilities, which is owned and operated by Easterseals Central Illinois and is located on Lake Bloomington. TPOC offers year round programs, including summer and day camps, in a completely accessible environment.

Indiana

981 Anderson Woods
4630 Adyeville Rd.
Bristow, IN 47515
812-639-1079
andersonwoods@psci.net
www.andersonwoods.org

Isaac Gatwood, Executive Co-Director
Megan Gatwood, Executive Co-Director
Anderson Woods is a private, nonprofit organization providing summer camp experiences for children and adults with special needs. The camp typically runs in June and July.

982 CHAMP Camp
494 S Emerson Ave.
Suite H-1
Greenwood, IN 46143
317-679-1860
Fax: 317-245-2291
brittany@champcamp.org
www.champcamp.org

Brittany Sichting, Contact
Emily Miller, Contact
CHAMP Camp is a one week summer camp experience for children and youth ages 6-18 who have tracheostomies or require respiratory assistance. The camp is held at Bradford Woods in Martinsville, Indiana, and activities include fishing, boating, canoeing, arts, swimming, and a 50 foot alpine tower climb.

983 Camp About Face
Riley Hospital For Children, Indiana Univ. Health
705 Riley Hospital Dr.
Indianapolis, IN 46202
317-944-5000
rileychildrens.org/support-services
Camp About Face is a one week summer program designed to benefit children and youth ages 8-18 with craniofacial anomalies. Camping activities include swimming, nature projects and camp outs that are supplemented by social work, medical support and educational sessions which help to build self-esteem and self-confidence.

984 Camp Brave Eagle
Indiana Hemophilia & Thrombosis Center
8326 Naab Rd.
Indianapolis, IN 46260
317-871-0000
www.campbraveeagle.org
Jennifer Maahs, Camp Director
Camp Brave Eagle is a summer camp for children and the siblings of children with bleeding disorders living in the state of Indiana. The camp is supervised by experienced medical staff.

985 Camp John Warvel
American Diabetes Association
8604 Allisonville Rd.
Suite 140
Indianapolis, IN 46250
317-352-9226
campsupport@diabetes.org
www.diabetes.org
A program of the American Diabetes Association, Camp John Warvel is a summer camp program for children with type 1 diabetes. The camp is designed to promote independence, confidence, and a healthy lifestyle through education, nutrition, and exercise. There is a 4:1 camper to staff ratio. The camp is held at Camp Crosley in North Webster, Indiana.

986 Camp Little Red Door
Little Red Door Cancer Agency
1801 N Meridian St.
Indianapolis, IN 46202-1411
317-925-5595
Fax: 317-925-5597
camp@littlereddoor.org
www.littlereddoor.org

Fred Duncan, Director & CEO
Mandy Pietrykowski, Chief Advancement Officer
Steve Williams, Chief Financial Officer
Camp Little Red Door is a one week summer camp for children and teens who have or have had cancer. The camp is held at Bradford Woods in Martinsville, Indiana with campers participating in traditional camp activities.

987 Camp Millhouse
25600 Kelly Rd.
South Bend, IN 46614
574-233-2202
Fax: 574-233-2511
campmillhouse@gmail.com
www.campmillhouse.org
Diana Breden, Executive Director
Melissa Swank, Camp Director
Camp Millhouse is a residential summer camp for children and adults with varying disabilities. Ages of campers range from 7 to 75+. The camp offers six week-long summer sessions as well as spring and fall weekend sessions. Activities include arts and crafts, swimming, ropes course, and sports. The camp offers low camper to staff ratios and 24-hour supervision and nursing staff.

988 Camp PossAbility
Camp PossAbility, Inc.
PO Box 370
Huntertown, IN 46748
260-341-5732
info@camppossability.org
www.camppossability.org
Sam Albro, President
Lauren E. Harmison, Founder & Vice President
Camp PossAbility is a one-week summer camp for young adults ages 18-40 with a traumatic spinal cord injury. The camp is held at Bradford Woods in Martinsville, Indiana.

989 Camp Quality Kentuckiana
PO Box 35474
Louisville, KY 40232
502-507-3235
kentuckiana@campqualityusa.org
www.campqualityusa.org/ki
Eddie Bobbitt, Executive Director
Charlie Obranowicz, Camp Director
Heather Barry, Camper Coordinator
Camp Quality is an international camping program for children with cancer. Camp Quality Kentuckiana, serves Kentucky and Indiana and offers children and their siblings summer camps and year round support programs. Volunteer doctors and nurses are at the camp 24 hours a day, and there is a 1:1 staff to camper ratio.

990 Camp Red Cedar
3900 Hursh Rd.
Fort Wayne, IN 46845
260-637-3608
Fax: 260-637-5483
redcedar@campredcedar.com
www.campredcedar.com
Carrie Perry, Director
Shelly Detcher, Assistant Director
Theresa Prentice, Facilities Manager
Camp Red Cedar is open to children and adults with or without disabilities. The camp offers summer residental and summer day camps along with year round theraputic and conventional horseback riding. Other activities include fishing, hiking, swimming, and arts and crafts.

991 Camp Riley
Riley's Children Foundation
30 S Meridian St.
Suite 200
Indianapolis, IN 46204-3509   317-634-4474
                                      877-867-4539
                                 Fax: 317-634-4478
                              riley@rileykids.org
              www.rileykids.org/about/camp-riley
Elizabeth Elkas, President & CEO
Meghan Miller, Chief Operations Officer
Karen Spataro, Chief Communications Officer
Camp Riley is an annual summer camp program for children and teens ages 8-18 with physical disabilities. The program offers camp activities in a safe and accessible environment. The camp is held at Bradford Woods in Martinsville, Indiana.

992 Happiness Bag
Happiness Bag, Inc.
3833 Union Rd.
Terre Haute, IN 47802   812-234-8867
                                Fax: 812-238-0728
                             info@happinessbag.org
                                www.happinessbag.org
Happiness Bag provides adaptive education and recreational services, including summer day camps and respite care programs, for children and adults with disabilities.

993 Hillcroft Services
501 W Air Park Dr.
Muncie, IN 47303   765-284-4166
                                    www.hillcroft.org
Debbie Bennett, President & CEO
Abby Halstead, Chief Financial Officer
Jessica Hammett, Chief Operations Officer
Offers a summer camp program for children with autism spectrum disorders.

994 Hoosier Burn Camp
PO Box 233
Battle Ground, IN 47920   765-567-0115
                                Fax: 765-567-0195
                          info@hoosierburncamp.org
                              www.hoosierburncamp.org
Mark Koopman, Executive Director
Abby James, Program Manager
Valerie McCain, Administrative Assistant
Hoosier Burn Camp is nonprofit organization that provides an annual summer camp and monthly events for children and teens ages 8-18 who have suffered a burn injury. The camp is held at Camp Tecumseh in Brookston, Indiana.

995 Indiana Deaf Camp
1434 S Wausau St.
Warsaw, IN 46580   260-602-6758
                                Fax: 317-844-1034
                                TTY: 574-306-4063
                              info@indeafcamps.org
                                www.indeafcamps.org
Barbara Stenacker, Executive Director
Curtis Sigafoose, Director
Indiana Deaf Camp is for children ages 4-17 who have hearing loss or are related to individuals with hearing loss.

Iowa

996 Camp Albrecht Acres
14837 Sherrill Rd.
PO Box 50
Sherrill, IA 52073   563-552-1771
                                Fax: 563-552-2732
                           office@albrechtacres.org
                               www.albrechtacres.org
Eric Veltstra, Executive Director
Cassi Banwarth, Director, Programming
Camp Albrecht Acres is a nonprofit organization offering a residential summer camp program for children and adults with special needs.

997 Camp Courageous of Iowa
12007 190th St.
PO Box 418
Monticello, IA 52310-0418   319-465-5916
                                Fax: 319-465-5919
                             info@campcourageous.org
                               www.campcourageous.org
Charlie Becker, Chief Executive Officer
A year round residential and respite care facility for individuals with special needs and their families. Campers range in age from 1-105 years old. Activities include traditional activities like canoeing, hiking, swimming, and crafts, plus adventure activities like caving and rock climbing.

998 Camp Hertko Hollow
4200 University Ave.
Suite 320
Des Moines, IA 50266   515-471-8523
                                     855-502-8500
                                Fax: 515-288-2531
                             www.camphertkohollow.com
Jessica Thornton, Executive Director
Deb Holwegner, Camp Director
Camp Hertko Hollow is an educational and recreational summer camp program for children and teens ages 6-17 with diabetes. Campers participate in traditional camp activities and learn about living with diabetes.

999 Camp Sunnyside
Easterseals Iowa
401 NE 66th Ave.
Des Moines, IA 50313   515-309-2375
                         campandrespite@easterealsia.org
                               www.easterseals.com/ia
Sherri Nielsen, President & CEO
Open to campers age 4 and up, with or without disabilities, Camp Sunnyside is owned and operated by Easterseals Iowa and offers week and day summer camps.

1000 Camp Tanager
Tanager Place
1614 W Mount Vernon Rd.
Mount Vernon, IA 52314   319-363-0681
                                Fax: 319-365-6411
                            campmail@tanagerplace.org
                                www.camptanager.org
Donald Pirrie, Camp Director
Camp Tanager offers a wide variety of programs, including medical camps in partnership with local Iowa hospitals. The week long medical programs are for children and teens ages 5-17 with chronic illnesses and disabilities such as hemophilia, diabetes and Tourette's syndrome.

Kansas

1001 Camp Discovery Kansas
American Diabetes Association
608 W Douglas Ave.
Wichita, KS 67203   316-684-6091
                             campsupport@diabetes.org
                                   www.diabetes.org
Lora Furstner, Contact
A program of the American Diabetes Association, Camp Discovery Kansas is for children and teens ages 8-16 with diabetes. Campers participate in traditional camp activities while receiving educational information on diabetes. The camp is held at Rock Springs 4-H Center in Junction City, Kansas.

1002 Camp Planet D
American Diabetes Association
608 W Douglas Ave.
Wichita, KS 67203   316-684-6091
                             campsupport@diabetes.org
                                   www.diabetes.org
Lora Furstner, Contact
A program of the American Diabetes Association, Camp Planet D is for children and teens ages 7-15 with diabetes. Campers participate in traditional camp activities while receiving educational in-

formation on diabetes. The camp is held at the Tall Oaks Conference Center in Linwood, Kansas.

1003 Camp Quality Kansas
11802 W. Pine
Wichita, KS 67278
316-304-3865
kansas@campqualityusa.org
www.campqualityusa.org/ks

Kandi LaMar, Executive Director
Brittney Reed, Psychosocial Coordinator & Personnel Chair
Camp Quality is an international camping program for children with cancer. Camp Quality Kansas offers children and their siblings summer camps and year round support programs. Volunteer doctors and nurses are at the camp 24 hours a day, and there is a 1:1 staff to camper ratio.

1004 Camp Sweet Betes
American Diabetes Association
608 W Douglas Ave.
Wichita, KS 67203
316-684-6091
campsupport@diabetes.org
www.diabetes.org

Lora Furstner, Contact
A program of the American Diabetes Association, Camp Sweet Betes is a day camp for children ages 5-8 with diabetes. Campers learn techniques for managing nutrition, exercise, and medication. The camp is held at Trinity Presbyterian Church in Wichita, Kansas.

Kentucky

1005 Camp Quality Kentuckiana
PO Box 35474
Louisville, KY 40232
502-507-3235
kentuckiana@campqualityusa.org
www.campqualityusa.org/ki

Eddie Bobbitt, Executive Director
Charlie Obranowicz, Camp Director
Heather Barry, Camper Coordinator
Camp Quality is an international camping program for children with cancer. Camp Quality Kentuckiana, serves Kentucky and Indiana and offers children and their siblings summer camps and year round support programs. Volunteer doctors and nurses are at the camp 24 hours a day, and there is a 1:1 staff to camper ratio.

1006 Kids Cancer Alliance
611 W Main St., Suite 300
PO Box 24337
Louisville, KY 40224
502-365-1538
info@kidscanceralliance.org
www.kidscanceralliance.org

Shelby Russell, Executive Director
Leah McComb, Program Director
Brandon Padgett, Program Coordinator
The Kids Cancer Alliance is a nonprofit organization that provides summer camps and support programs for children and the families of children with cancer. Camp programs include oncology and sibling camps, as well as teen and and family retreats.

1007 Lions Camp Crescendo
1480 Pine Tavern Rd.
PO Box 607
Lebanon Junction, KY 40150
502-264-0120
wibblesb@aol.com
www.lccky.org

Billie J. Flannery, Administrator
Organization dedicated to enhancing quality of life for youths, including those with disabilities, through the delivery of a traditional camping experience.

1008 The Center for Courageous Kids
1501 Burnley Rd.
Scottsville, KY 42164
270-618-2900
Fax: 270-618-2902
info@courageouskids.org
www.courageouskids.org

Joanie O'Bryan, President & CEO
Clint Cobb, Chief Operations Officer
Allysa Gooden, Director, Development

The Center for Courageous Kids is a year round medical camp for children who have chronic or life-threatening illnesses. Offers week-long summer camp sessions and family retreat weekend sessions.

Louisiana

1009 Camp Bon Coeur
300 Ridge Rd.
Suite K
Lafayette, LA 70506
337-233-8437
Fax: 337-233-4160
info@heartcamp.com
www.heartcamp.com

Susannah Craig, Executive Director
Chelsea Doyle, Summer Program Coordinator
Jessica Becnel, Family Support Group Coordinator
Camp Bon Coeur is a nonprofit organization offering summer camp sessions for children with congenital heart defects. Also offers weekend family camps, monthly support groups, and outings for individuals with heart defects and their families.

1010 Camp Challenge
PO Box 10591
New Orleans, LA 70181
504-347-2267
Fax: 866-295-3803
campdirector@campchallenge.org
www.campchallenge.org

Cathy Allain, Camp Director
R. Tony Ricard, Assistant Camp Director
Camp Challenge is a nonprofit organization offering a week long summer camp for young hematology and oncology patients, including children who have or have had cancer or sickle cell disorders. The camp has an on-site medical team available 24 hours a day. It is held at Louisiana Lions Camp in Leesville, Louisiana.

1011 Camp Pelican
PO Box 10235
New Orleans, LA 70181
888-617-1118
Fax: 866-295-3803
camppelican@gmail.com
www.camppelican.org

A joint venture between the Louisiana Pulmonary Disease Camp, Inc. and the Louisiana Lions League for Crippled Children, Camp Pelican is a week long overnight summer camp for children with pulmonary disorders, including severe asthma and cystic fibrosis, living in the state of Louisiana.

1012 Camp Quality Louisiana
1800 Forsythe Ave.
Suite 2, Box 307
Monroe, LA 71201
315-547-4319
louisiana@campqualityusa.org
www.campqualityusa.org/la

Alan Barth, Executive Director
Gay Nell Barth, Camp Director
Monica Mock, Activities Coordinator
Camp Quality is an international camping program for children with cancer. The Louisiana Camp is held at Kings Camp in Mer Rouge, Louisiana and offers children and their siblings summer camps and year round camping opportunities. Volunteer doctors and nurses are at the camp 24 hours a day, and there is a 1:1 staff to camper ratio.

1013 Louisiana Lions Camp
292 L. Beauford Dr.
Anacoco, LA 71403
337-239-6567
Fax: 337-239-9975
lalions@lionscamp.org
www.lionscamp.org

Raymond E. Cecil, Executive Director & Camp Director
Owned and operated by the Louisiana Lions League, Inc. the Louisiana Lions Camp is a no cost residential summer camp for children with intellectual and physical disabilities. Campers are able to experience traditional summer camp activities in a medically safe and fun environment. The Camp is also host to the American Diabetes Association, Camp Victory, and Camp Pelican.

1014 MedCamps of Louisiana
102 Thomas Rd.
Suite 615
West Monroe, LA 71291   318-329-8405
                              Fax: 318-329-8407
                              info@medcamps.com
                              www.medcamps.com

Caleb Seney, Executive Director
Kacie Hobson, Camp Director
MedCamps of Louisiana offers week-long residential summer camp programs for children with chronic illnesses and physical or developmental disabilities. Each week during the summer a different camp is held, specifically designed for a particular disability.

Maine

1015 Camp CaPella
PO Box 552
Holden, ME 04429   207-843-5104
                          www.campcapella.org
Deb Breindel, Director
Camp CaPella provides recreational and educational opportunities for children and adults with disabilities. The camp is located on Phillips Lake in Dedham, Maine and offers a variety of programs including day camps, overnight camps, family vacation packages, and travel camp.

1016 Camp Lawroweld
288 West Side Rd.
Weld, ME 04285   207-585-2984
                        bchase@nnec.org
                        www.camplawroweld.org
Trevor Schlisner, Director
Camp Lawroweld offers several camp programs including a week-long summer camp for individuals who are blind or visually impaired.

1017 Camp No Limits Maine
No Limits Foundation
114 Pine Tree Camp Road
Rome, ME 04963   207-569-6411
                        campnolimits@gmail.com
                        www.nolimitsfoundation.org
Mary Leighton, Founder & Executive Director
Kelsey Moody, Program Operations Manager
Alix Sandler, Marketing & Development Director
Camp No Limits Maine, a location of Camp No Limits, is a recreational and educational camp for youth who have experienced limb loss. Camp No Limits is a program of the nonprofit organization No Limits Foundation. The camp is held at Pine Tree Camp in Rome, Maine and is supported by Maine Adaptive Sports & Recreation.

1018 Camp Sunshine
35 Acadia Rd.
Casco, ME 04015   207-655-3800
                         Fax: 207-655-3825
                         info@campsunshine.org
                         www.campsunshine.org
Michael Katz, Executive Director
Maureen McAllister, Director, Operations
Michael Smith, Director, Development
Camp Sunshine is a free, year round camp for children and families of children with cancer, hematologic conditions, renal disease, systemic lupus, and solid organ transplantation. The camp also has bereavement programs for families.

1019 Camp sNOw Maine
No Limits Foundation
15 South Ridge Road
Newry, ME 04261   207-569-6411
                         campnolimits@gmail.com
                         www.nolimitsfoundation.org
Mary Leighton, Founder & Executive Director
Kelsey Moody, Program Operations Manager
Alix Sandler, Marketing & Development Director
Camp sNOw Maine is a location of Camp No Limits, a recreational and educational camp for youth who have experienced limb loss. Camp No Limits is a program of the nonprofit organization, No Limits Foundation. Partnered with Maine Adaptive Sports & Recreation, the camp includes winter activities including, skiing and snowboarding. The camp takes place in March. Unavailable in 2022 due to COVID-19 restrictions.

1020 Pine Tree Camp
Pine Tree Society
114 Pine Tree Camp Rd.
Rome, ME 04963   207-386-5990
                        Fax: 207-397-5324
                        ptcamp@pinetreesociety.org
                        www.pinetreesociety.org
Dawn Willard-Robinson, Camp Director
Mary Schafhauser, Assistant Camp Director
Lori Chesley, Coordinator, Camp Relations
Offering day camps, overnight camps, retreats, and specialized programs, Pine Tree Camp provides children and adults with disabilities the opportunity to participate in recreational activities, such as swimming, fishing, kayak, hiking, and boating. The camp is located in North Pond in Rome, Maine.

Maryland

1021 Camp Great Rock
Brainy Camps, Children's National
1 Inventa Pl.
4th Floor West
Silver Spring, MD 20910   202-476-5142
                    brainycamps@childrensnational.org
                    www.brainycamps.com/camps/camp-great-rock
Sandra Cushner-Weinstein, Director, Brainy Camps
Camp Great Rock is a one-week overnight summer camp for children and teens ages 7-17 with epilepsy. Campers participate in a variety of activities and receive educational information regarding epilepsy.

1022 Camp Littlefoot
The Treatment and Learning Centers
2092 Gaither Rd.
Suite 100
Rockville, MD 20850   301-424-5200
                             Fax: 301-424-8063
                             info@ttlc.org
                             www.ttlc.org
Patricia Ritter, Executive Director
Camp Littlefoot offers a variety of programs for children requiring speech-language and/or occupational therapy.

1023 Camp No Limits Maryland
No Limits Foundation
11 Horseshoe Point Lane
North East, MD 21901   207-569-6411
                              campnolimits@gmail.com
                              www.nolimitsfoundation.org
Mary Leighton, Founder & Executive Director
Kelsey Moody, Program Operations Manager
Alix Sandler, Marketing & Development Director
Camp No Limits Maryland, a location of Camp No Limits, is a recreational and educational camp for youth who have experienced limb loss. Camp No Limits, is a program of the nonprofit organization No Limits Foundation.

1024 Camp SunSibs
Johns Hopkins Children's Center
1800 Orleans St.
Baltimore, MD 21287   www.hopkinsmedicine.org
Joe Young, Director
A weekend camp for children ages 5-16 who have siblings diagnosed with cancer.

91

1025 Camp Sunrise
Johns Hopkins Children's Center
1800 Orleans St.
Baltimore, MD 21287   campsunriseappliations@gmail.com
                             www.hopkinsmedicine.org

Ashley Richards, Camp Director
Lauren Murphy, Camper Coordinator
Camp Sunshine is a week-long summer camp open to children and teens ages 4-18 who are currently being treated for cancer or who have undergone bone marrow transplants at Johns Hopkins Hospital.

1026 Deaf Camps, Inc.
Manidokan Outdoor Ministry Center
1600 Harpers Ferry Rd.
Knoxville, MD 21758   deafcampsinc@gmail.com
                            deafcampsinc.org

Louise Rollins, President
Erin Krug, Vice President
David Shepard, Secretary
Deaf Camps, Inc. is a volunteer-run nonprofit organization dedicated to providing camp experiences for deaf and hard of hearing children and children learning American Sign Language.

1027 Easterseals Camp Fairlee
Easterseals Delaware & Maryland's Eastern Shore
22242 Bay Shore Rd.
Chestertown, MD 21620   410-778-0566
                              Fax: 410-778-0567
                             fairlee@esdel.org
                          www.easterseals.com/de

Kenan J. Sklenar, President & CEO
Sallie Price, Camp Director
Easterseals Camp Fairlee provides year-round recreation and respite to children and adults with all types of disabilities. Best known for week long summer camp sessions June-August. Camp Fairlee was rebuilt in 2015 with new cabins, activity, center, health center and dining hall. Activities include, but are not limited to, swimming, wall climbing, zip lining, canoeing, kayaking, arts and crafts, indoor and outdoor games. Accredited by the American Camp Association.

1028 League at Camp Greentop
The League for People with Disabilities, Inc.
1111 E Cold Spring Lane
Baltimore, MD 21239   410-323-0500
                          info@leagueforpeople.org
                          www.leagueforpeople.org

David Greenberg, President & CEO
Margy Ryan, Senior Vice President, Finance
Shiketa Jenkins, Vice President, Workforce, Community & Youth Programs
A traditional sleepaway summer camp for youth and adults with disabilities. The League at Camp Greentop is located in Thurmont, Maryland, and has youth and all ages sessions, with campers participating in activities such as swimming, arts and crafts, sports, and games.

1029 Lions Camp Merrick
PO Box 56
Nanjemoy, MD 20662   301-870-5858
                             Fax: 301-246-9108
                          info@lionscampmerrick.org
                          www.lionscampmerrick.org

Heidi A. Fick, Executive Director
Donna Wadsworth, Office Administrator
A recreational camp for children ages 6-16 who are deaf, blind, or have type 1 diabetes. Camp activities include archery, canoeing, ropes courses, swimming, fishing, and games.

Massachusetts

1030 Camp Howe
557 East St.
PO Box 326
Goshen, MA 01032   413-268-7635
                              Fax: 413-268-8206
                            office@camphowe.com
                             www.camphowe.com

Terrie Campbell, Executive Director
Camp Howe provides camp programs for youth ages 7 to 17. The camp's ECHO Program offers one-week and two-week sessions for youth with physical and developmental disabilities.

1031 Camp Jabberwocky
200 Greenwood Ave. Ext.
PO Box 1357
Vineyard Haven, MA 02568   508-693-2339
                           info@campjabberwocky.org
                           www.campjabberwocky.org

Liza Gallagher, Executive Director
Kelsey Grousbeck, Director, Outreach
Camp Jabberwocky offers summer camp and family camp programs for individuals with physical and intellectual disabilities. The camp is located in Martha's Vineyard with campers usually staying between 1 and 4 weeks. Camp activities include day trips, horseback riding, barbecues, boating, biking, and spending time at the beach.

1032 Camp Starfish
636 Great Rd.
Suite 2
Stow, MA 01775   978-637-2617
                              Fax: 978-637-2617
                            info@campstarfish.org
                            www.campstarfish.org

Emily Golinsky, Interim Executive Director
Jamie Mahnken, Camp Director
Laura Petersen, Director, Staff Experience
Camp Starfish provides summer camps, day camps, and year round respite programs for children with emotional, behavioral, and learning disabilities. Camp Starfish has a 1:1 staff to camper ratio at all times.

1033 Eagle Hill School: Summer Program
Eagle Hill School
242 Old Petersham Rd.
PO Box 116
Hardwick, MA 01037   413-477-6000
                              Fax: 413-477-6837
                             www.eaglehill.school

PJ McDonald, Head of School
Michael Riendeau, Assistant Head of School, Academic Affairs
Kristyl Kelly, Assistant Head of School, Student Life
A program of Eagle Hill School, a school for students diagnosed with learning disabilities including ADHA. The Eagle Hill Summer session is a five week summer camp for students ages 10-16 with learning disabilities. The summer session incorporates education and recreation to address the specific academic and social skills of the student.

1034 Kamp for Kids at Camp Togowauk
Behavioral Health Network Inc.
417 Liberty St.
Springfield, MA 01104   413-246-9675
                             www.bhninc.org

Steve Winn, President & CEO
Anne Benoit, Program Manager
Kamp for Kids at Camp Togowauk is an integrated summer camp for youth with or without disabilities.

1035 Open Hearts Camp
The Edward J. Madden Open Hearts Camp
250 Monument Valley Rd.
Great Barrington, MA 01230   413-528-2229
                          hearts@openheartscamp.org
                          www.openheartscamp.org

David Zaleon, Executive Director
The Open Hearts Camp is a summer camp program divided into four age-specific sessions for children and teens who have had

open heart surgery. Campers must be in stable health and the program blends sports, recreation, arts and crafts and rest periods into a camper's day.

1036 Summer@Carroll
Carroll School
25 Baker Bridge Rd.
Lincoln, MA 01773

781-259-8342
summeradmissions@carrollschool.org
www.carrollschool.org

Kristin Curry, Director
Donna Brown, Assistant Director

A program of the Carroll School, an independent day school for elementary and high school students diagnosed with learning disabilities, Summer@Carroll is a 5 week day camp incorporating education and recreation for children with learning disabilities. Students participate in academic classes in the morning, splitting into smaller groups during the afternoon for recreational activities. Campers attending the day camp do not have to be students of the school during the regular school year.

1037 The Barton Center
The Barton Center for Diabetes Education, Inc.
30 Ennis Rd.
PO Box 356
North Oxford, MA 01537-0356

508-987-2056
Fax: 508-987-2002
info@bartoncenter.org
www.bartoncenter.org

Lynn Butler-Dinunno, Executive Director
Jenna Dufresne, Director, Health Services
Sarah Balko, Director, Camps & Programs

The Barton Center for Diabetes Education is a year round camp, retreat and conference center offering education, recreation, and support programs for children and teens with diabetes and their families. The center offers a variety of programs in Massachusetts, Connecticut, and New York.

1038 The Barton Center Camp Joslin
The Barton Center for Diabetes Education, Inc.
30 Ennis Rd.
PO Box 356
North Oxford, MA 01537-0356

508-987-2056
Fax: 508-987-2002
info@bartoncenter.org
www.bartoncenter.org

Lynn Butler-Dinunno, Executive Director
Jenna Dufresne, Director, Health Services
Sarah Balko, Director, Camps & Programs

A summer camp program of The Barton Center for Diabetes Education, Camp Joslin provides boys ages 6-16 with diabetes a traditional summer camp experience combined with diabetes education. Activities include sports, swimming, kayaking, canoeing, fishing, hiking, arts and crafts, and campfires.

1039 The Barton Center Clara Barton Camp
The Barton Center for Diabetes Education, Inc.
30 Ennis Rd.
PO Box 356
North Oxford, MA 01537-0356

508-987-2056
Fax: 508-987-2002
info@bartoncenter.org
www.bartoncenter.org

Lynn Butler-Dinunno, Executive Director
Jenna Dufresne, Director, Health Services
Sarah Balko, Director, Camps & Programs

A summer camp program of the Barton Center for Diabetes Education, Clara Barton Camp provides girls ages 6-16 with diabetes a traditional summer camp experience combined with diabetes education. Activities include sports, swimming, kayaking, canoeing, fishing, hiking, arts and crafts, and campfires.

1040 The Barton Center Danvers Day Camp
The Barton Center for Diabetes Education, Inc.
30 Ennis Rd.
PO Box 356
North Oxford, MA 01537-0356

508-987-2056
Fax: 508-987-2002
info@bartoncenter.org
www.bartoncenter.org

Lynn Butler-Dinunno, Executive Director
Jenna Dufresne, Director, Health Services
Sarah Balko, Director, Camps & Programs

A coed day camp for children and teens, ages 5-15, with type 1 diabetes. The camp is held in Danvers, Massachusetts at the St. John's Preparatory School. Campers get the opportunity to explore the 175-acre facility, play games, and construct art pieces.

1041 The Barton Center Family Camp
The Barton Center for Diabetes Education, Inc.
30 Ennis Rd.
PO Box 356
North Oxford, MA 01537-0356

508-987-2056
Fax: 508-987-2002
info@bartoncenter.org
www.bartoncenter.org

Lynn Butler-Dinunno, Executive Director
Jenna Dufresne, Director, Health Services
Sarah Balko, Director, Camps & Programs

The Barton Center Family Camp is offered for the families of youth with diabetes. Families participate in traditional camp activities and diabetes education sessions.

1042 The Barton Center Worcester Day Camp
The Barton Center for Diabetes Education, Inc.
30 Ennis Rd.
PO Box 356
North Oxford, MA 01537-0356

508-987-2056
Fax: 508-987-2002
info@bartoncenter.org
www.bartoncenter.org

Lynn Butler-Dinunno, Executive Director
Jenna Dufresne, Director, Health Services
Sarah Balko, Director, Camps & Programs

A coed day camp for children and teens ages 5-15 with diabetes. The camp is held in North Oxford, Massachusetts at the Clara Barton Birthplace Museum. Campers experience boating, canoeing, arts and crafts, and camp games.

1043 The Bridge Center
470 Pine St.
Bridgewater, MA 02324

508-697-7557
info@thebridgectr.org
www.thebridgectr.org

Karen Ellis, Finance Coordinator
Abby Ross, Year Round & Summer Camp Program Coordinator
Peggy O'Neill, Coordinator, Volunteers

A therapeutic recreational facility in Bridgewater, Massachusetts offering after-school programs, special events, school vacation full-week and summer day camp programs for individuals with disabilities.

Michigan

1044 Camp Barefoot
The Fowler Center for Outdoor Learning
2315 Harmon Lake Rd.
Mayville, MI 48744

989-673-2050
Fax: 989-673-6355
info@thefowlercenter.org
www.thefowlercenter.org

Lynn M. Seeloff, Camp Director
Lillia Sheline, Program Director

Offered to adults 18 or older with traumatic brain injuries/closed head injuries. A wide variety of activities are offered. The participants in Camp Barefoot request their week's activities, allowing each participant to design their own activity schedule.

1045 Camp Catch-A-Rainbow
YMCA Storer Camps
6941 Stony Lake Rd.
Jackson, MI 49201   517-536-8607
                                Fax: 517-536-4922
                            ccar@ymcastorercamps.org
                            www.ymcastorercamps.org
Katie Wilson, Camp Catch-A-Rainbow Coordinator
Camp Catch-A-Rainbow is a free camp for cancer survivors ages
4-17. The camp is held at YMCA Storer Camps in Jackson, Michigan.

1046 Camp Chris Williams
MI Coalition for Deaf & Hard of Hearing People
PO Box 16234
Lansing, MI 48901-6234   586-932-6090
                                campchris@michdhh.org
                        www.michdhh.org/camp-chris-williams
Val Boyer, Camp Director
A program of the Michigan Coalition for Deaf and Hard of Hearing, Camp Chris Williams is a one week summer camp for youths
ages 11-17 who are deaf or hard of hearing. Sessions are normally
held the first full week of August each year. Registration is online
only.

1047 Camp Grace Bentley
8250 Lakeshore Rd.
Burtchville Township, MI 48059   313-962-8242
                            campgracebentley@gmail.com
                                campgracebentley.org
Camp Grace Bentley offers day summer camp programs for children and teens ages 7-16 with physical and mental disabilities.
Each camper is screened before attending the camp to ensure the
camp can meet the needs of the camper. Activities include swimming, campfires, movie nights, team sports, arts and crafts,
karaoke night, and dances.

1048 Camp Midicha
American Diabetes Association
20700 Civic Center Dr.
Suite 100
Southfield, MI 48076   248-433-3830
                                campsupport@diabetes.org
                                www.diabetes.org
Camp Midicha is the Michigan summer camp program of the
American Diabetes Association for children with diabetes. The
camp is hosted at YMCA Camp Copneconic in Fenton, Michigan.

1049 Camp Quality North Michigan
PO Box 345
Boyne City, MI 49712   231-582-2471
                            mioffice@campqualityusa.org
                            www.campqualityusa.org/MI
Jean McDonough, Executive Director
Amy Smitter, Development Director
Camp Quality is an international camping program for children
with cancer. The Michigan Camp Quality is held in Lake Ann,
Michigan and offers children and their siblings summer camps
and year round camping opportunities. Volunteer doctors and
nurses are at the camp 24 hours a day, and there is a 1:1 staff to
camper ratio.

1050 Camp Quality South Michigan
PO Box 345
Boyne City, MI 49712   231-582-2471
                            mioffice@campqualityusa.org
                            www.campqualityusa.org/MI
Jean McDonough, Executive Director
Amy Smitter, Development Director
Camp Quality is an international camping program for children
with cancer. The South Michigan Camp Quality is held in Fenton,
Michigan and offers children and their siblings summer camps
and year round camping opportunities. Volunteer doctors and
nurses are at the camp 24 hours a day, and there is a 1:1 staff to
camper ratio.

1051 Echo Grove Camp
Salvation Army
1101 Camp Rd.
Leonard, MI 48367   248-628-3108
                                Fax: 248-628-7055
                        shayna.stubblefield@usc.salvationarmy.org
                                www.echogrove.org
Shayna Stubblefield, Program Director
The Salvation Army's Echo Grove Camp offers a structured
camping program for children, adults and seniors referred
through Corps Community Centers. In addition to outdoor recreation, camps may include religious, musical and skill-building
instruction.

1052 Indian Trails Camp
IKUS Life Enrichment Services
O-1859 Lake Michigan Dr. NW
Grand Rapids, MI 49534   616-677-5251
                                Fax: 616-677-2955
                                info@ikuslife.org
                                www.ikuslife.org
Scott Blakeney, Executive Director
Amy DeMott, Director, Programs & Services
Nikki Outhier, Director, Development
The Indian Trails Camp is a program of IKUS Life Enrichment
Services. The camp offers summer, day, and weekend respite programs for individuals of all ages with disabilities. Campers are
able to participate in adaptive recreation opportunities in a
barrier-free environment.

1053 St. Francis Camp On The Lake
10120 Murrey Rd.
Jerome, MI 49249   517-688-9212
                                Fax: 517-688-9298
                        director@saintfranciscamp.org
                            www.saintfranciscamp.org
Victoria Petty, Camp Director
St. Francis Camp on the Lake offers residential summer camps,
day camps, and respite care for children and adults with developmental and intellectual disabilities.

1054 Trail's Edge Camp
c/o Mott Respiratory Care, 8-714
1540 E Hospital Dr. SPC 4208
Ann Arbor, MI 48109-4208   director.trailsedgecamp@gmail.com
                                www.trailsedgecamp.org
Jeff Cain, Director
Betsy Howell, Activities Coordinator
Trail's Edge Camp is a one-week summer camp for children and
teens ages 5-18 who are ventilator dependent. Campers are able
to participate in camp activities such as games, horseback riding,
and fishing. The camp is limited to 32 campers and campers must
be able to communicate with other children through speech or
sign language.

Minnesota

1055 AuSM Summer Camp
Autism Society of Minnesota
2380 Wycliff St.
Suite 102
St. Paul, MN 55114   651-647-1083
                                Fax: 651-642-1230
                                camp@ausm.org
                                www.ausm.org
Ellie Wilson, Executive Director
Dawn Brasch, Senior Director, Finance & Operations
Kelly Thomalla, Senior Director, Integration & Advancement
A program of the Autism Society of Minnesota (AuSM), the Summer Camps are offered to children, teens, and adults with autism,
ages 6 and up, in a variety of formats including day and residential summer camp. The camp offers the following programs:
Camp Hand in Hand, for ages 9+, held at Camp Knutson in
Crosslake, Minnesota; Camp Discovery, for ages 10+, held at
True Friends/Courage North in Lake George, Minnesota; and
Wahode Day Camps, for ages 6-12, held at Camp Butwin in
Eagan, Minnesota.

Camps / Minnesota

1056   Camp Buckskin
PO Box 389
Ely, MN 55731
763-432-9177
info@campbuckskin.com
www.campbuckskin.com

Tom Bauer, Camp Co-Director
Mary Bauer, Camp Co-Director
Camp Buckskin is for campers ages 6-18 with underdeveloped social skills who may struggle to interact with others and make friends. The camp is also open to children who have been diagnosed with AD/HD, Aspergers, and/or a learning disability.

1057   Camp Confidence
Confidence Learning Center
1620 Mary Fawcett Memorial Dr.
East Gull Lake, MN 56401
218-828-2344
info@confidencelearningcenter.org
www.campconfidence.com

Jeff Olson, Executive Director
Bob Slaybaugh, Camp Director
Camp Confidence works to promote self-confidence and self-esteem for individuals with developmental and cognitive disabilities. Programs run year round with campers participating in hands on activities and outdoor recreation experiences.

1058   Camp Courage
True Friends
8046 83rd St. NW
Maple Lake, MN 55358
952-852-0101
800-450-8376
Fax: 952-852-0123
info@truefriends.org
www.truefriends.org

John Leblanc, President & CEO
Conor McGrath, Senior Director, Camp & Operations
Jon Salmon, Director, Programs
Camp is located in Maple Lake, Minnesota. Summer sessions for campers with a variety of disabilities. Camp Courage is owned and operated by True Friends.

1059   Camp Courage North
True Friends
37569 Courage North Dr.
Lake George, MN 56458
952-852-0101
800-450-8376
Fax: 952-852-0123
info@truefriends.org
www.truefriends.org

John Leblanc, President & CEO
Conor McGrath, Senior Director, Camp & Operations
Jon Salmon, Director, Programs
Camp is located in Lake George, Minnesota. Summer camp programs for individuals with disabilities. Camp Courage North is owned and operated by True Friends.

1060   Camp Eden Wood
True Friends
6350 Indian Chief Rd.
Eden Prairie, MN 55346
952-852-0101
800-450-8376
Fax: 952-852-0123
info@truefriends.org
www.truefriends.org

John Leblanc, President & CEO
Conor McGrath, Senior Director, Camp & Operations
Jon Salmon, Director, Programs
Offers resident camp programs for children, teenagers and adults with developmental, physical or multiple disabilities.

1061   Camp Heartland
One Heartland
26001 Heinz Rd.
Willow River, MN 55795
888-216-2028
helpkids@oneheartland.org
www.oneheartland.org

Patrick Kindler, Executive Director
Katie Donlin, Operations Manager
Kadien Bartels-Merkel, Program Director
A program of One Heartland, a nonprofit organization working to provide camping programs for children with serious illnesses or experiencing social isolation, Camp Heartland is a weeklong summer camp for children, ages 7-15, who are infected or affected by HIV/AIDS. The camp is held in Willow River, Minnesota.

1062   Camp Knutson
11148 Manhattan Pt. Blvd.
Crosslake, MN 56442
218-543-4232
camp.knutson@lssmn.org
www.lssmn.org/campknutson

Jared Griffin, Senior Camp Director
Caitlin Malin, Program Director
Camp Knutson is an accessible camp that hosts a variety of different programs for children with special needs such as skin disease, autism, down syndrome, heart disease, and children who have HIV/AIDS.

1063   Camp Odayin
Camp Odayin
3503 High Point Dr. N
Suite 250
Oakdale, MN 55128
651-351-9185
Fax: 651-351-9187
info@campodayin.org
www.campodayin.org

Sara Meslow, Executive Director
Alison Boerner, Assistant Director
Matt Olson, Finance Director
Camp Odayin provides camping experiences for youth and the families of youth with heart disease. Camp Odayin offers a variety of programs including residential, day, family, and winter camps as well as retreats.

1064   Camp Odayin Family Camp
Camp Odayin
3503 High Point Dr. N
Suite 250
Oakdale, MN 55128
651-351-9185
Fax: 651-351-9187
info@campodayin.org
www.campodayin.org

Sara Meslow, Executive Director
Alison Boerner, Assistant Director
Matt Olson, Finance Director
Camp Odayin's Family Camp is a two-night program for families with a child who has heart disease.

1065   Camp Odayin Residential Camp
Camp Odayin
3503 High Point Dr. N
Suite 250
Oakdale, MN 55128
651-351-9185
Fax: 651-351-9187
info@campodayin.org
www.campodayin.org

Sara Meslow, Executive Director
Alison Boerner, Assistant Director
Matt Olson, Finance Director
A program of Camp Odayin, the Residential Camp is for children in grades 1-11 with heart disease. Camps are hosted at Camp Lutherdale in Elkhorn, WI and Camp Knutson in Crosslake, MN.

1066   Camp Odayin Summer Camp
Camp Odayin
3503 High Point Dr. N
Suite 250
Oakdale, MN 55128
651-351-9185
Fax: 651-351-9187
info@campodayin.org
www.campodayin.org

Sara Meslow, Executive Director
Alison Boerner, Assistant Director
Matt Olson, Finance Director
Camp Odayin offers a variety of summer camp programs for children in grades 1-11 with heart disease. Camper eligibility is determined upon the recommendation of a pediatric cardiologist and the camp's medical director.

95

1067   Camp Odayin Winter Camp
Camp Odayin
3503 High Point Dr. N
Suite 250
Oakdale, MN 55128   651-351-9185
                                Fax: 651-351-9187
                            info@campodayin.org
                            www.campodayin.org

Sara Meslow, Executive Director
Alison Boerner, Assistant Director
Matt Olson, Finance Director

A winter camp program for youth in grades 1-12 with heart disease.

1068   Cristo Vive International: Minnesota Camp
Ironwood Springs Christian Ranch
7291 County 6 Rd. SW
Stewartville, MN 55976   218-910-8151
                            cvimncamp@gmail.com
                            www.cristovive.net

Kristin Munoz, Camp Coordinator

Christian camp with programming for individuals who are blind/deaf, physically or mentally challenged, have multiple disabilities, Down Syndrome, Autism/Asperger's, ADHD/ADD, Cerebral Palsy, and their families and siblings.

1069   Down Syndrome Camp
Down Syndrome Foundation
17186 Daniel Lane
Eden Prairie, MN 55346   651-321-2267
                    www.downsyndromefoundation.org

Angie Kniss, President & Founder
Nick Engbloom, Secretary
Ellie Wilson, Counselor Coordinator

A week-long coed summer camp for youth ages 10-21 who have Down Syndrome. The camp is held at Camp Knutson in Crosslake, Minnesota. The camp is fully accessible and activities include swimming, boating, fishing, tubing, paddleboarding, horseback riding, arts and crafts, and campfires. The camp's staff is trained to work with children and adults with special needs.

1070   True Friends
10509 108th St. NW
Annandale, MN 55302   952-852-0101
                                   800-450-8376
                                Fax: 952-852-0123
                            info@truefriends.org
                            www.truefriends.org

John Leblanc, President & CEO
Conor McGrath, Senior Director, Camp & Operations
Jon Salmon, Director, Programs

True Friends provides camp experiences for children and adults with disabilities. Programs are held at five locations: Camp Courage in Maple Lake, MN; Camp Eden Wood in Eden Prairie, MN; Camp Friendship in Annandale, MN; Camp Courage North in Lake George, MN; and True Friends' office in Plymouth, MN.

Mississippi

1071   Camp Dream Street
3863 Morrison Rd.
Utica, MS 39175   601-885-3793
                            info@dreamstreetms.org
                            www.dreamstreetms.org

Aimee Adler, Director
Ashley Rubinsky, Assistant Director

Dream Street is a five-day camp program for children ages 8-14 with physical disabilities. The camp offers activities such as swimming, arts and crafts, horseback riding and more.

Missouri

1072   Camp Barnabas
PO Box 3200
Spingfield, MO 65808   417-476-2565
                            info@campbarnabas.org
                            www.campbarnabas.org

John Tillack, Chief Executive Officer
Krystal Simon, Chief Operations Officer
Mike Mrosko, Camp Director

Camp Barnabas is a Christian camp for children, the siblings of children, and adults with special needs. The camp serves children and adults ages 7 and up.

1073   Camp Encourage
4025 Central St.
Kansas City, MO 64111   816-830-7171
                                Fax: 816-301-6228
                            info@campencourage.org
                            www.campencourage.org

Kelly Lee, Executive Director
Aimee Gorrow, Program Coordinator

Provides overnight and summer camp sessions for children and youth with autism spectrum disorders.

1074   Camp Hickory Hill
PO Box 1942
Columbia, MO 65205   573-445-9146
                        camphickoryhill@gmail.com
                        www.camphickoryhill.com

Jessica Bernhardt, Camp Director

Camp Hickory Hill is a residential summer camp for children ages 7-17 with diabetes. Campers participate in traditional summer camp activities as well as educational programs.

1075   Camp MITIOG
7615 N Platte Purchase Dr.
Suite 116
Kansas City, MO 64118   www.campmitiog.org

A week long summer camp for children with Spina Bifida. Camp MITIOG is held in Excelsior Springs, Missouri at the Lake Doniphan Conference and Retreat Center, which is a wheelchair accessible environment. Campers participate in activities such as swimming, fishing, canoeing, arts and crafts, nature classes, classes on self-help medical care and evening campfires.

1076   Camp No Limits Missouri
No Limits Foundation
13528 State Route AA
Potosi, MO 63664   207-569-6411
                        campnolimits@gmail.com
                        www.nolimitsfoundation.org

Mary Leighton, Founder & Executive Director
Kelsey Moody, Program Operations Manager
Alix Sandler, Marketing & Development Director

Camp No Limits Missouri, a location of Camp No Limits, is a recreational and educational camp for youth who have experienced limb loss. Camp No Limits is a program of the nonprofit organization No Limits Foundation. Unavailable in 2022 due to COVID-19 restrictions.

1077   Camp Quality Central Missouri
PO Box 953
Jefferson City, MO 65012   636-795-7229
                        cmo@campqualityusa.org
                        www.campqualityusa.org/cmo

Casey Bucher, Co-Director
Erin Carl, Co-Director

Camp Quality is an international camping program for children with cancer. The Central Missouri Camp is held in St.Clair, Missouri and offers children and their siblings summer camps and year round camping opportunities. Volunteer doctors and nurses are at the camp 24 hours a day, and there is a 1:1 staff to camper ratio.

1078 Camp Quality Greater Kansas City
3111 SE 3rd Terr.
Lee's Summit, MO 64063   816-244-6912
gkc@campqualityusa.org
www.campqualityusa.org/gkc
Crystal Davison, Executive Director
Rachael Slagle, Program Coordinator
Jacinda Farmer, Camp Director
Camp Quality Greater Kansas City is a local chapter of a nation-wide nonprofit dedicated to serving children with cancer and their families. They host a signature week-long summer camping experience for children with cancer and their siblings in addition to programs and support throughout the year for the entire family. Their mission is to promote hope while fostering life skills. Hosted at the Lake Maurer Retreat Center, each camper is paired 1:1 with a companion volunteer during camp.

1079 Camp Quality Northwest Missouri
1325 Village Dr.
St. Joseph, MO 64506   816-232-2267
nwmo@campqualityusa.org
www.campqualityusa.org/nwmo
Niccole Marshall, Executive Director
Lynette Bingaman, Office Manager
Camp Quality is an international camping program for children with cancer. The Northwest Missouri Camp is held in Stewartsville, Missouri and offers children and their siblings summer camps and year round camping opportunities. Volunteer doctors and nurses are at the camp 24 hours a day, and there is a 1:1 staff to camper ratio.

1080 Camp Quality Ozarks
PO Box 302
Joplin, MO 64802   417-455-6196
ozarks@campqualityusa.org
www.campqualityusa.org/oz
Kristin Patterson, Executive Director
Angee Tingle, Treasurer
Denise Dieckhoff, Secretary
Camp Quality is an international camping program for children with cancer. The Missouri Ozarks Camp is held in Neosho, Missouri and offers children and their siblings summer camps and year round camping opportunities. Volunteer doctors and nurses are at the camp 24 hours a day, and there is a 1:1 staff to camper ratio.

1081 Sunnyhill Adventures
6555 Sunlit Way
Dittmer, MO 63023   636-274-9044
sunnyhilladventures.org
Rob Darroch, Director
Summer camps and year-round programs are offered for youth and adults of all abilities.

1082 Wonderland Camp
18591 Miller Circle
Rocky Mount, MO 65072   573-392-1000
info@wonderlandcamp.org
www.wonderlandcamp.org
Jill Wilke, Executive Director
Stephanie Dehner, Director, Administration
Mike Clayton, Director, Fund Development & Communication
Wonderland Camp provides residential summer camps and year round weekend camps for children, teens, and adults with disabilities.

Montana

1083 Big Sky Kids Cancer Camps
Eagle Mount Bozeman
6901 Goldenstein Lane
Bozeman, MT 59715   406-586-1781
Fax: 406-586-5794
bigskykids@eaglemount.org
www.eaglemount.org
Kevin Sylvester, Executive Director
Shannon Stober, Senior Director, Programs
Trevor Olson, Director, Operations

Provides recreational opportunities for kids and young adults ages 5-23 with cancer. Big Sky offers skiing, swimming, fishing, ice skating, golf, cycling, and other outdoor activities.

1084 Camp Mak-A-Dream
PO Box 1450
Missoula, MT 59806   406-549-5987
Fax: 406-549-5933
info@campdream.org
www.campdream.org
Kim McKearnan, Executive Director
Jennifer Benton, Program Director
Camp Mak-A-Dream provides a cost-free summer camp experience to children, teens, young adults, women and families affected by cancer. Participants experience regular camp activities such as swimming and zip lining, as well as the chance to interact with ranch staff.

1085 Charles Campbell Childrens Camp
PO Box 23342
Billings, MT 59102   406-670-2496
campbellcamp@msn.com
billingslions.org/clubnews/campbell-camp
Doug Hanson, Director
Sue Hanson, Director
Camp is open to young adults with physical disabilities that include sight or hearing impairment, spina bifida, cerebral palsy, gross motor skill impairments and other disabilities. Campers enjoy hiking, swimming, fishing, dances, campfires and much more.

Nebraska

1086 Camp Floyd Rogers
PO Box 541058
Omaha, NE 68154   402-885-9022
director@campfloydrogers.com
www.campfloydrogers.com
Dylan Helberg, Camp Director
Carrie Busing, Operations Director
A camp for children ages 8-18 with diabetes. While at the camp, campers enjoy activities, participate in special events, engage in evening programs, and meet other children their own age with diabetes.

1087 Camp Kindle
Project Kindle
PO Box 81147
Lincoln, NE 68501   877-800-2267
eva@projectkindle.org
www.campkindle.org
Eva Payne, Founder & President
Mandy Nickolite, Vice President & Camp Director
Camp Kindle provides educational and recreational camp programs for children and youth with a chronic or life-threatening illness, disability, or life challenge.

1088 Camp Quality Heartland
PO Box 24322
Omaha, NE 68124   402-450-1674
heartland@campqualityusa.org
www.campqualityusa.org/htl
Stephanie Purcell, Executive Director
Laura Peitzmeier, Camp Director
Jordan Peitzmeier, Treasurer
Camp Quality is for children with cancer and their siblings. The camp offers a stress-free environment that offers exciting activities and fosters new friendships, while helping to give the children courage, motivation and emotional strength.

1089 Easterseals Nebraska Camp
Easterseals Nebraska
12565 West Center Rd.
Omaha, NE 68144   402-930-4053
Fax: 888-611-6396
campesn@ne.easterseals.com
www.easterseals.com/ne
James C. Summerfelt, President & CEO
Jami Biodrowski, Director, Camp & Respite

Offers a variety of camp and recreational programs to help people with disabilities gain independence in a safe and adapted environment.

1090   Kamp Kaleo
46872 Willow Springs Rd.
Burwell, NE 68823   308-346-5083
kampkaleo@gmail.com
www.kampkaleo.com

David Butz, Camp Administrator
Offers an overnight summer camp for individuals with developmental disabilities. Participants can expect to experience outdoor recreational activities such as canoeing, fishing, and swimming, and there is a strong focus on religious education.

1091   National Camps for Blind Children
Christian Record Services
5900 S 58th St.
Suite M
Lincoln, NE 68516   402-488-0981
Fax: 402-488-7582
info@christianrecord.org
www.christianrecord.org

Diane Thurber, President
Lonnie Kreiter, Vice President, Finance
National Camps for Blind Children is a program of Christian Record Services offering summer camps for individuals who are considered legally blind.

Nevada

1092   Camp Buck
Nevada Diabetes Association
18 Stewart St.
Reno, NV 89501   775-856-3839
800-379-3839
Fax: 775-348-7591
camp@diabetesnv.org
www.diabetesnv.org

Sarah Gleich, Executive Director
Nate Gibson, Director, Camps
Dakota Ostrenger, Director, Marketing
Co-ed summer camp for children ages 7-17 with diabetes. Campers participate in recreational and athletic activities as well as diabetes education.

1093   Camp Lotsafun
Amplify Life
480 Galletti Way
Bldg. 2
Sparks, NV 89431   775-827-3866
Fax: 775-827-0334
info@amplifylife.org
www.amplifylife.org

Jessica Daum, Executive Director
Luis Chavez Torres, Program Coordinator
Cindy Oesterle-Prescott, Office Manager
Provides therapeutic, educational, and recreational opportunities for individuals with developmental disabilities. Camp activities include swimming, kayaking, pet therapy, arts and crafts, drama and music. The camp is held at Eagle Lake, California.

1094   CampCare
PO Box 12155
Reno, NV 89510-2155   775-323-3737
cmoore@campcarenevada.org
www.campcarenevada.org

Carol Moore, Camp Director
The camp provides programs for individuals with special needs such as ADHD, autism and cerebral palsy.

1095   Discovery Day Camp
Nevada Blind Children's Foundation
95 S Arroyo Grande Blvd.
Henderson, NV 89012   702-735-6223
info@nvblindchildren.org
nvblindchildren.org/programs/day-camp

Emily Smith, Chief Executive Officer
Maribel Garcia, Director, Programs
Paula Farrell, Director, Finances & Facilities
A summer day camp program for children in grades K-12 who are visually impaired. Discovery Day Camp provides traditional camp activities that have been adapted to meet the needs of children with visual impairments.

New Hampshire

1096   Adam's Camp: New England
26 Shaker Rd.
Concord, NH 03301   508-901-9610
NewEngland@AdamsCamp.org
www.adamscampnewengland.org

Adrienne Evans, Executive Director
Offers both therapy and adventure camps for children and the families of children with special needs and developmental delays. Camps are available in New Hampshire and Massachusetts.

1097   Camp Allen
56 Camp Allen Rd.
Bedford, NH 03110   603-622-8471
Fax: 603-626-4295
michael@campallennh.org
www.campallennh.org

Michael Constance, Executive Director
Stephen Daley, Camp Director
Debra Schulte, Office Manager
A residential summer camp for individuals with disabilities. All of the activities are conducted by individual coordinators under the supervision of the Program Director. Activities include aquatics, arts, crafts, games and nature programs. All camp events, special events, evening programs, and field trips are scheduled throughout the summer and are structured to meet the individual abilities and needs of each camper.

1098   Camp Carefree
American Diabetes Association
Lions Camp Pride
154 Camp Pride Way
New Durham, NH 03855   campsupport@diabetes.org
www.diabetes.org

Phyllis Woestemeyer, Director
The camp is located at Lions Camp Pride in New Durham, New Hampshire. Camp Carefree is a American Diabetes Association summer camp for children with diabetes.

1099   Camp Connect
Easterseals New Hampshire
555 Auburn St.
Manchester, NH 03103   603-623-8863
www.easterseals.com/nh

Maureen Beauregard, President & CEO
A summer day camp for children in grades K-12 with Asperger Syndrome, Autism, Nonverbal Learning Disorder, and other social communication disorders. The camp has a large focus on continuing to address academic needs of the campers, but also incorporates music, drama, and arts and crafts.

1100   Camp Inter-Actions
Inter-Actions
170 West Rd.
Suite 6-B
Portsmouth, NH 03801   603-319-6120
campinfo@inter-actions.org
inter-actions.org

Debbie Gross, Camp Director
Camp Inter-Actions is a summer camp for children ages 8-15 who are blind or visually impaired. The camp is located in Kingston, New Hampshire and runs one, two, and three week sessions. Ac-

tivities include swimming, fishing, adapted sports/games, woodworking, pottery, and more.

1101 Camp Sno Mo
Easterseals New Hampshire
Hidden Valley Reservation
260 Griswold Ln.
Gilmanton Iron Works, NH 03837
603-364-5818
cellis@eastersealsnh.org
www.easterseals.com/nh

Maureen Beauregard, President & CEO
Chris Ellis, Camp Director
Camp Slo Mo is is a camp program for children with disabilities. Activities include water sports, team sports, hiking, archery, arts and crafts, and more offered in an accessible setting.

1102 Camp Wediko
Wediko Children's Services, New Hampshire Campus
11 Bobcat Blvd.
Windsor, NH 03244
603-478-5236
Fax: 603-478-2049
www.wediko.org

Edward Zadravec, Interim Executive Director
This program is a six-week residential program for youth ages 8-19 with social, emotional, and behavior challenges. This program serves children with disabilities such as ADHD, autism, mood disorders, and more.

1103 Camp Yavneh: Yedidut Program
Summer Office
18 Lucas Pond Rd.
Northwood, NH 03261
603-942-5593
info@campyavneh.org
www.campyavneh.org/yedidut

Bil Zarch, Executive Director
Miriam Loren, Director, Camper Care & Yedidut
Michelle Rosenhek Zelermyer, Director, Summer Camp
A residential Jewish summer camp program for children with disabilities. Traditional camp activities with a strong focus on Judaism and Jewish education.

New Jersey

1104 Camp Chatterbox
Children's Specialized Hospital
200 Somerset St.
New Brunswick, NJ 08901
908-301-5548
campchatterbox@childrens-specialized.org
csh.recdesk.com

Sara Barnhill, Clinical Coordinator
Camp Chatterbox is an overnight camp for people ages 5-22 who use augmentative communication devices. The camp offers recreational activities such as swimming, arts, and sports.

1105 Camp Deeny Riback
208 Flanders Netcong Rd.
Flanders, NJ 07836
973-929-2901
Fax: 973-463-3998
camps@jccmetrowest.org
cdr.jccmetrowest.org

Dana Gottfried, Director
Debra Scher, Assistant Director
Todd Seideman, Assistant Director
A Jewish summer camp for children of all ages. The camp integrates children with special needs through their Camp Friends program. The camp provide traditional outdoor camp activities.

1106 Camp Dream Street
Kaplen JCC on the Palisades
411 East Clinton Ave.
Tenafly, NJ 07670
201-569-7900
Fax: 201-569-7448
info@jccotp.org
www.jccotp.org

Jordan Shenker, Chief Executive Officer
Miriam Chilton, Chief Operating Officer
Kevin Cunningham, Chief Financial Officer

Dream Street is a camp program for children with cancer and other blood disorders. Activities include swimming, arts and crafts, horseback riding and more.

1107 Camp Jaycee
Camp Jaycee Administrative Office
985 Livingston Ave.
North Brunswick, NJ 08902
732-737-8279
Fax: 732-737-8279
info@campjaycee.org
www.campjaycee.org

Maureen Brennan, Camp Director
Nicole Goodwin, Coordinator, Camping Services
Camp Jaycee offers residential summer camp programs for adults with developmental and intellectual disabilities. The campsite is located in Effort, PA.

1108 Camp Jotoni
51 Old Stirling Rd.
Warren, NJ 07059
908-753-4244
www.campjotoni.org

Josh Burke, Director
Sponsored by the Arc of Somerset County, Camp Jotoni is a day and residential camp for children and adults with developmental disabilities. Campers are ages 5-21.

1109 Camp Merry Heart
Easterseals New Jersey
21 O'Brien Rd.
Hackettstown, NJ 07840
908-852-3896
Fax: 908-852-9263
recreaton@nj.easterseals.com
www.easterseals.com/nj

Brian Fitzgerald, President & CEO
An organized program of swimming, arts and crafts, boating, nature study and travel offered to campers with a variety of disabilities.

1110 Camp Nejeda
Camp Nejeda Foundation
910 Saddleback Rd.
PO Box 156
Stillwater, NJ 07875
973-383-2611
Fax: 973-383-9891
info@campnejeda.org
www.campnejeda.org

Bill Vierbuchen, Executive Director
Ginnie Ramberger, Registrar & Staff Coordinator
Jim Daschbach, Camp Director
For children with diabetes, ages 7-16. Provides an active and safe camping experience which enables the children to learn about and understand diabetes. Activities include boating, swimming, fishing, archery, and camping skills.

1111 Camp Quality New Jersey
PO Box 264
Adelphia, NJ 07710
908-556-6548
newjersey@campqualityusa.org
www.campqualityusa.org/nj

Kaitlin DeGennaro Wilson, Executive Director
Camp Quality is for children with cancer and their siblings. The camp offers a stress-free environment that offers exciting activities and fosters new friendships, while helping to give the children courage, motivation and emotional strength.

1112 Camp Sun'N Fun
The Arc Gloucester
1555 Gateway Blvd.
West Deptford, NJ 08096
856-629-4502
camp@thearcgloucester.org
www.thearcgloucester.org

Lisa Conley, Chief Executive Officer
Camp is located in Williamstown, New Jersey. Summer sessions for campers with developmental disabilities. Coed, ages 5+. Activities include swimming, arts and crafts, sports, games, music, dance and drama.

1113 Explorer's Club Camp
New Behavioural Network
2 Pin Oak Lane
Suite 250
Cherry Hill, NJ 08003
856-874-1616
Fax: 856-424-7660
nbh@nbngroup.com
www.newbehavioralnetwork.com/summer-camp
Explorer's Club Camp is a summer day camp program for children ages 4-17 who have ADHD, Austism Spectrum Disorder, and other behavior challenges. The camp's goal is to maintain progress made during the school year while giving campers a fun camp experience. Full and half day sessions offered.

1114 Happiness Is Camping
62 Sunset Lake Rd.
Hardwick, NJ 07825
908-362-6733
Fax: 908-362-5197
rich@happinessiscamping.org
www.happinessiscamping.org

Laura San Miguel, President
Julie McMahon, Secretary
Beth Fuchs, Treasurer
Located in Hardwick, New Jersey, Happiness is Camping is a week-long camp for kids with cancer and their siblings, ages 6-16. The camp is free for all attendees, and campers participate in a variety of traditional outdoor activities, including canoeing, fishing, swimming, archery, and more.

1115 Harbor Haven Summer Program
4 Hanover Rd.
Unit C3
Florham Park, NJ 07932
908-964-5411
Fax: 908-964-0511
info@harborhaven.com
www.harborhaven.com

Robyn Tanne, Director
Kim Van Woeart, Associate Director
Ryan Cox, Assistant Director
A seven-week summer program for children ages 3-15 with mild special needs. Harbor Haven offers traditional outdoor recreation activities and a daily academic period which reinforces math, reading, and language arts.

1116 Mane Stream
83 Old Turnpike Rd.
PO Box 305
Oldwick, NJ 08858
908-439-9636
Fax: 908-439-2338
info@manestreamnj.org
www.manestreamnj.org

Trish Hegeman, Executive Director
Jane Banta, Camp Director
Louisa Bartok, Manager, Marketing & Communications
A summer day camp for children with physical and cognitive challenges, their siblings, and non-disabled children. The camp is primarily focused on horsemanship lessons, with activities such as riding lessons, grooming, tacking, leading, basic horse care, and more. Eight week-long sessions available.

1117 Rising Treetops at Oakhurst
111 Monmouth Rd.
Oakhurst, NJ 07755
732-531-0215
Fax: 732-531-0292
info@risingtreetops.org
www.risingtreetops.org

Robert Pacenza, Executive Director
Charles Sutherland, Camp Director
Lori Schenck, Assistant Director, Services
A summer and day camp for adults and children with special needs, including autism and physical and intellectual disabilities. Campers experience traditional camp activities while gaining skills for greater independence.

1118 Round Lake Camp
NJY Camps
21 Plymouth St.
Fairfield, NJ 07004
973-575-3333
Fax: 973-575-4188
rlc@njycamps.org
www.roundlakecamp.org

Aryn Barer, Director
Round Lake Camp is for children ages 7-17 with learning differences and social communication disorders. Campers enjoy swimming, boating, sailing, mountain biking, and arts and crafts. The camp is located in Milford, PA.

New Mexico

1119 ADA Camp 180
American Diabetes Association
Fort Lone Tree Camp
307 Fort Lone Tree Rd.
Capitan, NM 88316
602-861-4731
campsupport@diabetes.org
www.diabetes.org
A program of the American Diabetes Association, Camp 180 provides camp experiences for children ages 8-12 and teens ages 13-16 with diabetes. The camp is held at Fort Lone Tree Camp in Capitan, New Mexico.

1120 Camp Enchantment
Rio Grande Community Development Corporation
318 Isleta Blvd. SW
Albuquerque, NM 87105
info@campenchantment.org
www.campenchantment.org

Shayna Rosenblum, Camp Director
A summer camp for children and teens ages 7-17 who have been diagnosed with cancer. The camp is held at Manzano Mountain Retreat in Torreon, NM. Activities include swimming, kayaking, dancing, archery, and more. The camping session is seven days.

1121 Camp Rising Sun
Center for Development and Disability
2300 Menaul Blvd. NE
Albuquerque, NM 87107
505-272-3000
800-270-1861
Fax: 505-272-5896
hsc.unm.edu/cdd

Paul Brouse, Camp Director
Held at the Manzano Mountain Retreat southeast of Albuquerque, Camp Rising sun is a summer camp designed specifially for children and teens with Autism Spectrum Disorder and their peers, ages 8-17. Activities include hiking, sports, photography, kayaking, campouts, and other nature activities.

New York

1122 ADA Camp Aspire
American Diabetes Association
809 Five Points Rd.
Rush, NY 14543
585-458-3040
www.diabetes.org
A program of the American Diabetes Association, Camp Aspire provides camp experiences for children with diabetes. The camp is held at the Rochester Rotary Sunshine Campus in Rush, New York.

1123 Autism Summer Respite Program
Commonpoint Queens
58-20 Little Neck Pkwy.
Little Neck, NY 11362
718-225-6750
larmband@commonpointqueens.org
www.commonpointqueens.org/summercamp

Lisa Armband, Contact
An afternoon camping program for children, teens, and young adults ages 5-21 with Autism and similar disabilities. Located at Sam Field Center.

1124 AutismUp: YMCA Summer Social Skills Program
AutismUp
50 Science Pkwy.
Rochester, NY 14620   585-248-9011
                                              Fax: 585-248-9159
                                          contact@autismup.org
                                                 autismup.org

Sarah Milko, Executive Director
Christina Hilton, Director, Finance & Operations
Lisa Ponticello, Director, Marketing & Development
This program is a collaboration between AutismUp and the
Greater Rochester YMCA. The Summer Social Skills Program is
a day camp held at Camp Arrowhead for children, 4-16, with Au-
tism Spectrum Disorders. Half day and full day sessions avail-
able, and campers are integrated into regular camp activities.

1125 Camp Abilities Brockport
The College at Brockport, State Univ of New York
350 New Campus Drive
Brockport, NY 14420   585-395-5361
                                          llieberman@brockport.edu
                                            www.campabilities.org

Lauren Lieberman, Camp Director
Alex Stribing, Assistant Director
Emily Gilbert, Aquatics Director
A one-week sports camp for children who are visually impaired,
blind or deaf blind. Children learn to be more physically active,
which in turn improves their health and well being.

1126 Camp Adventure
KiDS NEED MoRE
PO Box 305
Copiague, NY 11726   631-608-3135
                                              Fax: 631-532-4944
                                          info@kidsneedmore.org
                                                kidsneedmore.org

Melissa Firmes, President
John Ray, Treasurer
Jacqueline Lorenz, Secretary
Camp Adventure is a one-week sleep away camp for children and
teens ages 6-18 dealing with cancer and other life threatening illnesses. The camp takes place on Shelter Island at Quinipet Camp
and Retreat Center.

1127 Camp Anne
AHRC New York City
228 Four Corners Lane
Ancramdale, NY 12503   518-329-5649
                                              Fax: 518-329-5689
                                          michael.rose@ahrcnyc.org
                                              camping.ahrcnyc.org

Michael Rose, Camp Director
A day summer camp program for children and adults with intellectual and developmental disabilities. The camp offers activities
such as cooking, crafts, nature, sports, swimming, and more.
Camp Anne offers three 11-day sessions for adults ages 21-59,
and two 11-day sessions for childres ages 5-20. Each session can
accommodate 100 campers.

1128 Camp COAST
Empowering People's Independence (EPI)
2 Townline Circle
Rochester, NY 14623   585-442-4430
                                              Fax: 585-442-6964
                                                  info@epiny.org
                                                  www.epiny.org

Michael Radell, Camp Director
Camp COAST is a summer camp for young adults ages 18+ with
epilepsy and I/DD.

1129 Camp EAGR
Empowering People's Independence (EPI)
2 Townline Circle
Rochester, NY 14623   585-442-4430
                                              Fax: 585-442-6964
                                                  info@epiny.org
                                                  www.epiny.org

Michael Radell, Camp Director
Camp EAGR is a summer sleep-away camp for children with epilepsy and their siblings. Activities include swimming, horseback
riding, and rock climbing.

1130 Camp Good Days and Special Times
1332 Pitsford-Mendon Rd.
PO Box 665
Mendon, NY 14506   585-624-5555
                                                    800-785-2135
                                              Fax: 585-624-5799
                                          info@campgooddays.org
                                            www.campgooddays.org

Wendy Bleier-Mervis, Executive Director
Sheri Watkins, CFO & Director, Administration
The camp is dedicated to improving the quality of life for children
and adults affected by cancer or other life challenges. The camp
offers week-long sessions that are free of charge.

1131 Camp High Hopes
82 Pixley Rd.
Chenango Forks, NY 13746   607-226-5474
                                          joe@camphighhopes.org
                                            www.camphighhopes.org

Joe Brennan, Director
Hope Woodcock-Ross, Health Director
A week-long summer camp program for boys with hemophilia.
The camp has a 24-hour physician and nursing staff. Ages 7-17,
boys only.

1132 Camp Huntington
56 Bruceville Rd.
High Falls, NY 12440-5100   845-687-7840
                                                    855-707-2267
                                              Fax: 855-707-2267
                                          www.camphuntington.com

Daniel Falk, Executive Director
Dylan Sloan, Program Director
Margaret Short, Health Director
A co-ed residential summer camp specifically designed to focus
on adaptive and therapeutic recreation. Campers include those
with learning and developmental disabilities, ADD/HD, Autism
Spectrum Disorders, Asperger's, PDD, and other special needs.
Programs focus on recreation and social skills, independence,
and participation.

1133 Camp Kehilla
Henry Kaufmann Campgrounds
75 Colonial Springs Rd.
Wheatley Heights, NY 11798   516-484-1545
                                          jwasserman@sjjcc.org
                                              www.campkehilla.org

Joe Wasserman, Camp Director
Victoria Granatelli, Assistant Camp Director
A year-round camp for children, teens, and young adults with developmental disabilities and other neurodevelopmental conditions. Ages 5-21.

1134 Camp Little Oak
Aldersgate Camp & Retreat Center
7955 Brantingham Rd.
Greig, NY 13345   425-770-1801
                                                camplittleoak.org

Hannah Russell, Camp Director
A non-profit, week-long summer camp for girls diagnosed with a
bleeding disorder. The camp is held at Aldersgate Camp in Greig,
New York. Camp Little Oak runs traditional summer camp activities such as swimming, canoeing, and archery, as well as provides
education about blood disorders and conducts community service
projects.

1135 Camp Mark Seven
Mark Seven Deaf Foundation
144 Mohawk Hotel Rd.
Old Forge, NY 13420   315-207-5706
                                              TTY: 315-357-6089
                                          registrar@campmark7.org
                                              www.campmark7.org

Dave Staehle, Camp Director
A camp program for hard-of-hearing, deaf and hearing people.
Coed, open to all ages. The camp is located on the Fourth Lake in
the Adirondack Mountains.

1136 Camp Pa-Qua-Tuck
2 Chet Swezey Rd.
Center Moriches, NY 11934   631-878-1070
                                  www.camppaquatuck.com
Alyssa Pecorino, Executive Director
Melissa Locrotondo, Chief of Programming
Tommy Ryan, Director, Respite Camp
Camp Pa-Qua-Tuck is a residential camp for individuals with physical and developmental disabilities. The camp also offers Respite Camp, a weekend camp program for ages 6-40.

1137 Camp Ramapo
Ramapo for Children
Rt. 52/Salisbury Turnpike
PO Box 266
Rhinebeck, NY 12572   845-876-8403
                             Fax: 845-876-8414
                    office@ramapoforchildren.org
                      www.ramapoforchildren.org
Matthew McKnight, Camp Director
Lenora Sealey, Associate Camp Director
A residential summer camp for youth ages 6-16 with social, emotional, or learning challenges.

1138 Camp Reece
1782 S Johnsburg Rd.
Johnsburg, NY 12843-1909   212-289-4872
                                  info@campreece.org
                                  www.campreece.org
Duncan Lester, Executive Director
Octavia Man, Camp Director
Kiersten Twitchell, Camp Director
A sleep-away camp for children ages 10-17 with special needs. The camp is located at Skidmore College and offers activities such as photography, rafting, biking, sports, and more. The camp serves boys and girls with disabilities such as ADD/ADHD, learning disabilities, and high-functioning autism. There are two 3-week sessions or the full 6-week session available.

1139 Camp Sisol
Jewish Community Center of Greater Rochester/JCC
1200 Edgewood Ave.
Rochester, NY 14618   585-461-2000
                             Fax: 585-461-0805
                    bettertogether@jccrochester.org
                         www.jccrochester.org
Josh Weinstein, Chief Executive Officer
Coed, ages 5-16. Camp Sisol accommodates children with special needs.

1140 Camp Tova
92nd Street Y
1395 Lexington Ave.
New York, NY 10128   212-415-5573
                                  www.92y.org
Seth Pinsky, Chief Executive Officer
Alyse Myers, President
Lauren Wexler, Director, Camps
Camp Tova is a program for children with developmental disabilities. Campers participate in sports, arts, and outdoor activities and develop their creative, social, and physical skills.

1141 Camp Venture, Inc.
25 Smith St.
Suite 510
Nanuet, NY 10954   845-624-3860
                                  www.campventure.org
Matthew Shelley, Chief Executive Officer
Celia Solomita, Chief Financial Officer
Marie Pardi, Chief Program Officer
Camp Venture is a day camp for children ages 5-12 with and without developmental disabilities. Located in Stony Point, the camp also offers a young adult group for teens ages 13-21 with developmental disabilities. Children will experience regular camp activities while benefitting from group engagement.

1142 Camp Whitman on Seneca Lake
PO Box 24393
Rochester, NY 14624   315-201-0193
                             Fax: 315-531-4002
                    camp@campwhitman.org
                      www.campwhitman.org
Lea Kone, Camp Director
Provides camp opportunities for individuals with developmental disabilities. Campers are encouraged to participate in a full range of activities including games, sports, swimming, singing, and dancing.

1143 Clover Patch Camp
Center for Disability Services
55 Helping Hand Lane
Glenville, NY 12302   518-384-3042
                             Fax: 518-384-3001
                    cloverpatchcamp@cfdsny.org
                      www.cloverpatchcamp.org
Cindy Francis, Camp Director
Jackie Richards, Director, Residential Services
Clover Patch Camp is operated by the Center for Disability Services and is located in Glenville, New York. The camp is for individuals with a variety of disabilities. For ages 5+.

1144 Double H Ranch
97 Hidden Valley Rd.
Lake Luzerne, NY 12846   518-696-5676
                             Fax: 518-696-4528
                    myurenda@doublehranch.org
                      www.doublehranch.org
Max Yurenda, CEO & Executive Director
Kate Walsh, Camp Director
Alex Griffen, Assistant Camp Director, Programs
Summer residential camp and winter sports programs for children and young adults ages 6-16 who have cancer and other life threatening illnesses. The programs are free of charge and some of the recreational activities include bead making, arts and crafts, tennis, soccer, and volleyball.

1145 Friendship Circle Day Camp
Friendship Circle Upper East Side
419 E 77th St.
New York, NY 10075   office@friendshipcirclenyc.org
                          www.friendshipcirclenyc.org
Shlomo Gutnick, Executive Director
Sara Gutnick, Program Director
Dassy Chein, Program Coordinator
The Friendship Circle Day Camp allows children with special needs the opportunity to have a full camp experience. Campers participate in activities such as field trips, music, arts and crafts, and performances.

1146 Gow School Summer Programs
2491 Emery Rd.
South Wales, NY 14139   716-687-2004
                             Fax: 716-687-2003
                    summer@gow.org
                      www.gow.org
Matthew Fisher, Director
Co-ed summer programs for students ages 8-16 with dyslexia or similar learning disabilities. Offers a blend of morning academics, afternoon/evening traditional camp activities and weekend overnights.

1147 Kamp Kiwanis
New York District Kiwanis Foundation
9020 Kiwanis Rd.
Taberg, NY 13471   315-336-4568
                             Fax: 315-336-3845
                    kamp@kampkiwanis.org
                      www.kampkiwanis.org
Rebecca Lopez Clemence, Executive Director
Luke Clemence, Camp Director
Dori Gross, Assistant Camp Director
Kamp Kiwanis is a mainstream camp for underprivileged youth with and without special needs. Twenty campers with disabilities are integrated into weekly sessions. Programs are offered for children, teens, and adults.

1148 Katy Isaacson Elaine Gordon Lodge
AHRC New York City
653 Colgate Rd.
Box 37
East Jewett, NY 12424
518-589-6000
Fax: 518-589-6583
matthew.hatcher@ahrcnyc.org
camping.ahrcnyc.org

Matt Hatcher, Camp Director
An alternative and traditional summer day camp for adults and teens with intellectual and developmental disabilities. The lodge offers five 11-day sessions for adults ages 18-29, and one session for teens ages 13-17. Activities include boating, swimming, pony rides, sports, and more.

1149 Lisa Beth Gerstman Camp
Lisa Beth Gerstman Foundation
439 Oak St.
Suite 1
Garden City, NY 11530
516-594-4400
Fax: 516-594-7085
info@lisabethgerstman.org
www.lisabethgerstman.org

Harvey Gerstman, Co-Founder
Carol Gerstman, Co-Founder
Linda Gerstman, Co-Founder
A summer day camp for children with special needs. Activities include swimming, sports, and arts and crafts. Camps are located across the New York Metropolitan Area.

1150 Maplebrook School
5142 Route 22
Amenia, NY 12501
845-373-9511
Fax: 845-373-7029
admissions@maplebrookschool.org
www.maplebrookschool.org

Donna Konkolics, Head of School
Roger Fazzone, President
Jennifer Scully, Assistant Head, Postsecondary Studies
A coeducational boarding school which offers a six week camp for children with learning differences and ADD.

1151 Marist Brothers Mid-Hudson Valley Camp
1455 Broadway
PO Box 197
Esopus, NY 12429
845-384-6620
info@maristbrotherscenter.org
www.maristbrotherscenter.org

Jim Sheldon, Camp Director
Timothy Hagan, Director, Operations
Donnell Neary, Assistant Director
The camp provides week-long summer sessions for children who have a variety of special needs and illnesses, including cancer and physical, developmental, and mental disabilities. Each session is specific to the special need or illness.

1152 Mosholu Day Camp
Mosholu Montefiore Community Center
3450 Dekalb Ave.
New York, NY 10467
718-882-4000
frontdesk@mmcc.org
www.mmcc.org/camp

Rita Santelia, Chief Executive Officer
Shakil M. Khan, Chief Financial Officer
Jackina Farshtey, Chief of Staff
A day camp program for children in grades 1-10. The day camp offers specific programs for children and teens who are developmentally disabled. Camp Sunshine is for children ages 5-12, and Camp Elan is for children ages 12-16.

1153 Southampton Fresh Air Home
36 Barkers Island Rd.
Southampton, NY 11968
631-283-1594
Fax: 631-283-7596
www.sfah.org

Thomas Naro, Executive Director
David Billingham, Camp Director
Nathan Unwin, Assistant Camp Director
A residential camp facility accommodating physically challenged children. The Special Needs Summer Camp is for children and teens ages 8-18. One or three week sessions available, as well

as day camp. The SFAH provides adapted programs and activities that allow campers to develop physically, emotionally, and psychologically.

1154 Special Services Summer Day Camp
Commonpoint Queens
58-20 Little Neck Pkwy.
Little Neck, NY 11362
718-225-6750
larmband@commonpointqueens.org
www.commonpointqueens.org/summercamp

Lisa Armband, Contact
A day camp program for children and youth ages 5-21 with developmental disabilities. Activities include dancing, swimming, arts and crafts, and community-based field trips. The program is held at the Henry Kaufmann Campgrounds.

1155 Summit Camp
55 W 38th St.
4th Floor
New York, NY 10018
570-253-4381
info@summitcamp.com
www.summitcamp.com

Shepherd Baum, Director
Leah Love, Assistant Director
Thea Mullis, Travel Director
The camp is located in Honesdale, Pennsylvania, and is for children ages 8-19 who have a variety of developmental, social, or learning challenges. In addition to traditional camp activities, Summit Camp has a strong focus on social skills development and interpersonal growth.

1156 Sunshine Campus
809 Five Points Rd.
Rush, NY 14543
585-533-2080
www.sunshinecamp.org

Tracey Dreisbach, Executive Director
Brandi Koch, Camp Director
Jarod Alexander, Facility Director
The camp is located in Rush, New York. Camping sessions for children and young adults with a variety of disabilities. Ages 7-21. Campers experience a variety of traditional summer camp activities, including climbing wall, swimming, boating, hiking, and sports.

1157 VISIONS Vacation Camp for the Blind (VCB)
VISIONS Center on Blindness
111 Summit Park Rd.
Spring Valley, NY 10977
845-354-3003
888-245-8333
info@visionsvcb.org
www.visionsvcb.org

Krystal Findley-Jones, Director
A nonprofit agency that promotes the independence of people of all ages who are blind or visually impaired. Camp offers Braille classes, computers with large print and voice output, support groups, discussions, cooking classes, personal and home management training, and large print and Braille books.

1158 Wagon Road Camp
Children's Aid Society
117 W 124th St.
3rd Floor
New York, NY 10027
212-949-4800
www.childrensaidnyc.org

Phoebe Boyer, President & CEO
Vince Canziani, Camp Director
Wagon Road Day Camp is a co-ed program for children ages 6-13 with a variety of disabilities held in Chappaqua, New York. Activities include athletics, horsemanship, theater arts, nature studies, and arts and crafts.

1159 West Hills Day Camp
21 Sweet Hollow Rd.
Huntington, NY 11743
631-427-6700
Fax: 631-427-6504
info@westhillscamp.com
westhillsdaycamp.com

Susan Diamond, Director
Kimberly Doxey, Director
A summer day camp program for children with autism spectrum disorders an other related neurobiological disorders. Located on

Long Island, activities include swimming, climbing/ropes course, photography, arts and crafts, and more.

1160   **YMCA Camp Chingachgook on Lake George**
Capital District YMCA
1872 Pilot Knob Rd.
Kattskill Bay, NY 12844   518-656-9462
                                       Fax: 518-656-9362
                                   chingachgook@cdymca.org
                                   www.lakegeorgecamp.org

Jine Andreozzi, Executive Director
Mike Obermayer, Director, Summer Program
Carol Lewis, Office Manager
Offers sailing programs for people with disabilities.

North Carolina

1161   **Camp Carefree**
275 Carefree Lane
Stokesdale, NC 27357   336-427-0966
                                   directors@campcarefree.org
                                   www.campcarefree.org

Diane Samelak, Executive Director
Tony McCallum, Program Director
JeNai Davis, Program Director
A free, one-week camp for children with chronic illnesses. The camp also offers programs for siblings of ill children and children with a sick parent.

1162   **Camp Carolina Trails**
American Diabetes Association
1300 Baxter St.
Suite 150
Charlotte, NC 28204   704-373-9111
                                   campsupport@diabetes.org
                                   www.diabetes.org

The camp is for children ages 7-16 years of age who have diabetes. The camp is held on the YMCA's Camp Hanes campground in King, North Carolina. Activities include swimming, hiking, and field games. The camp employs a complete medical staff consisting of registered nurses, dieticians, and pediatric endoctrinologists.

1163   **Camp Dogwood**
7062 Camp Dogwood Dr.
PO Box 39
Sherrills Ford, NC 28673   828-478-2135
                                   tammy@nclionsinc.org
                                   nclionscampdogwood.org
Tammy Thomas, Camp Administrator
A recreational facility on Lake Norman offering 10 week-long sessions for adults who are blind and visually impaired. Ages 18 and up. Activities include swimming, tubing, local field trips, bowling, and more. Service dogs welcome.

1164   **Camp New Hope**
PO Box 154
Glendale Springs, NC 28629   336-982-3797
                                   campnewhopenc.com

Randy Brown, Executive Director
Camp New Hope is a privately owned facility for children with life-threatening medical conditions and their families. Families are able to enjoy fishing, canoeing, tubing, swimming, and more at their leisure.

1165   **Camp Royall**
250 Bill Ash Rd.
Moncure, NC 27559   919-542-1033
                                       Fax: 919-533-5324
                                   camproyall@autismsociety-nc.org
                                   www.autismsociety-nc.org/camp-royall
Sara Gage, Director
A week-long overnight and day camp for children and adults with autism. Campers participate in traditional camp activities such as swimming, boating, hiking, and arts and crafts. Counselor-to-camper ratio is 1:1 or 1:2, depending on the campers' needs.

1166   **Camp Sertoma**
Millstone 4-H Center
1296 Mallard Dr.
Ellerbe, NC 28338   sertomadeafcamp@gmail.com
                                   www.campsertomaclub.org
Sandy Waterman, Contact
Keith Russell, Camp Director, Millstone 4-H Center
Camp Sertoma is a camp program for deaf and hard of hearing youth. Activities include swimming, canoeing, fishing, hiking, hayrides, campfires, and games. Coed, ages 8-16.

1167   **Camp Tekoa**
United Methodist Camp Tekoa
PO Box 1793
Flat Rock, NC 28731-1793   828-692-6516
                                       Fax: 828-697-3288
                                   www.camptekoa.org

John Isley, Executive Director
Dave Bollen, Assistant Director
Karen Rohrer, Business Manager
Offers special needs camp programs for individuals with developmental disabilities.

1168   **SOAR Summer Adventures**
226 SOAR Lane
PO Box 388
Balsam, NC 28707   828-456-3435
                                       Fax: 801-820-3050
                                   admissions@soarnc.org
                                   www.soarnc.org

John Willson, Executive Director
A nonprofit adventure program working with disadvantaged youth diagnosed with learning disabilities in an outdoor, challenge-based environment. Focuses on esteem building and social skills development through rock climbing, backpacking, whitewater rafting, mountaineering, sailing, snorkeling, and more. Offers two week, one month, and semester programs. Locations include North Carolina, Florida, Wyoming, California, New York, Belize, Costa Rica, and the Caribbean.

1169   **Talisman Summer Camp**
64 Gap Creek Rd.
Zirconia, NC 28790   828-697-6313
                                   info@talismancamps.com
                                   www.talismancamps.com

Linda Tatsapaugh, Operations Director & Owner
Robiyn Mims, Admissions Director & Owner
Cory Greene, Camp Director
Talisman Summer Camp is located 40 minutes south of Asheville, North Carolina. Offers a program of hiking, rafting, climbing, and caving for young people with autism, ADHD and learning disabilities. Coed, ages 6-22.

1170   **Victory Junction**
4500 Adam's Way
Randleman, NC 27317   336-498-9055
                                   info@victoryjunction.org
                                   www.victoryjunction.org

Chad Coltrane, President & CEO
Lisa Weber, Chief Financial Officer
Frances Beasley, Chief Development Officer
The camp serves children with a variety of chronic medical conditions or serious illnesses, including Autism, Cancer, Craniofacial Anomalies, Diabetes, Sickle Cell, Spina Bifida and more. Victory Junction provides traditional camp activities and also includes a NASCAR themed area.

North Dakota

1171   **Camp Sioux**
American Diabetes Association
106 Solid Rock Circle
Park River, ND 58270   763-593-5333
                                   campsupport@diabetes.org
                                   www.diabetes.org

Camp Sioux, located in Park River, ND, is a week-long residential summer camp for children ages 8-15 who are living with diabetes. Programs encourage independence and self management with appropriate medical supervision to ensure the best possible experience for every camper. Nutrition activities, blood glucose monitoring, and injections/medications are integrated into the camp program.

Ohio

1172   Camp Arye
Jewish Community Center of Greater Columbus
1125 College Ave.
Columbus, OH 43209   614-231-2731
                                   Fax: 614-231-8222
                                   www.columbusjcc.org
Raeann Cronebach, Director
Ariana Solomon, Inclusion Coordinator
A Jewish summer camp for children and young adults with developmental, physical, emotional, mental and learning disabilities. Camp Arye is co-ed and for children in grades 1-7.

1173   Camp Cheerful
Achievement Centers For Children
15000 Cheerful Lane
Strongsville, OH 44136-5420   440-238-6200
                                    Fax: 440-238-1858
                                   www.achievementcenters.org
Sally Farwell, President & CEO
Scott Peplin, Executive Vice President & CFO
Deborah Osgood, Vice President, Development & Marketing
Camp Cheerful provides a number of day and overnight camping options for children and adults who have disabilities. The camp hosts traditional camp activities as well as year-round therapeutic horseback riding sessions and an accessible high ropes challenge course during the summer. The focus of activities is to increase the quality of life while encouraging confidence and independence.

1174   Camp Christopher: SumFun Day Camp
Catholic Charities Disability Services
Camp Christopher
930 N Hametown Rd.
Akron, OH 44333   330-376-2267
                                      800-296-2267
                            campchristopher@ccdocle.org
                            ccdocle.org/programs/sumfun-day-camp
Tess Flannery, Contact
A multi-week summer day camp for children, teens, and young adults ages 5-21 with developmental disabilities. Campers participate in regular camp activities while building confidence and social skills.

1175   Camp Echoing Hills
36272 County Rd. 79
Warsaw, OH 43844   740-327-2311
                                      www.ehvi.org
Lauren Unger, Camp Administrator
Summer camp for children and adults with physical, intellectual and developmental disabilities. The camp focuses on religion, social interaction, and skill development.

1176   Camp Emanuel
PO Box 752343
Dayton, OH 45475   937-477-5504
                            crawford@campemanuel.org
                            www.campemanuel.weebly.com
Brian Demarke, President
Stephanie Ackner, Vice President
Mary Foreman, Secretary
Camp Emanuel is a camp for hearing impaired and hearing youth. There are day sessions for children 5-14 and overnight resident sessions for children and teens 9-17. The camp aims to promote descision making, self-esteem, and acceptance by integrating non-hearing children with hearing children.

1177   Camp Hamwi
LifeCare Alliance - Central Ohio Diabetes Assoc.
1699 West Mound St.
Columbus, OH 43223   614-278-3130
                            amyer@lifecarealliance.org
                            www.lifecarealliance.org
Anthony Myer, Director, Youth & Family Program

A summer camp for kids with diabetes, ages 7-17. Sessions are divided by age group, with a Junior Challenge Week for ages 7-12 and a Senior Challenged week for ages 13-17. Activities include horseback riding, sports, swimming, and other outdoor activities.

1178   Camp Happiness
Catholic Charities Disability Services
7911 Detroit Ave.
Cleveland, OH 44102   216-334-2900
                                   Fax: 216-334-2905
                            ccdocle.org/programs/camp-happiness
Marilyn Scott, Director
Lauren Mailey, Program Administrator
Camp Happiness welcomes children and young adults ages 5-21 with intellectual and developmental disabilities. In addition to recreational services, Camp Happiness also provides educational and social services to help participants continue to practice and develop skills throughout the year.

1179   Camp Ho Mita Koda
14040 Auburn Rd.
Newbury, OH 44065   440-739-4095
                            info@camphomitakoda.org
                            www.camphomitakoda.org
Ian Roberts, Executive Director
Eric Brown, Camp Director
Camp Ho Mita Koda is a summer camp for children with type 1 diabetes. The camp aims to provide outdoor activities while also educating and building life skills for children with diabetes. Offers overnight camp, family camp, specialty camp, and leadership development programs.

1180   Camp Joy
10117 Old 3C Hwy.
PO Box 157
Clarksville, OH 45113   937-289-2031
                            info@camp-joy.org
                            camp-joy.org
Jen Eismeier, Executive Director
Casey Miller, Director, Operations
Jen Alvis, Director, Business Operations
A summer camp organization for children and teens with a variety of disabilities. Sessions for children, teens and young adults with asthma, HIV/AIDS, spina bifida, limb loss, cancer, blood diseases, and immune disorders.

1181   Camp Ko-Man-She
Diabetes Dayton
2555 S Dixie Dr.
Suite 112
Dayton, OH 45409   937-220-6611
                                   Fax: 937-224-0240
                            admin@diabetesdayton.org
                            www.diabetesdaytoncamp.com
Susan McGovern, Executive Director
Camp Ko-Man-She is located in Bellefontaine, Ohio, and is held annually for children with diabetes. The camp's goal is for children to socialize with other children who also have diabetes and to have fun outdoors in a medically supervised setting. Co-ed, ages 8-17.

1182   Camp Korelitz
American Diabetes Association
Camp Joy
10117 Old 3C Hwy.
Clarksville, OH 45113   513-759-9330
                            campsupport@diabetes.org
                            www.diabetes.org
A week-long residential camp for children ages 9-15 with diabetes. Camp Korelitz is a program of the American Diabetes Association, and is held at Camp Joy in Clarksville, Ohio. Activities include climbing walls, archery, and canoeing, as well as discussions and education about nutrition and diabetes.

1183   Camp Nuhop
1077 Township Rd. 2916
Perrysville, OH 44864   419-938-7151
                                      www.nuhop.org
Trevor Dunlap, Executive Director & CEO
Chris Clyde, Associate Director
Matt Poland, Director, Outdoor Education

A summer residential program for youth ages 6-18 with learning disabilities, behavioral disorders, or other neuroatypical disorders. Activities include outdoor education and team-building workshops. The staff-to-camper ratio is 3:7 or 3:8.

1184 Camp Oty'Okwa
24799 Purcell Rd.
South Bloomingville, OH 43152-9740   740-385-5279
rperkins@bbbscentralohio.org
campotyokwa.org

Rick Perkins, Camp Director
Matt Smith, Youth Camp Director
Emily Kridel, Environmental Education Director
Owned and operated by Big Brothers Big Sisters of Central Ohio, this summer camp accommodates children with disabilities such as ADD/ADHD, autism, learning disabilities, and behavioral or mood disorders.

1185 Camp Paradise
SHC, The Arc of Medina County
4283 Paradise Rd.
Seville, OH 44273   330-722-1900
shc@shc-medina.org
shc-medina.org/camp-paradise

Melanie Kasten-Krause, Executive Director
Shelly Wharton, Associate Executive Director
Michael Beh, Director, Finance
Camp Paradise is a summer camp for adults with developmental disabilities. The camp offers five weeks of themed programs. Day and residential camp available. Activities include music, art therapy, sports, swimming, bonfires, and more.

1186 Camp Quality Ohio
PO Box 358
Uniontown, OH 44685   234-738-2073
ohio@campqualityusa.org
www.campqualityusa.org/oh

Sarah Givens, Executive Director
Brian Krebs, Camp Director
Kelly Krebs, Camper Registrar
Camp Quality is for children with cancer and their siblings. The camp offers a stress-free environment that offers exciting activities and fosters new friendships, while helping to give the children courage, motivation and emotional strength.

1187 Camp Stepping Stone
Stepping Stones Inc. - Given Campus
5650 Given Rd.
Cincinnati, OH 45243   513-831-4660
Fax: 513-831-5918
steppingstonesohio.org

Chris Adams, Executive Director
Sam Allen, Director, Programs & Operations
Chris Brockman, Director, Facilities
A summer day camp program for youth with disabilities, ages 5-22. Activities include swimming, fishing, art, and music. Three separate three-week sessions are available. The camp is located at the Stepping Stones Given Campus in Cincinnati, Ohio.

1188 Camp Tiponi
Diabetes Dayton
2555 S Dixie Dr.
Suite 112
Dayton, OH 45409   937-220-6611
Fax: 937-224-0240
admin@diabetesdayton.org
www.diabetesdaytoncamp.com

Susan McGovern, Executive Director
A summer camp for youth with type 2 diabetes, prediabetes, or metabolic disorders. Campers participate in activities such as swimming, archery, hiking, and sports while gaining education and skills needed to maintain a healthy lifestyle. The camp is located at Camp Willson in Bellefontaine, Ohio.

1189 Courageous Acres
Courageous Community Services
12701 Waterville Swanton Rd.
Whitehouse, OH 43571   419-875-6828
Fax: 419-875-5598
info@ccsohio.org
www.ccsohio.org

Laura Kuhlenbeck, Executive Director
Courageous Acres is an accessible summer camp for children, teens, and adults with disabilities. Open to individuals ages 4+ in Northwest Ohio and Southeast Michigan.

1190 Flying Horse Farms
5260 State Route 95
Mt. Gilead, OH 43338   419-751-7077
Fax: 419-751-7010
info@flyinghorsefarms.org
flyinghorsefarms.org

Nichole E. Dunn, President & CEO
Rachel Escusa, Chief Advancement Officer
Stacey Kyser, Director, Development
Flying Horse Farms is a camp for children with serious illnesses, ages 7-15, and their families. The camp serves campers diagnosed with cancer, heart conditions, asthma, blood disorders, and more. Activities include swimming, fishing, and other traditional camp activities.

1191 Highbrook Lodge
Cleveland Sight Center
1909 E 101st St.
Cleveland, OH 44106   216-791-8118
Fax: 216-791-1101
TTY: 216-791-8119
info@clevelandsightcenter.org
www.clevelandsightcenter.org

Larry Benders, President & CEO
Kevin Krencisz, Chief Financial & Administrative Officer
Jassen Tawil, Director, Business Development & Customer Success
Camp is located in Chardon, Ohio. Summer sessions for children, adults and families who are blind or have low vision. Sessions include a wide range of outdoor camp activities. Camp activities focus on gaining independent skills, mobility, orientation and self-confidence in an accessible and traditional camp setting.

1192 Insight Horse Camp
Marmon Valley
7754 State Route 292 S
Zanesfield, OH 43360   937-593-8000
Fax: 937-593-6900
info@marmonvalley.com
marmonvalley.com

Matt Wiley, Executive Director
A coed resident camp program for children who are blind or visually impaired. The main focus of camp is on learning basic horsemanship skills. Campers also participate in traditional camp activities and Bible study discussions.

1193 Recreation Unlimited: Day Camp
Recreation Unlimited Foundation
7700 Piper Rd.
Ashley, OH 43003   740-548-7006
Fax: 740-747-2640
info@recreationunlimited.org
www.recreationunlimited.org

Paul L. Huttlin, Executive Director & CEO
Sarah Kelley, Camps Director
Camping sessions for children and teens, ages 5-22, with physical or developmental disabilities and their siblings. The camp provides a full day of traditional camp activities and aims to create an inclusive experience for all participants.

1194 Recreation Unlimited: Residential Camp
Recreation Unlimited Foundation
7700 Piper Rd.
Ashley, OH 43003   740-548-7006
Fax: 740-747-2640
info@recreationunlimited.org
www.recreationunlimited.org

Paul L. Huttlin, Executive Director & CEO
Sarah Kelley, Camps Director

Camping sessions for children and adults with a variety of physical and developmental disabilities. Two week long sessions for ages 8-22, one week long session for ages 18-35, and four week long sessions for ages 23 and up. The camp provides traditional outdoor recreation such as fishing, archery, exploration, campfires and more. A week long winter camp is offered for ages 18 and up.

1195 Recreation Unlimited: Respite Weekend Camp
Recreation Unlimited Foundation
7700 Piper Rd.
Ashley, OH 43003   740-548-7006
                                Fax: 740-747-2640
                        info@recreationunlimited.org
                        www.recreationunlimited.org
Paul L. Huttlin, Executive Director & CEO
Sarah Kelley, Camps Director
Camping sessions for children and adults with a variety of physical and developmental disabilities. There are seven weekend camps for youth ages 8-22 and eight weekend camps for adults ages 23 and up. Traditional outdoor activities are provided, along with lodging, meals, site nursing, and more.

1196 Recreation Unlimited: Specialty Camp
Recreation Unlimited Foundation
7700 Piper Rd.
Ashley, OH 43003   740-548-7006
                                Fax: 740-747-2640
                        info@recreationunlimited.org
                        www.recreationunlimited.org
Paul L. Huttlin, Executive Director & CEO
Sarah Kelley, Camps Director
Weekend and week-long camping sessions for youth and adults. The camps are dedicated to a specific disability or health concern and designed to meet the needs of certain groups.

1197 Rotary Camp
Rotary Club of Akron
4460 Rex Lake Dr.
Akron, OH 44319   330-644-4512
                                Fax: 330-644-1013
                        danr@akronymca.org
                        www.akronrotary.org
Dan Reynolds, Camp Director
Offers camping experiences for children and adults with disabilities. Rotary Camp provides traditional camping experiences while focusing on socialization and independence.

1198 St. Augustine Rainbow Camp
Disability Ministries at St. Augustine Parish
2486 W 14th St.
Cleveland, OH 44113   216-781-5530
                                Fax: 216-781-1124
                                TTY: 216-302-2375
                        augustine.rainbow.camp@gmail.com
                        www.staugustinecleveland.org
Rev. William O'Donnell, Administrator
Day camp for disabled and non-disabled youth ages 5-13. The camp serves youth from the deaf, hard-of-hearing, blind, and developmentally disabled communities of Greater Cleveland, as well as youth from the Tremont area.

1199 Stepping Stones: Camp Allyn
Stepping Stones Inc. - Allyn Campus
1414 Lake Allyn Rd.
Batavia, OH 45103   513-831-4660
                                Fax: 513-831-5918
                        steppingstonesohio.org
Chris Adams, Executive Director
Sam Allen, Director, Programs & Operations
Chris Brockman, Director, Facilities
An overnight residential camp for children and adults with disabilities. Coed, ages 16-65. Campers participate in crafts, swimming, hiking, and sports activities. The camp session lasts five days and is located at the Stepping Stones Allyn Campus in Batavia, Ohio.

1200 YMCA Outdoor Center Campbell Gard
4803 Augspurger Rd.
Hamilton, OH 45011   513-867-0600
                                Fax: 513-867-0127
                        campoffice@gmvymca.org
                        www.ccgymca.org
Pete Fasano, Executive Director
The camp is located in Hamilton, Ohio. Offers camp programs for youth with developmental disabilities. Runs overnight and day sessions for ages 7-22 and families.

Oklahoma

1201 Camp CANOE
Camp Fire Heart of Oklahoma
3309 E Hefner Rd.
Oklahoma City, OK 73131   405-478-5646
                        info@campfirehok.org
                        www.campfirehok.org
Penn Henthorn, Director, Programs & Camps
Camp CANOE is a summer day camp for children with autism and Down Syndrome. Camp CANOE focuses on skills such as self-reliance, confidence, communication, social skills, problem-solving, and more.

1202 Camp ClapHans
J.D. McCarty Center
2002 E Robinson St.
Norman, OK 73071   405-307-2865
                        camp@jdmc.org
                        www.campclaphans.com
Bobbie Hunter, Camp Director
A summer camp for children, teens, and young adults ages 8-18 with developmental disabilities. Activities include archery, arts and crafts, scavenger hunts, stargazing, and more. Sessions are four days and three nights, and are limited to 12 campers per session (6 boys and 6 girls).

1203 Camp Endres
Diabetes Solutions of Oklahoma, Inc.
3333 NW 63rd
Suite 100
Oklahoma City, OK 73116   405-843-4386
                                Fax: 888-665-2741
                        natalie@dsok.net
                        dsok.net/programs/camp-endres-day-camp
Kim Boaz-Wilson, Executive Director
Natalie Bayne, Camp Director
Camp Endres is a summer camp for individuals with diabetes. Programs include Day Camp (ages 4-10), Junior (ages 7-13), Senior (ages 14-18), Adult (ages 21+), and Family Camp sessions.

1204 Camp Lo-Be-Gon
American Diabetes Association
5401 S Harvard
Suite 120
Tulsa, OK 74135   918-492-3839
                                Fax: 918-492-4262
                        campsupport@diabetes.org
                        www.diabetes.org
A summer camp for youth ages 6-15 with diabetes. The camp is held at Camp Loughridge in Tulsa, Oklahoma.

1205 Camp Loughridge
4900 W 71st St.
Tulsa, OK 74131   918-446-4194
                        registrar@camploughridge.org
                        camploughridge.org
Jacob McIntosh, Executive Director
Loren Pirtle, Program Director
Camp Loughridge is a Christian summer day camp for children ages 6-10. The camp offers an Autism Inclusion program for children diagnosed with austism. Space is limited to two campers with autism per session.

1206 Camp Perfect Wings
Baptist General Convention of Oklahoma
3800 N May Ave.
Oklahoma City, OK 73112   405-942-3800
                                 www.oklahomabaptists.org

Becka Johnson, Camp Director
Camp program for children and adults with special needs, ages 8
and up. Activities include canoeing, pool games, low ropes challenges, and crafts. Held in spring/early summer.

Oregon

1207 Adventures Without Limits
1341 Pacific Ave.
Forest Grove, OR 97116   503-359-2568
                                Fax: 503-359-4671
                                info@awloutdoors.org
                                awloutdoors.com

Brad Bafaro, Founder & Executive Director
Jennifer Wilde, Director, Outreach & Development
Carrie Morton, Program Director
Adventures Without Limits facilitates inclusive outdoor adventures for people of all ages and ability levels. Trip activities include hiking, rafting, caving, rock climbing, kayaking,
snowshoeing, and more.

1208 B'nai B'rith Camp: Kehila Program
6443 SW Beaverton-Hillsdale Hwy.
Suite 234
Portland, OR 97221   503-496-7444
                            Fax: 503-452-0750
                            info@bbcamp.org
                            bbcamp.org

Michelle Koplan, Chief Executive Officer
Ben Charlton, Chief Program Officer
Bette Amir-Brownstein, Camp Director
The Kehila Program at B'nai B'rith Camp is a Jewish summer
camp program for children with special needs. This program is
run during the camp's Maccabee session.

1209 Camp Magruder
17450 Old Pacific Hwy.
Rockaway Beach, OR 97136   503-355-2310
                                  Fax: 503-355-8701
                                  troy@campmagruder.org
                                  www.campmagruder.org

Troy Taylor, Camp Director
Hope Montgomery, Program Director
Rik Gutzke, Facilities Manager
Camp is located in Rockaway Beach, Oregon. Sessions for teens
and adults with developmental disabilities through Camp Hope.

1210 Camp Meadowood Springs
77650 Meadowood Rd.
Weston, OR 97886   541-276-2752
                          Fax: 541-276-7227
                          camp@meadowoodsprings.org
                          www.meadowoodsprings.org

Michelle Nelson, Camp Director
This camp is designed to help children with communication disorders and learning differences. A full range of activities in recreational and clinical areas is available.

1211 Camp Millennium
2880 NW Stewart Pkwy.
Suite 200
Roseburg, OR 97471   541-677-0600
                            campmoregon@gmail.com
                            campmillennium.org

Mindy Bean, Camp Director
Steve Maine, Program Director
A week-long residential summer camp for children diagnosed
with cancer, ages 5-16. The camp is free to attend, and activities
include hiking, archery, horeseback riding, and more.

1212 Camp Starlight
PO Box 13107
Portland, OR 97213   503-964-1516
                            info@camp-starlight.org
                            camp-starlight.org

Melanie Smith-Wilusz, Camp Director
Kit Noble, Operations Director
Spike Huntington-Kline, Program Director
Camp Starlight is a week-long sleep-away summer camp for chil-
dren in Oregon and Washington whose lives are affected by
HIV/AIDS. There is a 1:1 staff-to-camper ratio. Activities in-
clude swimming, hiking, arts and crafts, archery, sports, and
games. The camp is free to attend.

1213 Camp Taloali
15934 N Santiam Hwy. SE
PO Box 32
Stayton, OR 97383   503-400-6547
                           campadmin@taloali.org
                           www.taloali.org

Randall Smith, Camp Administrator
Summer sessions for children who are deaf, hard of hearing, or
have a hearing impairment. Camp Taloali emphasizes communication, leadership, and social development.

1214 Camp Ukandu
601 SW 2nd Ave.
Suite 2300
Portland, OR 97204   503-276-2178
                            info@ukandu.org
                            www.ukandu.org

Jason Hickox, Executive Director
Ashley Light, Development Director
Kendra Gish, Program Director
Camp Ukandu is a summer camp for children and teens with cancer, ages 8-18, and their siblings. Activities include campfires,
horseback riding, rock walls, and more. The camp is free to
attend.

1215 Creating Memories
Creating Memories for Disabled Children
59895 Pollock Rd.
Joseph, OR 97846   541-398-0169
                          cmfdc777@yahoo.com
                          creatingmemoriesfordisabledchildren.com

Ken Coreson, Founder
Creating Memories for Disabled Children is a camp for children
and adults with disabilities. The camp's goal is to connect individuals with disabilities to nature. The camp offers a variety of
outdoor activities, including hiking and fishing. Attendance is
free.

1216 Easterseals Oregon Summer Camp
Easterseals Oregon
7300 SW Hunziker St.
Suite 103
Portland, OR 97223   503-228-5108
                            Fax: 503-228-1352
                            www.easterseals.com/oregon

Carol Salter, President & CEO
A camp program for children with disabilities. Activities include
boating and fishing, swimming, horseback riding, arts and crafts,
archery, sports and recreation, outdoor education, and campfires.

1217 Gales Creek Diabetes Camp
Gales Creek Camp Foundation
6950 SW Hampton St.
Suite 242
Tigard, OR 97223   503-968-2267
                          Fax: 503-992-6785
                          office@galescreekcamp.org
                          www.galescreekcamp.org

Robert Dailey, Executive Director
Maddie Ehl, Office & Programming Manager
Camp is located in Gales Creek, Oregon. Summer sessions for
children with Type 1 diabetes. Coed and family and pre-school
family camps also available. Gales Creek also helps teach campers about testing themselves, giving injections, and how to manage their own bodies.

1218 Hull Park and Retreat Center
Oral Hull Foundation for the Blind
43233 SE Oral Hull Rd.
PO Box 157
Sandy, OR 97055   503-668-6195
                              oralhull@gmail.com
                                    oralhull.org

Kerith Vance, Executive Director
The Oral Hull Foundation for the Blind provides recreational, educational, and social activities programs designed to fit the needs of guests with vision loss. Programs include week-long summer and winter retreats and three-night getaways for adults with vision impairments.

1219 Mt Hood Kiwanis Camp
10725 SW Barbur Blvd.
Suite 50
Portland, OR 97219   503-452-7416
                                    info@mhkc.org
                                    www.mhkc.org

Dave McDonald, Executive Director
Allan Cushing, Director, Operations
Skye Burns, Director, Development & Communications
Camp is located in Government Camp, Oregon. Summer sessions for children and adults with a variety of disabilities. Coed, ages 12 and up. Family and off-site adventure programs available.

1220 Strength for the Journey
Oregon-Idaho Conference UMC - Camp Registrar
1505 SW 18th Ave.
Portland, OR 97201   503-802-9214
                           registrar@gocamping.org
                          suttlelake.gocamping.org

Daniel Petke, Co-Director, Suttle Lake Camp
Jane Petke, Co-Director, Suttle Lake Camp
Camp is located near Sisters, Oregon at Suttle Lake Camp. Strength for the Journey is a program for adults living with HIV/AIDS.

1221 Suttle Lake Camp
29551 Suttle Lake Rd.
Sisters, OR 97759   541-595-6663
                          suttlelake@gocamping.org
                          suttlelake.gocamping.org

Daniel Petke, Co-Director
Jane Petke, Co-Director
Offers a variety of camp programs, including sessions for individuals with HIV/AIDS.

1222 Upward Bound Camp
40151 Gates School Rd.
Gates, OR 97346   503-897-2447
                               Fax: 503-897-4116
                        camp@upwardboundcamp.org
                          www.upwardboundcamp.org

Diane Turnbull, Executive Director
Upward Bound Camp is a Christian camp for children and adults with a variety of disabilities, ages 12 and up.

Pennsylvania

1223 Aces Adventure Weekend
Camp Hebron
957 Camp Hebron Rd.
Halifax, PA 17032   412-281-7244
                          www.easterseals.com/wcpenna
James G. Bennett, President & CEO
A weekend respite program for youth with high-functioning Austism, ages 11-22. Activities include canoeing, rock climbing, and cooking. The camp takes place at Camp Hebron in Halifax, Pennsylvania.

1224 Camp AIM
YMCA of Greater Pittsburgh
680 Andersen Dr.
Suite 400
Pittsburgh, PA 15220   412-227-3800
                            campaiminfo@gmail.com
                          www.ycamps.org/camp-aim

Kevin Bolding, President & CEO
Angela Schuettler, Chief Financial Officer
Carolyn Grady, Chief Development Officer
Camp AIM is a 6-week summer program for children, teens, and young adults with physical, cognitive, social/communication, and emotional/behavioral disabilities. The program combines life skills and social and recreational activities with music, art, physical education, and more. Ages 3-21.

1225 Camp Achieva
711 Bingham St.
Pittsburgh, PA 15203   412-995-5000
                                    888-272-7229
                               Fax: 412-995-5001
                               cscuilli@achieva.info
                                    www.achieva.info

Stephen H. Suroviec, President & CEO
Cathy Scuilli, Camp Director
Achieva provides life-long services such as early intervention therapies, in-home support, older adult protective services, and more, to individuals with disabilities. Offers summer day camp programs for youth up to age 21 with intellectual disabilities. The camp is located in Monaca, Pennsylvania.

1226 Camp Akeela
Camp Akeela Winter Address
314 Bryn Mawr Ave.
Bala Cynwyd, PA 19004   866-680-4744
                               Fax: 866-462-2828
                                www.campakeela.com

Eric Sasson, Camp Director
Debbie Sasson, Camp Director
Ben Jerez, Staffing Director
Camp Akeela is a co-ed, overnight camp for children and young adults ages 9-17 who have been diagnosed with Asperger's Syndrome or a non-verbal learning disability. The camp is located in Thetford Center, Vermont.

1227 Camp Amp
Easterseals Western & Central Pennsylvania, York
2550 Kingston Rd.
Suite 219
York, PA 17402   717-741-3891
                               Fax: 717-741-5359
                          www.easterseals.com/wcpenna
James G. Bennett, President & CEO
Dane Schick, Director, Camping & Recreation
Camp Amp is an overnight summer camp for children ages 7-17 with any disability or special need. The camp offers a mini session and a full week session. Activities include talent shows, sports, swimming, ropes course, hiking, and more. Camp Amp's goal is to foster independence and encourage socialization.

1228 Camp Can Do
Administrative Office
3 Unami Trail
Chalfont, PA 18914   717-273-6525
                              campcandoforever.org

Tom Prader, Director, Patient Camp
Stephanie Cole, Director, Patient Camp
Caitlyn McLarnon, Director, Sibling Camp
Camp Can Do is for children ages 8-17 who have been diagnosed with cancer in the last five years. The camp also offers a session for siblings of children with cancer.

1229 Camp Courage
American Diabetes Association
YMCA Camp Soles
134 Camp Soles Ln.
Rockwood, PA 15557   412-824-1181
                            campsupport@diabetes.org
                                    www.diabetes.org
A summer camp program of the American Diabetes Association. The camp is held at the YMCA Camp Soles, and is for children

ages 8-16 with diabetes. The camp runs traditional outdoor activities and employs on-site medical staff and dieticians.

1230 Camp Discovery
American Academy of Dermatology
PO Box 1968
Des Plaines, IL 60017   847-240-1280
                              866-503-7546
                              888-462-3376
                         Fax: 847-240-1859
                        www.campdiscovery.org

A program of the American Academy of Dermatology, Camp Discovery is a camp held in 5 locations across the United States for children with chronic skin conditions. Campers can participate in activities such as fishing, swimming, archery and horseback riding. The Pennsylvania camp is held in Millville, Pennsylvania at Camp Victory.
1993

1231 Camp Freedom
American Diabetes Association
150 Monument Rd.
Suite 100
Bala Cynwyd, PA 19004   610-828-5003
                          campsupport@diabetes.org
                             www.diabetes.org

Camp Freedom is a resident summer camp located in Schwenksville, Pennsylvania at Camp Kweebec. Sessions for children and teens with diabetes. Coed, ages 6-16.

1232 Camp Hot-to-Clot
National Hemophilia Foundation - Western PA
20411 Route 19
Unit 14
Cranberry Township, PA 16066-7512   724-741-6160
                                  Fax: 724-741-6167
                                  www.hemophilia.org

Brittani Spencer, President
Kara Dornish, Executive Director

Camp Hot-to-Clot is a summer camp for children ages 7-17 with bleeding disorders and their siblings. The camp is held at Camp Kon-O-Kwee in Fombell, PA. Activities include rock climbing, arts and crafts, field games, and more.

1233 Camp Lee Mar
Winter Address
805 Redgate Rd.
Dresher, PA 19025   215-658-1708
                         Fax: 215-658-1710
                             ari@leemar.com
                             www.leemar.com

Ari Segal, Director
Lynsey Trohoske, Assistant Director
Laura Leibowitz, Assistant Director

Seven week summer camp for children and young adults ages 7-21 with developmental, learning, communication, and other disabilities. The camp incorporates an Academic and Speech program with traditional camp activities.

1234 Camp Lily Lehigh Valley
Easterseals Eastern Pennsylvania
1501 Lehigh St.
Suite 201
Allentown, PA 18103   610-289-0114
                               camp@esep.org
                        www.easterseals.com/esep

Nancy Knoebel, President & CEO
Janine Noel, Camp Director

Camp Lily is a week-long day camp for children and young adults with a variety of disabilities. Coed, ages 8-21. The camp offers a variety of traditional camp activities and field trips so that campers can enhance their social skills and increase their independence. The camp takes place on the campus of Cedar Crest College.

1235 Camp Orchard Hill
640 Orange Rd.
Dallas, PA 18612   570-333-4098
                          Fax: 570-333-4058
                       office@camporchardhill.com
                        www.camporchardhill.com

Jim Payne, Executive Director
Derek Hodne, Program Director
Matt Chase, Facilities Director

Camp Orchard Hill provides day and overnight summer camps for ages 4-17. The camp is inclusive to children with mild to moderate special needs. Special needs campers participate alongside non-disabled campers in a multitude of outdoor activities.

1236 Camp Ramah in the Poconos
2100 Arch St.
Philadelphia, PA 19103   215-885-8556
                          Fax: 215-885-8905
                         info@ramahpoconos.org
                         www.ramahpoconos.org

Rabbi Joel Seltzer, Executive Director
Rachel Dobbs Schwartz, Camp Director
Bruce I. Lipton, Director, Finance & Operations

Camp Ramah is a Jewish summer camp that runs three separate programs for children with various disabilities and their families. There are two residential programs and one family program, the Tikvah Family Camp.

1237 Camp STAR
2504 Atlas St.
Pittsburgh, PA 15235   412-370-5481
                                 www.chp.edu

Cindy McCue, Camp Director

A week-long summer camp for children and teens ages 8-18 who are amputees. The camp is held at the YMCA Camp Kon-O-Kwee in Fombell, Pennsylvania. Activities include arts and crafts, zip lining, canoeing, rock climbing, and more. Campers are also able to learn about prosthetics, physical and recreational therapy, and limb care.

1238 Camp Setebaid
Setebaid Services, Inc.
PO Box 196
Winfield, PA 17889-0196   570-524-9090
                          Fax: 570-523-0769
                        info@setebaidservices.org
                        www.setebaidservices.org

Mark Moyer, Executive Director

Camping sessions for children with diabetes. The camp also hosts a family day for children with diabetes and their families.

1239 Camp Spencer Superstars
YMCA Camp Kon-O-Kwee
126 Nagel Rd.
Fombell, PA 16123   724-758-6238
                          Fax: 724-758-2705
                      campkon-o-kwee@ymcapgh.org
                          www.ycampkok.org

Charlie Deer, Camp Director

An overnight respite camp for adults, ages 18 and up, with special needs. The camp is fully inclusive and aims to encourage campers to develop social and life skills. Campers have access to all activities and programs, such as canoeing, bonfires, swimming, and more.

1240 Camp Victory
58 Camp Victory Rd.
PO Box 810
Millville, PA 17846   570-458-6530
                          www.campvictory.org

Jamie Huntley, Executive Director
Kate Stepnick, Camp Director

Camp Victory provides camping opportunities for children with chronic health problems or physical or mental challenges.

1241 Camp Wesley Woods: Exceptional Persons Camp
1001 Fiddlersgreen Rd.
Grand Valley, PA 16420   814-436-7802
                         info@wesleywoods.com
                         www.wesleywoods.com

Emily Reed, Chair

The Exceptional Persons Camp is a camp program for individuals with disabilities. Activities include swimming, games, sports, crafts, and Bible study.

1242 Camp Woodlands
The Woodlands Foundation
134 Shenot Rd.
Wexford, PA 15090   724-935-6533
www.woodlandsfoundation.org
Samantha Ellwood, Executive Director
Denise Balkovec, Deputy Director, Advancement & Operations
Clarissa Amond, Program Manager
Camp Woodlands is a camp for youth, teens, and adults with varying disabilities and chronic illness. The camp runs a number of programs for children, teens, adults, and seniors.

1243 Dragonfly Forest Summer Camp
YMCA Camp Speers
143 Nichecronk Rd.
Dingmans Ferry, PA 18328   570-828-2329
Fax: 570-828-2984
campspeers@philaymca.org
www.dragonflyforest.org
Dragonfly Forest Summer Camp program provides children with autism and medical needs such as asthma, sickle cell anemia and hemophilia the opportunity to enjoy an overnight camp experience in an environment that is safe and equipped to meet a variety of physical, medical, and psychological needs.

1244 Handi Camp
Handi Vangelism Ministries International
PO Box 122
Akron, PA 17501-0122   717-859-4777
Fax: 717-721-7662
info@hvmi.org
www.hvmi.org
Tim Sheetz, Founder
Mark Amey, Assistant Director, Handi Camp
Brian Robinson, Office Manager, Handi Camp
Christian overnight camping program for people with disabilities, ages 9-50, in Eastern Pennsylvania. Sponsored by Handi Vangelism Ministries International.

1245 Innabah Camps
United Methodist Church: Eastern Pennsylvania
712 Pughtown Rd.
Spring City, PA 19475   610-469-6111
Fax: 610-469-0330
www.innabah.org
Michael Hyde, Director
Samantha Wagaman, Assistant Director
Gina James, Office Manager
Innabah Camps runs a number of sessions for children, teens, and adults with developmental disabilities. The Challenge camps are for ages 12 and up.

1246 Mainstay Life Services Summer Program
Mainstay Life Services
200 Roessler Rd.
Pittsburgh, PA 15220   412-344-3640
Fax: 412-344-5486
info@mainstaylifeservices.org
mainstaylifeservices.org
Kim Sonafelt, Chief Executive Officer
Barbara Dyer, Coordinator, Community Services
Mainstay Life Services' summer respite and recreation program offers one or two week sessions on a college campus in Pittsburgh, Pennsylvania. The program is open to adults age 18 and over who live with families and caregivers.

1247 Outside In School Of Experiential Education, Inc.
PO Box 639
Greensburg, PA 15601   724-837-1518
Fax: 724-837-0801
www.myoutsidein.com
Michael C. Henkel, Executive Director
Camp programs primarily focus on substance abuse, but some services are available for special needs related to school/work. Programs are for boys ages 13-18.

1248 Phelps School Academic Support Program
583 Sugartown Rd.
Malvern, PA 19355   610-644-1754
Fax: 610-540-0156
admis@thephelpsschool.org
www.thephelpsschool.org
Charles A. McGeorge, Head of School
The Phelps School is a college preparatory day and boarding school dedicated to the individual boy. They serve students in grades 6 through 12/PG in a supportive and structured environment. Their supplemental Academic Support Program offers small (4:1) courses in reading, writing, and mathematics, as well as introductions to history and science, for young men with diagnosed learning differences. Also features a dedicated Executive Functioning Skill resource center.

1249 Sequanota Lutheran Conference Center and Camp
PO Box 245
Jennerstown, PA 15547   814-629-6627
contact@sequanota.com
www.sequanota.com
Rev. Nathan Pile, Executive Director
Angie Pile, Director, Business Management
Ann Ferry, Director, Hospitality
Runs Camp Bethesda, a summer camp for adults with developmental and intellectual disabilities. For ages 18 and up.

1250 Variety Club Camp and Developmental Center
2950 Potshop Rd.
PO Box 609
Worcester, PA 19490   610-584-4366
Fax: 610-584-5586
www.varietyphila.org
Dominique Bernardo, Chief Executive Officer
Nicholas Larcinese, Director, Programming
Kristin Podwojski, Director, Operations
Year-round camping and recreation facility for children with special needs and their families. Includes summer camping, aquatics, weekend retreats and other specialty programs. Coed, ages 5-21.

1251 West Penn Burn Camp
Allegheny Health Network
120 Fifth Ave.
Suite 2900
Pittsburgh, PA 15222   412-578-5295
www.ahn.org
Christine Perlick, Outreach Coordinator
Founded in 1986, West Penn Burn camp is a week-long overnight camp for children and teens, ages 7-17, who have burn injuries. The camp provides traditional camp activities as well as therapeutic services through the support and guidance of camp counselors. The camp is held at the YMCA Camp Kon-O-Kwee in Fombell, Pennsylvania.

1252 YMCA Camp Fitch
12600 Abels Rd.
North Springfield, PA 16430   814-922-3219
877-863-4824
Fax: 814-922-7000
registrar@campfitchymca.org
campfitchymca.org
Tom Parker, Executive Director
Joe Wolnik, Summer Camp Director
Brandy Duda, Outdoor Education Director
Camp is located in North Springfield, Pennsylvania. Camp programs include sessions for children with diabetes or epilepsy.

Rhode Island

1253 Camp Mauchatea
Rhode Island Lions Sight Foundation, Inc.
PO Box 19671
Johnston, RI 02919-0671   www.lions4sight.org
Robert P. Andrade, President
Earle U. Schahrff III, First Vice President
Steve Krohn, Secretary
Camp serving those who are blind/visually impaired. Campers enjoy developing and maintaining friendships with fellow camp-

ers. Some of the activities include boating and other water sports, as well as hiking and nature studies.

1254 Camp Ruggles
PO Box 353
Chepachet, RI 02814 401-567-8914
campruggles@gmail.com
www.campruggles.org

Jim Field, Executive Director
Ethan Roe, Assistant Director
Camp Ruggles is located in Glocester, RI and is a summer day camp for children with emotional and behavioral disabilities. The camp offers 240 hours of supervised therapeutic care for children ages 6-12.

1255 Canonicus Camp & Conference Center
54 Exeter Rd.
Exeter, RI 02822 401-294-6318
Fax: 401-294-7780
www.canonicus.org

Kathy Black, Director, Conferencing
Amanda Hosley, Director, Camping Ministries
Matt Black, Facilities Manager
Canonicus Camp offers camp and conference programs and facilities for children, adults, and groups with special needs. The camp is owned by the American Baptist Churches of Rhode Island.

1256 Hasbro Children's Hospital Asthma Camp
593 Eddy St.
Providence, RI 02903 401-444-8340
malsina@lifespan.org
www.hasbrochildrenshospital.org

Miosotis Alsina, Administrative Director
Camp for children with asthma, hosted by Canonicus Camp and Conference Center. Children learn about asthma and asthma management through interactive and educational activities. The camp also offers activities such as swimming, canoeing, and arts and crafts. Coed, ages 9-13.

South Carolina

1257 Burnt Gin Camp
SC Department of Health and Environmental Control
2100 Bull St.
Columbia, SC 29201 803-898-0784
Fax: 803-898-0613
campburntgin@dhec.sc.gov
www.scdhec.gov

Marie Aimone, Camp Director
A residential camp for youth who have physical disabilities and/or chronic illnesses. Camp Burnt Gun runs four six-day sessions for children ages 7-15; two six-day sessions for teenagers ages 16-20; and one four-day session for young adults ages 21-25. The camp is held in Wedgefield, South Carolina.

1258 Camp Adam Fisher
PO Box 2543
Columbia, SC 29202-2543 campadamfisher@gmail.com
www.campadamfisher.com

Scott McFarland, Camp Director
Maria McGregor Mullendore, Assistant Camp Director
Katherine Lewis, Medical Director
A week-long overnight camp for children with diabetes and their siblings, ages 6-17. Campers enjoy swimming, horseback riding, tubing, basketball, volleyball, and arts and crafts, while also learning how to manage their diabetes so they can live longer, healthier lives.

1259 Camp Courage
Prisma Health Children's Hospital
900 W Faris Rd.
2nd Floor
Greenville, SC 29605 864-455-8898
Fax: 864-455-5164
www.ghschildrens.org/programs

Ericka Turner, Camp Director
Camp Courage is a non-profit organization that provides a summer camp experience for children and teens with cancer or blood

disorders. Programs include week-long summer camps for children, weekend camp for siblings, fall carnival for patients and families, counselor training sessions, evening and weekend retreats, and monthly support groups. The camp is held at Pleasant Ridge Camp and Retreat Center.

1260 Camp Debbie Lou
726 Lucky Run
Latta, SC 29565 843-845-2617

Dean Richardson, Camp Director
For children between the ages of 4-14 who have been diagnosed with cancer and their families.

1261 Camp Luv-A-Lung
Prisma Health Children's Hospital
900 W Faris Rd.
2nd Floor
Greenville, SC 29605 864-455-8898
Fax: 864-455-5164
www.ghschildrens.org/programs

Jessica Herron, Contact
A summer camp for children ages 6-12 who have respiratory problems. The camp takes place at Pleasant Ridge Camp and Retreat Center in Marietta, South Carolina. Activities include swimming, archery, campfires, arts and crafts, and more.

1262 Camp Spearhead
Greenville County Recreation District
4806 Old Spartanburg Rd.
Taylors, SC 29687 864-467-3398
Fax: 864-288-6499
campspearhead@greenvillecounty.org
www.greenvillerec.com

Randy Murr, Therapeutic Recreation Manager
Camp for children with disabilities ages 8 and up. The camp is held at Pleasant Ridge Camp and Retreat Center in Marietta, South Carolina. Activities include canoeing, kayaking, swimming, archery, sports, and games.

South Dakota

1263 Camp Friendship
PO Box 1986
Rapid City, SD 57709-1986 www.campfriendshipsd.org
Held in the Black Hills of South Dakota, Camp Friendship is for individuals with physical and developmental disabilities. Activities include fishing, swimming, arts and crafts, campfires, and more. The camp consists of three sessions with two- and three-day overnight camps.

1264 Camp Gilbert
Camp Gilbert, Inc.
PO Box 89406
Sioux Falls, SD 57109-9406 605-610-8775
campgilbertinfo@gmail.com
www.campgilbert.com

Laura Parish, Camp Director
For children ages 8-18 with diabetes. Campers can enjoy a week of canoeing, swimming, sing-a-longs, crafts, and games, while also attending educational programs covering nutrition, exercise and lifestyle management.

1265 NeSoDak
Lutherans Outdoors in South Dakota
2001 S Summit Ave.
Sioux Falls, SD 57197 605-947-4440
800-888-1464
nesodak@losd.org
www.losd.org/nesodak

Vicki Foss, Director
Camp is located in Waubay, South Dakota. Hosts Camp Gilbert, a summer camp program for children with diabetes. Coed, ages 8-18.

Tennessee

1266 ACM Lifting Lives Music Camp
Vanderbilt Kennedy Center
110 Magnolia Circle
Nashville, TN 37203   615-322-8240
vkc.vumc.org

Jeffrey Neul, Director, IDDRC
Erik Carter, Co-Director, UCEDD
Elise McMillan, Co-Director, UCEDD
A camp for individuals with developmental disabilities where they can come to celebrate music by participating in songwriting workshops, recording sessions and live performances. For ages 18 and up. The program is specifically designed for people with Williams syndrome.

1267 All Days Are Happy Days Summer Camp
UTHSC Center on Developmental Disabilities
920 Madison Ave.
Suite 939
Memphis, TN 38103   901-448-6511
888-572-2249
Fax: 901-448-3844
TTY: 901-448-4677
www.uthsc.edu/cdd

Bruce Keisling, Executive Director
Week long camp for children ages 6-11 years of age who have been diagnosed with ADHD. The goal of the camp is to provide activities specifically designed for children with ADHD and to educate children and their parents on the treatment and management of ADHD and related behaviours.

1268 Bill Rice Ranch
627 Bill Rice Ranch Rd.
Murfreesboro, TN 37128   615-893-2767
800-253-7423
Fax: 615-898-0656
info@billriceranch.org
www.billriceranch.org

Wil Rice IV, President
Troy Carlson, Vice President
Matt Downs, Camp Director
Camping for hearing impaired children and youth ages 9-19. Also runs camps and retreats for deaf or hearing impaired adults.

1269 Camp Conquest
3934 West Union Rd.
Millington, TN 38053   901-545-2267
info@campconquest.com
www.campconquest.com
Becca Bryant, Camp Director
Camp Conquest is a Christian camp that provides life-changing experiences for children and adults with special needs, chronic illnesses, and disabilities. Activities include horseback riding, canoeing, ropes course, rock climbing wall, zip line, lake slide, swimming pool, and more.

1270 Camp Discovery
Tennessee Jaycees and Tennessee Jaycee Foundation
400 Camp Discovery Lane
Gainesboro, TN 38562   931-268-0239
director@jayceecamp.org
www.jayceecamp.org
Chester Lowe, Vice President
Serves children, teens, and adults ages 7 and up with disabilities. The camp is a project of the Tennessee Jaycees and the Tennessee Jaycee Foundation.

1271 Camp Joy
Lakeshore Camp and Retreat Center
1458 Pilot Knob Rd.
Eva, TN 38333   731-584-6102
Fax: 731-584-2267
office@lakeshorecamp.org
lakeshorecamp.org/summer-camp
Rev. Gary D. Lawson, Sr., Executive Director
Allison Doyle, Program Director
Katlyn White, Director, Communications
A summer camp for adults ages 31 and up with disabilities. The camp takes place at Lakeshore Camp and Retreat Center and runs regular camp activities such as swimming, arts and crafts, and other outdoor activities.

1272 Camp Koinonia
Koinonia Foundation of Tennessee
244 N Peters Rd.
Suite 211
Knoxville, TN 37923   865-888-7365
info@kftn.org
www.kftn.org/campkoinonia
Jacqui Pearl, Executive Director
Camp program for children and young adults ages 7-21 with disabilities. The camp offers recreational activities such as canoeing, music and games. The camp is operated by the Koinonia Foundation and the University of Tennessee's Therapeutic Recreation Program.

1273 Camp Oginali
Koinonia Foundation of Tennessee
244 N Peters Rd.
Suite 211
Knoxville, TN 37923   865-888-7365
info@kftn.org
www.kftn.org/campkoinonia
Jacqui Pearl, Executive Director
A weekend retreat for individuals ages 7 and up with Down syndrome. The camp is held every fall at Camp Montvale. Activities include fishing, low ropes courses, cooking, arts and crafts, and more.

1274 Camp Okawehna
Dialysis Clinic, Inc.
1633 Church St.
Suite 500
Nashville, TN 37203   615-327-3061
Fax: 605-341-8814
campo@dciinc.org
www.dciinc.org/camps
Andy Parker, Camp Director
Week-long summer camp for children ages 6-18 with kidney disease. Children who have had kidney transplants as well as children on hemodialysis and peritoneal dialysis are welcome.

1275 Camp Sugar Falls
American Diabetes Association
220 Great Circle Rd.
Nashville, TN 37228   615-298-3066
campsupport@diabetes.org
www.diabetes.org
Camp Sugar Falls is a day camp for children ages 6-17 who have diabetes and their siblings. Activities include education sessions, athletics and exercise. The camp is held at YMCA Camp Widjiwagan in Antioch, Tennessee.

1276 Camp Wonder
Lakeshore Camp and Retreat Center
1458 Pilot Knob Rd.
Eva, TN 38333   731-584-6102
Fax: 731-584-2267
office@lakeshorecamp.org
lakeshorecamp.org/summer-camp
Rev. Gary D. Lawson, Sr., Executive Director
Allison Doyle, Program Director
Katlyn White, Director, Communications
A summer camp for children and adults ages 14-30 with disabilities. The camp takes place at Lakeshore Camp and Retreat Center. Activities include swimming, crafts, games, and more traditional camp activities.

1277 Easterseals Tennessee Camping Program
Easterseals Tennessee
500 Wilson Pike Cir.
Suite 228
Brentwood, TN 37027   615-292-6640
Fax: 615-251-0994
www.easterseals.com/tennessee
Tim Ryerson, President & CEO
Offers overnight, day, and weekend programs for youths ages 7-16 and adults ages 16 and up with disabilities or traumatic brain injuries. The camps are held at the YMCA's Camp Widjiwagan.

1278 LeBonheur Cardiac Kids Camp
LeBonheur Children's Hospital
848 Adams Ave.
Memphis, TN 38103
866-870-5570
cardiac@lebonheur.org
www.lebonheur.org

Christopher Knott-Craig, MD, Co-Director, Heart Institute
Jeffrey Towbin, MD, Co-Director, Heart Institute
Camp for LeBonheur patients ages 10-17 who are being treated for a congenital heart condition or have a pacemaker. The camp provides recreational and educational activities while promoting healthy lifestyles.

Texas

1279 Camp Ailihpomeh
Texas Bleeding Disorders Camp Foundation
20212 Champion Forest Dr.
Suite 700-312
Spring, TX 77379
info@camp-ailihpomeh.org
www.camp-ailihpomeh.org

Grant Spikes, Camp Director
Amanda Wolgamott, Camp Administrator
A six-day overnight camp for boys ages 7-17 who have a bleeding disorder. The camp takes place at Camp John Marc and provides recreational and educational activities.

1280 Camp Aranzazu
5420 Loop 1781
Rockport, TX 78382
361-727-0800
Fax: 361-727-0818
info@camparanzazu.org
www.camparanzazu.org

Virginia Calton Ballard, Executive Director, Camp Aranzazu Foundation
Amelia Halsam, Camp Director
Lillian Anfosso, Finance & Administrative Director
A summer camp program for children with a variety of special needs and chronic illnesses, such as cancer, autism, asthma, cerebral palsy, Down Syndrome, epilepsy, and more. Activities center around emphasizing spiritual awareness, environmental awareness, team building and sports, the arts, and social skills.

1281 Camp Be An Angel
2003 Aldine Bender Rd.
Houston, TX 77032
281-219-3313
angel@beanangel.org
www.beanangel.org/camp

Marti Boone, Executive Director
Margaret Adsit, Development Director
Russ Massey, Program Director
Camp Be An Angel is a summer camp program for children with special needs under the age of 22 and their immediate families.

1282 Camp Blessing
7227 Camp Blessing Lane
Brenham, TX 77833
281-259-5789
info@campblessing.org
campblessing.org

Greg Anderson, Executive Director
Rachel Landon, Programs Coordinator
Dean Forland, Facilities Manager
A Christian summer camp for children and adults with special needs and their siblings. The camp serves individuals ages 7 and up with a physical, developmental, or intellectual disability. Camp Blessing offers traditional summer camp activities for campers of all levels of ability.

1283 Camp CAMP
Children's Association for Maximum Potential
PO Box 27086
San Antonio, TX 78227
210-671-5411
Fax: 210-671-5225
campmail@campcamp.org
www.campcamp.org

Susan Osborne, Chief Executive Officer
Brandon G. Briery, Chief Program Officer & Executive Camp Director
Sarah Coulombe, Chief Administrative Officer

Camping for children, teens, and adults ages 5-50 with a variety of disabilities and their siblings. The camp is held in Center Point, Texas. Activities are modified to include each camper's physical or developmental needs.

1284 Camp CPals
5501A Balcones
Suite 160
Austin, TX 78731
866-742-7284
info@cpathtexas.com
www.cpathtexas.com

Victoria Polega, President
Marielle Deckard, Secretary
Jamie Eppele, Director, Development
Camp CPals is an overnight weekend camp for campers of all ages with cerebral palsy. The camp's goal is to allow campers to gain confidence, independence, learn new skills, and meet other people with cerebral palsy. The camp is held in Burton, Texas.

1285 Camp Can-Do
YMCA Camp Carter
6200 Sand Springs Rd.
Fort Worth, TX 76114
817-738-9241
camper@ymcafw.org
www.ymcacampcarter.org

Holly Martin, Executive Camp Director
A week-long summer camp designed specifically for blind/visually impaired children, ages 6-12. The camp is held at the YMCA Camp Carter, and activities include hiking, canoeing, skeet shooting, and more.

1286 Camp Discovery
American Academy of Dermatology
PO Box 1968
Des Plaines, IL 60017
847-240-1280
866-503-7546
888-462-3376
Fax: 847-240-1859
www.campdiscovery.org

A program of the American Academy of Dermatology, Camp Discovery is a camp held in 5 locations across the United States for children with chronic skin conditions. Campers can participate in activities such as fishing, swimming, archery and horseback riding. The Texas camp is held in Burton, Texas at Camp For All.
1993

1287 Camp John Marc
4925 Greenville Ave.
Suite 400
Dallas, TX 75206
214-360-0056
mail@campjohnmarc.org
www.campjohnmarc.org

Kevin Randles, Executive Director
Megan White, Camp Director
Bre Loveless, Operations Manager
Year-round camping for children with a variety of chronic medical and physical challenges. Campers can participate in a number of traditional camp activities.

1288 Camp Neuron
Epilepsy Foundation Texas
2401 Fountain View Dr.
Suite 900
Houston, TX 77057
713-789-6295
888-548-9716
Fax: 713-789-5628
info@eftx.org
eftx.org

Donna Stahlhut, Chief Executive Officer
Camp Neuron offers an overnight camping experience for children and teens ages 8-14 with epilepsy or a diagnosed seizure disorder. There is no cost to attend the camp, and the camp is located at the Texas Lions Camp in Kerrville, Texas.

1289 Camp New Horizons North
American Diabetes Association
4100 Alpha Rd.
Dallas, TX 75244
972-392-1181
campsupport@diabetes.org
www.diabetes.org

Sherry Hill, Contact

A week-long summer camp program of the American Diabetes Association for children ages 5-12 and teens ages 13-17 with diabetes. The camp is held at Cross Creek Ranch in Parker, Texas.

1290   Camp New Horizons South
American Diabetes Association
4100 Alpha Rd.
Dallas, TX 75244   972-392-1181
                            campsupport@diabetes.org
                                    www.diabetes.org

Sherry Hill, Contact
A summer camp program of the American Diabetes Association for children ages 5-12 and teens ages 13-17 with diabetes. The camp is held at Southern Creek Ranch in Dallas, Texas.

1291   Camp No Limits Texas
No Limits Foundation
1220 Old San Antonio Rd
Buda, TX 78610   207-569-6411
                            campnolimits@gmail.com
                            www.nolimitsfoundation.org

Mary Leighton, Founder & Executive Director
Kelsey Moody, Program Operations Manager
Alix Sandler, Marketing & Development Director
Camp No Limits Texas, a location of Camp No Limits, is a recreational and educational camp for youth who have experienced limb loss. Camp No Limits is a program of the nonprofit organization No Limits Foundation. The weeklong camp is for children ages 5 and up, with campers participating in a variety of activities such as archery, kayaking, and fishing. The camp is held at Camp For All in Buda, Texas.

1292   Camp NoLoHi
American Diabetes Association
4100 Alpha Rd.
Dallas, TX 75244   972-392-1181
                            campsupport@diabetes.org
                                    www.diabetes.org

Sherry Hill, Contact
A summer camp program for children ages 5-13 and teens ages 14-17 with diabetes. The camp is held in Lubbock, Texas. Activities include swimming, fishing, outdoor games, and arts and crafts.

1293   Camp Quality Texas
18035 Melissa Springs Dr.
Tomball, TX 77375   713-553-7872
                            texas@campqualityusa.org
                            www.campqualityusa.org/TX

Falyne Kirkpatrick, Executive Director
Eric Pitts, Co-Camp Director
Lyndsey Gerhart, Co-Camp Director
Camp Quality is for children with cancer and their siblings. The camp offers a stress-free environment that offers exciting activities and fosters new friendships, while helping to give the children courage, motivation and emotional strength.

1294   Camp Rainbow
American Diabetes Association
4100 Alpha Rd.
Dallas, TX 75244   972-392-1181
                            campsupport@diabetes.org
                                    www.diabetes.org

A summer camp for children ages 4-17 with diabetes. A program of the American Diabetes Association, the camp is held at Victory Camp in Alvin, Texas.

1295   Camp Sandcastle
American Diabetes Association
4100 Alpha Rd.
Dallas, TX 75244   972-392-1181
                            campsupport@diabetes.org
                                    www.diabetes.org

A week long day camp for children ages 5-17 with type 1 diabetes. This camp is a program of the American Diabetes Association and is held at Camp Aranzazu in Rockport, Texas.

1296   Camp Spike 'n' Wave
Epilepsy Foundation Texas
2401 Fountain View Dr.
Suite 900
Houston, TX 77057   713-789-6295
                                        888-548-9716
                                    Fax: 713-789-5628
                                        info@eftx.org
                                            eftx.org

Donna Stahlhut, Chief Executive Officer
Camp Spike 'n' Wave is a residential camp for children and teens ages 8-14 with epilepsy or a seizure disorder. The camp is located at Camp For All in Burton, Texas, and runs activities such as swimming, boating, and sports. There is no cost to attend the camp.

1297   Camp Summit
17210 Campbell Rd.
Suite 180-W
Dallas, TX 75252   972-484-8900
                                    Fax: 972-620-1945
                            camp@campsummittx.org
                            www.campsummittx.org

Carla R. Weiland, President & CEO
Lisa Braziel, Director, Camp Operations & Strategy
Amanda Davis, Camp Director
Camp Summit offers camping for children and adults with a variety of disabilities. The program is coed, for ages 6-99.

1298   Camp Sweeney
PO Box 918
Gainesville, TX 76241   940-665-2011
                                    Fax: 940-665-9467
                            info@campsweeney.org
                            www.campsweeney.org

Ernie Fernandez, Camp Director
Bob Cannon, Program Director
Billie Hood, Business Manager
Camp Sweeney teaches self-care and self-reliance to children ages 5-18 with type 1 diabetes. Campers participate in activities such as swimming, fishing, horseback riding and arts and crafts while learning how to self manage their diabetes.

1299   Camp for All
6301 Rehburg Rd.
Burton, TX 77835   979-289-3752
                                    Fax: 979-289-5046
                            bdeans@campforall.org
                            www.campforall.org

Pat Prior Sorrells, President & CEO
Mary Beth Mosley, Development Director
April McIntosh, Human Resource & Finance Director
Camp For All is a fully accessible year-round camp facility located in Burton, Texas. The camp is for children and adults with a variety of disabilities. Some disabilities that the camp serves include autism, muscular dystrophy, spinal cord injuries, and more.

1300   Charis Hills Camp
498 Faulkner Rd.
Sunset, TX 76270   940-964-2145
                                    Fax: 940-964-2147
                            info@charishills.org
                            www.charishills.org

Rand Southard, Co-Director
Colleen Southard, Co-Director
Cara Krueger, Program Director
A Christian summer camp for children with learning disabilities, such as ADD/ADHD, Autism, Asperger's, and more. Campers will participate in traditional camp activities while also learning about Christ and improving social skills, self-esteem and confidence.

1301   Cristo Vive International: Texas Camp Conroe
702 Barbara Lane
Conroe, TX 77301   832-703-3733
                                    www.cristovive.net

Rachel Larson, Camp Coordinator
Christian camp with programming for individuals who are blind/deaf, physically or mentally challenged, have multiple disabilities, Down Syndrome, Autism/Asperger's, ADHD/ADD, Cerebral Palsy, and their families and siblings.

1302 **Cristo Vive International: Texas Camp Rio Grande Valley**
4300 S US Highway 281
Edinburg, TX 78539   956-532-8033
                                 www.cristovive.net
Mayra Green, Camp Coordinator
Christian camp with programming for individuals who are blind/deaf, physically or mentally challenged, have multiple disabilities, Down Syndrome, Autism/Asperger's, ADHD/ADD, Cerebral Palsy, and their families and siblings.

1303 **Dallas Academy**
950 Tiffany Way
Dallas, TX 75218   214-324-1481
                                 Fax: 214-327-8537
                                 www.dallas-academy.com
Elizabeth Murski, Head of School
Dallas Academy is a school for children with diagnosed learning differences such as autism, ADD/ADHD, dyslexia, and more. The academy offers a number of summer camps and programs.

1304 **Hill School of Fort Worth**
4817 Odessa Ave.
Fort Worth, TX 76133   817-923-9482
                                 Fax: 817-923-4894
                                 hillschool@hillschool.org
                                 www.hillschool.org
Roxann Breyer, Head of School
Matt Errico, Dean, Student Success
Jimmy Cessna, Registrar
Provides an alternative learning environment for students with learning differences. Hill School caters to individuals with disabilities by offering smaller class sizes and individualized learning programs. Offers an academic summer program during the month of June.

1305 **Kamp Kaleidoscope**
Epilepsy Foundation Texas
2401 Fountain View Dr.
Suite 900
Houston, TX 77057   713-789-6295
                                888-548-9716
                                Fax: 713-789-5628
                                info@eftx.org
                                eftx.org
Donna Stahlhut, Chief Executive Officer
Kamp Kaleidoscope is a residential camp for teens ages 15-19 with epilepsy or a seizure disorder. The camp takes place at the YMCA Collin County Adventure Camp in Anna, Texas, and is provided at no cost.

1306 **Texas Lions Camp**
PO Box 290247
Kerrville, TX 78029   830-896-8500
                                Fax: 830-896-3666
                                tlc@lionscamp.com
                                www.lionscamp.com
Stephen S. Mabry, President & CEO
Karen-Anne King, Vice President, Summer Camps
Milton Dare, Director, Development
Texas Lions Camp is a camp dedicated to serving children ages 7-16 in Texas with physical disabilities. While at camp, campers will participate in a variety of activities and be encouraged to become more independent and self-confident.

Utah

1307 **Action X-Treme Camp**
National Ability Center
1000 Ability Way
Park City, UT 84060   435-649-3991
                                Fax: 435-658-3992
                                info@discovernac.org
                                www.discovernac.org
Dan Glasser, Chief Executive Officer
Week-long overnight camp for teens with physical and visual disabilities. Activities include skiing, snowboarding, rock climbing, and more.

1308 **Camp Giddy-Up**
National Ability Center
1000 Ability Way
Park City, UT 84060   435-649-3991
                                Fax: 435-658-3992
                                info@discovernac.org
                                www.discovernac.org
Dan Glasser, Chief Executive Officer
Camp Giddy Up is a horsemanship camp, ages 8-18, for campers with and without disabilities. Campers will be participating in all activities related to horseback riding, including grooming, riding, and barn activities.

1309 **Camp Hobe**
PO Box 520755
Salt Lake City, UT 84152-0755   801-631-2742
                                www.camphobekids.org
Christina Beckwith, Executive Director
Ashley Clinger, Deputy Director
Nicole Bailey, Program Director
A summer camp for children with cancer (and similarly-treated disorders) and their siblings. The camp's goal is to allow kids to take part in a normal aspect of childhood in a safe and medically supervised environment. Camp Hob, offers a two-day session for ages 4-7, one five-day session for ages 7-12, and one five-day session for ages 12-19.

1310 **Camp ICANDO**
American Diabetes Association
Holladay, UT   campsupport@diabetes.org
                                www.diabetes.org
A summer camp program of the American Diabetes Association. Camp ICANDO is for children ages 5-12 with diabetes. The camp runs traditional camp activities and combines them with informal diabetes education.

1311 **Camp Kostopulos**
Kostopulos Dream Foundation
4180 E Emigration Canyon Rd.
Salt Lake City, UT 84108   801-582-0700
                                Fax: 801-583-5176
                                kdf@campk.org
                                www.campk.org
Mircea Divricean, President & CEO
Michael Divricean, Chief Operating Officer
Natalie Norris, Administrative Manager
Summer camping for children and adults ages 7 and up with disabilities. There are four types of summer camp programs offered: Day Camp, Residential Camp, Travel Trip Camp, and Partner Day Camps. There is also year round recreation on site and community based activities. Programs are designed to foster independence, confidence, physical fitness, and social and communication skills.

1312 **Camp Nah-Nah-Mah**
University of Utah Health Care Burn Camp Programs
50 N Medical Dr.
Salt Lake City, UT 84132   801-585-2847
                                healthcare.utah.edu/burncenter
Kristen Quinn, Camp Director
For children ages 6-13 who are burn survivors. Some of the activities include canoeing, rock climbing and archery. The camp takes place in Millcreek Canyon and is a five-day overnight camp.

1313 **Discovery Camp**
National Ability Center
1000 Ability Way
Park City, UT 84060   435-649-3991
                                Fax: 435-658-3992
                                info@discovernac.org
                                www.discovernac.org
Dan Glasser, Chief Executive Officer
Summer and winter camps for children ages 8-18 with and without physical and developmental disabilities. Also offers overnight camps for adults.

1314 FCYD Camp Utada
Foundation for Children and Youth with Diabetes
1995 W 9000 S
West Jordan, UT 84088   801-566-6913
                              www.fcydcamputada.org

Dave Okubo, MD, Co-Founder & Trustee
Elizabeth Elmer, Co-Founder & Trustee
Nathan Gedge, Co-Founder & Trustee
Camp Utada is a summer camp for children with diabetes. Coed, ages 1-18 and families.

1315 Kids Rock The World Day Camp
National Ability Center
1000 Ability Way
Park City, UT 84060   435-649-3991
                              Fax: 435-658-3992
                              info@discovernac.org
                              www.discovernac.org

Dan Glasser, Chief Executive Officer
A day camp program for children and teens ages 11-16 with diabetes. Activities include cycling, indoor climbing, arts and crafts, and more.

1316 Overnight Camps
National Ability Center
1000 Ability Way
Park City, UT 84060   435-649-3991
                              Fax: 435-658-3992
                              info@discovernac.org
                              www.discovernac.org

Dan Glasser, Chief Executive Officer
Overnight Camps are available for teens and young adults ages 15-24. Campers participate in traditional camp activities during the day. During the evenings, campers may attend campfires and sometimes sleep in tents.

1317 Pathfinders Camp
National Ability Center
1000 Ability Way
Park City, UT 84060   435-649-3991
                              Fax: 435-658-3992
                              info@discovernac.org
                              www.discovernac.org

Dan Glasser, Chief Executive Officer
Outdoor camp for children ages 8-14 with physical disabilities and their siblings and friends. Activities include adaptive cycling, rock climbing, paddle boarding, and more.

Vermont

1318 Camp Thorpe
PO Box 82
Brandon, VT 05733   802-247-6611
                              director@campthorpe.org
                              www.campthorpe.org

Heather Moore, Executive Director
Lyllie Harvey, Director, Operations
Karen Davidson, Assistant Director
Camp Thorpe is a residential summer camp for children, teens and adults with a range of social, behavioral, mental, and developmental disabilities. The camp offers two programs: Mountain Reach (ages 12-20) and Pine Haven (ages 21 and up).

1319 Silver Towers Camp
PO Box 166
Ripton, VT 05766   802-388-6446
                              Fax: 802-388-0219
                              www.vtelks.org/programs/silver-towers
Carolyn Ravenna, Camp Director
Two-week residential camp for individuals ages 6-75 with physical or mental disabilities. Activities include swimming, horseback riding, music, sing-a-longs, dancing, nature studies and more.

1320 Vermont Overnight Camp
The Barton Center for Diabetes Education, Inc.
30 Ennis Rd.
PO Box 356
North Oxford, MA 01537-0356   508-987-2056
                              Fax: 508-987-2002
                              info@bartoncenter.org
                              www.bartoncenter.org

Lynn Butler-Dinunno, Executive Director
Jenna Dufresne, Director, Health Services
Sarah Balko, Director, Camps & Programs
The Vermont Overnight Camp provides children and teens ages 6-16 with diabetes a traditional summer camp experience combined with diabetes education. Activities include sports, swimming, kayaking, canoeing, fishing, hiking, arts and crafts, and campfires. The camp is held at Camp Ta-Kum-Ta in South Hero, Vermont.

Virginia

1321 Camp Dickenson
Holston Conference of United Methodist Church
801 Camp Dickenson Lane
Fries, VA 24330   276-744-7241
                              office@campdickenson.com
                              www.campdickenson.com
Anthony Gomez, Camp Director
Camp Dickenson's Celebration Camp is a four-day camp for youth and adults with mild to moderate developmental disabilities. Activities include archery, hiking, swimming, and games.

1322 Camp Easterseals UCP
Easterseals UCP North Carolina & Virginia
900 Camp Easter Seals Rd.
New Castle, VA 24127   540-864-5750
                              camp@eastersealsucp.com
                              www.easterseals.com/ncva

Luanne Welch, President & CEO
Alex Barge, Camp Director
Summer camp, weekend respite, and family camp sessions for children and adults with disabilities and special needs. Therapeutic recreation activities including swimming, fishing, sports, horseback riding, rock climbing, and more.

1323 Camp Holiday Trails
400 Holiday Trails Lane
Charlottesville, VA 22903   434-977-3781
                              Fax: 866-342-7850
                              info@campholidaytrails.org
                              www.campholidaytrails.org

Tina LaRoche, Executive Director
McKenzie Markham, Program Director
Katrina Beitz, Director, Communications
Private, nonprofit camp for children with special health needs and various chronic illnesses. Coed, ages 7-17. Activities include canoeing, swimming, horseback riding, arts and crafts, drama, ropes course, etc. 24-hour medical supervision by doctor and nursing staff.

1324 Camp Jordan
Camp Hanover
3163 Parsleys Mill Rd.
Mechanicsville, VA 23111   804-779-2811
                              info@camphanover.org
                              www.camphanover.org

Doug Walters, Executive Director
Harry Zweckbronner, Associate Director, Programs
Lisa VanderPloeg, Office Manager
Camp Jordan is a sleepover camp session for children with diabetes in grades 6-12. The camp is a part of Camp Hanover, and activities include hiking, archery, campfires, paddle boards, and more.

1325 Camp Loud And Clear
Holiday Lake 4-H Educational Center
1267 4-H Camp Rd.
Appomattox, VA 24522   434-248-5444
                                          Fax: 434-248-6749
                                   info@holidaylake4h.com
                                        holidaylake4h.com

Preston Willson, President & CEO
Heather Benninghove, Center Director
Levi Callahan, Program Director
Camp Loud And Clear is a summer camp for youth ages 9-18 who
are deaf or have hearing loss. Activities include swimming, ar-
chery, Bible study, and more.

1326 Camps for Children & Teens with Diabetes
American Diabetes Association
2451 Crystal Dr.
Suite 900
Arlington, VA 22202   800-342-2383
                                campsupport@diabetes.org
                                          www.diabetes.org

Tracey D. Brown, Chief Executive Officer
Charlotte Carter, Chief Financial Officer
Charles Henderson, Chief Development Officer
The American Diabetes Association sponsors day camps, family
camps and resident camps for children and teens. These camps
provide an opportunity for children with diabetes to go to camp,
meet other children and gain a better understanding of their diabetes. Camps are located all across the country.

1327 Civitan Acres
Eggleston Services
1161 Ingleside Rd.
Suite A
Norfolk, VA 23502   757-625-2044
                                  info@egglestonservices.org
                                  www.egglestonservices.org

Paul J. Atkinson, President & CEO
Ron Fritch, Chief Financial Officer
Tasha Jones, Vice President, Rehabilitation Services
Offers a summer camp for adults and children with disabilities.
Sessions run for one week and aim to help campers improve their
emotional, intellectual, and physical dimensions of life.

1328 Loudoun County Adaptive Recreation Camps
Loudoun County Parks, Recreation & Community Svcs
PO Box 7800
Leesburg, VA 20177-7800   703-777-0343
                                          Fax: 703-771-5354
                                        prcs@loudoun.gov
                                          www.loudoun.gov

Steve Torpy, Director
Loudoun County's Adaptive Recreation Camps offer and promote integration opportunities for individuals with disabilities.
All camps are designed to meet the individual needs of the participants and aim to provide traditional summer camp experiences.

1329 Oakland School & Camp
128 Oakland Farm Way
Troy, VA 22974   434-293-9059
                                          Fax: 434-296-8930
                                information@oaklandschool.net
                                     www.oaklandschool.net

Carol Williams, Head of School
A highly individualized program that stresses improving reading
ability. Subjects taught are reading, English composition, math
and word analysis. Recreational activities include horseback riding, sports, swimming, tennis, crafts, archery and camping. For
girls and boys, ages 7-13. Students who attend the summer camp
often have a variety of learning disabilities, such as ADHD, dyslexia, visual/auditory processing disorders, and more.

Washington

1330 Camp Beausite NW
PO Box 1227
Port Hadlock, WA 98339   360-732-7222
                                        campbeausitenw.org

Raina Baker, Executive Director

The camp is located in Chimacum, Washington. Campers range
from 7-65 in age and includes those with developmental disabilities, cerebral palsy, autism, Down syndrome, and other physical
or mental disabilities. The camp offers five week-long overnight
summer camp sessions for adults and children.

1331 Camp Goodtimes
The Goodtimes Project
7400 Sand Point Way NE
Suite 101S
Seattle, WA 98115   206-556-3489
                                          Fax: 206-877-4437
                                info@thegoodtimesproject.org
                                   www.thegoodtimesproject.org

Bridget K. Dolan, Executive Director
Tanya Krohn, Director, Programming
Becky Felak, Program & Event Manager
A week-long residential summer camp for children ages 8-17 diagnosed with cancer and their siblings. The Goodtimes Project
also runs Kayak Adventure Camp for childhood cancer survivors,
aged 18-25.

1332 Camp Killoqua
15207 E Lake Goodwin Rd.
Stanwood, WA 98292   360-652-6250
                                    killoqua@campfiresnoco.org
                                       www.campkilloqua.org

Cassie Anderson, Camp Director, Outdoor Education & Operations
Pearl Verbon, Camp Director, Summer Camp, Rentals & Retreats
Camp Killoqua offers Inclusion Programs for all of its traditional
camp programs. The inclusion program allows campers ages 7-21
with mild to moderate developmental disabilities the chance to
participate in any Camp Killoqua session.

1333 Camp Korey
3616 Colby Ave.
PMB 247
Everett, WA 98201   425-440-0850
                                          Fax: 425-404-2158
                                        info@campkorey.org
                                            campkorey.org

Chris McReynolds, Co-President
Tim Rose, Co-President
Sue Colbourne, Vice President
A summer camp for children with life-altering medical conditions
and their families. The camp is free of charge and aims to allow
children to experience camp in a safe environment with specialized medical support.

1334 Camp Sealth
14500 SW Camp Sealth Rd.
Vashon, WA 98070-8222   206-463-3174
                                          Fax: 206-463-6936
                                     info@campfireseattle.org
                                          campfireseattle.org

Rick Taylor, Executive Director
Kristen Cook, Marketing & Development Director
Carrie Kishline, Summer Camp Director
Camp Sealth is a camp program for youth ages 5-17. The camp is
open to children with a variety of abilities and special needs.

1335 Easterseals Camp Stand by Me
Easterseals Washington
17809 S Vaughn Rd. NW
PO Box 289
Vaughn, WA 98394   253-884-2722
                                 campadmin@wa.easterseals.com
                                 www.easterseals.com/washington

Cathy Bisaillon, President & CEO
Angela Cox, Camp Director
Camp Stand by Me is a camp program for children and adults with
disabilities. Offers week-long summer sessions and weekend respite in the fall, winter, and spring.

1336 Prime Time, Inc.
6 S. 2nd St.
Suite 815
Yakima, WA 98901

509-248-2854
Fax: 509-248-5505
office@campprimetime.org
www.campprimetime.org

Bill Schorzman, Camp Manager
Merita Sletten, Office Manager
Camp Prime Time serves children with developmental disabilities or serious or terminal illnesses and their families.

1337 STIX Diabetes Programs
PO Box 8308
Spokane, WA 99203

509-484-1366
Fax: 509-955-1329
stix@stixdiabetes.org
www.stixdiabetes.org

Tonya Kobluk, Director, Administration & Camps
Cindy Schneider, Director, Community Outreach
Jill Strom, Director, Development
STIX Diabetes Programs is a non-profit organization providing camp experiences for children and teens with diabetes. STIX offers a three-day non-residential day camp for children ages 6-8; a week-long residential camp for youth ages 9-16; and an excursion-based Adventure Camp for teens ages 16-19.

West Virginia

1338 Mountaineer Spina Bifida Camp
534 New Goff Mountain Rd.
Charleston, WV 25313

info@drewsday.org
www.drewsday.org

Suzie Humphreys, Contact
A summer camp for individuals with spina bifida. Campers can participate in activities such as swimming, wheelchair hockey, baseball, and more.

Wisconsin

1339 Camp Daypoint
American Diabetes Association
375 Bishops Way
Brookfield, WI 53005

414-778-5500
campsupport@diabetes.org
www.diabetes.org

Becky Barnett, Camp Director
Camp Daypoint is a day camp for children ages 5-9 with diabetes. Activities include swimming, crafts, hikes, games, and more. The camp is held at YMCA Camp St. Croix in Hudson, Wisconsin.

1340 Camp Kee-B-Waw
Easterseals Wisconsin
1450 State Hwy. 13
Wisconsin Dells, WI 53965

608-254-8319
800-422-2324
Fax: 608-277-8333
TTY: 608-277-8031
camp@eastersealswisconsin.com
camp.eastersealswisconsin.com

Paul Leverenz, President & CEO
Carissa Peterson, Vice President, Camp & Respite Services
Stevie Thomas, Director, Camp Operations
Located at Camp Wawbeek, Camp Kee-B-Waw is a day camp for children ages 6-13 from Wisconsin Dells and surrounding communities.

1341 Camp Klotty Pine
Great Lakes Hemophilia Foundation
638 N 18th St.
Milwaukee, WI 53233

414-937-6782
888-797-4543
Fax: 414-257-1225
info@glhf.org
glhf.org

Karin Koppen, Camp Director

An overnight summer camp for children ages 7-15 who have been diagnosed with a bleeding disorder. The camp is held at Camp Lakotah in Wautoma, Wisconsin. The camp runs recreational camp activities such as archery, canoeing, and campfires, as well as education about their disorder and self-infusion instruction.

1342 Camp Needlepoint
American Diabetes Association
375 Bishops Way
Brookfield, WI 53005

414-778-5500
campsupport@diabetes.org
www.diabetes.org

Becky Barnett, Camp Director
Camp Needlepoint is a summer camp for children who have type 1 diabetes. Coed, ages 8-16. The camp takes place at the YMCA Camp St. Croix in Hudson, Wisconsin.

1343 Easter Seal Camp Wawbeek
Easterseals Wisconsin
1450 State Hwy. 13
Wisconsin Dells, WI 53965

608-254-8319
800-422-2324
Fax: 608-277-8333
TTY: 608-277-8031
camp@eastersealswisconsin.com
camp.eastersealswisconsin.com

Paul Leverenz, President & CEO
Carissa Peterson, Vice President, Camp & Respite Services
Stevie Thomas, Director, Camp Operations
Camp Wawbeek is a summer camp for children and adults with physical disabilities. Coed, ages 7 and up. During the summer, the camp runs six-day youth and teen sessions; six-day adult, young adult, and transition sessions; and weekend sessions from September to May.

1344 Lutherdale Bible Camp
Lutherdale Ministries
N7891 US Hwy. 12
Elkhorn, WI 53121

262-742-2352
Fax: 888-248-4551
info@lutherdale.org
www.lutherdale.org

Jeff Bluhm, Executive Director
David Box, Associate Director
Paul Degner, Operations & Facilities Manager
Lutherdale Bible Camp currently offers Team USA, a summer camp program for adults with developmental disabilities. Activities include talent show, parade, and campfires.

1345 Phantom Lake YMCA Camp
S110W30240 YMCA Camp Rd.
Mukwonago, WI 53149

262-363-4386
office@phantomlakeymca.org
www.phantomlakeymca.org

Karin Mulrooney, Chair
Sara Hacker, Secretary
Bill Canfield, Treasurer
Phantom Lake Camp offers day and residential camping sessions for children ages 3-17. All programs are open to individuals with disabilities.

1346 Timbertop Camp for Youth with Learning Disabilities
PO Box 423
Plover, WI 54467

715-869-6262
info@timbertopcamp.org
www.timbertopcamp.org

Pete Matthai, Camp Director
Timbertop Camp is a seven-day outdoor camp for children and youth with learning disabilities. Campers participate in traditional camp activities as well as activities that focus on enhancing cooperative abilities, interpersonal relationships, and self-esteem. The program includes nature exploration, canoeing, arts and crafts, archery, fishing, games, reading instruction, and campfires.

1347 **Wisconsin Badger Camp**
1250 US-151 BUS
PO Box 723
Platteville, WI 53818 608-348-9689
Fax: 608-348-9737
wiscbadgercamp@badgercamp.org
www.badgercamp.org

Brent Bowers, Executive Director
Austin Rist, Program Director
Steve Van Kooten, Camp Director
Wisconsin Badger Camp, established in 1966, is a summer camp that serves individuals with developmental disabilities. Badger Camp offers eight one-week sessions and one two-week session, with one week for children ages 3-13, one week for teens ages 14-21, and eight weeks for adults.

1348 **Wisconsin Elks/Easterseals Respite Camp**
Easterseals Wisconsin
1550 Waubeek Rd.
Wisconsin Dells, WI 53965 608-254-2502
800-422-2324
Fax: 608-277-8333
TTY: 608-277-8031
camp@easterealswisconsin.com
camp.easterealswisconsin.com

Paul Leverenz, President & CEO
Carissa Peterson, Vice President, Camp & Respite Services
Stevie Thomas, Director, Camp Operations
The Wisconsin Elks/Easterseals Respite Camp is a year-round camp for individuals with disabilities, including those with severe or multiple disabilities. Activities include arts and crafts, sports, games, high ropes course, and local field trips.

1349 **Wisconsin Lions Camp**
Wisconsin Lions Foundation
3834 County Rd. A
Rosholt, WI 54473 715-677-4969
877-463-6953
Fax: 715-677-4527
info@wisconsinlionscamp.com
www.wisconsinlionscamp.com

Evett Hartvig, Executive Director
Andrea Yenter, Camp Director
Phillip Potter, Assistant Camp Director
Provides camp programs for youth and adults in Wisconsin with disabilities, including autism, intellectual disabilities, diabetes, epilepsy, visual impairments, and hearing impairments. ACA accredited, located in central Wisconsin, near Stevens Point.

Wyoming

1350 **Camp Hope**
3920 W 45th St.
Casper, WY 82604 307-259-3327
Fax: 307-472-5008
camphopewyoming@gmail.com
www.camphopewy.net

Steve Johnson, Director
Nancy Johnson, Director
Camp Hope is a camp for children and young adults with diabetes. Activities include hiking, swimming, sports and games.

1351 **Eagle View Ranch**
SOAR
184 Uphill Rd.
PO Box 584
Dubois, WY 82513 307-455-3084
Fax: 801-820-3050
admissions@soarnc.org
www.soarnc.org

John Willson, Executive Director
Jeremy Neidens, Director, Eagle View Ranch
Camp for youth with ADHD and learning disabilities. Campers participate in a broad range of wilderness adventure experiences that help them to overcome challenges and develop problem-solving skills, effective communication strategies, and social skills.

Clothing

Clothing

1352 Adaptations by Adrian
PO Box 7
San Marcos, CA 92079-0007
760-744-3565
888-214-8372
Fax: 760-471-7560
adrians1@sbcglobal.net
www.adaptationsbyadrian.com
Fashions for the physically challenged child. Clothing offers Velcro closures, front pockets, concealed back openings and fashions for seated posture.

1353 Basic Rear Closure Sweat Top
Buck & Buck
3111 27th Ave S
Seattle, WA 98144-6502
206-722-4196
800-458-0600
Fax: 800-317-2182
info@buckandbuck.com
www.buckandbuck.com
Julie Buck, Owner
Top opens completely down the back for ease of dressing with snaps. *$19.00*

1354 Booties with Non-Skid Soles
Buck & Buck
3111 27th Ave S
Seattle, WA 98144-6502
206-722-4196
800-458-0600
Fax: 800-317-2182
info@buckandbuck.com
www.buckandbuck.com
Julie Buck, Owner
Acrylic knit or quilted cotton/poly and shearling inner. *$17.00*

1355 Buck and Buck Clothing
3111 27th Ave S
Seattle, WA 98144-6502
206-722-4196
800-458-0600
Fax: 800-317-2182
info@buckandbuck.com
www.buckandbuck.com
Julie Buck, Owner
Clothing for the disabled and elderly.
88 pages Yearly

1356 Budget Cotton/Poly Open Back Gown
Buck & Buck
3111 27th Ave S
Seattle, WA 98144-6502
206-722-4196
800-458-0600
Fax: 800-317-2182
info@buckandbuck.com
www.buckandbuck.com
Julie Buck, Owner
Short raglan sleeves, lace at neck and bodice over lapping snapback closure. *$14.00*

1357 Budget Flannel Open Back Gown
Buck & Buck
3111 27th Ave S
Seattle, WA 98144-6502
206-722-4196
800-458-0600
info@buckandbuck.com
www.buckandbuck.com
Julie Buck, Owner
3/4 raglan sleeve, lace at neck and bodice. *$17.00*

1358 Carolyn's Low Vision Products
3938 S. Tamiami Trail
Sarasota, FL 34231-3622
941-373-9100
800-648-2266
info@carolynscatalog.com
www.carolynscatalog.com
John Colton, Owner

A trusted leader in low-vision products. Free national mail-order catalog of items for visually impaired and blind people. Well versed in a variety of eye diseases that damage vision and have an expertise in helping customers making product purchasing decisions for their needs.

1359 Cotton Full-Back Vest
Buck & Buck
3111 27th Ave S
Seattle, WA 98144-6502
206-722-4196
800-458-0600
Fax: 800-317-2182
info@buckandbuck.com
www.buckandbuck.com
Julie Buck, Owner
Wide shoulder straps that don't slide off shoulders. *$5.00*

1360 Cotton/Poly House Dress
Buck & Buck
3111 27th Ave S
Seattle, WA 98144-6502
206-722-4196
800-458-0600
info@buckandbuck.com
www.buckandbuck.com
Julie Buck, Owner
Comes in short and long sleeves, assorted florals and plaids. *$36.00*

1361 Creative Designs
3704 Carlisle Ct
Modesto, CA 95356-924
209-523-3166
800-335-4852
robes4you@aol.com
www.robes4you.com
Barbara Arnold, Owner
Designer of the original Change-A-Robe and the new Handi-Robe, which allows the wearer to put it on without having to stand up. Robes are designed especially for physically challenged, disabled individuals, and wheelchair users. *$69.95*

1362 Dusters
Buck & Buck
3111 27th Ave S
Seattle, WA 98144-6502
206-722-4196
800-458-0600
info@buckandbuck.com
www.buckandbuck.com
Julie Buck, Owner
Three types: Floral, Budget Better. Snap front styles and gathered yokes, flannel $16.00-$24.00. *$36.00*

1363 Dutch Neck T-Shirt
Buck & Buck
3111 27th Ave S
Seattle, WA 98144-6502
206-722-4196
800-458-0600
Fax: 800-317-2182
info@buckandbuck.com
www.buckandbuck.com
Julie Buck, Owner
Stretchy neck makes it easy to get over the head. *$ 5.50*

1364 Exquisite Egronomic Protective Wear
Plum Enterprises
P.O. Box 85
Valley Forge, PA 19481-85
610-783-7377
800-321-7586
Fax: 610-783-7577
info@plument.com
www.plument.com
Janice Carrington, President/CEO
Egronomic Protective Wear; ProtectaCap custom-fitting headgear has earned an unparalleled reputation for quality, safety, and comfort. ProtectaCap+Plus technologically-advanced protective headgear closes the gap between hard and soft helmets. Comes with optional ProtectaChin Guard and new sporty design. Protectahip protective undergarment is the intelligent, innovative solution to the problem of hip injuries for both men and women.

1365 Flannel Gowns
Buck & Buck
3111 27th Ave S
Seattle, WA 98144-6502
206-722-4196
800-458-0600
info@buckandbuck.com
www.buckandbuck.com

Julie Buck, Owner
Comes in long or short with a deep button-front opening for ease of slipping on. Shorter long length. *$21.00*

1366 Flannel Pajamas
Buck & Buck
3111 27th Ave S
Seattle, WA 98144-6502
206-722-4196
800-458-0600
Fax: 800-317-2182
info@buckandbuck.com
www.buckandbuck.com

Julie Buck, Owner
$25.00

1367 Float Dress
Buck & Buck
3111 27th Ave S
Seattle, WA 98144-6502
206-722-4196
800-458-0600
info@buckandbuck.com
www.buckandbuck.com

Julie Buck, Owner
A safe bet for everyone from a size medium to a 3X. Gathered yoke front and back and literally yards of fabric for fullness. Comes in cotton or polyester. *$32.00*

1368 Foot Snugglers
Buck & Buck
3111 27th Ave S
Seattle, WA 98144-6502
206-722-4196
800-458-0600
Fax: 800-317-2182
info@buckandbuck.com
www.buckandbuck.com

Julie Buck, Owner
Quilted poly/cotton outers lined with plush shearling pile, provide a thick, comfortable cushion which helps minimize the pressure points on tender areas. *$.30*

1369 Headliner Hats
Designs for Comfort
PO Box 671044
Marietta, GA 30066-2429
770-565-8246
800-443-9226
Fax: 770-565-8425
headliner@mindspring.com
www.headlinerhats.com

Curt Maurer, President
A patented cap and hairpiece combination, the Headliner is both a quick, stylish coverup and an upbeat wig alternative for women experiencing hair care problems or hair loss. Ideal for social gatherings and outdoor activities as well as for sleeping and hospital stays. *$ 25.00*

1370 His & Hers
Wishing Wells Collection
Ste 965
11684 Ventura Blvd
Studio City, CA 91604-2699
818-840-6919
Fax: 818-760-3878
www.dawnwells.com

Dawn Wells, Owner
This sleep shirt is designed for him or her. *$21.99*

1371 Knee Socks
Buck & Buck
3111 27th Ave S
Seattle, WA 98144-6502
206-722-4196
800-458-0600
Fax: 800-317-2182
info@buckandbuck.com
www.buckandbuck.com

Julie Buck, Owner

Comes in regular and large size. $3.00 - $8.00

1372 M&M Health Care Apparel Company
Fashion Collection
1541 60th St
Brooklyn, NY 11219-5023
718-871-8188
800-221-8929
Fax: 718-436-2067
info@fashionease.com
www.fashionease.com

Abraham Klein, Owner
Specialized clothing for disabled people.

1373 Muu Muu
Buck & Buck
3111 27th Ave S
Seattle, WA 98144-6502
206-722-4196
800-458-0600
info@buckandbuck.com
www.buckandbuck.com

Julie Buck, Owner
Comes in long and short styles, assorted bright floral prints. $20.00-$22.00. *$31.00*

1374 Nightshirts
Buck & Buck
3111 27th Ave S
Seattle, WA 98144-6502
206-722-4196
800-458-0600
Fax: 800-317-2182
info@buckandbuck.com
www.buckandbuck.com

Julie Buck, Owner
Come in flannel or cotton patterns and prints in sizes S/M, 4XL, 2XL/3XL *$29.00*

1375 Open Back Nightgowns
Buck & Buck
3111 27th Ave S
Seattle, WA 98144-6502
206-722-4196
800-458-0600
Fax: 800-317-2182
info@buckandbuck.com
www.buckandbuck.com

Julie Buck, Owner
Come in cotton (sizes S-4X) or flannel (sizes S-3X). *$20.00*

1376 Panties
Buck & Buck
3111 27th Ave S
Seattle, WA 98144-6502
206-722-4196
800-458-0600
Fax: 800-317-2182
info@buckandbuck.com
www.buckandbuck.com

Julie Buck, Owner
Come in nylon or cotton, band leg for comfort. *$5.00*

1377 Polyester House Dress
Buck & Buck
3111 27th Ave S
Seattle, WA 98144-6502
206-722-4196
800-458-0600
info@buckandbuck.com
www.buckandbuck.com

Julie Buck, Owner
Comes in short and long sleeves, assorted florals. *$ 36.00*

1378 Printed Rear Closure Sweat Top
Buck & Buck
3111 27th Ave S
Seattle, WA 98144-6502
206-722-4196
800-458-0600
Fax: 800-317-2182
info@buckandbuck.com
www.buckandbuck.com

Julie Buck, Owner
Comes in assorted colors, plain or with animal motifs and snaps all the way down the back. *$28.00*

1379   Professional Fit Clothing
Ste 1
831 N Lake St
Burbank, CA 91502-1600

818-563-1975
800-422-2348
Fax: 818-563-1834
sales@professionalfit.com
www.professionalfit.com

Kurt Rieback, Owner
Professional fit clothing caters to homes that care for people with developmental disabilities and individuals who are physically challenged. Our clothing is fashionable, affordable and can be adapted to each person's special needs.

1380   Propet Leather Walking Shoes
Buck & Buck
3111 27th Ave S
Seattle, WA 98144-6502

206-722-4196
800-458-0600
Fax: 800-317-2182
info@buckandbuck.com
www.buckandbuck.com

Julie Buck, Owner
Two velcro straps, leather upper, shock-absorbing sole. *$58.00*

1381   Rear Closure Shirts
Buck & Buck
3111 27th Ave S
Seattle, WA 98144-6502

206-722-4196
800-458-0600
Fax: 206-722-1144
info@buckandbuck.com
www.buckandbuck.com

Julie Buck, Owner
Snaps down the back on T-shirts and dress shirts. *$ 33.00*

1382   Rear Closure T-Shirt
Buck & Buck
3111 27th Ave S
Seattle, WA 98144-6502

206-722-4196
800-458-0600
Fax: 800-317-2182
info@buckandbuck.com
www.buckandbuck.com

Julie Buck, Owner
Closes down the back with velcro snaps. *$10.00*

1383   Seersucker Shower Robe
Buck & Buck
3111 27th Ave S
Seattle, WA 98144-6502

206-722-4196
800-458-0600
Fax: 800-317-2182
info@buckandbuck.com
www.buckandbuck.com

Julie Buck, Owner
Totally covers a man or woman being wheeled to and from the shower or bath. A crisp, light weight shower robe. *$34.00*

1384   Side Velcro Slacks
Buck & Buck
3111 27th Ave S
Seattle, WA 98144-6502

206-722-4196
800-458-0600
Fax: 800-317-2182
info@buckandbuck.com
www.buckandbuck.com

Julie Buck, Owner
Slacks open down both sides from waist to hip with snap closures at sides. *$36.00*

1385   Side-Zip Sweat Pants
Buck & Buck
3111 27th Ave S
Seattle, WA 98144-6502

206-722-4196
800-458-0600
Fax: 800-317-2182
info@buckandbuck.com
www.buckandbuck.com

Julie Buck, Owner

Out-seam zippers un-zip 22-inch zippers down both sides to enable dressing a resident with severe leg contractures. *$25.00*

1386   Spec-L Clothing Solutions
849 Performance Drive
Stockton, CA 95206

714-427-0781
800-445-1981
Fax: 800-683-6510
www.clothingsolutions.com

Jim Lechner, Owner
The nation's leading designer and manufacturer of assistive clothing for men and women. Free 56 page catalog available.

1387   Specialty Care Shoppe
16126 E 161st St S
Bixby, OK 74008-7325

918-366-2901
Fax: 918-366-9445
www.specialtycareshoppe.com

K J Marshall, Owner
Catalog of attractive, affordable clothing and accessories for adults with special needs. Includes items for edema, incontinence, alzheimers, limited mobility, and hand impairment.

1388   Super Stretch Socks
Buck & Buck
3111 27th Ave S
Seattle, WA 98144-6502

206-722-4196
800-458-0600
Fax: 800-317-2182
info@buckandbuck.com
www.buckandbuck.com

Julie Buck, Owner
This sock has been improved to stretch laterally throughout the foot area as well as at the top. *$3.75*

1389   Support Plus
5581 Hudson Industrial Parkway
PO Box 2599
Hudson, OH 44236-0099

508-359-2910
866-229-2910
Fax: 800-950-9569
www.supportplus.com

Ed Janos, President
Offers a selection of support undergarments, braces and shoes for the physically challenged and medical professionals.

1390   TRU-Mold Shoes
42 Breckenridge St
Buffalo, NY 14213-1555

716-881-4484
800-843-6653
Fax: 716-881-0406
www.trumold.com

Husain Syed, Production Manager
Custom made, fully molded shoes, relieve pressure in sensitive areas by taking all of the weight off the painful areas.

1391   Thigh-Hi Nylon Stockings
Buck & Buck
3111 27th Ave S
Seattle, WA 98144-6502

206-722-4196
800-458-0600
Fax: 800-317-2182
info@buckandbuck.com
www.buckandbuck.com

Julie Buck, Owner
A sheer, full length stocking. *$4.50*

1392   Trunks
Buck & Buck
3111 27th Ave S
Seattle, WA 98144-6502

206-722-4196
800-458-0600
Fax: 800-317-2118
info@buckandbuck.com
www.buckandbuck.com

Julie Buck, Owner
Come in cotton or nylon, flare leg, full cut. *$5.00*

1393 **Velcro Booties**
Buck & Buck
3111 27th Ave S
Seattle, WA 98144-6502   206-722-4196
                                             800-458-0600
                                             Fax: 800-317-2182
                                             info@buckandbuck.com
                                             www.buckandbuck.com

Julie Buck, Owner
The high-domed toe, and extra-wide, non-skid sole design accommodates virtually every foot related problem. *$20.00*

1394 **Washable Shoes**
Buck & Buck
3111 27th Ave S
Seattle, WA 98144-6502   206-722-4196
                                             800-458-0600
                                             Fax: 800-317-2182
                                             info@buckandbuck.com
                                             www.buckandbuck.com

Julie Buck, Owner
Vinyl upper with velcro closure, nonskid sole. *$20.00*

1395 **Waterproof Bib**
Buck & Buck
3111 27th Ave S
Seattle, WA 98144-6502   206-722-4196
                                             800-458-0600
                                             Fax: 800-317-2182
                                             info@buckandbuck.com
                                             www.buckandbuck.com

Julie Buck, Owner
Made with 3 layers of fabric including waterproof backing, these attractive bibs will not soak through like most others, protecting clothing from stains. *$18.00*

1396 **Wishing Wells Collection**
Ste 965
11684 Ventura Blvd
Studio City, CA 91604-2699   818-840-6919
                                             Fax: 818-760-3878
                                             www.dawnwells.com

Dawn Wells, Owner
Lorraine Parker, General Manager
Features designs full of back overlap construction and all velcro closures clothing.

Computers

Assistive Devices

1397 Ability Research
PO Box 1721
Minnetonka, MN 55345-721
952-939-0121
Fax: 952-227-5809
info@abilityresearch.net
www.abilityresearch.net
Suzanne Severson, Administrator
Manufacturers and marketers of assistive technology equipment.

1398 Academic Software Inc
3504 Tates Creek Rd
Lexington, KY 40517-2601
859-552-1020
Fax: 253-799-4012
asistaff@acsw.com
www.acsw.com
Warren E Lacefield PhD, President
Penelope Ellis, Marketing Director
Sylvia P Lacefield, Graphic Artist
Employs a unique, goal-oriented approach to aid individuals in identifying adaptive devices with potential to support various physical limitations. Devices are categorized in seven databases: Existence, Travel, In-situ Motion, Environmental Adaptation, Communication, and Sports & recreation. ADLS provides its users with device descriptions, pictures and lists of sources for locating products and product information.

1399 Adaptivation
Ste 100
2225 W 50th St
Sioux Falls, SD 57105-6536
605-335-4445
800-723-2783
Fax: 605-335-4446
info@adaptivation.com
www.adaptivation.com
Jonathan Eckrich, President
Manufacturers of switches, voice output devices and enviromental controls.

1400 Analog Switch Pad
Academic Software
331 W 2nd St
Lexington, KY 40507-1113
859-233-2332
800-842-2357
Fax: 859-231-0725
Warren E Lacefield PhD, President
Penelope Ellis, Marketing Director
A touch-activated, force-adjustable, low-voltage DC, electronic switch designed to control battery-operated toys, environmental controls, and computer access interfaces. This device features a large activation area that is soft and compliant to the touch. Force sensitivity is adjusted by a small dial from approximately 1 ounce to 32 ounces activation pressure, applied over an area ranging from the size of a fingertip to the size of the entire switch surface.

1401 Arkenstone: The Benetech Initiative
480 S California Ave
Palo Alto, CA 94306-1609
650-644-3400
Fax: 650-475-1066
www.hrdag.org
Jim Fruthterman, CEO
Roberta G Brosnaha, General Manager/VP
Patrick Ball, Executive Director
Offers various models of ready-to-read personal computers for the disabled.

1402 Augmentative Communication Systems (AAC)
ZYGO-USA
48834 Kato Road
Suite 101A
Freemont, CA 94538
510-249-9660
800-234-6006
Fax: 510-770-4930
www.zygo-usa.com
Lawrence Weiss, President
Full range of AAC systems and assistive technology including computer-based systems and computer access programs and devices.

1403 Away We Ride IntelliKeys Overlay
Soft Touch Inc
12301 Central Ave NE
Ste 205
Blaine, NE 55434
763-755-1402
888-755-1402
sales@marblesoft.com
www.softtouch.com
Joyce Meyer, President
Four full color preprinted overlays to use with Away We Ride. Just put them on an IntelliKeys keyboard and you are ready to go.

1404 BIGmack Communication Aid
AbleNet, Inc.
2625 Patton Road
Roseville, MN 55113-1137
651-294-2200
800-322-0956
Fax: 651-294-2259
customerservice@ablenetinc.com
www.ablenetinc.com
Jennifer Thalhuber, President & CEO
Paul Sugden, CFO & Trustee
A single message communication aid, BIGmack has 2 minutes of memory and has a 5 inches in diameter switch surface. *$155.00*

1405 Close-Up 6.5
Norton- Lambert Corporation
PO Box 4085
Santa Barbara, CA 93140-4085
805-964-6767
www.norton-lambert.com
Jeannie Vesely, Marketing Coordinator
Remotely controls PC's via modem. Telecommute from your home or laptop PC to your office PC. Run applications, update spreadsheets, print documents remotely and access networks on remote PCs. Features: fast screen and file transfers, synchronize files, unattended transfers, multi-level security, transaction logs, automated installation. *$99.95*

1406 Concepts on the Move Advanced Overlay CD
Soft Touch Inc
12301 Central Ave NE
Ste 205
Blaine, MN 55434
763-755-1402
888-755-1402
Fax: 763-862-2920
sales@marblesoft.com
www.softtouch.com
Joyce Myer, President
Use this overlay CD with Concepts on the Move Advanced Preacademics. Overlays match the concepts and graphics in the program. Includes standard overlays with all the choices and SoftTouch's changeable format overlays. Print and laminate the blank templates. Then print and laminate the picture keys in all three sizes - small, medium and large. Includes Overlay Printer by IntelliTools for easy printing. *$115.00*

1407 Concepts on the Move Basic Overlay CD
Soft Touch Inc
12301 Central Ave NE
Ste 205
Blaine, MN 55434
763-755-1402
888-755-1403
Fax: 763-862-2920
sales@marblesoft.com
www.softtouch.com
Joyce Meyer, President
Use this Overlay CD with Concepts on the Move Basic Preacademics. Overlays match the concepts and graphics in the program. Includes standard overlays with all the choices and SoftTouch's changeable format overlays. Print and laminate the blank templates. Then print and laminate the picture keys in all three sizes - small, medium and large. It is easy and fast to place the images on the blank templates. *$115.00*

1408 Darci Too
WesTest Engineering Corporation
810 Shepard Ln
Farmington, UT 84025-3846

801-451-9191
Fax: 801-451-9393
larryk@westest.com
westest.com

Robert Lessmann, President
A universal device which allows people with physical disabilities to replace the keyboard and mouse on a personal computer with a device that matches their physical capabilities. DARCI TOO works with almost any personal computer and provides access to all computer functions. *$995.00*

1409 Eyegaze Computer System
LC Technologies Inc
10363A Democracy Lane
Fairfax, VA 22030

703-385-7133
800-393-4293
Fax: 703-385-7137
www.eyegaze.com

Nancy Cleveland, Medical Coordinator
Enables people with physical disabilities to do many things with their eyes that they would otherwise do with their hands.

1410 Five Green & Speckled Frogs IntelliKeys Overlay
Soft Touch Inc
12301 Central Ave NE
Ste 205
Blaine, MN 55434

763-755-1402
888-755-1403
Fax: 763-862-2920
sales@marblesoft.com
www.softtouch.com

Joyce Meyer, President
Seven full color preprinted overlays to use with Five Green and Speckled Frogs. Just put them on an IntelliKeys keyboard and you are ready to go. *$49.00*

1411 GW Micro
725 Airport North Office Park
Fort Wayne, IN 46825-6707

260-489-3671
Fax: 260-489-2608
www.gwmicro.com

Dan Weirich, Sales Executive
Marty Hord, Sales Manager
Computer hardware and software products for people with disabilities.

1412 InvoTek, Inc.
1026 Riverview Dr
Alma, AR 72921

479-632-4166
Fax: 479-632-6457
invotek.org

Thomas Jakobs, President
Diane Jakobs, Vice President, Operations
John Riggins, Chief Marketing Officer
InvoTek, Inc. is a research and development company that improves the quality of life for people who find it difficult or impossible to use their hands by giving them new, efficient ways to access computers.

1413 Jelly Bean Switch
AbleNet, Inc.
2625 Patton Road
Roseville, MN 55113-1137

651-294-2200
800-322-0956
Fax: 651-294-2259
customerservice@ablenetinc.com
www.ablenetinc.com

Jennifer Thalhuber, President & CEO
Paul Sugden, CFO & Trustee
A momentary touch switch made of shatterproof plastic, small and sensitive to 2-3 ounces of pressure, this switch is provided audible feedback when activated and is a compact version of the Big Red Switch. Choice of colors: red, blue, green and yellow. *$75.00*

1414 Large Print Keyboard Labels
Hooleon Corp
P.O.Box 589
Melrose, NM 88124-589

575-253-4503
800-937-1337
Fax: 928-634-4620
sales@hooleon.com
www.hooleon.com

Shannen Aikman, Admin Manager/Sales
Joan Crozier, President/Sales
Pressure sensitive labels for computer keyboards.

1415 MessageMate
Words+ Inc
42505 10th Street W
Lancaster, CA 93534-7059

661-723-6523
800-869-8521
Fax: 661-723-2114
www.words-plus.com

Jeff Dahlan, President
Ginger Woltosz, General Manager
Lightweight, hand-held communicator providing high-quality analog recording capability using either direct select keyboards or 1 to 2 switch access. Price ranges from $549.00 to $999.00. *$1550.00*

1416 Mouthsticks
Performance Health
28100 Torch Parkway
Suite 700
Warrenville, IL 60555-3938

630-393-6000
Fax: 630-393-7600
customsupport@performancehealth.com
www.performancehealth.com

Francis Dirksmeier, Chief Executive Officer
Greg Nulty, Chief Financial Officer
Jim Plewa, Chief Sales Officer
Wide offering of mouthsticks: BK 5380, 5381, 5383, 5385, 6002, or BK 5370 series). Designed for typing and page turning. Suitable for both personal and professional use. *$48.86*

1417 Old MacDonald's Farm IntelliKeys Overlay
Soft Touch Inc
12301 Central Ave NE
Ste 205
Blaine, MN 55434

763-755-1402
888-755-1403
Fax: 763-862-2920
sales@marblesoft.com
www.softtouch.com

Joyce Meyer, President
Extend your students' learning with more than 45 pre-made overlays that support all of the skills learned at the farm. Use with the IntelliKeys keyboard. Simply print and use. Print an extra set to make off computer activities, too. Note: Requires Overlay Maker or Overlay Printer by IntelliTools.

1418 Origin Instruments Corporation
854 Greenview Dr
Grand Prairie, TX 75050

972-606-8740
Fax: 972-606-8741
support@orin.com
www.orin.com

Origin Instruments develops and delivers access solutions for people who do not have the ability to control a computer or iOS Device (iPad, iPhone or iPod touch) with their hands.

1419 Perfect Solutions
2685 Treanor Ter
Wellington, FL 33414-6460

561-790-1070
800-726-7086
Fax: 561-790-0108
perfect@gate.net
www.perfectsolutions.com

Andrew Kramer, President
A computer for every student and it speaks! Wireless laptop computers starting at $299.00 are ideal for students to carry with them all day. Text-to-speech and web browsing are available. *$299.00*

1420 Phillip Roy, Inc.
P.O. Box 130
Indian Rocks Beach, FL 33785-130   727-593-2700
                                          800-255-9085
                                     Fax: 877-595-2685
                                          info@philliproy.com
                                          www.philliproy.com

Ruth Bragman, PhD, President
Phil Padol, Consultant
Offers multimedia materials appropriate for use with individuals
with disabilities. Programs range from preschool through the
adult level. Many of the programs are high interest topics/low vocabulary, ideal for transition and employability skills. Materials
are also available which focus on social and personal development. Lesson Plans, teacher's guides, pre/post assessment, and
other support materials are provided at no additional cost.

1421 SS-Access Single Switch Interface for PC's with MS-DOS
Academic Software
3504 Tates Creek Road
Lexington, KY 40517-2601   859-552-1020
                                          800-842-2357
                                     Fax: 253-799-4012
                                          asistaff@acsw.com
                                          www.acsw.com

Warren E Lacefield PhD, President
Penelope Ellis, Marketing Director
A general purpose single switch hardware and software interface
for DOS and the IBM and compatible PC family. It is designed to
be easy to install, simple to use, and compatible with the widest
possible range of computers and application software programs.
SS-ACCESS! connects to one of the PC serial ports and provides
a jack to connect an external switch. The DOS version of the software works by sending a user defined keystroke to the PC keyboard buffer whenever the switch is pressed. *$ 90.00*

1422 Simplicity
Words+
42505 10th Street W
Lancaster, CA 93534-7059   661-723-6523
                                          800-869-8521
                                     Fax: 661-723-2114
                                          info@words-plus.com
                                          www.words-plus.com

Jeff Dahlan, President
Ginger Wolosz, General Manager
Swing-down mount for portable computers and other devices is
made from high-quality aircraft aluminum. Simplicity contains
very few moving parts and installs in minutes, providing a positive, secure support for computer/device in both the stored and
overlap position. *$1199.00*

1423 Songs I Sing at Preschool IntelliKeys Overlay
Soft Touch
12301 Central Ave NE
Ste 205
Blaine, MN 55434   763-755-1402
                                          888-755-1403
                                     Fax: 763-862-2920
                                          sales@marblesoft.com
                                          www.softtouch.com

Joyce Meyer, President
Pre-made overlays for use with Songs I Sing at Preschool. Simply
print and use with an IntelliKeys keyboard. Print an extra set to
make off computer activities, too.

1424 Switch Basics IntelliKeys Overlay
Soft Touch
12301 Central Ave NE
Ste 205
Blaine, MN 55434   763-755-1402
                                          888-755-1403
                                     Fax: 763-862-2920
                                          sales@marblesoft.com
                                          www.softtouch.com

Joyce Meyer, President
Four preprinted overlays to use with Switch Basics. Just put them
on an IntelliKeys keyboard and you're ready to go.

1425 Teach Me Phonemics Blends Overlay CD
SoftTouch Inc.
12301 Central Ave NE
Ste 205
Blaine, MN 55434   763-755-1402
                                          888-755-1403
                                     Fax: 763-862-2920
                                          sales@marblesoft.com
                                          www.softtouch.com

Roxanne Butterfield, Marketing
Joyce Meyer, President
Teach Me Phonemics Blends Overlay CD contains over 40
IntelliKeys overlays for use with Teach Me Phonemics - Blends
program. Choose either 4-item or 9-item layout to match the presentation you use in the program. Print extra copies of the overlays for off computer activites, too.

1426 Teach Me Phonemics Medial Overlay CD
SoftTouch Incorporated
Ste C
17117 Oak Dr
Omaha, NE 68130-2193   402-330-1301
                                          877-763-8868
                                     Fax: 402-334-8478
                                          support@softtouch.com
                                          www.softtouch.com

Kip Fisher, Manager
Roxanne Butterfield, Marketing
Teach Me Phonemics Medial Overlay CD contains over 40
IntelliKeys overlays for use with Teach Me Phonemics - Medial
program. Choose either 4-item or 9-item layout to match the presentation you use in the program. Print extra copies of the overlays for off computer activites, too.

1427 Teach Me Phonemics Overlay Series Bundle
SoftTouch
Ste 401
4300 Stine Rd
Bakersfield, CA 93313-2352   661-396-8676
                                          877-763-8868
                                     Fax: 661-396-8760
                                          www.softtouch.com

Roxanne Butterfield, Marketing
Joyce Meyer, President
Teach Me Phonemics Overlay Series Bundle includes one copy of
each Teach Me Phonemics Overlay CD - Initial, Medial, Final and
- four CD's in all.

1428 Teach Me to Talk Overlay CD
Soft Touch
12301 Central Ave NE
Ste 205
Blaine, MN 55434   763-755-1402
                                          888-755-1403
                                     Fax: 763-862-2920
                                          sales@marblesoft.com
                                          www.softtouch.com

Joyce Meyer, President
For older version of Teach Me to Talk. Mac only version with red
label and PC only version with yellow label. More than 48
pre-made overlays that match the activities on Teach Me to Talk.
Simply print and use with an IntelliKeys keyboard. Print an extra
set to make off computer activities, too.

1429 Teach Me to Talk: USB-Overlay CD
Soft Touch
12301 Central Ave NE
Ste 205
Blaine, MN 55434   763-755-1402
                                          888-755-1403
                                     Fax: 763-862-2920
                                          sales@marblesoft.com
                                          www.softtouch.com

Joyce Meyer, President
Revised version of Teach Me to Talk Overlays for the newest version that is USB IntelliKeys compatible. This CD contains more
than 48 overlays that match the activities and updated graphics of
Teach Me to Talk. Includes Overlay Printer by IntelliTools for
easy printing.

1430 Teen Tunes Plus IntelliKeys Overlay
Soft Touch
12301 Central Ave NE
Ste 205
Blaine, MN 55434
763-755-1402
888-755-1403
Fax: 763-862-2920
sales@marblesoft.com
www.softtouch.com

Joyce Meyer, President
Seven full color, preprinted overlays to use with Teen Tunes Plus. Just put them on an IntelliKeys keyboard and you're ready to go. *$49.00*

1431 U-Control III
Words+
42505 10th St W
Lancaster, CA 93534-7059
575-253-4503
800-869-8521
Fax: 661-723-2114
www.words-plus.com

Jeff Dahlen, President
Ginger Wolosz, General Manager
Works with the Words+ system (EX Keys, Morse WSKE, Scanning WSKE, Talking Screen) to provide wireless, portable control of items which are already infrared-controlled such as a TV, VCR, CD player, etc. *$499.00*

1432 WinSCAN: The Single Switch Interface for PC's with Windows
Academic Software
3504 Tates Creek Rd
Lexington, KY 40517-2601
859-522-1020
Fax: 253-799-4012
asistaff@acsw.com
www.acsw.com

Warren E Lacefield, President
Penelope Ellis, Marketing Director/COO
A general purpose single-switch control interface for Windows. It provides single-switch users independent control access to educational and productivity software, multimedia programs, and recreational activities that run under Windows 3.1 and higher versions on IBM and compatible PC's. The user can navigate through Windows; choose program icons and run programs, games, and CD's; even surf the Internet with WinSCAN and his or her adaptive switch. *$349.00*

1433 Words+ IST (Infrared, Sound, Touch)
Words+
42505 10th St W
Lancaster, CA 93534-7059
575-253-4503
800-869-8521
Fax: 661-723-2114
www.words-plus.com

Jeff Dahlan, President
Ginger Wolosz, General Manager
A unique switch that is activated by slight movement or faint sound. The switch provides user control when connected to a device driven by a single switch. Individuals are currently accessing a wide variety of communication and computer systems with movement using the IST switch. *$395.00*

Braille Products

1434 Braille Keyboard Labels
Hooleon Corporation
PO Box 589
Melrose, NM 88124-589
928-634-7515
800-937-1337
Fax: 928-634-4620
sales@hooleon.com
www.hooleon.com

Barry Green, Sales Manager
Joan Crozier, President/Sales
Also large print keyboard labels and large print with Braille.

1435 Braille Paper
Maxi Aids
42 Executive Blvd.
Farmingdale, NY 11735-4710
631-752-0521
800-522-6294
Fax: 631-752-0689
TTY: 631-752-0738
sales@maxiaids.com
www.maxiaids.com

Elliot Zaretsky, Founder, President & CEO
Paper for braille embossing. Sizes include 8.5 by 11 inch and 11 by 11.5 inch.

1436 Brailon Plastic Sheets
Maxi Aids
42 Executive Blvd.
Farmingdale, NY 11735-4710
631-752-0521
800-522-6294
Fax: 631-752-0689
TTY: 631-752-0738
sales@maxiaids.com
www.maxiaids.com

Elliot Zaretsky, Founder, President & CEO
Brailon plastic sheets used with Thermoform machines to copy braille text and graphics.

1437 Brailon Thermoform Duplicator
American Thermoform Corporation
1758 Brackett St
La Verne, CA 91750-5855
909-593-6711
800-331-3676
Fax: 909-593-8001
pnunnelly@americanthermoform.com
www.americanthermoform.com

Patrick Nunnelly, VP
Gary Nunnelly, Owner
This copy machine, for producing tactile images, copies any brailled or embossed original, by a vacuum forming process. This model is for the reproduction of teaching aids and mobility maps.

1438 Duxbury Braille Translator
Duxbury Systems
Ste 6
270 Littleton Rd
Westford, MA 01886-3523
978-692-3000
Fax: 978-692-7912
info@duxsys.com
www.duxburysystems.com

Joe Sullivan, President
A complete line of easy to use word processing and Braille translation software available for Windows (including 64 bit windows). Applications for anyone wanting to produce or communicate with Braille; signs, note cards, textbooks, business communications and forms, telephone bills, etc. Simple to use, FREE technical support. Free one year upgrades. DBT is for producing Braille in English, Spanish, French, Portuguese, Italian, Latin, Greek, German and 125 other languages. *$600.00*

1439 Enabling Technologies Company
1601 NE Braille Pl
Jensen Beach, FL 34957-5345
772-225-3687
800-777-3687
Fax: 772-225-3299
info@brailler.com
www.brailler.com

Tony Schenk, President
Kate Schenk, Product Manager Western US
Greg Schenk, Sales & Marketing
Manufactures the most complete line of American made Braille embossers, including desktop or portable models capable of producing high quality single sided or interpoint Braille. Also carries a complete line of adaptive technology aids for the blind community at affordable prices.

1440   Freedom Scientific Blind/Low Vision Group
11800 31st Ct N
St Petersburg, FL 33716-1805   727-803-8000
                                      800-444-4443
                                  Fax: 727-803-8001
                          info@freedomscientific.com
                             www.freedomscientific.com

Brad Davis, VP Hardware Product Management
Dr Lee Hamilton, President/CEO
Developer and manufacturer of assistive technology products for
people who are blind or who have low vision. Innovative blindness products include: JAWS® screen reading software; the PAC
Mate Omni™, an accessible Pocket PC; the SARA™ scanning
and reading appliance; OpenBook™ scanning and reading software; FSReader™ DAISY player; FaceToFace™ deaf-blind
communications solution; and PAC Mate and Focus Braille Displays. *$16.95*

1441   Hooleon Corporation
PO Box 589
Melrose, NM 88124-589   928-634-7515
                                      800-937-1337
                                  Fax: 928-634-4620
                                 sales@hooleon.com
                                   www.hooleon.com

Kim Green, Manager
Joan Crozier, President/Sales
Large print and combination Braille adhesive keytop labels for
computer keyboards. Helps visually impaired computer users access correct key strokes either by sight or by touch. Raised Braille
meets ADA specifications and large print fills key top surface.

1442   Humanware
1 UPS Way
P.O. Box 800
Champlain, NY 12919   800-722-3393
                                  Fax: 888-871-4828
                               info@humanware.com
                                   humanware.com

Gilles Pepin, CEO
Humanware manufactures electronics to provide solutions that
empower the visually impaired.

1443   Large Print/Braille Keyboard Labels
Infogrip
Ventura, CA 93001   503-828-1221
                                      866-606-8551
                               support@infogrip.com
                                   www.infogrip.com

Liza Jacobs, President
Aaron Gaston, Vice President
Makes a standard keyboard more accessible for visually impaired
individuals with large print or Braille keyboard labels. Characters on the large print labels are .5 by .25 inches, about 3 times
larger than standard keyboard characters. Braille labels are available as clear labels with Braille dots or large print with Braille.
Each set includes all the keys used on a standard Windows keyboard. *$29.00*

1444   Raised Dot Computing
Duxbury Systems Incorporated
270 Littleton Rd.
Unit 6
Westford, MA 01886-3523   978-692-3000
                                  Fax: 978-692-7912
                                  info@duxsys.com
                              www.duxburysystems.com

Joe Sullivan, President
Peter Sullivan, VP of Software Development
Genevieve Sullivan, Treasurer
Software for the visually impaired.

1445   Touchdown Keytop/Keyfront Kits
Hooleon Corporation
P.O. Box 589
304 West Denby Ave
Melrose, NM 88124   575-253-4503
                                      800-937-1337
                                  Fax: 575-253-4299
                                Sales@Hooleon.com
                                   www.hooleon.com

Bob Crozier, Founder
Joan Crozier, President
Barry Green, Sales Manager
These kits enlarge the key legends of a computer and include
Braille for easy recognition.

Information Centers & Databases

1446   ATTAIN
Division of Disability Aging & Rehab Services
Ste 1400
32 E Washington St
Indianapolis, IN 46204-3552   317-232-1147
                                      800-528-8246
                                  Fax: 317-486-8809

Gary R Hand, Executive Director
Peter Bisbecos, Manager
Nonprofit organization that creates system change by expanding
the availability of community-based technology-related activities, outreach services, empowerment and advocacy activities
through the development of a comprehensive, consumer-responsive, statewide program to serve individuals with disabilities, of
all ages and all disabilities, their families, caregivers, educators
and service providers. Provides training, information and
referrals, system change and assessments for equipment needs.

1447   AbleData
103 W Broad St
Suite 400
Falls Church, VA 22046   301-608-8998
                                      800-227-0216
                                  Fax: 301-608-8958
                                  TTY: 301-608-8912
                           abledata@neweditions.net
                                   www.abledata.com

Katherine Belknap, Director
David Johnson, Publications Director
AbleData is an electronic database containing information on
assistive technology and rehabilitation equipment products for
children and adults with physical, cognitive and sensory disabilities. AbleData staff can perform database searches or the database can be searched via the website, informed consumer guides
or fact sheets.

1448   Aloha Special Technology Access Center
710 Green St
Honolulu, HI 96813-2119   808-523-5547
                                  Fax: 808-536-3765
                                 astachi@yahoo.com

Ali Silvert, President
Ms. Jacquely Brand, Founder
Computer technology center.

1449   Birmingham Alliance for Technology Access Center
Birmingham Independent Living Center
206 13th St S.
Birmingham, AL 35233-1317   205-251-2223
                                  Fax: 205-251-0605
                                  TTY: 205-251-2223
                                 www.drradvocates.org

Kathy Lovell, President
Phil Klebine, Vice President
Daniel Kessler, Executive Director
Computer technology center.

1450   Bluegrass Technology Center
409 Southland Drive
Lexington, KY 40503   859-294-4343
                                            800-209-7767
                                         Fax: 866-576-9625

Debbie Sharon, Acting Executive Director
Linnie Lee, Assistive Technology Specialist
Jean Isaacs, Assistive Technology Consultant
Provides assistive technology information, consulting and training for education, health professionals, consumers and parents of consumers. Maintains extensive lending library of assistive devices and adapted toys. Statewide training such as; AAC, how to obtain funding for assistive technology, augmentative and alternate communication, equipment implementation strategies, specific to hardware and software, etc.

1451   CITE: Lighthouse for Central Florida
215 East New Hampshire Street
Orlando, FL 32804   407-898-2483
                                         Fax: 407-898-0236
                                           csacca@lcf-fl.org
                       www.lighthousecentralflorida.org/Default.asp
Lee Nasehi, MSW, President/CEO
Donna Esbensen CPA,MBA, VP/CFO
Jeff Whitehead, MPA, MS, Director of Program Services
CITE promotes the independence of adults and children with blindness, low vision and other disabilities through technology, education, support and advocacy.

1452   Carolina Computer Access Center
P.O.Box 247
Cramerton, NC 28032   704-342-3004
                                         Fax: 704-342-1513

Linda Schilling, Executive Director
Nonprofit, community-based technology resource center for people with disabilities, providing information about and demonstration of the technology tools that enable individuals with disabilities to control and direct their own lives. Services and programs include: assessments, demonstrations, resource information, lending library, workshops and outreach.

1453   Center for Accessible Technology
3075 Adeline
Suite 220
Berkeley, CA 94703   510-841-3224
                                         Fax: 510-841-7956
                                            info@cforat.org
                                            www.cforat.org

Dmitri Belser, Executive Director
Eric Smith, Associate Director
A consumer-based technology resource and demonstration center for adults and children with disabilities, families, teachers, and professionals. The primary focus is on assistive technology for computer access. Seen by appointment only.

1454   Center for Applied Special Technology
40 Harvard Mills Square
Suite 3
Wakefield, MA 01880-3233   781-245-2212
                                         Fax: 781-245-5212
                                             cast@cast.org
                                            www.cast.org/

Anne Meyer, Founder
David H. Rose, Founder
Lisa Poller, Co-President
Expands opportunities for individuals with special needs through innovative use of computers and related technology. We pursue this mission through research and product development that further universal design for learning.

1455   Center for Assistive Technology & Inclusive Education Studies
2000 Pennington Rd.
P.O.Box 7718
Ewing, NJ 08628-0718   609-771-3016
                                         Fax: 609-637-5179
                                            caties@tcnj.edu
                                        caties.pages.tcnj.edu

Amanda Norvell, President
Matt Bender, VP
Regina Morin, Parliamentarian

Computer technology center offering resource time, workshops, technology, training and evaluations.

1456   Center on Evaluation of Assistive Technology
National Rehabilitation Hospital
102 Irving St NW
Washington, DC 20010   202-877-1000
                                       TTY: 202-726-3996
                                     justin.m.carter@medstar.net
                                        www.medstarhealth.org
Kenneth A. Samet, FACHE, President, CEO
Michael J. Curran, EVP, Chief Administrative and Financial Officer
Christine Swearingen, EVP, Planning, Marketing and Community Relations
The center develops ways of collecting, producing and distributing information to help users, prescribers and third-party payers make intelligent selections of devices.

1457   Compuserve: Handicapped Users' Database
5000 Arlington Centre Blvd
Columbus, OH 43220-2913   614-326-1002
                                            800-848-8990
                                         Fax: 614-538-4023
                                 webcenters.netscape.compuserve.com
This nationwide database with bulletin boards provides information for persons with disabilities and the issues and technologies that are of interest to them.

1458   Computer Access Center
P.O. Box 12464
Albuquerque, NM 87195   505-242-9588
                                              info@cac.org
                                              www.cac.org

Richard Barlow, Board of Director
Richard Rohr, Board of Director
Michael Poffenberger, Board of Director
Computer technology center.

1459   Computer Center for Visually Impaired People: Division of Continuing Studies
Baruch College
1 Bernard Baruch Way
Box H-648
New York, NY 10010   646-312-1420
                                         Fax: 646-312-5101
                                     www.baruch.cuny.edu/ccvip

Karen Gourgey, Director
Judith Gerber, Operations Manager
Lynette Tatum, Training Specialist
Offers courses, tutors, equipment and assistance.

1460   Computer Resources for People with Disabilities
Hunter House Publishers, Inc
424 Church Street
Suite 2240
Nashville, TN 37219   615-255-BOOK
                                     info@turnerpublishing.com
                                        www.hunterhouse.com

Kiran Rana, Publisher
Chris Alexander, Author
Sheila Alson, Author
Part One describes conventional and assistive technologies and gives strategies for accessing the Internet. Part Two features easy-to-use charts organized by key access concerns, and provides detailed descriptions of software, hardware, and communication aids. Part Three is a gold mine of Web resources, publications, support organizations, government programs, and technology vendors.

1461   Computer-Enabling Drafting for People with Physical Disabilities
County College of Morris
214 Center Grove Road
Randolph, NJ 07869-2086   973-328-5000
                                            888-226-8001
                                         Fax: 973-328-5067
                                              www.ccm.edu

Edward J Yaw, President
Dr. Dwight Smith, Vice President of Academic Affairs
Karen VanDerhoof, Vice President for Business and Finance

Since they opened in 1968, more than 40,000 graduates have passed through their halls. Many have become teachers, nurses, police officers, doctors and engineers. CCM has also been a community resource for those seeking to enhance their careers through additional education. They drafted a newsletter on Computer-Enabling Drafting for People with Physical Disabilities

1462 DIRLINE
National Library of Medicine
8600 Rockville Pike
Bethesda, MD 20894

301-594-5983
888-346-3656
Fax: 301-402-1384
TTY: 800-735-2258
www.nlm.nih.gov/

Dr. Donald A B. Lindberg, Director
Milton Corn, Deputy Director
Betsy Humphreys, Deputy Director
18,000 listings of organizations that serve as information resources, including libraries, professional associations and government agencies.

1463 Developmental Disabilities Council
626 Main Street, Suite A
P.O.Box 3455
Baton Rouge, LA 70821-3455

225-342-6804
800-450-8108
Fax: 225-342-1970
shawn.fleming@la.gov
www.laddc.org

Sandee Winchell, Executive Director
Shawn Fleming, Deputy Director
Derek White, Program Manager
The Louisiana Developmental Disabilities Council is made up of people from every region of the state who are appointed by the governor to develop and implement a five year plan to address the needs of persons with disabilities. Membership includes persons with developmental disabilities, parents, advocates, professionals, and representatives from public and private agencies.

1464 Employment Resources Program
330 South Grand Avenue West
Springfield, IL 62704

217-523-2587
800-447-4221
Fax: 217-523-0427
TTY: 217-523-2587
scil@scil.org
www.scil.org

Pete Roberts, Executive Director
Susanne Cooper, Program Director
Robin Ashton- Hale, Reintegration Coordinator
An information and referral service that encourages inquiries from professionals, individuals with disabilities, family members, organizations or anyone requesting information pertaining to disabilities. The staff at DRN uses both computer listings and in-house library files to provide the programs services. The DRN program is funded by a grant from the Illinois Department of Rehabilitation Services.

1465 Functional Skills Screening Inventory
Functional Resources
3905 Huntington Dr
Amarillo, TX 79019-4047

806-353-1114
Fax: 806-353-1114
www.winfssi.com

Ed Hammer, Owner
Heather Becker PhD, Owner
Assesses the individual's level of functional skills and identifies supports needed by educational, rehabilitation and residential programs serving moderately and severely disabled persons. Includes environmental assessments as well as profiles of jobs and training sites.

1466 High Tech Center
Sacramento State
6000 J Street
Sacramento, CA 95819

916-278-6011
sswd@csus.edu
www.csus.edu

Alexander Gonzalez, President
Judy Dean, Co-Director
Melissa Repa, Co-Director
The Center offers assessment and training in adaptive hardware/software for eligible students with disabilities at Sacramento State upon referral from the Office of Services to Students with Disabilities.

1467 Idaho Assistive Technology Project
121 W 3rd St
Moscow, ID 83843-2268

208-885-3557
Fax: 208-885-3628
www.idahoat.org

Ron Seiler, Project Director
Sue House, Information Specialist
A federally funded program managed by the center on disabilities and human development at the university of Idaho. The goal of the IATP is to increase the availability of assistive technology devices and services for Idahoans with disabilities. The IATP offers free trainings and technical assistance, a low-interest loan program, assistive technology assessments for children and agriculture workers, and free informational materials.

1468 Increasing Capabilities Access Network
525 W.Capitol
Little Rock, AR 72201

501-666-8868
800-828-2799
Fax: 501-666-5319
TTY: 501-666-8868
nfo@ar-ican.org
www.arkansas-ican.org

Bryen Ayres, Member of Advisory Council
Billy Altom, Member of Advisory Council
Adrienne Brown, Member of Advisory Council
A consumer responsive statewide systems change program promoting assistive technology for persons of all ages with disabilities. The program provides information on new and existing technology and maintains an equipment exchange free of charge. Training on assistive technology is also provided.

1469 International Center for the Disabled
340 E 24th St
New York, NY 10010-4019

212-585-6000
Fax: 212-585-6161
info@icdnyc.org
www.icdnyc.org

Jill Bowman, Manager
Les Halpert, CEO
The ICD is a comprehensive outpatient rehabilitation facility, providing medical rehabilitation, behavioral health and vocational services to children and adults with a broad range of physical, communication, emotional and cognitive disabilities.

1470 Kentucky Assistive Technology Service Network
200 Juneau Dr.
Suite 200
Louisville, KY 40243

502-429-4484
800-327-5287
Fax: 502-429-7114
www.katsnet.org

Derrick Cox, Manager
Statewide network of four regional assistive technology centers with a central coordinating office in Louisville and two regional centers in eastern Kentucky. Network services include but are not limited to assistive technology of services, loan of assistive devices, funding information and referral, assessment and evaluations, consultations on appropriate technologies, training, and technical assistance.

1471   Learning Independence Through Computers
2301 Argonne Drive
Baltimore, MD 21218   410-554-9134
                                        Fax: 410-261-2907
                                            info@linc.org
                                             www.linc.org

Theo Pinette, Executive Director
Sandy Fishman, Office and Computer Center Coordinator
Angela Tyler, Volunteer Services Manager
V-LINC creates technological solutions to improve the independence and quality of life for individuals of all ages with disabilities in Maryland. We do this through a mix of off-the-shelf computer software and equipment, and one-of-a-kind, customized assistive technology.

1472   MEDLINE
Dialog Corporation
2250 Perimeter Park Drive
Suite 300
Morrisville, NC 27560   800-334-2564
                                             919-804-6400
                                        Fax: 919-804-6410
                                           www.dialog.com

Tim Wahlberg, Genral Manager
Morten Nicholaisen, VP Global Sales and Account Mana
Libby Trudell, VP Strategic Initiatives
Bibliographic citations to biomedical literature.

1473   Maine CITE
University of Maine at Augusta
46 University Avenue
Augusta, ME 04330   207-621-3195
                                        Fax: 207-629-5429
                                        TTY: 877-475-4800
                                       iweb@mainecite.org
                                         www.mainecite.org

Robert McPhee, Member of Advisory Council
Deborah Gardner, Member of Advisory Council
Anita Dunham, Member of Advisory Council
Computer technology center.

1474   Maryland Technology Assistance Program
Maryland Department of Disabilities
2301 Argonne Drive
Rm T-17
Baltimore, MD 21218   410-554-9361
                                             800-832-4827
                                        Fax: 410-554-9237
                                        TTY: 866-881-7488
                                            www.mdtap.org

James McCarthy, Executive Director
Denise Schuler, Assistive Technology Specialist
Tanya Goodman, Loan Program Assistant Director
Assistive technology center. Information and referral, equipment display loans and demonstration, funding sources, alternative media, training, workshops and seminars. Rural outreach for individuals with disability in Maryland.

1475   Minnesota STAR Program
358 Centennial Office Building 658
Saint Paul, MN 55155- 1402   651-201-2640
                                             800-627-3529
                                             888-234-1267
                                        Fax: 651-282-6671
                                    star.program@state.mn.us

Chuck Rassbach, Program Director
Jennis Delisi, Program Staff
Jaoan Gillum, Program Staff
STAR's mission is to help all Minnesotans with disabilities gain access to and acquire the assistive technology they need to live, learn, work and lay. The Minnesota STAR program is federally funded by the Rehabilitation Services Administration.

1476   Mississippi Project START
2550 Peachtree Street
Jackson, MS 39216   601-987-4872
                                             800-852-8328
                                        Fax: 601-364-2349
                                        pgaltelli@mdrs.ms.gov
                                       www.msprojectstart.org

Patsy Galtelli, Executive Director
Dorothy Young, Project Director
Nekeba Simmons, Administrative Assistant
Project START is a Tech Act project established to bring about systems change in the field of assistive technology in the State of Mississippi. Activities include providing training opportunities for consumers and service providers on subjects such as state-of-the-art AT devices, their application and funding resources; referral information on AT evaluation centers; technical assistance to AT users; establishment of an AT equipment loan program and an Information and Referral Service.

1477   National Technology Database
American Foundation for the Blind/ AF B Press
2 Penn Plaza
Suite 1102
New York, NY 10121   212-502-7600
                                             800-232-5463
                                        Fax: 888-545-8331
                                          afbinfo@afb.net
                                              www.afb.org

Carl.R Augusto, President and CEO
Robin Vogel, Vice President, Resource Development
Kelly Bleach, Chief Administrative Officer
This database includes resources for visually impaired persons.
$99.00

1478   New Jersey Department of Labor & Workforce Development
Office of the Commissioner
1 John Fitch Plaza
P.O.Box 110
Trenton, NJ 08625-0110   609-292-7060
                                        Fax: 609-633-1359
                                        www.state.nj.us/labor

Harold J. Wirths, Commissioner
Aaron R. Fichtner, Ph.D., Deputy Commissioner
Frederick J. Zavaglia, Chief of Staff
Oversees various federal and state vocational rehabilitation services including sheltered workshops and independent living centers; adjudication of permanent disability claims filed with the Social Security Administration; oversees New Jersey's temporary disability program covering non-work related illnesses and injuries

1479   New Mexico Technology Assistance Program
625 Silver Ave SW
Suite 100 B
Albuquerque, NM 87102   505-841-4464
                                             877-696-1470
                                        Fax: 505-841-4467
                                      www.tap.gcd.state.nm.us

Tracy Agiovlasitis, Program Manager
Examines and works to eliminate barriers to obtaining assistive technology in New Mexico. Has established a statewide program for coordinating assistive technology services; is designed to assist people with disabilities to locate, secure, and maintain assistive technology.

1480   Northern Illinois Center for Adaptive Technology
3615 Louisiana Rd
Rockford, IL 61108   815-229-2163

Dave Grass, President
Computer technology center.

1481 OCCK
1710 W. Schilling Road
Salina, KS 67402-1160
785-827-9383
800-526-9731
Fax: 785-823-2015
TTY: 785-827-9383
occk@occk.com
www.occk.com

Shelia Nelson Stout, President, CEO
Carolee Miner, CEO
Computer technology center; training center for employment and independent living for people with disabilities; family support center. Kansas AgrAbility program coordinator, Kansas equipment exchange site.

1482 Options, Resource Center for Independent Living
318 3rd St. NW
East Grand Forks, MN 56721
218-773-6100
800-726-3692
Fax: 218-773-7119
options@myoptions.info
www.rcil.com

Burt Danovitz, Executive Director
The RCIL aggressively advocates for and defends the rights of persons with disabilities. RCIL believes in integration adn assisting people to reach their full potential, encouraging a culture of risk-taking, creativity and innovation through our programs and services. They monitor and assess the current legal climate around rights for persons with disabilities on an ongoing bases and are committed and deliberate in speaking about the problems and obstacles faced by persons with disabilities.

1483 Parents, Let's Unite for Kids
516 N 32nd St
Billings, MT 59101-6003
406-255-0540
800-222-7585
Fax: 406-255-0523
TTY: 406-657-2055
info@pluk.org

Roger Holt, Executive Director
Computer technology center. Parents, Let's Unite for Kids offers an assistive technology lab that is open to people of all ages. The lab is a computer and assistive technology demonstration site. There is no charge for services.

1484 Pennsylvania's Initiative on Assistive Technology
Temple University
1755 N. 13th St.
Student Center, Room 411 South
Philadelphia, PA 19122-6024
215-204-1356
800-204-7428
Fax: 215-204-6336
TTY: 866-268-0579
ATinfo@temple.edu
www.disabilities.temple.edu

Kim Singleton, Director
Pennsylvania's Initiative on Assistive Technology (PIAT) offers information and referral about assistive Technology (AT), device demonstrations, and awareness-level presentations. PIAT also operates Pennsylvania's AT Lending Library, a free, state-supported program that loans AT devices to Pennsylvanians of all ages.

1485 Rehabilitation Engineering and AssistiveTechnology Society of North America (RESNA)
2001 K Street NW
3rd Floor North
Washington, DC 20006
202-367-1121
Fax: 202-367-2121
info@resna.org
www.resna.org

Maureen Linden, President
Andrea Van Hook, Interim Executive Director
RESNA improves the potential of people with disabilities to achieve their goals through the use of technology. RESNA promotes research, development, education, advocacy and provision of technology; and by supporting the people engaged in these activities.

1486 SACC Assistive Technology Center
P.O.Box 1325
Simi Valley, CA 93062-1325
805-582-1881
www.semel.ucla.edu

Debi Schultze, CEO
SACC connects children, adults and seniors with special needs to computers, technologies and resources. We provide information and referral, assessments, tutoring, presentations and outreach awareness.

1487 South Dakota Department of Human Services: Computer Technology Services
Properties Plaza
500 East Capitol Avenue
Pierre, SD 57501
605-773-5990
800-265-9684
Fax: 605-773-5483
TTY: 605-773-6412
infodhs@state.sd.us
dhs.sd.gov

Dan Lusk, Division Director
Ted Williams, Director
Eric Weiss, Director
Computer technology center.

1488 Star Center
1119 Old Humboldt Rd
Jackson, TN 38305-1752
731-668-3888
888-398-5619
Fax: 731-668-1666
TTY: 731-668-9664
information@starcenter.tn.org
www.starcenter.tn.org

John Borden, CEO
Nation's largest assistive technology center dedicated to helping children and adults with disabilities achieve their goals for competitive employment, effective learning, returning to or starting school and independent living. Programs include: high-tech training, music therapy, art therapy, low vision evaluation, orientation and mobility evaluation and training, augmentative communication evaluation, vocational evaluations, assistive technology, job placement services and job skills training.

1489 Students with Disabilities Office
University of Texas at Austin
100 West Dean Keeton A5800
Austin, TX 78712-1100
512-471-5017
Fax: 512-471-7833
deanofstudents@austin.utexas.edu
deanofstudents.utexas.edu

Soncia Reagins-Lilly, Ed.D., Senior Associate VP for Student Affairs & Dean of Students
Douglas Garrard, Ed.D., Senior Associate Dean of Students
Wanda Brune, Administrative Associate

1490 TASK Team of Advocates for Special Kids
100 W Cerritos Ave
Anaheim, CA 92805
714-533-8275
866-828-8275
Fax: 714-533-2533
task@taskca.org
www.taskca.org

Marta Anchondo, Executive Director
Tom Bratkovich, Treasurer
Leana Way, Director
Computer technology center.

1491 Tech Connection
35 Haddon Avenue
Shrewsbury, NJ 07702
732-747-5310
Fax: 732-747-1896
info@frainc.org
www.frainc.org

Bill Sheeser, President
Nancy Phalanukom, Executive Director
Sue Levine, Program Administrator
Offers a noncommercial center to examine and try computers, adapted equipment, alternative input devices, and a variety of software. Program of Family Resource Associates and a member of the Alliance for Technology Access (ATA), a growing national coalition of computer resource centers, professionals, technol-

ogy developers and vendors, interacting with new technology to enrich the lives of people with disabilities. Tech Connection offers evaluations, for computer technology.

1492 Tech-Able
1451 Klondike Road, Suite D
Conyers, GA 30094 770-922-6768
Fax: 770-922-6769

Cassandra Baker, Executive Director
Pat Hanus, Program Assistant
Erika Ruffin-Mosley, Assistive Technology Trainer
Provide assistive technology to individuals with disabilities, toy-lending and software libraries, product demonstration, access to technology devices and fabrication of keyguards for keyboards. Low vision consultant on Thursdays; computer training for persons with disabilities.

1493 Technology Access Center of Tucson
P.O.Box 13178
Tucson, AZ 85732-3178 520-638-2733
Fax: 520-519-7954
tact1@qwestoffice.net
http://www.uacoe.arizona.edu/tact/
A resource center that provides assistive technology services for people with disabilities. Center personnel develop, provide and coordinate those services in communities throughout Middle Tennessee. Services are designed to assist people with disabilities to learn about, choose, acquire and use assistive technology devices. Services are offered to any child or adult with sensory, motor or cognitive disabilities, their family members, and professionals who serve them and employ them.

1494 Technology Assistance for Special Consumers
1856 Keats Dr NW.
Huntsville, AL 35810 256-859-8300
Fax: 256-859-4332
ucphuntsville.org/what-we-do/t-a-s-c/
Cheryl Smith, Chief Executive Officer
T.A.S.C. is a computer resource center with 10 computers, which are equipped with special adaptations for those who are blind, visually impaired, or severely physically disabled. The staff demonstrates and trains individuals on this equipment so that they can become more independent at home, school, and work. Over 2,500 pieces of educational software are available.

1495 Tidewater Center for Technology Access Special Education Annex
1415 Laskin Rd
Virginia Beach, VA 23451 757-424-2672
Fax: 757-263-2801
www.tcta.access.org
Pat Mc Gee, Manager
Myra Jessie Flint, Designee
Nonprofit organization providing persons with disabilities access, support, and knowledge—re: technology; organization contracts for consultations, workshops and training, or conventional and assistive technologies including computers, augmented communication devices and software; resources: extensive lending library of educational software; books and videotape library; yearly individual membership and corporate membership fees; working/presentation and evaluation fees available upon request.

1496 Vermont Assistive Technology Project: Department of Aging & Disabilities
Agency of Human Services
103 South Main Street
Weeks Building
Waterbury, VT 05671-2305 802-871-3353
800-750-6355
Fax: 802-871-3048
TTY: 802-241-1464
atp.vermont.gov
Amber Fulcher, Program Director
Sharon Alderman, Assistive Technology Reuse Coordinator
Emma Cobb, Assistive Technology Services Coordinator
Increase the awareness and change policies to insure assistive technology is available to all Vermonters with disabilities.

Keyboards, Mouses & Joysticks

1497 A4 Tech (USA) Corporation
5585 Brooks St
Montclair, CA 91763-4547 909-988-9633
www.a4tech.com
Robert C
Manufacturers of a cordless mouse, trackballs and joysticks that emulate mouse controls, flatbed scanners, modified keyboards, and other specialty mouses.

1498 Abacus
3150 Patterson Ave SE
Grand Rapids, MI 49512 616-698-0330
800-451-4319
Fax: 616-698-0325
www.abacuspub.com
Arnie Lee, President
Designs a mouse software program that permits programs written for one computer to be run on another computer.

1499 Ability Center of Greater Toledo
5605 Monroe St.
Sylvania, OH 43560 419-885-5733
Fax: 419-882-4813
www.abilitycenter.org
Tim Harrington, Executive Director
Ash Lemons, Associate Director
Debbie Andriette, Director, Human Resources
Manufactures keyboard wrist supports to help prevent repetitive motion disorders.

1500 Dreamer
TS Micro Tech
17109 Gale Ave
City of Industry, CA 91745-1810 626-939-8998
Fax: 626-839-8516
Steve Heung, Owner
An intelligent, add-on function keyboard providing single-keystroke access to multiple-keystroke functions.

1501 FlexShield Keyboard Protectors
Hooleon Corporation
P.O.Box 589
Melrose, NM 88124-589 928-634-7515
800-937-1337
Fax: 928-634-4620
Barry Green, Sales Manager
Joan Crozier, President
Transparent keyboard protectors allowing instant recognition of keytop legends. They have a matte finish to reduce glare. Also available are large print and braille keyboard labels and large print/braille combo labels.

1502 IntelliKeys
Intelli Tools
1720 Corporate Circle
Petaluma, CA 94954 707-773-2000
800-899-6687
Fax: 707-773-2001
info@intellitools.com
www.intellitools.com
Dayton Johnson, VP, Sales
Arjan Khalsa, CEO
Alternative, touch-sensitive keyboards; plugs into any Macintosh or Windows computer. *$395.00*

1503 IntelliKeys USB
Intelli Tools
1720 Corporate Circle
Petaluma, CA 94954 707-773-2000
800-899-6687
Fax: 707-773-2001
info@intellitools.com
www.intellitools.com
Dayton Johnson, VP, Sales
Arjan Khalsa, CEO
IntelliKeys alternative keyboard for USB computers and Windows 2000, Mac OSX. *$69.95*

1504 Key Tronic KB 5153 Touch Pad Keyboard
KeyTronic
N. 4424 Sullivan Road
Spokane Valley, WA 99216   509-928-8000
                                    Fax: 509-927-5555
                            EMSsales@keytronicems.com
                                       www.keytronic.com
Craig.D Gates, President/CEO
Ronald.F Klawitter, EVP of Administration and Chief Financial Officer
Douglas G. Burkhardt, Executive Vice President of Worldwide Operations
Integrates a regular full-function keyboard, a numeric keypad with a cursor key capability and a touch pad into one unit.

1505 King Keyboard
Infogrip
Ventura, CA 93001   503-828-1221
                                          866-606-8551
                                   support@infogrip.com
                                        www.infogrip.com
Liza Jacobs, President
Aaron Gaston, Vice President
Giant alternative keyboard that plugs directly into a computer - no special interface is required. The keys are 1.25 inches in diameter, slightly recessed, and provide both tactile and auditory feedback. The King has a built-in keyboard so that you can rest on its surface without activating keys. This keyboard allows you to control both keyboard and mouse functions, making it great for people who have difficulty maneuvering a standard mouse. *$130.00*

1506 Large Print Keyboard
Infogrip
Ventura, CA 93001   503-828-1221
                                          866-606-8551
                                   support@infogrip.com
                                        www.infogrip.com
Liza Jacobs, President
Aaron Gaston, Vice President
Standard Windows keyboard with large print keys. The keyboard and its keys are the same size as a standard keyboard; however, the print has been enhanced. The characters measure.5 by.25 inches, about 3 times larger than standard keyboard characters. *$130.00*

1507 Magic Wand Keyboard
In Touch Systems
11 Westview Road
Spring Valley, NY 10977   845-354-7431
                                          800-332-6244
                            sc@magicwandkeyboard.com
                           www.magicwandkeyboard.com
Jerry Crouch, President
Susan Crouch, VP
The magic wand keyboard allows your child to use a keyboard and mouse easily-no light beams, microphones, or sensors to wear of position. This miniature computer keyboard has zero-force keys that work with the slightest touch of a wand (hand-held of mouthstick). No strength required.

1508 McKey Mouse
In Touch Systems
11 Westview Road
Spring Valley, NY 10977   845-354-7431
                                          800-332-6244
                            sc@magicwandkeyboard.com
                           www.magicwandkeyboard.com
Jerry Crouch, President
Susan Crouch, VP
Microsoft compatible mouse for persons with little or no hand/arm movement; it's an option for the Magic Wand Keyboard and adds full mouse function without adding any extra devices.

1509 OnScreen
Infogrip
Ventura, CA 93001   503-828-1221
                                          866-606-8551
                                   support@infogrip.com
                                        www.infogrip.com
Liza Jacobs, President
Aaron Gaston, Vice President
OnScreen features word prediction/completion (with an editable dictionary), Key Dwell Timer (a timer that selects a key under the cursor), integrated Verbal Keys Feedback, Show and Hide Keys (turns on/off keys to prevent access and minimize confusion) a Smart Window (automatically re-positions the keyboard or panels off of the area in use). OnScreen also offers edit, numeric, macro, calculator and Windows enhancement capabilities. *$200.00*

1510 PortaPower Plus
Words+
42505 10th Street West
Lancaster, CA 93534-7059   661-723-7723
                                          800-869-8521
                                    Fax: 661-723-5524
                            info@simulations-plus.com
                             www.simulations-plus.com
Walter S Woltosz, M.S., M.A.S., President, CEO
John A. DiBella, Vice President, Marketing & Sales
John R. Kneisel, Chief Financial Officer
Rechargeable battery pack designed to give longer life and remote usage time to laptop computers and other portable battery-operated devices and accessories. Requires a 12 volt auto adapter. *$149.00*

1511 Unicorn Keyboards
Intelli Tools
1720 Corporate Circle
Petaluma, CA 94954   707-773-2000
                                          800-899-6687
                                    Fax: 707-773-2001
                                 info@intellitools.com
                                    www.intellitools.com
Dayton Johnson, VP, Sales
Arjan Khalsa, CEO
Alternative keyboards with membrane surface and large, user-defined keys. Large and small sizes are available. *$250.00*

Scanners

1512 Scanning WSKE
Words+
42505 10th Street West
Lancaster, CA 93534-7059   661-723-7723
                                          888-266-9294
                                    Fax: 661-723-5524
                            info@simulations-plus.com
                             www.simulations-plus.com
Walter S Woltosz, M.S., M.A.S., President, CEO
John A. DiBella, Vice President, Marketing & Sales
John R. Kneisel, Chief Financial Officer
A software and a hardware product designed to operate on an IBM compatible PC. The software provides dual word prediction, abbreviation expansion, five different methods of voice output, and access to commercial software applications.

1513 System 2000/Versa
Words+
42505 10th Street West
Lancaster, CA 93534-7059   661-723-7723
                                          800-869-8521
                                    Fax: 661-723-5524
                            info@simulations-plus.com
                             www.simulations-plus.com
Walter S Woltosz, M.S., M.A.S., President, CEO
John A. DiBella, Vice President, Marketing & Sales
John R. Kneisel, Chief Financial Officer
Provides all of the strategies currently being used in AAC, from dynamic display color pictographic language, to dual-word prediction text language, in a single system.

1514 Zygo-Usa
SVC Corporation
48834 Kato Road Suite 101-A
Fremont, CA 94538   510-249-9660
                                          800-234-6006
                                    Fax: 510-770-4930
                                       www.zygo-usa.com
Adam Weiss, Vp Sales & Marketing

ZYGO-USA has been involved in manufacturing and distributing assistive technologies since 1974. They specialize in augmentative and alternative computer access. They offer a wide range of technology products to our clients so they can achieve a greater independence and to enhance the quality of their lives. These soloutins improve and individual's ability to learn, work, and interact with family and friends.

Screen Enhancement

1515 Boxlight
Boxlight Corporation
151 State Highway 300, Suite A
P.O. Box 2609
Belfair, WA 98528
360-464-2119
866-972-1549
sales@boxlight.com
www.boxlight.com

Herb Myers, CEO/Founder
Sloan Myers, Founder
Hank Nance, President
BOXLIGHT is a global presentation solutions partner for trainers, educators and professional speakers. Solutions include projector sales, national rental service, technical support, repair, and presentation peripherals. For more information visit us online.

1516 FDR Series of Low Vision Reading Aids
Optelec U S
Breslau 4
Barendrecht, LT 92081-8358
886-783-444
800-826-4200
Fax: 886-783-400
info@optelec.com
in.optelec.com

Stephan Terwolbeck, President
Michiel van Schaik, VP
Janet Lennex, Director of Customer Excellence
The Low Vision Reading Aids features; high resolution, positive and negative display, a high-quality zoom lens, versatile swivel and a 12 inch or 19 inch high-resolution monitor, color or black and white, computer compatible, or portable.

1517 InFocus
AI Squared
130 Taconic Business Park Road
Manchester Center, VT 05255
802-362-3612
800-859-0270
Fax: 802-362-1670
sales@aisquared.com
www.aisquared.com

David Wu, CEO
Jost Eckhardt, VP of Engineering
Scott Moore, VP of Marketing
A memory-resident program that magnifies text and graphics - the entire screen, a single line or a portion of the screen.

1518 Portable Large Print Computer
Human Ware
1800, Michaud street
Drummondville, CA 94520-1213
819-471-4818
888-723-7273
Fax: 925-681-4630
ca.info@humanware.com
www.humanware.com/en-australia/home

Real Goulet, Chairman
Gilles Pepin, CEO
Michel Cote, Corporate Director
A portable large print computer which magnifies up to 64 times. It is linked to a PC and has a hand-held camera.

1519 ZoomText
A I Squared
130 Taconic Business Park Road
Manchester Center, VT 05255
802-362-3612
800-859-0270
Fax: 802-362-1670
sales@aisquared.com
www.aisquared.com

David Wu, CEO
Jost Eckhardt, VP of Engineering
Scott Moore, VP of Marketing
A RAM-resident program that enlarges screen characters up to eight times. It runs on IBM PC, XT, AT and PS/2.

Speech Synthesizers

1520 Artic Business Vision (for DOS) and Artic WinVision (for Windows 95)
Artic Technologies
3456 Rodchester Road
Troy, MI 48083
248-689-9883
Fax: 248-588-2650
info@ablezone.com

Dale McDaniel, Founder
Kathy Gargagliano, Founder
A speech processor for blind computer users featuring true interactive speech with spread sheets, word processors, database managers, etc. Now available with both Windows 3.1 and Windows 95 access. *$ 495.00*

1521 Computerized Speech Lab
Kay Elemetrics Corporation
3 Paragon Drive
Montvalle, NJ 07645
973-628-6200
800-289-5297
Fax: 201-391-2063
www.kaypentax.com

John Crump, President
Hardware/software for the acquisition, analysis/display, playback and storage of speech signals.

1522 DynaVox Technologies Speech Communication Devices
Dyna Vox Technologies
2100 Wharton St
Suite 400
Pittsburgh, PA 15203-1945
412-381-4883
866-396-2869
Fax: 412-381-5241
www.dynavoxtech.com

Ed Donnelly, CEO
Michelle Heying, President and COO
Kenneth Misch, CFO
Develops and manufactures speech communication devices that help individuals who are unable to speak due to speech, language and/or learning disabilities to communicate quickly and easily.

1523 Electronic Speech Assistance Devices
Luminaud, Inc.
8688 Tyler Blvd
Mentor, OH 44060
440-255-9082
800-255-3408
Fax: 440-255-2250
info@luminaud.com
www.luminaud.com

Thomas M. Lennox, President
Dorothy Lennox, Vice President
Offers a full line of speech aids, voice amplifiers, mini-vox amplifiers, laryngectomec products.

1524 Keywi
Hoffmann + Krippner Inc.
200 Westpark Drive
Suite 270
Peachtree City, GA 30269
770-487-1950
Fax: 770-487-1945
www.keywi-usa.com

Membrane keyboard and membrane switch technology

1525 Mega Wolf Communication Device
Wayne County Regional Educational Service Agency
33500 Van Born Rd
Wayne, MI 48184-2474 734-334-1300
Fax: 734-334-1620
www.resa.net

Lynda S. Jackson, President
Kenneth E. Berlinn, Vice President
James Petrie, Secretary
A low cost voice output communication device which is primarily intended to provide the power of speech to those individuals who are most severely challenged mentally and/or physically. The WOLF device is User programmable and uses the Texas Instruments' Touch and Tell case and touch panel; ADAMLAB electronics with synthesized (robotic) voice. For users able to point with approximately 6 ounces of pressure. *$400.00*

1526 Talking Screen
Words+
42505 10th St W
Lancaster, CA 93534-7059 661-723-7723
888-266-9294
Fax: 661-723-5524
info@simulations-plus.com
www.simulations-plus.com

Walter S Woltosz, M.S., M.A.S., Chairman, President and Chief Ex
John R. Kneisel, Chief Financial Officer
John DiBella, Vice President, Marketing and Sales
An augmentative communication program that allows the user to select graphic symbols on the display to produce speech output. Symbols can be used either singly or in sequence as picture abbreviations. *$1395.00*

1527 Turnkey Computer Systems for the Visually, Physically, and Hearing Impaired
E VA S
39 Canal St P.O. Box 371
Westerly, RI 02891-1511 401-596-3155
800-872-3827
Fax: 401-596-3979
TTY: 401-596-3500
contact@evas.com
www.evas.com

Gerald Swerdlick, Owner
Jerry Swerdlick, CEO
Offers clear speech with pleasant inflection and tonal quality as well as variable pitch, intonation and voices.

1528 Voice-It
V XI Corporation Incorporated
271 Locust Street
Denver, NH 03820 603-742-2888
800-742-8588
Fax: 603-742-5065
info@vxicorp.com
www.vxicorp.com

Michael Ferguson, President
Tom Manero, Chief Financial Officer
Phil Pane, Vice President Operations
Adds voice to popular spreadsheet and word processing applications on IBM PCs and compatibles, turning spreadsheets and word processing documents into talking documents.

1529 Window-Eyes
G W Micro
725 Airport North Office Park
Fort Wayne, IN 46825 260-489-3671
Fax: 260-489-2608
www.gwmicro.com

Dan Weirich, Owner/Vice President of Sales an
Doug Geoffray, Owner
Provides access to available software automatically reading information important to the user while ignoring the rest. A screen reader for the windows operative system.

1530 AIMS Multimedia
Discovery Education
8145 Holton Dr
Florence, KY 41042-3009 859-342-7200
Fax: 877-324-6830

Mike Wright, Director
Lynn Fassett, Administrative Assistant
Cindy Vogt, Human Resources Executive
AIMS Multimedia is a leader in the production and distribution of training and educational programs for the business and K-12 communities via YHS, interactive CD-ROM, DVD and Internet streaming video.

1531 Basic Math: Detecting Special Needs
Allyn & Bacon
One Liberty Square
Suite 1200
Boston, MA 02109-3988 617-261-0040
800-852-8024
Fax: 617-944-7273
samplingdept@pearson.com
www.greenellp.com

Thomas M Greene, Attorney at Law
Michael Tabb, Attorney at Law
Describes special mathematics needs of special learners.
180 pages
ISBN 0-205116-35-3

1532 Campaign Math
Mindplay
4400 E. Broadway Blvd
Suite 400
Tucson, AZ 85711-1726 520-888-1800
800-221-7911
Fax: 520-888-7904
mail@mindplay.com
www.mindplay.com

Judith Bliss, CEO
Brian Williams, Development Manager
Lisa Garcia, Director of Educational Services
A complete program on the electoral process as well as a math package which teaches ratios, fractions and percentages.

1533 Educational Activities Software
5600 W 83rd Street
Suite 300, 8200 Tower
Bloomington, MN 55437 866-243-8464
Fax: 239-225-9299
jwest@orchardlng.com
www.edmentum.com

Vin Riera, President & Chief Executive Officer
Rob Rueckl, Chief Financial Officer
Dave Adams, Chief Academic Officer
Comprehensive MATH SKILLS software tutorials teach concepts ranging from rounding and tables to measuring area. MAC/WIN compatible. *$369.00*
Per Unit

1534 Fraction Factory
Queue
80 Hathaway Drive
Stratford, CT 06615 800-232-2224
Fax: 800-775-2729
jdk@queueinc.com
qworkbooks.com

Anna Christopoulos, General Manager
Peter Uhrynowski, Comptroller
Steve Pernett, Director of Printing and Graphic
In 1980, Jonathan Kantrowitz started Queue, Inc. as an educational software company. After twenty thriving years publishing and distributing high-quality software to educators, Queue began transitioning from software to workbooks, focusing on state-specific test preparation.

1535 Information & Referral Services
Information + Referral Services
2590 N. Alvernon Way
Tucson, AZ 85712   520-323-1708
                                                      Fax: 520-325-8841
                                                           www.azinfo.org

Patti Caldwell, Executive Director
Chuck Palm, Treasurer
Ben Rensvold, Vice President
Provides information about health and human services for people
in Arizona over the telephone. Information specialists help callers clarify their needs, and provide referrals to the appropriate
service agency.

1536 King's Rule
WINGS for Learning
1600 Green Hills Rd
Scotts Valley, CA 95066-4981   831-426-2228
                                                      Fax: 831-464-3600

Ani Stocks, Owner
A software mathematical problem solving game. Students discover mathematical rules as they work their way through a castle
and generate and test a working hypothesis by asking questions.

1537 Learning About Numbers
C&C Software
5713 Kentford Cir
Wichita, KS 67220-3131   316-683-6056
                                                           800-752-2086
Carol Clark, President
Three programs use the power of computer graphics to provide
young children with a variety of experiences in working with
numbers. *$50.00*

1538 Math Rabbit
Learning Company
Ste 1900
100 Pine St
San Francisco, CA 94111-5205   415-659-2000
                                                           800-825-4420
                                                      Fax: 415-659-2020
                                                 thelearningco@hmhpub.com
                                                           www.hmhco.com

Linda K. Zecher, President, Chief Executive Officer and Director
Eric Shuman, Chief Financial Officer
William Bayers, Executive Vice President and General Counsel
Teaches early math concepts by matching objects to numbers,
then adding and subtracting up to 18.

1539 Math for Everyday Living
Educational Activities Software
5600 W 83rd Street
Suite 300, 8200 Tower
Bloomington, MN 55437   866-243-8464
                                                      Fax: 239-225-9299
                                                    jwest@orchardlng.com
                                                         www.edmentum.com

Vin Riera, President & Chief Executive Officer
Rob Rueckl, Chief Financial Officer
Dave Adams, Chief Academic Officer
Real life math skills are taught with this tutorial and practice soft-
ware program. Examples include Paying for a Meal (addition and
subtraction), Working with Sales Slips (multiplication), Unit
Pricing (division), Sales Tax (percent), Earning with Overtime
(fractions) plus more. Software: CD-ROM, Windows, MAC, and
DOS. *$159.00*

1540 Math for Successful Living
Siboney Learning Group
5600 W 83rd Street
Suite 300, 8200 Tower
Bloomington, MN 55437   866-243-8464
                                                      Fax: 239-225-9299
                                                    jwest@orchardlng.com
                                                         www.edmentum.com

Vin Riera, President & Chief Executive Officer
Rob Rueckl, Chief Financial Officer
Dave Adams, Chief Academic Officer
These programs include managing a checking account, budget-
ing, shopping strategies and buying on credit.

1541 Piece of Cake Math
Queue Inc
80 Hathaway Drive
Stratford, CT 06615   800-232-2224
                                                      Fax: 800-775-2729
                                                       jdk@queueinc.com
                                                        www.qworkbooks.com

Anna Christopoulos, General Manager
Peter Uhrynowski, Comptroller
Steve Pernett, Director of Printing and Graphic
In 1980, Jonathan Kantrowitz started Queue, Inc. as an educational software company. After twenty thriving years publishing
and distributing high-quality software to educators, Queue began
transitioning from software to workbooks, focusing on state-specific test preparation.

1542 Puzzle Tanks
WINGS for Learning
1600 Green Hills Rd
Scotts Valley, CA 95066-4981   831-426-2228
                                                      Fax: 831-464-3600
Ani Stocks, Owner
A mathematical problem solving game that involves multi-step
problems.

1543 Right Turn
WINGS for Learning
1600 Green Hills Rd
Scotts Valley, CA 95066-4981   831-426-2228
                                                      Fax: 831-464-3600
Ani Stocks, Owner
Requires students to predict, experiment and learn about the
mathematical concepts of rotation and transformation.

1544 RoboMath
4400 E. Broadway Blvd
Suite 400
Tucson, AZ 85711-1726   520-888-1800
                                                           800-221-7911
                                                      Fax: 520-888-7904
                                                       mail@mindplay.com
                                                          www.mindplay.com

Judith Bliss, CEO
Brian Williams, Development Manager
Lisa Garcia, Director of Educational Services
A complete program on the electoral process as well as a math
package which teaches ratios, fractions and percentages.

1545 Stickybear Math I Deluxe
Optimum Resource
1 Mathews Drive
Suite 107
Hilton Head Island, SC 29926-3689   843-689-8000
                                                      Fax: 843-689-8008
                                                      info@stickybear.com
                                                         www.stickybear.com

Richard Hefter, President
Sharpen basic addition and subtraction skills with this captivat-
ing series of math exercises. Grades Pre-K to 2. Available in as
single edition with sizing up to 30 users at a site. English/Span-
ish. *$59.95*

1546 Stickybear Math II Deluxe
Optimum Resource
1 Mathews Drive
Suite 107
Hilton Head Island, SC 29926-3689   843-689-8000
                                                      Fax: 843-689-8008
                                                      info@stickybear.com
                                                         www.stickybear.com

Richard Hefter, President
Multiplication and division, beginning with the elementary problems and developing into the more complex problems with re-
grouping. Grades 2-4. Available for single user through the 30
user site package. English/Spanish. *$59.95*

1547 Stickybear Math Splash
Optimum Resource
1 Mathews Drive
Suite 107
Hilton Head Island, SC 29926- 3689 843-689-8000
Fax: 843-689-8008
info@stickybear.com
www.stickybear.com

Richard Hefter, President
Unique multiple activities keep the learning level high while children acquire skills in addition, subtraction, multiplication and division. K-5th grade. Available as single edition up to 30 user site package. English/Spanish. *$59.95*

1548 Stickybear Math Word Problems
Optimum Resource
1 Mathews Drive
Suite 107
Hilton Head Island, SC 29926- 3689 843-689-8000
Fax: 843-689-8008
info@stickybear.com
www.stickybear.com

Richard Hefter, President
Hundreds of different word problems make it easy for students to practice basic math skills around analyzing and solving word problems. Grades 1-5. Available as single edition up to 30 user site package. English/Spanish. *$59.95*

1549 Stickybear Money
Optimum Resource
1 Mathews Drive
Suite 107
Hilton Head Island, SC 29926- 3667 843-689-8000
Fax: 843-689-8008
info@stickybear.com
www.stickybear.com

Chris Gintz, President
Teaches children to recognize US coins and paper money and introduces simple counting. K to 3rd grade. Bilingual. *$59.95*

1550 Stickybear Numbers Deluxe
Optimum Resource
1 Mathews Drive
Suite 107
Hilton Head Island, SC 29926- 3689 843-689-8000
Fax: 843-689-8008
info@stickybear.com
www.stickybear.com

Richard Hefter, President
Counting and number recognition are as easy as 1-2-3 with this award-winning program. Teaches number recognition of numbers 0-9 and 0-30. Pre-K to 2nd grade. Available as single edition up to 30 user site package. *$59.95*

1551 Tomorrow's Promise: Mathematics
Compass Learning
203 Colorado Street
Austin, TX 78701 512-478-9600
800-678-1412
866-586-7387
www.compasslearning.com

Eric Loeffel, President
Trey Chambers, Chief Financial Officer
Arthur Vanderveen, Vice President, Business Strategy and Development
By integrating interdisciplinary content and real-world application of skills, this product emphasizes the practical value of fundamental math skills. It helps your students develop a problem-solving aptitude for ongoing mathematics achievement.

Software: Miscellaneous

1552 Adventures in Musicland
Electronic Courseware Systems
1713 S State St
Champaign, IL 61820-7258 217-359-7099
800-832-4965
Fax: 217-359-6578
support@ecsmedia.com
http://ecsmedia.com.np/

G Peters, President
Jodie Varner, Marketing Manager
This unique set of music games features characters from Lewis Carroll's, Alice in Wonderland. Players learn through pictures, sounds, and animation which help develop understanding of musical tones, composers, and musical symbols. Games include MusicMatch, Melody Mixup, Picture Perfect and Sound Concentration. *$49.95*

1553 Ai Squared
130 Taconic Business Park Road
Manchester Center, VT 05255-669 802-362-3612
800-859-0270
Fax: 802-362-1670
sales@aisquared.com
http://www.aisquared.com

David Wu, CEO
Jost Eckhardt, VP of Engineering
Scott Moore, VP of Marketing
Developers of software for the visually impaired.

1554 All About You: Appropriate Special Interactions and Self-Esteem
P CI Educational Publishing
P.O.Box 34270
San Antonio, TX 78265-4270 210-377-1999
800-594-4263
800-471-3000
Fax: 888-259-8284

Lee Wilson, President and CEO
Randy Pennington, Executive VP
Jeff McLane, Founder
This game offers parents and game players a new line of communication when discussing various issues such as learning to be thoughtful, respecting the rights and feelings of others, how to make and keep friends and more. *$49.95*

1555 All Star Review
Tom Snyder Productions
100 Talcott Ave
Watertown, MA 02472-5703 800-342-0236
www.tomsnyder.com

Rick Abrams, Manager
Tom Synder, Founder
Bridget Dalton, Ed.D., Author
This package turns group review into a baseball game for small and large groups.

1556 Attainment Company
I ET Resources
504 Commerce Parkway
P.O. Box 930160
Verona, WI 53593- 0160 608-845-7880
800-327-4269
Fax: 800-942-3865
info@attainmentcompany.com
www.attainmentcompany.com

Autumn Garza, President
Don Bastian, CEO
Augmentative and alternative communication, software, videos, print and hands-on functional life skills and basic academic materials for development.

1557 Attention Getter
Soft Touch
12301 Central Ave NE Ste 205
4300 Stine Rd
Blaine, MN 55434   763-755-1402
                                    888-755-1402
                              Fax: 763-862-2920
                     support@marblesoft.com
                          www.softtouch.com

Joyce Meyer, President
The whimsical photos morph to another photo and then to a third photo in categories. Paired with interesting sounds and music, the photo animations are so engaging that the student is motivated to activate the computer to see and hear the next one. This is a perfect vehicle to achieve goals aimed at attention getting, activating a switch or intentionally. Compatible with USB IntelliKeys keyboards.

1558 Attention Teens
Soft Touch
12301 Central Ave NE Ste 205
Blaine, MN 55434   763-755-1403
                                    888-755-1403
                              Fax: 763-862-2921
                     support@marblesoft.com
                          www.softtouch.com

Joyce Meyer, President
Attention Teens (formerly known as Loony Teens) is a program for teens with disabilities who need powerful input to get their attention. Attention Teens is a computer program to do just this. Paired with interesting sounds and music, the photo animations are so engaging that the student is motivated to activate the computer to see and hear the next one. Compatible with USB IntelliKeys keyboards.

1559 Away We Ride
Soft Touch
12301 Central Ave NE Ste 205
4300 Stine Rd
Blaine, MN 55434   763-755-1404
                                    888-755-1404
                              Fax: 763-862-2922
                     support@marblesoft.com
                          www.softtouch.com

Joyce Meyer, President
Software for children and teens. For Macintosh and PC.

1560 Battenberg & Associates
11135 Rolling Springs Dr
Carmel, IN 46033-3629   317-843-2208

Jan Battenberg, Owner
Offers various software programs that develop the user's visual memory, sequencing skills, word recognition, hand-eye coordination and more.

1561 Behavior Skills: Learning How People Should Act
PCI Education Publishing
P.O.Box 34270
San Antonio, TX 78265-4270   210-377-1999
                                    800-471-3000
                              Fax: 888-828-
                          www.pcieducation.com

Jeff Clain, CEO
Erin Kinard, VP Product Development/Publisher
Helps players learn what behavior is acceptable and what behavior is not acceptable in the real world. *$49.95*

1562 Blocks in Motion
Don Johnston
26799 West Commerce Drive
Volo, IL 60073   847-740-0749
                                    800-999-4660
                              Fax: 847-740-7326
                       info@donjohnston.com
                          www.donjohnston.com

Don Johnston, Founder
Ruth Ziolkowski, President
Kevin Johnston, Director of Product Design
This unique art and motion program makes drawing, creating and animating fun and educational for all users. Based on the

Piagetian Theory for motor-sensory development, this program promotes the concept that the process is as educational and as much fun as the end result. *$79.00*

1563 Car Builder Deluxe
Optimum Resource
1 Mathews Drive
Suite 107
Hilton Head Island, SC 29926- 3689   843-689-8000
                              Fax: 843-689-8008
                          info@stickybear.com
                          www.stickybear.com

Richard Hefter, President
As design engineers, users build cars on screen, specifying chassis length, wheelbase, engine type, transmission, fuel tank size, suspension, steering, tires and brakes. All functional choices are interrelated and will affect the performance of the final design. Grades 3 & up. *$59.99*

1564 Center for Best Practices in Early Childhood
Horrabin Hall 32
Macomb, IL 61455   309-298-1634
                              Fax: 309-298-2305
                       jk-johanson@wiu.edu
                          www.wiu.edu/thecenter/

Linda Robinson, Assistant Director
The Center, part of the College of Education and Human Services at Western Illinois University, provides products, training materials, and information related to best practices for educators and families of young children with disabilities.

1565 Clock
Compass Learning
203 Colorado Street
Austin, TX 78701-3922   512-478-9600
                                    800-678-1412
                                    866-586-7387
                          www.compasslearning.com

Eric Loeffel, President
Trey Chambers, Chief Financial Officer
Arthur Vanderveen, Vice President, Business Strategy and Development
An extremely simple, easy-to-use program for children who are learning how to read the time of day from clocks and digital displays. Apple and MS-DOS and Mac available. *$39.95*

1566 Community Skills: Learning to Function in Your Neighborhood
Programming Concepts
8700 Shoal Creek Boulevard
Austin, TX 78757-6897   210-377-1999
                                    800-594-4263
                                    800-471-3000
                              Fax: 888-259-8284
                          www.proedinc.com

Lee Wilson, President and CEO
Randy Pennington, Executive VP
Jeff McLane, Founder
Offers parents and educators a functional way to teach community life skills. *$49.95*

1567 Companion Activities
Soft Touch
12301 Central Ave NE Ste 205
4300 Stine Rd
Blaine, MN 55434   763-755-1404
                                    888-755-1404
                              Fax: 763-862-2922
                     support@marblesoft.com
                          www.softtouch.com

Joyce Meyer, President
Print your own books, worksheets, flash cards, board games, matching games, bingo games, card games and many more. This CD offers numerous companion activities to different SoftTouch software titles. Activities range from very easy to difficult. Companion activities are great tools to reinforce learning. Use the work sheets - black and white and color - in the inclusion class for students with special needs.

1568 Concepts on the Move Advanced Preacademics
Soft Touch
12301 Central Ave NE Ste 205
P.O.Box 490215
Blaine, MN 55449   763-862-2920
                                          888-755-1402
                                    Fax: 763-862-2922
                               support@marblesoft.com
                                   www.marblesoft.com

Joyce Meyer, President
Choose from five concepts groups: categories, occupations, functions, goes with and prepositions. Use our Steps to Learning Design to choose how many concepts to present at one time and where to place each one in the scan array, on screen keyboard or IntelliKeys keyboard. Watch and listen as the concept morphs or changes and music plays. The words are also shown to reinforce emerging literacy skills. Compatible with USB IntelliKeys.

1569 Cooking Class: Learning About Food Preparation
Programming Concepts
8700 Shoal Creek Boulevard
Austin, TX 78757-6897   512-451-3246
                                          800-897-3202
                                          800-471-3000
                                    Fax: 800-397-7633
                                 general@proedinc.com
                                    www.proedinc.com

Jeff McLane, Founder
Lee Wilson, President and CEO
Randy Pennington, Executive VP
This game offers parents and educators a new way to teach basic preparation skills. Kitchen safety and sanitation are stressed throughout the game. *$49.95*

1570 Dilemma
Educational Activities Software
5600 West 83rd Street
Suite 300, 8200 Tower
Bloomington, MN 55437   800-447-5286
                                    Fax: 239-225-9299
                                   info@edmentum.com
                                    www.edmentum.com

Vin Riera, President/CEO
Dan Juckniess, SVP, Sales & Professional Services
Stacey Herteux, VP, Human Resources
Realistic stories with a choice of different gripping endings, color graphics, a built-in dictionary and a user controlled reading rate make these computer programs compelling enough to interest all students. Comprehension and vocabulary questions follow each story. *$159.00*

1571 Dino-Games
Academic Software
3504 Tates Creek Road
Lexington, KY 40517-2601   859-552-1020
                                          859-552-1040
                                    Fax: 253-799-4012
                                    asistaff@acsw.com
                                       www.acsw.com

Dr. Warren E Lacefield PhD, President
Penelope D. Ellis, COO, Sales & Marketing Director
Sylvia B. Lacefield, Graphic Artist
Dino-Games are single switch software programs for early switch practice. Dinosaur games provide practice in pattern recognition, cause and effect demonstration, directionality training, number concepts and problem solving. They are compatible with most popular switch interfaces and alternate keyboards. For Macintosh, IBM and compatibles. DINO-LINK is a matching game; DINO-MAZE is a series of maze games; DINO-FIND is a game of concentration; and DINO-DOT is a collection of dot-to-dot games.
$39.95 per game

1572 Directions: Technology in Special Education
DREAMMS for Kids
273 Ringwood Road
Freeville, NY 13068-5606   607-539-3027
                                    Fax: 607-539-9930
                                    janet@dreamms.org
                                     www.dreamms.org

Janet P. Hosmer, Editor/Publisher
Chester D. Hosmer, Jr., Technical Editor
Susan Lait, Regular Contributor
A CD containing all of 'Directions' past articles and information gathered from their newsletter which lists resources for assistive and adaptive computer ethnologies in the home, school and community. *$24.95*

1573 ESI Master Resource Guide
Educational Software Institute
4213 S 94th St
Omaha, NE 68127-1223   402-592-3300
                                          800-955-5570
                                    Fax: 402-592-2017

Lee Myers, President
Kathy Cavanaugh, Catalog Manager
Educational Software Institute (ESI) provides a one-stop shop to purchase software titles by all of the best publishers. The ESI Master Gold Book catalog and CD-ROM represents more than 400 software publishers, with information on more than 8,000 software titles. Take the confusion out of software selection by calling ESI for all of your software needs - including competitive prices, software previews, knowledgeable assistance, and the largest selection available all in one place.
Yearly

1574 EZ Keys
Words+
42505 10th Street West
Suite 109
Lancaster, CA 93534- 7059   661-723-7723
                                          888-266-9294
                                    Fax: 661-723-5524
                              info@simulations-plus.com
                               www.simulations-plus.com

Walter S Woltosz, M.S., M.A.S., Chairman, President and Chief Executive Officer
John A. Dibella, VP, Marketing & Sales
Virginia E. Woltosz. M.B.A., Secretary & Treasurer
A software and hardware product designed to operate on an IBM compatible PC. The software provides dual word prediction, abbreviation expansion, five different methods of voice output and access to commercial software applications. *$1395.00*

1575 Early Games for Young Children
Queue Incorporated
80 Hathaway Drive
Stratford, CT 06615   800-232-2224
                                    Fax: 800-775-2729
                                    jdk@queueinc.com
                                   www.qworkbooks.com

Anna Christopoulos, General Manager
Peter Uhrynowski, Comptroller
Steve Perrett, Director of Printing and Graphics
Software that includes nine activities that entertain preschoolers in honing basic math and language skills.

1576 Early Music Skills
Electronic Courseware Systems
1713 S State St
Champaign, IL 61820-7258   217-359-7099
                                          800-832-4965
                                    Fax: 217-359-6578
                                 support@ecsmedia.com
                                    www.ecsmedia.com

G Peters, President
Jodie Varner, Marketing Manager
A tutorial and drill program designed for the beginning music student. It covers four basic music reading skills: recognition of line and space notes; comprehension of the numbering system for the musical staff; visual and aural identification of notes moving up and down; and recognition of notes stepping and skipping up and down. *$ 39.95*

141

1577 **Eating Skills: Learning Basic Table Manners**
PCI Education Publishing
P.O.Box 34270
San Antonio, TX 78265-4270   210-377-1999
                                           800-594-4263
                                        Fax: 210-377-1121

Erin Kinard, VP Product Development/Publisher
Jeff Clain, CEO
Offers parents and educators a functional way to teach and reinforce basic table manners. *$49.95*

1578 **Electronic Courseware Systems**
1713 S State St
Champaign, IL 61820-7258   217-359-7099
                                          800-832-4965
                                       Fax: 217-359-6578
                                       support@ecsmedia.com
                                       www.ecsmedia.com

Jodie Varner, Manager
G Peters, President
Offers a complete library of instructional software for music, math, science and social studies.

1579 **Fall Fun**
Soft Touch
12301 Central Ave NE Ste 205
P.O.Box 490215
Blaine, MN 55449   763-862-2920
                                          888-755-1402
                                       Fax: 763-862-2922
                                       support@marblesoft.com
                                       www.marblesoft.com

Joyce Meyer, President
Your students can begin their day with the Pledge of Allegiance, Pumpkins, Owls, and Cats. Witches adorn Five Pumpkins Sitting on the Gate. Five Fat Turkeys out smart the pilgrims with song and antics. The owl and cat have songs of their own. A variety of activities reinforce concepts such as short, tall, first, second, third, same and different. Fall Fun includes cause and effect and easy to more difficult levels. Eight songs in all.

1580 **Five Green & Speckled Frogs**
Soft Touch
12301 Central Ave NE Ste 205
P.O.Box 490215
Blaine, MN 55449   763-862-2920
                                          888-755-1402
                                       Fax: 763-862-2922
                                       support@marblesoft.com
                                       www.marblesoft.com

Joyce Meyer, President
Laugh, learn and sing with Five Humorous Frogs. Activities start with cause and effect and progress to teach directionality and simple subtraction. This classic song makes learning numbers and number worlds easy. Selections can be set to 2, 3, 4, 5, or 6 on-screen choices. Two games are included. One teaches direction on a number line. If the child moves the frog in the correct direction, the frog gets a point. The other game teaches beginning subtraction.

1581 **Free and User Supported Software for the IBM PC: A Resource Guide**
McFarland & Company
960 NC Highway 88 W
P.O.Box 611
Jefferson, NC 28640-8813   336-246-4460
                                          800-253-2187
                                       Fax: 336-246-5018
                                       info@mcfarlandpub.com
                                       www.mcfarlandpub.com

Robert McFarland Franklin, Founder
Kenneth.J Ansley, Author
Victor.D Lopez, Author
A selection of word processing, database management, spreadsheets, and graphics programs are described and evaluated. Describes how the program works and its strengths and weaknesses. Rating charts cover such aspects as ease of use, ease of learning, documentation, and general utility. *$27.50*
224 pages Paperback
ISBN 0-89950 -99-0

1582 **GoalView: Special Education and RTI Student Management Information System**
Learning Tools International
2391 Circadian Way
Santa Rosa, CA 95407-5439   707-521-3530
                                          800-333-9954

Cathy Zier, President/CEO
Natalie Sipes, VP
Michael R. Paul, Director of IT/Senior Web Engine
A Web Based information system for students, educators and parents that enables accountability and achievement tracking; prepares IDEA compliant IEP's in minutes; provides over 250,000 education standards and special education goals and objectives in English and Spanish; generates Federal compliance reports; and creates IDEA GoalCard progress reports for students, schools and districts for every reporting period.

1583 **HELP**
V OR T Corporation
P.O.Box G (George)
Menlo Park, CA 94026   650-322-8282
                                          888-757-8678
                                       Fax: 650-327-0747
                                       custserv@vort.com
                                       vort.com

Tom Holt, Owner
A software version of HELP, covers over 650 skills in 6 developmental areas; cognitive, motor skills, language, gross motor, social and self-help.

1584 **Handbook of Adaptive Switches and Augmentative Communication Devices**
Academic Software
3504 Tates Creek Road
Lexington, KY 40517-2601   859-552-1020
                                          859-552-1040
                                       Fax: 253-799-4012
                                       asistaff@acsw.com
                                       www.acsw.com

Dr. Warren E Lacefield PhD, President
Penelope D. Ellis, COO, Sales & Marketing Director
Cindy L George, Author
This second edition contains physical descriptions and laboratory test data for a variety of commercially available pressure switches and augmentative communication devices and chapters on physical interaction, seating and positioning, and control access. It is an essential tool for assistive technology professionals and therapists who make decisions concerning physical access. *$60.00*
300 pages Hardcover

1585 **HandiWARE**
Microsystems Software
600 Worcester Rd
Framingham, MA 01702-5303   508-626-8511
                                          800-828-2600
                                       Fax: 508-879-1069
                                       infor@microsys.com
                                       www.handiware.com

Terri McGrath, Sales/Marketing
Bill Kilroy, Product Manager
Adapted access software, assists persons with physical, hearing and visual impairments in accessing computers running DOS and Windows. HandiWARE is a suite of 8 software programs which provide users with screen magnification, alternate keyboard access, word prediction, augmentative communication, hands free telephone access, a visual beep. $20.00-$595.00.

1586 **How to Write for Everyday Living**
Educational Activities Software
5600 West 83rd Street
Suite 300, 8200 Tower
Bloomington, MN 55437-585   800-447-5286
                                       Fax: 239-225-9299
                                       info@edmentum.com
                                       www.edmentum.com

Vin Riera, President/CEO
Dan Juckniess, SVP, Sales & Professional Services
Stacey Herteux, VP, Human Resources

An individualized Life Skills WRITING Software program emphasizing the reading, writing, communication and reference skills needed for real-life tasks: preparing a resume, an employment form, a business letter and envelope, a learner's permit, a social security application and banking forms. *$159.00*

1587 I KNOW American History
Soft Touch
12301 Central Ave NE Ste 205
P.O.Box 490215
Blaine, MN 55449-2352   763-862-2920
                                         888-755-1402
                                    Fax: 763-862-2922
                            support@marblesoft.com
                                www.marblesoft.com
Joyce Meyer, President
The new I KNOW programs is the way students practice attending, choice making and turn-taking while uncovering learning puzzles. Each press reveals more of the image while the narrator reads the text on the screen. Offers three levels of language: short phrases, short sentences and longer sentences to match the student's learning level. Choose from the five topic areas: American Symbols, Westward Movement, Early Colonial Americans, Industrial Revolution and Biographies.

1588 I KNOW American History Overlay CD
Soft Touch
12301 Central Ave NE Ste 205
P.O.Box 490215
Blaine, MN 55449-2352   763-862-2920
                                         888-755-1402
                                    Fax: 763-862-2922
                            support@marblesoft.com
                                www.marblesoft.com
Joyce Meyer, President
Use this Overlay CD with I KNOW American History program. Includes standard overlays and SoftTouch's changeable overlays. Includes Overlay Printer by IntelliTools. Use Overlay Maker by IntelliTools (not included) to modify the overlays or to make additional learning materials.

1589 Incite Learning Series
Don Johnston
26799 West Commerce Drive
Volo, IL 60073   847-740-0749
                                         800-999-4660
                                    Fax: 847-740-7326
                            info@donjohnston.com
                                www.donjohnston.com
Don Johnston, Founder
Ruth Ziolkowski, President
Kevin Johnston, Director of Product Design
A collection of original short films and a thought-provoking instruction model to engage every student in the critical thinking and feeling process. This research-based program was developed around the science of how students learn best using the theory of 'anchored instruction' and 'front-loading' standards-based curriculum. *$79.00*

1590 Innovation Management Group
179 Niblick Rd
Ste 454
Paso Robles, CA 93446   818-701-1579
                                         800-889-0987
                                    Fax: 818-936-0200
                            cs@imgpresents.com
                                www.imgpresents.com
Jerry Hussong, VP of Marketing
Publisher of the Assistive Technology Suite. The ultimate set of general purpose, adaptive computer access available today. Site License includes ALL computers and ALL active students and teachers at a single or multi-site location.

1591 IntelliPics Studio 3
Intelli Tools
1720 Corporate Cir
Petaluma, CA 94954-6924   707-773-2000
                                         800-547-6747
                                    Fax: 707-773-2001
Arjan Khalsa, CEO

Multimedia authoring tool for both students and teachers to create activities, games, quizzes, slide shows, reports and presentations. *$395.00*

1592 KIDS (Keyboard Introductory Development Series)
Electronic Courseware Systems
1713 S State St
Champaign, IL 61820-7258   217-359-7099
                                         800-832-4965
                                    Fax: 217-359-6578
                            support@ecsmedia.com
                                www.ecsmedia.com
G Peters, President
Jodie Varner, Marketing Manager
A four disk series for the very young. Zoo Puppet Theater reinforces learning correct finger numbers for piano playing; Race Car Keys teaches keyboard geography by recognizing syllables or note names; Dinosaurs Lunch teaches placement of the notes on the treble staff; and Follow Me asks the student to play notes that have been presented aurally. *$49.95*

1593 Keyboard Tutor, Music Software
Electronic Courseware Systems
1713 S State St
Champaign, IL 61820-7258   217-359-7099
                                         800-832-4965
                                    Fax: 217-359-6578
                            support@ecsmedia.com
                                www.ecsmedia.com
G Peters, President
Jodie Varner, Marketing Manager
Presents exercises for learning elementary keyboard skills including knowledge of names of the keys, piano keys matched to notes, notes matched to piano keys, whole steps and half steps. Each lesson allows unlimited practice of the skills. The program may be used with or without a midi keyboard attached to the computer. *$39.95*

1594 Keyboarding by Ability
Teachers Institute for Special Education
9933 NW 45th St
Sunrise, FL 33351-4744   954-235-7940
                                    Fax: 866-843-0765
                    Support@Special-Education-Soft.com
                            www.special-education-soft.com
Gary Byowitz, President
Allows the learning disabled or dyslexic student to acquire keyboarding skills through visually cued alphabetical approach designed and tested to meet the specific learning style needs of this unique population at every grade level. Package contains: IBM software, a set of lesson plans and instructional goals; supplemental graded data input exercises. *$369.00*

1595 Keyboarding for the Physically Handicapped
Teachers Institute for Special Education
9933 NW 45th Street
Sunrise, FL 33351   954-235-7940
                                    Fax: 866-843-0765
                    Support@Special-Education-Soft.com
                            www.special-education-soft.com
Jack Heller, Director/Owner
Gary Byowitz, President
Custom designed touch typing programs for any student. A person needs order by the number of usable fingers on each hand (not counting the thumb), and whether or not a one finger or a head-pointer edition is wanted. Package includes IBM software; a complete set of lesson plans and instructional goals. *$149.95*

1596 Keyboarding with One Hand
Teachers Institute for Special Education
P.O.Box 2300
Wantagh, NY 11793-140   Fax: 516-781-4070
                                jackheller@aol.com
Jack Heller, Director
This 22 lesson tutorial developed through 25 years of research, testing and teaching allows a student with one hand to acquire employable keyboarding skills using a touch system designed for the standard IBM PC keyboard. *$79.95*

1597 LPDOS Deluxe
Optelec U S
3030 Enterprise Court
STE C
Vista, CA 92081-8358
800-826-4200
Fax: 800-368-4111
info@optelec.com
us.optelec.com

Stephan Terwolbeck, President
Michiel van Schaik, VP
Janet Lennex, Director of Customer Excellence
Large print software programs. *$595.00*

1598 Large Print DOS
Optelec U S
3030 Enterprise Court
STE C
Vista, CA 92081-8358
800-826-4200
Fax: 800-368-4111
info@optelec.com
us.optelec.com

Stephan Terwolbeck, President
Michiel van Schaik, VP
Janet Lennex, Director of Customer Excellence

1599 Laureate Learning Systems
110 E Spring St
Winooski, VT 05404-1898
802-655-4755
800-562-6801
Fax: 802-655-4757
www.laureatelearning.com

Mary Wilson, Owner
Kathy Hollandsworth, Office Manager
Laureate publishes award-winning talking software for children and adults with disabilities. Programs cover cause and effect, language development, cognitive processing, and reading. High-quality speech, colorful graphics and amusing animation make learning fun. Accessible with touchscreen, single switch, keyboard and mouse. No reading required. Available on a hybrid CD-ROM for Windows and Macintosh. Visit our website for more information or call for a free catalog.

1600 Learning Company
Ste 400
222 3rd Ave SE
Cedar Rapids, IA 52401-1542
319-395-9626
888-242-6747
Fax: 319-395-0217
info@riverdeep.net
http://web.riverdeep.net
Barry O'Callaghan, Executive Chairman & Chief Executive Officer
Tony Mulderry, Executive Vice President, Corporate Development
Ciara Smyth, Executive Vice President, Global Business Operations
Software for children. For Macintosh or Windows (3.1 DOS or Windows 95, Windows 98 required). The Learning Company has been added to Riverdeep.

1601 Little Red Hen
Compass Learning
203 Colorado Street
Austin, TX 78701
512-478-9600
800-678-1412
866-586-7387
Fax: 619-622-7873
support@compasslearning.com
www.compasslearning.com
Eric Loeffel, President, CEO
Tammy Deal, VP, Human Resources
Eric Wasser, VP, Sales
Children learn about the rewards of hard work when they discover who the Little Red Hen's friends miss out on freshly baked bread. Puzzles, rhymes, story writing and other interactive exercises enhance the creative learning process. *$34.95*

1602 Looking Good: Learning to Improve Your Appearance
Programming Concepts
8700 Shoal Creek Boulevard
Austin, TX 78757-6897
512-451-3246
800-897-3202
800-471-3000
Fax: 800-397-7633
general@proedinc.com
www.proedinc.com
Jeff McLane, Founder
Lee Wilson, President and CEO
Randy Pennington, Executive VP
This game offers a creative way to discuss all areas of grooming. *$49.95*

1603 Monkeys Jumping on the Bed
Soft Touch
12301 Central Ave NE Ste 205
P.O.Box 490215
Blaine, MN 55449-2352
763-862-2920
888-755-1402
Fax: 763-862-2922
support@marblesoft.com
www.marblesoft.com

Joyce Meyer, President
This program combines a favorite preschool song with number and color activities. Children and adults will enjoy engaging music and delightful animation. Students with cognitive delays respond to upbeat music and interesting sounds. Large graphics help learners focus on the action. Several important concepts are presented in enjoyable activity formats. Students learn cause and effect in Let's Play and Just for Fun.

1604 Morse Code WSKE
Words+
42505 10th Street West
Suite 109
Lancaster, CA 93534- 7059
661-723-7723
888-266-9294
Fax: 661-723-5524
info@simulations-plus.com
www.simulations-plus.com
Walter S Woltosz, M.S., M.A.S., Chairman, President and Chief Executive Officer
John A. Dibella, VP, Marketing & Sales
Virginia E. Woltosz. M.B.A., Secretary & Treasurer
A software and hardware product designed to operate on an IBM compatible PC.

1605 Multi-Scan Single Switch Activity Center
Academic Software
3504 Tates Creek Road
Lexington, KY 40517-2601
859-552-1020
859-552-1040
Fax: 253-799-4012
asistaff@acsw.com
www.acsw.com
Dr. Warren E Lacefield PhD, President
Penelope D. Ellis, COO, Sales & Marketing Director
Cindy L George, Author
A single switch activity center containing four educational games: Match, Maze, Dot-to-Dot, and Concentration, along with six graphics libraries; Dinosaurs, Sports, Animals, Independent Living, Vocations, and Cosmetology. MULTI-SCAN allows you to select a graphic library, choose games for each user, and adjust the difficulty level and other settings for each game. Other features allow you to save the game setups under each user's name and print out individual performance reports after sessions. *$154.00*

1606 Muppet Learning Keys
WINGS for Learning
1600 Green Hills Rd
Scotts Valley, CA 95066-4981
831-426-2228
Fax: 831-464-3600

Ani Stocks, Owner
Designed to introduce children to the world of the computer as they become familiar with letters, numbers and colors.

1607 My Own Pain
Soft Touch
12301 Central Ave NE Ste 205
P.O.Box 490215
Blaine, MN 55449-2352 763-862-2920
888-755-1402
Fax: 763-862-2922
support@marblesoft.com
www.marblesoft.com

Joyce Meyer, President
Three activities - three levels. Press the switch and the paint brush chooses the color and paints the vehicle. Music reinforces the sounds when the picture is complete. A second activity allows the student to choose the color and paint the vehicle parts any color he or she wants. The third activity is a blueprint. Print the color that matches the one in the wire drawing. Color the drawing to complete the picture.

1608 NanoPac
4823 S Sheridan Rd
Suite 302
Tulsa, OK 74145-5717 918-665-0329
800-580-6086
Fax: 918-665-0361
TTY: 918-665-2310
www.nanopac.com

Silvio Cianfrone, President
NanoPac offers assistive technology for those with low vision, blindness and reading disabilities. Some of their products include voice recognition, environmental controls, text to speech, magnifiers and door openers.

1609 Old MacDonald's Farm Deluxe
Soft Touch
12301 Central Ave NE Ste 205
P.O.Box 490215
Blaine, MN 55449-2352 763-862-2920
888-755-1402
Fax: 763-862-2922
support@marblesoft.com
www.marblesoft.com

Joyce Meyer, President
Toddlers, preschoolers and early elementary students will be entertained and captivated by the six major activities and animations in the delightful program. Includes 18 real animation images or 9 cartoon like characters. The teacher or child can choose which animals they want to sing about. Some activities are designed for children within the normal population, others are designed for students with moderate and severe disabilities.

1610 Optimum Resource Educational Software
Optimum Resource
1 Mathews Drive
Suite 107
Hilton Head Island, SC 29926 843-689-8000
Fax: 843-689-8008
info@stickybear.com
www.stickybear.com

Richard Hefter, President
A complete topical curriculum of reading, math, keyboard skills and science programs that are age and skill specific. Programs include: Early Learning for Pre-K to 1st grade with introductions to numbers, language, shapes, and time; Language Arts from Pre-K to 12; Math for Pre-K to 12; two distinct Science programs; Tools for Educators provides Spelling and Math generators; and Bilingual programs for Pre-K through 9th grade. All are available as single user up to 30 user site packages.

1611 Optimum Resources/Stickybear Software
1 Mathews Drive
Suite 107
Hilton Head Island, SC 29926 843-689-8000
Fax: 843-689-8008
info@stickybear.com
www.stickybear.com

Richard Hefter, President
Publisher of award-winning educational software for thirty years. Programs in use by millions of students nationwide. *$59.95*

1612 Please Understand Me: Software Program and Books
Cambridge Educational
132 West 31st Street
17th Floor
New York, NY 10001 800-322-8755
Fax: 800-678-3633
custserv@films.com
www.films.com
Promotes self-understanding while helping each student understand they are different from others. *$69.00*
209 pages BiAnnual
ISBN 0-927368-56-x

1613 Pond
WINGS for Learning
1600 Green Hills Rd
Scotts Valley, CA 95066-4981 831-426-2228
Fax: 831-464-3600

Ani Stocks, Owner
Software game that teaches pattern recognition and encourages observation, trial and error and the interpretation of data.

1614 Print, Play & Learn #1 Old Mac's Farm
Soft Touch Incorporated
12301 Central Ave NE Ste 205
P.O.Box 490215
Blaine, MN 55449-2352 763-862-2920
888-755-1402
Fax: 763-862-2922
support@marblesoft.com
www.marblesoft.com

Joyce Meyer, President
Once your students have completed Old Mac's Farm, let them use the fun off-computer activities to continue learning. Over 25 activities with 250 sheets you print. Board games, dot-to-dot drawings, word puzzles, make a scene, flash cards. Concentration, sentence strips, worksheets and much more are available for teachers to expand their teaching goals. This CD is full of activities to print and use.

1615 Print, Play & Learn #7: Sampler
Soft Touch
12301 Central Ave NE Ste 205
P.O.Box 490215
Blaine, MN 55449-2352 763-862-2920
888-755-1402
Fax: 763-862-2922
support@marblesoft.com
www.marblesoft.com

Joyce Meyer, President
Print, Play and Learn Sampler gives you over 200 activities organized by training, easy, medium and hard levels so you can ready to help your student advance. Activities cover a wide range of basic knowledge, including colors, shapes, numbers, letters and much, much more. Note: Requires Overlay Maker or Overlay Printer by IntelliTools and a color printer.

1616 Puzzle Power: Sampler
Soft Touch
12301 Central Ave NE Ste 205
P.O.Box 490215
Blaine, MN 55449-2352 763-862-2920
888-755-1402
Fax: 763-862-2922
support@marblesoft.com
www.marblesoft.com

Joyce Meyer, President
Puzzle Power - Sampler offers a variety of puzzles in different themes. Each theme puzzle is followed by a puzzle of one item in this category. For example, first solve a puzzle for occupations. Then, solve a puzzle that is a baker. The pictures are large, clear and easily identifiable.

1617   Puzzle Power: Zoo & School Days
Soft Touch
12301 Central Ave NE Ste 205
P.O.Box 490215
Blaine, MN 55449-2352   763-862-2920
                                         888-755-1402
                                    Fax: 763-862-2922
                                    support@marblesoft.com
                                    www.marblesoft.com
Joyce Meyer, President
Here is a program for all of our students who need puzzle skills,
but cannot access commercial puzzles. Puzzle Power puzzles
start with just two pieces and progress to 16 pieces. The pictures
are large, clear and easily identifiable. Four different activities
enable all students to be successful. Automatic Placement: the
student just presses the switch or keyboard to place the pieces.
Magnet Mouse: all the student needs to do is move the mouse and
it drops into place.

1618   Rodeo
Soft Touch
12301 Central Ave NE Ste 205
P.O.Box 490215
Blaine, MN 55449-2352   763-862-2920
                                         888-755-1402
                                    Fax: 763-862-2922
                                    support@marblesoft.com
                                    www.marblesoft.com
Joyce Meyer, President
Rodeo action and familiar tunes for teens and preteens. Four activities invite students to learn, laugh, and sing as they go to the
rodeo with up to six age-peer friends. Age-appropriate graphics
with surprising animations reinforce the learning. The graphics
are large and colorful, the melodies familiar, and the words descriptive of the action on the screen.

1619   Shop Til You Drop
Soft Touch
12301 Central Ave NE Ste 205
P.O.Box 490215
Blaine, MN 55449-2352   763-862-2920
                                         888-755-1402
                                    Fax: 763-862-2922
                                    support@marblesoft.com
                                    www.marblesoft.com
Joyce Meyer, President
Designed specifically for preteens and teens with moderate and
severe disabilities, this program will become a staple for the
classroom. The student goes shopping and can choose which out-
fits to put together. They may choose to purchase the outfit - of
course, with mom's credit card. Another activity is a video arcade
game about money. Shop 'Til You Drop can be adjusted from a
single switch cause-and-effect program to row-and-column
scanning to direct choice.

1620   Songs I Sing at Preschool
Soft Touch
12301 Central Ave NE Ste 205
P.O.Box 490215
Blaine, MN 55449-2352   763-862-2920
                                         888-755-1402
                                    Fax: 763-862-2922
                                    support@marblesoft.com
                                    www.marblesoft.com
Joyce Meyer, President
Songs I Sing at Preschool offers many options for the teacher and
the student. Over the years, our software has used music because
our students really respond to the sounds and rhythms of songs.
Teachers select which songs to present, how many to present at
one time and where to place each song on the overlay, keyboard or
scan array.

1621   Stickybear Early Learning Activities
Optimum Resource
1 Mathews Drive
Suite 107
Hilton Head Island, SC 29926   843-689-8000
                                    Fax: 843-689-8008
                                    info@stickybear.com
                                    www.stickybear.com
Richard Hefter, President

Two modes of play allow youngsters to learn through prompted
direction or by the discovery method. Lively animation and
sound keep attention levels high as children learn writing, counting, shapes, opposites and colors. Stickybear Early Learning Activities is bilingual, so youngsters can build skills in both English
and Spanish. Pre-K to 1st grade. *$59.95*

1622   Stickybear Kindergarden Activities
Optimum Resource
1 Mathews Drive
Suite 107
Hilton Head Island, SC 29926   843-689-8000
                                    Fax: 843-689-8008
                                    info@stickybear.com
                                    www.stickybear.com
Richard Hefter, President
This dynamic new multifaceted program covers a wide range of
preschool skills that go far beyond the strictly academic. At
Stickybear's house, children discover the alphabet, numbers,
shapes, colors, plus - social skills, important safety messages and
delightful off-screen activities that foster creativity. Over three
hours of original music can be composed by a child and saved for
future use. *$59.95*

1623   Stickybear Science Fair Light
Optimum Resource
1 Mathews Drive
Suite 107
Hilton Head Island, SC 29926   843-689-8000
                                    Fax: 843-689-8008
                                    info@stickybear.com
                                    www.stickybear.com
Richard Hefter, President
The first in the new series of science-based programs Stickybear
Science Fair Light presents a content rich environment which allows students in grades 7-12 to explore, experiment with and understand light and it's properties. The program presents
experiments, both structured and free-form, which allow users to
work with prisms, lenses, color mixing, optical illusions and
more. *$59.95*

1624   Stickybear Town Builder
Optimum Resource
1 Mathews Drive
Suite 107
Hilton Head Island, SC 29926   843-689-8000
                                    Fax: 843-689-8008
                                    info@stickybear.com
                                    www.stickybear.com
Richard Hefter, President
Children learn to read maps, build towns, take trips and use a
compass in this simulation program. *$59.95*

1625   Stickybear Typing
Optimum Resource
1 Mathews Drive
Suite 107
Hilton Head Island, SC 29926   843-689-8000
                                    Fax: 843-689-8008
                                    info@stickybear.com
                                    www.stickybear.com
Richard Hefter, President
Sharpen typing skills with three challenging activities:
Stickybear Keypress, Stickybear Thump and Stickybear Stories.
Pre-K to 5th. *$59.95*

1626   Storybook Maker Deluxe
Compass Learning
203 Colorado Street
Austin, TX 78701   512-478-9600
                                        800-678-1412
                                        866-586-7387
                                    Fax: 619-622-7873
                                    support@compasslearning.com
                                    www.compasslearning.com
Eric Loeffel, President, CEO
Tammy Deal, VP, Human Resources
Eric Wasser, VP, Sales
Using Storybook Maker Deluxe and their imaginations, students
can create and publish stories filled with exciting graphics. Stu-
dents can write stories and watch as the text appears in the setting

they've chosen. Engaging sounds and music, plus lively animations, provide positive learning reinforcement throughout the program. *$44.95*

1627   Super Challenger
Electronic Courseware Systems
1713 S State St
Champaign, IL 61820-7258   217-359-7099
                                            800-832-4965
                                        Fax: 217-359-6578
                                        www.ecsmedia.com

Jodie Varner, Manager
G Peters, President
An aural-visual musical game that increases the player's ability to remember a series of pitches as they are played by the computer. The game is based on a 12-note chromatic scale, a major scale, and a minor scale. Each pitch is reinforced visually with a color representation of a keyboard on the display screen. Computer/software. *$39.95*

1628   Switch Basics
Soft Touch
12301 Central Ave NE Ste 205
P.O.Box 490215
Blaine, MN 55449-2352   763-862-2920
                                           888-755-1402
                                        Fax: 763-862-2922
                                      support@marblesoft.com
                                       www.marblesoft.com

Joyce Meyer, President
Discover whimsical animations and real life pictures while learning switch operations. Intriguing and humorous, nine different programs offer a multitude of learning experiences for all ages. Program options include: cause and effect, scanning, step scanning, row and column activities for one or two players. Watch the clouds roll away revealing African animals; visit the beauty salon or barber shop; work two to sixteen piece puzzles; or add swimming fish to a huge aquarium.

1629   Switch Interface Pro 5.0
Don Johnston
26799 West Commerce Drive
Volo, IL 60073   847-740-0749
                                           800-999-4660
                                        Fax: 847-740-7326
                                      info@donjohnston.com
                                       www.donjohnston.com

Don Johnston, Founder
Ruth Ziolkowski, President
Kevin Johnston, Director of Product Design
Allows individuals with physical disabilities to access the computer. Five ports accommodate multiple switches and emulate everything from a single-click to a return. Consequently, individuals gain access to the widest variety of switch-accessible software available. It requires no software and can be used with both Windows and Macintosh computers. *$79.00*

1630   Teach Me Phonemics Series Bundle
SoftTouch
Ste 401
4300 Stine Rd
Bakersfield, CA 93313-2352   661-396-8676
                                           877-763-8868
                                        Fax: 661-396-8760
                                      support@softtouch.com
                                       www.funsoftware.com

Joyce Meyer, President
Roxanne Butterfield, Marketing
The Teach Me Phonemics Series Bundle includes one copy of each Teach Me Phonemics program - Initial, Medial, Final and Blends - four CD's in all.

1631   Teach Me Phonemics Super Bundle
SoftTouch
Ste 401
4300 Stine Rd
Bakersfield, CA 93313-2352   661-396-8676
                                           877-763-8868
                                        Fax: 661-396-8760
                                       www.funsoftware.com

Roxanne Butterfield, Marketing
Joyce Meyer, President
Teach Me Phonemics Super Bundle includes all 4 Teach Me Phonemics programs and all 4 Teach Me Phonemics overlay CD's - eight CD's in all.

1632   Teach Me Phonemics: Blends
SoftTouch
Ste 401
4300 Stine Rd
Bakersfield, CA 93313-2352   661-396-8676
                                           877-763-8868
                                        Fax: 661-396-8760

Roxanne Butterfield, Marketing
Joyce Meyer, President
Teach Me Phonemics - Blends helps students explore words and hear the initial blend sounds. It features musical interludes and movement to engage the student. Teachers select the best combination options to motivate and engage the student. Options turn off and on the fly so you can quickly make changes to keep the student engaged.

1633   Teach Me Phonemics: Final
SoftTouch
Ste 401
4300 Stine Rd
Bakersfield, CA 93313-2352   661-396-8676
                                           877-763-8868
                                        Fax: 661-396-8760

Roxanne Butterfield
Joyce Meyer, President
Teach me Phonemics - Final helps students explore words and hear the final sounds. It features musical interludes and movement to engage the student. Options turn off and on the fly so you can quickly make changes to keep the student engaged.

1634   Teach Me Phonemics: Initial
SoftTouch
12301 Central Ave NE
Ste 205
Blaine, MN 55434   763-755-1402
                                           888-755-1403
                                        Fax: 763-862-2920
                                      sales@marblesoft.com
                                       www.softtouch.com

Roxanne Butterfield, Marketing
Joyce Meyer, President
Teach Me Phonemics - Initial helps students explore the words and hear the initial sounds. It features musical interludes and movement to engage the student. Teachers select the best combination options to motivate and engage the student. Options turn off and on the fly so you can quickly make changes to keep the student engaged.

1635   Teach Me Phonemics: Medial
SoftTouch
12301 Central Ave NE
Ste 205
Blaine, MN 55434   763-755-1402
                                           888-755-1403
                                        Fax: 763-862-2920
                                      sales@marblesoft.com
                                       www.softtouch.com

Roxanne Butterfield, Marketing
Joyce Meyer, President
Teach Me Phonemics - Medial helps students explore the words and hear the medial sounds. It features musical interludes and movement to engage the student. Teachers select the best combination options to motivate and engage the student. Options turn off and on the fly so you can quickly make changes to keep the student engaged.

1636 Teach Me to Talk
Soft Touch
12301 Central Ave NE Ste 205
P.O.Box 490215
Blaine, MN 55449-2352   763-862-2920
                                       888-755-1402
                                  Fax: 763-862-2922
                         support@marblesoft.com
                              www.marblesoft.com

Joyce Meyer, President
The first activity Teach Me to Talk is used as a springboard for the student to learn to speak the word. There are 150 real pictures. When a picture is chosen, it appears on a clear background with musical interludes, movement, written word and spoken word. It culminates by morphing to the corresponding black and white Mayer-Johnson symbol. The second activity Story Time, takes some of these nouns and puts them in four line poetry. This helps students hear the word in the midst of a sentence.

1637 Teen Tunes Plus
Soft Touch
12301 Central Ave NE Ste 205
P.O.Box 490215
Blaine, MN 55449-2352   763-862-2920
                                       888-755-1402
                                  Fax: 763-862-2922
                         support@marblesoft.com
                              www.marblesoft.com

Joyce Meyer, President
Introduce switch use to older students with disabilities. Large interesting graphics, a variety of musical interludes, and surprising animations are combined with calm soothing music and beautiful pictures in the software specifically designed for preteens and teens with severe cognitive delays and/or physical disabilities, and older students learning to use a switch.

1638 There are Tyrannosaurs Trying on Pants in My Bedroom
Compass Learning
203 Colorado Street
Austin, TX 78701-3922   512-478-9600
                                       800-678-1412
                                       866-586-7387
                                  Fax: 619-622-7873
                     support@compasslearning.com
                          www.compasslearning.com

Eric Loeffel, President, CEO
Tammy Deal, VP, Human Resources
Eric Wasser, VP, Sales
In this popular story, Saturday chores turn into fun-filled frolicking when dinosaurs come for a visit. Sounds, music and animation make learning about phonics and vocabulary dyno-mite. *$34.95*

1639 Three Billy Goats Gruff
Compass Learning
203 Colorado Street
Austin, TX 78701-3922   512-478-9600
                                       800-678-1412
                                       866-586-7387
                                  Fax: 619-622-7873
                     support@compasslearning.com
                          www.compasslearning.com

Eric Loeffel, President, CEO
Tammy Deal, VP, Human Resources
Eric Wasser, VP, Sales
Motivating exercises and creative activities provide hours of learning fun while young students follow the adventure of The Three Billy Goats Gruff in this animated version of the timeless tale. *$ 34.95*

1640 Three Little Pigs
Compass Learning
203 Colorado Street
Austin, TX 78701-3922   512-478-9600
                                       800-678-1412
                                       866-586-7387
                                  Fax: 619-622-7873
                     support@compasslearning.com
                          www.compasslearning.com

Eric Loeffel, President, CEO
Tammy Deal, VP, Human Resources
Eric Wasser, VP, Sales

Help young students build reading comprehension and writing skills with this interactive version of the children's classic, The Three Little Pigs. Animated storytelling and creative activities inspire children to read, write and rhyme. *$34.95*

1641 TouchCorders
Soft Touch
12301 Central Ave NE Ste 205
P.O.Box 490215
Blaine, MN 55449-2352   763-862-2920
                                       888-755-1402
                                  Fax: 763-862-2922
                         support@marblesoft.com
                              www.marblesoft.com

Joyce Meyer, President
TouchCorders are the flexible and easy-to-use communicator designed by Jo Meyer and Linda Bidabe for reach classroom use. TouchCorders are sensitive to touch at every angle and give the student kinesthetic feedback. With the unique Add 'n Touch system, Jo connects the puzzles bases of 2 or more TouchCorders on the fly to present vocabulary, sequencing, story telling, social stories, concepts and other curriculum and communication opportunities.

1642 TouchWindow Touch Screen
Riverdeep Incorporated
100 Pine Street
Suite 1900
San Francisco, CA 94111   415-659-2000
                                       800-542-4222
                                  Fax: 415-659-2020
                              info@riverdeep.net
                              www.riverdeep.net

Barry O'Callaghan, Executive Chairman & Chief Executive Officer
Tony Mulderry, Executive Vice President, Corporate Development
Ciara Smyth, Executive Vice President, Global Business Operations
Software for children. *$335.00*

1643 Turtle Teasers
Soft Touch
12301 Central Ave NE Ste 205
P.O.Box 490215
Blaine, MN 55449-2352   763-862-2920
                                       888-755-1402
                                  Fax: 763-862-2922
                         support@marblesoft.com
                              www.marblesoft.com

Joyce Meyer, President
Three Games, Three Levels from Easy, Medium to Hard. The Shell Game - easy: Watch one of the three turtles get the tomato. Then watch carefully as they switch positions and pop shut. Choose incorrectly and the frog disappears until the correct one is displayed. The Pond - medium: Watch the tomato disappear somewhere in the pond scene. Tomato Dump - hard: Hit the shell and it turns into the tomato, giving a score. There are different difficulty levels to equalize all students.

1644 What Was That!
Compass Learning
203 Colorado Street
Austin, TX 78701-3922   512-478-9600
                                       800-678-1412
                                       866-586-7387
                                  Fax: 619-622-7873
                     support@compasslearning.com
                          www.compasslearning.com

Eric Loeffel, President, CEO
Tammy Deal, VP, Human Resources
Eric Wasser, VP, Sales
In this bedtime story, noises in the night send three brother bears scurrying out of bed. Thoughtful questions test young readers' comprehension, while games, voice recording, writing practice and other playful activities stimulate their creativity.

1645 Wivik 3
Prentke Romich Company
1022 Heyl Road
Wooster, OH 44691
330-262-1984
800-262-1984
Fax: 330-263-4829
info@prentrom.com
www.prentrom.com

Dave Hershberger, President & CEO
Barry Romich, Co-Founder
On-screen keyboard provides access to any application in the latest Windows operating systems. Selections are made by clicking, dwelling or switch scanning. Enhancements include word prediction and abbreviation expansion.

1646 WordMaker
Don Johnston
26799 West Commerce Drive
Volo, IL 60073
847-740-0749
800-999-4660
Fax: 847-740-7326
info@donjohnston.com
www.donjohnston.com

Don Johnston, Founder
Ruth Ziolkowski, President
Kevin Johnston, Director of Product Design
The computer version of Dr Patricia Cunningham's book 'Systematic Sequential Phonics They Use.' The program systematically builds spelling and word decoding skills for struggling readers and writers. *$79.00*

1647 Write: Out Loud
Don Johnston
26799 West Commerce Drive
Volo, IL 60073
847-740-0749
800-999-4660
Fax: 847-740-7326
info@donjohnston.com
www.donjohnston.com

Don Johnston, Founder
Ruth Ziolkowski, President
Kevin Johnston, Director of Product Design
Write: Out Loud is an easy-to-use talking word processor that uses text-to-speech and revision and editing supports to help students write more effectively, more often and with more enthusiasm as they share creative thoughts on paper. *$79.00*

1648 You Tell Me: Learning Basic Information
Programming Concepts
8700 Shoal Creek Boulevard
Austin, TX 78757-6897
512-451-3246
800-897-3202
800-471-3000
Fax: 800-397-7633
general@proedinc.com
www.proedinc.com

Jeff McLane, Founder
Lee Wilson, President and CEO
Randy Pennington, Executive VP
This game teaches and reinforces basic information all individuals need to know. Questions asked in this game help prepare people to communicate personal identification information important to community survival. *$49.95*

Software: Professional

1649 Acrontech International
5500 Main St
Williamsville, NY 14221-6755
Fax: 716-854-4014
This company supplies software, audio mixers, and closed-caption televisions.

1650 DPS with BCP
V OR T Corporation
P.O.Box G (George)
Menlo Park, CA 94026
650-322-8282
888-757-8678
Fax: 650-327-0747
custserv@vort.com
vort.com

Tom Holt, Owner
This program uses unique DPS branching techniques to access goals and objectives.

1651 Descriptive Language Arts Development
Educational Activities Software
5600 West 83rd Street
Suite 300, 8200 Tower
Bloomington, MN 55437
888-351-4199
800-447-5286
Fax: 239-225-9299
info@edmentum.com
www.edmentum.com

Vin Riera, President/CEO
Dan Juckniess, SVP, Sales & Professional Services
Stacey Herteux, VP, Human Resources
This multimedia language arts development program provides instruction and application of fundamental English skills and concepts. *$395.00*

1652 Diagnostic Report Writer
Parrot Software
P.O. Box 250755
West Bloomfield, MI 48325
248-788-3223
800-727-7681
Fax: 248-788-3224
support@parrotsoftware.com
www.parrotsoftware.com

Dr. Frederic Weiner, Ph. D., CCC-SP, President, Owner
Creates a three page single-spaced diagnostic report for a child with a communication disorder from a list of questions; sections of the report include developmental and background history, oral peripheral exam, speech and language analysis, summary and recommendations.

1653 Draft: Builder
Don Johnston
26799 West Commerce Drive
Volo, IL 60073
847-740-0749
800-999-4660
Fax: 847-740-7326
info@donjohnston.com
www.donjohnston.com

Don Johnston, Founder
Ruth Ziolkowski, President
Kevin Johnston, Director of Product Design
A software-based graphic organizer that breaks down the writing process into manageable chunks to structure planning, organizing, and draft-writing. *$79.00*

1654 EZ Dot
CAPCO Capability Corporation
3910 S. Union Court
Spokane Valley, WA 99206-6345
509-927-8195
800-827-2182
Fax: 800-827-2182
info@skilltran.com
www.skilltran.com

Jeff Truthan, President
A critical software tool used in vocational counseling, job restructuring, recruitment and placement, better utilization of workers, and safety issues. This software offers occupational data by title, code, industry, GEO, DPT, or OGA. *$295.00*

1655 EZ Keys for Windows
Words+
Ste 109
42505 10th St W
Lancaster, CA 93534-7059

661-723-6523
800-869-8521
Fax: 661-723-2114
info@words-plus.com

Jean Dobbs, Editorial Director
Tim Gilmer, Editor
Josie Byzek, Managing Editor
A software and hardware product designed to operate on an IBM compatible PC. The software provides dual word prediction, abbreviation expansion, five different methods of voice output and access to commercial software applications. *$1395.00*

1656 Goals and Objectives
JE Stewart Teaching Tools
P.O.Box 15308
Seattle, WA 98115-308

206-262-9538
Fax: 206-262-9538

Jeff Stewart, Owner
Goals and Objectives software helps teachers make student plans including IEP's, IPP's and IHP's. The system provides curricula for all students and programs to develop and evaluate plans, print reports and make data forms. Systems are available for Windows and Macintosh for $139.

1657 Goals and Objectives IEP Program Curriculum Associates LLC
153 Rangeway Road
P.O.Box 2001
North Billerica, MA 01862-0901

978-667-8000
800-225-0248
Fax: 800-366-1158
www.curriculumassociates.com

Frank E. Ferguson, Chairman
Renee Foster, President & Publisher
Woody Palk, Senior Vice President, Sales
BRIGANCE CIBS-R standardized scoring conversion software, is a teacher's tool that prints goal and objective pages of the IEP. In less than two minutes per student, a teacher types student data into the computer.

1658 Nasometer
Kay Elemetrics Corporation
3 Paragon Drive
Montvale, NJ 07645

973-628-6200
800-289-5297
Fax: 201-391-2063
sales@kaypentax.com
www.kaypentax.com

John Crump, President
Steve Crump, Direct Sales
Measures the ratio of acoustic energy for the nasal and real-time visual cueing during therapy. Used clinically in the areas of cleft palate, motor speech disorders, hearing impairment and palatal prosthetic fittings.

1659 PSS CogRehab Software
Psychological Software Services
3304 W 75th St
Indianapolis, IN 46268-1664

317-257-9672
Fax: 317-257-9674
www.neuroscience.cnter.com

Odie L Bracy, Executive Director
PSS CogRehab Software is a comprehensive and easy-to-use multimedia cognitive rehabilitation software available, for clinical and educational use with head injury, stroke LD/ADD and other brain compromises. The packages include 64 computerized therapy tasks which contain modifiable parameters that will accommodate most requirements. Exercises include attention and executive skills, multiple modalities of visuosatial and memory skills, simple, complex, problem-solving skills.
$260 - $2500

1660 Parrot Easy Language Simple Anaylsis
Parrot Software
P.O.Box 250755
West Bloomfield, MI 48325

248-788-3223
800-727-7681
Fax: 248-788-3224
support@parrotsoftware.com
www.parrotsoftware.com

Dr. Frederic Weiner, Ph. D., CCC-SP, President, Owner
Designed for grammatical analysis of language samples. The user types and translates language samples of up to 100 utterances.

1661 SOLO Literacy Suite
Don Johnston
26799 West Commerce Drive
Volo, IL 60073

847-740-0749
800-999-4660
Fax: 847-740-7326
info@donjohnston.com
www.donjohnston.com

Don Johnston, Founder
Ruth Ziolkowski, President
Kevin Johnston, Director of Product Design
Places all of the right tools, and a wide-range of embedded learning supports, at their fingertips. SOLO includes word prediction, a text reader, graphic organizer and talking word processor, putting students in charge of their own learning and accommodations. Students of varying ages and abilities have access to, and make progress in, the general education curriculum. *$79.00*

1662 TOVA
Universal Attention Disorders
3321 Cerritos Avenue
Los Alamitos, CA 90720

562-594-7700
800-729-2886
Fax: 800-452-6919
info@tovatest.com
www.tovatest.com

Lawrence M. Greenberg, MD
A computerized assessment which, in conjunction with classroom behavior ratings, is a highly effective screening tool for ADD. TOVA includes software, complete instructions, and supporting data including norms.

1663 Visi-Pitch III
Kayelemetrics Corporation
3 Paragon Drive
Montvale, NJ 07645

973-628-6200
800-289-5297
Fax: 201-391-2063
sales@kaypentax.com

John Crump, President
Steve Crump, Direct Sales
Assists the speech/voice clinician in assessment and treatment tasks across an expansive range of disorders.

Software: Reading & Language Arts

1664 Choices, Choices 5.0
Tom Snyder Productions
100 Talcott Avenue
Watertown, MA 02472-5703

800-342-0236
www.tomsnyder.com

Tom Snyder, Founder
Bridget Dalton, Ed.D, Author
Peggy Healy Stearns, Ph.D., Author
Teaches students to take responsibility for their behavior. Helps students develop the skills and awareness they need to make wise choices and to think through the consequences of their actions.

1665 Co: Writer
Don Johnston
26799 West Commerce Drive
Volo, IL 60073
847-740-0749
800-999-4660
Fax: 847-740-7326
info@donjohnston.com
www.donjohnston.com

Don Johnston, Founder
Ruth Ziolkowski, President
Kevin Johnston, Director of Product Design
A software-based writing assistant that uses word prediction to cut through writing barriers and improve written expression. It is intended for students who struggle to write because of difficulty with spelling, syntax, and translating thoughts into writing. As students type, Co: Writer learns the context of the sentence and accurately 'predicts' words even when spelled phonetically or inventively. *$79.00*

1666 Community Exploration
Compass Learning
203 Colorado Street
Austin, TX 78701-3922
512-478-9600
800-678-1412
866-586-7387
Fax: 619-622-7873
support@compasslearning.com
www.compasslearning.com

Eric Loeffel, President, CEO
Tammy Deal, VP, Human Resources
Eric Wasser, VP, Sales
An award-winning learning adventure takes students who are learning English as a second language on a field trip to the make-believe town of Cornerstone. More than 50 community locations come to life with sound and animation. While exploring places in this typical American community where people live, work and play, students also enhance important English language skills. Offers an exciting approach for any age student who needs to improve their English language proficiency. 4-12. *$19.95*

1667 Conversations
Educational Activities Software
5600 West 83rd Street
Suite 300, 8200 Tower
Bloomington, MN 55437
888-351-4199
800-447-5286
Fax: 239-225-9299
info@edmentum.com
www.edmentum.com

Vin Riera, President/CEO
Dan Juckniess, SVP, Sales & Professional Services
Stacey Herteux, VP, Human Resources
Using American digitized voices, CONVERSATIONS provides 14 different dialogues in which the student can participate. The topics offer learners important information about American culture and the workplace. Available for DOS. *$195.00*

1668 Core-Reading and Vocabulary Development
Educational Activities
P.O.Box 87
Baldwin, NY 11510
516-223-4666
800-797-3223
Fax: 516-623-9282
www.edact.com

Alfred Harris, President
Carol Stern, VP
Students begin with 36 basic words and progress to more than 200. Reading and writing activities are coordinated and integrated throughout the program for more substantial permanent learning. Five units covering readability levels from pre-primer to grade three.
Full Program

1669 Friday Afternoon
203 Colorado Street
Austin, TX 78701-3922
512-478-9600
800-678-1412
866-586-7387
Fax: 619-622-7873
support@compasslearning.com
www.compasslearning.com

Eric Loeffel, President, CEO
Tammy Deal, VP, Human Resources
Eric Wasser, VP, Sales
Save hours of preparation time and dazzle your students with interesting new activities to supplement their classroom learning. With Friday afternoon, you'll produce flash cards, word puzzles, even customized bingo cards and more, all at the click of a mouse. MacIntosh diskette. *$99.95*

1670 How to Read for Everyday Living
Educational Activities Software
5600 West 83rd Street
Suite 300, 8200 Tower
Bloomington, MN 55437
888-351-4199
800-447-5286
Fax: 239-225-9299
info@edmentum.com
www.edmentum.com

Vin Riera, President/CEO
Dan Juckniess, SVP, Sales & Professional Services
Stacey Herteux, VP, Human Resources
Basic vocabulary and key words are taught and, when need, retaught using alternative teaching strategies. Passages that students read help put the vocabulary into context. Each lesson is followed by crossword and other puzzles check comprehension.

1671 Learning English: Primary
203 Colorado Street
Austin, TX 78701-3922
512-478-9600
800-678-1412
866-586-7387
Fax: 619-622-7873
support@compasslearning.com
www.compasslearning.com

Eric Loeffel, President, CEO
Tammy Deal, VP, Human Resources
Eric Wasser, VP, Sales
Four stories and rhymes help students familiarize themselves with essential English language concepts, recognize patterns in language and associate words with objects. *$49.95*

1672 Learning English: Rhyme Time
Compass Learning
203 Colorado Street
Austin, TX 78701-3922
512-478-9600
800-678-1412
866-586-7387
Fax: 619-622-7873
www.compasslearning.com

Eric Loeffel, President, CEO
Tammy Deal, VP, Human Resources
Eric Wasser, VP, Sales
Using classic children's rhymes in an animated multimedia program, students work on language skills, vocabulary and comprehension.

1673 Lexia I, II and III Reading Series
Lexia Learning Systems
200 Baker Ave Ext.
Concord, MA 01742
978-405-6200
800-435-3942
800-507-2772
Fax: 978-287-0062
info@lexialearning.com
www.lexialearning.com

Nick Gaehde, President and CEO
Paul More, Vice President, Finance
Collin Earnst, Vice President of Marketing
Lexia's software helps children and adults with learning disabilities master their core reading skills. Based on the Orton Gillingham method, Lexia Early Reading, Phonics Based Reading and SOS (Strategies for Older Students) apply phonics principles to help students learn essential sound-symbol

151

correspondence and decoding skills. The Quick Reading Tests generate detailed skill reports in only 5-8 minutes per student to provide data for further instruction. Price: $40-400 per workstation.

1674 Memory Castle
WINGS for Learning
1600 Green Hills Rd
Scotts Valley, CA 95066-4981   831-426-2228
Fax: 831-464-3600

Ani Stocks, Owner
Introduces a strategy to increase memory skills via an adventure Q198game. Set in a castle, the game requires memory, reading, spelling skills and more to win.

1675 On a Green Bus: A UKanDu Little Book
Don Johnston
26799 West Commerce Drive
Volo, IL 60073   847-740-0749
800-999-4660
Fax: 847-740-7326
info@donjohnston.com
www.donjohnston.com

Don Johnston, Founder
Ruth Ziolkowski, President
Kevin Johnston, Director of Product Design
This early literacy program that consists of several create-your-own 4-page animated stories that help build language experience on each page and then watch the page come alive with animation and sound. After completing the story, students can print it out to make a book which can be read over and over again. Because there are no wrong answers, all children can have a successful literacy experience. *$45.00*

1676 Open Book
Freedom Scientific
11800 31st Court North
St Petersburg, FL 33716   727-803-8000
800-444-4443
Fax: 727-803-8001
info@freedomscientific.com
www.freedomscientific.com

Lee Hamilton, President, CEO, and Chairman of
Mike Self, Sales Representative (Alabama)
Joseph McDaniel, Sales Representative (Alaska and
Software that reads scanned text allowed and includes other features that aid the vision-impaired. *$995.00*

1677 Optimum Resource Software
1 Mathews Drive
Suite 107
Hilton Head Island, SC 29926   843-689-8000
Fax: 843-689-8008
info@stickybear.com
www.stickybear.com

Richard Hefter, President
Optimum Resource publishes over 100 K-12 education curriculum software titles under its varietal brands, StickyBear, MiddleWare, High School and Tools for Teachers. Most programs are available in Bilingual English/Spanish, and are offered with options for the single user through 30 users.

1678 Parts of Speech
Optimum Resource
1 Mathews Drive
Suite 107
Hilton Head Island, SC 29926   843-689-8000
Fax: 843-689-8008
info@stickybear.com
www.stickybear.com

Richard Hefter, President
Designed to help students build grammar and vocabulary as they strengthen reading and writing ability. Grades 3 to 9. *$59.95*

1679 Programs for Aphasia and Cognitive Disorders
Parrot Software
P.O.Box 250755
West Bloomfield, MI 48325   248-788-3223
800-727-7681
Fax: 248-788-3224
support@parrotsoftware.com
www.parrotsoftware.com

Dr. Frederic Weiner, Ph. D., CCC-SP, President, Owner
Over 50 different computer programs that facilitate language, memory and attention training. Programs are available for MS DOS, WINDOWS and Apple II.

1680 Punctuation Rules
Optimum Resource
1 Mathews Drive
Suite 107
Hilton Head Island, SC 29926   843-689-8000
Fax: 843-689-8008
info@stickybear.com
www.stickybear.com

Richard Hefter, President
Punctuation Rules is designed to help students improve their punctuation skills. Students work with appropriate level sentences which follow common rules of punctuation. The program covers material ranging from categories of sentences to forming possessives and allows students to gain strength in their ability to correctly use periods, commas, apostrophes, question marks, colons, hyphens, quotation marks, exclamation points and more. Grades 3-9. Bilingual. *$59.95*

1681 Quick Reading Test, Phonics Based Reading, Reading SOS (Strategies for Older Students)
Lexia Learning Systems
200 Baker Ave Ext.
Concord, MA 01742   978-405-6200
800-435-3942
800-507-2772
Fax: 978-287-0062
info@lexialearning.com
www.lexialearning.com

Nick Gaehde, President and CEO
Paul More, Vice President, Finance
Collin Earnst, Vice President of Marketing
Lexia's software helps children and adults with learning disabilities master their core reading skills. Based on the Orton Gillingham method, Phonics Based Reading and S.O.S. (Strategies for the Older Student) apply phonics principles to help students learn essential sound-symbol correspondence and decoding skills. The Quick Reading Tests generate detailed phonemic skills reports in only 5-8 minutes per student to provide teachers with accurate data to focus their instruction. Price: $67-$500.

1682 Quick Talk
Educational Activities Software
5600 West 83rd Street
Suite 300, 8200 Tower
Bloomington, MN 55437   888-351-4199
800-447-5286
Fax: 239-225-9299
info@edmentum.com
www.edmentum.com

Vin Riera, President/CEO
Dan Juckniess, SVP, Sales & Professional Services
Stacey Herteux, VP, Human Resources
Students will learn and use new vocabulary immediately: high-frequency, everyday vocabulary words are introduced and used contextually using human speech, graphics and text. Voice-interactive program (MS-DOS). *$65.00*

1683   Race the Clock
Mindplay
4400 E. Broadway Blvd
Suite 400
Tucson, AZ 85711   520-888-1800
                                    800-221-7911
                                Fax: 520-888-7904
                                mail@mindplay.com
                                www.mindplay.com
Dan Figurski, Senior Vice President of Business
Chris Coleman, VP, Business Development
Judith Bliss, CEO
A matching game, uses the animation capabilities to teach verbs.
The player chooses a matching game from a menu.

1684   Read: Out Loud
Don Johnston
26799 West Commerce Drive
Volo, IL 60073   847-740-0749
                                    800-999-4660
                                Fax: 847-740-7326
                                info@donjohnston.com
                                www.donjohnston.com
Don Johnston, Founder
Ruth Ziolkowski, President
Kevin Johnston, Director of Product Design
An accessible text reader that provides access to the curriculum.
It features high-quality text to speech and study tools that help
students read with comprehension. *$79.00*

1685   Reader Rabbit
Learning Company
Ste 1900
100 Pine St
San Francisco, CA 94111-5205   415-659-2000
                                    800-825-4420
                                Fax: 415-659-2020
                                thelearningco@hmhpub.com
                                www.thelearningcompany.com
Linda K. Zecher, President and CEO
Eric Shuman, Chief Financial Officer
John K. Dragoon, Executive Vice President and Chi
Supports young students in building fundamental reading readi-
ness skills in a playful, multi-sensory environment.

1686   Reading Comprehension Series
Optimum Resource
1 Mathews Drive
Suite 107
Hilton Head Island, SC 29926- 3765   843-689-8000
                                Fax: 843-689-8008
                                info@stickybear.com
                                www.stickybear.com
Richard Hefter, President
The Reading Comprehension Series, includes seven volumes
packed with intriguing multi-level stories. Each volume will capture the interest of children ages 8-14 while teaching them crucial
reading comprehension skills. These open-ended programs are
versatile and easy to use, and Bilingual. *$59.95*

1687   Simon SIO
Don Johnston
26799 West Commerce Drive
Volo, IL 60073   847-740-0749
                                    800-999-4660
                                Fax: 847-740-7326
                                info@donjohnston.com
                                www.donjohnston.com
Don Johnston, Founder
Ruth Ziolkowski, President
Kevin Johnston, Director of Product Design
A researched and widely field-tested phonics program for begin-
ning readers, developed in collaboration with Dr. Ted
Hasselbring of Vanderbilt University. The program uses a per-
sonal tutor to deliver individualized instruction and corrective
feedback. *$79.00*

1688   Sound Sentences
Educational Activities Software
5600 West 83rd Street
Suite 300, 8200 Tower
Bloomington, MN 55437   888-351-4199
                                    800-447-5286
                                Fax: 239-225-9299
                                info@edmentum.com
                                www.edmentum.com
Vin Riera, President/CEO
Dan Juckniess, SVP, Sales & Professional Services
Stacey Herteux, VP, Human Resources
This sound-interactive program breaks away from traditional language instruction. Instead of formal concentration on verb and
basic vocabulary, students meet everyday English with colloquialisms they will hear in real life situations. They reinforce their
knowledge of sentence structure while acquiring the ability to
communicate in daily settings. (For MAC, MS-DOS and Windows). *$65.00*

1689   Spelling Rules
Optimum Resource
1 Mathews Drive
Suite 107
Hilton Head Island, SC 29926- 3765   843-689-8000
                                Fax: 843-689-8008
                                info@stickybear.com
                                www.stickybear.com
Richard Hefter, President
A curriculum based, easy-to-use program that provides students
with the practice they need to build strong spelling skills. Con-
cepts discussed include plurals, compounds, i-before-e, capital-
ization, and more. Grades 3 to 9. Bilingual. *$59.95*

1690   Start-to-Finish Library
Don Johnston
26799 West Commerce Drive
Volo, IL 60073   847-740-0749
                                    800-999-4660
                                Fax: 847-740-7326
                                info@donjohnston.com
                                www.donjohnston.com
Don Johnston, Founder
Ruth Ziolkowski, President
Kevin Johnston, Director of Product Design
Offers struggling readers a wide selection of engaging narrative
chapter books written at two readability levels (2-3rd and 4-5th
grade) and delivered in three media formats. Professionally-nar-
rated audio and computer supports help scaffold reading to ensure success. *$79.00*

1691   Start-to-Finish Literacy Starters
Don Johnston
26799 West Commerce Drive
Volo, IL 60073   847-740-0749
                                    800-999-4660
                                Fax: 847-740-7326
                                info@donjohnston.com
                                www.donjohnston.com
Don Johnston, Founder
Ruth Ziolkowski, President
Kevin Johnston, Director of Product Design
A reading series intended for students with multiple disabilities
who are in 3-12th grade, but reading at a beginning level. Dr. Ka-
ren Erickson developed this series, which combines switch-ac-
cessible software with three types of text. *$79.00*

1692   Stickybear Reading Comprehension
Optimum Resource
1 Mathews Drive
Suite 107
Hilton Head Island, SC 29926- 3765   843-689-8000
                                Fax: 843-689-8008
                                info@stickybear.com
                                www.stickybear.com
Richard Hefter, President
This multi-level reading comprehension program helps children
improve reading skills with 30 high-interest stories and question
sets created by the Weekly Reader editors. Children learn to recognize main ideas, define sequence, using context to identify
words, and more. Grades 2 to 4. Bilingual. *$59.95*

1693 Stickybear Reading Fun Park
Optimum Resource
1 Mathews Drive
Suite 107
Hilton Head Island, SC 29926- 3765   843-689-8000
Fax: 843-689-8008
info@stickybear.com
www.stickybear.com
Richard Hefter, President
Children discover and practice critical reading skills as the Stickybear family guides users through unique, action-packed activities, each with multiple levels of difficulty and skills that address both the auditory and visual needs of budding readers. Pre-K through 3rd grade. *$59.95*

1694 Stickybear Reading Room Deluxe
Optimum Resource
1 Mathews Drive
Suite 107
Hilton Head Island, SC 29926- 3765   843-689-8000
Fax: 843-689-8008
www.stickybear.com
Richard Hefter, President
Children build vocabulary and reading comprehension skills using hundreds of word/picture sets and thousands of put-together sentence parts. K-3rd grade. Bilingual, English/Spanish. *$59.95*

1695 Stickybear Spelling
Optimum Resource
1 Mathews Drive
Suite 107
Hilton Head Island, SC 29926- 3765   843-689-8000
Fax: 843-689-8008
www.stickybear.com
Richard Hefter, President
Children discover and practice critical spelling skills as they work with three unique action-packed activities, each with four graded levels of difficulty. The program is open-ended and teachers may add, change and modify the word lists for each individual. Stickybear Spelling contains more than 2000 recorded words. Levels may be set to allow students of different ages or abilities to compete effectively. Grades 2 through 4. *$59.95*

1696 Tomorrow's Promise: Language Arts
Compass Learning
13500 Evening Creek Drive North
Suite 600
San Diego, CA 92128   858-668-2586
866-475-0317
Fax: 858-408-2903
info@bridgepointeducation.com
www.bridgepointeducation.com
Andrew S. Clark, Founder, Chief Executive Officer
Diane Thompson, SVP, General Counsel
Charlene Dackerman, SVP, Human Resources
You'll strengthen students' grammar, usage and vocabulary skills and promote higher order thinking skills with this comprehensive Language Arts curriculum. It utilizes cross-curricular, thematic instruction engaging multimedia learning exercises that encourage writing, speaking and listening proficiency. Promotes higher order thinking skills. *$279.95*

1697 Tomorrow's Promise: Reading
Compass Learning
203 Colorado Street
Austin, TX 78701-3922   512-478-9600
800-678-1412
866-586-7387
Fax: 619-622-7873
www.compasslearning.com
Eric Loeffel, President, CEO
Tammy Deal, VP, Human Resources
Eric Wasser, VP, Sales
This multimedia curriculum balances thematic, interactive exploration with core skills development, increasing your students' early reading proficiency, building a solid literacy foundation and fostering a lifelong love for reading. *$279.95*

1698 Tomorrow's Promise: Spelling
Compass Learning
203 Colorado Street
Austin, TX 78701-3922   512-478-9600
800-678-1412
866-586-7387
Fax: 619-622-7873
www.compasslearning.com
Eric Loeffel, President, CEO
Tammy Deal, VP, Human Resources
Eric Wasser, VP, Sales
Lovable characters and engaging multimedia effects put young students on a fast-track to early spelling proficiency with fourteen activities and three games. A full year's instruction on each CD includes 30 world lists per grade, in story context, or create word lists to suit your needs. This program addresses students' multiple learning styles and rewards students as they progress through each stage of spelling skill acquisition. *$99.95*

1699 Vocabulary Development
Optimum Resource
1 Mathews Drive
Suite 107
Hilton Head Island, SC 29926- 3765   843-689-8000
Fax: 843-689-8008
www.stickybear.com
Richard Hefter, President
A featured program in the middle school series. Vocabulary Development is designed to help students increase vocabulary as they strengthen reading skills. Students relate their current knowledge of vocabulary to the context in which they discover an unfamiliar word. Utilizing a variety of contextual aids, this program illustrates synonyms, antonyms, prefixes, suffixes, homophones, multiple meanings and context clues, allowing students to apply experience and context. *$59.95*

1700 Whoops
Cornucopia Software
P.O.Box 6111
Albany, CA 94706   510-528-7000
supportstaff@practicemagic.com
www.practicemagic.com
Christina Morua, Manager
Checks spelling three ways. It checks words as they are typed, it checks an entire screen and highlights the errors and it reads ASCII text files from a disk and lists errors.

Software: Vocational

1701 Films Media Group
Infobase Publishing
132 W 31st St, 17th Floor
New York, NY 10001   800-322-8755
Fax: 800-678-3633
custserv@factsonfile.com
www.infobaselearning.com
Melinda Gallo, Senior Account Executive
Educational publisher of DVD programming for schools and libraries. *$64.86*
ISBN 0-927368-59-5

1702 Functional Literacy System
Conover Company
4 Brookwood Court
Appleton, WI 54914   920-231-4667
800-933-1933
Fax: 800-933-1943
support@conovercompany.com
www.conovercompany.com
Terry Schmitz, Founder and Owner
Mike, Vice President of Operations
Art Janowiak, Vice President of Sales
Assessment and skill building for basic functional literacy. This multimedia software program is adult in format and uses live action video taken in actual community settings to help learners become more capable of functioning independently. Twenty different programs are currently available. *$99.00*

1703 Learning Activity Packets
4 Brookwood Court
Appleton, WI 54914
920-231-4667
800-933-1933
Fax: 800-933-1943
support@conovercompany.com
www.conovercompany.com

Terry Schmitz, Founder and Owner
Mike, Vice President of Operations
Art Janowiak, Vice President of Sales
Demonstrates how basic academic skills relate to 30 major career areas. LAPs provide valuable diagnostics in applied academic applications and demonstrates to users the importance of academics as they relate to the workplace. Software. *$99.00*

1704 Microcomputer Evaluation of Careers & Academics (MECA)
Conover Company
4 Brookwood Court
Appleton, WI 54914
920-231-4667
800-933-1933
Fax: 800-933-1943
support@conovercompany.com
www.conovercompany.com

Terry Schmitz, Founder and Owner
Mike, Vice President of Operations
Art Janowiak, Vice President of Sales
A cost-effective, technology-based, career development system which provides users with opportunities to get their hands dirty. The MECA system utilizes work simulations and is built around common occupational clusters. Each cluster, or career area, consists of hands-on WORK SAMPLES which provide a variety of career exploration and assessment experiences, linked to LEARNING ACTIVITY PACKETS, which integrate basic academic skills into the career planning and placement process. *$580-$1,070.*

1705 OASYS
Vertek
12835 Bellevue-Redmond Road
Suite 310
Bellevue, WA 98005
425-455-9921
800-220-4409
Fax: 425-454-7264

Debra Callahan, Sales Representative, Northern California
Tim Whitney, Sales Representative, Ohio, Michigan
Beverly Duncan, Sales Representative, Florida
A software system that matches a person's skills and abilities to occupations and employers.

1706 Reading in the Workplace
Educational Activities Software
5600 West 83rd Street
Suite 300, 8200 Tower
Bloomington, MN 55437-585
888-351-4199
800-447-5286
Fax: 239-225-9299
info@edmentum.com
www.edmentum.com

Vin Riera, President/CEO
Dan Juckniess, SVP, Sales & Professional Services
Stacey Herteux, VP, Human Resources
A job-based, reading software program using real-life problems and solutions to capture students' attention and improve their vocabulary and comprehension skills. Units include: automotive, clerical, health care and construction. *$295.00*

1707 Stickybear Typing
Optimum Resource
1 Mathews Drive
Suite 107
Hilton Head Island, SC 29926- 3765
843-689-8000
Fax: 843-689-8008
www.stickybear.com

Richard Hefter, President
The award winning Stickybear Typing program allows users to sharpen typing skills and achieve keyboard mastery with three engaging and amusing multi-level activities. *$59.95*

1708 Work-Related Vocational Assessment Systems: Computer Based
Valpar International
P.O.Box 5767
Tucson, AZ 85703-767
262-797-0840
800-633-3321
Fax: 262-797-8488
sales@valparint.com
www.valparint.com

Neal Gunderson, President
Criterion-referenced to Department of Labor standards. Evaluate academic levels for reading, spelling, math and language, interests, personalities, cognitive and physical aptitudes.

1709 Workplace Skills: Learning How to Function on the Job
Programming Concepts
8700 Shoal Creek Boulevard
Austin, TX 78757-6897
512-451-3246
800-897-3202
Fax: 800-397-7633
general@proedinc.com
www.proedinc.com

Jeff McLane, Founder
Lee Wilson, President and CEO
Randy Pennington, Executive VP
Offers parents and educators a functional means by which to discuss all aspects of finding and keeping a job. *$49.95*

Word Processors

1710 Co:Writer: Talking Word Processor
Don Johnston
26799 West Commerce Drive
Volo, IL 60073
847-740-0749
800-999-4660
Fax: 847-740-7326
info@donjohnston.com
www.donjohnston.com

Don Johnston, Founder
Ruth Ziolkowski, President
Kevin Johnston, Director of Product Design
User-friendly talking word processor provides multi-sensory learning and positive reinforcements for writers of all ages and ability levels.

1711 DARCI
Wes Test Engineering Corporation
810 Shepard Lane
Farmington, UT 84025
801-451-9191
Fax: 801-451-9393
westest.com

Robert Lessmann, President
James Lynds
Provides transparent access to all computer functions by replacing the computer's keyboard with a smart joystick. *$975.00*

1712 Eye Relief Word Processing Software
SkiSoft Publishing Corporation
P.O.Box 364
Lexington, MA 02420-4
781-863-1876
www.skisoft.com

Ken Skier, President
Cynthia Skier, CFO
Large-type word processing program for visually-impaired PC users. *$295.00*

1713 IntelliTalk
Intelli Tools
24 Prime Parkway
Natick, MA 01760
707-773-2000
800-547-6747
Fax: 707-773-2001
customerservice@cambiumtech.com

Beth Davis, Director Sales Operations
Lori Castle, Supervisor
Arjan Khalsa, CEO
Talking word-processing program available for MacIntosh, Apple IIe, IBM compatible and Windows computers. *$39.95*

1714 Large Type
P.O.Box T
Hewitt, NJ 07421-2088
973-853-6585
800-736-2216
Fax: 928-832-2894
http://www.angelfire.com

Don Selwyn, Vice President
Rev. Tom Schwanda, President & Chairman
Robt. Fondiller, Ph.D., P.E, Vice President
Display enlargement programs for visually impaired users. Consist of a variety of programs for different needs, ranging from basic to full-featured.

1715 Pegasus LITE
Words+
Ste 109
42505 10th St W
Lancaster, CA 93534-7059
661-723-6523
800-869-8521
Fax: 661-723-2114
info@words-plus.com

Phil Lawrence, VP
Provides all of the strategies currently being used in AAC, from dynamic display color pictographic language, to dual-word prediction text language, in a single system. *$6995.00*

1716 Up and Running
Intelli Tools
24 Prime Parkway
Natick, MA 01760
707-773-2000
800-547-6747
Fax: 707-773-2001
customerservice@cambiumtech.com

Beth Davis, Director Sales Operations
Lori Castle, Supervisor
Arjan Khalsa, CEO
Instantly use hundreds of popular commercial software programs with this custom collection of setups and overlays. *$69.95*

Conferences & Shows

General

1717 AACRC Annual Conference
Association of Children's Residential Centers
648 N Plankinton Ave.
Suite 245
Milwaukee, WI 53203   414-403-1565
                                        877-332-2272
                          info@togetherthevoice.org
                             togetherthevoice.org
Kari Sisson, Executive Director
Amanda Prange, Training Coordinator
McKenzie Melchoir, Membership Services Specialist
August

1718 AADB National Conference
American Association of the Deaf-Blind
248 Rainbow Drive
Suite 14864
Livingston, TX 77399-2048   aadb-info@aadb.org
                                       www.aadb.org
Rene Pellerin, President
A week of general meetings, workshops, tours and evening recreational activities.

1719 AAIDD Annual Meeting
American Assn on Intellecutal/Devel. Disabilities
8403 Colesville Rd.
Suite 900
Silver Spring, MD 20910   202-387-1968
                                   Fax: 202-387-2193
                                      maria@aaidd.org
                                          aaidd.org
Maria Alfaro, Manager, Meetings & Website
This annual meeting offers workshops, symposia, multiperspective sessions, and social events over four days.
June

1720 AAO Annual Meeting
American Academy Of Opthamology
655 Beach St.
San Francisco, CA 94109-1336   415-561-8500
                                   Fax: 415-561-8533
                          www.aao.org/annual-meeting
David W. Parke II, Chief Executive Officer
Debra Rosencrance, VP, Meetings & Events
Offers the most comprehensive program with more than 2000 scientific presentations and six subspecialty day programs.
October/November

1721 ACA Annual Conference
American Counseling Association
P.O. Vox 31110
Alexandria, VA 22310-9998   800-347-6647
                                   Fax: 800-473-2329
                          www.counseling.org/conference
Richard Yep, Chief Executive Officer
Promotes the development of professional counselors, advances the counseling profession, and uses the profession and practice of counseling to promote respect for human dignity and diversity.
March/April

1722 ADA Annual Scientific Sessions
American Diabetes Association
2451 Crystal Dr.
Suite 900
Arlington, VA 22201   800-342-2383
                                   askada@diabetes.org
                                     www.diabetes.org
Tracey D. Brown, Chief Executive Officer
Linda Cann, SVP, Professional Services
Brings together physicians, scientists and other health care professionals from around the world to learn about the latest advances in basic and clinical science for diabetes.

1723 AER Annual International Conference
Assoc. for Educ. & Rehab of the Blind/Vis. Imp.
5680 King Centre Dr.
Suite 600
Alexandria, VA 22315   703-671-4500
                                   Fax: 703-671-6391
                               conference@aerbvi.org
                                     www.aerbvi.org
Neva Fairchild, President
Dedicated to rendering support and assistance to the professionals who work in all phases of education and rehabilitation of blind and visually impaired children and adults.
July

1724 AG Bell Global Listening and Spoken Language Symposium
Alexander Graham Bell Association
3417 Volta Pl., NW
Washington, DC 20007   202-337-5220
                                   Fax: 202-337-8314
                                   TTY: 202-337-5221
                                      info@agbell.org
                                  agbellsymposium.com
Emilio Alonso-Mendoza, Chief Executive Officer
A meeting of professionals who serve those who are deaf and hard of hearing.
June/July

1725 APSE National Conference
APSE
7361 Calhoun Place
Suite 680
Rockville, MD 20855   301-279-0060
                                   Fax: 301-279-0075
                                       info@apse.org
                                        www.apse.org
Erica Belois-Pacer, Director, Professional Development
Julie Christensen, Director, Policy & Advocacy
Erynn Pawlak, Director, Operations
A major conference on Supported Employment. The conference includes sessions presented by nationally recognized leaders in the field. Conference attendees come from all 50 states, Canada and several foreign countries and include professionals in supported employment, occupational therapy, rehabilitation technology and other related fields.
July

1726 ASHA Convention
American Speech-Language-Hearing Association
2200 Research Blvd.
Rockville, MD 20850-3289   301-296-5700
                                       800-638-8255
                                   Fax: 301-296-8580
                                 convention@asha.org
                                  convention.asha.org
Arlene A. Pietranton, Chief Executive Officer
Craig E. Coleman, VP, Planning
Exhibits by companies specializing in alternative and augmentative communication products, publishers, software and hardware companies, and hearing aid testing equipment manufacturers. Speech-Language Pathologists are professionals who identify, assess, and treat speech and language problems. Audiologists are hearing health care professionals who specialize in preventing, identifying and assessing hearing disorders as well as providing audiologic treatment including hearing aids and more.
November

1727 ASIA Annual Scientific Meeting
American Spinal Injury Association
9702 Gayton Rd.
Suite 306
Richmond, VA 23238   877-274-2724
                          asia.office@asia-spinalinjury.org
                               www.asia-spinalinjury.org
Patty Duncan, Executive Director
Carolyn Moffatt, Association Manager
Kim Ruff, Administrative Assistant

Professional association for physicians and other health professionals working in all aspects of spinal cord injury. Also holds an annual scientific that surveys the latest advancements in the field.
May

1728 ATIA Conference
Assistive Technology Industry Association
330 N Wabash Ave.
Suite 2000
Chicago, IL 60611-4267

312-321-5172
877-687-2842
Fax: 312-673-6659
info@atia.org
www.atia.org

David Dikter, Chief Executive Officer
Caroline Van Howe, Chief Operating Officer
Emily Schmitt, Marketing Manager
The ATIA Conference is the largest international conference showcasing excellence in assistive technology.

1729 Abilities Expo
299 N Euclid Ave.
2nd Floor
Pasadena, CA 91101

323-363-2099
info@abilities.com
abilities.com

David Korse, President & CEO
Caryn Bates, Director, Operations
Abilities Expo is a national event for people with disabilities, their families, caregivers, and healthcare professionals. Meets in Phoenix, Dallas, Chicago, Los Angeles, Miami, Houston, New York, and Toronto.

1730 American Academy for Cerebral Palsy and Developmental Medicine Annual Conference
555 East Wells
Suite 1100
Milwaukee, WI 53202

414-918-3014
Fax: 414-276-2146
info@aacpdm.org
www.aacpdm.org

Tamara Wagester, Executive Director
Erin Trimmer, Senior Meetings Manager
The Annual Meeting is a 3-day event, held in the Fall, designed to provide targeted opportunities for dissemination of information in the basic sciences, prevention, diagnosis, treatment, and technical advances as applied to persons with cerebral palsy and development disorders.
September

1731 American Academy of Audiology Conference
American Academy of Audiology
11480 Commerce Park Dr.
Suite 220
Reston, VA 20191

703-790-8466
Fax: 703-790-8631
infoaud@audiology.org
www.audiology.org

Patrick E. Gallagher, Executive Director
Kathryn Werner, Vice President, Public Affairs
Amy Miedema, Vice President, Communications & Membership
The American Academy of Audiology is the world's largest professional organization for audiologists. The Academy is dedicated to providing quality hearing care services through professional development, education, research, and increased public awareness of hearing and balance disorders.
March-April

1732 American Academy of Environmental Medicine Annual Conference
PO Box 195
Ashland, MO 65010

316-684-5500
Fax: 888-411-1206
www.aaemonline.org

Dane Mosher, President
Lauren Grohs, Executive Director
William A. Ingram, Secretary
The Academy is an association of physicians and other professionals engaged in investigating and coming up with preventive

strategies for medical care relating to environmentally triggered illnesses.

1733 American Board of Disability Analysts Annual Conference
1483 N. Mt. Juliet Rd.
Suite 175
Nashville, TN 37122

629-255-0870
Fax: 615-296-9980
office@eventsm3.com
www.americandisability.org

Bi-annual conference held for members to meet and discuss current events and attend seminars.

1734 Annual Conference on Dyslexia and Related Learning Disabilities
New York Branch International Dyslexia Association
1550 Deer Park Ave.
Suite C
Long Island, NY 11729

631-261-7441
www.lidyslexia.org

Concetta Russo, President
Caryl Deiches, Vice President
Carolyn McIntyre, Secretary
The International Dyslexia Association (IDA) is an organization focused on the complex issues of dyslexia and related language-based learning disabilities which make it difficult to learn to read and write.
March

1735 Annual TASH Conference
TASH
1101 15th St. NW
Suite 206
Washington, DC 20005

202-817-3264
Fax: 202-999-4722
info@tash.org
www.tash.org/conferences

Michael Brogioli, Executive Director
Linda Metchikoff-Hooker, Director, Special Events
Donald Taylor, Manager, Membership & Operations
Each year, the TASH Conference connects attendees to information and resources, facilitates connections between stakeholders within the disability movement, and helps attendees reignite their passion for an inclusive world.
December

1736 Arc National Convention, The
The Arc
1825 K St., NW
Suite 1200
Washington, DC 20006

202-534-3700
800-433-5255
Fax: 202-534-3731
convention.thearc.org

Peter Berns, Chief Executive Officer
Tanisha Forte, Director, Conference & Events
Experts and professionals gather from all over the world share best practices, struggles, successes and hopes for the future, and continue the conversation about protecting and promoting the human and civil rights for individuals with intellectual and developmental disabilities.
October

1737 Attention Deficit Disorders Association, Southern Region: Annual Conference
12345 Jones Rd.
Suite 287-7
Houston, TX 77070

281-897-0982
Fax: 281-894-6883
addaoffice@sbcglobal.net
www.adda-sr.org

Carlye Read, President
Barbara Beard, Vice President
Judy German, Treasurer
The Attention Deficit Disorders Association provides a resource network, supports individuals impacted by ADHHD and related condition and to advocate for the development of community resources.
February

1738   Blind Children's Center Annual Meeting
Blind Children's Center
4120 Marathon St.
Los Angeles, CA 90029-3584   323-664-2153
                    info@blindchildrenscenter.org
                    www.blindchildrenscenter.org
Sarah E. Orth, CEO
Fernanda Armenta-Schmitt, Director, Education & Family Services
A family-centered agency which serves children with visual impairments from birth to school-age. The center-based and home-based services help the children to acquire skills and build their independence. The Center utilizes its expertise and experience to serve families and professionals worldwide through support services, education and research.
September

1739   Blinded Veterans Association National Convention
Blinded Veterans Association
1101 King St.
Suite 300
Alexandria, VA 22314   800-669-7079
                    bva@bva.org
                    www.bva.org
Donald D. Overton, Jr., Executive Director
The convention has three functions: to serve as a platform for Association business, to educate blinded veterans about the resources available to them, and to provide a means whereby blinded veterans can support one another.
August

1740   CQL Accreditation
Council on Quality and Leadership
100 West Rd.
Suite 300
Towson, MD 21204   410-275-0488
                    info@thecouncil.org
                    www.c-q-l.org/accreditation
Mary Kay Rizzolo, President & CEO
Katherine Dunbar, VP, Accreditation
CQL Accreditation is a leader in working with human service organizations and systems to continuously define, measure and improve quality of life and quality of services.

1741   Centers of Excellence Leadership Conference
National Parkinson Foundation
200 SE 1st St.
Suite 800
Miami, FL 33131   800-473-4636
                    contact@parkinson.org
                    parkinson.org
John L. Lehr, CEO
James Beck, VP & Chief Scientific Officer
Yashnahia Cortorreal, VP & Chief Human Resources & Administration Pfficer
The mission of the National Parkinson Foundation is to make life better for people affected by Parkinson's through expert care, research, and education. The goal of the conference is to convene the medical directors, center coordinators and other leaders from the Centers of Excellence to discuss the latest research and best practices in care delivery and to highlight NPF's programs.
July/August

1742   Closing the Gap's Annual Conference
P.O. Box 68
Henderson, MN 56044   507-248-3294
                    Fax: 507-248-3810
                    www.closingthegap.com
Dolores Hagen, Co-Founder
Budd Hagen, Co-Founder
Topics cover a broad spectrum of technology as it is being applied to all disabilities and age groups in education, rehabilitation, vocation and independent living. People with disabilities, special educators, rehabilitation professionals, administrators, service/care providers, personnel managers, government officials, and hardware/software developers share their experiences and insights at this significant networking experience.
October/November

1743   Conference of the Association on Higher Education & Disability (AHEAD)
8015 West Kenton Circle
Suite 230
Huntersville, NC 28078   704-947-7779
                    Fax: 704-948-7779
                    www.ahead.org
Amanda Kraus, President
Stephan Smith, Executive Director
Howard Kramer, Conference Director
An annual conference focused on aiding and meeting the needs of persons with disabilities attending higher education institutions.

1744   Council for Exceptional Children Annual Convention and Expo
3100 Clarendon Blvd.
Suite 600
Arlington, VA 22201-5332   888-232-7733
                    TTY: 866-915-5000
                    service@cec.sped.org
                    cecconvention.org
Chad Rummel, Executive Director
Sharon Rodriguez, Governance & Executive Services Coordinator
Works to improve the educational success of children with disabilities and/or gifts and talents.
March/April

1745   Disability Matters
Springboard Consulting
4740 S Ocean Blvd.
Suite 505
Highland Beach, FL 33487   973-813-7260
                    Fax: 973-813-7261
                    info@consultspringboard.com
                    www.consultspringboard.com
Nadine Vogel, Chief Executive Officer
Elizabeth Ladu, Chief Financial Officer
Ivette Lopez, Chief of Staff
Features outstanding content as delivered by leading disability experts from corporations, academia, national non-profits and governments across North America. Conferences also take place in Europe and Asia-Pacific.

1746   Eye Bank Association of America Annual Meeting
Eye Bank Association of America
1101 17th St., NW
Suite 400
Washington, DC 20036   202-775-4999
                    Fax: 202-429-6036
                    www.restoresight.org
Kevin Corcoran, CAE, President & CEO
Genevieve Casaceli, Education & Programs Manager
Bernie Dellario, Director, Finance
A four day program, which includes a series of presentations in administrative, hospital development, scientific and technical fields that are relative to eye banking.
June

1747   IDF National Conference
Immune Deficiency Foundation
110 West Rd.
Suite 300
Towson, MD 21204   800-296-4433
                    Fax: 410-321-9165
                    info@primaryimmune.org
                    primaryimmune.org
Jorey Berry, President & Chief Executive Officer
Sarah Rose, Chief Financial Officer
Katherine Antilla, Vice President, Education
The four-day conference brings together primary immunodeficiency patients, caregivers and clinicians to participate in youth programs, panel discussions, educational sessions and networking opportunities.
June

1748 Lowe Syndrome Conference
Lowe Syndrome Association
P.O. Box 417
Chicago Ridge, IL 60415   216-630-7723
                                 www.lowesyndrome.org

Lisa Waldbaum, President
Jane Gallery, Treasurer
Tiffany Johnson, Director, Medical & Scientific Affairs
An international conference held approximately every two years
where family, friends, medical and other professionals gather to
exchange ideas and information.
June

1749 NACDD Annual Conference
1825 K St. NW
Suite 600
Washington, DC 20006   202-506-5813
                              info@nacdd.org
                              www.nacdd.org

Donna A. Meltzer, Chief Executive Officer
Erin Prangley, Director, Public Policy
NACDD is the national association for the 56 State and Territorial
Councils on Developmental Disabilities (DD Councils) which re-
ceive federal funding to support programs that promote self-de-
termination, integration, and inclusion for all Americans with
developmental disabilities.
July

1750 NADR Conference
National Association of Disability Representatives
1305 W 11th St.
Suite 222
Houston, TX 77008   202-822-2155
                           dmin@nadr.org
                           www.nadr.org

Michael Wener, President
Christopher Mazzulli, Vice President
Cliff Berkley, Secretary
NADR is an organization of Professional Social Security Claimants Representatives that focus on issues involving policies to
protect the interest of people with disabilities. NADR conducts
annual conventions open to members and non-members with educational seminars to keep practitioners up to date on Social Security rulings, regulatory changes, and practice improvements.
April

1751 NASW-NYS Chapter
NASW
188 Washington Ave.
Albany, NY 12210   518-463-4741
                          800-724-6279
                          Fax: 518-463-6446
                          info.naswnys@socialworkers.org
                          www.naswnys.org

Samantha Fletcher, Executive Director
Marcia Schwartzman Levy, President
Workshops, keynote speakers, and presentations offered at this
event will develop and enhance practice skills and knowledge in
the provision of quality mental health and community services.
March

1752 NEXT Conference & Exposition
American Physical Therapy Association
1111 North Fairfax St.
Alexandria, VA 22314-1488   703-684-2782
                                   800-999-2782
                                   Fax: 703-706-8536
                                   consumer@apta.org
                                   apta.org

Sharon L. Dunn, President
Matthew R. Hyland, Vice President
Kip Schick, Secretary
The American Physical Therapy Association is a national professional organization sponsors this annual conference. The goal is
to foster advancements in physical therapy practice, research,
and education.

**1753 National Association for the Dually Diagnosed
Conferences**
12 Hurley Ave.
Kingston, NY 12401   845-331-4336
                            info@thenadd.org
                            www.thenadd.org

Jeanne M. Farr, CEO
Michelle Jordan, Office Manager
Jeffrey Schmunk, Operations Manager
NADD is a non-for-profit membership organization designed to
promote awareness of, and services for, individuals who have
co-occuring intellectual disability and mental illness. NADD
provides training, consultation services, and publishes journals
and books. it also offers two conferences per year.

1754 National Council on the Aging Conference
251 18th St. S.
Suite 500
Arlington, VA 22202   571-527-3900
                             membership@ncoa.org
                             www.ncoa.org

James Knickman, Interim President & CEO
Donna Whitt, Senior Vice President, Chief Financial Officer
Kristin Kiefer, Chief Administrative Officer
Offers ideas and programs to increase program and administra-
tive skills through NCOA's professional development tracks and
offering of continuing education units.
May

1755 PVA Summit & Expo
Paralyzed Veterans of America
801 18th St. NW
Washington, DC 20006-3517   800-424-8200
                                   TTY: 800-795-4327
                                   summit@pva.org
                                   summitpva.org

Charles Brown, National President
Marcus Murray, National Secretary
Carl Blake, Executive Director
The annual 3-day medical conference brings together leaders
from medicine, health care, policy, and government to explore
and implement holistic strategies to strengthen the continuum of
care for patients with spinal cord injuries or related diseases.

1756 PWSA (USA) Conference
Prader-Willi Alliance Of New York
244 5th Ave.
Suite D-110
New York, NY 10001   800-442-1655
                            alliance@prader-willi.org
                            www.prader-willi.org/conference

Amy McDougall, President
Barbara McManus, Treasurer
Brian Burgin, 1st Vice President
Through conferences, publications, electronic communication
and networking (parent-to-parent, parent-to professional, and
professional-to-professional), the Prader-Willi Alliance provides a valuable resource for individuals and families sharing the
same concerns.
July

**1757 Pacific Rim International Conference on Disability And
Diversity**
Center on Disability Studies
1410 Lower Campus Rd.
Unit 171F
Honolulu, HI 96822   808-956-8816
                            prinfo@hawaii.edu
                            pacrim.coe.hawaii.edu

Patricia Morrissey, Director of the Center on Disability
The Pacific Rim International Conference on Disability and Diversity encourages and respects voices from diverse perspective
across numerous areas including voices from persons representing all disability areas, and experiences of family members and
supporters across all disability and diversity areas.

1758 **RESNA Annual Conference**
Rehab Engineering & Assistive Tech. North America
2001 K Street NW
3rd Floor North
Washington, DC 20006   202-367-1121
                                                Fax: 202-367-2121
                                                    info@resna.org
                                                    www.resna.org
Maureen Linden, President
Andrea Van Hook, Interim Executive Director
Sponsored by a multidisciplinary association for the advancement of rehabilitation and assistive technologies, this annual
conference brings together a large number of rehabilitation professionals, products and services from around the world and has
something to offer for both professionals and consumers. The
conference provides an informative and thought provoking forum for anyone with interests in rehabilitation technology.
June

1759 **Rehabilitation International World Congress**
866 United Nations Plaza
Office 422
New York, NY 10017   212-420-1500
                                                Fax: 212-505-0871
                                                   info@riglobal.org
                                                   www.riglobal.org
Teuta Rexhepi, Secretary General
Zhang Haidi, President
RI is a global network of people with disabilities, service provid-
ers, researchers, government agencies, and advocates protecting
and promoting the rights and inclusion of people with
disabilities.
Quadrennial

1760 **Southwest Conference On Disability**
University of New Mexico
2300 Menaul Blvd., NE
Albuquerque, NM 87107   505-272-3000
                                                Fax: 505-272-2014
                         HSC-swdisabilityconference@salud.unm.edu
                         www.cdd.unm.edu/apps/SWConf/pre sentation
The Center for Development and Disability (CDD), is New Mexico's University Center for Excellence in Developmental Disabilities Education, Research and Service that respond to the needs of
individuals with developmental disabilities and their families.

1761 **Tourette Association of America National Education
Conference**
42-40 Bell Blvd.
Suite 205
Bayside, NY 11361   888-486-8738
                                                support@tourette.org
                                                       tourette.org
Amanda Talty, President & CEO
This is a biannual conference that includes members of the TS
community and their families, educators, TS advocates, physi-
cians, researchers, allied professionals, and TSA staff members.
Attendees interact, socialize, share ideas, discuss issues of concern, and learn from experts.
1972

1762 **Young Onset Parkinson Conference**
National Parkinson Foundation & ADPF
200 SE 1st St.
Suite 800
Miami, FL 33131   800-473-4636
                                                Fax: 305-537-9901
                                                contact@parkinson.org
                                                www.parkinson.org
John L. Lehr, President and CEO
James Beck, Vice President, Chief Scientific Officer
*Yasnahia Cortorreal, Vice President, Human Resources & Adminis-
tration*
Purpose is to find the cause and cure for Parkinson's Disease and
related neurodegenerative disorders through research, education
and dissemination of current information to patients, care-givers
and families.
Annual

Construction & Architecture

Associations

1763 Adaptive Environments Center
200 Portland Street
Suite 1
Boston, MA 02114

617-695-1225
Fax: 617-482-8099
info@HumanCenteredDesign.org
www.humancentereddesign.org

Ralph Jackson, FAIA, President
Chris Pilkington, Vice President
Nancy Jenner, Treasurer

Develops educational programs and materials on universal design, Americans with Disabilities Act, home adaptation, and more. Central Adaptive Environments publication list also available.

1764 American Institute of Architects
1735 New York Ave. NW
Washington, DC 20006-5292

800-242-3837
memberservices@aia.org
www.aia.org

Robert A. Ivy, FAIA, EVP/Chief Executive Officer
Abigail Warnecke Gorman, Chief of Staff
Sarah Dodge, SVP, Advocacy & Relationships

The organization, with 200 chapters worldwide and 95,000 members, advocates for the value of architecture and ethical standards in the profession.

1765 American Society of Landscape Architects
636 Eye St. NW
Washington, DC 20001-3736

202-898-2444
888-999-2752
Fax: 202-898-1185
info@asla.org
www.asla.org

Roxanne Blackwell, Co-Interim EVP & CEO
Curt Millay, Co-Interim EVP & CEO
Susan Cahill-Aylward, Director, Information & Professional Practice

Professional organization for landscape architects in the U.S., with 15,000 members.

1766 Building Owners and Managers Association International
1101 15th St., NW
Suite 800
Washington, DC 20005

202-326-6300
Fax: 202-326-6377
info@boma.org
www.boma.org

Henry Chamberlain, President & COO
Patricia Areno, Senior Vice President
Luci Vallejo, Director, Executive Services

Conducts seminars nationwide and publishes resource guidebooks for building owners and managers on ADA requirements for commercial facilities and places of public accommodation.

1767 Department of Insurance/OSFM
North Carolina Department of Insurance
325 N. Salisbury St.
Raleigh, NC 27603

919-647-0014
Fax: 919-715-0067
tara.barthelmess@ncdoi.gov

Tara Barthelmess, Chief Accessibility Code Consultant

The Chief Accessibility Code Consultant interprets building code accessibility requirements for new and existing buildings undergoing construction or alteration. The position also receives and initiates investigation of accessibility-related complaints within the State of North Carolina whenever possible.

1768 Institute for Human Centered Design
Formerly Adaptive Environments
200 Portland St
Ste 1
Boston, MA 02214

617-695-1225
Fax: 617-482-8099
TTY: 617-695-1225
info@humancentereddesign.org
humancentereddesign.org

Valerie Fletcher, Executive Director
Gabriela Bonome-Sims, Director, Administration & Finance

Formerly known as Adaptive Environments, the Insititute focuses on collaborating and working with citizens to design communal places to be accessible for all, including those with disabilities.

1769 Mark Elmore Associates Architects
Ste 104
42 East St
Crystal Lake, IL 60014-4400

815-455-7260
800-801-7766
Fax: 815-455-2238
www.elmore-architects.com

Mark A Elmore, Owner

Architectural designs for accessible residential and commercial buildings. ADA compliance reviews.

1770 National Conference on Building Codes and Standards
505 Huntmar Park Drive
Suite 210
Herndon, VA 20170

703-437-0100
Fax: 703-481-3596
www.ncsbcs.org

Cynthia Wilk, President
Robert C. Wible, Executive Director
Debbie Becker, Administrative Assistant

Serves as a forum in the interchange of information and provides technical services, education and training to our members to enhance the public's social and economic well being through safe, durable, affordable, accessible and efficient buildings.

1771 National Council of Architectural Registration Boards (NCARB)
1401 H Street NW
Suite 500
Washington, DC 20006

202-879-0520
ncarb.org

Michael J. Armstrong, Chief Executive Officer
Mary S. de Sousa, Chief Operating Officer
Guillermo Ortiz de Zarate, Chief Innovation & Information Officer

Research service in print and online information. Large collection of books and periodicals on the building/architectural environments.

1772 National Institute of Building Sciences
1090 Vermont Ave. NW
Suite 700
Washington, DC 20005

202-289-7800
Fax: 202-289-1092
nibs@nibs.org
www.nibs.org

Lakisha Ann Woods, President & CEO
Rebecca Liko, Vice President, Finance & Controller
Sarah Swango, Senior Director, Business Development

The organization supports advances in building science and technology to improve the built environment. The U.S. Congress established it in the the Housing and Community Development Act of 1974.

1773 Overcoming Mobility Barriers International
1022 S 4st St
Omaha, NE 68105

402-342-5731
Fax: 402-342-5731

Kay Neil, Executive Director

Members are government officials, service consumers and providers, and other persons interested in removing mobility barriers for elderly, handicapped and disadvantaged persons. Advises and works in conjunction with other groups and government agencies to establish safety standards for special equipment used in retrofitting vehicles and works to retrain drivers in the use of nonconventional driving controls.

1774 PVA Architecture
Paralyzed Veterans of America
801 18th St. NW
Washington, DC 20006-3517   202-416-7645
                                    800-424-8200
                              TTY: 800-795-4327
                        pvaarchitecture@pva.org
                                  www.pva.org

Charles Brown, National President
Marcus Murray, National Secretary
Carl Blake, Executive Director
Provides architectural consulting services related to accessible designs. Experience includes product design and building codes and standards.

1775 United States Access Board
Ste 1000
1331 F St NW
Washington, DC 20004-1111   202-272-0080
                                    800-872-2253
                              Fax: 202-272-0081
                              TTY: 800-993-2822
                          info@access-board.gov
                            www.access-board.gov

Lance Robertson, Chair
Gregory S. Fehribach, Vice Chair
Offers information and technical assistance to the public on accessible design under the Americans with Disabilities Act and other laws. Guidance and publications are available free that address access to facilities, transit vehicles and information technology.

Publications & Videos

1776 Access Currents
United States Access Board
1331 F Street, NW
Suite 1000
Washington, DC 20004-1111   202-272-0080
                                    800-872-2253
                              Fax: 202-272-0081
                              TTY: 800-993-2822
                          info@access-board.gov
                            www.access-board.gov

Lance Robertson, Chair
Gregory S. Fehribach, Vice Chair
Offers information and referrals on architectural accessibility for architects, designers, government agencies, building owners and consumers. A list of free publications is available on request.
bi-monthly

1777 Access Equals Opportunity
Council of B BB s Foundation
3033 Wilson Blvd
Suite 600
Arlington, VA 22201   703-276-0100
                                       www.bbb.org

Beverly Baskin, Senior VP, Chief Mission Officer
Genie Barton, Vice President and Director, Onl
Rodney L. Davis, Senior VP Enterprise Programs
These six Title III compliance guides for existing small businesses offer creative cheap and easy suggestions for complying with the public accommodations section of the ADA. Each guide is industry specific for: retail stores, car sales/service, restaurants/bars, medical offices and fun/fitness centers. They include suggestions for readily achievable removal of architectural barriers; effective communication; and guidance for nondiscriminatory policies or procedures. *$2.50*

1778 Access for All
Hospital Audiences
548 Broadway
3rd Floor
New York, NY 10012   212-575-7676
                              Fax: 212-575-7669

David Sweeny, Executive Director
Jane Kleinsinger, Director of Operations
Jill Bernard, Marketing & Outreach Manager

Provides physical and program accessibility information for people with disabilities to New York City cultural institutions including theaters, museums, galleries, etc.

1779 Accessible Home of Your Own
Accent Special Publications
Bloomington, IL 61702-700
Raymond C Cheever, Publisher
Betty Garee, Editor
This guide includes 14 articles on the popular subject of how to make a disabled persons home more accessible. *$7.99*
52 pages Paperback 1990
ISBN 0-915708-29-9

1780 Adaptable Housing: A Technical Manual for Implementing Adaptable Dwelling
H UD U SE R
P.O.Box 23268
Washington, DC 20026-3268   202-708-3178
                                    800-245-2691
                              Fax: 202-708-9981
                              TTY: 800-927-7589
                        helpdesk@huduser.org
                              www.huduser.org

Patrick J. Tewey, Director, Budget, Contracts, and Program Control Division
Jacqueline D Buford, Director, Management and Administrative Services Division
Jean Lin Pao, General Deputy Assistant Secretary
An illustrated manual describing methods for implementing adaptability in housing. *$3.00*

1781 Architect Magazine
Hanley Wood Media Inc.
One Thomas Circle NW
Washington, DC 20003   202-452-0800
                       etters@architectmagazine.com
                          www.architectmagazine.com

Ned Cramer, Editor-in-Chief
Grieg O'Brien, Managing Editor
Official journal of the American Institute of Architects

1782 BOMA Magazine
Building Owners & Managers Association
1101 15th St., NW
Suite 800
Washington, DC 20005   202-326-6300
                              Fax: 202-326-6377
                                  info@boma.org
                                   www.boma.org

Henry Chamberlain, President & COO
Courtney McKay, Vice President, Communications & Marketing
Official magazine of the Building Owners & Managers Association.

1783 Consumer's Guide to Home Adaptation
Institute for Human Centered Design
200 Portland Street
Suite 1
Boston, MA 02114   617-695-1225
                              Fax: 617-482-8099
                              TTY: 617-695-1225
                    info@HumanCenteredDesign.org
                        www.humancentereddesign.org

Valerie Fletcher, Executive Director
Tzesika Iliovits, Project Manager, Inclusive Design Projects
A workbook that enables people with disabilities to plan the modifications necessary to adapt their homes. Describes how to widen doorways, lower countertops, etc. *$12.00*
52 pages Paperback
ISBN 0-970835-80-9

1784   Design for Acessibility
National Endowment for the Arts Office
400 7th Street, SW
Washington, DC 20506-0001
202-682-5400
Fax: 202-682-5715
webmgr@arts.gov
arts.gov

Jane Chu, Chairman
Joan Shigekawa, Senior Deputy Chairman
Mike Burke, Chief Information Officer
A handbook for compliance with Section 504 of the Rehabilitation Act of 1973 and the Americans with Disabilities Act of 1990 including technical assistance on making arts programs accessible to staff, performers and audience.
101 pages
ISBN 0-160042-83-6

1785   Directory of Accessible Building Products
N AH B Research Center
400 Prince George's Blvd
Upper Marlboro, MD 20774
301-249-4000
800-638-8556
Fax: 301-430-6180
www.homeinnovation.com

Michael Luzier, CEO & President
Michelle Desiderio, Vice President of Innovation Services
Tom Kenney, P.E, Vice President of Engineering & Research
Contains descriptions of more than 200 commercially available products designed for use by people with disabilities and age-related limitations. Paperback. *$5.00*
104 pages Yearly

1786   Do-Able Renewable Home
AARP Fulfillment
601 E Street NW
Washington, DC 20049
202-434-3525
888-687-2277
877-342-2277
Fax: 202-434-3443
member@aarp.org
www.aarp.org

John Wider, President, CEO, AARP Services Inc.
Lisa M. Ryerson, President, AARP Foundation
Robert R. Hagans, Jr., Executive Vice President & Chief Financial Officer
Describes how individuals with disabilities can modify their homes for independent living. Room-by-room modifications are accompanied by illustrations.

1787   ECHO Housing: Recommended Construction and Installation Standards
601 E Street NW
Washington, DC 20049
202-434-3525
888-687-2277
877-342-2277
Fax: 202-434-3443
member@aarp.org
www.aarp.org

John Wider, President, CEO, AARP Services Inc.
Lisa M. Ryerson, President, AARP Foundation
Robert R. Hagans, Jr., Executive Vice President & Chief Financial Officer
Illustrated design, construction, and installation standards for temporary dwelling units for elderly people on single family residential property.

1788   Electronic House: Enhanced Lifestyles with Electronics
Electronic House
111 Speen Street, Suite 200
P.O. Box 989
Framingham, MA 01701-2000
508-663-1500
800-375-8015
Fax: 508-663-1599
cheditorial@ehpub.com
electronichouse.com

Kenneth D. Moyes, President
Karen Bligh, Marketing Director
John Brillon, Web Creative Director
Dedicated to home automation. Featuring both extravagant and affordable smart homes that can be controlled with one touch. EH covers electronic systems that give homeowners more security, entertainment, convenience, and fun. Articles cover whole house control and subsystems like residential lighting, security, home theater, energy management and telecommunications. *$23.95*
84 pages BiMonthly
ISSN 0886-66 3

1789   Fair Housing Design Guide for Accessibility
National Council on Multifamily Housing Industry
1201 15th Street NW
Washington, DC 20005
202-266-8200
800-368-5242
Fax: 202-266-8400
www.nahb.com

Kevin Kelly, Chairman of the Board
Tom Woods, First Vice Chairman of the Board
Ed Brady, Second Vice Chairman of the Board
Specifically tailored to address the needs of architects and builders. The book includes a detailed technical analysis of the legislation's impact on multifamily design, highlights potential construction problems, and identifies possible solutions. *$29.95*

1790   Ideas for Making Your Home Accessible
Accent Books & Products
P.O.Box 700
Bloomington, IL 61702-0700
309-378-2961
800-787-8444
Fax: 309-378-4420
acmtlvng@aol.com
www.accentonliving.com

Raymond C Cheever, Publisher
Betty Garee, Editor
Offers over 100 pages of tips and ideas to help build or remodel a home. Includes many special devices and where to get them. *$7.50*
94 pages Paperback
ISBN 0-91570 -08-6

1791   Landscape Architecture Magazine
American Society of Landscape Architects
636 Eye St. NW
Washington, DC 20001-3736
202-898-2444
888-999-2752
Fax: 202-898-1185
landscapearchitecturemagazine.org

Bradford McKee, Editor
Michael D. O'Brien, Publisher
Official publication of the American Society of Landscape Architects.

1792   National Institute of Building Sciences
1090 Vermont Ave. NW
Suite 700
Washington, DC 20005
202-289-7800
Fax: 202-289-1092
nibs@nibs.org
www.nibs.org

Lakisha Ann Woods, President & CEO
Rebecca Liko, Vice President, Finance & Controller
Sarah Swango, Senior Director, Business Development
The organization supports advances in building science and technology to improve the built environment. The U.S. Congress established it in the the Housing and Community Development Act of 1974.

1793   Removing the Barriers: Accessibility Guidelines and Specifications
A PP A
1643 Prince Street
Alexandria, VA 22314
703-684-1446
Fax: 703-549-2772
webmaster@appa.org
www.appa.org

John F. Bernhards, Associate Vice President
E. Lander Medlin, Executive VP
Steve Glazner, Director of Knowledge Management

Offers site accessibility, building entrances, doors, interior circulation, restrooms and bathing facilities, drinking fountains and additional resources. *$45.00*
125 pages
ISBN 0-91335 -59-9

1794   Smart Kitchen/How to Design a Comfortable, Safe & Friendly Workplace
Ceres Press
P.O.Box 87
Woodstock, NY 12498-87   845-679-5573
                                             Fax: 845-679-5573
                                             cem620@aol.com
                                             healthyhighways.com

David Goldbeck, Owner
This book provides information about designing kitchens that may be helpful to people with disabilities as well as safe and energy efficient. *$16.95*
132 pages Paperback

1795   United Spinal Association
75-20 Astoria Blvd
Suite 120
East Elmhurst, NY 11370- 1177   718-803-3782
                                                800-444-0120
                                             Fax: 718-803-0414
                                             mkurtz@unitedspinal.org
                                             www.unitedspinal.org

Paul Tobin, President
Maria Kurtz, Executive Assistant
Information on spinal cord injury and laws and regulations concerning people with disabilities, including veterans.
Monthly

1796   Whole Building Design Guide
National Institute of Building Sciences
1090 Vermont Ave. NW
Suite 700
Washington, DC 20005   202-289-7800
                                             Fax: 202-289-1092
                                             nibs@nibs.org
                                             www.wbdg.org

Lakisha Ann Woods, President & CEO
Kristen Petersen, Managing Director, Marketing & Communications
Online portal with access to published materials on integrated whole-building design techniques and technologies, with an emphasis on integrated design and team efforts during planning and programming.

Education

Aids for the Classroom

1797 **ACT Assessment Test Preparation Reference Manual**
American College Testing Program
P.O. Box 414
Iowa City, IA 52243-0414   319-337-1270
     act.org

Marten Roorda, Chief Executive Officer
Suzana Delanghe, Chief Commercial Officer
Lucas Kuhlmann, Chief Technology Officer
This reference manual was developed as a resource for high
school teachers and counselors in assisting students with test
preparation. Offers accommodation for individuals with
disabilities.

1798 **AEPS Child Progress Record: For Children Ages Three
to Six**
Brookes Publishing
PO Box 10624
Baltimore, MD 21285-624   410-337-9580
     800-638-3775
     Fax: 800-638-3775
     custserv@brookespublishing.com
     www.brookespublishing.com

Paul Brooks, President
Melissa Behm, Executive VP
George Stamathis, VP and Publisher
This chart helps monitor change by visually displaying current
abilities, intervention targets, and child progress. In packages of
30. *$21.00*
8 pages Gate-fold
ISBN 1-557662-51-7

1799 **AEPS Curriculum for Three to Six Years**
Brookes Publishing
PO Box 10624
Baltimore, MD 21285-0624   410-337-9580
     800-638-3775
     Fax: 410-337-8539
     webmaster@brookespublishing.com
     www.brookespublishing.com

Paul H. Brookes, Chairman of the Board
Jeffrey D. Brookes, President
George S. Stamathis, VP/Publisher
Used after the AEPS® Test is completed and scored, this developmentally sequenced curriculum allows professionals to match the
child's IFSP/IEP goals and objectives with activity-based interventions — beginning with simple skills and moving on to more
advanced skills. *$ 65.00*
304 pages Spiral-bound
ISBN 1-557665-65-6

1800 **AEPS Data Recording Forms: For Children Ages Three
to Six**
Brookes Publishing
PO Box 10624
Baltimore, MD 21285-624   410-337-9580
     800-638-3775
     Fax: 800-638-3775
     custserv@brookespublishing.com
     www.readplaylearn.com

Paul Brooks, President
These forms can be used by child development professionals on
four separate occasions to pinpoint and then monitor a child's
strengths and needs in the six key areas of skill development measured by the AEPS Test. Packages of 10. *$24.00*
36 pages Saddle-stiched
ISBN 1-557662-49-5

1801 **AEPS Family Interest Survey**
Brookes Publishing
PO Box 10624
Baltimore, MD 21285-624   410-337-9580
     800-638-3775
     Fax: 800-638-3775
     custserv@brookespublishing.com
     www.brookespublishing.com

Paul Brooks, President
Tracy Gracy, Educational Sales Manager
This is a 30-item checklist that helps families to identify interests
and concerns to address in a child's IEP/IFSP. Comes in packages
of 30. *$15.00*
8 pages Saddle-stiched
ISBN 1-557660-98-0

1802 **Adaptivemall.com**
15 South Second Street
Dolgeville, NY 13329   315-429-7112
     800-371-2778
     Fax: 315-429-8862
     info@adaptivemall.com
     www.adaptivemall.com

Katie Bergeron Peglow,PT,MS, COO
Adaptivemall.comr help families find the best equipment to support their children at their highest functioning level.

1803 **Advanced Language Tool Kit**
School Specialty
625 Mt. Auburn Street, 3rd Floor
PO Box 9031
Cambridge, MA 02139-9031   617-547-6706
     800-225-5750
     Fax: 888-440-2665
     Feedback.EPS@schoolspecialty.com
     eps.schoolspecialty.com

Rick Holden, President, EPS
Jean S Osman, Co-Author
Paula D Rome, Author
Provides an overview o the structure, organization, and sound
units that are needed to develop skills for advanced reading and
spelling. The kit contains a teacher's manual and 3 pack of cards,
with features similar to the cards in the Language Tool Kit.
$60.00
ISBN 0-838885-48-9

1804 **All Kinds of Minds**
School Specialty
625 Mt. Auburn Street, 3rd Floor
PO Box 9031
Cambridge, MA 02139-9031   617-547-6706
     800-225-5750
     Fax: 888-440-2665
     Feedback.EPS@schoolspecialty.com
     eps.schoolspecialty.com

Rick Holden, President, EPS
Melvin D Levine, Author
A fictitious account of five different students who have learning
disabilities. *$33.00*
296 pages
ISBN 0-838820-90-5

1805 **American Sign Language Handshape Cards**
T J Publishers, Distributor
Ste 206
817 Silver Spring Ave
Silver Spring, MD 20910- 4617   301-585-4440
     800-999-1168
     Fax: 301-585-5930
     tjpubinc@aol.com

Angela K Thames, President
Jerald A Murphy, VP
Durable flashcards illustrate basic handshapes, classifiers and
the American manual alphabet. An instructional booklet describes games for differing skill levels to improve vocabulary, increase hand and eye coordination, sign recognition and usage.
$16.95

1806 Asthma Action Cards: Child Care Asthma/Allergy Action Card
Asthma and Allergy Foundation of America
8201 Corporate Drive
Suite 1000
Landover, MD 20785
202-466-7643
800-727-8462
Fax: 202-466-8940
info@aafa.org
www.aafa.org

Tom Flanigan, Chariman
William Mclin, President and CEO
Yolanda Miller, VP and CFO
Includes necessary information a provider needs to care for a young child who has asthma and allergies. The card includes a medication plan, a list of the child's specific signs and symptoms that indicate the child is having trouble breathing, and steps on how to handle an emergency situation.

1807 Asthma Action Cards: Student Asthma Action Card
Asthma and Allergy Foundation of America
1233 20th St NW
Suite 610
Washington, DC 20036-2330
202-833-1700
800-727-8462
Fax: 202-833-2351
info@aafa.org
www.swmlaw.com

Bill Mc Lin, Executive Director
Ben C Hadden, VP Finance & Treasurer
Bill Lin, Executive Director
Tool for communicating school aged children's and teen's asthma managment plan to school personnel. Includes sections for asthma triggers, daily medications, and emergency directions.

1808 Auditory-Verbal Therapy for Parents and Professionals
Alexander Graham Bell Association
3417 Volta Place, NW
Washington, DC 20007
202-337-5220
Fax: 202-337-8314
TTY: 202-337-5221
info@agbell.org
www.listeningandspokenlanguage.org
Meredith K. Sugar, Esq. (OH), President
Donald M. Goldberg, Immediate Past President
Ted A. Meyer, M.D., Ph.D. (SC, President-Elect, Secretary, Treasurer
A must-have for hearing health professionals, students entering hearing health fields and parents who want to explore the theory and practices of auditory-verbal therapy. *$54.95*
313 pages Paperback

1809 Autism Community Store
7800 E. Iliff Ave.
Suite J
Denver, CO 80231
303-309-3647
866-709-4344
Fax: 303-756-2311
support@autismcommunitystore.com
www.autismcommunitystore.com
Shannon Sullivan, Co-Founder
The Autism Community Store is a parent-owned autism and special needs resource, a special little shop helping families, teachers and therapists get hard-to-find products for kids with ASD, PDD-NOS, Aspergers, SPD, ADHD and other special needs at reasonable prices.

1810 Autism-Products.com
8776 E. Shea Blvd.
Suite 106-552
Scottsdale, AZ 85260
Fax: 815-550-1819
Kelly@Autism-Products.com
www.autism-products.com
Supplies products for children dealing with Austim.

1811 Beginning Reasoning and Reading
School Specialty
625 Mt. Auburn Street, 3rd Floor
PO Box 9031
Cambridge, MA 02139-9031
617-547-6706
800-225-5750
Fax: 888-440-2665
Feedback.EPS@schoolspecialty.com
eps.schoolspecialty.com
Rick Holden, President, EPS
Joanne Carlisle, Author
This workbook develops basic language and thinking skills that build the foundation for reading comprehension. Workbook exercises reinforce reading as a critical reasoning activity. *$10.45*
ISBN 0-838830-01-3

1812 Blue Skies: A Complete Multi-Media Curriculum on the Cloud
Phillip Roy, Inc.
P.O. Box 130
Indian Rocks Beach, FL 33785
727-593-2700
800-255-9085
Fax: 877-595-2685
info@philliproy.com
www.philliproy.com
Ruth Bragman, PhD, President
Phil Roy Padol, Consultant
A complete PDF duplicatable curriculum that indlues Life Skills Curriculum, Academic Curriculum, Vocational Curriculum, Special Educational Curriculum, and Parenting/Early Learning Curriculum. This curriculum was designed for students to learn to be successful. Lesson plans, teacher's guides, pre/post assessments, and other support materials provided. *$495.00*
ISBN 1-568184-12-8

1813 Buy!
JE Stewart Teaching Tools
PO Box 15308
Seattle, WA 98115-308
206-262-9538
Fax: 206-262-9538
Jeff Stewart, Owner
Teaches 50 words as they appear in commercial and community situations such as clinic, sale, receipt, price and cleaner. These words are functional at school, on the job and shopping. *$32.50*
116 pages
ISBN 1-877866-05-9

1814 Catalog for Teaching Life Skills to Persons with Development Disability
PCI Education Publishing
PO Box 34270
San Antonio, TX 78265-4270
210-377-1999
800-594-4263
Fax: 888-259-8284
Lee Wilson, President/CEO
Erin Kinard, VP Product Development/Publisher
Randy Pennington, VP, Sales & Marketing
Over 200 educational products that help individuals learn and maintain the life skills they need to succeed in an inclusive society.

1815 Classroom GOALS: Guide for Optimizing Auditory Learning Skills
Alexander Graham Bell Association
3417 Volta Pl. NW
Washington, DC 20007
202-337-5220
Fax: 202-337-8314
TTY: 202-337-5221
info@agbell.org
www.agbell.org
Emilio Alonso-Mendoza, Chief Executive Officer
This reader-friendly teacher's guide filled with tips, source materials and sample charts and plans is designed for educators who have yearned for a resource that explains how to incorporate auditory goals into academic learning for students with different degrees of hearing loss. *$34.95*
Paperback

1816 Classroom Notetaker: How to Organize a Program Serving Students with Hearing Impairments
Alexander Graham Bell Association
3417 Volta Pl. NW
Washington, DC 20007
202-337-5220
Fax: 202-337-8314
TTY: 202-337-5221
info@agbell.org
www.agbell.org

Emilio Alonso-Mendoza, Chief Executive Officer
This detailed manual for instructors, administrators and staff notetakers promotes classroom notetaking within long-term educational programs as absolutely vital for students who are deaf and hard of hearing from elementary school to college. *$24.95*
127 pages Paperback

1817 Community Services for the Blind and Partially Sighted Store: Sight Connection
9709 Third Ave NE
Ste 100
Seattle, WA 98115-2027
206-525-5556
800-458-4888
Fax: 206-525-0422
info@sightconnection.org
www.sightconnection.org

Miles Otoupal, Chair
Jonathan Avedovech, Vice Chair
David McBride, Treasurer
Over 400 products specifically designed to make life easier for people with vision loss.

1818 Community Signs
JE Stewart Teaching Tools
P.O.Box 15308
Seattle, WA 98115-308
206-262-9538
Fax: 206-262-9538

Jeff Stewart, Owner
Teaches 50 words like go, fire, rest room, men, women, danger and walk needed to successfully navigate our environment. *$ 32.50*

1819 Comprehensive Assessment of Spoken Language (CASL)
AGS
PO Box 99
Circle Pines, MN 55014-99
800-328-2560
Fax: 800-471-8457
agsmail@agsnet.com
www.agsnet.com

Kevin Brueggeman, President
Robert Zaske, Market Manager
CASL is an individually and orally administered research-based, theory-drive oral language assessment battery for ages 3 through 21. Fifteen tests measure language processing skills - comprehension, expression, and retrieval - in four language structure categories: lexical/semantic, syntactic, supralinguistic and pragmatic. *$299.95*

1820 Creative Arts Therapy Catalogs
MMB Music
9051 Watson Road
Suite 161
Saint Louis, MO 63126-1019
314-531-9635
800-543-3771
Fax: 314-531-8384
info@mmbmusic.com
www.mmbmusic.com

Marcia Goldberg, President
Catalogs of books, videos, recordings for the creative arts and wellness (music, art, dance, poetry, drama, therapies, photography).

1821 Cursive Writing Skills
School Specialty
625 Mt. Auburn Street, 3rd Floor
PO Box 9031
Cambridge, MA 02139-9031
617-547-6706
800-225-5750
Fax: 888-440-2665
Feedback.EPS@schoolspecialty.com
eps.schoolspecialty.com

Rick Holden, President, EPS
Diana Hanbury King, Author
Boosts writing achievement through handwriting skills. Handwriting instruction helps students become fluent writers, allowing them to focus on their thoughts and ideas rather than on letter and word formation. *$12.00*

1822 Different Roads to Learning
37 East 18th Street
10th Floor
New York, NY 10003
212-604-9637
800-853-1057
Fax: 212-206-9329
info@difflearn.com
www.difflearn.com

Julie Azuma, Founder
Its product line supports the social, academic and communicative development of children on the autism spectrum through Applied Behavior Analysis (ABA) and Verbal Behavior interventions

1823 Discount School Supply
PO Box 6013
Carol Stream, IL 60197-6013
800-627-2829
Fax: 800-879-3753
customerservice@discountschoolsupply.com
www.discountschoolsupply.com

Ron Elliott, Founder
Kelly Crampton, Chief Executive Officer
Discount School Supply offers the highest quality educational products at the lowest possible prices, supported by an extraordinary level of service.

1824 Do2learn
3204 Churchill Road
Raleigh, NC 27607
919-755-1809
Fax: 919-420-1978
www.do2learn.com

Do2learnprovides thousands of free pages with social skills and behavioral regulation activities and guidance, learning songs and games, communication cards, academic material, and transition guides for employment and life skills.

1825 Don Johnston
26799 West Commerce Drive
Volo, IL 60073
847-740-0749
800-999-4660
Fax: 847-740-7326
info@donjohnston.com
www.donjohnston.com

Don Johnston, Founder
Ruth Ziolkowski, President
Kevin Johnston, Director of Product Design
A provider of quality products and services that enable people with special needs to discover their potential and experience success. Products are developed for the areas of Physical Access, Augmentative Communication and for those who struggle with reading and writing.

1826 Dyslexia Training Program
School Specialty
625 Mt. Auburn Street, 3rd Floor
PO Box 9031
Cambridge, MA 02139-9031
617-547-6706
800-225-5750
Fax: 888-440-2665
Feedback.EPS@schoolspecialty.com
eps.schoolspecialty.com

Rick Holden, President, EPS
This 2-year, cumulative series of daily 1-hour video lessons and accompanying Student's Books and Teacher's Guides is a structured, multisensory sequence of alphabet, reading, spelling, cursive handwriting, listening, language history, and review

activities. Written by the Texas Scottish Rite Hospital for Children.

1827 ESpecial Needs
11704 Lackland Industrial Drive
St. Louis, MO 63146   314-692-2424
                                             877-664-4565
                                        Fax: 314-692-2428
                                        www.especialneeds.com
eSpecial Needs is a global supplier of equipment, programs, and curricula for physical education and recreation professionals, as well as products, equipment, and programs for professionals who deal with children and adults with physical and developmental disabilities.

1828 Encyclopedia of Basic Employment and Daily Living Skills
Phillip Roy, Inc.
13064 Indian Rocks Rd.
P.O. Box 130
Indian Rocks Beach, FL 33785   727-593-2700
                                             800-255-9085
                                        Fax: 877-595-2685
                                        info@philliproy.com
                                        www.PhillipRoy.com
Ruth Bragman, PhD, President
Phil Roy Padol, Consultant
Contains developmental skills for special education students. Contains lessons in 6 curriculum areas covering 80 objects with 541 lessons. Also includes objectives, instructional strategies, and assessment tasks. Curriculum is in PDF format and unlimited duplication is allowed after purchase. *$300.00*
ISBN 1-568184-15-8

1829 Exceptional Teaching Inc
Exceptional Teaching Inc
3994 Oleander Way
PO Box 2330
Castro Valley, CA 94546   510-889-7282
                                             800-549-6999
                                        Fax: 510-889-7382
                                        info@exceptionalteaching.com
                                        www.exceptionalteaching.com
Helene Holman, Owner/manager
Providing educational products for those with special needs via catalog and online store.

1830 Explode the Code
School Specialty
625 Mt. Auburn Street, 3rd Floor
PO Box 9031
Cambridge, MA 02139-9031   617-547-6706
                                             800-225-5750
                                        Fax: 888-440-2665
                                        Feedback.EPS@schoolspecialty.com
                                        eps.schoolspecialty.com
Rick Holden, President, EPS
Nancy M Hall, Author
Helps students build the essential literacy skills needed for reading success: phonological awareness, decoding, vocabulary, comprehension, fluency and spelling. *$6.20*
Grades K-4, 1-3

1831 Food!
JE Stewart Teaching Tools
PO Box 15308
Seattle, WA 98115-308   206-262-9538
                                        Fax: 206-262-9538
Jeff Stewart, Owner
Teaches 50 words like salt, pepper, hamburger, fruit, milk and soup, seen commonly on menus, packages and in directions used at home and at play. *$32.50*

1832 Fun for Everyone
AbleNet, Inc.
2625 Patton Road
Roseville, MN 55113-1137   651-294-2200
                                             800-322-0956
                                        Fax: 651-294-2259
                                        customerservice@ablenetinc.com
                                        www.ablenetinc.com
Jennifer Thalhuber, President & CEO
Paul Sugden, CFO & Trustee
Today, simple technology allows children and adults with disabilities to participate in leisure activities they were limited or excluded from in the past. *$20.00*

1833 Fundamentals of Autism
Slosson Educational Publications Inc.
538 Buffalo Road
East Aurora, NY 14052-280   716-652-0930
                                             800-655-3840
                                             888-756-7760
                                        Fax: 716-655-3840
                                        slossonprep@gmail.com
                                        www.slosson.com
Steven Slosson, President
John Slosson, VP
David Slosson, VP
The Fundamentals of Autism handbook provides a quick, user friendly, effective and accurate approach to help in identifying and developing educationally related program objectives for children diagnosed as autistic. These materials have been designed to be easily and functionally used by teachers, therapists, special education/learning disability resource specialists, psychologists and others who work with children diagnosed as autistic. *$56.00*
72 pages

1834 GO-MO Articulation Cards- Second Edition
Sage Publications
2455 Teller Road
Thousand Oaks, CA 91320   805-499-9774
                                             800-818-7243
                                        Fax: 800-583-2665
                                        info@sagepub.com
                                        www.sagepub.com
Blaise R Simqu, President & CEO
Tracey Ozmina, VP and COO
Chris Hickok, Senior VP and CFO
The most popular system used for remedying defective speech articulation in children and adults. This popular card set was the first and is still the best therapy tool of its kind, as it continues to produce results and maintains the interest of students of all ages.

1835 Gillingham Manaual
School Specialty
625 Mt. Auburn Street, 3rd Floor
PO Box 9031
Cambridge, MA 02139-9031   617-547-6706
                                             800-225-5750
                                        Fax: 888-440-2665
                                        Feedback.EPS@schoolspecialty.com
                                        eps.schoolspecialty.com
Rick Holden, President, EPS
Anna Gillingham, Author
Bessie W Stillman, Co-Author
Remedial training for children with specific disability in reading, spelling, and penmanship.
352 pages 69.95
ISBN 0-83880 -00-

1836 Guide to Teaching Phonics
School Specialty
625 Mt. Auburn Street, 3rd Floor
PO Box 9031
Cambridge, MA 02139-9031   617-547-6706
                                             800-225-5750
                                        Fax: 888-440-2665
                                        Feedback.EPS@schoolspecialty.com
                                        eps.schoolspecialty.com
Rick Holden, President, EPS
June Lyday Orton, Author

This flexible teacher's guide presents multisensory procedures developed in association with the late Dr. Samuel Orton. They consist of 100 phonograms for teaching phonetic elements and their sequences in words for reading, writing and spelling. Also contains coordinated Phonics Cards. *$19.25*
96 pages
ISBN 0-838802-41-9

1837 **Homemade Battery-Powered Toys**
Special Needs Project
324 State Street
Suite H
Santa Barbara, CA 93101-2364
818-718-9900
800-333-6867
Fax: 818-349-2027
editor@specialneeds.com
www.specialneeds.com

Hod Gray, Owner
Laraine Gray, Coordinator
Describes how to make simple switches and educational devices for severely handicapped children. *$7.50*

1838 **Idaho Assistive Technology Project**
University of Idaho
PO Box 444061
Moscow, ID 83844-4061
208-885-6097
800-432-8324
Fax: 208-885-6145
janicec@uidaho.edu
www.idahoat.org

Janice Carson, Project Director
Sue House, Information/Referral Specialst
A federally funded program managed by the Center on Disabilities and Human Development at the University of Idaho. The goal is to increase the availability of assistive technology devices and services for Idahoans with disabilities. *$15.00*

1839 **If It Is To Be, It Is Up To Me To Do It!**
AVKO Educational Research Foundation
3084 Willard Road
Birch Run, MI 48415-9404
810-686-9283
866-285-6612
Fax: 810-686-1101
webmaster@avko.org
www.avko.org

Don McCabe, President, Research Director Emeritus, Birch Run, Michigan
Linda Heck, VP, Clio, Michigan
Michael Lane, Treasurer, Clio, Michigan
A student and tutor's text, for use on dyslexics and non-dyslexics, by parents, spouses, or friends. *$29.95*
206 pages
ISBN 1-564007-42-1

1840 **Inclusive Play People**
Educational Equity Concepts
Fl 8
100 5th Ave
New York, NY 10011-6903
212-243-1110
Fax: 212-627-0407
TTY: 212-725-1803
www.iconcapital.com

Jacqueline Johnson, Manager
Six sturdy multiracial wooden figures that provide a unique variety of nonstereotyped work and family roles and are inclusive of disabled and nondisabled people of various ages. For block building and dramatic play. *$25.00*

1841 **Individualized Keyboarding**
AVKO Educational Research Foundation
3084 Willard Road
Birch Run, MI 48415-9404
810-686-9283
866-285-6612
Fax: 810-686-1101
webmaster@avko.org
www.avko.org

Don McCabe, President, Research Director Emeritus, Birch Run, Michigan
Linda Heck, VP, Clio, Michigan
Michael Lane, Treasurer, Clio, Michigan

Utilizes a multi-sensory approach to teach typing skills. It not only teaches typing skills, it also reinforces the reading patterns that are necessary for typing proficiency. *$14.95*
96 pages
ISBN 1-654004-01-5

1842 **Instruction of Persons with Severe Handicaps**
McGraw-Hill School Publishing
PO Box 182604
Columbus, OH 43272
877-833-5524
Fax: 614-759-3749
customer.service@mcgraw-hill.com
www.mcgraw-hill.com

Harold McGraw, President and CEO
Jack Callahan, Executive VP
John Berisford, Executive VP of HR
A complete introduction to the status of education as it pertains to people with severe handicaps.

1843 **Kaplan Early Learning Company**
1310 Lewisville Clemmons Rd
Lewisville, NC 27023
336-766-7374
800-334-2014
Fax: 800-452-7526
info@kaplanco.com
www.kaplanco.com

Hal Kaplan, President & CEO
Kaplan Early Learning Company is a international provider of products and services that enhance children's learning.

1844 **Keeping Ahead in School**
Educators Publishing Service
PO Box 9031
Cambridge, MA 2139-9031
617-547-6706
800-225-5750
Fax: 888-440-2665
feedback@epsbooks.com
www.epsbooks.com

Charles H Heinle, VP
Alexandra S Bigelow, Author
Gunnar Voltz, President
This book helps students not only understand their own strengths and weaknesses but also more fully appreciate their individuality. He suggests specific ways to approach work, bypass or overcome learning disorders, and manage other struggles that may beset students in school. *$24.75*
320 pages Paperback
ISBN 0-838820-69-7

1845 **KeyMath Teach and Practice**
AGS
P.O.Box 99
Circle Pines, MN 55014-99
800-328-2560
Fax: 800-471-8457
agsmail@agsnet.com
www.agsnet.com

Kevin Brueggeman, President
Robert Zaske, Market Manager
This set of materials provides all the tools needed to assess students' math skills...and the strategies to deal with problem areas. Three sets are available: Basic Concepts Package; Operations Package; and Applications Package. $219.95 each or $599.95 for whole set.

1846 **Lakeshore Learning Materials**
2695 E. Dominguez Street
Carson, CA 90895
310-537-8600
800-421-5354
Fax: 800-537-5403
lakeshore@lakeshorelearning.com
www.lakeshorelearning.com

Bo Kaplan, President/CEO
Josh Kaplan, VP Merchandising
Mat, Vice President of Operations
Offers books, resources, testing materials, assessment information and special education materials for the professional in the field of special education.
190 pages

1847   Language Parts Catalog
School Specialty
625 Mt. Auburn Street, 3rd Floor
PO Box 9031
Cambridge, MA 02139-9031   617-547-6706
                                          800-225-5750
                                   Fax: 888-440-2665
                   Feedback.EPS@schoolspecialty.com
                             eps.schoolspecialty.com
Rick Holden, President, EPS
Melvin D Levine, Author
Offers a humorous and informative explanation of the various aspects of language and how they operate. Laid out in the form of a catalog, the book presents various parts that can help students improve their language abilities. *$12.65*
ISBN 0-838819-80-X

1848   Language Tool Kit
School Specialty
625 Mt. Auburn Street, 3rd Floor
PO Box 9031
Cambridge, MA 02139-9031   617-547-6706
                                          800-225-5750
                                   Fax: 888-440-2665
                   Feedback.EPS@schoolspecialty.com
                             eps.schoolspecialty.com
Rick Holden, President, EPS
Paula D Rome, Author
Jean S Osman, Co-Author
Designed for use by a teacher or parents, teaches reading and spelling to students with specific language disability. *$43.25*
32 pages English Edition
ISBN 0-838885-20-3

1849   Language, Speech and Hearing Services in School
American Speech-Language-Hearing Association
10801 Rockville Pike
Rockville, MD 20852-3226   301-296-5700
                                          800-638-8255
                                   Fax: 301-296-8580
                            actioncenter@asha.org
                                    www.asha.org
Paul Rao, President
Robert Augustine, VP of Finance
Arlene Pietranton, Executive Director
Professional journal for clinicians, audiologists and speech-language pathologists. *$30.00*

1850   Learning American Sign Language
Harris Communications
15155 Technology Dr
Eden Prairie, MN 55344   800-825-6758
                                   Fax: 952-906-1099
                                   TTY: 952-388-2152
                             info@harriscomm.com
                                  www.harriscomm.com
Ray Harris, CEO
Offers over 700 titles on ASL including books, videotapes, CDs & DVDs. Free catalog available.
Video & Book

1851   Learning Resources
380 N. Fairway Drive
Vernon Hills, IL 60061   800-333-8281
                                   Fax: 888-892-8731
                          info@learningresources.com
                           www.learningresources.com
Learning Resourcesr is a global manufacturer of innovative, hands-on educational products. The Company's 1100+ high-quality products are sold in more than 80 countries, serving children and their families, preschool, kindergarten, primary, and middle-school markets.

1852   Learning to Sign in My Neighborhood
T J Publishers
2544 Tarpley Rd
Suite 108
Carrollton, TX 75006-2288   972-416-0800
                                          800-999-1168
                                   Fax: 301-585-5930
                                    tjpubinc@aol.com
Angela K Thames, President
Jerald A Murphy, VP
Beautifully illustrated coloring book lets children learn signs from kids just like themselves! Recommended for ages 4 and up, let children have fun while they learn signs for words typically used in day-to-day activities. *$3.50*
32 pages Softcover
ISBN 0-93266 -36-1

1853   Literacy Program
School Specialty
625 Mt. Auburn Street, 3rd Floor
PO Box 9031
Cambridge, MA 02139-9031   617-547-6706
                                          800-225-5750
                                   Fax: 888-440-2665
                   Feedback.EPS@schoolspecialty.com
                             eps.schoolspecialty.com
Rick Holden, President, EPS
Paula D Rome, Author
Jean S Osman, Co-Author
Written by the Texas Scottish Rite Hospital for Children. A one-year course that consists of 160 one-hour videotaped lessons accompanied by student workbooks, designed for high school students and adults who read below sixth grade level.

1854   Literature Based Reading
Oryx Press
4041 N Central Ave
Phoenix, AZ 85012-3330   602-265-2651
                                          800-279-6799
                                   Fax: 800-279-4663
Series offering children's books and activities to enrich the K-5 curriculum.

1855   Living an Idea: Empowerment and the Evolution of an Alternative School
Brookline Books
8 Trumbull Rd, Suite B-001
Northampton, MA 1060-4533   413-584-0184
                                          800-666-2665
                                   Fax: 413-584-6184
                                brbooks@yahoo.com
                             www.brooklinebooks.com
William H Walters, Author
Esther Wilder, Co-Author
This book is about the creation and 14 year evolution of a public alternative inner-city high school. The school lived an idea - empowerment. Students were encouraged to participate in shaping many aspects of their education, teachers were responsible for running the school, and parents invited to help govern. *$27.95*
ISBN 0-91479 -68-9

1856   Low Tech Assistive Devices: A Handbook for the School Setting
Therapro, Inc.
225 Arlington Street
Framingham, MA 02139-8723   508-872-9494
                                          800-257-5376
                                   Fax: 508-875-2062
                                info@therapro.com
                                    www.therapro.com
Karen Conrad Weihrauch, President & Owner
A how-to book with step by step directions and detailed illustrations for fabrication of frequently requested low-tech assistive devices. *$29.95*
320 pages Paperback

1857 MTA Readers
Educators Publishing Service
625 Mt. Auburn Street, 3rd Floor
PO Box 9031
Cambridge, MA 02139-9031
617-547-6706
800-225-5750
Fax: 888-440-2665
Feedback.EPS@schoolspecialty.com
www.epsbooks.com

Rick Holden, President, EPS
Illustrated readers for grades 1-3 that accompany the MTA Reading and Spelling Program (Multisensory Teaching Approach). Phonetic elements in a structured, but entertaining context.
48+ pages $4.65 - $11.65
ISBN 0-83882 -33-3

1858 Making School Inclusion Work: A Guide to Everyday Practice
Brookline Books
8 Trumbull Rd, Suite B-001
Northampton, MA 2445-4533
413-584-0184
800-666-2665
Fax: 413-584-6184
brbooks@yahoo.com
www.brooklinebooks.com

William H Walters, Author
Esther Wilder, Co-Author
This book tells the reader how to conduct a truly inclusive program, regardless of ethnic or racial background, economic level and physical or cognitive ability. *$24.95*
254 pages
ISBN 0-914791-96-4

1859 Making the Writing Process Work: Strategies for Composition and Self-Regulation
Brookline Books
8 Trumbull Rd, Suite B-001
Northampton, MA 2445-4533
413-584-0184
800-666-2665
Fax: 413-584-6184
brbooks@yahoo.com
www.brooklinebooks.com

William H Walters, Author
Esther Wilder, Co-Author
This book is geared toward students who have difficulty organizing their thoughts and developing their writing. The specific stategies teach students how to approach, organize, and produce a final written product.. *$24.95*
240 pages Paperback
ISBN 1-571290-10-9

1860 Manual Alphabet Poster
TJ Publishers
Ste 108
2544 Tarpley Rd
Carrollton, TX 75006-2288
972-416-0800
800-999-1168
Fax: 972-416-0944
TJPubinc@aol.com
www.TJpublishers.com

Pat O'Rourke, President
Poster presents the manual alphabet. *$4.50*

1861 Many Faces of Dyslexia
International Dyslexia Association
40 York Rd.
4th Floor
Baltimore, MD 21204-5243
410-296-0232
Fax: 410-321-5069
info@dyslexiaida.org
dyslexiaida.org

Margaret Byrd Rawson, Author
Provides information on the teaching and rehabilitation techniques for people with dyslexia. *$20.00*
269 pages Paperback

1862 Match-Sort-Assemble Job Cards
Exceptional Education
PO Box 15308
Seattle, WA 98115-308
206-262-9538

Jeff Stewart, Owner
Teaches workers to use a series of symbolic cues to control their own production cycles. *$565.00*
Class Set

1863 Match-Sort-Assemble Pictures
Exceptional Education
PO Box 15308
Seattle, WA 98115-308
206-262-9538

Jeff Stewart, Owner
People with profound, severe and moderate developmental disabilities have immediate access with MSA Pictures. Students work with pictures (and if necessary a template) to match, sort, assemble and disassemble parts that vary in shape, length and diameter. *$426.00*
Class Set

1864 Match-Sort-Assemble SCHEMATICS
Exceptional Education
PO Box 15308
Seattle, WA 98115-308
206-262-9538

Jeff Stewart, Owner
Students with moderate and mild developmental disabilities and those who have completed MSA Pictures are ready for MSA Schematics. It increases abstraction and displacement of instruction from the work clearly and simply. *$495.00*
Class Set

1865 Match-Sort-Assemble TOOLS
Exceptional Education
PO Box 15308
Seattle, WA 98115-308
206-262-9538
Fax: 475-486-4510

Jeff Stewart, Owner
Students and clients learn to use the tools required for many jobs in light industry. Mastery of the production cycle with independence, endurance and the ability to learn new tasks through pictures and schematics and basic hand functions will help clients acquire and maintain employment in a competitive field. *$595.00*
Class Set

1866 Meeting-in-a-Box
Asthma and Allergy Foundation of America
1233 20th St NW
Suite 610
Washington, DC 20036-7322
202-833-1700
800-7AS-THMA
Fax: 202-833-2351
info@aafa.org

Bill McLin, Executive Director
A series of self-contained, comprehensive kits that contain all the necessary components for a successful asthma presentation.

1867 More Food!
JE Stewart Teaching Tools
PO Box 15308
Seattle, WA 98115-308
206-262-9538
Fax: 206-262-9538

Jeff Stewart, Owner
Teaches 50 more words found in restaurants, grocery stores, cookbooks such as pizza, carrot, tacos, oysters and pineapple. These words are functional at home, going shopping and during leisure. *$32.50*

1868 More Work!
J E Stewart Teaching Tools
PO Box 15308
Seattle, WA 98115-308
206-262-9538
Fax: 206-262-9538

Jeff Stewart, Owner
Teaches 50 words as they appear on parts, tools, job instructions, signs and labels, such as fill, grasp, release, lock, search, position and select. These words are functional in school and on-the-job. *$32.50*

1869 Multisensory Teaching Approach
Educators Publishing Service
PO Box 9031
Cambridge, MA 2139-9031   617-367-2700
                                 800-225-5750
                                 Fax: 617-547-0412
                                 www.epsbooks.com
Comprehensive multisensory program in reading, writing, spelling, alphabet and dictionary skills for remedial and regular instruction. Based on Orton-Gillingham and Alphabetic Phonics. A complete program organized in kits, with additional classroom materials, supplementary materials, and handwriting programs.
$110 - $140
ISBN 0-83888 -10-9

1870 National Autism Resources
6240 Goodyear Rd.
Benicia, CA 94510   707-745-3308
                          877-249-2393
                          Fax: 877-259-9419
customerservice@nationalautismresources.com
www.nationalautismresources. com
National Autism Resources Inc. provides cost effective, research based therapeutic tools globaly that meet the needs of people on the autism spectrum across their lifespan since 2008.

1871 Peabody Articulation Decks
AGS
PO Box 99
Circle Pines, MN 55014-99   651-287-7220
                                   800-328-2560
                                   Fax: 763-786-9007
                                   agsmail@agsnet.com
                                   www.agsnet.com
Keith Powel, Special Education Transition Coo
Robert Zaske, Marketing Manager
Complete kit of playing-card sized PAD decks let students focus on the 18 most commonly misarticulated English consonants and blends. *$115.95*
ISBN 0-88671 -75-4

1872 Phonemic Awareness in Young Children: A Classroom Curriculum
Brookes Publishing
PO Box 10624
Baltimore, MD 21285-624   410-337-9580
custserv@brookespublishing.com
www.brookespublishing.com
Clary Creighton, Exhibits Coordinator
Tracy Gray, Educational Sales Manager
Paul Brooks, Owner
This is a supplemental, whole-class curriculum for improving pre-literacy listening skills. It contains activities that are fun, easy to use, and proven to work in any kindergarten classroom - general, bilingual, inclusive, or special education. This program takes only 15-20 minutes a day. *$24.95*
208 pages Spiral-bound
ISBN 1-557663-21-1

1873 Phonics for Thought
Educators Publishing Service
PO Box 9031
Cambridge, MA 2139-9031   617-367-2700
                                 800-225-5750
                                 Fax: 617-547-0412
                                 www.epsbooks.com
$8.00
Paperback

1874 Phonological Awareness Training for Reading
Sage Publications
2455 Teller Road
Thousand Oaks, CA 91320   805-499-9774
                                 800-818-7243
                                 Fax: 800-583-2665
                                 info@sagepub.com
                                 www.sagepub.com
Blaise R Simqu, President & CEO
Tracey Ozmina, Executive VP
Chris Hickok, Executive VP and CFO

Designed to increase the level of phonological awareness in young children. Can be taught individually or in small groups and takes about 12 to 14 weeks to complete if children are taught in short sessions three or four times a week. *$129.00*

1875 Play!
JE Stewart Teaching Tools
PO Box 15308
Seattle, WA 98115-308   206-262-9538
                               Fax: 206-262-9538
Jeff Stewart, Owner
Teaches 50 more words as they appear at recreation sites, on signs and labels and in newspapers and magazines, such as movie, visitor, ticket, gallery and zoo. These words are functional in school and at leisure. *$32.50*

1876 Power Breathing Program
Asthma and Allergy Foundation of America
8201 Corporate Drive
Suite 1000
Landover, MD 20785   202-466-7643
                            800-727-8462
                            Fax: 202-466-8940
                            info@aafa.org
                            www.aafa.org
Bill McLin, Executive Director
Devoloped the only asthma education program specifically designed for and pre-tested with teens. Teens with asthma have special challenges. This interactive program covers everything from the basics of asthma to dealing with their asthma in social situations, in college, and on the job. Includes everything you need to present this three-four session program. *$295.00*

1877 Primary Phonics
School Specialty
625 Mt. Auburn Street, 3rd Floor
PO Box 9031
Cambridge, MA 02139-9031   617-547-6706
                                  800-225-5750
                                  Fax: 888-440-2665
                                  Feedback.EPS@schoolspecialty.com
                                  eps.schoolspecialty.com
Rick Holden, President, EPS
Barbara W Makar, Author
A program of storybooks and coordinated workbooks that teaches reading for grades K-2. A structured phonetic approach. Contains 8 student workbooks, with 8 sets of 10 coordinated storybooks; consonant workbooks; initial consonant blend workbooks; picture dictionary, and coloring book.
ISSN 0838-83 0

1878 Reading for Content
School Specialty
625 Mt. Auburn Street, 3rd Floor
PO Box 9031
Cambridge, MA 02139-9031   617-547-6706
                                  800-225-5750
                                  Fax: 888-440-2665
                                  Feedback.EPS@schoolspecialty.com
                                  eps.schoolspecialty.com
Rick Holden, President, EPS
Carol Einstein, Author
A series of 4 books designed to help students improve their reading comprehension skills. Each book contains 43 reading passages followed by 4 questions. Two questions as for a recall of main ideas, and two ask the student to draw conclusions from what they have read. *$ 11.45*
96 pages

1879 Reading from Scratch
Educators Publishing Service
P.O.Box 9031
Cambridge, MA 2139-9031   617-367-2700
                                 800-225-5750
                                 Fax: 617-547-0412
                                 www.epsbooks.com
Contains multisensory reading and spelling material and oral and written lessons and exercises in syntax, grammar, and precomposition topics. Complete set.
$6.25 - $49.30
ISBN 0-83888 -75-5

1880   Recipe for Reading
School Specialty
625 Mt. Auburn Street, 3rd Floor
PO Box 9031
Cambridge, MA 02139-9031   617-367-2700
                                            800-225-5750
                                       Fax: 888-440-2665
                    Feedback.EPS@schoolspecialty.com
                              eps.schoolspecialty.com

Rick Holden, President, EPS
Nina Traub, Author
Frances Bloom, Co-Author
Contains comprehensive, multisensory, phonics-based reading
program presents a skill sequence and lesson structured designed
for beginning, at-risk, or struggling readers.

1881   Rewarding Speech
Speech Bin
PO Box 1579
Appleton, WI 54912-1579   772-770-0007
                                            888-388-3224
                                       Fax: 888-388-6344
                    customercare@schoolspecialty.com
                              www.speechbin.com

Jan J Binney, Senior Editor
Reproducible reward certificates for children. *$12.95*
32 pages

1882   SAYdee Posters
Speech Bin
PO Box 1579
Appleton, WI 54912-1579   772-770-0007
                                            888-388-3224
                                       Fax: 888-388-6344
                    customercare@schoolspecialty.com
                              www.speechbin.com

Jan J Binney, Senior Editor
Colorful speech and language posters. *$20.00*
24 pages
ISBN 0-93785 -47-5

1883   Sensation Products
74 Cotton Mill Hill
Unit A-350
Brattleboro, VT 5301   802-254-4480
                                       Fax: 802-254-4481
                              www.sensationproducts.com
Since 2000, Sensation Products has been the wholesale supplier
for school supply companies that serve Special Populations.

1884   Sensory University Toy Company, The
4992 Bristol Industrial Hwy
Buford, GA 30518   888-831-4701
                                       Fax: 770-904-6418
                              sales@sensoryuniversity.com
                              sensoryuniversity.com

Sensory University provides special needs products and toys for
the children treated in their facility. Over the years, the inventory
has increased to cover a full spectrum of educational items and
pediatric fitness products, as well as a library of over 100 titles
dedicated to improving the lives of children with many different
forms of developmental delay.

1885   Sequential Spelling: 1-7 with 7 Student Response Books
AVKO Educational Research Foundation
3084 Willard Rd
Birch Run, MI 48415-9404   810-686-9283
                                            866-285-6612
                                       Fax: 810-686-1101
                              webmaster@avko.org
                              www.avko.org

Deborah Wolf, President
Aaron Miller, Vice President
Sequential Spelling uses immediate student self-correction. It
builds from easier words of a word family such as all and then
builds on them to teach; all, tall, stall, install, call, fall, ball, and
their inflected forms such as: stalls, stalled, stalling, installing,
installment. *$89.95*
72 pages $8.95 each
ISBN 1-56400 -11-6

1886   Signing Naturally Curriculum
Harris Communications
15155 Technology Dr
Eden Prairie, MN 55344   800-825-6758
                                       Fax: 952-906-1099
                                       TTY: 952-388-2152
                              info@harriscomm.com
                              www.harriscomm.com

Ray Harris, CEO
A series based on the functional approach that is the most popular
and widely used sign language curriculum designed for teaching
American Sign Language. Book and videotape set for level 3.
Teacher's curriculum is also available. *$89.95*

1887   Small Wonder
AGS
PO Box 99
Circle Pines, MN 55014-99   651-287-7220
                                            800-328-2560
                                       Fax: 763-786-9007
                              agsmail@agsnet.com
                              www.agsnet.com

Kevin Brueggeman, President
Robert Zaske, Marketing Manager
This infant through toddler program offers a delightful array of
activities to teach babies about themselves, others, their sur-
roundings and the world outside. Level One - zero to 18 months;
Level Two 18-36 months. Discount price of $389.95 when both
levels ordered. *$229.95*
ISBN 0-91347 -62-5

1888   Solving Language Difficulties
School Specialty
625 Mt. Auburn Street, 3rd Floor
PO Box 9031
Cambridge, MA 02139-9031   617-547-6706
                                            800-225-5750
                                       Fax: 888-440-2665
                    Feedback.EPS@schoolspecialty.com
                              eps.schoolspecialty.com

Rick Holden, President, EPS
Amey Steere, Author
Caroline Z Peck, Co-Author
This basic workbook can be used in any corrective reading pro-
gram. It deals extensively with syllables, syllable division, pre-
fixes, suffixes and accent. *$9.75*
176 pages
ISBN 0-838803-26-1

1889   Speech Bin
Abilitations
PO Box 1579
Appleton, WI 54912-1579   772-770-0007
                                            800-513-2465
                                       Fax: 80- 51- 246
                              onlinehelp@schoolspecialty.com
                              www.speechbin.com

Jan J Binney, Senior Editor
Activities, worksheets and games to encourage practice of speech
and language skills. *$25.00*
128 pages
ISBN 0-93785 -42-4

1890   Speech-Language Delights
1965 25th Ave
Vero Beach, FL 32960-3062   772-770-0007

1891   Spell of Words
School Specialty
625 Mt. Auburn Street, 3rd Floor
PO Box 9031
Cambridge, MA 02139-9031   617-547-6706
                                            800-225-5750
                                       Fax: 888-440-2665
                    Feedback.EPS@schoolspecialty.com
                              eps.schoolspecialty.com

Rick Holden, President, EPS
Elsie T Rak, Author

Covers syllabication, word building along with prefixes, phonograms, word patterns, suffixes, plurals, and possessives. *$14.70*
128 pages Grades 7-Adult

1892   Spellbound
School Specialty
625 Mt. Auburn Street, 3rd Floor
PO Box 9031
Cambridge, MA 02139-9031   617-547-6706
                                             800-225-5750
                                             Fax: 888-440-2665
                    Feedback.EPS@schoolspecialty.com
                              eps.schoolspecialty.com
Rick Holden, President, EPS
Elsie T Rak, Author
This workbook begins with teaching simple, consistent rules and then moves on to those that are more difficult. By an inductive process, students use their own observations to confirm the spelling rules they learn. Each portion of the text is followed by exercises for drill and kinesthetic reinforcement. *$12.85*
144 pages Grades 7-Adult
ISBN 0-838801-65-X

1893   Spelling Dictionary
School Specialty
625 Mt. Auburn Street, 3rd Floor
PO Box 9031
Cambridge, MA 02139-9031   617-547-6706
                                             800-225-5750
                                             Fax: 888-440-2665
                    Feedback.EPS@schoolspecialty.com
                              eps.schoolspecialty.com
Rick Holden, President, EPS
Gregory Hurray, Author
Contains the most frequently used and misspelled words for students at these grade levels. Designed to be useable and reliable, to build research and writing skills, and to help teachers promote independent learning in a classroom setting *$6.35*
ISBN 0-838820-56-5

1894   Starting Over
School Specialty
625 Mt. Auburn Street, 3rd Floor
PO Box 9031
Cambridge, MA 02139-9031   617-547-6706
                                             800-225-5750
                                             Fax: 888-440-2665
                    Feedback.EPS@schoolspecialty.com
                              eps.schoolspecialty.com
Rick Holden, President, EPS
Joan Knight, Author
For students who are ready to try to learn to read again, or for those who are learning English as a second language. *$38.40*
ISBN 0-838881-65-5

1895   Studio 49 Catalog
MMB Music
9051 Watson Road
Suite 161
Saint Louis, MO 63126-1019   314-531-9635
                                             800-543-3771
                                             Fax: 314-531-8384
                              info@mmbmusic.com
                              www.mmbmusic.com
Marcia Goldberg, President
Michelle Greenlaw, VP
Percussion instruments for school, therapy, church and family.

1896   Syracuse Community-Referenced Curriculum Guide for Students with Disabilties
Brookes Publishing
PO Box 10624
Baltimore, MD 21285-624   410-337-9580
                                             800-638-3775
                                             Fax: 410-337-8539
                    custserv@brookespublishing.com
                              www.readplaylearn.com
Paul Brooks, President
Serving learners from kindergarten through age 21, this field-tested curriculum is a for professionals and parents devoted to directly preparing a student to function in the world. it examines the role of community living domains, functional academics, and embedded skills and includes practical implementation strategies and information for preparing students whose learning needs go beyond the scope of traditional academic programs. *$54.95*
416 pages Spiral-bound
ISBN 1-557660-27-1

1897   Teaching Individuals with Physical and Multiple Disabilities
McGraw-Hill, School Publishing
PO Box 182604
Columbus, OH 43272   877-833-5524
                                             Fax: 614-759-3749
                              www.mcgraw-hill.com
Harold McGraw, President and CEO
Jack Callahan, Executive VP
John Berisford, Executive VP of HR
Focuses on the functional needs of the handicapped and the teaching skills of background teachers that they need to help them reach the highest possible level of self-sufficiency.
410 pages

1898   Teaching Students Ways to Remember
Brookline Books
8 Trumbull Rd, Suite B-001
Northampton, MA 1060   800-666-2665
                                             Fax: 413-584-6184
                              brbooks@yahoo.com
                              www.brooklinebooks.com
Teaches techniques for improving or strengthening memory. *$21.95*
ISBN 0-914797-67-0

1899   Teaching Test-Taking Skills: Helping Students Show What They Know
Brookline Books
8 Trumbull Rd, Suite B-001
Northampton, MA 1060   800-666-2665
                                             Fax: 414-584-6184
                              brbooks@yahoo.com
                              www.brooklinebooks.com
Test-taking skills that, when used effectively, contribute to test-wise performance and help students work productively with test materials. *$21.95*
ISBN 0-914797-76-X

1900   Therapy Shoppe
P.O. Box 8875
Grand Rapids, MI 49518   616-696-7441
                                             800-261-5590
                                             Fax: 616-696-7471
                              info@therapyshoppe.com
                              www.therapyshoppe.com
Thousand's of extraordinary fidgets, sensory products, therapy toys, weighted and deep pressure specialties for autism and other special needs, occupational therapy supplies, unique classroom resources, and other innovative products for play, learning, self-regulation, handwriting, sensory integration, and sensory-motor skills development.

1901   To Teach a Dyslexic
AVKO Educational Research Foundation
3084 Willard Rd
Birch Run, MI 48415-9404   810-686-9283
                                             866-686-9283
                                             Fax: 810-686-1101
                              webmaster@avko.org
                              www.avko.org
Deborah Wolf, President
Aaron Miller, Vice President
A video available in DVD or video CD that shows Don McCabe working with a dyslexic teenager. The video helps teachers learn more about dyslexia and how to go about teaching a dyslexic student using the AVKO methodology and philosophy. This is a free video.
288 pages Paperback

1902 **Tools for Transition**
AGS
PO Box 99
Circle Pines, MN 55014-99 651-287-7220
800-328-2560
Fax: 763-786-9007
agsmail@agsnet.com
www.agsnet.com

Kevin Brueggeman, President
Robert Zaske, Marketing Manager
This program prepares students with learning disabilities for postsecondary education. *$129.95*

1903 **United Art and Education**
PO Box 9219
Fort Wayne, IN 46899-9219 260-478-1121
800-322-3247
Fax: 800-858-3247
www.unitednow.com

United Art Education founded in 1960 is committed to serve schools, organizations and individuals with quality products. Their goal is to make shopping fun for every customer, whether you're an art instructor, elementary teacher, school supply buyer, fine artist or parent.

1904 **VAK Tasks Workbook: Visual, Auditory and Kinesthetic**
Educational Tutorial Consortium
4400 S 44th St
Lincoln, NE 68516-1109 402-489-8133
Fax: 402-489-8160

T Elli Cross, Owner
A workbook emphasizing the multisensory approach to teaching vocabulary and spelling. It is intended for middle-grade and older students working with prefixes, roots, suffixes, homonyms, and the spelling of easily confused endings. Includes spelling posters. *$7.00*
96 pages Paperback

1905 **Volunteer Transcribing Services**
Ste 200
205 E 3rd Ave
San Mateo, CA 94401-4028 650-357-1571
Fax: 650-632-3510

Alanah Hoffman, Coordinator
VTS is a nonprofit California corporation that produces large print school books for visually impaired students in grades K-12.

1906 **Wordly Wise 3000**
School Specialty
625 Mt. Auburn Street, 3rd Floor
PO Box 9031
Cambridge, MA 02139-9031 617-547-6706
800-225-5750
Fax: 888-440-2665
Feedback.EPS@schoolspecialty.com
eps.schoolspecialty.com

Rick Holden, President, EPS
Kenneth Hodkinson, Author
Sandra Adams, Co-Author
Begins with a word list of 8-12 words, followed by clear, brief definitions and sentences that illustrate the meaning of the word. Books B and C often present more than one meaning of a word. Throughout all three books, drawings illustrate the meanings.
ISSN 0838-84 8

1907 **Work!**
JE Stewart Teaching Tools
PO Box 15308
Seattle, WA 98115-308 206-328-7664
Fax: 206-262-9538

Jan Gleason, Executive Director
Teaches 50 words as they appear on parts, tools, job instructions, signs, labels such as: hard hat, assembly, clamp, cut, drill, package and schedule. These words are functional in school and on-the-job. *$32.50*

1908 **Working Together & Taking Part**
A GS
PO Box 99
Circle Pines, MN 55014-99 651-287-7220
800-328-2560
Fax: 763-786-9007
agsmail@agsnet.com
www.agsnet.com

Kevin Brueggeman, President
Robert Zaske, Market Manager
Two programs to build children's social skills in grades 3-6 through folk literature. Has 31 activity-rich lessons, teaching skills like: following rules, accepting differences, speaking assertively and helping others. Discount price of $279.00 when ordering both. *$149.95*

Associations

1909 **AVKO Educational Research Foundation**
3084 Willard Rd
Birch Run, MI 48415-9404 810-686-9283
Fax: 810-686-1101
webmaster@avko.org
www.avko.org

Don McCabe, President
Linda Heck, Vice President
Comprised of individuals interested in helping others learn to read and spell. Develops and sells materials for teaching dyslexics or others with learning disabilities using a method involving audio, visual, kinesthetic and oral (multi-sensory) techniques.

1910 **Academy of Rehabilitative Audiology**
PO Box 2323
Albany, NY 12220-0323 ara@audrehab.org
www.audrehab.org

Karen Doherty, Ph.D, President
Brittney Carlson, Au.D, Ph.D, Treasurer
Ali Marinelli, Au.D, Ph.D, Secretary
The Academy of Rehabilitative Audiology provides professional education, research and programs for hearing handicapped persons. The primary purpose of the ARA is to promote excellence in hearing care through the provision of comprehensive rehabilitative and habilitative services.

1911 **Alternative Work Concepts**
PO Box 11452
Eugene, OR 97440 541-345-3043
Fax: 541-345-9669
www.alternativeworkconcepts.org

Liz Fox, Executive Director
To promote individualized, integrated, and meaningful employment opportunities in the community for adults with multiple disabilities; to improve the quality of life and provide continuous opportunities for personal growth for these individuals; and to assist businesses with workforce diversification.

1912 **American Migraine Foundation**
19 Mantua Rd.
Mount Royal, NJ 08061 856-423-0043
Fax: 856-423-0082
amf@talley.com
www.achenet.org

Lawrence C. Newman, MD, FAHS, Chair
Christine Lay, MD, FAHS, Vice-Chair
Nim Lalvani, MPH, Executive Director
Nonprofit, patient-health, professional partnership dedicated to advancing the treatment and management of headaches and to raising the public awareness of headache as valid, biologically based illness.

1913   American School Counselor Association
American Counselling Association
1101 King St.
Suite 310
Alexandria, VA 22314-2957   703-683-2722
                                          800-306-4722
                                   Fax: 703-997-7572
                               asca@schoolcounselor.org
                               www.schoolcounselor.org

Richard Wong, Executive Director
Kathleen Rakestraw, Director of Communications
Jennifer Walsh, Director of Education and Training
ASCA focuses on providing professional devlepoment, enhancing school counseling programs, and research effective school counseling practices. Mission is to promote excellence in professional school counseling and the development of all students.

1914   Association for Driver Rehabilitation Specialists
200 First Ave. NW
Suite 505
Hickory, NC 28601   866-672-9466
                                   Fax: 828-855-1672
                                        info@aded.net
                                        www.aded.net

Elizabeth Green, Executive Director
Adrienne Segundo, Credentialing Specialist
Keith Segundo, Director, Education
The Association for Driver Rehabilitation Specialists was established to support professionals working in the field of driver education and driver training and transportation equipment modifications for persons with disabilities through education and information dissemination.

1915   Association on Higher Education & Disability (AHEAD)
8015 West Kenton Circle
Suite 230
Huntersville, NC 28078   704-947-7779
                                   Fax: 704-948-7779
                                        www.ahead.org

Amanda Kraus, President
Stephan Smith, Executive Director
Oanh Huynh, Chief Financial Officer
AHEAD is a professional membership organization for individuals involved in the development of policy and in the provision of quality services to meet the needs of persons with disabilities involved in all areas of higher education, promoting full and equal participation.
4,000+ members

1916   CARF International
6951 East Southpoint Rd.
Tucson, AZ 85756-9407   520-325-1044
                                        888-281-6531
                                   Fax: 520-318-1129
                                   TTY: 520-495-7077
                                        info@carf.org
                                        carf.org

Brian J. Boon, President & Chief Executive Officer
Leslie Ellis-Lang, Managing Director, Child & Youth Services
Darren M. Lehrfeld, Chief Accreditation Officer
An independent, nonprofit accreditor of human service providers in the areas of aging services, behavioral health, child and youth services, DMEPOS, employment and community services, medical rehabilitation, and opioid treatment programs.
1966

1917   CEC Pioneers Division (CEC-PD)
Council for Exceptional Children (CEC)
3100 Clarendon Blvd.
Suite 600
Arlington, VA 22201-5332   888-232-7733
                                   TTY: 866-915-5000
                               cecpioneers@gmail.com
                           cecpioneers.exceptionalchildren.org
Chad Rummel, Executive Director
Exists to support the programs and activities of the Council for Exceptional Children.

1918   Center for Inclusive Design and Innovation
512 Means St. NW
Suite 250
Atlanta, GA 30318   404-894-8000
                                        866-279-2964
                                   Fax: 404-894-8323
                               cidi-support@design.gatech.edu
                                        cidi.gatech.edu

Eric Trevena, Senior Director, Operations
Carolyn Phillips, Director, Services & Learning
CIDI supports individuals with disabilities of any age within the State of Georgia and beyond through expert services, research, design and technological development, information dissemination, and educational programs.

1919   Council for Children with Behavioral Disorders (CCBD)
Council for Exceptional Children (CEC)
3100 Clarendon Blvd.
Suite 600
Arlington, VA 22201-5332   888-232-7733
                                   TTY: 866-915-5000
                                        service@cec.sped.org
                                        www.ccbd.net
Chad Rummel, Executive Director, CEC
Advocates for the education and welfare of youth with behavioral and emotional disorders.

1920   Council for Educational Diagnostic Services (CEDS)
Council for Exceptional Children (CEC)
3100 Clarendon Blvd.
Suite 600
Arlington, VA 22201-5332   888-232-7733
                                   TTY: 866-915-5000
                                        cedscec@gmail.com
                               ceds.exceptionalchildren.org
Chad Rummel, Executive Director
Focused on diagnostic and prescriptive procedures involving the education of gifted persons or those with disabilities.

1921   Council for Exceptional Children (CEC)
3100 Clarendon Blvd.
Suite 600
Arlington, VA 22201-5332   888-232-7733
                                   TTY: 866-915-5000
                               service@exceptionalchildren.org
                               www.exceptionalchildren.org
Chad Rummel, Executive Director
Laurie VanderPloeg, Associate Executive Director, Professional Affairs
Craig Evans, Chief Financial Officer
The Council for Exceptional Children aims to improve the educational success of individuals with disabilities and/or gifts and talents by advocating for appropriate policies, setting professional standards, and providing resources and professional development for special educators.

1922   Council of Administrators of Special Education (CASE)
Osigian Office Center
101 Katelyn Circle
Suite E
Warner Robins, GA 31088   478-333-6892
                                   Fax: 478-333-2453
                                        lpurcell@casecec.org
                                        www.casecec.org
Luann Purcell, Executive Director
Provides professional leadership and personal and professional development for special education administrators.

1923   Disability Research and Dissemination Center
Arnold School of Public Health, USC
Discovery 1 Bldg.
915 Greene St.
Columbia, SC 29208   info@disabilityresearchcenter.com
                               www.disabilityresearchcenter.com
Suzanne McDermott, Research & Administration
Margaret A. Turk, Training & Evaluation
Roberta S. Carlin, Dissemination
The DRDC was formed in 2012 and is a partnership between the University of South Carolina (USC), the State University of New York Upstate Medical University (SUNY Upstate), and the American Association on Health and Disability (AAHD). Its five core

areas are Administration, Research, Research Translation, Evaluation, and Dissemination & Policy.

1924   Division for Communication, Language, and Deaf/Hard of Hearing (DCD)
Council for Exceptional Children (CEC)
3100 Clarendon Blvd.
Suite 600
Arlington, VA 22201-5332
888-232-7733
TTY: 866-915-5000
service@cec.sped.org
dcdcec.org

Chad Rummel, Executive Director, CEC
Dedicated to improving education for deaf/hard of hearing students, and those with communicative disabilities.

1925   Division for Culturally and Linguistically Diverse Exceptional Learners (DDEL)
Council for Exceptional Children (CEC)
3100 Clarendon Blvd.
Suite 600
Arlington, VA 22201-5332
888-232-7733
TTY: 866-915-5000
ddel.exceptionalchildren@gmail.com
ddel.exceptionalchildren.org

Chad Rummel, Executive Director
Serves culturally and linguistically diverse students with disabilities.

1926   Division for Early Childhood (DEC)
PO Box 662089
Los Angeles, CA 90066
310-428-7209
Fax: 855-678-1989
dec@dec-sped.org
www.dec-sped.org

Peggy Kemp, Executive Director
Diana Stanfill, Associate Director
Brittany Clark, Operations Manager
Serves educators who work with children with special needs from birth through age 8.

1927   Division for Early Childhood of the Council for Exceptional Children
Council for Exceptional Children
3100 Clarendon Blvd.
Suite 600
Arlington, VA 22201-5332
888-232-7733
TTY: 866-915-5000
service@cec.sped.org
www.dec-sped.org

Peggy Kemp, Executive Director
Diana Stanfill, Associate Director
Brittany Clark, Operations Coordinator
Promotes policies and advances evidence-based practices that support families and enhance the optimal development of young children who have or are at risk for developmental delays and disabilities.

1928   Division for Learning Disabilities (DLD)
Council for Exceptional Children (CEC)
3100 Clarendon Blvd.
Suite 600
Arlington, VA 22201-5332
888-232-7733
TTY: 866-915-5000
service@cec.sped.org
www.teachingld.org

Chad Rummel, Executive Director, CEC
Seeks to enhance services, research, and legislation for persons with learning disabilities.

1929   Division for Physical, Health & Multiple Disabilities: Complex and Chronic Conditions
Council for Exceptional Children (CEC)
3100 Clarendon Blvd.
Suite 600
Arlington, VA 22201-5332
888-232-7733
TTY: 866-915-5000
cecdphmd@gmail.com
ccc.exceptionalchildren.org

Chad Rummel, Executive Director

Dedicated to quality education for all individuals with physical disabilities, multiple disabilities, and special health care needs.

1930   Division for Research (CEC-DR)
Council for Exceptional Children (CEC)
3100 Clarendon Blvd.
Suite 600
Arlington, VA 22201-5332
888-232-7733
TTY: 866-915-5000
service@cec.sped.org
www.cecdr.org

Chad Rummel, Executive Director, CEC
Seeks to advance research into education for the gifted and/or disabled.

1931   Division of International Special Education and Services (DISES)
Council for Exceptional Children (CEC)
3100 Clarendon Blvd.
Suite 600
Arlington, VA 22201-5332
888-232-7733
TTY: 866-915-5000
info@dises-cec.org
dises-cec.org

Chad Rummel, Executive Director, CEC
Dedicated to special education programs in other countries.

1932   Division of Visual and Performing Arts Education (DARTS)
Council for Exceptional Children (CEC)
3100 Clarendon Blvd.
Suite 600
Arlington, VA 22201-5332
888-232-7733
TTY: 866-915-5000
cecdartswebmaster@gmail.com
darts.exceptionalchildren.org

Chad Rummel, Executive Director
Promotes art, music, drama, and dance for students with disabilities.

1933   Division on Autism and Developmental Disabilities (DADD)
Council for Exceptional Children (CEC)
3100 Clarendon Blvd.
Suite 600
Arlington, VA 22201-5332
888-232-7733
TTY: 866-915-5000
service@cec.sped.org
www.daddcec.com

Chad Rummel, Executive Director, CEC
Seeks to improve quality of life for individuals with autism and other intellectual disabilities, especially youth.

1934   Division on Career Development and Transition (DCDT)
Council for Exceptional Children (CEC)
3100 Clarendon Blvd.
Suite 600
Arlington, VA 22201-5332
888-232-7733
TTY: 866-915-5000
jrazeghi@gmu.edu
www.exceptionalchildren.org

Chad Rummel, Executive Director
Dedicated to assisting disabled students with their transition from school to adult life.

1935   Division on Visual Impairments and Deafblindness (DVIDB)
Council for Exceptional Children (CEC)
3100 Clarendon Blvd.
Suite 600
Arlington, VA 22201-5332
888-232-7733
TTY: 866-915-5000
dvidbwebmaster@gmail.com
dvidb.exceptionalchildren.org

Chad Rummel, Executive Director
Dedicated to assisting students with visual impairments or deafblindness.

1936 Filomen M. D'Agostino Greenberg Music School
111 E 59th St.
New York, NY 10022   315-842-4489
music@fmdgmusicschool.org
fmdgmusicschool.org
Leslie Jones, Executive Director
Dalia Sakas, Director, Music Studies
Amanda Wheeler, Director, Administration
Formerly affiliated with the Lighthouse Guild, the Filomen M.
D'Agostino Greenberg Music School is the only community mu-
sic school in the US for people who are blind or visually impaired,
offering instruction and an accessible music technology center.

1937 HEAL: Health Education AIDS Liaison
New York, NY   347-867-4497
michaelellner2@gmail.com
www.healaids.com
Michael Ellner, President
Barnett J. Weiss, Board Member
Roberto Giraldo, Board Member
Nonprofit, community-based educational organization providing information, hope, and support to people who are HIV positive or living with AIDS. The men and women at HEAL are health
professionals, people living with life threatening diseases, and
volunteers.

1938 Incight
111 SW Columbia St
Suite 940
Portland, OR 97201   971-244-0305
scott@incight.org
incight.org
Scott Hatley, Executive Director
Vail Horton, Director, Results
Hannah Rankin, Director, Results
Incight in a non-profit organization that supports people with disabilities in the areas of education, employment, and independent
living. Incight offers programs that address workplace
descrimination, college application process and recreational
needs of those they serve.

**1939 Innovations in Special Education Technology Division
(ISET)**
Council for Exceptional Children (CEC)
3100 Clarendon Blvd.
Suite 600
Arlington, VA 22201-5332   888-232-7733
TTY: 866-915-5000
service@cec.sped.org
www.isetcec.org
Chad Rummel, Executive Director, CEC
Advocates for technology and media to assist gifted persons and
those with disabilities.

1940 International Childbirth Education Association
110 Horizon Dr.
Suite 210
Raleigh, NC 27615   919-674-4183
Fax: 919-459-2075
info@icea.org
www.icea.org
Katesha Phillips, Executive Director
Jenna Westheimer, Membership & Certification Coordinator
Allison Winter, Marketing Coordinator
The Association offers teaching certificates, seminars, continu-
ing education workshops, and mail order center.

1941 International Dyslexia Association
40 York Rd.
4th Floor
Baltimore, MD 21204   410-296-0232
Fax: 410-321-5069
info@dyslexiaida.org
dyslexiaida.org
Sonja Banks, Chief Executive Officer
David Holste, Chief Financial Officer
*Jason Marshall, Interim Chief Communications & Engagement
Officer*
Provides free information and referral services for diagnosis and
tutoring for parents, educators, physicians, and individuals with
dyslexia. Membership includes yearly journal and quarterly

newsletter, and Pennsylvania newsletter; discounts to
conferences and events.

1942 Job Accommodation Network
PO Box 6080
Morgantown, WV 26506-6080   304-293-7186
800-526-7234
Fax: 304-293-5407
TTY: 877-781-9403
jan@askjan.org
askjan.org
Deborah Hendricks, Director
Anne Hirsch, Associate Director
JAN's mission is to facilitate the employment and retention of
workers with disabilities by providing employers, employment
providers, people with disabilities, their family members, and
other interested parties with information on job accommodations,
self-employment, and small business opportunities and related
subjects.

1943 LD Online
2775 S. Quincy St.
Arlington, VA 22206   Fax: 703-998-2060
ldonline@weta.org
ldonline.org
Noel Gunther, Executive Director
Christian Lindstrom, Director, Learning Media
Lydia Breiseth, Director, Colorin Colorado
LD OnLine seeks to help children and adults reach their full potential by providing accurate and up-to-date information and advice about learning disabilities and ADHD. The site features
hundreds of helpful articles, multimedia, monthly columns by
noted experts, first person essays, children's writing and artwork,
a comprehensive resource guide, very active forums, and a Yellow Pages referral directory of professionals, schools, and
products.

1944 Lighthouse Guild
250 West 64th Street
New York, NY 10023   800-284-4422
www.lighthouseguild.org
Calvin W. Roberts, President & CEO
James M. Dubin, Chairman
Lawrence E. Goldschmidt, Vice Chairman & Treasurer
Lighthouse Guild is a not-for-profit vision & healthcare organization, addressing the needs of people who are blind or visually
impaired, including those with multiple disabilities or chronic
medical conditions.

1945 Michigan Psychological Association
124 W Allegan St.
Suite 1900
Lansing, MI 48933   517-347-1885
Fax: 517-484-4442
www.michiganpsychologicalassociation.org
Antu Segal, President
Valencia Montgomery, Treasurer
Cynthia S. Rodriguez, Secretary
Nonprofit organization of over 1000 psychologists, working to
advance psychology as a science and a profession and to promote
the public welfare by encouraging the highest professional standards, offering public education and providing a public service,
and by participating in the public policy process on behalf of the
profession and health care consumers.

**1946 National Association for Adults with Special Learning
Needs**
P.O. Box 716
Bryn Mawr, PA 19010   naasln.org
Richard Cooper, Co-President
Joan Hudson-Miller, Co-President
Frances A. Holthaus, Vice President
NAASLN is an association for those who serve adults with spe-
cial learning needs. NAASLN members include educators, train-
ers, employers and human service providers.

1947   National Association of Colleges and Employers
62 Highland Ave.
Bethlehem, PA 18017   610-868-1421
                                        admin@naceweb.org
                                        naceweb.org

Jennifer Lasater, President
Shawn Vanderziel, Executive Director
A national association with services for career planning, placement and recruitment professionals.

1948   National Association of Parents with Children in Special Education
3642 E Sunnydale Dr.
Chandler Heights, AZ 85142   800-754-4421
                                        Fax: 800-424-0371
                                        contact@napcse.org
                                        www.napcse.org
George Giuliani, President
NAPCSE is a national membership organization dedicated to rendering all possible support and assistance to parents whose children receive special education services, both in and outside of school.

1949   National Association of State Directors of Special Education
1000 Diagonal Rd.
Suite 600
Alexandria, VA 22314   703-519-3800
                                        Fax: 703-519-3808
                                        www.nasdse.org
John Eisenberg, Executive Director
Valerie Williams, Director, Government Relations
Joanne Cashman, Member Services
NASDSE focuses on improving educational services and outcomes for children and youth with disabilities throughout the United States, the Department of Defense, the federated territories and the Freely Associated States of Palau, Micronesia and the Marshall Islands.

1950   National Center for Homeopathy
1120 Route 73
Suite 200
Mount Laurel, NJ 08054   856-437-4752
                                        Fax: 856-439-0525
                                        www.homeopathycenter.org
Deb Dupnik, Executive Director
Natascha Williams, Meeting Manager
Steve Clark, Membership Coordinator
The National Center for Homeopathy (NCH) is a non-profit organization dedicated to promoting health through homeopathy by advancing the use and practice of homeopathy.

1951   National Council on Rehabilitation Education (NCRE)
1099 E. Champlain Dr.
Suite A-137
Fresno, CA 93720   559-906-0787
                                        info@ncre.org
                                        ncre.org
David A. Rosenthal, Ph.D, CRC, President
Mona Robinson, Ph.D, CRC, First Vice President
Allison Fleming, Ph.D, CRC, Second Vice President
Members include academic institutions and organizations, professional educators, researchers, and students. Assists in the documentation of the effect of education in improving services to persons with disabilities; determines the skills and training necessary for effective rehabilitation services; develops role models, standards and uniform licensure and certification requirements for rehabilitation personnel.

1952   National Education Association of the United States
1201 16th St. NW
Washington, DC 20036-3290   202-833-4000
                                        Fax: 202-822-7974
                                        www.nea.org
Lily Eskelsen Garcia, President
Becky Pringle, Vice President
Princess R. Moss, Secretary/Treasurer
The National Education Association (NEA) is committed to advancing the cause of public education.

1953   National Society for Experiential Education
19 Mantua Rd.
Mount Royal, NJ 08061   856-423-3427
                                        Fax: 856-423-3420
                                        nsee@talley.com
                                        www.nsee.org
Haley Burst, Executive Director
Wendy Stevens, Meeting Manager
Arianna B., Program Manager
National nonprofit organization which advocates experiential learning and works with college administrators and high school and college internship programs.

1954   Servcies for Students with Disabilities (SSD)
College Board
P.O. Box 7504
London, KY 40742-7504   212-713-8333
                                        844-255-7728
                                        Fax: 866-360-0114
                                        ssd@info.collegeboard.org
                                        www.collegeboard.com
David Coleman, Chief Executive Officer
Jeremy Singer, President
Tracy MacMahon, Senior Vice President, Operations
National, nonprofit association dedicated to preparing, inspiring and connecting students to college and opportunity. Provide the accomodations students with disabilities need to complete test and other evaluations.

1955   Society for Disability Studies
P.O. Box 5570
Eureka, CA 95502   510-206-5767
                                        sds@disstudies.org
                                        www.disstudies.org
Devva Kasnitz, Ph.D, Interim Executive Director
SDS is a scholarly association of more than 400 artists, scholars and activists who promote Disability Studies, recognizing disability as a complex and valuable aspect of human experience.

1956   Teacher Education Division (TED)
Council for Exceptional Children (CEC)
3100 Clarendon Blvd.
Suite 600
Arlington, VA 22201-5332   888-232-7733
                                        TTY: 866-915-5000
                                        service@cec.sped.org
                                        tedcec.org
Chad Rummel, Executive Director, CEC
Sharon Rodriguez, Governance & Executive Services Coordinator
Advocates for continual professional development of professionals in special education and related fields.

1957   The AG Academy for Listening and Spoken Language
Alexander Graham Bell Association
3417 Volta Pl. NW
Washington, DC 20007   202-337-5220
                                        Fax: 202-337-8314
                                        TTY: 202-337-5221
                                        academy@agbell.org
                                        agbellacademy.org
Jenna Voss, Chair
Emilio Alonso-Mendoza, Chief Executive Officer
Listening and Spoken Language Specialsts (LSLST) work with infants and children who are deaf or hard of hearing and their families seeking a listening and spoken language outcome in a variety of settings: home-based intervention, public schools, independent schools, private therapy, clinical centers for the deaf and hard of hearing, audiological and cochlear implant centers.

1958   The Association for the Gifted (TAG)
Council for Exceptional Children (CEC)
3100 Clarendon Blvd.
Suite 600
Arlington, VA 22201-5332   888-232-7733
                                        TTY: 866-915-5000
                                        tag.cec@gmail.com
                                        cectag.com
Chad Rummel, Executive Director, CEC
Sharon Rodriguez, Governance & Executive Services Coordinator
Serves parents and professionals working with gifted and talented children.

1959   **United Cerebral Palsy**
1825 K St. NW
Suite 600
Washington, DC 20006-5638   202-776-0406
                                             www.ucp.org
Armando Contreras, President & CEO
Anita Porco, Vice President, Affiliate Network
Michael Ludgardo, Manager, Development
United Cerebral Palsy (UCP) educates, advocates and provides
support services to ensure a life without limits for people with a
spectrum of disabilities. UCP and its nearly 68+ affiliates have a
mission to advance the independence, productivity and full citizenship of people with a broad range of disabilities by providing
services and support to children and adults.

Directories

1960   **ADDitude Directory**
108 West 39th St.
Suite 805
New York, NY 10018   646-366-0830
                                        Fax: 646-366-0842
                           customerservice@additudemag.com
                                    directory.additudemag.com
The ADDitude Directory is a comprehensive directory that contains listings from some of the nation'sleading specialists in attention deficit disorder (ADD/ADHD) and learning disabilities.

1961   **BOSC: Directory of Facilities for People with Learning
Disabilities**
Books on Special Children
PO Box 3378
Amherst, MA 1004-3378   413-256-8164
                                        Fax: 413-256-8896
Michael Young, President
Directory of schools, independent living programs, clinics and
centers, colleges and vocational programs, agencies and commer-
cial products. Five sections in special post binder that can be up-
dated annually. Hardcover. *$70.00*
300+ pages Yearly
ISSN 0961-3888

1962   **Community Resource Directory**
5300 Hiatus Road
Sunrise, FL 33351   954-745-9779
                                             800-963-5337
                              webmaster@adrcbroward.org
                                     www.adrcbroward.org
The document contains over 355 pages of updated information regarding programs and services for elder residents of Broward.

1963   **Complete Learning Disabilities Resource Guide**
Grey House Publishing
4919 Route 22
P.O. Box 56
Amenia, NY 12501   518-789-8700
                                             800-562-2139
                                        Fax: 518-789-0556
                                    books@greyhouse.com
                                       www.greyhouse.com
Leslie Mackenzie, Publisher
Laura Mars, Editorial Director
Jessica Moody, Vice President, Marketing
A comprehensive educational guide offering over 6,000 listings
on associations and organizations, schools, government agencies, testing materials, camps, products, books, newsletters, legal
information, classroom materials and more. Includes separate
chapters on ADD and Literacy, as well as informative articles.
$165.00
800 pages Annual

1964   **Complete Mental Health Resource Guide**
Sedgwick Press/Grey House Publishing
4919 Route 22
P.O. Box 56
Amenia, NY 12501   518-789-8700
                                             800-562-2139
                                        Fax: 518-789-0556
                                    books@greyhouse.com
                                       www.greyhouse.com
Leslie Mackenzie, Publisher
Laura Mars, Editorial Director
Jessica Moody, Vice President, Marketing
This directory offers comprehensive information covering the
field of behavioral health, with critical information for both the
layman and the mental health professional. It covers, in depth, 22
specific mental disorders, and includes informative descriptions
and a complete list of resources. *$165.00*
800 pages Annual

1965   **Complete Resource Guide for Pediatric Disorders**
Sedgwick Press/Grey House Publishing
4919 Route 22
P.O. Box 56
Amenia, NY 12501   518-789-8700
                                             800-562-2139
                                        Fax: 518-789-0556
                                    books@greyhouse.com
                                       www.greyhouse.com
Leslie Mackenzie, Publisher
Laura Mars, Editorial Director
Jessica Moody, Vice President, Marketing
An annual directory for professionals, parents and caregivers.
Provides valuable information on more than 200 pediatric condi-
tions, disorders, diseases and disabilities, including informative
descriptions and a wide variety of resources, from associations to
publications. *$165.00*
1000 pages Annual

1966   **Complete Resource Guide for People with Chronic
Illness**
Grey House Publishing
4919 Route 22
P.O. Box 56
Amenia, NY 12501   518-789-8700
                                             800-562-2139
                                        Fax: 518-789-0556
                                    books@greyhouse.com
                                       www.greyhouse.com
Leslie Mackenzie, Publisher
Laura Mars, Editorial Director
Jessica Moody, Vice President, Marketing
This directory is structured around the 80 most prevalent chronic
illnesses. Each chronic illness chapter includes an informative
description, plus a comprehensive listing of resources and support services available for people diagnosed with chronic illness
and their network of supportive individuals. *$165.00*
1000 pages Annual

1967   **Directory Of Services For People With Disabilities**
117 W. Duval St.
Suite 205
Jacksonville, FL 32202-4111   904-630-4940
                                        Fax: 904-630-3476
                                        TTY: 904-630-4933
                                    disabledservices@coj.net
                                             www.coj.net
The agencies listed in this guide can be of great assistance to per-
sons with disabilities and their family members.

1968 **Directory for Exceptional Children**
Prorter Sargent
2 LAN Drive
Suite 100
Westford, MA 01886   978-692-5092
                                            800-342-7470
                                       Fax: 978-692-4714
                                       info@carnegiecomm.com
                                       www.carnegiecomm.com
Joe Moore, President, CEO
Mark Cunningham, SVP, Enrollment Marketing
Melissa Rekos, SVP, Digital Services
Supports parents and professionals seeking the optimal educational, therapeutic or clinical environment for special-needs youth. *$75.00*
1120 pages Trienniel
ISBN 0-875581-50-1

1969 **Educators Resource Guide**
Grey House Publishing
4919 Route 22
PO Box 55
Amenia, NY 12501   518-789-8700
                                            800-562-2139
                                       Fax: 845-373-6390
                                       books@greyhouse.com
                                       www.greyhouse.com
Leslie Mackenzie, Publisher
Laura Mars, Editorial Director
Jessica Moody, Vice President, Marketing
Gives education professionals immediate access to Associations and Organizations, Conferences and Trade Shows, Educational Research Centers, Employment Opportunities and Teaching Abroad, School Library Services, Scholarships, Financial Resources and much more. *$ 145.00*
650 pages Annual

1970 **Greater Milwaukee Area Health Care Guide for Older Adults**
PO Box 285
Germantown, WI 53022   262-253-0901
                                       Fax: 262-253-0903
                                       info@seniorresourcesonline.com
                                       www.seniorresourcesonline.com
Gary Knippen, President
This directory is designed for older adults, family members and professionals looking for health care options in Milwaukee, Ozaukee, Washington and Waukesha counties. The directory is comprehensive with all providers included at no charge.

1971 **Greater Milwaukee Area Senior Housing Options**
PO Box 285
Germantown, WI 53022   262-253-0901
                                       Fax: 262-253-0903
                                       info@seniorresourcesonline.com
                                       www.seniorresourcesonline.com
Gary Knippen, President
This directory is designed for older adults, family members and professionals looking for senior housing options in Milwaukee, Ozaukee, Washington and Waukesha counties. The directory is comprehensive with all providers included at no charge.

1972 **Indiana Directory of Disability Resources**
225 S. University Street
ABE Bldg.
West Lafayette, IN 47907-2093   765-494-5013
                                            800-825-4264
                                       bng@ecn.purdue.edu
                                       engineering.purdue.edu/~bng/IDDR/
The purpose of the Indiana Directory of Disability Resources (IDDR) is to provide Hoosiers with a useful guide to disability services and to increase the public's awareness of the available resources.

1973 **Nevada's Care Connection**
3416 Goni Road
Suite D-132
Carson City, NV 89706   702-486-3600
                                       cpasquale@adsd.nv.gov
                                       www.nevadaadrc.com
Cheyenne Pasquale, ADRC Project Manager

Nevada's Care Connection: Aging and Disability Resource Center (ADRC) program provides information and access to programs and services that benefit Nevada's seniors, people with disabilities and caregivers.

1974 **Northeast Wisconsin Directory of Servicesfor Older Adults**
PO Box 285
Germantown, WI 53022   262-253-0901
                                       Fax: 262-253-0903
                                       info@seniorresourcesonline.com
                                       www.seniorresourcesonline.com
Gary Knippen, President
This directory is designed for older adults, family members and professionals looking for housing and health care options in Brown, Calumet, Door, Fond du Lac, Green Lake, Kewaunee, Manitowoc, Marinette, Marquette, Oconto, Outagamie, Shawano, Sheboygan, Waupaca, Waushara and Winnebago counties.

1975 **ODHH Directory of Resources and Services**
1521 N. 6th Street
Harrisburg, PA 17102   717-783-4912
                                       TTY: 717-783-4912
                                       RA-LI-OVR-ODHH@pa.gov
ODHH is the office for the Deaf & Hard of Hearing's one-stop listing of resources and services for people who are deaf or hard of hearing.

1976 **Responding to Crime Victims with Disabilities**
2000 M Street NW
Suite 480
Washington, DC 20036   202-467-8700
                                       Fax: 202-467-8701
                                       www.victimsofcrime.org
Philip M. Gerson, Chair
G. Morris Gurley, Vice-Chair
Mai Fernandez, Executive Director
The mission of the National Center for Victims of Crime is to forge a national commitment to help victims of crime rebuild their lives. It is dedicated to serving individuals, families, and communities harmed by crime.

1977 **Selective Placement Program Coordinator Directory**
1900 E Street, NW
Washington, DC 20415-1000   202-606-1800
                                       www.opm.gov
Selective Placement Program Coordinator (SPPC) who helps management recruit, hire and accommodate people with disabilities

1978 **South Central Wisconsin Directory of Services for Older Adults**
PO Box 285
Germantown, WI 53022   262-253-0901
                                       www.seniorresourcesonline.com
Gary Knippen, President
This directory is designed for older adults, family members and professionals looking for housing and health care options in Columbia, Dane, Dodge, Grant, Green, Iowa, Jefferson, Juneau, Lafayette, Richland, Rock, Sauk, and Walworth counties.

1979 **Southeast Wisconsin Directory of Services for Older Adults**
PO Box 285
Germantown, WI 53022   262-253-0901
                                       www.seniorresourcesonline.com
Gary Knippen, President
This directory is designed for older adults, family members and professionals looking for housing and health care options in Kenosha, Racine and Walworth counties.

1980 **Teaching Special Students in Mainstream**
Books on Special Children
P.O.Box 305
Congers, NY 10920-305   845-638-1236
                                       Fax: 845-638-0847
Overview of mainstream, team of professionals managing classroom behavior, tips for teachers, social acceptance and handling of specific differences. *$33.00*
515 pages Softcover

Educational Publishers

1981 AFB Press
American Foundation for the Blind / AFB Press
2 Penn Plaza
Suite 1102
New York, NY 10121   212-502-7600
                                  Fax: 888-545-8331
                                  afbinfo@afb.net
                                  www.afb.org

Carl R. Augusto, President and CEO
Paul Schroeder, Vice President, Programs and Policy
Rick Bozeman, Chief Financial Officer
Develops, publishes, and sells a wide variety of informative books, pamphlets, periodicals, and videos for students, professionals, and researchers in the blindness and visual impairment fields, for people professionally involved in making the mainstream community accessible, and for blind and visually impaired people and their families; publication and video orders.

1982 Academic Therapy Publications
Academic Therapy Publications / High Noon Books
20 Leveroni Ct.
Novato, CA 94949-5746   415-883-3314
                                  800-422-7249
                                  Fax: 888-287-9975
                                  sales@academictherapy.com
                                  www.academictherapy.com

Jim Arena, President
Stacy Frauwirth, Assessment Project Manager
Holly Melton, Head Writer & Senior Project Manager
Academic Therapy Publications produces and distributes psychological and educational tests used by professionals involved in special education and learning differences in the K-12 school system as well as adult services.

1983 AccessText Network
512 Means St. NW
Suite 250
Atlanta, GA 30318   866-271-4968
                                  membership@accesstext.org
                                  www.accesstext.org

Dawn Evans, AccessText Network Coordinator
AccessText is a conduit between the publishing world and colleges and universities across the country, with a shared mission to ensure students with disabilities have equal access to their textbooks in an accessible format and in a timely manner.

1984 American Counseling Association (ACA)
P.O. Box 31110
Alexandria, VA 22310-9998   800-347-6647
                                  Fax: 800-473-2329
                                  www.counseling.org

Richard Yep, Chief Executive Officer
Offers tools and books for counseling professionals.

1985 Association of University Centers on Disabilities (AUCD)
AUCD
1100 Wayne Ave.
Suite 1000
Silver Spring, MD 20910   301-588-8252
                                  Fax: 301-588-2842
                                  aucdinfo@aucd.org
                                  www.aucd.org

John Tschida, Executive Director
Michele Lunsford, Director, Communications, Events & Development
Dawn Rudolph, Senior Director, Technical Assistance & Network Engagement
AUCD is a membership organization consisting of University Centers for Excellence in Developmental Disabilities (UCEDD), Leadership Education in Neurodevelopmental Disabilities (LEND) Programs, and Intellectual and Developmental Disability Research Centers (IDDRC). AUCD supports its members through advocacy, technical assistance, information dissemination, networking, and leadership.

1986 Brookes Publishing Company
PO Box 10624
Baltimore, MD 21285-0624   410-337-9580
                                  800-638-3775
                                  Fax: 410-337-8539
                                  webmaster@brookespublishing.com
                                  www.brookespublishing.com

Paul H. Brookes, Chairman of the Board
Jeffrey D. Brookes, President
George S. Stamathis, VP/Publisher
Publishes highly respected resources in early childhood, early intervention, inclusive and special education, developmental disabilities, learning disabilities, communication and language, behavior and mental health.

1987 Brookline Books
8 Trumbull Rd
B-001
Northampton, MA 01060   413-584-0184
                                  800-666-2665
                                  Fax: 413-584-6184
                                  brbooks@yahoo.com
                                  www.brooklinebks.com

Offering books ranging from non-fiction to poetry that both share vital stories about disability and education, and present strategies and possible solutions in situations related to general education or to specific circumstances.

1988 Brooks/Cole Publishing Company
511 Forest Lodge Rd
Pacific Grove, CA 93950-5040   831-373-0728
                                  800-354-9706
                                  Fax: 831-375-6414

Offers books in Special Education for those preparing to be special educators and for in-service professionals.

1989 BurnsBooks Publishing
680 Ridge Road
Middletown, CT 6457   860-344-0233
                                  Fax: 860-344-0233
                                  burnsbookspub@aol.com
                                  www.burnsbookspublishing.com

urnsBooks create confidence and overcome anxiety in the new reader through the use of carefully controlled vocabulary, larger print, and greater spaces between sentences.

1990 Charles C Thomas Publisher LTD
2600 S 1st Street
Springfield, IL 62704-4730   217-789-8980
                                  800-258-8980
                                  Fax: 217-789-9130
                                  books@ccthomas.com
                                  www.ccthomas.com

Michael P. Thomas, President
Publishes specialty titles and textbooks in medicine, dentistry, nursing, and veterinary medicine, as well as a complete line in the behavioral sciences, criminal justice, education, special education, and rehabilitation. Aims to accommodate the current needs for information.

1991 DisabilityAdvisor.com
37 North Orange Ave.
Suite 500
Orlando, FL 32801   321-332-7800
                                  888-393-1010
                                  Fax: 888-985-6060
                                  www.disabilityadvisor.com

Joseph E. Ram, Publisher
Kay Derochie, Editor
Jackie Booth, Ph.D., Editor
DisabilityAdvisor.com provides free information on federal and state disability benefits programs and other resources for readers and their families. This includes disabled children and students, military veterans, injured workers and disabled seniors. Readers are encouraged to submit their questions and comments online. The website also offers information on managing finances, education, parenting, relationships and other issues of interest to the disabled and their friends and families.

1992 Dolphin Computer Access
231 Clarksville Road
Suite 7
Princeton Junction, NJ 8550

866-797-5921
Fax: 609-799-0475
info@dolphinusa.com
www.yourdolphin.com

Noel Duffy, Managing Director
Dolphin helps vision and print impairments

1993 Gallaudet University Press
800 Florida Avenue, NE
Washington, DC 20002-3695

202-651-5488
Fax: 202-651-5489
gupress@gallaudet.edu
gupress.gallaudet.edu

David F Armstrong, Executive Director
Publishes scholarly trade books and journals about deaf people and their language, history, and culture for deaf people, parents of deaf children, professionals, educators and the general public. Produces spring and fall catalogs.

1994 Greenwood Publishing Group
88 Post Rd W
Westport, CT 06880-4208

203-226-3571
Fax: 203-222-1502
webmaster@greenwood.com
greenwood.com

Wayne Smith, President
Kirstin Olsen, Author
ABC-CLIO and Greenwood Press are recognized as industry-leading providers of the highest-quality reference materials. These imprints offer authoritative reference scholarship and innovative coverage of history and humanities topics across the secondary and higher education curriculum.

1995 Grey House Publishing
4919 Route 22
P.O. Box 56
Amenia, NY 12501

518-789-8700
800-562-2139
Fax: 518-789-0556
books@greyhouse.com
www.greyhouse.com

Leslie Mackenzie, Publisher
Laura Mars, Editorial Director
Jessica Moody, Vice President, Marketing
Grey House Publishing publishes directories, handbooks and reference works for public, high school and academic libraries and the business and health communities. Most titles are available as online databases.

1996 Hammill Institute on Disabilities
8700 Shoal Creek Blvd.
Austin, TX 78757-6897

512-451-3521
Fax: 512-451-3728
info@hammill-institute.org
hammill-institute.org

The Institute was organized for charitable, scientific, and educational purposes to enhance the well-being of people with disabilities, their parents and caretakers. The Institute publishes journals and monographs on the subject in collaboration with other associations.

1997 Harbor House Law Press
PO Box 480
Hartfield, VA 23071

804-758-8400
Fax: 202-318-3239
webmaster@wrightslaw.com
www.harborhouselaw.com

Harbor House Law Pressdevelops user-friendly publications about special education law and advocacy.

1998 High Noon Books
Academic Therapy Publications / High Noon Books
20 Leveroni Ct
Novato, CA 94949-5746

800-422-7249
888-287-9975
products@academictherapy.com
www.highnoonbooks.com

Jim Arena, President
Holly Melton, Head Writer & Senior Project Manager
High Noon Books produces and distributes a variety of phonic-based and high-interest/low level chapter books, ebooks, and audio for beginning, at-risk, and struggling readers.

1999 Information from HEATH Resource Center
National Clearinghouse on Postsecondary Education
2134 G Street, N.W.
Washington, DC 20052

202-939-9320
800-544-3284
Fax: 202-833-5696
www.HEATH-resource-center.org

The HEATH Resource Center operates the national clearinghouse on postsecondary education for individuals with disabilities. Support from the US Department of Education enables the Center, a program of the America Council on Education, to serve as an information exchange on educational support services; adaptations; and opportunities at American campuses, vocational-technical schools, adult education programs, independent living centers, and other postsecondary training entities.

2000 Lynne Rienner Publishers
1800 30th St.
Ste. 314
Boulder, CO 80301

303-444-6684
Fax: 303-444-0824
www.rienner.com

Lynne Rienner Publishers founded in 1984 publishes in the fields of international studies and comparative politics (all world regions), US politics, and sociology and criminology (with a US focus).

2001 MAPCON Technologies
8191 Birchwood Court
Suite A
Johnston, IA 50131-2930

515-331-3358
800-223-4791
Fax: 515-331-3373
www.mapcon.com

Joel Tesdall, President/CEO
Diane Wiand, Client Solutions Advocate
Lora Whicker, Accounting
MAPCON is a computerized maintainance management software.

2002 McGraw-Hill Company
PO Box 182605
Columbus, OH 43218

800-338-3987
Fax: 609-308-4480
customer.service@mheducation.com
www.mcgraw-hill.com

David Levin, President, CEO
Ellen Haley, President, CTB
Peter Cohen, President, School Education
Offers a catalog of testing resources and materials for the special educator.

2003 National Association of School Psychologists
4340 East West Hwy.
Suite 402
Bethesda, MD 20814

301-657-0270
866-331-6277
Fax: 301-657-0275
TTY: 301-657-4155
www.nasponline.org

Kathleen Minke, Executive Director
Laura Benson, Chief Operating Officer
Represents over 25,000 school psychologists and related professionals. It serves its members and society by advancing the profession of school psychology and advocating for the rights, welfare, education and mental health of children, youth and their families.

2004 National Center for Learning Disabilities
32 Laight St
2nd Floor
New York, NY 10013   212-545-7510
                                          888-575-7373
                                   Fax: 212-545-9665
                                          info@ncld.org
                                          www.ncld.org

Frederic M Poses, Chairman
Mimi Corcoran, President & CEO
Rashonda Ambrose, Director of Strategic Partnerships
Contains features, articles, human interest news and other practical material to benefit children and adults with learning disabilities and their families, as well as educators and other helping professionals. The center also offers online forums and other resources on their website.
Quarterly

2005 PEAK Parent Center
917 East Moreno Ave.
Suite 140
Colorado Springs, CO 80903   719-531-9400
                                   Fax: 719-531-9452
                                          info@peakparent.org
                                          www.peakparent.org

Michele Williers, Executive Director
Pam Christy, Director, Parent Training & Information
PEAK Parent Center is Colorado's federally-designated Parent Training and Information Center (PTI). As a PTI, PEAK supports and empowers parents, providing them with information and strategies to use when advocating for their children with disabilities. PEAK works one-on-one with families and educators helping them realize new possibilities for children with disabilities by expanding knowledge of special education and offering new strategies for success.
1986

2006 PRO-ED
8700 Shoal Creek Boulevard
Austin, TX 78757-6897   512-451-3246
                                          800-897-3202
                                   Fax: 512-451-8542
                                          info@proedinc.com
                                          www.proedinc.com
PRO-ED Inc. is a publisher of standardized tests, books, curricular resources, and therapy materials. PRO-ED Inc's products are used by professionals, parents, and students around the world.

2007 Peytral Publications
P.O. Box 1162
Minnetonka, MN 55345   952-949-8707
                                   TTY: 952-906-9777
                                          www.peytral.com
An independent publisher and distributor of special education materials which promote Success for All Learners.

2008 Prufrock Press
PO Box 8813
Waco, TX 76714   254-756-3337
                                          800-998-2208
                                   Fax: 800-240-0333
                                          jmcintosh@prufrock.com
                                          www.prufrock.com

Joel McIntosh, Publisher
Lacy Compton, Senior Editor
Rachel Taliaferro, Editor
Publishes books, textbooks, teaching materials supporting the education of gifted, advanced, and twice-exceptional learners.

2009 Research Press
P.O. Box 7886
Champaign, IL 61826   217-352-3273
                                          800-519-2707
                                   Fax: 217-352-1221
                                          orders@researchpress.com
                                          www.researchpress.com

Robert W. Parkinson, Founder
Dr Richard M Foxx, Author
Jeffrey S. Allen, Author
Research Press is an independent, family-owned business founded in 1968 by Robert W. Parkinson (1920-2001). During the past 40 years, the company has earned a solid reputation for publishing practical and effective educational and mental health resources. Authors from the early years include well-known names in the field of psychology, such as B.F. Skinner, Albert Ellis, Gerald Patterson, Wesley Becker, John Guttmann, Richard Foxx, Arnold Lazarus, and Joseph Cautela.

2010 Research Press Company
2612 N. Mattis Ave.
Champaign, IL 61822   217-352-3273
                                          800-519-2707
                                   Fax: 217-352-1221
                                          www.researchpress.com
Research Press is an independent, family-owned business founded in 1968 by Robert W. Parkinson

2011 Sage Publications
2455 Teller Road
Thousand Oaks, CA 91320   805-499-0721
                                          800-818-7243
                                   Fax: 800-583-2665
                                          info@sagepub.com
                                          www.sagepub.com

Sara Miller McCune, Founder, Publisher & Executive Chairman
Blaise R Simqu, President/CEO
Chris Hickok, Senior Vice President & Chief Financial Officer
Publishes books, text books, journals, reference books, and databases mainly related to psychology, special education and speech, language and hearing.

2012 Special Needs Project
Special Needs Project
324 State Street
Suite H
Santa Barbara, CA 93101-2364   818-718-9900
                                          800-333-6867
                                   Fax: 818-349-2027
                                          editor@specialneeds.com
                                          www.specialneeds.com

Hod Gray, Owner
Publishes child development textbooks, books about aspergers syndrome, autism, and other disabilities.

2013 Supporting Success for Children with Hearing Loss
15619 Premiere Drive
Suite 101
Tampa, FL 33624   850-363-9909
                                   Fax: 480-393-4331
                          accounting@successforkidswithhearingloss.com
                                   successforkidswithhearinglo ss.com
Karen Anderson, PhD, Director
Improving the Outcomes of Children with Hearing Loss

2014 Woodbine House
6510 Bells Mill Road
Bethesda, MD 20817   800-843-7323
                                          info@woodbinehouse.com
                                          www.woodbinehouse.com
Woodbine House is a publisher specializing in books about children with special needs.

State Agencies: Alabama

2015 Alabama Department of Education: Division of Special Education Services
50 North Ripley St
P.O. Box 302101
Montgomery, AL 36104   334-242-9700
                                   Fax: 334-262-2677
                                          www.alsde.edu

Crystal Richardson, Program Coordinator
Provides technical assistance to all education agencies serving Alabama's gifted children as well as children with disabilities.

State Agencies: Alaska

2016 **Alaska Department of Education: Special Education**
State of Alaska
801 West 10th St
Ste 200, P.O.Box 110500
Juneau, AK 99811-0500
907-465-8693
Fax: 907-465-2806
TTY: 907-465-2815
sped@alaska.gov
www.education.alaska.gov/TLS/SPED
Dr. Susan McCauley, Division Director
Paul Prussing, Deputy Director
Cassidy Jones, Special Education Programs Manager
Administers special educational programs to the disabled residents of Alaska, through the Division of Teaching & Learning Support.

State Agencies: Arkansas

2017 **Arkansas Department of Special Education**
1401 West Capitol Ave, Victory Bldg
Suite 450
Little Rock, AR 72201
501-682-4221
Fax: 501-682-3456
TTY: 501-682-4222
spedsupport@arkansas.gov
arksped.k12.ar.us
Tom Hicks, Interim Associate Director
Ella Albert, Management Project Analyst
Howie Knoff, Director
Provides oversight of all educational programs for children and youth with disabilities, ages 3 to 21. Provides technical assistance to all public agencies providing educational services to this population.

State Agencies: California

2018 **California Department of Education: Special Education Division**
1430 N Street
Sacramento, CA 95814-5901
916-319-0800
Fax: 916-327-3516
scheduler@cde.ca.gov
www.cde.ca.gov
Tom Torlakson, State Superintendent of Public Instruction and Director of E
Fred Balcom, Director
Gordon Jackson, Director
Information and resources to serve the unique needs of persons with disabilities so that each person will meet or exceed high standards of achievement in academic and nonacademic skills.

State Agencies: Colorado

2019 **Colorado Department of Education: Special Education Service Unit**
Colorado Department of Education
201 E Colfax Ave
Denver, CO 80203-1704
303-866-6600
Fax: 303-830-0793
www.cde.state.co.us
Ed Steinberg, Commissioner
Provides consultation on materials and educational services for visually handicapped children, supervises volunteer services, transcribes textbooks for visually handicapped students.

State Agencies: Connecticut

2020 **Connecticut Department of Education: Bureau of Special Education**
165 Capitol Avenue
Hartford, CT 06106
860-713-6543
Fax: 860-713-7014
www.sde.ct.gov
Anne Louise Thompson, Bureau Chief
Lisa Spooner, Administrative Assistant
Regina Gaunichaux, Secretary
The State Board of Education believes each student is unique and needs an educational environment that provides for, and accommodates, his or her strengths and areas of needed improvement.

2021 **Department of Rehabilitation Services & Bureau of Education And Services for the Blind**
State of Connecticut Agency
184 Windsor Ave
Windsor, CT 06095-4536
860-602-4000
800-842-4510
Fax: 860-602-4020
TTY: 860-602-4221
brian.sigman@ct.gov
www.ct.gov/besb
The Bureau of Education and Services for the Blind (BESB), within the Department of Rehabilitation Services provides resources, comprehensive low vision services, specialized education services, life skills training, case management, and vocational services to individuals of all ages who are legally blind and to children who are visually impaired.

State Agencies: Delaware

2022 **Department of Public Instruction: Exceptional Children & Special Programs Division**
Department of Education
Ste 2
401 Federal St
Dover, DE 19901-3639
302-739-5471
Fax: 302-739-2388
www.doe.k12.de.us
Martha Toomey, Executive Director

State Agencies: DC

2023 Administration for Community Living
330 C St. SW
Washington, DC 20201   202-401-4634
                                        www.acl.gov

Anjali Forber-Pratt, Director
Alison Barkoff, Principal Deputy Administrator
Vicki Gottlich, Director, Center for Policy & Evaluation
ACL's mission is to maximize the independence and well-being of people with disabilities so that they can participate fully in society. ACL achieves its goals by funding services provided by community-based organizations and investing in research, education and innovation.

2024 District of Columbia Public Schools: Special Education Division
1200 First Street, NE
Washington, DC 20002-4210   202-442-5885
                                        202-442-5517
                                   Fax: 202-442-5026
                                        www.dcps.dc.gov

Paul L Vance MD, Superintendent
Committed to providing a continuum of services that offers students with disabilities the opportunity to actively participate in the learning environment of their neighborhood school.

2025 Federal Emergency Management Agency
500 C Street S.W.
Washington, DC 20472   202-646-2500
                                        800-621-3362
                                   TTY: 800-427-5593
                                        www.fema.gov

W. Craig Fugate, Administrator
Michael Coen, Jr., Chief of Staff
Joseph Nimmich, Deputy Administrator
FEMA's mission is to support the citizens and first responders to ensure that as a nation we work together to build, sustain and improve our capability to prepare for, protect against, respond to, recover from and mitigate all hazards.

2026 Lab School of Washington
4759 Reservoir Rd NW
Washington, DC 20007-1921   202-965-6600
                                        www.labschool.org

Mimi W. Dawson, Chair
Mac Bernstein, Vice Chair
Mike Tongour, Secretary
The Lab School six week summer session includes individualized reading, spelling, writing, study skills and math programs. A multisensory approach addresses the needs of bright learning disabled children. Related services such as speech/language therapy and occupational therapy are integrated into the curriculum. Elementary/Intermediate; Junior High/High School.

2027 National Clearinghouse on Family Support and Children's Mental Health
Ste 800
1 Dupont Cir NW
Washington, DC 20036-1149   202-939-9320
                                        800-544-3284
                                   Fax: 202-833-4760
                                        ncfy.acf.hhs.gov/

State Agencies: Florida

2028 Florida Department of Education: Bureau of Exceptional Education And Student Services
325 West Gaines Street
Turlington Building, Suite 1514
Tallahassee, FL 32399   850-245-0505
                                   Fax: 850-245-9667
                        Monica.Verra-Tirado@fldoe.org
                                        www.fldoe.org/ese

Monica Verra-Tirado, Ed.D., Bureau Chief
Gerard Robinson, Commissioner
Randy Hanna, Chancellor

Administers programs for students with disabilities and for gifted students. Coordinates student services throughout the state and participates in multiple inter-agency efforts designed to strengthen the quality and variety of services to students with special needs.

2029 Florida State College at Jacksonville Services for Students with Disabilities
501 W State St
Jacksonville, FL 32202   904-633-8100
                                        888-873-1145
                                   Fax: 904-633-5955
                                        info@fscj.edu
                                        fscj.edu

Randle P DeFoor, Chair
Cynthia A Bioteau, President
Richard Turner, Associate Vice President of Enrollment Management
Florida State College ensures acessibility of its services, activities, facilities and academic programs to students with disabilities. Special accmmodations are provided to anyone with a physical, mental or learning disability.

State Agencies: Hawaii

2030 Hawaii Department of Education: Special Needs
Hawaii Department of Education
3430 Leahi Ave
Honolulu, HI 96815-4246   808-941-3894
                                   Fax: 808-941-3894

Margaret Donovan MD, State Administrator
Provides consultation on educational services for local schools, offers psychological testing and evaluation, maintains resource rooms in district schools and more for the blind and handicapped throughout the state.

State Agencies: Illinois

2031 Illinois State Board of Education: Department of Special Education
100 N 1st St
Springfield, IL 62777   217-782-5589
                                   Fax: 217-782-0372
                                        www.isbe.net

Elizabeth Hanselman, Asst Superintendent Special Ed.
Mission is to advance the human and civil rights of people with disabilities in Illinois. Statewide advocacy organization providing self-advocacy assistance, legal services, education and public policy initiatives. Designated to implement the federal protection and advocacy system; has broad statutory power to enforce the rights of people with physical and mental disabilities, including developmental disabilities and mental illnesses.

State Agencies: Indiana

2032 Indiana Department of Education: Special Education Division
Indiana Department of Education
South Tower, Suite 600
115 W. Washington Street
Indianapolis, IN 46204-2731   877-851-4106
                                        webmaster@doe.in.gov
                                        www.doe.in.gov/

Robert A Marra, Manager
Tony Bennett, Chair
Provides consultation on educational services for local schools, offers psychological testing and evaluation, maintains resource rooms in district schools and more for the blind and handicapped throughout the state.

State Agencies: Iowa

2033   **Iowa Department of Public Instruction: Bureau of Special Education**
400 E 14th St
Des Moines, IA 50319-9000   515-457-2000
Fax: 515-242-6019
www.educateiowa.gov/

Tom Kuehl, CEO
Jason Glass, Director
Jeff Berger, Administrative Services

State Agencies: Kansas

2034   **Kansas State Board of Education: Special Education Services**
900 SW Jackson Street
Topeka, KS 66612-1212   785-296-3201
800-203-9462
Fax: 785-296-7933
TTY: 785-296-6338
contact@ksde.org
www.ksde.org

Ethan Erickson, Director
Kathy Gosa, Director
Denise Kahler, Director
Provides leadership and support for exceptional learners receiving special education services throughout Kansas schools and communities.

State Agencies: Kentucky

2035   **Kentucky Department of Education: Divisionof Exceptional Children's Services**
500 Mero St
Capital Tower Plaza
Frankfort, KY 40601   502-564-4770
Fax: 502-564-7749
www.education.ky.gov

Darlene Jesse, Director
Provides consultation on educational services for local schools, offers psychological testing and evaluation, maintains resource rooms in district schools and more for the blind and handicapped throughout the state.

State Agencies: Louisiana

2036   **Louisiana Department of Education: Office of Special Education Services**
Louisiana Department of Education
1201 North Third Street
Baton Rouge, LA 70802   225-342-0090
877-453-2721
Fax: 225-342-0193
www.doe.state.la.us

David Elder, Manager
Kim Fitch, Director Human Resources
George Nelson, President

State Agencies: Massachusetts

2037   **Getting Ready for the Outside World (G.R.O.W.)**
Riverview School
551 Route 6A East Sandwich
Cape Cod, MA 2537-1448   508-888-0489
Fax: 508-833-7001
admissions@riverviewschool.org
www.riverviewschool.org

Janice James, Vice Chairman
Deborah Cowan, Vice Chair
James Shallcross, Treasurer
Riverview School's G.R.O.W. Program is a unique ten month transitional prgoram (1-3 years) for young adults with complex language, learning and cognitive disabilities. This post secondary program is designed to further develop academic, vocational and independent living skills, to enable students to function as independently as possible.

2038   **Massachusetts Department of Education: Program Quality Assurance**
Massachusetts Department of Education
75 Pleasant Street
Malden, MA 2148-4906   781-388-3300
Fax: 617-388-3476
boe@doe.mass.edu
www.doe.mass.edu/pqa/

Pamela Kaufamann, Administrator

State Agencies: Maryland

2039   **Agency for Healthcare Research and Quality**
540 Gaither Road
Rockville, MD 20850   301-427-1364
www.ahrq.gov
Richard G. Kronick, PhD, Director, Director
Sharon B. Arnold, PhD, Deputy Director
The Agency for Healthcare Research and Quality's (AHRQ) mission is to produce evidence to make health care safer, higher quality, more accessible, equitable, and affordable, and to work within the U.S. Department of Health and Human Services and with other partners to make sure that the evidence is understood and used.

2040   **Center for Mental Health Services**
5600 Fishers Lane
Rockville, MD 20857   877-726-4727
TTY: 800-487-4889
samhsainfo@samhsa.hhs.gov
www.samhsa.gov
Tom Coderre, Acting Deputy Assistant Secretary
Sonia Chessen, Chief of Staff
Trina Dutta, Senior Advisor
The Center for Mental Health Services leads federal efforts to promote the prevention and treatment of mental disorders.

2041   **Centers for Medicare & Medicaid Services**
7500 Security Blvd.
Baltimore, MD 21244   410-786-3000
877-267-2323
TTY: 866-226-1819
www.cms.gov

Chiquita Brooks-LaSure, Administrator
Jonathan Blum, Principal Deputy Administrator
Karen Jackson, Deputy Chief Operating Officer
US federal agency which administers Medicare, Medicaid, and the State Children's Health Insurance Program.

2042 Maryland State Department of Education: Division of Special Education
200 West Baltimore Street
Baltimore, MD 21201-2595   410-767-0100
                                 888-246-0016
                            Fax: 410-333-8165
                    www.marylandpublicschools.org
Nancy S Grasmick, State Superintendent
Dr. Lillian Lowery, Superintendent of Schools
James V. Foran, Assistant State Superintendent
Collaborates with families, local early intervention systems, and local school systems to ensure that all children and youth with disabilities have access to appropriate services and educational opportunities to which they are entitled under federal and state laws.

2043 National Human Genome Research Institute
National Institutes of Health
Building 31, Room 4B09
31 Center Drive, MSC 2152
Bethesda, MD 20892-2152   301-402-0911
                            Fax: 301-402-2218
                            lbrody@mail.nih.gov
                            www.genome.gov
Eric D. Green, M.D., Ph.D., Director
Lawrence Brody, Ph.D., Director
Bettie Graham, Ph.D., Director
The National Human Genome Research Institute began as the National Center for Human Genome Research (NCHGR), which was established in 1989 to carry out the role of the National Institutes of Health (NIH) in the International Human Genome Project (HGP).

2044 National Institute of General Medical Sciences
45 Center Drive MSC 6200
Bethesda, MD 20892-6200   301-496-7301
                            info@nigms.nih.gov
                            www.nigms.nih.gov
Jon R. Lorsch, Ph.D., Director
Judith H. Greenberg, Ph.D., Deputy Director
Ann Hagan, Ph.D., Associate Director
The National Institute of General Medical Sciences (NIGMS) supports basic research that increases understanding of biological processes and lays the foundation for advances in disease diagnosis, treatment and prevention.

State Agencies: Michigan

2045 Michigan Department of Education: Special Education Services
608 W. Allegan Street
PO Box 30008
Lansing, MI 48909   517-373-3324
                            Fax: 517-373-7504
                    DHS-OCS-PEP@michigan.gov
                    www.michigan.gov/mde
John C. Austin, President
Kathleen N. Straus, President of the State Board
Michelle Fecteau, Executive Director
Oversees the administrative funding of education and early intervention programs and services for young children and students with disabilities.

2046 Services for Students with Disabilities
University of Michigan
G-664 Haven Hall
505 South State St.
Ann Arbor, MI 48109-1045   734-763-3000
                            Fax: 734-936-3947
                            TTY: 734-615-4461
                            ssdoffice@umich.edu
                            www.ssd.umich.edu
Stuart Segal, Director
Offers information to students of the University of Michigan and their parents.

State Agencies: Minnesota

2047 Community Supports for People with Disabilities (CSP)
South Central Technical College (SCTC)
1920 Lee Blvd
North Mankato, MN 56003-2504   507-389-7200
                                 800-722-9359
                            online@southcentral.edu
                            www.southcentral.edu
Christensen Tami, Executive Director
Keith Stover, President
Human services program available as a physical or online program, designed for those wanting to earn a certificate, diploma or associate degree as a Direct Support Professional for use in the health and human services industries. The program comprises eight courses relating to professional services and support for people with disabilities.

2048 Professional Development Programs
6303 Osgood Ave. N.
Ste 104
Stillwater, MN 55082   651-439-8865
                                 877-439-8865
                            Fax: 877-259-5906
                            www.pdppro.com
Cindy Lacosse, VP
Lori Lacrosse, President
Sponsors cutting edge and popular continuing education workshops and symposia of interest to professionals who provide services to children and adults with special needs.

State Agencies: Missouri

2049 Missouri Department of Elementary and Secondary Education: Special Education Programs
205 Jefferson St
PO Box 480
Jefferson City, MO 65102   573-751-5739
                            Fax: 573-526-4404
                            TTY: 800-735-2966
Stephen Barr, Assistant Commissioner
The Office of Special Education administers state and federal funds to support services for students and adults with disabilities.

State Agencies: Mississippi

2050 Mississippi Department of Education: Office of Special Services
359 North West Street
P.O. Box 771
Jackson, MS 39201   601-359-3513
                            Fax: 601-987-3892
Dr Tom Burnham, Superintendent
Key priorities are: reading, early literacy, student achievement, teachers/teaching, leadership/principals, safe and orderly schools, parent relations/community involvement, and technology.

State Agencies: Montana

2051 Department of Public Health Human Services
PO Box 4210
Helena, MT 59604-4210   406-444-5622
                            Fax: 406-444-1970
                            www.dphhs.mt.gov
Anna Whitin Sorrell, Director
Bernie Jacobs, Chief Legal Counsel
Deb Sloat, Human Resources Office
Provides consultation on educational services for local schools, offers psychological testing and evaluation, maintains resource rooms in district schools and more for the blind and handicapped throughout the state.

State Agencies: North Carolina

2052 National Institute of Environmental Health Sciences
111 T.W. Alexander Drive
Research Triangle Park, NC 27709   919-541-4580
birnbaumls@niehs.nih.gov
www.niehs.nih.gov
Linda S. Birnbaum, Ph.D., Director
Richard Woychik, Ph.D., Deputy Director
Sheila A. Newton, Ph.D., Policy, Planning, and Evaluation
The mission of the NIEHS is to discover how the environment affects people in order to promote healthier lives.

**2053 North Carolina Department of Public Instruction:
Exceptional Children Division**
301 N Wilmington St
Raleigh, NC 27601   919-807-3300
Fax: 919-715-1569
www.ncpublicschools.org
June St. Clair Atkinson, Ed.D, State Superintendent of Public Instruction
Mike McLaughlin, Senior Policy Advisor to the State Superintendent
Rachel Beaulieu, Legislative & Community Affairs Director
The mission is to assure that students with disabilities develop mentally, physically, emotionally, and vocationally through the provision of an appropriate individualized education in the least restrictive environment.

State Agencies: North Dakota

**2054 North Dakota Department of Education: Special
Education**
600 E. Boulevard Avenue, Dept. 201
Floors 9, 10, and 11
Bismarck, ND 58505-0440   701-328-2260
866-741-3519
Fax: 701-328-2461
TTY: 701-328-4920
mdanderson@nd.gov
www.dpi.state.nd.us
Kirsten Baesler, State Superintendent
Jerry Coleman, Director, School Finance & Organization
Linda Schloer, Child Nutrition & Food Distribution, Director
Provides consultation on educational services for local schools, offers psychological testing and evaluation, maintains resource rooms in district schools and more for the blind and handicapped throughout the state.

State Agencies: Nebraska

**2055 Nebraska Department of Education: Special Populations
Office**
1200 N Street, Suite 400
PO Box 98922
Lincoln, NE 68509   402-471-2186
877-253-2603
Fax: 402-471-2909
NDEQ.moreinfo@Nebraska.gov
deq.ne.gov
Rod Gangwish Shelton, Council Member
Douglas Anderson Aurora, Council Member
Mark Whitehead Lincoln, Council Member
Assists school districts in establishing and maintaining effective special education programs for children with disabilities (date of diagnosis through the school year when a child reaches 21). Major function: provide technical assistance to school districts and to parents of children with disabilities, assist programs in meeting state and federal special education regulations. Also responsible for assuring that the rights of children with disabilities and their parents are protected.

State Agencies: New Hampshire

2056 Institute on Disability
University of New Hampshire
10 West Edge Drive
Suite 101
Durham, NH 03824   603-862-4320
Fax: 603-862-0555
contact.iod@unh.edu
www.iod.unh.edu
Charles E. Drum, Director & Professor
Andrew Houtenville, Director of Research
Matthew Gianino, Director of Communications
Provides coherent university-based focus for the improvement of knowledge, policies, and practices related to the lives of persons with disabilities and their families.

**2057 New Hampshire Department of Education: Bureau for
Special Education Services**
101 Pleasant Street
Concord, NH 03301-3860   603-271-3494
Fax: 603-271-1953
Lori.Temple@doe.nh.gov
www.education.nh.gov
Santina Thibedeau, Administrator
Virginia Barry, Commissioner
Linda Breden, Secretary
The mission of Special Education is to improve educational outcomes for children and youth with disabilities by providing and promoting leadership, technical assistance and collaboration statewide. Provides oversight and implementation of federal and state laws that ensure a free appropriate public education for all children and youth with disabilities in New Hampshire.

State Agencies: New Jersey

**2058 New Jersey Department of Education: Office of Special
Education Program**
New Jersey Department of Education
PO Box 500
Trenton, NJ 8625-500   609-292-0147
Fax: 609-984-8422
www.nj.gov/education/specialed/info/
Barbara Gantwerk, Director
Alfred Murray, Executive Director

2059 New Jersey Speech-Language-Hearing Association
174 Nassau St
Suite 337
Princeton, NJ 08542   888-906-5742
Fax: 888-729-3489
info@njsha.org
njsha.org
Mary Faella, President
Robynne Kratchman, Vice President
Joan Warner, Treasurer
The New Jersey Speech-Language-Hearing Association offers services to audiologists, speech-language pathologists, and scientists studying in these fields. Services include resources, advocacy, information and programs to help foster professional development.

2060 The Arc of New Jersey
985 Livingston Ave
North Brunswick, NJ 08902   732-246-2525
Fax: 732-214-1834
info@arcnj.org
arcnj.org
Joanne Bergin, President
Thomas Baffuto, Executive Director
Celine Fortin, Associate Executive Director
The Arc of New Jersey is committed to enhancing the quality of life of children and adults with intellectual and developmental disabilities and their families, through advocacy, empowerment, education and prevention.

State Agencies: New Mexico

2061 New Mexico State Department of Education
300 Don Gaspar Ave
Santa Fe, NM 87501-2744   505-827-6508
Fax: 505-827-6696
www.sde.state.nm.us

Bill Trant, Assistant Director
Judy Parks, Assistant Director
Provides consultation on educational services for local schools, offers psychological testing and evaluation, maintains resource rooms in district schools and more for the blind and handicapped throughout the state.

State Agencies: Nevada

2062 Nevada Department of Education: Special Eduction Branch
700 E Fifth St
Carson City, NV 89701-5096   775-687-9800
Fax: 775-687-9101
www.doe.nv.gov

Nick Gakalatos, Manager
The Office of Special Ed and School Improvement Program of the Nevada State Department of Education is responsible for management of state and federal programs providing educational opportunities for students with diverse learning needs. Included are such programs as: special education/disabled (IDEA); disadvantaged/at-risk programs (Title I/IASA); early childhood programs (Title I/ESEA); early childhood programs; migrant education; English language learners; NRS 395 student placement program.

State Agencies: New York

2063 New York State Education Department
1606 One Commerce Plz
Albany, NY 12234   518-474-5930
Fax: 518-486-6880
www.nysed.gov

Bernard Margolis, Manager
Provides vocational rehabilitation and educational services for eligible individuals with disabilities throughout New York State. Services include evaluation, counseling, job placement, and referral to other agencies.

State Agencies: Ohio

2064 Ohio Department of Education: Division of Special Education
Ohio Department of Education
25 S Front St
Columbus, OH 43215-4183   614-995-1545
877-644-6338
Fax: 614-728-1097
TTY: 888-886-0181
www.ode.state.oh.us

Mike Armstrong, Manager
Provides technical assistance to educational agencies for the development and implementation of educational services to meet the needs of students with disabilities and/or those who are gifted. Provides information to parents. Administers state and federal funds allocated to educational agencies for the provision of services to students with disabilities and/or those who are gifted.

2065 The Arc of Allen County
546 S Collett St
Lima, OH 45805   419-225-6285
Fax: 419-228-7770
info@thearcofohio.org
www.arcallencounty.org

Brad Perrott, Executive Director
Vicki Alves, Day Service Manager
Lisa Hengstler, Office Assistant
Offers services to people with intellectual and developmental disabilities. Some programs include day care, educational training, human rights advocacy, and information and referral.

State Agencies: Oklahoma

2066 Oklahoma State Department of Education
2500 N Lincoln Blvd
Oklahoma City, OK 73105-4599   405-521-3301
Fax: 405-521-6205

Misty Kimbrough, Manager
Sandy Garrett, Administrator
Janet Barresi, State Superintendent
Provides consultation on educational services for local schools, offers psychological testing and evaluation, maintains resource rooms in district schools and more for the blind and handicapped throughout the state.

State Agencies: Oregon

2067 Oregon Department of Education: Office of Special Education
Oregon Department of Education:
255 Capitol St NE
Salem, OR 97310-1300   503-945-5600
Fax: 503-378-2897
www.dpeducation.com

Bruce Goldberg, Manager
Heidi Cockrell, Executive Assistant
Katy Coba, Executive Director
State agency ensuring provision of special education services to children with disabilities from birth to age 21.

State Agencies: Pennsylvania

2068 Pennsylvania Department of Education: Bureau of Special Education
333 Market St
Harrisburg, PA 17126-333   717-783-6788
Fax: 717-783-6139
TTY: 717-783-8445
00specialed@psupen.psu.edu
www.pde.state.pa.us

Linda Rhen, Administrator
John Tommasini, Assistant Director
Provides effective and efficient administration of the Commonwealth of Pennsylvania's resources dedicated to enabling school districts to maintain high standards in the delivery of special education services and programs for all exceptional students.

State Agencies: Rhode Island

2069 Rhode Island Department of Education: Office of Special Needs
255 Westminster St
Providence, RI 2903   401-222-4600
Fax: 401-784-9513
www.ride.ri.gov

Al Moscola, Manager
Alfred Moscola, Manager
Provides consultation on educational services for local schools, offers psychological testing and evaluation, maintains resource

rooms in district schools and more for the blind and handicapped throughout the state.

State Agencies: South Carolina

2070 South Carolina Assistive Technology Program (SCATP)
Center for Disability Resources
8301 Farrow Rd
Columbia, SC 29208-3245
803-935-5263
800-915-4522
Fax: 800-935-5342
www.sc.edu/scatp

Carol Page, Program Director
Mary Bechter, Program Coordinator
SCATP is a federally funded project concerned with getting technology into th hands of people with disabilities so that they might live, work, learn and be a more independent part of the community.

2071 South Carolina Department of Education: Office of Exceptional Children
1429 Senate St
Suite 808
Columbia, SC 29201-3730
803-734-8224
Fax: 803-734-4824
sdeservicedesk@sde.ok.gov
www.scschools.com

Susan Durant, State Director
Provides consultation on educational services for local schools, offers psychological testing and evaluation, maintains resource rooms in district schools and more for the blind and handicapped throughout the state.

State Agencies: South Dakota

2072 South Dakota Department of Education & Cultural Affairs: Office of Special Education
700 Governors Dr
Pierre, SD 57501-2291
605-773-3804
Fax: 605-773-6041

Chelle Somsen, Manager
Dorothy Liegl, Manager

State Agencies: Tennessee

2073 Tennessee Department of Education
710 James Robertson Pkwy
Nashville, TN 37243-1219
615-741-2731
888-212-3162
Fax: 615-741-1791

Ruth S Letson, Manager
Kevin Huffman, Commissioner
Provides consultation on educational services for local schools, offers psychological testing and evaluation, maintains resource rooms in district schools and more for the blind and handicapped throughout the state.

State Agencies: Texas

2074 Texas Education Agency
1701 N Congress Ave
Austin, TX 78701-1494
512-463-8532
Fax: 512-463-8057
www.tealighthouse.org

Shirley J Neeley, Commissioner of Education
Provides consultation on educational services for local schools, offers psychological testing and evaluation, maintains resource rooms in district schools and more for the blind and handicapped throughout the state.

2075 Texas Education Agency: Special Education Unit
1701 Congress Ave
PO Box 420637
Austin, TX 77242-637
512-463-8532
Fax: 512-463-8057
info@tdea.org
www.tdea.org

Gene Lenz, Deputy Associate Commissioner
Shirley Neeley, Administrator

2076 Texas School of the Deaf
1102 S Congress Ave
Austin, TX 78704-1791
512-462-5353
800-332-3873
Fax: 512-462-5424
ercod@tsd.state.tx.us
tsd.state.tx.us

Claire Bugen, Superintendent
Russell West, Residential Services Director
Gary Bego, Business and Operations Director
Ensures that students excel in an environment where they learn, grow and belong. Supports deaf students, families and professionals in Texas by providing resources through outreach services.

State Agencies: Utah

2077 Utah State Office of Education: At-Risk and Special Education Service Unit
Utah State Office of Education
250 East 500 South
P.O.Box 144200
Salt Lake City, UT 84114-4200
801-538-7500
Fax: 801-538-7521
webmaster@schools.utah.gov
schools.utah.gov

Sandra Cox, Financial Analyst
Mark Peterson, Director
Glenna Gallo, State Director of Special Educat
Provides consultation on educational services for local schools, offers psychological testing and evaluation, maintains resource rooms in district schools and more for the blind and handicapped throughout the state.

State Agencies: Virginia

2078 National Science Foundation
4201 Wilson Blvd
Arlington, VA 22230
703-292-5111
TTY: 703-292-5090
info@nsf.gov
www.nsf.gov

France A. Cérdova, Director
Richard O. Buckius, Chief Operating Officer
Michael Van Woert, Executive Officer/Director
NSF is the only federal agency whose mission includes support for all fields of fundamental science and engineering, except for medical sciences.

2079 Virginia Department of Education: Divisionof Pre & Early Adolescent Education
Virginia Department Of Education
James Monroe Building, 101, N. 14th
P.O.Box 2120
Richmond, VA 23219
804-236-3631
Fax: 804-236-3635
webmaster@doe.virginia.gov
www.pen.k12.va.us

Dr. Steven R Staples, Superintendent of Public Instruction
Kent Dickey, Deputy Superintendent, Finance & Operations
Chris Sorensen, Director, Budget
Provides consultation on educational services for local schools, offers psychological testing and evaluation, maintains resource rooms in district schools and more for the blind and handicapped throughout the state.

State Agencies: Washington

2080 Superintendent of Public Instruction: Special Education Section
Old Capitol Building, 600 Washingto
P.O. Box 47200
Olympia, WA 98504-7200   360-725-6000
                               Fax: 360-586-0247
                               TTY: 360-664-3631
                               www.k12.wa.us
Randy I. Dorn, State Superintendent of Public I
Alan Burke, Deputy Superintendent
Robert Butts, Assistant Superintendent
Provides leadership, service and support for the development and implementation of research-based curriculum to assure that all learners achieve at all levels.

State Agencies: West Virginia

2081 West Virginia Department of Education: Office of Special Education
Rm 6
1900 Kanawha Blvd E
Charleston, WV 25305-0001   304-558-3660
                                   Fax: 304-558-3741
                                   wvde.state.wv.us
Liza Cordeiro, Executive Director
Mary Nunn, Assistant Director
Marshall Patton, Executive Director
Provides consultation on educational services for local schools, offers psychological testing and evaluation, maintains resource rooms in district schools and more for the blind and handicapped throughout the state.

State Agencies: Wyoming

2082 Wyoming Department of Education
2300 Capitol Avenue
Hathaway Building, 2nd Floor
Cheyenne, WY 82002-2060   307-777-7690
                                 Fax: 307-777-6234
                                 edu.wyoming.gov
Cindy Hill, WDE Superintendent
Deb Lindsey, Division Administrator, Assessment
Teri Wigert, Division Administrator, Support Systems & Resources
Mission is to lead, model, and support continuous improvement of education for everyone in Wyoming.

Magazines & Journals

2083 Adapted Physical Activity Programs
Human Kinetics
1607 N. Market Street
P.O.Box 5076
Champaign, IL 61820   800-747-4457
                             Fax: 217-351-1549
                             info@hkusa.com
                             www.humankinetics.com
Patty Lehn, Publicity Manager
Lori Cooper, Marketing Manager
Bill Dobrik, Sales Associate
Human Kinetics produces a variety of resources for adapted physical education practitioners, including books on activities, a research journal and higher education references. *$24.00*
Quarterly
ISSN 0736-58 9

2084 Advance for Providers of Post-Acute Care
Merion Publications
2900 Horizon Drive
King of Prussia, PA 19406   610-278-1400
                                   800-355-5627
                                   Fax: 610-278-1421
                                   webmaster@advanceweb.com
                                   advanceweb.com
Timothy Baum, MS, CRNP, Author
A free magazine for providers of post-acute care.

2085 American Journal of Occupational Therapy (AJOT)
American Occupational Therapy Association
6116 Executive Blvd.
Suite 200
North Bethesda, MD 20852-4929   301-652-6611
                                       800-729-2682
                                       customerservice@aota.org
                                       ajot.aota.org
Sherry Keramidas, Executive Director
Neil Harvison, Chief Officer, Knowledge Division
Matthew Clark, Chief Officer, Innovation & Engagement
Official peer-reviewed publication of the American Occupational Therapy Association.
6 issues/year

2086 American Journal on Intellectual and Developmental Disabilities (AJIDD)
AAIDD
8403 Colesville Rd.
Suite 900
Silver Spring, MD 20910   202-387-1968
                                 Fax: 202-387-2193
                                 books@aaidd.org
                                 aaidd.org
Frank Symons, PhD, Editor
American Journal on Intellectual and Developmental Disabilities (AJIDD)is a scientific, scholarly, and archival multidisciplinary journal for reporting original contributions to knowledge of intellectual disability, its causes, treatment, and prevention.
Bimonthly

2087 Behavioral Disorders
Council for Exceptional Children
3100 Clarendon Blvd.
Suite 600
Arlington, VA 22201-5332   888-232-7733
                                  TTY: 866-915-5000
                                  services@exceptionalchildren.org
                                  www.exceptionalchildren.org
Bryan G. Cook, Editor
Provides professionals with a means to exchange information and share ideas related to research, empirically tested educational innovations and issues and concerns relevant to students with behavioral disorders.
Quarterly

2088 CEC Catalog
Council for Exceptional Children
3100 Clarendon Blvd.
Suite 600
Arlington, VA 22201-5332   888-232-7733
                                  TTY: 866-915-5000
                                  service@exceptionalchildren.org
                                  www.exceptionalchildren.org/store
Chad Rummel, Executive Director
Laurie VanderPloeg, Associate Executive Director, Professional Affairs
Craig Evans, Chief Financial Officer
Catalog from the Council for Exceptional Children offering books, guides, materials, and specialty items for special educators.

2089   Career Development and Transition for Exceptional Individuals
2455 Teller Road
Thousand Oaks, CA 91320
800-818-7243
Fax: 800-583-2665
journals@sagepub.com
cde.sagepub.com

Blaise R. Simqu, President/ CEO
Tracey A. Ozmina, EVP/ COO
Chris Hickok, SVP/ CFO
Career Development and Transition for Exceptional Individuals (CDTEI) specializes in the fields of secondary education, transition, and career development for persons with documented disabilities and special needs.

2090   Case Manager Magazine
Elsevier Health
3251 Riverport Lane
Maryland Heights, MO 63043
314-447-8070
800-222-9570
textbook@elsevier.com

Thomas Reller, Vice President Global Corporate
Harald Boersma, Senior Manager Corporate Relatio
Ylann Schemm, Corporate Relations Manager
This national magazine is for medical case managers, social workers, counselors and home health professionals who work with people with serious injury or illness. It is a membership benefit of CMSA, the national association for case managers. *$55.00*
84 pages BiMonthly

2091   Catalyst
The Catalyst
Ste 275
1259 El Camino Real
Menlo Park, CA 94025-4208
800-647-0314
Sue Swezey, Editor
Digest of news and information on the use of computers in special education. *$15.00*
20 pages Quarterly

2092   Challenge Magazine
451 Hungerford Drive
Suite 100
Rockville, MD 20850
301-217-0960
Fax: 301-217-0968
Info@dsusa.org
www.disabledsportsusa.org

Kirk Bauer, Executive Director
Claire Duffy, Program Coordinator
Orlando Gill, Field Representative
Challenge Magazine is a publication of Disabled Sports USA, providing adaptive sports information to adults and children with disabilities, including those who are visually impaired, amputees, spinal cord injured (paraplegic and quadriplegic), and those who have multiple sclerosis, head injury, cerebral palsy, autism and other related intellectual disabilities.

2093   Clinical Connection
American Advertising Dist of Northern Virginia
708 Pendleton St
Alexandria, VA 22314-1819
703-549-5126
Fax: 703-548-5563
Kathie Harrington, M.A., CCC, Author
Covers speech language pathology.

2094   College and University
AACRAO
One Dupont Circle NW
Suite 520
Washington, DC 20036
202-293-9161
Fax: 202-872-8857
reillym@aacrao.org
aacrao.org

Brad Myers, President
Dan Garcia, President Elect
Adrienne McDay, Past President
Scholarly research journal. American Association of Collegiate Registrars and Admissions Offers (AACRAO) is a nonprofit, voluntary, professional, educational association of degree-granting, postsecondary institutions, government agencies, private educa-

tional organizations and education-oriented businesses in the United States and abroad. $80 per year US; $90 per year international.
30 pages Quarterly
ISSN 0010-0889

2095   Communication Disorders Quarterly
2455 Teller Road
Thousand Oaks, CA 91320
800-818-7243
Fax: 800-583-2665
journals@sagepub.com
cde.sagepub.com

Blaise R. Simqu, President/ CEO
Tracey A. Ozmina, EVP/ COO
Chris Hickok, SVP/ CFO
Communication Disorders Quarterly (CDQ) presents cutting edge information on typical and atypical communication — from oral language development to literacy.

2096   Continuing Care
Stevens Publishing Corporation
14901 Quorum Dr,
Suite 425
Dallas, TX 75254
972-687-6700
Fax: 972-687-6750
info@1105media.com
1105media.com

Neal Vitale, President & Chief Executive Officer
Richard Vitale, Senior Vice President & Chief Financial Officer
Mike Valenti, Executive Vice President
A national magazine for case management and discharge planning professionals published monthly except for December.
$119.00
34 pages Monthly

2097   Counseling & Values
American Counseling Association
P.O. Box 31110
Suite 600
Alexandria, VA 22310-9998
800-347-6647
Fax: 800-473-2329
ahconley@vcu.edu
www.counseling.org

Richard Yep, Chief Executive Officer
Abigail H. Conley, Editor
Counseling and Values is the official journal of the Association for Spiritual, Ethical, and Religious Values in Counseling (ASERVIC), a member association of the American Counseling Association. Counseling and Values is a professional journal of theory, research, and informed opinion concerned with the relationships among psychology, philosophy, religion, social values, and counseling. *$20.00*
Bi-annual

2098   Counseling Psychologist
American Psychological Association
2455 Teller Road
Thousand Oaks, CA 91320
805-499-0721
800-818-7243
Fax: 800-583-2665
info@sagepub.com
www.sagepub.com

Sara Miller McCune, Founder, Publisher & Executive Chairman
Blaise R Simqu, President/CEO
Chris Hickok, Senior Vice President & Chief Financial Officer
Thematic issues in the theory, research and practice of counseling psychology. *$78.00*
Bi-Monthly

2099   Counselor Education & Supervision
American Counseling Association
P.O. Box 31110
Alexandria, VA 22310
800-347-6647
Fax: 800-473-2329
acesjournal@gmail.com
www.counseling.org

Richard Yep, Chief Executive Officer
James S. Korcuska, Editor

Dedicated to the growth and development of the counseling profession and those who are served. *$14.00*
Quarterly

2100   Disability & Society
711 3rd Avenue
8th Floor
New York, NY 10017   212-216-7800
                                           800-634-7064
                                      Fax: 212-564-7854
                                      www.routledge.com
Len Barton, Author
The study of disability has traditionally been influenced mainly by medical and psychological models. The aim of this new text, Disability and Society, is to open up the debate by introducing alternative perspectives reflecting the increasing sociological interest in this important topic.

2101   Disability Studies Quarterly
552 Park Hall
Buffalo, NY 14260-4130   marembis@buffalo.edu
                                           dsq-sds.org
Michael Rembis, Interim Editor-in-Chief
Tanja Aho, Interim Managing Editor
Disability Studies Quarterly (DSQ) is the journal of the Society for Disability Studies (SDS). It is a multidisciplinary and international journal of interest to social scientists, scholars in the humanities, disability rights advocates, creative writers, and others concerned with the issues of people with disabilities.

2102   Disability and Health Journal
American Association on Health and Disabiity
110 N Washington St.
Suite 407
Rockville, MD 20850   301-545-6140
                                      Fax: 301-545-6144
                                      contact@aahd.us
                            www.aahd.us/disability-and-health-journal
Monika Mitra, Editor
Margaret A. Turk, Editor
Disability and Health Journal is a scientific, scholarly and multidisciplinary journal for reporting original contributions that advance knowledge in disability and health.

2103   Early Intervention
Early Childhood Intervention Clearinghouse
51 Gerty Drive
Room 20
Champaign, IL 61820-7469   217-333-1386
                                           877-275-3227
                                      Fax: 217-244-7732
                                      Illinois-eic@illinois.edu
                                      www.eiclearinghouse.org
Susan Fowler, Director
Features articles, conference calendar, material reviews and news concerning early childhood intervention and disability.
4 pages Quarterly

2104   Emerging Horizon
PO Box 278
Ripon, CA 95366-0278   209-599-9409
                                      emerginghorizons.com
Travel information for wheel chair users and slow walkers.

2105   Exceptional Children (EC)
Council for Exceptional Children
3100 Clarendon Blvd.
Suite 600
Arlington, VA 22201-5332   888-232-7733
                                      TTY: 866-915-5000
                            service@exceptionalchildren.org
                            www.exceptionalchildren.org
John Wills Lloyd, Editor
William Therrien, Editor
Peer-reviewed journal with articles including research, literature surveys and position papers concerning exceptional children, special education and mainstreaming.
Quarterly

2106   Focus on Autism and Other Developmental Disabilities
Sage Publications
2455 Teller Road
Thousand Oaks, CA 91320   805-499-0721
                                           800-818-7243
                                      Fax: 800-583-2665
                                      info@sagepub.com
                                      www.sagepub.com
Sara Miller McCune, Founder, Publisher & Executive Chairman
Blaise R. Simqu, President & CEO
Chris Hickok, Senior Vice President & Chief Financial Officer
Practical management, treatment and planning strategies; a must for persons working with individuals with autism and other developmental disabilities. *$43.00*
64 pages Quarterly

2107   Focus on Exceptional Children
Love Publishing Company
9101 East Kenyon Avenue
Suite 2200
Denver, CO 80237   303-221-7333
                                      Fax: 303-221-7444
                                      lpc@lovepublishing.com
                                      www.lovepublishing.com
Steve Graham, Consulting Editor
Ron Nelson, Consulting Editor
Eva Horn, Consulting Editor
Contains research and theory-based articles on special education topics, with an emphasis on application and intervention, of interest to teachers, professors and administrators. *$36.00*
Monthly

2108   HerbalGram
American Botanical Council
6200 Manor Rd.
Austin, TX 78723-4345   512-926-4900
                                           800-373-7105
                                      Fax: 512-926-2345
                                      abc@herbalgram.org
                                      herbalgram.org
Mark Blumenthal, Founder, Executive Director & Editor
Tyler Smith, Editor
Hannah Bauman, Associate Editor
Official quarterly journal of the American Botanical Council.

2109   HomeCare Magazine
Cahaba Media Group
1900-28th Ave S.
Ste 200
Birmingham, AL 35209   205-212-9402
                                      cahabamedia.com
Wally Evans, Publisher
Greg Meineke, Vice President, Sales
Stephanie Gibson Lepore, Editor
The business magazine of the home medical equipment industry offering information on legislation and regulations affecting the homecare industry, monthly profiles of suppliers, operational tips, newest products in the industry, advice on sales, government regulations. *$ 65.00*
120 pages Monthly

2110   I Wonder Who Else Can Help
AARP
601 E Street NW
Washington, DC 20049   202-434-3525
                                           888-687-2277
                                           877-342-2277
                                      Fax: 202-434-3443
                                      member@aarp.org
                                      www.aarp.org
John Wider, President, CEO, AARP Services Inc.
Lisa M. Ryerson, President, AARP Foundation
Robert R. Hagans, Jr., Executive Vice President & Chief Financial Officer
Contains information about crisis counseling, needs and resources, written in lay terms.

2111 Inclusion
AAIDD
8403 Colesville Rd.
Suite 900
Silver Spring, MD 20910   202-387-1968
                                 Fax: 202-387-2193
                                 books@aaidd.org
                                 aaidd.org
Colleen Thoma, Co-Editor
LaRon Scott, Co-Editor
Inclusionis an open submission ejournal. Inclusion is published
quarterly in an online-only format, enabling timely dissemina-
tion of emerging and promising research, policy, and practices.
Quarterly

2112 Intellectual and Developmental Disabilities (IDD)
AAIDD
8403 Colesville Rd.
Suite 900
Silver Spring, MD 20910   202-387-1968
                                 Fax: 202-387-2193
                                 books@aaidd.org
                                 aaidd.org
James R. Thompson, Editor
Intellectual and Developmental Disabilities (IDD) is a peer re-
viewed multidisciplinary journal disseminating information on
policies, practices, and concepts relating to intellectual and de-
velopmental disabilities.
Bimonthly

2113 Intervention in School and Clinic
Sage Publications
2455 Teller Road
Thousand Oaks, CA 91320   805-499-0721
                                 800-818-7243
                                 Fax: 800-583-2665
                                 info@sagepub.com
                                 www.sagepub.com
Sara Miller McCune, Founder, Publisher & Executive Chairman
Blaise R. Simqu, President & CEO
Chris Hickok, Senior Vice President & Chief Financial Officer
A hands-on, how-to resource for teachers and clinicians working
with students for whom minor curriculum and environmental
modifications are ineffective. *$35.00*
64 pages

2114 Journal of Addictions & Offender Counseling
American Counseling Association
P.O. Box 31110
Alexandria, VA 22310-9998   703-823-9800
                                 800-347-6647
                                 Fax: 800-473-2329
                                 jaoc.iaaoc@utoledo.edu
                                 www.counseling.org
Richard Yep, Chief Executive Officer
John M. Laux, Editor
Official journal of the International Association of Addictions
and Offender Counselors, a member association of the American
Counseling Association. Contains information on programs, the-
ory, and research into addictions and offender counseling. *$25.00*
Bi-annual

2115 Journal of Applied School Psychology
Haworth Press
711 Third Avenue
New York, NY 10017   212-216-7800
                                 800-354-1420
                                 Fax: 212-244-1563
                                 subscriptions@tandf.co.uk
                                 www.haworthpress.com
This journal disseminates the latest and the highest quality information to all professionals who provide special services in the
schools and related educational settings. Haworth Press are now
acquired by the Taylor & Francis Journals. *$60.00*
BiAnnually

2116 Journal of Counseling & Development
American Counseling Association
P.O. Box 31110
Alexandria, VA 22310-9998   800-347-6647
                                 Fax: 800-473-2329
                                 jcd@unt.edu
                                 www.counseling.org
Richard Yep, Chief Executive Officer
Matthew Lemberger-Truelove, Editor
Publishes practice, theory, and research articles across 18 differ-
ent counseling and development specialty areas. Sections include
research, assessment and diagnosis, theory and practice, and
trends. *$35.00*
128 pages Quarterly

2117 Journal of Disability Policy Studies
2455 Teller Road
Thousand Oaks, CA 91320   800-818-7243
                                 Fax: 800-583-2665
                                 journals@sagepub.com
                                 cde.sagepub.com
Blaise R. Simqu, President/ CEO
Tracey A. Ozmina, EVP/ COO
Chris Hickok, SVP/ CFO
Journal of Disability Policy Studies (DPS) addresses compelling
variable issues in ethics, policy and law related to individuals
with disabilities.

2118 Journal of Emotional and Behavioral Disorders
Sage Publications
2455 Teller Road
Thousand Oaks, CA 91320   805-499-0721
                                 800-818-7243
                                 Fax: 800-583-2665
                                 info@sagepub.com
                                 www.sagepub.com
Sara Miller McCune, Founder, Publisher & Executive Chairman
Blaise R. Simqu, President & CEO
Chris Hickok, Senior Vice President & Chief Financial Officer
An international, multidisciplinary journal featuring articles on
research, practice and theory related to individuals with emotional and behavioral disorders and to the professionals who
serve them. *$39.00*
64 pages Quarterly

2119 Journal of Learning Disabilities
Sage Publications
2455 Teller Road
Thousand Oaks, CA 91320   805-499-0721
                                 800-818-7243
                                 Fax: 800-583-2665
                                 info@sagepub.com
                                 www.sagepub.com
Sara Miller McCune, Founder, Publisher & Executive Chairman
Blaise R. Simqu, President & CEO
Chris Hickok, Senior Vice President & Chief Financial Officer
An international, multidisciplinary publication containing arti-
cles on practice, research and theory related to learning disabili-
ties. Published bi-monthly. *$49.00*
Magazine

2120 Journal of Midwifery & Women's Health (JMWH)
American College of Nurse Midwives
8403 Colesville Rd.
Suite 1230
Silver Spring, MD 20910   240-485-1800
                                 Fax: 240-485-1818
                                 membership@acnm.org
                                 midwife.org
Melissa Avery, Editor-in-Chief
Laura Bolte, Managing Editor
Ira Kantrowitz-Gordon, Deputy Editor
Official journal of the American College of Nurse Midwives.

2121 Journal of Motor Behavior
Heldref Publications
325 Chestnut Street
Suite 800
Philadelphia, PA 19106
215-625-8900
800-354-1420
Fax: 215-625-2940
customer.service@taylorandfrancis.com
www.heldref.org

Emilli Pawlowsky, Marketing Manager
Laura Rosse, Assistant Marketing Manager
Douglas Kirkpatrick, Publisher
A professional journal aimed at psychologists, therapists and educators who work in the areas of motor behavior, psychology, neurophysiology, kinesiology, and biomechanics. Offers up-to-date information on the latest techniques, theories and developments concerning motor control. Titles previously published by Heldref Publications will be joining the T&F portfolio. *$77.00*
115 pages Quarterly

2122 Journal of Musculoskeletal Pain
Haworth Press
711 Third Avenue
New York, NY 10017
212-216-7800
800-354-1420
Fax: 212-244-1563
subscriptions@tandf.co.uk
www.haworthpress.com
This journal serves as a central resource for the dissemination of information about musculoskeletal pain. Haworth Press are now acquired by the Taylor & Francis Journals. *$75.00*
110 pages Quarterly

2123 Journal of Positive Behavior Interventions
2455 Teller Road
Thousand Oaks, CA 91320
800-818-7243
Fax: 800-583-2665
journals@sagepub.com
cde.sagepub.com

Blaise R. Simqu, President/ CEO
Tracey A. Ozmina, EVP/ COO
Chris Hickok, SVP/ CFO
Journal of Positive Behavior Interventions (PBI) offers sound, research-based principles of positive behavior support for use in school, home and community settings with people with challenges in behavioral adaptation.

2124 Journal of Postsecondary Education & Disability (JPED)
AHEAD
8015 West Kenton Circle
Suite 230
Huntersville, NC 28078
704-947-7779
Fax: 704-948-7779
jped@ahead.org
www.ahead.org

Stephan Smith, Executive Director
Ezekiel Kimball, Executive Editor
Ryan Wells, Executive Editor
An annual publication dedicated to the advancement of full participation in higher education for persons with disabilities. The journal focuses on a variety of related topics that emphasize research, issues, and trends related to the theory and practice of postsecondary disability services.
Quarterly

2125 Journal of Prosthetics and Orthotics
330 John Carlyle Street
Suite 210
Alexandria, VA 22314
703-836-7114
Fax: 703-836-0838
info@abcop.org
www.abcop.org

Catherine Carter, Executive Director
Debbie Ayres, Director, Marketing & Public Relations
Stephen Fletcher, CPO, LPO, Director, Clinical Resources
Provides the latest research and clinical thinking in orthotics and prosthetics, including information on new devices, fitting techniques and patient management experiences. Each issue contains

research-based information and articles reviewed and approved by a highly qualified editorial board. *$60.00*
64 pages Quarterly
ISSN 1040-88 0

2126 Journal of Reading, Writing and Learning Disabled International
Hemisphere Publishing Corporation
7625 Empire Drive
Florence, KY 41042-2919
800-634-7064
Fax: 800-248-4724
orders@taylorandfrancis.com
www.taylorandfrancis.com
Articles on reading, writing and learning disabilities, including mainstreaming issues. *$9.00*

2127 Journal of Rehabilitation
National Rehabilitation Association (NRA)
PO Box 150235
Alexandria, VA 22315
703-836-0850
888-258-4295
journalofrehab@email.arizona.edu
nationalrehab.org/journal-of-rehabilitation
Wendy Parent-Johnson, Editor
Official journal of the National Rehabilitation Association.
Quarterly

2128 Journal of School Health Association
Suite 403
4340 East West Highway
Bethesda, MD 20814
301-652-8072
Fax: 301-652-8077
info@ashaweb.org
ashaweb.org

Jeffrey K. Clark, President
Stephen Conley, Executive Director
Julie Greenfield, Marketing and Conferences Direct
This is a monthly journal which offers information to professionals and parents on school health. Membership dues, $95.00.

2129 Journal of Special Education
Sage Publications
2455 Teller Road
Thousand Oaks, CA 91320
805-499-0721
800-818-7243
Fax: 800-583-2665
info@sagepub.com
www.sagepub.com

Sara Miller McCune, Founder, Publisher & Executive Chairman
Blaise R. Simqu, President & CEO
Chris Hickok, Senior Vice President & Chief Financial Officer
Internationally known as the prime research journal in special education. JSE provides research articles of special education for individuals with disabilities, ranging from mild to severe. Published quarterly. *$39.00*
Magazine

2130 Journal of Vocational Behavior
Academic Press, Journals Division

The Journal of Vocational Behavior publishes empirical and theoretical articles that expand knowledge of vocational behavior and career development across the life span. Research presented in the journal encompasses the general categories of career choice, implementation, and vocational adjustment and adaptation. The articles are also valuable for applications in counseling and career development programs in colleges and universities, business and industry, government, and the military. *$7.00*

2131 Learning Disabilities: A Contemporary Journal
179 Bear Hill Rd.
Suite 104
Waltham, MA 02451
978-897-5399
Fax: 978-897-5355
help@ldworldwide.org
www.ldw-ldcj.org

Matthias Grunke, Editor
Teresa Allissa Citro, Editor
Marco G. P. Hessels, Associate Editor

Learning Disabilities: A Contemporary Journal (LDCJ) is a peer-reviewed forum for research, practice, and opinion regarding learning disabilities (LD) and associated disorders.

2132 Learning Disabilities: A Multidisciplinary Journal
Learning Disabilities Association of America
461 Cochran Rd.
Suite 245
Pittsburgh, PA 15228 412-341-1515
Fax: 412-344-0224
info@ldaamerica.org
www.ldaamerica.org
Cindy Cipoletti, Executive Director
The journal is a vehicle for disseminating the most current thinking on learning disabilities and to provide information on research, practice, theory, issues, and trends regarding learning disabilities from the perspectives of varied disciplines involved in broadening the understanding of learning disabilities.

2133 Learning Disability Quarterly
2455 Teller Road
Thousand Oaks, CA 91320 800-818-7243
Fax: 800-583-2665
journals@sagepub.com
ldq.sagepub.com
Blaise R. Simqu, President/ CEO
Tracey A. Ozmina, EVP/ COO
Chris Hickok, SVP/ CFO
Learning Disability Quarterly (LDQ) publishes high-quality research and scholarship concerning children, youth, and adults with learning disabilities.

2134 MDA/ALS Newsmagazine
Muscular Dystrophy Association
161 N Clark
Suite 3550
Chicago, IL 60601 800-572-1717
alsn.mda.org
Donald S. Wood, President & Chief Executive Officer
Presents news related to muscular dystrophy and other neuromuscular diseases including research, personal profiles, fundraising activities and patient services.

2135 Movement Disorders
555 East Wells Street
Suite 1100
Milwaukee, WI 53202- 3823 414-276-2145
Fax: 414-276-3349
info@movementdisorders.org
www.movementdisorders.org
Matthew B. Stern, President
Oscar S. Gershanik, President-Elect
Francisco Cardoso, Secretary
Movement Disorders, the official Journal of the International Parkinson and Movement Disorder Society (MDS), is a highly read and referenced journal covering all topics of the field - both clinical and basic science.

2136 People & Families
PO Box 700
Trenton, NJ 8625-700 609-292-345
800-792-8858
Fax: 609-292-7114
TTY: 609-777-3238
njcdd@njcdd.org
www.njcdd.org
Kevin T. Jonathan, Waller
Editor
People & Families, the NJCDD's nationally recognized magazine, focuses on issues of importance to the developmental disabilities community in New Jersey.

2137 Psychiatric Staffing Crisis in Community Mental Health
Nat l Council for Community Behavioral Healthcare
76 Ninth Avenue
New York, NY 10011 201-559-3882
800-THE-BOOK
amilevoj@bn.com
www.barnesandnoble.com
Andy Milevoj, Vice President, Investor Relations
Mary Ellen Keating, SVP, Corporate Communications & Public Affairs
Carolyn Brown, Director of Corporate Communications
Find out some of the simple, low-cost ways you can increase workplace satisfaction among staff psychiatrists and compete successfully for their talents. *$20.00*

2138 Quest Magazine
Muscular Dystrophy Association
161 N Clark
Suite 3550
Chicago, IL 60601 800-572-1717
ResourceCenter@mdausa.org
www.mda.org/quest
Donald S. Wood, President & Chief Executive Officer
Magazine of the Muscular Dystrophy Association.

2139 Readings: A Journal of Reviews and Commentary in Mental Health
American Orthopsychiatric Association
3524 Washington Avenue
P.O. Box 1048
Sheboygan, WI 53081-1048 920-457-5051
800-558-7687
Fax: 920-457-1485
info@americanortho.com
www.americanortho.com
Michael Bogenschuetz, President
Randy Benz, Chief Executive Officer
Charles Achter, Assistant Controller
Reviews of recent books in mental health and allied disciplines. Includes essay reviews and brief reviews. *$25.00*
32 pages Quarterly

2140 Rehab Pro
1926 Waukegan Rd
Suite 1
Glenview, IL 60025-1770 847-657-6964
Fax: 847-657-6963
carlw@tcag.com
www.rehabpro.org
Carl Wangman, Executive Director
The magazine is to promote the profession and to inform the public about the activities of the national organization, its state chapter affiliates, and the work of its special interest sections.
38 pages BiMonthly

2141 Remedial and Special Education
Sage Publications
2455 Teller Road
Thousand Oaks, CA 91320 805-499-0721
800-818-7243
Fax: 800-583-2665
info@sagepub.com
www.sagepub.com
Sara Miller McCune, Founder, Publisher & Executive Chairman
Blaise R. Simqu, President & CEO
Chris Hickok, Senior Vice President & Chief Financial Officer
A professional journal that bridges the gap between theory and practice. Emphasis is on topical reviews, syntheses of research, field evaluation studies and recommendations for the practice of remedial and special education. Published six times a year. *$39.00*
64 pages

2142 **Structural Integration: The Journal of the Rolf Institute**
5055 Chaparral Ct.
Suite 103
Boulder, CO 80301
303-449-5903
Fax: 303-449-5978
www.rolf.org

Christina Howe, Executive Director
Mary Contreras, Director, Admissions & Recruitment
Samantha Sherwin, Director, Financial Aid & Compliance
Professional journal consisting of articles on research, practice building, faculty perspectives, reviews, and other topics relating to the field of Rolfing Structural Integration.

2143 **Teaching Exceptional Children (TEC)**
Council for Exceptional Children
3100 Clarendon Blvd.
Suite 600
Arlington, VA 22201-5332
888-232-7733
TTY: 866-915-5000
service@exceptionalchildren.org
www.exceptionalchildren.org

Dawn Rowe, Academic Editor
Journal designed for teachers of gifted students and students with disabilities, featuring practical methods and materials for classroom use.
61 pages BiMonthly

Newsletters

2144 **APA Access**
750 First Street, NE
Washington, DC 20002-4242
202-336-5500
800-374-2721
rllowman@gmail.com
www.apa.org

Rodney L. Lowman, PhD, Chair
Barry Anton, PhD, President
Bonnie Markham, PhD, PsyD, Treasurer
Exclusively for APA members, APA Access provides a helpful insider's view of the latest APA news. Each monthly issue highlights an array of current topics, such as advocacy updates, continuing education opportunities, press releases, previews of Monitor on Psychology articles, APA publishing news, new APA products and a calendar of events.

2145 **Alert**
Association on Handicapped Student Service Program
P.O.Box 21192
Columbus, OH 43221
614-365-5216
Fax: 614-365-6718
Keeps members informed about Association activities, current legislative issues, innovative programs, and more. *$30.00*

2146 **Children's Mental Health and EBD E-news**
PACER Center
8161 Normandale Blvd.
Bloomington, MN 55437
952-838-9000
800-537-2237
Fax: 952-838-0199
pacer@pacer.org
www.pacer.org

Paula F. Goldberg, Executive Director
Newsletter providing resources for parents with children affected by mental health and emotional or behavioral issues.

2147 **Counseling Today**
American Counseling Association
P.O. Box 31110
Alexandria, VA 22310
800-347-6647
Fax: 800-473-2329
ct.counseling.org

Richard Yep, Chief Executive Officer
Aims to serve individuals active in professional counseling, as well as other citizens, community leaders and policy makers who appreciate the importance of the role of professional counselors in today's society. The publication features news and articles on professional counseling developments, resources, strategies, regulations, and more.
Monthly

2148 **Disability Compliance for Higher Education**
LRP Publications
P.O. Box 24668
West Palm Beach, FL 33416-4668
561-622-2423
800-341-7874
Fax: 561-622-1375
custserve@lrp.com
lrp.com

Kenneth F. Kahn, Owner and President
Ed Chase, Vice President
The only newsletter that is dedicated to the exclusive coverage of disability issues that affect colleges and universities. *$195.00*
8 pages Monthly

2149 **Disability Pride Newsletter**
900 Rebecca Avenue
Pittsburgh, PA 15221
800-633-4588
Fax: 412-371-9430
lgray@trcil.org

Rachel Rogan, CEO
Gregory Daigle, Chief Financial Officer
Lisa Wilson, HR Program Manager
Three Rivers Center for Independent Living (TRCIL) is a non-residential, non-profit, community-based human service organization. There purpose is to assist people with disabilities to lead self-directed and productive lives within the community.

2150 **Disability Resources Monthly**
Disability Resources
4 Glatter Ln
South Setauket, NY 11720-1032
631-585-0290
Fax: 631-585-0290

Avery Klauber, Executive Director
A newsletter that monitors, reviews and reports on resources for independent living. A monthly newsletter that features short topical articles, news items and reviews of books, pamphlets, periodicals, videotapes, on-line services, organizations and other resources for and about people with disabilities. It is intended primarily for librarians, social workers, educators, rehabilitation specialists, disability advocates, ADA coordinators and other health and social service professionals. *$33.00*
4 pages Monthly
ISSN 1070-72 0

2151 **Early Childhood Reporter**
LRP Publications
P.O. Box 24668
West Palm Beach, FL 33416-4668
561-622-2423
800-341-7874
Fax: 561-622-1375
custserve@lrp.com
www.lrp.com

Kenneth F. Kahn, Owner and President
Ed Chase, Vice President
Monthly reports with information on federal, state, and local legislation affecting the implementation of early intervention and preschool programs for children with disabilities. *$145.00*
12-16 pages $10 shipping

2152 **FYI**
AAIDD
8403 Colesville Rd.
Suite 900
Silver Spring, MD 20910
202-387-1968
Fax: 202-387-2193
aaidd.org

Margaret A. Nygren, Executive Director & Chief Executive Officer
Kathleen McLane, Director, Publications Program
A monthly newsletter that provides news about AAIDD resources, educational opportunities, and activities.

2153 **Family Engagement**
PACER Center
8161 Normandale Blvd.
Bloomington, MN 55437 952-838-9000
800-537-2237
Fax: 952-838-0199
pacer@pacer.org
www.pacer.org

Paula F. Goldberg, Executive Director
E-newsletter providing parents and professionals with resources for supporting family engagement with schools.

2154 **Fellow Insider**
AAIDD
8403 Colesville Rd.
Suite 900
Silver Spring, MD 20910 202-387-1968
Fax: 202-387-2193
aaidd.org

Margaret A. Nygren, Executive Director & Chief Executive Officer
Kathleen McLane, Director, Publications Program
Quarterly newsletter for Fellows of the American Association on Intellectual and Developmental Disabilities.

2155 **Field Notes**
AAIDD
8403 Colesville Rd.
Suite 900
Silver Spring, MD 20910 202-387-1968
Fax: 202-387-2193
aaidd.org

Margaret A. Nygren, Executive Director & Chief Executive Officer
Kathleen McLane, Director, Publications Program
A monthly newsletter providing summaries of studies published in peer reviewed journals, along with links to the original articles.

2156 **Gram Newsletter, The**
PO Box 1114
Claremont, CA 91711 909-621-1494

Arline Krieger, President
Pam Hamilton, 1st Vice-President
EunMi Cho, 3rd Vice-President
The Learning Disabilities Association of California's (LDA-CA's) quarterly newsletter, The GRAM, provides LDA-CA members with timely information.

2157 **Growing Readers**
LD Online
2775 S. Quincy St.
Arlington, VA Fax: 703-998-2060
ldonline@weta.org
www.ldonline.org

Noel Gunther, Executive Director
Christian Lindstrom, Director, Learning Media
Monthly tips for raising strong readers and writers, written especially for parents. Used by schools and PTAs in parent newsletters, and by libraries and community literacy organizations.

2158 **Healthline**
CV Mosby Company
1600 John F. Kennedy Boulevard
Suite 1800
Philadelphia, PA 19103-2822 215-239-3900
800-523-1649
Fax: 215-239-3990
www.us.elsevierhealth.com
Health and fitness information for healthcare professionals and the general public alike.
Monthly

2159 **Help Newsletter**
Learning Disabilities Association of Arkansas
P.O. Box 23514
Little Rock, AR 72221 501-666-8777
Fax: 501-666-8777
www.ldaarkansas.org

Nathan Green, President
Rebecca Walker, VP
Becca Green, Past President, Treasurer

Information on how to overcome obstacles and to achieve in spite of learning disabilities. *$30.00*
8 pages Quarterly

2160 **HerbalEGram**
American Botanical Council
6200 Manor Rd.
Austin, TX 78723-4345 512-926-4900
800-373-7105
Fax: 512-926-2345
abc@herbalgram.org
herbalgram.org

Mark Blumenthal, Founder, Executive Director & Editor
Hannah Bauman, Assistant Editor
Electronic newsletter of the American Botanical Council, with current editions available to members only.

2161 **Insights**
135 Parkinson Avenue
Staten Island, NY 10305 800-223-2732
Fax: 718-981-4399
apda@apdaparkinson.org
www.apdaparkinson.org

Fred Greene, Chairman
Patrick McDermott, 1st Vice Chairman
Jerry Wells, Esq., Secretary
APDA was founded in 1961 with the dual purpose to Ease the Burden - Find the Cure for Parkinson's disease.

2162 **Inspiring Possibilities**
PACER Center
8161 Normandale Blvd.
Bloomington, MN 55437 952-838-9000
800-537-2237
Fax: 952-838-0199
pacer@pacer.org
www.pacer.org

Paula F. Goldberg, Executive Director
From PACER's National Parent Center on Transition and Employment, the e-newsletter provides news and updates for youth with disabilities transitioning from school to the workforce.

2163 **LD Monthly Report**
LD Online
2775 S. Quincy St.
Arlington, VA Fax: 703-998-2060
ldonline@weta.org
www.ldonline.org

Noel Gunther, Executive Director
Christian Lindstrom, Director, Learning Media
LD OnLine seeks to help children and adults reach their full potential by providing accurate and up-to-date information and advice about learning disabilities and ADHD.

2164 **MA Report**
National Allergy and Asthma Network
Ste 200
3554 Chain Bridge Rd
Fairfax, VA 22030-2709 703-385-4403
Fax: 703-352-4354

Offers information on medical breakthroughs, patient care, public awareness, activities and events focusing on the allergy and asthma patient. This newsletter is the only Monthly Asthma Report that a patient will need to keep fully informed with medical articles written by experts in the field.
Monthly

2165 **Member Update**
AAIDD
8403 Colesville Rd.
Suite 900
Silver Spring, MD 20910 202-387-1968
Fax: 202-387-2193
aaidd.org

Margaret A. Nygren, Executive Director & Chief Executive Officer
Kathleen McLane, Director, Publications Program
A weekly newsletter providing updates on professional development opportunities, including conferences and webinars, job postings, calls for papers, and opportunities to join advisory committees and provide comments on federal initiatives.

2166 National Bullying Prevention Center Newsletter
PACER Center
8161 Normandale Blvd.
Bloomington, MN 55437   952-838-9000
       800-537-2237
       Fax: 952-838-0199
       pacer@pacer.org
       www.pacer.org
Paula F. Goldberg, Executive Director
Provides resources from PACER's National Bullying Prevention
Center (NBPC). Publishes information on bullying prevention as
well as news on anti-bullying events. Published quarterly and
during National Bullying Prevention Month in October.

2167 O&P Almanac
American Orthotic & Prosthetic Association
330 John Carlyle Street
Suite 200
Alexandria, VA 22314   571-431-0876
       Fax: 571-431-0899
       info@aopanet.org
       www.aopanet.org
Anita Liberman-Lampear, MA, President
Charles H. Dankmeyer, Jr, CPO, President-Elect
James Campbell, CO, Ph.D., Vice President
Offers in-depth coverage on orthotics and prosthetics to current
professional, government, business and reimbursement activities
affecting the orthotics and prosthetics industry. *$59.00*
80 pages Monthly

2168 Occupational Therapy in Health Care
Haworth Press
711 Third Avenue
New York, NY 10017   212-216-7800
       800-354-1420
       Fax: 212-244-1563
       subscriptions@tandf.co.uk
       www.haworthpress.com
Each issue focuses on significant practices and concerns involving occupational therapy and therapists. Haworth Press are now
acquired by the Taylor & Francis Journals. *$75.00*

**2169 Ohio Coalition for the Education of Children with
Disabilities**
165 W Center St, 3rd Floor, Chase B
Suite 302
Marion, OH 43302   740-382-5452
       800-374-2806
       Fax: 740-383-6421
       ocecd@ocecd.org
       www.ocecd.org
Martha Lause, Manager
Lee Ann Derugen, Co-Director
Margaret Burley, Executive Director
Forum is a newsletter reporting on educational, legislative and
other developments affecting persons with disabilities.
8 pages

2170 PACER E-News
PACER Center
8161 Normandale Blvd.
Bloomington, MN 55437   952-838-9000
       800-537-2237
       Fax: 952-838-0199
       pacer@pacer.org
       www.pacer.org
Paula F. Goldberg, Executive Director
E-newsletter providing information on special events and other
news. Published monthly.

2171 PACER Partners
PACER Center
8161 Normandale Blvd.
Bloomington, MN 55437   952-838-9000
       800-537-2237
       Fax: 952-838-0199
       pacer@pacer.org
       www.pacer.org
Paula F. Goldberg, Executive Director
Published by PACER's Development Office, the newsletter con-
nects families, friends, donors, and the staff of PACER.

2172 PACESETTER
PACER Center
8161 Normandale Blvd.
Bloomington, MN 55437   952-838-9000
       800-537-2237
       Fax: 952-838-0199
       pacer@pacer.org
       www.pacer.org
Paula F. Goldberg, Executive Director
Provides resources and information on special education and
PACER programs. PACER's main newsletter.

2173 SAMHSA News
US Department of Health and Human Services
5600 Fishers Lane
Rockville, MD 20857   877-726-4727
       TTY: 800-487-4889
       samhsainfo@samhsa.hhs.gov
       www.samhsa.gov
Tom Coderre, Acting Assistant Secretary
Sonia Chessen, Chief of Staff
Trina Dutta, Senior Advisor
This quarterly agency newsletter reports on information on sub-
stance abuse, mental health treatment and prevention programs of
the Substance Abuse and Mental Health Services Administration.
Quarterly

2174 Sibling Information Network Newsletter
AJ Pappanikou Center
270 Farmington Avenue
Suite 181
Farmington, CT 06030   860-679-1500
       866-623-1315
       Fax: 860-679-1571
       TTY: 860-679-1502
       contact.us.ucedd@uchc.edu
       www.uconnucedd.org
Mary Beth Bruder, PhD, UCEDD/LEND Director
Gerarda Hanna, J.D., M.Ed., Associate UCEDD Director
*Gabriela Freyre-Calish, MSW, Coordinator, Director, Cultural
Diversity*
Contains information aimed at the varying interested of our mem-
bership. Program descriptions, requests for assistance, confer-
ence announcements, literature summaries and research reports.
$8.50

2175 Sibpage
AJ Pappanikou Center
270 Farmington Avenue
Suite 181
Farmington, CT 06030   860-679-1500
       866-623-1315
       Fax: 860-679-1571
       TTY: 860-679-1502
       contact.us.ucedd@uchc.edu
       www.uconnucedd.org
Mary Beth Bruder, PhD, UCEDD/LEND Director
Gerarda Hanna, J.D., M.Ed., Associate UCEDD Director
*Gabriela Freyre-Calish, MSW, Coordinator, Director, Cultural
Diversity*
Developed specifically for children containing games, recipes,
pen pals, and articles written by siblings relating to developmen-
tal disabilities.
4 pages

2176 Special Edge
Resources in Special Education
Fl 4
1107 9th St
Sacramento, CA 95814-3616   916-492-9999
       877-493-7833
       Fax: 916-492-4004
Virigina Reynolds, President
Provides education news, collaborative programs, amendments
to the laws, tools for accommodations, resource information, a
calendar of events, and more.
BiMonthly

2177 Special Education Report
LRP Publications
360 Hiatt Dr
Dept. 150F
Palm BeachGardens, FL 33418   800-341-7874
                                     Fax: 561-622-2423
                                     custserve@lrp.com
                                     lrp.com
Current, pertinent information about federal legislation, regulations, programs and funding for educating children with disabilities. Covers federal and state litigation on the Individuals with Disabilities Education Act and other relevant laws. Looks at innovations and research in the field.

2178 Topics in Early Childhood Special Education
Sage Publications
2455 Teller Road
Thousand Oaks, CA 91320   805-499-0721
                                 800-818-7243
                                 Fax: 800-583-2665
                                 info@sagepub.com
                                 www.sagepub.com
Sara Miller McCune, Founder, Publisher & Executive Chairman
Blaise R. Simqu, President & CEO
Chris Hickok, Senior Vice President & Chief Financial Officer
Designed for professionals helping young children with special needs in areas such as assessment, special programs, social policies and developmental aids. *$43.00*
Quarterly

2179 Treatment Review
AIDS Treatment Data Network
57 Willoughby St.
2nd Floor
Brooklyn, NY 11201   347-473-7400
                            800-734-7104
                            TTY: 212-925-9560
                            info@housingworks.org
                            www.housingworks.org
Charles King, Chair
Linney Smith, Vice Chair
Earl Ward, Vice Chair
Individual members receive treatment education, counseling, referrals and case management support. Services are available in both English and Spanish. The Treatment Review newsletter includes descriptions of approved, alternative and experimental treatments, as well as announcements of seminars and forums on treatments and clinical trials.
Quarterly

2180 VIP Newsletter
Blind Children's Fund
6761 West US 12
P.O. Box 363
Three Oaks, MI 49128   989-779-9966
                              Fax: 269-756-3133
                              www.blindchildrensfund.org
Karla B. Kwast, Executive Director
Jeremy Murphy, President
Robert R. Storrer Jr., Vice President
Provides parents and professionals with information, materials and resources that help them successfully teach and nurture blind, visually and multi-impaired infants and preschoolers. *$10.00*

Professional Texts

2181 7 Steps for Success
Council for Exceptional Children
3100 Clarendon Blvd.
Suite 600
Arlington, VA 22201-5332   888-232-7733
                                  TTY: 866-915-5000
                                  service@exceptionalchildren.org
                                  www.exceptionalchildren.org
Elizabeth C. Hamblet, Author
A book helping young adults with disabilities transitioning from high school to college.

2182 A Guide to Teaching Students With Autism Spectrum Disorders
Council for Exceptional Children
3100 Clarendon Blvd.
Suite 600
Arlington, VA 22201-5332   888-232-7733
                                  TTY: 866-915-5000
                                  service@exceptionalchildren.org
                                  www.exceptionalchildren.org
Monica E. Delano, Co-Author
Darlene E. Perner, Co-Author
This book is a resource for all special educators and general educators who work with students with autism spectrum disorders (ASD). The underlying premise is that students with ASD should be explicitly taught a full range of social, self-help, language, reading, writing and math skills, as are their typically developing classmates.

2183 A Teacher's Guide to Isovaleric Acidemia
150 North 18th Avenue
Phoenix, AZ 85007   602-542-1025
                           Fax: 602-542-0883
                           www.azdhs.gov
Will Humble, Director
Thomas Salow, Manager
Resource book for preschool teachers and school staff on isovaleric academia basics and classroom activities. *$2.50*

2184 A Teacher's Guide to Methylmalonic Acidemia
Arizona State Department of Health Services
150 North 18th Avenue
Phoenix, AZ 85007   602-542-1025
                           Fax: 602-542-0883
                           www.azdhs.gov
Will Humble, Director
Thomas Salow, Manager
Resource book for preschool teachers and school staff on methylmalonic academia basics and classroom activities. *$2.50*

2185 A Teacher's Guide to PKU
Arizona Department of Health Services
150 North 18th Avenue
Phoenix, AZ 85007   602-542-1025
                           Fax: 602-542-0883
                           www.azdhs.gov
Will Humble, Director
Thomas Salow, Manager
Resource book for preschool teachers and school staff on PKU basics, NutraSweet warning, and classroom activities. *$2.50*
13 pages

2186 AD/HD and the College Student: The Everything Guide to Your Most Urgent Questions
750 First Street, NE
Washington, DC 20002-4242   202-336-5500
                                   800-374-2721
                                   rllowman@gmail.com
                                   www.apa.org
Patricia O. Quinn, MD, Author
Whether you are looking for information or facing an urgent situation, AD/HD and the College Studentprovides answers to your most pressing questions. Organized in a question-and-answer format, this guide is loaded with helpful information, practical tips, and resources.

2187 ADD Challenge: A Practical Guide for Teachers
2612 N. Mattis Ave.
P.O. Box 7886
Champaign, IL 61822   217-352-3273
                             800-519-2707
                             Fax: 217-352-1221
                             orders@researchpress.com
                             www.researchpress.com
Robert W. Parkinson, Founder
Steven B. Gordon, Author
Dr Richard M Foxx, Author
Research Press is an independent, family-owned business founded in 1968 by Robert W. Parkinson (1920-2001).

2188 ADHD Coaching: A Guide for Mental Health Professionals
750 First Street, NE
Washington, DC 20002-4242
202-336-5500
800-374-2721
rllowman@gmail.com
www.apa.org

Frances Prevatt, PhD, Co-Author
Abigail Levrini, PhD, Co-Author
This book describes the underlying principles as well as the nuts and bolts of ADHD coaching. Step-by-step details for gathering information, conducting the intake, establishing goals and objectives, and working through all stages of coaching are included, along with helpful forms and a detailed list of additional resources.

2189 ADHD in the Classroom: Strategies for Teachers
Guilford Publication
72 Spring Street
New York, NY 10012
212-431-9800
800-365-7006
Fax: 212-966-6708
info@guilford.com
www.guilford.com

Bob Matloff, President
Seymour Weingarten, Editor-in-Chief
Russell A. Barkley, Author
Designed specifically to help teachers with their ADHD students, thereby providing a better learning environment for the entire class. *$95.00*
ISBN 0-898629-85-3

2190 ADHD in the Schools: Assessment and Intervention Strategies
72 Spring Street
New York, NY 10012
212-431-9800
800-365-7006
Fax: 212-966-6708
info@guilford.com
www.guilford.com

Bob Matloff, President
Seymour Weingarten, Editor-in-Chief
George J. DuPaul, Author
The landmark volume emphasizes the need for a team effort among parents, community-based professionals, and educators. Provides practical information for educators that is based on empirical findings. Chapters Focus on how to identify and assess students who might have ADHD, the relationship between ADHD and learning disabilities; how to develop and supplement classroom-based programs. Communication strategies to assist physicians and the need for community-based treatments *$36.00*
269 pages Paperback
ISBN 0-898622-45-X

2191 AEPS Curriculum for Birth to Three Years
Brookes Publishing
P.O.Box 10624
Baltimore, MD 21285-0624
410-337-9580
800-638-3775
Fax: 410-337-8539
custserv@brookespublishing.com
readplaylearn.com
Directly linked to IEP/IFSP goals developed for a child from the AEPS test measure, the AEPS curriculum provides a complete set of learning activities to facilitate children's acquisition of functional skills. *$59.95*
496 pages
ISBN 1-557660-96-4

2192 Access to Health Care
World Institute on Disability
3075 Adeline St.
Suite 155
Berkeley, CA 94703
510-225-6400
Fax: 510-225-0477
wid@wid.org
www.wid.org
Marcie Roth, Executive Director & Chief Executive Officer
Katherine Zigmont, Senior Director, Operations & Deputy Director
Reggie Johnson, Senior Director, Marketing & Communications

Policy bulletins focusing on the capacity of the private and public health insurance systems to respond to the health care needs of persons with disabilities or chronic illness.

2193 Activity-Based Approach to Early Intervention, 2nd Edition
Brookes Publishing
P.O.Box 10624
Baltimore, MD 21285-0624
410-337-9580
800-638-3775
Fax: 410-337-8539
webmaster@brookespublishing.com
www.brookespublishing.com
Paul H. Brookes, Chairman of the Board
Jeffrey D. Brookes, President
George S. Stamathis, VP/Publisher
Activity-based intervention shows how to use natural and relevant events to teach infants and young children, of all abilities, effectively and efficiently. *$24.00*
240 pages
ISBN 1-55766 -87-5

2194 Adapted Physical Education for Students with Autism
Charles C. Thomas
2600 S First St
Springfield, IL 62704-4730
217-789-8980
800-258-8980
Fax: 217-789-9130
books@ccthomas.com
www.ccthomas.com
Kimberly Davis, Author
Focuses on the physical education needs and curriculum for autistic children. Available in cloth, paperback and hardcover. *$27.95*
142 pages Paper
ISBN 0-398060-85-1

2195 Adapting Early Childhood Curricula for Children with Special Needs (9th Edition)
Pearson Higher Education
330 Hudson St
New York, NY 10013
212-641-2400
www.pearsonhighered.com
Ruth E. Cook, Author
M. Diane Klein, Author
Deborah Chen, Author
This highly readable, well researched, and current resource uses a developmental focus, rather than a disability orientation, to discuss typical and atypical child development and curricular adaptations, and encourage the treatment of students as children first, without regard to their learning differences. *$102.67*
528 pages Loose-Leaf or Access Code Card 1915
ISBN 0-134019-41-3

2196 Adapting Instruction for the Mainstream: A Sequential Approach to Teaching
McGraw-Hill School Publishing
P.O. Box 182605
Columbus, OH 43218
800-338-3987
Fax: 609-308-4480
customer.service@mheducation.com
mcgraw-hill.com
David Levin, President, CEO
Ellen Haley, President, CTB
Peter Cohen, President, School Education
This text gives both regular and special education teachers everything they need to help mildly handicapped students succeed in the mainstream.
226 pages

2197 Adaptive Education Strategies Building on Diversity
Brookes Publishing Company
P.O.Box 10624
Baltimore, MD 21285-0624   410-337-9580
                                        800-638-3775
                                    Fax: 410-337-8539
                        webmaster@brookespublishing.com
                            www.brookespublishing.com
Paul H. Brookes, Chairman of the Board
Jeffrey D. Brookes, President
George S. Stamathis, VP/Publisher
Based on more than two decades of systematic research, this comprehensive manual provides a road map to the effective implementation of adaptive education. *$35.00*
304 pages Paperback
ISBN 1-557880-84-0

2198 Adolescents and Adults with Learning Disabilities and ADHD
370 Seventh Avenue
Suite 1200
New York, NY 10001-1020   800-365-7006
                                    Fax: 212-966-6708
                                       info@guilford.com
                                       www.guilford.com
No%ol Gregg, PhD, Author
Most of the literature on learning disabilities and attention-deficit/hyperactivity disorder (ADHD) focuses on the needs of elementary school-age children, but older students with these conditions also require significant support.

2199 Advanced Sign Language Vocabulary: A Resource Text for Educators
Charles C. Thomas
2600 S First St
Springfield, IL 62704-4730   217-789-8980
                                        217-258-8980
                                    Fax: 217-789-9130
                                   books@ccthomas.com
                                       www.ccthomas.com
Elizabeth E. Wolf, Author
Janet R. Coleman, Author
This book is a collection of advanced sign language vocabulary for use by educators, interpreters, parents or anyone wishing to enlarge their sign vocabulary. *$53.95*
202 pages Spiralbound
ISBN 0-398057-22-2

2200 Advances in Cardiac and Pulmonary Rehabilitation
Haworth Press
711 Third Avenue
New York, NY 10017   212-216-7800
                                        800-354-1420
                                    Fax: 212-244-1563
                              subscriptions@tandf.co.uk
                                  www.haworthpress.com
Enhance your rehabilitation program with this authoritative volume. Haworth Press are now acquired by the Taylor & Francis Journals. *$34.95*
74 pages Hardcover
ISBN 0-866869-86-3

2201 Aging Brain
Taylor & Francis Group
Ste 800
325 Chestnut St
Philadelphia, PA 19106-2608   215-625-8900
                                        800-354-1420
                                    Fax: 215-625-2940
                         www.taylorandfrancisgroup.com
Elderly treatment.
225 pages Paperback
ISBN 0-85066 -78-0

2202 Aging and Disability: Crossing Network Lines
Springer Publishing
11 West 42nd Street
15th Floor
New York, NY 10036   212-431-4370
                                        877-687-7476
                                    Fax: 212-941-7842
                            marketing@springerpub.com
                                       springerpub.com
Theodore C. Nardin, CEO/Publisher
Jason Roth, VP/Marketing Director
Annette Imperati, Marketing/Sales Director
Michelle Putnam has set forth this volume to reflect the current research, facilitate collaboration across service networks, and encourage movement toward more effective service policies. Professional stakeholders evaluate the bridges and barriers to crossing network lines, and chapter on current websites, agencies, and coalitions provides the much needed tools to bring collaboration into practice.

2203 Aging and Rehabilitation II: The State ofthe Practice
Springer Publishing Company
11 W 42nd St
15th Fl
New York, NY 10036-8002   212-431-4370
                                        877-687-7476
                                    Fax: 212-941-7842
                                   cs@springerpub.com
                                   www.springerpub.com
Ted Nardin, chief Executive Officer
Jason Roth, Vice President, Marketing & Sales
Kathy Weiss, Senior Sales Director
Current, multidisciplinary investigations of various practice issues. Leading experts in the field use a practical perspective to provide specific comments on interventions. The scope of this work encompasses the autonomy of elderly disabled, mobility, mental health and value issues, as well as basic aspects in rehabilitation of the elderly. *$8.95*
348 pages Hardcover 1990
ISBN 0-826170-80-3

2204 Alphabetic Phonics Curriculum
Educators Publishing Service
625 Mount Auburn Street
3rd Floor
Cambridge, MA 02138- 3039   617-547-6706
                                        800-225-5750
                       Feedback.EPS@schoolspecialty.com
                                       www.epsbooks.com
Rick Holden, President, EPS
Ungraded multisensory curriculum for teaching phonics and the structure of language. Uses Orton-Gillingham approach to teach handwriting, spelling, reading, reading comprehension, and oral and written expression. program includes basic manual, workbooks, tests, teachers' guides, drill cards and all cards. *$28.15*
ISSN 8388-42

2205 Alternative Educational Delivery Systems
National Association of School Psychologists
4340 East West Highway
Suite 402
Bethesda, MD 20814   301-657-0270
                                        866-331-NASP
                                    Fax: 301-657-0275
                                    TTY: 301-657-4155
                               webmaster@naspweb.org
                                       nasponline.org
Stephen E. Brock, President
Todd A. Savage, President-Elect
Laura Benson, Chief Operating Officer
A book offering information to the professional on how to enhance educational options for all students.

2206 Alternative Teaching Strategies
Special Needs Project
324 State Street
Suite H
Santa Barbara, CA 93101-2364

818-718-9900
800-333-6867
Fax: 818-349-2027
editor@specialneeds.com
www.specialneeds.com

Hod Gray, Owner
Offers help for teachers who teach behaviorally troubled students.

2207 Antecedent Control: Innovative Approaches to Behavioral Support
Brookes Publishing
P.O.Box 10624
Baltimore, MD 21285-0624

410-337-9580
800-638-3775
Fax: 410-337-8539
webmaster@brookespublishing.com
www.brookespublishing.com

Paul H. Brookes, Chairman of the Board
Jeffrey D. Brookes, President
George S. Stamathis, VP/Publisher
This book explains the theory and methodology of antecedent control. The treatment techniques in this book are effective for both children and adults.
416 pages Paperback
ISBN 1-55766-34-3

2208 Anxiety-Free Kids: An Interactive Guide for Parents and Children
Prufrock Press
PO Box 8813
Waco, TX 76714-8813

800-998-2208
Fax: 800-240-0333
info@prufrock.com
www.prufrock.com

Joel McIntosh, Publisher & Marketing Director
Lacy Compton, Senior Editor
Rachel Taliaferro, Editor
Offers parents strategies that help children happy and worry-free, methods that relieve a child's excessive anxieties and phobias, and tools for fostering interaction and family-oriented solutions. *$19.95*
280 pages Paperback
ISBN 1-593633-43-1

2209 Applied Rehabilitation Counseling (Springer Series on Rehabilitation)
Springer Publishing Company
11 W 42nd St
15th Fl
New York, NY 10036-8002

212-431-4370
877-687-7476
Fax: 212-941-7842
cs@springerpub.com
www.springerpub.com

Ted Nardin, Chief Executive Officer
Jason Roth, Vice President, Marketing & Sales
Kathy Weiss, Senior Sales Director
This comprehensive text describes current theories, techniques, and their applications to specific disabled populations. Perspectives on varying counseling approaches such as psychodynamic, existential, gestalt, behavioral and psychoeducational orientations are systematically outlined in an easy-to-follow format. Practical applications for counseling are emphasized with attention given to strategies, goal-setting and on-going evaluations. *$43.95*
404 pages Paperback 1986
ISBN 0-826153-71-2

2210 Art-Centered Education and Therapy for Children with Disabilities
Charles C. Thomas
2600 S First St
Springfield, IL 62704-4730

217-789-8980
800-258-8980
Fax: 217-789-9130
books@ccthomas.com
www.ccthomas.com

Frances E. Anderson, Author
This book has been written to help both the regular education, and art and special education teachers, both pre- and in-service, better understand some of the issues and realities of providing education and remediation to children with disabilities. The book is also offered as model concept that has govern the author's personal and professional career of over thirty years. *$41.95*
284 pages Paperback
ISBN 0-398060-06-1

2211 Assessing the Handicaps/Needs of Children
Books on Special Children
P.O.Box 3378
Amherst, MA 01004-3378

413-256-8164
Fax: 413-256-8896

Papers on treatment, rehab and social support in assessing the needs of developmentally disabled children. *$66.00*
260 pages Hardcover
ISBN 0-12218 -02-0

2212 Assessment & Management of Mainstreamed Hearing-Impaired Children
Sage Publications
2455 Teller Road
Thousand Oaks, CA 91320

805-499-0721
800-818-7243
Fax: 800-583-2665
info@sagepub.com
www.sagepub.com

Sara Miller McCune, Founder, Publisher & Executive Chairman
Blaise R. Simqu, President & CEO
Chris Hickok, Senior Vice President & Chief Financial Officer
The theoretical and practical considerations of developing appropriate programming for hearing-impaired children who are being educated in mainstream educational settings are presented in this book.

2213 Assessment Log & Developmental Progress Charts for the Carolina Curriculum
Brookes Publishing
P.O.Box 10624
Baltimore, MD 21285-0624

410-337-9580
800-638-3775
Fax: 410-337-8539
webmaster@brookespublishing.com
www.brookespublishing.com

Paul H. Brookes, Chairman of the Board
Jeffrey D. Brookes, President
George S. Stamathis, VP/Publisher
This 28-page booklet allows the progress of children with skills in the 12-36 month development range to be easily recorded. Available in packages of 10. *$23.00*
28 pages Saddle-stiched
ISBN 1-557662-21-5

2214 Assessment and Remediation of Articulatoryand Phonological Disorders
McGraw-Hill School Publishing
PO Box 182604
Columbus, OH 43218

877-833-5524
800-338-3987
Fax: 609-308-4480
customer.service@mheducation.com
www.mcgraw-hill.com

David Levin, President/Chief Executive Officer
David Stafford, Senior Vice President/General Counsel
Maryellen Valaitis, Senior Vice President Human Resources
Offers comprehensive coverage of articulation disorders.

2215 Assessment in Mental Handicap: A Guide to Assessment Practices & Tests
Brookline Books
8 Trumbull Rd
Suite B-001
Northampton, MA 01060   413-584-0184
                                800-666-2665
                           Fax: 413-584-6184
                           brbooks@yahoo.com
                           www.brooklinebooks.com

Esther Wilder, Co-Author
Helps professionals understand the rationale and uses for assessment practices, and provides details of appropriate instruments within each type: adaptive behavior scales, assessment of behavioral disturbances, early development and Plagetian tests. *$20.00*
Hardcover
ISBN 0-91479-31-X

2216 Assessment of Children and Youth
Longman Education/Addison Wesley
1185 Avenue of the Americas
New York, NY 10036-2601   212-997-8500
                                 866-203-6215
                           TTY: 800-231-5469
                                 www.hess.com

Dr. Mark R. Williams, Chairman of the Board
Gregory P. Hill, President/COO
John B. Hess, Chief Executive Officer
Introductory text for preservice and in-service special educators on assessment, based on the principle that every child is unique. Comprehensive coverage of both formal and informal assessment instruments. *$50.00*
640 pages Paperback
ISBN 0-80131-02-5

2217 Assessment of Individuals with Severe Disabilities
Brookes Publishing Company
PO Box 10624
Baltimore, MD 21285-0624   410-337-9580
                                  800-638-3775
                            Fax: 410-337-8539
                            custserv@brookespublishing.com
                            www.brookespublishing.com
Paul H. Brookes, Chairman
Jeffrey D. Brookes, President
Melissa A. Behm, ExecutiveVice President
This expanded text offers instructors guidelines to design a comprehensive educational assessment for individuals with severe disabilities. *$34.00*
432 pages Paperback
ISBN 1-557660-67-0

2218 Assessment of the Technology Needs of Vending Facilitiy Managers In Tennessee
Mississippi State University
108 Herbert - South
Room 150/PO Drawer 6189
Mississippi State Univers, MS 39762-6189   662-325-2001
                                             800-675-7782
                                       Fax: 662-325-8989
                                       TTY: 662-325-2694
                                       nrtc@colled.msstate.edu
                                       www.blind.msstate.edu
Jacqui Bybee, Research and Training Coordinato
Michele Capella McDonnall, Ph.D., Research Professor/Interim Director
Jessica Thornton, Business Manager
This report summarizes the results and recommendations of a survey conducted of vending facility managers throughout the state of Tennessee who participate in the Randolph-Sheppard program. *$15.00*
39 pages Paperback

2219 Assessment: The Special Educator's Role
Brookes Publishing Company
PO Box 10624
Baltimore, MD 21285-0624   410-337-9580
                                  800-638-3775
                            Fax: 410-337-8539
                            custserv@brookespublishing.com
                            www.brookespublishing.com
Paul H. Brooks, Chairman
Jeffrey D. Brookes, President
Melissa A. Behm, ExecutiveVice President
Aimed at students with little or no classroom experience in assessment, the book focuses on the integration of dynamic, curriculum-based and norm-referenced data for diagnostic decisions and program planning.
580 pages Casebound
ISBN 0-53421-32-1

2220 Assistive Technology in the Schools: A Guide for Idaho Educators
Idaho Assistive Technology Project
University of Idaho
1187 Alturas Dr.
Moscow, ID 83843- 8331   205-885-3557
                                800-432-8324
                          Fax: 208-885-6102
                          idahoat@uidaho.edu
                          www.idahoat.org

LaRhae Rhoads, Author
Ron Seiler, Author
Michelle Doty, Author
This manual is designed to provide educators, parents, students with disabilities and related service providers with assistance in identifying, selecting, and acquiring assistive technology (AT) devices and services.

2221 Asthma Management and Education
Asthma and Allergy Foundation of America
8201 Corporate Drive
Suite 1000
Landover, MD 20785   202-466-7643
                            800-727-8462
                            info@aafa.org
                            www.aafa.org

Lynn Hanessian, Chair
Mitchell Grayson, MD, Chair, Research
Barbara Corn, Chair, Governance
One session, two hour program developed to educate allied health professionals about up-to-date asthma care and patient education, information and materials. Includes hands on experience with peak flow meters and demonstrations of medical devices.

2222 Aston-Patterning
PO Box 3568
Incline Village, NV 89450-3568   775-831-8228
                                   Fax: 775-831-8955
                                   office@astonkinetics.com
                                   www.astonkinetics.com

J Aston, Owner
Angelina Calafiore, Office Manager
Integrated system of movement education, body assessment, environmental modification and fitness training.

2223 Attention Deficit Disorder in Children
Charles C. Thomas
2600 S First St
Springfield, IL 62704-4730   217-789-8980
                                    800-258-8980
                              Fax: 217-789-9130
                              books@ccthomas.com
                              www.ccthomas.com

CC Thomas has been producing a strong list of specialty titles and textbooks in the biomedical sciences since 1927.

2224 Aural Habilitation
Alexander Graham Bell Association
3417 Volta Pl NW
Washington, DC 20007-2737   202-337-5220
Fax: 202-337-8314
TTY: 202-337-5221
info@agbell.org
www.listeningandspokenlanguage.org
Meredith K. Sugar, Esq. (OH), President
Ted A. Meyer, M.D., Ph.D, President-Elect/Secretary-Treasurer
Emilio Alonso-Mendoza, Chief Executive Officer
This classic text for professionals, educators and parents discusses verbal learning and aural habilitation of young children with hearing losses to ensure that each child is educated in the best setting. It discusses communication, normal development of spoken language, speech audiologic assessment, hearing aids and use of residual hearing, and program designs for individualized needs, including the assessment and planning of IEPs. *$26.95*
324 pages

2225 Behavior Analysis in Education: Focus on Measurably Superior Instruction
Brookes Publishing Company
PO Box 10624
Baltimore, MD 21285-0624   410-337-9580
800-638-3775
Fax: 410-337-8539
custserv@brookespublishing.com
www.brookespublishing.com
Paul H. Brookes, Chairman
Jeffrey D. Brookes, President
Melissa A. Behm, ExecutiveVice President
Designed to disseminate measurably superior instructional strategies to those interested in advancing sound, pedagogically effective, field-tested educational practices, this book is intended for graduate-level courses and seminars in special education and/or psychology focusing on behavior analysis and instruction.
512 pages Casebound
ISBN 0-53422-60-9

2226 Behavior Modification
Sage Publications
2455 Teller Rd
Thousand Oaks, CA 91320-2218   805-499-0721
800-818-7243
Fax: 800-583-2665
info@sagepub.com
www.sagepub.com
Sara Miller McCune, Founder, Publisher and Executive Chairman
Blaise R. Simqu, President & CEO
Chris Hickok, Senior Vice President & Chief Financial Officer
Describes in detail for replication purposes assessment and modification techniques for problems in psychiatric, clinical, educational and rehabilitation settings. *$53.00*
640 pages Quarterly

2227 Behind Special Education
Love Publishing Company
9101 E Kenyon Ave
Suite 2200
Denver, CO 80237-1854   303-221-7333
Fax: 303-221-7444
lpc@lovepublishing.com
www.lovepublishing.com
This new work is a critical analysis of the nature of disability, special education, school organization and reform progress. *$24.95*
ISBN 0-89108-17-4

2228 Biomedical Concerns in Persons with Down's Syndrome
Paul H Brookes Publishing Company
PO Box 10624
Baltimore, MD 21285-0624   410-337-9580
800-638-3775
Fax: 410-337-8539
custserv@brookespublishing.com
www.brookespublishing.com
Paul H. Brookes, Chairman
Jeffrey D. Brookes, President
Melissa A. Behm, ExecutiveVice President

Written by leading authorities and spanning many disciplines and specialties, this comprehensive resource provides vital information on biomedical issues concerning individuals with Down's Syndrome. *$45.00*
336 pages Hardcover
ISBN 1-557660-89-1

2229 Breaking Barriers
AbleNet, Inc.
2625 Patton Road
Roseville, MN 55113-1137   651-294-2200
800-322-0956
Fax: 651-294-2259
customerservice@ablenetinc.com
www.ablenetinc.com
Jennifer Thalhuber, President & CEO
Paul Sugden, CFO & Trustee
A practical resource for parents, caregivers, teachers and therapists. *$15.00*

2230 Building Skills for Independence in the Mainstream
15619 Premiere Drive
Suite 101
Tampa, FL 33624   850-363-9909
Fax: 480-393-4331
accounting@successforkidswithhearingloss.com
successforkidswithhearinglo ss.com
Karen L. Anderson, Director/ Co-Author
Gale Wright, Co-Author
Building Skills for Independence in the Mainstream was developed as a Guide for DHH professionals to support their work with classroom teachers and with students to develop the skills needed for independence with hearing aids and self-advocacy.

2231 Building Skills for Success in the Fast-Paced Classroom
15619 Premiere Drive
Suite 101
Tampa, FL 33624   850-363-9909
Fax: 480-393-4331
accounting@successforkidswithhearingloss.com
successforkidswithhearinglo ss.com
Karen L. Anderson, PhD, Co-Author
Kathleen A. Arnoldi, MA
The purpose of this book is to provide resources that will assist these students in optimizing their achievement through improved access and self-advocacy. The information contained in this book targets the expanded core curriculum, or those skills that must be mastered in order to benefit from the core curriculum. This book is meant to be a practical ready-to-go resource for professionals who work with school-age children with hearing loss.

2232 Building the Healing Partnership: Parents, Professionals and Children with Chronic Illnesses
Brookline Books
8 Trumbull Rd
Ste B-001
Northampton, MA 01060   413-584-0184
800-666-2665
Fax: 413-584-6184
brbooks@yahoo.com
www.brooklinebks.com
Patricia Tanner Leff, Author
Elaine H. Walizer, Author
Successful programs understand that the disabled child's needs must be considered in the context of a family. This book was specifically written for practitioner's who must work with families but who have insufficient training in family systems assessment and intervention. It is a valuable blend of theory and practice with pointers for applying the principles. *$24.95*
312 pages Paperback 1992
ISBN 0-914797-60-3

2233 CAI, Career Assessment Inventories for the Learning Disabled
Academic Therapy Publications
20 Leveroni Crt
Novato, CA 94949-5746　　　　　　　415-883-3314
　　　　　　　　　　　　　　　　　800-422-7249
　　　　　　　　　　　　　Fax: 888-287-9975
　　　　　　　　　　　sales@academictherapy.com
　　　　　　　　　　　www.academictherapy.com
Carol Weller, Author
Mary Buchanan, Author
Takes personality, ability and interest into account in pointing learning disabled students of all ages toward intelligent and realistic career choices. Contains binder with paperback teaching guide plus 50 interest inventories and 50 abilities inventories.
64 pages 1983
ISBN 0-878793-50-X

2234 Caring for Children with Chronic Illness
11 W 42nd St
15th Floor
New York, NY 10036-8002　　　　　　212-431-4370
　　　　　　　　　　　　　　　　　877-687-7476
　　　　　　　　　　　　　Fax: 212-941-7842
　　　　　　　　　　　cs@springerpub.com
　　　　　　　　　　　www.springerpub.com
Ursula Springer, President
Theodore C. Nardin, CEO/Publisher
Jason Roth, VP/Marketing Director
A critical look at the current medical, social, and psychological framework for providing care to children with chronic illnesses. Emphasizing the need to create integrated, interdisciplinary approaches, it discusses issues such as the roles of families, professionals, and institutions in providing health care, the impact of a child's illness on various family structures, financing care, the special problems of chronically ill children as they become adolescents and more. *$36.95*
320 pages Hardcover
ISBN 0-82615-00-1

2235 Carolina Curriculum for Infants and Toddlers with Special Needs (3rd Edition)
Brookes Publishing
P.O. Box 10624
Baltimore, MD 21285-0624　　　　　　410-337-9580
　　　　　　　　　　　　　　　　　800-638-3775
　　　　　　　　　　　　　Fax: 410-337-8539
　　　　　　　　　　　custserv@brookespublishing.com
　　　　　　　　　　　www.brookespublishing.com
Nancy M. Johnson-Martin, Author
Susan M. Attermeier, Author
Bonnie J. Hacker, Author
This book includes detailed assessment and intervention sequences, daily routine integration strategies, sensorimotor adaptations, and a sample 24-page assessment log that shows readers how to chart a child's individual progress.
504 pages Spiral-bound

2236 Carolina Curriculum for Preschoolers with Special Needs
Brookes Publishing
PO Box 10624
Baltimore, MD 21285-0624　　　　　　410-337-9580
　　　　　　　　　　　　　　　　　800-638-3775
　　　　　　　　　　　　　Fax: 410-337-8539
　　　　　　　　　　　custserv@brookespublishing.com
　　　　　　　　　　　www.brookespublishing.com
Paul H. Brookes, Chairman
Jeffrey D. Brookes, President
Melissa A. Behm, ExecutiveVice President
This curriculum provides detailed teaching and assessment techniques, plus a sample 28-page assessment log that shows readers how to chart a child's individual progress. This guide is for children between 2 and 5 in their developmental stages who are considered at risk for developmental delay or who exhibit special needs. *$34.00*
352 pages Spiral-bound
ISBN 1-55766-32-8

2237 Challenge of Educating Together Deaf and Hearing Youth: Making Manistreaming Work
Charles C. Thomas
2600 S First St
Springfield, IL 62704-4730　　　　　　217-789-8980
　　　　　　　　　　　　　　　　　800-258-8980
　　　　　　　　　　　　　Fax: 217-789-9130
　　　　　　　　　　　books@ccthomas.com
　　　　　　　　　　　www.ccthomas.com
Those who have this challenge of education: teachers, administrators, other professionals, parents, and concerned individuals will benefit from this book. Also available in cloth. *$51.35*
198 pages Hardcover
ISBN 0-398063-91-5

2238 Challenged Scientists: Disabilities and the Triumph of Excellence
Greenwood Publishing Group
130 Cremona Drive
Santa Barbara, CA 93117　　　　　　805-968-1911
　　　　　　　　　　　　　　　　　800-368-6868
　　　　　　　　　　　　　Fax: 866-270-3856
　　　　　　　　　　　CustomerService@abc-clio.com
　　　　　　　　　　　www.abc-clio.com
This volume points out how the increasing need for scientists in this country can be lessened by utilizing a long overlooked pool of scientific talent in those persons who are scientifically oriented but who happen to have physical or sensory disabilities. Hardcover. $49.95-$55.00.
208 pages
ISBN 0-275938-73-5

2239 Child Care and the ADA: A Handbook for Inclusive Programs
Brookes Publishing
PO Box 10624
Baltimore, MD 21285-0624　　　　　　410-337-9580
　　　　　　　　　　　　　　　　　800-638-3775
　　　　　　　　　　　　　Fax: 410-337-8539
　　　　　　　　　　　custserv@brookespublishing.com
　　　　　　　　　　　www.brookespublishing.com
Paul H. Brookes, Chairman
Jeffrey D. Brookes, President
Melissa A. Behm, ExecutiveVice President
This book is designed for educators and administrators in child care settings. It offers a straightforward discussion of the Americans with Disabilities Act including children with disabilities in community programs. *$25.95*
240 pages Paperback
ISBN 1-55766-85-5

2240 Child with Disabling Illness
Lippincott, Williams & Wilkins
16522 Hunters Green Pkwy
Hagerstown, MD 21740　　　　　　301-223-2300
　　　　　　　　　　　　　　　　　800-638-3030
　　　　　　　　　　　　　Fax: 301-223-2400
　　　　　　　　　　　orders@lww.com
　　　　　　　　　　　www.lww.com
$108.50
700 pages

2241 Childhood Behavior Disorders: Applied Research & Educational Practice
Sage Publications
2455 Teller Road
Thousand Oaks, CA 91320-2218　　　　805-499-0721
　　　　　　　　　　　　　　　　　800-818-7243
　　　　　　　　　　　　　Fax: 800-583-2665
　　　　　　　　　　　info@sagepub.com
　　　　　　　　　　　www.sagepub.com
Sara Miller McCune, Founder, Publisher, Chairperson
Blaise R. Simqu, President/CEO
Chris Hickok, Senior Vice President & Chief Fi
The only comprehensive overview of childhood behavior disorders. This book gives you the how and why for helping children with behavior disorders.

2242 Childhood Disablity and Family Systems(Routledge Library Editions) (Volume 5)
Routledge (Taylor & Francis Group)
711 Third Ave
New York, NY 10017
212-216-7800
800-634-7064
Fax: 202-564-7854
enquiries@taylorandfrancis.com
www.routledge.com

Michael Ferrari, Editor
Marvin B. Sussman, Editor
Focuses on what the presence of a disabled child means to a family. Those professionals involved in teaching, research, and direct care with families having disabled children will value the coverage of such topics as the contemporary context of disability, ethical issues, family effects, and care systems. First published in 1987 by Haworth Press, the book is now published under Routledge. *$140.00*
256 pages Hardcover 1916
ISBN 1-138101-55-9

2243 Children and Youth Assisted by Medical Technology in Educational Settings, 2nd Edition
Brookes Publishing
PO Box 10624
Baltimore, MD 21285-0624
410-337-9580
800-638-3775
Fax: 410-337-8539
custserv@brookespublishing.com
www.brookespublishing.com

Paul H. Brookes, Chairman
Jeffrey D. Brookes, President
Melissa A. Behm, ExecutiveVice President
Contains detailed daily care guidelines and emergency-response techniques, including information on working with a range of students who have the HIV infection, that rely on ventilators, that utilize tube feeding, or require catheterization. Also covers every aspect of planning for inclusive classrooms, including information on personnel training, entrance planning and transition, legal requirements, and transportation issues. *$52.00*
432 pages Spiral-bound
ISBN 1-55766 -36-3

2244 Children's Needs Psychological Perspective
National Association of School Psychologists
4340 East West Hwy.
Suite 402
Bethesda, MD 20814
301-657-0270
866-331-6277
Fax: 301-657-0275
TTY: 301-657-4155
www.nasponline.org

Kathleen Minke, Executive Director
Laura Benson, Chief Operating Officer
This monograph was developed with the recognition that many factors beyond the classroom and the child's own personal characteristics influence school success.
637 pages

2245 Choices: A Guide to Sex Counseling with Physically Disabled Adults
Krieger Publishing Company
1725 Krieger Dr
Malabar, FL 32950
321-724-9542
800-724-0025
Fax: 321-951-3671
info@krieger-publishing.com
www.krieger-publishing.com

Maureen E. Neistadt, Author
Provides rehabilitation professionals with the basic information necessary for limited sexuality counseling of physically disabled adults. *$20.90*
132 pages
ISBN 0-898749-03-4

2246 Choosing Options and Accommodations for Children
Brookes Publishing
PO Box 10624
Baltimore, MD 21285-0624
410-337-9580
800-638-3775
Fax: 410-337-8539
custserv@brookespublishing.com
www.brookespublishing.com

Bridging the gap between the philosophy and practice of inclusive education, this important manual provides a practical assessment and planning process for the inclusion of students with disabilities in general education classrooms. *$29.00*
192 pages
ISBN 1-55766 -06-5

2247 Cirriculum Development for Students with Mild Disabilities
Charles C. Thomas
2600 S First St
Springfield, IL 62704-4730
217-789-8980
800-258-8980
Fax: 217-789-9130
books@ccthomas.com
www.ccthomas.com

Carroll J. Jones, Author
This book was designed to provide the foundation from which to write cirrocumuli that will provide academic and social skills for Individual Education Programs (IEPs). *$38.95*
258 pages Spiral-Paper
ISBN 0-398070-18-2

2248 Clinical Alzheimer Rehabilitation
Springer Publishing
11 W 42nd St
15th Floor
New York, NY 10036-8002
212-431-4370
877-687-7476
Fax: 212-941-7842
cs@springerpub.com
www.springerpub.com

Theodore C. Nardin, CEO/Publisher
Jason Roth, VP/Marketing Director
Annette Imperati, Marketing/Sales Director
This comprehensive and easy-to-read guidebook contains the latest research on dementia and AD in the elderly population, including the causes and risk factors of AD, diagnosis information, and symptoms and progressions of the disease. Significant emphasis is given to the physical, mental, and verbal rehabilitation challenges of patients with AD. The authors outline specific rehabilitation goals for the physical therapist, speech-language pathologist, and general caregiver.

2249 Clinical Management of Childhood Stuttering, 2nd Edition
Sage Publications
2455 Teller Road
Thousand Oaks, CA 91320-2218
805-499-0721
800-818-7243
Fax: 800-583-2665
info@sagepub.com
www.sagepub.com

Sara Miller McCune, Founder, Publisher, Chairperson
Blaise R. Simqu, President/CEO
Chris Hickok, Senior Vice President/CFO
Updates and integrates recent findings in childhood stuttering into a broad range of therapeutic strategies for assessing and treating the young dysfluent child. *$38.00*
336 pages

2250 Cognitive Approaches to Learning Disabilities
Sage Publications
2455 Teller Road
Thousand Oaks, CA 91320-2218
805-499-0721
800-818-7243
Fax: 800-583-2665
info@sagepub.com
www.sagepub.com

Sara Miller McCune, Founder, Publisher, Chairperson
Blaise R. Simqu, President/CEO
Chris Hickok, Senior Vice President/CFO

The first to bridge the gap between cognitive psychology and information processing theory in understanding learning disabilities. *$39.00*
495 pages Hardcover

2251   Cognitive Strategy Instruction That Really Improves Children's Academic Skills
Brookline Books
8 Trumbull Rd
Suite B-001
Northampton, MA 01060   413-584-0184
                               800-666-2665
                               Fax: 413-584-6184
                               brbooks@yahoo.com
                               www.brooklinebooks.com
Esther Isabe Wilder, Author
A concise and focused work that summarily presents the few procedures for teaching strategies that aid academic subject matter learning: decoding reading comprehension, vocabulary, math, spelling and writing. Learning unrelated facts and science. Completely revised in 1995. *$27.95*
Paperback
ISBN 1-571290-07-9

2252   Collaborating for Comprehensive Services for Young Children and Families
Brookes Publishing Company
PO Box 10624
Baltimore, MD 21285-0624   410-337-9580
                                  800-638-3775
                                  Fax: 410-337-8539
                                  custserv@brookespublishing.com
                                  www.brookespublishing.com
Paul H. Brookes, Chairman
Jeffrey D. Brookes, President
Melissa A. Behm, ExecutiveVice President
Taking collaboration a step beyond basic implementation, this useful book shows agency and school leaders how to coordinate their efforts to stretch human services dollars while still providing quality programs. Provides the building blocks needed to establish a local interagency coordinating council. *$37.00*
272 pages
ISBN 1-557661-03-0

2253   Collaborative Teams for Students with Severe Disabilities
Brookes Publishing
PO Box 10624
Baltimore, MD 21285-0624   410-337-9580
                                  800-638-3775
                                  Fax: 410-337-8539
                                  custserv@brookespublishing.com
                                  www.brookespublishing.com
Paul H. Brookes, Chairman
Jeffrey D. Brookes, President
Melissa A. Behm, ExecutiveVice President
How can educators, parents and therapists work together to ensure the best possible educational experience for students with severe disabilities? This resource describes how a collaborative team can successfully create exciting learning opportunities for students, while teaching them to participate fully at home, school, work and play. *$ 30.00*
304 pages
ISBN 1-55766 -88-3

2254   Communicating with Parents of Exceptional Children
Love Publishing Company
9101 E Kenyon Ave
Suite 2200
Denver, CO 80237-1854   303-221-7333
                               Fax: 303-221-7444
                               lpc@lovepublishing.com
                               www.lovepublishing.com
Roger L. Kroth, Author
Denzil Denzil Edge, Author
This book shows how teachers can facilitate parent involvement with children's education. It presents the mirror model of parent involvement, family, dynamics, how to listen actively to parents,

values and perceptions, problem-solving, parent conferences and training groups. *$19.95*
ISBN 0-89108 -67-4

2255   Communication & Language Acquisition: Discoveries from Atypical Development
Brookes Publishing
PO Box 10624
Baltimore, MD 21285-0624   410-337-9580
                                  800-638-3775
                                  Fax: 410-337-8539
                                  custserv@brookespublishing.com
                                  www.brookespublishing.com
Paul H. Brookes, Chairman
Jeffrey D. Brookes, President
Melissa A. Behm, ExecutiveVice President
This text demonstrates how the study of language acquisition in children with atypical development promotes advances in basic theory. *$44.00*
352 pages Hardcover
ISBN 1-557662-79-7

2256   Communication Skills for Working with Elders
Springer Publishing Company
11 W 42nd St
15th Floor
New York, NY 10036-8002   212-431-4370
                                 877-687-7476
                                 Fax: 212-941-7842
                                 cs@springerpub.com
                                 www.springerpub.com
Ursula Springer, President
Theodore C. Nardin, CEO/Publisher
Jason Roth, VP/Marketing Director
How aging and illness affects communication. *$17.95*
160 pages Softcover
ISBN 0-82615 -20-7

2257   Communication Unbound
Teachers College Press
Ste 2115
14781 Memorial Dr
Houston, TX 77079-5210   415-738-4323
                                Fax: 415-738-4329
                                tcc.orders@aidcvt.com
                                www.pearsonhighered.com
Complete title is 'Communication Unbound: How Facilitated Communication is Challenging the Traditional Views of Autism and Ability/Disability'. Reveals the wonder of expression by people who have been trapped in silence and diminished by presumptions of their incompetence. *$18.95*
240 pages Paperback
ISBN 0-087737-21-4

2258   Complete Handbook of Children's Reading Disorders: You Can Prevent or Correct LDs
Gallery Bookshop
319 Kasten Street
PO Box 270
Mendocino, CA 95460-270   707-937-2215
                                 Fax: 707-937-3737
                                 info@gallerybookshop.com
                                 www.gallerybooks.com
Tony Miksak, Owner
The complete handbook of children's reading disorders. *$34.95*
732 pages Paperback
ISBN 0-80772 -83-3

2259   Computer Access/Computer Learning
Special Needs Project
324 State Street
Suite H
Santa Barbara, CA 93101-2364   818-718-9900
                                      800-333-6867
                                      Fax: 818-349-2027
                                      editor@specialneeds.com
                                      www.specialneeds.com
Mark Darrow, Founder,The Prolotherapy Institu
A resource manual in adaptive technology and computer training. *$22.50*

2260 Consulting Psychologists Press
1055 Joaquin Rd
Suite. 200
Mountain View, CA 94043-1243 650-969-8901
800-624-1765
Fax: 650-969-8608
custserv@cpp.com

Carl E. Thoresen, Chairman
Jeffrey Hayes, President and Chief Executive Officer
Andrew Bell, Vice President of International
Catalog offering job assessment software, career development reports, educational assessment information and books for the professional.

2261 Counseling Persons with Communication Disorders and Their Families
Sage Publications
2455 Teller Road
Thousand Oaks, CA 91320-2218 805-499-0721
800-818-7243
Fax: 800-583-2665
info@sagepub.com
www.sagepub.com

Sara Miller McCune, Founder, Publisher, Chairperson
Blaise R. Simqu, President & CEO
Chris Hickok, Senior Vice President & Chief Fi
A learning manual for speech-language pathologists and audiologists on how to deal with the emotional issues facing them in their work with clients with communication disorders and their families. *$ 29.00*
187 pages

2262 Counseling in the Rehabilitation Process
Charles C. Thomas
2600 S First St
Springfield, IL 62704-4730 217-789-8980
800-258-8980
Fax: 217-789-9130
books@ccthomas.com
www.ccthomas.com

Gerald L. Gandy, Author
E. Davis Martin Jr, Author
Richard E. Hardy, Author
This text provides the reader with a comprehensive overview and introduction to the field of rehabilitation counseling and services, and also has applicability in the growing field of community counseling. *$51.95*
358 pages paper 1999
ISBN 0-398069-70-4

2263 Creating Positive Classroom Environments: Strategies for Behavior Management
Brooks / Cole Publishing Company
511 Forest Lodge Rd
Pacific Grove, CA 93950-5040 831-373-0728
800-354-9706
Fax: 831-375-6414
bc-info@brookscole.com
www.cengage.com
A hands-on text that offers an approach to classroom management that encourages situation-specific decision making. Presenting research-based information on how to establish an effective behavior management system in both regular and special education settings, the book centers on ways to help students manage their own behavior, rather than on ways their behavior can be managed by teachers, peers, parents or other adults.
448 pages Paperbound
ISBN 0-53422 -54-4

2264 Cristine M. Trahms Program for Phenylketonuria
University of Washington
PO Box 357920
Seattle, WA 98195 206-598-1800
877-685-3015
Fax: 206-598-1915
pku@u.washington.edu
www.depts.washington.edu/pku
C. Ronald Scott, MD, Professor, Pediatrics, Division
Clinical program for children and adults with phenylketonuria.

2265 Critical Voices on Special Education: Problems & Progress Concerning the Mildly Handicapped
State University of New York Press
22 Corporate Woods Boulevard
3rd Floor
Albany, NY 12211-2504 518-472-5000
866-430-7869
Fax: 518-472-5038
info@sunypress.edu
www.sunypress.edu

James Peltz, Associate Director
Janice Vunk, Assistant to the Director
Scott B Sigmon, Editor
Problems and progress concerning the mildly handicapped.
$24.95
265 pages Paperback 1990
ISBN 0-79140 -20-3

2266 Cultural Diversity, Families and the Special Education System
Teachers College Press
1234 Amsterdam Ave
New York, NY 10027-6602 212-678-3929
800-575-6566
Fax: 212-678-4149
tcpress@tc.columbia.edu
www.teacherscollegepress.com

Beth Harry, Author
This timely and thought-provoking book explores the quadruple disadvantage faced by the parents of poor, minority, handicapped children whose first language is not that of the school they attend.
$22.95
296 pages Paperback
ISBN 0-807731-19-6

2267 Curriculum Decision Making for Students with Severe Handicaps
Teachers College Press
1234 Amsterdam Ave
New York, NY 10027-6602 212-678-3929
800-575-6566
Fax: 212-678-4149
www.teacherscollegepress.com
The inclusion of severely handicapped students within the scope of public education has brought about many changes for teachers in special education, this book helps the professional to distinguish which avenues are the best to take. *$17.95*
192 pages Paperback
ISBN 0-807728-61-6

2268 Deciphering the System: A Guide for Families of Young Disabled Children
Brookline Books
8 Trumbull Rd
Ste B-001
Northampton, MA 01060 413-584-0184
800-666-2665
Fax: 413-584-6184
brbooks@yahoo.com
www.brooklinebks.com

Paula Beckman, Author
This book informs parents of disabled children (0-5) of their rights and the service system, e.g., ways to manage the cumulating information, tips on IEP and IFSP meetings and the educational assessment process, and how parents can work with multiple service providers. It includes contributions from both parents and professionals who have experience with the service system. *$21.95*
208 pages Paperback 1999
ISBN 0-914797-87-5

2269 Defining Rehabilitation Agency Types
Mississippi State University
108 Herbert - South
Room 150 Industrial Education Depar
Mississippi State, MS 39762-6189   662-325-2001
                                     800-675-7782
                              Fax: 662-325-8989
                              TTY: 662-325-2694
                              nrtc@colled.msstate.edu
                              www.blind.msstate.edu

Jacqui Bybee, Research Associate II
Michele Capella McDonnall, Ph.D., Research Professor/Interim Director
Jessica Thornton, Business Manager
Relationships of participant selection and cost factors of service delivery across rehabilitation agency types. A national survey of state agencies for the blind was conducted to examine factors that define the characteristics of different agencies; similar programs were grouped together. Classification criteria were developed to distinguish agencies into logical groups based on line of authority, funding and operating procedures. *$10.00*
15 pages Paperback

2270 Designing and Using Assistive Technology: The Human Perspective
Brookes Publishing
PO Box 10624
Baltimore, MD 21285-0624   410-337-9580
                             800-638-3775
                      Fax: 410-337-8539
                      custserv@brookespublishing.com
                      www.brookespublishing.com

Paul H. Brookes, Chairman
Jeffrey D. Brookes, President
Melissa A. Behm, ExecutiveVice President
Presented here is a holistic perspective on how and why people choose and use AT. Features personal insights and the latest research on design and development. *$31.00*
352 pages Paperback
ISBN 1-55766 -14-9

2271 Developing Cross-Cultural Competence:Guideto Working with Young Children & Their Families
Brookes Publishing
PO Box 10624
Baltimore, MD 21285-0624   410-337-9580
                             800-638-3775
                      Fax: 410-337-8539
                      custserv@brookespublishing.com
                      www.brookespublishing.com

Paul H. Brookes, Chairman
Jeffrey D. Brookes, President
Melissa A. Behm, ExecutiveVice President
This enlightening book perceptively and sensitively explores cultural, ethnic, and language diversity in human services. For those who work with families whose infants and young children may have or be at risk for a disability or chronic illness. (Second Edition) *$ 32.00*
448 pages Paperback
ISBN 1-55766 -31-9

2272 Developing Individualized Family Support Plans: A Training Manual
Brookline Books
Suite B-001
8 Trumbull Rd
Northampton, MA 01060   413-584-0184
                          800-666-2665
                   Fax: 413-584-6184
                   brbooks@yahoo.com
                   www.brooklinebooks.com

Esther Wilder, Co-Author
This manual provides in-service training coordinators, administrators, supervisors and university personnel with a compact package of functional and practical methods to train professionals about implementing family-centered individualized family support plans (IFSP'S). Also, case studies provide concrete examples to aid in learning to write IFSP's. *$24.95*
ISBN 0-914797-69-7

2273 Developing Staff Competencies for Supporting People with Disabilities
Brookes Publishing
PO Box 10624
Baltimore, MD 21285-0624   410-337-9580
                             800-638-3775
                      Fax: 410-337-8539
                      custserv@brookespublishing.com
                      www.brookespublishing.com

Paul H. Brookes, Chairman
Jeffrey D. Brookes, President
Melissa A. Behm, ExecutiveVice President
This timely second edition, now in a new easier to read format, gives service providers helpful strategies for increasing effectiveness and maintaining well-being while working in the rewarding yet challenging field of human services. *$34.00*
480 pages Paperback
ISBN 1-55766 -07-3

2274 Development of Language
McGraw-Hill, School Publishing
220 E Danieldale Rd
Desoto, TX 75115-2490   800-648-2970
                   Fax: 800-593-4418
                   www.mhschool.com
An organizational book based on the developmental stages of language.
464 pages

2275 Developmental Disabilities of Learning
Gallery Bookshop
319 Kasten Street
PO Box 270
Mendocino, CA 95460-270   707-937-2215
                      Fax: 707-937-3737
                      info@gallerybookshop.com
                      www.gallerybooks.com

Tony Miksak, Owner
Manual for professionals on developmental and learning disabilities in the growing child. *$25.00*
224 pages Illustrated

2276 Developmental Disabilities: A Handbook for Occupational Therapists
Haworth Press
711 Third Avenue
New York, NY 10017   212-216-7800
                       800-354-1420
                Fax: 212-244-1563
                subscriptions@tandf.co.uk
                www.haworthpress.com
Provides broad coverage of the spectrum of problems confronted by patients with developmental disabilities and the many kinds of occupational therapy services these individuals need. Experts identify exemplary institutional and community service programs for treating patients with autism, cerebral palsy, epilepsy, and other conditions. Haworth Press are now acquired by the Taylor & Francis Journals. *$ 74.95*
268 pages Hardcover
ISBN 0-866569-59-6

2277 Developmental Disabilities: A Handbook for Interdisciplinary Practice
Brookline Books
8 Trumbull Rd
Suite B-001
Northampton, MA 01060   413-584-0184
                          800-666-2665
                   Fax: 413-584-6184
                   brbooks@yahoo.com
                   www.brooklinebooks.com

Esther Wilder, Co-Author
Successful interdisciplinary team practice for persons with developmental disabilities that require each team member to understand and respect the contributions of the others. This handbook explains the professions most often represented on interdisciplinary teams: their natures, concerns and roles in the interdisciplinary context. *$29.95*
256 pages
ISBN 1-571290-03-6

2278   Developmental Variation and Learning Disorders
Educators Publishing Service
PO Box 9031
Cambridge, MA 02139-9031   617-367-2700
                                            800-225-5750
                                       Fax: 617-547-0412
                                   eps@schoolspecialty.com
                                       www.epsbooks.com

Rick Holden, President
Discusses seven major areas of development and four major areas
of academic proficiency and then ties this information together
by examining factors that predispose a child to dysfunction and
disability, offering guidelines to assessment and management,
and analyzing long-range outcomes and factors that promote re-
siliency for parents, educators and clinicians. *$69.00*
640 pages Cloth
ISBN 0-838819-92-3

2279   Digest of Neurology and Psychiatry
Institute of Living: Hartford Hospital
80 Seymour Street
Hartford, CT 06106-3309   860-545-5000
                                           800-673-2411
                                      Fax: 860-545-5066
                                       www.harthosp.org

Douglas Elliot, Chair of the Board
Stuart K. Markowitz, MD, FACR, President/SVP
*Gerald J. Boisvert, HHC Regional Vice President / Chief Financial
Officer,*
Abstracts and reviews of selected current literature in psychiatry,
neurology and related fields.

2280   Disability Funding News
8204 Fenton St
Silver Spring, MD 20910-4502   301-588-6380
                                           800-666-6380
                                      Fax: 301-588-6385
                                   www.cdpublications.com

Mike Gerecht, Publisher

2281   Disability Studies and the Inclusive Classroom
711 3rd Avenue
8th Floor
New York, NY 10017   212-216-7800
                                           800-634-7064
                                      Fax: 212-564-7854
                                       www.routledge.com

Susan Baglieri, Co-Author
Arthur Shapiro, Co-Author
This book's mission is to integrate knowledge and practice from
the fields of disability studies and special education. Parts I & II
focus on the broad, foundational topics that comprise disability
studies (culture, language, and history) and Parts III & IV move
into practical topics (curriculum, co-teaching, collaboration,
classroom organization, disability-specific teaching strategies,
etc.) associated with inclusive education.

2282   Disability and Rehabilitation
Taylor & Francis
7625 Empire Dr
Florence, KY 41042-2919   800-634-7064
                                      Fax: 800-248-4724
                                 orders@taylorandfrancis.com
                                   www.taylorandfrancis.com
An international, multidisciplinary journal seeking to encourage
a better understanding of all aspects of disability, and to promote
the rehabilitation process. *$395.00*
Monthly
ISSN 0963-82 8

2283   Disability, Sport and Society
711 3rd Avenue
8th Floor
New York, NY 10017   212-216-7800
                                           800-634-7064
                                      Fax: 212-564-7854
                                       www.routledge.com

Nigel Thomas, Co-Author
Andy Smith, Co-Author
Disability sport is a relatively recent phenomenon, yet it is also
one that, particularly in the context of social inclusion, is attracting increasing political and academic interest. The purpose of
this important new text - the first of its kind - is to introduce the
reader to key concepts in disability and disability sport and to examine the complex relationships between modern sport, disability and other aspects of wider society.

**2284   Disabled Rights: American Disability Policy and the
Fight for Equality**
3240 Prospect Street, NW
Suite 250
Washington, DC 20007   202-687-5889
                                      Fax: 202-687-6340
                                   gupress@georgetown.edu
                                     press.georgetown.edu/

Jacqueline Vaughn Switzer, Author
Disabled Rights explains how people with disabilities have been
treated from a social, legal, and political perspective in the
United States.

**2285   Divided Legacy: A History of the Schism in Medical
Thought, The Bacteriological Era**
North Atlantic Books
2526 Martin Luther King Jr. Way
Berkeley, CA 94704   510-549-4270
                                           800-337-2665
                                      Fax: 510-549-4276
                                orders@northatlanticbooks.com
                                   www.northatlanticbooks.com

Alla Spector, Director of Finance & Office Operations
Doug Reil, Executive Director/Associate Publisher
Ed Angel, Director of Office Administration
Concluding volume of Coulter's history of medical philosophy,
from ancient times to today. Covers the origins of bacteriology
and immunology in world medicine; describes the clash between
orthodox and alternative medicine.

2286   Dual Relationships in Counseling
American Counseling Association
P.O. Box 31110
Alexandria, VA 22310-9998   800-347-6647
                                      Fax: 800-473-2329
                                       www.counseling.org

Richard Yep, Chief Executive Officer
Discusses issues involving dual relationships in counseling.

**2287   Early Communication Skills for Children with Down
Syndrome**
Woodbine House
6510 Bells Mill Rd
Bethesda, MD 20817-1636   301-897-3570
                                           800-843-7323
                                      Fax: 301-897-5838
                                    info@woodbinehouse.com
                                     www.woodbinehouse.com

Nancy Gray Paul, Acquisitions Editor
Libby Kumin, Author
An expert shares her knowledge of speech and language development in young children with Down syndrome. Intelligibility,
hearing loss, apraxia and other factors that affect communications are discussed. It also covers speech-language assessments
and alternative communication options and literacy. *$19.95*
368 pages
ISBN 1-890627-27-5

**2288   Early Intervention: Implementing Child & Family
Services for At-Risk Infants and Toddlers**
PRO-ED Inc.
8700 Shoal Creek Blvd
Austin, TX 78757-6897   512-451-3246
                                           800-897-3202
                                      Fax: 800-397-7633
                                       general@proedinc.com
                                       www.proedinc.com

Marci J. Hanson, Author
Eleanor W. Lynch, Author
New directions and recent legislation have produced a need for
this guide which is designed for professionals facing the chal-

lenge of program development for disabled and at-risk infants, toddlers and their families. *$68.20*
394 pages Paperback 1995
ISBN 0-890796-21-1

2289 Ecology of Troubled Children
Brookline Books Publications
8 Trumbull Rd
Suite B-001
Northampton, MA 01060

413-584-0184
800-666-2665
Fax: 413-584-6184
brbooks@yahoo.com
www.brooklinebooks.com

Esther Isabe Wilder, Author
Designed for frontline mental health clinicians working with children with serious emotional disturbances; shows how to make children's' worlds more supportive by changing the places, activities and people in their lives. *$15.95*
256 pages
ISBN 1-571290-57-5

2290 Educating Children with Disabilities: A Transdisciplinary Approach
Brookes Publishing
PO Box 10624
Baltimore, MD 21285-0624

410-337-9580
800-638-3775
Fax: 410-337-8539
custserv@brookespublishing.com
www.brookespublishing.com

Paul H. Brookes, Chairman
Jeffrey D. Brookes, President
Melissa A. Behm, ExecutiveVice President
Widely respected textbook presents you with the strategies you need for developing an inclusive curriculum, integrating health care and educational programs and addressing needs and concerns. *$38.00*
512 pages
ISBN 1-557662-46-0

2291 Educating Children with Multiple Disabilities: A Transdisciplinary Approach
Brookes Publishing
PO Box 10624
Baltimore, MD 21285-0624

410-337-9580
800-638-3775
Fax: 410-337-8539
custserv@brookespublishing.com
www.brookespublishing.com

Paul H. Brookes, Chairman
Jeffrey D. Brookes, President
Melissa A. Behm, ExecutiveVice President
Emphasizing transdisciplinary cooperation between teachers, therapists, nurses and parents, this book describes a general model and specific techniques for effectively educating children with multiple disabilities. *$29.00*
496 pages Paperback
ISBN 1-557662-46-0

2292 Educating Individuals with Disabilities: IDEIA 2004 and Beyond (1st Edition)
Springer Publishing Company
11 W 42nd St
15th Fl
New York, NY 10036-8002

212-431-4370
877-687-7476
Fax: 212-941-7842
cs@springerpub.com
www.springerpub.com

Ted Nardin, Chief Executive Officer
Jason Roth, Vice President, Marketing & Sales
Kathy Weiss, Director, Sales
Discusses how learning-disabled students are identified and assessed today, in light of the 2004 Individuals with Disabilities Education Improvement Act. Grigorenko's interdisciplinary collection is the first to comprehensively review the IDEIA 2004 Act and distill the changes professionals working with learning-disabled students face. The text takes an overarching per-

spective, first discussing the IDEIA in its historical, political, and legal context. *$100.00*
512 pages Hardcover 1908
ISBN 0-826103-56-1

2293 Educating Students Who Have Visual Impairments with Other Disabilities
Brookes Publishing
PO Box 10624
Baltimore, MD 21285-0624

410-337-9580
800-638-3775
Fax: 410-337-8539
custserv@brookespublishing.com
www.brookespublishing.com

Paul H. Brookes, Chairman
Jeffrey D. Brookes, President
Melissa A. Behm, ExecutiveVice President
This introductory text provides techniques for facilitating functional learning in students with a wide range of visual impairments and multiple disabilities. With a concentration on educational needs and learning styles, the authors of this multidisciplinary volume demonstrate functional assessment and teaching adaptations that will improve students' inclusive learning experiences. *$49.95*
552 pages Paperback
ISBN 1-557662-80-0

2294 Educating all Students in the Mainstream
Brookes Publishing Company
PO Box 10624
Baltimore, MD 21285-0624

410-337-9580
800-638-3775
Fax: 410-337-8539
custserv@brookespublishing.com

Paul H. Brookes, Chairman
Jeff Brookes, President
Melissa A. Behm, ExecutiveVice President
Incorporating the research and viewpoints of both regular and special educators, this textbook provides an effective approach for modifying, expanding, and adjusting regular education to meet the needs of all students. *$34.00*
304 pages
ISBN 1-557660-22-0

2295 Educational Audiology for the Limited Hearing Infant and Preschooler
Charles C. Thomas
2600 S First St
Springfield, IL 62704-4730

217-789-8980
800-258-8980
Fax: 217-789-9130
books@ccthomas.com
www.ccthomas.com

Donald Goldberg, Author
Nancy Coleffe-Schenck, Author
Doreen Pollack, Author
Offers information on current concepts and practices in audio-logic screening and evaluation, development of the listening function, development of speech, development of language, the role of parents, parent education, mainstreaming of the limited-hearing child, and program modifications for the severely learning disabled child. Also includes information on auditory assessment, sensory aides, cochlear implants, acoupedics and auditory verbal programs. *$79.95*
430 pages Paperback
ISBN 0-398067-51-1

2296 Educational Care
Educators Publishing Service
625 Mount Auburn St
3rd Floor
Cambridge, MA 02138-3039

617-547-6706
800-225-5750
Feedback.EPS@schoolspecialty.com
www.eps.schoolspecialty.com

Paula Fabbro, Sales Consultant
Leo Micale, Sales Consultant
Kristen Colson, Sales Consultant
This book, written for both parents and teachers, is based on the view that education should be a system of care that is able to look

after the specific needs of individual students. Using case studies, it analyzes various types of learning disorders and then suggests ways to help students with these problems. *$31.50*
325 pages
ISBN 0-838819-87-7

2297 Educational Intervention for the Student
Charles C. Thomas
2600 S First St
Springfield, IL 62704-4730
217-789-8980
800-258-8980
Fax: 217-789-9130
books@ccthomas.com
www.ccthomas.com
CC Thomas has been producing a strong list of specialty titles and textbooks in the biomedical sciences since 1927.

2298 Educational Prescriptions
Educators Publishing Service
625 Mount Auburn St
3RD Floor
Cambridge, MA 02138-3039
617-547-6706
800-225-5750
Feedback.EPS@schoolspecialty.com
Paula Fabbro, Sales Consultant
Leo Micale, Sales Consultant
Kristen Colson, Sales Consultant
This book provides specific recommendations for the classroom management of students who are experiencing subtle developmental and/or learning difficulties. Intended for regular classroom teachers, specific examples of accommodations teachers can make are provided for grades 1-3 and 4-6. *$13.50*
64 pages
ISBN 0-838819-90-7

2299 Effective Instruction for Special Education
Sage Publications
2455 Teller Road
Thousand Oaks, CA 91320-2218
805-499-0721
800-818-7243
Fax: 800-583-2665
info@sagepub.com
www.sagepub.com
Sara Miller McCune, Founder, Publisher, Chairperson
Blaise R. Simqu, President/CEO
Chris Hickok, Senior Vice President/CFO
This exciting and wide-ranging book provides special educators with effective methods for teaching students with mild and moderate learning and behavioral problems, as well as for teaching remedial students in general. *$37.00*
419 pages Paperback

2300 Effectively Educating Handicapped Students
Longman Publishing Group
9th Fl
Upper Saddle River, NJ 07458-1813
201-236-3281
800-922-0579
Fax: 201-236-3290
www.pearsoned.com
For educators and other professionals who work with deaf and hearing impaired students in preschool and elementary programs. A developmental approach provides the foundation for several intervention methods including preparation for instruction, language, speech, audition and speechreading.
468 pages Paperback
ISBN 0-801303-17-6

2301 Emotional Problems of Childhood and Adolescence
McGraw-Hill School Publishing
PO Box 182604
Columbus, OH 43218
877-833-5524
800-338-3987
Fax: 609-308-4480
customer.service@mheducation.com
www.mcgraw-hill.com
David Levin, President/Chief Ex
David Stafford, Senior Vice President/General Counsel
Maryellen Valaitis, Senior Vice President Human Resources
For future special educators, psychologists and others who work with emotionally disturbed children and adolescents.

2302 Enabling & Empowering Families: Principles & Guidelines for Practice
Brookline Books
8 Trumbull Rd
Suite B-001
Northampton, MA 01060
413-584-0184
800-666-2665
Fax: 413-584-6184
brbooks@yahoo.com
www.brooklinebooks.com
Esther Wilder, Co-Author
This book was written for practitioners who must work with families but who have insufficient training in family systems assessment and intervention. The authors' system enables professionals to help the family identify its needs, locate the formal and informal resources to meet these needs and develop the abilities to effectively access these resources. *$24.95*
220 pages
ISBN 0-914797-59-X

2303 Evaluation and Educational Programming of Students with Deafblindness & Severe Disabilities
Charles C. Thomas
2600 S First St
Springfield, IL 62704-4730
217-789-8980
800-258-8980
Fax: 217-789-9130
books@ccthomas.com
www.ccthomas.com
Carroll J. Jones, Author
Subtitle: Sensorimotor Stage. This second edition offers a very complete package of information on the special education of deaf-blind students; including detailed diagnostic information to assist the instructor in evaluating the physical, social, mental status of the student, as well as the educational progress. *$50.95*
265 pages Spiral-Paper 2001
ISBN 0-398072-16-2

2304 Evaluation and Treatment of the Psychogeriatric Patient
Haworth Press
711 Third Avenue
New York, NY 10017
212-216-7800
800-354-1420
Fax: 212-244-1563
subscriptions@tandf.co.uk
www.haworthpress.com
This pertinent book assists occupational therapists and other health care providers in developing up-to-date psychogeriatric programs and understands details of treating the cognitively impaired elderly. Haworth Press are now acquired by the Taylor & Francis Journals. *$74.95*
111 pages Hardcover
ISBN 1-560240-52-0

2305 Exceptional Children in Focus
McGraw-Hill School Publishing
PO Box 182604
Columbus, OH 43218
877-833-5524
800-338-3987
Fax: 609-308-4480
customer.service@mheducation.com
www.mcgraw-hill.com
David Levin, President/Chief Ex
David Stafford, Senior Vice President/General Counsel
Maryellen Valaitis, Senior Vice President Human Resources
Combines a light, personal look at the problems of special educators experiences with the basic facts of exceptionality.
288 pages

2306 Exceptional Lives: Special Education in Today's Schools, 4th Edition
Pearson Education
1 Lake St
Upper Saddle River, NJ 07458-1813
201-236-3281
800-922-0579
Fax: 201-236-3290
www.pearsoned.com
Comprehensive coverage is built upon six guiding principles: 1) high expectations for individuals with disabilities and their educators, 2) inclusion for all students, 3) relationships and friend-

ships as essential outcomes of collaboration, 4) positive contributions by students with disabilities, 5) the importance of choice and self-advocacy for students with disabilities, and 6) full citizenship for all students with disabilities. Emphasizes the daily lives of students and educators. *$90.00*
592 pages
ISBN 0-131126-00-8

2307 Facilitating Self-Care Practices in the Elderly
Haworth Press
711 Third Avenue
New York, NY 10017 212-216-7800
800-354-1420
Fax: 212-244-1563
subscriptions@tandf.co.uk
www.haworthpress.com
This up-to-date book is a synthesis of current knowledge from published sources and expert consultants relating to three commonly occurring problems in home health care practice: self-administration of medications, family caregiving issues, and teaching the elderly. Haworth Press are now acquired by the Taylor & Francis Journals. *$74.95*
185 pages Hardcover
ISBN 1-560240-13-X

2308 Family-Centered Early Intervention with Infants and Toddlers
Brookes Publishing
PO Box 10624
Baltimore, MD 21285-0624 410-337-9580
800-638-3775
Fax: 410-337-8539
custserv@brookespublishing.com
www.brookespublishing.com
Paul H. Brookes, Chairman
Jeffrey D. Brookes, President
Melissa A. Behm, ExecutiveVice President
This informative text provides professionals with insight and practical guidelines to help fulfill the federal requirements for provision of early intervention services. *$37.00*
368 pages Hardcover
ISBN 1-557661-24-3

2309 Feeding Children with Special Needs
Arizona Department of Health Services
150 North 18th Avenue
Phoenix, AZ 85007-2607 602-542-1025
Fax: 602-542-0883
www.azdhs.gov
Will Humble, Director
Jeff Bloomberg, J.D., Manager
Robert Lane, Esq., Administrative Counsel
Guide designed to help develop a greater awareness of the special challenges involved in the nutrition and feeding concerns for children with special health care needs, and ways to approach the issues. *$5.00*

2310 Focal Group Psychotherapy
New Harbinger Publications
5674 Shattuck Ave
Oakland, CA 94609-1662 510-652-0215
800-748-6273
Fax: 800-652-1613
customerservice@newharbinger.com
www.newharbinger.com
Matthew McKay, Founder
Patrick Fanning, Co-Founder/Writer
Guide to leading brief, theme-based groups. This book offers an extensive week-by-week description of the basic concepts and interventions for 14 theme or focal groups for: codependency, rape victims, shyness, survivors of incest, agoraphobia, survivors of toxic parents, depression, child molesters, anger control, domestic violence offenders, assertiveness, alcohol and drug abuse, eating disorders, and parent training. *$59.95*
544 pages Cloth
ISBN 1-879237-18-0

2311 Free Hand: Enfranchising the Education of Deaf Children
TJ Publishers

Margaret Walworth, Author
Donald F. Moores, Author
Terrence J. O'Rourke, Author
A select group of nationally prominent educators, linguists and researchers met at Hofstra University to consider the most vital and controversial question in education of the deaf: what role should ASL play in the classroom? Become part of that discussion with A Free Hand. *$16.95*
204 pages Softcover
ISBN 0-93266 -40-X

2312 Friendship 101
Council for Exceptional Children
3100 Clarendon Blvd.
Suite 600
Arlington, VA 22201-5332 888-232-7733
TTY: 866-915-5000
service@exceptionalchildren.org
www.exceptionalchildren.org
Juliet E. Hart Barnett, Co-Author & Editor
Kelly J. Whalon, Co-Author & Editor
Book and webinar for general special educators who work with children with autism spectrum disorder (ASD). Presents evidence-based practices shown to enhance social competence in children with ASD.

2313 Functional Assessment Inventory Manual
Stout Vocational Rehab Institute
655 15th St. NW
Suite 800
Washington, DC 20005 715-232-1411
800-538-3742
Fax: 715-232-2356
botterbuschd@uwstout.edu
www2.epa.gov
Gina McCarthy, Administrator
Gwen Keyes Fleming, Chief of Staff
Bob Perciasepe, Deputy Administrator
The Functional Assessment is a systematic enumeration of a client's vocationally relevant strengths and limitations. *$12.00*
96 pages Paperback
ISBN 0-916671-53-4

2314 Get Ready for Jetty!: My Journal About ADHD and Me
750 First Street, NE
Washington, DC 20002-4242 202-336-5500
800-374-2721
rllowman@gmail.com
www.apa.org
Jeanne Kraus, Author
Jetty writes about these things as well as her recent ADHD diagnosis in her journal.

2315 Getting Around Town
Council for Exceptional Children
3100 Clarendon Blvd.
Suite 600
Arlington, VA 22201-5332 888-232-7733
TTY: 866-915-5000
service@exceptionalchildren.org
www.exceptionalchildren.org
M. Sherril Moon, Co-Author
Emily M. Luedtke, Co-Author
Elizabeth Halloran-Tornquist, Co-Author
This bookprovides examples of possible IEP goals and field-tested lesson plans for individual students or entire classes across all age and grade levels. *$34.95*

2316 Global Perspectives on Disability: A Curriculum
Mobility International USA
132 E Broadway
Suite 343
Eugene, OR 97401 541-343-1284
Fax: 541-343-6812
TTY: 541-343-1284
clearinghouse@miusa.org
www.miusa.org
Susan Sygall, Chief Executive Officer
Cindy Lewis, Director, Programs

Designed for secondary and higher education instructors. Includes five lesson plans covering disability awareness, disability rights and international perspectives on disability. Available in alternative formats.

2317 **Glossary of Terminology for Vocational Assessment/Evaluation/Work**
Rehabilitation Resource University
University of Wisconsin-Stou
Menomonie, WI 54751
715-232-2236
Fax: 715-232-2356
gundlachj@uwstout.edu
Ronald Fry, Manager
Jennifer Gundlach Klatt, Program Assistant
This glossary contains 254 terms and their definitions. Primary focus is on the terminology related to the practice and professionals of vocational assessment, vocational evaluation and work adjustment. *$9.50*
40 pages Softcover

2318 **Graduate Technological Education and the Human Experience of Disability**
Haworth Press
711 Third Avenue
New York, NY 10017
212-216-7800
800-354-1420
Fax: 212-244-1563
subscriptions@tandf.co.uk
www.haworthpress.com
This book examines graduate schools of theology and their limited familiarity with the study of disability — and the presence of people with disabilities in particular — on their campuses. This text offers critical research and illuminates new pathways for theologia and practice in the community of faith. It offers suggestions for incorporating disability studies into theological education and religious life.Haworth Press are now acquired by the Taylor & Francis Journals. *$34.95*
115 pages Hardcover
ISBN 0-789060-08-6

2319 **HIV Infection and Developmental Disabilities**
Brookes Publishing
PO Box 10624
Baltimore, MD 21285-0624
410-337-9580
800-638-3775
Fax: 410-337-8539
custserv@brookespublishing.com
www.brookespublishing.com
Paul H. Brookes, Chairman
Jeffrey D. Brookes, President
Melissa A. Behm, ExecutiveVice President
A resource for service providers pinpointing the most crucial medical, legal and educational issues to control HIV infection. *$47.00*
320 pages
ISBN 1-557660-83-2

2320 **Handbook for Implementing Workshops for Siblings of Special Children**
Special Needs Project
324 State Street
Suite H
Santa Barbara, CA 93101-2364
818-718-9900
800-333-6867
Fax: 818-349-2027
editor@specialneeds.com
www.specialneeds.com
Mark Darrow, Founder,The Prolotherapy Institu
Based on three years of professional experience, this handbook provides guidelines and techniques for those who wish to start and conduct workshops for siblings. *$40.00*

2321 **Handbook for Speech Therapy**
Psychological & Educational Publications
PO Box 520
Hydesville, CA 95547
800-523-5775
Fax: 800-447-0907
psych-edpublications@suddenlink.net
Basic handbook for beginning speech teachers, shows how speech sounds are made, what their individual characteristics are,

how they relate to each other, what the most common errors are, and how to correct those errors.
143 pages paperback

2322 **Handbook for the Special Education Administrator**
Edwin Mellen Press
PO Box 450
Lewiston, NY 14092-1205
716-754-2266
Fax: 716-754-4056
jrupnow@mellenpress.com
www.mellenpress.com
Arthur R. Crowell, Author
Bonnie Crogan, Marketing
Irene Miller, Accounting
Organization and procedures for special education. *$ 49.95*
96 pages Hardcover
ISBN 0-88946 -22-9

2323 **Handbook of Acoustic Accessibility**
15619 Premiere Drive
Suite 101
Tampa, FL 33624
850-363-9909
Fax: 480-393-4331
accounting@successforkidswithhearingloss.com
successforkidswithhearinglo ss.com
Joseph J. Smaldino, Co-Author
Carol Flexer, Co-Author
Most students with hearing loss are educated in mainstream education classrooms the majority of each school day.Communication - between peers and with teachers - is the coin of education and upon which a wealth of knowledge is built.Unfortunately for students with hearing loss, the typical classroom environment is hazardous for listening and interferes with access to all classroom communication.

2324 **Handbook of Developmental Education**
Greenwood Publishing Group
130 Cremona Drive
Santa Barbara, CA 93117
805-968-1911
800-368-6868
Fax: 866-270-3856
CustomerService@abc-clio.com
www.abc-clio.com
This comprehensive handbook has brought together the leading practitioners and researchers in the field of developmental education to focus on the developmental learning agenda. Hardcover.
400 pages $65 - $75
ISBN 0-275932-97-4

2325 **Handbook on Supported Education for Peoplewith Mental Illness**
Brookes Publishing
PO Box 10624
Baltimore, MD 21285-0624
410-337-9580
800-638-3775
Fax: 410-337-8539
custserv@brookespublishing.com
www.brookespublishing.com
Paul H. Brookes, Chairman
Jeffrey D. Brookes, President
Melissa A. Behm, ExecutiveVice President
Here you will find all necessary information that mental health professionals need in order to provide supported education services. There are specific suggestions on how to help people with mental illness return to or remain in college, trade school, or GED programs. Also addressed are funding and legal issues, accommodations, and specific interventions.
208 pages Paperback
ISBN 1-55766 -52-1

2326 **Head Injury Rehabilitation: Children**
Taylor & Francis
47 Runway Dr
Ste G
Levittown, PA 19057-4738
267-580-2622
Fax: 215-785-5515
Rehabilitation guide for the help of children or adolescents that have suffered brain injury.
460 pages Cloth
ISBN 0-85066 -67-1

2327 Health Care Management in Physical Therapy
Charles C. Thomas
2600 S First St
Springfield, IL 62704-4730   217-789-8980
                                    800-258-8980
                                Fax: 217-789-9130
                                books@ccthomas.com
                                www.ccthomas.com
CC Thomas has been producing a strong list of specialty titles and
textbooks in the biomedical sciences since 1927.

2328 Health Care for Students with Disabilities
Brookes Publishing Company
PO Box 10624
Baltimore, MD 21285-0624   410-337-9580
                                  800-638-3775
                              Fax: 410-337-8539
                          custserv@brookespublishing.com
                          www.brookespublishing.com

Paul H. Brookes, Chairman
Jeffrey D. Brookes, President
Melissa A. Behm, ExecutiveVice President
This practical guidebook provides detailed descriptions of the 16
health-related procedures most likely to be needed in the class-
room by students with disabilities. *$25.00*
304 pages Paperback
ISBN 1-557660-37-9

**2329 Helping Learning- Disabled Gifted Children Learn
Through Compensatory Active Play**
Charles C. Thomas
2600 S First St
Springfield, IL 62704-4730   217-789-8980
                                    800-258-8980
                                Fax: 217-789-9130
                                books@ccthomas.com
                                www.ccthomas.com

James Harry Humphrey, Author
$36.95
156 pages Hardcover 1990
ISBN 0-398056-95-1

2330 Helping Students Grow
American College Testing Program
500 ACT Drive
PO Box 168
Iowa City, IA 52243-0168   319-337-1000
                              info@keytrain.com
                              www.act.org
Jon Whitmore, Chief Executive Officer
Tom J. Goedken, Chief Financial Officer/Senior Vice President
Patricia C. Steinbrech, Chief Information Officer
Designed to assist counselors in using the wealth of information
generated by the ACT Assessment.

2331 Home Health Care Provider: A Guide to Essential Skills
Springer Publishing
11 W 42nd St
15th Floor
New York, NY 10036-8002   212-431-4370
                                 877-687-7476
                             Fax: 212-941-7842
                             cs@springerpub.com
                             www.springerpub.com
Theodore C. Nardin, CEO/Publisher
Jason Roth, VP/Marketing Director
Annette Imperati, Marketing/Sales Director
This book is designed to foster quality care to home care recipients. Prieto provides information, tips, and techniques on personal care routines as well as additional responsibilities,
including home safety and maintenance, meal planning, errand
running, caring for couples, and making use of recreational time.
The book focuses on the psycho-social needs of home care recipients, stressing the need to maintainthe house as a home, and sustaining the recipient's way of life throughout caregiving.

2332 How to Teach Spelling/How to Spell
Educators Publishing Service
625 Mount Auburn St
3rd Floor
Cambridge, MA 02138-3039   617-547-6706
                                  800-225-5750
                          Feedback.EPS@schoolspecialty.com
Paula Fabbro, Sales Consultant
Leo Micale, Sales Consultant
Kristen Colson, Sales Consultant
This is a comprehensive resource manual based on the
Orton-Gillingham approach to reading and spelling. It recom-
mends what and how much to teach at each grade level at the be-
ginning of each lesson or section. There are four student manuals
that accompany this. *$22.50*
Teachers Manual
ISBN 0-838818-47-1

**2333 Human Exceptionality: School, Community,and Family
(12th Edition)**
Cengage Learning
20 Channel Center St
Boston, MA 02210   617-289-7700
                          617-289-7844
                          www.cengage.com/us
Michael L. Hardman, Author
M. Winston Egan, Author
Clifford J. Drew, Author
An evidence-based testament to the critical role of cross-professional collaboration in enhancing the lives of exceptional individuals and their families. This text's unique lifespan approach
combines powerful research, evidence-based practices, and inspiring stories, engendering passion and empathy and enhancing
the lives of individuals with exceptionalities.
544 pages Hardcover

**2334 I Can't Hear You in the Dark: How to Lean and Teach
Lipreading**
Charles C. Thomas
2600 S First St
Springfield, IL 62704-4730   217-789-8980
                                    800-258-8980
                                Fax: 217-789-9130
                                books@ccthomas.com
                                www.ccthomas.com
Betty Woerner Carter, Author
The goal of this text is to improve communication and strengthen
relationships with others. *$40.95*
226 pages Spiral-Paper 1997
ISBN 0-398067-89-2

2335 I Heard That!
3417 Volta Pl NW
Washington, DC 20007-2737   202-337-5220
                              Fax: 202-337-8314
                              TTY: 202-337-5221
                              info@agbell.org
                          www.listeningandspokenlanguage.org
Meredith K. Sugar, Esq. (OH), President
Ted A. Meyer, M.D., Ph.D, President-Elect/Secretary-Treasurer
Emilio Alonso-Mendoza, Chief Executive Officer
Provides a framework for teachers, clinicians and parents when
writing objectives and designing activities to develop listening
skills in children with hearing loss from newborn to 3 years.
$7.95
36 pages

2336 I Heard That!2
Alexander Graham Bell Association
3417 Volta Pl NW
Washington, DC 20007-2737   202-337-5220
                              Fax: 202-337-8314
                              TTY: 202-337-5221
                              info@agbell.org
                          www.listeningandspokenlanguage.org
Meredith K. Sugar, Esq. (OH), President
Ted A. Meyer, M.D., Ph.D, President-Elect/Secretary-Treasurer
Emilio Alonso-Mendoza, Chief Executive Officer

Provides a framework for teachers, clinicians and parents when writing objectives and designing activities to develop listening skills in children who are deaf or hard of hearing. *$7.95*

36 pages

2337   If It Is To Be, It Is Up To Us To Help!
AVKO Educational Research Foundation
3084 Willard Rd
Ste W
Birch Run, MI 48415-9404   810-686-9283
                                             866-285-6612
                                         Fax: 810-686-1101
                                             www.avko.org

Don Mc Cabe, President
Ted A. Meyer, M.D., Ph.D, Vice-President
Michael Lane, Treasurer

A book of lesson plans for an Adult Community Education Course for Volunteer Tutors. Contains information on how to go about establishing such a course and how to secure cooperation from local and national organizations. Free as an e-book for Foundation members. *$ 14.95*

ISBN 1-56400 -42-1

2338   Images of the Disabled, Disabling Images
ABC-CLIO
130 Cremona Dr
Santa Barbara, CA 93117   805-968-1911
                                             800-368-6868
                                         Fax: 866-270-3856
                              customerservice@abc-clio.com
                                         www.abc-clio.com

Alan Gartner, Author

Combines an examination of the presentation of persons with disabilities in literature, film and the media with an analysis of the ways in which these images are expressed in public policy concerning the disabled. *$84.00*

227 pages Hardcover 1986

ISBN 0-275921-78-6

2339   Implementing Family-Centered Services in Early Intervention
Brookline Books
8 Trumbull Rd
Suite B-001
Northampton, MA 01060   413-584-0184
                                             800-666-2665
                                         Fax: 413-584-6184
                                         brbooks@yahoo.com
                                     www.brooklinebooks.com

This book describes a team-based decision-making workshop for implementing family-centered services in early interventions. Unlike a training curriculum, it focuses on the decisions that teams must make as they seek to become family-centered. *$19.95*

180 pages Paperback

ISBN 0-91479 -62-

2340   Including All of Us: An Early Childhood Curriculum About Disability
Educational Equity Concepts
381 Park Ave South
Suite 701
New York, NY 10016   212-243-1110
                                         Fax: 212-367-4640
                                         lcolon@fhi360.org
                                             www.fhi360.org

Frank Schneiger, President
Antonia Cottrell Martin, Founder and President
Merle Froschl, Director, Educational Equity

The first nonsexist, multicultural, mainstreamed curriculum. Step-by-step activities incorporate disability into three curriculum areas: Same/Different (hearing impairment), Body Parts (visual impairment), and Transportation (mobility impairment). *$14.95*

144 pages

ISBN 0-93162 -00-4

2341   Including Students with Severe and Multiple Disabilites in Typical Classrooms
Brookes Publishing
PO Box 10624
Baltimore, MD 21285-0624   410-337-9580
                                             800-638-3775
                                         Fax: 410-337-8539
                           custserv@brookespublishing.com
                                   www.brookespublishing.com

Paul H. Brookes, Chairman
Jeffrey D. Brookes, President
Melissa A. Behm, ExecutiveVice President

This straightforward and jargon free resource gives instructors the guidance needed to educate learners who have one or more sensory impairments in addition to cognitive and physical disabilities. *$32.95*

224 pages Paperback

ISBN 1-55766 -39-8

2342   Including Students with Special Needs: A Practical Guide for Classroom Teachers
Allyn & Bacon
75 Arlington St
Suite 300
Boston, MA 02116-3988   ab_webmaster@abacon.com
                      www.pearson.com/us/higher-education.html

Focuses on educating students with special needs in inclusive settings based on substantive administrative backing, support for general education teachers, and an understanding that sometimes not all needs can be met in a single location.

544 pages

ISBN 0-20528 -85-4

2343   Inclusive & Heterogeneous Schooling: Assessment, Curriculum, and Instruction
Brookes Publishing
PO Box 10624
Baltimore, MD 21285-0624   410-337-9580
                                             800-638-3775
                                         Fax: 410-337-8539
                           custserv@brookespublishing.com
                                   www.brookespublishing.com

Paul H. Brookes, Chairman
Jeff Brookes, President
Melissa A. Behm, ExecutiveVice President

Presents methods for successfully restructuring classrooms to enable all students, particularly those with disabilities, to flourish. Provides specific strategies for assessment, collaboration, classroom management, and age-specific instruction. *$34.95*

448 pages Paperback

ISBN 1-55766 -02-9

2344   Independent Living Approach to Disability Policy Studies
World Institute on Disability
3075 Adeline St.
Suite 155
Berkeley, CA 94703   510-225-6400
                                         Fax: 510-225-0477
                                             wid@wid.org
                                             www.wid.org

Marcie Roth, Executive Director & Chief Executive Officer
Katherine Zigmont, Senior Director, Operations & Deputy Director
Reggie Johnson, Senior Director, Marketing & Communications

A collection of essays and bibliographies aiming to build a framework for understanding how the relationship between public policy, disability studies and disability policy studies will impact the future.

2345 **Information & Referral Center**
Mississippi State University
108 Herbert - South
Room 150/PO Drawer 6189
Mississippi State Univers, MS 39762-6189   662-325-2001
800-675-7782
Fax: 662-325-8989
TTY: 662-325-2694
nrtc@colled.msstate.edu
www.blind.msstate.edu
Jacqui Bybee, Research and Training Coordinato
Michele Capella McDonnall, Ph.D., Research Professor/Interim Director
Jessica Thornton, Business Manager
A comprehensive website that includes information about client assistance programs, vocational rehabilitation agencies, low vision clinics and information about blindness and low vision.
$25.00
150 pages

2346 **Instructional Methods for Students**
Allyn & Bacon
75 Arlington St
Suite 300
Boston, MA 02116-3988   ab_webmaster@abacon.com
www.home.pearsonhighered.com
Instructional methods for students with learning and behavior problems.
450 pages
ISBN 0-205087-35-3

2347 **Interactions: Collaboration Skills for School Professionals**
Longman Education/Addison Wesley
75 Arlington St
Suite 300
Boston, MA 02116-3988   ab_webmaster@abacon.com
Shows school professionals how to develop and use the skills necessary for effective collaboration among teachers, school support staff, and parents of children with special needs. *$35.00*
270 pages Paperback
ISBN 0-80131 -21-2

2348 **International Journal of Arts Medicine**
MMB Music
9051 Watson Road
Suite 161
Saint Louis, MO 63126   314-531-9635
800-543-3771
Fax: 314-531-8384
info@mmbmusic.com
www.mmbmusic.com
Norm Goldberg, Founder/chairman
Exploration of the creative arts and healing. Presents peer-reviewed articles clearly written by educators in the creative arts, as well as internationally prominent physicians, therapists and health care professionals.

2349 **Interpreting Disability: A Qualitative Reader**
Teachers College Press
1234 Amsterdam Avenue
New York, NY 10027   212-678-3929
800-575-6566
Fax: 212-678-4149
tcpress@tc.columbia.edu
www.tcpress.com
Brian Ellerbeck, Executive Acquisitions Editor
Marie Ellen Larcada, Senior Acquisitions Editor
Emily Spangler, Acquisitions Editor
This book offers a collection of exemplary qualitative research affecting people with disabilities and their families. Instead of focusing upon methodological details, the chapters illustrate the variety of styles and formats that interpretive research can adopt in reporting its results. *$24.95*
328 pages Paperback
ISBN 0-807731-21-8

2350 **Intervention Research in Learning Disabilities**
Gallery Bookshop
319 Kasten Street
PO Box 270
Mendocino, CA 95460-270   707-937-2215
Fax: 707-937-3737
info@gallerybookshop.com
www.gallerybooks.com
Tony Miksak, Owner
Based on the Symposium on Intervention Research, this volume presents 12 papers addressing issues in intervention research, academic interventions, social and behavioral interventions, and postsecondary interventions. *$30.00*
347 pages

2351 **Introduction to Learning Disabilities**
Allyn & Bacon
75 Arlington St
Suite 300
Boston, MA 02116-3988   www.pearsonhighered.com
Presents the current state of research in the area of learning disabilities, as well as intervention ideas and programs. Includes updated material on the 1997 re-authorization of IDEA (Individuals with Disabilities Education Act) and expanded coverage of ADHD and its relationship to learning disabilities. Presents the latest information on the characteristics of persons with learning disabilities, causes, and educational interventions.
608 pages
ISBN 0-20529 -43-4

2352 **Introduction to Special Education: Teaching in an Age of Challenge, 4th Edition**
Allyn & Bacon
75 Arlington St
Suite 300
Boston, MA 02116-3988   www.pearsonhighered.com
Provides an applied approach to children with disabilities through the use of specific research and suggestions to focus on how the educational practices impact the lives of children, their families, and their teachers.
640 pages cloth
ISBN 0-20526 -94-4

2353 **Introduction to the Profession of Counseling**
McGraw-Hill School Publishing
PO Box 182604
Columbus, OH 43218   877-833-5524
800-338-3987
Fax: 609-308-4480
customer.service@mheducation.com
www.mcgraw-hill.com
David Levin, President/Chief Executive Officer
David Stafford, Senior Vice President/General Counsel
Maryellen Valaitis, Senior Vice President Human Resources
Offers information, theories and techniques for counseling numerous cases from drug addiction to special populations.
464 pages

2354 **Issues and Research in Special Education**
Teachers College Press
PO Box 20
Williston, VT 05495-0020   800-575-6566
Fax: 802-664-7626
tcp.orders@aidcvt.com
www.teacherscollegepress.com
Provides up-to-date research and discourse on a wide range of topics affecting professionals in the field of special education.
$38.00
264 pages Hardcover
ISBN 0-807731-95-1

2355 **Kendall Demonstration Elementary School Curriculum Guides**
Gallaudet University Bookstore
800 Florida Ave NE
Washington, DC 20002-3695
202-651-5488
800-621-2736
Fax: 202-651-5489
TTY: 888-630-9347
gupress@gallaudet.edu
www.gupress.gallaudet.edu
Dr. T Alan Hurwitz, President
Edward Bosso, Vice President for Administration
Dr. Lynne Murray, Vice President for Development
KDES is a day school serving students from birth through age 15, beginning with the Parent-Infant Program and ending in grade 8. Students come from the Washington, D.C., metropolitan area.

2356 **Language Arts: Detecting Special Needs**
Allyn & Bacon
75 Arlington St
Suite 300
Boston, MA 02116-3988
617-848-7500
800-852-8024
Fax: 617-944-7273
www.home.pearsonhighered.com
Bill Barke, Chairman/CEO
Nancy Forfyth, President
Kevin Stone, Vice President, National Sales M
Describes special language arts needs of special learners.
180 pages paperback
ISBN 0-205116-36-1

2357 **Language Learning Practices with Deaf Children**
Sage Publications
2455 Teller Road
Thousand Oaks, CA 91320
805-499-9774
800-818-7243
Fax: 800-583-2665
books.claim@sagepub.com
www.sagepub.com
Sara Miller McCune, Founder, Publisher, Chairperson
Stephen P. Quigley, Co-Author
Susan Rose, Co-Author
This new edition describes the variety of language-development theories and practices used with deaf children without advocating anyone. *$38.00*
321 pages Hardcover

2358 **Language and Communication Disorders in Children**
McGraw-Hill School Publishn
PO Box 182604
Columbus, OH 43218
877-833-5524
800-338-3987
Fax: 609-308-4480
customer.service@mheducation.com
www.mcgraw-hill.com
David Levin, President/Chief Executive Officer
David Stafford, Senior Vice President/General Counsel
Maryellen Valaitis, Senior Vice President Human Resources
Comprehensive coverage encompassing all aspects of children's language disorders.
512 pages

2359 **Learning Disabilities, Literacy, and Adult Education**
Brookes Publishing
PO Box 10624
Baltimore, MD 21285-0624
410-337-9580
800-638-3775
Fax: 410-337-8539
custserv@brookespublishing.com
www.brookespublishing.com
Paul H. Brookes, Chairman
Jeffrey D. Brookes, President
Melissa A. Behm, ExecutiveVice President
This book focuses on adults with severe learning disabilities and the educators who work with them. Described are the characteristics, demographics, and educational and employment status of

adults with LD and the laws that protect them in the workplace and in educational settings.
450 pages Paperback
ISBN 1-55766 -47-5

2360 **Learning Disabilities: Concepts and Characteristics**
McGraw-Hill School Publishing
220 E Danieldale Rd
Desoto, TX 75115-2490
972-224-4772
800-442-9685
Fax: 972-228-1982
Harold McGraw III, Chairman/ President/ Chief Ex
Jack F. Callahan, Executive Vice President, Chief
James A. McLoughlin, Co-Author
Covers the conceptual basis of learning disabilities, identification, etiology and diagnosis.
448 pages

2361 **Learning Disability: Social Class and the Cons of Inequality In American Education**
Greenwood Publishing Group
130 Cremona Drive
Santa Barbara, CA 93117
805-968-1911
800-368-6868
Fax: 866-270-3856
CustomerService@abc-clio.com
www.abc-clio.com
James Carrier, Author
Presents a detailed historical description of the social and educational assumptions integral to the idea of learning disability.
167 pages $43.95 - $47.95
ISBN 0-313253-96-X

2362 **Learning and Individual Differences**
National Association of School Psychologists
4340 East West Hwy.
Suite 402
Bethesda, MD 20814
301-657-0270
866-331-6277
Fax: 301-657-0275
TTY: 301-657-4155
www.nasponline.org
Kathleen Minke, Executive Director
Laura Benson, Chief Operating Officer

2363 **Learning to Feel Good and Stay Cool: Emotional Regulation Tools for Kids With AD/HD**
750 First Street, NE
Washington, DC 20002-4242
202-336-5500
800-374-2721
rllowman@gmail.com
www.apa.org
Judith M. Glasser, PhD, Co-Author
Kathleen G. Nadeau, PhD, Co-Author
Packed with practical advice and fun activities, this book will show you how to Understand your emotions, Practice healthy habits to stay in your Feel Good Zone, Feel better when you get upset, Know the warning signs that you are heading into your Upset Zone, Problem-solve so upsets come less often

2364 **Learning to See: American Sign Language asa Second Language**
Gallaudet University Press
800 Florida Ave NE
Washington, DC 20002-3695
202-651-5206
800-621-2736
Fax: 800-621-8476
TTY: 888-630-9347
clerc.center@gallaudet.edu
www.gupress.gallaudet.edu
Dr. T Alan Hurwitz, President
Edward Bosso, Vice President for Administration
Phyliss Wilcox, Co-Author
This important book has been updated to help teachers teach American Sign Language as a second language, including information on Deaf culture, the history and structure of ASL, teaching methods and issues facing educators. *$19.95*
160 pages Softcover

2365   Let's Write Right: Teacher's Edition
AVKO Educational Research Foundation
3084 Willard Rd
Ste W
Birch Run, MI 48415-9404   810-686-9283
                                          866-285-6612
                                     Fax: 810-686-1101

Barry Chute, President
Julie Guyette, Vice President
Don Mc Cabe, Research Director
A manuscript and cursive writing program designed not only to
teach handwriting but help with reading and spelling patterns as
well. Teaches students to learn to read cursive as manuscript is being taught and ease the transition to cursive by using a
D'Nealian-like script. Exercises involve phoically consistent
patterns to help reinforce fluency with spelling and handwriting.
$39.95
164 pages

**2366   Library Manager's Guide to Hiring and Serving
         Disabled Persons**
McFarland & Company
960 NC Hwy 88 W
Jefferson, NC 28640   336-246-4460
                                          800-253-2187
                                     Fax: 336-246-5018
                             infoinso@mcfarlandpub.com
                               www.mcfarlandbooks.com

Kieth C. Wright, Author
Judith F. Davie, Author
Information for library staff on hiring and serving disabled per-
sons. *$27.50*
171 pages Library binding 1990
ISBN 0-899505-16-3

**2367   Life-Span Approach to Nursing Care for Individuals
         with Developmental Disabilities**
Brookes Publishing
PO Box 10624
Baltimore, MD 21285-0624   410-337-9580
                                          800-638-3775
                                     Fax: 410-337-8539
                           custserv@brookespublishing.com
                              www.brookespublishing.com

Paul H. Brookes, Chairman
Jeffrey D. Brookes, President
Melissa A. Behm, ExecutiveVice President
This reference book was written by and for nurses. This guide addresses fundamental nursing issues such as health promotion, infection control, seizure management, adaptive and assistive
technology, and sexuality. Also offered are in-depth case studies,
helpful charts and tables, and problem-solving strategies. *$49.95*
464 pages Hardcover
ISBN 1-557661-51-0

**2368   Mainstreaming Deaf and Hard of Hearing Students:
         Questions and Answers**
Gallaudet University Bookstore
800 Florida Ave NE
Washington, DC 20002-3600   202-651-5000
                                          800-451-1073
                                     Fax: 202-651-5489
                                     TTY: 888-630-9347
                              clerc.center@gallaudet.edu
                               www.gupress.gallaudet.edu

Dr. T Alan Hurwitz, President
Debra S. Lipkey, University Budget Director
Donald Beil, Chief of Staff
This booklet presents mainstreaming as one educational option
and suggests some considerations for parents, teachers and administrators. *$6.00*
40 pages

**2369   Mainstreaming Exceptional Students: A Guide for
         Classroom Teachers**
Allyn & Bacon
75 Arlington St
Suite 300
Boston, MA 02116-3988   617-848-7500
                                          800-852-8024
                                     Fax: 617-944-7273
                              www.home.pearsonhighered.com

Nancy Forfyth, President
Bill Barke, CEO
Jane B. Schulz, Co-Author
Covers the various categories of exceptional students and dis-
cusses educational strategies and classroom management.
464 pages paperback
ISBN 0-20515 -24-6

2370   Mainstreaming: A Practical Approach for Teachers
McGraw-Hill School Publishing
PO Box 182604
Columbus, OH 43218   877-833-5524
                                          800-338-3987
                                     Fax: 609-308-4480
                           customer.service@mheducation.com
                                   www.mcgraw-hill.com

David Levin, President/Chief Executive Officer
David Stafford, Senior Vice President/General Counsel
Maryellen Valaitis, Senior Vice President Human Resources
Provides teachers, administrators and school psychologists with
the background, techniques and strategies they need to offer appropriate services for mildly handicapped students in the mainstream classroom.

2371   Managing Diagnostic Tool of Visual Perception
Gallery Bookshop
319 Kasten Street
PO Box 270
Mendocino, CA 95460-270   707-937-2215
                                     Fax: 707-937-3737
                              info@gallerybookshop.com
                                www.gallerybooks.com

Constantine Mangina, Author
For diagnosing specific perceptual learning abilities and disabili-
ties. *$14.00*
ISBN 0-80580 -83-4

2372   Medical Rehabilitation
Lippincott, Williams & Wilkins
227 S 6th St
Suite 227
Philadelphia, PA 19106-3713   215-545-5630
                                          800-777-2295
                                     Fax: 215-732-9988
                                       www.lpub.com

Cheryl Murkey, Manager
Information for the professional on new techniques and treatments in the medical rehabilitation fields. *$80.50*
368 pages Illustrated
ISBN 0-88167 -85-5

**2373   Meeting the ADD Challenge: A Practical Guide for
         Teachers**
Research Press
PO Box 7886
Champaign, IL 61826-9177   217-352-3273
                                          800-519-2707
                                     Fax: 217-352-1221
                                rp@researchpress.com
                                www.researchpress.com

Robert W. Parkinson, Founder
Dr. Michael Asher, Co-Author
Dr. Steven B Gordon, Co-Author
$24.95
ISBN 0-878223-45-9

2374 **Mental & Physical Disability Law Digest**
A BA Commission on Mental and Physical Disability
1050 Connecticut Ave. N.W.
Suite 400
Washington, DC 20036-1019   202-662-1000
                                   800-285-2221
                              Fax: 202-442-3439
                              cmpdl@abanet.org
                              www.americanbar.org
Robert M. Carlson, Chair, House of Delegates:
James R. Silkenat, President
William C. Hubbard, President-Elect
Provides comprehensive, summary and analysis of federal and
state disability and state disability laws from mental disability
law and disability discrimination law perspectives. *$60.00*
376 pages
ISBN 1-590310-05-5

2375 **Mental Health Concepts and Techniques for the
Occupational Therapy Assistant**
Lippincott, Williams & Wilkins
227 S 6th St
Suite 227
Philadelphia, PA 19106-3713   215-521-8300
                                     800-777-2295
                                Fax: 301-824-7390
                                www.lpub.com
J Lippincott, CEO
This text offers clear and easily understood explanations of the
various theoretical and practiced health models. *$36.00*
344 pages
ISBN 0-88167 -53-X

2376 **Mental Health and Mental Illness**
Lippincott, Williams & Wilkins
227 S 6th St
Suite 227
Philadelphia, PA 19106-3713   215-592-5400
                                     800-777-2295
                                Fax: 301-824-7390
                                www.lpub.com
Kathy Sykes, Manager
Concise, comprehensive and completely up to date, this book
presents the most current theory in mental health nursing for the
student and the new practitioner. *$28.95*
480 pages
ISBN 0-39755 -73-7

2377 **Mentally Ill Individuals**
Mainstream
Ste 830
3 Bethesda Metro Ctr
Bethesda, MD 20814-6301   301-961-9299
                                 800-247-1380
                            Fax: 301-654-6714
Charles Moster
Mainstreaming mentally ill individuals into the workplace. *$2.50*
12 pages

2378 **Midland Treatment Furniture**
Performance Health
28100 Torch Parkway
Suite 700
Warrenville, IL 60555-3938   630-393-6000
                               Fax: 630-393-7600
                        customersupport@performancehealth.com
                        www.performancehealth.com
Francis Dirksmeier, Chief Executive Officer
Greg Nulty, Chief Financial Officer
Jim Plewa, Chief Sales Officer
This catalog has the biggest selection of OT/PT products any-
where. Whether you deal with larger or smaller caseloads, you
need treatment furniture you can count on. Midland Treatment
Furniture from SPR is designed and built to stand up to the heavi-
est use. From tilt tables and traction packages to mat platforms
and parallel bars, you'll find the complete line of Midland Treatment Furniture inside this brochure. All products are assembled
from premium materials and carefully crafted.
Free

2379 **Multisensory Teaching of Basic Language Skills: Theory
and Practice**
Brookes Publishing
PO Box 10624
Baltimore, MD 21285-0624   410-337-9580
                                  800-638-3775
                             Fax: 410-337-8539
                             custserv@brookespublishing.com
                             www.brookespublishing.com
Paul H. Brookes, Chairman
Jeffrey D. Brookes, President
Melissa A. Behm, ExecutiveVice President
This book presents specific multisensory methods for helping
students who are having trouble learning to read due to dyslexia
or other learning disabilities. Recommended techniques are offered for teaching alphabet skills, composition, comprehension,
handwriting, math, organization and study skills, phonological
awareness, reading and spelling. *$59.00*
608 pages Hardcover
ISBN 1-557663-49-1

2380 **Music, Disability, and Society**
1852 North 10th Street
Philadelphia, PA 19122   215-926-2140
                                800-621-2736
                           www.temple.edu/tempress
Alex Lubet, Author
In Music, Disability, and Society, Alex Lubet challenges the rigid
view of technical skill and writes about music in relation to disability studies. He addresses the ways in which people with disabilities are denied the opportunity to participate in music.

2381 **Occupational Therapy Across Cultural Boundaries**
Haworth Press
711 Third Avenue
New York, NY 10017   212-216-7800
                            800-354-1420
                       Fax: 212-244-1563
                       subscriptions@tandf.co.uk
                       www.taylorandfrancisgroup.com
Derek Mapp, Non-Executive Chairman
Roger Horton, CEO
*Emma Blaney, Group HR Director - Head of Corporate Responsi-
bility*
Examines the concept of culture from a unique perspective, that
of individual occupational therapists who have worked in environments very different from those in which they were educated
or had worked previously. Journal publications formerly published by Haworth Press are now listed on the Taylor & Francis
Journals website. *$74.95*
107 pages Hardcover
ISBN 1-560242-23-X

2382 **Occupational Therapy Approaches to Traumatic Brain
Injury**
Routledge (Taylor & Francis Group)
711 Third Ave
New York, NY 10017   212-216-7800
                            800-634-7064
                       Fax: 212-564-7854
                       enquiries@taylorandfrancis.com
                       www.routledge.com
Laura H. Krefting, Author
Jerry A. Johnson, Author
Focusing on the disabled individual, the family, and the societal
responses to the injured, this comprehensive book covers the
spectrum of available services from intensive care to transitional
and community living. Formerly published by Haworth Press, titles are now listed on Routledge/Taylor Francis Group. *$140.00*
137 pages Hardcover
ISBN 1-560240-64-4

2383   Overcoming Dyslexia in Children, Adolescents and Adults
Sage Publications
2455 Teller Road
Thousand Oaks, CA 91320   805-499-9774
                                     800-818-7243
                                Fax: 800-583-2665
                           books.claim@sagepub.com
                                 www.sagepub.com
Sara Miller McCune, Founder, Publisher, Chairperson
Blaise R Simqu, President/CEO
Tracey A. Ozmina, Executive Vice President & Chief
This book describes some forms of dyslexia in detail and then relates those problems to the social, emotional and personal development of dyslexic individuals. *$34.00*
350 pages Paperback

2384   Oxford Textbook of Geriatric Medicine
Oxford University Press
198 Madison Ave
New York, NY 10016-4308   212-726-6000
                                     800-445-9714
                                Fax: 919-677-1303
                             custserv.us@oup.com
                                    global.oup.com
Rebecca Seger, Director, Institutional Sales, Americas
Lesa Moran Owen, Library Sales Operations Manager
Lenny Allen, Director, Institutional Accounts
This comprehensive text brings together extensive experience in clinical geriatrics with a strong scientific base in research. *$125.00*
784 pages

2385   Pain Centers: A Revolution in Health Care
Lippincott Williams And Wilkins
227
227 S 6th St
Philadelphia, PA 19106-3713   215-521-8300
                                     800-777-2295
                                Fax: 301-824-7390
                                     www.lpub.com
J Lippincott, CEO
$103.00
280 pages

2386   Parental Concerns in College Student Mental Health
Haworth Press
711 Third Avenue
New York, NY 10017   212-216-7800
                                     800-354-1420
                                Fax: 212-244-1563
                           subscriptions@tandf.co.uk
                          www.taylorandfrancisgroup.com
Derek Mapp, Non-Executive Chairman
Roger Horton, CEO
Emma Blaney, Group HR Director - Head of Corporate Responsibility
An instructive guide for parents and mental health professionals regarding the most important issues about psychological development in college students. Journal publications formerly published by Haworth Press are now listed on the Taylor & Francis Journals website. *$74.95*
204 pages Hardcover
ISBN 0-866567-20-8

2387   Parents and Teachers
Alexander Graham Bell Association
3417 Volta Pl NW
Washington, DC 20007-2737   202-337-5220
                                     866-337-5220
                                Fax: 202-337-8314
                                TTY: 202-337-5221
                                   info@agbell.org
                     www.listeningandspokenlanguage.org
Kathleen S. Treni, M.Ed., M.A., President
Meredith K. Knueve, Esq., Secretary-Treasurer
Alexander T. Graham, Executive Director/CEO
This excellent book offers in-depth guidance to parents and teachers whose partnership can foster language in school-aged children with hearing impairments. The first section examines roles of parents, teachers, professionals and children in language acquisition, residual hearing and audiological management, language development stages and readying children for preschool. The second portion of the book presents specific objectives and teaching strategies to use at school and at home. *$27.95*
386 pages

2388   Patient and Family Education
Springer Publishing Company
11 W 42nd St
15th Floor
New York, NY 10036-8002   212-431-4370
                                     877-687-7476
                                Fax: 212-941-7842
                               cs@springerpub.com
                                www.springerpub.com
Dr. Ursula Springer, President
Ted Nardin, CEO
James C. Costello, Vice President, Journal Publishi
This guide outlines the actual clinical content needed to develop, implement and maintain patient education programs. Conveniently arranged in one-hour long lesson plans, each disease or condition is organized in an easy-to-follow format. *$26.95*
272 pages Softcover
ISBN 0-82615 -41-7

2389   Person to Person: Guide for Professionals Working with the Disabled
Paul H Brookes Publishing Company
PO Box 10624
Baltimore, MD 21285-0624   410-337-9580
                                     800-638-3775
                                Fax: 410-337-8539
                          custserv@brookespublishing.com
                            www.brookespublishing.com
Paul H. Brookes, Chairman
Jeffrey D. Brookes, President
Melissa A. Behm, ExecutiveVice President
This second edition of an already-popular book helps professionals approach interactions with a people-first, disability second attitude. *$29.00*
288 pages Paperback
ISBN 1-557661-00-6

2390   Personality and Emotional Disturbance
Taylor & Francis
Ste G
47 Runway Dr
Levittown, PA 19057-4738   267-580-2622
                                Fax: 215-785-5515
Richard Roberts, CEO
The brain injured person has unique needs. Recent findings have highlighted that it is the personality, behavioral and emotional problems which most prohibit a return to work, create the greatest burden for the long-term care and rehabilitation of physical and cognitive functions. *$72.00*
260 pages Cloth
ISBN 0-85066 -71-3

2391   Phenomenology of Depressive Illness
Human Sciences Press
233 Spring St
New York, NY 10013-1522   212-229-2859
                                     877-283-3229
                                Fax: 212-463-0742
                                   ainy@aveda.com
                                     www.aveda.edu
Provides the reader with a detailed knowledge of the clinical characteristics of depressive disorders that will permit judgement of the general ability of the various theoretical models of depressive disorders. *$42.95*
263 pages Cloth
ISBN 0-89885 -69-9

2392 Physical Disabilities and Health Impairments: An Introduction
McGraw-Hill School Publishing
PO Box 182604
Columbus, OH 43218   877-833-5524
800-338-3987
Fax: 609-308-4480
customer.service@mheducation.com
www.mcgraw-hill.com
David Levin, President/Chief Executive Officer
David Stafford, Senior Vice President/General Counsel
Maryellen Valaitis, Senior Vice President Human Resources
A comprehensive text which presents a wealth of up-to-date medical information for teachers.

2393 Physical Education and Sports for Exceptional Students
McGraw-Hill Company
2460 Kerper Blvd
Dubuque, IA 52001-2224   800-338-3987
Fax: 614-755-5654
www.mhhe.com/hper/physed
Michael Horvat, Author
Harold McGraw III, Chairman, President and Chief Ex
Jack F. Callahan, Executive Vice President, Chief
Physical education for exceptional students and teaching students with learning and behavior exceptionalities.
Cloth

2394 Physical Management of Multiple Handicaps: A Professional's Guide
Brookes Publishing Company
PO Box 10624
Baltimore, MD 21285-0624   410-337-9580
800-638-3775
Fax: 410-337-8539
custserv@brookespublishing.com
www.brookespublishing.com
Paul H. Brookes, Chairman
Jeffrey D. Brookes, President
Melissa A. Behm, ExecutiveVice President
Comprehensive guide, takes a transdisciplinary approach to therapeutic/technological management of persons with multiple handicaps. *$36.00*
352 pages Hardcover
ISBN 1-557660-47-6

2395 Physically Handicapped in Society
Ayer Company Publishers
Ste 322
400 Bedford St
Manchester, NH 03101-1195   603-669-9307
888-267-7323
Fax: 603-669-7945
www.ayerpub.com
Kathy Train, Office Manager
Ellie Phipps, Customer Service
A group of 39 books. Biographies that offer studies on attitudes, sociological and psychological. Please write or call for catalog. *$965.00*
Hardcover
ISBN 0-40513 -00-3

2396 Practicing Rehabilitation with Geriatric Clients
Springer Publishing Company
11 W 42nd St
15th Floor
New York, NY 10036-8002   212-431-4370
877-687-7476
Fax: 212-941-7842
cs@springerpub.com
www.springerpub.com
Dr. Ursula Springer, President
Ted Nardin, CEO
James C. Costello, Vice President, Journal Publishi
Physical therapy in the geriatric client, psychological and psychiatric considerations in the rehabilitation of the elderly. *$32.95*
256 pages Hardcover
ISBN 0-82616 -80-5

2397 Pragmatic Approach
Educators Publishing Service
625 Mount Auburn St
3RD Floor
Cambridge, MA 02138-3039   617-547-6706
800-225-5750
Fax: 617-547-0285
Paula Fabbro, Sales Consultant
Leo Micale, Sales Consultant
Kristen Colson, Sales Consultant
Monograph on evaluation of children's performances on Slingerland Pre-Reading Screening Procedures to Identify First Grade Academic Needs. *$6.00*
56 pages
ISBN 0-838816-85-1

2398 Preschoolers with Special Needs: Children At-Risk, Children with Disabilities
Allyn & Bacon
75 Arlington St
Suite 300
Boston, MA 02116-3988   617-848-7500
800-852-8024
Fax: 617-944-7273
www.home.pearsonhighered.com
Bill Barke, CEO
Janet W. Lerner, Co-Author
Barbara Lowenthal, Co-Author
Explores ways of providing preschool children with special needs and their families with a learning environment that will help them develop and learn. Emphasizes the needs of preschoolers age three to six and provides information to teachers and others who work with young children in all settings. Current models of curricula, which incorporate new features from research and practical exprexiences with children who have special needs, are described and discussed. *$59.00*
336 pages cloth
ISBN 0-205358-79-9

2399 Preventing Academic Failure - Teachers Handbook
Educators Publishing Service
625 Mount Auburn St
3rd Fl
Cambridge, MA 02138-3039   617-547-6706
800-225-5750
Fax: 617-547-0285
eps.schoolspecialty.com
The PAF Teacher Handbook is a detailed guide for using the PAF program. It includes ungraded multisensory curriculum coordinating Orton-Gillingham and Merrill Linguistic reading techniques for language disabled students. Resource offers lessons on teaching phonics, spelling and reading to reinforce the development of language skills. A separate handwriting program is available. *$67.25*
Paperback
ISBN 0-838852-71-8

2400 Preventing School Dropouts
Sage Publications
2455 Teller Road
Thousand Oaks, CA 91320   805-499-9774
800-818-7243
Fax: 800-583-2665
books.claim@sagepub.com
www.sagepub.com
Sara Miller McCune, Founder, Publisher, Chairperson
Blaise R Simqu, President/ CEO
Tracey A. Ozmina, Executive Vice President & Chief
For secondary teachers, special education and regular, who have difficulty teaching youth in their classes. Presented are 120 tactics, specific instructional techniques, for helping adolescents to stay in school. Each tactic is written in a format that includes five sections. *$38.00*
509 pages

2401 **Prevocational Assessment**
Exceptional Education
P.O.Box 15308
Seattle, WA 98115-308   206-262-9538
                                          Fax: 475-486-4510

Jeff Stewart, Owner
Use the PACG to assess your students in nine areas (attendance
and endurance, learning and behavior, communication skills, social skills, grooming and eating and toileting) covering 46 specific workshop experiences. *$12.00*
16 pages Complete Set
ISBN 1-87786 -23-7

2402 **Primary Special Needs and the National Curriculum**
7625 Empire Drive
Florence, KN 41042-2919   800-634-4724
                                 orders@taylorandfrancis.com

Ann Lewis, Author
This new edition of Ann Lewis's widely acclaimed text has been
substantially revised and updated to take into account the recent
revisions to the National Curriculum and the guidance of the
Code of Practice.

2403 **Progress Without Punishment: Approaches for Learners
with Behavior Problems**
Teachers College Press
1234 Amsterdam Ave
New York, NY 10027-6602   212-678-3929
                                          800-575-6566
                                          Fax: 212-678-4149
                                   tcpress@tc.columbia.edu
                               www.teacherscollegepress.com

Anne M. Donnellan, Author
In this volume, the authors argue against the use of punishment,
and instead advocate the use of alternative intervention procedures. *$17.95*
184 pages Paperback
ISBN 0-807729-11-6

2404 **Promoting Postsecondary Education for Students with
Learning Disabilities**
Sage Publications
2455 Teller Road
Thousand Oaks, CA 91320   805-499-9774
                                          800-818-7243
                                          Fax: 800-583-2665
                                   books.claim@sagepub.com
                                          www.sagepub.com

Sara Miller McCune, Founder, Publisher, Chairperson
Stan F. Shaw, Co-Author
Joan M. McGuire, Co-Author
Primarily designed for postsecondary service providers who are
responsible for serving college students with learning disabilities. *$41.00*
440 pages

2405 **Psychiatric Mental Health Nursing**
Lippincott, Williams & Wilkins
227 S 6th St
Suite 227
Philadelphia, PA 19106-3713   215-521-8300
                                          800-777-2295
                                          Fax: 301-824-7390

J Lippincott, CEO
This text emphasizes and contrasts the roles of the generalist
nurse and the psychiatric nurse specialist. *$52.00*
1120 pages Illustrated

2406 **Psychoeducational Assessment of Visually Impaired and
Blind Students**
Sage Publications
2455 Teller Road
Thousand Oaks, CA 91320   805-499-9774
                                          800-818-7243
                                          Fax: 800-583-2665
                                   books.claim@sagepub.com
                                          www.sagepub.com

Sara Miller McCune, Founder, Publisher, Chairperson
Blaise R Simqu, President/CEO
Tracey A. Ozmina, Executive Vice President & Chief

Professional reference book that addresses the problems specific
to assessment of visually impaired and blind children. Of particular value to the practitioner are the extensive reviews of available
tests, including ways to adapt those not designed for use with the
visually handicapped. *$29.00*
140 pages Paperback
ISBN 0-890791-08-2

2407 **Psychological and Social Impact of Illness and Disability**
Springer Publishing
11 W 42nd St
15th Floor
New York, NY 10036-8002   212-431-4370
                                          877-687-7476
                                          Fax: 212-941-7842
                                   cs@springerpub.com
                                          www.springerpub.com

Dr. Ursula Springer, President
Ted Nardin, CEO
Ph.D. Orto Arthur E. Dell, Editor
The newest edition of Psychological and Social Impact of Illness
and Disability continues the tradition of presenting a realistic
perspective on life with disabilities and then improves upon its predecessors with the inclusion of illness as a major influence on client care needs. Further broadening the scope of this edition is the
inclusion of personal perspectives and stories from those living
with illness or disabilities. These stories offer a look into what it
is like to cope with these issues.

2408 **Reading and Deafness**
Sage Publications
2455 Teller Road
Thousand Oaks, CA 91320   805-499-9774
                                          800-818-7243
                                          Fax: 800-583-2665
                                   books.claim@sagepub.com
                                          www.sagepub.com

Sara Miller McCune, Founder, Publisher, Chairperson
Beverly J Trezek, Co-Author
Peter V. Paul, Co-Author
Three areas are looked at in this book: deaf children's prereading
development of real-world knowledge, cognitive abilities and
linguistic skills. *$39.00*
422 pages

2409 **Readings on Research in Stuttering**
Longman Publishing Group
1 Penn Plaza
Suite 2222
New York, NY 10119   646-556-8401
                                          Fax: 646-556-8415
                                   coffee@rothfos.com
                                          www.rothfos.com

Dan Dwyer, CEO
Thomas Minogue, CFO
Maria Tanpinco-Queyquep, Traffic Manager
Collection of the key journal articles published on stuttering over
the past decade, addressing trends in recent research in the field.
231 pages Paperback
ISBN 0-801304-10-5

2410 **Recreation Activities for the Elderly**
Springer Publishing Company
11 W 42nd St
15th Floor
New York, NY 10036-8002   212-431-4370
                                          877-687-7476
                                          Fax: 212-941-7842
                                   cs@springerpub.com
                                          www.springerpub.com

Dr. Ursula Springer, President
Ted Nardin, CEO
James C. Costello, Vice President, Journal Publishi
Included in this volume are simple crafts that utilize easily ob-
tainable, inexpensive materials, hobbies focusing on collections,
nature, and the arts' and games emphasizing both mental and
physical activity. *$23.95*
240 pages Softcover
ISBN 0-82616 -30-1

2411 Reference Manual for Communicative Sciences and Disorders
Pro- Ed Publications
8700 Shoal Creek Blvd
Austin, TX 78757-6897
512-451-3246
800-897-3202
Fax: 512-451-8542
info@proedinc.com
www.proedinc.com

Raymond D. Kent, Author
An indispensable guide to standards and values essential in the assessment of communication disorders. *$54.00*
393 pages

2412 Rehabilitation Interventions for the Institutionalized Elderly
Haworth Press
711 Third Avenue
Floor 8th
New York, NY 10017
212-216-7800
800-354-1420
Fax: 212-564-7854
subscriptions@tandf.co.uk

Derek Mapp, Non-Executive Chairman
Roger Horton, CEO
Emma Blaney, Group HR Director - Head of Corporate Responsibility
Gerontology professionals offer suggestions to enrich the quality of rehabilitation services offered to the institutionalized elderly. This volume examines up to the minute ideas, some that would have been unlikely even a few years ago, that focus exclusively on rehabilitation services for the institutionalized elderly. Journal publications formerly published by Haworth Press are now listed on the Taylor & Franc *$44.95*
77 pages Hardcover
ISBN 0-866568-33-6

2413 Rehabilitation Nursing for the Neurological Patient
Springer Publishing Company
11 W 42nd St
15th Fl
New York, NY 10036-8002
212-431-4370
877-687-7476
Fax: 212-941-7842
cs@springerpub.com
www.springerpub.com

Ted Nardin, Chief Executive Officer
Jason Roth, Vice President, Sales & Marketing
Kathy Weiss, Director, Sales
Reviews the physiology, pathophysiology, & nursing management of problems frequently encountered in neuro- rehabilitation and reviews the pathphysiology of specific disabilities & the related nursing interventions. *$32.95*
229 pages Hardcover 1992
ISBN 0-826176-60-7

2414 Rehabilitation Resource Manual: VISION
Resources for Rehabilitation
22 Bonad Rd
Winchester, MA 01890-1302
781-368-9094
Fax: 781-368-9096
info@rfr.org
www.rfr.org

Marshall E. Flax, MS, Author
A desk reference that enables service providers, librarians and others to make effective referrals. Includes guidelines on establishing self-help groups, information on research and service organizations, and chapters on assistive technology, for special population groups and by eye condition. *$44.95*
Biennial

2415 Rehabilitation Technology
CRC Press
6000 Broken Sound Pkwy NW
Ste 300
Boca Raton, FL 33487
800-634-7064
Fax: 800-374-3401
orders@crcpress.com
www.crcpress.com

Glenn E. Hedman, Author

Learn how the use of technological devices can enhance the lives of disabled children. Informs physical therapists, occupational therapists, and rehabilitation technologists about the devices that are available today and provides important background information on these devices. CRC Press is part of the Taylor & Francis Group. *$39.95*
173 pages Hardcover 1990
ISBN 1-560240-33-4

2416 Report Writing in Assessment and Evaluation
Stout Vocational Rehab Institute
University of Wisconsin-Stout
712 South Broadway
Menomonie, WI 54751
715-232-1478
Fax: 715-232-2356
giffordj@uwstout.edu
www.uwstout.edu

Charles W. Sorensen, Chancellor
Judy Gifford, Director
Stephen W. Thomas, Author
This examines questions of who are you writing for and what does the referral source want. Defines characteristics of good reports, common problems, writing in different settings, types of reports, getting ready to write, and writing prescriptive recommendations. *$ 17.75*
188 pages Softcover

2417 Resource Room, The
State University of New York Press
22 Corporate Woods Boulevard
3rd Floor
Albany, NY 12210-2314
518-472-5000
866-430-7869
Fax: 518-472-5038
info@sunypress.edu
www.sunypress.edu

Barry Edwards McNamara, Author
Provides teachers and administrators with helpful, practical information and explores the role of the resource room teacher as it relates to three major functions: assessment, instruction and consultation. It will also assist supervisors and administrators in evaluating their resource programs. *$28.95*
148 pages Paperback
ISBN 0-887069-84-0

2418 Resources for Rehabilitation
22 Bonad Rd
Winchester, MA 01890-1302
781-368-9094
Fax: 781-368-9096
info@rfr.org
www.rfr.org

Provides training and information to professionals and the public about disabilities and resources available to help. Publishes resource guides, professional publications and patient/client educational materials. Conducts custom designed training programs and workshops.

2419 Restructuring High Schools for All Students: Taking Inclusion to the Next Level
Brookes Publishing
PO Box 10624
Baltimore, MD 21285-0624
410-337-9580
800-638-3775
Fax: 410-337-8539
custserv@brookespublishing.com
www.brookespublishing.com

Paul H. Brookes, Chairman
Jeffrey D. Brookes, President
Melissa A. Behm, ExecutiveVice President
Details the process of creating an inclusive, collaborate community of learners and teachers at the secondary level. *$29.95*
304 pages Paperback
ISBN 1-557663-13-0

2420 Restructuring for Caring and Effective Education: Administrative Guide
Brookes Publishing
PO Box 10624
Baltimore, MD 21285-0624   410-337-9580
800-638-3775
Fax: 410-337-8539
custserv@brookespublishing.com
www.brookespublishing.com

Paul H. Brookes, Chairman
Jeffrey D. Brookes, President
Melissa A. Behm, ExecutiveVice President
In this empowering book, leading general and special education schools reform experts synthesize the major school restructuring initiatives and describe the processes and rationale for changing the organizational structure and instructional practices of schools. *$ 29.00*
384 pages Paperback
ISBN 1-55766 -91-3

2421 Scoffolding Student Learning
Brookline Books
8 Trumbull Rd
Suite B-001
Northampton, MA 01060   413-584-0184
800-666-2665
Fax: 413-584-6184
brbooks@yahoo.com
www.brooklinebooks.com

Paul H. Brookes, Chairman
Jeffrey D. Brookes, President
Melissa A. Behm, ExecutiveVice President
Collection of papers on the theory and practice of scoffolding—an interactive style of instructions that helps students develop more powerful thinking tools. *$21.95*
180 pages Paperback
ISBN 1-571290-36-2

2422 Selective Nontreatment of Handicapped
Oxford University Press
2001 Evans Rd
Cary, NC 27513-2009   919-677-0977
800-445-9714
Fax: 919-677-1303
custserv.us@oup.com
www.global.oup.com

Lesa Moran Owen, Library Sales Operations Manager
Rebecca Seger, Director, Institutional Sales, Americas
Lenny Allen, Director, Institutional Accounts
Information on selective nontreatment of handicapped newborns, moral dilemmas in neonatal medicine. *$17.95*
304 pages Paperback

2423 Semiotics and Dis/ability: Interogating Categories of Difference
State University of New York Press
22 Corporate Woods Boulevard
3rd Floor
Albany, NY 12210-2314   518-472-5000
866-430-7869
Fax: 518-472-5038
info@sunypress.edu
www.sunypress.edu

James Peltz, Associate Director
Linda Rogers, Editor
Examines the ways the words disability and difference and socially and culturally constructed. *$25.95*
265 pages Paperback 1990
ISBN 0-791449-06-6

2424 Service Coordination for Early Intervention: Parents and Friends
Brookline Books
8 Trumbull Rd
Suite B-001
Northampton, MA 01060   413-584-0184
800-666-2665
Fax: 413-584-6184
brbooks@yahoo.com
www.brooklinebooks.com

Deborah D. Hatton, Co-Author
R. A. McWilliam, Co-Author
P. J. Winton, Co-Author
This book helps administrators and professionals to structure early intervention and ongoing services so that professionals work collaboratively with parents to promote the health, well-being and development of children with special needs. *$19.95*
110 pages Paperback
ISBN 0-91479 -91-3

2425 Services for the Seriously Mentally Ill: A Survey of Mental Health Centers
Nat'l Council for Community Behavioral Healthcare
12300 Twinbrook Pkwy
Ste 320
Rockville, MD 20852-1606   301-984-6200
Fax: 301-881-7159

Linda Rosenberg, CEO
Dale K Klatzker, Board Chair
This ground-breaking report documents what administrators and practitioners have maintained for many years: community mental health organizations devote a significant percentage of the human and financial resources to serving the seriously mentally ill. *$30.00*

2426 Sexuality and Disability
Springer Publishing
11 W 42nd St
15th Fl
New York, NY 10036-8002   212-431-4370
Fax: 212-460-1575
www.springer.com

Sigmund Hough, Editor-in-Chief
A journal devoted to the psychological and medical aspects of sexuality in rehabilitation and community settings. The journal features original scholarly articles that address the psychological and medical aspects of sexuality in the field of rehabilitation, case studies, clinical practice reports, and guidelines for clinical practice.
Quarterly

2427 Shop Talk
PO Box 7886
Champaign, IL 61826-9177   217-352-3273
800-519-2707
Fax: 217-352-1221
rp@researchpress.com
www.researchpress.com

Robert W. Parkinson, Founder
Philip Roth, Author

2428 Signed English Schoolbook
Gallaudet University Press
800 Florida Ave NE
Washington, DC 20002-3600   202-651-5488
800-451-1073
Fax: 202-651-5489
TTY: 888-630-9347
clerc.center@gallaudet.edu
www.gupress.gallaudet.edu

Harry Bornstein, Co-Author
Karen L. Saulnier, Co-Author
Dr. T Alan Hurwitz, President
The Signed English Schoolbook provides vocabulary for teachers and others who serve school-age children and adolescents and covers the full range of school activities. *$13.95*
184 pages Softcover

2429 Social Skills for Students With Autism Spectrum Disorders and Other Developmental Disorders
Council for Exceptional Children
3100 Clarendon Blvd.
Suite 600
Arlington, VA 22201-5332   888-232-7733
                                       TTY: 866-915-5000
                               service@exceptionalchildren.org
                                  www.exceptionalchildren.org
Laurence R. Sargent, Co-Author
Toni Cook, Co-Author
Darlene E. Perner, Co-Author
A book teaching children to understand their own behaviours.
$24.95

2430 Social Studies: Detecting and Correcting Special Needs
Allyn & Bacon
75 Arlington St
Suite 300
Boston, MA 02116-3988   617-848-7500
                                           800-852-8024
                                      Fax: 617-944-7273
                               www.home.pearsonhighered.com
Harry Bornst Barke, CEO
Nancy Forfyth, President
Lana J. Smith, Co-Author
Describes social studies and special needs for special learners.
180 pages
ISBN 0-205121-51-9

2431 Social and Emotional Development of Exceptional Students: Handicapped
Charles C. Thomas
2600 S First St
Springfield, IL 62704-4730   217-789-8980
                                           800-258-8980
                                      Fax: 217-789-9130
                                   books@ccthomas.com
                                     www.ccthomas.com
Michael P. Thomas, President
Carroll J. Jones, Author
Sixteen years after the passage of P.L. 94-142, the dream of special educators to educate the handicapped and nonhandicapped children and youth together resulting in increased academic gains and age-appropriate school skills for handicapped children and youth has not yet materialized. This book helps eliminate an existing void by providing teachers with understandable information regarding the social and emotional development of exceptional students. Also in cloth at $41.95 (ISBN# 0-398-05781-8) *$29.95*
218 pages Softcover
ISBN 0-398061-94-7

2432 Special Education Today
LifeWay Christian Resources Southern Baptist Conv.
One LifeWay Plaza
Nashville, TN 37234   615-251-2000
                                           800-458-2772
                                      Fax: 615-532-9412
                                     www.lifeway.com
Thom S. Rainer, President/CEO
Brad Waggoner, Executive Vice President
Eric Geiger, Vice President, Church Resources Division
This unique quarterly publications ministers to people with special education needs and to their families, the church, and other caregivers. It offers a variety of helps and encouragement, including: What's working in churches, Suggestions for adapting teaching techniques, inspirational stories about people who have disabilities, Parenting and family issues, Ideas for reaching, witnessing, worship, and recreation. *$4.25*
36 pages Quarterly

2433 Special Education for Today
Allyn & Bacon
75 Arlington St
Suite 300
Boston, MA 02116-3988   617-848-7500
                                           800-852-8024
                                      Fax: 617-944-7273
                               www.home.pearsonhighered.com
See search r Barke, CEO
Michael S. Rosenberg, Co-Author
David L. Westling, Co-Author
An undergraduate introduction to special education covering all major areas of exceptionality. Contains pedagogical features designed to make the book accessible to the undergraduate.
576 pages hardcover
ISBN 0-138264-53-8

2434 Speech and the Hearing-Impaired Child
Alexander Graham Bell Association
3417 Volta Pl NW
Washington, DC 20007-2737   202-337-5220
                                           866-337-5220
                                      Fax: 202-337-8314
                                      TTY: 202-337-5221
                                         info@agbell.org
                             www.listeningandspokenlanguage.org
Meredith K. Sugar, Esq. (OH), President
Ted A. Meyer, M.D., Ph.D, President-Elect/Secretary-Treasurer
Emilio Alonso-Mendoza, Chief Executive Officer
This textbook for professionals deals with basic theoretical issues in the acquisition of speech and the form of language (phonetics and phonology) in children with hearing losses. It provides a systematic framework to develop and evaluate speech target behaviors and their underlying subskills. *$29.95*
402 pages Paperback

2435 Speech-Language Pathology and Audiology: An Introduction
McGraw-Hill School Publishing
PO Box 182604
Columbus, OH 43218   877-833-5524
                                           800-338-3987
                                      Fax: 609-308-4480
                               customer.service@mheducation.com
                                     www.mcgraw-hill.com
David Levin, President/Chief Executive Officer
David Stafford, Senior Vice President/General Counsel
Maryellen Valaitis, Senior Vice President Human Resources
Offers classroom-tested coverage of clinical objectives and functioning.
301 pages

2436 Spinal Cord Dysfunction
Oxford University Press
2001 Evans Rd
Cary, NC 27513-2009   919-677-0977
                                           800-451-7556
                                      Fax: 919-677-1303
                                   humanres@oup-usa.org
Lesa Moran Owen, Library Sales Operations Manager
Rebecca Seger, Director, Institutional Sales, Americas
Lenny Allen, Director, Institutional Accounts
Offers information on restoration of function after spinal cord damage as seen from the point of view of identification of impaired or absent function in the nerve cells and processes which survive after the initial insult, intact but with impaired functions.
$95.00
368 pages

2437 Steps to Success: Scope & Sequence for Skill Development
15619 Premiere Drive
Suite 101
Tampa, FL 33624   850-363-9909
                                      Fax: 480-393-4331
                         accounting@successforkidswithhearingloss.com
                                  successforkidswithhearinglo ss.com
Lynne H. Price, Author
Steps to Success is a curriculum for students who are deaf or hard of hearing in grades kindergarten through 12.

2438 Strategies for Teaching Learners with Special Needs
McGraw-Hill School Publishing
PO Box 182604
Columbus, OH 43218
877-833-5524
800-338-3987
Fax: 609-308-4480
customer.service@mheducation.com
www.mcgraw-hill.com
David Levin, President/Chief Executive Officer
David Stafford, Senior Vice President/General Counsel
Maryellen Valaitis, Senior Vice President Human Resources
This is a text that helps special educators develop the full range of teaching competencies needed to be effective.
560 pages

2439 Strategies for Teaching Students with Learning and Behavior Problems
Allyn & Bacon
75 Arlington St
Suite 300
Boston, MA 02116-3988
617-848-7500
800-852-8024
Fax: 617-944-7273
www.home.pearsonhighered.com
Bill Barke, CEO
Nancy Forfyth, President
Sharon R. Vaughn, Co-Author
Provides descriptions of methods and strategies for teaching students with learning and behvior problems, managing professional roles, and collaborating with families, professionals, and paraprofessionals.
544 pages
ISBN 0-205113-89-3

2440 Students with Acquired Brain Injury: The School's Response
Brookes Publishing
PO Box 10624
Baltimore, MD 21285-0624
410-337-9580
800-638-3775
Fax: 410-337-8539
custserv@brookespublishing.com
www.brookespublishing.com
Ann Glang, Editor
Bonnie Todis, Editor
Paul H. Brooks, Chairman of the Board
This book is designed for school professionals and describes a range of issues that this population faces and presents proven means of addressing them in ways that benefit all students. Included topics are hospital-to-school transitions, effective assessment strategies, model programs in public schools, interventions to assist classroom teachers, and ways to involve family members in the educational program. *$29.95*
424 pages Paperback
ISBN 1-55766 -85-1

2441 Students with Mild Disabilities in the Secondary School
Longman Group
75 Arlington St
Suite 300
New York, NY 10036-2601
212-782-3300
800-852-8024
www.home.pearsonhighered.com
William Hitchings, Co-Author
Michael Horvath, Co-Author
Bonnie Schmalle, Co-Author
Provides methods and strategies for curriculum delivery to students with mild disabilities at the secondary school level.
2313G pages Paperback
ISBN 0-801301-66-1

2442 Supporting and Strengthening Families
Brookline Books
8 Trumbull Rd
Suite B-001
Northampton, MA 01060
413-584-0184
800-666-2665
Fax: 413-584-6184
brbooks@yahoo.com
www.brooklinebooks.com
Carl J Dunst, Author
A collection of papers addressing the theory, methods, strategies, and practices involved in adopting an empowerment and family-centered resources approach to supporting families and strengthening individual and family functioning. *$30.00*
252 pages Paperback
ISBN 0-91479 -94-8

2443 TESTS
Slosson Educational Publications
538 Buffalo rd
PO Box 280
East Aurora, NY 14052
716-652-0930
888-756-7766
Fax: 800-665-3840
slossonprep@gmail.com
www.slosson.com
Steven W. Slosson, President
Dr. Georgina Moynihan, Office Personnel
Slosson Educational Publications, Inc. offers educators an extensive selection of testing products, along with books on autism. ADED and other special needs materials. Our catalog includes 30 pages of speech-language testing and language rehabilitation products. The behavioral conduct. Special needs section includes checklist and scales on aberrant/disruptive behavior, tapes on ADD, as well as products for dyslexia and remediation of reversals.

2444 Teacher's Guide to Including Students with Disabilities in Regular Physical Education
Brookes Publishing
PO Box 10624
Baltimore, MD 21285-0624
410-337-9580
800-638-3775
Fax: 410-337-8539
custserv@brookespublishing.com
www.brookespublishing.com
Martin E. Block, Author
Melissa A. Behm, Executive Vice President
Paul H. Brooks, Chairman of the Board
Provides simple and creative strategies for meaningfully including children with disabilities in regular physical education programs. *$39.00*
288 pages Paperback
ISBN 1-557661-56-1

2445 Teachers Working Together
Brookline Books
8 Trumbull Rd
Suite B-001
Northampton, MA 01060
413-584-0184
800-666-2665
Fax: 413-584-6184
brbooks@yahoo.com
www.brooklinebooks.com
Carol Davis, Co-Author
Alice Yang, Co-Author
This collection of papers describes collaboraborative efforts for such classroom settings as preschools, elementary, middle and high schools, for content area teaching and into the transition to work. Each chapter describes actual practice and analyzes what is required to accomplish this collaboration. *$19.95*
Paperback
ISBN 1-57139 -66-4

2446 Teachig Students with Special Needs in Inclusive Classrooms
SAGE Publications
2455 Teller Rd
Thousand Oaks, CA 91320
800-818-7243
Fax: 800-583-2665
orders@sagepub.com
us.sagepub.com

Diane P. Bryant, Author
Brian P. Bryant, Author
Deborah D. Smith, Author

Using the research-validated ADAPT framework, Teaching Students with Special Needs in Inclusive Classrooms helps future teachers determine how, when, and with whom to use proven academic and behavioral interventions to obtain the best outcomes for students with disabilities. This book will provide the skills and inspiration that teachers need to make a positive difference in the educational lives of struggling learners.

2447 Teaching Adults with Learning Disabilities
Krieger Publishing Company
1725 Krieger Drive
Malabar, FL 32902
321-724-9542
800-724-0025
Fax: 321-951-3671
info@krieger-publishing.com
www.krieger-publishing.com

Dale R. Jordan, Author
R Krieger, Owner

Designed to teach literacy providers and classroom instructors how to recognize specific learning disability (LD) patterns and block reading, spelling, writing and arithmetic skills in students of all ages. One of the major problems faced by literary providers is keeping low-skill adults involved in basic education programs long enough to increase their literacy skills to the level of success. Shows instructors in adult education how to modify teaching strategies. *$25.50*
160 pages
ISBN 0-894649-10-8

2448 Teaching Children With Autism in the General Classroom
Prufrock Press
PO Box 8813
Waco, TX 76714-8813
254-756-3337
800-998-2208
Fax: 254-756-3339
gbates@prufrock.com
www.prufrock.com

Joel McIntosh, Publisher & Marketing Director
Ginny Bates, Customer Service and Office Manager
Lacy Compton, Senior Editor

Provides an introduction to inclusionary practices that serve children with autism, giving teachers the practical advice they need to ensure each students receives the quality education he or she deserves. *$39.95*
350 pages Paperback
ISBN 1-593633-64-6

2449 Teaching Disturbed and Disturbing Students: An Integrative Approach
Sage Publications
2455 Teller Road
Thousand Oaks, CA 91320
805-499-9774
800-818-7243
Fax: 800-583-2665
books.claim@sagepub.com
www.sagepub.com

Sara Miller McCune, Founder, Publisher, Chairperson
Blaise R Simqu, President & CEO
Tracey A. Ozmina, Executive Vice President & Chief

Using an integrative approach, this text provides teachers with step-by-step details of how to implement and use the methods and theories discussed in each chapter. *$37.00*
465 pages

2450 Teaching Every Child Every Day: Integrated Learning in Diverse Classrooms
Brookline Books
8 Trumbull Rd
Suite B-001
Northampton, MA 01060
413-584-0184
800-666-2665
Fax: 413-584-6184
brbooks@yahoo.com
www.brooklinebooks.com

Karen R. Harris, Editor
Steve Graham, Editor
Don Deshler, Editor

Collection of articles addressing various issues in teaching to diverse classrooms—varied in need for special educational services, English proficiency, and socioeconomic and racial backgrounds. *$19.95*
224 pages Paperback
ISBN 0-57129-40-0

2451 Teaching Infants and Preschoolers with Handicaps
Mc Graw-Hill, School Publishing
PO Box 182604
Columbus, OH 43218
877-833-5524
800-338-3987
Fax: 609-308-4480
customer.service@mheducation.com
www.mcgraw-hill.com

David Levin, President/Chief Executive Officer
David Stafford, Senior Vice President/General Counsel
Maryellen Valaitis, Senior Vice President Human Resources

Builds a solid background in early childhood special education.
380 pages

2452 Teaching Language-Disabled Children: A Communication/Games Intervention
Brookline Books
8 Trumbull Rd
Ste B-001
Northampton, MA 01060
413-584-0184
800-666-2665
Fax: 413-584-6184
brbooks@yahoo.com
www.brooklinebks.com

Susan Conant, Author

Offers practitioners specific teaching methods for helping students play communication games. *$22.95*
185 pages Hardcover 1983
ISBN 0-914797-38-7

2453 Teaching Learners with Mild Disabilities: Integrating Research and Practice
Brooke Publishing
PO Box 10624
Baltimore, MD 21285-0624
410-337-9580
800-638-3775
Fax: 410-337-8539
custserv@brookespublishing.com
www.brookespublishing.com

Ruth Lyn Meese, Author
Melissa A. Behm, Executive Vice President
Paul H. Brooks, Chairman of the Board

The authors illustrate interactions among regular teachers, special education teachers and students with mild disabilities through the use of hypothetical case studies of students and teachers.
496 pages Paperbound
ISBN 0-53421-02-0

2454 Teaching Mathematics to Students with Learning Disabilities
Sage Publications
2455 Teller Road
Thousand Oaks, CA 91320
805-499-9774
800-818-7243
Fax: 800-583-2665
www.sagepub.com

Sara Miller McCune, Founder, Publisher, Chairperson
Blaise R Simqu, President & CEO
Nancy S. Bley, Co-Author

New trends in school mathematics have surfaced in the teaching world. Problem-solving, estimation and the use of computers are receiving considerably greater emphasis than in the past and these areas are included in the new text. *$38.00*
486 pages Paperback

2455   Teaching Mildly and Moderately Handicapped Students
Allyn & Bacon
75 Arlington St
Suite 300
Boston, MA 02116-3988   617-848-7500
                                         800-852-8024
                                    Fax: 617-944-7273
                              www.home.pearsonhighered.com
Bill Barke, CEO
Nancy Forfyth, President
B. R. Gearheart, Author
A cross-categorical text providing teaching ideas and techniques. Focuses on the theme of learning as a constructive process in which the learner interacts with the environment, constructing new systems of knowledge, Behavioral techniques and research are also presented.
hardcover
ISBN 0-138939-00-4

2456   Teaching Reading to Children with Down Syndrome: A Guide for Parents and Teachers
Woodbine House
6510 Bells Mill Rd
Bethesda, MD 20817-1636   301-897-3570
                                         800-843-7323
                                    Fax: 301-897-5838
                                info@woodbinehouse.com
                                www.woodbinehouse.com
Irvin Shapell, Publisher
Patricia Logan Oelwein, Author
Beth Binns, Special Marketing Manage
Guide includes lessons customized to meet the unique interests and learning style of each child. *$16.95*
371 pages Paperback
ISBN 0-933149-55-7

2457   Teaching Reading to Disabled and Handicapped Learners
Charles C. Thomas
2600 S First St
Springfield, IL 62704-4730   217-789-8980
                                         800-258-8980
                                    Fax: 217-789-9130
                                    books@ccthomas.com
                                    www.ccthomas.com
Michael P. Thomas, President
Freddie W. Litton, Author
Harold D. Love, Author
Designed as a text for undergraduate and graduate students, this resource aims to help the many children, adolescents, and adults who encounter difficulty with reading. It guides prospective and present special education teachers in assisting and teaching handicapped learners to read. The text integrates traditional methods with newer perspectives to provide and effective reading program in special education. *$43.95*
252 pages Paperback 1996
ISBN 0-398062-48-X

2458   Teaching Reading to Handicapped Children
Love Publishing Company
9101 E Kenyon Ave
Suite 2200
Denver, CO 80237-1854   303-221-7333
                                    Fax: 303-221-7444
                                lpc@lovepublishing.com
                                www.lovepublishing.com
Charles H. Hargis, Author
The author covers skills teaching through letter sound association, word identification, synthetic and analytic methods and others, plus testing and assessment. *$24.95*
ISBN 0-89108-13-5

2459   Teaching Self-Determination to Students with Disabilities
Brookes Publishing
PO Box 10624
Baltimore, MD 21285-0624   410-337-9580
                                         800-638-3775
                                    Fax: 410-337-8539
                              custserv@brookespublishing.com
                              www.brookespublishing.com
Michael L. Wehmeyer, Co-Author
Martin Agran, Co-Author
Paul H. Brooks, Chairman of the Board
Basic skills for successful transition. This teacher-friendly source will help educators prepare students with disabilities with the specific skills they need for a satisfactory, self-directed life once they leave school. *$34.95*
384 pages Paperback
ISBN 1-55766-02-5

2460   Teaching Students with Learning Problems
McGraw-Hill School Publishing
PO Box 182604
Columbus, OH 43218   877-833-5524
                                         800-338-3987
                                    Fax: 609-308-4480
                              customer.service@mheducation.com
                              www.mcgraw-hill.com
David Levin, President/Chief Executive Officer
David Stafford, Senior Vice President/General Counsel
Maryellen Valaitis, Senior Vice President Human Resources
Expanded coverage of learning strategies, generalization training, self-monitoring techniques, and techniques for increasing the time students spend on academic tasks.
608 pages

2461   Teaching Students with Learning and Behavior Problems
Sage Publications
2455 Teller Road
Thousand Oaks, CA 91320   805-499-9774
                                         800-818-7243
                                    Fax: 800-583-2665
                                    www.sagepub.com
Sara Miller McCune, Founder, Publisher, Chairperson
Blaise R Simqu, President & CEO
Sharon R. Vaughn, Co-Author
$65.00
444 pages Paperback
ISBN 0-890799-28-4

2462   Teaching Students with Mild and Moderate Learning Problems
Allyn & Bacon Longman College Faculty
75 Arlington St
Suite 300
Boston, MA 02116-3988   617-367-0025
                                         800-852-8024
                                    Fax: 617-367-2155
                              www.home.pearsonhighered.com
Bill Barke, CEO
John Langone, Author
Kevin Stone, Vice President, National Sales M
Provides teachers with skills for assisting students with mild to moderate handicaps in making successful transitions in school and community environments.
496 pages
ISBN 0-205123-62-7

2463   Teaching Students with Moderate/Severe Disabilities, Including Autism
Charles C. Thomas
2600 S First St
Springfield, IL 62704-4730   217-789-8980
                                         800-258-8980
                                    Fax: 217-789-9130
                                    books@ccthomas.com
                                    www.ccthomas.com
Michael P. Thomas, President
Elva Duran, Author
This resource and guide was written to help teachers, parents, and other caregivers provide the best educational opportunities for their students with moderate and severe disabilities. The author

addresses functional language and other language intervention strategies, vocational training, community based instruction, transition and postsecondary programming, the adolescent student with autism, students with multiple disabilities, parent and family issues, and legal concerns. *$58.95*
416 pages Paperback
ISBN 0-398067-01-5

2464 Teaching Students with Special Needs in Inclusive Settings
Allyn & Bacon
75 Arlington St
Suite 300
Boston, MA 02116-3988   617-848-7500
                               800-852-8024
                          Fax: 617-944-7273

Tom E.C. Smith, Co-Author
Edward A. Polloway, Co-Author
James Patton, Co-Author
This text is intended to be a survey text providing practical guidance to general education teachers. It will help them to meet the diverse needs of students with disabilities.
544 pages
ISBN 0-20527 -16-6

2465 Teaching Young Children to Read
Brookline Books
8 Trumbull Rd
Suite B-001
Northampton, MA 01060   413-584-0184
                               800-666-2665
                          Fax: 413-584-6184
                          brbooks@yahoo.com
                          www.brooklinebooks.com
Dolores Durkin, Author
John P.
Detailed instructions on teaching reading to preschoolers. Gradually develops full fluency. *$16.95*
192 pages Paperback
ISBN 0-57129 -48-6

2466 Teaching the Bilingual Special Education Student
Ablex Publishing Corporation
P.O.Box 811
Stamford, CT 06904-811   Fax: 201-767-6717
This book focuses on teaching those students who are bilingual, handicapped and in need of special instruction. It responds to the complex and practical issues of teaching these students in an effective way.
ISBN 0-89391 -23-4

2467 Teaching the Learning Disabled Adolescent: Strategies and Methods
Love Publishing Company
9101 E Kenyon Ave
Ste 2200
Denver, CO 80237-1813   303-221-7333
                          Fax: 303-221-7444
                          lpc@lovepublishing.com
                          www.lovepublishing.com
Gordon R. Alley, Author
This book gives expert strategies and methods for teaching learning disabled adolescents how, rather than what, to learn. *$39.95*
360 pages Hardcover 1979
ISBN 0-891080-94-5

2468 Technology and Handicapped People
Springer Publishing Company
11 W 42nd St
15th Floor
New York, NY 10036-8002   212-431-4370
                               877-687-7476
                          Fax: 212-941-7842
                          cs@springerpub.com
                          www.springerpub.com
Dr. Ursula Springer, President
Ted Nardin, CEO
James C. Costello, Vice President, Journal Publishi

Important information for concerned professionals about new rehabilitation techniques and treatments for handicapped people.
$29.95
224 pages Hardcover
ISBN 0-82614 -10-8

2469 Textbooks and the Student Who Can't Read Them: A Guide for Teaching Content
Brookline Books
8 Trumbull Rd
Suite B-001
Northampton, MA 01060   413-584-0184
                               800-666-2665
                          Fax: 413-584-6184
                          brbooks@yahoo.com
                          www.brooklinebooks.com
Based on a careful analysis of 10 textbook programs, the author concisely and sensibly indicate s the procedures that facilitate teachers' use of regular grade level textbooks with low-reading students. *$21.95*
Paperback
ISBN 0-91479 -57-3

2470 The Education of Children with Acquired Brain Injury
David Fulton Publishers (Routledge)
711 Third Ave
New York, NY 10017   212-216-7800
                          Fax: 212-564-7854
                          orders@taylorandfrancis.com
                          www.routledge.com
Sue Walker, Author
Beth Wicks, Author
Teachers have to be aware of their pupils' special educational needs. Find out what an acquired brain injury is and how to maximize learning opportunities for those with the condition with this book.
128 pages

2471 The Fundamentals of Special Education: A Practical Guide for Every Teacher
Corwin Press Inc.
2455 Teller Rd
Thousand Oaks, CA 91320   805-499-9734
                               800-233-9936
                          Fax: 805-499-5323
                          order@corwin.com
                          us.corwin.com
Bob Algozzine, Author
Jim Ysseldyke, Author
This guide highlights major concepts in special education-from disability categories, identification issues, and IEPs to appropriate learning environments and the roles general and special educators play.
104 pages

2472 The K&W Guide to Colleges for Studentswith Learning Disablties (13th Edition)
The Princeton Review - Penguin Random House
1745 Broadway
New York, NY 10019   212-782-9000
                          customerservice@penguinrandomhouse.com
                          www.penguinrandomhouse.com
An updated guide to the more than 900 colleges with programs for the learning disabled. *$31.99*
848 pages Paperback 1916
ISBN 1-101920-38-6

2473 There's a Hearing Impaired Child in My Class
Gallaudet University Bookstore
800 Florida Ave NE
Washington, DC 20002-3600   202-651-5000
                               800-451-1073
                          Fax: 202-651-5489
                          TTY: 888-630-9347
                          clerc.center@gallaudet.edu
Debra Nussbaum, Author
Dr. T Alan Hurwitz, President
Edward Bosso, Vice President for Administratio

This complete package provides basic facts about deafness, practical strategies for teaching hearing impaired children, and the question-and-answer information for all students. *$16.95*
44 pages

2474   Toward Effective Public School Program for Deaf Students
Teachers College Press
525 W 120th St
New York, NY 10027-6605   212-678-3000
                                            800-575-6566
                                          Fax: 212-678-4149
                                webcomments@tc.columbia.edu
                                          www.tc.columbia.edu
Susan H. Fuhrman, Ph.D., President of the College
Harvey Spector, Vice President for Finance and Administration
Suzanne M. Murphy, Vice President for Development and External Affairs
This book translates research and data into useable recommendations and possible courses of action for organizing effective public school programs for deaf students. *$22.95*
272 pages Paperback
ISBN 0-807731-59-5

2475   Treating Adults with Physical Disabilities: Access and Communication
World Institute on Disability
3075 Adeline St.
Suite 155
Berkeley, CA 94703   510-225-6400
                                          Fax: 510-225-0477
                                               wid@wid.org
                                               www.wid.org
Marcie Roth, Executive Director & Chief Executive Officer
Katherine Zigmont, Senior Director, Operations & Deputy Director
Reggie Johnson, Senior Director, Marketing & Communications
A training curriculum for medical professionals who want to improve the quality of care for people with disabilities and chronic illnesses. Also covers architectural, communication, attitudinal and economic policy barriers to quality health care and specific skills to increase good communication and rapport.

2476   Treating Cerebral Palsy for Clinicians by Clinicians
Sage Publications
2455 Teller Road
Thousand Oaks, CA 91320   805-499-9774
                                            800-818-7243
                                          Fax: 800-583-2665
                                           www.sagepub.com
Sara Miller McCune, Founder, Publisher, Chairperson
Blaise R Simqu, President & CEO
Tracey A. Ozmina, Executive Vice President & Chief
A clinical manual for professionals beginning to work with persons who have cerebral palsy. *$31.00*
312 pages

2477   Treating Disordered Speech Motor Control
Sage Publications
2455 Teller Road
Thousand Oaks, CA 91320   805-499-9774
                                            800-818-7243
                                          Fax: 800-583-2665
                                           www.sagepub.com
Sara Miller McCune, Founder, Publisher, Chairperson
Blaise R Simqu, President & CEO
Deanie Vogel, Author
This book about neuromotor disturbances of speech production is aimed at practicing professionals and advanced graduate students interested in the neuropathologies of communication. *$36.00*
410 pages

2478   Treating Families of Brain Injury Survivors
Springer Publishing Company
11 W 42nd St
15th Floor
New York, NY 10036-8002   212-431-4370
                                            877-687-7476
                                          Fax: 212-941-7842
                                          cs@springerpub.com
                                          www.springerpub.com
Dr. Ursula Springer, President
Ted Nardin, CEO
James C. Costello, Vice President, Journal Publishi
Provides the mental health practitioner with a comprehensive program for helping families of head injury survivors cope with the change in their lives. Includes background on medical aspects of head injury, family structure functioning and special needs of various family members.
220 pages
ISBN 0-82616 -20-1

2479   Understanding and Teaching Emotionally Disturbed Children & Adolescents
Sage Publications
2455 Teller Road
Thousand Oaks, CA 91320   805-499-9774
                                            800-818-7243
                                          Fax: 800-583-2665
                                           www.sagepub.com
Sara Miller McCune, Founder, Publisher, Chairperson
Blaise R Simqu, President & CEO
Tracey A. Ozmina, Executive Vice President & Chief
The teacher's handbook provides information that will change misconceptions about children who are frequently labeled as emotionally disturbed. It also gives information about a wide variety of intervention methods and approaches for use in educational settings. *$41.00*
620 pages Hardover

2480   Using the Dictionary of Occupational Titles in Career Decision Making
Stout Vocational Rehab Institute
University of Wisconsin Stou
Menomonie, WI 54751   715-232-2470
                                          Fax: 715-232-5008
                                            luij@uwstout.edu
John Lui, Contact Person
This is a self-study manual for learning how to use the 1991 U.S. Department of Labor's Dictionary of Occupational Titles. It gives the DOT user a tool to understand the DOT and then put its information to work. Shows how to quickly obtain information about the work performed in 12,741 occupations listed and described in the DOT and the worker requirements for those occupations. *$24.00*
142 pages Softcover

2481   VBS Special Education Teaching Guide
Life Way Christian Resources Southern Baptist Conv
1 Lifeway Plz
Nashville, TN 37234-1001   615-251-2000
                                           www.lifeway.com
Tom Hellam, VP of Executive Communications a
Thom Rainer, President & CEO
This book contains teaching plans for five bible study sessions with reproducible handouts for learners. The plans use multisensory, experiential-based learning activities designed for adults and older youth who have developmental disabilities. Suggestions for Bible learning, crafts, recreation, snacks and theme interpretation are included. Designed primarily for Vacation Bible School, but may be used in camp/retreat settings. *$9.95*
56 pages Yearly

2482 Vermont Interdependent Services Team Approach (VISTA)
Brookes Publishing
PO Box 10624
Baltimore, MD 21285-624
410-337-9580
800-638-3775
Fax: 410-337-8539
custserv@brookespublishing.com
www.brookespublishing.com
Paul Kelly, National Textbook Sales Manager
Tracy Gray, Educational Sales Manager
Paul Brooks, President
A guide to coordinating educational support services. This manual enables IEP team members to fulfill the related services provisions of IDEA as they make effective support services decisions using a collaborative team approach. *$27.95*
176 pages Spiral bound
ISBN 1-55766-30-4

2483 What School Counselors Need to Know
Council for Exceptional Children
3100 Clarendon Blvd.
Suite 600
Arlington, VA 22201-5332
888-232-7733
TTY: 866-915-5000
service@exceptionalchildren.org
www.exceptionalchildren.org
Barbara E. Baditoi, Co-Author
Pamelia E. Brott, Co-Author
This book provides counselors (and school administrators) with essential information to make the most of their participation in providing special education services. *$25.95*

2484 When You Have a Visually Impaired Student in Your Classroom: A Guide for Teachers
American Foundation for the Blind
2 Penn Plaza
Suite1102
New York, NY 10121
212-502-7600
800-232-5463
Fax: 888-545-8331
afbinfo@afb.net
afb.org
Carl Augusto, President
This guide provides information on students' abilities and needs, resources and educational team members, federal special education requirements, and technology materials used by students. *$9.95*
84 pages
ISBN 0-891283-93-5

2485 Working Bibliography on Behavioral and Emotional Disorders
Natl. Clearinghouse for Alcohol & Drug Information
1 Choke Cherry Road
Rockville, MD 20857
301-468-2600
877-SAM-SA 7
Fax: 301-468-6433
Lizabeth J Foster, Librarian/Info. Resource Manager
Pamela S. Hyde, Administrator
NCADI is a service of the U.S. Substance Abuse and Mental Health Services Administration. As the national focal point for information on alcohol and other drugs, NCADI collects, prepares, classifies, and distributes information about alcohol, tobacco and other drugs, prevention strategies and materials, research, treatment, etc.
40 pages

2486 Working Together with Children and Families: Case Studies
Brookes Publishing Company
PO Box 10624
Baltimore, MD 21285-624
410-337-9580
800-638-3775
Fax: 410-337-8539
custserv@brookespublishing.com
www.brookespublishing.com
Paul Kelly, National Textbook Sales Manager
Tracy Gray, Educational Sales Manager
Paul Brooks, Owner

Early interventionists will be able to bridge the gap between theory and practice with this edited collection of case studies.
$23.00
336 pages
ISBN 1-557661-23-5

2487 Working with Visually Impaired Young Students: A Curriculum Guide for 3 to 5 Year Olds
Charles C. Thomas
2600 S First St
Springfield, IL 62704-4730
217-789-8980
800-258-8980
Fax: 217-789-9130
books@ccthomas.com
www.ccthomas.com
Michael P. Thomas, President
Ellen Trief, Editor
The first step in the education process of a visually impaired child is the early identification and treatment by an eye care specialist. This book is geared to the age of birth through 3-years. Available in cloth, paperback and hardcover. *$42.95*
194 pages Paperback
ISBN 0-398068-75-2

Testing Resources

2488 ADD-SOI Center, The
2007 Cedar Avenue
Manhattan Beach, CA 90266
310-546-6500
Fax: 310-546-9068
ADDSOI@aol.com
www.addsoi.com
The ADD-SOI Center provides services and assessments for ADD (Attention Deficit Disorder), ADHD, and SOI at our Manhattan Beach, California facility.

2489 AEPS Child Progress Report: For Children Ages Birth to Three
Brookes Publishing
PO Box 10624
Baltimore, MD 21285-624
410-337-9580
800-638-3775
Fax: 410-337-8539
custserv@brookespublishing.com
www.brookespublishing.com
Paul Kelly, National Textbook Sales Manager
Tracy Gray, Educational Sales Manager
Paul Brooks, Owner
This chart helps monitor change by visually displaying current abilities, intervention targets, and child progress. In packages of 30. *$18.00*
6 pages Gate-fold
ISBN 1-55766 -65-0

2490 AEPS Data Recording Forms: For Children Ages Birth to Three
Brookes Publishing
PO Box 10624
Baltimore, MD 21285-624
410-337-9580
800-638-3775
Fax: 410-337-8539
custserv@brookespublishing.com
readplaylearn.com
Paul Brooks, Owner
Melissa Behm, Executive Vice President
These forms can be used by child development professionals on four separate occasions to pinpoint and then monitor a child's strengths and needs in the six key areas of skill development measured by the AEPS Test. Packages of 10. *$23.00*
36 pages Saddle-stiched
ISBN 1-55766 -97-2

2491 AEPS Measurement for Birth to Three Years
Brookes Publishing
PO Box 10624
Baltimore, MD 21285-624   410-337-9580
                                            800-638-3775
                                       Fax: 410-337-8539
                            custserv@brookespublishing.com
                                 www.brookespublishing.com
Paul Kelly, National Textbook Sales Manager
Tracy Gray, Educational Sales Manager
Paul Brooks, Owner
This dynamic volume explains the Assessment, Evaluation and
Programming System, provides the complete AEPS Test and par-
allel assessment/evaluation tools for families and includes the
forms and plans needed for implementation. *$39.00*
352 pages

2492 AEPS Measurement for Three to Six Years
Brookes Publishing
PO Box 10624
Baltimore, MD 21285-624   410-337-9580
                                            800-638-3775
                                       Fax: 410-337-8539
                            custserv@brookespublishing.com
                                 www.brookespublishing.com
Paul Kelly, National Textbook Sales Manager
Tracy Gray, Educational Sales Manager
Paul Brooks, Owner
Resources in early childhood, early intervention, inclusive and
special education, developmental disabilities, learning disabili-
ties, communication and language, behavior, and mental health.
$57.00
400 pages Spiral-bound
ISBN 1-55766 -87-1

2493 AIR: Assessment of Interpersonal Relations
Sage Publications
2455 Teller Road
Thousand Oaks, CA 91320   805-499-0721
                                            800-818-7243
                                       Fax: 800-583-2665
                                         info@sagepub.com
                                           www.sagepub.com
Sara Miller McCune, Founder, Publisher, Chairperson
Blaise R Simqu, President & CEO
A thoroughly researched and standardized clinical instrument assessing the quality of adolescents' interpersonal relationships in
a hierarchical fashion, including global relationship quality and
relationship quality with three domains: Family, Social and Academic. *$89.00*

2494 ALST: Adolescent Language Screening Test
Sage Publications
2455 Teller Road
Thousand Oaks, CA 91320   805-499-0721
                                            800-818-7243
                                       Fax: 800-583-2665
                                         info@sagepub.com
                                           www.sagepub.com
Sara Miller McCune, Founder, Publisher, Chairperson
Blaise R Simqu, President & CEO
Provides speech/language pathologists and other interested pro-
fessionals with a rapid thorough method for screening adoles-
cents (ages 11-17). *$119.00*

**2495 Adaptive Mainstreaming: A Primer for Teachers and
Principals, 3rd Edition**
Longman Publishing Group
1330 Avenue of the Americas
New York, NY 10019   212-641-2400
                                            800-745-8489
                                           www.pearson.com
Glen Moreno, Chairman
Marjorie Scardino, Chief Executive Officer
An introduction to education for handicapped and gifted stu-
dents. Presents research-based rationales for teaching excep-
tional students in the least restrictive environment. Provides

historical perspectives, offers realistic descriptions of prevailing
practices in the field, and reviews trends and new directions.
366 pages Paperback
ISBN 0-582285-04-6

2496 Ages & Stages Questionnaires
Brookes Publishing
PO Box 10624
Baltimore, MD 21285-624   410-337-9580
                                            800-638-3775
                                       Fax: 410-337-8539
                            custserv@brookespublishing.com
                                 www.brookespublishing.com
Paul Kelly, National Textbook Sales Manager
Tracy Gray, Educational Sales Manager
Paul Brooks, Owner
ASQ is an economical and field-tested system for identifying
whether infants and young children may require further developmental evaluation and offers a screening and tracking program
that helps early intervention professionals, service coordinators,
and administrators maximize financial resources while promoting the health and growth of the children they serve. Set includes
11 color-coded, reproducible questionnaires, 11 reproducible,
age appropriate scoring sheets. *$135.00*

2497 American College Testing Program
500 Act Drive
PO Box 168
Iowa City, IA 52243-168   319-337-1000
                                       Fax: 319-339-3021
                                                  act.org
John Whitmore, CEO
Mark D Musik, President Emeritus
An independent, nonprofit organization that provides a variety of
educational services to students and their parents, to high schools
and colleges, and to professional associations and government
agencies.

2498 Assessing Students with Special Needs
Longman Publishing Group
10 Bank Street
9th Floor
White Plains, NY 10606-1933   914-993-5000
                                           www.ablongman.com
Joanne Dresner, President
Step-by-step guide to informal, classroom assessment of students
with special needs.
174 pages Paperback
ISBN 0-801301-77-7

**2499 Assessment Log & Developmental Progress Charts for
the CCPSN**
Brookes Publishing
P.O.Box 10624
Baltimore, MD 21285-624   410-337-9580
                                            800-638-3775
                                       Fax: 410-337-8539
                            custserv@brookespublishing.com
                                 www.brookespublishing.com
Paul Kelly, National Textbook Sales Manager
Tracy Gray, Educational Sales Manager
Paul Brooks, Owner
This 28-page booklet allows readers to actually chart the ongoing
progress of each preschool child. Available in packages of 10.
$22.00
28 pages Saddle-stiched
ISBN 1-55766 -39-5

2500 Assessment of Learners with Special Needs
Allyn & Bacon
75 Arlinton Street
Ste 300
Boston, MA 2116-3988   617-848-7500
                                            800-852-8024
                                       Fax: 617-944-7273
                                           www.ablongman.com
Bill Barke, CEO
Thomas Longman, Founder
The central goal of this book is to help teachers become sophisti-
cated, informed test consumers in terms of choosing, using and

interpreting commercially prepared tests for their special needs students.
508 pages Casebound
ISBN 0-205227-33-3

2501 Benchmark Measures
Educators Publishing Service
PO Box 9031
Cambridge, MA 2139
617-547-6706
800-225-5750
Fax: 888-440-2665
feedback@epsbooks.com
www.epsbooks.com

Charles H Heinle, VP
Alexandra S Bigelow, Author
Gunnar Voltz, President
Ungraded test containing three sequential levels that assess alphabet and dictionary skills, reading, handwriting and spelling, and correspond to the first three schedules of the Alphabetic Phonics curriculum. The tests can be used at any level to measure a student's general knowledge of phonics. *$64.40*
Kit

2502 Brain Clinic, The
19 West 34th Street
Penthouse
New York, NY 10001
212-268-8900
nurosvcs@aol.com
thebrainclinic.com

Dr. James Lawrence Thomas, Director
The brain clinic offers diagnosis and Treatment of ADD, Learning Disabilities, Migraines, and Traumatic Brain Injury.

2503 CREVT: Comprehensive Receptive and Expressive Vocabulary Test
Sage Publications
2455 Teller Road
Thousand Oaks, CA 91320
805-499-0721
800-818-7243
Fax: 800-583-2665
info@sagepub.com
www.sagepub.com

Sara Miller McCune, Founder, Publisher, Chairperson
Blaise R Simqu, President & CEO
A new, innovative, efficient measure of both receptive and expressive oral vocabulary. The CREVT has two subtests and is based on the most current theories of vocabulary development, suitable for ages 4 through 17. *$174.00*
Complete Kit

2504 Carolina Curriculum for Preschoolers with Special Needs
Brookes Publishing
P.O.Box 10624
Baltimore, MD 21285-624
410-337-9580
800-638-3775
Fax: 410-337-8539
custserv@brookespublishing.com
www.brookespublishing.com

Paul Kelly, National Textbook Sales Manager
Tracy Gray, Educational Sales Manager
Paul Brooks, Owner
This curriculum provides detailed teaching and assessment techniques, plus a sample 28-page Assessment Log that shows readers how to chart a child's individual progress. This guide is for children between 2 and 5 in their developmental stages who are considered at risk for developmental delay or who exhibit special needs. *$35.95*
352 pages Spiral-bound
ISBN 1-557660-32-8

2505 Center For Personal Development
405 North Wabash Ave.
Suite 208 & 1114
Chicago, IL 60611
312-755-7000
Fax: 312-755-7001
info@chicagotherapist.com
www.chicagotherapist.com

Steven Nakisher, Licensed Clinical Psychologist
Cara McCanse, Licensed Clinical Psychologist
Sarah Krcmarik, Staff Psychotherapist
The Center for Personal Development was founded in 1998 to provide a diverse range of high-quality mental health services.

2506 Center for Human Potential
525 East 100 South
Suite 120
Salt Lake City, UT 84102
801-483-2447
801-486-8705
www.c4hp.com

C. Brendan Hallett Psy.D., Clinical Director
Michael DeCaria, Ph.D., Licensed Clinical Psychologist
Annice Julian, Psy.D., Licensed Clinical Psychologist
Center for Human Potentialis a human services company that helps individuals, businesses and organizations reach their potential by achieving balance in the fundamental areas of life: Emotional, Physical, Mental, Spiritual and Financial. We offer individual, couples, and family counseling to help with a number of issues.

2507 Center for Neuropsychology, Learning & Development
1955 Pauline Blvd
Suite 100A
Ann Arbor, MI 48103
734-994-9466
Fax: 734-994-9465
www.cnld.org

Roger E. Lauer, Clinical Director
Jodene Goldenring Fine, Ph.D., Licensed Psychologist
CNLD was founded over 20 years ago to serve Southeast Michigan and the greater Ann Arbor community by providing quality mental health care for children, adolescents, adults and families.

2508 Center for Student Health and Counseling
1825 SW Broadway
Portland, OR 97201
503-725-3000
800-547-8887
Fax: 503-725-4882
askadm@pdx.edu
www.pdx.edu/shac/ldadhd

Portland State University's mission is to enhance the intellectual, social, cultural and economic qualities of urban life by providing access throughout the life span to a quality liberal education for undergraduates and an appropriate array of professional and graduate programs especially relevant to metropolitan areas.

2509 Children's Assessment Center, The
2500 Bolsover St.
Houston, TX 77005
713-986-3300
Fax: 713-986-3553
info@cac.hctx.net
cachouston.org

Brady E. Crosswell, Chairman
Gail Prather, President
Elaine Stolte, Executive Director
The Children's Assessment Center (CAC)provides a safe haven to sexually abused children and their families.

2510 Cognitive Solutions Learning Center
2409 N. Clybourn Ave.
Chicago, IL 60614
773-755-1775
Fax: 773-439-5499
info@helpforld.com
www.helpforld.com/index.php/about-us/

Dr. Ari Goldstein, Founder
Jason Almodovar, M.S.Ed., Office Manager
Cognitive Solution offers a broad range of services, including learning disability and attention deficit disorder assessment and remediation, executive functions training, and the latest neurofeedback technologies.

2511 DAYS: Depression and Anxiety in Youth Scale
Sage Publications
2455 Teller Road
Thousand Oaks, CA 91320   805-499-0721
                                 800-818-7243
                           Fax: 805-376-9443
                           info@sagepub.com
                           www.sagepub.com
Sara Miller McCune, Founder, Publisher, Chairperson
Blaise R Simqu, President & CEO
A unique battery of three norm-references scales useful in identifying major depressive disorder and overanxious disorders in children and adolescents. *$129.00*
Complete Kit

2512 DOCS: Developmental Observation Checklist System
Pro- Ed Publications
8700 Shoal Creek Blvd
Austin, TX 78757-6897   512-451-3246
                               800-897-3202
                         Fax: 800-397-7633
                         general@proedinc.com
                         www.proedinc.com
Donald D Hammill, Owner
Courtney King, Marketing Coordinator
A three-part system for the assessment of very young children with respect to general development, adjustment behavior and parent stress and support. *$124.00*

2513 Dennis Developmental Center
1 Children's Way
Little Rock, AR 72202-3591   501-364-1100
                               TTY: 501-364-1184
                               www.archildrens.org
Arkansas Children's Hospital (ACH) is the a pediatric medical center in Arkansas.

2514 Developmental Services Center
Therapeutic Nursery Program
4525 Lee St NE
Washington, DC 20019   202-388-3216
                         Fax: 202-576-8799
Alice Anderson
Offers assessment information and evaluation for developmentally delayed students.

2515 Frames of Reference for the Assessment of Learning Disabilities
Brookes Publishing
P.O.Box 10624
Baltimore, MD 21285-624   410-337-9580
                                 800-638-3775
                           Fax: 410-337-8539
                           custserv@brookespublishing.com
                           www.brookespublishing.com
Paul Kelly, National Textbook Sales Manager
Tracy Gray, Educational Sales Manager
Paul Brooks, Owner
New views on measurement issues. Here you'll find an in=depth look at the fundamental concerns facing those who work with children with learning disabilities - assessment and identification. *$55.00*
672 pages Hardcover
ISBN 1-55766 -38-3

2516 How to Conduct an Assessment
FSSI
3905 Huntington Dr
Amarillo, TX 79109-4047   806-353-1114
                           Fax: 806-353-1114
Ed Hammer, Owner
The Functional Skills Screening Inventory,this behavioral checklist allows for parents and professionals to observe critical behaviors in individuals with multiple disabilities (7 years to adult years).

2517 Inclusive & Heterogeneous Schooling: Assessment, Curriculum, and Instruction
Brookes Publishing
P.O.Box 10624
Baltimore, MD 21285-624   410-337-9580
                                 800-638-3775
                           Fax: 410-337-8539
                           custserv@brookespublishing.com
                           www.brookespublishing.com
Paul Kelly, National Textbook Sales Manager
Tracy Gray, Educational Sales Manager
Paul Brooks, Owner
Presents methods for successfully restructuring classrooms to enable all students, particularly those with disabilities, to flourish. Provides specific strategies for assessment, collaboration, classroom management, and age-specific instruction. *$34.95*
448 pages Paperback
ISBN 1-557662-02-9

2518 Infant & Toddler Convection of Fairfield: Falls Church
Joseph Willard Health Center
3750 Old Lee Hwy
Fairfax, VA 22030-1806   703-246-7180
                           Fax: 703-246-7307
Susan Sigler, Program Coordinator
Allan Phillips, Director Early Intervention
Offers assessments, evaluations and educational/therapeutic infant programs for parents infants and toddlers birth to age 3.
Sliding Scale

2519 K-BIT: Kaufman Brief Intelligence Test
AGS
Ste 1000
5910 Rice Creek Pkwy
Shoreview, MN 55126-5023   651-287-7220
                                 800-328-2560
                           Fax: 800-471-8457
                           agsmail@agsnet.com
                           www.agsnet.com
Kevin Brueggeman, President
Robert Zaske, Market Manager
Quick and easy-to-use, KBIT assesses verbal and non-verbal abilities through two reliable subtests - vocabulary and matricies. *$ 124.95*
Ages 4-90

2520 K-FAST: Kaufman Functional Academic Skills Test
AGS
Ste 1000
5910 Rice Creek Pkwy
Shoreview, MN 55126-5023   651-287-7220
                                 800-328-2560
                           Fax: 800-471-8457
                           agsmail@agsnet.com
                           www.agsnet.com
Robert Zaske, Market Manager
Helps assess a person's capacity to function effectively in society regarding functional reading and math skills. *$99.95*
Ages 15-85+

2521 K-SEALS: Kaufman Survey of Early Academic and Language Skills
AGS
5910 Rice Creek Pkwy
Shoreview, MN 55126-5025   651-287-7220
                                 800-328-2560
                           Fax: 800-471-8457
                           agsmail@agsnet.com
                           www.agsnet.com
Kevin Brueggeman, President
Robert Zaske, Market Manager
An individually administered test of children's of both expressive and receptive skills, pre-academic skills and articulation. K-SEALS offers reliable scores usually in less than 25 minutes. *$ 179.95*
Ages 3-0; 6-11

2522 KLST-2: Kindergarten Language Screening Test Edition, 2nd Edition
Sage Publications
2455 Teller Road
Thousand Oaks, CA 91320
805-499-9774
800-818-7243
Fax: 800-583-2665
info@sagepub.com
www.sagepub.com

Paul Kelly, National Textbook Sales Manager
Blaise R Simqu, President & CEO
Identifies children who need further diagnostic testing to determine whether or not they have language deficits that will accelerate academic failure. *$94.00*

2523 Kaufman Test of Educational Achievement(K-TEA)
AGS
PO Box 99
Circle Pines, MN 55014-99
800-328-2560
Fax: 800-471-8457
agsmail@agsnet.com
www.agsnet.com

Robert Zaske, Marketing Manager
Kevin Brueggeman, President
K-TEA is an individually administered diagnostic battery that measures reading, mathematics, and spelling skills. Setting the standards in achievement testing today, K-TEA Comprehensive provides the complete diagnostic information you need for educational assessment and program planning. The Brief Forum is indispensable for school and clinical psychologists, special education teachers when a quick a measure of achievement is needed. *$249.95*

2524 Learning House
264 Church Street
Guilford, CT 6437
203-453-3691

Susan Santora, Founder and Director
Learning House is a professional community committed to enhancing the lives of individuals with dyslexia and other learning disabilities in safe and supportive surroundings.

2525 LearningRx
5085 List Drive
Suite 200
Colorado Springs, CO 80919
719-264-8808
www.learningrx.com

Dr. Ken Gibson, Founder
LearningRx is a brain training program.

2526 Life Centered Career Education: A Contemporary Based Approach
Council for Exceptional Children
3100 Clarendon Blvd.
Suite 600
Arlington, VA 22201-5332
888-232-7733
TTY: 866-915-5000
service@exceptionalchildren.org
www.exceptionalchildren.org

Chad Rummel, Executive Director
Laurie VanderPloeg, Associate Executive Director, Professional Affairs
Craig Evans, Chief Financial Officer
Provides a framework for building 97 functional skill competencies appropriate for preparing for adult life and special education students. *$28.00*
175 pages

2527 Measure of Cognitive-Linguistic Abilities(MCLA)
Speech Bin
PO Box 1579
Appleton, VA 54912-1579
772-770-0007
888-388-3224
Fax: 888-388-6344
onlinehelp@schoolspecialty.com
www.speechbin.com

Jan J Binney, Senior Editor

A diagnostic test of cognitive-linguistic abilities of adolescents and adults with traumatically induced brain injuries. High level. Normed. *$89.00*
100 pages
ISBN 0-93785 -72-

2528 Miriam
501 Bacon Avenue
St. Louis, MO 63119-1512
314-968-3893
Fax: 314-962-0482
athorp@miriamstl.org
www.miriamstl.org/learning-center

Andrew Thorp, Executive Director
Sarah Scott, Development Director
Carol Faust, Business Manager
Miriam improves the quality of life for children with learning disabilities and their families through innovative and comprehensive programs.

2529 Neuropsychology Assessment Center
One University Place
Chester, PA 19013
610-499-4273
www.widenernac.org

Mary F. Lazar, PsyD, Director
Wendy M. Sarkisian, PsyD, Assistant Director
Located in the Philadelphia area, the Neuropsychology Assessment Center (NAC) specializes in neuropsychological evaluations for the investigation of a variety of psychological conditions.

2530 ONLINE
West Virginia Research and Training Center
P.O.Box 1004
Institute, WV 25112-1004
304-766-9495
800-624-8284
Fax: 304-766-2689
www.icdi.wvu.edu

Clifford Lantz, President
A quarterly newsletter offering information about hardware technology, software (commercial and home grown); applications that work and bonuses such as an exchange program for copyright-free software. *$25.00*
Quarterly

2531 OWLS: Oral and Written Language Scales LC/OE & WE
AGS
P.O.Box 99
Circle Pines, MN 55014-99
800-328-2560
Fax: 800-471-8457
www.agsnet.com

Kevin Brueggeman, President
Robert Zaske, Market Manager
One kit provides an assessment of listening comprehension while the other assesses oral expression tasks: semantic, syntactic, pragmatic, and supralinguistic aspects of language. Written Expression may be administered individually or in small groups. *$249.95*

2532 PAT-3: Photo Articulation Test
Sage Publications
2455 Teller Road
Thousand Oaks, CA 91320
805-499-9774
800-818-7243
Fax: 800-583-2665
info@sagepub.com
www.sagepub.com

Paul Kelly, National Textbook Sales Manager
Blaise R Simqu, President & CEO
This test consists of 72 color photographs. The first 69 photos test consonants and all but one vowel and one diphthong. The remaining pictures test connected speech and the remaining vowel and diphthong. *$144.00*
Complete Kit

2533 Peabody Early Experiences Kit (PEEK)
AGS
P.O.Box 99
Circle Pines, MN 55014-99   800-328-2560
Fax: 800-471-8457
www.agsnet.com

Kevin Brueggeman, President
Robert Zaske, Market Manager
1,000 activities and all the materials you need to build youngsters' cognitive, social and language skills. Manuals, puppets, manipulatives, picture card deck, picture mini decks and more to teach early development concepts. *$789.95*

2534 Peabody Individual Achievement Test-Revised Normative Update (PIAT-R-NU)
AGS
P.O.Box 99
Circle Pines, MN 55014-99   800-328-2560
Fax: 800-471-8457
www.agsnet.com

Kevin Brueggeman, President
Robert Zaske, Market Manager
PIAT-R-NU is an efficient individual measure of academic achievement. Reading, mathematics, and spelling are assessed in a simple, non-threatening format that requires only a pointing response for most items. This multiple choice format makes the PIAT-R ideal for assessing individuals who hesitate to give a spoken response, or have limited expressive abilities. *$289.98*

2535 Peabody Language Development Kits (PLDK)
AGS
P.O.Box 99
Circle Pines, MN 55014-99   800-328-2560
Fax: 800-471-8457
www.agsnet.com

Kevin Brueggeman, President
Robert Zaske, Market Manager
The main goals of the Peabody Kit language program are to stimulate overall language skills in Standard English and, for each level of the program, advance children's cognitive skills about a year. *$ 649.95*
Level P
ISBN 0-88671 -25-1

2536 Pediatric Early Elementary (PEEX II) Examination
Educators Publishing Service
625 Mount Auburn Street
3rd Floor
Cambridge, MA 2138- 3039   617-547-6706
800-225-5750
Fax: 888-440-2665
feedback@epsbooks.com
www.epsbooks.com

Charles H Heinle, VP
Alexandra S Bigelow, Author
Gunnar Voltz, President
Assesses the second-fourth grade child's performance on thirty-two tasks in six specific areas of development: fine-motor function, language, gross-motor function, memory, visual processing, and delayed recall. At three points during the exam, the child is rated on selective attention and behavior and effect. *$15.40 - $93*
ISBN 0-83888 -80-6

2537 Pediatric Exam of Educational-PEERAMID Readiness at Middle Childhood
Educators Publishing Service
625 Mount Auburn Street
3rd Floor
Cambridge, MA 2138- 3039   617-547-6706
800-225-5750
Fax: 888-440-2665
feedback@epsbooks.com
www.epsbooks.com

Charles H Heinle, VP
Alexandra S Bigelow, Author
Gunnar Voltz, President
Assesses the 4th-10th grade child's performance on thirty-one tasks in six specific areas: minor neurological indicators, fine-motor function, language, gross-motor function, temporal-sequential organization, and visual processing. Complete set. *$15.40 - $109*
ISBN 0-83888 -99-3

2538 Pediatric Examination of Educational Readiness
Educators Publishing Service
625 Mount Auburn Street
3rd Floor
Cambridge, MA 2139- 3039   617-547-6706
800-225-5750
Fax: 888-440-2665
feedback@epsbooks.com
www.epsbooks.com

Charles H Heinle, VP
Alexandra S Bigelow, Author
Gunnar Voltz, President
Assesses the Pre-1st grade child's performance on twenty-nine tasks in six specific areas of development: orientation, gross-motor, visual-fine motor, sequential, linguistic and preacademic learning. The child is rated on ten dimensions of selective attention/activity processing efficiency and adaptation. Complete set. *$12.85 - $86.40*
ISBN 0-83888 -80-1

2539 Pediatric Extended Examination at-PEET Three
Educators Publishing Service
625 Mount Auburn Street
3rd Floor
Cambridge, MA 2138- 3039   617-547-6706
800-225-5750
Fax: 888-440-2665
feedback@epsbooks.com
www.epsbooks.com

Charles H Heinle, VP
Alexandra S Bigelow, Author
Gunnar Volta, President
Assesses the preschool-age child's performance on twenty-eight tasks in five basic areas of development: gross-motor, language, visual-fine motor, memory, and intersensory integration. Complete set.
$13.75 - $126
ISBN 0-83888 -79-4

2540 Pre-Reading Screening Procedures
Educators Publishing Service
625 Mount Auburn Street
3rd Floor
Cambridge, MA 2138- 3039   617-547-6706
800-225-5750
Fax: 888-440-2665
feedback@epsbooks.com
www.epsbooks.com

Charles H Heinle, VP
Alexandra S Bigelow, Author
Gunnar Voltz, President
This revised group test, for grades K-1, evaluates auditory, visual and kinesthetic strengths in order to identify children who may have some form of dyslexia or specific language disability. *$ 18.00*
Grades K-1
ISBN 0-83885 -23-4

2541 Preparing for ACT Assessment
American College Testing Program
500 Act Drive
PO Box 168
Iowa City, IA 52243-168   319-337-1000
Fax: 319-339-3021
act.org

Richard L Ferguson, CEO
Designed to help high school students ready themselves for the ACT Assessment's subject area tests, explains the purposes of the four tests, describes their content and format, provides tips and exercises to improve student's test-taking skills and includes a complete sample text with scoring key.

2542 Psycho-Educational Assessment of Preschool Children
National Association of School Psychologists
Ste 105
4340 East West Hwy
Bethesda, MD 20814-4468

301-657-0270
866-331-NASP
Fax: 301-657-0275
ADMIN@SOELIN.COM
soelin.com

Susan Gorin, Executive Director
This is a contributed text on assessing specific skills of preschool children.
592 pages

2543 RULES: Revised
Speech Bin
PO Box 1579
Appleton, VA 54912-1579

772-770-0007
888-388-3224
Fax: 888-388-6344
customercare@schoolspecialty.com
www.speechbin.com

Jan J Binney, Senior Editor
Treatment program for young children who have phonological disorders. *$43.95*
280 pages
ISBN 0-93785 -51-3

2544 Receptive-Expressive Emergent-REEL-2 Language Test, 2nd Edition
Sage Publications
2455 Teller Road
Thousand Oaks, CA 91320

805-499-9774
800-818-7243
Fax: 800-583-2665
info@sagepub.com
www.sagepub.com

Paul Kelly, National Textbook Sales Manager
Blaise R Simqu, President & CEO
A revision of the popular scale used for the multidimensional analysis of emergent language. The REEL-2 is specifically designed for use with a broad range of at risk infants and toddlers in the new multidisciplinary programs developing under P.L. 99-457. *$79.00*

2545 Regents' Center for Learning Disorders
103 Hooper Street
Athens, GA 30602

706-542-4589
Fax: 706-583-0001
rcld@uga.edu
rcld.uga.edu

Tasha Falkingham, Office Manage
Karen Myers, Budget Analyst
Trish Foels, Staff Clinician, Psychologist
Provide assessment, training, research, andresources related to students who have learning disorders (e.g., Attention-Deficit/Hyperactivity Disorder, Autism Spectrum Disorders, Learning Disabilities, Emotional Disorders, and Traumatic Brain Injury) that impact their functioning in the academic environment.

2546 Schmieding Developmental Center
519 Latham Drive
Lowell, AR 72745

479-750-0125
Fax: 479-750-0323
www.archildrens.org

Mary Ann Scott, PhD, Program Director
Damon Lipinski, PhD, Program Director
Jerie Beth Karkos, MD, Medical Director
Arkansas Children's Hospital (ACH) is the a pediatric medical center in Arkansas.

2547 Slingerland Screening Tests
Educators Publishing Service
625 Mount Auburn Street
3rd Floor
Cambridge, MA 2138- 3039

617-547-6706
800-435-7728
Fax: 888-440-2665
feedback@epsbooks.com
www.epsbooks.com

Charles H Heinle, VP
Alexandra S Bigelow, Author
Gunnar Voltz, President
These tests, by Beth Slingerland, for individuals or groups of children, grades 1-6, identify children who show indications of having specific language disability in reading, handwriting, spelling or speaking. Form D evaluates personal orientation in time and space as well as the ability to express ideas in writing.
$14.80 - $27.45
ISBN 0-83882 -02-2

2548 Special Needs Advocacy Resource Book
Prufrock Press
PO Box 8813
Waco, TX 76714-8813

800-998-2208
Fax: 800-240-0333
info@prufrock.com
www.prufrock.com

Joel McIntosh, Publisher & Marketing Director
Rich Weinfield, Author
Michelle Davis, Author
Subtitle: What You Can Do Now to Advocate for Your Exceptional Child's Education. This is a unique hadnbook that teaches parents how to work with schools to achieve optimal learning situations and accommodations for their child's needs. *$19.95*
328 pages
ISBN 1-593633-09-7

2549 Speech Bin
PO Box 1579
Appleton, VA 54912-1579

772-770-0007
888-388-3224
Fax: 888-388-6344
customercare@schoolspecialty.com
www.speechbin.com

Jan J Binney, Senior Editor
Catalog offering test materials, assessment information, books and special education resources for speech-language pathologists, occupational and physical therapists, audiologists, and other rehabilitation professionals in schools, hospitals, clinics and private practices.
ISSN 4773-324

2550 Stuttering Severity Instrument for Children and Adults
Psychological & Educational Publications
P.O.Box 520
Hydesville, CA 95547-520

707-768-1807
800-523-5775
Fax: 800-447-0907

Morrison Gardner, President
With this tool teachers can determine whether to schedule a child for therapy or to evaluate the effects of treatment.

2551 TLC Speech-Language/Occupational TherapyCamps
2092 Gaither Rd.
Suite 100
Rockville, MD 20850

301-424-5200
Fax: 301-424-8063
TTY: 301-424-5203
info@ttlc.org
www.ttlc.org

Patricia Ritter, Executive Director
TLC provides small group summer programs for children with special needs. Offers speech-language and occupational therapy summer camps for children ages 3-7.

2552 Taking Part: Introducing Social Skills to Young Children
AGS
P.O.Box 99
Circle Pines, MN 55014-99   800-328-2560
                                    Fax: 800-471-8457
                                    www.agsnet.com

Kevin Brueggeman, President
Robert Zaske, Market Manager
The first social skills curriculum to be linked directly to an assessment tool. More than 30 lessons correlate with the skills assessed by the Social Skills Rating System, a multirater approach to assessing prosocial and problem behaviors. *$149.95*

2553 Teaching of Reading: A Continuum from Kindergarten through College, The
AVKO Educational Research Foundation
3084 Willard Rd
Birch Run, MI 48415-9404   810-686-9283
                                    866-285-6612
                                    Fax: 810-686-1101
                                    avko.org

Don Mc Cabe, Executive Director
A textbook for teaching teachers how to teach language arts with lessons about dyslexia, phonics, learning to write, the connection between reading and spelling, and diagnostic and prescriptive tests. Free as an e-book for Foundation members. *$49.95*
364 pages

2554 Test Critiques: Volumes I-X
Sage Publications
2455 Teller Road
Thousand Oaks, CA 91320   805-499-9774
                                    800-818-7243
                                    Fax: 800-583-2665
                                    info@sagepub.com
                                    www.sagepub.com

Paul Kelly, National Textbook Sales Manager
Blaise R Simqu, President & CEO
Provides the professional and nonprofessional with in-depth, evaluative studies of more than 800 of the most widely used of these assessment instruments. *$649.00*

2555 Test of Early Reading Ability Deaf or Hard of Hearing
Pro- Ed Publications
8700 Shoal Creek Blvd
Austin, TX 78757-6816   512-451-3246
                                    800-897-3202
                                    Fax: 800-397-7633
                                    general@proedinc.com
                                    www.proedinc.com

Donald D Hammill, Owner
Courtney King, Marketing Coordinator
This adaptation of the TERA-2 for simultaneous communication of American Sign Language is the ONLY individually administered test of reading designed for children with moderate to profound sensory hearing loss. *$169.00*
Complete Kit

2556 Test of Language Development: Primary
Sage Publications
2455 Teller Road
Thousand Oaks, CA 91320   805-499-9774
                                    800-818-7243
                                    Fax: 800-583-2665
                                    info@sagepub.com
                                    www.sagepub.com

Paul Kelly, National Textbook Sales Manager
Blaise R Simqu, President & CEO
TOLD P:2 and TOLD 1:2 are the most popular tests of spoken language used by clinicians today. They are used to identify children who have language disorders and to isolate the particular types of disorders they have. Primary Edition for ages 1-4 to 8-11: Intermediate Edition for ages 8-6 to 12-11.

2557 Test of Mathematical Abilities, 2nd Edition
Sage Publications
2455 Teller Road
Thousand Oaks, CA 91320   805-499-9774
                                    800-818-7243
                                    Fax: 800-583-2665
                                    info@sagepub.com
                                    www.sagepub.com

Paul Kelly, National Textbook Sales Manager
Blaise R Simqu, President & CEO
The latest version was developed for use in grades 3 through 12. It measures math performance on the two traditional major skill areas in math as well as attitude, vocabulary and general application of math concepts in real life. *$84.00*

2558 Test of Nonverbal Intelligence, 3rd Edition
Sage Publications
2455 Teller Road
Thousand Oaks, CA 91320   805-499-9774
                                    800-818-7243
                                    Fax: 800-583-2665
                                    info@sagepub.com
                                    www.sagepub.com

Paul Kelly, National Textbook Sales Manager
Blaise R Simqu, President & CEO
A language-free measure of intelligence, aptitude and reasoning. The administration of the test requires no reading, writing, speaking or listening on the part of the test subject. The items included in this test are problem-solving tasks that increase in difficulty. Each item presents a set of figures in which one or more components is missing. The test items include one or more of the characteristics of shape, position, direction, rotation, contiguity, shading, size, movement or pattern. *$229.00*
Complete Kit

2559 Test of Phonological Awareness
Sage Publications
2455 Teller Road
Thousand Oaks, CA 91320   805-499-9774
                                    800-818-7243
                                    Fax: 800-583-2665
                                    info@sagepub.com
                                    www.sagepub.com

Paul Kelly, National Textbook Sales Manager
Blaise R Simqu, President & CEO
Measures young children's awareness of the individual sounds in words. Children who are sensitive to the phonological structure of words in oral language have a much easier time learning to read than children who are not. *$143.00*

2560 Test of Written Spelling, 3rd Edition
Pro- Ed Publications
8700 Shoal Creek Blvd
Austin, TX 78757-6897   512-451-3246
                                    800-897-3202
                                    Fax: 800-397-7633
                                    general@proedinc.com
                                    www.proedinc.com

Donald D Hammill, Owner
Courtney King, Marketing Coordinator
This revised edition assesses the student's ability to spell words whose spellings are readily predictable in sound-letter patterns, words whose spellings are less predictable and both types of words considered together. *$74.00*

2561 Texas Scottish Rite Hospital for Children
2222 Welborn Street
Dallas, TX 75219   214-559-5000
                                    Fax: 800-421-1121
                                    tsrhdv@tsrh.org
                                    www.tsrhc.org

Robert L. Walker, President/ CEO
Mark G. Bateman, SVP, Public Relations
Leslie A. Clonch, Jr., Vice President/ CIO
TSRHC treats children with orthopedic conditions, such as scoliosis, clubfoot, hand disorders, hip disorders and limb length differences, as well as certain related neurological disorders and learning disorders, such as dyslexia.

2562 Woodcock Reading Mastery Tests
Pearson
5601 Green Valley Dr
Bloomington, MN 55437-1099 800-627-7271
Fax: 800-232-1223
pearsonassessments@pearson.com
www.pearsonassessments.com

Christine Carlson, Product Manager
Doug Kubach, President & CEO
The Woodcock Reading Mastery Tests - Revised provides an interpretive system and age range to help you assess reading skills of children and adults. Two forms, G and II, make it easy to test and retest, or you can combine the results of both forms for a more comprehensive assessment. Revised with recent updates.
$329.95

2563 Young Children with Special Needs: A Developmentally Appropriate Approach
Allyn & Bacon
75 Arlington Street
Ste 300
Boston, MA 2116-3988 617-848-7500
800-852-8024
Fax: 617-944-7273
www.ablongman.com

Bill Barke, CEO
Thomas Longman, Founder
This book is designed to prepare students in making curriculum decisions in order to care for and foster the development of young children with special needs in normal early childhood settings.
270 pages
ISBN 0-20518 -94-X

Treatment & Training

2564 ABLE Program MCC-Longview
3200 Broadway
Kansas City, MO 64111-2105 816-604-1000
Fax: 816-672-2719
joan.bergstrom@mcckc.edu
mcckc.edu/ABLE

Joan Bergstrom, Director
Kay Owens, Administrative Assistant
Intensive support services program for post secondary students with neurological disabilities. The ABLE Program can be reached at http://mcckc.edu/ABLE

2565 Academy for Guided Imagery
30765 Pacific Coast Hwy
Ste 355
Malibu, CA 90265-3643 800-726-2070
Fax: 800-727-2070
info@acadgi.com
www.acadgi.com

David E Bresler, President
The Academy aims to teach people to access and use the power of the mind/body connection for healing, and to further understanding of the imagery process in human life and development. They provide systematic training and guidance to health professionals who are interested in the use of Guided Imagery in their practice. The Academy's Imagery Store offers guided imagery CDs, DVDs and books for self-healing.

2566 Adventist HealthCare
820 West Diamond Avenue
Suite 600
Gaithersburg, MD 20878 301-315-3030
Fax: 301-315-3000
www.adventisthealthcare.com

David E. Weigley, M.B.A., Chairman
Robert T. Vandeman, Vice-Chair
Terry Forde, Secretary
dventist HealthCare, based in Gaithersburg, Md., is a not-for-profit organization of dedicated professionals who work together to provide excellent wellness, disease management and health-care services to the community.

2567 Asthma & Allergy Education for Worksite Clinicians
Asthma and Allergy Foundation of America
8201 Corporate Drive
Suite 1000
Landover, VA 20785 202-466-7643
800-727-8462
Fax: 202-466-8940
info@aafa.org
aafa.org

Bill Mc Lin, President & CEO
Helen Taylor, Information Specialist
Developed to teach health professionals in the worksite about asthma and allergies and ultimately improve the health of the employees who have theses de\iseases. The program gives worksite clinicians the knowledge and tools they need to give employees guidance on how to control environmental factors both in the home and in the workplace, self-manage thier asthma and/or allergies and to determaine if ti is necessary for employees to see an allergist if symptoms persist.

2568 Asthma & Allergy Essentials for Children's Care Provider
Asthma and Allergy Foundation of America
8201 Corporate Drive
Suite 1000
Landover, VA 20785 202-466-7643
800-727-8462
Fax: 202-466-8940
info@aafa.org
aafa.org

Bill Mc Lin, President & CEO
Helen Taylor, Information Specialist
Course gives child care providers the tools and knowledge they need to care for children with asthma and allergies. During the interactive, three hour program, a trained health professional teaches providers how to recognize the signs and symptoms of an asthma or allergy episode, how to institute environmental control measures to prevent these episodes, and how to properly use medication and the tools for asthma management. In areas of the country serviced by AAFA's 14 chapters.

2569 Asthma Care Training for Kids (ACT)
Asthma and Allergy Foundation of America
8201 Corporate Drive
Suite 1000
Landover, VA 20785 202-466-7643
Fax: 202-466-8940
info@aafa.org
www.aafa.org

Bill Mc Lin, President & CEO
Helen Taylor, Information Specialist
Interactive program for children ages seven to 12 and their families. Children and their families attend three group sessions seperately to learn their own unique styles and then come together at the end of each session to share their knowledge.

2570 Ayurvedic Institute
PO Box 23445
Albuquerque, NM 87292-1445 505-291-9698
800-863-7721
Fax: 505-294-7572
ayurveda.com

Wynn Werner, Administrator
Directed by Dr. Vasant Lad, trains people in Ayurveda.

2571 Brooks Rehabilitation Hospital
3599 University Blvd S
Jacksonville, FL 32216 904-345-7600
Fax: 904-345-7619
www.brookshealth.org

Gary W. Sneed, Chairman
Michael Spigel, President/ COO
Douglas M. Baer, Chief Executive Officer
Brooks Rehabilitation provides the most advanced therapy and medical care.

2572 Center for Parent Information and Resources
35 Halsey St
4th Floor
Newark, NJ 07102 973-642-8100
www.parentcenterhub.org

Debra A. Jennings, Director
Myriam Alizo, Project Assistant
Lisa K□pper, Product Development Coordinator
The Center for Parent Information and Resources (CPIR) serves as a central resource of information and products to the community of Parent Training Information (PTI) Centers and the Community Parent Resource Centers (CPRCs), so that they can focus their efforts on serving families of children with disabilities.

2573 Center for Spinal Cord Injury Recovery
261 Mack
Detroit, MI 48201 866-724-2368
Fax: 313-745-9064
krodgers@dmc.org
www.centerforscirecovery.org

Krystal Rodgers, Administrative Assistant
The Center for SCI Recoveryr (CSCIR)provides long-term, high intensity, non-traditional, activity based therapy to maximize recovery.

2574 Cottage Rehabilitation Hospital
400 W. Pueblo Street
Santa Barbara, CA 93105 805-682-7111
mzate@sbch.org
www.cottagehealth.org
Cottage Health is a not-for-profit hospital system that includes Santa Barbara Cottage Hospital, Cottage Children's Hospital, Cottage Rehabilitation Hospital, Santa Ynez Valley Cottage Hospital, and Goleta Valley Cottage Hospital.

2575 Courage Kenny Rehabilitation Institute
Allina Health
800 E 28th St.
Minneapolis, MN 55407 612-863-4495
www.allinahealth.org
Courage Kenny Rehabilitation Institute was created in 2013 by the merger of Sister Kenny Rehabilitation Institute and Courage Center. A part of Allina Health, the Institute offers rehabilitation and community services for children and adults with injuries and disabilities.

2576 Harriet & Robert Heilbrunn Guild School
JGB Audio Library for the Blind
15 W 65th St
New York, NY 10023-6601 212-769-6200
800-284-4422
Fax: 212-769-6266
www.JGB.org

Allen R Morse, JD, PhD, President & CEO
Ken Stanley, Manager
A Jewish Guild for the blind.

2577 Howard School, The
1192 Foster St NW
Atlanta, GA 30318-4329 404-377-7436
Fax: 404-377-0884
admissions@howardschool.org
howardschool.org

Marifred Cilella, Head Of School
The Howard School educates students 5 years old through 12th grade with language learning disabilities and learning differences. Small student/teacher ratios allow for instruction that is personalized to complement the individual learning styles and to help each student understand his/her learning process. Students gain the tools and strategies needed to become independent, life-long learners.

2578 Kennedy Krieger Institute
707 North Broadway
Baltimore, MD 21205 443-923-9200
800-873-3377
888-554-2080
www.kennedykrieger.org

Jennifer Accardo, M.D., Neurologist
Adrianna Amari, Ph.D., Training & Research Coordinator
Roberta L. Babbitt, Ph.D, Program Director

Kennedy Krieger Institute is an internationally recognized institution dedicated to improving the lives of children and young adults with pediatric developmental disabilities and disorders of the brain, spinal cord and musculoskeletal system, through patient care, special education, research, and professional training.

2579 Kessler Institute for Rehabilitation
1199 Pleasant Valley Way
West Orange, NJ 07052 973-731-3600
877-322-2580
Fax: 973-243-6819
www.kessler-rehab.com

Sue Kida, President
Provides physical medicine and rehabilitation through the integration of highly specialized care, treatment, technology, education, research, and advocacy.

2580 Lake Michigan Academy
West Michigan Learning Disabilities Foundation
2428 Burton St SE
Grand Rapids, MI 49546-4806 616-464-3330
Fax: 616-285-1935

Amy Barto, Executive Director
Is a private day school for children with learning disabilities.

2581 Levinson Medical Center
98 Cutter Mill Road
Suite 90
Great Neck, NY 11021 516-482-2888
800-334-7323
Fax: 516-482-2480
drlevinson@aol.com
www.dyslexiaonline.com

Dr. Harold Levinson, Psychiatrist, Neurologist
Carolyn Malman, Office Manager
Lisa Danziger, Patient Coordinator
Medical center groundbreaking medical treatment offers rapid and often dramatic help to suffering dyslexic/ADHD children and adults

2582 Mad Hatters: Theatre That Makes a World of Difference
P.O.Box 50002
Kalamazoo, MI 49005-2 Fax: 269-385-5868
Bobbe A Luce, Executive Director
A nationally-known theater which has presented effective and innovative programs to more than 175,000 people in over 1,150 performances in the past 15 years. Our presentations and training programs are a proven method of changing attitudes and behaviors. The Mad Hatters is a leader in the field of sensitivity training to build community and foster the inclusion of all people in society. Fees: $500-$4000 per program, depending on topic and audience.

2583 MedStar National Rehabilitation Network
102 Irving Street NW
Washington, DC 20010 202-877-1000
www.medstarnrh.org
At MedStar National Rehabilitation Network, they treat adults and children with disabling illness or injury.

2584 Missouri Rehabilitation Center
One Hospital Drive
Columbia, MO 65212 573-882-4141
www.muhealth.org
University of Missouri Health Care offers a full spectrum of care, ranging from primary care to highly specialized, multidisciplinary treatment for patients with the most severe illnesses and injuries.

2585 Neuroxcel
401 Northlake Blvd.
North Palm Beach, FL 33048 866-391-6247
www.neuroxcel.com
Neuroxcelr Corporation is a Palm Beach, FL-based post rehabilitation Inclusive Fitness Strength and Conditioning Training Center, committed to improving the lives of individuals with a spinal cord injury (SCI), stroke, neurological conditions and various other special populations.

2586 Ramapo Training
Ramapo for Children
Rt. 52/Salisbury Turnpike
PO Box 266
Rhinebeck, NY 12572
845-876-8403
Fax: 845-876-8414
office@ramapoforchildren.org
www.ramapoforchildren.org

Adam Weiss, Chief Executive Officer
Bruce Kuziola, Chief Financial & Administrative Officer
Adam St. Bernard Jacobs, Director, Development & Communications

Ramapo Training was established to provide staff training and program support for educational and recreational programs, especially those that serve children-at-risk and those with special needs.

2587 Sandhills School
1500 Hallbrook Dr
Columbia, SC 29209-4021
803-695-1400
Fax: 803-695-1214
info@sandhillsschool.org
www.sandhillsschool.org

Anne Vickers, Head of School
Erika Senneseth, Asst Head of School
Angela Daniel, Director of Development

Exists to provide educational programs and intellectual development for average to above average students, six to 15, who learn differently and to promote the development of self-awareness, joy in learning and a vision of themselves as life-long learners.

2588 Senior Program for Teens and Young Adults with Special Needs
Camp J CC
6125 Montrose Rd
Rockville, MD 20852-4860
301-881-0100
Fax: 301-881-6549
jcccamp@jccgw.org
www.jccgw.org

Scott Cohen, President
Mindy Burger, Vice President for Development

The senior Program is a transitional program for teens and young adults with severe learning disabilities and multiple disabilities. Socialization, recreation and independent living skills are enhanced in a fun enviroment. Activities include art, music, recreational swim and more.

2589 Spinal Cord Injury Center
132 S. 10th Street
375 Main Building
Philadelphia, PA 19107
215-955-6579
Fax: 215-955-5152

Marilyn P. Owens, RN, BSN, Project Coordinator
Brittany Hayes, Research Coordinator
Jacqueline Robinson, Administrative Assistant

SCI provides medical care for their injuries, along with emotional, social, vocational and psychological rehabilitation to cope with the changes in their bodies and in their lifestyles that often result from the injury.

2590 Stanford Health Care
300 Pasteur Drive
Stanford, CA 94304
650-498-3333
800-756-9000
stanfordhealthcare.org

Amir Dan Rubin, President and CEO
Raj Behal, MD, Chief Quality Officer
James Hereford, Chief Operating Officer

Stanford Health Care provides patients with the very best in diagnosis and treatment.

2591 Teacher of Students with Visual Impairments
3635 Coal Mountain Rd.
Cumming, GA 30028   c.willings@teachingvisuallyimpaired.com
www.teachingvisuallyimpaired.com
Teaching Students with Visual Impairments.

2592 The Glenholme School
Devereux Advanced Behavioral Health Connecticut
81 Sabbaday Ln.
Washington, CT 06793
860-868-7377
Fax: 860-868-7894
info@theglenholmeschool.org
www.theglenholmeschool.org

The Glenholme School is an independent, co-educational special needs boarding and day school for young people, ages ten to adult in middle school, high school, postgraduate, transitional living for career development. The positive atmosphere provides guidance for students with special needs to achieve competent social and academic levels. The comprehensive learning environment supports the success of students with various learning disabilities, from Asperger's to Tourette's.

2593 UAB Spain Rehabilitation Center
1720 2nd Ave South
Birmingham, AL 35294
205-934-4011
TTY: 205-934-4642
www.uab.edu

Ray L. Watts, M.D., President
G. Allen Bolton Jr., VP, Financial Affairs

UAB's missionis to be a research university and academic health center that discovers, teaches and applies knowledge for the intellectual, cultural, social and economic benefit of Birmingham, the state and beyond.

2594 University of Maryland Rehabilitation and Orthopaedic Institute
Uni of MD Rehab & Ortho Institute
2200 Kernan Drive
Baltimore, MD 21207
410-448-2500
888-453-7626
TTY: 800-735-2258
www.umrehabortho.org

Cynthia A. Kelleher, MPH, MBA, Interim President and CEO
John P. Straumanis, VP, Medical Affairs
W. Walter Augustin, III, CPA, VP of Financial Services

University of Maryland Rehabilitation & Orthopaedic Institute (formerly Kernan Hospital), a committed provider of orthopaedic surgery and the largest inpatient rehabilitation hospital and provider of rehabilitation services in the state of Maryland, has been serving the Baltimore community for over 100 years.

2595 Vanguard School, The
Valley Forge Specialized Educational Services
1777 N Valley Rd
Paoli, PA 19301
610-296-6700
Fax: 610-640-0132
www.vanguardschool-pa.org

Tim Lanshe, Director of Education
James Kirkpatrick, CFO
Peg Osborne, Admissions Director

An Approved Private School (APS) for students aged 4-21 years with exceptionalities including autism spectrum disorder, mild emotional disturbances and/or neurological impairments.

2596 Worthmore Academy
3535 Kessler Boulevard East Dr
Indianapolis, IN 46220-5154
317-902-9896
877-700-6516
Fax: 317-251-6516
bjackson@worthmoreacademy.org
www.worthmoreacademy.org

Brenda Jackson, Director
Alyssa Blaire Cook, Assistant Director

A place where children with learning disabilities receive individualized instruction to help remediate his or her condition. The most common learning disabilities we work with are Dyslexic, A.D.D, A.D.H.D, Autism Spectrum (including Asperger's Syndrome), and communication disorders.

Exchange Programs

General

2597 A Guide to International Educational Exchange
Mobility International USA
132 E Broadway
Suite 343
Eugene, OR 97401　　　　541-343-1284
Fax: 541-343-6812
TTY: 541-343-1284
clearinghouse@miusa.org
www.miusa.org

Susan Sygall, Chief Executive Officer
Cindy Lewis, Director, Programs
A Guide to International Educational Exchange, Community Service and Travel for People with Disabilities includes information travel and international programs, as well as personal experience stories from people with disabilities who have had successful international experiences.
600 pages

2598 American Institute for Foreign Study
River Plaza 9 W Broad St
Stamford, CT 6902-3788　　　　203-399-5000
866-906-2437
Fax: 203-399-5590
info@aifs.com
www.aifs.com

William L Gertz, CEO
Organizes cultural exchange programs throughout the world for more than 50,000 students each year and arranges insurance coverage for our own participants as well as participants of other organizations. Also provides summer travel programs overseas and in the US ranging from one week to a full academic year.

2599 American Universities International Programs
307 S College Ave
Fort Collins, CO 80524-2801　　　970-495-0084
888-730-2847
Fax: 970-495-0114
info@auip.com
www.auip.com

Laurie Klith, Executive Director
Study abroad organization sending students to universities in Australia and New Zealand.

2600 American-Scandinavian Foundation
58 Park Ave
38 Street
New York, NY 10016-3007　　　212-779-3587
Fax: 212-686-1157
info@amscan.org
scandinaviahouse.org

Edward Gallagher, President
Promotes international understanding through educational and cultural exchange between the United States and Denmark, Finland, Iceland, Norway and Sweden.

2601 Antioch College
One Morgan Place
Yellow Springs, OH 45387-1635　　　937-319-6082
Fax: 937-319-6085

Mark Roosevelt, President
Thomas Brookley, CFO & COO
Gariot Louima, Chief Communications Officer
Education abroad offers numerous programs which can be included in undergraduate and graduate study programs.

2602 Army and Air Force Exchange Services
PO Box 660202
Dallas, TX 75266-202　　　214-312-2011
800-527-2345
Fax: 800-446-0163
TTY: 800-423-2011
www.aafes.com

James Moore, Senior VP
MG Bruce Casella, Commander/CEO

Brings a tradition of value, service, and support to its 11.5 million authorized customers at military installations in the United States, Europe and in the Pacific.

2603 Association for International Practical Training
10400 Little Patuxent Pkwy
Suite 250
Columbia, MD 21044-3519　　　410-997-2200
Fax: 410-992-3924
aipt@aipt.org
aipt.org

Elizabeth Chazottes, CEO
Nonprofit organization dedicated to encouraging and facilitating the exchange of qualified individuals between the US and other countries so they may gain practical work experience and improve international understanding.

2604 Basic Facts on Study Abroad
International Education
809 United Nations Plz
New York, NY 10017-3503　　　212-883-8200
Fax: 212-984-5452
publications@un.org
iie.org

Allen E Goodman, CEO
Peggy Blumenthal, Executive Vice President
Information book including foreign study planning, educational choices, finances and study abroad programs. *$35.00*
30 pages

2605 Beaver College
Arcadia University
450 S Easton Rd
Glenside, PA 19038-3215　　　215-572-2901
888-232-8379
Fax: 215-572-2174

Lorna Stern, Deputy Director
One of the largest college-based study abroad programs in the country. Prices from $8000.00 semester to $22000.00 a year.

2606 Buffalo State (SUNY)
1300 Elmwood Ave
South Wing 410
Buffalo, NY 14222-1095　　　716-878-4620
Fax: 716-878-3054
intleduc@buffalostate.edu

Lee Ann Grace, Asst Dean Int'l/Exchange Program
Provides international educational exchange opportunities for students of university age and older through its Office of International Education.

2607 Building Bridges: Including People with Disabilities in International Programs
Mobility International USA
132 E Broadway
Suite 343
Eugene, OR 97401　　　541-343-1284
Fax: 541-343-6812
TTY: 541-343-1284
clearinghouse@miusa.org
www.miusa.org

Susan Sygall, Chief Executive Officer
Cindy Lewis, Director, Programs
Empowers people with disabilities around the world through international exhange and international development to achieve their human rights. The international exchange programs usually last two-four weeks and are held throughout the year in the US and abroad. Activities include living with homestay families, leadership seminars, disability rights workshops, cross cultural learning and teambuilding activities such as river rafting and challenging courses.

2608 Davidson College, Office of Study Abroad
Davidson College
PO Box 7171
Davidson, NC 28035-7171　　　704-894-2000
Fax: 704-894-2005
kocampbell@davidson.edu
www3.davidson.edu

Carol Quillen, President

Recognizes the value of study abroad for both the devlopment of worl understanding and the development of the student as a broadminded, objective and mature individual.

2609   High School Students Guide to Study, Travel, and Adventure Abroad
300 Fore Street
Portland, ME 4101   207-553-4000
                                        Fax: 207-553-4299
                                          contact@ciee.org
                                             www.ciee.org

Robert E. Fallon, CEO & President
Kenton Keith, Senior Vice President for Progra
This guide provides high school students with all the information they need for a successful trip abroad. Included are sections to help students find out if they're ready for a trip abroad, make the necessary preparations and get the most from their experience. Over 200 programs are described including language study, summer camps, homestays, study tours and work camps. The program descriptions include information for people with disabilities.
ISSN 0312-11

2610   IPSL Institute of Global Learning
4110 SE Hawthorne Blvd.
Suite 200
Portland, OR 97214   503-395-4775
                                        Fax: 503-954-1881
                                            info@ipsl.org
                                               ipsl.org

Thomas Morgan, President
Arianne Newton, Director, Programs
IPSL is an educational organization servicing students, colleges, universities, service agencies and related organizations around the world by fostering programs that link volunteer service and academic study. IPSL is a registered Social Benefit Corporation that is committed to its mission and dedicated to promoting an ethic of service. They invest over 83% of our revenues directly back into the communities where they serve.

2611   International Christian Youth Exchange
134 W 26th St
New York, NY 10001-6803   212-206-7307
                                        Fax: 212-633-9085

Ed Gragert
Offers participants a unique experience to learn about another culture and make friends from different countries.

2612   International Student Exchange Programs (I SEP)
1655 N Fort Myer Drive
Suite 400
Arlington, VA 22209   703-504-9960
                                        Fax: 703-243-8070
                                            info@isep.org
                                             www.isep.org

Dr. Thomas Hochstettler, Chair
Dr. Tony Atwater, President
ISEP is a network of 275 post-secondary institutions in the United States and 38 other countries cooperating to provide affordable international educational experiences for a diverse student population.

2613   International University Partnerships
University of Pennsylvania
1011 South Dr
Indiana, PA 15705-1046   724-357-2100
                                        Fax: 724-357-6213
                                               iup.edu

David Werner, President
Offers a variety of international educational exchange programs to students who wish to study overseas.

2614   Lake Erie College
391 W. Washington St.
Painesville, OH 44077   440-296-1856
                                              800-533-4996
                                        Fax: 440-375-7005
                                          admissions@lec.edu
                                              www.lec.edu

Michael Victor, President
Michael Keresman III, Director

Sends students abroad for a term or longer to develop intellectual awareness and individual maturity.

2615   Lane Community College
4000 E 30th Ave
Eugene, OR 97405   541-463-3100
                                        Fax: 541-463-5201
                                          asklane@lanecc.edu
                                             www.lanecc.edu

Margaret Hamilton, Ph.D, President
Lane Community College offers a wide variety of instructional programs including transfer credit programs, career and technical degree and certificate programs, continuing education noncredit courses, ESL, GED programs, and customized training for local businesses. The college offers support services for those with disabilities through their Center for Accessible Resources.

2616   Lions Clubs International
300 W 22nd St
Oak Brook, IL 60523-8842   630-571-5466
                                        Fax: 630-571-8890
                                           www.lionsclubs.org

Joe Preston, International President
Jitsuhiro Yamada, First Vice President
Robert E. Corlew, Second Vice President
Over 46,000 individual clubs in over 194 countries and geographical areas which provide community service and promote better international relations. Clubs work with local communities to provide needed and useful programs for sight, diabetes and hearing, and aid in study abroad.

2617   Lisle
900 County Road 269
Leander, TX 78641-1633   512-259-4404

Barbara E Bratton, Owner
Educational organization which works toward world peace and better quality of human life through increased understanding between persons of similar and different cultures.

2618   National 4-H Council
7100 Connecticut Ave
Chevy Chase, MD 20815-4934   301-961-2800
                                        Fax: 301-961-2894
                                               www.4-h.org

Donald Floyd, President
Jennifer Sirangelo, Executive Vice President
4-H opened the door for young people to learn leadership skills and explore ways to give back. 4-H revolutionized how youth connected to practical, hands-on learning experiences while outside of the classroom.

2619   New Directions for People with Disabilities
5276 Hollister Ave.
Suite 207
Santa Barbara, CA 93111   805-967-2841
                                              888-967-2841
                                        Fax: 805-964-7344
                                       hello@newdirectionstravel.org
                                      www.newdirectionstravel.org

Dee Duncan, Executive Director
A nonprofit organization providing local, national, and international travel vacations and holiday programs for people with mild to moderate developmental disabilities.
1985

2620   People to People International
911 Main Street
Suite 2110
Kansas City, MO 64105-2246   816-531-4701
                                        Fax: 816-561-7502
                                            ptpi@ptpi.org
                                             www.ptpi.org

Mary Eisenhower, CEO
Roseanne Rosen, Senior Vice President of Operati
Brian Hueben, Senior Director, Administration
Exchanges international understanding and friendship through educational, cultural and humantarian activities involving the exchange of ideas and experiences directly among people of different countries and diverse cultures. Is also dedicated to enhancing

cross cultural communication within each communityand across communities and nations.

2621 Rotary Youth Exchange
Rotary International
1560 Sherman Ave
Evanston, IL 60201-4818   847-866-3000
                                 866-976-8279
                                 Fax: 847-328-4101
                                 youthexchange@rotary.org
                                 www.rotary.org

Kalyan Banerjee, International President
Noel A Bajat, Vice President
Kenneth R Boyd, Director
This worldwide organization of business and professional leaders provides humanitarian service, encourages high ethical standards in all vocations, and helps build goodwill and peace in the world. Approximately 1.2 million Rotarians belong to more than 31,000 Rotary clubs located in 167 countries for exchange opportunities.

2622 Scandinavian Exchange
24 Dickinson Street
Amherst, MA 1002   413-253-9737
                                Fax: 413-253-5282
                                howery@scandinavianseminar.org
                                www.scandinavianseminar.org

Jacqueline D Waldman, CEO
William Kaufmann, Chair
Student exchange program founded in 1949.

2623 Sister Cities International
915 15th Street, NW
4th Floor
Washington, DC 20005   202-347-8630
                                Fax: 202-393-6524
                                info@sister-cities.org
                                sister-cities.org

Patrick Madden, President
Jim Doumas, Executive Vice President, & Inte
A non profit citizen diplomacy network creating and strengthening partnerships between US and international communities in an effort to increase global cooperation at the municipal level, to promote cultural understanding and to stimulate economic development. Encourages local community development and volunteer action by motivating and empowering private citizens, municipal officials and business leaders to conduct long term programs of mutual benefits including exchange situations.

2624 State University of New York
1400 Washington Ave
Albany, NY 12222-100   518-442-3300
                                Fax: 518-442-5383
                                ugadmissions@albany.edu
                                www.albany.edu

George Philip, President
Alain Kaloyeros, Senior Vice President & CEO
Susan Phillips, Provost & VP for Academic Affai
Offers over 150 international educational exchange programs in 37 different countries. Broad mission of excellence in undergraduate and graduate education, research and public service engages 17,000 diverse students in nine schools and colleges across three campuses.

2625 University of Minnesota at Crookston
2900 University Ave
Crookston, MN 56716-5000   218-281-6510
                                800-862-6466
                                Fax: 218-281-8050
                                UMCinfo@umn.edu
                                www.crk.umn.edu

Charles Casey, CEO
Eric Kaler, President
The University of Minnesota, Crookston (UMC) is a public, baccalaureate, coeducational institution and a coordinate campus of the University of Minnesota

2626 University of Oregon
5000 N Willamette Blvd
Portland, OR 97203-5798   503-943-8000
                                Fax: 503-725-3067
                                webmaster@up.edu
                                up.edu

Patricia Esley, Manager
Rev.E.Willia Beauchamp, President
James Lyons, VP University Relations
Study/cultural experience is available in Tokyo and other Japanese cities as part of the Japan Studies Program at the University.

2627 Western Washington University
516 High St
Bellingham, WA 98225-5996   360-650-3000
                                Fax: 360-650-3022
                                www.wwu.edu

Bruce Shepard, President
Paul Dunn, Senior Executive Asst. to the Pr
Barbara Stoneberg, Assistant to the President

2628 World Experience Teenage Exchange Program
2440 S Hacienda Blvd
Suite 116
Hacienda Heights, CA 91745-4763   626-330-5719
                                   800-633-6653
                                   Fax: 626-333-4914

Kerry Gonzales, President
Marge Archaumbault, President
Offers a quality and affordable program for over two decades and continues to provide students and host families a youth exchange program based on individual attention, with the help of an international network of overseas directors and USA coordinators.

2629 World of Options
Mobility International USA
132 E Broadway
Suite 343
Eugene, OR 97401   541-343-1284
                                Fax: 541-343-6812
                                TTY: 541-343-1284
                                clearinghouse@miusa.org
                                www.miusa.org

Susan Sygall, Chief Executive Officer
Cindy Lewis, Director, Programs
Empowering people with disabilities around the world through international exchange and international development to achieve their human rights.
338 pages

2630 Youth for Understanding International Exchange
6400 Goldsboro Road
Suite 100
Bethesda, MD 20817-5841   240-235-2100
                                800-833-6243
                                Fax: 240-352-2104
                                admissions@yfu.org
                                yfu.org

Rachel Andreson, Founder
Samantha Brizzolara, Chair
Youth for Understanding (YFU) International Exchange, an educational, nonprofit organization, prepares young people for the opportunities and responsabilities in a changing, independent world. With YFU, students can choose a year, semenster, or summer program in one or more than 35 countries worldwide. More than 200,000 young people from more than 50 nations in Asia, Europe, North and South America, Africa and the Pacific have participated in YFU exchanges.

Foundations & Funding Resources

Alabama

2631 Alabama Power Foundation
PO Box 2641
Birmingham, AL 35203
205-257-2508
powerofgood.com

Myla Calhoun, President
Hallie Bradley, Manager, Community Initiatives
Brandon Glover, Manager, Strategic Initiatives
Honoring its mission to strengthen the communities the company serves, the foundation focuses its efforts on organizations that support education, civic activities, health services, the environment and the arts. By supporting the state's educational system from pre-K to universities, the foundation is investing in Alabama's future and the well-being of its residents.

2632 Andalusia Health Services
700 River Falls Street
PO Box 667
Andalusia, AL 36420
334-222-2030
Fax: 334-222-7844
chrissie@andalusiachamber.com
www.andalusiachamber.com

Janna McGlamory, President
Debbie Marcum, Vice President
Ashley Eiland, Executive Vice President
Only offers grants to the residents of Covington County in Alabama who are pursuing a degree in a medical field.

2633 Arc Of Alabama, The
557 S Lawrence St
Montgomery, AL 36104-4611
334-262-7688
866-243-9557
Fax: 334-834-9737
www.thearcofal.org/#!contact/c1d94

Larry Bailey, President
Sherron Culpepper, 1st Vice President
Bruce Koppenhoeffer, 2nd Vice President
The Arc of Alabama, Inc. is a volunteer-based membership organization made up of individuals with intellectual, developmental and other disabilities, their families, friends, interested citizens, and professionals in the disability field.

2634 Rapahope Children's Retreat Foundation
205 Lambert Ave.
Suite A
Mobile, AL 36604
251-476-9880
info@rapahope.org
www.rapahope.org

Melissa McNichol, Executive Director
Roz Dorsett, Assistant Director
Rapahope is an organization that offers a one week long summer camp for children who have, or who have had cancer. For children ages 7-17, the camp offers a wide range of summer camp activities, including but not limited to, swimming, kayaking, horseback riding, and arts. The camp is offered at no cost to campers or their families.

Alaska

2635 Arc of Alaska
The Arc of Anchorage
2211 Arca Dr
Anchorage, AK 99508-3462
907-277-6677
800-258-2232
Fax: 907-272-2161
TTY: 907-277-0735
info@thearcofanchorage.org

Rod Shipley, President
Dave Falsey, Vice President
Meredith Parham, Secretary
The Arc helps Alaskans who experience developmental disabilities, behavioral health concerns or deafness achieve lives of dignity and independence as valued members of our community.

2636 Rasmuson Foundation
301 West Northern Lights Blvd.
Suite 400
Anchorage, AK 99503
907-297-2700
877-366-2700
Fax: 907-297-2770
www.rasmuson.org

Edward B. Rasmuson, Chairman
Cathryn Rasmuson, Vice Chair
Diane Kaplan, President & CEO
The Rasmuson Foundation invests both in individuals and well managed organizations dedicated to improving the quality of life for Alaskans.

Arizona

2637 American Foundation Corporation
4518 North 32nd Street
Phoenix, AZ 85018
602-955-4770
Fax: 602-955-4700
www.americanfoundation.org

Ben L. Schaub, Founder and CEO
The American Foundation can be your sponsor, and help your company set up a corporate foundation in a public charity or support organization format.

2638 Arizona Autism Resources
The Arc of Arizona
PO Box 90714
Phoenix, AZ 85066
602-234-2721
800-433-5255
Fax: 602-234-5959
arc@arcarizona.org
www.arcarizona.org

Robert Snyder, President
Michael Leyva, Vice President
Jon Meyers, Executive Director
The Arc is committed to securing for all people with developmental disabilities the opportunity to choose and realize their goals in regard to where they live, learn, work and play.

2639 Arizona Community Foundation
2201 E Camelback Road
Suite 405B
Phoenix, AZ 85016
602-381-1400
800-222-8221
Fax: 602-381-1575
info@azfoundation.org
www.azfoundation.org

Ron Butler, Chair
Shelly Cohn, Vice Chair
Steven G. Seleznow, President & CEO
The mission of the Arizona Community Foundation is to empower and align philanthropic interests with community needs and build a legacy of living.

2640 Arizona Instructional Resource Center for Students who are Blind or Visually Impaired, The
Foundation For Blind Children
1235 E. Harmont Drive
Phoenix, AZ 85020
602-678-5800
800-322-4870
Fax: 602-678-5819
mashton@SeeItOurWay.org
www.seeitourway.org

Dee Nortman, CFO
Marc Ashton, Chief Executive Officer
Barbra Smith, Chief of Staff
The Foundation for Blind Children contracts with the Arizona Department of Education to provide statewide media services for students between pre-kindergarten and 12th grade who have a visual impairment or are blind andEneed their instructional materials in a specialized medium such as braille, large print, or electronic files as well as adaptive equipment.

2641 Civitan Foundation
12635 N. 42nd Street
Phoenix, AZ 85032 602-953-2944
www.civitanfoundationaz.com
Dawn Trapp, Executive Director
The foundation aims to enhance the quality of life for children
and adults with developmental disabilities through programs
such as camp, employment opportunities, adult learning, respite,
and summer programs for teens.
1968

2642 Margaret T Morris Foundation
PO Box 592
Prescott, AZ 86302-592 928-445-6633
Fax: 928-445-6633

Susan Rheem, Executive Director

Arkansas

2643 Arc of Arkansas
2004 Main St
Little Rock, AR 72206-1526 501-375-7770
Fax: 501-372-4621
www.arcark.org
Willie Jones, President
Steve Hitt, Chief Executive Officer
Roger Williams, Chief Financial Officer
Serving people with disabilites and their families for over fourty
years.

2644 Winthrop Rockefeller Foundation
225 East Markham Street
Suite 200
Little Rock, AR 72201 501-376-6854
Fax: 501-374-4797
webfeedback@wrfoundation.org
www.wrfoundation.org
Phillip N. Baldwin, Chair
David Rainey, Ed.D., Vice chair
Sherece Y. West-Scantlebury, Ph.D, President & CEO
Mission is to improve the quality of life in Arkansas. It focuses its
grantmaking efforts in three areas: education, economic development and civic affairs. Education projects funded in the past have
included grants to schools that are working to involve teachers
and parents in making decisions about what happens at their
schools, projects that work to remove prejudice from the educational process and more. Major grants are made to support the
development of new programs.

California

2645 AIDS Healthcare Foundation
6255 Sunset Blvd.
21st Floor
Los Angeles, CA 90028 323-860-5200
www.aidshealth.org
Michael Weinstein, President
Peter Reis, Senior Vice President
Scott Carruthers, Chief Pharmacy Officer
The Los Angeles-based AIDS Healthcare Foundation (AHF) is a
global nonprofit organization providing medicine and advocacy
to people all around the world. AHF is currently the largest provider of HIV/AIDS medical care in the U.S.

2646 Ahmanson Foundation
9215 Wilshire Blvd
Beverly Hills, CA 90210 310-278-0770
info@theahmansonfoundation.org
www.theahmansonfoundation.org
William H. Ahmanson, President
Karen Ahmanson Hoffman, Managing Director & Secretary
Kristen K. O'Connor, CFO & Treasurer
The Foundation primarily gives in Southern California with major emphasis in Los Angeles County. The Foundation focuses on
the arts and humanities, education, mental health and support for
a broad range of social welfare programs.

2647 Alice Tweed Touhy Foundation
205 E Carrillo Street
Suite 219
Santa Barbara, CA 93101-7186 805-962-6430

Jeanne Mc Kay, Manager
Rehabilitation, recreation and building funds are given to organizations only within the Santa Barbara area.

2648 Alternating Hemiplegia of Childhood Foundation
2000 Town Center
Suite 1900
Southfield, MI 48075 313-663-7772
Fax: 313-733-8987
sharon@ahckids.org
ahckids.org
Lynn Egan, President
Joshua Marszalek, Vice President
Gene M Andrasco, Treasurer
Non-profit organization dedicated to promoting professional and
public awareness of Alternating Hemiplegia of Childhood
(AHC) and providing current information to affected individuals
and their families. The foundation also supports ongoing medical
research into the cause, treatment and potential cure of AHC and
maintains a registry of families, affected chidren and physicians
who are familiar with AHC.

2649 Arc of California
1225 8th Street
Suite 350
Sacramento, CA 95815 916-552-6619
800-698-6619
Fax: 916-441-3494
www.thearcca.org
Tony Anderson, Executive Director
Richard Fitzmaurice, President
Betsy Katz, Secretary
Advocates for people with intellectual and all developmental disabilities since 1953. The ARC of California is committed to securing for all people with developmental disabilities, in
partnership with thier families, legal guardians or conservators
the opportunity to choose and realize their goals of where and
how they learn, live, work and play.

2650 Atkinson Foundation
1660 Bush Street
Suite 300
San Mateo, CA 94109 415-561-6540
Fax: 650-357-1101
sangeles@pfs-llc.net
www.atkinsonfdn.org
Elizabeth Curtis, Administrator
Stacey Angels, Grants Manager
The Foundation focuses and awards grants to community service
and civic organizations serving the residents of San Mateo
County, California through programs that benefit children,
youth, seniors, the disadvantaged and those in need of rehabilitation. Grants are also made to local churches and schools, and
overseas for sustainable development, health education and family planning. No grants to individuals or for research, travel, special events, annual campaigns, media and publications.

2651 Baker Commodities Corporate Giving Program
4020 Bandini Blvd
Vernon, CA 90058 323-268-2801
Fax: 323-268-5166
info@bakercommodities.com
Jim Andreoli, President
Baker Commodities has been one of the nation's leading providers of rendering, and grease removal services. Baker Commodities, Inc. is a completely sustainable company, recycling animal
by-products and kitchen waste into valuable products that can be
used to feed livestock, power vehicles, and act as a base for
everyday items.

2652 Bank of America Foundation
315 Montgomery St
Fl 8
San Francisco, CA 94104-1803   415-622-8248
888-488-9802
Fax: 704-386-6444
www.bankamerica.com/foundation
Ilana Orin, Manager
The Foundation will consider grants in four categories including: Health & Human Services, which provides support to health & human service organizations primarily through grants to the United Way campaigns; Education, with the focus on preparing people to become productive employees and participating citizens; Conservation & Environment, the improvement of California communities for the benefit of their citizens; and Culture & The Arts, supporting the leading performing and visual arts groups.

2653 Blind Babies Foundation
1814 Franklin Street
Suite 300
Oakland, CA 94612   510-446-2229
Fax: 510-446-2262
www.blindbabies.org
Dottie Bridge, President
Sharon Sacks, PhD, 1st Vice President
Clare Friedman, PhD, 2nd Vice President
Founded in 1949, the foundation provides home-based early intervention services to families with young children with vision impairment in the Northern and Central regions of California.

2654 Bothin Foundation
1660 Bush Street
Suite 300
San Francisco, CA 94109   415-561-6540
Fax: 415-561-6477
ccasey@pfs-llc.net
Lyman H. Casey, President
A. Michael Casey, Vice President & Treasurer
Devon Laycox, Vice President
The Bothin Foundation makes grants for capital, building, and equipment needs to organizations providing direct services to low-income, at risk children, youth and families, the elderly, and the disabled in San Francisco, Marin, Sonoma, and San Mateo counties.

2655 Briggs Foundation
1969 Lancewood Ln
Carlsbad, CA 92009-6826   760-704-6481
Fax: 760-704-6483
Blaine A Briggs, President
Private non-operating foundation.

2656 Burns-Dunphy Foundation
5 3rd Street
Suite 528
San Francisco, CA 94103-3213   415-421-6995
Fax: 415-882-7774
Walter Gleason
Cressey Nakagawa
Grants are given to promote wellness for the visually impaired, physically and mentally disabled and to promote research in these areas.

2657 California Community Foundation
221 S. Figueroa Street
Suite 400
Los Angeles, CA 90012   213-413-4130
Fax: 213-383-2046
info@ccf-la.org
www.calfund.org
Cynthia A. Telles, Chairman
Antonia Hernandez, President & CEO
John E. Kobara, EVP & COO
Areas of funding priority include grants for the disabled, child welfare, rehabilitation, developmentally disabled, employment projects, research and computer projects. Giving is limited to the greater Los Angeles area.

2658 California Endowment
1000 N Alameda St
Los Angeles, CA 90012   213-628-1001
800-449-4149
Fax: 213-703-4193
questions@calendow.org
Zac Guevara, Vice Chair
Robert Ross, President & CEO
Martha Jimenez, EVP/ Counsel
California Endowment's mission is to expand access to affordable, quality health care for underserved individuals and communities, and to promote fundamental improvements in the health status of all Californians.

2659 Carrie Estelle Doheny Foundation
707 Wilshire Boulevard
Suite 4960
Los Angeles, CA 90017   213-488-1122
Fax: 213-488-1544
doheny@dohenyfoundation.org
www.dohenyfoundation.org
Robert A. Smith,III, President
Nina Shepherd, CAO/ CFO
Pam Thomas, Grants Administrator
The Foundation primarily funds local, not-for-profit organizations endeavoring to advance education, medicine and religion, to improve the health and welfare of the sick, aged, incapacitated, and to aid the needy.

2660 Coeta and Donald Barker Foundation
3740 Cahuenga Blvd
Studio City, CA 91604   760-340-1162
818-980-3630
Fax: 818-980-2709
info@scga.org
www.scga.org
Nancy Harris, President
Kevin Heaney, Executive Director
Andrea Fredlin, Admin Asst., Club Services
It is an independent organization that gives its attention to organizations that are charitable or nonprofit under the laws of the state of Oregon or California.

2661 Conrad N Hilton Foundation
30440 Agoura Road
Agoura Hills, CA 91301   818-851-3700
Fax: 310-694-9051
cnhf@hiltonfoundation.org
hiltonfoundation.org
Steven M. Hilton, Chairman, President & CEO
Barron Hilton, Chairman Emeritus
Donald H Hubbs, Director Emeritus
Our grant-making style is to initiate and develop major long-term projects and then seek out the organizations to implement them. As a consequence of this proactive approach, the Foundation does not generally consider unsolicited proposals. Our major projects currently include: blindness prevention and treatment, support the work of the Catholic Sisters, drug abuse prevention among youth, support of the Conrad N. Hilton College of Hotel and Restaurant Management, and much more.

2662 Crescent Porter Hale Foundation
1660 Bush Street
Suite 300
San Francisco, CA 94109   415-561-6540
Fax: 415-561-5477
evalentine@pfs-llc.net
www.crescentporterhale.org
E. William Swanson, President
Sr. Estela Morales, MSW, Vice President
Eunice Valentine, Executive Director
Serves organizations in the San Francisco Bay Area who are involved in the following areas of concern: education in the fields of art and music; private elementary, high school and university education; capital funding; and other worthwhile programs which can be demonstrated as serving broad community purposes, leading toward the improvement of the quality of life.

2663 David and Lucile Packard Foundation
343 Second Street
Los Altos, CA 94022   650-917-7142
                                            Fax: 650-948-5793
                                    communications@packard.org
                                              www.packard.org

Susan Packard Orr, Chairman
Julie E. Packard, Vice Chairman
Nancy Packard Burnett, Vice Chairman
This foundation provides grants to nonprofit organizations in the
following areas: conservation; population; science; children,
familes, and communities; arts and organizational effectiveness;
and philanthropy. It provides national and international grants
and also has a special focus on the Northern California Counties.

2664 Deutsch Foundation
5454 Beethoven St
Los Angeles, CA 90066   310-862-3000
                                                 877-340-7700
                                            Fax: 310-862-3100
                                              deutschinc.com

Linda Sawyer, Chairman
Kim Getty, President, North America
Val Difebo, CEO, Deutsch NY
Learning disabled, visually impaired, mental health, eye re-
search, child welfare, speech and hearing impaired, physically
disabled and independence projects are funded through this
Foundation. Giving is limited to California.

2665 Dream Street Foundation
324 S. Beverly Dr.
Suite 500
Beverly Hills, CA 90212   424-333-1371
                                            Fax: 310-388-0302
                                 www.dreamstreetfoundation.org

Patty Grubman, Founder
Provides nationwide camping programs for children and young
adults with cancer, chronic and life threatening illnesses.

2666 East Bay Community Foundation
De Domenico Building
200 Frank H Ogawa Plaza
Oakland, CA 94612   510-836-3223
                                            Fax: 510-836-7418
                                          jwhead@eastbaycf.org
                                                 www.ebcf.org

Sherry M. Hirota, Chair
Ingrid Lamirault, Vice Chair
Peter Garcia, Vice Chair
A collection of funds created by many people, organizations and
businesses, the Foundation helps those people and groups to support effective nonprofit organizations to the East Bay and
beyond.

2667 Evelyn and Walter Hans Jr
114 Sansome Street
Suite 600
San Francisco, CA 94104   415-856-1400
                                            Fax: 415-856-1500
                                                www.haasjr.org

Walter J. Haas, Chair
Ira S. Hirschfield, President & Trustee
Michael Blake, VP of Finance
A private foundation interested in programs which assist people
who are hungry, homeless, or at risk of homelessness; enable
older adults to maintain independent lives in the community and
support Hispanic community development in San Francisco's
Mission District. The Foundation also encourages proposals for
corporate social responsibility efforts within the business
community.

2668 Family Caregiver Alliance
785 Market St.
Suite 750
San Francisco, CA 94103   415-434-3388
                                                 800-445-8106
                                            Fax: 415-434-3508
                                             info@caregiver.org
                                              www.caregiver.org

Ping Hao, MBA, President
Jacquelyn Kung, Vice President
Kathleen Kelly,MPA, Executive Director
To improve the quality of life for caregivers and those they care
for through information, services, and advocacy.

2669 Financial Aid for the Disabled and Their Families
Reference Service Press
2310 Homestead Rd.
Suite C1 #219
Los Altos, CA 94024   650-861-3170
                                            Fax: 650-861-3171
                                          info@rspfunding.com
                                            www.rspfunding.com

Gail Schlachter, President
R David Weber, Editor-in-Chief
Mike Fields, Database and Website Manager
This directory, which Children's Bookwatch calls invaluable de-
scribes more than 1,100 financial aid opportunities available to
support persons with disabilities and members of their families.
Updated ever 2 years. $39.50
300 pages
ISBN 1-588410-31-5

2670 Firemans Fund Foundation
Firemans Fund Insurance Companies
777 San Marin Dr
Novato, CA 94998   415-899-2000
                                                 800-227-1700
                                            Fax: 415-899-3600

Lori Dickerson Fouche, President & CEO
Jill Paterson, Chief Financial Officer
Eleanor Barnard, Chief Distribution & Sales
Provides discretionary grants to the disabled only in Marin and
Sonoma counties in the San Francisco Bay area.

2671 Fred Gellert Foundation
1038 Redwood Highway
Building B, Suite 2
Mill Valley, CA 94941   415-381-7575
                                            Fax: 415-381-8526
                          foundationcenter.org/grantmaker/fredgellert/
Fred Gellert, Founder
Patty Oday, Administrator
Focuses on organizations and programs serving residents of San
Mateo and San Francisco and Marin counties in California, with
the exception of environmentally concerned organizations.

2672 Gallo Foundation
P.O. Box 1130
Modesto, CA 95353-1130   209-579-3204
                                                 877-687-9463
                                            Fax: 209-341-3307
                                               www.ejgallo.com

John Gallo, Senior VP Operations
Physically and mentally disabled, child welfare, Special Olympics, United Cerebral Palsy and Easter Seal Society are among the
grants provided by this foundation.

2673 Glaucoma Research Foundation
251 Post Street
Suite 600
San Francisco, CA 94108   415-986-3162
                                                 800-826-6693
                                            Fax: 415-986-3763
                                         question@glaucoma.org
                                              www.glaucoma.org

Andrew Iwach, MD, Board Chair
Robert L. Stamper, MD, Vice Chair
Thomas M. Brunner, President/CEO
A national organization dedicated to protecting the sight of peo-
ple with glaucoma through research and education. The Founda-
tion conducts and supports research that contributes to improved

patient care and a better understanding of the disease process. Provides education, advocacy and emotional support to patients and their families.

2674 Harden Foundation
1636 Ercia Street
Salinas, CA 93906 831-442-3005
Fax: 831-443-1429
joe@hardenfoundation.org
www.hardenfoundation.org
Patricia Tynan Chapman, President
C. Bill Elliott, Vice President/Treasurer
Joseph C. Grainger, Executive Director
Founded to assist charitable organizations in the Salinas Valley.

2675 Henry J Kaiser Family Foundation
2400 Sand Hill Rd
Menlo Park, CA 94025-6941 650-854-9400
Fax: 650-854-4800
www.kff.org
Drew Altman, President/CEO
Gary Claxton, Vice President
Esther Dicks, Vice President
A non-profit, private operating foundation focusing on the major health care issues facing the US, with a growing role in global health. Kaiser develops and runs its own research and communications programs, sometimes in partnership with other non-profit research organizations or major media companies.

2676 Henry W Bull Foundation
Santa Barbara Bank & Trust
P.O. Box 2340
Santa Barbara, CA 93120 202-720-7871
Fax: 805-884-1404
info@coreprojects.com
www.activistfacts.com/about/
Janice Gibbons, VP/Senior Trust Officer
Grant given to a wide range of organizations that include those which provide services for the disabled; arts, education, services for elderly and youth grants awarded two times a year. Grant size ranges from $500 to $5,000. Proposal deadlines April 1, Sept 1.

2677 Irvine Health Foundation
18301 Von Karman Avenue
Suite 440
Irvine, CA 92612-0120 949-253-2959
Fax: 949-253-2962
info@ihf.org
www.ihf.org
Timothy L. Strader, Sr., Chairman
Carol Mentor McDermott, Vice Chairman
Edward B. Kacic, President
Mission is to improve the physical, mental and emotional well-being of all Orange County residents.

2678 Joseph Drown Foundation
1999 Avenue of the Stars
Suite 2330
Los Angeles, CA 90067 310-277-4488
Fax: 310-277-4573
staff@jdrown.org
www.jdrown.org
Norman C Obrow, President
Giving is focused primarily in California. No support for religious purposes or to individuals. Goal is to assist individuals in becoming successful, self-sustaining, contributing citizens.

2679 Kenneth T and Eileen L Norris Foundation
11 Golden Shore
Suite 450
Long Beach, CA 90802 562-435-8444
Fax: 562-436-0584
grants@ktn.org
www.norrisfoundation.org
Lisa D Hanson, Chairman
Ronald R Barnes, Executive Director & Trustee
Walter J Zanino, Controller
The Foundation is primarily focused on medicine and education. To a lesser extent the foundation contributes to community programs including visually impaired, autism, mentally and physically disabled, deaf and mental health in the Southern California

area. Average grant size in this area is $5,000-$10,000. Grants are also given in the area of culture and youth.

2680 Koret Foundation
33 New Montgomery Street
Suite 1090
San Francisco, CA 94105-4526 415-882-7740
Fax: 415-882-7775
info@koretfoundation.org
www.koretfoundation.org
Susan Koret, Board Chair
Anita L. Friedman, President
Michael J. Boskin, President
Koret seeks to fund outstanding examples of innovative approaches to community challenges and opportunities.

2681 LA84 Foundation
2141 W Adams Blvd
Los Angeles, CA 90018 323-730-4600
Fax: 323-730-9637
info@la84.org
www.la84.org
Frank M. Sanchez, Chair
Anita L. DeFrantz, President
F. Patrick Escobar, VP, Grants & Programs
The LA84 Foundation was established to manage Southern California's share of the surplus from the highly successful 1984 Olympic Games in Los Angeles and offers sports programs, a premier sports library and meeting facilities. The foundation currently serves two million youth in eight Southern California counties.

2682 LJ Skaggs and Mary C Skaggs Foundation
1221 Broadway
21st Floor
Oakland, CA 94612-1837 510-451-3300
Fax: 510-451-1527
skaggs@fablaw.com
Philip M Jelley, President
Jayne C Davis, Vice President
Robert N Janopaul, Director
The Foundation presently makes grants under four program categories: performing arts, social concerns, projects of historic interest and special projects.

2683 Legler Benbough Foundation
2550 Fifth Avenue
Suite 132
San Diego, CA 92103 619-235-8099
Fax: 619-235-8077
peter@benboughfoundation.org
Peter K. Elsworth, President
John G. Rebelo, Jr., Treasurer
Nbob Kelly, Director
The mission of the foundation is to improve the quality of life of the people of San Diego. The foundation focuses on three target areas for funding, one in the area of providing economic opportunity, one in the area of enhancing cultural opportunity, and one that provides focus for health, education and welfare funding.

2684 Levi Strauss Foundation
1155 Battery St
San Francisco, CA 94111-1264 415-501-7208
800-872-5384
Fax: 415-544-3490
www.levistrauss.com/levi-strauss-foundation
Chip Bergh, President & CEO
Roy Bagattini, EVP/President
Lisa Collier, EVP/President
Has a funding initiative to support organizations which provide services for people with AIDS, and/or educational programs which help prevent the further spread of the HIV virus. The Foundation will assist in the development and enhancement of such services only in those communities where Levi Strauss & Co. has plants and distribution centers.

2685   Louis R Lurie Foundation
555 California Street
Suite 5100
San Francisco, CA 94104-1707   415-392-2470
Fax: 415-421-8669
www.foundationcenter.org/grantmaker/lurie
Nancy Terry, Foundation Administrator
Visually impaired, hard-of-hearing and physically disabled in the
San Francisco Bay Area and Metropolitan Chicago areas only.

2686   Luke B Hancock Foundation
360 Bryant St
Palo Alto, CA 94301-1409   650-321-5536
Fax: 650-321-0697
Ruth Ramel, Director
Has concentrated its resources over the past year on programs
which provide job training and employment for at-risk youth.
Consortium funding with other foundations in areas where there
is unmet need; emergency and transitional funding; and selected
funding for music education.

2687   Marin Community Foundation
5 Hamilton Landing
Suite 200
Novato, CA 94949   415-464-2500
Fax: 415-464-2555
info@marincf.org
www.marincf.org
Cleveland Justis, Chair
Thomas Peters, Ph.D., President & CEO
Sid Hartman, CFO/COO
Mission is to encourage and apply philanthropic contributions to
help improve the human condition, embrace diversity, promote a
humane and democratic society, and enhance the communities
quality of life, now and for future generations.

2688   Mary A Crocker Trust
57 Post Street
Suite 610
San Francisco, CA 94104-5023   650-576-3384
Fax: 415-982-0141
staff@mactrust.org
www.mactrust.org
Established in 1889, the Foundation is interested in Bay Area programs such as environment, education and community relations.

2689   MedicAlert Foundation International
5226 Pirrone Crt
Salida, CA 95368   800-432-5378
customer_service@medicalert.org
www.medicalert.org
Barton G. Tretheway, CAE, Chairt
David Leslie, President & CEO
Melody Howard, Vice President Of Call Center Operations
A trusted emergency support network dedicated to educating
emergency responders and medical personnel for facing everyday emergency situations, as well as providing emergency care
services for members.

**2690   National Center on Caregiving at Family Caregiver
Alliance (FCA)**
785 Market Street
Suite 750
San Francisco, CA 94103   415-434-3388
800-445-8106
Fax: 415-434-3508
info@caregiver.org
www.caregiver.org
Ping Hao, MBA, President
Jacquelyn Kung, Vice President
Kathleen Kelly, MPA, Executive Director
FCA offers programs at national, state and local levels to support
and sustain caregivers. The National Center on Caregiving
(NCC) program works to advance the development of high-quality, cost-effective policies and programs for caregivers in every
state of the country. Uniting research, public policy and services,
the NCC serves as a central source of information on caregiving
and long term care issues for policy makers, service providers,
media, funders and family caregivers.

2691   National Foundation of Wheelchair Tennis
940 Calle Amanecer
Suite B
San Clemente, CA 92673-6218   714-361-3663
Fax: 714-361-6603
www.nfwt.org
Bill Butler
Founded in January of 1980, the intention of this foundation is to
assist the newly physically disabled individual to realize his full
potential in society by enhancing his esteem, independence productivity and physical capabilities regardless of age, sex, creed or
disability extent.

2692   Parker Foundation
2604-B El Camino Real
Suite 244
Carlsbad, CA 92008   760-720-0630
Fax: 760-720-1239
mail@theparkerfoundation.org
www.theparkerfoundation.org
Judy McDonald, President
Gordon Swanson, Vice President
Ann Davies, Secretary
The assets are directed to projects which will contribute to the
betterment of any aspect of the people of San Diego County, Cali-
fornia and solely to entities which, among other things, are orga-
nized exclusively for charitable purposes and are operating in
San Diego County, California.

2693   Pasadena Foundation
301 East Colorado Boulevard
Suite 810
Pasadena, CA 91101-2824   626-796-2097
Fax: 626-583-4738
pcfstaff@pasadenacf.org
www.pasadenacf.org
David M. Davis, Chair
Judy Gain, Vice Chair
Jennifer Fleming DeVoll, Executive Director
The mission of the Pasadena Foundation is to improve the quality
of life for citizens of the Pasadena area through support of non-
profit organizations that provide services beneficial to the
community.

2694   RC Baker Foundation
P.O. Box 6150
Orange, CA 92863-6150   714-750-8987

F L Scott, Manager
Established in 1952, for general philanthropic purposes. The
bulk of assistance and support has been to religious, scientific,
educational institutions and youth organizations.

2695   Ralph M Parsons Foundation
888 West Sixth Street
Suite 700
Los Angeles, CA 90017   213-362-7600
Fax: 213-482-8878
www.rmpf.org
James A. Thomas, Chairman
Elizabeth Lowe, Vice Chairman
Wendy Garen, President & CEO
The Foundation is concerned with the encouragement and sup-
port of projects and programs deemed beneficial to mankind in
several major areas of interest such as: education; social impact;
civic and cultural; health and special products. Only funds in Los
Angeles County.

2696   Robert Ellis Simon Foundation
312 S Canyon View Drive
Los Angeles, CA 90049-3812   310-275-7335

Joan Willens
Mental health and visually impaired grants are the main concerns
of this organization.

2697 San Francisco Foundation
One Embarcadero Cente
Suite 1400
San Francisco, CA 94111   415-733-8500
Fax: 415-477-2783
info@sff.org
www.sff.org
Sandra R Hernandez, CEO
Nick Hodges, VP for Philanthropic Services
Bobbie Chapman, Director of Business Development
The Foundation's purpose is to improve life, promote greater equality of opportunity and assist those in need or at risk in the San Francisco Bay Area. The Foundation strives to protect and enhance the unique resources of the Bay Area, committed to equality of opportunity for all and the elimination of any injustice, seeks to enhance human dignity and seeks to establish mutual trust, respect and communication among the Foundation.

2698 Santa Barbara Foundation
1111 Chapala Street
Suite 200
Santa Barbara, CA 93101   805-963-1873
Fax: 805-966-2345
info@sbfoundation.org
www.sbfoundation.org
Eileen Sheridan, Chair
James Morouse, Vice Chair
Ronald Gallo, President & CEO
The Foundations mission is to enrich the lives of the people of Santa Barbara County through philanthropy. The Foundation awards grants to nonprofits within the County in the areas of education, health, human services, personal development, cluture, recreation, community enhancement and environment. No support is given to individuals except through student aid.

2699 Seany Foundation
3530 Camino del Rio N
Suite 101
San Diego, CA 92108   858-551-0922
www.theseanyfoundation.org
Paula Lutzky, Chief Financial Officer
Emily Brody, Director, Marketing & Media
Tiana LaCerva, Director, Special Events
Funds programs dedicated to bringing joy to children with cancer and their families.

2700 Sidney Stern Memorial Trust
860 Via de la Paz
PO Box 457
Pacific Palisades, CA 90272   310-459-2117
info@sidneysternmemorialtrust.org
www.sidneysternmemorialtrust.org
Betty Hoffenberg, Director
A Southern California-based foundation providing grants to non-profit organizations for various projects. The foundation gives priority to the following areas of interest: education, health and science, community service projects, youth, services to the mentally and emotionally disabled, the arts, organizations and activities serving California. The Board prefers to make contributions to organizations that use the funds directly in the furtherance of their charitable and public purposes.

2701 Sierra Health Foundation
1321 Garden Hwy
Sacramento, CA 95833   916-922-4755
Fax: 916-922-4024
info@sierrahealth.org
www.sierrahealth.org
Jose Hermocillo, Chair
David W. Gordon, Vice Chair
Chet P. Hewitt, President & CEO
The Foundation strives to establish a collaborative relationship with its grantees, and with other funders and foundations, through an open dialogue. The Foundation approaches each grant as a partnership, with opportunities for the grantee and grantor to work cooperatively to enhance the effectiveness of the grant project.

2702 Silicon Valley Community Foundation
2400 West El Camino Real
Suite 300
Mountain View, CA 94040-1498   650-450-5400
Fax: 650-450-5401
info@siliconvalleycf.org
www.siliconvalleycf.org
C.S. Parker, Chair
Samuel Johnson,Jr., Vice Chair
Emmitt D. Carson, Ph.D, President & CEO
Serving all of San Mateo & Santa Clara counties, Silicon Valley Foundation has more than $1.5B in assets under management and 1500 philanthropic funds. The community provides grants through donor advised and corporate funds in addition to its own Community Endowment Fund. In addition, the community foundation serves as a regional center for philanthropy, providing donors simple and effective ways to give locally & globally.

2703 Sonora Area Foundation
362 S Stewart Street
Sonora, CA 95370   209-533-2596
Fax: 209-533-2412
www.sonora-area.org
Jim Johnson, President SAF
Roger Francis, Vice President
Edward B. Wyllie, Executive Director
The Sonora Area Foundation strengthens its community through assisting donors, making grants, and providing leadership.

2704 Stella B Gross Charitable Trust C/O Bank of The West Trust Department
PO Box 1121
San Jose, CA 95108-1121   408-947-5203
Gabe Padilla, Trust Admin
Organization must be federal and state tax-exempt and reside within the bounds of Santa Clara County, California to be eligible.

2705 Teichert Foundation
3500 American River Dr
Sacramento, CA 95864   916-484-3011
Fax: 916-484-6506
www.teichert.com
Frederick Teichert, LHD, Executive Director
Awards grants to community organizations and provides employee matching grants. Teichert Foundation expresses the companie's commitment to build and preserve a healthy and prosperous region.

2706 WM Keck Foundation
550 South Hope Street
Suite 2500
Los Angeles, CA 90071- 2617   213-680-3833
Fax: 213-614-0934
info@wmkeck.org
www.wmkeck.org
Allison Keller, Executive Director & CFO
Maria Pellegrini, Ph.D, Executive Director of Programs
Thomas Everhart, Ph.D, Senior Scientific Advisor
Created to support accredited colleges and universities with particular emphasis on the sciences, engineering and medical research. The Foundation also maintains a Southern California Grant Program that provides support for non-profit organizations in the field of civic and community services, health care, precollegiate education and the arts.

2707 Wayfinder Family Services
5300 Angeles Vista Blvd.
Los Angeles, CA 90043   323-295-4555
800-352-2290
Fax: 323-296-0424
www.wayfinderfamily.org
Miki Jordan, Chief Executive Officer
Jay Allen, President & Chief Operating Officer
Fernando Almodovar, Chief Financial Officer
Formerly Junior Blind of America, Wayfinder provides programs and services for children and adults who are blind or visually impaired and their families to achieve independence and self-esteem. Programs include; Camp Bloomfield, Visions: Adventures in Learning, Infant-Family Program, Early Childhood Program,

255

Special Education School, Children's Residential Program, Davidson Program for Independence, and Student Transition and Enrichment Program, Vision Screening and After School enrichment.

2708 **Whittier Trust**
Whittier Trust Company
1600 Huntington Dr
South Pasadena, CA 91030
626-441-5111
Fax: 626-441-0420
hrdept@whittiertrust.com
www.whittiertrust.com

Michael J Casey, Chairman
David A Dahl, President & CEO
Brian H Flynn, Senior Vice President, Business Development
Whittier Trust offers financial services and expertise in the area of family wealth management. Some of their other areas of consultation include philanthropic advising, investment management, legal services and real estate.

2709 **Willam G Gilmore Foundation**
1660 Bush Street
Suite 300
San Francisco, CA 94109
415-561-0650
Fax: 415-561-5477

William N Hancock, Owner

Colorado

2710 **AV Hunter Trust**
650 South Cherry Street
Suite 535
Glendale, CO 80246- 1897
303-399-5450
Fax: 303-399-5499
afreeman@pfs-llc.net
www.avhuntertrust.org

Mary K. Anstine, President
George C. Gibson, Vice President
Barbara L. Howie, Executive Director
Donated nearly $50 million to nonprofit organizations serving those who captured Mr. Hunter's attention and sparked his compassion. Trust gives aid, comfort, support, or assistance to children or aged people or indigent adults.

2711 **Adolph Coors Foundation**
215 St. Paul Street
Suite 300
Denver, CO 80206
303-388-1636
Fax: 303-388-1684
www.coorsfoundation.org

John W. Jackson, Executive Director
Jeanne L. Bistranin, Senior Program Officer
Carrie C. Tynan, Program Officer
Applicant organizations must be classified as 501 and must operate within the United States. The areas covered by the Foundation are health, education, youth, community services, civic and cultural and public affairs.

2712 **Arc of Colorado**
1580 Logan Street
Suite 730
Denver, CO 80203
303-864-9334
800-333-7690
Fax: 303-864-9330
mrymer@thearcofco.org
www.thearcofco.org

Randy Patrick, President
Tonna Kelly, Vice President
Marijo Rymer, Executive Director
A private not-for-profit, membership-based, grassroots association. The Arc of Colorado is the state office whith local units located in various areas throughout the state.

2713 **Bonfils-Stanton Foundation**
Daniels and Fisher Tower
1601 Arapahoe St.
Suite 500
Denver, CO 80202
303-825-3774
Fax: 303-825-0802
webinfo@bonfils-stanton.org
bonfils-stantonfoundation.org

Gary P. Steuer, President/CEO
Gina A. Ferrari, Director, Grants Program
Ann M. Hovland, CFO/Treasurer
Grants limited to Colorado 501 (c)(3) organizations and are evaluatied based on alignment with these Foundation objectives: 1) The Bonfils-Stanton Foundation supports cultural organizations that consistently demonstrate artistic excellence, visionary leadership, and adaptive capacity; and 2) They idenitfy and nurture grassroots innovative organizations and initiative that enhance the values, spirit, and diversity of Denver's cultural community.

2714 **Comprecare Foundation**
PO Box 740610
Arvada, CO 80006
303-432-2808
Fax: 303-432-2808
www.comprecarefoundation.org

Milton W. Bollman, Chairman of the Board
Dr. Ellen Mangione, MD, MPH, Vice Chairman
James R. Gilsdorf, Executive Director
The purpose of the Comprecare Foundation is to encourage, aid or assist specific health related programs and to make grants to support the activities of organizations which are designed to advance and promote health care education, the delivery of health care services, and the improvement of community health and welfare.

2715 **Denver Foundation**
55 Madison Street
8th Floor
Denver, CO 80206
303-300-1790
Fax: 303-300-6547
information@denverfoundation.org
www.denverfoundation.org

Sandra Shreve, Chair
Ginny Bayless, Vice Chair and Chair-Elect
David M Miller, President & CEO
Neighbors helping neighbors, that's what the foundation is for. As Denver's only community foundation we've been accepting charitable donations since 1925. Those funds have been given back to the community in ongoing grants to nonprofit organizations - organizations that touch nearly every meaningful artistic, cultural, civic, health and human services interest of metro Denver's citizens.

2716 **El Pomar Foundation**
10 Lake Circle
Colorado Springs, CO 80906
719-633-7733
800-554-7711
Fax: 719-577-5702
grants@elpomar.org
www.elpomar.org

William J. Hybl, Chairman/CEO
William Ward, Vice Chair
R. Thayer Tutt, Jr., President/CIO
Mission of El Pomar is to enhance, encourage and promote the current and future well being of the people of Colorado through grantmaking and community stewardship.

2717 **Helen K and Arthur E Johnson Foundation**
1700 Broadway
Suite 1100
Denver, CO 80290-1718
303-861-4127
800-232-9931
Fax: 303-861-0607
www.johnsonfoundation.org

Ms. Lynn H. Campion, Chairman
Ms. Berit K. Campion, Vice Chair
John H Alexander Jr, President
A nonprofit, grantmaking private foundation incorporated under the laws of the State of Colorado in 1948. The Foundation is a general purpose foundation whose grant program consists of a wide variety of creative efforts to solve problems and to enrich

the quality of life. The areas of interest are: education, youth, health, community services, civic and culture and senior citizens. Grants limited to the state of Colorado.

2718   Listen Foundation
6950 E Belleview Ave.
Suite 203
Greenwood Village, CO 80111   303-781-9440
info@listenfoundation.org
www.listenfoundation.org

Allison Biever, President
David Kelsall, MD, Medical Director
The Listen Foundation provides access to Listening and Spoken Language Therapy (LSL) for children are deaf and hard of hearing.

Connecticut

2719   Aetna Foundation
151 Farmington Ave
Hartford, CT 06156   860-273-0123
800-872-3862
www.aetnahealthinsurance.com

Mark T Bertolini, Chairman/CEO
Karen S. Rohan, President
William J. Casazza, EVP & General Counsel
The Aetna Foundation is the independent charitable and philanthropic arm of Aetna Inc. The Foundation helps build healthy communities by promoting volunteerism, forming partnerships and funding initiatives that improve the quality of life where our employees and customers live and work.

2720   Arc of Connecticut
43 Woodland Street
Suite 260
Hartford, CT 6105-2300   860-246-6400
Fax: 860-246-6406
arcct@aol.com
www.arcct.com

Leslie Simoes, Interim Executive Director
The Arc of Connecticut is an advocacy organization committed to protecting the rights of people with intellectual, cognitive, and developmental disabilities and to promoting opportunities for their full inclusion in the life of thier communities.

2721   Community Foundation of Southeastern Connecticut
68 FederalStreet
PO Box 769
New London, CT 06320   860-442-3572
877-442-3572
Fax: 860-442-0584
maryam@cfect.org
www.cfect.org

Susan Pochal, Chair
Dianne E. Williams, Vice Chair
Maryam Elahi, President & CEO
Provides donors with an easy and convenient way to give back to our community with joy and impact. We make grants to nonprofit organizations and support their efforts to strengthen our community.

2722   Connecticut Mutual Life Foundation
140 Garden St
Hartford, CT 6154   860-727-3000

Astrida Olds, Executive Director
Distinguished throughout its long history by unusual commitment to high principles of corporate purpose and business ethics. That commitment has been reflected not only in the firm belief that normal business functions must be carried out with a sense of responsibility beyond that required by the marketplace. Maintains an ongoing program of corporate contributions, a nationwide matching gifts plan for all employees on behalf of private and public education, skills training programs, and more.

2723   Cornelia de Lange Syndrome Foundation
302 West Main Street
#100
Avon, CT 06001   860-676-8166
800-753-2357
Fax: 860-676-8337
info@cdlsusa.org
www.cdlsusa.org

Robert Boneberg, Esq., President
Richard Haaland, Ph.D., Vice President
David Harvey, Vice President
Provides information about birth defects caused by Cornelia de Lange Syndrome.

2724   Fidelco Guide Dog Foundation
103 Vision Way
Bloomfield, CT 06002   860-243-5200
Fax: 860-769-0567
admissions@fidelco.org
www.fidelco.org

Karen C. Tripp, Chair
G. Kenneth Bernhard, Esq., Vice Chair
Gregg Barratt, Chief of Staff
The Fidelco Guide Dog Foundation creates increased freedom and independence for men and women who are blind by providing them with guide dogs.

2725   GE Foundation
General Electric Company
3135 Easton Tpke
Fairfield, CT 6828   203-373-3216
Fax: 203-373-3029
gefoundation@ge.com
www.ge.com

Jeffrey R. Immelt, Chairman/ CEO
Daniel C. Heintzelman, Vice Chair
Jeffrey S. Bornstein, SVP & CFO, GE
Believes that our greatest national resource is the work force. If we are to successfully compete in the global arena, then we become involved in improving the education of all of our citizens. The Foundation sets examples for others to emulate helping people with their international grant program to higher education and to health care for children in developing countries.

2726   Hartford Foundation for Public Giving
10 Columbus Blvd
8th Floor
Hartford, CT 06106   860-548-1888
Fax: 860-524-8346
lindakelly@hfpg.org
www.hfpg.org

Yvette Melendez, Chair
Bonnie J. Malley, Vice Chair
Linda J. Kelly, President
Developmentally disabled, housing, deaf, recreation and education grants.

2727   Hartford Insurance Group
1 Hartford Plz
Hartford, CT 6155-1708   860-547-5000
www.thehartford.com

Christopher Swift, Chairman/ CEO
Doug Elliot, President
Beth Bombara, Chief Financial Officer
Giving is primarily in the Hartford, CT area and in communities where the company has a regional office. No support is available for political or religious purposes. Grants are given in the areas of education, health and United Way organizations.

2728   Henry Nias Foundation
20 Carmen Rd
Milford, CT 6460-7508   203-874-2787

Charles D Fleischman, President
Giving limited to NY metropolitan area. Arts, cultural programs, medical school/education, and children and youth.

2729 Jane Coffin Childs Memorial Fund for Medical Research
333 Cedar St, SHM
L300
New Haven, CT 6510-3206   203-785-4612
                                  Fax: 203-785-3301
                                  www.jccfund.org

Dr Randy Schekman, Director
The Fund awards fellowships to suitably qualified individuals for full time postdoctoral studies in the medical and related sciences bearing on cancer.

2730 John H and Ethel G Nobel Charitable Trust
Bankers Trust Company
1 Fawcett Pl
PO Box 1297
New York, NY 1008-1297   203-629-7120
                                 Fax: 203-629-7170

Paul J Bisset, VP

2731 Scheuer Associates Foundation
960 Lake Ave
Greenwich, CT 6831-3032   203-622-5002
                                 Fax: 203-622-5002

Thomas Scheuer, President

2732 Swindells Charitable Foundation Trust
Shawmut Bank
1221SW YamhillStreet
Suite 100
Portland, OR 97205-2303   503-222-0689
                                 Fax: 503-222-0726
                                 dwecker@swindellstrust.org
                                 www.swindellstrust.org

Maggie Willard, President
Grants made to charitable organizations or societies incorporated for the relief of sick and suffering poor children and/or the relief of sick suffering and indigent aged men and women and/or the support of public charitable hospitals. Geographic area includes Hartford, CT area primarily. Application is required, deadlines are Feb. 1 and Aug. 1.

Delaware

2733 Arc of Delaware
2 S Augustine Street
Suite B
Wilmington, DE 19804-2504   302-996-9400
                                    Fax: 302-996-0683
                                    TTY: 800-232-5460
                                    eraign@arcde.org
                                    www.thearcofdelaware.org

Bill Seufert, President
Becky Hill, Vice President
Merry Jones, Vice President
The Arc of Delaware is a non-profit organization of volunteers and staff who work together to improve the quality of life for people with disabilitiesand their families. We strive to include all children and adults with cognitive, intellectual and developmental disabilities in every community.

2734 Longwood Foundation
100 W 10th St
Suite 1109
Wilmington, DE 19801-1694   302-683-8200
                                    Fax: 302-654-2323
                                    www.longwoodfoundation.com

ThŠre du Pont, President
Peter Morrow, Executive Director
Offers grants to the mentally and physically disabled - capital, program, education and housing grants in the state of Delaware.

District of Columbia

2735 Alexander and Margaret Stewart Trust
Brawner Building
888 17th Street NW
Suite 1250
Washington, DC 20006-3321   202-333-1277
                                    Fax: 202-333-3128
                                    aplatt@projectsinternational.com
                                    www.projectsinternational.com

Chas W. Freeman, Chairman
Peter J.C, Young, President
Imtiaz T. Ladak, Chief Financial Officer
Grants are given only to the Washington, DC area organizations providing care or treatment to cancer patients or those with childhood afflictions.

2736 American Hotel and Lodging Association Foundation
1201 Eye St. NW.
Suite 1100
Washington, DC 20005   202-289-3100
                               Fax: 202-289-3199
                               ahleffoundation@ahla.com
                               www.ahlafoundation.org

Rosanna Maietta, President
Shelly Weir, Senior VP, Career Development
Kara Filer, VP, Donor Relations & Development
Programs include apprenticeship, community-based initiatives for youth, hospitality certification, funding for employee education, and a career center.

2737 Arc of the District of Columbia
415 Michigan Avenue, NE
Suite 150
Washington, DC 20017- 2144   202-636-2950
                                     Fax: 202-635-7086
                                     www.arcdc.net

Robert A. Anderson, President
Mary Lou Meccariello, Executive Director
Michael Gonzales, Chief Operating Officer
Advocating for and providing services to persons with developmental disabilities.

2738 Eugene and Agnes E Meyer Foundation
The Meyer Foundation
1250 Connecticut Ave NW
Suite 800
Washington, DC 20036- 2620   202-483-8294
                                     Fax: 202-328-6850
                                     meyer@meyerfdn.org
                                     www.meyerfoundation.org

Joshua Bernstein, Chair
Deborah Ratner Salzberg, Vice Chair
Nicky Goren, President & CEO
Awards grants to projects dealing with the learning disabled, blind, mental health and vocational training in the Washington metropolitan area.

2739 Federal Student Aid Information Center
US Department of Education
400 Maryland Ave SW
Washington, DC 20202   202-275-5446
                               800-872-5327
                               www.ed.gov

Arne Duncan, Secretary of Education
Tony Miller, Deputy Secretary
Martha Kanter, Under Secretary
Answers questions about Federal student aid from students, parents and Members of Congress, as well as financial aid administrators.

2740 GEICO Philanthropic Foundation
1 Geico Plz
Washington, DC 20076   301-986-3000
                               800-841-3000
                               Fax: 301-986-2851
                               www.geico.com

Tony M Nicely, CEO
Hospitals, physically disabled and Special Olympics.

2741 Jacob and Charlotte Lehrman Foundation
1836 Columbia Rd NW
Washington, DC 20009-2002   202-328-8400
                                  Fax: 202-338-8405
                                  www.lehrmanfoundation.org

Elizabeth Berry, Director
Robert Lehrman, Trustee
Samuel Lehrman, Trustee
The Jacob & Charlotte Lehrman Foundation supports and seeks
to enrich Jewish life in Washington DC, Israel and around the
world. It is committed to making Washington a better place for all
people and supports the arts, education and undeserved children,
the environment, and healthcare.

2742 John Edward Fowler Memorial Foundation
79 Fifth Avenue
16th Street
New York, NY 10003-3076   212-620-4230
                                 800-424-9836
                                 Fax: 212-807-3677
                                 www.foundationcenter.org
Bradforth K. Smith, President
Lisa Philp, Vice President
Lawrence T. McGill, Vice President
Although not a program priority, the foundation does offer grants
to the physically disabled in the Washington, DC area only.

2743 Joseph P Kennedy Jr Foundation
1133 19th Street NW
12th Floor
Washington, DC 20036-3604   202-393-1250
                                   Fax: 202-824-0351
Rebecca Salon, President
Steven Eidelman, Executive Director
Has two firm objectives: to seek the prevention of developmental
disabilities, and to improve the way society deals with its citizens
who are already affected. The Foundation uses its funds in areas
where a multiplier effect can be achieved through development of
innovative models for the prevention and amelioration, through
provision of seed money that encourages new researchers, and
thorough use of the Foundation's influence to promote public
awareness.

2744 Kiplinger Foundation
1100 13th Street, NW
Suite 750
Washington, DC 20005-3938   202-887-6400
                                   800-544-0155
                                   Fax: 202-778-8976
                                   www.kiplinger.com
Knight Kiplinger, VP
Limited to the greater Washington, DC area, the grants focus primarily on education, social welfare, cultural activities and community programs. Matching grants to eligible secondary or
higher education institutions are provided on behalf of employ-
ees and retirees of Kiplinger Washington Editors, Inc. The
Foundation does not fund scholarships.

2745 Morris and Gwendolyn Cafritz Foundation
1825 K St NW
Ste 1400
Washington, DC 20006-1271   202-223-3100
                                   800-544-0155
                                   Fax: 202-296-7567
                                   info@cafritzfoundation.org
                                   www.cafritzfoundation.org
Calvin Cafritz, Chairman/President/ CEO
John E. Chapoton, Vice Chairman and Treasurer
Ed McGeogh, Vice President - Asset Managemen
Grants are awarded to only 501(c)(3) organizations that are in the
DC area. Grants are not awarded for capitol purposes, special
events, endowments, or to individuals.

2746 Paul and Annetta Himmelfarb Foundation
4545 42nd St NW
Ste 203
Washington, DC 20016-4623   202-966-3796

M Preston, Executive Director
Primary areas of interest include health, children, human need,
and Israel.

2747 Public Welfare Foundation
1200 U St NW
Washington, DC 20009-4443   202-965-1800
                                   info@publicwelfare.org
                                   www.publicwelfare.org
Lydia M. Marshall, Chair
Mary E. McClymont, President
Phillipa Taylor, Chief Financial and Administrati
The foundation's funding is specifically targeted to economically
disadvantaged populations. Proposals must fall within one of the
following categories: criminal justice, disadvantaged elderly,
disadvantaged youth, environment, health and population and reproductive health, human rights and global security, and community economic developmental and participation. Proposals
should be addressed to the Review Committee.

Florida

2748 Able Trust
3320 Thomasville Road
Suite 200
Tallahassee, FL 32308   850-224-4493
                               Fax: 850-224-4496
                               TTY: 850-224-4493
                               info@abletrust.org
                               www.abletrust.org
Susanne Homant, President
Guenevere Crum, Senior Vice President
Kathryn McManus, MA, Chief Development Director
The Able Trust is a non-profit, public/private partnership that
supports non-profit vocational rehabilitation programs through-
out Florida with fundraising, grant making and public awareness
of disability issues.

2749 American Academy of Pain Medicine Foundation
American Academy of Pain Medicine
1705 Edgewater Dr.
Suite 7778
Orlando, FL 32804   800-917-1619
                           Fax: 407-749-0714
                           info@painmed.org
                           painmed.org/aapm-foundation
W. Michael Hooten, President
The Foundation supports AAPM's core purpose to optimize the
health of patients in pain and eliminate the major health problem
of pain by advancing the practice and the specialty of pain
medicine.
1911

2750 Arc of Florida
2898 Mahan Dr
Ste 1
Tallahassee, FL 32308-5462   850-921-0460
                                    800-226-1155
                                    info@arcflorida.org
                                    www.arcflorida.org
Pat Young, President
Dick Bradley, Vice President Administration
Linda Bloom, Vice President Advocacy
Advocates for all people with developmental disabilities,
through education, awareness, research, advocacy and the sup-
port of families, friends and community.

2751 Bank of America Client Foundation
50 Central Avenue
Suite 750
Sarasota, FL 34236-5900   941-951-4103
                                 maryann.l.smith@ustrust.com
                                 www.fdnweb.org/boacf/
Maryann L. Smith, Vice President, Senior Trust Off
Committed to creating meaningful change in the communities we
serve through our philanthropic efforts, associate volunteerism,
community development activities and investing, support of arts
and culture programming and environmental initiatives.

259

2752   Barron Collier Jr Foundation
2600 Golden Gate Pkwy
Naples, FL 34105-3227   239-262-2600
Fax: 239-262-1840
ContactUs@BarronCollier.com
www.barroncollier.com

Karen V. Triplett, Director of Property Management
Jose Medina, Facilities Manager

Barron Collier Companies - dedicated to the responsible development, management and stewardship of its extensive land holdings and other assets in the businesses of agriculture, real estate, and mineral management.

2753   Camiccia-Arnautou Charitable Foundation
Ste 402
980 N Federal Hwy
Boca Raton, FL 33432-2712   561-368-5757
Fax: 561-368-8505

Ronda Gluck, President

2754   Chatlos Foundation
PO Box 915048
Longwood, FL 32791-5048   407-862-5077
info@chatlos.org
www.chatlos.org

Bill Chatlos, Trustee

Funds nonprofit organizations in the USA and around the globe. Funding is provided in the following areas of giving: Bible Colleges/Seminaries, Religious Causes, Medical Concerns, Liberal Arts Colleges and Social Concerns. Category of placement is determined by the organizations overall mission rather than the project under consideration. The Foundation does not make scholarship grants directly to individuals but rather to educational institutions which in turn select recipients.

2755   Edyth Bush Charitable Foundation
199 E Welbourne Ave
Ste 100
Winter Park, FL 32789-4365   407-647-4322
888-647-4322
Fax: 407-647-7716
dodahowski@edythbush.org
www.edythbush.org

Gerald F. Hilbrich, Chairman
Herbert W. Holm, Vice Chairman
David A. Odahowski, President/CEO

Funding is resrticted to 501c3 nonprofit organizations located and operating in Orange, Osceola, Seminole and Lake Counties, Florida. Visit www.edythbush.org for a list of funding policies.

2756   FPL Group Foundation
700 Universe Blvd
Juno Beach, FL 33408-2657   561-694-4000
888-488-7703
Fax: 561-694-4620
PoweringFlorida@FPL.com
www.fpl.com

Maria V. Fogarty, Senior Vice President, Internal
James L. Robo, President and Chief Operating Of
Joseph T. Kelliher, Executive Vice President, Federa

The company consistently outperforms national averages for service reliability while customer bills are below the national average. A clean energy leader, FPL has one of the lowest emissions profiles and one of the leading energy efficiency programs among utilities nationwide. FPL is a subsidiary of Juno Beach, Fla.-based NextEra Energy, Inc.

2757   Jefferson Lee Ford III Memorial Foundation
9600 Collins Ave
Bal Harbour, FL 33154-2202   305-868-2609
Fax: 305-868-2640

Sanford L King, Director
Yvonne Quatrale, President

Disabled children, hearing and speech center. Grants are only given to tax exempt organizations, no individual grants are offered.

2758   Jessie Ball duPont Fund
40 East Adams Street
Ste 300
Jacksonville, FL 32202-3302   904-353-0890
800-252-3452
Fax: 904-353-3870
contactus@dupontfund.org
www.dupontfund.org

Sherry P. Magill, President
Mark D. Constantine, Vice President for Strategy, Pol
Barbara Roole, Senior Program Officer

Established under the terms of the will of the late Jessie Ball duPont. The fund is a national foundation having a special though not exclusive interest in issues affecting the South. The Fund works with the approximately 325 individual institutions to which Mrs. duPont personally contributed during the five-year period, 1960 through 1964.

2759   Lost Tree Village Charitable Foundation
8 Church Lane
North Palm Beach, FL 33408-2908   561-622-3780
Fax: 561-841-6773
info@losttreefoundation.org
www.losttreefoundation.org

Pam Rue, Executive Director
Teresa Elu, Executive Assistant
Bob Heon, Controller

The Lost Tree Village Charitable Foundation is dedicated to building a stronger community and improving the quality of life for all local residents. Grants are awarded annually to local non-profit health and human service organizations providing information, expertise and assistance to those in need. Applications are only accepted from organizations located in Palm Beach and Southern Martin Counties. Visit the website for guidelines and further information.

2760   Miami Foundation, The
40 NW 3rd Street
Suite 405
Miami, FL 33128   305-371-2711
Fax: 305-371-5342
info@miamifoundation.org
www.miamifoundation.com

Javier Alberto Soto, President and CEO
Rebecca Mandelman, VP for Strategy and Engagement

The Foundation approaches all of its program activities with a focus on building the community. We conduct acticvities and support efforts that build community assets and relationships among individuals, organizations, and communities that connect people with resources and opportunities to improve their quality of life.

2761   Mount Sinai Medical Center
4300 Alton Road
Miami Beach, FL 33140-6574   305-674-2121
305-674-2777
www.msmc.com/foundation

Wayne Chaplin, Chairman
Steven D. Sonenreich, President & CEO
Jason Loeb, Foundation President
Autism Research

2762   National Parkinson Foundation
200 SE 1st Street
Suite 800
Miami, FL 33131-1494   800-473-4636
contact@parkinson.org
www.parkinson.org

John L. Lehr, President & CEO
James Beck, SVP & Chief Scientific Officer
Yasnahia Cortorreal, VP & chief Human Resources & Administration Officer

The mission of the NPF is to improve the quality of care for people with Parkinson's disease through research, education, and outreach.

2763   Publix Super Markets Charities
Publix Super Market Corporation Office
PO Box 407
Lakeland, FL 33802-0407   800-242-1227
                                           www.publix.com
Gino DiGrazia, Vice President of Finance
Maria Brous, Director of Media & Community R
Kimberly Reynolds, Media & Community Relations
In addition to giving to thousands of local projects, Publix annually supports five organizations in companywide campaigns: Special Olympics, March of Dimes, Children's Miracle Network, United Way and Food for All

2764   The Cherab Foundation
2301 NE Savannah Rd
Suite 1771
Jensen Beach, FL 34957   772-335-5135
                                           help@cherab.org
                                           cherabfoundation.org
Lisa Geng, Founder & President
Jolie Abreu, Vice President
The Cherab Foundation is a world-wide nonprofit organization working to improve the communication skills and education of all children with speech and language delays and disorders. The Cherab Foundation is committed to assisting with the development of new therapeutic approaches, preventions, and cures to neurologically-based speech disorders.

Georgia

2765   Arc Of Georgia
100 Edgewood Ave NE
Ste 1675
Atlanta, GA 30303-3068   678-733-8969
                                           888-401-1581
                                           Fax: 678-733-8970
                                           info@thearcofgeorgia.org
                                           www.thearcofgeorgia.org
Torin Togut, President
David Glass, Vice President
Julie Lee, Secretary
The Arc of Georgia advocates for the rights and full participation of all children and adults with intellectual and developmental disabilities. Together with our network of members and other local Chapters, we improve systems of supports and services, connect families, inspire communities, and influence public policy.

2766   Community Foundation for Greater Atlanta
50 Hurt Plz SE
Ste 449
Atlanta, GA 30303-2915   404-688-5525
                                           Fax: 404-688-3060
                                           info@cfgreateratlanta.org
                                           www.cfgreateratlanta.org
Suzanne Boas, Board Chair
Alicia Philipp, President
Robert Smulian, Vice President of Philanthropic
The Community Foundation for Greater Atlanta is a creative, cost-effective and tax-efficient way for people to invest in our community. We help donors and their families meet their charitable goals by educating them or critical issues and by matching them with organizations that serve their interests. By working with donors and the community, we improve the quality of life for residents in our region.

2767   Florence C and Harry L English Memorial Fund
Sun Trust Bank Atlanta
PO Box 4418
Mail Code 041
Atlanta, GA 30302   404-588-8250
                                           Fax: 404-724-3082
Anil T. Cheriyan, Chief Information Officer
Kenneth J. Carrig, Chief Human Resources Officer
Rilla S. Delorier, Chief Marketing and Client Exper
Grants only made to Metro Atlanta non-profit organizations; no grants to churches or individuals.

2768   Georgia Power
96 Annex
Atlanta, GA 30308-3374   404-506-6526
                                           888-655-5888
                                           www.georgiapower.com
W. Paul Bowers, Chairman/ President/ CEO
John L. Pemberton, Senior VP/SPO,
Georgia Power is an investor-owned, tax-paying utility that serves 2.25 million customers in all but four of Georgia's 159 counties.

2769   Grayson Foundation
1701 Willa Place Drive
Kernersville, NC 2728   336-650-9914
                                           graysonfoundation@gmail.com
                                           www.graysonfoundation.net
Donna Sherrell, Finance- Public Relations
Tricia Gladstone, Behavior Analyst-Finance Public
Roger Sherrell, Information Technology-Web Manag
Grayson Foundation enhances the quality of public educationfor the students of the Grayson cluster of schools by providing funds which enrich and extend educational oppurtunities.

2770   Harriet McDaniel Marshall Trust in Memory of Sanders McDaniel
Sun Trust Bank Atlanta
96 Annex
PO Box 4418
Atlanta, GA 30396   404-588-8250
                                           888-891-0938
                                           Fax: 404-724-3082
Anil T. Cheriyan, Chief Information Officer
Kenneth J. Carrig, Chief Human Resources Officer
Rilla S. Delorier, Chief Marketing and Client Exper
Grants only made to Metro Atlanta non-profit organizations, no grants to churches or individuals.

2771   IBM Corporation
1 New Orchard Rd
Armonk, NY 10504-1772   914-499-1900
                                           800-425-3333
                                           TTY: 804-068-4225
                                           response@in.ibm.com
                                           www.ibm.com
Samuel J Palmisano, Chairman
Virginia M. Rometty, President and Chief Executive Of
Rodney C. Adkins, Senior Vice President
Manages disability programs (which leverage IBM resources through partnerships) designed to train persons with disabilities and assist them in gaining employment. Also, disseminates information regarding products and resources for persons with disabilities with those of other companies and organizations.

2772   John H and Wilhelmina D Harland Charitable Foundation
3565 Piedmont Road, NE
Two Piedmont Center, Suite 710
Atlanta, GA 30305-1502   404-264-9912
                                           Fax: 404-266-8834
                                           info@harlandfoundation.org
                                           www.harlandfoundation.org
Margaret C. Reiser, President
Winifred S. Davis, Vice President/Treasurer
Robert E. Reiser, Secretary
The Harland Charitable Foundation was established in 1972 by John H. and Wilhelmina D. Harland to support worthy local causes in Atlanta, with a particular interest in improving the welfare of children and youth as well as support of community services and arts and culture.

2773   Lettie Pate Whitehead Foundation
191 Peachtree Street NE
Suite 3540
Atlanta, GA 30303- 2951   404-522-6755
                                           Fax: 404-522-7026
                                           fdns@woodruff.org
                                           www.woodruff.org
James B. Williams, Chairman
James M. Sibley, Vice Chairman
Lawrence L. Gellerstedt, President /CEO

Non-profit organization dedicated to the support of needy women in nine southeastern states.

2774   Rich Foundation
222 Summer Street
Stamford, CT 06901   203-359-2900
                                      Fax: 203-328-7980
                                      info@fdrich.com
                                      www.fdrich.com

A private foundation under section 509(a) of the Internal Revenue Code designed primariliy for the benefit of the residents and charitable organizations of lower Fairfield County.

2775   SunTrust Bank, Atlanta Foundation
Sun Trust Bank Atlanta
PO Box 4418
Mail Code 041
Atlanta, GA 30302   404-588-8250
                                      Fax: 404-724-3082
                                      www.suntrust.com

Anil T. Cheriyan, Chief Information Officer
Kenneth J. Carrig, Chief Human Resources Officer
Rilla S. Delorier, Chief Marketing and Client Exper

Hawaii

2776   Arc of Hawaii
3989 Diamond Head Rd
Honolulu, HI 96816-4413   808-737-7995
                                      Fax: 808-732-9531
                                      info@thearcinhawaii.org
                                      www.thearcinhawaii.org

Thomas Huber, President
Lee Moriwaki, Vice President
Duane Bartholomew, Secretary

The Arc is a national, grassroots organization of and for people with intellectual and related developmental disabilities. With more then 140,000 members in 1000 local and state chapters. The Arc is the largest volunteer organization devoted soley to working on behalf of people with intellectual disabilities.

2777   Atherton Family Foundation
827 Fort Street Mall
Honolulu, HI 96813-2817   808-566-5524
                                      888-731-3863
                                      Fax: 808-521-6286
                                      foundations@hcf-hawaii.org

Patricia R. Giles, Vice President
Judith M. Dawson, President
Frank C. Atherton, Vice President and Treasurer

Supports educational projects, programs and institutions as the highest priority, with the enterprises of a religious nature and those concerned with health and social services given careful attention. The Foundation is one of the largest private resources in the State devoted exclusively to the support of activities of a charitable nature.

2778   GN Wilcox Trust
Bank of Hawaii
PO Box 3170
Honolulu, HI 96802-3170   808-649-8580
                                      800-272-7262
                                      Fax: 808-538-4006
                                      stafford.kiguchi@boh.com
                                      www.boh.com

Paul Boyce, AVP and Grants Administrator
Elaine Moniz, Trust Specialist
William L. Carpenter, Senior Vice President

Benefits the people of Hawaii by funding programs that support social services, education, culture, the arts, youth services, religion, health and rehabilitation.

2779   Hawaii Community Foundation
827 Fort Street Mall
Honolulu, HI 96813-2817   808-537-6333
                                      888-731-3863
                                      Fax: 808-521-6286
                                      info@hcf-hawaii.org
                                      www.hawaiicommunityfoundation.org

Kelvin Taketa, President/CEO
Chris van Bergeijk, Vice President/Chief Operating O
Joseph Martyak, Vice President of Communications

The Hawaii Community Foundation is a public, statewide, charitable services and grantmaking organization supported by donor contributions for the benefit of Hawaii's people.

2780   McInerny Foundation Bank Of Hawaii, Corporate Trustee
PO Box 3170
Honolulu, HI 96802-3170   808-649-8580
                                      800-272-7262
                                      Fax: 808-538-4006
                                      stafford.kiguchi@boh.com
                                      www.boh.com

Paula Boyce, Avp And Grants Administrator
Elaine Moniz, Trust Specialist
William L. Carpenter, Senior Vice President

Although the Trust is broad-purposed, it does not make grants to churches or individuals, nor for endowments, reserve purposes, deficit financing, or for the purchase of real estate.

2781   Sophie Russell Testamentary Trust Bank Of Hawaii
PO Box 3170
Honolulu, HI 96802-3170   808-649-8580
                                      800-272-7262
                                      Fax: 808-538-4006
                                      stafford.kiguchi@boh.com
                                      www.boh.com

Paula Boyce, Asst. Vice President
Elaine Moniz, Trust Specialist
William L. Carpenter, Senior Vice President

Supports qualified tax-exempt charitable organizations, in the State of Hawaii only. Offers grants to the Humane Society and institutions giving nursing care and serving the physically and mentally handicapped.

Illinois

2782   Alzheimer's Association
225 N Michigan Ave
Fl 17
Chicago, IL 60601-7633   312-335-8700
                                      800-272-3900
                                      Fax: 866-699-1246
                                      TTY: 312-335-5886
                                      info@alz.org
                                      www.alz.org

Stewart Putnam, Chair
Christopher Binkley, Vice Chair
Harry Johns, President /CEO

Mission is to eliminate Alzheimer's disease through the advancement of research, to provide and enhance care and support for all affected, and to reduce the risk of dementia through the promotion of brain health.

2783   American National Bank and Trust Company
33 N La Salle St
PO Box 191
Danville, VA 24543-0191   312-661-6000
                                      800-240-8190
                                      Fax: 815-961-7745
                                      www.amnb.com

Charles H. Majors, Chairman/ CEO
Jeffrey V. Haley, President
Charles T. Canaday, Jr., Senior Vice President

Supports the endeavors of organizations working to meet the critical needs of the city and its surrounding communities. Success is greatly affected by the well-being of the communities the company serves, thus the foundation seeks to fulfill the social obligations both through financial funding and human resources. The

Foundation funding categories include organizations and programs involved in economic development, education, community and social services, healthcare and culture and the arts.

2784   Amerock Corporation
P.O.Box 7018
Rockford, IL 61125-7018   815-963-9631
                                       800-435-6959
                                  Fax: 800-618-6733
                                  www.amerock.com
Robert Bailey, President
Grants are given to organizations promoting wellness, health and rehabilitation of the visually impaired and physically disabled.

2785   Arc of Illinois
The Illinois Life Span Project
20901 S La Grange Rd
Ste 209
Frankfort, IL 60423-3213   815-464-1832
                                       800-588-7002
                                  Fax: 815-464-5292
                                  www.thearcofil.org
Brain Rubin, President
Therese Devine, Vice President
Tony Paulauski, Executive Director
The Arc of Illinois is committed to empowering persons with disabilities to achieve full participation in community life thru informed choices.

2786   Benjamin Benedict Green-Field Foundation
18313 Greenleaf Ct
Tinley Park, IL 60487-2176   708-444-4241
                                  Fax: 708-614-0496
                                  www.greenfieldfoundation.org
Colin Fisher, Chairman of the Board
Kathryn Groenendal, President
Dan Jarke, Vice President
A privately endowed grantmaking organization trying to improve the qaulity of life for children and the elderly in the city of chicago.

2787   Blowitz-Ridgeway Foundation
1701 E Woodfield Rd
Suite 201
Schaumburg, IL 60173-5127   847-330-1020
                                  Fax: 847-330-1028
                                  laura@blowitzridgeway.org
                                  www.blowitzridgeway.org
Daniel L Kline, President
Pierre R. LeBreton, Ph.D., Vice-President
Thomas P. Fitzgibbon, Treasurer
Provides limited program, capital and research grants to organizations aiding the physically and mentally disabled, and agencies serving children and youth. Grants generally limited to Illinois.

2788   Chaddick Institute for Metropolitan Development
2352 N. Clifton Ave.
Suite 130
Chicago, IL 60614-2302   773-325-7310
                                  Fax: 312-362-5506
                                  lasadvising@depaul.edu
                                  las.depaul.edu
Joseph P Scwieterman PhD, Director
Marisa Schulz, LEED AP, Assistant Director
Justin Kohls, Program Manager
Advances the principals of effective land use, transportation, and community planning. Offers planners, attorneys, developers, and entrepreneurs a forum to share expertise on difficult land-use issues through workshops, conferences, and policy studies.

2789   Chicago Community Trust
225 North Michigan Avenue
Suite 2200
Chicago, IL 60601- 4501   312-616-8000
                                  Fax: 312-616-7955
                                  www.cct.org
Frank M. Clark, Chairman
Terry Mazany, President /CEO
Jamie Phillippe, Vice President-Development and D
A community foundation established in 1915, which receives gifts and bequests from individuals, families or organizations interested in providing through the community foundation, financial support for the charitable agencies or institutions which serve the residents of metropolitan Chicago.

2790   Chicago Community Trust and Affiliates
225 North Michigan Avenue
Suite 2200
Chicago, IL 60601- 4501   312-616-8000
                                  Fax: 312-616-7955
                                  TTY: 312-853-0394
                                  www.cct.org
Frank M. Clark, Chairman
Terry Mazany, President /CEO
Jamie Phillippe, Vice President-Development and D
Provides critical charitable resources in the arts, community and economic development, education, health and wellness, hunger and homeless alleviation, legal services, programs for youth, the elderly, and people with disabilities, and services to assure that basic human needs are met for all members of our community.

2791   Community Foundation of Champaign County
307 W University Ave
Champaign, IL 61820-3411   217-359-0125
                                  Fax: 217-352-6494
                                  www.cfeci.org
Brooke Didier Starks, Chair
Tom Costello, Vice-Chair
Joan M. Dixon, President /CEO
A network of cultural resource providers and educational organizations who collaborate in the creation, coordination, and promotion of cultural resource programs for Champaign County Schools.

2792   Dr Scholl Foundation
1033 Skokie Blvd
Ste 230
Northbrook, IL 60062-4109   847-559-7430
                                  www.drschollfoundation.com
Pamela Scholl, President
The Foundation is dedicated to providing financial assistance to organizations committed to improving our world. Grants are made annually after an executive review by the staff and all the directors.

2793   Duchossois Foundation
Chamberlain Group
845 N Larch Ave
Elmhurst, IL 60126-1114   630-279-3600
                                  Fax: 630-530-6091
                                  employment@duch.com
                                  www.duch.com
Richard L. Duchossois, Chairman
Robert L. Fealy, President /COO
Craig J. Duchossois, Chief Executive Officer
Established in 1984, the foundation returns dollars to the communities supporting its facilities and employees. Within these following areas, organizations are carefully selected on the basis of community needs and the organization's value and performance. Areas aimed at include: medical research, children/youth programs and cultural institutions.

2794   Evenston Community Foundation
1560 Sherman Ave
Suite 535
Evanston, IL 60201-5910   847-492-0990
                                  Fax: 847-492-0904
                                  info@evanstonforever.org
                                  www.evanstonforever.org
Sara Schastok, Phd., President and CEO
Gwen Jessen, Vice President for Philanthropy
Marybeth Schroeder, Vice President for Programs
The Foundation is a publicly supported plilanthropic organization dedicated to enriching Evanston and the lives of its people, now and in the future. The Foundation builds and manages its own and other community endowments, addresses Evanston's changing needs through grant making, and provides leadership on important community needs.

2795   Field Foundation of Illinois
200 S Wacker Dr
Ste 3860
Chicago, IL 60606-5848   312-831-0910
                                      Fax: 312-831-0961
                                   byoung@fieldfoundation.org
                                    www.fieldfoundation.org

Lyle Logan, Board Chair
Aurie A. Pennick, Executive Director and Treasurer
Sarah M. Linsley, Secretary
The Field Foundation seeks to provide support for community, civic and cultural organizations in the Chicago area, enabling both new and established programs to test innovations, to expand proven strengths or to address specific, time-limited operational needs.

2796   Francis Beidler Charitable Trust
53 W Jackson Blvd
Ste 530
Chicago, IL 60604-3422   312-922-3792
                                      Fax: 312-922-3799

Francis Beidler, Owner
Children/youth, services. Community development, business promotion, crime and violence prevention. Federated giving programs, higher education, human services and family planning.

2797   Fred J Brunner Foundation
9300 King St
Franklin Park, IL 60131-2114   847-678-3232
                                      Fax: 847-678-0642

Fred J Brunner, CEO
General disability grants.

2798   George M Eisenberg Foundation for Charities
Ste 480
2340 S Arlington Heights Rd
Arlington Heights, IL 60005-4507   847-981-0545
                                      Fax: 847-941-0548

James Marousis, Manager

2799   Grover Hermann Foundation
233 S Wacker Dr
Suite 6600
Chicago, IL 60606-6473   312-258-5500
                                      Fax: 312-258-5600
                                   rsafer@schiffhardin.com
                                    www.schiffhardin.com
Ronald S. Safer, Managing Partner, Executive Comm
Provides funds for educational, health, public policy, community and religious organizations throughout the United States. Its major interests are in higher education and health.

2800   John D and Catherine T MacArthur Foundation
Office of Grants Management
140 S Dearborn St
Chicago, IL 60603-5285   312-726-8000
                                      Fax: 312-920-6258
                                      TTY: 312-920-6285
                                   4answers@macfound.org
                                    www.macfound.org
Marjorie M. Scardino, Chair
Julia Stasch, Interim President
Cecilia A. Conrad, Vice President-MacArthur Fellows
The Foundation supports creative people and effective institutions committed to building a more just, verdant, and peaceful world. In addition, we work to defend human rights, advance global conservation, & security, make cities better places, and understand how technology is affecting children and society.

2801   Les Turne Amyotrophic Laterial Sclerosis Foundation
5550 Touhy Ave
Ste 302
Skokie, IL 60077-3254   847-679-3311
                                          888-257-1107
                                      Fax: 847-679-9109
                                   info@lesturnerals.org
                                    www.lesturnerals.org

Ken Hoffman, President
Andrea Paul Backman, Executive Director
Shari Diamond, RN, BSN, Director of Patient Services

Voluntary health organization dedicated to raising funds for ALS research, patient services and public awareness. Provides educational materials for affected individuals and family members, health care professionals, and the general public. Program services include referrals and counseling; audio-visual aids and periodic newsletters. Offers support groups and patient networking to affected individuals, family members, and caregivers.

2802   Little City Foundation
1760 W Algonquin Rd
Palatine, IL 60067-4799   847-358-5510
                                      Fax: 847-358-3291
                                   info@littlecity.org
                                    www.littlecity.org
Matthew B. Schubert, President
B. Timothy Desmond, Executive Vice President
David Rose, Vice President
We offer innovative and personalized programs to fully assist and empower children & adults with autism and other intellectual and developmental disabilities. With a commitment to attaining a greater quality of life for Illinois most vulnerable citizens, we actively promote choice, person-centered planning and a holistic approach to health and wellness. 'ChildBridge' services include in-home personal & family supports, clinical behavior intervention, 24/7 residential services and much more.

2803   MAGIC Foundation for Children's Growth
6645 North Ave
Oak Park, IL 60302-1057   708-383-0808
                                          800-362-4423
                                      Fax: 708-383-0899
                                   ContactUs@magicfoundation.org
                                    www.magicfoundation.org
Rich Buckley, Chairman
Ken Dickard, Vice Chairman
Mary Andrews, CEO and Co-Founder
This is a national nonprofit organization providing support and education regarding growth disorders in children and related adult disorders, including adult GHD. Dedicated to helping children whose physical growth is affected by a medical problem by assisting families of afflicted children through local support groups, public education/awareness, newsletters, specialty divisions and programs for the children.

2804   McDonald's Corporation Contributions Program
2111 McDonalds Dr
Oak Brook, IL 60523-5500   630-623-3000
                                          800-244-6227
                                      Fax: 630-623-5700
                                    www.mcdonalds.com
Don Thompson, President and Chief Executive Of
Tim Fenton, Chief Operating Officer
Peter J. Bensen, Executive Vice President and Chi

2805   Michael Reese Health Trust
150 N Wacker Dr
Ste 2320
Chicago, IL 60606-1608   312-726-1008
                                      Fax: 312-726-2797
                                    www.healthtrust.net
Herbert S. Wander, Chairman
The Hon. How Carroll, Vice Chairman
Walter R. Nathan, Secretary
The trust seeks to improve the health of people in Chicago's metropolitan communities through effective grantmaking in health care, health education, and health research.

2806   National Eye Research Foundation
910 Skokie Blvd
Ste 207a
Northbrook, IL 60062-4033   847-564-9400
                                          800-621-2258
                                      Fax: 847-564-0807
                                   info@nerf.org
                                    www.subway.com
Joel Tenner, Manager
Dedicated to improving eye care for the public and meeting the professional needs of eye care practitioners; sponsors eye research projects on contact lens applications and eye care problems. Special study sections in such fields as orthokertology, primary eyecare, pediatrics, and through continuing education

programs. Provides eye care information for the public and professionals. Educational materials including pamphlets. Program activities include education and referrals.

2807 National Foundation for Ectodermal Dysplasias
6 Executive Dr
Suite 2
Fairview Heights, IL 62208-1360   618-566-2020
                                    Fax: 618-566-4718
                                    info@nfed.org
                                    www.nfed.org

Anil Vora, President
George Barbar, Vice President
Mary Fete, Executive Director
To empower and connect people touched by ectodermal dysplasias through education, support, and research.

2808 National Headache Foundation
820 N Orleans St
Ste 411
Chicago, IL 60610-3131   312-274-2650
                                    888-643-5552
                                    Fax: 312-640-9049
                                    info@headaches.org
                                    www.headaches.org

Seymour Diamond, M.D., Executive Chairman
Roger K. Cady, M.D., Associate Executive Chairman
Arthur H. Elkind, M.D., President
Foundation exists to enhance the healthcare of headache sufferers. It is a source of help to sufferers' families, physicians who treat headache sufferers, allied healthcare professionals and to the public.

2809 OMRON Foundation OMRON Electronics
1 Commerce Dr
Schaumburg, IL 60173-5330   847-843-7900
                                    800-556-6766
                                    Fax: 847-884-1866
                                    aoisales@omron.com
                                    www.omron247.com

Tastu Goto, CEO
Supports local community projects through direct donations and matching employee-directed contributions.

2810 Parkinson's Disease Foundation
1359 Broadway
Suite 1509
New York, NY 10018-2331   212-923-4700
                                    800-457-667
                                    Fax: 212-923-4778
                                    info@pdf.org
                                    www.pdf.org

Howard D. Morgan, Chair
Constance Woodruff Atwell, Ph.D., Vice Chair
Robin Anthony Elliott, President
International voluntary not-for-profit organization dedicated to patient services; education of affected individuals, family members, and healthcare professionals; and promotion and support of research for Parkinson's Disease and related disorders. Offers an extensive referral service to guide affected individuals to proper diagnosis and clinical care. Provides referrals to genetic counseling and support groups; promotes patient advocacy; and offers a variety of educational and support materials
Quarterly

2811 Peoria Area Community Foundation
331 Fulton St
Ste 310
Peoria, IL 61602-1449   309-674-8730
                                    Fax: 309-674-8754
                                    jim@communityfoundationci.org
                                    www.communityfoundationci.org

Donna Maracci, Chair
David Wynn, Vice Chair
Mark Roberts, CEO
Established to meet a wide variety of social, cultural, educational and other charitable needs throughout Central Illinois.

2812 Polk Brothers Foundation
20 W Kinzie St
Ste 1110
Chicago, IL 60654-5815   312-527-4684
                                    Fax: 312-527-4681
                                    questions@polkbrosfdn.org
                                    www.polkbrosfdn.org

Sandra P. Guthman, Chair
Raymond F. Simon, Vice Chair
Gordon S. Prussian, Secretary
The Polk Brothers Foundation seeks to improve the quality of life for the people of Chicago. We partner with local nonprofit organizations that work to reduce the impact of poverty and provide area residents with better access to quality education, preventive health care and basic human services.

2813 Retirement Research Foundation
8765 W Higgins Rd
Ste 430
Chicago, IL 60631-4170   773-714-8080
                                    Fax: 773-714-8089
                                    info@rrf.org
                                    www.rrf.org

Nathaniel P. McParland, M.D., Chairman
Ruth Ann Watkins, Secretary
Downey R. Varey, Treasurer
A private philanthropy with primary interest in improving the quality of life of older persons in the United States.

2814 Sears-Roebuck Foundation
3333 Beverly Rd
Hoffman Estates, IL 60179   847-286-2500
                                    800-932-3188
                                    Fax: 800-326-0485
                                    www.sears.com

W Bruce Johnson, CEO
Has a special interest in projects that address women, families, and diversity, but awards most of its funding to disease-specific charities and United Way in the Chicago area.

2815 Siragusa Foundation
1 E Wacker Dr
Ste 2910
Chicago, IL 60601-1912   312-755-0064
                                    Fax: 312-755-0069
                                    www.siragusa.org

John E. Hicks, Chair & President
Ross D. Siragusa, Vice Chair
John R. Siragusa, Treasurer
The Siragusa Foundation, is a private family foundation that is committed to honoring its founder by sustaining and developing Chicago's extraordinary nonprofit resources.

2816 Square D Foundation
1415 S Roselle Rd
Palatine, IL 60067-7337   847-397-2600
                                    Fax: 847-925-7500
                                    www.schneider-electric.com

Makes donations for operating support, capital development needs, and special projects to nonprofit organizations that have been granted exemption from the Federal Income Tax. The Foundation has a strong commitment to the following areas: health and welfare, education, civic and community affairs, and culture and the arts. Support of higher education is also made for scholarships, endowments for facility and acquisition or expansion of equipment or facilities, through Matching Gift Program.

2817 WP and HB White Foundation
540 W Frontage Rd
Ste 3240
Northfield, IL 60093-1232   847-446-1441

Margaret Blandford, Executive Director
The Foundation's funds are allocated on a continuing basis within the metropolitan area of Chicago where our founder's business prospered. The Foundation helps organizations specializing in the visually impaired, mental health, youth and recreation.

2818 Washington Square Health Foundation
875 N Michigan Ave
Ste 3516
Chicago, IL 60611-1957   312-664-6488
                               Fax: 312-664-7787
                               washington@wshf.org
                               www.wshf.org
William N. Werner, MD, MPH, Board Chair
Howard Nochumson, Executive Director/President
William B. Friedeman, Secretary
Grants funds in order to promote and maintain access to adequate healthcare for all people in the Chicagoland area regardless of race, sex, creed or financial need.

2819 Wheat Ridge Ministries
1 Pierce Pl
Ste 250 E
Itasca, IL 60143-2634   630-766-9066
                               800-762-6748
                               Fax: 630-766-9622
                               www.wheatridge.org
Kevin Boettcher, Chair
Richard Herman, President
Brain Becker, Senior Vice President
Weat Ridge supports more then 100 new health-related ministries each year through a variety of grant programs

Indiana

2820 Arc of Indiana
107 N Pennsylvania St
Suite 800
Indianapolis, IN 46204- 2423   317-977-2375
                                      800-382-9100
                                      Fax: 317-977-2385
                                      thearc@arcind.org
                                      www.arcind.org
Kerry Fletcher, President
Marlene Lu, Vice President
Mike Foddrill, Treasurer
Arc of Indiana is commited to people with cognitive and developmental disabilities realizing their goals of learning, living, working, and playing in the community.

2821 Ball Brothers Foundation
222 S Mulberry St
Muncie, IN 47305-2802   765-741-5500
                               Fax: 765-741-5518
                               info@ballfdn.org
                               www.ballfdn.org
James A. Fisher, Chairman/ CEO
Jud Fisher, President/Chief Operating Office
Frank B. Petty, Vice Chairman
The Ball Brothers Foundation is dedicated to the stewardship legacy of the Ball brothers and to the pursuit of improving the quality of the Muncie, Delaware County, east Central Indiana and Indiana, through philanthropy and leadership.

2822 Community Foundation of Boone County
102 N. Lebanon
Suite 200
Lebanon, IN 46052   317-873-0210
                           Fax: 317-873-0219
                           info@communityfoundationbc.org
                           www.communityfoundationbc.org
Marc Applegate, Chairman of the Board
Ray Ingham, Vice Chair
Mike Harlos, Treasurer
The Community Foundation of Boone County provides pathways for connecting people who care with causes that matter for now and in the future.

2823 John W Anderson Foundation
402 Wall St
Valparaiso, IN 46383-2562   219-462-4611
                                   Fax: 219-531-8954
                                   andersonfnd@aol.com
Bruce Wargo, Manager

Physically and mentally disabled, recreation and youth agencies in Northwest Indiana area.

Iowa

2824 Arc of Iowa
114 S. 11th Street
Ste 302
West Des Moines, IA 50265- 3259   515-402-1618
                                         800-362-2927
                                         Fax: 515-330-2195
                                         casey@thearcofiowa.org
                                         www.thearcofiowa.org
Casey Westhoff, Executive Director
The Arc of Iowa exists to ensure that people with intellectual disabilities and developmental disabilities receive the services, supports and opportunities necessary to fully realize their right to live, work and enjoy life in the community without discrimination.

2825 Hall-Perrine Foundation
115 3rd St SE
Ste 803
Cedar Rapids, IA 52401-1222   319-362-9079
                                     Fax: 319-362-7220
                                     www.hallperrine.org
William Whipple, Chairman
Jack Evans, President
Darrel Morf, Vice President
This foundation is dedicated tio improving the quality of life for peole in Linn County, IA by responding to the changing social, economic, and cultural needs of the community.

2826 Mid-Iowa Health Foundation
3900 Ingersoll Ave
Ste 104
Des Moines, IA 50312-3535   515-277-6411
                                   Fax: 515-271-7579
                                   info@midiowahealth.org
                                   www.midiowahealth.org
Becky Miles-Polka, Chairman
Rob Hayes, Vice Chair
Suzanne Mineck, President
Mission is to serve as a partner and catalyst for improving the health of vulnerable people in greater Des Moines.

2827 Principal Financial Group Foundation
711 High St
Des Moines, IA 50392   515-247-5111
                              800-986-3343
                              Fax: 515-235-5724
Larry Zimpleman, Chairman/ President/ CEO
Daniel J. Houston, President - Retirement, Insuranc
James P. McCaughan, President - Principal Global Inv
The Principal Financial Group is a leading global financial company offering businesses, individuals and industrial clients a wide range of financial products and services.

2828 Siouxland Community Foundation
505 5th St
Suite 412
Sioux City, IA 51101-1507   712-293-3303
                                   Fax: 712-293-3303
                                   office@siouxlandcommunityfoundation.org
                                   www.siouxlandcommunityfoundation.org
Richard J. Dehner, President
Robert F. Meis, Vice President
Marilyn J. Hagberg, Secretary
The Siouxland Community Foundation strives to enhance the quality of life in the greater Siouxland tri-state area by seeking charitable gifts to build permanent endowments as charitable capital for the community, providing a flexable vehicle to receive and distribute gifts of any size, making grants in response to community needs, and providing services that will help shape the well-being of Siouxland.

Kansas

2829   Arc of Kansas
2701 SW Randolph Ave
Topeka, KS 66611-1536
785-232-0597
Fax: 785-232-3770
info@tarcinc.org
www.tarcinc.org

Barbara Duncan, President
Matthew Bergman, Vice President
Travis Stryker, Secretary
Organzation works to ensure that the estimated 7.2 million Americans with intellectual and developmental disabilities have the services and supports they need to grow, develop, and live in communities across the nation.

2830   Hutchinson Community Foundation
1 North Main, Suite 501
PO Box 298
Hutchinson, KS 67504-0298
620-663-5293
Fax: 620-663-9277
info@hutchcf.org
www.hutchcf.org

Aubrey Abbot Patterson, President and Executive Director
Terri L. Eisiminger, Vice President of Administration
Janet Hamilton, Community Investment Officer
Connects donors to community needs and opportunities, increases philanthropy and provides community leadership.

2831   Richard W Higgins Charitable Foundation
Marshall & Ilsley Trust of Florida
2520 South Iowa
Ste 100
Lawrence, KS 66046-2713
877-202-9234
www.applebees.com

Ken Krei, President
Jessica James, Executive Chef
Patrick Humphrey, Executive Chef
Gives primarily for medical research with geographical focus on New York and Florida.

Kentucky

2832   Arc of Kentucky
706 E. Main Street
Suite A
Frankfort, KY 40601-2408
502-875-5225
800-281-1272
Fax: 502-875-5226
arcofky@aol.com
arcofky.org

James Cheely, President
Patty Dempsey, Executive Director
Ellen Nicholson, Secretary
The Arc of Kentucky works to ensure a quality of life for children and adults with intellectual and developmental disabilities to help in securing a positive future. The Arc values services and supports that enhance the quality of life through independence, friendship, choice and respect for individuals with intellectual and developmental disabilities.

Louisiana

2833   Arc of Louisiana
606 Colonial Dr
Ste G
Baton Rouge, LA 70714-6535
225-383-1033
866-966-6260
Fax: 225-383-1092
info@thearcla.org
www.thearcla.org

Larry Pete, President
Henry Friloux, Vice President
Kelly Serrett, Executive Director

The Arc of Louisiana advocates for and with individuals with intellectual and developmental disabilities and their families that they shall live to their fullest potential.

2834   Baton Rouge Area Foundation
402 N 4th St
Baton Rouge, LA 70802-5506
225-387-6126
877-387-6126
Fax: 225-387-6153
mverma@braf.org
www.braf.org

C. Kris Kirkpatrick, Chair
S. Dennis Blunt, Vice Chair
John G. Davies, President/CEO
The Foundation provides grants to nonprofits to make lives better in the region. It also takes on projects, often with parters, to remake Baton Rouge.

2835   Community Foundation of Shreveport-Bossier
401 Edwards St
Ste 105
Shreveport, LA 71101-5551
318-221-0582
Fax: 318-221-7463
info@cfnla.org
www.cfnla.org

Janie D. Richardson, Chairman
Thomas H. Murphy, Vice Chairman
Terry C. Davis, Ph.D, Secretary
Provides a variety of charitable funds and gift options to help our partners achieve their vision for a stronger, more vibrant community. By bringing together fund donors, their financial advisors and non profit agencies, the Foundation is a powerful catalyst for building charitable giving and effecting positive change in our area

Maine

2836   BCR Foundation
83 Mussey Rd.
Scarborough, ME 04074
207-883-8000
800-227-6111
Fax: 207-883-0100
solutions@bcr.net

Specializes on the delivery of a variety of telecommunications products and services to include digital and VoIP telephone systems, voicemail systems, computer-telephone applications, and the installation of data, voice and video cabling.

2837   No Limits Foundation
265 Centre Dr.
Wales, ME 04280
207-569-6411
info@nolimitsfoundation.org
www.nolimitsfoundation.org

Mary Leighton, Founder & Executive Director
Kelsey Moody, Program Operations Manager
Alix Sandler, Marketing & Development Director
Non-profit organization offering camps for children with limb loss and differences.

2838   UNUM Charitable Foundation
Maine Association of Non Profits
565 Congress St
Ste 301
Portland, ME 04101-3308
207-871-1885
Fax: 207-780-0346
Manp@NonprofitMaine.org
www.nonprofitmaine.org

Doug Woodbury, Board President
Ted Scontras, Board Vice President
Joan Smith, Board Treasurer
The Foundation encourages projects that: stimulate others in the private or public sector to participate in problem solving; advance innovative and cost-effective approaches for addressing defined, recognized needs; and demonstrate ability to obtain future project funding, if needed. The foundation generally limits its consideration of capital campaign requests to the Greater Portland, Maine area.

Maryland

2839 American Health Assistance Foundation
22512 Gateway Center Dr
Clarksburg, MD 20871-2005
301-948-3244
800-437-2423
Fax: 301-258-9454
info@brightfocus.org
www.brightfocus.org

Stacy Pagos Haller, President / CEO
Donna Callison, Vice President of Development
Michael Buckley, Vice President of Public Affairs
The American Health Assistance Foundation (AHAF) is a registered non-profit organization that funds research into cures for Alzheimer's disease, macular degeneration and glaucoma, and provides the public with informarnion about risk factors, preventative lifestyles, availiable treatments and coping strategies.

2840 American Occupational Therapy Foundation
4720 Montgomery Lane
Suite 202
Bethesda, MD 20814-3449
240-292-1079
Fax: 240-396-6188
aotf@aotf.org
aotf.org

Diana L. Ramsay, Chair
Wendy J. Coster, Vice Chair
Scott Campbell, CEO
AOFT provides advanced research, education and public awareness for occupational therapy, so that all people may participate fully in life regardless of their physical, social, mental or developmental circumstances.

2841 Arc of Maryland
121 Cathedral St, 2B
PO Box 1747
Annapolis, MD 21401- 1747
410-571-9320
888-272-3449
Fax: 410-974-6021
info@thearcmd.org
www.thearcmd.org

Richard Dean, President
Aileen O'Hare, Vice President
Annette Hinkle, Treasurer
The Arc of Maryland works to create a world where children and adults with cognitive and developmental disabilities have and enjoy equal rights and opportunities.

2842 Baltimore Community Foundation
2 E Read Street
Floor 9
Baltimore, MD 21202-6903
410-332-4171
Fax: 410-837-4701
questions@bcf.org
www.bcf.org

Raymond L. Bank, Chair
Tedd Alexander, Vice Chair
Laura L. Gamble, Vice Chair
Makes grants in Baltimore City and Baltimore County; see website for how to apply. BCF is governed by a 30-member board of trustees, made up of a cross section of Baltimore.

2843 Candlelighters Childhood Cancer Foundation
10920 Connecticut Ave.
PO Box 498
Kensington, MD 20895- 0498
301-962-3520
855-858-2226
Fax: 301-962-3521
staff@acco.org
www.acco.org

Naomi Bartley, President
Janine Lynne, Vice President
Ken Phillips, Treasurer
An international organization providing information and support, and advocacy to parents of children with cancer and survivors of childhood cancer.Health and Education professionals also welcome as members.Network of local support groups. Information on disabilities related to treatment of childhood cancer. Publications.

2844 Children's Fresh Air Society Fund
Baltimore Community Foundation
2 E Read St
Baltimore, MD 21202-2470
410-332-4171
Fax: 410-837-4701
grants@bcf.org
bcf.org

Tom E. Wilcox, President
Danista Hunte, Vice President, Community Invest
Ralph M. Serpe, CFRE, Vice President, Development
Makes grants to nonprofit camps to provide tuition for disadvantaged and disabled Maryland children to attend summer camp. See website for how to apply.

2845 Clark-Winchcole Foundation
3 Bethesda Metro Ctr
Suite 550
Bethesda, MD 20814-5358
301-654-3607

Laura Phillips, President
Supported tax-exempt charitable organizations operating in the metropolitan area of Washington, DC in the following areas: deaf, higher education and physically disabled.

2846 Columbia Foundation
10630 Little Patuxent Parkway
Century Plaza, Suite 315
Columbia, MD 21044
410-730-7840
Fax: 410-997-6021
www.cfhoco.org

Bruce Harvey, Chair
Joseph Maranto, Vice Chair
Barb Van Winkle, Secretary
The Columbia Foundation serves as a catalyst for building a more caring, creative and effective community in Howard County by promoting and creating opportunities for personal and corporate philanthropy, managing endowments, anticipating and responding to community needs, and strategically granting funds.

2847 Corporate Giving Program
Ryland Group
11000 Broken Land Pkwy
Columbia, MD 21044
410-715-7022
800-267-0998
Fax: 410-715-7909

Bruce N Haas, President
Contributions of equipment, volunteers and financial support to organizations working to meet the challenges and needs of modern society.

2848 Cystic Fibrosis Foundation
6931 Arlington Rd
2nd floor
Bethesda, MD 20814-5200
301-951-4422
800-344-4823
Fax: 301-951-6378
info@cff.org
www.cff.org

Catherine C. McLoud, Board Chair
Robert J. Beall, Ph.D., President/Chief Executive Office
C. Richard Mattingly, Executive Vice President/Chief O
The mission of the Cystic Fibrosis Foundation, a nonprofit donor-supported organization is to assure the development of the means to cure and control cystic fibrosis and to improve the quality of life for those with the disease.

2849 Foundation Fighting Blindness
7168 Columbia Gateway Dr.
Suite 100
Columbia, MD 21046
410-423-0600
800-683-5555
TTY: 410363713951
info@FightBlindness.org
www.blindness.org

William T. Schmidt, Chief Executive Officer
Valerie Navy-Daniels, Chief Development Officer
Stephen M. Rose, PhD, Chief Research Officer
The Foundation Fighting Blindness (FFB) works to promote research in order to prevent, treat and restore vision. FFB is currently the world's leading private funder of retinal disease research, funding over 100 research grants and 150 researchers.

2850 George Wasserman Family Foundation
Grossberg Company
6707 Democracy Blvd
Suite 300
Bethesda, MD 20817-1176 301-571-4977
Fax: 301-571-6250

Helen Salud, Manager
Anthony Cpa, Partner

2851 Giant Food Foundation
8301 Professional Pl
Ste 115
Landover, MD 20785-2351 301-341-4100
888-469-4426
jmiller@giantfood.com
www.giantfood.com

Anthony Hucker, President
Brian Beatty, Md. Director of Marketing and Ex
Stefanie Cain, Md. District Director
Offers grants in the areas of mental health, recreation, community and cultural programs, art, and educational programs for the health and prosperity of the greater Washington area.

2852 Harry and Jeanette Weinberg Foundation
7 Park Center Ct
Owings Mills, MD 21117-4200 410-654-8500
Fax: 410-654-4900
cdemchak@hjweinberg.org
hjweinbergfoundation.org

Ellen M. Heller, Chair
Barry I. Schloss, Treasurer
Alvin Awaya, Vice-President
The Harry & Jeanette Weinberg Foundation, Inc. is dedicated to assisting the poor, primarily through operating and capital grants to direct service organizations located in Baltimore, Hawaii, Northeastern Pennsylvania, New York, Israel and the Former Soviet Union. These grants are focused on meeting basic needs such as shelter, nutrition, health & socialization & on enhancing an individual's ability to meet those needs. Within that focus, emphasis is placed on the elderly & Jewish community.

2853 Immune Deficiency Foundation
110 West Rd.
Suite 300
Towson, MD 21204 800-296-4433
Fax: 410-321-9165
info@primaryimmune.org
primaryimmune.org

Jorey Berry, President & Chief Executive Officer
Sarah Rose, Chief Financial Officer
Katherine Antilla, Vice President, Education
The Immune Deficiency Foundation is the national patient organization dedicated to improving the diagnosis, treatment, and quality of life of persons with primary immunodeficiency diseases through advocacy, education, and research.

2854 Kennedy Krieger Institute
707 North Broadway
Baltimore, MD 21205 443-923-9200
800-873-3377
888-554-9400
TTY: 443-923-2645
findaspecialist@kennedykrieger.org
www.kennedykrieger.org

Gary W. Goldstein, MD
Internationally recognized for improving the lives of children and adolescents with disorders and injuries of the brain, spinal cord and musculoskeletal system, the Kennedy Krieger Institute serves more than 20,000 individuals each year through inpatient and outpatient clincs, home and community services and school-based programs. Kennedy Krieger provides a wide range of services for children and young adults with developmental concerns mid to severe, and is home to a team of investigators.

2855 Miracle-Ear Children's Foundation
5000 Cheshire Ln N
Minneapolis, MN 55446-3706 763-268-4000
800-464-8002
Fax: 763-268-4365
www.miracle-ear.com/en-us/

Nonprofit organization that provides hearing aids to children whose families to not qualify for public assistance. Provides hearing aid fittings and follow-up care and services free of charge through Miracle-Ear Hearing Centers. Provides information on alternative communication. Offers educational materials and brochures.

2856 National Federation of the Blind
200 E. Wells St.
at Jernigan Place
Baltimore, MD 21230 410-659-9314
Fax: 410-685-5653
nfb@nfb.org
nfb.org

Mark A. Riccobono, President
John Berggren, Executive Director, Operations
Anil Lewis, Executive Director, Blindness Initiatives
The National Federation of the Blind (NFB) works to help blind people achieve self-confidence, self-respect and self-determination and to achieve complete integration into society on a basis of equality. The Federation provides public educations, information and referral services, scholarships, literature and publications, adaptive equipment, advocacy services, legal services, employment assistance and more.

2857 Optometric Extension Program Foundation
2300 York Road
Suite 113
Timonium, MD 21093 410-561-3791
Fax: 949-250-8157
Kelin.Kushin@oep.org
www.oepf.org

Paul A. Harris, OD, President
Robin Lewis, OD, Vice President
Kelin Kushin, Executive Director
Vision care for learning disabilities and head trauma patients.

2858 Sjogren's Syndrome Foundation
6707 Democracy Blvd
Suite 325
Bethesda, MD 20817-1164 301-530-4420
800-475-6473
Fax: 301-530-4415
tms@sjogrens.org
www.sjogrens.org

Kenneth Economou, Chairman of the Board
Stephen Cohen, OD, Chairman-Elect
Vidya Sankar, DMD, MHS, Treasurer
Provides patients practical information and coping strategies that minimize the effects of Sjogren's syndrome. In addition, the Foundation is the clearinghouse for medical information and is the recognized national advocate for Sjogren's syndrome. *$25.00 Monthly*

2859 The ACNM Foundation, Inc.
American College of Nurse Midwives
8403 Colesville Rd.
Suite 1230
Silver Spring, MD 20910 240-485-1800
Fax: 240-485-1818
membership@acnm.org
midwife.org

Holly Powell Kennedy, President
Mary K. Collins, Vice President
Susan DeJoy, Treasurer
Charitable foundation of the American College of Nurse Midwives.

Massachusetts

2860 Abbot and Dorothy H Stevens Foundation
P.O. Box 111
North Andover, MA 01845 978-688-7211
Fax: 978-686-1620

Josh Miner, Executive Director
Established in 1953, Purpose is giving primarily to the arts, education, conservation, and health and human services.

2861 **Arc of Massachusetts, The**
217 South St
Waltham, MA 02453-2710   781-891-6270
                                  Fax: 781-891-6271
                              arcmass@arcmass.org
                                  www.arcmass.org

Leo Sarkissian, Executive Director
Joshua Komyerox, Government Affairs Director
Brenda Asis, Development Director
Quarterly newsletter for The Arc of Massachusetts is Advocate.

2862 **Arc of Northern Bristol County**
141 Park St
Attleboro, MA 02703-3020   508-226-1445
                                     888-343-3301
                                  Fax: 508-226-1476
                                  info@arcnbc.org
                                       arcnbc.org

Richard Harwood, Chairperson
Valerie Zagami, Vice Chairperson
Paul Oliveira, Treasurer
Mission is to strive for the right of all people with developmental
disabilities to be valued as individuals, to experience choice, and
to be fully included in all aspects of community life

2863 **Boston Foundation**
75 Arlington St
10th Fl
Boston, MA 02116-3992   617-338-1700
                                  Fax: 617-338-1604
                                          tbf.org

Michael Keating, Esq., Chair
Catherine D'Amato, Vice Chair
Paul S. Grogan, President & CEO
The Foundation's grantmaking, special initiatives and civic leadership promote innovation across a broad range of compelling
community issues, from educational excellence to affordable
housing to workforce development and the arts.

2864 **Boston Globe Foundation**
P.O. Box 55819
Boston, MA 02205-5819   617-929-2000
                                  bostonglobe.com

Mary Jacobus, President
The mission of the Boston Globe Foundation is to empower community-based organizations to effect real change in the ares of
greatest need, where the Globe is uniquely postioned to add the
most value. Priority focus areas: strengthen the reading, writing
and critical thinking of young people, while fostering their inherent love of learning. Strengthen the roads that link people to culture. Strengthen the civic fabric of the city. Be responsive to the
needs of our immediate community.

2865 **Bushrod H Campbell and Ada F Hall Charity Fund**
Palmer & Dodge
111 Huntington Ave
Boston, MA 02199-7610   617-239-0540
                                  Fax: 617-227-4420

Brenda Taylor, Foundation Administrator
The fund's areas of interest include organizations and/or their
projects supporting aid to the elderly, healthcare and population
control. Medical research grants are administered through the
Medical Foundation. No grants are awarded to individuals and
the geographical area of support is limited to organizations located in Massachusetts within the area of Boston and Route 128.

2866 **Clipper Ship Foundation**
77 Summer St
8th Floor
Boston, MA 02110-1006   617-391-3088
                                  Fax: 617-426-7087
                          hblaisdell@gmafoundations.com
                              clippershipfoundation.org

Ron Ancrum, President
Makes grants to federally tax-qualified non-profit organizations
offering human services to individuals living in Greater Boston
and the cities of Lawrence and Brockton.

2867 **Community Foundation of Western Massachusetts**
1500 Main Street, Suite 2300
P.O. Box 15769
Springfield, MA 01115-5769   413-732-2858
                                  Fax: 413-733-8565
                          wmass@communityfoundation.org
                              www.communityfoundation.org

Katie Allan Zobel, President and CEO
Nancy Reiche, M.S.W., Vice President for Programs
Donna Roseman David, Chief Financial Officer/Chief Ad
Provides a simple way to achieve the charitable objectives of donors most effectively; supports nonprofit organizations that offer
programs in the arts, education, human services, healthcare,
housing, and the environment; and works to improve the quality
of life in our region.

2868 **Frank R and Elizabeth Simoni Foundation**
1401 Boston Providence Tpke
Norwood, MA 02062-5053   781-762-3449
                                  Fax: 781-769-6166

Matthew Mac Donald, President
Ann Mac Donald, Secretary
Robert Mac Donald, Clerk

2869 **Friendly Ice Cream Corp Contributions Program**
1855 Boston Rd
Wilbraham, MA 01095-1002   413-543-3544
                                     800-966-9970
                                  Fax: 413-731-4467
                                       friendlys.com

John Maguire, Chief Financial Officer
Steve Weigel, EVP, Chief Operating Officer
Pat Hickey, EVP, Chief Financial Officer

2870 **Greater Worcester Community Foundation**
370 Main St
Ste 650
Worcester, MA 01608-1738   508-755-0980
                                  Fax: 508-755-3406
                              info@greaterworcester.org
                                  greaterworcester.org

Gerald Gaudette III, Chair
Warner S. Fletcher, Vice Chair
Thomas J. Bartholomew, Treasurer
By focusing on the entire community rather then on any specific
issue, the community foundation is able to address matters of
greater importance to the people of the region. The Foundation
has built a permanent, flexable endowment and has distributed
grants and awards to a broad range of organizations and people
throughout the region.

2871 **Hyams Foundation**
50 Federal St
9th Floor
Boston, MA 02110   617-426-5600
                                  Fax: 617-426-5696
                              info@hyamsfoundation.org
                                  hyamsfoundation.org

Martella Wilson-Taylor, Chair
Angela Brown, Director of Programs
Mike Givens, Communications Manager
The mission of the foundation is to increase economic and social
stregnth within low-income communities in Boston and Chelsea,
Massachusetts. Some areas they provide funding to include com-
munity identified issues, racial justice and transitional funding.

2872 **Raytheon Company Contributions Program**
870 Winter St
Waltham, MA 02451-1449   781-522-3000
                                  Fax: 781-860-2172
                                       raytheon.com

Thomas A. Kennedy, Chief Financial Officer
David C. Wajsgras, Senior Vice President and Chief
Keith J. Peden, Senior Vice President - Human Re
Industry leader in defense and government electronics, space, in-
formation technology, technical services, and business aviation
and special mission aircraft.

2873 TJX Foundation
TJX Companies
770 Cochituate Rd
Framingham, MA 01701-4666 508-390-1000
Fax: 508-390-2091
www.tjx.com

Carol Meyrowitz, CEO
The purpose of the TJX Foundation's Giving Program is to support qualified, tax-exempt nonprofit organizations that provide services which promote and improve the quality of life for children, women and families in need.

2874 The Beveridge Family Foundation, Inc.
3 Upland Ln.
West Newbury, MA 01985 800-229-9667
administrator@beveridge.org
www.beveridge.org

Ward Slocum Caswell, President
Philip Caswell, Chairman and Vice President
Ruth S. DuPont, Treasurer
The mission of The Frank Stanley Beveridge Foundation, Inc. is to preserve and enhance the quality of life by embracing and perpetuating Frank Stanley Beveridge's philanthropic vision through grantmaking initiatives in support of The Stanley Park of Westfield, Inc. and programs in youth development, health, education, religion, art, and environment primarily in Hampden and Hampshire Counties, Massachusetts.

2875 Vision Foundation
8901 Strafford Cir
Knoxville, TN 37923-1500 865-357-4603
Fax: 865-690-9322

Gordon Adams, President
Offers counseling, support groups, seminars and transportation for the blind providing 600 members.

Michigan

2876 Ann Arbor Area Community Foundation
301 N Main St
Ste 300
Ann Arbor, MI 48104-1296 734-663-0401
Fax: 734-663-3514
info@aaacf.org
aaacf.org

Michelle Crumm, Chair
Tim Wadhams, Vice Chair
Neel Hajra, President & CEO
Interested in funding projects which will improve the quality of life for citizens of the Ann Arbor area. Eligible projects generally fall within these categories: education, culture, social service, community development, environmental awareness and health and wellness. The Foundation aims to support creative approaches to community needs and problems by making grants which will benefit the widest possible range of people.

2877 Arc of Michigan
State of Michigan
1325 S Washington Ave
Lansing, MI 48910-1652 517-487-5426
800-292-7851
Fax: 517-487-0303
dhoyle@arcmi.org
arcmi.org

Shari Fitzpatrick, President
Kim Brown, Vice President
Bob Altizer, Secretary
The Arc Michigan empowers local chapters to assure that citizens with disabilities are valued and that they and their families participate fully in and contribute to the life of their community.

2878 Berrien Community Foundation
2900 S State St
Ste 2e
Saint Joseph, MI 49085-2467 269-983-3304
Fax: 269-983-4939
bcf@BerrienCommunity.org
berriencommunity.org

Hillary Bubb, Chair
Mabel Mayfield, Vice Chair
Lisa Cripps-Downey, President
The Foundation is a union of numerous gifts, bequests and other contributions that form permanent endowments and other funds.

2879 Blind Children's Fund
P.O. Box 187
Grand Ledge, MI 48837 517-488-4887
www.blindchildrensfund.org

Carrie L Owens, Board President
Diana Popp, Executive Director
Provides parents and professionals information materials and resources to help them teach and nurture blind and visually impaired children so they may reach their potential.

2880 Community Foundation of Monroe County
P.O. Box 627
28 S. Macomb St.
Monroe, MI 48161-627 734-242-1976
Fax: 734-242-1234
info@cfmonroe.org
cfmonroe.org

Kathleen Russeau, MBA, Executive Director
Michele Sandiefer, Office Manager
Julie Rhinehart, YAC Coordinator
The mission of the Community Foundation of Monroe County is to encourage and facilitate philanthropy in Monroe County.

2881 Cowan Slavin Foundation
7881 Dell Rd
Saline, MI 48176-9744 734-944-1439
Fax: 734-944-3529

David Bovee, Owner

2882 Daimler Chrysler
Automobility Program
P.O. Box 5080
Troy, MI 48007-5080 800-255-9877
Fax: 855-409-0475
rebates@chrysler.com
Provides a cash reimbursement to assist in reducing the cost of adaptive driving equipment and conversion aids installed on new model Daimler Chrysler LLC vehicles. Up to a maximum of $1000 on Dodge Caravan, Grand Caravan, and Chrysler Town and Country vans and up to $750 on all other vehicles.

2883 Frank & Mollie S VanDervoort Memorial Foundation
4646 Okemos Rd
Okemos, MI 48864-1795 517-349-7232

Ann L Gessert, Secretary

2884 Fremont Area Community Foundation
4424 W. 48th Street
PO Box B
Fremont, MI 49412-176 231-924-5350
Fax: 231-924-5351
tfacf.org

Robert Zeldenrust, Chair
William Johnson, Vice Chair
Carla Roberts, President & CEO
A local nonprofit organization serving the residence of Newaygo County. We connect the needs of the community with those who have the conviction to make a lasting impact. Our mission is to improve the quality of life for the people of Newaygo County.Zeldenrust

2885   Grand Rapids Foundation
185 Oakes St SW
Grand Rapids, MI 49503-4008   616-454-1751
                                          Fax: 616-454-6455
                                          grfound@grfoundation.org
                                          grfoundation.org
Paul M. Keep, Chair
Laurie Finney Beard, Vice Chair
Diana R. Sieger, President
Grand Rapids Community Foundation leads the community in making positive, sustainable change. Through our grantmaking and leadership initiatives we help foster academic achievement, build economic prosperity, achieve healthy ecosystems, encourage healthy people, support social enrichment, and create vibrant neighborhoods.

2886   Granger Foundation
6267 Aurelius Rd
Lansing, MI 48911-2187   517-393-1670
                                          Fax: 517-393-1382
                                          grangerconstruction.com
Alton Granger, Chairman
Glenn D. Granger, President & CEO
The primary purpose of the Granger Foundation is to enhance the quality of life within the Greater Lansing, Michigan Area. Our mission is to support Christ-centered activities. We also support efforts that enhance the lives of youth in our community.

2887   Harvey Randall Wickes Foundation
4800 Fashion Square Blvd
Suite 472
Saginaw, MI 48604- 2677   989-799-1850
                                          Fax: 989-799-3327
                                          www.tgci.com
James Finkbeiner
Grants for rehabilitation.

2888   Havirmill Foundation
3505 Greenleaf Blvd
Ste 203
Kalamazoo, MI 49008-2580   269-375-1193
                                          millenniumrestaurants.com
Ken Miller, CEO, Principal Partner
Matthew Burian, President
Bob Lewis, Operating Partner

2889   Kelly Services Foundation
999 W Big Beaver Rd
Troy, MI 48084-4782   248-362-4444
                                          Fax: 248-244-4588
                                          kfirst@kellyservices.com
                                          kellyservices.com
George S. Corona, Chief Operating Officer
Carl T. Camden, President & CEO
Terence E. Adderley, Executive Chairman

2890   Kent County Arc
2922 Fuller Ave. NE
Ste 201
Grand Rapids, MI 49505   616-459-3339
                                          Fax: 401-737-8907
                                          info@arckent.org
                                          www.arckent.org
Pam Cross, President
Tim Lundgren, Vice-President
Tammy Finn, Executive Director
Providing individuals with disabilties meaningful opportunities throughout their communities.

2891   Kresge Foundation
3215 W Big Beaver Rd
Troy, MI 48084-2818   248-643-9630
                                          Fax: 248-643-0588
                                          info@kresge.org
                                          kresge.org
Rip Rapson, President and CEO
Amy B. Coleman, VP/ CFO
Ariel H. Simon, Vice President, Chief Program
This foundation offers challenge grants for capital projects, most often for construction or renovation of buildings, but also for the purchase of major equipment and real estate. As challenge grants,

they are intended to stimulate new, private gifts in the midst of an organized fund raising effort. Offers special opportunities to build capacity, both in providing enhanced facilities in which to present programs and in generating private support. Only charitable organizations may apply.

2892   Lanting Foundation
1575 S Shore Dr
Holland, MI 49423-4436   616-335-2033
Arlyn Lanting, Partner

2893   Rollin M Gerstacker Foundation
PO Box 1945
Midland, MI 48641-1945   989-631-6097
                                          www.gerstackerfoundation.org
Gail E. Lanphear, Chairperson
Lisa J. Gerstacker, President
E. N. Brandt, Vice President /Secretary
The Rollin M. Gerstacker Foundation was founded by Mrs. Eda U. Gerstacker in 1957, in memory of her husband. Its primary purpose is to carry on, indefinitely, financial aid to charities of all types supported by Mr. and Mrs. R.M. Gerstacker during their lifetimes. These charities are concentrated in the states of Michigan and Ohio.

2894   Steelcase Foundation
PO Box 1967
GH-4E
Grand Rapids, MI 49501-1967   616-246-4695
                                          Fax: 616-475-2200
                                          foundation@Steelcase.com
                                          steelcase.com
Julie Ridenour, President
The Foundation focuses on the areas of human service, health, education, community development, the arts and the environment; giving particular concern to people who are disadvantaged, disabled, young and elderly as they attempt to improve the quality of their lives.
1951

Minnesota

2895   Arc of Minnesota
800 Transfer Road
Suite 7A
St. Paul, MN 55114   651-523-0823
                                          800-582-5256
                                          Fax: 651-523-0829
                                          mail@arcmn.org
                                          www.arcmn.org
John Rentschler, President
Lisa Schoneman, Vice President
Amy Hewitt, Secretary
Your membership in The Arc of Minnesotta benefits persons with developmental disabilities and their families as they live, learn, work and play. Please join today!

2896   Burnett Foundation
P.O. Box 633
Northfield, MN 55057-6881   817-877-3344
                                          tomburnettfamilyfoundation@msn.com
                                          www.tomburnettfoundation.org
V Neils Agather, Executive Director

2897   Deluxe Corporation Foundation
Deluxe Corporation
3680 Victoria St N
Shoreview, MN 55126-2966   651-483-7111
                                          800-328-0304
                                          Fax: 651-483-7270
                                          feedback@deluxe.com
                                          ww.deluxe.com
Lee J Schram, CEO
Terry D. Peterson, CFO /Senior VP
Malcolm J. McRoberts, Senior Vice President, Small Bus
Funds programs such as schools, museums, programs for the disadvantaged. We believe programs and services like these represent the heart and soul of our communities.

2898 General Mills Foundation
P.O. Box 9452
Minneapolis, MN 55440-9452   800-248-7310
                                    Fax: 763-764-8330
                    corporate.response@genmills.com
                                    generalmills.com

Kendall J. Powell, Chairman / CEO
Ann W.H. Simonds, Senior Vice President/ Chief Mar
Keith A Woodward, Vice President, Treasurer

2899 Hugh J Andersen Foundation
342 5th Ave N
Suite 200
Bayport, MN 55003-4502   651-439-1557
                                    888-439-9508
                                    Fax: 651-439-9480
                                    contact@srinc.biz
                                    www.srinc.biz

Brad Kruse, Program Director
Established in 1962, this fund is a nonprofit charitable corporation classified as a private foundation. The Foundation was established as a general charitable fund, but now identifies projects that build individual and community capacity to be a priority. Giving is focused primarily in the counties of Washington, Minnesota, & St, Croix, Polk and Pierce of Wl. Grants are given in the areas of human services, health, education, arts and culture, community services and the environment.

2900 James R Thorpe Foundation
5866 Oakland Avenue
Minneapolis, MN 55417-5418   763-250-9304
                    info@jamesrthorpefoundation.org
                    www.jamesrthorpefoundation.org

Tim Thorpe, President
Robert C. Cote, Treasurer
Kerrie Blevins, Foundation Manager
Foundation based on values of respect and compassion, and is dedicated to making the greater Minneapolis area better for all its citizens.

2901 Jay and Rose Phillips Family Foundation
615 First Ave. NE
Ste. 330
Minneapolis, MN 55413   612-623-1654
                                    Fax: 612-623-1653
                    info@phillipsfamilyfoundationmn.org

Patrick Troska, Executive Director
Joel Luedtke, Senior Program Officer
Tracy Lamparty, Grants and Operations Manager

2902 Minneapolis Foundation
80 S 8th St
800 IDS Center
Minneapolis, MN 55402-2100   612-672-3878
                                    866-305-0543
                                    Fax: 612-672-3846
                    email@mplsfoundation.org
                    www.mplsfoundation.org

Sandra L. Vargus, President and CEO
Jean M. Adams, Chief Operating Officer/Chief Fi
Teresa Morrow, Vice President, External Relatio
Provides a variety of charitable fund and gift options to help Minnesotans make a difference.

2903 Ordean Foundation
424 W Superior St
Duluth, MN 55802-1591   218-726-4785

Steve Mangan, Executive Director
Grants are given for a variety of purposes including: treatment and rehabilitation for persons who are chronically or temporarily mentally ill, persons whose physical capacity is impaired by injury or illness, promotes mental and physical health of the elderly, provides for youth guidance programs designed to avoid delinquency, and provides relief, aid and charity to people with no or low incomes. Grants are only offered to certain cities and townships near and around St. Louis County/Duluth.

2904 Otto Bremer Foundation
445 Minnesota St
Ste 2250
Saint Paul, MN 55101-2161   651-227-8036
                                    888-291-1123
                                    Fax: 651-312-3665
                                    obf@ottobremer.org
                                    www.ottobremer.org

Kari Suzuki, Director of Operations
Diane Benjamin, Executive Director
Danielle Cheslog, Grants Manager
Mission is to assist people in achieving full economic, civic and social participation in and for the betterment of their communities.

2905 Rochester Area Foundation
400 South Broadway
Suite 300
Rochester, MN 55904   507-282-0203
                                    Fax: 507-282-4938
                                    info@rochesterarea.org
                                    rochesterarea.org

JoAnn Stormer, President
Max Evans, Administration/Communications
Ann Fahy-Gust, Grants and Impact Officer
The mission of the Rochester Area Foundation is to strengthen community philanthropy by promoting responsible and informed giving and to assist donors in meeting their charitable objectives.

Mississippi

2906 Arc of Mississippi
704 North President Street
Jackson, MS 39202   601-355-0220
                                    800-717-1180
                                    Fax: 601-355-0221
                                    info@arcms.org
                                    www.arcms.org

Kim Duffy, President
Ronnie Raggio, Senior Vice-President
Shirley Miller, Secretary
The Arc is Committed to securing for all people with developmental disabilities the opportunity to choose and realize their goals of where and how they learn live work and play.

Missouri

2907 Allen P & Josephine B Green Foundation
1055 Broadway
Suite 130
Kansas City, MO 64105   816-627-3420
                                    Fax: 816-268-3420
                    greenfoundation@gkccf.org
                                    www.greenfdn.org

Matthew Fuller, Manager of Community Investment
While the Foundation makes grants in a variety of fields, in the past its major support was in the field of medical research. During a 20-year period, 1951-71, it contributed over $900,000 to research in Parkinson's and related diseases of the nervous system; $600,000 for research in pediatric neurology and lesser amounts in other areas of medical research, but the board is now trending in other directions. Grants are limited to Missouri and none are offered to individuals.

2908 Anheuser-Busch
1 Busch Pl
Saint Louis, MO 63118-1852   314-577-2000
                                    800-342-5283
                                    Fax: 314-577-2900
                                    anheuser-busch.com

August A Busch Iv, President
Supports education, helped fund health and human services organizations, provided disaster relief, and worked to preserve the environment.

2909   Arc of the US Missouri Chapter
PO Box 7823
Columbia, MO 65205   573-552-7648
                                     www.arcofmissouri.org

chapter #42

2910   Greater Kansas City Community Foundation & Affiliated Trusts
1055 Broadway Blvd
Suite 130
Kansas City, MO 64105-1595   816-842-0944
                                     866-719-7886
                                     Fax: 816-842-8079
                                     info@gkccf.org
                                     www.growyourgiving.org

William S. Berkley, Past Chair
Dr. Jim Hinson, Vice Chair
William H. Coughlin, President
Mission is to improve the quality of life in Greater Kansas City by increasing charitable giving, connecting donors to community needs they care about, and providing leadership on critical community issues.

2911   Greater St Louis Community Foundation
319 N 4th St
Ste 300
Saint Louis, MO 63102-1906   314-588-8200
                                     Fax: 314-588-8088

Stephen J. Rafferty, Chair
Thomas R. Collins, Vice Chair & Secretary
Amelia A.J. Bond, President & CEO
To improve the quality of life across the region by helping individuals, families and businesses make a difference through charitable giving.

2912   H&R Block Foundation
1 H and R Block Way
Kansas City, MO 64105-1905   816-854-4363
                                     Fax: 816-854-8025
                                     foundation@hrblock.com
                                     www.blockfoundation.org

Henry W. Bloch, Chairman/ Treasurer/ Director
Thomas M. Bloch, Vice Chairman & Director
David P. Miles, President
A charitable organization under the not-for-profit corporation law of the state of Missouri. Grants are made only to organizations which are tax exempt from Federal Income taxation and which are not classified as private foundations. Major emphasis is placed in the metropolitan areas of Kansas City, Missouri: and Columbus, Ohio. The goal is to provide proportionately significant support of relatively few activities, as opposed to minor support for a great many.

2913   James S McDonnell Foundation
1034 S Brentwood Blvd
Suite 1850
Saint Louis, MO 63117- 1284   314-721-1532
                                     Fax: 314-721-7421
                                     info@jsmf.org
                                     jsmf.org

Susan M Fitzpatrick, President
John T. Bruer, President Emeritus
Cheryl A. Washington, Grants Manager
The Foundation supports scientific, educational, and charitable causes locally, nationally and internationally.

2914   Lutheran Charities Foundation of St Louis
8860 Ladue Road
Suite 200
Saint Louis, MO 63124   314-231-2244
                                     Fax: 314-727-7688
                                     info@lutheranfoundation.org
                                     www.lutheranfoundation.org

Karl A. Dunajcik, Chairperson of the Board
Ann L. Vazquez, President/ CEO
Melinda K. McAliney, Program Director
Seeks the improved care of people in the greater St. Louis metropolitan region. Lutheran Foundation of St. Louis manages the endowment established upon the sale of the Lutheran Medical Center and provides grant awards for health, human care, Lu-

theran congregations' community service programs, and Lutheran education.

2915   RA Bloch Cancer Foundation
1 H and R Block Way
Kansas City, MO 64105-1905   816-854-5050
                                     800-433-0464
                                     Fax: 816-854-8024
                                     hotline@blochcancer.org
                                     www.blochcancer.org

Vangie Rich, Executive Director
Rosanne Wickman, Hotline Director
Provides a hotline that matches newly diagnosed cancer patients with someone who has survived the same kind of cancer. Offers free infomration, resources and support groups, and distributes lists of multidisciplinary second opinion centers. Also supplies three books at no charge: Fighting Cancer; Cancer... There's Hope; and A Guide for Cancer Supporters. All services and books are free of charge.

2916   Victor E Speas Foundation
10434 Indiana Ave
Kansas City, MO 64137-1532   816-868-9300
                                     mo.grantmaking@ustrust.com
                                     www.bankofamerica.com

Latricia Scott Adams, President
VCC is a membership-based organization that brings together area volunteer managers and others interested in volunteerism for mutual support, exchange of ideas and information, and educational programs of timely interest.

Nebraska

2917   Arc of Nebraska
215 Centennial Mall South
Suite 508
Lincoln, NE 68508   402-475-4407
                                     888-519-6524
                                     Fax: 402-475-0214
                                     info@arc-nebraska.org
                                     www.arc-nebraska.org

Debbie Salomon, President
David Rowe, 1st Vice President
Kadi Holmberg, 2nd Vice President
Arc of Nebraska is commited to helping children and adults with disabilities secure the oppurtunity to choose and realize their goals of where and how they learn, live, work, and play.

2918   Cooper Foundation
1248 O St
Suite 870
Lincoln, NE 68508-1493   402-476-7571
                                     Fax: 402-476-2356
                                     info@cooperfoundation.org
                                     cooperfoundation.org

Jack Campbell, Chair
Brad Korell, VP Business Development
Art Thompson, President
Serves only Nebraska with the primary interest in education, arts and humanities and the human services area.

2919   Mosaic
4980 S 118th St
Omaha, NE 68137-2200   402-896-9988
                                     877-366-7242
                                     Fax: 402-896-1511
                                     info@mosaicinfo.org
                                     www.mosaicinfo.org

Linda Timmons, President / CEO
Cindy Schroeder, Chief Financial Officer
Raul Saldivar, Chief Operating Officer
Headquarters for the faith-based organization providing services to people with disabilities in communities nationwide, and in conjunction with international partners. Mosaic was born of a merger of these two Lutheran organizations: Bethpage and Martin Luther Homes Society.

2920 Slosburg Family Charitable Trust
10040 Regency Cir
Ste 200
Omaha, NE 68114-3734 402-391-7900
Fax: 402-391-2991
richdale.com

David Slosburg, Owner

2921 Union Pacific Foundation
1400 Douglas Street
Omaha, NE 68179 402-544-5000
888-870-8777
888-877-7267
Fax: 402-501-0021
www.up.com

John J. Koraleski, Executive Chairman
Lance M. Fritz, President & COO of Union Pacific
Eric L. Butler, EVP, Marketing and Sales
The Union Pacific Foundation is the philanthropic arm of the Union Pacific Corporation and Union Pacific Railroad. Union Pacific believes that the quality of life in the communities in which its employees live and work is an integral part of its own success.

Nevada

2922 EL Wiegand Foundation
165 W Liberty St
Suite 200
Reno, NV 89501-1955 775-333-0310
Fax: 775-333-0314
www.thewiegandfoundationinc.com
Kristen A Avansino, President/Executive Director

2923 Nell J Redfield Foundation
PO Box 61
Reno, NV 89504-0061 775-323-1373
Fax: 775-323-4476
redfieldfoundation@yahoo.com
Jerry Smith, Manager
Gerald C. Smith, V.P. and Secy

2924 William N Pennington Foundation
441 W Plumb Ln
Reno, NV 89509-3766 775-333-9100
Fax: 775-333-9111
William Pennington, Owner

New Hampshire

2925 Agnes M Lindsay Trust
660 Chestnut St
Manchester, NH 03104-3550 603-669-1366
866-669-1366
Fax: 603-665-8114
admin@lindsaytrust.org
lindsaytrust.org
Susan E. Bouchard, Administrative Director
Ernest E. Dion, CPA, Trustee
Alan G. Lampert, Esq., Trustee
Funding for health and wefare organizations, special needs, mental health, blind, deaf and cultural programs to organizations, specifically for capital needs, not operating funds, located in the New England states of Maine, Massachusetts, New Hampshire and Vermont. We highly recommend you visit our web site.

2926 Foundation for Seacoast Health
100 Campus Dr
Ste 1
Portsmouth, NH 03801-5892 603-422-8200
Fax: 603-422-8206
ffsh@communitycampus.org
ffsh.org
Debra S. Grabowski, Executive Director
Kathleen Taylor, Finance Director
Eligio Santana, Facility Manager
Giving limited to Portsmouth, Rye, New Castle, Greenland, Newington, North Hampton, NH; and Kittery, Eliot, and York, ME.

New Jersey

2927 American Migraine Foundation
19 Mantua Rd.
Mount Royal, NJ 08061 856-423-0043
Fax: 856-423-0082
amf@talley.com
www.achenet.org
Lawrence C. Newman, MD, FAHS, Chair
Christine Lay, MD, FAHS, Vice-Chair
Nim Lalvani, MPH, Executive Director
Nonprofit, patient-health, professional partnership dedicated to advancing the treatment and management of headaches and to raising the public awareness of headache as valid, biologically based illness.

2928 Arc of New Jersey
985 Livingston Ave
N Brunswick, NJ 08902-1843 732-246-2525
Fax: 732-214-1834
arcnj.org
Robert Hage, President
Joanne Bergin, First Vice President
Kevin Sturges, Second Vice President
The Arc of New Jersey is committed to enhancing the quality of life of children and adults with intellectual and developmental disabilities and their families, through advocacy, empowerment, education and prevention.

2929 Arnold A Schwartz Foundation
15 Mountain Blvd
Warren, NJ 7059-5611 908-757-7800
Fax: 908-757-8039
Steven A Kunzman, President

2930 Campbell Soup Foundation
1 Campbell Pl
Camden, NJ 08103-1701 800-257-8443
media@campbellsoup.com
campbellsoup.com
Denise M. Morrison, President/ CEO
Anthony P. DiSilvestro, Senior Vice President and Chief
Mark Alexander, President
Goal of this foundation is to match the company's assets with community needs in order to help forge solutions to community challenges. The Foundation believes that involvement at the community level can play a catalytic role in improving the quality of life. Giving is located in the areas of education, nutrition and health, cultural and youth related programs. The major focus of the foundation is on nutrition and health related matters, and places a high priority on Camden, New Jersey areas.

2931 Children's Hopes & Dreams Wish Fulfillment Foundation
280 US Highway 46
Dover, NJ 07801-2084 706-482-2248
Fax: 706-482-2289
Provides continual support for children and their families through the International Pen-Pal Program and the Kid's Kare Packages program. All services are free. Fulfills the last dreams of children with life threatening illnesses.

2932 Community Foundation of New Jersey
35 Knox Hill Road Morristown
PO Box 338
Morristown, NJ 07963-0388 973-267-5533
800-659-5533
Fax: 973-267-2903
info@cfnj.org
www.cfnj.org
Hans Dekker, President
Madeline Rivera, Program Officer
Susan I. Soldivieri, Chief Financial Officer
The Community Foundation of New Jersey is an alliance of families, businesses, and foundations that work together to create lasting differences in lives and communities today and tomorrow.

2933 FM Kirby Foundation
17 DeHart Street
PO Box 151
Morristown, NJ 07963-0151   973-538-4800
                        www.fdncenter.org/grantmaker/kirby
S. Dillard Kirby, President and Director
Jefferson W Kirby, Vice President and Director
Alice Kirby Horton, Assistant Secretary and Director
Family foundation, grants made to a wide range of nonprofit organizations in education, health and medicine, the arts and humanities, civic and public affairs, as well as religious, welfare and youth organizations.

2934 Fannie E Rippel Foundation
14 Maple Avenue
Suite 200
Morristown, NJ 07960   973-540-0101
                              Fax: 973-540-0404
                          info@rippelfoundation.org
                          www.rippelfoundation.org
Laura K Landy, President/ CEO
Chana Fitton, Chief Operating Officer
John D. Campbell, Chairman
Core purposes: research and treatment related to cancer and heart disease, the health of women and the elderly, and the quality of our nation's hospitals.

2935 Fund for New Jersey
One Palmer Square East
Suite 303
Princeton, NJ 08542   609-356-0421
                              fundfornj.org
Kiki Jamieson, President
Lucy Vandenberg, Senior Program Officer
Laura Mandell, Office Manager
Our grants promote projects that share a high purpose of furthering effective democracy through a range of methods encompassing education, advocacy, public policy analysis, and community problem-solving.

2936 Merck Company Foundation
2000 Galloping Hill Road
Kenilworth, NJ 07033   908-740-4000
                              merck.com
Kenneth C. Frazier, Chairman
Robert M. Davis, Executive Vice President and Chi
Willie A. Deese, EVP and President, Merck Manufac
Mission of the foundation is to support organizations and innovative programs in alignment with four strategic profiles: Improving access to quality health care and the appropriate use of medicines and vaccines, building capacity in the biomedical and health sciences, promoting environments that support innovation, economic growth and development in and ethical and fair context, and supporting communities where Merck employees work and live.

2937 Nabisco Foundation
7 Campus Dr
Parsippany, NJ 07054-4413   973-682-7096
                                   Fax: 973-503-3018
Henry Sandbach, Director

2938 Ostberg Foundation
PO Box 1098
Alpine, NJ 07620-1098   201-569-6800
                               Fax: 201-767-8006

2939 Prudential Foundation
Prudential Financial
751 Broad St
15th Floor
Newark, NJ 07102-3714   973-802-6000
                               Fax: 973-802-7486
                     community.resources@prudential.com
                               prudential.com
John R Strangfeld, Chairman and CEO
Mark B. Grier, Vice Chairman
Charles Lowrey, Executive Vice President, Chief
Gives priority to national programs that further our objectives and programs serving areas where The Prudential has a substan-

tial employee presence. Places special emphasis on the home state of New Jersey and the headquarters city, Newark.

2940 Robert Wood Johnson Foundation
Route 1 and College Road East
P.O. Box 2316
Princeton, NJ 08543-2316   609-452-8701
                                  877-843-7953
                             Fax: 888-727-1966
                                  mail@rwjf.org
                                  rwjf.org
Roger S. Fine, Chairman
Risa Lavizzo-Mourey, President and CEO
Robin E. Mockenhaupt, Chief of Staff
Our mission is to assure that all Americans have access to basic health care at reasonable cost, improve care and support for people with chronic health conditions, promote healthy communities and lifestyles and also, reduce the personal, social and economic harm caused by substance abuse.

2941 Victoria Foundation
31 Mulberry Street
5th Floor
Newark, NJ 07102-1397   973-792-9200
                               Fax: 973-792-1300
                          info@victoriafoundation.org
                          www.victoriafoundation.org
Frank Alvarez, President
Margaret H. Parker, Vice President
Gary M. Wingens, Treasurer
Desire is to help individuals in need reach their potential remains. Provides emergency coal for needy families and treated rheumatic fever in children.

New Mexico

2942 Arc of New Mexico
3655 Carlisle NE
Albuquerque, NM 87110-1644   505-883-4630
                                    800-358-6493
                               Fax: 505-883-5564
                               rcostales@arcnm.org
                                    arcnm.org
John Hall, President
Dolores Harden, Senior Vice President
Elaine Palma, Secretary
Our mission is to improve the quality of life for individuals with developmental disabilities of all ages by advocating for equal opportunities and choices in where and how they learn, live, work, play and socialize. The Arc of New Mexico promotes self-determination, healthy families, effective community support systems and partnerships.

2943 Frost Foundation
511 Armijo St
Suite A
Santa Fe, NM 87501-2899   505-986-0208
                                 info@frostfound.org
                                 frostfound.org
Mary Amelia Whited-Howell, President
Philip B. Howell, Executive Vice President
Taylor F. Moore, Secretary/Treasurer
The Frost Foundation was created to be operated excusively for educational, charitable, and religious purposes.

2944 McCune Charitable Foundation
345 E Alameda St
Santa Fe, NM 87501-2229   505-983-8300
                                 Fax: 505-983-7887
                            mccune@nmmccune.org
                                 nmmccune.org
Sarah McCune Losinger, Chair
Wendy Lewis, Executive Director
Henry Rael, Program Officer
Dedicated to enriching the health, education, environment, and cultural and spiritual life of New Mexicans.

2945 Santa Fe Community Foundation
501 Halona Street
Santa Fe, NM 87505 505-988-9715
Fax: 505-988-1829
foundation@santafecf.org
www.santafecf.org

Suzanne Ortega Cisneros, Chair
Barry Herskowitz, Vice Chair
Kenneth Romero, Secretary

New York

2946 AFB Center on Vision Loss
American Foundation for the Blind
2 Penn Plaza
Suite 1102
New York, NY 10121-4524 212-502-7600
Fax: 888-545-8331
afbinfo@afb.net
afb.org

Carl R Augusto, President & CEO
Kelly Bleach, Chief Administrative Officer
Rick Bozeman, Chief Financial Officer
National nonprofit organization that expands possibilities for people with vision loss.

2947 Altman Foundation
521 5th Ave
Fl 35
New York, NY 10175-3500 212-682-0970
Fax: 212-682-1648
info@altman.org
altmanfoundation.org

Karen L. Rosa, President
Jeremy Tennenbaum, Chief Financial Officer
Ann E. Maldonado, Office Manager
For the benefit of such charitable and educational institutions in the City of New York as said directors shall approve. Foundation grants support programs and institutions that enrich the quality of life in the city, with a particular focus on initiatives that help individuals, families and communities benefit from the services and opportunities that will enable them to achieve their full potential.

2948 Ambrose Monell Foundation
1 Rockefeller Plz
Suite 301
New York, NY 10020-2002 212-586-0700
Fax: 212-245-1863
www.monellvetlesen.org

Ambrose K. Monell,, President and Treasurer
Eugene P. Grisanti, Vice-President
George Rowe, Vice-President
Voluntary aiding and contributing to religious, charitable, scientific, literary, and educational uses and purposes, in New York, elsewhere in the US and throughout the world.

2949 American Chai Trust
41 Madison Ave
Suite 400
New York, NY 10010-2202 212-889-0575
Fax: 212-743-8120
info@perlmanandperlman.com
www.perlmanandperlman.com

2950 American Foundation for Suicide Prevention (AFSP)
199 Water St.
11th Floor
New York, NY 10038 212-363-3500
888-333-2377
Fax: 212-363-6237
info@afsp.org
afsp.org

Robert Gebbia, Chief Executive Officer
Christine Yu Moutier, Chief Medical Officer
Stephanie Rogers, Senior Vice President, Communications & Marketing
The American Foundation for Suicide Prevention is a voluntary health organization that gives those affected by suicide a nationwide community empowered by research, education, and advocacy to take action against this disease. AFSP achieves their goal by funding scientific research, educating the public about mental health and suicide prevention, and supporting survivors of suicide loss and all those affected by suicide.

2951 American Foundation for the Blind
2 Penn Plaza
Suite 1102
New York, NY 10121 800-232-5463
www.afb.org

Kirk Adams, President & CEO
Darren M. Davis, Executive Administrator Executive Office
The American Foundation for the Blind (AFB) is a national nonprofit that is dedicated to removing barriers, creating solutions, and expanding possibilities for the blind and visually impaired. The AFB is focused on spreading access to technology, elevating the quality of information and tools for professional who serve people with vision loss, and the promotion of independent living for those with vision loss.

2952 Arthur Ross Foundation
20 E 74th St
Ste 4c
New York, NY 10021-2654 212-737-7311
Fax: 212-650-0332

Arthur Ross, President

2953 Artists Fellowship
47 5th Ave
New York, NY 10003-4303 212-255-7740
info@artistsfellowship.org
www.artistsfellowship.org

Babette Bloch, President
Private, charitable foundation that assists professional fine arts and their families in times of emergency, disability, or bereavement.

2954 Bodman Foundation
767 3rd Ave
4th Floor
New York, NY 10017-2023 212-644-0322
Fax: 212-759-6510

John N. Irwin III, Chairman
Russell P. Pennoyer, President
Peter Frelinghuysen, Vice President
Foundation concentrates their grant programs in New York City, but foundation also makes some grants in Northern New Jersey. Funding is concentrated in six program areas: Arts & Culture, Education, Employment, Health, Public Policy and Youth and Families.

2955 Brain & Behavior Research Foundation
747 Third Ave.
33rd Floor
New York, NY 10017 646-681-4888
800-829-8289
info@bbrfoundation.org
bbrfoundation.org

Jeffrey Borenstein, President & Chief Executive Officer
Louis Innamorato, Vice President, Finance & Chief Financial Officer
Lauren Duran, Vice President, Communications, Marketing & PR
The Brain & Behavior Research Foundation is a nonprofit organization committed to alleviating the suffering caused by mental illness by awarding grants in the field of mental health research.
1987

2956 Brooklyn Home for Aged Men
P.O.Box 280062
Brooklyn, NY 11228 718-745-1638
Fax: 718-745-0813
www.brooklynhome.org

Catherine M. Birdseye, Co-President
William E. Spaulding, Co-President
Andelusia Wheeler, Co-President
The Brooklyn Home For Aged Men has served the community for more than one hundred years. Although originally set up as a residence for men, it later accepted women and couples as well.

2957   Cancer Care
275 7th Avenue
22nd Floor
New York, NY 10001-6754   212-712-8400
                                        800-813-4673
                                   Fax: 212-712-8495
                                   info@cancercare.org
                                   www.cancercare.org

Patricia J. Goldsmith, Chief Executive Officer
John Rutigliano, Chief Operating Officer
Sue Lee, Senior Director of Development
A national non-profit organization that provides free, professional support services to anyone affected by cancer: people with cancer, caregivers, children, loved ones, and the bereaved.

2958   Children's Tumor Foundation
120 Wall Street
16th Floor
New York, NY 10005-3904   212-344-6633
                                        800-323-7938
                                   Fax: 212-747-0004
                                        info@ctf.org
                                           ctf.org

Linda Halliday Martin, Chairperson
Colin Bryar, Vice Chairperson
Annette Bakker, PhD, President and Chief Scientific Officer
A nonprofit 501 (c)(3) medical foundation, dedicated to improving the health and well-being of individuals and families affected by neurofibromatosis. The Foundation sponsors medical research, clinical services, public education programs and patient support services. It is the central source for up-to-date and accurate information about NF. It also assists patients and families with referrals to NF clinics and healthcare professionals specializing in NF. The goal is to find a cure for NF.

2959   Commonwealth Fund
1 E 75th St
New York, NY 10021-2692   212-606-3800
                                   Fax: 212-606-3500
                                        info@cmwf.org
                                   www.commonwealthfund.org
Benjamin K. Chu, Chairman
Cristine Russell, Vice Chairman
Donald Moulds, Executive Vice President for Pro
A private foundation with the broad charge to enhance the common good. Carries out this mandate by supporting efforts that help people live healthy and productive lives, and by assisting certain groups with serious and neglected problems. Supports independent research on health and social issues and makes grants to improve heathcare practice and policy.

2960   Community Foundation for Greater Buffalo
726 Exchange Street,
Suite 525
Buffalo, NY 14210   716-852-2857
                                   Fax: 716-852-2861
                                        mail@cfgb.org
                                           cfgb.org

Marsha Joy Sullivan, Chair
William Joyce, Vice Chair
Gary L. Mucci,, Secretary
Mission is connecting people, ideas, and resources to improve lives in Western New York

2961   Community Foundation of Herkimer & Oneida Counties
2608 Genesee Street
Utica, NY 13502-4728   315-735-8212
                                   Fax: 315-735-9363
                                   info@foundationhoc.org
                                        foundationhoc.org

Alicia Dicks, President/CEO
Gilles Lauzon, Director of Finance
Elayne Johnson, Director of Fund Administration
Mission of the foundation is to improve the lives of the residents of Herkimer and Oneida Counties.

2962   Community Foundation of the Capitol Region
Six Tower Place
Albany, NY 12203-3749   518-446-9638
                                   Fax: 518-446-9708
                                        info@cfgcr.org
                                        www.cfgcr.org

Karen Bilowith, President/CEO
Mindy Derosia, Development Officer
Shelly Connolly, Program Assistant
Mission is to strengthen our community by attracting charitable endowments both large and small, maximizing benefits to donors, making effective gtants, and providing leadership to address community needs.

2963   Comsearch: Broad Topics
Foundation Center
79 5th Ave
New York, NY 10003-3034   212-620-4230
                                        800-424-9836
                                   Fax: 212-807-3677
                                   communications@foundationcenter.org
                                        www.fdncenter.org

Bradford K. Smith, President
Lisa Philip, Vice President for Strategic Phi
Jen Bokoff, Director of GrantCraft
Subset publications of The Foundation Grants Index, are printouts of actual foundation grants, covering 26 key areas of grantmaking. This tool is designed for fundraisers who wish to examine grantmaking activities in a broad field of interest.
$55.00

2964   DE French Foundation
Ste 503
120 Genesee St
Auburn, NY 13021-3672   315-252-3634

Walter Lowe, Owner

2965   Dana Foundation
Dana Alliance for Brain Initiatives
505 Fifth Avenue
6th floor
New York, NY 10017   212-223-4040
                                   Fax: 212-317-8721
                                        danainfo@dana.org
                                        www.dana.org

Edward F Rover, President /Chairman
Burton M. Mirsky, Executive Vice President, Financ
Barbara Rich, Ed.D., EVP, Communications; Assistant S
A private philanthropy with principal interests in brain science, immunology, and arts education.

2966   David J Green Foundation
Ste 12
599 Lexington Ave
New York, NY 10022-6030   212-317-8820
                                   Fax: 212-371-5099

Valerie Ventolora, Manager
Michael Greene, Manager

2967   Easterseals New York
633 3rd Ave.
New York, NY 10017   212-943-4364
                                   www.easterseals.com/newyork
Marianne Gribbon, Senior Director, Childhood Services
Robert Lambert, Director, Workforce & Veterans Services
Offers resources and expertise that allow children and adults with disabilities to live with dignity and independence. Provides programs and solutions that enhance the lives of people with disabilities, while heightening community awareness and acceptance.

2968   Edna McConnel Clark Foundation
415 Madison Ave
Tenth Floor
New York, NY 10017-7949   212-551-9100
                                   Fax: 212-421-9325
                                        info@emcf.org
                                           emcf.org

Nancy Roob, President
Woodrow C. McCutchen, Vice President, Senior Portfolio
Kelly Fitzsimmons, Vice President, Chief Program an

Helps young people, ages 9-24, from low-income backgrounds become independent, productive adults.

2969 Edward John Noble Foundation
Fl 19
32 E 57th St
New York, NY 10022-8562
212-759-4212
Fax: 212-888-4531

June Noble Larkin, Owner
June Larkin, Owner

2970 Epilepsy Foundation of Long Island
1500 Hempstead Turnpike
East Meadow, NY 11554
516-739-7733
888-672-7154
Fax: 516-739-1860
efli.org

Thomas Hopkins, President & CEO
Paul Giotis, Chief Operating Officer
Lawrence Boord, Chief Financial Officer
Provides education, counseling and residential care to Long Island residents with epilepsy and related conditions.

2971 Episcopal Charities
1047 Amsterdam Avenue
New York, NY 10025-1747
212-316-7575
episcopalcharities@dioceseny.org
episcopalcharities-newyork.org

John Talty, President
Lorraine A. LaHuta, Vice President
Evan A. Davis, Secretary
Provides funding and support to a broad range of community-based human service programs throughout the Diocese of New York. These programs, sponsored by Episcopal congregations, serve disadvantaged individuals, youth and families on a non-sectarian basis.

2972 Esther A & Joseph Klingenstein Fund
125 Park Ave.
Suite 1700
New York, NY 10017
212-492-6181
www.klingfund.org

Supports, in the early stages of their careers, young investigators engaged in basic or clinical research that may lead to a better understanding of neurological and psychiatric disorders.

2973 Fay J Lindner Foundation
189 Wheatley Road
Brookville, NY 11545
516-686-4440
www.fayjlindnercenter.org

Terrence Ullrich, President
Dr. Robert Steinberger, Vice President
Thomas F. Moore, Treasurer

2974 Ford Foundation
320 E 43rd St
New York, NY 10017-4890
212-573-5000
Fax: 212-351-3677
office-of-communications@fordfoundation.org
www.fordfound.org

Darren Walker, President
Kenneth T Monterio, Vice President, Secretary and Ge
Alfred Ironside, Vice President/Communications
A resource for innovative people and institutions worldwide. Goals are to: strenghthen democratic values; reduce poverty and injustice; promote international cooperation; and advance human achievement. While not specific to disabilities, the Ford Foundation operates on several levels that indirectly assist and support those with disabilities through human and civil rights issues, social justice support, economic fairness and opportunity, and access to education involvements.

2975 Fortis Foundation
28 Liberty Street
New York, NY 10005-1401
212-859-7197
Fax: 212-859-7010
ir.assurant.com

Elaine D. Rosen, Chair
Howard L. Carver, Director
Melissa Kivett, Senior Vice President, Investor

2976 Foundation Center
79 5th Ave
16th Street
New York, NY 10003-3076
212-620-4230
800-424-9836
Fax: 212-807-3677
communications@foundationcenter.org
foundationcenter.org

Bradford K Smith, President
Lisa Philip, VP, Strategic Philanthropy
Jen Bokoff, Director of GrantCraft
The Foundation Center publishes Foundation Directory Online, with key facts on the US grantmakers and their grants.

2977 Foundation Center Library Services
Foundation Center
79 5th Ave
16th Street
New York, NY 10003-3076
212-620-4230
800-424-9836
Fax: 212-807-3677
communications@foundationcenter.org
foundationcenter.org

Bradford K Smith, President
Lisa Philip, VP, Strategic Philanthropy
Jen Bokoff, Director of GrantCraft
The Center disseminates current information on foundation and corporate giving through our national collections in New York City and Washington D.C., our field offices in San Francisco and our network of over 180 cooperating libraries in all 50 states and abroad.

2978 Foundation for Advancement in Cancer Therapy
PO Box 1242
Old Chelsea Station
New York, NY 10113-1242
212-675-6349
info@rethinkingcancer.org
www.rethinkingcancer.org

Ruth Sackman, Founder
A clearinghouse for information regarding alternative cancer therapies, emphasizing nutritional and metabolic approaches.

2979 Gebbie Foundation
215 Cherry St
Jamestown, NY 14701-5207
716-487-1062
Fax: 716-484-6401
info@gebbie.org
www.gebbie.org

Gregory J Edwards, CEO
Daniel Kathman, President
Jonathan Taber, Vice President
Giving in Chautauqua County, and secondly, in neighboring areas of western New York. Giving is offered in other areas only when the project is consonant with program objectives that cannot be developed locally.

2980 Gladys Brooks Foundation
1055 Franklin Avenue
Suite 208
Garden City, NY 11530
www.gladysbrooksfoundation.org
Jessica L Rutledge, Director
The purpose of this Foundation is to provide for the intellectual, moral and physical welfare of the people of this country by establishing and supporting nonprofit libraries, educational institutions, hospitals and clinics. The Foundation will make grants only to private, publicly supported, nonprofit, tax-exempt organizations.

2981 Glickenhaus Foundation
546 5th Ave
New York, NY 10036-5000
212-953-7800
info@glickenhaus.com

Seth M. Glickenhaus, Senior Partner and Chief Investm

2982 Guide Dog Foundation for the Blind
371 East Jericho Turnpike
Smithtown, NY 11787-2976
631-930-9000
800-548-4337
Fax: 631-930-9009
info@guidedog.org
www.guidedog.org

James C. Bingham, Chair
Alphonce J. Brown, Vice Chair
Barbara J. Kelly, Secretary
Providing mobility through the use of trained guide or service dogs to individuals who are blind or with other special needs.

2983 Hearing Health Foundation (HHF)
575 Eighth Ave.
Suite 1201
New York, NY 10018
212-257-6140
866-454-3924
Fax: 212-257-6139
TTY: 888-435-6104
info@hhf.org
hearinghealthfoundation.org
Timothy Higdon, President & Chief Executive Officer
Noemi Disla, Director, Finance, Operations & Administration
Christopher Geissler, Director, Program & Research Support
Hearing Health Foundation promotes hearing health and advocates for the prevention and cure of hearing loss and tinnitus through research.
1958

2984 Hearst Foundations
300 W 57th St
Fl 26
New York, NY 10019-3741
212-649-2000
Fax: 212-887-6855
hearst.com

Steven R. Swartz, President and Chief Executive Of
National philanthropic resources for organziations and institutions working in the fields of education, health, culture and social services. Our goal is to ensure that people of all backgrounds have the opportunity to build healthy, productive and inspiring lives.

2985 Henry and Lucy Moses Fund
405 Lexington Ave
New York, NY 10174-1299
212-554-7800
Fax: 212-554-7700
www.mosessinger.com

Irving Sitnick, President
Provides legal services to many prominent industries, individuals and families in the New York City area.

2986 Herman Goldman Foundation
Fl 18
61 Broadway
New York, NY 10006-2708
212-797-9090

Alan Nisselson, President
A private nonoperating foundation.

2987 Kenneth & Evelyn Lipper Foundation
Fl 6
101 Park Ave
New York, NY 10178
212-883-6333

Kenneth Lipper, Director

2988 Long Island Alzheimer's Foundation
5 Channel Drive
Port Washington, NY 11050-2216
516-767-6856
Fax: 516-767-6864
www.liaf.org

Paul Eibeler, Chairman
Fred Jenny, Executive Director
Sean Phillips, Director of Development

2989 Louis and Anne Abrons Foundation
First Manhattan Company
399 Park Avenue
New York, NY 10022-7001
212-756-3300
Fax: 212-223-4175
firstmanhattan.com

David Manischewitz, CEO
Sam Colin, Senior Managing Director
Allan Glick, Senior Managing Director

2990 Margaret L Wendt Foundation
Ste 277
40 Fountain Plz
Buffalo, NY 14202-2200
716-855-2146
Fax: 716-855-2149

Robert J Kresse, Manager

2991 Merrill Lynch & Company Foundation
250 Vesey St
New York, NY 10080
212-449-1000
800-637-7455
Fax: 212-449-7969
ml.com

Brian T Moynihan, CEO
John Theil, Head
Andy M Sieg, Managing Director
Ongoing support for the arts, health, human services, and civic issues. Merrill Lynch's philanthropic priority is a sustained investment in education. Q992

2992 Metzger-Price Fund
Ste 2300
230 Park Ave
New York, NY 10169
212-867-9500
Fax: 212-599-1759

Isaac A Saufer, Secretary/Treasurer

2993 Milbank Foundation for Rehabilitation
116 Village Boulevard
Suite 200
New York, NY 08540
609-951-2283
Fax: 609-951-2281
fdnweb.org/milbank

Jeremiah M. Bogert, Chairman & Secretary
Jeremiah Milbank III, President and Treasurer
Carl Helstrom, Executive Director
Awarding grants from trust funds based on a competitive selection process or the preferences of the foundation managers and granters. The foundations mission is to integrate people with disabilities into all aspects of american life. Current priorities include, but are not limited to: consumer-focused initiatives that enable people with disablties to lead fulfilling,independent lives; innovative policy research and education on market-based approaches to health care and rehabilitation...

2994 Morgan Stanley Foundation
1585 Broadway
New York, NY 10036-8293
212-761-4000
Fax: 212-761-0086
mediainquiries@morganstanley.com
morganstanley.com
James P. Gorman, Chairman and Chief Executive Off
Thomas Nides, Vice Chairman
Jeff Brodsky, Chief Human Resources Officer
Our overachieving mission is threefold: build the potential of individuals and families, encourage and support our employees charitable efforts, and strengthen relationships with our communities.

2995 National Foundation for Facial Reconstruction
333 East 30th St.
Lobby Office
New York, NY 10016-4974
212-263-6656
Fax: 212-263-7534
info@myface.org
myface.org
Barbara H. Zuckerberg, President
John R. Gordon, Chairman
Sondra Neuschotz, Secretary
A nonprofit organization whose major purposes are to provide facilities for the treatment and assistance of individuals who are un-

able to afford private reconstructive surgical care, to train and educate professionals in this surgery, to encourage research in the field and to carry on public education.

2996   National Hemophilia Foundation
7 Penn Plaza
Suite 1204
New York, NY 10001   212-328-3700
                                         888-463-6643
                                    Fax: 212-328-3777
                                    info@hemophilia.org
                                    www.hemophilia.org

Leonard Valentino, President & CEO
Dawn Rotellini, Chief Operating Officer
Kevin Mills, Chief Scientific Officer
Dedicated to finding better treatments and cures for bleeding and clotting disorders and to preventing the complications of these disorders through education, advocacy and research.

2997   Neisloss Family Foundation
Ste 7
1737 Veterans Hwy
Central Islip, NY 11749-1533   631-234-1600
                                    Fax: 631-234-1066
Stanley Neisloss, President/Owner

2998   New York Community Trust
909 3rd Ave
22nd Floor
New York, NY 10022-4752   212-686-0010
                                    Fax: 212-532-8528
                                    aw@nyct-cfi.org
                                    nycommunitytrust.org
Lorie A Slutsky, President
Carolyn M Weiss, CFO
Mary Z. Greenebaum, Chief Investment Officer
Our goal is to out charitable money to work, making grants to the city's nonprofit community and building an endowment to tackle future problems.

2999   New York Foundation
10 E 34th St
10th Floor
New York, NY 10016-4327   212-594-8009
                                    info@nyf.org
                                    nyf.org
Marlene Provizer, Chair
Roger Schwed, Vice Chair
Sue A Kaplan, Secretary
Grants are given that involve New York City or a particular neighborhood of the city. Emphasize advocacy and community organizing. Address a critical need or disadvantaged population, particularly youth or the elderly. Are strongly identified with a particular community. Require an amount of funding to which a Foundation grant would make a substantial contribution. And can show a clear role for the Foundation's funds.

3000   Northern New York Community Foundation
120 Washington St
Suite 400
Watertown, NY 13601-3376   315-782-7110
                                    Fax: 315-782-0047
                                    info@nnycf.org
                                    www.nnycf.org
Joseph W. Russell, President
Linda S. Merrell, Vice President
Jacquelyn A. Schell, Secretary
Raises, manages and administers an endowment and collection of funds for the benefit of the community

3001   Parkinson's Disease Foundation
1359 Broadway
Room 1509
New York, NY 10018-7867   212-923-4700
                                         800-457-6676
                                    Fax: 212-923-4778
                                    info@pdf.org
                                    www.pdf.org
Howard D Morgan, Chair
Constance Atwell, Vice Chair
Isobel Konecky, Secretary

The Parkinson's Disease Foundation is a leading national presence in Parkinson's disease research, education and public advocacy. We are working for the nearly one million people in the US who live with Parkinson's by funding promising scientific research to find the causes of and a cure for Parkinson's while supporting people with Parkinson's, their families and caregivers through educational programs and support services.

3002   Peter and Elizabeth C. Tower Foundation
2351 North Forest Rd.
Suite 106
Getzville, NY 14068-1225   716-689-0370
                                    Fax: 716-689-3716
                                    info@thetowerfoundation.org
                                    thetowerfoundation.org
Tracy A. Sawicki, Executive Director
Donald W. Matteson, Chief Program Officer
Charles E. Colston Jr., Program Officer
The Peter and Elizabeth C. Tower Foundation supports community programming that results in children, adolescents, and young adults affected by substance use disorders, learning disabilities, mental illness, and intellectual disabilities achieving their full potential.
1990

3003   Reader's Digest Foundation
Readers Digest Association
Readers Digest Rd
Pleasantville, NY 10570   914-238-1000
                                    Fax: 914-238-4559
                                    letters@rd.com
                                    rd.com
Mary G Berner, CEO
Dedicated to creating opportunities and promoting efforts that encourage individuals to make a positive difference in their communities, and to supporting programs designed to help young people learn, grow and enrich their lives.

3004   Research to Prevent Blindness
645 Madison Ave
Floor 21
New York, NY 10022-1010   212-752-4333
                                         800-621-0026
                                    Fax: 212-688-6231
                                    www.rpbusa.org
Diane S. Swift, Chair
Brian F. Hofland PhD, President
David H Brenner, Vice President and Secretary
National voluntary health foundation supported by foundations, corporations and voluntary gifts and bequests from individuals. Established to stimulate basic and applied research into the causes, prevention and treatment of blinding eye diseases.

3005   Rita J and Stanley H Kaplan Foundation
Rm 306
866 United Nations Plz
New York, NY 10017-1822   212-688-1047
                                    Fax: 212-688-6907
                                    www.kaplanfoundation.org
Nancy Kaplan Belsky, President
Susan B. Kaplan, Vice President
Scott Kaplan Belsky, Secretary & Treasurer

3006   Robert Sterling Clark Foundation
135 E 64th St
New York, NY 10065-7045   212-288-8900
                                    Fax: 212-288-1033
                                    rscf@rsclark.org
                                    rsclark.org
James Allen Smith, Chairman
Vincent McGee, President
Clara Miller, Treasurer
Giving primarily in New York with emphasis on advocacy, research, and public education aimed at informing New York City of state policies.

3007   Skadden Fellowship Foundation
4 Times Sq
New York, NY 10036-6518   212-735-3000
                                           Fax: 212-735-2000
                                           info@skadden.com
                                           www.skadden.com

Alan C Myers, Director
William Schumann, Legal Assistant
The aim of the Foundation is to give Fellows the freedom to pursue public intrest work, thus the Fellows create their own projects at public interest organizations with at least 2 lawyers on staff before they apply.

3008   St George's Society of New York
216 E 45th St
Suite 901
New York, NY 10017-3304   212-682-6110
                                           Fax: 212-682-3465
                                           info@stgeorgessociety.org
                                           stgeorgessociety.org

John Shannon, Almoner
Anna Titley, Director of Operations and Commu
Samantha Hamilton, Director of Development and Memb
St George's Society provides monthly stipends to the elderly and the handicapped.

3009   Stanley W Metcalf Foundation
Ste 503
120 Genesee St
Auburn, NY 13021-3672   315-252-3634

Walter Lowe, Owner

3010   Stonewall Community Foundation
446 West 33rd Street
New York, NY 10001-1913   212-367-1155
                                           Fax: 212-367-1157
                                           stonewall@stonewallfoundation.org
                                           www.stonewallfoundation.org

Dante Mastri, President
Neill Coleman, Vice President
Chris Davis, Secretary
Mission is to promote the well being of lesbian, gay, bisexual, and transgender (LGBT) individuals and strengthen the LGBT community. We do this by increasing resources; targeting those resources strategically to areas of greatest need; and by serving as a catalyst and clearinghouse for ideas and solutions. Through grant-making donor-advised funds, endowment funds and charitable education, Stonewall supports LGBT organizations and helps donors realize their philanthropic goals.

3011   Surdna Foundation
330 Madison Ave
30th Floor
New York, NY 10017-5016   212-557-0010
                                           grants@surdna.org
                                           surdna.org

Jocelyn Downie, Chairperson
Peter B Benedict, Vice Chairperson
Lawrence S.C Griffth, Secretary & Treasurer
The Foundation makes grants in the areas of environment, community revitalization, effective citizenry, the arts and the nonprofit sector.

3012   The Adaptive Sports Foundation
100 Silverman Way
PO Box 266
Windham, NY 12496   518-734-5070
                                           Fax: 518-734-6740
                                           info@adaptivesportsfoundation.org
                                           www.adaptivesportsfoundation.org

Robert W Stubbs, Chair
Todd Munn, Executive Director
Pam Greene, Program Director
The Adaptive Sports Foundation is a non-profit organization providing programs for children and adults with physical and cognitive disabilities. Programs center around outdoor physical activities and sports, including skiing and snowboarding, canoeing and cycling.

3013   Tisch Foundation
Fl 19
655 Madison Ave
New York, NY 10065-8043   212-521-2930
                                           Fax: 212-521-2983

Mark J Krinsky, VP

3014   Van Ameringen Foundation
509 Madison Avenue
New York, NY 10022-5501   212-758-6221
                                           Fax: 212-688-2105
                                           info@vanamfound.org
                                           www.vanamfound.org

Kenneth A. Kind, President / Treasurer
Steadman Westergaard, Vice President and Secretary
Eleanor Sypher, Executive Director
From its beginning the Foundation has sought to stimulate prevention, education, and direct care in the mental health field with an emphasis on those individuals and populations having an impoverished background and few opportunities, for whom appropriate intervention would produce positive change.

3015   Verizon Foundation
1 Verizon Way
Basking Ridge, NJ 07920-1097   866-247-2687
                                           Fax: 908-630-2660
                                           www.verizon.com

Lowell C McAdam, Chairman & CEO
Roy H Chestnutt, Executive Vice President
James J Gerace, Chief Communications Officer
Mission is to improve education, literacy, family safety and healthcare by supporting Verizon's commitment to deliver technology that touches life. We focus our philanthropic efforts on 3 areas: Education, Safety and Health. & Volunteerism.

3016   Western New York Foundation
11 Summer St
Third Floor
Buffalo, NY 14209-2256   716-839-4225
                                           Fax: 716-883-1107
                                           bgosch@wnyfoundation.org
                                           www.wnyfoundation.org

Jennifer S. Johnson, Chairman
James A. W. McLeod, President
John N. W. Walsh III, Vice President
The Western New York Foundation makes grants in the seven counties of Western New York State: Erie, Niagra, Genesee, Wyoming, Allegany, Cattaraugus and Chautauqua

3017   William T Grant Foundation
570 Lexington Avenue
18th Floor
New York, NY 10022-6837   212-752-0071
                                           Fax: 212-752-1398
                                           info@wtgrantfdn.org
                                           wtgrantfoundation.org

Adam Gamoran, President
Vivian Tseng, Vice President, Program
Deborah McGinn, Vice President, Finance and Admi
Purpose is to further the understanding of human behavior through research. The mission focuses on improving the lives of youth ages 8 to 25 in the United States.

North Carolina

3018   Arc of North Carolina
343 East Six Forks Rd.
Suite 320
Raleigh, NC 27609   919-782-4632
                                           800-662-8706
                                           Fax: 919-782-4634
                                           info@arcnc.org
                                           www.arcnc.org

Adonis Brown, President
Robert Rusty Bradstock, Senior Vice President
Rhonda Schandevel, Secretary
Committed to securing for all people with developmental disabilities the opportunity to choose and realize their goals of where and how they learn, live, work, and play.

3019 Bob & Kay Timberlake Foundation
1660 E Center Street Ext
Lexington, NC 27292-1309

336-243-7777
800-776-0822
Fax: 336-249-2469
bobtimberlake.com

Daniel Timberlake, President

3020 Duke Endowment
800 East Morehead Street
Charlotte, NC 28202-4012

704-376-0291
Fax: 704-376-9336
dukeendowment.org

Eugene W. Cochrane Jr., President
Arthur E. Morehead IV, Vice President/General Counsel
Susan L. McConnell, Director of Higher Education
Mission is to serve the people of North Carolina and South Carolina by supporting selected programs of higher education, health care, children's welfare, and spiritual life.

3021 First Union Foundation
301 S College St
Charlotte, NC 28288

704-383-0525
Fax: 704-374-2484

Judy Allison, Director

3022 Foundation for the Carolinas
220 N. Tryon Street
Charlotte, NC 28202

704-973-4500
800-973-7244
Fax: 704-973-4599
mmarsicano@fftc.org
fftc.org

Michael Marsicano, Ph.D., President & CEO
Brian Collier, Executive Vice President
Debra S. Watt, SVP, Information Technology
Giving primarily to organizations serving the citizens of North and South Carolina.

3023 Kate B Reynolds Charitable Trust
128 Reynolda Village
Winston Salem, NC 27106-5123

336-397-5500
800-485-9080
Fax: 336-723-7765
kbr.org

Karen McNeil-Miller,, President
Lori Fuller, Director, Evaluation and Learnin
Joel Beeson, Director, Operations
Mission is to improve the quality of life and quality of health for the financially needy of North Carolina. Grants resricted to the state of North Carolina only.

3024 Mary Reynolds Babcock Foundation
2920 Reynolda Rd
Winston Salem, NC 27106-3016

336-748-9222
Fax: 336-777-0095
info@mrbf.org
mrbf.org

Jennifer Barksdale, Finance Officer
Toshawia Bruner, Office Assistant
Lavastian Glenn, Network Officer
For 1994, this foundation is committed to an extensive educational and planning process to better understand the Southeast and to articulate the role the foundation seeks to play in the region into the twenty-first century.

3025 Triangle Community Foundation
324 Blackwell St
Suite 1220
Durham, NC 27701-3690

919-474-8370
Fax: 919-941-9208
info@trianglecf.org
trianglecf.org

Lacy M. Presnell, Chair
Pat Nathan, Secretary
C. Perry Colwell, Assistant Secretary
Triangle Community Foundation connects philanthropic resources with community needs, creates opportunity for enlightned change and encourages philanthropy as a way of life.

North Dakota

3026 Alex Stern Family Foundation
4141 28th South Avenue
Suite 102
Fargo, ND 58104-8403

701-271-0263
Fax: 701-271-0408
alexsternfamilyfoundation.org

Don Scott, Executive Director
Rondi McGovern, Trustee
Dan Carey, Trustee
The Foundation supports the arts, social welfare/human services, education, youth recreation, civic projects and health issues for the benefit of the greater Fargo-Moorhead area.

3027 Arc of North Dakota
2500 DeMers Avenue
Grand Forks, ND 58201-2420

701-772-6191
877-250-2022
Fax: 701-772-2195
thearc@arcuv.com
www.thearcuppervalley.com

Peggy Johnson, President
Joan Karpenko, First Vice President
Ruth Jenny, Secretary
Mission is to work in partnership with our constituents, members and affiliated chapters to ensure that children and adults with intellectual and developmental disabilities have the supports, benefits, and services they need, and are accepted, respected and fully included in their communities.

3028 North Dakota Community Foundation
309 N Mandan Street
309 N Mandan Street, Suite 2
P.O.Box 387
Bismarck, ND 58502-0387

701-222-8349
kdvorak@ndcf.net
www.ndcf.net

Kevin J Dvorak, CFP, President & CEO
Amy N. Warnke, CFRE, Development Director East
Kara L. Geiger, Development Director West
The mission of the North Dakota Community Foundation is to improve the quality of life for North Dakota's citizens through charitable giving and promothing philanthropy.

Ohio

3029 Akron Community Foundation
345 W Cedar St
Akron, OH 44307-2407

330-376-8522
Fax: 330-376-0202
jpetures@akroncf.org

Mark Alio, Chair
Steven Cox, Vice Chair
Dr. Sandra Selby, Secretary
Mission is to improve the quality of life in the Greater Akron area by building permanent endowments, and providing philanthropic leadership that enables donors to make lasting investments in the community.

3030 Albert G and Olive H Schlink Foundation
49 Benedict Avenue, Suite C
Norwalk, OH 44857

curtis@hwak.com
www.schlinkfoundation.org

3031 Arc of Ohio
1335 Dublin Rd
Suite 100-A
Columbus, OH 43215-7037

614-487-4720
800-875-2723
Fax: 614-487-4725
info@thearcofohio.org
thearcofohio.org

Gary Tonks, Executive Director
John Hannah, President
Connie Calhoun, Vice President
The mission of The Arc of Ohio is to advocate for human rights, personal dignity and community participation of individuals with

developmental disabilities, through legislative and social action, information and education, local chapter support and family involvement.

3032   Bahmann Foundation
8041 Hosbrook Rd
Suite 210
Cincinnati, OH 45236-2909
513-891-3799
Fax: 513-891-3722
info@bahmann.org
www.bahmann.org

John Gatch, Executive Director
The mission of the Bahmann Foundation is to reduce isolation of low-income older adults through technology.

3033   Cleveland Foundation
1422 Euclid Ave
Suite 1300
Cleveland, OH 44115-2063
216-861-3810
Fax: 216-861-1729
Hello@CleveFdn.org
clevelandfoundation.org

James A. Ratner, Chairman
Paul J. Dolan, Vice Chairman
Ronald B. Richard, President and CEO
In general, grants are made in (but not restriced to) the areas of arts and culture, community development, economic development, education, environment, health and human services.

3034   Columbus Foundation and Affiliated Organizations
1234 E Broad St
Columbus, OH 43205-1453
614-251-4000
Fax: 614-251-4009
info@columbusfoundation.org
columbusfoundation.org

Doug F. Kridler, President & CEO
Raymond J. Biddiscombe, CPA, Senior Vice President - Finance
Lisa Schweitzer Courtice, P, EVP - Community Research and Gra
The Columbus Foundation offers a range of charitable fund types that can be used for individuals, families and businesses.

3035   Eleanora CU Alms Trust
Fifth Third Bank
Department 00864
9990 Montgomery Rd
Cincinnati, OH 45263
513-793-2200

Robert W Laclair, President
Giving is limited to Cincinnati, OH.

3036   Eva L And Joseph M Bruening Foundation
Foundation Management Services
1422 Euclid Ave
Suite 966
Cleveland, OH 44115-1952
216-621-2901
Fax: 216-621-8198
www.fmscleveland.com

Janet E. Narten, Founder
Cristin N. Slesh, President
Valerie Schramm, Operations Assistant
Charitable foundation providing grants to noprofit organizations located inCuyahoga county Ohio. No grant are awarded to inviduals.

3037   Fred & Lillian Deeks Memorial Foundation
P.O.Box 1118
Cincinnati, OH 45201-1118
937-339-2329
Fax: 937-339-1861

3038   GAR Foundation
277 East Mill Street
Akron, OH 44308
330-576-2926
Fax: 330-294-5315
info@garfdn.org

Christine Amer Mayer, President
Kirstin S. Toth, Senior Vice President
Candace Campbell Jackson, Consulting Program Officer
The mission of the Foundation is to strengthen communities in our region through discerning and creative support of worthy organizations.

3039   George Gund Foundation
1845 Guildhall Building
45 Prospect Avenue, West
Cleveland, OH 44115-1008
216-241-3114
Fax: 216-241-6560
info@gundfdn.org
gundfoundation.org

Geoffrey Gund, President & Treasurer
Ann L. Gund, Vice President
David T. Abbott, Executive Director
The George Gund Foundation was established in 1952 as a private, nonprofit institution with the sole purpose of contributing to human well-being and the progress of society.

3040   Greater Cincinnati Foundation
200 West Fourth St.
Cincinnati, OH 45202-2775
513-241-2880
Fax: 513-852-6886
info@gcfdn.org
www.gcfdn.org

Kathryn e. Merchant, President/CEO
Terri Masur, Executive Assistant
Elizabeth Reiter Benson, APR, Vice President for Communic
Offers a wide variety of giving tools to help people achieve their charitable goals and create lasting good work in their communities.

3041   HCR Manor Care Foundation
333 N. Summit St.
P.O.Box 10086
Toledo, OH 43699-0086
419-252-5500
Fax: 419-252-6404
foundation@hcr-manorcare.com
hcr-manorcare.com

Paul A Ormond, Chairman, President and CEO
An independent, not-for-profit corporation that provides funding for organizations and programs that address the needs of the elderly and individuals requiring post-acute care services.

3042   HWH Foundation
Canton, OH
330-818-1300
contacthwh@hwhfoundation.org
www.hwhfoundation.org

Elizabeth Lacey Hoover, Chairman
Colton Hoover Chase, Vice Chairman
Mark Butterworth, Executive Director
The Herbert W Hoover Foundation funds unique opportunities that provide solutions to issues related to the Community, Education and the Environment.

3043   Harry C Moores Foundation
100 South Third Street
Columbus, OH 43215-4291
614-227-2300
Fax: 614-227-2390
info@bricker.com
bricker.com

Kurtis A Tunnell, Managing Partner
Ahmad Sino, Chief Information Officer
Steve P Odum, Chief Financial Officer

3044   Helen Steiner Rice Foundation
1301 Western Ave.
Cincinnati, OH 45203
513-287-7022
800-877-2665
helensteinerrice.com

Virginia J. Ruehlmann, Creative Consultant
Dorothy C. Lingg, Office Manager
Willis D. Gradison, Jr., Board of Trustee
Non-profit corporation whose purpose is to award grants to worthy charitable programs that aid the poor, the needy, and the elderly.

3045   Nationwide Foundation
One Nationwide Plaza
Columbus, OH 43215-2220
614-249-7111
800-882-2822
Fax: 614-249-5721
www.nationwide.com

Kirt A. Walker, President and COO Nationwide Fin
Mark A. Pizzi, President and Chief Operating Of
Stephen S. Rasmussen, Chief Executive Officer, Nationw

The Nationwide Foundation is an independent corporation funded by Nationwide Companies to help positively impact the quality of life in communities where our associates, agents and their families live and work.

3046 Nordson Corporate Giving Program
28601 Clemens Rd
Westlake, OH 44145-1148   440-892-1580
                                   Fax: 440-892-9507
                                   kladiner@nordson.com
                                   nordson.com

Michael F. Hilton, President and Chief Executive O
Gregory A. Thaxton, Senior Vice President, Chief Fin
John J. Keane, Senior Vice President, Advanced
Nordson Corporation encourages individual financial support of nonprofit organizations, colleges, and universities

3047 Parker-Hannifin Foundation
6035 Parkland Blvd
Cleveland, OH 44124-4141   216-896-3000
                                         800-272-7537
                                   Fax: 216-896-4000
                                   parker.com

Donald E. Washkewicz, Chairman, Chief Executive Office
Lee C. Banks, Executive Vice President and Ope
Robert P. Barker, Executive Vice President, Operat
To be a leading worldwide manufacturer of components and systems for the builders and users of durable goods.

3048 Reinberger Foundation
30000 Chagrin Blvd.
Suite 300
Cleveland, OH 44124-4439   216-292-2790
                                   Fax: 216-292-4466
                                   info@reinbergerfoundation.org
                                   www.reinbergerfoundation.org

Karen R. Hooser, President
Sally R. Dyer, Trustee
Richard H. Oman, Trustee
Committed to enhancing the quality of life for individuals from all walks of life. To achieve this goal, proposals in the areas of the arts, education, healthcare, and social service are favored.

3049 Robert Campeau Family Foundation
7 West Seventh Street
Cincinnati, OH 45202-2424   513-579-7000
                                   Fax: 513-579-7555

Terry J Lundgren, Chairman and Chief Executive Officer

3050 Sisler McFawn Foundation
P.O.Box 149
Akron, OH 44309   330-849-8887
                                   Fax: 330-996-6215

Charlotte M Stanley, Grants Manager
Our trust restricts giving to certain programs and types of organizations. You can see recent giving has been by referring to the list of grants approved and paid during the past year. Call foundation office to request a guidelines brochure and list.

3051 Stark Community Foundation
400 Market Ave North
Suite 200
Canton, OH 44702-1557   330-454-3426
                                   Fax: 330-454-5855
                                   info@starkcf.org
                                   www.starkcommunityfoundation.org

Mark Samolczyk, President
Patricia Quick, VP/ CFO
Chris Decker, Finance and Systems Officer
Stark Community Foundation is dedicated to promoting the betterment of Stark County and enhancing the quality of life of all its citizens.

3052 Stocker Foundation
201 Burns Road
Elyria, OH 44035   440-366-4884
                                   Fax: 440-366-4656
                                   contact@stockerfoundation.org
                                   stockerfoundation.org

Brenda Norton, President
Dawn Dobras, Treasurer
Patricia O'Brien, Executive Director

The Stocker Foundation seeks creative ideas and projects that are catalysts for constructive change in the community through arts and culture, community needs, education, health social services and women's issues.

3053 Toledo Community Foundation
300 Madison Avenue
Suite 1300
Toledo, OH 43604-1583   419-241-5049
                                   Fax: 419-242-5549
                                   toledocf@toledocf.org
                                   www.toledocf.org

David F. Waterman, Chair
Dr. Anthony Armstrong, Vice Chair
Rita N.A. Mansour, Secretary
The Toledo Community Foundation is a public, charitable foundation which exists to improve the quality of life in the region.

3054 William J and Dorothy K O'Neill Foundation
7575 Northcliff Ave.
Suite 205
Cleveland, OH 44144   216-831-4134
                                   Fax: 216-378-0594
                                   info@oneill-foundation.org
                                   www.oneillfdn.org

Leah S Gary, President & CEO
Symone R McClain, Manager of Grants & Office Opera
Timothy M. McCue, MPH, Senior Program Officer

3055 Youngstown Foundation
100 Federal Plaza East, Suite 101
P.O.Box 1162
Youngstown, OH 44503-1162   330-744-0320
                                   Fax: 330-744-0344
                                   Jan@youngstownfoundation.org
                                   www.youngstownfoundation.org

Jan Strasfeld, Executive Director
Crissi Jenkins, Program Coordinator
Rena Colarossi, Admin. Assistant
Funds proposals that provide direct services to children with medically diagnosed disabilities. Grants are awarded to Ohio non-profit agencies that are qualified under the Internal Revenue Service Code 501 (c) (3) for the care of such children in the greater Youngstown Area.

Oklahoma

3056 Anne and Henry Zarrow Foundation
401 S Boston Ave
Suite 900
Tulsa, OK 74103-4012   918-295-8004
                                   Fax: 918-295-8049
                                   bmajor@zarrow.com
                                   www.zarrow.com

A broad-based funding foundation. However, ares of emphasis include Jewish causes, the indignant, the disenfranchised and the homeless. The Foundation meets on a quarterly basis, in the months of February, April, September and November. Proposals are due on the first day of the following months:January, April, August and October. Any proposals recieved after the due date will be held until the next quarter's meeting.

3057 Sarkeys Foundation
530 East Main St
Norman, OK 73071-5823   405-364-3703
                                   Fax: 405-364-8191
                                   angela@sarkeys.org
                                   sarkeys.org

Kim Henry, Executive Director
Lori Sutton, Facilities Manager
Angella Holladay, Director of Grants Management
Improves the quality of life in Oklahoma. Offers contributions in the areas of social services, arts and cultural programs, educational funding and health care and medical research. Funding only in agencies in the state of Oklahoma.

Oregon

3058 Arc of Oregon
2405 Front Street NE
Suite 120
Salem, OR 97301-4342
503-581-2726
877-581-2726
Fax: 503-363-7168
www.thearcoregon.org

Marcie Ingledue, Executive Director
Tiffany Tombleson, Administrative Assistant
Paula Boga, OSNT Program Director
Guardianship, Advocacy and Planning Services. Oregon special needs trust; information and referral.

3059 Cambia Health Foundation
100 SW Market St.
Suite E15B
Portland, OR 97201
503-225-4813
cambiahealthfoundation.org

Peggy Maguire, President & Chair
Rob Coppedge, Chief Executive Officer
Anjie Vannoy, Vice President, Finance & Controller
Cambia Health Foundation is the corporate foundation of Cambia Health Solutions dedicated to transforming the way people experience health care to create a more person-focused and economically sustainable health care system.
1907

3060 Chiles Foundation
1614 Mahan Center Boulevard
Suite 104
Tallahassee, Fl 32308
805-385-7800
Fax: 805-385-7808
kchiles@lawtonchiles.org
chilesfoundation.org

Kitty Chiles, Executive Director
Bud Chiles, President
Dr. Wil J. Blechman, Board Member
Giving in Oregon, with emphasis on Portland, and the Pacific Northwest.

3061 Jackson Foundation
P.O.Box 3168
Portland, OR 97208-3168
503-275-4414
march.voyles@usbank.com
www.thejacksonfoundation.com
Robert H Depew, Vice President & Senior Trust Of
Libby Voyles, Trust Relationship Associate
Purpose is to respond to the requests deemed appropriate to promote the welfare of the public of the city of Portland or the State of Oregon or both.

3062 Leslie G Ehmann Trust
P.O.Box 3168
Portland, OR 97208-3168
503-275-5929
800-522-9100
Fax: 503-275-4117

William Dolan, Trustee

Pennsylvania

3063 Air Products Foundation
7201 Hamilton Blvd
Allentown, PA 18195-9642
610-481-4911
Fax: 610-481-5900
gigmrktg@airproducts.com
www.airproducts.com

Seifi Ghasemi, Chairman & CEO
M. Scott Crocco, Senior Vice President and Chief
Guillermo Novo, Senior Vice President
Giving primarily in areas of company operations throughout the US.

3064 Arc of Pennsylvania
301 Chestnut Street
Suite 403
Harrisburg, PA 17101-2535
717-234-2621
800-692-7258
Fax: 717-234-2622
info@thearcpa.org
thearcpa.org

Maureen Cronin, Executive Director
Pam Klipa, Government Relations Director
Gwen Adams, Operations Director
The Arc's mission is to work to include all children and adults with cognitive, intellectual, and developmental disabilities in every community. We promote active citizenship and inclusion in every community.

3065 Arcadia Foundation
105 E Logan St
Norristown, PA 19401-3058
202-747-0876

Marilyn L Steinbright, President
Robert Carmona-Borjas, Founder

3066 Brachial Plexus Palsy Foundation
210 Springhaven Cir
Royersford, PA 19468-1178 www.brachialplexuspalsyfoundation.org
Nonprofit organization dedicated to raising funds for support of families who hae children with brachial plexus injuries. Supports medical facilities that research and treat such injuries, holds fund-raising events to support further research, has support groups, and produces educational materials including a newsletter, Outreach, and brochures.

3067 Columbia Gas of Pennsylvania Corporate Giving
650 Washington Rd
Pittsburgh, PA 15228-2702
412-572-7104
Fax: 412-572-7140
www.columbiagaspamd.com/html/
Rosemary Martinelli, Manager Corporation

3068 Connelly Foundation
100 Front Street,
Suite 1450
West Conshohocken, PA 19428-2873
610-834-3222
Fax: 610-834-0866
info@connellyfdn.org
connellyfdn.org

Josephine C. Mandeville, Chair & President
Emily C Riley, Executive Vice President
Lewis W Bluemle, Senior Vice President
Seeks to foster learning and to improve the quality of life in the Greater Philadelphia area. The Foundation supports local non-profit organizations in the fields of education, health and human services, arts and culture and civic enterprise.

3069 Dolfinger-McMahon Foundation
30 South 17th Street
Philadelphia, PA 19103-4196
215-979-1768
www.dolfingermcmahonfoundation.org
Sheldon M. Bonovitz, Trustee
David E. Loder, Trustee
Frank G. Cooper, Counsel

3070 Heinz Endowments
Howard Heinz Endowment
625 Liberty Ave
30 Dominion Tower
Pittsburgh, PA 15222- 3115
412-281-5777
Fax: 412-281-5788
bobbyvagt@heinz.org
heinz.org

Grant Oliphant, President
Edward Kolano, Vice President Finance and Admin
Ann C. Plunkett, Director, Human Resources
Mission is to help our region thrive as a whole community-economically, ecologically, educationaly, and culturaly while advancing the state of knowledge and practice in the fields in which we work.

3071 Henry L Hillman Foundation
310 Grant Street
Suite 2000
Pittsburgh, PA 15219   412-338-3466
foundation@hillmanfo.com
hillmanfamilyfoundations.org
David K Roger, President
Lisa R Johns, Treasurer and Senior Program Off
Lauri K. Fink, Senior Program Officer
Established with a broad purpose to improve the quality of life in
Pittsburgh and southwestern Pennsylvania.

3072 Jewish Healthcare Foundation of Pittsburgh
650 Smithfield Street
Suite 2400
Pittsburgh, PA 15222- 3915   412-594-2550
Fax: 412-232-6240
info@jhf.org
jhf.org
Karen Wolk Feinstein, PhD, President and Chief Executive Of
Carla Barricella, Communications Director
Lindsey Kirstatter Hartle, Accounting Manager
The mission of the JHF is to support and foster the provision of
healthcare services, healthcare education, and, when appropriate, medical and scientific research, and to respond to the
health-related needs of elderly, underprivileged, indigent, and
undeserved persons in both the Jewish and general community
throughout Western Pennsylvania.

3073 Juliet L Hillman Simonds Foundation
310 Grant Street
Suite 2000
Pittsburgh, PA 15219   412-338-3466
Fax: 412-338-3520
foundation@hillmanfo.com
hillmanfamilyfoundations.org
David K. Roger, President
Lisa R. Johns, Treasurer and Senior Program Off
Lauri K. Fink, Senior Program Officer

3074 Oberkotter Foundation
1600 Market St
Suite 3600
Philadelphia, PA 19103-7212   215-751-2601
Fax: 215-751-2678
info@oberkotterfoundation.org
oberkotterfoundation.org
George H Nofer, Executive Director
Mildred L. Oberkotter, M.S.W., Trustee
Bruce A. Rosenfield, J.D., Trustee
The Oberkotter Foundation focuses its efforts on supporting families who have chosen listening and spoken language for their
child and on opportunities for children learning listening and
spoken language to develop their social, emotional, language and
educational skills.

3075 PECO Energy Company Contributions Program
Fl 7toorh
2301 Market St
Philadelphia, PA 19103-1338   215-841-4000
800-494-4000
Fax: 215-841-6830
www.peco.com
Denis P O'Brien, SVP/ CEO
Michael A. Innocenzo, SVP/ COO
Phillip S. Barnett, SVP/ CFO/ Treasurer

3076 PNC Bank Foundation
249 5th Ave
Pittsburgh, PA 15222-2707   412-762-2000
Fax: 412-762-7829
marianna.hallett@pnc.com
www.pncbank.com
Samuel R Patterson, Senior VP
The PNC Foundation's priority is to form partnerships with community-based nonprofit organizations within the markets PNC
serves in order to enhance educational opportunities for children,
particularly underserved pre-K children though our signature,
PNC Grow Uo Great Program, and to promote the growth of targeted communities through economic development initiatives.

3077 Philadelphia Foundation
1234 Market St
Suite 1800
Philadelphia, PA 19107-3704   215-563-6417
Fax: 215-563-6882
philafound.org
R Andrew Swinney, President
Pat Meller, Vice President for Finance & Adm
Andrea Congo, Executive Assistant
The Philadelphia Foundation improves our community by ad-
vancing change, leading on issues of importance, forging mean-
ingful relationships and providing knowledge, resources and
stewardship.

3078 Pittsburgh Foundation
Five PPG Place
Suite 250
Pittsburgh, PA 15222-5405   412-391-5122
Fax: 412-391-7259
oliphantg@pghfdn.org
pittsburghfoundation.org
Maxwell King, President and CEO
Jonathan Brelsford, Vice President of Investments
Jay Donato, Senior Investment Analyst
The Pittsburgh Foundation works to improve the quality of life in
the Pittsburgh region by evaluating and addressing community is-
sues, promoting responsible philanthropy, and connecting do-
nors to the critical needs of the community.

3079 Shenango Valley Foundation
7 West State Street
Suite 301
Sharon, PA 16146-2713   724-981-5882
866-901-7204
Fax: 724-983-9044
comm-foundation.org
Lawrence E. Haynes, Executive Director
Amy Atkinson, Associate Director
Shelly Mason, Chief Financial Officer
Mission is to promote the betterment of our region and enhance-
ment of the quality of life for all of its citizens.

3080 Staunton Farm Foundation
650 Smithfield Street
Suite 210
Pittsburgh, PA 15222- 3907   412-281-8020
Fax: 844-281-8020
office@stauntonfarm.org
stauntonfarm.org
Joni S. Schwager, Executive Director
Bethany Hemingway, Program Officer
Jason Fate, Office Manager
Dedicated to improving the lives of people who live with mental
illness.

3081 Stewart Huston Charitable Trust
50 South First Avenue
Coatesville, PA 19320-3418   610-384-2666
Fax: 610-384-3396
admin@stewarthuston.org
stewarthuston.org
Scott G. Huston, Executive Director
Charles L. Huston III, Trustee
Shelton P Sanford, Trustee
The purpose of the Trust is to provide funds, technical assistance
and collaboration on behalf of non-profit organizations engaged
exclusively in religious, charitable or educational work; to extend opportunities to deserving needs persons and, in general, to
promote any of the above causes.

3082 Teleflex Foundation
155 S Limerick Rd
Limerick, PA 19468-1603   610-948-5100
Fax: 610-948-5101
teleflex.com
Jeffrey P Black, CEO
The Teleflex Foundation strives to create an impact on the quality
of life in Teleflex communities and build supportive relationships among our stakeholders. The Foundation places a priority
on progrmas that have the commitmenet and volunteer involvement of Teleflex communities.

3083 USX Foundation
600 Grant St
Pittsburgh, PA 15219-2702   412-433-1121
Fax: 412-433-6847
www.ussteel.com

CD Mallick, General Manager
Patricia Funaro, Program Manager
Giving primarily in areas of company operations located within
the United States.

3084 William B Dietrich Foundation
Duane Morrs Llt
30 S 17th St
Philadelphia, PA 19103-4001   215-979-1000
Fax: 215-979-1020
www.duanemorris.com

William B Dietrich, President

3085 William Talbott Hillman Foundation
310 Grant Street
Suite 2000
Pittsburgh, PA 15219   412-338-3466
Fax: 212-792-2677
foundation@hillmanfo.com
hillmanfamilyfoundations.org

David K. Roger, President
Lisa R. Johns, Treasurer and Senior Program Off
Lauri K. Fink, Senior Program Officer

**3086 William V and Catherine A McKinney Charitable
Foundation**
20 Stanwix St
Pittsburgh, PA 15222-4802   412-644-8332
Fax: 412-644-6058
verizon.com

William M Schmidt, Senior Vice President

Rhode Island

3087 Arc South County Chapter
2 Barber Avenue
Warwick, RI 02886-3549   401-480-9355
paul@pence.com
www.riroads.com
Developmentally disabled center/service assistance to individuals with developmental disabilities.

3088 Arc of Blackstone Valley
500 Prospect St.
Wing B, Suite 203
Pawtucket, RI 02860- 4332   401-727-0150
800-257-6092
Fax: 401-727-1545
contact@bvcriarc.org
www.bvcriarc.org

Kathleen O'Neill, President
Thomas E. Hodge, Vice President
John J. Padien III, Chief Executive Officer
A private nonprofit organization providing residential, developmental, employment and recreational programs and services to
more then 400 individuals with intellectual and related
disabilities

3089 Arc of Northern Rhode Island
The Homestead Group Administrative Offices
68 Cumberland St
Suite 200
Woonsocket, RI 02895-3323   401-765-3700
Fax: 401-765-1124
arcofnri.org

The mission of the Homestead Group is to help the people we support lead the lives they want and deserve

3090 Champlin Foundations
2000 Chapel View Boulevard
Suite 350
Cranston, RI 02920   401-944-9200
Fax: 401-944-9299

Jonathan K. Farnum, Distribution Committee
John Gorham, Distribution Committee
Dione D. Kenyon, Distribution Committee
Giving in the Rhode Island area. Champlin does not give grants to
individuals, only to RI tax-exempt organizations.

3091 CranstonArc
The Keystone Group
PO Box 20130
Cranston, RI 02920-942   401-941-1112
Fax: 401-383-8751
info@accesspointri.org
www.accesspointri.org

Thomas Kane, President & CEO
Kevin McHale, Chief Operating Officer
Maureen Russo, Director of Human Resources
Mission is to empower persons with differing abilites to claim
and enjoy their right to dignity and respect through their lives.

3092 Down Syndrome Society of Rhode Island
4635 Post Road
Warwick, RI 02818   401-463-5751
Fax: 401-463-5337
TTY: 800-745-5555
coordinatordssri@verizon.net
www.dssri.org

Claudia M. Lowe, Coordinator
Marilyn Blanche
Jeff DiMillio
The Down Syndrome Society of Rhode Island (DSSRI) is dedicated to promoting the rights, dignity and potential of all individuals with Down syndrome through advocacy, education, public
awareness, and support.

3093 Frank Olean Center
93 Airport Rd
Westerly, RI 02891-3420   401-596-2091
Fax: 401-596-3945
info@oleancenter.org
oleancenter.org

Joan Gradilone, President
Tony Vellucci, Executive Director
Rick Harley, Vice President
A non-profit organization representing and providing services
and supports to persons with developmental disabilities and their
families throughout Southern Rhode Island and Southeastern
Connecticut.

3094 Horace A Kimball and S Ella Kimball Foundation
23 Broad Street
Westerly, RI 02891-1879   401-348-1238
Fax: 401-364-3565
www.hkimballfoundation.org

Thomas F Black III, President
Norman D. Baker, Jr., Secretary and Treasurer
Edward C. Marth, Foundation Trustees
Makes grants almost exclusively to Rhode Island operatives
(charities) or those benefitting Rhode Island residents and
causes.

3095 James L. Maher Center
120 Hillside Avenue
Newport, RI 02840   401-846-0340
Fax: 401-849-4267
www.mahercenter.org

Jack Casey, President
William Maraziti, Executive Director
Barbara Burns, President
The mission is to advance independence and opportunity for chil-
dren and adults with developmental disabilities and their
families.

3096 Rhode Island Arc
99 Bald Hill Rd
Cranston, RI 02920-2647　　　401-463-9191
Fax: 401-463-9244
riarc@compuserve.com

Mary Lou Mc Caffray, Executive Director

3097 Rhode Island Foundation
One Union Station
Providence, RI 02903-1758　　　401-274-4564
Fax: 401-331-8085
info@rifoundation.org
rifoundation.org

Neil Steinberg, President & CEO
Wendi DeClercq, Executive Assistant
James S. Sanzi, Esq., Vice President of Development
The Rhode Island Foundation works to build a better Rhode Island as a philanthropic resource, for people, communities, organizations, and programs.

South Carolina

3098 Arc of South Carolina
1202 12th Street
Cayce, SC 29033　　　803-748-5020
Fax: 803-445-1026
TheArc@ArcSC.org
www.arcsc.org

Margie Williamson, Executive Director
Caroline Kistler, Project Director
Carly Prince, Case Manager
The Arc of South Carolina advocates for and alongside people with cognitive, intellectual and developmental disabilities and their families.

3099 Center for Disability Resources
University of South Carolina School of Medicine
Department of Pediatrics
8301 Farrow Rd.
Columbia, SC 29208　　　803-935-5231
Fax: 803-935-5059
david.rotholz@uscmed.sc.edu
uscm.med.sc.edu/cdrhome
A University Affiliated Program which develops model programs designed to serve persons with disabilities and to train students in fields related to disabilities.

3100 Colonial Life and Accident Insurance Company Contributions Program
1200 Colonial Life Blvd W
Columbia, SC 29210-7670　　　803-798-7000
Fax: 803-731-2618

Randy Horn, President and Chief Executive Of
Bill Deeham, Senior Vice President of Sales
Tim Arnold, Senior Vice President of Sales a

Tennessee

3101 Arc of Anderson County
728 Emory Valley Road, Suite 42
P.O.Box 4823
Oak Ridge, TN 37831-4823　　　865-481-0550
arc@arcaid.org
www.thearcandersoncounty.com
Sally Browning, President
Dargie Arwood, Executive Director
Ginny Miceli, President
The Arc of Anderson County provides support and advocacy to people with cognitive, intellectual and developmental disabilities. The Arc provides support, information and training for families and caregivers of adults and children with these disabilities.

3102 Arc of Davidson County
111 N Wilson Blvd
Nashville, TN 37205-2411　　　615-248-4112
Fax: 615-322-9184
arcdc.org
Kate Deitzer, President
Cynthia Gardner, Vice President
Thom Druffel, Treasurer
Provides services to adults and children with intellectual and developmental disabilities.

3103 Arc of Hamilton County
4613 Brainerd Rd
Chattanooga, TN 37411-3826　　　423-624-6887
800-624-6887
Fax: 423-624-3974
arcofhamilton@aol.com
thearchc.org
Shawn Ellis, Executive Director
Provides assistance to individuals and families with developmental disabilities, in the form of advocacy, information, and support coordination

3104 Arc of Tennessee
151 Athens Way
Suite 100
Nashville, TN 37228-1367　　　615-248-5878
800-835-7077
Fax: 615-248-5879
info@thearctn.org
thearctn.org
John Lewis, President
John Shouse, Vice President
Donna Lankford, Secretary
Advocacy, information, referral and support for people with intellectual and developmental disabilities and their families.

3105 Arc of Washington County
110 East Mountcastle Drive
Johnson City, TN 37601-7557　　　423-928-9362
Fax: 423-928-7431
kim@arcwc.org
www.arcwc.org
Malessa Fleenor, Executive Director
Kim Reid, Human Resources, Quality Assuran
Kim Wheeler, Respite Coordinator
Is a non-profit organization that serves individuals with disabilities and their families. They have an independent support coordination service, as well as, early intervention, family support and respite services.

3106 Arc of Williamson County
129 W Fowlkes St
Suite 151
Franklin, TN 37064-3562　　　615-790-5815
Fax: 615-790-5891
sbbarc@thearcwc.org
thearcwc.org
Donna Isbell, President
Steve Cassidy, Vice President
Ashley Coulter, Secretary
The Arc is a family-based organization committed to securing for all people with intellectual, developmental, or other disabilities the opportunity to choose and realize their goals of where and how they live, learn, work, and play.

3107 Arc-Diversified
453 Gould Dr
Cookeville, TN 38506　　　931-432-5981
800-239-9029
Fax: 931-432-5987

3108 Benwood Foundation
736 Market St
Suite 1600
Chattanooga, TN 37402-4812 423-267-4311
Fax: 423-267-9049
info@benwood.org
benwood.org

Sarah Morgan, President
Kristy Huntley, Program & Financial Officer
Connie Perrin, Accounting & Grants Manager
Benwood Foundation seeks to stimulate creative and innovative efforts to build and strengthen the Chattanooga community.

3109 Community Foundation of Greater Chattanooga
1270 Market St
Chattanooga, TN 37402-2713 423-265-0586
Fax: 423-265-0587
info2@cfgc.org
cfgc.org

Peter T. Cooper, President
Rebecca Underwood, Vice President, Finance & Admini
Marty Robinson, Vice President, Donor Relations
A non-profit organization which receives, holds, invests and distributes assets contributed by individuals and organizations for the benefit of Chattanooga, its citizens and its institutions.

3110 Education and Auditory Research Foundation
PO Box 330867
Nashville, TN 37203-7506 615-627-2724
800-545-4327
Fax: 615-627-2728
www.earfoundation.org

Michael Glasscock, President
Provides the general public support services promoting the integration of the hearing and balance impaired into mainstream society; to provide practicing ear specialists continuing medical education courses and related programs specifically regarding rehabilitation and hearing preservation; to educate young people and adults about hearing preservation and early detection of hearing loss, enabling them to prevent at an early age hearing and balance disorders.

3111 International Paper Company Foundation
6400 Poplar Ave
Memphis, TN 38197 901-419-9000
800-207-4003
Fax: 901-419-4439
internationalpaper.comm@ipaper.com
internationalpaper.com

Mark S Sutton, Chairman & CEO
David J Bronczek, President & CEO
C. Cato Ealy, Senior Vice President, Corporate
The Foundation's primary focus is education-specifically environmental education, iliteracy programs for young children and minority career development opportunities for college bound youth.

3112 Montgomery County Arc
1825 K Street
NW, Suite 1200
Washington, DC 20006-2145 202-534-3700
800-433-5255
Fax: 202-534-3731
info@thearc.org
www.thearc.org

Ronald Brown, President
Elise McMillan, Vice President
Peter V Berns, Chief Executive Officer
Organization works to ensure that the estimated 7.2 million Americans with intellectual and developmental disabilities have the services and supports they need to grow, develop and live in communities across the nation.

Texas

3113 Abell-Hangar Foundation
P.O.Box 430
Midland, TX 79702-0430 432-684-6655
Fax: 432-684-4474
abell-hanger.org

David L Smith, Executive Director
The Foundation makes grants to nonprofit organizations, which are involved in such undertakings for public welfare, including but not limited to, education, health services, human services, arts and cultural activities and community or social benefit.

3114 Albert & Bessie Mae Kronkosky Charitable Foundation
112 East Pecan
Suite 830
San Antonio, TX 78205-1574 210-475-9000
888-309-9001
Fax: 210-354-2204
kronkosky.org

Palmer Moe, Managing Director
Mission is to produce profound good that is tangible and measurable in Bandera, Bexar, Comal, and Kendall counties in Texas by implimenting the Kronkosky's charitable purposes.

3115 American Express Foundation
P.O. Box 981540
El Paso, TX 79998-1540 800-528-4800
TTY: 800-221-9950
americanexpress.com

Kenneth I Chenault, Chairman and Chief Executive Off
L. Kevin Cox, Chief Human Resources Officer
Marc D. Gordon, Executive Vice President and Chi
Grants are awarded in the three program areas: Community Service, Cultural Heritage, and Economic Independence. Most grants are made for projects operating where the company has a major employee or market presence.

3116 Arc of Texas, The
8001 Centre Park Dr
Suite 100
Austin, TX 78754-5118 512-454-6694
800-252-9729
Fax: 512-454-4956
www.thearcoftexas.org

Charlie Huber, President
John Schneider, Vice President
Amy Mizcles, Executive Director
The Arc of Texas creates opportunities for all people with intellectual and developmental disabilities to actively participate in their communities and make the choices that affect their lives in a positive manner.

3117 BA and Elinor Steinhagen Benevolent Trust
Chase Bank of Texas
700 North St.
Suite D
Beaumont, TX 77701-3928 409-832-6565
Fax: 409-832-7532
www.setxnonprofit.org

Jean Moncla, CTFA, President
Ivy Pate, Treasurer
Chester Jourdan, Executive Director

3118 Brown Foundation
P.O.Box 130646
Houston, TX 77219-0646 713-523-6867
Fax: 713-523-2917
bfi@brownfoundation.org
brownfoundation.org

Nancy Pittman, Executive Director
The purpose of the Brown Foundation is to distribute funds for public charitable purposes, principally for support, encouragement and assistance to education, the arts and community service.

3119 CH Foundation
P.O.Box 94038
Lubbock, TX 79493-4038   806-792-0448
                                Fax: 806-792-7824
                                ksanford@chfoundation.com
                                www.chfoundationlubbock.com

Kay Sanford, Executive Director
Heather Hocker, Grants Administrator
Cheryl Sanford, Administrative Assistant

Mission of the CH foundation is to significantly improve human services and cultural and educational opportunities for the residents of the South Plain of Texas.

3120 Cockrell Foundation
1000 Main St
Suite 3250
Houston, TX 77002-6338   713-209-7500

Ernest H. Cockrell, President
Nancy Williams, Executive Vice President

Purpose is for giving for higher education at the University of Texas at Austin; support also for cultural programs, social services, youth services and health care. Limitations are giving in Houston, Texas and no grants are awarded to individuals.

3121 Communities Foundation of Texas
5500 Caruth Haven Ln
Dallas, TX 75225-8146   214-750-4222
                                Fax: 214-750-4210
                                jsmith@cftexas.org
                                cftexas.org

Brent E. Chrisopher, President and Chief Executive Of
Elizabeth W. Bull, Senior Vice President and Chief
Jeverley R. Cook, Ph.D., Executive Director, W.W. Caruth,

Mission is to improve lives, we serve the community by investing wisely and making effective charitable grants.

3122 Community Foundation of North Texas
306 West 7th
Suite 1045
Fort Worth, TX 76102-4906   817-877-0702
                                Fax: 817-632-8711
                                cfntx.org

Nancy E. Jones, President
Rob Miller, Director of Finance
Vicki Andrews, Director of Operations/Donor Ser

Community Foundation is a tax exempt organization that provides stewardship for many individual charitable funds. With its specialized services, Community Foundation of North Texas gives donors efficient charitable fund administration.

3123 Cullen Foundation
601 Jefferson St
40th Floor
Houston, TX 77002-7900   713-651-8837
                                Fax: 713-651-2374
                                cullenfdn.org

Isaac Arnold, Jr, President
Wilhelmina E Robertson, Vice President and Secretary
Meredith T Cullen, Assistant Secretary

Grants are restricted to Texas-based organizations for programs in Texas, primarily in the Houston area.

3124 Curtis & Doris K Hankamer Foundation
Ste 530
9039 Katy Fwy
Houston, TX 77024-1656   713-461-8140

Gregory A Herbst, Manager

3125 Dallas Foundation
3963 Maple Avenue
Ste. 390
Dallas, TX 75219-4447   214-741-9898
                                Fax: 214-741-9848
                                info@dallasfoundation.org
                                dallasfoundation.org

Mary M Jalonick, President & CEO
Gary W. Garcia, Senior Director of Development
Dawn Townsend, Director of Marketing & Communic

Serves as a leader, catalyst and resource for philanthropy by providing donors with a flexible means of making gifts to charitable causes that enhance our community.

3126 David D & Nona S Payne Foundation
P.O.Box 174
Pampa, TX 79066-174   806-665-0063
Vanessa G Buzzard, Director

The David & Nona S Payne Foundation was established in August 1980. Mrs Payne established the foundation and did much of her charitable giving in honor of her late husband.

3127 El Paso Natural Gas Foundation
P.O.Box 2511
Houston, TX 77252-2511   713-420-2600
                                Fax: 713-420-5312
                                foundation@elpaso.com
                                www.kindermorgan.com

Douglas Foshee, CEO

Focuses on the areas in locations where we have significant facilities or concentrated employees. Primary area of focus is Civic and Community, Education and Health and Human Services. Secondary area of focus is Arts and Culture and Environment.

3128 Epilepsy Foundation of Southeast Texas
2401 Fountain View Dr
Suite 900
Houston, TX 77057-4821   713-789-6295
                                888-548-9716
                                info@eftx.org
                                www.epilepsy.com/texas

Donna Stahlhut, CEO
Rebecca Moreau, Program Director
Amanda Walker Rockwell, Senior Development Coordinator

The Epilepsy Foundation of Southeast Texas is a non-profit organization devoted to improving the lives of people with epilepsy in Texas. Services offered by the foundation include public education programs, medical care, therapy and recreation programs.

3129 Epilepsy Foundation: Central and South Texas
10615 Perrin Beitel Rd
Suite 602
San Antonio, TX 78217   210-653-5353
                                888-606-5353
                                Fax: 210-653-5355
                                staff@efcst.org
                                www.efcst.org

Ariel Robbins, Program Manager

The Epilepsy Foundation of Central & South Texas is a voluntary health organization serving people with epilepsy. Services offered include youth programs, seizure clinics, support groups, referrals and more.

3130 Harris and Eliza Kempner Fund
2201 Market St
12th Floor
Galveston, TX 77553-1529   409-765-6671
                                Fax: 409-765-9098
                                kempnercapital.com

Diana L. Bartula, Vice President, Chief Compliance
V. Delynn Greene, Vice President, Head Trader, Ope

Mission is to further the vision and heritage of the Kemper Family's commitment to philanthropy and sense of responsibility to society.

3131 Hillcrest Foundation
Bank of America
P.O.Box 830241
Dallas, TX 75283   214-209-1965

Daniel Kelly, VP

3132 Hoblitzelle Foundation
5556 Caruth Haven Lane
Suite 200
Dallas, TX 75225-8020   214-373-0462
                                kstone@hoblitzelle.org
                                www.hoblitzelle.org

William T Solomon, Chairman
Caren H. Prothro, Vice Chairman
J. McDonald Williams, Treasurer

Grants made by the directors are usually focused on specific, non-recurring needs of the educational, social service, medical, cultural, and civic organizations in Texas, particularly in the Dallas area.

3133 **Hogg Foundation for Mental Health**
3001 Lake Austin Blvd.
Austin, TX 78703   512-471-5041
hogg-operations@austin.utexas.edu
hogg.utexas.edu
Octavio N. Martinez Jr., Executive Director
Vicky Coffee, Director, Programs
Crystal Viagran, Director, Finance & Operations
The Hogg Foundation for Mental Health is a nonprofit organization that is dedicated to the advancement of mental wellness for the people of Texas through outreach programs, conferences, seminars, research grants, and more.

3134 **Houston Endowment**
600 Travis St
Suite 6400
Houston, TX 77002-3003   713-238-8100
Fax: 713-238-8101
houstonendowment.org
Ann B Stern, President
Sheryl L Johns, Vice President for Admin
F. Xavier Pena, Vice President for Finance and G
A private philanthropic foundation that improves life for people of the greater Houston area through its contributions to charitable organizations and educational institutions.

3135 **John G & Marie Stella Kennedy Memorial Foundation**
555 N Carancahua
Suite 1700, Tower II
Corpus Christi, TX 78401-0851   361-887-6565
Fax: 361-887-6582
Judge J. A. Garcia, President and Director
Marc A. Cisneros, Chief Executive Officer
Sylvia Whitmore, Chief Operating Officer
To advance and nurture activities that contribute to the foundation's core, Catholic values.

3136 **John S Dunn Research Foundation**
3355 West Alabama
Suite 990
Houston, TX 77098-1722   713-626-0368
Fax: 713-626-3866
jsdrf@swbell.net
johnsdunnfoundation.org
J. Dickson Rogers, President
Dan S. Wilford, Vice President
John R. Wallace, Secretary and Treasurer

3137 **Lola Wright Foundation**
515 Congress Avenue
10th Floor
Austin, TX 78701   512-397-2001
amber.carden@ustrust.com
fdnweb.org/lolawright
Wilford Flowers, President and Director
Paul Hilgers, Vice-President and Director
Ron Oliveira, Secretary and Director

3138 **Meadows Foundation**
3003 Swiss Ave
Dallas, TX 75204-6049   214-826-9431
800-826-9431
Fax: 214-827-7042
www.mfi.org
Linda P Evans, President and CEO
Tom Gale, Vice President and Chief Investm
Paula Herring, Vice President and Treasurer
The Meadows Foundation exists to assist people and institutions of Texas improve the quality and circumstances of life for themselves and future generations.

3139 **Moody Foundation**
2302 Post Office St
Suite 704
Galveston, TX 77550-1994   409-797-1500
colleent@moodyf.org
moodyf.org
Frances Moody-Dahlderg, Chairman & Executive Director
Jamie G. Williams, Human Resources Director
Garrik Addison, Chief Financial Officer
Created for the perpetual benefit of present and future generations.

3140 **Pearle Vision Foundation**
2534 Royal Ln
Dallas, TX 75229-3884   214-821-7770
www.pearlevision.com
Leo Priolo Jr, Owner
Organization dedicated to sight preservation through vision research and education.

3141 **San Antonio Area Foundation**
303 Pearl Parkway
Suite 114
San Antonio, TX 78215   210-225-2243
Fax: 210-225-1980
info@saafdn.org
saafdn.org
Marie Smith, Chair
G.P. Singh, Vice Chair
Michelle R. Scarver, Secretary
The San Antionio Area Foundation aspires to significantly enhance the quality of life in our community by providing outstanding service to donors, producting significant asset growth, strengthning community collaboration and managing an exemplary grants program.

3142 **Shell Oil Company Foundation**
40 Bank Street
London, TX 77252-2463   281-544-7171
Fax: 713-241-3329
info@shellfoundation.org
www.shellfoundation.org
Malcolm Brinded, Chairman
Ben van Beurden, Trustee
William Kalema, Trustee
A not-for-profit foundation funded by donations from Shell Oil Company and other participating Shell companies and subsidiaries.

3143 **South Texas Charitable Foundation**
P.O.Box 2459
Victoria, TX 77902   512-573-4383
Rayford L Keller, Secretary

3144 **Sterling-Turner Foundation**
5850 San Felipe Street
Suite 125
Houston, TX 77057-3292   713-237-1117
Fax: 713-223-4638
jeannie.arnold@stfdn.org
www.sterlingturnerfoundation.org
T. R. Reckling, President
Isla C. Reckling, Treasurer
Patricia Stilley, Executive Director
Sterling Turner Foundation is a private trust which can assist any Section 501 (c) (3) organization in the state of Texas. The Foundation is not permitted to assist any individuals

3145 **TLL Temple Foundation**
109 Temple Blvd
Lufkin, TX 75901-7321   936-639-5197
Wayne Corley, Executive Director

3146 **William Stamps Farish Fund**
Ste 1250
1100 Louisiana St
Houston, TX 77002-5232   713-757-7313
Terry Ward, Manager

Utah

3147 Arc of Utah
18585 Coastal Hwy # 19
Rehoboth Beach, DE 19971
801-364-5060
800-371-3060
Fax: 801-364-6030
gacosta@dunndunn.com
www.bewitchedtattoos.com
Kathy Scott, Executive Director
The Arc of Utah advocates for and with cognitive, intellectual and developmental disabilities and their families through awareness, outreach, education, support and public policy.

3148 Marriner S Eccles Foundation
79 S Main St
Salt Lake City, UT 84111-1929
801-532-0934

Shannon K Toronto

3149 Questar Corporation Contributions Program
333 South State Street
P.O. Box 45433
Salt Lake City, UT 84145-0433
801-324-5000

Ronald W Jibson, President & CEO
Craig C Wagstaff, Executive vice president
Micheal Dunn, Executive vice president
Focuses on promoting a healthy environment by investing in and fulfilling its corporate responsibility to support the well-being of communitites where Questar and its subsidiaries conduct business.

Vermont

3150 Vermont Community Foundation
3 Court Street
Middlebury, VT 05753
802-388-3355
Fax: 802-388-3398
info@vermontcf.org
www.vermontcf.org
Stuart Comstock-Gay, President
Nina McDonnell, Grants Administrator
Janet McLaughlin, Special Projects Director
Helps build and manage charitable funds created by individuals, families, groups, organizations, and institutions to improve the quality of life in Vermont.

Virginia

3151 Arc of Virginia
2147 Staples Mill Road
Richmond, VA 23230
804-649-8481
Fax: 804-649-3585
info@thearcofva.org
www.thearcofva.org
Howard Cullum, President
Shareen Young-Chavez, President-Elect
Marisa Laios, Vice President
The Arc of Virginia advocates for individuals with developmental disabilities and their families, so they may all lead productive and fulfilling lives.

3152 Beacon Tree Foundation
9201 Arboretum Pkwy.
Suite 140
N. Chesterfield, VA 23236
800-414-6427
info@beacontree.org
beacontree.org
Beacon Tree Foundation is dedicated to being an advocate for the family, providing education about treatment and financial resources to help heal children and teens struggling with mental health issues and to provide hope for the future.

3153 Camp Foundation
P.O.Box 813
Franklin, VA 23851
757-562-3439

Bobby B Worrell, CEO

3154 Community Foundation of Richmond & Central Virginia
7501 Boulder View Drive
Suite 110
Richmond, VA 23225- 4047
804-330-7400
Fax: 804-330-5992
info@tcfrichmond.org
tcfrichmond.org
Darcy Oman, President
Bobby Thalhimer, Senior Advisor
Molly Dean Bittner, Vice President
The Community Foundation provides effective stewardship of philanthropic assets entrusted to its care by donors who wish to enhance the quality of community life.

3155 John Randolph Foundation
112 North Main Street
P.O.Box 1606
Hopewell, VA 23860- 1161
804-458-2239
Fax: 804-458-3754
lsharpe@johnrandolphfoundation.org
www.johnrandolphfoundation.org
Lisa H. Sharpe, Executive Director
M. Stephen Cates, Director of Finance and Accounti
Kiffy Werkheiser, Development Program Officer
The John Randolph Foundation is a community-based Foundation working to improve the health and quality of life for residents of Hopewell and surrounding areas through Grants and Scholarships.

3156 National Right to Work Legal Defense Foundation
8001 Braddock Rd.
Springfield, VA 22160
703-321-8510
800-336-3600
Fax: 703-321-9319
nrtw.org
Raymond LaJeunesse, Vice President & Legal Director
Byron S. Andrus, Staff Attorney
Matthew B. Gilliam, Staff Attorney
The National Right to Work Legal Defense Foundation is a non-profit, charitable organization. Its mission is to eliminate coercive union power and compulsory unionism abuses through strategic litigation, public information, and education programs.
1968

3157 Norfolk Foundation
101 W. Main Street,
Suite 4500
Norfolk, VA 23510-2103
757-622-7951
Fax: 757-622-1751
mbrunson@hamptonroadscf.org
www.hamptonroadscf.org
Deborah M DiCroce, Ed.D., President and CEO
Tim McCarthy, Chief Financial Officer
Kay A. Stine, CFRE, Vice President for Development
The mission of the Norfolk Foundation is to inspire philanthropy and transform the quality of life in southeastern Virginia.

3158 Robey W Estes Family Foundation
Robey W Estes Jr
3901 West Broad Street
P.O. Box 25612
Richmond, VA 23230-5612
866-378-3748
estes-express.com
Robey W Estes Jr, President and CEO

3159 Virginia Beach Foundation
Suite 4500
101 W. Main Street,
Virginia Beach, VA 23454
757-422-5249
Fax: 757-422-1849
mbrunson@hamptonroadscf.org
www.hamptonroadscf.org
Deborah M DiCroce, President
Tim McCarthy, Chief Financial Officer

Mission is to stimulate the establishment of endowments to serve the people of Virgina Beach now and in the future. Respond to changing, emerging, community needs. Provide a vehicle and a service for donors with varied interests. Serve as a resource, broker, catalyst and leader in the community.

Washington

3160 Arc of Washington State
2638 State Avenue NE
Olympia, WA 98506-4880
360-357-5596
888-754-8798
Fax: 360-357-3279
info@arcwa.org
arcwa.org

Cindy O'Neill, Board President
Sue Elliott, Executive Director
Angie Ziska, Secretary
Mission is to advocacte for the rights and full participation of all people with intellectual and developmental disabilities.

3161 Ben B Cheney Foundation
3110 Ruston Way
Suite A
Tacoma, WA 98402-5308
253-572-2442
Info@benbcheneyfoundation.org
benbcheneyfoundation.org

Bradbury F. Cheney, President
Piper Cheney, Vice President
Carolyn J. Cheney, Secretary Treasurer
The Foundation makes grants in communities where the Cheney Lumber Company was active. The Foundation's goal is to improve the quality of life in those communities by making grants to a wide range of activities.

3162 Community Foundation of North Central Washington
9 South Wenatchee Ave
Wenatchee, WA 98801-3332
509-663-7716
Fax: 888-317-8314
info@cfncw.org
www.cfncw.org

Beth Stipe, Executive Director
Kristy Harris, Chief Financial Officer
Lila R. Edlund, Director of Administration
Assists donors by helping identify their specific charitable and goals and provide grants and scholarships that help groups and people address critical issues in North Central Washington

3163 Glaser Progress Foundation
1601 Second Avenue
Suite 1080
Seattle, WA 98101-9223
206-728-1050
Fax: 206-728-1123

Martin Collier, Executive Director
Mitchell Fox, Program Officer
Melessa Rogers, Operations Manager
The Glaser Prograss Foundation focuses on four program areas: measuring progress, animal advocacy, independent media and global HIV/AIDS.

3164 Greater Tacoma Community Foundation
950 Pacific Avenue
Suite 1100
Tacoma, WA 98402-4423
253-383-5622
Fax: 253-272-8099
info@gtcf.org
www.gtcf.org

Rose Lincoln Hamilton, President and CEO
Shirley Brockmann, CPA, Vice President Finance & Adminis
Elyse Rowe, Chief of Strategy and Community
Mission is fostering generosity by connecting people who care with causes that matter, forever enriching our community.

3165 Inland Northwest Community Foundation
421 West Riverside Avenue
Suite 606
Spokane, WA 99201- 0405
509-624-2606
888-267-5606
Fax: 509-624-2608
admin@inwcf.org
www.inwcf.org

Mark Hurtubise, Ph.D., J.D., President and CEO
Troy Braga, CPA, Controller
P J Watters, Director of Gift Planning
Serving 20 counties throughout Eastern Washington and Northern Idaho, mission is to foster vibrant and sustainable communities in the Inland Northwest.

3166 Medina Foundation
801 2nd Ave
Suite 1300
Seattle, WA 98104-1517
206-652-8783
Fax: 206-652-8791
info@medinafoundation.org
www.medinafoundation.org

Jennifer Teunon, Executive Director
Jessica Case, Program Officer
Aana Lauckhart, Program Officer
A family foundation that works to foster positive change in the Greater Puget Sound area. The Foundation strives to improve the human condition by supporting organizations that provide critical services to those in need.

3167 Norcliffe Foundation
999 3rd Ave
Suite 1006
Seattle, WA 98104-4001
206-682-4820
Fax: 206-682-4821
arline@thenorcliffefoundation.com
www.thenorcliffefoundation.com

Arline Hefferline, Foundation Manager
Nora P. Kenway, President
Geographic area of funding limited to the Puget Sound Region in and around Seattle, Washington.

3168 Stewardship Foundation
1145 Broadway
Suite 1500
Tacoma, WA 98402-1278
253-620-1340
Fax: 253-572-2721
info@stewardshipfdn.org
www.stewardshipfdn.org

William T. Weyerhaeuser, Chair
Gail T. Weyerhaeuser, Vice Chair and Treasurer
Chi- Dooh, Director
Christian, evangelical organizations - national or international impact.

3169 Weyerhaeuser Company Foundation
33663 Weyerhaeuser Way South
Federal Way, WA 98003
253-924-2345
800-525-5440
www.weyerhaeuser.com

Daniel S Fulton, President & CEO
Patricia M Bedient, EVP & CFO
Sandy D McDade, SVP & General Counsel
Although the foundation does fund programs for disabled persons from time to time, it is not a specific priority for the foundation. Since it was formed in 1948, the foundation has given more than $81.1 million to nonprofit organizations and is one of the oldest funds for corporate philanthropy in the country. Nearly all of its contributions have been made within the communities where Weyerhaeuser employees live and work and awards approximately 600 grants annually.

West Virginia

3170 Arc Of West Virginia, The
912 Market Street
Parkersburg, WV 26101-4737
304-422-3151

chapter #54

3171 **Bernard McDonough Foundation**
311 Fourth Street
Parkersburg, WV 26101-5315   304-424-6280
                                    Fax: 304-424-6281
                            www.mcdonoughfoundation.org
Robert W Stephens, Ed.D., President
Mary Riccobene, Vice President
Francis C. McCusker, Treasurer
Directors and officers continue the legacy of the McDonoughs by
providing grants that create a healthier, more educated and cultur-
ally appreciative citizenry.

3172 **High Technology Foundation**
1000 Galliher Dr.
Suite 1000
Fairmont, WV 26554   304-363-5482
                            877-363-5482
                            info@wvhtf.org
                            www.wvhtf.org

Michael I. Green, Chairman
James L. Estep, President & Chief Executive Officer
High Technology Foundation is dedicated to maximizing economic development in West Virginia through the high-technology business sector.
1990

Wisconsin

3173 **Arc of Dunn County**
2602 Hils Court
Menomonie, WI 54751-4160   715-235-7373
                                  Fax: 715-233-3565
                            www.arcofdunncounty.org
Rebecca Cooper, Executive Director
Kathy Lausted, Guardianship Director
Advocating for the rights of citizens with disabilities.

3174 **Arc of Eau Claire**
4800 Golf Road
Suite 450
Eau Claire, WI 54701-6130   715-833-1735
                                   Fax: 715-833-1215
                            frcec@frcec.org
                            www.frcec.org
Brook Steele, President
Melanie Koehler, Vice President
Dr. Jennifer Eddy, Secretary
Mission is to provide programs and services that build on family
strengths through prevention, education, support and networking
in collaboration with other resources in the community.

3175 **Arc of Fox Cities**
211 E. Franklin St.
Suite A
Appleton, WI 54911   920-735-0943
                            Fax: 920-725-1531
                            info@arcfoxcities.com
                            arcfoxcities.com
Laura McCormick, President
Todd Klauer, Vice President
Bryan Mueller, Secretary
Mission statement is to utilize advocacy, respect and concern to
empower all people with disabilities to have the opportunity to
choose and realize their goal of a full life and a secure future.

3176 **Arc of Racine County**
6214 Washington Ave
Suite C-6
Racine, WI 53404-3350   262-634-6303
                            info@thearcofracine.org
                            www.thearcofracine.org
Peggy Foreman, Executive Director
Alison Henry, Program Manager
Ross Gietzel, Program Assistant
The Arc of Racine's mission is to advocate for and provide infor-
mation and services to improve lives.

3177 **Arc of Wisconsin Disability Association**
2800 Royal Ave
Suite 202
Monona, WI 53713-1518   608-222-8907
                               877-272-8400
                               Fax: 608-222-8908
                               arcw@att.net
John Beisbier, President
Donna Auchue, Vice President
Tina Beauprey, Secretary
The Arc-Wisconsin strives to be a major force in advocating and
promoting self-determined quality of life opportunities for
poeple with developmental and related disabilities and their
families.

3178 **Arc-Dane County**
6602 Grand Teton Plz
Madison, WI 53719-1091   608-833-1199
                                Fax: 608-833-1307
                            arcdanecounty@gmail.com
                            arcdanecounty.org
Ken Hobbs, President
John Leemkuil, Vice President
Mark Lederer, Secretary
The Arc-Dane County is a non-profit organization whose primary
objective is to support children and adults with developmental
disabilities and their families through advocacy to assure these
individuals are offered the same opportunities and have the rights
due all people. The Arc-Dane County provides numerous services through education, overall support, and legislation that assists those individuals with developmental disabilities be it
within their homes, communities, or at work.

3179 **Faye McBeath Foundation**
101 W. Pleasant Street
Suite 210
Milwaukee, WI 53212- 3157   414-272-2626
                                   Fax: 414-272-6235
P. Michael Mahoney, Chair
Mary T. Kellner, Vice Chair
Gregory M. Wesley, Secretary
A private independent foundation providing grants to tax exempt
nonprofit organizations principally the metropolitan Milwaukee
area.

3180 **Helen Bader Foundation**
233 North Water Street
4th Floor
Milwaukee, WI 53202- 5761   414-224-6464
                                   Fax: 414-224-1441
                            info@hbf.org
                            www.hbf.org
Daniel J. Bader, President/CEO
Lisa G. Hiller, VP, Administration
Maria Lopez Vento, VP, Programs and Partnerships
Strives to be a philanthropic leader in improving the quality of
life of the diverse communities in which it works. The Foundation makes grants, convenes partners, and shares knowledge to
affect emerging issues in key areas.

3181 **Johnson Controls Foundation**
5757 N Green Bay Ave
P.O. Box 591
Milwaukee, WI 53201- 4408   414-524-1200
                                   800-333-2222
                                   Fax: 414-524-2077
                            johnsoncontrols.com
Stephen A Molinaroli, Chairman, President and CEO
Dr. Breda Bolzenius, Vice President, Vice Chairman
Kim Metcalf-Kupres, Vice President and Chief Marketi
Organized and directed to be operated for charitable purposes
which include the distribution and application of financial sup-
port to soundly managed and operated organizations or causes
which are fundamentally philanthropic.

3182 Lynde and Harry Bradley Foundation
1241 N Franklin Pl
Milwaukee, WI 53202-2901   414-291-9915
                                   Fax: 414-291-9991
                                   www.bradleyfdn.org

Dennis J. Kuester, Chairman
David V. Uihlein, Vice Chairman
Michael W. Grebbe, President and CEO
The Foundation's programs support limited, competent government; a dynamic marketplace for economic, intellectual and cultural activity; a vigorus defense at home and abroad, of American ideas and institutions; and scholarly studies and academic achievement.

3183 Milwaukee Foundation
101 W Pleasant St
Suite 210
Milwaukee, WI 53212-3963   414-272-5805
                                   Fax: 414-272-6235
                         info@greatermilwaukeefoundation.org
                         www.greatermilwaukeefoundation.org
Ellen M Gilligan, President and CEO
Marcus White, Vice President
Kathryn J. Dunn, Vice President
Guided by three tenets- helping donors create personal legacies of giving that last beyond their lifetimes, investing donor funds for maximum return with minimal risk, and playing a leadership role tackling the communities most challenging needs.

3184 Northwestern Mutual Life Foundation
720 E Wisconsin Ave
Milwaukee, WI 53202-4703   414-271-1444
                                   www.northwesternmutual.com
John E Schlifske, Chairman and CEO
Gregory C. Oberland, President
Michael G. Carter, Executive Vice President and CFO

3185 Patrick and Anna M Cudahy Fund
70 E. Lake St.,
Suite 1120
Chicago, Il 60601   312-422-1442
                                   Fax: 312-641-5736
                         laurenkrieg@cudahyfund.org
                         cudahyfund.org
Janet S Cudahy MD, President
Lauren Krieg, Executive Director
A general purpose foundation which primarily supports organizations in Wisconsin and the metropolitan Chicago area. Interests are social service, youth, and education with some giving for the arts, and other areas.

3186 SB Waterman & E Blade Charitable Foundation
Marshall & Ilsley Trust Company
111 E. Kilbourn Ave.,
Milwaukee, WI 53202-2980   414-287-8700
                                   Fax: 414-765-8200
Thomas C Boettcher, Director
Giving primarily to health associations. Geographical focus is Wisconsin.

Wyoming

3187 Arc of Natrona County
314 W. Midwest Ave
P.O. Box 393
Casper, WY 82601   307-577-4913
                                   800-433-5255
                                   Fax: 307-577-4014
                                   info@thearc.org
                                   arcofnatronacounty.org
Beau Covert, President
Dr. Nathan Edwards, Vice President
Kelley Reimer, Treasurer
Organization works to ensure that the estimated 7.2 million Americans with intellectual and developmental disabilities have the services and supports they need to grow, develop and live in communities across the nation.

Funding Directories

3188 Chronicle Guide to Grants
318 S. Lee Street
Alexandria, DC 20037-1146   202-466-1200
                                   800-287-6072
                                   Fax: 202-452-1033
                                   help@philanthropy.com
                                   heideninc.com
Phil Semas, Manager
Edward J. Heiden, President
A computerized research tool, on floppy disks or a CD-ROM, for immediate use on any IBM compatible personal computer. Offers electronic listings of 10,000 grants from hundreds of foundations, with a subscription that offers 1,000 plus new listings every two months. Each listing offers grant information as well as names, addresses and phone numbers of the grant-making organizations. $295.00

3189 College Student's Guide to Merit and Other No-Need Funding
Reference Service Press
5000 Windplay Dr
Suite 4
El Dorado Hills, CA 95762-9319   916-939-9620
                                   Fax: 916-939-9626
                                   info@rspfunding.com
                                   www.rspfunding.com
Gail Schlachter, Founder
R. David Weber, Editor
Sandy Hirsh, Editor
More than 1,200 funding opportunities for currently-enrolled or returning college students are described in this directory. $32.50
450 pages
ISBN 1-588410-41-2

3190 Community Health Funding Report
CD Publications
8204 Fenton St
Silver Spring, MD 20910-4502   301-588-6380
                                   800-666-6380
                                   Fax: 301-588-6385
                                   www.cdpublications.com
Michael Gerecht, President
The once twice-monthly report is now web-based to allow for breaking news updates and up the the minute information about funding, including: public and private grant announcements; reports on successful health programs nationwide; interviews with grant officials; plus national news on health policy topics affecting various organizations. $439.00
Web-based

3191 Directory of Financial Aids for Women
Reference Service Press
2310 Homestead Rd
Suite C1 #219
Los Altos, CA 94024   650-861-3170
                                   Fax: 650-861-3171
                                   info@rspfunding.com
                                   www.rspfunding.com
Gail Schlachter, Founder
R. David Weber, Editor
Sandy Hirsh, Editor
Funding programs listed support study, research, travel, training, career development, or innovative effort at any level; descriptions of more than 1,700 funding programs - representing billions of dollars in financial aid set aside for women; also an annotated bibliography of 60 key directories that identify even more financial aid opportunities and a set of indexes that let you search the directory by title, sponser, researching, tenability, subject, and deadline. $45.00
578 pages Biennial
ISBN 1-588410-00-5

3192 Disability Funding News
8204 Fenton St
Silver Spring, MD 20910-4502   301-588-6380
                                      800-666-6380
                                 Fax: 301-588-6385
                             www.cdpublications.com

Michael Gerecht, President

3193 FC Search
Foundation Center
79 fifth Avenue
New York, NY 10003-3034   212-620-4230
                                     800-424-9836
                                Fax: 212-807-3677
                       order@foundationcenter.org
                            foundationcenter.org

Bradford K Smith, President
Lisa Philip, Vice President for Strategic Phi
Jen Bokoff, Director of GrantCraft
Provides access to the Foundation Center's comprehensive database of funders in a convenient CD-ROM format. *$1845.00*

3194 Federal Grants & Contracts Weekly
LRP Publications
360 Hiatt Drive
Palm Beach Gardens, FL 33418-1718   800-341-7874
                                 Fax: 561-622-2423
                                  custserve@lrp.com
                                      www.lrp.com

Kelly Sullivan, Editor
Kenneth F. Kahn, President
The latest funding announcements of federal grants for project opportunities in research, training and services. Provides profiles of key programs, tips on seeking grants, updates on legislation and regulations, budget developments and early alerts to upcoming funding opportunities. *$340.00*
Weekly

3195 Financial Aid for Asian Americans
Reference Service Press
2310 Homestead Rd
Suite C1 #219
Los Altos, CA 94024   650-861-3170
                                 Fax: 650-861-3171
                                 info@rspfunding.com
                                 www.rspfunding.com

Gail Schlachter, Founder
R. David Weber, Editor
Sandy Hirsh, Editor
This is the source to use if you are looking for financial aid for Asian Americans; nearly 1,000 funding opportunities are described. *$35.00*
336 pages
ISBN 1-588410-02-1

3196 Financial Aid for Hispanic Americans
Reference Service Press
2310 Homestead Rd
Suite C1 #219
Los Altos, CA 94024   650-861-3170
                                 Fax: 650-861-3171
                                 info@rspfunding.com
                                 www.rspfunding.com

Gail Schlachter, Founder
R. David Weber, Editor
Sandy Hirsh, Editor
Nearly 1,300 funding programs open to Americans of Mexican, Puerto Rican, Central American, or other Latin American heritage are described here. *$37.50*
472 pages
ISBN 1-588410-03-X

3197 Financial Aid for Native Americans
Reference Service Press
2310 Homestead Rd
Suite C1 #219
Los Altos, CA 94024   650-861-3170
                                 Fax: 650-861-3171
                                 info@rspfunding.com
                                 www.rspfunding.com

Gail Schlachter, Founder
R. David Weber, Editor
Sandy Hirsh, Editor
Detailed information is provided on 1,500 funding opportunities open to American Indians, Native Alaskans, and Native Pacific Islanders. *$37.50*
562 pages
ISBN 1-588410-04-8

3198 Financial Aid for Research and Creative Activities Abroad
Reference Service Press
2310 Homestead Rd
Suite C1 #219
Los Altos, CA 94024   650-861-3170
                                 Fax: 650-861-3171
                                 info@rspfunding.com
                                 www.rspfunding.com

Gail Schlachter, Founder
R. David Weber, Editor
Sandy Hirsh, Editor
Described here are 1,200 funding programs (scholarships, fellowships, grants, etc.) available to support research, professional, or creative activities abroad. *$45.00*
378 pages
ISBN 1-588410-82-5

3199 Financial Aid for Veterans, Military Personnel and their Dependents
Reference Service Press
2310 Homestead Rd
Suite C1 #219
Los Altos, CA 94024   650-861-3170
                                 Fax: 650-861-3171
                                 info@rspfunding.com
                                 www.rspfunding.com

Gail Schlachter, Founder
R. David Weber, Editor
Sandy Hirsh, Editor
According to Reference Book Review, this directory (with its 1,100 entries) is the most comprehensive guide available on the subject. *$40.00*
392 pages
ISBN 1-588410-43-9

3200 Financial Aid for the Disabled and Their Families
Reference Service Press
2310 Homestead Rd
Suite C1 #219
Los Altos, CA 94024   650-861-3170
                                 Fax: 650-861-3171
                                 info@rspfunding.com
                                 www.rspfunding.com

Gail Schlachter, Founder
R. David Weber, Editor
This directory, which Children's Bookwatch calls invaluable describes more than 1,100 financial aid opportunities available to support persons with disabilities and members of their families. Updated every 2 years. *$37.50*
508 pages Every other yr.
ISBN 1-588410-01-3

3201 Foundation & Corporate Grants Alert
LRP Publications
360 Hiatt Drive
Palm Beach Gardens, FL 33418-1718   800-341-7874
                                 Fax: 561-622-2423
                                  custserve@lrp.com
                                      www.lrp.com

Kelly Sullivan, Editor
Kenneth F. Kahn, President

A complete guide to foundation and corporate grant opportunities for nonprofit organizations. Tracks developments and trends in funding and provides notification of changes in foundations' funding priorities. *$245.00*
Monthly
ISSN 1062-46 6

3202 Foundation 1000
Foundation Center
79 fifth Avenue
New York, NY 10003-3076

212-620-4230
800-424-9836
Fax: 212-807-3691
order@foundationcenter.org
www.foundationcenter.org

Bradford K Smith, President
Lisa Philip, Vice President for Strategic Phi
Jen Bokoff, Director of GrantCraft
Offers comprehensive information on the 1000 largest foundations in the US. *$195.00*

3203 Foundation Directories
Foundation Center
79 fifth Avenue
New York, NY 10003-3034

212-620-4230
800-424-9836
Fax: 212-807-3677
order@foundationcenter.org
foundationcenter.org

Bradford K Smith, President
Lisa Philip, Vice President for Strategic Phi
Jen Bokoff, Director of GrantCraft
Lists key facts on the top 20,000 US foundations. *$ 125.00*
ISBN 0-87954 -36-1

3204 Foundation Grants to Individuals
Foundation Center
79 fifth Avenue
New York, NY 10003-3034

212-620-4230
800-424-9836
Fax: 212-807-3677
order@foundationcenter.org
foundationcenter.org

Bradford K Smith, President
Lisa Philip, Vice President for Strategic Phi
Jen Bokoff, Director of GrantCraft
The only publication that provides extensive coverage of foundation funding prospects for individual grantseekers. *$40.00*
Biennially

3205 From the State Capitals: Public Health
Wakeman/Walworth
P.O.Box 7376
Alexandria, VA 22307-376

703-768-9600
Fax: 703-768-9690

Mark Willen, Editor
Digest of state and municipal health care financing and cost containment measures, includes medical legislation, disease control, etc. *$245.00*
6 pages

3206 Grant Guides
Foundation Center
79 fifth Avenue
New York, NY 10003-3034

212-620-4230
800-424-9836
Fax: 212-807-3677
order@foundationcenter.org
foundationcenter.org

Bradford K Smith, President
Lisa Philip, Vice President for Strategic Phi
Jen Bokoff, Director of GrantCraft
Provides descriptions of actual foundation grants awarded in various subject fields. *$35.00*
ISBN 0-87954 -90-6

3207 Guide to Funding for International and Foreign Programs
79 fifth Avenue
New York, NY 10003-3034

212-620-4230
800-424-9836
Fax: 212-807-3677
order@foundationcenter.org
foundationcenter.org

Bradford K Smith, President
Lisa Philip, Vice President for Strategic Phi
Jen Bokoff, Director of GrantCraft
Grantmakers featured in this guide provide funding for international relief, disaster assistance, human rights, civil liberties, community development, conferences, and education. *$190.00*

3208 Guide to US Foundations their Trustees, Officers and Donors
Foundation Center
79 fifth Avenue
New York, NY 10003-3034

212-620-4230
800-424-9836
Fax: 212-807-3677
order@foundationcenter.org
foundationcenter.org

Bradford K Smith, President
Lisa Philip, Vice President for Strategic Phi
Jen Bokoff, Director of GrantCraft
Provides crucial facts on grantmaking. Each entry includes contact information, current assets, annual contributions, officers, donors and more. *$135.00*

3209 High School Senior's Guide to Merit and Other No-Need Funding
Reference Service Press
2310 Homestead Rd
Suite C1 #219
Los Altos, CA 94024

650-861-3170
Fax: 650-861-3171
info@rspfunding.com
www.rspfunding.com

Gail Schlachter, Founder
R. David Weber, Editor
Sandy Hirsh, Editor
Here's your guide to 1,100 funding programs that never look at income level when making awards to college bound high school seniors. *$29.95*
400 pages
ISBN 1-588410-44-X

3210 How to Pay for Your Degree in Business & Related Fields
Reference Service Press
2310 Homestead Rd
Suite C1 #219
Los Altos, CA 94024

650-861-3170
Fax: 650-861-3171
info@rspfunding.com
www.rspfunding.com

Gail Schlachter, Founder
R. David Weber, Editor
Sandy Hirsh, Editor
If you need funding for an undergraduate or graduate degree in business or related fields, this is the directory to use (500+ funding programs described). *$30.00*
290 pages
ISBN 1-588411-45-1

3211 How to Pay for Your Degree in Education& Related Fields
Reference Service Press
2310 Homestead Rd
Suite C1 #219
Los Altos, CA 94024

650-861-3170
Fax: 650-861-3171
www.rspfunding.com

Gail Schlachter, Founder
R. David Weber, Editor
Sandy Hirsh, Editor

Here's hundreds of funding opportunities available to support undergraduate and graduate students preparing for a career in education, guidance etc. *$30.00*

250 pages

ISBN 1-588411-46-x

3212   National Directory of Corporate Giving
Foundation Center
79 fifth Avenue
New York, NY 10003-3034

212-620-4230
800-424-9836
Fax: 212-807-3677
order@foundationcenter.org
foundationcenter.org

Bradford K Smith, President
Lisa Philip, Vice President for Strategic Phi
Jen Bokoff, Director of GrantCraft
Offers over 2,000 corporate funders, current giving reviews and profiles of sponsoring companies. *$195.00*

3213   Older Americans Report
Business Publishers
2222 Sedwick Drive
Durham, NC 27713-1995

240-514-0600
800-223-8720
Fax: 800-508-2592
custserv@bpinews.com
www.bpinews.com

Leonard Eiser, Publisher
Follows all programs and funding sources in education, housing, job training, therapy, Social Security Supplemental Security Income, Medicare, Medicaid and more of importance to persons with disabilities. Also covers the latest on the Americans with Disabilities Act. Publishes a newsletter. *$327.00*

3214   Student Guide
US Department of Education
400 Maryland Avenue SW
Washington, DC 20202

202-401-2000
800-872-5327
Fax: 202-401-0689
TTY: 800-437-0833
customerservice@inet.ed.gov
ed.gov

Arne Duncan, Secretary of Education
Jim Shelton, Deputy Secretary
Ted Mitchell, Under Secretary
Describes the major student aid programs the US Department of Education administers and gives detailed information about program procedures.

74 pages

Government Agencies

Federal

3215 Administration on Aging
Administration for Community Living
330 C St. SW
Washington, DC 20201 202-401-4634
acl.gov/about-acl/administration-aging
Edwin Walker, Deputy Assistant Secretary for Aging
Administers the Older Americans Act of 1965 to assist states and local communities in developing programs and services for older persons.

3216 Administration on Children, Youth and Families
330 C St. SW
Washington, DC 20201 202-401-4634
www.acf.hhs.gov/acyf
Elizabeth Darling, Acting Commissioner
Responsible for federal programs that support social services for children, youth, and families; protective services for at-risk youth; and adoption services for children with special needs.

3217 Administration on Disabilities
Administration for Community Living
330 C St. SW
Washington, DC 20201 202-401-4634
acl.gov
Anjali Forber-Pratt, Director
Alison Barkoff, Principal Deputy Administrator
Vicki Gottlich, Director, Center for Policy & Evaluation
Ensures that individuals with disabilities and their families participate in the design of and have access to culturally competent services, supports, and other assistance and opportunities that promote independence, productivity, and integration and inclusion into the community.

3218 Americans with Disabilities Act Information and Technical Assistance
US Department of Justice
950 Pennsylvania Ave. NW
9th Floor
Washington, DC 20530 202-307-0663
800-514-0301
Fax: 202-307-1197
TTY: 800-514-0383
www.ada.gov
Rebecca B. Bond, Chief
Anne Raish, Principal Deputy Chief
Christina Galindo-Walsh, Deputy Chief
The ADA assures that Americans with disabilities have the same opportunities as all Americans. To this end, the Justice Department produces publications and conducts programs to increase compliance of the ADA nationwide.

3219 Centers for Medicare & Medicaid Services
7500 Security Blvd.
Baltimore, MD 21244 410-786-3000
877-267-2323
TTY: 866-226-1819
www.cms.gov
Chiquita Brooks-LaSure, Administrator
Jonathan Blum, Principal Deputy Administrator
Karen Jackson, Deputy Chief Operating Officer
Responsible for administering Medicare, Medicaid, and the Children's Health Insurance Program. Formerly the Health Care Financing Administration.

3220 Civil Rights Division/Disability Rights Section
US Department of Justice
950 Pennsylvania Ave. NW
9th Floor
Washington, DC 20530 202-307-0663
800-514-0301
Fax: 202-307-1197
TTY: 800-514-0383
www.ada.gov
Rebecca B. Bond, Chief
Anne Raish, Principal Deputy Chief
Christina Galindo-Walsh, Deputy Chief
The US Department of Justice answers questions about the Americans with Disabilities Act (ADA) and provides free materials by mail and fax through the ADA Information Line.

3221 Committee for Purchase from People Who Are Blind or Severely Disabled
1401 S. Clark St.
Suite 715
Arlington, VA 22202-3259 703-603-2100
800-999-5963
Fax: 703-328-2909
info@abilityone.gov
www.abilityone.gov
Kimberly Zeich, Acting Executive Director & Chief Executive Officer
Irene Glaeser, Acting Deputy Executive Director & Chief Operating Officer
Kelvin Wood, Chief of Staff
A federal agency that administers the Javits-Wagner-O'Day Program, directing federal agencies to purchase products and services from nonprofit agencies that employ people who are blind or have other severe disabilities. Provides a wide range of vocational options to individuals with severe disabilities.

3222 Equal Opportunity Employment Commission
131 M St. NE
Washington, DC 20507 800-669-4000
TTY: 800-669-6820
info@eeoc.gov
www.eeoc.gov
Charlotte A. Burrows, Chair
Janet Dhillon, Commissioner
Keith E. Sonderling, Commissioner
This agency is responsible for enforcing workplace anti-discrimination laws, including the Americans with Disabilities Act (ADA) and the Rehabilitation Act.

3223 Federal Communications Commission
45 L St. NE
Washington, DC 20554 202-418-0500
888-225-5322
Fax: 866-418-0232
fccinfo@fcc.gov
fcc.gov
Jessica Rosenworcel, Chairwoman
Brendan Carr, Commissioner
Geoffrey Starks, Commissioner
Enforces ADA telecommunications provisions which require that companies offering telephone service to the general public must offer telephone relay services to individuals who use text telephones or similar devices. Also enforces closed captioning rules, hearing compatibility and access to equipment and services for people with disabilities.

3224 Health Resources and Services Administration (HRSA)
US Department of Health and Human Services
5600 Fishers Lane
Rockville, MD 20857 301-443-3376
877-464-4772
TTY: 877-897-9910
www.hrsa.gov
Diana Espinosa, Deputy Administrator
Jordan Grossman, Chief of Staff
Carole Johnson, Administrator
The Health Resources and Services Administration provides programs for people with HIV/AIDS, pregnant women, mothers, and other individuals in need of high quality primary health care.

3225 National Cancer Institute
9609 Medical Center Dr.
Rockville, MD 20850   800-422-6237
                              TTY: 800-332-8615
                              nciinfo@nih.gov
                              www.cancer.gov

Norman E. Sharpless, Director
Douglas R. Lowy, Principal Deputy Director
James Doroshow, Deputy Director, Clinical & Translational
Research
The National Cancer Institute conducts and supports research, training, health information dissemination, and programs related to cancer, cancer rehabilitation, and the care of cancer patients.
1975

3226 National Coalition of Federal Aviation Employees with Disabilities
Federal Aviation Administration
6500 South MacArthur, AML-4023
RRF Building-185
Oklahoma City, OK 73169   405-954-6877
                              greg.brooks@faa.gov
                              www.ncfaed.org

Gregory A. Brooks, National President
NCFAED works on improving work conditions for employees; expanding National Coalition to serve all FAA employees; promoting equal opportunity for people with disabilities in the FAA workplace; assisting the FAA in its commitment to remove physical and attudinal barriers which inhibit opportunities for people with disabilities; and aligning with internal and external organizations to attract future generations of people with disabilities to the FAA as employees.

3227 National Council on Disability
1331 F St. NW
Suite 850
Washington, DC 20004   202-272-2004
                              Fax: 202-272-2022
                              TTY: 202-272-2074
                              www.ncd.gov

Anne Sommers McIntosh, Executive Director
Joan M. Durocher, General Counsel & Director, Policy
Lisa Grubb, Director, Administration, Finance & Operations
Federal agency led by members appointed by the President of the United States and confirmed by the United States Senate. The overall purpose of the National Council is to promote policies, programs, practices and procedures that guarantee equal opportunities to persons with disabilities.

3228 National Eye Institute
National Institutes of Health
31 Center Dr.
MSC 2510
Bethesda, MD 20892-2510   301-496-5248
                              2020@nei.nih.gov
                              www.nei.nih.gov

Michael F. Chiang, Director
Santa Tumminia, Deputy Director
Melanie Reagan, Acting Executive Officer
As part of the federal government's National Institutes of Health (NIH), the National Eye Institute finances intramural and extramural research on eye diseases and visual disorders.

3229 National Institute of Arthritis and Musculoskeletal and Skin Diseases
National Institutes of Health
31 Center Dr., MSC 2350
Building 31, Room 4C02
Bethesda, MD 20892-2350   301-496-8190
                              877-226-4267
                              Fax: 301-480-2814
                              TTY: 301-565-2966
                              www.naims.nih.gov

Lindsey A. Criswell, Director
Robert H. Carter, Deputy Director
Rick Phillips, Acting Associate Director, Management &
Operations
The mission of the National Institute of Arthritis and Musculoskeletal and Skin Diseases is to advance understanding and treatment of diseases of the bones, joints, muscles, and skin

by supporting research, training scientists, and disseminating information on such diseases.

3230 National Institute of Diabetes and Digestive and Kidney Diseases
National Institutes of Health
31 Center Dr.
Bethesda, MD 20892   800-860-8747
                              TTY: 866-569-1162
                              healthinfo@niddk.nih.gov
                              www.niddk.nih.gov

Griffin P. Rodgers, Director
Gregory G. Germino, Deputy Director
Camille Hoover, Executive Officer
The National Institute of Diabetes and Digestive and Kidney Diseases conducts and supports research, training, and science-based information dissemination on diabetes, digestive diseases, and kidney, urologic, and hematologic diseases.

3231 National Institute of Mental Health
National Institutes of Health
6001 Executive Blvd.
Room 6200, MSC 9663
Bethesda, MD 20892-9663   866-615-6464
                              TTY: 866-415-8051
                              nimhinfo@nih.gov
                              www.nimh.nih.gov

Joshua A. Gordon, Director
Shelli Avenevoli, Deputy Director
The mission of the National Institute of Mental Health is to advance the prevention, recovery, and cure of mental illnesses through basic and clinical research.

3232 National Institute of Neurological Disorders and Stroke
National Institutes of Health
PO Box 5801
Bethesda, MD 20824   800-352-9424
                              www.ninds.nih.gov

Nina Schor, Deputy Director
The mission of the National Institute of Neurological Disorders and Stroke is to reduce the burden of neurological disease by supporting neuroscience research, funding and conducting training and career development programs, and disseminating scientific information on neurological health.

3233 National Institute on Aging
31 Center Dr., MSC 2292
Building 31, Room 5C27
Bethesda, MD 20892   800-222-2225
                              TTY: 800-222-4225
                              niaic@nia.nih.gov
                              www.nia.nih.gov

Richard J. Hodes, Director
Lisa Mascone, Deputy Director, Management
Luigi Ferrucci, Scientific Director
The National Institute on Aging (NIA) is the primary federal agency engaged in researching Alzheimer's disease, providing resources to scientists and educating the public on the results of studies.

3234 National Institute on Deafness and Other Communication Disorders
National Institutes of Health
31 Center Dr.
MSC 2320
Bethesda, MD 20892-2320   301-827-8183
                              800-241-1044
                              TTY: 800-241-1055
                              nidcdinfo@nidcd.nih.gov
                              www.nidcd.nih.gov

Debara L. Tucci, Director
Judith A. Cooper, Deputy Director
Timothy J. Wheeles, Executive Officer
The National Institute on Deafness and Other Communication Disorders supports and conducts research to help prevent, detect and diagnose disabilities that affect hearing, balance, taste, smell, voice, speech, and communication.
1988

3235 National Institute on Disability, Independent Living, and Rehabilitation Research (NIDILRR)
Administration for Community Living
330 C St. SW
Washington, DC 20201   202-401-4634
acl.gov

Anjali Forber-Pratt, Director
Alison Barkoff, Principal Deputy Administrator
Vicki Gottlich, Director, Center for Policy & Evaluation
Serving as the federal government's disability research agency, NIDILRR provides research, training, and technical assistance to maximize the full inclusion of individuals with disabilities into society; promotes the use of rehabilitation technology for individuals with disabilities; and ensures the distribution of practical scientific and technological information in usable formats.

3236 Office of Disability Employment Policy
US Department of Labor
200 Constitution Ave. NW
Washington, DC 20210   202-693-7880
866-633-7365
odep@dol.gov
www.dol.gov/agencies/odep

Melissa Turner, Executive Officer
Taryn M. Williams, Assistant Secretary
Jennifer Sheehy, Deputy Assistant Secretary
Non-regulatory federal agency that promotes and develops policies that increase employment opportunities for people with disabilities.

3237 Office of Fair Housing and Equal Opportunity
US Department of Housing & Urban Development
451 7th St. SW
Washington, DC 20410   202-708-1112
TTY: 202-708-1455
www.hud.gov/program_offices

Marcia L. Fudge, Secretary
Adrianne Todman, Deputy Secretary
Jenn Jones, Chief of Staff
The Office of Fair Housing and Equal Opportunity (FHEO) enforces and develops laws and policies that eliminate housing discrimination and ensure that all Americans have equal access to housing. The laws enforced by FHEO include Titles II and III of the Americans with Disabilities Act and Section 504 of the Rehabilitation Act.

3238 Office of Retirement and Disability Policy (ORDP)
Social Security Administration

800-772-1213
TTY: 800-325-0778
www.ssa.gov/policy

Stephen G. Evangelista, Acting Deputy Commissioner
Dawn S. Wiggins, Associate Commissioner
Natalie T. Lu, Associate Commissioner
Serves as the principal advisor to the Commissioner of Social Security on major policy issues, including those relating to disability policy.

3239 Office of Special Education Programs
US Department of Education
400 Maryland Ave. SW
Washington, DC 20202   202-401-2000
800-872-5327
TTY: 800-730-8913
www.ed.gov/about/offices/list/osers/osep
Valerie C. Williams, Director
David Cantrell, Deputy Director
Assists infants, toddlers, children and youth with disabilities by providing leadership and financial support to states and local districts.

3240 President's Committee on People with Intellectual Disabilities
Administration for Community Living
330 C St. SW
Washington, DC 20201   202-401-4634
acl.gov

Anjali Forber-Pratt, Director
Alison Barkoff, Principal Deputy Administrator
Vicki Gottlich, Director, Center for Policy & Evaluation

Established by the presidential executive order to advise the President of the United States and the Secretary of Health and Human Services on issues concerning citizens with intellectual disabilities. PCPID is overseen and supported by the Administration for Community Living (ACL).

3241 Rehabilitation Services Administration
US Department of Education
400 Maryland Ave. SW
Washington, DC 20202   202-401-2000
800-872-5327
TTY: 800-730-8913
www2.ed.gov

The Rehabilitation Services Administration (RSA) oversees formula and discretionary grant programs that help individuals with physical or mental disabilities obtain employment and live more independently through the provision of such supports as counseling, medical and psychological services, job training and other individualized services.

3242 Social Security Administration

800-772-1213
TTY: 800-325-0778
www.ssa.gov

Stephen G. Evangelista, Acting Deputy Commissioner
Dawn S. Wiggins, Associate Commissioner
Natalie T. Lu, Associate Commissioner
Administers old age, survivors, and disability insurance programs under Title II of the Social Security Act. Also administers the federal income maintenance program under Title XVI of the Social Security Act. Maintains network of local/regional offices nationwide.

3243 Substance Abuse and Mental Health Services Administration (SAMHSA)
US Department of Health and Human Services
5600 Fishers Lane
Rockville, MD 20857   877-726-4727
TTY: 800-487-4889
samhsainfo@samhsa.hhs.gov
www.samhsa.gov

Tom Coderre, Acting Deputy Assistant Secretary
Sonia Chessen, Chief of Staff
Trina Dutta, Senior Advisor
SAMHSA aims to advance substance use and mental health services and improve the lives of people living with mental and substance use disorders.

3244 US Department of Education: Office for Civil Rights
400 Maryland Ave. SW
Washington, DC 20202-1100   800-421-3481
800-872-5327
TTY: 800-730-8913
ocr@ed.gov
www2.ed.gov/about/offices/list/ocr
Prohibits discrimination in programs and activities funded by the Department of Education. Investigates complaints and provides technical assistance to individuals and entities with rights and responsibilities under Section 504.

3245 US Department of Labor: Office of Federal Contract Compliance Programs
200 Constitution Ave. NW
Washington, DC 20210   866-487-2365
TTY: 877-889-5627
webmaster@dol.gov
www.dol.gov/agencies/ofccp

Jenny R. Yang, Director
Dariely Rodriguez, Chief of Staff
Michele Hodge, Deputy Director
Prohibits contractors and subcontractors from discriminating against applicants or employees.

3246 US Department of Transportation
1200 New Jersey Ave. SE
Washington, DC 20590   202-366-4000
                                         855-368-4200
                                         TTY: 711
                                         www.dot.gov

Pete Buttigieg, Secretary
Polly Trottenberg, Deputy Secretary
Laura Schiller, Chief of Staff
Enforces ADA provisions that require nondiscrimination in public and private mass transportation systems and services.

3247 US Department of Veterans Affairs
                                         800-698-2411
                                         TTY: 711
                                         www.va.gov

Denis McDonough, Secretary
Tanya J. Bradsher, Chief of Staff
The Department of Veterans Affairs provides programs for veterans and their families. Programs include health care, rehabilitation services, compensation for disabilities, veterans benefits, and more.

3248 US Office of Personnel Management
1900 E St. NW
Washington, DC 20415-1000   202-606-1800
                                        TTY: 800-877-8339
                                        opm.gov

Kiran Ahuja, Director
Provides human resources leadership and support to federal agencies. Administers a merit system for federal employment that includes recruiting, examining, training, and promoting people on the basis of knowledge and skills, regardless of sex, race, religion or other factors.

Alabama

3249 Alabama Council For Developmental Disabilities
RSA Union Building
RSA Union Building
PO Box 301410
Montgomery, AL 36130- 1410   334-242-3973
                                        800-232-2158
                                        Fax: 334-242-0797
                                        Myra.Jones@mh.alabama.gov
                                        www.acdd.org

Stefan Eisen, Jr., Chair, Parent Advocate
Sophia Whitted, Fiscal Manager
Elmyra Jones-Banks, Executive Director
Serves as an advocate for Alabama's citizens with developmental disabilities and their families; to empower them with the knowledge and opportunity to make informed choices and exercise control over their own lives; and to create a climate for positive socialchange to enable them to be respected, independent and productive integrated members of society.

3250 Alabama Department of Public Health
The RSA Tower, 201 Monroe Street
PO Box 303017
Montgomery, AL 36130-3017   334-206-5300
                                        800-ALA-1818
                                        www.adph.org

Kathy Vincent, Staff Assistant
Donald E Williamson, Administrator
Provides professional services for the improvement and protection of the public's health through disease prevention and the assurance of public health services to resident and transient populations of the state regardless of social circumstances or the ability to pay.

3251 Alabama Department of Rehabilitation Services
602 S. Lawrence St.
Montgomery, AL 36104   334-293-7500
                                         800-441-7607
                                         Fax: 334-293-7383
                                         TTY: 800-499-1816
                                         www.rehab.alabama.gov

Michelle K. Glaze, District 1, Mobile
Jimmy Varnado, District 2, Montgomery
Eddie Williams, District 5, Hunstville
To enable Alabama's children and adults with disabilities to achieve their maximum potential.

3252 Alabama Department of Senior Services
201 Monroe Street
RSA Tower Suite 350
Montgomery, AL 36140   334-242-5743
                                         877-425-2243
                                         Fax: 334-242-5594
                                         Ageline@adss.alabama.gov

Irene Collins, Executive Director
Thomas Ray Edwards, Board Chairman
Dr. Horace Patterson, Vice-Chair
The mission of the Alabama Department of Senior Services is to promote the independence and dignity of those we serve through a comprehensive and coordinated system of quality services

3253 Alabama Disabilities Advocacy Program
University of Alabama
P.O.Box 870395
Tuscaloosa, AL 35487-0395   205-348-4928
                                        800-826-1675
                                        Fax: 205-348-3909
                                        adap@adap.ua.edu

Anita Davidson, Legal Assistant
Janet Owens, Accounting Specialist
James Tucker, Director
The federally mandate statewide protection and advocacy system serving eligible individuals with disabilities in Alabama. ADAP has five program components: Protection and Advocacy for persons with developmental disabilities (PADD), Protection and Advocacy for Individuals with Mental Illness (PAIMT), Protection and Advocacy of Individual Rights (PAIR), Protection and Advocacy for Assistive Technology (PAAT) and Protection & Advocacy For Beneficiaries of Social Security (PABSS).

3254 Alabama Division of Rehabilitation and Crippled Children
602 S Lawrence Street
Montgomery, AL 36104   334-293-7500
                                         800-441-7607
                                         Fax: 334-293-7383
                                         www.rehab.state.al.us

Cary F Boswell, Commissioner
Steven Kayes, Board Member
Jimmie Varnado, Board Member

3255 Alabama Governor's Committee on Employment of Persons with Disabilities
602 S. Lawrence St.
Montgomery, AL 36104   334-293-7500
                                         800-441-7609
                                         Fax: 334-293-7383
                                         TTY: 800-499-1816
                                         www.rehab.alabama.gov

Jane E. Burdeshaw, Commissioner
The Alabama Governor's Committee on Employment of People with Disabilities (AGCEPD) is a program of the Alabama Department of Rehabilitation Services (ADRS).

3256 Alabama State Department of Human Resources
Childcare Services Division
50 North Ripley Street
Montgomery, AL 36130   334-242-1310
                                         Fax: 334-353-1115
                                         barry.spear@dhr.alabama.gov
                                         www.dhr.state.al.us

Nancy T. Buckner, Commissioner
Nancy Jinright, Chief of Staff/Ethics Officer
John Hardy, Communications

Partners with communities to promtoe family stability and provide for the safety and self-sufficiency of vulnerable Alabamians.

3257   Client Assistance Program: Alabama
400 South Union Street
Suite 465
Montgomery, AL 36104

334-263-2749
800-288-3231
Fax: 334-230-9765
rachel.hughes@rehab.alabama.gov
www.sacap.alabama.gov

Rachel Hughes, Director/Advocate

3258   Disability Determination Service: Birmingham
P.O.Box 830300
Birmingham, AL 35283-0300

205-989-2100
800-292-8106
Fax: 205-989-2295
ssa.gov

Tommy Warren, Executive Director
Janet Cox, Owner

3259   Social Security: Mobile Disability Determination Services
PO Box 2371
Mobile, AL 36652-2371

251-433-2820
800-292-6743
Fax: 251-436-0599
www.ssa.gov

Tommy Warren, Executive Director
Jack Miller, Office Manager

3260   South Central Alabama Mental Health (SCAMHC)
19815 Bay Branch Rd.
Andalusia, AL 36420

334-222-2523
877-530-0002
www.scamhc.org

Quasi-governmental organization established by local government entities, providing a range of services to approximately 4,500 mentally ill, substance abuse, and developmentally disabled individuals in Butler, Coffee, Covington and Crenshaw Counties.

3261   Workers Compensation Board Alabama
649 Monroe Street
Montgomery, AL 36131

334-242-2868
800-528-5166
Fax: 334-353-8262
webmaster@labor.alabama.gov
labor.alabama.gov/wc

Charles DeLamar, Director
Al Pelham, Supervisor
Sandy Hallmark, Supervisor

The Workers' Compensation Division is responsible for the administration of the Alabama Workers' Compensation Law to ensure proper payment of benefits to employees injured on the job and encourage safety in the work place

Alaska

3262   ATLA
2217 E Tudor Rd
Ste 4
Anchorage, AK 99507-1068

907-563-2599
800-723-2852
Fax: 907-563-0699
www.atla.biz

Kathy Privratsky, Executive Director
Mystie Rail, Commissioner
Margaret Cisco, AT Specialist

Assistive Technology sales and services. ATLA is Alaska's only assistive technology resource center.

3263   Alaska Commission on Aging
150 Third Street #103
PO Box 110693
Juneau, AK 99811- 0693

907-465-3250
Fax: 907-465-1398
dhss.alaska.gov/acoa

Mary Shields, Chair
Rolf Numme, Vice Chair
Denise Daniello, Executive Director

Works to promote and protect the health and well-being of Alaskans.

3264   Alaska Department of Handicapped Children
Ste 314
1231 Gambell St
Anchorage, AK 99501-4664

907-346-1995

Gregory Lee, CEO

3265   Alaska Division of Vocational Rehabilitation:
801 W. 10th Street,
Suite A
Juneau, AK 99801-1878

907-465-2814
800-478-2815
Fax: 907-465-2856
dawn.duval@alaska.gov
labor.alaska.gov

Dianne Blummer, Commissioner
David G Stone, Deputy commissioner
John Cannon, Director

Provides comprehensive services to people with disabilities to assist in achieving an employment outcome.

3266   Client Assistance Program: Alaska
2900 Boniface Pkwy
Ste 100
Anchorage, AK 99504-3195

907-333-2211
800-478-0047
Fax: 907-333-1186
www.icdri.org/legal/AlaskaCAP.htm

Pam Stratton, Executive Director

We provide informatory referral to other programs in Alaska that are funded under the Rehabilitation Act of 1973 as amended; Individual assistance or advocacy, if an individual with disability has applied for or received services from an agency funded under the Rehabilitation Act and has concerns or questions we will work with them to help resolve their concerns with the agency.

3267   Department Of Health & Social Services - Division Of Behaviorial Health
350 Main Street
Suite 214
Juneau, AK 99801-1149

907-465-3370
800-465-4828
Fax: 907-465-2668
www.alaska.gov

Albert E. Wall, Director
Stacy Toner, Division Operations Manager
Liz Clement, Program Coordinator

The division plans for and provides appropriate prevention, treatment and support for families impacted by mental disorders or developmental disabilities while maximizing self-determination. Community based services are provided by grantees. Inpatient services are provided in two division operated facilities.

3268   Governor's Committee on Employment and Rehabilitation of People with Disabilities
Division of Vocational Rehabilitation (DVR)
801 W 10th Street
Suite A
Juneau, AK 99801-1878

907-465-2814
800-478-2815
Fax: 907-465-2815
dawn.duval@alaska.gov
www.labor.state.ak.us/dvr

Cheryl Walsh, Executive Director

Carries on a continuing program to promote the employment and rehabilitation of citizens with disabilities in the State of Alaska. Advocates for a comprehensive statewide system for access to assistive technology. Obtains and maintains cooperation with public and private groups and individuals in this field.

3269 Governor's Council on Disabilities and Special Education
3601 C Street
Suite 740
Anchorage, AK 99524-0249
907-269-8990
888-269-8990
Fax: 907-269-8995
GCDSE@alaska.gov
www.hss.state.ak.us/gcdse/

Patrick Reinhart, Executive Director
Rich Sanders, Planner III
Britteny M Howell, M.A., ABD, Research Analyst III
The Governor's Council on Disabilities & Special Education was created to meet Alaska's diverse needs.

3270 Protection & Advocacy System: Alaska
Disability Law Center of Alaska
3330 Arctic Blvd
Ste 103
Anchorage, AK 99503-4580
907-565-1002
800-478-1234
Fax: 907-565-1000
akpa@dlcak.org

Deborah Smith, President
James M Shine Sr
Deals with rights of the disabled. Works in conjunction with agencies, law offices and family members.

3271 Protection & Advocacy for Persons with Developmental Disabilities: Alaska
Advocacy Services of Alaska
Ste 101
615 E 82nd Ave
Anchorage, AK 99518-3100
907-222-2652
866-275-7273
Fax: 907-677-8777
TTY: 866-232-4525

Greg Schomaker, Manager

3272 Workers Compensation Division
Department of Labor & Workforce Development
PO Box 115512
Juneau, AK 99811-5512
907-465-2790
Fax: 907-465-2797
workerscomp@alaska.gov
www.labor.state.ak.us/wc

Clark Bishop, Commissioner
Trena Heikes, Division Director
Michael Monagle, Director
The Division of Workers' Compensation is the agency charged with the administration of the Alaska Workers' Compensation Act (Act). The Act provides for the payment by employers or their insurance carriers of medical, disability and reemployment benefits to injured workers

Arizona

3273 Arizona Department of Economic Security
1717 W Jefferson
Phoenix, AZ 85007
602-542-4791
www.azdes.gov

Michael Trailor, Director
The Department of Economic Security is a human service agency providing services in six areas: Aging and Community Services, Benefits and Medical Eligibility, Child Support Enforcement, Children and Family Services, Developmental Disabilities and Employment and Rehabilitation Services.

3274 Arizona Department of Health Services
150 North 18th Avenue
Ste 330
Phoenix, AZ 85007-3243
602-542-1025
Fax: 602-542-0883
www.azdhs.gov

Will Humble, Director
Neal Young, Director
Lynne Smith, Chief Exeuctive Officer

The mission of Children's Rehabilitative Services is to improve the quality of life for children by providing family-centered medical treatment, rehabilitation, and related support services to enrolled individuals who have certain medical, handicapping, or potentially handicapping conditions.

3275 Arizona Division of Aging and Adult Services
1789 West Jefferson Street
Site Code 950A
Phoenix, AZ 85007-3202
602-542-4446
Fax: 602-542-6655
www.azdes.gov

Rex Critchfield, Manager
Neal Young, Director
Lynne Smith, Chief Executive Officer
The Division supports at-risk Arizonans to meet their basic needs and to live safely, with dignity and independence.

3276 Arizona Rehabilitation State Services for the Blind and Visually Impaired
4620 N 16th St, B-106
Ste 100
Phoenix, AZ 85016-5121
602-266-9579
Fax: 602-264-7819
www.azdes.gov

Paul Howell, Vocational Rehab Supervisor
Suzanne Sayre f, Rehab Counselor for Blind
Offers clients a conservation program, eye examinations, treatments, counseling, social work, psychological testing and evaluation, professional training, computer training and more for the visually impaired. The staff includes 56 full time employees.

3277 Developmental Disability Council: Arizona
2828 N Country Club Rd
Ste 100
Tucson, AZ 85716-3202
602-542-4049
800-889-5893
Fax: 602-542-5320
www.cpes.com

David A Berns, Manager
Nebal Chavez, Executive Director
Susan Madison, Manager
The mission of the GovernorOs Council on Developmental Disabilities is to bring together persons with disabilities representing Arizona cultural diversity and their families and other community members, to protect rights, eliminate barriers, and jointly promote equal opportunities

3278 Governor's Council on Developmental Disabilities
1700 West Wasington Street
Suite 420
Phoenix, AZ 85007
520-325-9688
877-665-3176
Fax: 520-325-3561
lclausen@azdes.gov
azgovernor.gov/DDPC/

Larry Clausen, Executive Director
Shelly Adams, Executive Secretary
The purpose of the council is to advocate for and assure that individuals with developmental disabilities and their families participate in the design of and have access to culturally competent services, supports and provides opportunities to become integrated and included in the community.

3279 International Dyslexia Association: Arizona Branch
Meredith Puls AZ-IDA
985 W. Silver Spring Place
Oro Valley, AZ 85755-6548
480-941-0308
arizona.ida@gmail.com

Meredith Puls, President
Rebekah Dyer, Vice President
Melissa A. L. Pallister, Treasurer
Provides free information and referral services for diagnosis and tutoring for parents, educators, physicians, and individuals with dyslexia. Membership includes yearly journal and quarterly newsletter, and Pennsylvania newsletter; discounts to conferences and events.

3280   Protection & Advocacy for Persons with Disabilities: Arizona
Arizona Center for Disability Law
5025 E Washington St
Suite 202
Phoenix, AZ 85034
602-274-6287
800-927-2260
Fax: 602-274-6779
TTY: 602-274-6287
center@azdisabilitylaw.org
www.azdisabilitylaw.org

Anthony DiRienzi, President
Art Gode, Vice President
J. J. Rico, Executive Director
The Center provides disability-related legal information and advice to individuals who need their services and assistance. In addition to limited legal representation, their goal is to provide efficient, streamlined services to educate people with disabilities and their support on how to enforce their legal rights through self-advocacy. Guides and documents are available online by selecting Self-Advocacy Materials button on the homepage.

3281   Social Security: Phoenix Disability Determination Services
Social Security Admission
4000 North Central Avenue
Suite 1800
Phoenix, AZ 85714
520-638-2000
800-772-1213
TTY: 800-325-0778
www.ssa.gov

The Social Security Administration functions as the principal agency of the United States federal government that administers Social Security, or more specifically, the federal Old-Age, Survivors, and Disability Insurance (OASDI) program. The OASDI pays retirement, disability, and survivorsO benefits to qualifying individuals.

3282   Social Security: Tucson Disability Determination Services
4710 South Palo Verde Road
Tucson, AZ 85714-2030
520-638-2000
800-772-1213
TTY: 800-325-0778
www.ssa.gov

The Social Security Administration functions as the principal agency of the United States federal government that administers Social Security, or more specifically, the federal Old-Age, Survivors, and Disability Insurance (OASDI) program. The OASDI pays retirement, disability, and survivorsO benefits to qualifying individuals.

Arkansas

3283   Arkansas Assistive Technology Projects
Increasing Capabilities Access
900 W.7th Street
Little Rock, AR 72201-4538
501-666-8868
800-828-2799
Fax: 501-666-5319
info@ar-ican.org

Eddie Schmeckenbecher, Supervisor
Essie Hardin, Secretary
Bryan Ayres, Advisory Counsel
A consumer responsive, statewide program promoting assistive technology devices and sources for persons of all ages with all disabilities. Referral and information services provide information about devices, where to obtain them and their cost.

3284   Arkansas Division of Aging & Adult Services
Department of Human Services
PO Box 1437
Slot-S-530
Little Rock, AR 72203-1437
501-682-2441
Fax: 501-682-8155
aging.services@arkansas.gov
www.state.ar.us/dhs/aging

Craig Cloud, Director
Stephenie Blocker, Assistant Director
Brad Nye, Assistant Director
The division provides services geared for adults and the elderly including supervised living, home delivered meals, adult day care, senior centers, personal care, household chores, and adult protective services.

3285   Arkansas Division of Developmental Disabilities Services
Donaghey Plaza
PO Box 1437
Little Rock, AR 72203-1437
501-682-1001
Fax: 501-682-8820

Charlie Green, Manager
State agency to assist persons with developmental disabilities and their family in obtaining appropriate assistance and services.

3286   Arkansas Division of Services for the Blind
Department Of Health and Human Services
700 Main St
Little Rock, AR 72203-4608
501-682-5463
800-960-9270
Fax: 501-682-0366
TTY: 800-285-1131
humanservices.arkansas.gov/dsb

Terry Sheeler, Chairman
Dickie Walker, Vice Chairman
Sandy Edwards, Secretary
State program which offers services in the areas of health, counseling, social work, self help and education for the visually and multihandicapped. The staff includes 4 full time and 13 part time members including mobility specialists and rehabilitation teachers.

3287   Arkansas Governor's Developmental Disabilities Council
5800 West 10th Street
Suite 805
Little Rock, AR 72204- 1763
501-661-2589
855-627-7580
Fax: 501-661-2399
ddcouncil.org

Regina Wilson, Executive Director
Teresa Sandar, Family Services Coordinator
Lee Russell, Information Oficer
A federally-funded state agency established to bring the perspective of individuals with developmental disabilities and his or her family or natural support system to policy makers and make improvements to the service system.

3288   Baptist Health Rehabilitation Institute
Baptist Heath
9601 Baptist Health Dr.
Little Rock, AR 72205-7299
501-202-1839
888-BAP-TIST
Fax: 501-202-7352
www.baptist-health.com

Ellen Callaway, Director, Rehabilition Therapy
Acute rehab facility serving patients with ortho, spinal cord injury, brain injury, CVA, arthritis, cardiac and generalized weakness; JCAHO and CARF accredited; 17 outpatient therapy centers throughout central Arkansas.

3289   Children's Medical Services
P.O.Box 1437
Little Rock, AR 72203-1437
501-682-8207
800-482-5850
Fax: 501-682-8247
www.cms-kids.com

Nancy Holder, Program Director
Iris Fehr, Nursing Director
A collection of programs for eligible children with special needs. Each one of our programs and services are family-centered and designed to help children with a variety of conditions and needs.

3290 President's Committee on People with Disabilities: Arkansas
7th & Main St
Little Rock, AR 72203

3291 Social Security: Arkansas Disability Determination Services
701 Pulaski Street
Little Rock, AR 72201-3990
501-682-3030
800-772-1213
Fax: 501-682-7553
www.socialsecurity.gov

Arthur Boutiette, COO

California

3292 California Department of Aging
1300 National Drive
Suite 200
Sacramento, CA 95834-1992
916-419-7500
Fax: 916-928-2267
TTY: 800-735-2929
webmaster@aging.ca.gov
aging.ca.gov

Lora Connoly, Director
Diane Paulsen, Chief Deputy Director
Anna Esparza, Executive Assistant
The Department contracts with the network of Area Agencies on Aging, who directly manage a wide array of federal and state-funded services that help older adults find employment; support older and disabled individuals to live as independently as possible in the community; promote healthy aging and community involvement; and assist family members in their vital care giving role

3293 California Department of Handicapped Children
714 P Street
Rm 323
Sacramento, CA 95814-6401
916-445-4171

Maridee Gregory
Diana Bonta, Chief Executive Officer

3294 California Department of Rehabilitation
721 Capitol Mall
Sacramento, CA 95814-3510
916-324-1313
800-952-5544
TTY: 916-558-5807
externalaffairs@dor.ca.gov

Joe Xavier, Director
David Supkofl, Manager
Assists people with disabilities, particularly those with severe disabilities, in obtaining and retaining meaningful employment and living independently in their communities. The department develops, purchases, provides and advocates for programs and services in vocational rehabilitation, habilitation and independent living with a priority on serving persons with all disabilities, especially those with the most severe disabilities.

3295 California Governor's Committee on Employment of People with Disabilities
Employment Development Department
800 Capitol Mall
PO Box 826880
Sacramento, CA 94280-0001
916-654-8055
800-695-0350
Fax: 916-654-9821
TTY: 916-654-9820
www.edd.ca.gov

Charlie Kaplan, Staff Director
GCEPD works to eliminate the barriers that preclude equal consideration for employment opportunities for people with disabilities. The Governor's Committee is responsible for providing leadership to increase the numbers of people with disabilities in the California workforce.

3296 California Protection & Advocacy: (PAI) A Nonprofit Organization
Protection and Advocacy (PA I)
1831 K Street
Sacramento, CA 95811-4114
916-504-5800
800-776-5746
Fax: 916-504-5802
SERVICES@DISABILITYRIGHTSCA.ORG
www.disabilityrightsca.org

Catherine Blakemore, Executive Director
Andrew Mudryk, Deputy Director
Alan Gildestein, Managing Attorney
Advancing the human and legal rights of people with disabilities.

3297 California State Council on Developmental Disabilities
1507 21st Street
Suite 210
Sacramento, CA 95811-5297
916-322-8481
866-802-0514
Fax: 916-443-4957
council@scdd.ca.gov
www.scdd.ca.gov

April Lopez, Chairperson
Jenny Ning Yang, Interim Vice-Chairperson
Tammy Eudy, Office Assistant
The State Council on Developmental Disabilities (SCDD) is established by state and federal law as an independent state agency to ensure that people with developmental disabilities and their families receive the services and supports they need.

3298 Client Assistance Program: California
CA Health and Human Services Agency Dept of Rehab
721 Capitol Mall
PO Box 944222
Sacramento, CA 95814
916-324-1313
800-952-5544
Fax: 916-558-5391
TTY: 916- 558-580
capinfo@dor.ca.gov
www.dor.ca.gov

Tony P Sauer, Director
We have a three-pronged mission to provide services and advocacy that assist people with disabilities to live independently, become employed and have equality in the communities in which they live and work.

3299 International Dyslexia Association: Central California Branch
4594 E Michigan Ave
Fresno, CA 93703-1556
559-251-9385
800-222-3123
Fax: 599-252-1216
info@dyslexiaida.org
dyslexiaida.org

Joy Moody, President
Provides free information and referral services for diagnosis and tutoring for parents, educators, physicians, and individuals with dyslexia. Membership includes yearly journal and quarterly newsletter, and Pennsylvania newsletter; discounts to conferences and events.

3300 Long Beach Department of Health and Human Services
2525 Grand Avenue
Long Beach, CA 90815-1765
562-570-4000
Fax: 562-570-4049
www.longbeach.gov/health/

Ron Arias, Executive Director
Michael Johnson, Manager
The Long Beach Department of Health and Human Services (Health Department) has been improving the health of the Long Beach community for over a century.

3301 Los Angeles County Department of Health Services
313 N Figueroa Street
Los Angeles, CA 90012-2602
213-240-8101
800-427-8700
Fax: 213-250-4013

Mitchell H Katz, MD, Director
Hal F. Yee, Jr., M.D., Ph.D., Chief Medical Officer
Allan Wecker, Chief Financial Officer

Los Angeles County Department of Health Services is one of the US's largest publicly supported health systems. The system is the main provider of health care for the area's poor and uninsured. It provides general medical and surgical care and is affiliated with the medical school at USC. The system also manages the Emergency Medical Services (EMS) Agency and the Community Health Plan HMO, a low-cost managed care plan for members of Medicaid and other state-funded programs.

3302 Social Security: California Disability Determination Services
3164 Garrity Way
Richmond, CA 94806-1983 800-772-1213
TTY: 800-325-0778
www.ssa.gov

Sally Keen, San Francisco Regional PDF Coord

3303 Social Security: Fresno Disability Determination Services
Social Security
1052 C St
Fresno, CA 93706-3245 559-487-5391
800-772-1213
Fax: 510-970-2947
TTY: 800-325-0778
www.ssa.gov

Sally Keen, Regional PDF Coordinator

3304 Social Security: Oakland Disability Determination Services
P.O. Box 24225
Oakland, CA 94623-1225 510-622-3506
800-772-1213
TTY: 800-325-0778
www.ssa.gov

3305 Social Security: Sacramento Disability Determination Services
P.O. Box 997121
Suite A
Sacramento, CA 95899-7121 916-515-4400
800-772-1213
Fax: 916-263-5310
TTY: 916-381-9445
ssa.gov

3306 Social Security: San Diego Disability Determination Services
P.O. Box 85326
San Diego, CA 92186-5326 619-278-4300
800-772-1213
Fax: 619-278-4303
TTY: 800-325-0778
www.ssa.gov

Colorado

3307 Colorado Department of Aging & Adult Services
1575 Sherman St
10th Floor
Denver, CO 80203-1702 303-866-5700
Fax: 303-620-2696
cdhs.communications@state.co.us
Reggie Bicha, Executive Director
A department providing services to the elderly.

3308 Colorado Developmental Disabilities Council
1120 Lincoln
Suite 706
Denver, CO 80203 720-941-0176
Fax: 720-941-8490
cddpc.email@state.co.us
coddc.org

Katherine Carol, Chairperson
Irene Aguilar, Colorado Senate
Marcia Tewell, Executive Director
The mission is to advocate in collaboration with and on behalf of people with developmental disabilities for the establishment and

implementation of public policy which will further their independence, productivity and integration.

3309 Colorado Division of Mental Health
3824 W. Princeton Circle
Denver, CO 80236-3111 303-866-7400
Fax: 303-866-7428
colorado.gov

Patrick K. Fox, Director
Administration of public health program

3310 Colorado Health Care Program for Children with Special Needs
4300 Cherry Creek Drive south
Denver, CO 80246-1530 303-692-2370
800-886-7689
Fax: 303-753-9249
cdphe.psdrequests@state.co.us
www.colorado.gov/cdphe/hcp

Christopher Stanley, Board member
Angie Goodger, HCP Consultant
Kelsey Minor, HCP Consultant
Provides information and state aid to children with disabilities.

3311 Division of Workers' Compensation Dapartment of Labor & Employment
633 17th Street
Suite 201
Denver, CO 80202-3660 303-318-8700
800-388-5515
888-390-7936
Fax: 303-575-8882
cdle_workers_compensation@state.co.us
www.colorado.gov/cdle
Ellen Golombek, Executive Director
Infomation regarding Division Rules and procedures for Claimants, Employers, Adjusters, and parties to claim.

3312 Eastern Colorado Services for the Disabled
P. O. Box 1682
617 South 10th Avenue
Sterling, CO 80751-3168 970-522-7121
Fax: 970-522-1173
rhonda@ecsdd.org
www.easterncoloradoservices.org
Rhonda Roth, Executive Director
Traci Schrade, Finance Director
Melissa Dassaro, Case Management Director
Case coordination, infant stimulation, family support, residential and vocational programs.

3313 International Dyslexia Association: Rocky Mountain Branch
740 Yale Rd.
Boulder, CO 80305-5010 303-721-9425
855-5ID- RMB
Fax: 303-721-9425
ida_rmb@yahoo.com
www.dyslexia-rmbida.org

Karen Leopold, President
Lynn Kuhn, Secretary
Yona Sammartino, Administrative Director
Provides free information and referral services for diagnosis and tutoring for parents, educators, physicians, and individuals with dyslexia. Membership includes yearly journal and quarterly newsletter, and Pennsylvania newsletter; discounts to conferences and events.

3314 Legal Center for People with Disabilities& Older People
455 Sherman St
Ste 130
Denver, CO 80203-4403 303-722-0300
800-288-1376
Fax: 303-722-0720
TTY: 303-722-3619

John R. Posthumus, President
Stephen P. Rickles, Vice President
Nancy Tucker, Secretary
Uses the legal system to protect and promote the rights of people with disabilities and older people in Colorado through direct legal representation, advocacy, education and legislative analysis.

The Legal Center is Colorado's Protection and Advocacy System. We are also the State Ombudsman for nursing homes and assisted living facilities. Call for a free publications and products list.

Connecticut

3315 Connecticut Board of Education and Servicefor the Blind
184 Windsor Avenue
Windsor, CT 06095-4536
860-602-4000
800-842-4510
Fax: 860-602-4020
TTY: 860-602-4221
brian.sigman@CT.GOV
www.ct.gov/besb/site/default.asp
Amy Porter, Commissioner
Offers rehabilitative services and information for persons with legal blindness and childrenwhonare visually impaired that are residents of Connecticut.

3316 Connecticut Commission on Aging
210 Capitol Avenue
Hartford, CT 06106
860-240-5200
Fax: 860-240-5204
Julia Evans Starr, Executive Director
Deborah Migneault, Senior Policy Analyst
Alyssa Norwood, Project Manager
Advocates on beha;f of elderly persons in Connecticut by regularly monitoring their status, assessing the impact of current and propsed initiatives, and conducting activities which promote the interests of these individuals and report to the Governor and the Legislature.

3317 Connecticut Department of Children and Youth Services
505 Hudson Street
Hartford, CT 06106
860-550-6300
Fax: 860-724-2001
Commissioner.dcf@ct.gov
www.ct.gov
Gary Scappini, Manager
Bruce Douglas, Executive Director

3318 Connecticut Developmental Disabilities Council
263 Farmington Avenue
Farmington, CT 6030
860-679-1561
800-653-1134
Fax: 860-679-1571
TTY: 860-679-1502
ctkasa.org
Ed Preneta, Executive Director
Kids As Self Advocates (KASA) is a national grassroots network that helps youth with special needs and their friends become self-advocates, helps other people in the community understand what it's like to live with special health care needs.

3319 Connecticut Office of Protection and Advocacy for Persons with Disabilities
60B Weston Street
Suite B
Hartford, CT 06120-1551
860-297-4300
800-842-7303
Fax: 860-566-8714
TTY: 860-297-4320
www.ct.gov/opapd
Craig B Henrici, Executive Director
Alexandria Bode, Board Member
Thomas Behrendt, Board Member
Provides information, referrals, advocacy assistance & limited legal services to people with disabilities in the state of Connecticut whose civil rights have been violated or who are experiencing the difficulty securing relevant support services. P & A supports the development of community advocacy groups by providing training & technical assistance. P & A is responsible for investigating abuse & neglect of all individuals with intellectual disability ages 18-59.

3320 Social Security: Hartford Area Office
960 Main Street
2nd Floor
Hartford, CT 06103-1228
877-619-2851
800-772-1213
Fax: 860-566-1795
TTY: 860-525-4967
www.ssa.gov
Jan Gilbert, Professional Relations Coord.

Delaware

3321 Delaware Assistive Technology Initiative(DATI)
461 Wyoming Road
Newark, DE 19716-0269
302-831-0354
Fax: 302-831-4690
TTY: 800-870-3284
dati@asel.udel.edu
www.dati.org
Beth Mineo, Project Director
Joann McCafferty, Staff Assistant
The Delaware Assistive Technology Initiative (DATI) connects Delawareans who have disabilities with the tools they need in order to learn, work, play and participate in community life safely and independently. DATI services include: Equipment demonstration centers in each county; no-cost, short-term equipment loans that let you try before you buy; Equipment Exchange Program; AT workshops and other training sessions; advocacy for improved AT access policies and funing and several more.

3322 Delaware Client Assistance Program
United Cerebral Palsy Association
254 E Camden Wyoming Ave
Camden, DE 19934-1303
302-698-9336
800-640-9336
Fax: 302-698-9338
icdri.org/legal/DelawareCAP.htm
Melissa Shahan, Executive Director
Provides advocacy services for persons involved with programs covered under the Rehabilitation Act of 1973 as amended, information and referrals on ADA, Title I.

3323 Delaware Department of Health and Social Services
Administration Building D HS S Campus
1901 N Du pont Highway
Main Building
New Castle, DE 19720-1160
302-255-9040
800-464-4357
Fax: 302-255-4429
TTY: 302-744-4556
dhssinfo@state.de.us
www.dhss.delaware.gov
Rita Landgraf, Cabinet Secretary
Henry Smith III, Deputy secretary
Provides most of the human services available through Delaware State Government, including Medicaid, the Children's Health Insurance Program, food stamps, welfare-to-work, vaccines for children, child support enforcement, public health programs, and general services for the aging. Also for individuals with developmental and physical disabilities, visual impairments, mental illness and other vulnerable populations.

3324 Delaware Department of Public Instructing
Townsend Building
401 Federal Street
Dover, DE 19901-1402
302-735-4000
800-433-5292
Fax: 302-739-4654
deeds@doe.k12.de.us
http://www.doe.k12.de.us
Mark T. Murphy, Secretary of Education
David J. Blowman, Deputy Secretary
Mary Kate McLaughlin, Chief of Staff
A publicly funded, state agency that gives information about local facilities and administers supplemental funds for visually handicapped students in local schools. It also maintains special teachers of sight conservation and braille programs for both children and adults.

3325 Delaware Developmental Disability Council
410 Federal Street 2nd Floor
Suite 2
Dover, DE 19901- 3640   302-739-3333
    800-464-4357
    Fax: 302-739-2015
    pat.maichle@state.de.us

Barbara Monaghan, Council Chair
Patricia L. Maichle, Senior Administrator
Kristin Cosden, Social Service Administrator
Working to ensure that people with developmental disabilities enjoy the same quality of life as the rest of society.

3326 Delaware Division for the Visually Impaired
1901 North Dupont Highway
New Castle, DE 19720-1160   302-255-9800
    Fax: 302-255-4441
    dhssinfo@state.de.us
    www.dhss.delaware.gov/dvi/

Rita Landgraf, Secretary
Henry Smith, Deputy Secretary
Betsy Deldeo, Office Manager
State agency serving the visually impaired persons from birth, with or without other handicaps. Services offered include vocational rehabilitation, independent living, orientation and mobility, technology assessment, transition from school to work.

3327 Delaware Protection & Advocacy for Persons with Disabilities
Arc of Delaware
144 E Market St
Georgetown, DE 19947-1411   302-856-6019
    Fax: 302-856-6133

Becky Allen, Executive Director

3328 Delaware Workers Compensation Board
Industrial Accident Board de dept
4425 North Market Street
Wilmington, DE 19802-1307   302-761-8085
    Fax: 302-761-6601
    www.delawareworks.com

James Cagle, Manager
The Office of Workers' Compensation administers and enforces state laws, rules and regulations regarding industrial accidents and illnesses.

3329 Social Security: Wilmington Disability Determination
U S Department of Health and Human Services
1528 S 16th Street
Wilmington, NC 28401-3908   866-964-6227
    800-772-1213
    Fax: 910-254-3444
    TTY: 910-815-4695
    www.socialsecurity.gov

J Allen Murphy, Founder
Vickie O'Brien, Manager

3330 The Division for the Visually Impaired
Herman M. Holloway, Sr. Campus
1901 N Dupont Hwy
New Castle, DE 19720   302-255-9800
    Fax: 302-255-4441
    dhssinfo@state.de.us
    dhss.delaware.gov

Alan Wingrove, General Manager
Romy Mikhail, Customer Service, Quality & ISO Manager
The Division for the Visually Impaired provides educational, vocational and technical support to people with visual impairments. Some programs offered include education, employment support, guidance for living independently and using assistive devices, business enterprise programs, volunteer opporunities and more.

District of Columbia

3331 District of Columbia Department of Handicapped Children
D C General Hospital
Bldg 10
1900 Massachusetts Ave SE
Washington, DC 20003- 2542   202-541-6337
    Fax: 202-675-7694

Jacqueline Mcmorris, Acting Chief
Nayab Ali, MD

3332 District of Columbia Office on Aging
500 K Street NE
Washington, DC 20002-2714   202-724-5622
    Fax: 202-724-4979
    TTY: 202-724-8925
    dcoa@dc.gov
    dcoa.dc.gov

John M Thompson, Executive Director
Deborah Royster, General Counsel
Tanya Reid, Executive Assistant
Serves the District of Columbia residents 60 years of age and older. Contact the Information and Assistance Unit for more information about innovative programs and services offered by the Office.

3333 Information, Protection & Advocacy for Persons with Disabilities
IPACHI
220 I Street, N.E.
Suite 130
Washington, DC 20002   202-547-0198
    Fax: 202-547-2083
    jbrown@uls-dc.org
    www.acf.HHS.gov/programs/add/states/pas.html

Jane Brown, Executive Director
Ronald Tyson, Information/Referral
Offers services and support for persons with disabilities in the Washington, DC area.

3334 Information, Protection and Advocacy Center for Handicapped Individuals
220 I Street, N.E.
Suite 130
Washington, DC 20002-2340   202-547-0198
    Fax: 202-547-2083
    jbrown@uls-dc.org
    www.acf.hhs.gov/programs/add/states/pas.html

Jane Brown, Executive Director
Serves all persons with disabilities in the DC, Maryland and Virginia areas offering them legal representation and advocacy, information and referrals and several publications.

3335 International Dyslexia Association of DC
40 York Rd., 4th Floor
Baltimore, MD 21204-1016   410-296-0232
    800-222-3123
    Fax: 410-321-5069
    info@dyslexiaida.org
    dyslexiaida.org

Ruth R Tifford LCSW, President
Provides free information and referral services for diagnosis and tutoring for parents, educators, physicians, and individuals with dyslexia. Membership includes yearly journal and quarterly newsletter, and Pennsylvania newsletter; discounts to conferences and events.

3336 Public Technology Institute
660 North Capitol St. NW
Suite 400
Washington, DC 20001   202-626-2400
    info@pti.org
    www.pti.org

Alan R. Shark, Executive Director
Leonard Scott, Director, Public Safety Technology Programs
Susan Cable, Program Manager, Citizen-Engaged Communities
Supports local government executives and elected officials through research, education, consulting services, and recogni-

tion programs. Research includes how technology can better benefit people with disabilities.
28 pages

3337 Wage and Hour Division of the Employment Standards Administration
US Department of Labor
200 Constitution Ave NW
Washington, DC 20210-1
202-693-5000
866-487-2365
Fax: 202-219-8822
TTY: 877-889-5627
webmaster@dol.gov
www.dol.gov
Hilda Solis, Secretary of Labor
Seth Harris, Deputy Secretary
Elizabeth Kim, Executive Secretariat Director
Administers regulations governing the employment of individuals with disabilities in sheltered workshops and the disabled workers industries.

3338 Washington Hearing and Speech Society
2150 N 107th St, Suite 205
Seattle, WA 98133-2633
206-209-5271
Fax: 206-367-8777
office@wslha.org
www.wslha.org
Paul Diez, President
Judith Bernier, Secretary
Julie Leonardo, Treasurer
Offers individuals with hearing or speech impairments, in the DC area, speech, reading classes, audiological services and new aids.

3339 Well Mind Association of Greater Washington
18606 New Hampshire Ave
Ashton, MD 20861-9789
301-774-6617
Fax: 301-946-1402
Holistic mental health information and publications, public lectures in the Washington D.C. area, and nationwide referrals.

3340 Workers Compensation Board: District of Columbia
4058 Minnesota Avenue, NE,
Washington, DC 20019-5626
202-724-7000
202-698-4817
Fax: 202-673-6993
does@dc.gov
Deborah A Carroll, Director
The Workers' Compensation Program processes claims and monitors the payment of benefits to injured private-sector employees in the District of Columbia

Florida

3341 ARC Gateway
3932 North 10th Avenue
Pensacola, FL 32503-2807
850-434-2638
Fax: 850-438-2180
info@arc-gateway.org
www.arc-gateway.org
Peter Mougey, President
Patricia Young, Vice President
Lynn Erickson, Secretary
ARC Gateway is a non-profit organization that serves children who have or are at risk of developmental disabilities as well as adults with developmental disabilitie

3342 Assistive Technology Educational Network of Florida
1207 S Mellonville Avenue
Sanford, FL 32771-2240
800-558-6580
Fax: 407-320-2379
Diane_Penn@scps.k12.fl.us
www.icdri.org/Assistive%20Technology/aten.htm
Dee Wright, Executive Secretary
Diane Penn, MA, Technology Specialist
Provides state-wide information, awareness and training for students, family members, teachers and other professionals in the area of assisted technology; a quarterly newsletter and a network of specialists (Local Assistive Technology Specialists) trained by ATEN to provide support at the district level.

3343 Bureau Of Exceptional Education And Student Services
325 West Gaines Street Suite 614
Tallahassee, FL 32399
850-245-0475
Fax: 850-245-0953
Monica.Verra-Tirado@fldoe.org
www.fldoe.org
Pam Stewart, Education Commissioner
Monica Verra Tirado, Bureau Chief
Chatherine Aponte Gray, Administrative Assistant
Provides consultative services for the establishment and operation of school programs for visually impaired students. Provides assistance for in-service teacher training through state or regional workshops or technical assistance to individual programs.

3344 Department of Health & Rehabilitative Services
1317 Winewood Blvd
Building 1
Tallahassee, FL 32399-700
850-487-1111
Fax: 850-922-2993
www.dcf.state.fl.us
David Wilkins, Secretary
Ramin Kouzehkanani, Deputy Secretary
John Bryant, Manager
The Florida Department of Children and Families has adopted an integrated approach to programs and services as we work to help improve the lives of individuals and families.

3345 Disability Rights Florida
2473 Care Dr.
Suite 200
Tallahassee, FL 32308
850-488-9071
800-342-0823
Fax: 850-488-8640
TTY: 800-346-4127
www.disabilityrightsflorida.org
Peter Sleasman, Executive Director
Ann Siegel, Legal Director
Cherie E. Hall, Director, Operations
A federally mandated Protection & Advocacy (P&A) organization working to ensure the safety, well-being and success of people with disabilities.

3346 Division of Workers Compensation
200 East Gaines Street
Tallahassee, FL 32399-0318
850-413-3089
877-693-5236
Fax: 850-413-2950
Tanner.Holloman@myfloridacfo.com
Tanner Holloman, Division Director
Andrew Sabolic, Assistant Director
Terry Kester, Chief Information Officer
To actively ensure the self-execution of the workers' compensation system through education and informing all stakeholders of their rights and responsibilities, leveraging data to deliver exceptional value to our customers and stakeholders, and holding parties accountable for meeting their obligations.

3347 Florida Adult Services
1317 Winewood Boulevard
Building 1, Room 202
Tallahassee, FL 32399-700
850-488-2881
800-962-2873
800-273-8255
Fax: 850-922-4193
www.myflfamilies.com
Robert Anderson, State Director
Jan Chaney, Administrative Assistant
Roy Car, Data/Systems
The Florida Department of Children and Families has adopted an integrated approach to programs and services as we work to help improve the lives of individuals and families.

3348 Florida Department of Handicapped Children
4030 Esplanade Way
Suite 380
Tallahassee, FL 32399-7016
850-488-4257
866-273-2273
Fax: 850-245-1075
www.apd.myflorida.com
Mike Gresham, Executive Director
John Bryant, Manager

The APD works in partnership with local communities and private providers to assist people who have developmental disabilities and their families.

3349 Florida Department of Mental Health and Rehabilitative Services
1317 Winewood Blvd
Building 1
Tallahassee, FL 32399-700
850-487-1111
Fax: 850-922-2993
www.dcf.state.fl.us

David Wilkins, Secretary
Ramin Kouzehkanani, Deputy Secretary

3350 Florida Developmental Disabilities Council
124 Marriott Drive
Suite 203
Tallahassee, FL 32301-2981
850-488-4180
800-580-7801
Fax: 850-922-6702
TTY: 888-488-863
fddc@fddc.org
fddc.org

Sylvia James Miller, Council Chair & Parent Advocate
Tricia Riccardi, Council Vice-Chair
Debra Dowds, Executive Director
To advocate and promote meaningful participation in all aspects of life for Floridians with developmental disabilities.

3351 Florida Division of Vocational Rehabilitation
4070 Esplanade Way
Building 1
Tallahassee, FL 32399- 7016
850-245-3399
800-451-4327
Fax: 850-245-3316
TTY: 850-488-2867
rehabworks.org

Bill Palmer, Manager
Linda Parnell, Manager
Aleisa Mckinlay, Director
State agency serving individuals with physical or mental disabilities that interfere with them keeping or maintaining employment.

3352 International Dyslexia Association: Florida Branch
40 York Rd., 4th Floor
Baltimore, MD 21204-3896
410-296-0232
800-222-3123
Fax: 410-321-5069
ear228@aol.com
dyslexiaida.org

Kristen Penczek, Executive Director
David Holste, Director Of Operations
Stacy Friedman, Manager of Operation
Provides free information and referral services for diagnosis and tutoring for parents, educators, physicians, and individuals with dyslexia. Membership includes yearly journal and quarterly newsletter, and Pennsylvania newsletter; discounts to conferences and events.

3353 Social Security Administration
2002 Old Saint Augustine Rd
Suite B12
Tallahassee, FL 32301-4861
850-942-8978
800-772-1213
Fax: 850-942-8980
ssa.gov

Carrie Tucker, Operations Supervisor
Sheila Lee, Management Support Specialist
Administers the Title II and Title XVII disability programs. To be insured for Title II benefits, applicants must have worked in covered employment for at least five of the last ten years prior to becoming disabled. To be eligible for Title XVII disability benefits, applicants must meet an income and resource test.

3354 Social Security: Miami Disability Determination
Social Security
11401 W Flagler St
Miami, FL 33174-1023
305-226-0449
800-772-1213
TTY: 800-325-0778
www.ssa.gov

Robert L Meekins, Deputy General for Executive Ope

3355 Social Security: Orlando Disability Determination
Social Security
P.O. Box 144040
Orlando, FL 32814-2231
407-648-6673
800-342-2065
TTY: 407-245-7057
www.ssa.gov

John C Massolio Jr, Founder
Neil Bush, President

3356 Social Security: Tampa Disability Determination
Social Security Administration
PO Box 340572
Tampa, FL 33694-572
813-878-2906
800-772-1213
www.dbsatampabay.org

John Balcomb, President
Carol Yaros, 1st Vice President
Cheryl McGhan, 2nd Vice President
The Depression and Bipolar Support Alliance Tampa Bay, is a nonprofit and all volunteer organization for individuals, family and friends of those who have been diagnosed with bipolar disorder, depression and other affective disorders.

Georgia

3357 ADA Technical Assistance Program
Southeast Disability & Business Technical Assist.
1419 Mayson Street NE
Atlanta, GA 30324
404-541-9001
800-949-4232
Fax: 404-541-9002
ADAsoutheast@law.syr.edu
www.sedbtac.org

Pamela Williamson, Project Director
Cheri Hofmann, Information Specialist
Cyndi Smith, Office Assistant
One of ten regional centers funded by NIDRR, to provide information and technical assistance to assist in voluntary compliance with the Americans with Disabilities Act, and accessible education-based information technology.

3358 Division of Birth Defects and Developmental Disabilities
1600 Clifton Road
Atlanta, GA 30333-4027
404-498-3800
800-232-4636
TTY: 888-232-6348
cdcinfo@cdc.gov
www.cdc.gov

Coleen A Boyle, Director
The mission of CDC's National Center on Birth Defects and Developmental Disabilities (NCBDDD) is to promote the health of babies, children and adults and to enhance the potential for full, productive living.

3359 Georgia Advocacy Office
One West Court Square
Suite 625
Decatur, GA 30030
404-885-1234
800-537-2329
Fax: 404-378-0031
info@thegao.org
thegao.org

Ruby Moore, Executive Director
Crystal Rasa, Program Manager
Mona Givens, Director of Investigation
Protection and advocacy services for Georgians with disabilities.

3360 Georgia Client Assistance Program
Division of Rehabilitation Services
2 Peachtree Street NW
Suite 29-250
Atlanta, GA 30303- 3141   404-656-4507
800-822-9727
Fax: 404-651-6880
dhs.georgia.gov/

Mark Trail, Manager
Robertiena Fletcher, Chair
Franklin G Auman, Vice Chair
Helps eligible persons with complaints, appeals and understanding available benefits under the 1992 Rehabilitation Act Amendments and Title I of the Americans with Disabilities Act. CAP investigates complaints, mediates conflict, represents complainants in appeals, provides legal services if warranted, advocates for due process, identifies and recommends solutions to system problems, advises of benefits available under the 1992 Rehab Act Amendments and Americans with Disabilities Act.

3361 Georgia Council On Developmental Disabilities
2 Peachtree St N.W.
26th Floor, Suite 246
Atlanta, GA 30303-3141   404-657-2126
888-275-4233
Fax: 404-657-2132
TTY: 404-657-2133
eric.jacobson@gcdd.ga.gov
www.gcdd.org

Eric E. Jacobson, Executive Director
Caitlin Childs, Organizing Director
Dottie Adams, Family/Individual Support Dir.
The Georgia Council on Developmental Disabilities collaborates with Georgia's citizens, public and private advocacy organizations and policymakers to positively influence public policies that enhance the quality of life for people with disabilities and their families. GCDD provides this through education and advocacy activities, program implementation, funding and public policy analysis and research.
Quartlery

3362 Georgia Department of Aging
2 Peachtree Street NW
33rd Floor
Atlanta, GA 30303-3142   404-657-5258
866-552-4464
Fax: 404-657-5285
dhs.georgia.gov/

Stephen Dolinger, President
Andrea Fuller-Ruffin, Administrator
The Division of Aging Services (DAS) works to continuously improve the effectiveness and efficiency of services.

3363 Georgia Department of Handicapped Children
2600 Skyland Dr NE
Atlanta, GA 30319-3640   404-679-1625
Fax: 404-679-1630

Ron Jackson, Manager
Frank Koues, Auditor

3364 Georgia Division of Mental Health, Developmental Disabilities & Addictive Diseases
Two Peachtree Drive NW
24th Floor
Atlanta, GA 30303-3142   404-657-2252
800-715-4225
Fax: 404-657-2310
mhddad.dhr.georgia.gov

Kimberly Ryan, Board Member
David Glass, Board member
Ellice P. Martin, Board Member
MHDDAD provides treatment and support services to people with mental illnesses and addictive diseases, and support to people with developmental disabilities. MHDDAD serves people of all ages with the most severe and likely to be long-term conditions.

3365 Georgia State Board of Workers' Compensation
270 Peachtree St NW
Atlanta, GA 30303-1299   404-656-3875
800-533-0682
Fax: 404-657-1767
sbwc.georgia.gov

Frank McKay, Chairman
Elizabeth Gobeil, Director
Delece A. Brooks, Executive Director
To provide superior access to the Georgia Workers' Compensation program for injured workers and employers in a manner that is sensitive, responsive, and effective and to insure efficient processing and swift, fair resolution of claims, while encouraging workplace safety and return to work.

3366 International Dyslexia Association: Georgia Branch
1951 Greystone Rd.
Atlanta, GA 30318   404-256-1232
info@idaga.org
www.idaga.org

Jennifer Kopp, President
jennings Miller, Vice-President
Robert Moore, Treasurer
Provides free information and referral services for diagnosis and tutoring for parents, educators, physicians, and individuals with dyslexia. Membership includes yearly journal and quarterly newsletter, and Pennsylvania newsletter; discounts to conferences and events.

3367 Social Security: Atlanta Disability Determination
401 W Peachtree St NW
Suite 2860 Flr 28
Atlanta, GA 30308-3538   800-772-1213
TTY: 800-325-0778
www.socialsecurity.gov

3368 Social Security: Decatur Disability Determination
2853 Candler Rd
Suite 8
Decatur, GA 30034-1421   800-772-1213
TTY: 800-325-0778
ssa.gov

Hawaii

3369 Assistive Technology Resource Centers of Hawaii
200 North Vineyard Boulevard
Suite 430
Honolulu, HI 96817-5362   808-532-7110
800-645-3007
Fax: 808-532-7120
TTY: 808-532-7113
atrc-info@atrc.org
www.atrc.org

Barbara Fischlowitz-Leong, Executive Director
Jodi Asato, Deputy Director
Edna Kaahaaina, Office Manager
Provides information and referral to anyone interested in assistive technology devices and services. Operates equipment loan. Bank Provides training to consumer and professional groups including self-advocacy skills for consumers and family members. Works to ensure that schools, vocational rehabilitation agencies and health insurers provide assessments, funding and training in the use of assistive technology devices and services for their clients. Low-interest loan programs available.

3370 Diabetes Network of East Hawaii
1221 Kilauea Ave
Suite 70
Hilo, HI 96720-4264   808-935-1673
Fax: 808-935-6760

Steve Fukunada, Manager

313

3371   Disability and Communication Access Board
1010 Richards St
Suite 118
Honolulu, HI 96813   808-586-8121
                                            Fax: 808-586-8129
                                            dcab@doh.hawaii.gov
                                            hawaii.gov/health/dcab

Francine Wai, Executive Director
Bill-Wayne Nakamatsu, Parking Program Specialist
Provides ADA coordination for state & county government; reviews state & county construction documents to appropriate federal & state accessibility guidelines; credentials American sign language interpreters; coordinates parking for persons with disabilites; coordinates information & referral for consumers, parents and others seeking disability related information.

3372   Hawaii Assistive Technology Training and
200 North Vineyard Boulevard
Suite 430
Honolulu, HI 96817-5362   808-532-7110
                                               800-645-3007
                                            Fax: 808-532-7120
                                            atrc-info@atrc.org
                                            www.atrc.org

Barbara Fischlowitz-Leong, Executive Director

3373   Hawaii Department for Children With Special Needs
Department of Health
741 Sunset Avenue
Honolulu, HI 96816-2343   808-733-9070
                                            Fax: 808-733-9068
                                            patricia.heu@doh.hawaii.gov
                                            health.hawaii.gov

Patricia Heu, Manager
Karen Mak, Manager
Children with Special Health Needs Branch(CSHNB) is working to assure that all children and youth with special health care needs (CSHCN) will reach optimal health, growth, and development, by improving access to a coordinated system of family-centered health care services and improving outcomes, through systems development, assessment, assurance, education, collaborative partnerships, and family support.

3374   Hawaii Department of Health, Adult Mental Health Division
P.O.Box 3378
Honolulu, HI 96801-3378   808-586-4686
                                            Fax: 808-586-4745
The Adult Mental Health Division is one part of theHawaii State Department of Health,State of Hawaii. The Mission of the Department of Health is to protect and improve health and the environment for all people in Hawaii.

3375   Hawaii Department of Human Services
Hawaii Department of Human Serv
P.O. Box 339
Honolulu, HI 96813   808-586-4892
                                            Fax: 808-586-4890
                                            dhs@dhs.hawaii.gov
                                            humanservices.hawaii.gov

Rachael Wong, Director
Pankaj Bhanot, Deputy Director
Lisa Nakao, Admin Assis. & Legislative Coor.
To provide timely, efficient and effective programs, services and benefits for the purpose of achieving the outcome of empowering Hawaii's most vulnerable people; and to expand their capacity for self-sufficiency, self-determination, independence, healthy choices, quality of life, and personal dignity.

3376   Hawaii Disability Compensation Division Department of Labor and Industrial Relations
830 Punchbowl Street
Room 209
Honolulu, HI 96813-5095   808-586-9200
                                            Fax: 808-586-9219
                                            dlir.director@hawaii.gov
                                            hawaii.gov/labor

Walter Kawamura, Administrator
Clyde Imada, Workers Comp Chief
The Disability Compensation Division (DCD) administers the Workers' Compensation (WC) law, the Temporary Disability In-

surance (TDI) law, and the Prepaid Health Care (PHC) law. All employers with one or more employees, whether working full-time or part-time, are directly affected.

3377   Hawaii Disability Rights Center
1132 Bishop Street
Suite 2102
Honolulu, HI 96813-3701   808-949-2922
                                               800-882-1057
                                            Fax: 808-949-2928
                                            info@hawaiidisabilityrights.org
                                            hawaiidisabilityrights.org

John Dellera, Executive Director
Ann Collins, Director Of Operations
IT IS THE POLICY OF HDRCto advocate for as many people with disabilities in the State of Hawaii, on as wide a range of disability rights issues, as our resources allow; and to resolve rights violations with the lowest feasible level of intervention; but, if necessary, to also provide full legal representation to protect the rights of people with disabilities, consistent with authorizing statutes and Center priorities.

3378   Hawaii Executive Office on Aging
250 South Hotel Street
Suite 406
Honolulu, HI 96813-2831   808-586-0100
                                               800-468-4644
                                            Fax: 808-586-0185
                                            hawaii.gov/health/eoa

Noemi Pendleton, Manager
Virginia Pressler, Director
Keith Y. Yamamoto, Deputy Director
State unit on aging responsible for policy formulation, program development, planning, information dissemination, advocacy and other activities, for persons age 60 and over.

3379   Hawaii State Council on Developmental Disabilities
919 Ala Moana Blvd
Suite113
Honolulu, HI 96814-4920   808-586-8100
                                            Fax: 808-586-7543

Waynette K Y Cabral, Executive Administrator
Joe Shacter, Planner
Debbie Miyasaka Gushiken, Community & Legislative Liaison
The mission of the council is to support people with developmental disabilities to control their own destiny and determine the quality of life they desire. The Council: engages in analysis and policy development; provides training in legislative advocacy and leadership development for individuals with disabilities and their families; demonstrates new approaches to services and supports; informs policymakers about developmental disability issues; and fosters interagency collaboration.

3380   International Dyslexia Association: Hawaii Branch
913 Alewa Dr.
Honolulu, HI 96817-1610   808-538-7007
                                            hida@dyslexia-hawaii.org

Charles Bering, President
Deborah Knight, Vice President
Laurie Moore, Treasurer
Provides free information and referral services for diagnosis and tutoring for parents, educators, physicians, and individuals with dyslexia. Membership includes yearly journal and quarterly newsletter. Call for conference dates.

3381   Social Security: Honolulu Disability Determination
Social Security
300 Ala Moana Blvd
Honolulu, HI 96850-1   808-541-3600
                                               800-772-1213
                                            TTY: 800-825-0778
                                            hivrsbd@kestrok.com
                                            www.ssa.gov

Neil Shim, Administrator

3382 State Planning Council on Developmental Disabilities
919 Ala Moana Blvd
Room 101
Honolulu, HI 96814-4920

808-586-8121
Fax: 808-586-8129
TTY: 808-586-8121
dcab@doh.hawaii.gov
hawaii.gov/health/dcab

Michael Okamoto, Chairperson
Peter Fritz, Vice Chairperson
Francine Wai, Executive Director
Consists of 25 Hawaii residents appointed by the governor. The council addresses the needs of the people with developmental disabilities: specifically, develops a state plan that sets the priorities for persons with developmental disabilities.

Idaho

3383 Idaho Commission on Aging
341 W Washington
Boise, ID 83702-1

208-334-3833
800-926-2588
Fax: 208-334-3033
ICOA@aging.idaho.gov
www.idahoaging.com

Sam Haws, Administrator
Cathy Hart, State Ombudsman
Jeff Weller, Deputy Administrator
There number one priority is to provide the best possible service through this single point of entry website where people of all incomes and ages can obtain information on a full range of long-term care support programs and services.

3384 Idaho Council on Developmental Disabilities
Health and Wellfare
700 W. State Street
Suite 119
Boise, ID 83702-5868

208-334-2178
800-544-2433
Fax: 208-334-3417
info@icdd.idaho.gov
icdd.idaho.gov

Jim Baugh, Council Member
Christine Pisani, Executive Director
Tracy Warren, Program Specialist/Planner
The mission of the Idaho Council on Developmental Disabilities is to promote the capacity of people with developmental disabilities and their families to determine, access, and direct the services and/or support they need to live the lives they choose, and to build the communities ability to support their choices.

3385 Idaho Department of Handicapped Children
Statehouse
Boise, ID 83720-1

208-334-8000

Thomas Bruck, Chief
Sandy Frazier, Manager

3386 Idaho Disability Determinations Service
PO Box 21
Boise, ID 83707-0021

208-327-7333
800-626-2681
Fax: 208-327-7331
TTY: 800-377-3529
labor.idaho.gov

Roger B Madsen, Director
Rogelio Valdez, Executive Director
Under contract with the Social Security Administration, makes determinations of medical eligibility for disability benefits.

3387 Idaho Industrial Commission
P.O. Box 83720
Boise, ID 83720-0041

208-334-6000
800-950-2110
Fax: 208-334-2321
mholbrook@iic.idaho.gov
www.iic.idaho.gov

Mindy Montgomery, Manager
Beth Kilian, Commission Secretary

Free rehabilitation services to workers' who have suffered on the job injuries in Idaho. Field offices throughout the state.

3388 Idaho Mental Health Center
1720 Westgate Dr
Boise, ID 83704-7164

208-334-0808
800-926-2588
Fax: 208-334-0828

Richard Armstrong, Director
Darrell Kerby, Chairperson
Tom Stroschein, Vice Chair
The State of Idaho provides state funded and operated community based mental health care services through Regional Behavioral Health Centers (RBHC) located in each of the seven geographical regions of the state. Each RBHC provides mental health services through a system of care that is both community-based and consumer-guided.

Illinois

3389 Attorney General's Office: Disability Rights Bureau & Health Care Bureau
100 W Randolph Street
Chicago, IL 60601-3218

312-814-3000
877-305-5145
Fax: 312-793-0802
TTY: 800-964-3013
illinoisattorneygeneral.gov

Lisa Madigan, Manager
Raymond Throlkeld, Chief Health Care Bureau
Information on Illinois' Comprehensive Health Insurance Plan and architectural accessibility. Enforcement of Illinois' access law and standards and other disability rights laws. Information on initiatives such as: Opening the Courthouse Doors to People with Disabilities; the abuse, neglect or financial exploitation of people with disabilities and voter accessibility. Other information and referrals.

3390 Client Assistance Program (CAP)
Illinois State Board of Education
100 South Grand Ave. E.
Springfield, IL 62794

217-524-0695
800-641-3929
888-460-5111
Fax: 217-524-1184
dhs.cap@illinois.gov
www.dhs.state.il.us

James T. Dimas, Secretary
Francisco Alvarado, Manager
Quinetta L. Wade, Rehabilitation Services
The Client Assistance Program (CAP) helps people with disabilities receive quality Vocational Rehabilitation services by advocating for their interests and helping them identify resources, understand procedures, resolve problems, and protect their rights in the rehabilitation process, and employment.

3391 Equip for Equality
20 North Michigan Avenue
Suite 300
Chicago, IL 60602- 4861

312-341-0022
800-537-2632
Fax: 312-541-7544
TTY: 800-610-2779
contactus@equipforequality.org
equipforequality.org

Zena Naiditch, President/CEO
Barry C Taylor, Vice President
Lia Burkey, Administrative Assistant
Equip for equality is an independent, private, not-for-profit organization designated by the Governor in 1985 to implement the federally mandated Protection and Advocacy (P&A) System in Illinois. The mission of Equip for Equality is to advance the human and civil rights of children and adults with disabilities in Illinois.

3392 **Equip for Equality - Carbondale Office**
300 East Main St
Suite 18
Carbondale, IL 62901
618-457-7930
800-758-0559
Fax: 618-457-7985
TTY: 800-610-2779
contactus@equipforequality.org
equipforequality.org

Zena Naiditch, President/CEO
Barry C Taylor, Vice President
Lia Burkey, Administrative Assistant
Equip for equality is an independent, private, not-for-profit organization designated by the Governor in 1985 to implement the federally mandated Protection and Advocacy (P&A) System in Illinois. The mission of Equip for Equality is to advance the human and civil rights of children and adults with disabilities in Illinois.

3393 **Equip for Equality - Moline Office**
1515 Fifth Ave
Suite 420
Moline, IL 61265
309-786-6868
800-758-6869
Fax: 309-797-8710
TTY: 800-610-2779
contactus@equipforequality.org
equipforequality.org

Zena Naiditch, President/CEO
Barry C Taylor, Vice President
Lia Burkey, Administrative Assistant
Equip for equality is an independent, private, not-for-profit organization designated by the Governor in 1985 to implement the federally mandated Protection and Advocacy (P&A) System in Illinois. The mission of Equip for Equality is to advance the human and civil rights of children and adults with disabilities in Illinois.

3394 **Equip for Equality - Springfield Office**
1 West Old State Capitol Plaza
Suite 816
Springfield, IL 62701
217-544-0464
800-758-0464
Fax: 217-523-0720
TTY: 800-610-2779
contactus@equipforequality.org
equipforequality.org

Zena Naiditch, President/CEO
Barry C Taylor, Vice President
Lia Burkey, Administrative Assistant
Equip for equality is an independent, private, not-for-profit organization designated by the Governor in 1985 to implement the federally mandated Protection and Advocacy (P&A) System in Illinois. The mission of Equip for Equality is to advance the human and civil rights of children and adults with disabilities in Illinois.

3395 **Illinois Assistive Technology Project**
1 West Old State Capitol Plaza
Suite 100
Springfield, IL 62701-1200
217-522-7985
800-852-5110
Fax: 217-522-8067
TTY: 217-522-9966
iatp@iltech.org
iltech.org

Wilhelmina Gunther, Executive Director
Shelly Lowe, Finance/Personnel Manager
Yvonne Miller, Administrative Assistant
Directed by and for people with disabilities and their family members. As a federally mandated program, IATP strives to break down barriers and change policies that make getting and using technology difficult. IATP offers solutions to help people find what is available in products and services that will best meet their needs, where to find it, and how to get it.

3396 **Illinois Council on Developmental Disability**
State of Illinois Center
100 W Randolph St
16-100
Chicago, IL 60601-3218
312-814-2121
800-843-6154
Fax: 312-814-7441
www2.illinois.gov

Sheila T. Romano, Executive Director
Dennis Sienko, Manager
The Illinois Council on Developmental Disabilities (ICDD) is dedicated to leading change in Illinois so that all people with developmental disabilities are able to exercise their rights to freedom and equal opportunity.

3397 **Illinois Department of Mental Health and Developmental Disabilities**
Suite 3b
314 E Madison
Springfield, IL 62701
217-782-6680
Fax: 217-524-3834

Karen Perrin, Manager
Lori Stone, Director

3398 **Illinois Department of Rehabilitation**
100 South Grand Avenue East
Springfield, IL 62762-1304
217-782-6680
800-843-6154
Fax: 217-524-3834
TTY: 800-447-6404
DHS.WEBBITS@ILLINOIS.GOV
www.dhs.state.il.us/page.aspx?item=29736

Robert Kilbury, Director
Timothy Martin, Manager
DHS's Division of Rehabilitation Services is the state's lead agency serving individuals with disabilities. DRS works in partnership with people with disabilities and their families to assist them in making informed choices to achieve full community participation through employment, education, and independent living opportunities.

3399 **Illinois Department on Aging**
One Natural Resources Way
Suite 100
Springfield, IL 62702-1271
217-785-2870
800-252-8966
Fax: 217-785-4477
TTY: 888-206-1327
www2.illinois.gov

John K. Holton, Director
Jennifer Reif, Deputy Director
Matthew Ryan, Chief of Staff
The MISSION of the Illinois Department on Aging is to serve and advocate for older Illinoisans and their caregivers by administering quality and culturally appropriate programs that promote partnerships and encourage independence, dignity, and quality of life.

3400 **International Dyslexia Association: Illinois Branch**
751 Roosevelt Rd.
Suite 116
Glen Ellyn, IL 60137
630-469-6900
Fax: 630-469-6810
www.readibida.org

Jo Ann Paldo, President
Foley Burckardt, Vice President
Joan Budovec, Treasurer
Provides free information and referral services for diagnosis and tutoring for parents, educators, physicians, and individuals with dyslexia in Illinois. Membership includes yearly journal and quarterly newsletter.

3401 **Social Security: Springfield Disability Determination**
3112 CONSTITUTION DR
Springfield, IL 62704-1323
877-279-9504
800-772-1213
TTY: 800-325-0778
ssa.gov

3402 Workers Compensation Board Illinois
100 W Randolph St
Ste 8-200
Chicago, IL 60601-3227   312-814-6611
                                      866-352-3033
                                      Fax: 312-814-6523
                                      infoquestions.wcc@illinois.gov
                                      www2.illinois.gov

Joann Fratianni, Chairman
The Illinois Workers' Compensation Commission resolves disputes between employees and employers regarding work-related injuries and illnesses.

Indiana

3403 Indiana Client Assistance Program
4701 N. Keystone Avenue
Suite 222
Indianapolis, IN 46204-1191   317-722-5555
                                      800-622-4845
                                      Fax: 317-722-5564
                                      TTY: 317-722-5555
                                      www.icdri.org/legal/IndianaCAP.htm

Michael Burks, Chairman
Wen Lu, Secretary and Treasurer

3404 Indiana Developmental Disability Council
402 West Washington Street
Room E145
Indianapolis, IN 46204-2801   317-232-7770
                                      Fax: 317-233-3712
                                      www.in.gov

Katrina Gossett, Chair
Dawn Adams JD, Agency representative
Suellen Jackson-Boner, Executive Director
The Indiana Governor's Council is an independent state agency that facilitates change. Our mission is to promote public policy which leads to the independence, productivity and inclusion of people with disabilities in all aspects of society

3405 Indiana Protection & Advocacy Services Commission
4701 N. Keystone Avenue
Suite 222
Indianapolis, IN 46205-1561   317-722-5555
                                      800-622-4845
                                      Fax: 317-722-5564
                                      ExecutiveDirector@ipas.in.gov
                                      www.in.gov/ipas

Dawn Adams, Executive Director
Milo Gray, Client & Legal Services Director
Gary Richter, Support Services Director
An independent state agency established to protect and promote the rights of individuals with disabilities through empowerment and advocacy.

3406 Indiana State Commission for the Handicapped
P.O.Box 1964
Indianapolis, IN 46206   317-233-1292

3407 International Dyslexia Association: Indiana Branch
Fisher, IN 46038   317-926-1450
                                      www.ida-indiana.org
Kim Haughee, President
Sara Silvey, Vice President
Ginger Lentz, Secretary
The Indiana Branch was formed to help the members of the learning disabilities community in Indiana. Promotes understanding and facilitate treatment of the Specific Language Disability (Dyslexia) in children and adults, promotes teacher training and educational intervention strategies for dyslexic students and to foster effective teaching, supports research in the field and early identification of dyslexia, serves as a clearinghouse for information and to actively disseminate knowledge.

Iowa

3408 Governor's Developmental Disability Council
617 East Second Street
Des Moines, IA 50309-1831   515-281-9082
                                      800-452-1936
                                      Fax: 515-281-9087
                                      http://idaction.com/

Becky Harker, Executive Director
Rik Shannon, Public Policy Manager
Janet Shoeman, Program Planner/Contract Manager
The Council identifies, develops and promotes public policy and support practices through capacity building, advocacy, and systems change activities. The purpose is to ensure that people with developmental disabilities and their families are included in planning, decision making, and development of policy related to services and supports that affect their quality of life and full participation in communities of their choice.

3409 International Dyslexia Association: Iowa Branch
P.O. Box 11188
Cedar Rapids, IA 52410-1188   765-507-9432
                                     info@iowaida.org
                                     ia.dyslexiaida.org

Denise Little, President
Tricia Krsek, Vice President
Genevieve Monthie, Secretary
The purpose of the Iowa Branch of IDA is to increase awareness of dyslexia and promote services that address the importance of diagnosis and remediation for those not meeting their reading potential. Providese services and assistance in a way that promotes unity, support, and cooperation among those who work with these individuals so that all communities in Iowa benefit from the skills and talents of its citizens.

3410 Iowa Child Health Specialty Clinics
100 Hawkins Drive
Room 247 CDD
Iowa City, IA 52242-1016   319-356-1117
                                     866-219-9119
                                     Fax: 319-356-3715
                                     kathy-colbert@uiowa.edu
                                     www.chsciowa.org

Jeffrey Lobas, Director
Brian Wilkes, Director Of Operations
Child Health Specialty Clinics has a mission to improve the health, development, and well-being of Iowa's children and youth with special health care needs in partnership with families, service providers, and communities.

3411 Iowa Commission of Persons with Disabilities
Department of Human Rights
Lucas State Office Bldg, 2nd Floor
Des Moines, IA 50319- 2006   515-242-6171
                                     888-219-0471
                                     Fax: 515-242-6119
                                     TTY: 888-219-0471
                                     www.state.ia.us/dhr/pd

Jill Fulitano-Avery, Administrator
To equalize opportunities for full participation in employment and other areas of the state's economic, educational, social and political life for Iowans with disabilities.

3412 Iowa Compass
Center for Disabilities & Development
100 Hawkins Dr
Suite S295
Iowa City, IA 52242-1011   800-779-2001
                                     TTY: 877-686-0032
                                     iowa-compass@uiowa.edu
                                     www.iowacompass.org

Michael Lightbody, Project Director
Carolyn Petitgout, CRS, Admin Services Coordinator & Database Editor
Iowa Compass offers free information and program referrals to thousands of unique local, state and national organizations serving people with complex health related conditions and disabilities.
BiMonthly

3413 Iowa Department for the Blind
State Of Iowa
524 4th Street
Des Moines, IA 50309-2364
515-281-1333
800-362-2587
Fax: 515-281-1263
TTY: 515-281-1355
information@blind.state.ia.us
www.IDBonline.org

Richard Sorey, Director
Jodi Aldini, Library Support Staff
Julie Aufdenkamp, Transition Specialist, Transitio
Mission is to be the means for persons who are blind to obtain univeral access and full participation as citizens in whatever roles they may choose.

3414 Iowa Department of Human Services
1305 E Walnut St
Des Moines, IA 50319-114
515-242-6510
800-972-2017
Fax: 515-281-4597

Terry E Branstad, Governor
Charles M Palmer, Director
Sally Titus, Deputy Director
Help individuals and families to achieve stable and healthy lives.

3415 Iowa Department on Aging
510 E 12th Street
Suite 2
Des Moines, IA 50319-9025
515-725-3333
800-532-3213
Fax: 866-236-1430
www.aging.iowa.gov

Donna K. Harvey, Director
Danika Welch, Executive Secretary
Joel Wulf, Administrator

3416 Iowa Protection & Advocacy for the Disabled
400 East Court Avenue
Suite 300
Des Moines, IA 50309
515-278-2502
800-779-2502
Fax: 515-278-0539
info@DRIowa.org
disabilityrightsiowa.org

Christine Glosser, President
Todd Lantz, Vice President
Jane Hudson, Executive Director
Disability Rights IOWA aims to defend and promote the human and legal rights of Iowans who have disabilities and mental illness.

3417 Social Security: Des Moines Disability Determination
Social Security Administration
Riverpoint Office Complex
455 SW 5TH ST STE F
Des Moines, IA 50309-2115
515-284-4260
800-772-1213
Fax: 515-284-4394
TTY: 800-325-0778
ssa.gov

Leroy Brown, Manager

3418 Workers Compensation Board Iowa
1000 East Grand Avenue
Des Moines, IA 50319-0209
515-281-5387
Fax: 515-281-6501
www.iowaworkforce.org

Joseph S Cortese II, Commissioner
Janna E. Martin, Commissioner
Sandy Breckenridge, Administrative Secretary
The Workers' Compensation Act is a part of the Iowa Code designed to provide certain benefits to employees who receive injury (85), occupational disease (85A) or occupational hearing loss (85B) arising out of and during the course of their employment.

Kansas

3419 Beach Center on Families and Disability
University of Kansas
1200 Sunnyside Ave.
Room 3134
Lawrence, KS 66045-7534
785-864-7600
866-783-3378
beachcenter@ku.edu
www.beachcenter.org

Michael Wehmeyer, Director
A federally funded center that conducts research and training in the factors that contribute to the successful functioning of families with members who have disabilities.

3420 International Dyslexia Association: Kansas/Missouri Branch
16628 Bond St.
Overland Park, KS 66221
816-945-2665
ksmoida@gmail.com
ksmo.dyslexiaida.org

Cathy Denesia, President
Holly Aranda, Vice President
Nora Wolf, Treasurer
Provides free information and referral services for diagnosis and tutoring for parents, educators, physicians, and individuals with dyslexia in Illinois. Membership includes yearly journal and quarterly newsletter.

3421 Kansas Advocacy and Protective Services
214 SW 6th Ave.,
Ste 100
Topeka, KS 66603-3726
785-273-9661
877-776-1541
Fax: 785-273-9414
TTY: 877-335-3725
www.drckansas.org/

Rocky Nichols, Executive Director
Debbie White, Deputy Director
Lane Williams, Deputy Director
Protection and advocacy for persons with disabilities.

3422 Kansas Client Assistance Program
635 SW Harrison
Suite 100
Topeka, KS 66603
785-273-9661
877-776-1541
Fax: 785-273-9414
TTY: 877-335-3725
rocky@drckansas.org
www.icdri.org/legal/KansasCAP.htm

3423 Kansas Commission on Disability Concerns
900 SW Jackson
Suite 100
Topeka, KS 66612-1246
785-296-1722
800-295-5232
Fax: 785-296-1795
KCDCoffice@ks.gov
kcdcinfo.ks.gov

Martha Gabehart, Executive Director
Kerrie Bacon, Employment Liaison
The Kansas Commission on Disability Concerns provides disability-related supports and information to the people of Kansas. The commission offers legislative advocacy, education and resource networking to ensure full and equal citizenship for all Kansans with disabilities.

3424 Kansas Department on Aging
503 S Kansas Ave
New England Building
Topeka, KS 66603- 3404
785-296-4986
800-432-3535
Fax: 785-296-0256
TTY: 785-291-3167
wwwmail@kdads.ks.gov
www.kdads.ks.gov

Kathy Greenlee, Manager
Barbara Conant, Public Information Officer
Kari Bruffett, Secretary

Services and information for Kansas seniors, over age 60.

3425 Kansas Developmental Disability Council
Disability Rights Center of Kansas
915 SW Harrison
DSOB Rm 141
Topeka, KS 66612-3726

785-296-2608
877-431-4604
Fax: 785-296-2861
TTY: 877-335-3725
sgieber@kcdd.org
www.kcdd.org/

Steve Gieber, Executive Director
Craig Knutson, Public Policy Coordinator
Charline Cobbs, Senior Administrative Assistant
The purpose of the Kansas Council on Developmental Disabilities (KCDD) is to support people of all ages with developmental disabilities so they have the opportunity to make choices regarding both their participation in society, and their quality of life.

Kentucky

3426 Kentucky Cabinet for Health and Family Services
275 E Main St.
Frankfort, KY 40621

502-564-5497
800-372-2973
Fax: 502-564-9523
chfs.ky.gov

Jeffrey D. Howard, Commissioner
Oversees program areas relating to aging, behavioral/developmental health, children with special needs, family resources, medicaid, public health, and more.

3427 Kentucky Council on Developmental Disability
1151 So. Fourth Street
Louisville, KY 40203

502-584-1239
800-372-2973
Fax: 502-584-1261
info@councilondd.org
councilondd.org

Richard Bush, President
Dave Fowler, Treasurer
Missy Kinnaird, Secretary
Implementation of Developmental Disabilities Planning Council responsible under P.L. 101-496.

3428 Kentucky Office for the Blind
275 E Main St
Frankfort, KY 40621

502-564-4754
800-321-6668
Fax: 502-564-2951
TTY: 502-564-2929
blind.ky.gov

Cora McNabb, Executive Director
Deanna Doll, Vocational Rehabilitation Counselor
Tonisha Everhart, Vocational Rehabilitation Counselor
Provides career services and assistance to adults with severe visual handicaps who want to become productive in the home or work force. The office also runs a Client Assistance Program established to provide advice, assistance and information available from rehabilitation programs to persons with handicaps.

3429 Kentucky Office of Aging Services
Cabinet for Health Services
275 East Main Street
Suite 1E-B
Frankfort, KY 40621

502-564-6930
Fax: 502-564-4595
TTY: 888-642-1137
David.Boswell@ky.gov

Deborah Anderson, Commissioner
Chris Harbeck, Executive Secretary
Marnie Mountjoy, Staff Assistant
The Kentucky Office of Aging Services is the state agency directly responsible for programs and services for people with disabilities. Efforts are made to fully integrate the service response information that considers broad farmiliar implications.

3430 Kentucky Protection & Advocacy
100 Fair Oaks Ln 3rd Fl
Frankfort, KY 40601-1108

502-564-2967
800-372-2988
Fax: 502-564-0848
kypa.net

Marsha Hockensmith, Executive Director
Protection and advocacy, Kentucky's federally-mandated protection and advocacy system, protects & promotes the disability rights of individuals through free legally-based advocacy, technical assistance, and education.

3431 Social Security: Frankfort Disability Determination
Social Security
140 Flynn Avenue
Frankfort, KY 40601

866-964-1724
800-772-1213
Fax: 502-226-4519
TTY: 502-226-4519
www.ssa.gov

Stephen Jones, Director
Burton Sisk, Manager

3432 Social Security: Louisville Disability Determination
Social Security
601 W Broadway
Room 101
Louisville, KY 40202-2227

866-716-9671
800-772-1213
TTY: 502-582-5238
ssa.gov

Louisiana

3433 Louisiana Assistive Technology Access Network
3042 Old Forge Dr.
P O Box 14115
Baton Rouge, LA 70898

225-925-9500
800-270-6185
Fax: 225-925-9560
www.latan.org/

Jim Parks, President & CEO
Sandee Winchell, Executive Director
An information and training resource on Assistive Technology for the State of Louisiana. LATAN operates three regional centers to provide better access for consumers.

3434 Louisiana Center for Dyslexia and Related Learning Disorders
PO Box 2050
Thibodaux, LA 70310-1

985-448-4214
Fax: 985-448-4423
karen.chauvin@nicholls.edu
www.nicholls.edu

Karen Chauvin, Director
Jason Talbot, Assessment & Research Coor
Ashley D Munson, Senior Program Coordinator
Provides free information and referral services for diagnosis and tutoring for parents, educators, physicians and individuals with dyslexia. The voice of our membership is heard in 48 countries. Membership includes yearly journal and quarterly newsletter. Call for conference dates.

3435 Louisiana Department of Aging
Office of Elderly Affairs
PO Box 629
Baton Rouge, LA 70821-0629

225-342-9500
Fax: 225-342-5568
robin.wagner@la.gov
new.dhh.louisiana.gov/

Tara LeBlanc, Assistant Secretary
Robin Wagner, Deputy Assistant Secretary
Kirsten Clebart, Director
Serves as a focal point for Louisiana's senior citizens and administers a broad range of home and community based services through a network of 37 Area Agencies on Aging. Serve as the focal point for the development, implementation, and administration of the public policy for the state of Louisiana, and address the needs of the state's elderly citizens.

3436   Louisiana Department of Health - Mental Health Services
PO Box 629
Baton Rouge, LA 70821-0629   225-342-9500
                                               888-342-6207
                                          Fax: 225-342-5568
                                               ldhinfo@la.gov
                                               new.dhh.louisiana.gov
Rebekah Gee, Ph.D, Secretary
Michelle Alletto, Deputy Secretary
Jimmy Guidry, Ph.D, State Health Officer
The Office of Behavioral Health's mental health services provide a variety of treatments for people who have different types of mental illnesses.Also offered are treatment clinics and family support services.

3437   Louisiana Developmental Disability Council
PO Box 3455
626 Main Street, Suite A
Baton Rouge, LA 70821-3455   225-342-6804
                                               800-450-8108
                                          Fax: 225-342-1970
                                               shawn.fleming@la.gov
                                               www.laddc.org
Sandra Sam Beech, Chairperson
Brenda Cosse, Vice Chairperson
Sandee Winchell, Executive Director
The Council's mission is to lead and promote advocacy, capacity building, and systemic change toimprove the quality of life for individualswith developmental disabilities and their families.

3438   Louisiana Learning Resources System
2525 Wyandotte St
Baton Rouge, LA 70805-6464   225-355-6197
                                          Fax: 225-357-3508
Bobbie Robertson, Administrator
Provides consultation on educational seOrvices for local schools, offers psychological testing and evaluation, maintains resource rooms in district schools and more for the blind and handicapped throughout the state.

3439   Social Security: Baton Rouge Disability Determination
Department of Social Services
5455 Bankers Ave
Baton Rouge, LA 70808   866-613-3070
                                               800-772-1213
                                          Fax: 225-219-9399
                                          TTY: 225-382-2090
                                               adren.wilson@dss.state.la.us
                                               www.ssa.gov
Shirley Williams, Director
Ann Williamson, Manager

3440   Workers Compensation Board Louisiana
1001 North 23rd Street
Post Office Box 94094
Baton Rouge, LA 70804-9094   225-342-3111
                                               800-259-5154
                                          Fax: 225-342-7960
                                               owd@lwc.la.gov
                                               www.laworks.net
Curt Eysink, Executive Director
Carey Foy, Deputy Executive Director
Renee Ellender Roberie, Chief Financial Officer
The Louisiana Workforce Commission's vision is to make Louisiana the best place in the country to get a job or grow a business, and our goal is to be the country's best workforce agency.

Maine

3441   Maine Assistive Technology Projects
University of Maine at Augusta
Georgia Institute of Technology
490 Tenth Street
Atlanta, GA 30332-0156   404-894-4960
                                          Fax: 404-894-9320
                                               catea@coa.gatech.edu
                                               assistivetech.net

A statewide program promoting assistive technology devices and services for persons of all ages with all disabilities.

3442   Maine Bureau of Elder and Adult Services
11 State House Station
41 Anthony Avenue
Augusta, ME 04333   207-287-9200
                                               800-262-2232
                                          Fax: 207-287-9229
                                               www.maine.gov
Ricker Hamilton, Director
AnnMarie Stevens, Administrative Assistant
Lois Emerson, Office Specialist I
Adult Protective Services (APS), is responsible for providing or arranging for services to protect incapacitated and/or dependent adults in danger.

3443   Maine Department of Health and Human Services
221 State Street
Augusta, ME 04333-0040   207-287-3707
                                          Fax: 207-287-3005
                                               www.maine.gov/dhhs
Mary C. Mayhew, Commissioner
Sam Adolphsen, Chief Operating Officer
Ricker Hamilton, Deputy Commissioner of Programs
Provision of an array of services to people with nental illness, substance abuse issues, children with special needs and people with developmental disabilities.

3444   Maine Developmental Disabilities Council
225 Western Avenue
Suite 4
Augusta, ME 04330   207-287-4213
                                               800-244-3990
                                          Fax: 207-287-8001
                                               nancy.e.cronin@maine.gov
                                               www.maineddc.org
Nancy Cronin, Executive Director
Rachel Dyer, Associate Director
Erin Howes, Office Manager
The MDDC is a partnership of people with disabilities, their families, and agencies which identifies barriers to community inclusion, self-determination, and independence, and acts to effect positive change.

3445   Maine Division for the Blind and Visually Impaired
21 Enterprise Dr
Suite 2
Augusta, ME 04333-0073   207-624-5120
                                               800-760-1573
                                          Fax: 207-624-5133
                                          TTY: 800-633-0770
                                               mdol@maine.gov
                                               www.maine.gov/rehab/dbvi
Harold Lewis, Director
Sandra Cavanaugh, Executive Director
Works to bring about full access to employment, independence and community integration for people with disabilities in Maine.

3446   Maine Office of Elder Services
State of Maine
11 State House Station
41 Anthony Avenue
Augusta, ME 04333   207-287-9200
                                               800-262-2232
                                          Fax: 207-287-9229
                                          TTY: 800-606-0215
                                               mdol@maine.gov
James Martin, Director
Gary Wolcott, Associate Director
Romaine Turyn, Aging Service Manager
The Office of Elder Services (OES), an Office within the Maine Department of Health and Human Services, promotes programs and services for older adults, their families and for people with disabilities.

3447 Maine Workers' Compensation Board
27 State House Station
Augusta, ME 04333
207-287-3751
888-801-9087
Fax: 207-287-7198
TTY: 877-832-5525
www.maine.gov/wcb

Paul H Sighinolfi, Executive Director
Lindsay Lizzotte, Secretary Specialist
Gary Koocher, Management Representative
The general mission of the Maine Workers' Compensation Board is to serve the employees and employers of the State fairly and expeditiously by ensuring compliance with the workers' compensation laws, ensuring the prompt delivery of benefits legally due, promoting the prevention of disputes, utilizing dispute resolution to reduce litigation and facilitating labor-management cooperation.

3448 Social Security: Maine Disability Determination
330 Civic Center Dr
Suite 4
Augusta, ME 04330-6325
866-882-5422
800-772-1213
TTY: 207-623-4190
ssa.gov

Louis Tepin, Manager
This office makes the medical determination about whether a consumer is disabled and, therefore, medically eligible for Social Security benefits. Legally, an individual is considered disabled if he or she is unable to do any substantial gainful work activity because of a medical condition (or conditions), that has lasted, or can be expected to last for at least 12 months, or that is expected to result in death.

Maryland

3449 Health Resources & Services Administration: State Bureau of Health
5600 Fishers Lane
Rockville, MD 20857
301-443-3376
877-464-4772
TTY: 877-897-9910
www.hrsa.gov

Diana Espinosa, Deputy Administrator
Jordan Grossman, Chief of Staff
Carole Johnson, Administrator
Through appropriated funds, supports education programs, credentialing analysis, and development of human resources needed to staff the U.S. health care system.

3450 International Dyslexia Association: Maryland Branch
International Dyslexia Association
P.O. Box 233
Brookland, MD 21022-0233
800-509-4980
md.dyslexiaida.org

Annette Fallon, President
Karen Fallon, Vice President
Timothy Yearick, Secretary
Nonprofit organization providing free information and referral services for diagnosis and tutoring for parents, educators, physicians, and individuals with dyslexia. Membership includes yearly journal and quarterly newsletter. Call for conference dates.

3451 Maryland Client Assistance Program Division of Rehabilitation Services
2301 Argonne Drive
Baltimore, MD 21218-1628
410-554-9442
888-554-0334
Fax: 410-554-9362
TTY: 443-798-2840
dors@maryland.gov
dors.maryland.gov

Suzanne R. Page, DORS Director
Helps individuals with disabilities understand the rehabilitation process and receives appropriate and quality services from the Division of Rehabilitation Services and other programs and facilities providing services under the Rehabilitation Act of 1973.

3452 Maryland Department of Aging
State Office Building
301 West Preston Street
Suite 1007
Baltimore, MD 21201- 2393
410-767-1100
800-243-3425
Fax: 410-333-7943
www.mdoa.state.md.us/

Stuart Rosenthal, Chair
Sharonlee J. Vogel, Vice-Chair
Rona E. Kramer, Secretary
The Department of Aging protects the rights and quality of life of older persons in Maryland. To meet the needs of senior citizens, the Department administers programs throughout the State, primarily through local area agencies on aging.

3453 Maryland Department of Handicapped Children
201 W Preston St
Unit 50
Baltimore, MD 21201-2301
410-335-6470
www.msa.md.gov

Judson Force, Director
Children's Medical Services is a joint federal/state/local program which assists in obtaining specialized medical, surgical and related habilitative/rehabilitative evaluation and treatment services for children with special health care needs and their families. To be eligible for the program's services, an individual must be a resident of Maryland, younger than 22 years, have or be suspected of having an eligible medical condition and meet both medical and financial criteria.

3454 Maryland Developmental Disabilities Council
217 E Redwood Street
Suite 1300
Baltimore, MD 21202-3313
410-767-3670
800-305-6441
Fax: 410-333-3686
www.md-council.org

Brian Cox, Executive Director
Catherine Lyle, Deputy Director
Rachel London, Director, Children & Family Poli
A public policy organization comprised of people with disabilities and family members who are joined by state officials, service providers and other designated partners. The Council is an independent, self-governing organization that represents the interests of people with developmental disabilities and their families.

3455 Maryland Division of Mental Health
201 W. Preston Street
Baltimore, MD 21201
410-767-6500
877-463-3464
dhmh.healthmd@maryland.gov

Norma Pinette, Executive Director
Van T. Mitchell, Secretary
Our Public Health Services Division oversees vital public services to Maryland residents including infectious disease and environmental health concerns, family health services and emergency preparedness and response activities.

3456 Maternal and Child Health Bureau - Health Resources and Services Administration
5600 Fishers Lane
Rockville, MD 20857
301-443-3376
877-464-4772
TTY: 877-897-9910
www.hrsa.gov

Diana Espinosa, Deputy Administrator
Jordan Grossman, Chief of Staff
Carole Johnson, Administrator
Offers information, books and pamphlets to professionals, parents and children facing health issues or disabilities.

3457 Social Security: Baltimore Disability Determination
711 West 40th Street
Ste 415 Rotunda Mall
Baltimore, MD 21211-2120
800-772-1213
TTY: 800-325-0778
ssa.gov

This office makes the medical determination about whether a consumer is disabled and, therefore, medically eligible for Social Security benefits. Legally, an individual is considered disabled if he or she is unable to do any substantial gainful work activity because of a medical condition (or conditions), that has lasted, or can be expected to last for at least 12 months, or that is expected to result in death.

3458 Workers Compensation Board Maryland
10 East Baltimore Street
Baltimore, MD 21202-1641

410-864-5100
800-492-0479
Fax: 410-333-8122
info@wcc.state.md.us
www.wcc.state.md.us

R. Karl Aumann, Chairperson
Mary K. Ahearn, Chief Executive Officer
David E. Jones, Chief Financial Officer

Massachusetts

3459 Center for Public Representation
22 Green Street
Northampton, MA 01060-3708

413-586-6024
Fax: 413-586-5711
info@cpr-ma.org
centerforpublicrep.org

Bob Agoglia, President
Nickie Chandler, Clerk/Treasurer
Bob Riedel, Director
The Center seeks to improve the quality of lives of people with mental illness and other disabilities through the systemic enforcement of their legal rights while promoting improvements in services for citizens with disabilities

3460 Massachusetts Assistive Technology Partnership
Children s Hospital Boston
1295 Boylston St
Suite 310
Boston, MA 02215-3407

617-355-7820
800-848-8867
Fax: 617-355-6345

Marylyn Howe, Project Director
Pat Hill, Training Coordinator
A statewide program promoting assistive technology devices and services for persons with all disabilities.

3461 Massachusetts Client Assistance Program
Massachusetts Office on Disability
1 Ashburton Pl
Suite 1305
Boston, MA 02108-1518

617-727-7440
800-322-2020
www.mass.gov/anf/employment-equal-access-disa
Barbara Lybarger, Assistant Director
Myra Berloff, Director
Michael Dumont, Assistant Director
Provides advocacy and information services.

3462 Massachusetts Department of Mental Health
25 Staniford St.
Boston, MA 02114-2503

617-626-8000
TTY: 617-727-9842
dmhinfo@massmail.state.ma.us
www.mass.gov/dmh

Joan Mikula, Commissioner
The Massachusetts Department of Mental Health, as the State Mental Health Authority, assures and provides access to services and supports to meet the mental health needs of individuals of all ages, enabling them to live, work and participate in their communities. The Department establishes standards to ensure effective and culturally competent care to promote recovery. The Department sets policy, promotes self-determination, protects human rights and supports mental health training and research.

3463 Massachusetts Developmental Disabilities Council
100 Hancock Street
Second Floor, Suite 201
Quincy, MA 02169-4398

617-770-7676
Fax: 617-770-1987
TTY: 617-770-9499
www.state.ma.us/mddc/

Daniel Shannon, Executive Director
Faith Behum, Disability Policy Specialist
Kristin Britton, Director of Public Policy
Group of citizens which analyzes needs of people with severe, lifelong disabilities and works to improve public policy. MDDC produces several publications and has committees and a grants program to study and advocate for changes in the service system.

3464 Social Security: Boston Disability Determination
110 Chauncy Street
Boston, MA 02111

617-727-7600
800-772-1213
TTY: 800-882-2040
www.socialsecurity.gov

Michael F. Bertrand, Commissioner

3465 Workers Compensation Board Massachusetts
Rm 211
1 Ashburton Pl
Boston, MA 02108-1518

617-626-7122
Fax: 617-727-1090
www.state.ma.us/dia

Russell Gilfus, Manager
The Massachusetts Workers' Compensation system is in place to make sure that workers are protected by insurance if they are injured on the job or contract a work-related illness. Under this system, employers are required by Massachusetts General Laws c. 152, 25A to provide workers' compensation (WC) insurance coverage to all their employees.

Michigan

3466 Department of Blind Rehabilitation
Western Michigan University
1903 W Michigan Ave
Kalamazoo, MI 49008-5218

269-387-3455
Fax: 269-387-3567
g.dennis@wmich.edu
www.wmich.edu/visionstudies

James Leja, Chair
Charles Adams, Faculty Specialist I
Gayla Dennis, Office Coordinator
The Department of Blindness and Low Vision Studies at Western Michigan University is recognized internationally as the oldest, largest and best program of its kind. It originated in 1961 with a graduate degree in Orientation and Mobility, responding to the need for professionals to rehabilitate the many military personnel blinded during World War Two and the Korean War.

3467 Michigan Association for Deaf and Hard of Hearing
5236 Dumond Court
Suite C
Lansing, MI 48917-6001

517-487-0066
800-968-7327
Fax: 517-487-0202
TTY: 517-487-2586
info@madhh.org
www.madhh.org

Nancy Asher, Executive Director
Pat Walton, Office Manager
MADHH is a statewide collaboration agency dedicated to improving the lives of people who are deaf and hard of hearing through leadership in education, advocacy & services. Interpreter IC print-out, assistive devices available.

3468 Michigan Association for Deaf, and Hard of Hearing
5236 Dumond Court
Suite C
Lansing, MI 48917-6001   517-487-0066
    800-968-7327
    Fax: 517-487-2586
    www.madhh.org
Nancy Asher, Executive Director
Pat Walton, Office Manager
MADHH is a statewide collaboration agency dedicated to improving the lives of people who are deaf and hard of hearing through leadership in education, advocacy and services.

3469 Michigan Client Assistance Program
4095 Legacy Pkwy
Ste 500
Lansing, MI 48911-4264   517-487-1755
    800-288-5923
    Fax: 517-487-0827
    TTY: 800-288-5923
    molson@mpas.org
    www.mpas.org
Kate Pew Wolters, President
Thomas Landry, 1st Vice President
John McCulloch, 2nd Vice President
The Client Assistance Program (CAP) assists people who are seeking or receiving services from Michigan Rehabilitation Services, Consumer Choice Programs, Michigan Commission for the Blind, Centers for Independent Living, and Supported Employment and Transition Programs. The CAP program is part of Michigan Protection and Advocacy Service, Inc.

3470 Michigan Coalition for Staff Development and School Improvement
12236 6 1/2 Mile Road
MCES
Battle Creek, MI 49014-1062   269-967-2086
    800-444-2014
    Fax: 517-371-1170
TheMichigan Coalition of Essential Schools(MCES) has serviced over 60 public and private schools in the state over the past 14 years. Our experienced staff, consisting of K-12 educators in the classroom and building and district leadership, is poised and ready to help schools build and sustain capacity for whole school change and increased student achievement.

3471 Michigan Commission for the Blind - Gaylord
Ste 102
209 W 1st St
Gaylord, MI 49735-1386   989-732-2448
    800-292-4200
    Fax: 989-731-3587
    www.michigan.gov
Judy Terwilliger, Manager
The mission of the Michigan Commission for the Blind (MCB) is to provide opportunity to individuals who are blind or visually impaired to achieve employability and/or function independently in society. The MCB vision is that someday it will be said that Michigan is a great place for blind people to live, learn, work, raise a family, and enjoy life

3472 Michigan Commission for the Blind
Michigan Dept Of Energy, Labor & Economic Growth
PO Box 30652
Lansing, MI 48909-8152   517-373-2062
    800-292-4200
    Fax: 517-335-5140
    TTY: 517-373-4025
    turneys@michigan.gov
    www.michigan.gov/mcb
Patrick Cannon, State Director
The Michigan Commision for the blind is a state government agency that provides state and federally funded training and other services to individuals who are legally blind (blind and visually impaired). Services are provided to people of all ages throughout the state of Michigan toward the goal of employment and/or independence.

3473 Michigan Commission for the Blind Training Center
PO Box 30652
Lansing, MI 48909   517-373-2062
    800-292-4200
    Fax: 517-335-5140
    TTY: 517-373-4025
    mossc@michigan.gov
    www.michigan.gov/mcb
Cheryl L Heibeck, Director
Bruce Schultz, Assistant Director
Residential facility that provides instruction to legally blind adults in braille, computer operation and assistive technology, handwriting, cane travel, cooking, personal management, industrial arts and also crafts. During training students will develop career plans which may include work experience, internships, volunteer opprtunities and even part-time paid employment.

3474 Michigan Commission for the Blind: Escanaba
305 Ludington St
State Office Bldg., 1st Floor
Escanaba, MI 49829-4029   906-786-8602
    800-323-2535
    Fax: 906-786-4638
    michigan.gov/mcb
Bernie Kramer, Manager
The mission of the Michigan Commission for the Blind (MCB) is to provide opportunity to individuals who are blind or visually impaired to achieve employability and/or function independently in society. The MCB vision is that someday it will be said that Michigan is a great place for blind people to live, learn, work, raise a family, and enjoy life

3475 Michigan Commission for the Blind: Flint
125 E Union St
Seventh Floor
Flint, MI 48502-2041   810-760-2030
    800-292-4200
    Fax: 810-760-2032
Debbie Wilson, Manager
Vocational and Independent living skills training for individuals who are legally blind.

3476 Michigan Commission for the Blind: Grand Rapids
250 Ottawa Avenue
Grand Rapids, MI 49503-4029   906-786-8602
    800-323-2535
    Fax: 906-786-4638
    michigan.gov/mcb
Bernie Kramer, Manager
The mission of the Michigan Commission for the Blind (MCB) is to provide opportunity to individuals who are blind or visually impaired to achieve employability and/or function independently in society. The MCB vision is that someday it will be said that Michigan is a great place for blind people to live, learn, work, raise a family, and enjoy life

3477 Michigan Council of the Blind and Visually Impaired (MCBVI)
Neal Freeling
350 Ottawa Ave NW
Grand Rapids, MI 49503-2316   616-356-0180
    800-292-4200
    Fax: 616-356-0199
    michigan.gov/mcb
Bernie Kramer, Manager
MCBVI is a diverse group of very friendly people from around the state working together to improve the lives of all citizens who are blind or visually impaired.

3478 Michigan Department of Handicapped Children
3423 N Martin Luther King Jr Blvd
Lansing, MI 48906-2934   517-484-9312
    Fax: 517-484-9836
Alan Curtiss, President
Bobbie Butler, Manager

3479 Michigan Developmental Disabilities Council
201 Townsend Street
Suite 120
Lansing, MI 48910-1646 517-335-3158
Fax: 517-335-2751
TTY: 517-335-3171
mdch-dd-council@michigan.gov
www.michigan.gov/ddcouncil
Nick Lyon, Director
Nancy Grijalva, Assistant
Tim Becker, Chief Deputy Director
The Michigan DD Council is a group of citizens from across the state. Its membership is made up of: people with developmental disabilities; people from families who have, among their members, people with developmental disabilities; and professionals from state and local agencies charged with assisting people with developmental disabilities.

3480 Michigan Office of Services to the Aging
P.O.Box 30676
Lansing, MI 48909-8176 517-373-8230
Fax: 517-373-4092
OSAInfo@michigan.gov
www.michigan.gov/osa
Wendi Middleton, Division Director
Kari Sederburg, Director
Carol Dye, Senior Executive Assistant
State unit on aging; allocates and monitors state and federal funds for the Older American Act services: nutrition, community services, administers home and community based waiver, develops programs through Area Agencies on Aging, advocates on behalf of seniors with legislature, governor, state departments, federal government, responsible for state planning of aging services, develops formula for distribution of state and federal funds.

3481 Michigan Protection & Advocacy Service
4095 Legacy Pkwy
Ste 500
Lansing, MI 48911-4264 517-487-1755
800-288-5923
Fax: 517-487-0827
molson@mpas.org
www.mpas.org
Kate Pew Wolters, President
Thomas Landry, 1st Vice President
John McCulloch, 2nd Vice President
People with disabilities have to deal with a wide variety of issues. TThey try to answer any questions you may have relating to disability. They have experience in the following areas: discrimination in education, employment, housing, and public places; abuse and neglect; Social Security benefits; Medicaid, Medicare and other insurance; housing; Vocational Rehabilitation; HIV/AIDS issues; and many other disability-related topics

3482 Michigan Rehabilitation Services
300 N. Washington Sq.
Lansing, MI 48913 517-335-4590
888-784-7328
Fax: 517-373-0059
TTY: 517-373-4035
zimmermanng@michigan.org
www.michigan.org
George Zimmermann, Vice President
Michelle Begnoche, Communications Specialist
Bonnie Fink, Travel Consultant Coordinator
A state and federally funded program that helps persons with disabilities prepare for and fund a job that matches their interests and abilities. Assistance is also available to workers with disabilities who are having difficulty keeping a job. A person is eligible for MRS services if he or she has a disability, is unemployed and needs vocational rehabilitation services to prepare for and find a job or independent living services.

3483 Social Security Administration
1100 West High Rise
6401 Security Blvd.
Baltimore, MD 21235-3878 517-393-3876
800-772-1213
Fax: 517-393-4686
TTY: 800-325-0778
jennifer.bower@ssa.gov
ssa.gov
Tiffany L. Flick, Executive Secretary
Michael J. Astrue, Commissioner
Carolyn W. Colvin, Deputy Commissioner
We deliver services through a nationwide network of over 1,400 offices that include regional offices, field offices, card centers, teleservice centers, processing centers, hearing offices, the Appeals Council, and our State and territorial partners, the Disability Determination Services. We also have a presence in U.S. embassies around the globe. For the public, we are the face of the government. The rich diversity of our employees mirrors the public we serve.

3484 State of Michigan Workers' Compensation Agency
PO Box 30016
Lansing, MI 48909-7516 888-396-5041
Fax: 517-322-1808
wcinfo@michigan.gov
www.michigan.gov/wca/
Mark C. Long, Director
Jack A. Nolish, Deputy Director
Julie Lenneman, Administrative Assistant
Michigan's injured workers and their employers are governed by the Workers' Disability Compensation Act. This Act was first adopted in 1912 and provides compensation to workers who suffer an injury on the job and protects employers' liability. The mission of the Workers' Compensation Agency is to efficiently administer the Act and provide prompt, courteous and impartial service to all customers.

Minnesota

3485 International Dyslexia Association: Upper Midwest Branch
International Dyslexia Association
5021 Vernon Ave. S
Suite 159
Minneapolis, MN 55436-2102 612-486-4242
info.umw@dyslexiaida.org
umw.dyslexiaida.org
Tom Strewler, President
Donna Burns, Member at Large
Jennifer Bennett, Secretary
The Upper Midwest Branch of the International Dyslexia Association serves the residents of Minnesota, North Dakota, South Dakota, and Winnipeg, Canada. They offer local educational conferences about dyslexia and related subjects, Orton-Gillingham training for teachers, tutors, and parents, quarterly speaker series, member discounts on conferences, information line, and tutor referral.

3486 Minnesota Assistive Technology Project
STAR
358 Centennial Office Building
658 Cedar Street
Saint Paul, MN 55155-1402 651-201-2640
888-234-1267
800-627-3529
Fax: 651-282-6671
star.program@state.mn.us
Chuck Rassbach, Program Director
Kim Moccia, Program Coordinator
Jennie Delisi, Resource Specialist
A statewide program promoting assistive technology devices and services for persons of all ages with all disabilities.

3487   Minnesota Board on Aging
P.O. Box 64976
Saint Paul, MN 55164-0976   651-431-2500
                                             800-882-6262
                                             800-333-2433
                                        Fax: 651-431-7453
                                        TTY: 800-627-3529
                                             www.mnaging.org

Don Samuelson, Chair
Jean Wood, Executive Director
Leonard Axelrod, Board Member

A state unit on aging for the state of Minnesota. Funds 14 area agencies on aging throughout the state that provide services at the local level. The mission is to keep older people in the homes or places of residence for as long as possible.

3488   Minnesota Children with Special Needs, Minnesota Department of Health
P.O.Box 64882
Saint Paul, MN 55164-0882   651-201-3650
                                             800-728-5420
                                        Fax: 651-201-3655
                                        TTY: 651-201-5797
                                        health.cyshn@state.mn.us

Dr. Edward Ehlinger, Commissioner
Daniel L. Pollock, Deputy Commissioner
Jeanne F. Ayers, Assistant Commissioner

Minnesota Children with Special Health Needs (MCSHN) provides leadership through partnerships with families and other key stakeholders to improve the access and quality of all systems impacting children and youth with special health care needs and their families.

3489   Minnesota Department of Human Services: Behavioral Health Division
P.O. Box 64981
Saint Paul, MN 55164   651-431-2225
                                             800-366-5411
                                        Fax: 651-431-7418
                                        dhs.info@state.mn.us
                                        mn.gov/dhs/adult-mental-health

Emily Piper, Commissioner
Charles E. Johnson, Deputy Commissioner
Amy Dellwo, Acting Chief of Staff

Oversees the provision of services to people with mental illness in the state of Minnesota. Services are provided on the local level through a network of 87 county social service departments.

3490   Minnesota Department of Labor & Industry Workers Compensation Division
443 Lafayette Rd N
Saint Paul, MN 55155-4301   651-284-5005
                                             800-342-5354
                                        TTY: 651-297-4198
                                        dli.communications@state.mn.us
                                        doli.state.mn.us

Ken Petersom, Commissioner
Jessica Looman, Deputy Commissioner
James Honerman, Communications

To reduce the impact of work related injuries for employees and employers. Advice is given and questions answered on the toll-free number.

3491   Minnesota Disability Law Center
430 1st Avenue North
Suite 300
Minneapolis, MN 55401- 1780   612-334-5970
                                             800-292-4150
                                        Fax: 612-334-5755
                                        TTY: 612-332-4668
                                        website@mylegalaid.org
                                        mylegalaid.org/about/our-work/disability-law

Mary L. Knoblauch, Chair
Cathy Haukedahl, Executive Director
Andrea Kaufman, Director of Development

Provides free, civil, legal assistance to Minnesotans with disabilities on issues related to their disability.

3492   Minnesota Governor's Council on Developmental Disabilities
370 Centennial Office Building
658 Cedar St.
Saint Paul, MN 55155   651-296-4018
                                             877-348-0505
                                        Fax: 651-297-7200
                                        TTY: 800-627-3529
                                        admin.dd@state.mn.us
                                             mn.gov/mnddc

John Hoffman, Chair
Colleen Wieck, PhD, Executive Director
Andrei Hahn, Planner

The mission of the Minnesota Governor's Council on Developmental Disabilities is to provide information, education, and training that will lead to increased independence, productivity, integration and inclusion for people with developmental disabilities and their families.

3493   Minnesota Protection & Advocacy for Persons with Disabilities
Minnesota Disability Law Center
2324 University Avenue West
Suite 101B
Saint Paul, MN 55114-1742   651-228-9105
                                             800-292-4150
                                        Fax: 651-222-0745
                                        statesupport@mnlegalservices.org

Mary Kaczorek, Supervising Attorney
Ann Conroy, Office Manager
Elsa Marshall, Education for Justice Coordinato

Provide public legal information on legal issues impacting the rights of low-income Minnesotans

3494   Minnesota State Council on Disability(MSCOD)
121 E 7th Place
Suite 107
Saint Paul, MN 55101-2114   651-361-7800
                                             800-945-8913
                                        Fax: 651-296-5935
                                        council.disability@state.mn.us
                                             www.disability.state.mn.us

Joan Willshire, Executive Director
Linda Gremillion, Business Operations Manager
Margot Imdieke Cross, Accessibility Specialist

The MSCOD collaborates, advocates, advises and provide technical information to expand opportunities, increase the quality of life and empower all persons with disabilities. This mission is accomplished by: providing information, referral and technical assistance to thousands of individuals every year via email, letter or telephone; through trainings on a variety of disability related topics; through publications and its web site; and through its advocacy and advisory work.

3495   Minnesota State Services for the Blind
2200 University Avenue West
Suite 240
Saint Paul, MN 55114-1840   651-539-2300
                                             800-652-9000
                                        Fax: 651-649-5927
                                        TTY: 651-642-0506
                                        star.program@state.mn.us
                                        http://mn.gov/deed/job-seekers/blind-visual-i

Richard Strong, Executive Director
Kenneth Trebelhorn, Council Member
Jan Bailey, Chair

State agency serving blind and visually impaired persons with rehabilitation, information access, assistive technology, training and job placement services. Extensive older blind program.

3496   Social Security: St. Paul Disability Determination
5210 Perry Robinson
Lansing, MI 48911-3878   877-512-5944
                                              800-772-1213
                                        Fax: 517-393-4686
                                        TTY: 800-325-0778
                                        jennifer.bower@ssa.gov
                                             www.ssa.gov

Karena L. Kilgore, Executive Secretary
Carolyn W. Colvin, Commissioner
Carolyn W. Colvin, Deputy Commissioner

We deliver services through a nationwide network of over 1,400 offices that include regional offices, field offices, card centers, teleservice centers, processing centers, hearing offices, the Appeals Council, and our State and territorial partners, the Disability Determination Services. We also have a presence in U.S. embassies around the globe. For the public, we are the face of the government. The rich diversity of our employees mirrors the public we serve.

Mississippi

3497 International Dyslexia Association: Louisiana Branch
1217 N. 32nd Ave.
Hattiesburg, MS 39401
601-467-1662
carla.carlos4dys@gmail.com
la.dyslexiaida.org

Carla Carlos, President
Lisa Best, Treasurer
Gale Pick, Secretary
Provides free information and referral services for diagnosis and tutoring for parents, educators, physicians, and individuals with dyslexia in Illinois. Membership includes yearly journal and quarterly newsletter.

3498 Mississippi Assistive Technology Division
1281 Highway 51
PO Box 1698
Jackson, MS 39215-1698
601-853-5160
800-443-1000
Fax: 601-853-5158
www.mdrs.ms.gov

Jean Massey, Superintendent of Education
Carey Wright, Superintendent of Education
Jack Virden, Chairman
A statewide program promoting assistive technology devices and services for persons of all ages with all disabilities.

3499 Mississippi Client Assistance Program
Mississippi Department of Rehabilitation Services
500-G East Woodrow Wilson Drive
P.O. Box 4958
Jackson, MS 39296
601-982-7051
Fax: 601-982-1951
www.msdisabilities.com

Dr. Ken Cleveland, President
Presley Posey, Executive Director
Dr. Michael Ogburn, Executive Director
Advocacy program for clients/client applicants for state of MS vocational services.

3500 Mississippi Department of Mental Health
1101 Robert E Lee Bldg
239 North Lamar Street
Jackson, MS 39201
601-359-1288
877-240-8513
Fax: 601-359-6295
TTY: 601-359-6230
www.dmh.ms.gov

Sampat Shivengi, M.D., Chair
George N. Harrison, Vice Chair
Edwin C. Legrand, Executive Director
Administers Mississippi's public programs of serving persons with mental illness, developmental disabilities, alcohol and substance abuse problems, and alzheimer's disease and related dementia.

3501 Mississippi Division of Aging and Adult Services
Mississippi Department Of Human Services
750 North State Street
Jackson, MS 39202-3033
601-355-5536
800-345-6347
877-882-4916
Fax: 601-359-3664
www.mdhs.state.ms.us/

Donald R. Taylor, Executive Director
Julia M. Todd, Director
Judy Collins, Director
Protects the rights of older citizens while expanding their opportunities and access to quality services.

3502 Mississippi State Department of Health
Children s Medical Program
570 East Woodrow Wilson Drive
Post Office Box 1700
Jackson, MS 39216-1700
601-576-7400
866-458-4948
Fax: 601-364-7447
web@HealthyMS.com
www.msdh.state.ms.us

Larry Clark, Director
Vickey Berryman, Director, Bureau of Licensure
Jim Craig, Director, Office of Health Pro
Financial assistance to families of children with physical handicaps. Rehabilitative in nature and has as its goal the correction or reduction of physical handicaps. Eligibility determined by diagnosis and provided to children from birth to age twenty-one. Financial eligibility is determined by factors of family income, family size, estimated cost of treatment and family liabilities. Categories include, but are not limited to: orthopedic, congenital heart defects, cerebral palsy, etc.

3503 Mississippi: Workers Compensation Commission
1428 Lakeland Dr
P.O. Box 5300, 39296-5300
Jackson, MS 39216-4718
601-987-4200
866-473-6922
Fax: 601-987-4220
www.mwcc.state.ms.us

Liles Williams, Chairman
John Junkin, Commissioner
Debra Gibbs, Commissioner
Our goal is to provide the public with useful information regarding Workers' Compensation in the state of Mississippi.

Missouri

3504 Institute for Human Development
University of Missouri-Kansas City
215 W. Pershing Road
6th floor
Kansas City, MO 64108- 2639
816-235-1770
800-444-0821
Fax: 888-503-3107
TTY: 800-452-1185
beckmanncc@umkc.edu
www.ihd.umkc.edu

Carl F. Calkins, Ph.D., Director
Kay Conklin, Training Director
Cindy Beckmann, Assistant to the Director
A statewide program promoting person-centered planning and services for persons of all ages with all disabilities.

3505 Missouri Division Of Developmental Disabilities
Missouri Department Of Mental Health
1706 E. Elm St.
P.O.Box 687
Jefferson City, MO 65102
573-751-4122
800-364-9687
Fax: 573-751-8224
ddmail@dmh.mo.gov
www.dmh.mo.gov

Jay Nixon, Governor
Keith Schafer, Ed.D., Director
Bob Bax, Deputy Director
The Missouri Department of Mental Health was first established as a cabinet-level state agency by the Omnibus State Government Reorganization Act, effective July 1, 1974. State law provides three principal missions for the department: (1) the prevention of mental disorders, developmental disabilities, substance abuse, and compulsive gambling; (2) the treatment, habilitation, and rehabilitation of Missourians who have those conditions; and (3) the improvement of public understanding and attitudes

3506 Missouri Protection & Advocacy Services
925 S Country Club Dr
Jefferson City, MO 65109-4510

573-893-3333
866-777-7199
Fax: 573-893-4231
TTY: 800-735-2966
moadvocacy.org

Joe Wrinkle, Chair
Barbara H. French, Vice Chair
Shawn De Loyola, Executive Director

MO P&A potects the rights of individuals with disabilities by providing advocacy and legal services for disability related issues. As Missouri's Protection and Advocacy system, Mo P&A investigates allegations of abuse, neglect, death, and violations of rights against individuals with disabilities. Those who contact Mo P&A can receive information, referrals, advocacy services or legal counsel provided through one of nine federally-funded programs.

3507 Missouri Rehabilitation Services for the Blind
615 Howerton Court
PO Box 2320
Jefferson City, MO 65102-2320

573-751-3221
800-592-6004
Fax: 573-751-3091
askrsb@dss.mo.gov
www.dss.mo.gov/fsd/rsb/

Mark Laird, Executive Director
Ronald J. Levy, Director
Brian Kinkade, Deputy Director

Offers services for the totally blind, legally blind, visually impaired, including counseling, educational, recreational, rehabilitation, computer training and professional training services.

3508 Social Security: Jefferson City Disability Determination
129 SCOTT STATION ROAD
Jefferson City, MO 65101-4421

877-405-9803
800-772-1213
Fax: 517-393-4686
TTY: 800-325-0778
jennifer.bower@ssa.gov
www.ssa.gov

Karena L. Kilgore, Executive Secretary
Carolyn W. Colvin, Commissioner
Carolyn W. Colvin, Deputy Commissioner

We deliver services through a nationwide network of over 1,400 offices that include regional offices, field offices, card centers, teleservice centers, processing centers, hearing offices, the Appeals Council, and our State and territorial partners, the Disability Determination Services. We also have a presence in U.S. embassies around the globe. For the public, we are the face of the government. The rich diversity of our employees mirrors the public we serve.

3509 Workers Compensation Board Missouri
Department of Labor and Industrial Realtions
421 East Dunkin Street
P.O. Box 58
Jefferson City, MO 65102-0058

573-751-4231
800-775-2667
800-320-2519
Fax: 573-751-4945
workerscomp@labor.mo.gov
labor.mo.gov/DWC/

Butch Albert, Chairman
James Avery, Commissioner
Curtis E. Chick, Commissioner

The Missouri Division of Workers' Compensation administers the programs providing services to all stake holders including workers who have been injured on the job or been exposed to occupational disease arising out of and in the course of employment. The Division makes sure that an injured worker receives benefits that he/she is entitled to under the Missouri Workers' Compensation law. The Division's Administrative Law Judges have the authority to approve settlements or issue awards after a hear

3510 Addictive & Mental Disorders Division
555 Fuller Ave
PO Box 202905
Helena, MT 59620-2905

406-444-3964
Fax: 406-444-4435
http://www.dphhs.mt.gov/amdd/

Lou Thompson, Administrator
Joan Cassidy, Chemical Dependency Bureau Chief
E. Lee Simes, Medical Director

The mission of the Addictive and Mental Disorders Division (AMDD) of the Montana Department of Public Health and Human Services is to implement and improve an appropriate statewide system of prevention, treatment, care, and rehabilitation for Montanans with mental disorders or addictions to drugs or alcohol.

3511 Disability Rights Montana
1022 Chestnut Street
Helena, MT 59601-890

406-449-2344
800-245-4743
Fax: 406-449-2418
TTY: 406-449-2344
advocate@disabilityrightsmt.org
www.disabilityrightsmt.org/janda3/

Bernadette Franks-Ongoy, Executive Director
Kelli Kaufman, Director of Finance & Administra
Steve Heaverlo, Director of Programs/Advocacy Sp

Protects and advocates the human and legal rights of Montanans with mental and physical disabilities while advancing dignity, equality, and self-determination. Designated federal P&A, with AT, CAP, PADD, PAIMI and PAIR programs. Advocacy and legal services for abuse, neglect, rights violations, access, discrimination in employment, accommodations and housing, and assistance with vocational rehabilitation/visual services.

3512 MonTECH
029 McGill Hall
University of Montana
Missoula, MT 59803

406-243-5751
877-243-5511
Fax: 406-243-4730
montech@ruralinstitute.umt.edu
montech.ruralinstitute.umt.edu

Anna Goldman, Program Director
Chris Clasby, Program Coordinator
Leslie Mullette

Specializing in Assistive Technology and oversee a variety of AT related grants and contracts. The overall goal is to develop a comprehensive, statewide system of assistive technology related assistance. Striving to ensure that all people in Montana with disabilities have equitable access to assistive technology devices and services in order to enhance their independence, productivity and quality of life.

3513 Montana Blind & Low Vision Services
111 N Last Chance Gulch, Suite 4C
PO Box 4210
Helena, MT 59604-4210

406-444-2590
877-296-1197
Fax: 406-444-3632
dphhs.mt.gov

Lou Thompson, Administrator
Joan Cassidy, Chemical Dependency Bureau Chief
E. Lee Simes, Medical Director

Mission: promoting work and independence for Montanans with disabilities.

3514 Montana Council on Developmental Disabilities
2714 Billings Ave
Helena, MT 59601-9767

406-443-4332
866-443-4332
Fax: 406-443-4192
www.mtcdd.org

Deborah Swingley, CEO/Executive Director
Dee Burrell, Contract Manager

The Council is made up of Montanans both with and without developmental disabilities, who believe in improving the lives of Montana's citizens who have a disability. We concentrate on issues related to self-determination, education, employment, transportation, housing, recreation, health care, community inclusion and the overall quality of life of people with developmental disabilities. As a Council we are committed to both question, and action as we work to discover and promote creative ways t

3515 Montana Department of Aging
Room 210
111 Sanders
Helena, MT 59604
406-444-7734
Fax: 406-444-3465
www.agingcare.com

Keith Messmer, Manager
Jeff Sturm, President

3516 Montana Department of Handicapped Children
111 North Sanders Street
Helena, MT 59620
406-444-7734
Fax: 406-444-3465
dphhs.mt.gov

Keith Messmer, Manager

3517 Montana Protection & Advocacy for Persons with Disabilities
1022 Chestnut Street
Helena, MT 59601-820
406-449-2344
800-245-4743
Fax: 406-449-2418
TTY: 406-449-2344
advocate@disabilityrightsmt.org
www.disabilityrightsmt.org/janda3/

Susie McIntyre, President
Will Warberg, Sales and Marketing Manager
Bernadette Franks-Ongoy, Executive Director
Disability Rights Montana is the federally-mandated civil rights protection and advocacy system for Montana. We have the legal authority to represent almost any person with a disability.

3518 Montana State Fund
P.O.Box 4759
Helena, MT 59604-4759
406-495-5000
800-332-6102
Fax: 406-495-5020
TTY: 406-495-5030
www.montanastatefund.com

Elizabeth Best, Chairman
Montana State Fund is committed to the health and economic prosperity of Montana through superior service, leadership and caring individuals, working in an environment of teamwork, creativity and trust.

3519 Social Security: Helena Disability Determination
10 W 15th St
Ste 1600
Helena, MT 59626-9704
406-441-1270
800-772-1213
TTY: 406-441-1278
www.socialsecurity.gov

Karena L. Kilgore, Executive Secretary
Carolyn W. Colvin, Commissioner
Carolyn W. Colvin, Deputy Commissioner
Social Security offers online information and services to third parties who do business with them.

Nebraska

3520 Nebraska Advocacy Services
134 S 13th St
Suite 600
Lincoln, NE 68508-1930
402-474-3183
800-422-6691
Fax: 402-474-3274
info@disabilityrightsnebraska.org
www.disabilityrightsnebraska.org

Jill Flagel, Chairperson
Mary Angus, Vice-Chairperson
Timothy F. Shaw, Chief Executive Officer
Offers protection and advocacy services to people with developmental disabilities or mental illness. Direct assistance provided if

issue within broad case priorities. Sliding scale fee. Information and referral at no cost.

3521 Nebraska Client Assistance Program
301 Centennial Mall South
P. O. Box 94987
Lincoln, NE 68509-4987
402-471-3656
800-742-7594
Fax: 402-471-3656
victoria.rasmussen@nebraska.gov
www.cap.state.ne.us/

The Nebraska Client Assistance Program (CAP) is a free service to help you find solutions if you are having problems with Vocational Rehabilitation, Nebraska Commission for the Blind and Visually Impaired or Centers for Independent Living.

3522 Nebraska Commission for the Blind & Visually Impaired
4600 Valley Rd
Suite 100
Lincoln, NE 68510-4844
402-471-2891
877-809-2419
Fax: 402-471-3009
kathy.stephens@nebraska.gov
ncbvi.state.ne.us

Pearl Van zandt, Executive Director
Carlos Servan, Deputy Director
Bob Deaton, Deputy Director
Offers services for the totally blind, legally blind, visually impaired, and more with health, counseling, educational, recreational, rehabilitation, computer training and professional training services.

3523 Nebraska Department of Health & Human Services of Medically Handicapped Children's Prgm
301 Centennial Mall S
5TH Floor
Lincoln, NE 68508-2529
402-471-3121
800-383-4278
Fax: 402-471-3577
dhhs.ne.gov

Kerry Winterer, Chief Executive Officer
Amy Borer, Admininstrative Assistant,Divisi
Dan Howell, CEO,Beatrice State Developmental
Maternal and child health, Title V, children with special health care needs; community based, statewide programs to facilitate diagnoses and care of children with disabilities and chronic medical conditions.

3524 Nebraska Department of Health and Human Services, Division of Aging Services
P.O.Box 95026
301 Centennial Mall South
Lincoln, NE 68509-5026
402-471-2115
800-942-7830
Fax: 402-471-3577
dhhs.ne.gov

Kerry Winterer, Chief Executive Officer
Amy Borer, Admininstrative Assistant,Divisi
Dan Howell, CEO,Beatrice State Developmental
The Council focuses on persons who experience a severe disability that occurs before the individual attains the age of 22, which includes persons with physical disabilities, mental/behavioral health conditions and persons that are served by the current state developmental disabilities system.

3525 Nebraska Department of Mental Health
4545 South 86th Street
Lincoln, NE 68526-2529
402-483-6990
888-210-8064
Fax: 402-483-7045
www.nmhc-clinics.com

Jill Zlomke McPherson, Executive Director
Thomas I. McPherson, Technical Coordinator
Lee Zlomke, Clinical Director
Nebraska Mental Health Centers is a family mental health clinic for people from all walks of life. Among the many services we provide are psychological evaluations, individual and group counseling, substance abuse care, neuropsychological services, domestic violence group intervention and help for victims of domestic violence, treatment for eating disorders, an ADHD clinic, Women's Counseling and much more.

3526 Nebraska Planning Council on Developmental Disabilities
Department of Health and Human Services
P.O.Box 95026
Lincoln, NE 68509-5026   402-471-2115
                                     Fax: 402-471-3577
                                     TTY: 402-471-9570
             dhhs.ne.gov/developmental_disabilities/Pages/
Mary Gordon, Executive Director
Kerry Winterer, Chief Executive Officer
Amy Borer, Admininstrative Assistant,Divisi
The Council focuses on persons who experience a severe disability that occurs before the individual attains the age of 22, which includes persons with physical disabilities, mental/behavioral health conditions and persons that are served by the current state developmental disabilities system.

3527 Nebraska Workers' Compensation Court
State of Nebraska
P.O.Box 98908
Lincoln, NE 68509-8908   402-471-6468
                                          800-599-5155
                                     Fax: 402-471-8231
                                          www.wcc.ne.gov/
Glenn W. Morton, Administrator
Susan K. Davis, Public Information Manager
Jacqueline J Boesen, General Counsel
It is the web site of the Nebraska Workers' Compensation Court. The court maintains this web site to enhance public access and provide general information regarding workers' compensation in Nebraska.

3528 Social Security: Lincoln Disability Determination
Department of Education
P.O.Box 94987
Lincoln, NE 68509-4987   402-471-2295
                                          800-772-1213
                                     TTY: 402-471-3659
                                          www.socialsecurity.gov
Karena L. Kilgore, Executive Secretary
Carolyn W. Colvin, Commissioner
Carolyn W. Colvin, Deputy Commissioner
Social Security offers online information and services to third parties who do business with them.

Nevada

3529 Aging and Disability Services Division
3416 Goni Rd
Suite D 132
Carson City, NV 89706-8008   775-687-4210
                                          800-992-0900
                                     Fax: 775-687-0574
                                          adsd@adsd.nv.gov
                                          adsd.nv.gov
Jane Gruner, Administrator
Tina Gerber-Winn, Deputy Administrator
Michele Ferral, Deputy Administrator
Provides services for seniors in Nevada including community based care. advocacy and volunteer programs. Call write or e-mail for more information.

3530 Nevada Assistive Technology Project
Ste 32
3656 Research Way
Carson City, NV 89706-7932   775-687-4452
                                          888-337-3839
                                     Fax: 775-687-3292
Todd Butterworth, Manager
Serves all ages and all disabilities through partnerships with community organizations. The NATP provides training, advocacy, funding, information and referral services, a newsletter and weekly television show.

3531 Nevada Bureau of Vocational Rehabilitation
500 East Third Street
Carson City, NV 89713   775-684-0400
                                     Fax: 775-684-4184
                                     TTY: 775-684-0360
                                          detr.state.nv.us
Maureen Cole, Administrator
Melaine Mason, Deputy Administrator, Operations
Janice John, Deputy Administrator, Programs
Bureau of Vocational Rehabilitation is a state and federally funded program designed to help people with disabilities become employed and to help those already employed perform more successfully through training, counseling and other support methods.

3532 Nevada Community Enrichment Program (NCEP)
2550 University Avenue
Suite 330N
Saint Paul, MN 55114   651-645-7271
                                          800-466-7722
                                     Fax: 651-645-0541
                                     TTY: 800-627-352
                                          info@accessiblespace.org
Mark E. Hamel, Esq., Chair
Kay Knutson, Vice Chair
John W. Adams, MBA, Secretary
Comprehensive neurological rehabilitation and life skills training.

3533 Nevada Developmental Disability Council
896 W. Nye Ln.
Suite 202
Carson City, NV 89703   775-687-8619
                                     Fax: 775-684-8626
                                          www.nevadaddcouncil.org
Jodi Thornley, Chairman
Santa Perez, Vice Chairman
Sherry Manning, Executive Director
The mission of the Nevada Developmental Disabilities Council is to provide resources at the community level which promote equal opportunity and life choices for people with disabilities through which they may positively contribute to Nevada society.

3534 Nevada Disability Advocacy and Law Center -Sparks/Reno Office
2820 West Charleston
Boulevard #11
Las Vegas, NV 89102   702-257-8150
                                          888-349-3843
                                     Fax: 702-257-8170
                                          lasvegas@ndalc.org
                                          www.ndalc.org
Reggie Bennettr, Secretary/Treasurer
Jana Spoor, President
John Miller, Vice President
Nevada's protection and advocacy system for the human legal and service rights of individuals with disabilities. NDALC has offices in Reno/Sparks and Las Vegas, with services provided statewide.

3535 Nevada Division for Aging: Las Vegas
175 Berkeley Street
Boston, MA 02116   888-398-8924
                                          libertymutual.com
Michael J. Babcockrs, Director
Marian L. Heard, Director
Martn P. Slark, Director
Develops, coordinates and delivers a comprehensive support service system in order for Nevada' senior citizens to lead independent, meaningful and dignified lives.

3536 Nevada Division of Mental Health and Developmental Services
5865 Lakeshore Road
Buford, GA 30518   770-945-4441
                                     Fax: 678-482-1965
Keith Mixon, CEO/President
Offers treatment, prevention, education, habitation and rehabilitation for mental disorders. Works with advocacy groups, families, agencies and the community.

3537 Social Security: Carson City Disability Determination
1170 Harvard Way
Reno, NV 89502-2107   775-784-5221
                                             800-772-1213
                                        Fax: 775-784-5501
                                       TTY: 800-325-0778
                                        www.socialsecurity.gov
Karena L. Kilgore, Executive Secretary
Carolyn W. Colvin, Commissioner
Carolyn W. Colvin, Deputy Commissioner
Social Security offers online information and services to third
parties who do business with them.

3538 State of Nevada Client Assistance Program
1631 W. Craig Rd.
Suite # 9-162
North Las Vegas, NV 89032-3767   702-635-4020
                                             800-633-9879
                                             800-633-9879
                                        Fax: 702-642-7020
                                       TTY: 800-633-9879
To provide information to and safegaurd rights of applicants and
clients or individuals who seek services such as vocational rehabilitation or independent living from agencies which provide
those services under the Rehabilitation Act, and to provide information to individuals about the employment discrimination title
of the Americans with Disabilities Act.

3539 Workers Compensation Board Nevada
1301 North Green Valley Parkway
Suite 200
Henderson, NV 89074   702-486-9000
                                        Fax: 775-687-6305
                                        dirweb.state.nv.us

New Hampshire

3540 New Hampshire Workers Compensation Board
46 Donovan St
Concord, NH 03301-2624   603-225-2841
                                             800-698-2364
                                        Fax: 603-226-6903
                                        www.nhprimex.org
Ty Gagne, CEO
Jonathan Kipp, Operations Manager
Julie Converse, Director of Finance
Primex3 stands ready to provide our school, municipal, and
county government members with the most comprehensive
coverages and services available to New Hampshire local
government.

**3541 New Hampshire Assistive Technology Partnership
Project**
Department of Education
10 West Edge Drive
Suite 101
Durham, NH 03824   603-862-4320
                                        Fax: 603-862-0555
                                        atinnh.org
Jan Nisbet, Director
Mary Schuh, Associate Director
Eve Fralick, Associate Director
The goal of the New Hampshire Assistive Technology Partner-
ship Project is to increase access to assistive technology through
the creation and support of consumer driven systems for the pro-
vision of state-of-the-art assistive technology products and services for citizens with disabilities in the state of New Hampshire.

3542 New Hampshire Bureau of Developmental Services
Department of Health and Human Services
129 Pleasant St
Concord, NH 03301-3852   603-271-5034
                                        Fax: 603-271-5166
                                        www.dhhs.nh.gov
Matthew Ertas, Director
Peggy Sue Greenwood, Administrative Assistant
Developmental Services promotes opportunities for normal life
experiences for persons with developmental disabilities and
aquired brain disorders in all areas of community life: employment, housing, recreation, social relationships and community
association. Services and supports are organized throught a central state office and ten private nonprofit community area agencies. Family support is provided to families of children with
chronic health conditions or are developmentally disabled.

3543 New Hampshire Client Assistance Program
121 South Fruit Street
Suite 101
Concord, NH 03301-8518   603-271-2773
                                             800-852-3405
                                        Fax: 603-271-2837
                                        Disability@nh.gov
                                        www.state.nh.us/disability/caphomepage.html
Bill Hagy, Ombudsman
John Richards, Executive Director
Jillian Shedd, Accessibility Coordinator
The Commission's goal is to remove the barriers, architectural,
attitudinal or programmatic, that bar persons with disabilities
from participating in the mainstream of society.

3544 New Hampshire Commission for Human Rights
64 South Street
Concord, NH 03301-8501   603-225-3431
                                             800-735-2964
                                        Fax: 603-224-3766
                                        webmaster@nh.gov
                                        www.nh.gov
Peggy Mc Allister, Executive Director
Enforces New Hampshire law against discrimination in housing,
employment or public accomodations. Disability discrimination
is prohibited under New Hampshire law. Takes formal charges
and investigates them.

3545 New Hampshire Department of Mental Health
129 Pleasant Street
Concord, NH 03301-3852   603-226-0111
                                        Fax: 603-271-5058
                                        www.dhhs.nh.gov
Donald Shumway, Director
Paul Garmon
Tim Rourke, Religious Leader

3546 New Hampshire Developmental Disabilities Council
2 1/2 Beacon Street
21 Fruit Street
Concord, NH 03301- 4447   603-271-3236
                                             800-852-3345
                                             800-852-3236
                                        Fax: 603-271-1156
                                       TTY: 800-735-2964
                                        nhddc.org
Kristen McGraw, Chairman
Katherine Epstein, Vice-Chair
Carol Stamatakis, Executive Director
Offers information, referral and support services to disabled per-
sons. A federally funded state agency.

3547 New Hampshire Division of Elderly and Adult Services
Bureau of Elderly & Adult Services
129 Pleasant St
Concord, NH 03301-3852   603-271-4680
                                             800-351-1888
                                        Fax: 603-271-4643
                                        pio@dhhs.state.nh.us
                                        www.dhhs.state.nh.us
Nicholas A. Toumpas, Comissioner
Mary Maggioncaida, Administrator
Marilee Nihan, Deputy Commissioner
The Bureau of Elderly and Adult Services provides a variety of
social and long-term supports to adults age 60 and older and to
adults between the ages of 18 and 60 who have a chronic illness or
disability. These services range from home care, meals on wheels,
care management, transportation assistance and assisted living to
nursing home care.

3548   New Hampshire Governor's Commission on Disability
121 South Fruit Street
Suite 101
Concord, NH 03301-8518   603-271-2773
                                           800-852-3405
                                      Fax: 603-271-2837
                                      Disability@nh.gov
                                      www.nh.gov/disability
Paul Van Blarigan, Chairman
Charles J. Saia, Executive Director
Michael Coe, Accessibility Coordinator
The Commission's goal is to remove the barriers, architectural, attitudinal or programmatic, that bar persons with disabilities from participating in the mainstream of socie

3549   New Hampshire Protection & Advocacy for Persons with Disabilities
Disabilities Rights Center, Inc
64 North Main Street
Suite 2, 3rd Floor
Concord, NH 03301-4913   603-228-0432
                                           800-834-1721
                                      Fax: 603-225-2077
                                      TTY: 800-834-1721
                                      advocacy@drcnh.org
                                           drcnh.org
Paul Levy, President
Joanne Malloy, Vice President
Richard Cohen, Executive Director
Legal services for individuals with disabilities; I & R.

3550   Social Security: Concord Disability Determination
Ste 100
70 Commercial St
Concord, NH 03301-5005   603-224-1939
                                           800-772-1213
                                      TTY: 800-325-0778
                                           www.ssa.gov
Karena L. Kilgore, Executive Secretary
Carolyn W. Colvin, Commissioner
Carolyn W. Colvin, Deputy Commissioner
Social Security offers online information and services to third parties who do business with them.

3551   Workers Compensation Board New Hampshire
PO Box 2076
95 Pleasant Street
Concord, NH 03301   603-271-3176
                                           800-272-4353
                                      Fax: 603-271-2668
                                      workerscomp@labor.state.nh.us
                                           www.nh.gov/labor
Kathryn J. Barger, Director, Workers' Compensation
George N. Copadis, Commissioner of Labor
David M. Wihby, Deputy Commissioner
The Department of Labor monitors Employers, Workers Compensation, and Insurance Carriers to insure that they are in compliance with NH Labor laws. These laws range from minimum wage, overtime, safety issues and workers compensation.

New Jersey

3552   Division of Developmental Disabilities
210 South Broad Street
3rd Floor
Trenton, NJ 08608   609-292-9742
                                           800-922-7233
                                      Fax: 609-777-0187
                                      TTY: 609-633-7106
                                      advocate@drnj.org
                                           www.njpanda.org
James W Smith Jr, Executive Director
New Jersey's designated protection and advocacy system for poeple with disabilities and provides legal, nonlegal individual and systems advocacy.

3553   International Dyslexia Association: New Jersey Branch
P.O. Box 32
Long Valley, NJ 07853   908-876-1179
                                      Fax: 908-876-3621
                                      njida@msn.com
                                      nj.dyslexiaida.org
Patricia Barden, President
Provides free information and referral services for diagnosis and tutoring for parents, educators, physicians, and individuals with dyslexia in Illinois. Membership includes yearly journal and quarterly newsletter.

3554   New Jersey Commission for the Blind and Visually Impaired
153 Halsey St, Fl 6
PO Box 47017
Newark, NJ 7101-4701   973-648-3333
                                           877-685-8878
                                      Fax: 973-693-5046
                                      www.state.nj.us/humanservices/cbvi
Daniel B. Frye, J.D., Executive Director
Bernice Davis, Executive Assistant
Edward Szajdecki, Manager
The mission of the New Jersey Commission for the Blind and Visually Impaired is to promote and provide services in the areas of education, employment, independence and eye health through informed choice and partnership with persons who are blind or visually impaired, their families and the community. Serves Bergen, Essex, Hudson, Morris, Passaic, Sussex and Warren Counties.

3555   New Jersey Department of Aging
210 South Broad Street
3rd Floor
Trenton, NJ 08608   609-292-9742
                                           800-922-7233
                                      Fax: 609-777-0187
                                      TTY: 609-633-7106
                                      advocate@drnj.org
                                           www.drnj.org
Walter Anthony Woodberry, Chairman
Andrew McGeady, Vice Chairman
Linda K. Soley, Treasurer

3556   New Jersey Department of Health/Special Child Health Services
New Jersey Department of Health and Senior Service
P.O.Box 360
Trenton, NJ 08625-0360   609-777-7778
                                      Fax: 609-292-3580
                                      www.nj.gov/health/fhs/sch/
Jennifer Velez, ESQ, Commissioner
Provides services for New Jersey children that will prevent or reduce the effects of a developmental delay, chronic illness or behavioral disorder.

3557   New Jersey Division of Mental Health Services
Department Human Services
222 South Warren Street
P.O. Box 700
Trenton, NJ 8625- 700   609-292-3717
                                           800-382-6717
                                      Fax: 609-341-3333
                                      www.state.nj.us/humanservices
Jennifer Velez, ESQ, Commissioner
Lynn A. Kovich, Assistant Commissioner
Oversees the public mental health system for the state of New Jersey. Operates six regional and specialty psychiatric hospitals, and contracts with over 125 not-for-profit agencies to provide a comprehensive system of community mental health services throughout all counties in the state.

3558   New Jersey Governor's Liaison to the Office of Disability Employment Policy
1 John Fitch Plaza
P. O.Box 110
Trenton, NJ 08625-110   609-659-9045
                                            Fax: 609-633-9271
                            Constituent.Relations@dol.state.nj.us
                                            lwd.state.nj.us/labor
Harold J. Wriths, Commissioner
Frederick J. Zavaglia, Chief of Staff
Aaron R. Fichtner, Ph.D., Deputy Commissioner
The Division of Vocational Rehabilitation Services provides vocational rehabilitation services to prepare and place in employment eligilbe individuals with disabilities who, because of their disabling conditions, would otherwise be unable to secure and/or mantain employment

3559   New Jersey Protection & Advocacy for Persons with Disabilities
210 South Broad Street
3rd Floor
Trenton, NJ 08608   609-292-9742
                                                800-922-7233
                                            Fax: 609-777-0187
                                            TTY: 609-633-7106
                                            advocate@drnj.org
                                                www.drnj.org
Walter Anthony Woodberry, Chairman
Andrew McGeady, Vice Chairman
Linda K. Soley, Treasurer

3560   Regional ADA Technical Assistance Center
United Cerebral Palsy Associations of New Jersey
201 Dolgen Hall
Ithaca, NY 14853   607-255-6686
                                                800-949-4232
                                            Fax: 607-255-2763
                                        northeastada@cornell.edu
                                            www.northeastada.org
LaWanda H. Cook, Ph.D., Extension Associate/Training Spe
Hannah Rudstam, Ph.D., Director of Training
Erin Sember-Chase, Project Coordinator and Technic

3561   Social Security Administration
1100 West High Rise
6401 Security Blvd.
Baltimore, MD 21235   800-772-1213
                                            TTY: 800-325-0778
                                                www.ssa.gov
Karena L. Kilgore, Executive Secretary
Carolyn W. Colvin, Commissioner
Carolyn W. Colvin, Deputy Commissioner
Social Security disability is a social insurance program that workers and employers pay for with their Social Security taxes. Eligibility is based on your work history, and the amount of your benefit is based on your earnings. Social Security also has a disability program for people with limited income and resources- the Supplemental Security Income (SSI) program. For more information on these federal programs, please call our nationwide toll-free number.

New Mexico

3562   New Mexico Aging and Long-Term Services Department
2550 Cerrillos Rd
P.O. Box 27118
Santa Fe, NM 87505-3260   505-476-4799
                                                866-451-2901
                                            Fax: 505-476-4836
                                        www.nmaging.state.nm.us
Miles Copeland, Deputy Secretary
Retta Ward, Secretary
Jason Sanchez, Administrative Services Division
Information and services for seniors, people with disabilities and their families.

3563   New Mexico Client Assistance Program
1720 Louisiana Blvd NE
Site 204
Albuquerque, NM 87110- 7070   505-256-3100
                                                800-432-4682
                                            Fax: 505-256-3184
                                                info@drnm.org
                                                www.drnm.org
Katie Toledo, Chairperson
Cyndy Costanza, Vice Chairperson
Jeanne A. Hamrick, President
The mission of Disability Rights New Mexico (DRNM) is to protect, promote and expand the legal and civil rights of persons with disabilities. DRNM is an independent, private nonprofit agency operating federally mandated and other advocacy programs in pursuit of this mission.

3564   New Mexico Commission for the Blind (NMCFTB)
2905 Rodeo Park Dr E
Bldg 4, Suite 100
Santa Fe, NM 87505   505-476-4479
                                                888-513-7968
                                            www.cfb.state.nm.us
Arthur A. Schreiber, Chairman
Shirley Lansing, Commissioner
Robert Reidy, Commissioner
Offers services for the totally blind, legally blind, visually impaired, and more with health, counseling, educational, recreational, rehabilitation, computer training and professional training services.

3565   New Mexico Department of Health: Children's Medical Services
1190 S Saint Francis Dr
Santa Fe, NM 87505-4173   505-841-6100
                                                800-797-3260
                                            Fax: 505-827-2530
Gloria Bonner, Program Manager
Susan Baum, Medical Director
Freida Adams, Nurse Coordinator
Title V MCH Program for children with special health care needs from birth to age 21 years. Services provided include: diagnosis, medical intervention, clinics and service coordination.

3566   New Mexico Governor's Committee on Concerns of the Handicapped
491 Old Santa Fe Trl
Santa Fe, NM 87501-2753   505-476-0412
                                                877-696-1470
                                            Fax: 505-827-6328
                                            gcd@state.nm.us
                                            www.gcd.state.nm.us/
Susan Gray, Chair
Curtiss Wilson, Vice Chair
Jim Parker, Director

3567   New Mexico Protection & Advocacy for Persons with Disabilities
1720 Louisiana Blvd NE
Site 204
Albuquerque, NM 87110- 7070   505-256-3100
                                                800-432-4682
                                            Fax: 505-256-3184
                                                info@drnm.org
                                                www.drnm.org
Katie Toledo, Chairperson
Cyndy Costanza, Vice Chairperson
Jeanne A. Hamrick, President
The mission of Disability Rights New Mexico (DRNM) is to protect, promote and expand the legal and civil rights of persons with disabilities. DRNM is an independent, private nonprofit agency operating federally mandated and other advocacy programs in pursuit of this mission.

3568 New Mexico Technology Assistance Program
625 Silver Ave SW
Suite 100 B
Albuquerque, NM 87102
505-841-4464
877-696-1470
Fax: 505-841-4467
www.tap.gcd.state.nm.us
Tracy Agiovlasitis, Program Manager
Examines and works to eliminate barriers to obtaining assistive technology in New Mexico. Has established a statewide program for coordinating assistive technology services; is designed to assist people with disabilities to locate, secure, and maintain assistive technology.

3569 New Mexico Workers Compensation Administration
2410 Centre Avenue SE
P.O.Box 27198
Albuquerque, NM 87125-7198
505-841-6000
800-255-7965
Fax: 505-841-6009
www.workerscomp.state.nm.us/
Ned S. Fuller, Director
Robert E. Doucette, Executive Deputy Director
Darin A. Childers, General Counsel
Regulates workers' compensation in New Mexico.

3570 Social Security: Santa Fe Disability Determination
6401 Security Blvd.
Baltimore, MD 21235
800-772-1213
TTY: 800-325-0778
www.socialsecurity.gov
Karena L. Kilgore, Executive Secretary
Carolyn W. Colvin, Commissioner
Carolyn W. Colvin, Deputy Commissioner

3571 Southwest Branch of the International Dyslexia Association
International Dyslexia Association
3915 Carlisle Blvd. NE
Albuquerque, NM 87107
505-255-8234
800-222-3123
Fax: 505-262-8547
swida@southwestida.org
Carolee Dean, President
Claudia Gutierrez, Vice President
Michelle Wick, Recording Secretary
Provides free information and referral services for diagnosis and tutoring for parents, educators, physicians, and individuals with dyslexia. The voice of our membership is heard in 48 countries. Membership includes yearly journal and quarterly newsletter. Call for conference dates.

3572 Workers Compensation Board New Mexico
2410 Centre Avenue SE
P.O.Box 27198
Albuquerque, NM 87125-7198
505-841-6000
800-255-7965
Fax: 505-841-6009
www.workerscomp.state.nm.us/
Ned S. Fuller, Director
Robert E. Doucette, Executive Deputy Director
Darin A. Childers, General Counsel
Regulates workers' compensation in New Mexico.

New York

3573 Albany County Department for Aging and Albany Social Services
112 State Street
Room 900
Albany, NY 12207-2304
518-447-7000
Fax: 518-447-7188
aging@albanycounty.com
albanycounty.com
George Brown, Commissioner
Judy L. Coyne, Commissioner
Kathleen M. Dalton, Ph.D., Commissioner

The Point of Entry access line provides information and assistance and comprehensive referrals, and or assessments for the elderly, adults and children with disabilities, their family, or service providers.

3574 Jawonio
260 N Little Tor Road
New City, NY 10956-2627
845-708-2000
Fax: 845-634-7731
TTY: 845-639-3521
www.jawonio.org
Jill A. Warner, Executive Director & CEO
Matthew Shelly, Chief Program Officer
Diana Hess, Chief Communications Officer
A dedicated community resource providing services to more than 500 children and adults annually. Provide early intervention, day care and pre-school special ed to our children. Job training, day habilitation, recreation, medical and service coordination for adults.

3575 Jawonio Vocational Center
260 N Little Tor Rd
New City, NY 10956-2627
845-708-2000
Fax: 845-634-7731
TTY: 845-639-3521
jawonio.org
Jill A. Warner, Executive Director & CEO
Matthew Shelly, Chief Program Officer
Diana Hess, Chief Communications Officer
A dedicated community resource providing services to more than 500 children and adults annually. Provide early intervention, day care and pre-school special ed to our children. Job training, day habilitation, recreation, medical and service coordination for adults.

3576 NYS Commission on Quality of Care & Advocacy for Persons with Disabilities
401 State St
Schenectady, NY 12305-2300
518-388-2892
Fax: 518-388-2890
Andrew M. Cuomo, Governor
Roger Bearden, Chair
Bruce Blower, Member

3577 NYSARC
393 Delaware Ave
Delmar, NY 12054-3094
518-439-8311
800-724-2094
Fax: 518-439-1893
info@nysarc.org
nysarc.org
Laura J. Kennedy, President
Patricia Campanella, Senior Vice President
Joseph M. Bognanno, Vice President

3578 National Alliance on Mental Illness of New York State
99 Pine Street
Suite 302
Albany, NY 12207-1336
518-462-2000
800-950-3228
Fax: 518-462-3811
info@naminys.org
www.naminys.org
Sherry Grenz, President
Wend Burch, Executive Director
Sharon Clairmont, Finance & Business Office Dir.

3579 New State Office of Mental Health Agency
Office of Mental Health
44 Holland Ave
Albany, NY 12229
518-474-4403
800-597-8481
Fax: 518-474-2149
www.omh.ny.gov
Mike Hogan, Commissioner
Promoting the mental health of all New Yorkers with a particular focus on providing hope and recovery for adults with serious mental illness and children with serious emotional disturbances.

3580 New York Client Assistance Program
855 Central Avenue
Suite 110
Albany, NY 12206
518-459-6422
Fax: 518-459-7847
TTY: 518-459-6422
www.nls.org

3581 New York Department of Handicapped Children
Department of Heath Education
Corning Tower
Empire State Plaza
Albany, NY 12237
518-456-0665
866-881-2809
Fax: 518-456-1126
www.health.ny.gov

Andrew M. Cuomo, Governor
Dr James B. Crucetti, MD, MPH, Commissioner
Howard Zucker, Acting Commissioner

3582 New York State Commission for the Blind
52 Washington St
Rensselaer, NY 12144-2796
518-473-7793
866-871-3000
Fax: 518-486-7550
www.ocfs.state.ny.us

Madeline Raciti, Manager
Offers services for the totally blind, legally blind, visually impaired, and more with health, counseling, educational, recreational, rehabilitation, computer training and professional training services.

3583 New York State Commission on Quality of Care
401 State St
Schenectady, NY 12305-2300
518-388-2892
Fax: 518-388-2890

Andrew M. Cuomo, Governor
Roger Bearden, Chair
Bruce Blower, Member

3584 New York State Congress of Parents and Teachers
1 Wembley Ct
Albany, NY 12205-6258
518-452-8808
877-569-7782
Fax: 518-452-8105
pta.office@nyspta.org
nyspta.org

Bonnie Russell, President
Gracemarie Rozea, First Vice President
Judy Van Harren, Secretary
Parent Teacher Association and PTA are registered service marks of the National Congress of Parents and Teachers (National PTA). Only those groups chartered by the New York State PTA are entitled to use the name PTA. Any other use constitutes trademark infringement.

3585 New York State Office of Advocates for Persons with Disabilities
Ste 1001
1 Empire State Plz
Albany, NY 12223-1100
518-449-7860
800-522-4369
Fax: 518-473-6005

Gary O'Brien, Chair Commissioner
Provides information and referral services; administers NYS Tech Art Project; promotes implementation of disability-related laws.

3586 New York State Office of Mental Health
44 Holland Ave
Albany, NY 12229-1
518-474-4403
800-597-8481
Fax: 518-474-2149
www.omh.state.ny.gov in

Michael Hogan, Ph.D.
Promoting the mental health of all New Yorkers with a particular focus on providing hope and recovery for adults with serious mental illness and children with serious emotional disturbances.

3587 New York State TRAID Project
New York State Commisionon Qualityof Careand Advoc
Ste 1001
1 Empire State Plz
Albany, NY 12223-1100
518-449-7860
800-522-4369
Fax: 518-473-6005

Cliff Sigfride, Manager

3588 Parent to Parent of New York State
500 Balltown Rd
Schenectady, NY 12304-2247
518-381-4350
800-305-8817
Fax: 518-393-9607
mjuda@ptopnys.org
parenttoparentnys.org

Louise Nitto, President
Jim Costello, Vice President
Elizabeth Smithmeyer, Secretary
Parent to Parent of NYS, which began in 1994, is a statewide not for profit organization established to support and connect families of individuals with special needs. The 13 offices, located throughout NYS, are staffed by Regional Coordinators, who are parents or close relatives of individuals with special needs.

3589 Protection and Advocacy Agency of NY
401 State St
Schenectady, NY 12305-2303
518-388-2892
Fax: 518-388-2890

Andrew M. Cuomo, Governor
Roger Bearden, Chair
Bruce Blower, Member

3590 Regional Early Childhood Director Center
89 Washington Ave.
Room 580 EBA
Albany, NY 12234
518-474-2925
800-222-5627
accesadm@mail.nysed.gov
www.acces.nysed.gov
Provides information, support and referral assistance to parents and professionals who are concerned with chilren with special needs or handicapping condition between the ages of birth to five.

3591 Schools And Services For Children With Autism Spectrum Disorders.
116 E 16th St
5th Floor
New York, NY 10003-2164
212-677-4650
Fax: 212-254-4070

Ellen Miller-Wachtel, Chairman
Shon E. Glusky, President
Owen P. J. King, Treasurer
This publication fun resource for children provides extreme coverage of services for children with autism, asbergez syndrome, and/or PDD.

3592 Singeria/Metropolitan Parent Center
2082 Lexington Ave.
4th Floor
New York, NY 10035
212-643-2840
866-867-9665
Fax: 212-496-5608
intake@sinergiany.org
sinergiany.org

Len Torres, President
Johnny C. Rivera, Vice President
Paola Jordan, Treasurer

3593 Social Security: Albany Disability Determination
1 Clinton Ave
Albany, NY 12207
518-431-4051
800-772-1213
TTY: 518-431-4050
www.ssa.gov

Karena L. Kilgore, Executive Secretary
Carolyn W. Colvin, Commissioner
Carolyn W. Colvin, Deputy Commissioner

3594 State Agency for the Blind and Visually Impaired
52 Washington St
Rensselaer, NY 12144-2834
518-473-7793
866-871-3000
Fax: 518-486-7550
info@ocfs.state.ny.us
www.ocfs.state.ny.us

3595 State Education Agency Rural Representative
89 Washington Avenue
Albany, NY 12234
518-474-3852
Fax: 518-473-2860
RegentsOffice@mail.nysed.gov
www.nysed.gov

Merryl H. Tisch, Chancellor
Anthony S. Bottar, Vice Chancellor

3596 State Mental Health Representative for Children and Youth
44 Holland Ave
Albany, NY 12229
518-473-6328
www.rcybc.ca

David Woodlock, Deputy Commissioner

3597 United We Stand of New York
98 Moore St
Brooklyn, NY 11206-3326
718-302-4313
Fax: 718-302-4315
uwsofny@aol.com

Lourdes Rivera-Putz, Executive Director
Lourdes Figueroa, Intake/Receptionist
Carmen Soltero, Outreach/Trainer
Assists families with improving the quality of life for all individuals with disabilities.

3598 University Afiliated Program/Rose F Kennedy Center
1971
1300 Morris Park Avenue
Bronx, NY 10461
718-430-2000
www.einstein.yu.edu

Maris D. Rosenberg, Interim Director
Christine M. Baric, Assistant Director
John J. Foxe, Director

3599 University of Rochester Medical Center
601 Elmwood Ave
Rochester, NY 14642
585-275-8762
Fax: 585-275-3366
phil_davidson@urmc.rochester.edu
www.rochester.edu

Brad Berk, MD, PhD, CEO

3600 VESID
New York State Education Department
89 Washington Ave.
Room 580 EBA
Albany, NY 12234
800-222-5627
Fax: 518-474-8802
accesadm@mail.nysed.gov
www.acces.nysed.gov/vr/
Dr Rebecca Cort, Deputy Commissioner
Vocational and educational services for individuals with disabilities.

3601 VSA Arts of New York City
2700 F Street, NW
Washington, DC 20566
202-467-4600
800-444-1324
Fax: 717-225-6305
bbvsanyc@msn.com

David M. Rubenstein, Chairman
Deborah F. Rutter, President
Christoph Eschenbach, Music Director
Provides art, educational and creative expression experiences to thousands of children, youth, and adults with disabilities who reside in the five boroughs of New York City. It provides opportunities for people with disabilities to demonstrate their accomplishments in the arts and foster increased understanding and acceptance.

3602 Westchester Institute for Human Development
Cedarwood Hall
Valhalla, NY 10595
914-493-8150
info@WIHD.org
www.wihd.org

William H. Bave, Chairman
Pamela Thornton, Vice Chairman
Ansley Bacon PhD, President/CEO
WIHD advances policies and practices that foster the healthy development and ensure the safety of all children, strengthen families and communities, and promote health and well-being among people of all ages with disabilities and special health care needs.

3603 Workers Compensation Board New York
PO Box 5205
328 State Street
Schenectady, NY 12305-2318
518-462-8880
877-632-4996
Fax: 518-473-1415
www.wcb.ny.gov

Andrew M. Cuomo, Governor
Robert E. Beloten, Chairman
Richard A. Bell, Commissioner

North Carolina

3604 Developmental Disability Services Section
Building 325n
Albemarle
Raleigh, NC 27699
919-420-7901
Fax: 919-420-7917
www.dhhs.state.nc.us/mhddsas/
Diana Simmons, Human Resources Manager
Ureh N. Lekwauwa, Chief, Clinical Policy
Courtney Cantrell, Acting Director
Makes policies and monitors public services and supports to people with mental illness, developmental disabilities and substance abuse throughout North Carolina.

3605 International Dyslexia Association: North Carolina Branch
NC
nc.dyslexiaida.org
Kris Cox, President
Provides free information and referral services for diagnosis and tutoring for parents, educators, physicians, and individuals with dyslexia in Illinois. Membership includes yearly journal and quarterly newsletter.

3606 North Carolina Workers Compensation Board
4340 Mail Service Center
Raleigh, NC 27699-4340
919-807-2501
800-688-8349
Fax: 919-508-8210
infospec@ic.nc.gov
www.ic.nc.gov
Julian Bunn, Owner

3607 North Carolina Assistive Technology Project
1110 Navaho Dr
Suite 101
Raleigh, NC 27609-7322
919-872-2298
Fax: 919-850-2792
Ricki Cook, Project Director
Annette Lauber, Funding Specialist
Jacquelyne Gordon, Consumer Resource Specialist
The North Carolina Assistive Technology Project exists to create a statewide, consumer-responsive system of assistive technology services for all North Carolinians with disabilities. The project's activities impact children and adults with disabilities across all aspects of their lives.

3608 North Carolina Children & Youth Branch
North Carolina Publc of Health
1928 Mail Service Ctr
Raleigh, NC 27699-1900
919-839-6262
Fax: 919-733-8034
Lawrence J Wheeler, Manager
Cathy Kluttz, Unit Manager Special Service
Dianne Tyson, Help Line Manager

3609 **North Carolina Client Assistance Program**
2806 Mail Service Ctr
Raleigh, NC 27699-2806
919-855-3600
800-215-7227
Fax: 919-715-2456
nccap@dhhs.nc.gov
cap.state.nc.us

John Marens, Director
Diane Rawdarowicz, Client Advocate
Sharon Wisner, Client Advocate
A federally funded program designed to assist individuals with disabilities in understanding and using rehabilitation services. CAP serves as an integral part of the rehabilitation system by advising and informing individuals of all services and benefits available to them through programs authorized under both the Rehabilitation Act and Title 1 of the Americans with Disabilities Act.

3610 **North Carolina Developmental Disabilities**
3125 Poplarwood Court
Suite 200
Raleigh, NC 27604-7368
919-850-2901
800-357-6916
Fax: 919-850-2915
Info@nccdd.org
www.nc-ddc.org

Caroline Valand, Executive Director
A planning council established to assure that individuals with developmental disabilities and their families participate in the planning of and have access to culturally competent services, supports, and other assistance and opportunities that promote independence, productivity, and integration and inclusion into the community; and to promote, through systemic change, capacity building and advocacy activities, a consumer and family-centered comprehensive system.

3611 **North Carolina Division of Aging**
2101 Mail Service Ctr
Raleigh, NC 27699-2001
919-855-4800
Fax: 919-733-0443
ncdhhs.gov

Dennis Streets, Manager
Jim Slate, Director
Laketha Miller, Controller

3612 **North Carolina Industrial Commission**
4340 Mail Service Center
Raleigh, NC 27699-4340
919-807-2501
800-688-8349
Fax: 919-508-8210
infospec@ic.nc.gov
www.ic.nc.gov

J Howard Bunn Jr, Chairman
Peg Dorer, Executive Director

3613 **Social Security Administration**
4701 Old Wake Forest Rd
Raleigh, NC 27609-4919
877-803-6311
800-772-1213
800-325-0778
Fax: 919-790-2860
TTY: 919-790-2773
www.socialsecurity.gov

Karena L. Kilgore, Executive Secretary
Carolyn W. Colvin, Commissioner
Carolyn W. Colvin, Deputy Commissioner
Provides information on how to obtain social security through a disability.

North Dakota

3614 **Division of Mental Health and Substance Abuse**
600 East Boulevard Avenue
Dept 325
Bismarck, ND 58505- 0250
701-328-2310
800-472-2622
Fax: 701-328-2359
dhseo@nd.gov
www.nd.gov/humanservices

Dennis Goetz, Executive Director
Kerry Wicks, Executive Director
Andrew J. McLean, Medical Director
The Department of Human Services' Mental Health and Substance Abuse Services Division provides leadership for the planning, development, and oversight of a system of care for children, adults, and families with severe emotional disorders, mental illness, and/or substance abuse issues.

3615 **North Dakota Workers Compensation Board**
50 E Front Ave
Bismarck, ND 58504
701-328-3800
800-777-5033
Fax: 701-329-9911
TTY: 701-328-3786

Brent Edison, Director

3616 **North Dakota Client Assistance Program**
400 East Broadway
Suite 409
Bismarck, ND 58501-4071
701-328-2950
800-472-2670
Fax: 701-328-3934
panda@nd.gov
www.ndpanda.org/cap

Dennis Lyon, CEO
Janelle Olson, Advocate
Paula Rustad, Office Assistant
CAP assists clients and client applicants of North Dakota Vocational Rehabilitation services, Tribal Vocational Rehabilitation, or Independent Living services.

3617 **North Dakota Department of Human Resources**
1237 W Divide Ave
Suite 6
Bismarck, ND 58501-1208
701-328-5300
800-451-8693
Fax: 701-328-5320
dhsaging@nd.gov
www.nd.gov

Shane Goettle, Manager

3618 **North Dakota Department of Human Services**
600 E Boulevard Ave
Dept 325
Bismarck, ND 58505-0250
701-328-2310
800-472-2622
Fax: 701-328-2359
dhseo@nd.gov
www.nd.gov/dhs

Carol K Olson, Executive Director
Dennis Goetz, Executive Director
Kerry Wicks, Executive Director
Provides services that help vulnerable North Dakotans of all ages to maintain or enhance their quality of life, which may be threatened by lack of financial resources, emotional crises, disabling conditions, or an inability to protect themselves.

3619 **Protection & Advocacy Project**
1984
400 East Broadway
Suite 409
Bismarck, ND 58501-4071
701-328-2950
800-472-2670
Fax: 701-328-3934
panda@nd.gov
ndpanda.org

Teresa Larsen, Executive Director
Janelle Olson, Advocate
Paula Rustad, Office Assistant

The Protection and Advocacy is a state agency whose purpose is to advocate for and protect the rights of people with disabilities. The Protection and Advocacy Project has programs to serve people with developmental disabilities, mental illnesses and other types of disabilities. The projects programs and services are free to eligible individuals.

3620 **Social Security: Bismarck Disability Determination**
1680 E Capitol Ave
Bismarck, ND 58501-5603 701-250-4200
800-772-1213
TTY: 701-250-4620
ssa.gov

Karena L. Kilgore, Executive Secretary
Carolyn W. Colvin, Commissioner
Carolyn W. Colvin, Deputy Commissioner

3621 **Workers Compensation Board North Dakota**
1600EastCenturyAvenue
Suite1
Bismarck, ND 58503-649 701-328-3800
800-777-5033
Fax: 701-328-3820
www.workforcesafety.com

Sandy Blunt, CEO

Ohio

3622 **Epilepsy Council of Greater Cincinnati**
Ste 550
895 Central Ave
Cincinnati, OH 45202-5700 513-721-2905
877-804-2241
Fax: 513-721-0799
ecgc@fuse.net

Kathy Stewart, Executive Director

3623 **International Dyslexia Association: Central Ohio Branch**
P.O. Box 1601
Westerville, OH 43086 614-899-5711
coh.dyslexiaida.org

Mike McGovern, President
Blythe Wood, Vice President
Chris Lowe, Secretary
Provides free information and referral services for diagnosis and tutoring for parents, educators, physicians, and individuals with dyslexia. Membership includes yearly journal and quarterly newsletter.

3624 **Ohio Bureau for Children with Medical Handicaps**
Ohio Department of Health
246 N. High St
P.O.Box 1603
Columbus, OH 43215-1603 614-466-3543
800-755-4769
Fax: 614-728-3616
bcmh@odh.ohio.gov
www.odh.ohio.gov

John R. Kasich, Governor
James Bryant Md, Bureau Chief
Alvin Jackson, MD, Director
Provides funding for the diagnosis, treatment and coordination of services for eligible Ohio children, under age 21, with medical handicaps; conducts quality assurance activities to establish standards of care and determine unmet needs of children with handicaps and their families; collaborates with public health nurses to increase access to care; and assists families to access and use third party resources. Conducts a separate program for adults with cystic fibrosis.

3625 **Ohio Bureau of Worker's Compensation**
30 W Spring St
Columbus, OH 43215-2256 800-335-0996
Fax: 877-321-9481
TTY: 800-292-4833
ombudsperson@bwc.state.oh.us
www.bwc.ohio.gov

Stephen Buehrer, Administrator/CEO
Dale Hamilton, Chief Operating Officer (COO)
Kevin Abrams, Chief of Employers Services
To provide a quality, customer-focused workers' compensation insurance system for Ohio's employers and employees.

3626 **Ohio Client Assistance Program**
50 W. Broad St.
Suite 1400
Columbus, OH 43215-5923 614-466-7264
800-282-9181
Fax: 614-752-4197
TTY: 614-728-2553
www.olrs.ohio.gov

Donald Bishop, Executive Director

3627 **Ohio Department of Aging**
1982
50 W Broad St
Fl 9
Columbus, OH 43215-3363 614-466-5500
866-243-5678
888-243-5678
Fax: 614-466-5741
TTY: 614-466-6191
www.aging.ohio.gov

Bonnie Kantor-Burman, Director
John Ratliff, Public Information Officer
The department serves and represents about 2 million Ohioans age 60 & older. They advocate for the needs of all older citizens with emphasis on improving the quality of life, helping senior citizens live active, healthy, & independent lives, & promoting positive attitudes toward aging & older people. Committed to helping the frail elderly who choose to remain at home by providing home & community based services, their goal is to promote the level of choice, independence & self-care.

3628 **Ohio Department of Mental Health**
30 E Broad St
8th Floor
Columbus, OH 43215-3414 614-466-4775
877-275-6364
Fax: 614-752-8410

Michael Hogan, Director
Christine Vincenty, Manager

3629 **Ohio Developmental Disabilities Council**
899 E Broad St, Ste 203
Columbus, OH 43205 614-466-5205
800-766-7426
Fax: 614-466-0298
www.ddc.ohio.gov

Carolyn Knight, Executive Director
Mark Seifarth, Chair
Robert Shuemak, Vice Chair
The Ohio Developmental Disabilities Council is one of 55 councils found in all states and territories which provides funding for systems change grant projects. The DD Council is a planning and advocacy agency that seeks to improve the lives of Ohioans with disabilities.

3630 **Ohio Developmental Disability Council (ODDC)**
899 E Broad St, Ste 203
Columbus, OH 43205 614-466-5205
800-766-7426
Fax: 614-466-0298
www.ddc.ohio.gov

Carolyn Knight, Executive Director
Mark Seifarth, Chair
Robert Shuemak, Vice Chair

3631 Ohio Governor's Council on People with Disabilities
400 E Campus View Blvd
Columbus, OH 43235-4685   614-438-1200
                                   800-282-4536
                                   gcpd.ohio.gov

Jacqueline Romer-Sensky, Chairman
Jack Licate, Vice Chairman
Kevin Miller, Executive Director
The Governor's Council on People with Disabilities exists to: Advise the Governor and General Assembly on statewide disability issues, promote the value of diversity, dignity and the quality of life for people with disabilities, be a catalyst to create systemic change promoting awareness of disability-related issues that will ultimately benefit all citizens of Ohio, Educate and advocate for: partnerships at the local, state and national level, promotion of equality, access and independence.

3632 Ohio Rehabilitation Services Commission
400 E Campus View Blvd
Columbus, OH 43235-4604   614-438-1200
                                   800-282-4536
                                   ohio.gov

Kevin Miller, Executive Director
RSC is Ohio's state agency that provides vocational rehabilitation (VR) services to help people with disabilities become employed and independent. We also offer a variety of services to Ohio businesses, resulting in quality jobs for individuals who have disabilities.

3633 Ohio Women, Infants, & Children Program - Ohio Department of Health
246 N High St
Columbus, OH 43215-2406   614-644-8006
                              Fax: 614-564-2470

Michele Frizzell, Chief, Bureau of Nutrition Svcs.

3634 Social Security: Columbus Disability Determination
90 E Washington Bridge Rd
Suite 140
Worthington, OH 43085   614-888-5339
                                  800-772-1213
                             TTY: 614-288-0226
                                  www.socialsecurity.gov

Karena L. Kilgore, Executive Secretary
Carolyn W. Colvin, Commissioner
Carolyn W. Colvin, Deputy Commissioner

Oklahoma

3635 Oklahoma Workers Compensation Board
Department of Labor
3017 N. Stiles, Suite 100
Oklahoma City, OK 73105   405-521-6100
                                   888-269-5353
                              Fax: 405-521-6018
                                   labor.info@labor.ok.gov
                                   www.ok.gov/odol

Jim Marshall, Chief of Staff
Mark Costello, Commissioner of Labor
Lizzette McNeill, Communications Director

3636 Oklahoma Client Assistance Program/Office of Disability Concerns
2401 NW 23rd Street
Suite 90
Oklahoma City, OK 73107- 2431   405-521-3756
                                  800-522-8224
                             Fax: 405-522-6695
                                  www.ok.gov

Todd Lamb, Governor
Gary Jones, Auditor and Inspector
E. Scott Pruitt, Attorney General
CAP informs and advises applicants and consumers about the vocational rehabilitation process and services available under the Federal Rehabilitation Act, including services provided by DVR and DVS. CAP staff can help you communicate concerns to the DVR/DVS and assist you with administrative, mediation, fair hearing, legal and other solutions

3637 Oklahoma Department of Human Services Aging Services Division
25 Sigourney Street, 10th Floor
Hartford, CT 06106   405-521-3646
                                   866-218-6621
                                   800-522-7233
                              Fax: 860-424-5301

Margaret Ger Murkette, MSW, Director
Ed Lake, Director

3638 Oklahoma Department of Labor
3017 N. Stiles
Suite 100
Oklahoma City, OK 73105-5206   405-521-6100
                                   888-269-5353
                              Fax: 405-521-6018
                                   www.labor.ok.gov

Mark Castello, Commissioner
Jim Marshall, Chief of Staff
Stacy Bonner, Deputy Commissioner

3639 Oklahoma Department of Mental Health & Substance Abuse Services
1200 NE 13th Street
P.O.Box 53277
Oklahoma City, OK 73152-3277   405-522-3908
                                   800-522-9054
                              Fax: 405-522-3650
                              TTY: 405-522-3851
                                   www.odmhsas.org

J. Andy Sullivan, Chairperson
Gail Henderson, Vice-Chair
Terri White, Commissioner
State agency providing mental helath, substance abuse and domestic violence services.

3640 Oklahoma Department of Rehabilitation Services
3535 NW 58th St.
Suite 500
Oklahoma City, OK 73112-4824   405-951-3400
                                   800-845-8476
                              Fax: 405-951-3529
                                   www.oklahoma.gov/okdrs.html

Melinda Fruendt, Executive Director
The Oklahoma Department of Rehabilitation Services (DRS) provides assistance to Oklahomans with disabilities through vocational rehabilitation, employment, independent living, residential and outreach programs, and the determination of medical eligibility for disability benefits.

3641 Workers Compensation Board Oklahoma
1915 N Stiles Ave
Oklahoma City, OK 73105-4918   405-522-8600
                                   800-522-8210

Leroy E Young, D.O., Chairman
Joyce Sanders, Supervisor
Michael J. Harkey, Vice Presiding Judge

Oregon

3642 International Dyslexia Association: Oregon Branch
International Dyslexia Association
P.P. Box 2609
Portland, OR 97208-2609   503-228-4455
                                   info@orbida.org
                                   or.dyslexiaida.org

Jane Cooper, President
Danielle Thompson, Vice President
Anne Mauboussin, Treasurer
Provides free information and referral services for diagnosis and tutoring for parents, educators, physicians, and individuals with dyslexia. Membership includes yearly journal and quarterly newsletter.

3643 Office of Vocational Rehabilitation Services (OVRS)
500 Summer St NE
Salem, OR 97301-1063   503-945-5944
Fax: 503-378-2897
TTY: 503-945-6214
www.oregon.gov/dhs

Erinn Kelley-Siel, Director
Gene Evans, Communication Director
Eric Moore, Chief Financial Officer
The mission of OVRS to assist Oregonians with disabilities to achieve and maintain employment and independence.

3644 Oregon Advocacy Center
620 SW 5th Ave
5th Floor
Portland, OR 97204-1428   503-243-2081
800-452-6094
Fax: 503-243-1738
TTY: 800-556-5351

Robert Joondeph, Executive Director
Barbara Herget, Operations Director
The protection and advocacy system for Oregon.

3645 Oregon Client Assistance Program
620 SW 5th Ave
5th Floor
Portland, OR 97204-1420   503-243-2081
Fax: 503-243-1738
TTY: 800-556-5351

Robert Joondeph, Executive Director

3646 Oregon Department of Mental Health
500 Summer St NE
Salem, OR 97301-1063   503-945-5944
Fax: 503-378-2897
TTY: 503-945-6214
www.oregon.gov/DHS

Erinn Kelley-Siel, Director
Gene Evans, Communication Director
Eric Moore, Chief Financial Officer
Sets out the purpose and guides the activities of our large, complex organization. Vision is for better outcomes for clients and communities through collaboration, integration and shared responsibility.

3647 Oregon Technology Access for Life
2225 Lancaster Drive NE
Salem, OR 97305-1396   503-361-1201
800-677-7512
Fax: 503-370-4530
TTY: 503-361-1201
www.accesstechnologiesinc.org

Laurie Brooks, President
A statewide program promoting assistive technology devices and services for persons of all ages with all disabilities.

3648 Social Security: Salem Disability Determination
90 E Washington Bridge Rd
Suite 140
Worthington, OH 43085-3772   614-888-5339
800-722-1213
TTY: 614-288-0226
www.socialsecurity.gov

Karena L. Kilgore, Executive Secretary
Carolyn W. Colvin, Commissioner
Carolyn W. Colvin, Deputy Commissioner

3649 Vocational Rehabilitation Agency: Oregon Commission for the Blind
535 SE 12th Avenue
Portland, OR 97214-2408   971-673-1588
888-202-5463
Fax: 503-234-7468
ocb.mail@state.or.us
www.oregon.gov/blind

Dacia Johnson, Executive Director
A resource for visually impaired Oregonians, as well as their families, friends, and employers. Nationally recognized programs and staff that make a difference in people's lives every day.

3650 Washington County Disability, Aging and Veteran Services
Ste 208
180 E Main St
Hillsboro, OR 97123-4054   503-640-3489
Fax: 503-693-6124

Jeff Hill, Director
Janet Long, Support Staff
Provides services to individuals through the Older Americans Act, state in home care services and represent, veterans in benefit claims process with Federal VA.

Pennsylvania

3651 Disability Rights of Pennsylvania (DRP)
Harrisburg Office
301 Chestnut St
Suite 300
Harrisburg, PA 17101   717-839-5235
800-692-7443
Fax: 717-236-0192
TTY: 877-375-7139
ldo@disabilityrightspa.org
www.disabilityrightspa.org

Jeneice Davis, Chairman
Peri Jude Radecic, CEO
Kelly Darr, Legal Director
The Disability Rights of Pennsylvania is a statewide, non-profit corporation dedicated to advancing and protecting the civil rights of adults and children with disabilities by ensuring access to community services, a full and inclusive education and the freedom to live free of discrimination, abuse and neglect.

3652 International Dyslexia Association: Pennsylvania Branch
1062 E. Lancaster Ave.
Suite 15A
Rosemont, PA 19010   610-527-1548
855-220-8885
www.pbida.org

Lisa Goldstein, President
Tracy Bowes, Office Manager
Provides free information and referral services for diagnosis and tutoring for parents, educators, physicians, and individuals with dyslexia. Membership includes yearly journal and quarterly newsletter, and Pennsylvania newsletter.

3653 Mental Health Association in Pennysylvania
1414 N Cameron St
1st Floor
Harrisburg, PA 17103-1049   717-346-0549
855-220-8885
Fax: 717-236-0192
www.mhapa.org

Julia Walker, Esq., President
Michael Brody, President & CEO
Marge Dailey, Director of Human Resources
The Mental Health Association in Pennysylvania is a non-profit providing services to those struggling with mental health issues. Services include advocacy, education and public policy.

3654 Pennsylvania Workers Compensation Board
651 Boas Street
Room 1700
Harrisburg, PA 17121-2510   717-787-5279
Fax: 717-772-0342
dli.state.pa.us

Joseph Brimmeier, CEO

3655 Pennsylvania Bureau of Blindness & Visual Services
Department of Pennsylvania
1521 N 6th St
Harrisburg, PA 17102   717-787-3201
800-622-2842
Fax: 717-787-3210
www.dli.state.pa.us

David Denotaris, Director
Jennifer Cave, Clerk Typist 3
Offers services for the totally blind, legally blind, visually impaired, and more with health, counseling, educational, recre-

ational, rehabilitation, computer training and professional training services.

3656 Pennsylvania Client Assistance Program
1515 Market Street
Suite 1300
Philadelphia, PA 19102- 1819
215-557-7112
888-745-2357
Fax: 215-557-7602
www.equalemployment.org

Stephen S. Pennington, Executive Director
Jamie C Ray, Assistant Director
Margaret Passio-McKenna, Senior Advocate

The Pennsylvania Client Assistance Program is dedicated to ensuring that the rehabilitation system in Pennsylvania is open and responsive to your needs. CAP help is provided to you at no charge, regardless of income. CAP helps people who are seeking services from the Office of Vocational Rehabilitation, Blindness and Visual Services, Centers for Independent Living and other programs funded under federal law.

3657 Pennsylvania Department of Aging
555 Walnut St
5th Floor
Harrisburg, PA 17101-1919
717-783-1550
Fax: 717-783-6842
aging@pa.gov
www.aging.state.pa.us

Nora Eisenhower, Manager

3658 Pennsylvania Department of Children with Disabilities
P.O. Box 2675
Harrisburg, PA 17105-2675
717-787-2600
Fax: 717-772-0323
www.pachildren.state.pa.US

Tom Corbett, Governor
Shelly Yanoff, Commission Chair

3659 Pennsylvania Developmental Disabilities Council
605 South Drive
Room 561
Harrisburg, PA 17120
717-789-6057
877-685-4452
TTY: 717-705-0819
www.paddc.org

Amy High, Vice Chairperson
Graham Mulholland, Executive Director
Sandra Amador Dusek, Deputy Director

3660 Public Interest Law Center of Philadelphia
United Way Building, 2nd Floor
1709 Benjamin Franklin Parkway
Philadelphia, PA 19103-5153
215-627-7100
Fax: 215-627-3183
pilcop.org

Eric J. Rothschild, Chair
Brian T. Feeney, Vice Chair
Jennifer R. Clarke, Executive Director

A non-profit, public interest law firm with a Disabilities Project specializing in class action suits brought by individuals and organizations.

3661 Social Security: Harrisburg Disability Determination
Suite 160
90 E Washington Bridge Rd
Worthington, OH 17101-1925
614-888-5339
800-722-1213
TTY: 614-288-0226
ssa.gov

Karena L. Kilgore, Executive Secretary
Carolyn W. Colvin, Commissioner
Carolyn W. Colvin, Deputy Commissioner

3662 Workers Compensation Board Pennsylvania
651 Boas Street
Room 1700
Harrisburg, PA 17121-2510
717-787-5279
Fax: 717-772-0342
www.dli.state.pa.us

Tom Corbett, Governor
Julia K. Hearthway, Secretary
Joseph Brimmeier, CEO

Rhode Island

3663 Department of Behavioral Healthcare, Developmental Disabilities and Hospitals
The Hazard Building
41 West Rd.
Cranston, RI 02920
401-462-3201
www.bhddh.ri.gov

Rebecca Boss, Director
Michelle Place, Assistant to the Director

State department responsible for creating and administering systems of care for individuals with disabilities, specifically focused on mental health and mental illness, developmental disabilities, substance abuse and long term hospital care.

3664 Rhode Island Department Health
3 Capitol Hl
Providence, RI 02908-5097
401-222-3855
Fax: 401-222-6548

Mary Salerno, Manager
Patricia Nolan, Executive Director
Pamela Corcoran, Disability Health Program

3665 Rhode Island Department of Elderly Affairs
74 West Road
Hazard Bldg, 2nd Floor
Cranston, RI 02920- 3001
401-462-3000
Fax: 401-462-0740

Corrine Russo, Manager

3666 Rhode Island Department of Mental Health
Cottage 405 Court B
Cranston, RI 02920
401-462-2003
Fax: 401-462-2008
www.butler.org

George W. Shuster, Chairman
Dennis D. Keefe, President & CEO
Reed Cosper, Manager

3667 Rhode Island Developmental Disabilities Council
400 Bald Hill Rd
Suite 515
Warwick, RI 02886-1692
401-737-1238
Fax: 401-737-3395
TTY: 401-737-1238
riddc@riddc.org
www.riddc.org

Charles Zawacki, Chairperson, Individual & Family
John Susa, Chairperson, Executive Committee
Anne Frank, Chairperson, Individual & Family

The Rhode Island Developmental Disabilities Council works to make Rhode Island a better place for people with developmental disabilities to live, work, go to school, and be part of their community.

3668 Rhode Island Disability Law Center
275 Westminster St
Suite 401
Providence, RI 02903-3434
401-831-3150
800-733-5332
Fax: 401-274-5568
TTY: 401-831-5335
info@ridlc.org
www.ridlc.org

Raymond A Marcaccio, Esq., Chair
Raymond L Bandusky, Executive Director
Darby Castigliego, Director of Finance & Administration

The Rhode Island Disability Law Center (RIDLC) provides free legal assistance to persons with disabilities. Services include individual representation to protect rights or to secure benefits and services, self-help information, educational programs and administrative and legislative advocacy.

3669 Rhode Island Governor's Commission on Disabilities
John O Pastore Center
Warwick City Hall
3275 Post Road
Warwick, RI 02920-3049 401-738-2000
Fax: 401-462-0106
www.warwickri.gov

Bob Cooper, Executive Secretary
The Commision is responsible for: coordinating compliance by
state agencies with federal and state disablity right laws; approv-
ing or modifying state and local goverment agency's open meeting accessibility for persons with disabilities transition plans;
assisting local boards of canvassers to ensure accessible polling
places locations; aproving or rejecting requests to waive the state
building code's standards for accessibility at facilities to be
leased by state agencies...

3670 Rhode Island Parent Information Network
1210 Pontiac Avenue
Cranston, RI 02920 401-270-0101
800-464-3399
Fax: 401-270-7049
info@ripin.org
ripin.org

Kathleen DiChiara, Chairman
Ammala Douangsavanh, Vice Chairman
Stephen Brunero, Executive Director
A nonprofit organization established by parents and concerned
professionals providing culturally appropriate information,
training and support for families and professionals designed to
improve educational and life outcomes for all children. Serving
the State of Rhode Island.

**3671 Rhode Island Services for the Blind and Visually
Impaired**
40 Fountain St
Providence, RI 02903-1830 401-421-7005
800-752-8088
Fax: 401-421-9259
TTY: 401-421-7016
www.ors.ri.gov

Kathleen Grygiel, Administrator
Ronald Racine, Associate Director
Laurie DiOrio, Acting Associate Director
Offers services for the totally blind, legally blind, visually impaired, and more with health, counseling, educational, recreational, rehabilitation, computer training and professional
training services.

3672 Services for the Blind and Visually Impaired
40 Fountain St
Providence, RI 02903-1830 401-421-7005
Fax: 401-222-1328
TTY: 401-421-7016
www.ors.ri.gov

Kathleen Grygiel, Administrator
Ronald Racine, Associate Director
Laurie DiOrio, Acting Associate Director
Offers services for the blind and visually impaired.

3673 Social Security: Providence Disability Determination
Social Security
40 Fountain Street
6th Floor
Providence, RI 02903-3246 401-222-3182
800-772-1213
Fax: 401-222-3868
TTY: 401-273-6648
Deborah.A.Cannon@ssa.gov
www.ssa.gov

Karena L. Kilgore, Executive Secretary
Carolyn W. Colvin, Commissioner
Carolyn W. Colvin, Deputy Commissioner
We deliver services through a nationwide network of over 1,400
offices that include regional offices, field offices, card centers,
teleservice centers, processing centers, hearing offices, the Appeals Council, and our State and territorial partners, the Disability Determination Services. We also have a presence in U.S.
embassies around the globe. For the public, we are the face of the

government. The rich diversity of our employees mirrors the
public we serve.

3674 Workers Compensation Board Rhode Island
1 Dorrance Plz
Providence, RI 02903-3973 401-458-5000
Fax: 401-222-3121

George E Healy Jr, Manager
George Healy Jr, Manager

South Carolina

3675 Protection & Advocacy for People with Disabilities
Ste 208
3710 Landmark Dr
Columbia, SC 29204-4034 803-782-0639
866-275-7273
Fax: 803-790-1946
TTY: 866-232-4525
info@pandasc.org
protectionandadvocacy-sc.org

Gloria Prevost, Executive Director
Anne Trice, Director of Administration
J. Ashley Twombley, Chair
An independent, nonprofit organization responsible for safe
guarding rights of South Carolinians with disabilities and other
handicapped individuals without regard to age, income, severity
of disability, sex, race, or religion.

3676 Social Security: West Columbia Disability Determination
P.O. Box 60
Columbia, SC 29171-0060 803-896-6400
800-772-1213
Fax: 803-822-4318
TTY: 800-325-0078
www.socialsecurity.gov

Karena L. Kilgore, Executive Secretary
Carolyn W. Colvin, Commissioner
Carolyn W. Colvin, Deputy Commissioner
We deliver services through a nationwide network of over 1,400
offices that include regional offices, field offices, card centers,
teleservice centers, processing centers, hearing offices, the Appeals Council, and our State and territorial partners, the Disability Determination Services. We also have a presence in U.S.
embassies around the globe. For the public, we are the face of the
government. The rich diversity of our employees mirrors the
public we serve.

3677 South Carolina Assistive Technology Project
Midlands Center
8301 Farrow Road
Columbia, SC 29203 803-935-5263
800-915-4522
Fax: 803-935-5342
TTY: 803-935-5263
jjendron@usit.net
www.sc.edu/scatp/

Carol Page, Ph.D, CCC-SLP, A, Program Director
Janet Jendron, Program Coordinator
Mary Alice Bechtler, Program Coordinator
A statewide program promoting assistive technology devices and
services for persons of all ages with all disabilities. Recently a
statewide AT resource, demonstrations and equipment loan center and lab annual expo and training and workshops on a variety
of disabilities and technology topics.

3678 South Carolina Client Assistance Program
Governor's Office oe Executive Policy & Programs
1205 Pendleton St
Columbia, SC 29201-3756 803-734-0285
800-868-0040
Fax: 803-734-0546
TTY: 803-734-1147
cap@oepp.sc.gov

Denise Riley Pensmith, MSW, Executive Director
Cindy Popenhagen, Administrative Assistant
The Client Assistance Program (CAP) helps citizens of the State
by acting as advocates regarding services provided by the Vocational Rehabilitation Department (VR), Commission for the

Blind, and all Independent Living programs and projects funded under the Rehabilitation Act of 1973. As advocates, CAP staff can investigate, negotiate, mediate, and pursue administrative, and other remedies to ensure that clients' rights are protected.

3679 South Carolina Commission for the Blind (SCCB)
1430 Confederate Ave.
Columbia, SC 29201-79 803-898-8731
publicinfo@sccb.sc.gov
www.sccb.state.sc.us

Goal is to help individuals with visual impairments prepare for and obtain appropriate employment.

3680 South Carolina Department of Children with Disabilities
2600 Bull St
Columbia, SC 29201-1708 803-434-4260

Miroslav Cuturic, Director
Peter Getz, Administrator

3681 South Carolina Department of Mental Health
Office of Administration
PO Box 485
Columbia, SC 29202 803-898-8581
800-273-8255
TTY: 800-647-2066
webmaster@scdmh.org
scdmh.net

Mark W. Binkley, Interim State Director
The S.C. Department of Mental Health gives priority to adults, children, and their families affected by serious mental illnesses and significant emotional disorders. We are committed to eliminating stigma and promoting the philosophy of recovery, to achieving our goals in collaboration with all stakeholders, and to assuring the highest quality of culturally competent services possible.

3682 South Carolina Developmental Disabilities Council
Office of the Governor
1205 Pendleton St
Suite 461
Columbia, SC 29201-3756 803-734-0465
Fax: 803-734-1409
TTY: 803-734-1147
jvancleave@oepp.sc.gov
www.scddc.state.sc.us

Valarie Bishop, Executive Director
Cheryl English, Program Information Coordinator
Kimberly Johnson Fontanez, Grants Administrator
The mission of the South Carolina Developmental Disabilities Council is to provide leadership in advocating, funding and implementing initiatives which recognize the inherent dignity of each individual, and promote independence, productivity, respect and inclusion for all persons with disabilities and their families.

3683 Workers Compensation Board: South Carolina
PO Box 1715
Columbia, SC 29202-1715 803-737-5700
Fax: 803-737-5768
www.state.sc.us/wcc

Gary Cannon, Executive Director
Kim Balleutine, Admin. Assistant

South Dakota

3684 Children's Special Health Services Program
600 E Capitol Ave
Pierre, SD 57501-2536 605-773-3361
800-738-2301
Fax: 605-773-5683
DOH.info@state.sd.us
www.doh.sd.gov

Dianne Weyer, Manager
Barb Hemmelman, Program Manager
Health KiCC is a program, funded through federal and state monies, that provides financial assistance for medical appointments, procedures, treatments, medications and travel reimbursement for children with certain chronic health conditions.

3685 Division of Labor and Management
South Dakota Department of Labor
700 Governors Dr
Pierre, SD 57501-2291 605-773-3101
Fax: 605-773-6184
dlr.sd.gov

Sara Minton, Executive Director
Pamela S Roberts, Secretary
Marcia Hultman, Deputy Secretary of Labor and D
Our mission is to promote economic opportunity and financial security for individuals and businesses through quality, responsive and expert services; fair and equitable employment solutions; and safe and sound business practices.

3686 Health KiCC
South Dakota Department of Health
600 E Capitol Ave
Pierre, SD 57501-2536 605-773-3361
800-738-2301
Fax: 605-773-5683
DOH.info@state.sd.us
www.doh.sd.gov

Dianne Weyer, Manager
Health KiCC is a program, funded through federal and state monies, that provides financial assistance for medical appointments, procedures, treatments, medications and travel reimbursement for children with certain chronic health conditions.

3687 South Dakota Advocacy Services
221 S Central Ave
Ste. 38
Pierre, SD 57501-2479 605-224-8294
800-658-4782
Fax: 605-224-5125
sdas@sdadvocacy.com
sdadvocacy.com

Sandy Stocklin Hook, Partners Coordinator
Designated protection and advocacy progam for South Dakota providing legal, administrative, mediation and other services to elgible persons with disabilities in the state.

3688 South Dakota Department of Aging
700 Governors Dr
Pierre, SD 57501-2291 605-773-3656
866-854-5465
Fax: 605-773-4085

Marilyn Kinsman, Division Director
Lynne Valenti, Deputy Secretary
Amy Iversen-Pollreisz, Deputy Secretary
The Division of Adult Services and Aging (ASA) provides home and community service options to individuals 60 years of age and older and 18 years of age and older with physical disabilities, regardless of income.

3689 South Dakota Department of Human Services
Hillsview Plaza
3800 E Hwy 34
Pierre, SD 57501 605-773-5990
Fax: 605-773-5483
infodhs@state.sd.us
dhs.sd.gov

Shawnie Rechtenbaugh, Secretary
Provides resources for individuals with developmental disabilities, including rehabilitation services, services for the blind and visually impaired, and long-term services and supports.

3690 South Dakota Department of Social Services Division of Behavioral Health
700 Governors Dr.
Pierre, SD 57501 605-367-5236
855-878-6057
Fax: 605-773-7076
DSSbh@state.sd.us
dss.sd.gov/behavioralhealth

Laurie Gill, Secretary
Brenda Tidbull-Zeltinger, Deputy Secretary
Tiffany Wolfgang, Division Director
South Dakota's state mental health authority.

3691 South Dakota Division of Rehabilitation
700 Governors Dr
Pierre, SD 57501-2291   605-773-3101
                                           Fax: 605-773-6184
                                              www.sdjobs.org
Sara Minton, Executive Director
Pamela S Roberts, Secretary
Marcia Hultman, Deputy Secretary of Labor and D
Offers diagnosis, evaluation and physical restoration services,
counseling, social work, educational and professional training,
employment and rehabilitation services for the disabled.

3692 Workers Compensation Board: South Dakota
700 Governors Dr
Pierre, SD 57501-2291   605-773-3101
                                           Fax: 605-773-6184
                                              www.sdjobs.org
Sara Minton, Executive Director
Marcia Hultman, Secretary
Lyle Harter, Director of Administrative Servi
Our mission is to promote economic opportunity and financial se-
curity for individuals and businesses through quality, responsive
and expert services; fair and equitable employment solutions;
and safe and sound business practices.

Tennessee

3693 Disability Determination Services
400 Deaderick St
Nashville, TN 37243-1403   800-342-1117
                                 DHS.CustomerService@tn.gov
                                             www.tennessee.gov
Thea Smith, Human Resources Program Specialist
Wendy Davis, Finance & Administration
Cherrell Campbell-Street, Assistant Commissioner
The Disability Determination Services is a branch of the Division
of Rehabilitation Services in the Department of Human Services.
Its main responsibility is to process Social Security and Supple-
mental Security Income disability claims.

3694 International Dyslexia Association: Tennessee Branch
Knoxville, TN   865-207-4918
                                     msamwood@bellsouth.net
                                                www.tnida.org
Emily Dempster, President
Erin Alexander, Senior Vice President
Nikki Davis, Secretary
The Tennessee Branch of the International Dyslexia Association
(TN-IDA) was formed to increase awareness about Dyslexia in
the state of Tennessee. TN-IDA supports efforts to provide infor-
mation regarding appropriate language arts instruction to those
involved with language-based learning differences and to encourage the identity of these individuals at-risk for such
disorders as soon as possible.

3695 Tennessee Assistive Technology Projects
Citizens Plaza State Office Buildin
511 Union St.
Nashville, TN 37219-1403   615-313-5183
                                                800-732-5059
                                         TTY: 615-313-5695
                                             TN.TTAP@tn.gov
                                                   www.tn.gov
Bill Haslam, Governor
Raquel Hatter, Commissioner
Beth White, Manager
A statewide program promoting assistive technology devices and
services for persons of all ages with all disabilities.

3696 Tennessee Client Assistance Program
Tennessee Protection and Advocacy
P.O.Box 121257
Nashville, TN 37212-1257   615-298-1080
                                                800-342-1660
                                           Fax: 615-298-2046
Shirley Shea, Executive Director
Doris Lopez, Assistant Executive Director

3697 Tennessee Commission on Aging and Disability
502 Deaderick Street
9th Floor
Nashville, TN 37243-860   615-741-2056
                                           Fax: 615-741-3309
                                          www.tn.gov/aging.html
Richard M. Honn, Executive Director
Ryan Ellis, Aging Info. & Data Director
Kathy Zamata, Aging Program Director

3698 Tennessee Council on Developmental Disabilities
500 James Robertson Pkwy
1st Floor
Nashville, TN 37243   615-532-6615
                                           Fax: 615-532-6964
                                                tnddc@tn.gov
                                                  tn.gov/cdd
Wanda Willis, Executive Director
Lynette Porter, Deputy Director
Alicia Cone, Director of Grant Program
The council is a state agency that leads initiatives to improve disability policies by educating policymakers and the public about
best practices in disability services, facilitating collaboration
across organizations, and producing educational publications on
the subject.

3699 Tennessee Department of Children with Disabilities
511 Union St.
Nashville, TN 37219-9004   615-741-9701
                                                800-861-1935
                                           Fax: 615-253-5216
                                                   www.tn.gov
Ruth S Letson, Manager
Haticile Buchanan, Manager
Mary Beth Franklyn, CS Program Director
Tennessee's children thrive in safe, healthy and stable families.
Families thrive in healthy, safe and strong communities. Tennes-
see's citizens benefit from the best child welfare and juvenile jus-
tice agency in the country.

3700 Tennessee Department of Mental Health
500 Deaderick Street
Nashville, TN 37243-3400   615-532-6597
                                                800-560-5767
                                           Fax: 615-532-6514
Doug Varney, Commissioner
Grant Lawrence, Director Office of Communication
Bob Grunow, Deputy Commissioner
TDMH is the state's mental health and substance abuse authority.
Its mission is to plan for and promote the availability of a comprehensive array of quality prevention, early intervention, treat-
ment, habilitation, and rehabilitation services and supports based
on the needs and choices of individuals and families served. Responsible for policy, and oversight, and for advocacy of the
consumer within the state.

3701 Tennessee Division of Rehabilitation
400 Deaderick St
Nashville, TN 37243-1403   615-313-4700
                                                800-270-1349
                                         TTY: 615-313-5695
                                            http://www.tn.gov
Patsy Matthews, Commissioner
Randall Beasley, Manager
Raquel Hatter, Commissioner
Offers rehabilitation, medical and therapeutic information and
referrals to the disabled.

3702 Workers Compensation Division Tennessee
Dept of Labor & Workforce Development
220 French Landing Drive
1st Floor
Nashville, TN 37243- 1002   615-741-6642
                                                800-332-2667
                                           Fax: 615-532-1468
                                               wc.info@tn.gov
                                    www.tn.gov/labor-wfd/wcomp.html
Karla Davis, Commissioner
Alisa Malone, Deputy Commissioner
Stephanie Mitchell, General Counsel

We administer the workers' compensation system and promote a better understanding of the program's benefits by informing employees and employers of their rights and responsibilities. Workers' Compenstation administers a mediation program for disputed claims, encourage workplace safety, participate in a public awareness campaign concerning fraud, and oversee an information awareness program for educating the public on laws and regulations which define workers' compensation requirements. We ensure

Texas

3703 Disability Policy Consortium
2222 West Braker Lane
Austin, TX 78758-1024

512-454-4816
800-252-9108
Fax: 512-323-0902
disabilitytx.org

Mary Faithful, Executive Director
Roberta Rosenberg-Roque, Manager
An independent group of statewide advocacy organizations that strives to achieve the development and full implementation of public policy that promotes and supports the rights, inclusion, integration and independence of Texans with disabilities.

3704 Disability Rights Texas
2222 West Braker Lane
Austin, TX 78758-1024

512-454-4816
866-362-2851
www.disabilityrightstx.org

Mary Faithfull, Executive Director
Patty Anderson, Deputy Director
A federally designated legal protection and advocacy agency (P&A) for people with disabilities in Texas. Helps people with disabilities understand and exercise their rights under the law, ensuring their full and equal participation in society.

3705 Division of Special Education
1701 Congress Ave.
Austin, TX 78701-1402

512-463-9414
Fax: 512-463-9838
teainfo@tea.state.tx.us
www.tea.state.tx.us

Cory Green, Federal & State Education Policy
Donna Bahorich, Chair
Ruban Cortez Jr., Secretary
The Texas Education Agency is the state agency that oversees primary and secondary public education. It is headed by the commissioner of education. The mission of TEA is to provide leadership, guidance and resources to help schools meet the educational needs of all students

3706 Easterseals Central Texas
2324 Ridepoint Dr.
Suite F1
Austin, TX 78754

512-615-6800
Fax: 512-615-7121
www.easterseals.com/centraltx

Tod Marvin, President
Easterseals provides a wealth of programs and services to help promote independence and create opportunities for people with disabilities.

3707 Easterseals North Texas
1424 Hemphill St.
Fort Worth, TX 76104

888-617-7171
www.easterseals.com/northtexas

Tod Marvin, President
Jennifer Friesen, Vice President, Programs & Services
Easterseals provides a wealth of programs and services to help promote independence and create opportunities for people with disabilities.

3708 El Valle Community Parent Resource Center
Ste J
530 S Texas Blvd
Weslaco, TX 78596-6262

956-969-0215
800-680-0255
Fax: 956-968-7102

Robert Garza, Owner

3709 Grassroots Consortium
Greenroots Consortium
6202 Belmark St
Houston, TX 77087-6324

713-643-9576
Fax: 713-643-6291
Speckids@aol.com

Agnes A Johnson, Director

3710 International Dyslexia Association: Austin Branch
Austin, TX

512-452-7658
aus.dyslexiaida.org

Mary Bach, President
Karen Monteith, Vice President
Herman H. Klare, Treasurer
Provides free information and referral services for diagnosis and tutoring for parents, educators, physicians, and individuals with dyslexia in Illinois. Membership includes yearly journal and quarterly newsletter.

3711 National Alliance on Mental Illness (Texas)
P.O. Box 300817
Austin, TX 78703

512-693-2000
Fax: 512-693-8000
officemanager@namitexas.org
namitexas.org

John Dornheim, President
Holly Doggett, Executive Director
Greg Hansch, Public Policy Director
NAMI Texas is the state headquarters of the National Alliance on Mental Illness, a national nonprofit that aims to improve the lives of all persons affected by mental illness. NAMI Texas oversees over 25 local affiliates throughout the state. NAMI Texas raises awareness about mental illness through the dissemination of information, and seeks to address the mental health needs of Texans through education and support programs for persons with mental illness, families, friends, and professionals.

3712 Parent Connection
1020 Riverwood Ct
Conroe, TX 77304-2811

936-756-8321
800-839-8876
parentCNCT@aol.com
http://www.parentingaspergerscommunity.com/pu

Dave Angel, Founder
Includes parenting help and Aspergers advice, including parenting tips, tricks and techniques to help your child with Aspergers. Our worldwide membership base is helping parents to understand their child with Aspergers better and make their home & family life a better place to be.

3713 Parents Supporting Parents Network
8001 Centre Park Drive
Suite 100
Austin, TX 78754

512-454-6694
800-252-9729
Fax: 512-454-4956
secretary@thearcoftexas.org
www.thearcoftexas.org

Charlie Huber, President
John Schneider, Vice-President
Nancy Lepley, Treasurer
Since our founding in 1950 by a group of parents of children with intellectual and developmental disabilities, The Arc at the local, state and national level has been instrumental in the creation of virtually every program, service, right, and benefit that is now available to more than half a million Texans with intellectual and developmental disabilities. Today, The Arc continues to advocate for including people with intellectual and developmental disabilities in all aspects of society.

3714 Partners Resource Network
Ste B
1090 Longfellow Dr
Beaumont, TX 77706-4819   409-898-4684
                                                  800-866-4726
                                             Fax: 409-898-4869
                                 partnersresource@sbcglobal.net
                                                  partnerstx.org

Janice Meyer, Executive Director
Statewide network of three parent training and information centers.

3715 Social Security: Austin Disability Determination
P.O. Box 149198
Austin, TX 78714-9198   512-437-8311
                                                  800-772-1213
                                                  800-252-9627
                                             Fax: 512-437-8595
                                             TTY: 512-916-5958
                                               dan.tippit@ssa.gov
                                                  www.ssa.gov

Karena L. Kilgore, Executive Secretary
Carolyn W. Colvin, Commissioner
Carolyn W. Colvin, Deputy Commissioner
We deliver services through a nationwide network of over 1,400 offices that include regional offices, field offices, card centers, teleservice centers, processing centers, hearing offices, the Appeals Council, and our State and territorial partners, the Disability Determination Services. We also have a presence in U.S. embassies around the globe. The rich diversity of our employees mirrors the public we serve.

3716 Statewide Information at Texas School for the Deaf
1102 S Congress Ave
Austin, TX 78704-1728   512-462-5353
                                             Fax: 512-462-5353
                                          webmaster@tsd.state.tx.us
                                                  www.tsd.state.tx.us

Sonia Karimi Bridges, Video Communication Specialist
Avonne Brooker-Rutowski, Program Specialist
David Coco, Program Specialist
Welcome to Texas School for the Deaf, a place where students who are deaf or hard of hearing including those with additional disabilities, have the opportunity to learn, grow and belong in a culture that optimizes individual potential and provides accessible language and communication across the curriculum. Our educational philosophy is grounded in the belief that all children who are deaf and hard of hearing deserve a quality language and communication-driven program that provides education tog

3717 Texas Advocates Supporting Kids with Disabilities
P.O.Box 162685
Austin, TX 78716-2685   512-310-2102
                                             Fax: 512-310-2102
                                               ASKTASK@aol.com

3718 Texas Commission for the Blind
P.O. Box 149198
Austin, TX 78714-9198   512-459-8575
                                                  800-252-5204
                                             Fax: 512-424-4730
                                                  www.dars.state.tx.us

Canzata Crowder, Manager
Offers services for the totally blind, legally blind, and visually impaired, with counseling, educational, recreational, rehabilitation, computer training and professional training services.

3719 Texas Commission for the Deaf and Hard of Hearing
D AR S
P.O. Box 149198
Austin, TX 78714-9198   512-407-3250
                                                  800-628-5115
                                             Fax: 512-424-4730
                                             TTY: 512-407-3251
                                                  www.dars.state.tx.us

Veronda L. Durden, Commissioner
Glenn Neal, Deputy Commissioner
David Myers, Executive Director

3720 Texas Council for Developmental Disabilities
6201 E Oltorf St
Suite 600
Austin, TX 78741-7509   512-437-5432
                                                  800-262-0334
                                             Fax: 512-437-5434
                                             TTY: 512-437-5431
                                               tcdd@tcdd.texas.gov
                                                  txddc.state.tx.us

Mary Durheim, Chairman
Andrew D. Crim, Vice Chairman
Roger Webb, Executive Director
The Texas Council for Developmental Disabilities is a 27-member board dedicated to ensuring that all Texans with developmental disabilities, about 411,479 individuals, have the opportunity to be independent, productive and valued members of their communities. The mission of the Texas Council for Developmental Disabilities is to create change so that all people with disabilities are fully included in their communities and exercise control over their own lives.

3721 Texas Department of Human Services
701 W 51st St
P.O. Box 149030
Austin, TX 78751-2312   512-438-3011
                                                  888-834-7406
                                             Fax: 512-472-0603
                                             TTY: 888-425-6889
                                               mail@dads.state.tx.us
                                                  www.dads.state.tx.us

Jon Weizenbaum, Commissioner
Kristi Jordan, Associate Commissioner
Chris Adams, Deputy Commissioner

3722 Texas Department on Aging
701 W 51st St
P.O. Box 149030
Austin, TX 78751-2312   512-438-3011
                                                  800-252-9240
                                                  www.dads.state.tx.us

Jon Weizenbaum, Commissioner
Kristi Jordan, Associate Commissioner
Chris Adams, Deputy Commissioner

3723 Texas Federation of Families for Children's Mental Health
Ste 505
7701 N Lamar Blvd
Austin, TX 78752-1000   512-407-8844
                                                  866-893-3264
                                             Fax: 512-407-8266
                                                  www.txffcmh.org

Patti Derr, Executive Director
Pat Calley, Chairperson
S Barron, Operations Director

3724 Texas Governor's Committee on People with Disabilities
1100 San Jacinto Blvd
P.O. Box 12428
Austin, TX 78701- 1935   512-463-2000
                                             Fax: 513-463-5745
                                 www.governor.state.tx.us/disabilities
Angela English, LPC, LMFT, Executive Director
Erin Lawler, JD, MS, Accessibility and Disability Rig
Nancy Van Loan, Executive Assistant
The Governor's Committee on People with Disabilities is within the office of the Governor. The committee's mission is to further opportunities for persons with disabilities to enjoy full and equal access to lives of independence, productivity, and self-determination. The committee is composed of 12 members appointed by the governor and of nonvoting ex officio members.

3725   Texas Health and Human Services (HHS)
Brown-Heatly Building
4900 N Lamar Blvd.
Austin, TX 78751-3247   512-424-6500
                                            TTY: 512-424-6597
                                               hhs.texas.gov

Courtney N. Phillips, Executive Commissioner
Cecile Young, Chief Deputy Executive Commissioner
John Hellerstedt, Commissioner, Department of State Health
Services
Responsible for health services in the state of texas, including
mental health and substance abuse treatment.

3726   Texas Respite Resource Network
P.O. Box 149030
710 West 51st Street
Austin, TX 78714- 9030   512-438-5555
                                            Fax: 512-438-4374
                                               archrespite.org

Jill Kagan, Program Director
Liz Newhouse, Assistant Director
Mike Mathers, Executive Director
A state clearinghouse and technical assistance network for respite in Texas. TRRN identifies, initiates and improves respite
options for families caring for individuals with disabilities on the
local, state and national levels. TRRN provides training/techni-
cal assistance to programs/groups wanting to establish respite
services.

3727   Texas Technology Access Project
Center for Disabilities Studies
10100 Burnet Rd
Austin, TX 78758-4445   512-232-0740
                                                 800-828-7839
                                            Fax: 512-232-0761
                                            TTY: 512-232-0762
                                       rogerlevy@austin.utexas.edu
                                         techaccess.edb.utexas.edu

Roger Levy, Program Director
Darlene West, Assistive Technology Coordinator
Steve Thomas, Operations and External Relation
Their mission is to increase access for people with disabilities to
assistive technology that provides them more control over their
immediate environments and an enhanced ability to function
independently.

3728   Texas UAP for Developmental Disabilities
University of Texas
1 University Station
Austin, TX 78712   512-471-3434
                                                 800-828-7839
                                                 www.utexas.edu

Gregory L. Fences, President
Judith H. Langlois, Executive Vice President and Pr
Gregory J. Vincent, Vice President
Welcome to The University of Texas at Austin. Founded in 1883,
UT is one of the largest and most respected universities in the nation. Ours is a diverse learning community, with students from every state and more than 100 countries. We're a university with
world talent and Texas traditions. Discover more about us online
and come visit our beautiful campus in person.

3729   Texas Workers Compensation Commission
333 Guadalupe
P.O. Box 149104
Austin, TX 78701-1645   512-676-6000
                                                 800-578-4677
                                                 800-252-3439
                                            Fax: 512-804-4401
                                            TTY: 512-322-4238
                                       WebStaff@tdi.state.tx.us
                                               www.tdi.texas.gov

Robert Shipe, Executive Director
Rod Bordelon, Commissioner
Workers' compensation is a state-regulated insurance program
that pays medical bills and replaces some lost wages for employees who are injured at work or who have work-related diseases or
illnesses.

3730   United Cerebral Palsy of Texas
National Cerebral Palsy of American
Ste 145
1016 La Posada Dr
Austin, TX 78752-3828   512-472-8696
                                                 800-798-1492
                                            Fax: 512-472-8026

Jean Langendorf, Executive Director
Offers a unique array of programs and services designed for one
specific purpose: to ensure that people with cerebral palsy and
similar disabilities have the opportunity to participate fully and
equally in every aspect of our society.

Utah

3731   Access Utah Network
Ste 100
155 S 300 W
Salt Lake City, UT 84101-1288   801-533-4636
                                                 800-333-8824
                                            Fax: 801-533-3968

Mark L. Smith, Information Specialist
Access Utah Network is Utah's prime source for information and
referral for individuals with disabilities and their caregivers
since 1990. Our operators can provide you with the information
you need to find accessible housing, assistive technology and financial and social supports needed to live independently with a
disability. Call us or explore our web site today to see how Access
Utah Network can help you become more independent.

3732   Social Security: Salt Lake City Disability Determination
Social Security
P.O. Box 144032
Salt Lake City, UT 84111-4032   801-321-6500
                                                 800-772-1213
                                                 800-221-3493
                                            Fax: 801-321-6599
                                            TTY: 801-524-5047
                                           Dave.Carlson@ssa.gov
                                                   www.ssa.gov

Karena L. Kilgore, Executive Secretary
Carolyn W. Colvin, Commissioner
Carolyn W. Colvin, Deputy Commissioner
We deliver services through a nationwide network of over 1,400
offices that include regional offices, field offices, card centers,
teleservice centers, processing centers, hearing offices, the Appeals Council, and our State and territorial partners, the Disability Determination Services. We also have a presence in U.S.
embassies around the globe. The rich diversity of our employees
mirrors the public we serve.

3733   Utah Assistive Technology Projects
Utah State University
6855 Old Main Hl
Logan, UT 84322-6855   435-797-3824
                                                 800-524-5152
                                            TTY: 435-797-2355
                                                 www.uatpat.org

Sachin Pavithran, Program Director
Alma Burgess, UATP Data Collection Coordinator
Clay Christensen, Lab Coordinator
A statewide program promoting assistive technology devices and
services for persons of all ages with all disabilities.

3734   Utah Client Assistance Program
205 N 400 W
Salt Lake City, UT 84103-1125   801-363-1347
                                                 800-662-9080
                                            Fax: 801-363-1437
                                        www.disabilitylawcenter.org

Bryce Fifield Ph.D, President
Jared Fields, Vice President
Barbara M. Campbell, Treasurer
Since 1979, the Disability Law Center (DLC) has helped thousands of Utahns with disabilities and their families. The DLC has
broad statutory powers to safeguard the human and civil rights of
persons with disabilities. We provide self-advocacy assistance,
legal services, disability rights education, and public policy ad-

vocacy on behalf of the more than 400,000 Utah residents with disabilities. Our services are available statewide and without regard for ability to pay.

3735 Utah Department of Aging and Adult Services
195 North 1950 West
Salt Lake City, UT 84116

801-538-3910
877-424-4640
Fax: 801-538-4395
debooth@utah.gov

Nels Holmgren, Director
Michael S. Styles, Assistant Director
Michelle Benson, Director
The department administers a wide variety of home and community-based services for Utah residents who are 60 or older. Programs and services are primarily delivered by a network of 12 Area Agencies on Aging which reach all geographic areas of the state. Their goal is to provide services that allow people to remain independent.

3736 Utah Department of Human Services: Division of Services for People with Disabilities
195 North 1950 West
Salt Lake City, UT 84116

801-538-4171
844-275-3773
dhsinfo@utah.gov
dspd.utah.gov

Information and referral services for people with disabilities, including DD/MR, brain injury and physical disabilities throughout the state of Utah.

3737 Utah Division Of Substance Abuse & Mental Health
Utah Department of Human Services
195 No. 1950 West
Salt Lake City, UT 84116-1550

801-538-4171
Fax: 801-538-4016
WWW.DHS.UTAH.GOV

Lana Stohl, Executive Director

3738 Utah Division of Services for the Disabled
195 North 1950 West
Salt Lake City, UT 84116

801-538-3910
877-424-4640
Fax: 801-538-4395

Paul T. Smith, Division Director
Clay Hiatt, Fiscal Management
Offers services for the totally blind, legally blind, visually impaired, and more with health, counseling, educational, recreational, rehabilitation, computer training and professional training services.

3739 Utah Governor's Council for People with Disabilities
155 S 300 W
Suite 100
Salt Lake City, UT 84101-1288

801-533-4636
Fax: 801-533-3968
www.gcpd.org/

Mark Smith, Manager
Angela Allen, Administrative Secretary

3740 Utah Labor Commission
160 E 300 S
3rd Floor
Salt Lake City, UT 84114-6600

801-530-6800
800-222-1238
Fax: 801-530-6390
laborcom@utah.gov
laborcommission.utah.gov

Jaceson R Maughan, Commissioner
Alison Adams-Perlac, Director
Britton Beims, Employment Discrimination Investigation
The Utah Labor Commission is a regulatory agency that works to ensure safety in the workplace. The commission also offers services related to workplace injuries, wage issues, descrimination and industrial accidents.

3741 Utah Protection & Advocacy Services for Persons with Disabilities
Disability Law Center
205 N 400 W
Salt Lake City, UT 84103-1125

801-363-1347
800-662-9080
Fax: 801-363-1437
www.disabilitylawcenter.org

Bryce Fifield Ph.D, President
Jared Fields, Vice President
Barbara M. Campbell, Treasurer
Since 1979, the Disability Law Center (DLC) has helped thousands of Utahns with disabilities and their families. The DLC has broad statutory powers to safeguard the human and civil rights of persons with disabilities. We provide self-advocacy assistance, legal services, disability rights education, and public policy advocacy on behalf of the more than 400,000 Utah residents with disabilities. Our services are available statewide and without regard for ability to pay.

Vermont

3742 Disability Law Project
57 N Main St
Rutland, VT 05701-3246

800-889-2047
Fax: 802-775-0022
nbreiden@vtlegalaid.org
vtlegalaid.org

Nanci Smith, President
Jessica Porter, Vice President/Secretary
John Holme, Treasurer
Legal services (protection and advocacy) for people with disabilities on legal issues arising from disability. Statewide. Adults and children. Employment, education, discrimination, housing, public benefits, health care.

3743 Disability Rights Vermont
141 Main Street
Suite 7
Montpelier, VT 05602-2916

802-229-1355
800-834-7890
Fax: 802-229-1359
TTY: 800-889-2047
info@disabilityrightsvt.org
www.disabilityrightsvt.org

Sarah Wendell-Launderville, President
David Gallagher, Vice president
Crocker Paquin, Treasurer
Advocacy and legal services for people with mental illness on legal issues arising, out of disabilities. Children and adults.

3744 Social Security: Vermont Disability Determination Services
Ste 6
93 Pilgrim Park Rd
Waterbury, VT 05676-1729

802-241-2463
800-734-2463
800-772-1213
Fax: 802-241-2492
www.ssa.gov

Karena L. Kilgore, Executive Secretary
Carolyn W. Colvin, Commissioner
Carolyn W. Colvin, Deputy Commissioner
We deliver services through a nationwide network of over 1,400 offices that include regional offices, field offices, card centers, teleservice centers, processing centers, hearing offices, the Appeals Council, and our State and territorial partners, the Disability Determination Services. We also have a presence in U.S. embassies around the globe. The rich diversity of our employees mirrors the public we serve.

3745 Vermont Assistive Technology Projects
103 S Main St
Weeks Building
Waterbury, VT 05671-2305　　　　　800-750-6355
　　　　　　　　　　　　　　　　　800-750-6355
　　　　　　　　　　　　　　Fax: 802-871-3048
　　　　　　　　　　　　　　TTY: 802-241-1464
　　　　　　　　　　　　　　　　atp.vermont.gov
Amber Fulcher, Program Director
Sharon Alderman, Assistive Technology Reuse Coord
Emma Cobb, Assistive Technology Services Co
Increase awareness and change policies to insure assistive technology (AT) is available to all Vermonters with disabilities. Our Commitment is to enable Vermonters with disabilities to have greater independence, productivity, and confidence. To provide them with a clear and direct avenue toward integration and inclusion within the work force and community.

3746 Vermont Client Assistance Program
57 N Main St
Rutland, VT 05701-3246　　　　　802-775-0021
　　　　　　　　　　　　　　　800-769-7459
　　　　www.vocrehabvermont.org/html/clientassistance
Patrick Flood, Commissioner
The Client Assistance Program (CAP) is an independent advocacy program to help if you are applying for or receiving services from one of the following sources: Division of Vocational Rehabilitation (VR); Vermont Center for Independent Living (VCIL); Division for the Blind and Visually Impaired (DBVI); Vermont Association of Business, Industry & Rehabilitation (VABIR); Vermont Association for the Blind and Visually Impaired (VABVI); Supported Employment Programs; Transition Programs.

3747 Vermont Department of Aging
103 S Main St
Weeks Building
Waterbury, VT 05671-1601　　　　　802-241-2401
　　　　　　　　　　　　　　Fax: 802-871-3281
　　　　　　　　　　　　　　TTY: 802-241-3557
　　　　　　　　　　　　　　　dail.vermont.gov
Susan Wehry, Commissioner
Marybeth McCaffrey, Director
Linda Henzel, Executive Staff Assistant

3748 Vermont Department of Developmental and
103 S Main St
Weeks Building
Waterbury, VT 05671-1601　　　　　802-241-2401
　　　　　　　　　　　　　　Fax: 802-871-3281
　　　　　　　　　　　　　　TTY: 802-241-3557
　　　　　　　　　　　　　　　dail.vermont.gov
Jonathan Wood, Manager

3749 Vermont Department of Disabilities, Aging and Independent Living
Aging and Disabilities
103 S Main St
Waterbury, VT 05671-1601　　　　　802-241-2401
　　　　　　　　　　　　　　Fax: 802-241-2325
　　　　　　　　　　　　　　　dail.vermont.gov
Susan Wehry, Commissioner
Camille George, Deputy Commissioner

3750 Vermont Department of Health: Children with Special Health Needs
Vermont Department Of Health
108 Cherry Street
Burlington, VT 05402-70　　　　　802-863-7200
　　　　　　　　　　　　　　　800-464-4343
　　　　　　　　　　　　　　Fax: 802-865-7754
　　　　　　　　　　　　　　　healthvermont.gov
Harry Chen, M.D., Commissioner
Barbara Cimaglio, Deputy Commissioner for Alcohol
Tracy Dolan, Deputy Commissioner for Public H
Multidisciplinary clinics and family support for children with chronic conditions, birth to age 21 years.

3751 Vermont Developmental Disabilities Council
103 S Main St
Waterbury, VT 05671-9800　　　　　082-241-2220
Cynthia D LaWare, Secretary
The mission of VTDDC is to facilitate connections and to promote supports that bring people with developmental disabilities into the heart of Vermont Communities.

3752 Vermont Division for the Blind & Visually Impaired
Agency of Human Svcs Dept Disabilities, Aging & IL
103 S Main St
Weeks Building
Waterbury, VT 5671-2304　　　　　802-871-3038
　　　　　　　　　　　　　　　800-405-5005
　　　　　　　　　　　　　　　888-405-5005
　　　　　　　　　　　　　　Fax: 802-871-3048
　　　　　　　　　　　　　　www.dbvi.vermont.gov
Fred Jones, Director
Scott Langley, Counselor
Heather Allen, Administrative Assistant
Offers services for the totally blind, legally blind, visually impaired, and more with health, counseling, educational, recreational, rehabilitation, computer training and professional training services.

3753 Vermont Division of Disability & Aging Services
103 S Main St
Weeks Building
Waterbury, VT 05671-1601　　　　　802-241-2401
　　　　　　　　　　　　　　Fax: 802-871-3281
　　　　　　　　　　　　　　TTY: 802-241-3557
　　　　　　　　　　　　　　　www.dail.vermont.gov
Susan Wehry, Commissioner
Marybeth McCaffrey, Director
Linda Henzel, Executive Staff Assistant
Provides services to adults and children with developmental disabilities all to the aging.

3754 Workers Compensation Board Vermont
Department of Labor
5 Green Mountain Drive
PO Box 488
Montpelier, VT 05601- 0488　　　　　802-828-2286
　　　　　　　　　　　　　　Fax: 802-828-2195
　　　　　　　　　　　　　　　labor.vermont.gov
J. Stephen Monahan, Director of Workers' Compensation & Safety
Welcome to the Vermont Department of Labor's website. VDOL's primary focus is to provide services that assist businesses, workers, and job seekers.

Virginia

3755 Aging and Disability Services
2100 Washington Blvd
4th Floor
Arlington, VA 22204　　　　　703-228-1700
　　　　　　　　　　　　　TTY: 703-228-1788
　　　　　　　　　　　　　arlaaa@arlingtonva.us
　　　　　　　　　　　aging-disability.arlingtonva.us
Anita Friedman, Director, Department of Human Services
The Aging and Disability Services Division offers care coordination, home care, and supportive services to the aging residents of Arlington. Services are provided to adults over 60, adults with developmental disabilities and their caregivers.

3756 International Dyslexia Association: Virginia Branch
3126 West Cary St.
Suite 102
Richmond, VA 23221　　　　　866-893-0583
　　　　　　　　　　　　　va.dyslexiaida.org
Lisa Snidery, President
Lisa Harrah, Vice President
Robin Hegner, Secretary
Provides free information and referral services for diagnosis and tutoring for parents, educators, physicians, and individuals with dyslexia in Illinois. Membership includes yearly journal and quarterly newsletter.

3757 Virginia Department for the Blind and Vision Impaired (DBVI)
397 Azalea Ave.
Richmond, VA 23227
804-371-3140
800-622-2155
www.vdbvi.org

Raymond E. Hopkins, Commissioner
Rick L. Mitchell, Deputy Commissioner, Services
Matt Koch, Deputy Commissioner, Enterprises
Offers services for the totally blind, legally blind, visually impaired, and more with health, counseling, educational, recreational, rehabilitation, computer training and professional training services.

3758 Virginia Department of Mental Health
P.O.Box 1797
Richmond, VA 23218-1797
804-786-3921
Fax: 804-371-6638
TTY: 804-371-8977
www.dbhds.virginia.gov

Debra Ferguson, Commissioner
John Pezzoli, Deputy Commissioner
Daniel Herr, Assistant Commissioner of Behavi
Available to citizens statewide, Virginia's public mental health, intellectual disability and substance abuse services system is comprised of 16 state facilities and 40 locally-run community services boards (CSBs) The CSBs and facilities serve children and adults who have or who are at risk of mental illness, serious emotional disturbance, intellectual disabilities, or substance abuse disorders.

3759 Virginia Developmental Disability Council
103 S Main St
Waterbury, VT 05671-9800
082-241-2220

Cynthia D LaWare, Secretary
The mission of VTDDC is to facilitate connections and to promote supports that bring people with developmental disabilities into the heart of Vermont Communities.

3760 Virginia Office Protection and Advocacy for People with Disabilities
1512 Willow Lawn
Suite 100
Richmond, VA 23230-3034
804-225-2042
800-552-3962
Fax: 804-662-7057
info@dLCV.org
disabilitylawva.org

Coleen Miller, Executive Director
LaToya Blizzard, Deputy Director
Mickie Chapman, IT Specialist
Through zealous and effective advocacy and legal representation to: protect and advance legal, human, and civil rights of persons with disabilities; combat and prevent abuse, neglect, and discrimination; and promote independence, choice, and self-determination by persons with disabilities.

3761 Virginia Office for Protection & Advocacy
5005 Mitchelldale
Suite #100
Houston, TX 77092-3034
713-574-5287
866-964-2867
Fax: 281-476-7800
info@dLCV.org

V Coleen Miller, Executive Director
Rusty Hill, Administrative Assistant
LaToya Blizzard, Deputy Director for Fiscal and O
An independent state agency that helps ensure that the rights of persons with disabiltiies in the Commonwealth are protected. The mission of DRVD is to provide zealous and effective advocacy and legal representation to protect and advance legal, human and civil rights of persons with disabilities, combat and prevent abuse, neglect and discrimination, and promote independence, choice and self-determination by persons with disabilities.

3762 Virginia Office for Protection and Advocacy
5005 Mitchelldale
Suite #100
Houston, TX 77092-3034
713-574-5287
866-964-2867
Fax: 281-476-7800
info@dLCV.org

V Coleen Miller, Executive Director
Rusty Hill, Administrative Assistant
LaToya Blizzard, Deputy Director for Fiscal and O
An independent state agency that helps ensure that the rights of persons with disabiltiies in the Commonwealth are protected. The mission of DRVD is to provide zealous and effective advocacy and legal representation to protect and advance legal, human and civil rights of persons with disabilities, combat and prevent abuse, neglect and discrimination, and promote independence, choice and self-determination by persons with disabilities.

3763 Virginia's Developmental Disabilities Planning Council
Stae Agency
1100 Bank Street
7th Floor
Richmond, VA 23219-3426
804-786-0016
800-846-4464
Fax: 804-662-7662
TTY: 800-811-7893
info@vbpd.virginia.gov
www.vaboard.org

Korinda Rusinyak, Chairman
Charles Meacham, Vice Chairman
Dennis Manning, Secretary
To create a Commonwealth that advances opportunities for independence, personal decision-making and full participation in community life for individuals with developmental disabilities.

Washington

3764 DSHS/Aging & Adult Disability Services Administration
P.O.Box 45130
Olympia, WA 98504-5130
360-902-7797
800-737-0617
Fax: 360-902-7848
TTY: 800-737-7931

Dan Murphy, Director
Bea Rector, Project Director
Tamarra Paradee, Executive Secretary
The Aging and Disability Services Administration assists children and adults with developmental delays or disabilities, cognitive impairment, chronic illness and related functional disabilities to gain access to needed services and supports by managing a system of long-term care and supportive services that are high quality, cost effective, and responsive to individual needs and preferences.

3765 Disability Rights: Washington
315 5th Avenue South
Suite 850
Seattle, WA 98104-2691
206-324-1521
800-562-2702
Fax: 206-957-0729
TTY: 206-957-0728
info@dr-wa.org
www.disabilityrightswa.org

Mark Stroh, Executive Director
David Carison, Director of Legal Advocacy
Emily Cooper, Staff Attorney
WPAS is a private, non-profit right protection agency for persons with disabilities residin in Washington state. Our advocacy services include information referral, technical assistance, training, publications and systemic advocacy.

3766 International Dyslexia Association: Washington State Branch
P.O. Box 27435
Seattle, WA 98165
info@wabida.org
wabida.org

Kristie English, President
Jessica Ruger, Vice President
Beverly Wolf, Treasurer
Provides free information and referral services for diagnosis and tutoring for parents, educators, physicians, and individuals with dyslexia in Arkansas, Idaho, Montana and Washington state. Membership includes yearly journal and quarterly newsletter.

3767 Social Security: Olympia Disability Determination
Social Security
P.O. Box 9303-MS-45550
Olympia, WA 98507
360-664-7356
800-772-1213
800-562-6074
Fax: 360-586-0851
TTY: 800-325-0778
Jennifer.Elsen@ssa.gov
www.ssa.gov

Karena L. Kilgore, Executive Secretary
Carolyn W. Colvin, Commissioner
Carolyn W. Colvin, Deputy Commissioner
We deliver services through a nationwide network of over 1,400 offices that include regional offices, field offices, card centers, teleservice centers, processing centers, hearing offices, the Appeals Council, and our State and territorial partners, the Disability Determination Services. We also have a presence in U.S. embassies around the globe. The rich diversity of our employees mirrors the public we serve.

3768 WA Department of Services for the Blind
4565 7th Avenue SE
PO Box 40959
Lacey, WA 98504-0959
206-906-5500
800-552-7103
info@dsb.wa.gov
www.dsb.wa.gov

Michael MacKillop, Acting Executive Director
Vocational rehabilitation for the blind.

3769 Washington Client Assistance Program
2531 Rainier Ave S
Seattle, WA 98144-5328
206-721-5999
800-544-2121
888-721-6072
Fax: 206-721-4537
TTY: 206-721-6072
www.washingtoncap.org

Jerry Johnson, Executive Director
Bob Huven, rehabilitation coordinator
Advocacy and information assistance for persons of disability seeking services through vocational rehabilitation or other program under the 1973 Rehabilitation Act as commented. We provide counseling.

3770 Washington Developmental Disability
2600 Martin Way E
Suite F
Olympia, WA 98506-4974
360-586-3560
800-634-4473
Fax: 360-586-2424
Ed.Holen@ddc.wa.gov
www.ddc.wa.gov

Diana Zottman, Chairman
Ed Holen, Executive Director
Brain Dahl, Support Coordinator
Developmental Disabilities Council members are appointed by the Governor to plan comprehensive services for the State of Washington's citizens with developmental disabilities.

3771 Washington Governor's Committee on Disability Issues & Employment
605 Woodland Square Loop SE
Lacey, WA 98503
360-438-3168
Fax: 928-447-6579
gcdetz@gmail.com
www.gcde.org

Martin Haule, Director
Toby Olson, Manager

3772 Washington Office of Superintendent of Public Instruction
600 Washington St. S.E.
P. O. Box 47200
Olympia, WA 98504-7200
360-725-6000
TTY: 360-644-3631
www.k12.wa.us

Randy Dorn, State Superintendent
Gil Mendoza, Deputy Superintendent
JoLynn Berge, Assistant Superintendent
The Office of Superintendent of Public Instruction (OSPI) is the primary agency charged with overseeing K-12 education in Washington state. OSPI works with the state's 296 school districts to administer basic education programs and implement education reform on behalf of more than one million public school students.

3773 Washington State Developmental Disabilities Council
2600 Martin Way E
Suite F
Olympia, WA 98506-4974
360-586-3560
800-634-4473
Fax: 360-586-2424
Ed.Holen@ddc.wa.gov
www.ddc.wa.gov

Diana Zottman, Chairman
Ed Holen, Executive Director
Brain Dahl, Support Coordinator
Developmental Disabilities Council members are appointed by the Governor to plan comprehensive services for the State of Washington's citizens with developmental disabilities.

3774 Workers Compensation Board Washington
State of Washington
7273 Linderson Way SW
Tumwater, WA 98501-5414
360-902-5800
800-547-8367
Fax: 360-902-5798
TTY: 360-902-5797
www.lni.wa.gov

Judy Schurke, Director
Lisa Rodriguez, Executive Assistant
Vickie Kennedy, Special Assistant
&I is a diverse state agency dedicated to the safety, health and security of Washington's 3.2 million workers. We help employers meet safety and health standards and we inspect workplaces when alerted to hazards. As administrators of the state's workers' compensation system, we are similar to a large insurance company, providing medical and limited wage-replacement coverage to workers who suffer job-related injuries and illness. Our rules and enforcement programs also help ensure workers are pai

West Virginia

3775 Bureau of Employment Programs Division of Workers' Compensation
State of West Virginia
407 Virginia Street East
Charleston, WV 25301-2531
304-357-0101
800-628-4265
Fax: 304-357-0788
helpdesk@kanawha.us
kanawha.us

Patricia Starkey, Manager
Vern Cormick, Manager
Michael ' Campbell, Director of IT

Kanawha County today is an exciting technology center that is earning recognition in information technology, medical research, chemical synthesis research, and telecommunications.

3776 Disability Determination Section
Ste 500
500 Quarrier St
Charleston, WV 25301-2913   304-343-5055
                                                         800-772-1213
                                                         800-344-5033
                                                    Fax: 304-353-4212
                                                            www.ssa.gov

Karena L. Kilgore, Executive Secretary
Carolyn W. Colvin, Commissioner
Carolyn W. Colvin, Deputy Commissioner
We deliver services through a nationwide network of over 1,400 offices that include regional offices, field offices, card centers, teleservice centers, processing centers, hearing offices, the Appeals Council, and our State and territorial partners, the Disability Determination Services. We also have a presence in U.S. embassies around the globe. The rich diversity of our employees mirrors the public we serve.

3777 Social Security: Charleston Disability Determination
Social Security
500 Quarrier Street
Suite 500
Charleston, WV 25301-2913   304-343-5055
                                                         800-772-1213
                                                         800-344-5033
                                                    Fax: 304-353-4212
                                                            www.ssa.gov

Karena L. Kilgore, Executive Secretary
Carolyn W. Colvin, Commissioner
Carolyn W. Colvin, Deputy Commissioner
We deliver services through a nationwide network of over 1,400 offices that include regional offices, field offices, card centers, teleservice centers, processing centers, hearing offices, the Appeals Council, and our State and territorial partners, the Disability Determination Services. We also have a presence in U.S. embassies around the globe. The rich diversity of our employees mirrors the public we serve.

3778 West Virginia Advocates
1207 Quarrier St
Suite 400
Charleston, WV 25301-1826   304-346-0847
                                                         800-950-5250
                                                    Fax: 304-346-0867
                                              kellie.l.aikman@wv.gov
                                                       wvadvocates.org

Terry Dilcher, President
John Galloway, Treasurer
Don Neurman, Secretary
West Virginia Advocates, Inc. (WVA) is the federally mandated protection and advocacy system for people with disabilities in West Virginia. WVA is a private, nonprofit agency. Our services are confidential and free of charge.

3779 West Virginia Client Assistance Program
West Virginia Advocates
1900 Kanawha Blvd E
Room 9
Charleston, WV 25305-1   304-558-3780
                                                    Fax: 304-558-4092

Clarice Hausch, Executive Director

3780 West Virginia Department of Aging
1900 Kanawha Blvd. East
Charleston, WV 25305   304-558-3317
                                                         877-987-3646
                                                    Fax: 304-558-5609
                                               www.wvseniorservices.gov

Robert E. Roswall, Commissioner
Nel Kimble
The information we offer is tailored to those who are seeking to locate programs and services for themselves or their loved ones and also for professionals who may be looking for up-to-date information relating to the field of aging.

3781 West Virginia Department of Children with Disabilities
Children with Special Health Care Needs
One Davis Square
Suite 100 East
Charleston, WV 25301- 1757   304-558-0684
                                                    Fax: 304-558-1130
                                              DHHRSecretary@wv.gov
                                                         www.dhhr.wv.gov

Douglas M. Robinson, Deputy Commissioner
Virginia Mahan, Executive Secretary
Karen Villanueva-Matkovich, General Counsel
The Bureau for Public Health directs public health activities at all levels within the state to fulfill the core functions of public health: the assessment of community health status and available resources; policy development resulting in proposals to support and encourage better health; and assurance that needed services are available, accessible, and of acceptable quality.

3782 West Virginia Department of Health
One Davis Square
Suite 100 East
Charleston, WV 25301   304-558-0684
                                                    Fax: 304-558-1130
                                              DHHRSecretary@wv.gov
                                                         www.dhhr.wv.gov

Douglas M. Robinson, Deputy Commissioner
Virginia Mahan, Executive Secretary
Karen Villanueva-Matkovich, General Counsel
The Bureau for Public Health directs public health activities at all levels within the state to fulfill the core functions of public health: the assessment of community health status and available resources; policy development resulting in proposals to support and encourage better health; and assurance that needed services are available, accessible, and of acceptable quality.

3783 West Virginia Developmental Disabilities Council
110 Stockton St
Charleston, WV 25387   304-558-0416
                                                    . Fax: 304-558-0941
                                                    TTY: 304-558-2376
                                                 dhhrwvddc@wv.gov
                                                         www.ddc.wv.gov

Diana Zottman, Chairman
Ed Holen, Executive Director
Brain Dahl, Support Coordinator
Working to assure that West Virginians with developmental disabilities receive the services, supports, and other forms of assistance they need to exercise self-determination and achieve independence, productivity, integration, and inclusion in the community.
6-8 pages Quarterly Newsl

3784 West Virginia Division of Rehabilitation Services
107 Capitol Street
Charleston, WV 25301-2609   304-356-2060
                                                         800-642-8207
                                                         www.wvdrs.org

Donna L. Ashworth, Acting Director
Kay Goodwin, Cabinet Secretary
DRS' mission is to enable and empower individuals with disabilities to work and to live independently.

Wisconsin

3785 Disability Rights Wisconsin: Milwaukee Office
Ste 3230
6737 W Washington St
Milwaukee, WI 53214-5651   414-773-4646
                                                         800-708-3034
                                                    Fax: 414-773-4647
                                                    TTY: 888-758-6049
                                                            info@drwi.org
                                                   disabilityrightswi.org

Ted Skemp, President
Beth Moss, Vice President
Susan Gramling, Secretary
The protection and advocacy agency for people with disabilities in Wisconsin. DRW provides guidance, advice, investigation, ne-

gotiation and in some cases legal representation to people with disabilities and their families. Local and state level systems advocacy and training are also provided.

3786 International Dyslexia Association: Wisconsin Branch
1616 Graham Ave.
Eau Claire, WI 54701   608-355-0911
                                        wi.dyslexiaida.org

Tammy Tillotson, President
Kimberly Chan, Treasurer
Pattie Huse, Secretary
Provides free information and referral services for diagnosis and tutoring for parents, educators, physicians, and individuals with dyslexia in Illinois. Membership includes yearly journal and quarterly newsletter.

3787 Social Security: Madison Field Office
6011 Odana Rd
Madison, WI 53719-1101   866-770-2262
                                        800-772-1213
                                        Fax: 608-270-1021
                                        TTY: 800-325-0778
                                        wi.fo.madison@ssa.gov
                                        www.ssa.gov

3788 West Virginia Department of Health
One Davis Square
Suite 100 East
Charleston, WV 25301   304-558-0684
                                        800-441-4576
                                        Fax: 304-558-1130
                                        DHHRSecretary@wv.gov
                                        www.dhhr.wv.gov

Rocco S. Fucillo, Cabinet Secretary
Susan Shelton Perry, Deputy Secretary for Legal Servi
Ellen Cannon, Privacy Officer
The Department of Health and Family Services operates the federal Title V Maternal and Child Health Block Grant Program for Children with Special Health Care Needs. The program provides program monitoring, consultation and technical assistance to five regional CSHCN centers throughout Wisconsin; a Birth Defects Monitoring and Surveillance Program and a Universal Newborn Hearing Screening Program.

3789 Wisconsin Board for People with Developmental Disabilities (WBPDD)
201 W Washington Ave
Suite 111
Madison, WI 53703-2796   608-266-7826
                                        888-332-1677
                                        Fax: 608-267-3906
                                        TTY: 608-266-6660
                                        wcdd.org

Jennifer Ondrejka, Manager
Joshua Ryf, Office Manager
Statewide systems advocacy group for people with developmental disabilities in Wisconsin.

3790 Wisconsin Bureau of Aging
State Office of Wisconsin
1 West Wilson Street
Madison, WI 53703   608-266-1865
                                        Fax: 608-267-3203
                                        TTY: 888-701-1251
                                        DHSwebmaster@wisconsin.gov

Donna Mc Dowell, Executive Director
Gail Schwersenska, Section Chief
Dennis G. Smith, Secretary
Keeps and updates information and printed materials on senior housing directories, nursing home listings, and home care agencies.

3791 Wisconsin Coalition for Advocacy: Madison Office
16 N Carroll St
Suite 400
Madison, WI 53703-2762   608-267-0214
                                        800-928-8778
                                        Fax: 608-267-0368

Kim Hogan, Intake Specialist
Mr Lynn Breedlove, Executive Director

The protection and advocacy agency for people with disabilities in Wisconsin. WCA provides guidance, advice, investigation, negotiation and in some cases legal representation to people with disabilities and their families. Local and state level systems advocacy and training are also provided.

3792 Wisconsin Governor's Committee for People with Disabilities
1 West Wilson Street
Madison, WI 53703   608-266-1865
                                        877-865-3432
                                        Fax: 608-266-3386
                                        TTY: 888-701-1251
                                        DHSwebmaster@wisconsin.gov

Donna Mc Dowell, Executive Director
Gail Schwersenska, Section Chief
Dennis G. Smith, Secretary
To advise the Governor and state agencies on problems faced by people with disabilities; to review legislation affecting people with disabilities; to promote effective operation of publicly-administered or supported programs serving people with disabilities; to promote the collection, dissemination and incorporation of adequate information about persons with disabilities for purposes of public planning at all levels of government.

3793 Workers Compensation Board Wisconsin
Room C100, 201 E. Washington Avenue
P. O. Box 7901
Madison, WI 53707-7901   608-266-1340
                                        Fax: 608-267-0394
                                        dwd.wisconsin.gov/wc

Reggie Newson, Secretary
Jonathan Barry, Deputy Secretary
John Metcalf, Division Administrator
The Worker's Compensation Division administers programs designed to ensure that injured workers receive required benefits from insurers or self-insured employers; encourage rehabilitation and reemployment for injured workers; and promote the reduction of work-related injuries, illnesses, and deaths.

Wyoming

3794 Social Security: Cheyenne Disability Determination
Social Security
821 W Pershing Blvd
Cheyenne, WY 82002-1   307-777-7341
                                        800-438-5788
                                        Fax: 307-637-0247
                                        Jeff.Graham@ssa.gov
                                        ssa.gov

Karena L. Kilgore, Executive Secretary
Carolyn W. Colvin, Commissioner
Carolyn W. Colvin, Deputy Commissioner
We deliver services through a nationwide network of over 1,400 offices that include regional offices, field offices, card centers, teleservice centers, processing centers, hearing offices, the Appeals Council, and our State and territorial partners, the Disability Determination Services. We also have a presence in U.S. embassies around the globe. The rich diversity of our employees mirrors the public we serve.

3795 WY Department of Health: Mental Health and Substance Abuse Service Division
401 Hathaway Building
Cheyenne, WY 82002-1   307-777-7656
                                        800-535-4006
                                        Fax: 307-777-7439
                                        TTY: 307-777-5581
                                        www.health.wyo.gov

Thomas O. Forslund, Director
Lee Clabots, Deputy Director
Bob Peck, Chief Financial Officer
State office responsible for purchase of service and program development policy.

3796   Workers Compensation Board Wyoming
350 South Washington Street
PO Box 1068
Afton, WY 83110-3004   307-886-9260
                              Fax: 307-886-9269

3797   Wyoming Client Assistance Program
Protection and Advocacy System
2nd Fl
320 W 25th St
Cheyenne, WY 82001-3069   307-632-2682
                              877-854-5041
                              Fax: 307-638-0815
                              wypanda@vcn.com
                                        ap.org

Jeanne Thobro, Manager
Jeanne A Thobro, Executive Director

3798   Wyoming Department of Aging
State Department of Wyoming
401 Hathaway Building
Cheyenne, WY 82002-1   307-777-7656
                              800-442-2766
                              Fax: 307-777-7439
                              wyaging@wyo.gov
                              health.wyo.gov

Thomas O. Forslund, Director
Lee Clabots, Deputy Director
Bob Peck, Chief Financial Officer
The Wyoming Department of Health's Aging Division is committed to providing care, ensuring safety and and promoting independent choices for Wyoming's older adults

3799   Wyoming Developmental Disability Council
122 W 25th St
1st. Fl. West, Herschler Building,
Cheyenne, WY 82002   307-777-7230
                              800-438-5791
                              Fax: 307-777-5690
                              wgcdd@wyo.gov

Shannon Buller, Executive Director
Von Maul, Administrative Assistant
Sam Janney, Public Information Officer
Our purpose is to assure that individuals with developmental disabilities and their families participate in and have access to needed community services, individualized supports and other forms of assistance that promote independence, productivity, integration and inclusion in all facets of community life.

3800   Wyoming Protection & Advocacy for Persons with Disabilities
7344 Stockman Street
Cheyenne, WY 82009   307-632-3496
                              Fax: 307-638-0815
                              wypanda@wypanda.com
                              wypanda.com

Tori Rosenthal, President
Jeanne A Thobro, Executive Director
Wyoming Protection & Advocacy System, Inc. (P&A), established in 1977, is the official non-profit corporation authorized to implement certain mandates of several federal laws. Enacted by Congress, these laws provide various protection and advocacy services.

Independent Living Centers

Alabama

3801 Birdie Thornton Center
2350 Hine Street
Athens, AL 35611   256-232-0366
                                Fax: 256-230-9398

Kristy Allen King, Program Director
Heather Mereidth, Program Professional, QMRP
Rabieb Clem, Senior Aid
The Birdie Thornton Center is devoted to providing care, education, and training to adults with developmental delays and disabilities.

3802 Independent Living Center of Mobile
5301 Moffett Rd
Suite 110
Mobile, AL 36618-2926   251-460-0301
                                 Fax: 251-341-1267
                                 TTY: 251-460-2872
                                 Michaeld@ilcmobile.org
                                 ilcmobile.org

Michael Davis, Executive Director
Darmita Flood, Administrative Assistant
Barbara Hattier, ILS/Transportation Coordinator
Helping people with disabilities become independent.

3803 Independent Living Resources Of Greater Birmingham: Alabaster
120 Plaza Cir, Suite C
P. O. Box 2048
Alabaster, AL 35007-7034   205-685-0570
                                 Fax: 205-251-0605
                                 TTY: 205-685-0570
                                 www.ilrgb.org

Kathy Lovell, President
Phil Klebine, Vice President
Susan Parker, Secretary
The mission of this Independent Living Center is to empower people with disabilities to fully participate in the community.

3804 Independent Living Resources of Greater Birmingham: Jasper
300 Birmingham Ave
PO Box 434
Jasper, AL 35502-3811   205-387-0159
                                 Fax: 205-387-0162
                                 TTY: 205-387-0159
                                 www.ilrgb.org

Kathy Lovell, President
Phil Klebine, Vice President
Susan Parker, Secretary
The purpose of this Independent Living Center is to empower people with disabilities to fully participate in the community.

3805 Independent Living Resources of Greater Birmingham
1418 6th Avenue North
Birmingham, AL 35203-1317   205-251-2223
                                 Fax: 205-251-0605
                                 TTY: 205-251-2223

Kathy Lovell, President
Phil Klebine, Vice President
Susan Parker, Secretary
The mission of this Independent Living Center is to empower people with disabilities to fully participate in the community.

3806 Montgomery Center for Independent Living
600 S Court St
Montgomery, AL 36104-4106   334-240-2520
                                 Fax: 334-240-6869
                                 TTY: 334-240-2520
                                 mcil@bellsouth.net
                                 www.cilmontgomery.org

Scott Renner, Executive Director
Barbara F. Crozier, President
Kenneth Marshall, Vice President

Encourgaes people with disabilities to support one another in reaching their own independent living goals.

3807 State of Alabama Independent Living/Homebound Service (SAIL)
Alabama Department of Rehabilitation Services
602 S. Lawrence St.
Montgomery, AL 36104   www.rehab.alabama.gov
The following services are provided to Alabamians with significant disabilities: specialized in-home education and counseling; attendant care; training; and medical services.

Alaska

3808 Access Alaska: ADA Partners Project
1217 East 10th Ave
Suite 105
Anchorage, AK 99501-2044   907-248-4777
                                 800-770-4488
                                 888-462-1444
                                 Fax: 907-263-1942
                                 TTY: 907-248-8799
                                 info@accessalaska.org
                                 accessalaska.org

Lorali Simon, President
Mike O'Neill, Vice President
Jim Duffield, Treasurer
Assisting Alaskans with disabilities to live independently in the community of their choice.

3809 Access Alaska: Fairbanks
526 Gaffney Rd
Suite 100
Fairbanks, AK 99701-4914   907-479-7940
                                 800-770-7940
                                 Fax: 907-474-4052
                                 TTY: 907-474-8619
                                 info@accessalaska.org
                                 accessalaska.org

Lorali Simon, President
Mike O'Neill, Vice President
Jim Duffield, Treasurer
A local non profit agency using its resources to actively promote a society where persons with disabilities can live and work independently in the community of their choice.

3810 Access Alaska: Mat-Su
1075 Check St,
Suite 109
Wasilla, AK 99654-6937   907-357-2588
                                 800-770-0228
                                 Fax: 907-357-5585
                                 info@accessalaska.org
                                 accessalaska.org

Lorali Simon, President
Mike O'Neill, Vice President
Jim Duffield, Treasurer
Provides independent living services to persons with significant disabilities. Mission is to encourage and promote the total integration of persons with disabilities into the community of their choice. Services include independent living skills training, information and referral, advocacy, peer support, and at home modifications.

3811 Alaska SILC
Ste 206
1217 East 10th Ave
Anchorage, AK 99501-1760   907-248-4777
                                 800-770-4488
                                 888-294-7452
                                 Fax: 907-263-1942
                                 info@accessasilc.org
                                 www.alaskasilc.org

Jim Beck, Executive Director
Lorali Simon, President
Mike O'Neill, Vice President
The Alaska Statewide Independent Living is committed to promoting a philosophy of consumer control, peer support, self help, self determination, equal access, and individual and systems ad-

vocacy, in order to maximize leadership, empowerment, independence, productivity, and to support full inclusion and integration of individuals with disabilities into the mainstream of American society.

3812 Arctic Access
P.O.Box 930
Kotzebue, AK 99752-930

907-412-0695
877-442-2393
TTY: 907-442-2393

Roger Wright Jr, Executive Director
Russell Williams, Jr,, Elder & Disability Resource Coor
Audrey Aanes
The Arctic Access Independent Living Center provides services and opportunities for elders and others with disabilities so they may remain in their village and be as active as possible with their families and commuties in the North West Arctic and Bering Straits Regions of Alaska.

3813 Hope Community Resources
540 W Intl Airport Rd
Anchorage, AK 99518-1105

907-561-5335
800-478-0078
Fax: 907-564-7429
info@hopealaska.org
hopealaska.org

Robert Owens, President
John Dittrich, Vice President
Eugene 'Gene' Bates, Treasurer
Provider of services to individuals who experience a disability.

3814 Kenai Peninsula Independent Living Center
265 E. Pioneer Suite 201
P.O.Box 2474
Homer, AK 99603- 2474

907-235-7911
800-770-7911
Fax: 907-235-6236
peninsulailc.org

Candy Norman, President
Mike Harmer, Vice President
Offers peer counseling, disability education and awareness, attendant care registry and information on accessible housing.

3815 Kenai Peninsula Independent Living Center: Seward
201 Third Avenue, Suite 101Bs
P. O. Box 3523
Seward, AK 99664-3523

907-224-8711
Fax: 907-224-7793
www.peninsulailc.org

Candy Norman, President
Mike Harmer, Vice President
Offers peer counseling, disability, education and awareness, attendant care registry and information on accessible housing.

3816 Keni Peninsula Independent Living Center: Central Peninsula
47255 Princeton Avenue
Suite 8
Soldotna, AK 99669

907-262-6333
Fax: 907-260-4495
www.peninsulailc.org

Candy Norman, President
Mike Harmer, Vice President
Offers peer counseling, disability education and awareness, attendant care registry and information on accessible housing.

3817 Southeast Alaska Independent Living
3225 Hospital Drive
Suite 300
Juneau, AK 99801-7863

907-586-4920
800-478-7245
Fax: 907-586-4980
TTY: 907-523-5285
info@sailinc.org
sailinc.org

Robert Purvis, President
Jeff Irwin, Vice President
Suzanne Williams, Secretary
To empower consumers with disabilities by providing services and information to support them in making choices that will positively affect their independence and productivity in society.

3818 Southeast Alaska Independent Living: Ketchikan
602 Dock St
Suite 107
Ketchikan, AK 99901-6574

907-225-4735
888-452-7245
Fax: 907-247-4735
ketchikan@sailinc.org
www.sailinc.org

Robert Purvis, President
Jeff Irwin, Vice President
Suzanne Williams, Secretary
To empower consumers with disabilities by providing services and information to support them in making choices that will positively affect their independence and productivity in society.

3819 Southeast Alaska Independent Living: Sitka
514 Lake St
Suite C
Sitka, AK 99835-7405

907-747-6859
888-500-7245
Fax: 907-747-6783
sitka@sailinc.org
www.sailinc.org

Robert Purvis, President
Jeff Irwin, Vice President
Suzanne Williams, Secretary
To empower consumers with disabilities by providing services and information to support them in making choices that will positively affect their independence and productivity in society.

Arizona

3820 ASSIST! to Independence
P.O.Box 4133
Tuba City, AZ 86045-4133

928-283-6261
888-848-1449
Fax: 928-283-6284
TTY: 928-283-6672
assist01@frontiernet.net
www.assisttoindependence.org

Michael Blatchford, Executive Director
Priscilla Lane, IL Services Coordinator/Dep Dir
A community based, American Indian owned and operated non-profit agency that was established by and for people with disabilities and chronic health conditions to help fill some of the gaps in service delivery.

3821 Arizona Bridge to Independent Living
5025 E Washington St
Suite 200
Phoenix, AZ 85034-7439

602-256-2245
800-280-2245
Fax: 602-254-6407
www.abil.org

Mary Slaughter, Chairman
Brad Wemhaner, Vice Chairman
Michael Somsan, Secretary
ABIL offers and promotes programs designed to empower people with disabilities to take personal responsibility so they may achieve or continue independent lifestyles within the community.

3822 Arizona Bridge to Independent Living: Phoenix
1229 E.Washington St.
Suite D405
Phoenix, AZ 85034

602-296-0551
800-280-2245
Fax: 602-256-0184
TTY: 602-296-0591
www.abil.org

Mary Slaughter, Chairman
Brad Wemhaner, Vice Chairman
Michael Somsan, Secretary
ABIL offers and promotes programs designed to empower people with disabilities to take personal responsibility so they may achieve or continue independent lifestyles within the community.

3823   Arizona Bridge to Independent Living: Mesa
2150 S Country Club Dr
Suite 10
Mesa, AZ 85210-6879   480-655-9750
                                               800-280-2245
                                          Fax: 480-655-9751
                                          TTY: 480-655-9750
                                               www.abil.org

Mary Slaughter, Chairman
Brad Wemhaner, Vice Chairman
Michael Somsan, Secretary
ABIL offers and promotes programs designed to empower people
with disabilities to take personal responsibility so they may
achieve or continue independent lifestyles within the community.

3824   Community Outreach Program for the Deaf
268 W Adams St
Tucson, AZ 85705-6534   520-792-1906
                                          Fax: 520-770-8554
                                          TTY: 520-792-1906
                                          request@copdaz.org
                                               copdaz.org

Anne Levy, Executive Director
A non-profit organization, which has been serving the needs of
people in Southern Arizona who are deaf or hard of hearing.

3825   DIRECT Center for Independence
1001 N Alvernon Way
Tucson, AZ 85711   520-624-6452
                                               800-342-1853
                                          Fax: 520-792-1438
                                          direct@directilc.org
                                               www.directilc.org

Vicki Cuscino, President
A non-consumer directed, community-based advocacy organization, that promotes independent living and offers a variety of programs for all people with disabilities which encourage them to
achieve their full potential and to participate in the community.

**3826   New Horizons Independent Living Center: Prescott
Valley**
8085 E Manley Dr
Prescott Valley, AZ 86314-6154   928-772-1266
                                               800-406-2377
                                          Fax: 928-772-3808
                                          TTY: 928-772-1266

Deborah Henderson, Office Manager
Liz Toone, Executive Director
Nick Perry, President
To provide services and advocacy which empower and enable
people with disabilities to self-determine the goals and activities
of their lives.

**3827   Services Maximizing Independent Living and
Empowerment (SMILE)**
1931 South Arizona Ave
Suite 4
Yuma, AZ 85364-5721   928-329-6681
                                               855-209-8363
                                          Fax: 928-329-6715
                                          TTY: 928-782-7458
                                          info@smile-az.org
                                               www.smile-az.org

Laura Duval, Executive Director
Brenda Howard, Finance Manager/ Admin Assistant
Shawnnita Miranda, Advocate/ Home modification Mana
SMILE continually advocates for the Independent Living Philosophy, both individually and system wide. The Board and staff
constantly strives to improve the system by writing letters, training staff, providing services, and creating public awareness as to
the services and opportunities open to people who have
disabilities.

3828   Sterling Ranch: Residence for Special Women
Sterling Ranch
P.O.Box 36
Skull Valley, AZ 86338-36   928-442-3289
                                          Fax: 928-442-9272
                                               www.sterlingranch.info

Russell Dryer, Executive Director
Trent Nichel, Manager

A nonprofit residence for women with developmental disabilities
which has been in operation since 1947. As a small facility (19
residents) the orientation is personal and family-like. Offers activities that range from gardening, quilting, academics, sign-language, crafts and a myriad of field trips and excursions. Private
rooms and spacious living on 4 1/2 acres.

Arkansas

3829   Arkansas Independent Living Council
11324 Arcade Drive
Suite 7
Little Rock, AR 72212   501-372-0607
                                               800-772-0607
                                          Fax: 501-372-0598
                                          arkansasilc@att.net
                                               www.ar-silc.org

Sha Stephens, Executive Director
Cheryl, Director
Brenda Stinebuck, Chair
A non-profit organization promoting independent living for peo-
ple with disabilities.

3830   Delta Resource Center for Independent Living
11324 Arcade Drive
Little Rock, AR 72212-6249   501-372-0607
                                               800-772-0607
                                          Fax: 501-372-0598
                                          drcilar@yahoo.com
                                               www.ar-silc.org

Sha Stephens, Executive Director
Katy Morris, Director
Cheryl, Director
Provides services, support, and advocacy which enables people
with severe disabilities to live as independently as possible
within their family and community.

3831   Mainstream
300 S Rodney Parham Rd.
Suite 5
Little Rock, AR 72205   501-280-0012
                                               800-371-9026
                                          Fax: 501-280-9267
                                          TTY: 501-280-9262
                                               www.mainstreamilrc.com

Rita Byers, Executive Director
A non-residential, consumer-driven independent living resource
center for persons with disabilities. Mainstream operates with the
conviction that people with disabilities have the right and responsibility to make choices, to control their lives and to participate
fully and equally in the community. Mainstream offers the following services free of charge: Advocacy, Peer Support, Training
and Education, Information and Referral, Ramp program, and
more.
1988

3832   Our Way: The Cottage Apt Homes
9175 Greenback Lane
Orangevale, CA 95662-6616   501-225-5030
                                               888-879-9584
                                          Fax: 501-225-5190
                                               rentthecottages.com

Katrina Williams, Manager
Crystal Brown, Assistant Manager
Advocacy and information services. One bedroom apartments for
mobility impaired and elderly 62 years or older persons.
Based on income

3833   Sources for Community IL Services
1918 N Birch Ave
Fayetteville, AR 72703-2408   479-442-5600
                                               888-284-7521
                                          Fax: 479-442-5192
                                          TTY: 479-251-1378
                                          jmather@arsources.org
                                               www.arsources.org

Brent Williams, PhD, President
Elise Burt, Treasurer
Burke Fanari, Secretary

Provides services, support, and advocacy for individuals with disabilities, their families and the community.

3834   Spa Area Independent Living Services
621 Albert Pike
Hot Springs, AR 71913   501-624-7710
                                               800-255-7549
                                          Fax: 501-624-7003

Dejan S. Vojnovic, President
Joseph E. Anderson, Vice President - Real Estate
Bryan S. Cox, Vice President - Technology
Provides services and advocacy by and for persons with all types of disabilities. The goal is to assist individuals with disabilities to achieve thier maximum potential within their families and communities.

California

3835   Access Center of San Diego
8885 Rio San Diego Dr
Suite 131
San Diego, CA 92108-1625   619-293-3500
                                               800-300-4326
                                          Fax: 619-293-3508
                                          TTY: 619-293-7757
                                              info@a2isd.org
                                              www.a2isd.org

Louis Frick, Executive Director
Derek Parker, Chair
Jacquelyn E. Nash, Vice Chair
Access to Independence is an independent living center (ILC), a nonresidential, cross-disability, non-profit corporations that provide services to people with disabilities to help maximize their independence and fully integrate into their communities. Access to Independence is one of 391 ILCs across the country and one of 29 serving Californians. Like all ILCs, Access to Independence offers required federal and state programs and services to people of all disability types and ages at no charge.

3836   Access to Independence
8885 Rio San Diego Drive
Suite 131
San Diego, CA 92108- 1625   619-293-3500
                                               800-300-4326
                                          Fax: 619-293-3508
                                          TTY: 619-293-7757
                                              info@a2isd.org
                                              www.a2isd.org

Louis Frick, Executive Director
Derek Parker, Chair
Jacquelyn E. Nash, Vice Chair
A community resource for people with disabilities to lead independent lives.

3837   Access to Independence of Imperial Valley
101 Hacienda Drive
Suite 13
Calexico, CA 92231-2875   760-768-2044
                                               866-976-3515
                                          Fax: 760-768-4977
                                          TTY: 619-293-7757
                                              info@a2isd.org
Louis Frick, Executive Director
Derek Parker, Chair
Jacquelyn E. Nash, Vice Chair
A community resource for people with disabilities to lead independent lives.

3838   Access to Independence of North County
209 E Broadway
Vista, CA 92084-6005   760-643-0447
                                          Fax: 760-435-9206
                                              info@a2isd.org
Louis Frick, Executive Director
Derek Parker, Chair
Jacquelyn E. Nash, Vice Chair
A community resource for people with disabilities to lead independent lives.

3839   Beaumont Senior Center: Community Access Center
1310 Oak Valley Parkway
Beaumont, CA 92223-2218   951-769-8524
                                          Fax: 951-769-8519
                                          TTY: 909-769-2794
Laurie Hoirup, Director
A non profit organization; one of 29 similar programs throughout the state of California CAC is a community resource, advocate, and educator for Riverside County residents with disabilities.

3840   California Foundation For Independent Living Centers
1234 H Street
Suite 100
Sacramento, CA 95814-1912   916-325-1690
                                          Fax: 916-325-1699
                                          TTY: 916-325-1695
                                              cfilc@cfilc.org
                                              www.cfilc.org
Robert Hand, Chairperson
Ana Acton, Vice Chairperson
Tink Miller, Executive Director
Community Rehabilitation Services, Inc. (CRS) is a private, non-profit agency established in 1974 to assist persons with disabilities within the East/North East areas of Los Angeles County to enhance their options for living independently. Any person who is 18 yrs of age or more with physical, sensory, mental/emotional or developmental disabilities can work with us to become more self-sufficient. Our intake procedures provide an orientation to the staff, facilities and services at CRS.

3841   California Foundation for Independent Living Centers
1235 H Street
Suite 100
Sacramento, CA 95814-1913   916-325-1690
                                          Fax: 916-325-1699
                                          TTY: 916-325-1695
                                              cfilc@cfilc.org
                                              www.cfilc.org
Robert Hand, Chairperson
Ana Acton, Vice Chairperson
Tink Miller, Executive Director
CFILC's mission is to support independent living centers in their local communities through advocating for systems change and promoting access and integration for people with disabilities.

3842   California State Independent Living Council (SILC)
1235 H Street
Suite 100
Sacramento, CA 95814-4010   916-325-1690
                                               866-866-7452
                                          Fax: 916-325-1699
                                          TTY: 866-745-2889
                                              www.calsilc.org
Susan M. Madison, Chairman
Eli Gelardin, Vice Chairman
Liz Pazdral, Executive Director
To maximize options for independence for persons with disabilities

3843   Center for Independence of the Disabled
Suite 103
2001 Winward Way
San Mateo, CA 94404-3062   650-645-1780
                                          Fax: 650-645-1785
                                          TTY: 650-522-9313
                                          http://www.cidsanmateo.org
Brad Friedman, Co-President
Laura Whitsitt Hillyard, Co-President
Thomas J. Devine, Vice President
Increase the social, educational, and economic participation of persons with disabilities in San Mateo County, and to encourage, support, and provide options for self determination, equal access and freedom of choice.

3844 Center for Independence of the Disabled- Daly City
Ste 256
355 Gellert Blvd
Daly City, CA 94015-2675

650-991-5124
Fax: 650-757-2075
TTY: 650-991-5182
dalycity5@aol.com
www.cidbelmont.org

Kent Mickelson, Director
The Daly City Branch office fulfills its mission by serving disabled consumers in Brisbane, Colma, Daly City, El Granada, Half Moon Bay, Montara, Moss Beach, Pacifica, Pescadero, Princeton and South San Francisco. Our mission is to increase the social, educational, economic, social and political participants of persons with disabilities in San Mateo county, California.

3845 Center for Independent Living
Suite 103
2001 Winward Way
San Mateo, CA 94404

650-645-1780
Fax: 650-645-1785
TTY: 510-522-9313
bburgess@cilberkeley.org
www.cidsanmateo.org

Beatrice Burgess, Interim Executive Director
Jody Yarborough, President
Michael Levinson, Vice President
The Center for Independent Living, Inc (CIL) is a national leader in helping people with disabilities live independently and become productive members of society. Advocates for greater accessibility in communities, designing techniques in independent living and providing direct services to people with disabilities.
1972

3846 Center for Independent Living: East Oakland
Suite 100
3075 Adeline Street
Berkeley, CA 94703-2403

510-841-4776
Fax: 510-841-6168
info@cilberkeley.org
www.cilberkeley.org

Melissa Male, Chair
Bea Worthen, Vice-Chair
Paul Hippolitus, Secretary
A national leader in helping people with disabilities live independently and become productive, fully participating members of society.

3847 Center for Independent Living: Oakland
Suite 100
3075 Adeline Street
Berkeley, CA 94703-1285

510-841-4776
Fax: 510-841-6168
TTY: 510-444-1837
info@cilberkeley.org
cilberkeley.org

Melissa Male, Chair
Bea Worthen, Vice-Chair
Paul Hippolitus, Secretary
A national leader in supporting disabled people in their efforts to lead independent lives.

3848 Center for Independent Living: Tri-County
2822 Harris Street
Eureka, CA 95503

707-445-8404
877-576-5000
Fax: 707-445-9751
TTY: 707-445-8405
aa@tilinet.org
www.tilinet.org

Gail Pascoe, President
Linda Arnold, Vice President
Kevin O'Brien, Treasurer

3849 Center for Independent Living:Fresno
3475 Wesy Shaw Ave
Suite 101
Fresno, CA 93711

559-276-6777
Fax: 559-276-6778
TTY: 559-276-6779

Bob Hand, Manager

3850 Center for Independent Living; Oakland
1904 Franklin Street
Suite 320
Oakland, CA 94612-2324

510-763-9990
Fax: 510-763-4910
TTY: 510-536-2271
info@cilberkeley.org
cilberkeley.org

Melissa Male, Chair
Bea Worthen, Vice-Chair
Hank Stratford, Treasurer
Independent living center to maximise the options for independence for persons with disabilities.

3851 Center of Independent Living: Visalia
121 E Main
Suite 101
Visalia, CA 93291-6262

559-622-9276
Fax: 559-622-9638

Fran Phillips, Executive Directorram Manager
Renee Ezelle, Manager

3852 Central Coast Center for IL: San Benito
1234 H Street
Suite 100
Sacramento, CA 95814-1914

916-325-1690
Fax: 916-325-1699
TTY: 916-325-1695
www.cfilc.org

Ana Acton, Chairperson
Larry Grable, Vice Chairperson
Nayana Shah, Treasurer
To advocate for barrier-free access and equal opportunity for people with disabilities to participate in the community life by increasing the capacity of Independent Living Centers to achieve their missions.

3853 Central Coast Center for Independent Living
318 Cayuga St.
Suite 208
Salinas, CA 93901-2600

831-757-2968
Fax: 831-757-5549
TTY: 831-757-3949
cccil.org

Jennifer L. Williams, President
Elsa Quezada, Executive Director
Brenda Cardoza, Information and Referral Special
CCCIL promotes the independence of people with disabilities by supporting their equal and full participation in community life. CCCIL provides advocacy, education and support to all people with disabilities, their families and the community.

3854 Central Coast Center: Independent Living - Santa Cruz Office
1350 - 41st Avenue
Suite 101
Capitola, CA 95010-3930

831-462-8720
Fax: 831-462-8727
TTY: 831-462-8729
www.cccil.org

Jennifer L. Williams, President
Elsa Quezada, Executive Director
Brenda Cardoza, Information and Referral Special
CCCIL promotes the independence of people with disabilities by supporting their equal and full participation in community life. CCCIL provides advocacy, education and support to all people with disabilities, their families and the community.

3855 Central Coast for Independent Living
1111 San Felipe Rd
Suite 107
Hollister, CA 95023-2814

831-636-5196
Fax: 831-637-0478
TTY: 831-637-6235
www.cccil.org

Jennifer L. Williams, President
Elsa Quezada, Executive Director
Brenda Cardoza, Information and Referral Special
CCCIL promotes the independence of people with disabilities by supporting their equal and full particpation in community life.

CCCIL provides advocacy, education and support to all people with disabilities, their families and the community.

3856 Central Coast for Independent Living: Watsonville
18 W. Beach St.
Suite Y
Watsonville, CA 95076-4371

831-724-2997
Fax: 831-724-2915
TTY: 831-786-0915
www.cccil.org

Jennifer L. Williams, President
Elsa Quezada, Executive Director
Brenda Cardoza, Information and Referral Special

An advocacy and information center organized by and for people with disabilities that strives to make our communities more accessible and to empower people with disabilities with information and skills to live fulfilling lives in our communities.

3857 Communities Actively Living Independent and Free
634 S Spring St
2nd Floor
Los Angeles, CA 90014-3921

213-627-0477
Fax: 213-627-0535
TTY: 213-623-9502
info@calif-ilc.org

Lillibeth Navarro, Founder & Executive Director
Alex San Martin, Temporary Chair
Fernando Roldan, Board Secretary

Envisions a culturally diverse independent living center designed to empower the Disability Community.

3858 Community Access Center
6848 Magnolia Ave
Suite 150
Riverside, CA 92506-2858

951-274-0358
Fax: 951-274-0833
TTY: 951-274-0834
execdir@ilcac.org
www.ilcac.org

Mark Dyer, President
Janet Newcomer, Vice President
Perry Halteman, Secretary

A non-profit organization; one of 29 similar programs throughout the state of California. CAC is a community resource, advocate, and educator for Riverside County residents with disabilities.

3859 Community Access Center: Indio Branch
83233 Indio Blvd
Indio, CA 92201-4748

760-347-4888
Fax: 760-347-0722
TTY: 760-347-6802
pmgr3@ilcac.org
www.ilcac.org

Mark Dyer, President
Janet Newcomer, Vice President
Perry Halteman, Secretary

To empower persons with disabilities to control their own lives, create an accessible community and advocate to achieve complete social, economic, and political integration. We implement this vision by providing information, supportive services and independent living skills training.

3860 Community Access Center: Perris
371 Wilkerson Ave
Perris, CA 92570-2241

951-443-1158
Fax: 951-443-2608
TTY: 951-443-1158
www.ilcac.org

Mark Dyer, President
Janet Newcomer, Vice President
Perry Halteman, Secretary

Community Access Center empowers persons with disabilities to control their own lives, create an accessible community and advocate to achieve complete social, economic, and political integration. CAC also implements this vision by providing information, supportive services and independent living skills training.

3861 Community Rehabilitation Services
844 E. Mission Road
Suite A & B
San Gabriel, CA 91776- 2759

323-266-0453
Fax: 626-614-1590
TTY: 323-266-3016

Frances Garcia, Executive Director

CRS is an independent living center that provides free services to persons with disabilities in the areas of advocacy, housing and independent living skills; assistive technology, employment, personal assistant services, peer counseling and information and referral.

3862 Community Resources for Independence: Mendocino/Lake Branch
Ste B
415 Talmage Rd
Ukiah, CA 95482-7486

707-463-8875
Fax: 707-463-8878
TTY: 707-463-4498

Tanner Silva, Manager

A non-profit corporation established by a group of disabled and non-disabled individuals to advance the rights of persons with disabilities to equal justice, access, opportunity and participation in the communities.

3863 Community Resources for Independence: Napa
Ste 208
1040 Main St
Napa, CA 94559-2605

707-258-0270
Fax: 707-258-0275
TTY: 707-257-0274

Tyler Stanley, Manager
Matthew Shultz, Independent Living Advocate

A non-profit corporation established by a group of disabled and non-disabled individuals to advance the rights of persons with disabilities to equal justice, access, opportunity and participation in the communities.

3864 Community Resources for Independent Living: Hayward
3311 Pacific Ave
Livermore, CA 94550-5013

925-371-1531
Fax: 925-373-5034
TTY: 925-371-1533
info@cril-online.org
crilhayward.org

Sheri Burns, Executive Director
Michael Galvan, PhD., Program Director
April Monroe, Finance Director

CRIL offers independent living services at no charge to persons with disabilities living in southern and eastern Alameda county. CRIL is also a resource for disability awareness education and training, advocacy and technical advice.

3865 Community Resources for Independent Living
39155 Liberty St
Suite A100
Fremont, CA 94538-1503

510-794-5735
crilhayward.org

Sheri Burns, Executive Director
Michael Galvan, PhD., Program Director
April Monroe, Finance Director

Community Resources for Independent Living is a peer-based disability organization that advocates and provides resources for people with disabilities to improve lives and make communities fully accessible.

3866 DRAIL (Disability Resource Agency for Independent Living)
501 W Weber Ave
Ste 200-A
Stockton, CA 95203-6239

209-477-8143
Fax: 209-477-7730
TTY: 209-465-5643
barry@drail.org
www.drail.org

Terry Gray, President
Michael Kim Cornelius, Treasurer
Adeline Bagwell, Secretary

A non-profit corporation that is community based, consumer controlled, consumer choice, cross disability center for independent living.

3867 Dayle McIntosh Center: Laguna Niguel
24031 El Toro Road
Suite 300
Laguna Hills, CA 92653-3632   949-460-7784
                                               800-422-7444
                                          Fax: 949-334-2302
                                          TTY: 800-735-2929
                                               www.daylemc.org

Libby Partain, President
Cindy McLeroy, Vice President
Eva Casas-Sarmiento, Secretary

DMC advances empowerment and inclusion of all persons with disabilities. DMC is the largest Independent Living Center in California, and was named in memory of a young woman with a severe physical disability who worked to found the center.

3868 Disability Resource Agency for Independent Living: Modesto
920-12th Street
Modesto, CA 95354-543   209-521-7260
                                          Fax: 209-521-4763
                                          TTY: 209-576-2409
                                               larry@drail.org
                                               www.drail.org

Terry Gray, President
Michael Kim Cornelius, Treasurer
Adeline Bagwell, Secretary

A non-profit corporation that is community based, consumer controlled, consumer choice, cross disability center for independent living.

3869 Disability Services & Legal Center
521 Mendocino Ave.
Santa Rosa, CA 95401-1649   707-528-2745
                                          Fax: 707-528-9477
                                          TTY: 707-528-2151
                                               www.disabilityserviceandlegal.org

Adam Brown, Chairman
Shirley Johnson-Foell, Board President
Jack Geary, Board Member

A non-profit corporation established by a group of disabled and non-disabled individuals to advance the rights of persons with disabilities to equal justice, access, opportunity and participation in the communities.

3870 Disabled Resources Center
2750 E Spring St
Suite 100
Long Beach, CA 90806-2263   562-427-1000
                                          Fax: 562-427-2027
                                          TTY: 562-427-1366
                                               info@drcinc.org
                                               drcinc.org

C. Timothy Lashlee, President
Dora Hogan, Vice President
Finola Campbell, Treasurer

To empower people with disabilities to live independently in the community, to make their own decisions about their lives and to advocate on their own behalf.

3871 FREED Center for Independent Living
2059 Nevada City Hwy
Suite 102
Grass Valley, CA 95945- 3227   530-477-3333
                                               800-655-7732
                                          Fax: 530-477-8184
                                          TTY: 530-477-8194
                                               freed.org

Ana Acton, Executive Director

To eliminate barriers to full equality for people with disabilities through programs which promote independent living.

3872 FREED Center for Independent Living: Marysville
508 J St
Marysville, CA 95901-5636   530-742-4476
                                          TTY: 530-742-4474
                                               freed.org

Claudia Hallis, Manager

To eliminate barriers to full equality for people with disabilities through programs which promote independent living.

3873 First Step Independent Living
1174 Nevada St
Redlands, CA 92374-2893   800-362-0312

Independent living center, empowers people with disabilities to become active, productive, members of the community.

3874 Independent Living Center of Kern County
5251 Office Park Dr
Suite 200
Bakersfield, CA 93309   661-325-1063
                                               877-688-2079
                                               800-529-9541
                                          Fax: 661-325-6702
                                          TTY: 661-325-6702
                                               info@ilcofkerncounty.org
                                               www.ilcofkerncounty.org

Jimmie Soto, Executive Director
Tammy Hartsch, Finance Manager
Harvey Clowers, Special Projects and AT Coordina

A consumer-based consumer-directed non-profit agency assisting persons with disabilities to live independently in their community. The ILCKC presently offers a wide range of services to a growing population of persons with disabilities.

3875 Independent Living Center of Lancaster
606 East Avenue K4
Lancaster, CA 93535-2844   661-942-9726
                                          Fax: 661-945-5690
                                          TTY: 661-723-2509
                                               www.ilcsc.org

Taura Jacob, Manager
Marcy Hernandez
Niyanta Dave

ILCSC is a non-profit, consumer based, non-residential agency providing a wide range of services to a growing population of people with disabilities. ILCSC is dedicated to empowering persons with disabilities to exercise indpendence-pofessionally, personally and creatively-while striving to educate the community on their needs.

3876 Independent Living Resource Center
7425 El Camino Real
Suite R
Atascadero, CA 93422-4656   805-464-3203
                                          Fax: 805-462-1166
                                          TTY: 805-462-1162
                                               info@ilrc-trico.org
                                               www.ilrc-trico.org

Kit McMillion, President
Larry Laborde, Vice President
Dani Anderson, Executive Director

To assist and encourage individuals to achieve their optimal level of self-sufficiency while eliminating the architectural, communication and attitudinal barriers which prevent them from full participation in the community.

3877 Independent Living Resource Center: Santa Barbara
423 W Victoria St
Santa Barbara, CA 93101-3619   805-284-9051
                                          Fax: 805-963-1350
                                          TTY: 805-963-0595
                                               info@ilrc-trico.org
                                               www.ilrc-trico.org

Kit McMillion, President
Larry Laborde, Vice President
Dani Anderson, Executive Director

To assist and encourage individuals to achieve their optimal level of self-sufficiency while eliminating the architectural, communication and attitudinal barriers which prevent them from full participation in the community.

3878   Independent Living Resource Center: San Francisco
825 Howard Street
San Francisco, CA 94103-4128   415-543-6222
                                                  Fax: 415-543-6318
                                                  TTY: 415-543-6698
                                                  info@ilrcsf.org
                                                  ilrcsf.org

Juma Byrd, President
Kolya Kirienko, Vice President
Ben MacMullan, Treasurer
To ensure that people with disabilities are full social and economic partners, both within their families and in a fully accessible community.

3879   Independent Living Resource Center: Santa Maria Office
327 East Plaza Dr
Suite 3A
Santa Maria, CA 93454-6930   805-354-5948
                                                  Fax: 805-349-2416
                                                  TTY: 805-925-0015
                                                  info@ilrc-trico.org
                                                  www.ilrc-trico.org

Kit McMillion, President
Larry Laborde, Vice President
Dani Anderson, Executive Director
To assist and encourage individuals to achieve their optimal level of self-sufficiency while eliminating the architectural, communication and attitudinal barriers which prevent them from full participation in the community.

3880   Independent Living Resource Center: Ventura
1802 Eastman Ave
Suite 112
Ventura, CA 93003-5759   805-256-1036
                                                  Fax: 805-650-9278
                                                  TTY: 805-650-5993
                                                  info@ilrc-trico.org
                                                  www.ilrc-trico.org

Kit McMillion, President
Larry Laborde, Vice President
Dani Anderson, Executive Director
An organization of, by and for persons with disabilities who reside or work in the service area. Purpose is to assist and encourage individuals to achieve their optimal level of self-sufficiency while eliminating the architectural, communication and attitudinal barriers which prevent them from full participation in the community.

3881   Independent Living Resource of Contra Coast
1850 Gateway Blvd
Suite 120
Concord, CA 94520-3293   925-363-7293
                                                  Fax: 925-363-7296
                                                  www.ilrscc.org

Sarah BirdwelL, Board President
Kathy Mitsopoulos, Board Vice President
Teri Ruggiero, Board Secretary
Offers workshops, services are accessible to individuals with cognitive disabilities, physical disabilities, deaf and hard of hearing, emotional disabilities, visual impairments, learing disabilities and seniors.

3882   Independent Living Resource of Fairfield
470 Chadbourn Rd
Ste. B
Fairfield, CA 94534   707-435-8174
                                                  Fax: 707-435-8177
                                                  www.ilrscc.org

Sarah BirdwelL, Board President
Kathy Mitsopoulos, Board Vice President
Teri Ruggiero, Board Secretary
To empower people with disabilities to: control their own lives, provide advocacy and support for individuals with disabilities to live independently, create an accessible community free of physical and attitudinal barriers.

3883   Independent Living Resource: Antioch
3727 Sunset Lane
#103
Antioch, CA 94509-1761   925-754-0539
                                                  TTY: 925-755-0934
                                                  www.ilrscc.org

Sarah BirdwelL, Board President
Kathy Mitsopoulos, Board Vice President
Teri Ruggiero, Board Secretary
Non-profit organizations run and controlled by persons with disabilities. They are non-residential, community-based centers where people with disabilities can receive assistance with a variety of daily living issues and learn the skills they need to take controll of their lives from people who have had similar experiences living with a disability.

3884   Independent Living Resource: Concord
1850 Gateway Blvd
Suite 120
Concord, CA 94520-3293   925-363-7293
                                                  Fax: 925-363-7296
                                                  gilc@ilrccc.org
                                                  www.ilrscc.org

Sarah BirdwelL, Board President
Kathy Mitsopoulos, Board Vice President
Teri Ruggiero, Board Secretary
To empower people with disabilities to: control their own lives, provide advocacy and support for individuals with disabilities to live independently, create an accessible community free of physical and attitudinized barriers.

3885   Independent Living Resources (ILR)
Bldg 2a
101 Broadway
Richmond, CA 94804-1945   510-233-7400
                                                  info@ilrccc.org

Marvin Dyson, Manager
Provides services to meet the diverse needs of people who have a variety of disabilities in all age groups.

3886   Independent Living Service Northern California: Redding Office
169 Hartnell Ave
Suite 128
Redding, CA 96002-1849   530-242-8550
                                                  800-464-8527
                                                  Fax: 530-241-1454
                                                  TTY: 530-242-8550
                                                  actionctr.org

Lauri Evans, President
Frank Smith, Vice President
Evan Levang, Executive Director
Independent Living Services of Northern California is a private non profit organization that provides support services to help empower community members with disabilities.

3887   Independent Living Services of Northern California
Jennifer Roberts Building
1161 East Ave
Chico, CA 95926-1018   530-893-8527
                                                  800-464-8527
                                                  Fax: 530-893-8574
                                                  TTY: 530-893-8527
                                                  actionctr.org

Lauri Evans, President
Frank Smith, Vice President
Evan Levang, Executive Director
Independent Living Services of Northern California is a private, non profit organization that provides support services to help empower community members with disabilities.

3888   Marin Center for Independent Living
710 4th St
San Rafael, CA 94901-3213   415-459-6245
                                                  Fax: 415-459-7047
                                                  TTY: 415-459-7027
                                                  marincil.org

Chris Schultz, President
Joe Brnnett, Vice President
Eli Gelardin, Executive Director

A non-profit organization that provides advocacy and services for seniors and persons with disabilities.

3889 Mother Lode Independent Living Center(DRAIL: Disability Resource Agency for Independent Living)
67 Linoberg St
Suite A.
Sonora, CA 95370-4646
209-532-0963
Fax: 209-532-1591
TTY: 209-288-3309
barry@drail.org
www.drail.org

Terry Gray, President
Michael Kim Cornelius, Treasurer
Adeline Bagwell, Secretary
DRAIL is a non-profit, community based, consumer controlled, cross disability center for independent living.

3890 Placer Independent Resource Services
11768 Atwood Rd
Suite 29
Auburn, CA 95603
530-885-6100
800-833-3453
Fax: 530-885-3032
TTY: 530-885-0326
lbrewer@pirs.org
pirs.org

Eldon Luce, President
Michael Cummings, Vice President
Dan Roye, Director
A non profit independent living center whose mission is to advocate, empower, educate and provide services for people with disabilities that would enable them to live more independently.

3891 Resources for Independent Living
420 i St, Level B.
Suite 3
Sacramento, CA 95814-2319
916-446-3074
Fax: 916-446-2443
leonc@ril-sacramento.org
www.ril-sacramento.org

Ramona Garcia, Board Chairperson
Francisco Godoy, Vice Chairperson
Joanne Bodine, Treasurer
Promoting the socio-economic independence of persons with disabilities by providing peer-supported, consumer-directed independent living services and advocacy.

3892 Rolling Start
570 W 4th St
Suite 107
San Bernardino, CA 92401-1438
909-884-2129
Fax: 909-386-7446
TTY: 909-884-7396

John Anaya, Chairperson
Kathi Pryor, Treasurer
Francis Bates, Executive Director
Empowers and educates people with disabilities to achieve the independent life of their choice.

3893 Rolling Start: Victorville
17330 Bear Valley Road
Suite A102
Victorville, CA 92395
760-843-7959
Fax: 760-843-7977
TTY: 760-951-8175

John Anaya, Chairperson
Kathi Pryor, Treasurer
Francis Bates, Executive Director
Empowers and educates people with disabilities to achieve the independent life of their choice.

3894 Services Center For Independent Living
107 S Spring Street
Claremont, CA 91711-549
909-621-6722
800-491-6722
Fax: 909-445-0727
TTY: 949-445-0726
www.scil-ilc.org

Larry Grable, Executive Director
Janice Ornelas, Independent Living Specialist
Angela Nwokike, System Change Advocate
Dedicated to expanding access, information and resources to help increase independence and enhance the quality of life for the East San Gabriel Valley residents with disabilities.

3895 Silicon Valley Independent Living Center
25 N. 14th St.
Suite 1000, 10th floor
San Jose, CA 95112
408-894-9041
Fax: 669-231-4795
info@svilc.org
svilc.org

Patricia Kokes, President
Richard A. Wentz, Vice President
Gabe Lopez, Treasurer
A private, consumer-driven, nonprofit corporation that offers quality services to individuals with disabilities in Silicon Valley.

3896 Silicon Valley Independent Living Center: South County Branch
7881 Church Street
Suite C
Gilroy, CA 95020-7346
408-843-9100
Fax: 408-842-4791
TTY: 408-842-2591
info@svilc.org
svilc.org

Patricia Kokes, President
Richard A. Wentz, Vice President
Gabe Lopez, Treasurer
A private, consumer-driven, non-profit corporation that offers quality services to individuals with disabilities in Silicon Valley.

3897 Southern California Rehabilitation Services
7830 Quill Dr
Suite D
Downey, CA 90242-3440
562-862-6531
Fax: 562-923-5274
TTY: 562-869-0931
scrs-ilc.org

Lisa Hayes, President
Michael Strong, Vice President
Carol Trees, Secretary/Treasurer
Empowers persons with disabilities to achieve their personalized goals through community education and individualized services that provide the knowledge, skills, and confidence building to maximize their quality of life.

3898 Through the Looking Glass
3075 Adeline St.
Ste. 120
Berkeley, CA 94703
510-848-1112
800-644-2666
Fax: 510-848-4445
TTY: 510-848-1005
tlg@lookingglass.org
www.lookingglass.org

Maureen Block, J.D., Board President
Thomas Spalding, Board Treasurer
Alice Nemon, D.S.W., Board Secretary
To create, demonstrate and encourage non-pathological and empowering reesources and model early intervention services for families with disability issues in parent or child which integrate expertise derived from personal disability experience and disability culture.

3899 Tri-County Independent Living Center
2822 Harris Street
Eureka, CA 95503
707-445-8404
877-576-5000
Fax: 707-445-9751
TTY: 707-445-8405
aa@tilinet.org
www.tilinet.org

Gail Pascoe, President
Linda Arnold, Vice President
Kevin O'Brien, Treasurer
Promotes the philosophy of independent living, to connect individuals to services, and to create and accessible community, so that people with disabilities can have control over their lives and full access to the communities in which they live.

3900 Westside Center for Independent Living
12901 Venice Blvd
Los Angeles, CA 90066-3509
310-390-3611
888-851-9245
Fax: 310-390-4906
TTY: 310-398-9204
www.wcil.org

David Geffen, President
Chris Knauf, 1st Vice President
Brenda Green, Secretary
The Westside Center for Independent Living (WCIL) helps people living with disabilities maintain self-sufficient and productive lives through non-residential peer support services and training programs. Independent Living promotes self-determination, community living, full participation in community life and access to the same opportunities and resources available to people without disabilities.

Colorado

3901 Atlantis Community
201 S Cherokee St
Denver, CO 80223-1836
303-733-9324
Fax: 303-733-6211
TTY: 303-733-0047
info@atlantiscommunity.org

David Hays, Manager
Provide direct services, and to empower people with disabilities integrating, with full and equal rights, into all parts of society including employment, affordable, accessible, housing, transportation, recreation, communication, education, and public places while exercising and exerting choice and self determination.

3902 Center for Independence
740 Gunnison Ave
Grand Junction, CO 81501-3222
708-588-0833
Fax: 708-588-0406
center-for-independence.org

Linda Taylor, Executive Director
The Center for Independence works to promote community solutions and to empower individuals with disabilities to live independently.

3903 Center for People with Disabilities
615 Main St
Longmont, CO 80501-4983
303-772-3250
Fax: 303-772-5125
TTY: 303-772-3250
info@cpwd.org
www.cpwd-ilc.org

Dale Gaar, Board President
Deborah.A Conley, Board Vice President
Nancy Phares-Zook, Board Secretary
Provides resources, information, and advocacy to assist people with disabilities in overcoming barriers to independent living.

3904 Center for People with Disabilities: Pueblo
1304 Berkley Ave
Pueblo, CO 81004-3002
719-546-1271
800-659-3656
Fax: 719-546-1374
ivaleneamidei@yahoo.com
www.ilcpueblo.org

Larry Williams, Executive Director
One of the 10 centers for independent living in Colorado founded under Title VII of the Rehabilitation Act of 1973 as amended in 1978. All new centers under this Independent Living (CIL) Title of the Act received initial and ongoing grants through this new Federal Program created by the Act.

3905 Center for People with Disabilities: Boulder
1675 Range St
Boulder, CO 80301-2722
303-442-8662
888-929-5519
Fax: 303-442-0502
info@cpwd.org
www.cpwd-ilc.org

Dale Gaar, Board President
Deborah.A Conley, Board Vice President
Nancy Phares-Zook, Board Secretary
Providing resources, information and advocacy to people with disabilities. Assist people with disabilities in transitioning from nursing homes to independent living in the community. Also provide personal assistance services.

3906 Colorado Springs Independence Center
729 South Tejon Street
Colorado Springs, CO 80903
719-471-8181
Fax: 719-471-7829
TTY: 719-471-2076
www.theindependencecenter.org

Billy A., Chair Elect
Billy B., Secretary
To empower persons with disabilities to maximize their independence within the community and to remove barriers which impact their quality of life, while encouraging them to live independently in their community.

3907 Connections for Independent Living
1331 8th Avenue
Greeley, CO 80631-4027
970-352-8682
800-887-5828
Fax: 970-353-8058
TTY: 970-352-8682
pattid4z@yahoo.com
www.connectionsforindependentliving.org

Beth Danielson, Executive Director
Michael Stevens, Director of Services
Alicia Garza, Director
Certified IL Center, I and R advocacy, peer support, skills training, sign language interpretations, reader services, housing. Cross-disability, all ages.

3908 Denver CIL
Ste 100
777 Grant St
Denver, CO 80203-3501
303-837-1020
Fax: 303-837-0859
www.denverhousing.org

Greg Beran, Owner
Ismael Guerrero, Executive Director
Joshua Crawley, Agency Counsel
Provides resources, information, and advocacy to assist people with disabilities in overcoming barriers to independent living.

3909 Disability Center for Independent Living
4821 East 38th Avenue
Denver, CO 80207-1232
303-320-1345
Fax: 303-320-1345
TTY: 303-322-2330
avillasenor.dcil@gmil.com
www.accil.net

Larry Williams, Executive Director
John Wooster, Consultant
Anthony Gonzales, Housing Coordinator
Independent living center providing quality services for people with disabilities.

3910 Disabled Resource Services
1017 Robertson Street
Unit B
Fort Collins, CO 80524-3915   970-482-2700
Fax: 970-449-6972
TTY: 970-407-7060
disabledresourceservices.org

George Tremblay, Chairman
John Weins, Vice Chairman
Nancy Jackson, Executive Director
To empower individuals with disabilities to achieve their maximum level of independence and to gain personal dignity within society. Disabled Resource Services, as a private non-profit state certified center for independent living, is dedicated to working with individuals with all types of disabilities in Larimer County to promote their independence and equality through services which support advocacy, awareness and access to their community.

3911 Disbled Resource Services
640 E Eisenhower Blvd
Loveland, CO 80537-3954   970-667-0816
Fax: 970-593-6582
disabledresourceservices.org

George Tremblay, Chairman
John Weins, Vice Chairman
Nancy Jackson, Executive Director
To empower individuals with disabilities to achieve their maximum level of independence and to gain personal dignity within society.

3912 Greeley Center for Independence
2780 28th Ave
Greeley, CO 80634-7803   970-339-2444
800-748-1012
Fax: 970-339-0033
gciinc@gciinc.org
www.gciinc.org

Chari Armagost, Chief Financial Officer
Sarita Reddy, PH. D, Executive Director
Rob Rabe, Director of Outpatient Service
Provides places of growth, transition and encouragement, where people with temporary and permanent disabilities can reach toward their maximum potential of personal independence and wellness.

3913 Independent Life Center
P.O.Box 612
Craig, CO 81626-612   970-826-0833
888-526-0833
Fax: 970-826-0832
TTY: 970-826-0833

Larry Williams, Executive Director
John Wooster, Consultant
Anthony Gonzales, Housing Coordinator
Provides resources, information, and advocacy to assist people with disabilities in overcoming barriers to independent living.

3914 Southwest Center for Independence
3473 Main Avenue
#23
Durango, CO 81301-5474   970-259-1672
866-962-2158
Fax: 970-259-0947
TTY: 970-259-1672
swindependence.org/

Martha Mason, Executive Director
Mariellen Walz, Chair
Patricia Ziegler, Assistant Director
Empowering individuals with disabilities and their families to achieve their maximum level of independence in work, play and other areas of life.

3915 Southwest Center for Independence: Cortez
2409 East Empire Street
PO Box 640
Cortez, CO 81321-9164   970-570-8001
866-962-2158
Fax: 970-565-7169
director@swilc.org
swindependence.org/

Mariellen Walz, Chair
Johnny Bulson, Vice Chair
Jason Armstrong, Treasurer
Empowers individiuals with disabilities and their families to achieve their maximum level of independence in work, play and other areas of life.

Connecticut

3916 Center for Disability Rights
764-B Campbell Ave
764 Campbell Ave
W Haven, CT 06516- 3786   203-934-7077
Fax: 203-934-7078
TTY: 203-934-7079
info@cdr-ct.org
cdr-ct.org

Marc Gallucci, Executive Director
Chris Zurcher, Consumer Relations
Dana Canevari, I&R Specialist
Resources, information, and advocacy to assist people with disabilities in overcoming barriers to independent living.

3917 Center for Independent Living SC
26 Palmers Hill Rd
Stamford, CT 06902-2113   203-353-8550
Fax: 203-353-1423
TTY: 203-353-8550

Dana Canevari, Director
Provides resources, information, and advocacy to assist people with disabilities in overcoming barriers to independent living.

3918 Chapel Haven
1040 Whalley Ave
New Haven, CT 06515-1740   203-397-1714
Fax: 203-937-2466
admissions@chapelhaven.org
chapelhaven.org

Michael Storz, President
The only combined state-accredited special education facility and independent living facility for adults with cognitive disabilities.

3919 Connecticut State Independent Living Council
151 New Park Ave
Hartford, CT 06106   860-523-0126
Fax: 860-523-5603
info@ctsilc.org
ctsilc.org

Katherine Pellerin, President
Keith Mullinar, Vice President
Alexia Bouckoms, Treasurer
The mission of the council is to promote equal access, opportunities, and social inclusion for people with disabilities in all spheres of society.

3920 Disabilities Network of Eastern Connecticut
19 Ohio Avenue
Suite 2
Norwich, CT 06360-2111   860-823-1898
Fax: 860-886-2316
CFerry@dnec.org
dnec.org

Katherine Pellerin, President
Robert Davidson, Vice President
Jane O'Friel, Secretary/Treasurer
Dedicated to supporting and advancing the rights of individuals with disabilities. The goal is to creat a completely inclusive society where people live together in communities regardless of their abilities.

3921   Disability Resource Center of Fairfield County
80 Ferry Blvd
Suite 205
Stratford, CT 06615-6079   203-378-6977
                                    Fax: 203-375-2748
                                    TTY: 203-378-3248
                                    www.accessinct.org

Ethel M R, President
Thomas D, Vice-President
Anthony Lacava, Executive Director
A crosss-disability resource and advocacy organization for people with disabilities that has provided unique, consumer-directed services both for individuals and for the communities of Fairfield County.

3922   Independence Northwest Center for Independent Living
1183 New Haven Rd
Suite 200
Naugatuck, CT 06770-5033   203-729-3299
                                    Fax: 203-729-2839
                                    TTY: 203-729-1281
                            info@independencenorthwest.org
                            www.independencenorthwest.org

Maureen Mayo, President
Tom Ford, Vice President
Charles Marino, Treasurer
Provides services in such areas as peer counseling, advocacy, independent living skills training and information and referral.

3923   New Horizons Village
37 Bliss Rd
Unionville, CT 06085   860-673-8893
                                    Fax: 860-675-4369
                        Michael.Shaw@NewHorizonsVillage.com
                                    newhorizonsvillage.com

Carolyn Fields, Administrator
A 68 unit apartment complex designed for people who have severe physical disabilities.

Delaware

3924   Freedom Center for Independent Living
400 N Broad St
Middletown, DE 19709-1089   302-376-4399
                                        866-687-3245
                                    Fax: 302-376-4395
                                    TTY: 302-376-4397
                                    info@fcilde.org
                                    fcilde.org

Hersernest Cole, Executive Director
Lillian Evans, Independent Living Specialist
Protects the Civil Rights and promote the empowerment of persons with disabilities and their families through our independent living philosophy.

3925   Independent Living
Apt 210
1800 N Broom St
Wilmington, DE 19802-3854   302-429-6693
                                    Fax: 302-429-8031
                                    TTY: 302-429-8034
Susan Cycyk, Executive Director
Providing skilled support and caring guidance to adults with disabilities. Our case management services include: daily living skills training, medical coordination, transportation assistance, financial management, housing assistance, and vocational/educational planning.

3926   Independent Resource Georgetown
Ste 37
410 S Bedford St
Georgetown, DE 19947-1850   302-854-9330
                                    Fax: 302-854-9408
                                    TTY: 302-854-9340

Larry Henderson, Director
Pat Boyd, Manager
Provides independent living services to persons who experience a significant disability. Offers skills training, individually and in small groups, peer support/peer counseling and information and

referral services. Strives to remove the architectural and attitudnal barriers through individual and systems advocacy.

3927   Independent Resources: Dover
154 South Governor's Avenue
Dover, DE 19904-7311   302-735-4599
                                    Fax: 302-735-5623
                                    TTY: 302-735-5629
                        lhenderson@independentresources.org
                                    www.iri-de.org

Tes DelTufo, Office Director
Carolyn Miller, IL Specialist
Debbie Justice, IL Specialist
Private, non-profit, consumer-controlled, community based organization providing services and advocacy by and for persons with all types of disabilities. Their goal is to assist individuals with disabilities to achieve their maximum potential within their families and communities.

3928   Independent Resources: Wilmington
6 Denny Rd
Suite 101
Wilmington, DE 19809-3444   302-765-0191
                                    Fax: 302-765-0195
                                    TTY: 302-765-0194
                                    www.iri-de.org

Larry D Henderson, Executive Director
Phyllis Farrare, Director of Operations
Private, non-profit, consumer-controlled, community based organization providing services and advocacy by and for persons with all types of disabilities. Their goal is to assist individuals with disabilities to achieve their maximum potential within their families and communities.

3929   Mosaic Of De
4980 S. 118TH ST
Omaha, NE 68137   302-456-5995
                                        877-366-7242
                                    Fax: 402-896-1511
                                    info@mosaicinfo.org
                                    mosaicinfo.org

Terry Olson, Executive Director
Linda Timmons, President and CEO
Raul Saldivar, Chief Operating Officer
Provides services to adults with developmental disabilities who reside in homes and apartments. Services are designed to provide them with opportunities for choices and participation in the life of their communities. Supports are geared to assist each individual in becoming more independent in activities of daily living, vocational skills, community mobility and transportation, and recreation and leisure activities.

District of Columbia

3930   District of Columbia Center for Independent Living
1400 Florida Ave NE
Washington, DC 20002-5032   202-388-0033
                                    Fax: 202-398-3018
                                    info@dccil.org
                                    dccil.org

Rev. Patric Hailes Fears, President
Dr. John Thompson, Vice President
Carl Bartels, Treasurer
Mission is to maximize the leadership, empowerment, independence, and productivity of individuals with disabilities, and to integrate these individuals into the mainstream of American society.

3931   National Council on Independent Living (NCIL)
P.O. Box 31260
Washington, DC 20006   202-207-0334
                                        844-778-7961
                                    Fax: 202-207-0341
                                    TTY: 202-207-0340
                                    ncil@ncil.org
                                    www.ncil.org

Darrell Lynn Jones, Interim Executive Director
Jenny Sichel, Director, Operations
Denise Law, Coordinator, Member Services

A national cross-disability grassroots organization, NCIL advances independent living and the rights of people with disabilities through consumer-driven advocacy.

Florida

3932 Ability 1st
1300 E. Green Street
Pasadena, CA 91106   626-396-1010
                                  877-768-4600
                            Fax: 626-396-1021
                            info@abilityfirst.org
                            abilityfirst.org

Steve Brockmeyer, Chairman
John Kelly, Vice Chairman
Lori.E Gangemi, President
To empower persons with disabilities to live independently and participate actively in their community.

3933 Adult Day Training
Goodwill Industries - Suncoast
10596 Gandy Blvd N
St Petersburg, FL 33702-1422   727-523-1512
                                   888-279-1988
                             Fax: 727-563-9300
                             TTY: 727-579-1068
                gw.marketing@goodwill-suncoast.com
                          www.goodwill-suncoast.org
Deborah A. Passerini, President & Chief Executive Officer
Tracey Boucher, Corporate Treasurer & Chief Financial Officer
Kris Rawson, Vice President for Mission Services & Chief Mission Officer
An innovative program which uses job skills to teach self-help, daily living, communication, mobility, travel, decision-making, behavioral and social skills. This focus provides concrete, transferable experiences to help prepare individuals for greater community inclusion by achieving the highest possible degree of independence in their daily life, increasing their confidence and supporting their successful transitions to less structured, self-sufficient environments.

3934 CIL of Central Florida
720 N Denning Dr
Winter Park, FL 32789-3020   407-623-1070
                             Fax: 407-623-1390
                             info@cilorlando.org
                             cilorlando.org
Jason Vennings, Development Director
Kim Byerly, Chair
Cheryl Stone, Secretary
A private, non-profit organization dedicated to helping people with disabilities achieve their self-determined goals for independent living.

3935 Caring and Sharing Center for Independent Living
12552 Belcher Rd S
Largo, FL 33773-3014   727-539-7550
                                   866-539-7550
                             Fax: 727-539-7588
                www.disabilityachievementcenter.org
Barbara Dandro, Treasurer
Mary Bucca, Secretary
Patricia Bell, Director
Empowering people with disabilities.

3936 Caring and Sharing Center: Pasco County
12552 Belcher Rd S
Largo, FL 33773-3014   727-539-7550
                                   866-539-7550
                             Fax: 727-539-7588
                www.disabilityachievementcenter.org
Barbara Dandro, Treasurer
Mary Bucca, Secretary
Patricia Bell, Director
Empowering people with disabilities.

3937 Center for Independent Living in Central Florida
720 N Denning Dr
Winter Park, FL 32789-3095   407-623-1070
                             Fax: 407-623-1390
                             info@cilorlando.org
                             cilorlando.org
Jason Vennings, Development Director
Kim Byerly, Chair
Cheryl Stone, Secretary
In partnership with the community, promotes personal right snad responsiblities among people with all disabilities.

3938 Center for Independent Living of Broward
4800 N State Road 7
Suite 102
Lauderdale Lakes, FL 33319-5811   954-722-6400
                                   888-722-6400
                             Fax: 954-735-1958
                             cilb@cilbroward.org
                             www.cilbroward.org
Craig Lilienthal, President
Christopher Sharp, VP
Shea Smith, Treasurer
Offers assistance to people with disabilities in fulfilling the goals of independence and self-sufficiency.

3939 Center for Independent Living of Florida Keys
103400 Overseas Hwy
Suite 243
Key Largo, FL 33037-2849   305-453-3491
                                   877-335-0187
                             Fax: 305-453-3488
                             TTY: 305-453-3491
                             cilkeys@cilkeys.org
                             www.cilofthekeys.org
Brenda K Pierce, Executive Director
Offers assistance to persons with disabilities in acquiring independent living and self-advocacy skills in order to obtain and maintain independence and self-sufficiency.

3940 Center for Independent Living of N Florida
1823 Buford Ct
Tallahassee, FL 32308-4465   850-575-9621
                             Fax: 850-575-5740
                             TTY: 850-575-5245
                             cilnf@nettally.com
                             www.ability1st.info
Judith Barrett, Executive Director
Offers assistance to persons with disabilities in acquiring independent living and self-advocacy skills in order to obtain and maintain independence and self-sufficiency

3941 Center for Independent Living of NW Florida
3600 N Pace Blvd
Pensacola, FL 32505-4240   850-595-5566
                                   877-245-2457
                             Fax: 850-595-5560
                             cil-drc@cil-drc.org
                             cil-drc.org
James Hicks, President
Kathleen Wilks, Secretary
John Bouchard, Treasurer
Provides services such as information and referral, peer counseling, housing, advocacy, training, independent living skills training, free wheelchairs, loan locker, assistive technology.

3942 Center for Independent Living of North Central Florida
3445 NE 24th Street
Ocala, FL 34470-9214   352-368-3788
                                   877-232-8261
                             Fax: 352-629-0098
                             www.cilncf.org
Joe Dyke, President
Robert Miller, Vice President
David Christie, Treasurer
Empowers people with disabilities to exert their individual rights to live as independently as possible, make personal life choices and achieve full community inclusion.

3943 **Center for Independent Living of North Central Florida**
222 SW 36th Ter
Gainesville, FL 32607-2863 352-378-7474
800-265-5724
Fax: 352-378-5582
TTY: 352-372-3443
www.cilncf.org

Joe Dyke, President
Robert Miller, Vice President
David Christie, Treasurer
Empowering people with disabilities to exert their individual rights to live as independently as possible, make personal life choices and achieve full community inclusion.

3944 **Center for Independent Living of S Florida**
6660 Biscayne Blvd
Miami, FL 33138-6285 305-751-8025
Fax: 305-751-8944
TTY: 305-751-8891
soflacil.org

Alvin W. Roberts, President
Gregg Goldfarb, Vice President
Timothy Werner, Ph.D, Secretary
A community based non for profit, independent living center serving people of all ages with any type of disability. Services: Basic education, GED preperation, American sign language advocacy, peer support, information and referral, independent living skills training, housing assistance, transportation assistance, home modiifications, transition from nursing facility to the community assisatnace filing ADA complaints, accessibility surveys, diability awareness traing.

3945 **Center for Independent Living of SW Florida**
2321 Bruner Ln
Fort Myers, FL 33912-1904 239-277-1447
800-435-7352
Fax: 239-277-1647
Ronald J Muschong, Interim Executive Director
Helping people with disabilities achieve independence and self-determination in their lives.

3946 **Coalition for Independent Living Options: Okeechobee**
1680 SW Bayshore Boulevard
Suite 231
Port St. Lucie, FL 34984 772-878-3500
Fax: 772-878-3344
www.cilo.org

Scott Shoemaker, President
Sharon D'Eusanio, Vice President
Joseph Fields Jr., Esquire, Secretary
Private non-profit promoting independences for people with disabilities in Palm Beach, Martin, St. Lucie & Okeechobee Counties. Services include advocacy, independent living skills & training, peer support, after school & summer programs for teens, crime victim support services, and veterans transition services.

3947 **Coalition for Independent Living Options: Fort Pierce**
6800 Forest HIll Boulevard
West Palm Beach, FL 33413 561-966-4288
Fax: 561-966-0441
www.cilo.org

Scott Shoemaker, President
Sharon D'Eusanio, Vice President
Joseph Fields Jr., Esquire, Secretary
Private non-profit promoting independences for people with disabilities in Palm Beach, Martin, St. Lucie & Okeechobee Counties. Services include advocacy, independent living skills & training, peer support, after school & summer programs for teens, crime victim support services, and verterans transition services.

3948 **Coalition for Independent Living Options**
6800 Forest HIll Boulevard
West Palm Beach, FL 33413-3310 561-966-4288
Fax: 561-966-0441
www.cilo.org

Scott Shoemaker, President
Sharon D'Eusanio, Vice President
Joseph Fields Jr., Esquire, Secretary
Private non-profit promoting independences for people with disabilities in Palm Beach, Martin, St. Lucie & Okeechobee Counties. Services include advocacy, independent living skills &

training, peer support, after school & summer programs for teens, crime victim support services, and verterans transition services.

3949 **Coalition for Independent Living Options: Stuart**
1680 SW Bayshore Boulevard
Suite 231
Port St. Lucie, FL 34984 772-878-3500
Fax: 772-878-3344
www.cilo.org

Scott Shoemaker, President
Sharon D'Eusanio, Vice President
Joseph Fields Jr., Esquire, Secretary
Private non-profit promoting independences for people with disabilities in Palm Beach, Martin, St. Lucie & Okeechobee Counties. Services include advocacy, independent living skills & training, peer support, after school & summer programs for teens, crime victim support services, and verterans transition services.

3950 **Disability Resource Center**
300 W. 5th St.
Panama City, FL 32401-4704 850-769-6890
Fax: 850-769-6891
outreach@drcpc.org
www.drcpc.org

Robert Cox, Executive Director
Becky Cadwell, Independent Living Specialist
They are commiteed to collaborating with other disability/consumer-focused organizations in their community

3951 **Lakeland Adult Day Training**
3033 Drane Field Rd
Suite 5
Lakeland, FL 33811-3305 863-701-1351
TTY: 863-701-1356
gw.marketing@goodwill-suncoast.com
www.goodwill-suncoast.org

Oscar J. Horton, Chairman
Martin W. Gladysz, Vice Chairman
Heather Ceresoli, Vice Chairman
An innovative program which uses job skills to teach self-help, daily living, communication, mobility, travel, decision-making, behavioral and social skills. This focus provides concrete, transferable experiences to help prepare individuals for greater community inclusion by achieving the highest possible degree of independence in their daily life, increasing their confidence and supporting their successful transitions to less structured, self-sufficient environments.

3952 **Lighthouse Central Florida**
215 E New Hampshire St
Orlando, FL 32804-6403 407-898-2483
Fax: 407-895-5255
lvaneepoel@lcf-fl.org
www.lighthousecentralflorida.com

Alex B. Hull, Chair
David Stahl, Vice Chair
Paul Prewitt, Secretary
Promote the independence and success of people living with vision impairment.

3953 **Miami-Dade County Disability Services and Independent Living (DSAIL)**
701 NW 1st Court
Miami, FL 33136-1647 786-469-4600
Fax: 305-547-7355
www.miamidade.gov

Michael Moxam, Manager
Lucia Davis-Raiford, Director
Offers information and referral services serving all types of disabilities with the goal of assisting the disabled acquiring independence and control over their lives. Teaches independent living skills, job readiness and placement, home health care, sensitivity training, training in ASL and Braille, counsel people with disabilities or wide range of problems.

3954 **Ocala Adult Day Training**
2920 W Silver Springs Blvd
Ocala, FL 34475-5654   352-629-0456
                                    TTY: 352-629-0874
gw.marketing@goodwill-suncoast.com
www.goodwill-suncoast.org

Oscar J. Horton, Chairman
Martin W. Gladysz, Vice Chairman
Heather Ceresoli, Vice Chairman
An innovative program which uses job skills to teach self-help, daily living, communication, mobility, travel, decision-making, behavioral and social skills. This focus provides concrete, transferable experiences to help prepare individuals for greater community inclusion by achieving the highest possible degree of independence in their daily life, increasing their confidence and supporting their successful transitions to less structured, self-sufficient environments.

3955 **Pinellas Park Adult Day Training**
7601 Park Blvd
Pinellas Park, FL 33781-3704   727-541-6205
                                    TTY: 727-544-5835
gw.marketing@goodwill-suncoast.com
www.goodwill-suncoast.org

Oscar J. Horton, Chairman
Martin W. Gladysz, Vice Chairman
Heather Ceresoli, Vice Chairman
An innovative program which uses job skills to teach self-help, daily living, communication, mobility, travel, decision-making, behavioral and social skills. This focus provides concrete, transferable experiences to help prepare individuals for greater community inclusion by achieving the highest possible degree of independence in their daily life, increasing their confidence and supporting their successful transitions to less structured, self-sufficient environments.

3956 **SCCIL at Titusville**
571-W Haverty Court
Rockledge, FL 32955   321-633-6011
                                    Fax: 321-633-6472
                                    TTY: 706-724-6324
jilldunham9@gmail.com
www.virtualcil.net

Jill Dunham-Schuller, Executive Director
Directory of Independent Living Centers throughout the United States.

3957 **Self Reliance**
8901 N Armenia Ave
Tampa, FL 33604-1041   813-375-3965
                                    Fax: 813-375-3970
                                    TTY: 813-375-3972
bruehl@self-reliance.org
www.self-reliance.org

Finn Kavanagh, Executive Director
Michele Pineda, Director of Finance & Operations
Gary Martoccio, Programs Director
A cross disability agency providing services to both children and adults with disabilities to identify and overcome barriers to independence in their lives. Self Reliance also promotes independence through empowering persons with disabilities and improving the communities in which they live.

3958 **Space Coast Center for Independent Living**
571 Haverty Court, Suite W.
Rockledge, FL 32955   321-633-6011
                                    Fax: 321-633-6472
spacecoastcil.org

Michael Lavoie, President
Howard Fetes, VP
Jason Miller, Treasurer/Secretary
Provides overall services for individuals with al types of disabilities. Offers peer support, advocacy, skills training, accessibility surveys, support groups, transportation, specialized equipment and sign language interpreter referral services and home modifications.

3959 **Suncoast Center for Independent Living, Inc.**
3281 17th Street
Sarasota, FL 34235   941-351-9545
                                    Fax: 941-316-9320
Info@scil4u.org
www.scil4u.org

Kevin Sanderson, Chair
Michael Fluker, Executive Director
Vicke Mack, Treasurer
Helping people with disabilities live independently.

3960 **disAbility Solutions for Independent Living**
119 S Palmetto Ave
Suite 180
Daytona Beach, FL 32114- 4369   386-255-1812
                                        866-310-1039
                                    Fax: 386-255-1814
                                    TTY: 386-252-6222
info@dsil.org
www.dsil.org

Julie M Shaw, Executive Director
To maximize the leadership, empowerment, independence and productivity of individuals with disabilities, to promote and attain integration and full inclusion of individuals with disabilities in all aspects of our society; accomplished through consumer control, peer support, education, self-determination, equal access and individual and systems advocacy

Georgia

3961 **Arms Wide Open**
5036 Snapfinger Woods Dr.
Suite 205
Decatur, GA 30035- 1677   678-404-7696
                                    Fax: 770-498-2778
kenmorris@armswideopen.org
www.armswideopen.org

Ken Morris, Director
Arms Wide Open operates a durable medical equipment loan program and a life care program. The mission of Arms Wide Open is to provide support services to the aged, disabled and chronically ill for the purpose of helping them to avoid institutional placement.

3962 **Bain, Inc. Center For Independent Living**
316 W Shotwell St.
Bainbridge, GA 39819-3906   229-246-0150
                                        888-830-1530
                                    Fax: 229-246-1715
                                    TTY: 888-830-1530
www.baincil.org

Virginia Harris, Executive Director
Malissa Thompson, Program Manager
Tomonia Becon, Nursing Home Transition Coordina
A non-residential Center for Independent Living serving eleven counties throughout Southwest. BAIN is a non-profit, community based resource and advocacy center run by and for individuals with disabilities.

3963 **DisAbility LINK**
1901 Montreal Rd.
Suite 102
Tucker, GA 30084   404-687-8890
                                    Fax: 404-687-8298
                                    TTY: 711
www.disabilitylink.org

Kim Gibson, Executive Director
Ken Mitchell, Disability Rights & Peer Support Training Advocate
Joseph Bryant, Financial Director
Committed to promoting the rights of all people with disabilities.

3964 **Disability Connections**
170 College St
Macon, GA 31201-1656   478-741-1425
                                        800-743-2117
                                    Fax: 478-755-1571
disabilityconnections.com

Jerilyn Leverett, Executive Director

A private non-profit organization that looks to enable all people with disabilities to attain and have access to all opportunities in life.

3965   Division of Rehabilitation Services
Georgia Department of Labor
410 Mall Blvd
Suite B
Savannah, GA 31406-4869

912-356-2226
Fax: 912-356-2875
TTY: 912-356-2940
dol.state.ga.us

Mark Bultler, Commissioner
Jody Lane, Manager
George Foley, Manager
Vocational rehabilitation services.

3966   Living Independence for Everyone (LIFE)
5105 Paulsen Street
Suite 143-B
Savannah, GA 31405

912-920-2414
800-948-4824
Fax: 912-920-0007
www.lifecil.com

Mark Schreiber, President
Stuart Klugler, Vice President
John Paul Berlon, Secretary
The Southeast's Regional disability resource center that offers a wide range of resources, education, and advocacy to the community to help level the playing field for people with disabilities to create a world in which everyone can fully participate.

3967   Multiple Choices Center for Independent Living
145 Barrington Dr.
Athens, GA 30605-3133

706-850-4025
www.multiplechoices.us

Doug Hatch, President
Donald Veater, VP
Elllen Des Jardines, Secretary
To break down all barriers to inclusion by enhancing the equality of life and empowering people with disabilities through advocacy, education and training.

3968   North District Independent Living Program
Ste 209
311 Green St NW
Gainesville, GA 30501-3364

770-535-5930

Sharon McCurry, Coordinator
Cindy Hanna, Executive Director
Information and referral, advocacy, peer counseling, service coordination and ADA consultation.

3969   Southwest District Independent Living Program
P.O.Box 1606
Albany, GA 31702-1606

229-430-4170
Fax: 229-430-4466

Bill Layton, Director
Diane Davis, Executive Director
Offers peer counseling, disability education and awareness, attendant care registry, and information on accessible home for the disabled.

3970   Statewide Independent Living Council of Georgia
315 West Ponce de Leon Avenue
Suite 600
Decatur, GA 30030-2617

770-270-6860
888-288-9780
Fax: 770-270-5957
shellys5@hotmail.com
silcga.org

Steve Oldaker, President
Angela Denise Davis, Vice President
Mark Schreiber, Treasurer
Founded to ensure that people with disabilities have opportunities to live as independently as possible.

3971   Walton Options for Independent Living
948 Walton Way
Augusta, GA 30901-519

706-724-6262
877-821-8400
Fax: 706-724-6729
TTY: 706-724-6262
tjohnston@waltonoptions.org
www.waltonoptions.org

Tiffany Cilford, Executive Director
Ann Campbell-Kelly, Special Projects Coordinator
Alyson Schwartz, Special Projects Coordinator
Services include individual and systems advocacy, peer support, skills training (including basic computer and return to work skills), information and referral services and transition from institutions back to the community.

Hawaii

3972   Center For Independent Living- Kauai
State Office Building 3060 Eiwa Str
Lihue, HI 96766-6529

808-274-3484
Fax: 808-245-3485
kauaiddc@pixi.com

Humberto Blanco, Administrator
Teri Yamashiro, IL Specialist
Offers peer counseling, disability education, attendant care registry, outreach services and advocacy.

3973   Hawaii Center For Independent Living
1055 Kinoole Street
Suite 105le St
Hilo, HI 96720-3872

808-935-3777
800-420-6928
TTY: 808-935-7888
www.cil-hawaii.org

Gordon Fuller, Executive Director
Provides an array of support services for people with all types of disabilities of any age.

3974   Hawaii Center for Independent Living-Maui
220 Imi Kala Street
Suite 103
Wailuku, HI 96793-1209

808-242-4966
866-303-4245
800-420-6928
Fax: 808-244-6978
TTY: 808-242-4968
www.cil-hawaii.org

Clytie Nishihara, Manager
T Lay, Administrative Assistant
Offers disability education and awareness, advocacy and counseling.

3975   Hawaii Centers for Independent Living
200 N. Vineyard Blvd Bldg. A501
Honolulu, HI 96817-3950

808-522-5400
800-420-6928
Fax: 808-522-5427
www.cil-hawaii.org

Cheryl Mizusaawa, Executive Director
M.J. (Kimo) Keawe, COO & Executive Director
Our staff and Board of directors are excellent advocates with the disabled community. We will connect you with resources to make your own choices for housing, employment, and personal care and to find assistive devices and technology to improve quality of life. On both the islands of Oahu and Hawaii, we have an independent living specialist who is fluent in American sign language and is well known in the deaf community.

3976   Kauai Center for Independent Living
4340 Nawiliwili Rd.
Lihue, HI 96766-6529

808-246-4800
800-420-6928
Fax: 808-245-7218
www.cil-hawaii.org

Laurao Tobosa, Program Coordinator
Provides a variety of support services for people with all types of disabilities.

Idaho

3977 American Falls Office: Living Independently for Everyone (LIFE)
250 S. Skyline
Idaho Falls, ID 83402-4508 208-529-8610
Fax: 208-529-6804
diane@idlife.org
www.idlife.org

Dean Nilson, Executive Director
Tina Noreen, Programs Coordinator
Mickey Palmer, Fiscal Intermediary Manager
Enables people with disabilities to manage their own lives, make their own choices, and give information and knowledge to assist in living with dignity and bravado.

3978 Dawn Enterprises
280 Cedar Street P.O.Box 388
Blackfoot, ID 83221-388 208-785-5890
Fax: 208-785-3095
dawnent.org

Donna Butler, Executive Director
Teresa Oakes, Assistant Director/Fiscal Coordi
To assist individuals of Southeastern Idaho with mental, physical or social disabilities in achieving independence through employment training, skill training, social development, or living enhancements up to each individual's maximum capability.

3979 Disability Action Center NW
505 N Main St
Moscow, ID 83843-2615 208-883-0523
800-475-0070
Fax: 208-883-0524
www.dacnw.org

Larry Topp, President
Jean Coil, Vice President
Mark Leeper, CEO
A non-profit community partnership working to promote the independence and equality of all individuals with disabilities in all aspects of society. $45.00

3980 Disability Action Center NW: Coeur D'Alene
7560 N Government Way
Suite 1
Coeur D Alene, ID 83815- 4069 208-664-9896
800-854-9500
Fax: 208-666-1362
www.dacnw.org

Larry Topp, President
Jean Coil, Vice President
Mark Leeper, CEO
A non-profit community partnership working to promote the independence and equality of all individuals with disabilities in all aspects of society.

3981 Disability Action Center NW: Lewiston
330 5th Street
Suite A1
Lewiston, ID 83501-2086 208-746-9033
800-746-9033
Fax: 208-746-1004
www.dacnw.org

Larry Topp, President
Jean Coil, Vice President
Mark Leeper, CEO
A non-profit community partnership working to promote the independence and equality of all individuals with disabilities in all aspects of society.

3982 Idaho Falls Office: Living Independently for Everyone (LIFE)
250 S. Skyline
Idaho Falls, ID 83402-3702 208-529-8610
800-631-2747
Fax: 208-232-2753
www.idlife.org

Dean Nielson, Executive Director
Tina Noreen, Programs Coordinator
Mickey Palmer, Fiscal Intermediary Manager
Enables people with disabilities to manage their own lives, make their own choices, and give information and knowledge to assist in living with dignity and bravado.

3983 LIFE: Fort Hall
1333 Moursund
Houston, TX 77019 713-520-0232
Fax: 713-520-5785
TTY: 713-520-0232
www.ilru.org

Lex Frieden, Director
Enables people with disabilities to manage their own lives, make thier own choices, and give information and knowledge to assist in living with dignity and bravado.

3984 Living Independence Network Corporation
1878 W Overland Rd
Boise, ID 83705-3142 208-336-3335
Fax: 208-384-5037
info@lincidaho.org
lincidaho.org

Roger Howard, Executive Director
A non-profit organization empowering people with disabilities to achieve their desired level of independence.

3985 Living Independence Network Corporation: Twin Falls
1182 Eastland Dr North
Suite C
Twin Falls, ID 83301-8972 208-733-1712
Fax: 208-733-7711
info@lincidaho.org
www.lincidaho.org

Melva Heinrich, Executive Director
A non-profit organization empowering people with disabilities to achieve their desired level of independence.

3986 Living Independence Network Corporation: Caldwell
1609 Kimball Ave
Ste. 201
Caldwell, ID 83605-6965 208-454-5511
Fax: 208-454-5515
TTY: 208-454-5511
info@lincidaho.org
www.lincidaho.org

Heidi Caldwell, Executive Director
A non-profit organization empowering people with disabilities to achieve their desired level of independence.

3987 Living Independent for Everyone (LIFE): Pocatello Office
640 Pershing Ave
PO Box 4185
Pocatello, ID 83201-3702 208-232-2747
800-631-2747
Fax: 208-232-2753
TTY: 208-232-2747
tracy@idlife.org
www.idlife.org

Dean Nielson, Executive Director
Mickey Palmer, Fiscal Intermediary Manager
Tina Noreen, Programs Coordinator
Enables people with disabilities to manage thier own lives, make their own choices, and give information and knowledge to assist in living with dignity and bravado.

3988 Living Independently for Everyone (LIFE): Blackfoot Office
Living Independently for Everyone (LIFE): Pocate
570 W. Pacific
P.O.Box 86
Blackfoot, ID 83221-86 208-785-9648
Fax: 208-785-2398
lori@idlife.org
www.idlife.org

Dean Nielson, Executive Director
Tina Noreen, Programs Coordinator
Mickey Palmer, Fiscal Intermediary Manager
Enable people with disabilities to manage their own lives, make their own choices, and give information and knowledge to assist in living with dignity and bravado.

3989 Living Independently for Everyone: Burley
2311 Park Ave
Suite 7
Burley, ID 83318-2170   208-678-7705
                                    Fax: 208-678-7771
                                         www.idlife.org

Dean Nielson, Executive Director
Mickey Palmer, Fiscal Intermediary Manager
Tina Noreen, Programs Coordinator
Enables people with disabilities to manage their own lives, make their own choices, and give information and knowledge to assist in living with dignity and bravado.

3990 Southwestern Idaho Housing Authority
1108 W Finch Dr
Nampa, ID 83651-1732   208-467-7461
                                    Fax: 208-463-1772

David W Patten, Manager
Offers housing for rent and section/8

Illinois

3991 Access Living of Metropolitan Chicago
115 W Chicago Ave
Chicago, IL 60654-3209   312-640-2100
                                         800-613-8549
                                    Fax: 312-640-2101
                                    TTY: 312-640-2102
                                        accessliving.org

Marca Bristo, CEO
Bhuttu Mathews, Disability Resources Coordinator
Gary Arnold, Public Relations Coordinator
Established in 1980, access living is a change agent commited to fostering an incusive society that enables Chicagoans with disabilities to live fully engaged and self-directed lives. Nationally recognized as a leading force in the disability community. Access Living challenges stereotypes, protects civil rights, and champions social reform.

3992 Center on Deafness
3444 Dundee Rd
Northbrook, IL 60062-2258   847-559-0110
                                    Fax: 847-559-8199
                                    TTY: 847-559-9493
                                    www.centerondeafness.org

Bonnie Simon, Executive Director
Donna Gomez, Residential Services/ Adult Plac
Brandi Buie, School Intake
COD is dedicated to providing quality services for persons who are deaf or hard of hearing and their families, through educational, vocational, and residential services in a therapuetic, community-based environment

3993 Community Residential Alternative
Coleman Tri- County Services
22 Veterans Drive, ST. A
P.O. Box 869
Harrisburg, IL 62946-2017   618-252-0275
                                    Fax: 618-252-2389
                                    TTY: 618-269-4211
                                    cts.62946@frontier.com
                                    colemantricounty.tripod.com

Samantha Austin, Executive Director
Six bed group home that provides a residential alternative for the developmentally disabled adult. This program is designed to promote independence in daily living skills, economic self-sufficiency, and integration into the community.

3994 Division of Rehabilitation Services
Department of Human Services
100 South Grand Avenue East
Springfield, IL 62762-2625   217-782-2093
                                         800-843-6154
                                    Fax: 217-524-2471
                                    DHS.WebBits@illinois.gov
                                        www.dhs.state.il.us

Carol Adams, President
Provides medical, therapeutic and counseling services for the disabled, as well as employment services.

3995 DuPage Center for Independent Living
3130 Finley Rd.
Ste. 500
Downers Grove, IL 60515-5877   630-469-2300
                                    Fax: 630-469-2606
                                    TTY: 630-469-2300
                                         www.dupagecil.org

Charles Stack, Board President
Bette Lawrence Water, Vice President
John Lausas, Treasurer
A non residential, community based, not for profit agency wich provides advocacy and services to persons with disabilities in DuPage County.

3996 Fite Center for Independent Living
1230 Larkin Ave
Elgin, IL 60123-6200   847-695-5818
                                    Fax: 847-695-5892

Linda Bradford-Foster, Chairman, Board Treasurer
Gracia Bittner, Board Secretary
Provides services to people with disabilities in Kane, Kendall and McHenry counties. Our non-residential agency provides independent living skills training, advocacy, systemic + individual peer counseling, information and referral and housing services. Also provides technical assistance to businesses and agencies to work with people with disabilities. Locations in Elgin and Aurora. Please call for further details.

3997 Illinois Department of Rehab Services
Department of Human Services
100 South Grand Avenue East
Springfield, IL 62762-1   217-782-2093
                                         800-843-6154
                                    Fax: 217-524-2471
                                    DHS.WebBits@illinois.gov
                                        www.dhs.state.il.us

Carol Adams, President
Karen Perrin, Manager
The state's lead agency serving individuals with disabilities. DRS works in partnership with people with disabilities and their families to assist them in making informed choices to achieve full community participation through employment, education, and independent living opportunities.

3998 Illinois Valley Center for Independent Living
18 Gunia Dr
La Salle, IL 61301-9780   815-224-3126
                                         800-822-3246
                                    Fax: 815-224-3576
                                         ivcil@ivcil.com
                                              ivcil.com

John Hurst, President
Gary Rydleski, Vice President
Sue Faber, Secretary
A nonprofit service and advocacy organization that assists persons with disabilities in opening doors to their independence.

3999 Illinois and Iowa Center for Independent Living
501 11th St.
PO Box 6156
Rock Island, IL 61231-6156   309-793-0090
                                         877-541-2505
                                         855-744-8918
                                    Fax: 309-793-5198
                                         www.iicil.com

Liz Sherwin, Executive Director
Alfonso Ayew-Ew, Blind Independent Living Skill S
Eddie Williams, CommunityReintegration Advocate
To create and maintain independence options for people with disabilities by advocating for civil rights, providing services, and promoting full participation of disabled individuals in all aspects of the community.

4000 Impact Center for Independent Living
2735 E Broadway
Alton, IL 62002-1859
618-462-1411
888-616-4261
Fax: 618-474-5309
staff@impactcil.org
impactcil.org

Susy Woods, President
Judy O'Malley, Vice President
Bishop Samuel White, Treasurer
Promotes pride and respect for people with disabilities by sharing the tools that are necessary to take control of one's own life.

4001 Jacksonville Area CIL: Havana
220 W Main St
Havana, IL 62644-1138
309-543-6680
877-759-2187
Fax: 309-543-6711
info@jacil.org
www.jacil.org

Phil Foxworth, President
Mark Arnold, Vice President
Ruth Lanier, Secretary
Committed to enabling persons with disabilities to gain effective control and director of their own lives in the home, in the workplace and in the community.

4002 Jacksonville Area Center for Independent Living
15 Permac Road
Jacksonville, IL 62650-2071
217-245-8371
Fax: 217-245-1872
TTY: 217-245-8371
info@jacil.org
www.jacil.org

Phil Foxworth, President
Mark Arnold, Vice President
Ruth Lanier, Secretary
Committed to enabling persons with disabilities to gain effective control and direction of their own lives in the home, in the workplace and in the community.

4003 LIFE Center for Independent Living
2201 Eastland Dr
Suite 1
Bloomington, IL 61704
309-663-5433
888-543-3245
Fax: 309-663-7024
TTY: 309-663-5433
rickielee@lifecil.org
www.lifecil.org

Rickielee Benecke, Executive Director
Jill Doran, Associate Director
Brianne Anderson, Office Manager
A community-based, not-for-profit, non-residential organization that promotes disability rights, equal access, and full community participation for persons with disabilities.

4004 LINC-Monroe Randolph Center
Ste 4
1514 S Main St
Red Bud, IL 62278-1382
618-282-3700
Fax: 618-282-2740
TTY: 618-282-3700

Violete Nast, Manager

4005 Lake County Center for Independent Living
377 N Seymour Ave
Mundelein, IL 60060-2322
847-949-4440
Fax: 847-949-4445
TTY: 847-949-0641
lindsey@lccil.org
www.lccil.org

Kelli Brooks, Executive Director
Andy Balint, Director of Finance
Lety Cruz, Bilingual Program Assistant
Lake County Center for Indepdendent Living is a disability rights organization governed and staffed by a majority of people with disabilities. LCCIL offers services and advocacy that promote a fully accessible society, which expects participation by persons with disabilities.

4006 Life Center for Independent Living: Pontiac
318 West Madison Street
Pontiac, IL 61764-1785
815-844-1132
Fax: 815-844-1148
lifecil@lifecil.org
lifecil.org

Gail Kear, Executive Director
Jill Doran, Associate Director
Brianne Anderson, Office Manager
A community-based, not-for-profit, non-residential organization that promotes disability rights, equal access, and full community participation for persons with disabilities.

4007 Living Independently Now Center (LINC)
120 E a St
Belleville, IL 62220-1401
618-235-9988
Fax: 618-233-3729
TTY: 618-235-9988
info@lincinc.org
www.lincinc.org

Linda Conley, President
Ron Tialdo, Vice-President
Lynn Jarman, Executive Director
Empowers persons with disabilities to live independently and to promote accessibility and inclusion in all areas.

4008 Living Independently Now Center: Sparta
Western Egyptian Building
207 West 4th Street
Waterloo, IL 62298
618-317-4028
info@lincinc.org
www.lincinc.org

Linda Conley, President
Ron Tialdo, Vice-President
Lynn Jarman, Executive Director
Empowers persons with disabilities to live independently and to promote accessibility and inclusion in all areas.

4009 Living Independently Now Center: Waterloo
Western Egyptian Building
207 West 4th Street
Waterloo, IL 62298-1336
618-317-4028
info@lincinc.org
www.lincinc.org

Linda Conley, President
Ron Tialdo, Vice-President
Lynn Jarman, Executive Director
Empowers persons with disabilities to live independently and to promote accessibility and inclusion in all areas.

4010 Mosaic: Pontiac
4980 S. 118th St.
Omaha, NE 68137
877-366-7242
Fax: 402-896-1511
www.mosaicinfo.org

Max Miller, Chairperson
James Zils, Vice Chairperson
Lisa Negstad, 2nd Vice Chairperson
A faith-based organization serving people with developmental disabilities.

4011 Opportunities for Access: A Center for Independent Living
4206 Williamson Pl
Suite 3
Mount Vernon, IL 62864-6705
618-244-9212
Fax: 618-244-9310
TTY: 618-244-9575
ofacil.org

Michael Egbert, Executive Director
Serves, trains and provides information to persons with disabilities, family members and significant others and service providers. Services include: advocacy, information and referral, peer support, skills training, volunteer programs and other related services. Services are free. A cross disability community based, non-residential, nonprofit organization serving Clay, Clinton, Edwards, Effingham, Fayette, Hamilton, Jasper, Jefferson, Marion, Wabash, Washington, Wayne and White Counties.

4012 Options Center for Independent Living: Bourbonnais
22 Heritage Dr
Suite 107
Bourbonnais, IL 60914-2510   815-936-0100
                                 Fax: 815-936-0117
                                 TTY: 815-936-0132
                                 www.optionscil.org

Mark Mantarian, President
Ronald D. Smith, Vice President
Dina Raymond, Co-Secretary
A non-residential, not-for-profit, community-based organization that promotes independent living for people with disabilities.

4013 Options Center for Independent Living: Watseka
103 Laird Ln
Suite 103
Watseka, IL 60970   815-432-1332
                                 Fax: 815-432-1360
                                 TTY: 815-432-1361

Mark Mountain, President
Ronald D. Smith, Vice President
Dina Raymond, Co-Secretary
A non-residential, not-for-profit, community-based organization that promotes independent living for people with disabilities.

4014 PACE Center for Independent Living
1317 E Florida Ave
Urbana, IL 61801-6007   217-344-5433
                                 Fax: 217-344-2414
                                 TTY: 217-344-5024
                                 info@pacecil.org
                                 pacecil.org

Evelyn Brown, President
Fred Neubert, Vice President
Nancy McClellan-Hickey, Executive Director
Promotes the full participation of people with disabilities in the rights and responsibilities of society. Provides services, which assist people with disabilities in achieving or maintaining independence.

4015 Progress Center for Independent Living
7521 Madison St
Forest Park, IL 60130-1407   708-209-1500
                                 Fax: 708-209-1735
                                 TTY: 708-209-1826
                                 info@progresscil.org
                                 www.progresscil.org

Anne Gunter, Independent Living Advocate
Kim Liddell, Independent Living Advocate
Horacio Esparza, Executive Director
A community-based, non-profit, non-residential, service and advocacy organization operated for people with disabilities, by people with disabilities.

4016 Progress Center for Independent Living: Blue Island
12940 Western Ave
Blue Island, IL 60406-3766   708-388-5011
                                 Fax: 708-388-5016
                                 TTY: 708-389-8250
                                 info@progresscil.org
                                 www.progresscil.org

Horacio Esparza, Executive Director
Anne Gunter, Independent Living Advocate
Kim Liddell, Independent Living Advocate
A community-based, non-profit, non residential, service and advocacy organization operated for people with disabilities, by people with disabilities.

4017 Regional Access & Mobilization Project
202 Market St
Rockford, IL 61107-3954   815-968-7467
                                 Fax: 815-968-7612
                                 TTY: 815-968-2401
                                 rampcil.org

Shari Snyder, President
Tina Kaatz, Vice President
Craig Fetty, Secretary
To promote an accessible society that allows and expects full participation by people with disabilities.

4018 Regional Access & Mobilization Project: Belvidere
530 S State St
Suite 103
Belvidere, IL 61008-3711   815-544-8404
                                 Fax: 815-544-1896
                                 TTY: 815-544-8404
                                 rampcil.org

Shari Snyder, President
Tina Kaatz, Vice President
Craig Fetty, Secretary
Promote an accessible society that allows and expects full participation by people with disabilities.

4019 Regional Access & Mobilization Project: De Kalb
115 N First Street
Dekalb, IL 60115-3055   815-756-3202
                                 Fax: 815-756-3556
                                 TTY: 815-756-4263
                                 rampcil.org

Shari Snyder, President
Tina Kaatz, Vice President
Craig Fetty, Secretary
Promotes an accessible society that allows and expects full partiipation by persons with disabilities.

4020 Regional Access & Mobilization Project: Freeport
2155 W Galena Ave
Freeport, IL 61032-3013   815-233-1128
                                 Fax: 815-233-0743
                                 TTY: 815-233-1128
                                 rampcil.org

Shari Snyder, President
Tina Kaatz, Vice President
Craig Fetty, Secretary
Promotes an accessible society that allows and expects full partiipation by persons with disabilities.

4021 Soyland Access to Independent Living(SAIL)
2449 E Federal Dr
Decatur, IL 62526-2160   217-876-8888
                                 800-358-8080
                                 Fax: 217-876-7245
                                 TTY: 217-876-8888
                                 jwooters@decatursail.com
                                 www.decatursail.com

Jeri J Wooters, Executive Director
Betty Watkins, Rural Outreach Coordinator
A community-based, non-residential Center for Independent Living whose purpose is to promote and practice independent living for all people with disabilities.

4022 Soyland Access to Independent Living: Charleston
757 Windsor Rd
Charleston, IL 61920-7474   217-345-7245
                                 Fax: 217-345-7226
                                 TTY: 217-345-7245
                                 triplec@consolidated.net
                                 www.decatursail.com

Betty Watkins, Rural Outreach Coordinator
Jeri J Wooters, Executive Director
A community-based, non-residential Center for Independent Living whose purpose is to promote and practice independent living for all people iwth disabilities.

4023 Soyland Access to Independent Living: Shelbyville
1810 W.S. 3rd ST P.O.Box 650
Shelbyville, IL 62565-650   217-774-4322
                                 Fax: 217-774-4368
                                 TTY: 217-774-4322
                                 sailsel@consolidated.net
                                 www.decatursail.com

Jeri J Wooters, Executive Director
Betty Watkins, Rural Outreach Coordinator
A community-based, non-residential Center for Independent Living whose purpose is to promote and practice independent living for all people with disabilities.

4024   Soyland Access to Independent Living: Sullivan
1102 W Jackson St
Sullivan, IL 61951-1067   217-728-3186
                                            Fax: 217-728-2299
                                            TTY: 217-728-3186
                                        sulsail@wireless111.com
                                            www.decatursail.com

Betty Watkins, Rural Outreach Coordinator
Jeri J Wooters, Executive Director

A community-based, non-residential Center for Independent Living whose purpose is to promote and practice independent living for all people with disabilities.

4025   Springfield Center for Independent Living
330 South Grand Ave W
Springfield, IL 62704-3716   217-523-4032
                                                 800-447-4221
                                            Fax: 217-523-0427
                                            TTY: 217-523-4032
                                                scil@scil.org
                                                     scil.org

Pete Roberts, Executive Director
Susan Coopers, Program Director
Denise Groesch, Reintegration Coordinator

To increase opportunities for equality, integration and independence for all persons with disabilities through advocacy, services, and public education.

4026   Stone-Hayes Center for Independent Living
39 N Prairie St
Galesburg, IL 61401-4613   309-344-1306
                                                 888-347-4245
                                            Fax: 309-344-1305
                                            TTY: 309-344-1306

Vanya Peterson, Executive Director
Michael Bohnenkamp, Associate Director
John Hunigan, Office Manager

The purpose of INCIL is to facilitate the collaboration of all Centers for Independent Living in Illinois for promoting, through the Independent Living Movement, equal opportunities and civil rights for all persons with disabilities.

4027   West Central Illinois Center for Independent Living
639 York St.
Suite 204
Quincy, IL 62301-1065   217-223-0400
                                            Fax: 217-223-0479
                                            TTY: 217-223-0475
                                               info@wcicil.org
                                               www.wcicil.org

Glenda Hackemack, Executive Director
Dale Winner, Information & Referral Coordinat
Dustin Gorde Director of Community, Jenny

A not-for-profit advocacy center funded by state and federal grants to provide services to people with disabilities.

4028   West Central Illinois Center for Independent Living: Macomb
440 N Lafayette St
Macomb, IL 61455-1512   309-833-5766
                                            Fax: 309-833-4690
                                            TTY: 217-223-0475
                                               info@wcicil.org
                                               www.wcicil.org

Glenda Hackemack, Executive Director
Dale Winner, Information & Referral Coordinat
Dustin Gorde Director of Community, Jenny

A not-for-profit advocacy center funded by state and federal grants to provide services to people with disabilities.

4029   Will Grundy Center for Independent Living
2415 W Jefferson St
Suite A
Joliet, IL 60435-6464   815-729-0162
                                            Fax: 815-729-3697
                                            TTY: 815-729-2085
                                               will-grundycil.org

Elaine Sommer, President
Chris Boyk, Vice President
Dianne Mundle, Treasurer

A cross-disability, community based organization that strives for equality and empowerment of persons with disabilities in the Will and Grundy County areas.

Indiana

4030   Assistive Technology Training and Information Center (ATTIC)
1721 Washington Ave
Vincennes, IN 47591-4823   812-886-0575
                                                 877-96A-8842
                                            Fax: 812-886-1128
                                          inbox@atticindiana.org
                                            www.atticindiana.org

Patricia Stewart, Executive Director
Rebecca Anderson, Assistant Director
Mark Schmitt, Fiscal Controller

ATTIC provides support, information and education for individuals with disabilities and for families of children with special needs, and the professionals who assist these families. All disabilities, all ages.

4031   DAMAR Services
6067 Decatur Blvd.
Indianapolis, IN 46241   317-856-5201
                                            Fax: 317-856-2333
                                               info@damar.org
                                                   damar.org

Gail Shiel, Chairman
Rick Torbeck, Vice Chairman
Jim Dalton, Psy.D., HSPP, President and CEO

Builds better futures for children and adults facing life's greatest developmental and behavioral challenges.

4032   Everybody Counts Center for Independent Living
3616 Elm St
Room 3
East Chicago, IN 46410-7097   219-229-5055
                                                 888-769-3636
                                            Fax: 219-769-5326
                                            TTY: 219-756-3323
                                      info@everybodycounts.org
                                          everybodycounts.org

Teresa Torres, Executive Director
Emma Lewis Sullivan, On Loan Consultant
Mark Torres, Systems Manager

A nonprofit corporation dedicated to the achievement of maximum independence and enhanced quality of life for persons with disabilities.

4033   Four Rivers Resource Services
Hwy. 59 South
P.O. Box 249
Linton, IN 47441-249   812-847-2231
                                            Fax: 812-847-8836
                                             fourrivers@frrs.org
                                                    frrs.org

Stephen Sacksteder, Executive Director
Robin Duncan, Chief Financial Officer
Dean Dorrell, Information Systems Director

FRRS is established to enable individuals with disabilities and other challenges to attain self independence and natural interdependence, inclusion in normal life experiences and opportunities, and general life enrichment, by working in partnership with them, their families and the communities in and around Greene, Sullivan, Daviess, and Martin Counties.

4034   Future Choices Independent Living Center
309 N High St
Muncie, IN 47305-1618   765-741-8332
                                                 866-741-3444
                                            Fax: 765-741-8333
                                               futurechoices.org

Beth Y. Quarles, President

Provides unlimited options for minorities, youth, and Hoosiers with disabilities.

4035   Independent Living Center of Eastern Indiana (ILCEIN)
1818 W Main St
Richmond, IN 47374-3822

765-939-9226
877-939-9226
Fax: 765-935-2215
www.ilcein.org

Jim McCormick, Executive Director
Dean Turner, Administrative Director
Ann Barnhart, Compliance Manager
Serving Fayette, Franklin, Henry, Decatur, Rush, Union and Wayne Counties.

4036   Indianapolis Resource Center for Independent Living
5302 East Washington Street
Indianapolis, IN 46219

317-926-1660
866-794-7245
Fax: 317-926-1687
info@abilityindiana.org
www.abilityindiana.org

Judy Townsend, President
Dave Trulock, Vice President
Jacqueline Troy, Treasurer
Provides services, support and information to people with disabilities to help insure equal access to all aspects of community life.

4037   League for the Blind and Disabled
5821 S Anthony Blvd
Fort Wayne, IN 46816-3701

260-441-0551
800-889-3443
Fax: 260-441-7760
TTY: 800-889-3443
the-league@the-league.org
the-league.org

David A. Nelson, CEO/President
Catherine Collins, Chair
Anne Palmer, Administrative Assistant
To provide and promote opportunities that empower people with disabilities to achieve their potential.

4038   Martin Luther Homes of Indiana
Mosaic
26 N Brown Ave
Terre Haute, IN 47803-1523

812-235-3399
Fax: 812-235-1590

Providing a wide array of services to assist individuals and families in achieving positive life goals. Services to persons with disabilities and other special needs include community living options, training and employment options, spiritual growth and development options, training and counseling support.

4039   Ruben Center for Independent Living
5302 East Washington Street
Indianapolis, IN 46219-3227

317-926-1660
Fax: 317-926-1687
TTY: 219-397-6496
info@abilityindiana.org
www.abilityindiana.org

Judy Townsend, President
Dave Trulock, Vice President
Jacqueline Troy, Treasurer
An independent living center providing support, information and education.

4040   SILC, Indiana Council on Independent Living (ICOIL)
P.O.Box 7083
Indianapolis, IN 46207-7083

317-232-1303
800-545-7763
Fax: 317-232-6478

Nancy Young, Program Director
Richard Simers, SILC Chairperson

4041   Southern Indiana Center for Independent Living
1494 W. Main Street
PO Box 308
Mitchell, IN 47446-1943

812-277-9626
800-845-6914
Fax: 812-277-9628
sicilindiana.org

Al Tolbert, Executive Director
Darlene Webster, Independent Living Center Direct

SICIL is a consumer controlled, community based, cross-disability, non-residential and not for profit organization that promotes and practices the philosophy of independent living: consumer control, peer support, self-help, self-determination, equal access, and individual and community advocacy. SICIL also promotes accesible and affordable housing, recreation and transportation.

4042   Wabash Independent Living Center & Learning Center (WILL)
1 Dreiser Square
Terre Haute, IN 47807

812-298-9455
877-915-9455
Fax: 812-299-9061
TTY: 877-915-9455
info@thewillcenter.org
www.thewillcenter.org

Don Rogers, Chairman
Jody Pomfret, Vice Chairman
Kevin Burke, Treasurer
To empower people with disabilities to ensure that they have full and complete access to community resources to promote their independence

Iowa

4043   Black Hawk Center for Independent Living
2800 Falls Ave.
P.O. Box 2275
Waterloo, IA 50701-2275

319-291-7755
888-291-7754
Fax: 319-291-7781
TTY: 800-735-2942

To create and maintain independence options by working with people with disabilities.

4044   Central Iowa Center for Independent Living
655 Walnut St
Suite 131
Des Moines, IA 50309-3930

515-243-1742
888-503-2287
Fax: 515-243-5385

Bob Jeppesen, Executive Director
Frank Strong, Associate Director
Crystal Toman, Office Coordinator
CICIL is a community based, non-profit, non-residential program serving persons with disabilities. CICIL assists all persons, regardless of disability in making choices about their own lives and in experiencing success in achieving independence.

4045   Evert Conner Rights & Resources CIL
730 S Dubuque St
Iowa City, IA 52240-4202

319-338-3870
800-982-0272
Fax: 319-354-1799

Scott Gill, Executive Director
Provides community services like disability awareness training and classroom presentations. Individual services include independent living skills training and peer counseling. All services are custom designed to support the independence of people with disabilities in their own community.

4046   Hope Haven
1800 19th St
PO Box 70
Rock Valley, IA 51247-1098

712-476-2737
Fax: 712-476-3110
hopehaven.org

Dr. Kent Eric Eknes, President
Ron Boote, Vice President
David Vanningen, Executive Director
Unleashes the potential in people through work and life skills so that they may enjoy a productive life in their community.

4047 League of Human Dignity, Center for Independent Living
1520 Avenue M
Council Bluffs, IA 51501-1185 712-323-6863
Fax: 712-323-6811
Cinfo@leagueofhumandignity.com
www.leagueofhumandignity.com
Carrie England, Director
League of Human Dignity actively promotes the full integration of individuals with disabilities into society. To this end, the League will advocate their needs and rights, and provide quality services to involve these persons in becoming and remaining independent citizens.

4048 Martin Luther Homes of Iowa
P.O. Box 2316
Princeton, NJ 08543-2316 877-843-7953
Fax: 563-568-3992
www.rwjf.org
Mary Lynn ReVoir, Project Director
Fred Naumann III, Communications
Richard Wicks, Executive Director

4049 South Central Iowa Center for Independent Living
117 1st Ave W
Oskaloosa, IA 52577-3243 641-672-1867
800-651-7911
Fax: 641-672-1867
brookie43@gmail.com
www.iowasilc.org/cilinfo.html
Deb Philpot, Executive Director
Provides services, support, information and referral to people with disabilities to help insure equal access to all aspects of community life.

4050 Three Rivers Center for Independent Living
900 Rebecca Avenue
Pittsburgh, PA 15221-2938 412-371-7700
800-633-4588
Fax: 412-371-9430
TTY: 412-371-6230
lgray@trcil.org
Stanley A. Holbrook, President & Executive Director
Lisa Wilson, HR Program Manager
Rachel Rogan, Director of Waiver Services
Providing a wide array of services to assist individuals and families in achieving positive life goals.

Kansas

4051 Advocates for Better Living For Everyone(A.B.L.E.)
Ste C
521 Commercial St
Atchison, KS 66002 913-367-1830
888-845-2879
Fax: 913-367-1830
Ken Gifford, President & CEO
A not for profit agency providing services within the State of Kansas. ABLE looks to assist people with disabilities as well as any other member of the community to live an integrated, quality life with dignity, respect, and independence.

4052 Center for Independent Living SW Kansas: Liberal
1023 N Kansas Ave
Suite 2
Liberal, KS 67901-2655 620-624-5500
800-327-4048
Fax: 620-624-6576
TTY: 620-624-5500
www.cilswks.org
Victor Otero, Manager
Crystal Tharp, Independent Living Advocate
Dedicated to helping people achieve full participation in society.

4053 Center for Independent Living Southwest Kansas
P.O.Box 2090
Garden City, KS 67846-2090 620-276-1900
800-736-9443
Fax: 620-271-0200
Troy Horton, Executive Director
Dedicated to helping people achieve full participation in society.

4054 Center for Independent Living Southwest Kansas: Dodge City
2601 Central Ave
Dodge City, KS 67801-6200 620-227-6660
800-326-1366
Fax: 620-227-8185
TTY: 620-227-6660
Mary Jane Sandoval, Independent Living Advocate
Dedicated to helping people achieve full participation in society

4055 Coalition for Independence
4911 State Ave
Kansas City, KS 66102-1749 913-321-5140
866-201-3829
Fax: 913-321-5182
TTY: 913-321-5216
cfi-kc.org
Clarence Smith, Executive Director
Laarni Sison, Executive Assistant
Claire Marr, Lead Independent Living Speciali
Facilitates positive and responsible independence for all people with disabilities by acting as an advocate for individuals with disabilities, providing services, and promoting accessibility and acceptance.

4056 Cowley County Developmental Services
P.O.Box 618
Arkansas City, KS 67005-618 620-442-5270
866-442-5270
Fax: 620-442-5623
Bill Brooks, Executive Director
Provides services for persons with developmental disabilities in Cowley County..

4057 Independence
2001 Haskell Ave
Lawrence, KS 66046-3249 785-841-0333
888-824-7277
Fax: 785-841-1094
comment@independenceinc.org
independenceinc.org
Karen McGrath, President
Bruce Passman, Vice President
Sandra London, Lieb
Provides advocacy, services, and education for people with disabilities and our communities.

4058 Independent Connection
1710 W. Schilling Road
P.O.Box 1160
Salina, KS 67402- 1160 785-827-9383
800-526-9731
Fax: 785-823-2015
TTY: 785-827-9383
www.occk.com
Shelia Nelson-Stout, President/CEO
Deanna L. Lamer, Senior Director,Human Resources
Tasha Suppes, Human Resources Coordinator
Dedicated to helping people with physical or mental disabilities remove barriers to employment, independent living, and full participation in their communities.

4059 Independent Connection: Abilene
Suite 221
300 N. Cedar St.
Abilene, KS 67410 785-263-2208
Fax: 785-263-3795
TTY: 785-263-2208
www.occk.com
Shelia Nelson-Stout, President/CEO
Deanna L. Lamer, Senior Director,Human Resources
Tasha Suppes, Human Resources Coordinator

Dedicated to helping people with physical or mental disabilities remove barriers to employment, independent living, and full participation in their communities.

4060   Independent Connection: Beloit
501 W 7th St
Beloit, KS 67420-2107

785-738-5423
Fax: 785-738-3320
TTY: 785-738-5423
www.occk.com

Shelia Nelson-Stout, President/CEO
Deanna L. Lamer, Senior Director,Human Resources
Tasha Suppes, Human Resources Coordinator
Dedicated to helping people with physical or mental disabilities remove barriers to employment, independent living, and full participation in their communities.

4061   Independent Connection: Concordia
1502 Lincoln St
Concordia, KS 66901-4830

785-243-1977
Fax: 785-243-4524
TTY: 785-243-1977
www.occk.com

Shelia Nelson-Stout, President/CEO
Dedicated to helping people with physical or mental disabilities remove barriers to employment, independent living, and full participation in their communities.

4062   Independent Living Resource Center
3033 W 2nd St N
Wichita, KS 67203-5357

316-942-6300
800-479-6861
Fax: 316-942-2078
ilrcks.org

Jean Shuler, President
Angie Schmidt, Vice Chairman
Derrick Prichard, Secretary/Treasurer
Empower people with disabilities to lead independent lives by providing advocacy, education and direct services. Serve people with all types of disabilities; permanent or temporary, physical disabilities, mental disabilities, and developmental disabilities.

4063   Kansas Services for the Blind & Visually Impaired
2601 SW East Circle Dr N
Topeka, KS 66606-2445

785-296-3738
800-547-5789
Fax: 785-291-3138
srskansas.org

Dennis Ford, Manager
Michael Donnelly, Director
Helps persons who are blind or visually to improve their quality of life. KSBVI provides people with an array of services and experiences aimed at overcoming not only the physical difficulties brought on by the loss of vision, but also the fear of change associated with vision loss. KSBVI can also help with job search and retention activities; life skills training; access to medical services; and technical assistance..

4064   LINK: Colby
505 N Franklin Ave
Suite G
Colby, KS 67701-2342

785-462-7600
800-736-9418
TTY: 785-462-7600
brianatwell@linkinc.org
www.linkinc.org

Brian Atwell, Executive Director
Promotes and supports the civil rights of people with disabilities and empowers them to achieve a life of independence and equality..

4065   Living Independently in Northwest Kansas: Hays
2401 E 13th St
Hays, KS 67601-2663

785-625-6942
800-596-5926
Fax: 785-625-2334
TTY: 785-625-6942
brianatwell@linkinc.org
www.linkinc.org

Brian Atwell, Executive Director

Promotes and supports the civil rights of people with disabilities and empowers them to achieve a life of independence and equality.

4066   Prairie IL Resource Center
103 W 2nd St
Pratt, KS 67124-2644

620-672-9600
Fax: 620-672-9601
info@pilr.org
www.pilr.org

Dave Mullins, President
Stephanie Guthrie, Vice President
Chris Owens, Executive Director
To achieve the full inclusion and acceptance of people with disabilities through education and advocacy

4067   Prairie Independent Living Resource Center
17th S Main St
Hutchinson, KS 67501

620-663-3989
888-715-6818
Fax: 620-663-4711
TTY: 620-663-9920
info@pilr.org
www.pilr.org

Dave Mullins, President
Stephanie Guthrie, Vice President
Chris Owens, Executive Director
To achieve the full conclusion and acceptance of people with disabilities through education and advocacy

4068   Resource Center for Independent Living
104 S. Washington Ave.
Iola, KS 66749-8805

620-365-8144
877-944-8144
Fax: 620-365-7726
rcilinc.org

Chad Wilkins, Executive Director
Committed to working with individuals, families, and communities to promote independent living and individual choice to persons with disabilities.

4069   Resource Center for Independent Living, Inc. (RCIL)
409 Columbia St.
Utica, NY 13503-210

315-797-4642
800-580-7245
Fax: 315-797-4747
TTY: 315-797-5837
rcilinc.org

Chad Wilkins, Executive Director
Committed to working with individuals, families, and communities to promote independent living and individual choice to persons with disabilities. As a center for independent living in Kansas, we provide advocacy, peer counseling, information and referral, independent living skills training and deinstitutionalization. In addition to these services, we also provide HOBS payroll services and a variety of programs benefiting individuals with disabilities.

4070   Resource Center for Independent Living: Emporia
215 West Sixth Avenue
Suite 202
Emporia, KS 66801-2886

620-342-1648
888-261-4024
Fax: 620-342-1821
info@rcilinc.org
rcilinc.org

Deone Wilson, Executive Director
Beth Combes, Information & Outreach Coordinat
Amy Richardson, Targeted Case Manager
Committed to working with individuals, families, and communities to promote independent living and individual choice to persons with disabilities.

4071   Resource Center for Independent Living: Arkansas City
P.O. Box 257
1137 Laing
Osage City, KS 66523   785-528-3105
                                        800-580-7245
                                    Fax: 785-528-3665
                                    TTY: 785-528-3106
                                    info@rcilinc.org
                                        rcilinc.org

Deone Wilson, Executive Director
Tania Harrington, Director of Quality Assurance
Adam Burnett, Director of Core Services
Committed to working with individuals, families, and communities to promote independent living and individual choice to persons with disabilities.

4072   Resource Center for Independent Living: Burlington
P.O. Box 257
1137 Laing
Osage City, KS 66523   785-528-3105
                                        800-580-7245
                                    Fax: 785-528-3665
                                    TTY: 785-528-3106
                                    info@rcilinc.org
                                        rcilinc.org

Deone Wilson, Executive Director
Tania Harrington, Director of Quality Assurance
Adam Burnett, Director of Core Services
Committed to working with individuals, families, and communities to promote independent living and individual choice to persons with disabilities.

4073   Resource Center for Independent Living: Coffeyville
P.O. Box 257
1137 Laing
Osage City, KS 66523   785-528-3105
                                        800-580-7245
                                    Fax: 785-528-3665
                                    TTY: 785-528-3106
                                    info@rcilinc.org
                                        rcilinc.org

Deone Wilson, Executive Director
Tania Harrington, Director of Quality Assurance
Adam Burnett, Director of Core Services
Committed to working with individuals, families, and communities to promote independent living and individual choice to persons with disabilities.

4074   Resource Center for Independent Living: El Dorado
615 1/2 N Main St
El Dorado, KS 67042-2027   316-322-7853
                                        800-960-7853
                                    Fax: 316-322-7888
                                    info@rcilinc.org
                                        rcilinc.org

Macy Gaines, Independent Living Specialist
Doris Hammons, Targeted Case Manager
Shirley Mullin, Targeted Case Manager
Committed to working with individuals, families, and communities to promote independent living and individual choice to persons with disabilities.

4075   Resource Center for Independent Living: Ft Scott
P.O. Box 257
1137 Laing
Osage City, KS 66523   785-528-3105
                                        800-580-7245
                                    Fax: 785-528-3665
                                    TTY: 785-528-3106
                                    info@rcilinc.org
                                        rcilinc.org

Deone Wilson, Executive Director
Tania Harrington, Director of Quality Assurance
Adam Burnett, Director of Core Services
Committed to working with individuals, families, and communities to promote independent living and individual choice to persons with disabilities.

4076   Resource Center for Independent Living: Ottawa
233 W 23rd Street
Ottawa, KS 66067-3533   785-242-1805
                                        800-995-1805
                                    Fax: 785-242-1448
                                        rcilinc.org

Chad Wilkins, Executive Director
Committed to working with individuals, families, and communities to promote independent living and individual choice to persons with disabilities.

4077   Resource Center for Independent Living: Overland Park
Ste 100
10200 W 75th St
Shawnee Mission, KS 66204-2242   913-362-6618
                                        877-439-2847
                                    Fax: 913-677-2742
                                        rcilinc.org

Chad Wilkins, Executive Director
RCIL is committed to working with individuals, families, and communities to promote independent living and individual choice to persons with disabilities.

4078   Resource Center for Independent Living: Topeka
1507 S.W. 21stStreet
Suite 203
Topeka, KS 66604-2356   785-267-1717
                                        877-719-1717
                                    Fax: 785-267-1711
                                    info@rcilinc.org
                                        rcilinc.org

Rosie Cooper, Director of Independent Living S
Stuart Jones, Assistive Technology Specialist
Mikel McCary, Assistive Technology Specialist
Committed to working with individuals, families, and communities to promote independent living and individual choice to persons with disabilities.

4079   Southeast Kansas Independent Living (SKIL)
1801 Main
P.O. Box 957
Parsons, KS 67357-957   620-421-5502
                                        800-688-5616
                                    Fax: 620-421-3705
                                    TTY: 620-421-0983
                                    skil@skilonline.com
                                    www.skilonline.com

Nancy Varner, Chairman
Janet Spillman, Vice Chairman
Shari Coatney, CEO/President
To empower, integrate and maximize independence for all persons with disabilities.

4080   Southeast Kansas Independent Living: Independence
107 East Main
P.O.Box 944
Independence, KS 67301-944   620-331-1006
                                        866-927-1006
                                    Fax: 620-331-1257
                                    TTY: 620-331-1006
                                    skilindy@skilonline.com
                                    www.skilonline.com

Nancy Varner, Chairman
Janet Spillman, Vice Chairman
Shari Coatney, CEO/President
To empower, integrate and maximize independence for all persons with disabilities.

4081   Southeast Kansas Independent Living: Chanute
2 W. Main
P.O.Box 645
Chanute, KS 66720-645   620-431-0757
                                        866-927-0757
                                    Fax: 620-431-7274
                                    TTY: 620-431-0757
                                    skilchanute@skilonline.com
                                    www.skilonline.com

Nancy Varner, Chairman
Janet Spillman, Vice Chairman
Shari Coatney, CEO/President

To empower, integrate and maximize independence for all persons with disabilities.

4082   Southeast Kansas Independent Living: Columbus
123 N. Kansas
P.O. Box 478
Columbus, KS 66725-1801
620-429-3600
866-927-3600
Fax: 620-429-1027
skilcolumbus@skilonline.com
www.skilonline.com

Nancy Varner, Chairman
Janet Spillman, Vice Chairman
Shari Coatney, CEO/President
To empower, integrate and maximize independence for all persons with disabilities.

4083   Southeast Kansas Independent Living: Fredonia
623 Monroe
P.O.Box 448
Fredonia, KS 66736-448
620-378-4881
866-927-4881
Fax: 620-378-4851
TTY: 620-378-4881
skilfredonia@skilonline.com
www.skilonline.com

Nancy Varner, Chairman
Janet Spillman, Vice Chairman
Shari Coatney, CEO/President
To empower, integrate and maximize independence for all persons with disabilities.

4084   Southeast Kansas Independent Living: Hays
510 W. 29thStreet, Suite A
PO Box 366
Hays, KS 67601-366
785-628-8019
800-316-8019
Fax: 785-628-3116
TTY: 785-628-3128
skilhays@skilonline.com
www.skilonline.com

Nancy Varner, Chairman
Janet Spillman, Vice Chairman
Shari Coatney, CEO/President
To empower, integrate and maximize independence for all persons with disabilities.

4085   Southeast Kansas Independent Living: Pittsburg
1403 N. Broadway
P.O.Box 1706
Pittsburg, KS 66762-1706
620-231-6780
866-927-6780
Fax: 620-232-9915
TTY: 620-231-6780
skilpittsburg@skilonline.com
www.skilonline.com

Nancy Varner, Chairman
Janet Spillman, Vice Chairman
Shari Coatney, CEO/President
To empower, integrate and maximize independence for all persons with disabilities.

4086   Southeast Kansas Independent Living: Sedan
113 West Main
P.O.Box 340
Sedan, KS 67361-340
620-725-3990
866-906-3990
Fax: 620-725-3942
TTY: 620-725-3990
skilsedan@skilonline.com
www.skilonline.com

Nancy Varner, Chairman
Janet Spillman, Vice Chairman
Shari Coatney, CEO/President
To empower, integrate and maximize independence for all persons with disabilities.

4087   Southeast Kansas Independent Living: Yates Center
119 W. Butler
P.O.Box 129
Yates Center, KS 66783-129
620-625-2818
866-927-2818
Fax: 620-625-2585
www.skilonline.com

Nancy Varner, Chairman
Janet Spillman, Vice Chairman
Shari Coatney, CEO/President
To empower, integrate and maximize independence for all persons with disabilities.

4088   Three Rivers Independent Living Center
504 Miller Drive
P.O.Box 408
Wamego, KS 66547-0408
785-456-9915
800-555-3994
Fax: 785-456-9923
TTY: 785-456-9915
reception@threeriversinc.org
www.threeriversinc.org

Audrey Schremmer-Philips, Executive Director
Keyna Steinbrock, IL Specialist
Erica Christie, Director of Supports & Services
A nonprofit organization promoting the self reliance of individuals with disabilities through education, advocacy, training and support.

4089   Three Rivers Independent Living Center: Clay
719 5th Street
P.O.Box 33
Clay Center, KS 67432-0033
785-632-6117
Fax: 785-632-6117
TTY: 785-632-6117
reception@threeriversinc.org
www.threeriversinc.org

Audrey Schremmer-Philips, Executive Director
Keyna Steinbrock, IL Specialist
Erica Christie, Director of Supports & Services
A non-profit organization promoting the self reliance of individuals with disabilities through, education, advocacy, training and support.

4090   Three Rivers Independent Living Center: Manhattan
401 Houston St.
Manhattan, KS 66502
785-776-9294
800-432-2703
Fax: 785-776-9479
reception@threeriversinc.org
www.threeriversinc.org

Audrey Schremmer-Philips, Executive Director
Keyna Steinbrock, IL Specialist
Erica Christie, Director of Supports & Services
A non profit organization promoting the self reliance of individuals with disabilities through education, advocacy, training and support.

4091   Three Rivers Independent Living Center: Seneca
416 Main St
Seneca, KS 66538-1926
785-336-0222
Fax: 785-336-0288
reception@threeriversinc.org
www.threeriversinc.org

Audrey Schremmer-Philips, Executive Director
Keyna Steinbrock, IL Specialist
Erica Christie, Director of Supports & Services
A non profit organization promoting the self reliance of individuals with disabilities through education, advocacy, training and support.

4092   Three Rivers Independent Living Center: Topeka
P.O.Box 4152
Topeka, KS 66604-4152
785-273-0249
Fax: 785-273-0249
reception@threeriversinc.org
www.threeriversinc.org

Audrey Schremmer-Philips, Executive Director
Keyna Steinbrock, IL Specialist
Erica Christie, Director of Supports & Services

A non profit organization promoting the self reliance of individuals with disabilities through education, advocacy, training and support.

4093 Topeka Independent Living Resource Center
501 SW Jackson St
Suite 100
Topeka, KS 66603-3300

785-233-4572
Fax: 785-233-1561
TTY: 785-233-4572
tilrcweb@tilrc.org
tilrc.org

Mike Oxford, Executive Director
Evan Korynta, Operations Manager
Angie Harter, Independent Living Advocacy Staf
A civil and human rights organization that advocates for justice, equality and essential services for a fully integrated and accessible society for all people with disabilities.

4094 Whole Person: Nortonville
7301 Mission Road
Suite 135
Prairie Village, KS 66208- 3006

913-262-1294
877-767-8896
Fax: 913-262-2392
info@thewholeperson.org
www.thewholeperson.org

Rick O'Neal, President
Jim Atwater, Vice President
MIchelle Ford, Secretary
Assists people with disabilities to live independently and encourages change within the community to expand opportunities for independent living.

4095 Whole Person: Nortonville, The
7301 Mission Road
Suite 135
Prairie Village, KS 66208- 3006

913-262-1294
877-767-8896
Fax: 913-262-2392
info@thewholeperson.org
www.thewholeperson.org

Rick O'Neal, President
Jim Atwater, Vice President
MIchelle Ford, Secretary
Assists people with disabilities to live independently and encourages change within the community to expand opportunities for independent living.

4096 Whole Person: Prairie Village
7301 Mission Rd
Prairie Village, KS 66208-3006

913-262-1294
Fax: 913-262-2392
info@thewholeperson.org
www.thewholeperson.org

Rick O'Neal, President
Jim Atwater, Vice President
MIchelle Ford, Secretary
Assists people with disabilities to live independently and encourages change within the community to expand opportunities for independent living.

4097 Whole Person: Prairie Village, The
7301 Mission Road
Suite 135
Prairie Village, KS 66208- 3006

913-262-1294
877-767-8896
Fax: 913-262-2392
info@thewholeperson.org
www.thewholeperson.org

Rick O'Neal, President
Jim Atwater, Vice President
MIchelle Ford, Secretary
Assists people with disabilities to live independently and encourages change within the community to expand opportunities for independent living.

4098 Whole Person: Tonganoxie
7301 Mission Road
Suite 135
Prairie Village, KS 66208- 3006

913-262-1294
877-767-8896
Fax: 913-262-2392
info@thewholeperson.org
www.thewholeperson.org

Rick O'Neal, President
Jim Atwater, Vice President
MIchelle Ford, Secretary
Assists people with disabilities to live independently and encourages change within the community to expand opportunities for independent living.

Kentucky

4099 Center for Accessible Living
501 S. 2nd Street
Ste 200
Louisville, KY 40202-2121

502-589-6620
888-813-8497
Fax: 502-589-3980
TTY: 502-589-6690
www.calky.org

Jan Day, CEO
Michael Markiewicz, Chief Financial Officer
Jeanne M. Gallimore, Branch Director
To assist the individuals with disabilities who seek to live independently.

4100 Center for Accessible Living: Murray
1051 N 16th St
Suite C
Murray, KY 42071-8511

270-753-7676
888-261-6194
Fax: 270-753-7729
TTY: 270-767-0549
www.calky.org

Jeanne M. Gallimore, Branch Director
Susan Tharpe, Coordinator of Services
Jan Day, CEO
To assist the individuals with disabilities who seek to live independently.

4101 Center for Independent Living: Kentucky Department for the Blind
Independent Living Office
Rear
409 N Miles St
Elizabethtown, KY 42701-1834

270-766-5126

Buel E Stalls Jr, Office Manager and IL Specialist
Nancy Bachuss, Manager
Offers peer counseling, attendant care registry and other services to the community as they relate to the blind community. The Murray office is an independent living regional office which covers 20 far western counties of Kentucky..

4102 Disability Coalition of Northern Kentucky
Ste 219
525 W 5th St
Covington, KY 41011-1293

859-431-7668
Fax: 859-431-7688
TTY: 800-648-6057

Kitt Heeg, Executive Director
Empowering people with disabilities through education, networking, and positive attitudes..

4103 Disability Resource Initiative
624 Eastwood St
Bowling Green, KY 42103-1602

270-796-5992
877-437-5045
Fax: 270-796-6630

Marilyn Mitchell, Executive Director
Tracy Cole, Independent Living Specialist
Steve Burchett, IT Specialist

One of the most important premises in Independent Living is that people with disabilities are the most knowledgable about their own needs. Because of this all of their services are designed to be consumer-driven. Within each service, Center Staff work with both participant and provider to achieve and maintain an Independent Lifestyle.

4104 Independence Place
1093 S. Broadway
Suite 1218
Lexington, KY 40504-1787
859-266-2807
877-266-2807
Fax: 859-335-0627
TTY: 800-648-6056
info@independenceplaceky.org
www.independenceplaceky.org

Michael Fein, Chairman
Carla Webster, Vice Chairwoman
Pamela Roark-Glisson, Executive Director
To assist people with disabilities to achieve their full potential for community inclusion through improving access, choice and equal opportunity.

4105 Pathfinders for Independent Living
105 E Mound St
Harlan, KY 40831-2355
606-573-5777
877-340-PATH
Fax: 606-573-5739
TTY: 606-573-5777

Sandra Goodwyn, Executive Director
Andrew Saylor, Director of IT (Internal) and Fi
Stacy Marple, Director of IT (External)
They publish a newsletter called LifeLine 4-5 times a year. Most articles are written by Sandra Goodwyn. Editor is Andrew Saylor. Serves people with disabilities to maintain as much independence as they desire

4106 SILC Department of Vocational Rehabilitation
209 Saint Clair St
Frankfort, KY 40601-1817
502-564-4440
800-372-7172
Fax: 502-564-6745
sarahf.richardson@ky.gov

Sarah Richardson, SILC Liaison
We recognize and respect the contributions of all individuals as a necessary and vital part of a productive society..

Louisiana

4107 New Horizons: Central Louisiana
Ste 18
2406 Ferrand St
Monroe, LA 71201-3236
318-323-4374
800-428-5505
Fax: 318-323-5445
nhilc@nhilc.org
www.nhilc.org

Alan Loosley, President
Sharon Geddes, Vice-President
Clint Snell, Vice-President for Finance
A private, non-profit, non-residential, consumer-controlled, community-based organization that enables people with disabilities to live independently.

4108 New Horizons: Northeast Louisiana
3717 Government Street
Suite 7
Alexandria, LA 71301-4037
318-484-3596
888-361-3596
Fax: 318-484-3640
nhilc@nhilc.org
www.nhilc.org

Alan Loosley, President
Sharon Geddes, Vice-President
Clint Snell, Vice-President for Finance
A private, non-profit, non-residential, consumer controlled, community based organization that enables people with disabilities to live independently.

4109 New Horizons: Northwest Louisiana
1111A Hawn Avenue
Shreveport, LA 71106-6144
318-671-8131
877-219-7327
Fax: 318-688-7823
www.nhilc.org

Alan Loosley, President
Sharon Geddes, Vice-President
Clint Snell, Vice-President for Finance
A private, non-profit, non-residential, consumer-controlled, community based organization that enables people with disabilities to live independently.

4110 Resources for Independent Living: Baton Rouge
New Orleans Resources for Independent Living
3233 South Sherwood Forest Blvd.
Suite 101A
Baton Rouge, LA 70816
225-753-4772
877-505-2260
Fax: 225-753-4831
www.noril.org

Yavonka G. Archaga, Executive Director
Alisha S. Hammond, Assistant Director
Rosie Calvin, Program Manager
RIL provides quality services to individuals with disabilities to assist with living independent. RIL also offers services to inculde information and referral, advocacy, peer support and independent living skills training.

4111 Resources for Independent Living: Metairie
2001 21st Street Kenner
Kenner, LA 70062
504-522-1955
877-505-2260
Fax: 504-522-1954

Yavonka G. Archaga, Executive Director
Alisha S. Hammond, Assistant Director
Rosie Calvin, Program Manager
RIL provides quality services to individuals with disabilities to assist with living independently. RIL also offers an array of services to include information and referral, advocacy, peer support and independent living skills training.

4112 Southwest Louisiana Independence Center: Lake Charles
2016 Oak Park Boulevard
Lake Charles, LA 70601-5391
337-477-7198
888-403-1062
Fax: 337-477-7198
TTY: 337-477-7198
www.slic-la.org

SILC provides Information and Referral, Advocacy, Peer Counseling and other Independent Living Services, to develop community options for persons with significant disabilities in Southwest and Central Louisiana, and to assist them in achieving and maintaining self-sufficient, productive lives.

4113 Southwest Louisians Independence Center: Lafayette
850 Kaliste Saloom Rd
Suite 118
Lafayette, LA 70508-4230
337-269-0027
888-516-5009
Fax: 337-233-7660
www.slic-la.org

SLIC provides Information and Referral, Advocacy, Peer Counseling and other Independent Living Services, to develop community options for persons with significant disabilities in Southwest and South Central Louisiana, and to assist them in achieving and maintaining self-sufficient, productive lives. PCA provider services

4114 Volunteers of America of Greater New Orleans
4152 Canal St.
New Orleans, LA 70119
504-482-2130
Fax: 504-482-1922
voagno.org

Robert C. Rhoden, Chair
Wayne M. Baquet, Chair Elect
James M. Le Blanc, President/CEO
Volunteers of America Greater New Orleans offers many services that aim to improve the lives of children, youth, and families.

4115 W Troy Cole Independent Living Specialist
Ste H
1900 Lamy Ln
Monroe, LA 71201-9200   318-323-4374

Katherine Carnell, Manager

Maine

4116 Alpha One: Bangar
3300 Ponce de Leon Blvd.
Coral Gables, FL 33134   305-567-9888
                                                     877-228-7321
                                                 Fax: 305-567-1317
                                            info@alpha-1foundation.org
                                                     www.alpha1.org

John W. Walsh, President & CEO, Co-founder
Marcia F. Ritchie, Vice President/ COO
Marsha A. Carnes, Director of Program Evaluation
Committed to being a leading enterprise providing the community with information, services and products that create opportunities for people with disabilities to live independently. Provides many services including adaptive and mobility equipment selection, peer support, advocacy, information and referral services, adapted drive evaluation and training, and consumer directed personal assistance.

4117 Alpha One: South Portland
127 Main St
South Portland, ME 04106-2647   207-767-2189
                                                     800-640-7200
                                                 Fax: 207-799-8346
                                                 TTY: 207-767-5387
                                                www.alphaonenow.com

Dennis Stubbs, Chairman
Bob McPhee, Vice-Chairman
Darlene Stewart, Independent Living Specialist
Committed to being a leading enterprise providing the community with information, services and products that create opportunities for people with disabilities to live independently. Offers adaptive equipment loan program, independent living skills instruction, adapted driver evaluation and training, information and referral services, peer support, advocacy, access design consultation, and more.

4118 Motivational Services
71 Hospital Street
P.O.Box 229
Augusta, ME 04332-0229   207-626-3465
                                                 Fax: 207-626-3469
                                                 TTY: 207-621-2542
                                                 www.mocomaine.com

Connie Dunn, President
Grace Leonard, Vice President/Secretary
Faith Madore, Treasurer
Improving the lives of people with disabilities through housing, employment and community support.

4119 Shalom House
106 Gilman St
Portland, ME 04102-3034   207-874-1080
                                                 Fax: 207-874-1077
                                                 TTY: 207-842-6888
                                            generalmail@shalomhouseinc.org
                                                 shalomhouseinc.org

Megan Lewis, Human Resources Manager
Mary Haynes-Rodgers, Executive Director
Kristine Lausier, Quality Assurance Administrator
Offers hope for adults living with severe mental illness by providing a choice of quality housing and support services that help people lead stable and fulfilling lives in the community.

Maryland

4120 Broadmead
13801 York Rd
Cockeysville, MD 21030-1899   410-527-1900
                                                     877-STA-HOME
                                                    www.broadmead.org

Ann H. Heaton, Chair
John E. Howl, Chief Executive Officer
Patricia Gordon, Chief Financial Officer/Treasure
To provide continuing care services to a diverse group of seniors in a warm, congenial community founded and operated in the spirit of the Religious Society of Friends.

4121 Eastern Shore Center for Independent Living
309 Sunburst Highway
Suite 13
Cambridge, MD 21613-2050   410-221-7701
                                                     800-705-7944
                                                 Fax: 410-221-7714
                                                 TTY: 410-221-4150
                                                 www.autismspeaks.org

Liz Feld, President
Alec M. Elbert, Chief Strategy & Dev Officer
Jamitha Fields, VP, Community Affairs
ESCIL provides services to people with all disabilities regardless of age, religion, gender, ethnicity, race or national origin. In addition to the core services of information and referral, skills training, peer support and advocacy, ESCIL also offers assistance with accessibility modifications, Americans with Disabilities Act education and training, housing referrals and counseling, transportation referral and information, Brailling capabilities, Personal Attendent Services referral, and more.

4122 Freedom Center
14 W. Patrick Street
Suite 10
Frederick, MD 21701   301-846-7811
                                                 Fax: 301-846-9070
                                        advocate@thefreedomcenter-md.org
                                                 thefreedomcenter-md.org

Jamey George, Executive Director
Russell Holt, President
Patrick Mcmurtray, Vice-President
A walk in center for independent living, provides services and supports to empower individuals with disabilities to lead self-directed, independent, and productive lives in a barrier-free community.

4123 Housing Unlimited
Ste G1
1398 Lamberton Dr
Silver Spring, MD 20902-3435   301-592-9314
                                                 Fax: 301-592-9318
                                        information@housingunlimited.org
                                                 www.housingunlimited.org

Nancy Cohen, President Emerita
Russell Phillips, President
Robyn S. Raysor, Vice President
To address the housing crisis for adults with psychiatric disabilities who reside in Montgomery County, Maryland.

4124 Independence Now
12301 Old Columbia Pike
Suite 101
Silver Spring, MD 20904-1656   301-277-2839
                                                 Fax: 301-625-9777
                                                    info@innow.org
                                                       innow.org

Robert Watson, President
Sarah Sorensen, Executive Director
Todd Thorpe, Director of Operations
A nonprofit organization created by people with disabilities and provides services that promote independence and the inclusion of people with disabilities in their communities.

4125 Independence Now: The Center for Independent Living
12301 Old Columbia Pike
Suite 101
Silver Spring, MD 20904
301-277-2839
Fax: 301-625-9777
info@innow.org
innow.org

Robert Watson, President
Sarah Sorensen, Executive Director
Todd Thorpe, Director of Operations
A nonprofit organization created by people with disabilities to provide services that promote independence and the inclusion of people with disabilities within their communities.

4126 Making Choices for Independent Living
Ste 202
1118 Light St
Baltimore, MD 21230-4152
410-234-8195
888-560-2221

Jimmie Joku Cooper, Owner
Provides services to help empower people with disabilities to lead self-directed, independent and productive lives in the community and protect their civil rights.OUTOF ORDER.

4127 Resources for Independence
30 N. Mechanic Street
Unit B
Cumberland, MD 21502-2705
301-784-1774
800-371-1986
Fax: 301-784-1776
www.rficil.org

Lori Magruder, Executive Director
John Michaels, Assistant Director
Robert Cannon, Benefits Counselor
Private, non-profit, consumer-controlled, community-based organization providing services and advocacy by and for persons with all type of disabilities. Their goal is to create opportunities for independence, and to assist individuals with disabilities to achieve their maximum level of independent functioning within their families and communities.

4128 Southern Maryland Center for LIFE
P.O.Box 657
Charlotte Hall, MD 20622-657
301-884-4498
Fax: 301-884-6099
www.somd.com

Marie Robinson, Executive Director
Carrie Lanthier, Administrative Assistant
A non-profit community based organization which provides services to disabled people who live or work in the tri-county area. Our mission is to empower people with disabilities to lead self-directed, independent, and productive lives in their community.

Massachusetts

4129 Adlib
215 North St
Pittsfield, MA 01201-4644
413-442-7047
800-232-7047
Fax: 413-443-4338
adlib@adlibcil.org
adlibcil.org

Linda Febles, President
Michael Hinkley, Vice President
Allison Bedard, Treasurer
Offers information and referral services, independent living skills training, peer counseling, individual and group advocacy services available to all people with disabilities. Access consultation provided to businesses, agencies and institutions in accordance to the Americans with Disabilities Act.

4130 Arc of Cape Cod
P.O.Box 428
171 Main Street
Hyannis, MA 02601-428
508-790-3667
Fax: 508-775-5233
info@arcofcapecod.org
www.arcofcapecod.org

Provides adults with developmental disabilities a full range of individual supports to assist them in becoming valued members of their community.

4131 Boston Center for Independent Living
5th Floor
60 Temple Place
Boston, MA 02111-1324
617-338-6665
Fax: 617-338-6661
TTY: 617-338-6662
www.bostoncil.org

Sergio Goncalves, Chairman
Linda Landry, Vice Chairman
Stacey Zelbow, Treasurer
A frontline civil rights organization led by people with disabilities that advocates to eliminate discrimination, isolation and segregation by providing advocacy, information and referral, peer support, skills training, and PCA services in order to enhance the independence of people with disabilities.

4132 Cape Organization for Rights of the Disabled (CORD)
106 Bassett Ln.
Hyannis, MA 02601
508-775-8300
800-541-0282
Fax: 508-775-7022
TTY: 508-775-8300
cordinfo@cilcapecod.org
www.cilcapecod.org

Coreen Brinckerhoff, CEO & Chair
Mike Magnant, President & COO
Gretchen Arvanitopoulos, Vice President
The Cape Organization for the Rights of the Disabled is dedicated to advancing independence, productivity, and integration of people with disabilities into mainstream society. CORD is the Center for Independent Living (CIL) and is a member of the Aging and Disability Resources Consortium (ADRC) serving Cape Cod and the Islands.

4133 Center for Living & Working: Fitchburg
76 Summer Street
Suite 110
Fitchburg, MA 01420-5785
978-345-1568
TTY: 978-345-1568
centerlwA@centerlw.org
www.centerlw.org

Cindy Purcell, Board President
Mary Ann Donovan, Treasurer
Ed Roth, Secretary
The Center for Living and Working is a non-profit Independent Living Center which takes its direction from persons with disabilities. The Center advocates to empower persons with disabilities to take active roles in their lives and in their community in which they live. Also provides comprehensive and innovative programs and services in order to maximize individual independence and opportunities.

4134 Center for Living & Working: Framingham
484 Main St
Suite 345
Worcester, MA 01608-1824
508-798-0350
Fax: 508-797-4015
TTY: 508-755-1003
opsearch@centerlw.org
www.centerlw.org

Cindy Purcell, Board President
Mary Ann Donovan, Treasurer
Ed Roth, Secretary
The Center for Living and Working is a non-profit Independent Living Center which takes its direction from persons with disabilities. The Center advocates to empower persons with disabilities to take active roles in their lives and in their community in which they live. Also provides comprehensive and innovative programs and services in order to maximize individual independence and opportunities.

4135 **Center for Living & Working: Worcester**
484 Main St
Suite 345
Worcester, MA 01608-1824
508-798-0350
Fax: 508-797-4015
TTY: 508-755-1003
opsearch@centerlw.org
www.centerlw.org

Cindy Purcell, Board President
Mary Ann Donovan, Treasurer
Ed Roth, Clerk/Secretary
The Center for Living and Working is a non-profit Independent Living Center which takes its direction from persons with disabilities. The Center advocates to empower persons with disabilities to take active roles in their lives and in their community in which they live. Also provides comprehensive and innovative programs and services in order to maximize individual independence and opportunities.

4136 **Developmental Evaluation and Adjustment Facilities**
215 Brighton Ave
Allston, MA 02134-2013
617-254-4041
800-886-5195
Fax: 617-254-7091
info@deafinconline.org
deafinconline.org

Sharon L. Applegate, Executive Director
Kelly Kim, President
John Sullivan, Treasurer
Encourages and empowers deaf, hard of hearing, deafblind and late-deafened individuals to lead independent and productive lives.

4137 **Independence Associates**
100 Laurel Street
1st Suite 122
East Bridgewater, MA 02301-4012
508-583-2166
800-649-5568
Fax: 508-583-2165
info@iacil.org
iacil.org

Mark Lewis, President
James Clark, Treasurer
Anita Ashdon, Secretary
Provides comprehensive services which will enhance the range of acceptable options available to the consumer and improve the quality of life of persons with disabilities; to work on behalf of the objective of the disablility rights and independent living movement.

4138 **Independent Living Center of Stavros: Greenfield**
55 Federal St
Greenfield, MA 01301-2546
413-774-3001
www.stavros.org

Glenn Hartmann, President
Nancy Bazanchuk, Vice President
Donna M. Bliznak, Treasurer
Promoting independence and access in the communities for persons with disabilities and deaf people.

4139 **Independent Living Center of Stavros: Springfield**
210 Old Farm Road
Amherst, MA 01002-2704
413-256-0473
800-804-1899
Fax: 413-256-0190
www.stavros.org

Glenn Hartmann, President
Nancy Bazanchuk, Vice President
Donna M. Bliznak, Treasurer
Promoting independence and access in the communities for persons with disabilities and deaf people.

4140 **Independent Living Center of the North Shore & Cape Ann**
27 Congress St
Suite 107
Salem, MA 01970-5577
978-741-0077
888-751-0077
Fax: 978-741-1133
ilcnsca.org

Mary Margaret Moore, Executive Director
Marion A Dawicki, President
Patricia Cox, Vice President
A service and advocacy center run by and for people with disabilities that supports the struggle of people who have all types of disabilities to live independently and participate fully in community life.

4141 **MetroWest Center for Independent Living**
280 Irving Street
Framingham, MA 01702-7306
508-875-7853
Fax: 508-875-8359
TTY: 508-875-7853
info@mwcil.org
mwcil.org

Youcef J. Bellil, President
Michael Kennedy, Vice President
Edward J. Carr, Treasurer
To help individuals with disabilities become productive and contributing members of the community and to eliminate barriers within the community that impede this process.

4142 **Multi-Cultural Independent Living Center of Boston**
329 Centre Street
Jamaica Plain, MA 02130-1232
617-942-8060
Fax: 617-942-8630
TTY: 617-288-2707
info@milcb.org
milcb.org

Derrick Dominique, Executive Director
Ana Ortiz, Director of Services
Eleanor Slaughter, Senior IL Advocate
Seeks to create opportunities for people with disabilities and their families in unserved/under-served populations and cultures who reside in Boston's inner city.

4143 **Northeast Independent Living Program**
20 Ballard Rd
Lawrence, MA 01843-1018
978-687-4288
Fax: 978-689-4488
TTY: 978-687-4288
help@nilp.org
nilp.org

June Cowen, Executive Director
Nanette Goodwin, Assistant Director
Lisa DiGiuseppe, Director of Finance
A consumer controlled Independent Living Center providing Advocacy and Services to people with all disabilities in the greater Merrimack Valley who wish to live as independently as possible in the commuity.

4144 **Renaissance Clubhouse**
176 Walker St
2nd Floor
Lowell, MA 01854-3126
978-454-7944
Fax: 978-937-7867
renclub1@gmail.com

Elaine Walker, Executive Director
Pammy Sadoie, Assistant Director
Offers daily structure, assistance wtih jobs, retirement, and housing.

4145 **Southeast Center for Independent Living**
66 Troy Street
Suite 3
Fall River, MA 02720-3023
508-679-9210
Fax: 508-677-2377
TTY: 508-679-9210
scil@secil.org
secil.org

Lisa M Pitta, Executive Director
Damase Cote, President
Paul Remy, Vice President

The Philosophy of Independent Living, maintains that individuals with disabilities have the right to choose services and make decisions for themselves. This belief is the foundation and guiding principle of all of SCIL's policies and operations. SCIL provides training, information and support to help consumers achieve individual goals, experience personal growth and participate fully in community life.

4146 Student Independent Living Experience Massachusetts Hospital School
560 Harrison Avenue
Suite 600
Boston, MA 02118-2447 617-338-6409
800-843-5879
TTY: 800-328-3202
www.mass.gov
Offers young adults with disabilities an opportunity to participate in a group learning situation, where they will develop independent and transitional living skills through a residential or non-residential model.

Michigan

4147 Ann Arbor Center for Independent Living
3941 Research Park Drive
Ann Arbor, MI 48108-6852 734-971-0277
Fax: 734-971-0826
www.annarborcil.org

Carolyn Grawi, Executive Director
Chris Baty, Theater Coordinator
Bryan Wilkinson, Director of Operations and Sales
AACIL assists people with disabilities and their families in living full and productive lives. AACIL assures the equality of opportunity, full participation, independent living and economic self-sufficiency of people with disabilities in the community.

4148 Arc Michigan
1325 S Washington Ave
Lansing, MI 48910-1652 517-487-5426
800-292-7851
Fax: 517-487-0303
dhoyle@arcmi.org
arcmi.org

Donald Teegarden, President
Laurel Robb, Vice President
Dohn Hoyle, Executive Director
Exists to empower local chapters of The ARC to assure that citizens with developmental disabilities are valued and that they and their families can participate fully in and contribute to the life of their community.

4149 Arc/Muskegon
601 Terrace Street
Suite 101
Muskegon, MI 49440-2197 231-777-2006
Fax: 231-777-3507
info@arcmuskegon.org
www.arcmuskegon.org

Tim Michalski, President
Brenda McCarthy Wiener, Vice President
Margaret O'Toole, Executive Director
Offers information and referral, advocacy services and peer counseling.

4150 Bad Axe: Blue Water Center for Independent Living
614 N Port Crescent Street
P.O. Box 29
Bad Axe, MI 48413-1207 989-269-5421
810-987-9337
Fax: 989-269-5422
info@bwcil.org
www.bwcil.org

Karen Massaro-Mundt, President
Chuck Wanninger, Treasurer
Jim Whalen, Executive Director
A non-profit, consumer-based organization that advocates, informs and supports persons with disabilities in the community.

4151 Bay Area Coalition for Independent Living
Ste 17
701 S Elmwood Ave
Traverse City, MI 49684-3185 231-929-4865
Fax: 231-929-4896
steve@bacil.org

Steve Wade, Director

4152 Capital Area Center for Independent Living
2812 N. Martin Luther King Jr. Blvd
Lansing, MI 48906 517-999-2760
877-652-3777
Fax: 517-999-2767
TTY: 800-649-3777
www.cacil.org

Mark Pierce, Executive Director
Jeffrey Gass, Financial Manager
Justine Bond, Independent Living Specialist
CACIL provide training, mentoring, and referrals to help people with disabilities and their families live productive lives.

4153 Caro: Blue Water Center for Independent Living
1184 Cleaver Rd
Caro, MI 48723-1143 989-673-3678
810-987-9337
Fax: 989-673-3656
info@bwcil.org
www.bwcil.org

Karen Massaro-Mundt, President
Chuck Wanninger, Treasurer
Jim Whalen, Executive Director
A non-profit, consumer-based organization that advocates, informs and supports persons with disabilities in the community.

4154 Center for Independent Living of Mid-Michigan
3941 Research Park Drive
Ann Arbor, MI 48108-6832 734-971-0277
Fax: 734-971-0826
www.annarborcil.org

Carolyn Grawi, Executive Director
Chris Baty, Theater Coordinator
Bryan Wilkinson, Director of Operations and Sales
Comprised of over 51 percent of people with disabilities, and advocates for the rights of people with disabilities in the Mid-Michigan area. Call for information on disability issues or for assistance in obtaining services, within your community..

4155 Community Connections of Southwest Michigan
5671 N. Skeel Ave.
Suite 8
Oscoda, MI 48750 989-569-6001
800-578-4245
Fax: 269-925-7141

Kathy Ellis, Director
An advocacy organization that teaches and empowers people with disabilities to make choices about living life to the fullest, controlling and directing their own lives and asserting their rights and responsibilites within their Berrien County communities..

4156 Cristo Rey Handicappers Program
1717 N High St
Lansing, MI 48906-4529 517-372-4700
Fax: 517-372-8499
www.cristo-rey.org

Marlene M Berens, Manager
To care for the spiritual and social needs of individuals and families by offering services that encourage self-sufficiency and recognize the dignity of the human person..

4157 Detroit Center for Independent Living
1042 Griswold
Suite 2
Port Huron, MI 48060 810-987-9337
810-987-9337
Fax: 810-987-9548
info@bwcil.org
www.bwcil.org

Karen Massaro-Mundt, President
Chuck Wanninger, Treasurer
Jim Whalen, Executive Director

BWCIL is a consumer-based organization designed to serve persons with disabilities who have physical, psychiatric, sendory, cognitive, and multiple disabilities through the provision of advocacy, information and referral, service provision, and the promotion of needed services so to maximize the individual's optimal level of independence.

4158 Disability Advocates of Kent County
3600 Camelot Drive SE
Grand Rapids, MI 49546-8103
616-949-1100
Fax: 616-949-7865
contact@dakc.us
disabilityadvocates.us

David Bulkowski, JD, Executive Director
Denise Borges, Employment Specialist
Jackson Botsford, Accessibility Specialist

Exists to advocate, assist, educate and inform on independent living options for persons with disabilities and to create a barrier-free society for all.

4159 Disability Connection
27 E. Clay Avenue
Muskegon, MI 49442
231-722-0088
866-322-4501
Fax: 231-722-0066
dcilmi.org

John Wahlberg, President
Michael Hamm, Vice President
Tamera Collier, Executive Director

To advocate, educate, empower, and provide resources for persons with disabilities and promote accessible communities.

4160 Disability Network Southwest Michigan
517 E Crosstown Pkwy
Kalamazoo, MI 49001-2867
269-345-1516
Fax: 269-345-0229
info@dnswm.org
www.dnswm.org

Cameron J. Lambe, Chair
Cheri Stoltzner, Vice Chair
Joel W Cooper, President

To educate and empower people with disabilities to create change intheir own lives, and to advocate for social change to create inclusive communities. As a center for independent living, they are part of the disability rights movement.

4161 Disability Network of Mid-Michigan
1705 S. Saginaw Road
Midland, MI 48640-6825
989-835-4041
800-782-4160
Fax: 989-835-8121
dnmm.org

Tom Provoast, President
Dr. Barbara Gibson, Vice President
David Emmel, Executive Director

To promote and encourage independence for all people with disabilities.

4162 Disability Network of Oakland & Macomb
16645 15 Mile Rd
Clinton Township, MI 48035-2206
586-268-4160
800-284-2457
Fax: 586-285-9942
info@dnom.org
dnom.org

Andrew Maurer, Chairperson
Randy Charon, Vice Chairperson
Kellie Boyd, Executive Director

Commited to advancing personal choice, independence, and positive social change for persons with disabilities through advocacy, education and outreach.

4163 Disability Network/Lakeshore
426 Century Lane
Holland, MI 49423-2200
616-396-5326
800-656-5245
Fax: 616-396-3220
TTY: 616-396-5326
info@dnlakeshore.org
dnlakeshore.org

Michelle Chaney, President
Amber Marcy, Vice President
Brian Dykhuis, Treasurer

A cross-disability, community-based organization providing advocacy, education, and information and referral to persons with disabilities in Ottawa and Allegan counties.

4164 Grand Traverse Area Community Living Management Corporation
935 Barlow St
Traverse City, MI 49686-4250
231-932-9030
www.gtaclmc.org

Mary Jean Brick, Administrative Director

We are a training home for individuals with developmental disabilities over the age of 18

4165 Great Lakes/Macomb Rehabilitation Group
Apt 104
4 E Alexandrine St
Detroit, MI 48201-2032
313-832-3371
Fax: 313-832-3850

Jeannie Meece-Brooks, Contact
Independent living center.

4166 JARC
30301 Northwestern Hwy
Suite 100
Farmington Hills, MI 48334-3277
248-538-6611
877-767-7781
Fax: 248-538-6615
jarc@jarc.org
jarc.org

Ronald Applebaum, President
Richard A. Loewenstein, Chief Executive Officer
Randy P. Baxter, Chief Financial Officer

A nonprofit, nonsecretarian agency dedicated to enabling people with disabilities to live full, dignified lives in the community, and to providing support and advocacy for their families.

4167 Lapeer: Blue Water Center for Independent Living
392 West Nepessing Street
Lapeer, MI 48446-2192
810-664-9098
810-987-9337
Fax: 810-664-0937
info@bwcil.org
www.bwcil.org

Karen Massaro-Mundt, President
Chuck Wanninger, Treasurer
Jim Whalen, Executive Director

A non-profit, consumer-based organization that advocates, informs and supports persons with disabilities in the community.

4168 Livingston Center for Independent Living
3075 E Grand River Ave
Suite 108
Howell, MI 48843-6585
517-545-1741
Fax: 517-548-1751
www.virtualcil.net

Dan Durci, Director
Independent living skills training and empowerment training for persons with disabilities..

4169 Michigan Commission for the Blind: Independent Living Rehabilitation Program
235 S. Grand Ave.
P.O. Box 30037
Lansing, MI 48909-1254
989-758-1765
800-292-4200
Fax: 989-758-1405
www.michigan.gov

Debbie Wilson, Manager
Patrick Cannon, Agency Director

Rehabilitation teaching, independent living skills for persons over 55 with severe vision loss.

4170 Michigan Commission for the Blind: Detroit
Ste 4-450
3038 W Grand Blvd
Detroit, MI 48202-6012
313-456-1646
Fax: 313-456-1645
mcnealg@michigan.gov

Gwen McNeal, Supervisor
Shawnese Laury-Johnson, Assistant East Region Manager
Promotes the inclusion of people with legal blindness into our communities on a full and equal basis through empowerment, education, participation, and choice..

4171 Monroe Center for Independent Living
1285 N Telegraph Rd
Monroe, MI 48162-3368
734-242-5919
mrawlings@aacil.org
monroecil.tripod.com

Linda Maier, Manager
To act as a catalyst for personal and social change through the empowerment of people with disabilities; and, to replace the perception of disability as tragic with a disability culture promoting pride, power and personal style.

4172 Port Huron: Blue Water Center for Independent Living
1042 Griswold St
Suite 2
Port Huron, MI 48060-5431
810-987-9337
810-987-9337
Fax: 810-987-9548
info@bwcil.org

Karen Massaro-Mundt, President
Chuck Wanninger, Treasurer
Jim Whalen, Executive Director
A non-profit, consumer-based organization that advocates, informs and supports persons with disabilities in the community.

4173 Sandusky: Blue Water Center for Independent Living
103 East Sanilac Road
Suite 3
Sandusky, MI 48471-1615
810-648-2555
810-987-9337
Fax: 810-648-2583
info@bwcil.org

Karen Massaro-Mundt, President
Chuck Wanninger, Treasurer
Jim Whalen, Executive Director
A non-profit, consumer-based organization that advocates, informs and supports persons with disabilities in the community.

4174 Southeastern Michigan Commission for the Blind
4450 Grandy St
Detroit, MI 48207
313-456-0334
877-932-6424
Fax: 313-456-1645
www.michigan.gov

Patrick Cannon, Executive Director
Pat Bragg, Manager
Vocational rehabilitation agency. Personal adjustment vocational assessment and training, job placement and follow-up services.

4175 Superior Alliance for Independent Living(SAIL)
1200 Wright Street
Suite A
Marquette, MI 49855
906-228-5744
800-379-7245
Fax: 906-228-5573
TTY: 906-228-5744
www.upsail.com

Elgie Dow, President
Aaron Andres, Vice President
Amy Maes, Executive Director
Promotes the inclusion of people with disabilities into our communities on a full and equal basis through empowerment, education, participation and choice.

4176 disAbility Connections
409 Linden Ave
Jackson, MI 49203-4065
517-782-6054
Fax: 517-782-3118
www.disabilityconnect.org

Michael Jackson, President
James Gorse, Vice President
Lesia Pikaart, Executive Director
Supporting Jackson County residents in their efforts to lead independent, fulfilling, productive lives.

Minnesota

4177 Access North Center for Independent Living of Northeastern MN
1309 East 40th Street
Hibbing, MN 55746
218-262-6675
800-390-3681
Fax: 218-262-6677
info@accessnorth.net
www.accessnorth.net

Donald Brunette, Executive Director
Patty Baratto, Administrative Assistant
Assists individuals to live independently, pursue meaningful goals, and have equal opportunities and choices. Other offices are located in Duluth, Brainerd, Walker & Aitkin.

4178 Accessible Space, Inc.
2550 University Avenue West
Suite 330N
Saint Paul, MN 55114-1085
651-645-7271
800-466-7722
Fax: 651-645-0541
TTY: 800-627-3529
info@accessiblespace.org
www.accessiblespace.org

Mark E. Hamel, Esq., Chairman
Kay Knutson, Vice Chairman
Steve Schugel, Treasurer
Accessible, rent-subsidized apartments for very low-income adults with qualifying physical disabilities as well as seniors. Accessible Space, Inc., sponsors, develops and manages housing & ASI apartments are rent based on income and are located across the country.

4179 Courage Center
800 E. 28th St.
Minneapolis, MN 55407-4298
612-863-4200
866-880-3550
Fax: 763-520-0577
TTY: 763-520-0245
couragekenny@allina.com
www.allinahealth.org

Jan Malcolm, CEO
Alice Johnson, Chief Financial Officer
Stephen Bariteau, Chief Development Officer
A nonprofit rehabilitation and resource center that advances the lives of children and adults experiencing barriers to health and independence. Specialize in treating brain injury, spinal cord injury, stroke, chronic pain, autism and disabilities experienced since birth.

4180 Freedom Resource Center for Independent Living: Fergus Falls
125 W Lincoln Avenue
Suite 7
Fergus Falls, MN 56537-2152
218-998-1799
800-450-0459
Fax: 218-998-1798
freedom@freedomrc.org
www.freedomrc.org

Nate Aalgaard, Executive Director
Angie Bosch, Office Coordinator
Mark Mark Bourdon Bourdon, Program Director
Freedom Resource Center assists people in working towards goals they establish for themselves.

4181 Metropolitan Center for Independent Living
Ste 16
1600 University Ave W
Saint Paul, MN 55104-3825   651-646-8342
                                Fax: 651-603-2006
                                TTY: 651-603-2001
                        homeramps@gmail.com
MCIL is dedicated to the full promotion of independent living
philosophy by supporting individuals with disabilities in their
personal efforts to pursue self-directed lives.

**4182 Minnesota Association of Centers for Independent
Living**
215 North Benton Drive
Sauk Rapids, MN 56379   320-529-9000
                                    888-529-0743
                                Fax: 320-529-0747
                    ilicil@independentlifestyles.org
                        independentlifestyles.org

Cara Ruff, Executive Director
Jay Keller, Board Chairman
Pamela Kotzenmacher, Treasurer
A non-profit organization whose purpose is to advocate for the in-
dependent living needs of people with disabilities who are citi-
zens of the State of Minnesota

4183 OPTIONS
Ste B
123 S Main St
Crookston, MN 56716-1970   218-281-5722
                                Fax: 218-281-5722
                                TTY: 218-281-5722

Gordie Haug, Manager
Provides people with disabilities advocacy, information, skills
training and peer mentoring relationships to help them achieve
their personal goals of how and where they live their lives.

**4184 Options Interstate Resource Center for Independent
Living**
2200 2nd Street SW
Rochester, MN 55902-1887   507-285-1815
                                    800-726-3692
                                Fax: 218-773-7119
                                TTY: 218-773-6100
                        options@myoptions.info
                            www.macil.org

Vicki Dalle Molle, President
Randy Sorensen, Executive Director
Located in Minnesota, but also serves North Dakota..

4185 Perry River Home Care
330 High Way Pen S
Saint Cloud, MN 56304   320-255-1882
                                Fax: 320-255-5137

Berna Florentine, CEO
Ken Figge, President
Courtney Salzi, Administrator
Offers skilled nursing services RN, LPN, TV Therapy, Pediatrics,
Rehabilitation Services, PT, OT, ST, Paraprofessional staff,
Home Health Aides, Homemakers, Personal Care Attendants,
Companions, Live-ins, Sleep overs, Respite care, Extended
hours.

4186 SMILES
820 Winnebago Ave
Suite 1
Fairmont, MN 56031-3619   507-345-7139
                                    888-676-6498
                                Fax: 507-235-3488
                            www.smilescil.org

Brain Koch, President
Doug Robinson, Vice President
Alan Augustin, Executive Director
A nonprofit organization committed to providing a wide array of
services that assist individuals with disabilities that live independently, pursue meaningful goals, and enjoy the same opportunities and choices as all persons.

4187 SMILES: Mankato
709 S. Front Street
Suite 7
Mankato, MN 56001-3887   507-345-7139
                                    888-676-6498
                                Fax: 507-345-8429
                        smiles@smilescil.org
                            smilescil.org

Brain Koch, President
Doug Robinson, Vice President
Alan Augustin, Executive Director
A nonprofit organization committed to providing a wide array of
services that assist individuals with disabilities that live independently, pursue meaningful goals, and enjoy the same
oportunities and choices as all persons.

**4188 Southeastern Minnesota Center for Independent Living:
Red Wing**
2200 2nd Street SW
Rochester, MN 55902   507-285-1815
                                    888-460-1815
                                Fax: 507-288-8070
                        semcil@semcil.org
                            www.semcil.org

Brian Koch, President
Doug Robinson, Vice President
Alan Augustin, Executive Director
Non profit organization that assists people with disabilities to be-
come independent and productive community members.

**4189 Southeastern Minnesota Center for Independent Living:
Rochester**
2200 Second Street SW
Rochester, MN 55902-3980   507-285-1815
                                    888-460-1815
                                Fax: 507-288-8070
                        semcil@semcil.org
                            www.semcil.org

Brain Koch, President
Doug Robinson, Vice President
Alan Augustin, Executive Director
A non profit organization that assists people with disabilities to
become independent and productive community members.

4190 Southwestern Center for Independent Living
2864 S Nettleton Ave
Suite 700
Springfield, MO 65807   417-886-1188
                                    800-676-7245
                                Fax: 417-886-3619
                                TTY: 417-886-1188
                        scil@swcil.org
                            www.swcil.org

Randy Custer, Board President
Emilio Vela, CEO
Shannon Porter, Deputy Director
SWCIL is a private, non-profit community-based organization
providing independent living services to assist people with disabilities in obtaining and maintaining the greatest control over
their lives. Services are available in southwestern Minnesota to
persons of all ages, with any disability. Services include community access, education & outreach, mental health counseling,
youth services, transition services and more.

4191 Vinland Center Lake Independence
3675 Ihduhapi Road
Loretto, MN 55357-308   763-479-3555
                                    866-956-7612
                                Fax: 763-479-2605
                        vinland@vinlandcenter.org
                            www.vinlandcenter.org

Gerald Seck, President
Mary Roehl, Executive Director
Colleen Larson, Operations Manager
A Minnesota based rehabilitation center which offers services in
three distinct service areas: vocational rehabilitation; inclusive
community programs; and for people with cognitive disabilities,
specially adapted chemical dependency treatment.

Mississippi

4192 Alpha Home Royal Maid Association for the Blind
PO Drawer 30
Hazlehurst, MS 39083-30
601-894-1771
Fax: 601-894-2993

Howard Becker, Director
Offers attendant care registry, information on accessible housing and referrals.

4193 Gulf Coast Independent Living Center
18 JM Tatum Industrial Drive
Hattiesburg, MS 39401-8341
601-544-4860
Fax: 601-582-2544

Albert Holifield, Executive Director
Independent living center.

4194 Jackson Independent Living Center
1981 Hollywood Dr
Jackson, TN 38305-2131
731-668-2211
800-848-0298
Fax: 731-668-0406
TTY: 601-351-1585
information@jcil.tn.org
www.j-cil.com/contact-us.html

Denea Smith, Director
Timothy Jackson
Provides services to consumers with severe disabilities.

4195 LIFE of Mississippi
1304 Vine St
Jackson, MS 39202-3429
601-969-4009
800-748-9398
Fax: 601-969-1662
TTY: 800-748-9398
www.lifeofms.com

Augusta Smith, Executive Director
Margie Moore, Project Coordinator
Densie Smith, Assistant
To empower people wit significant disabilities to be as independent and as fully involved in their communities as they can and want to be.

4196 LIFE of Mississippi: Biloxi
2030 Pass Road
Suite C
Biloxi, MS 39531
228-388-2401
Fax: 228-338-2413
www.lifeofms.com

Augusta Smith, Executive Director
Ruby Jackson, I.L. Specialist
Kim Allison, IL Specialist/ B2I
To empower people with significant disabilities to be as independent and as fully involved in their communities as they can and want to be.

4197 LIFE of Mississippi: Greenwood
502a W Park Ave
Greenwood, MS 38930-2906
662-453-9940
Fax: 662-453-9934
www.lifeofms.com

Augusta Smith, Executive Director
Pam Wraggs, I.L. Specialist
Ruth Elliott, IL Specialist Assistant
To empower people with significant disabilities to be as independent and as fully involved in their communities as they can and want to be.

4198 LIFE of Mississippi: Hattiesburg
710 Katie Ave
Hattiesburg, MS 39401-4377
601-583-2108
www.lifeofms.com

Augusta Smith, Executive Director
Margie Moore, Project Coordinator
Densie Smith, Assistant
To empower people with significant disabilities to be as independent and as fully involved in their communities as they can and want to be.

4199 LIFE of Mississippi: McComb
915-A S. Locust Street
McComb, MS 39648-4817
601-684-3079
www.lifeofms.com

Augusta Smith, Executive Director
Margie Moore, Project Coordinator
Densie Smith, Assistant
To empower people with significant disabilities to be as independent and as fully involved in their communities as they can and want to be.

4200 LIFE of Mississippi: Meridian
Ste 103a
2440 N Hills St
Meridian, MS 39305-2653
601-485-7999
www.lifeofms.com

Augusta Smith, Executive Director
Margie Moore, Project Coordinator
Densie Smith, Assistant
To empower people with significant disabilities to be as independent and as fully involved in their communities as they can and want to be.

4201 LIFE of Mississippi: Oxford
Ste 5
404 Galleria Dr
Oxford, MS 38655-4383
662-234-7010
www.lifeofms.com

Augusta Smith, Executive Director
Margie Moore, Project Coordinator
Densie Smith, Assistant
To empower people with significant disabilities to be as independent and as fully involved in their communities as they can and want to be.

4202 LIFE of Mississippi: Tupelo
1051 Cliff Gookin Blvd
Tupelo, MS 38801-6739
662-844-6633
Fax: 662-844-6803
www.lifeofms.com

Emily Word, Regional Coordinator
Ronnie Jernigan, I.L. Specialist/HOT
Wayne Lauderdale, I.L. Specialist
To empower people with significant disabilities to be as independent and as fully involved in their communities as they can and want to be.

Missouri

4203 Access II Independent Living Center
101 Industrial Parkway
Gallatin, MO 64640-1280
660-663-2423
888-663-2423
Fax: 660-663-2517
access@accessii.org
www.accessii.org

Heather Swymeler, Executive Director
Brandy Gannan, Program Manager
Amber Wells, Financial Director
The mission of Access II is to remove architectural and attitudinal barriers that limit the independence of persons with disabilities, promote a positive change in attitudes about disability and persons with disabilities, and encourage greater independence for persons with disabilities in our communities. As a Center for Independent Living, Access II is comitted to the provision of a full range of independent living services.

4204 Bootheel Area Independent Living Services
PO Box 326
Kennett, MO 63857-326
573-888-0002
888-449-0949
Fax: 573-888-0708
TTY: 573-888-0002
tshaw@bails.org
www.bails.org

Tim Shaw, Executive Director
BAILS goal is to foster an open, barrier free society flor all people regardless of their disability. BAILS service area is predomi-

nantly rural and includes the Southeast Missouri counties of: Dunklin, New Madrid, Pemiscot and Stoddard.

4205   Coalition for Independence: Missouri Branch Office
6724 Troost Ave
Ste. 408
Kansas City, MO 66131   816-822-7432
                                            Fax: 816-363-3469
                                            TTY: 913-321-5126

Clarenece Smith, Executive Director
Coalition For Independence (CFI) is to facilitate positive and responsible independence for all people with disabilities by acting as an advocate for individuals with disabilities, providing services, and promoting accessibility and acceptance.

4206   Delta Center for Independent Living
PO Box 550
Suite #107
St. Peters, MO 63376-5608   636-926-8761
                                                 866-727-3245
                                            Fax: 636-447-0341
                                            info@dcil.org
                                            www.dcil.org

Jennifer Mueller-Sparrow, President
Don Whalen, Vice President
Otis Pitts, Secretary
A non profit corporation which assists people with significant disabilities who want to live more independently.

4207   Disability Resource Association
130 Brandon Wallace Way
Festus, MO 63028-1726   636-931-7696
                                            Fax: 636-931-4863
                                            TTY: 636-937-9016
                                    dra@disabilityresourceassociation.org
                                    www.disabilityresourceassociation.org
Craig Henning, Executive Director
Nancy Pope, Assistant Director
Suzan Weller, Director/Resource Developer
Independent Living Cener.

4208   Easterseals Midwest
11933 Westline Industrial Dr.
St. Louis, MO 63146   800-200-2119
                                            Fax: 314-394-4007
                                            info@esmw.org
                                    www.easterseals.com/midwest
Wendy Sullivan, Chief Executive Officer
Jeff Arledge, Chief Financial Officer
Tom Barry, Chief Development Officer
Easterseals Midwest helps people with disabilities live and work with dignity in their communities. Programs include community living and independent supported living arrangement services, with support in the following areas: housing, health and safety, money management, nutrition, transportation, and more.

4209   Independent Living Center of Southeast Missouri
511 Cedar St
Poplar Bluff, MO 63901-7301   573-686-2333
                                                 888-890-2333
                                            Fax: 573-686-0733
                                            TTY: 573-776-1178
                                            info@ilcsemo.org
                                            www.ilcsemo.org
Bruce Lynch, Executive Director
Debbie Hardin, Independent Living Director
To make Southeast Missouri barrier free for all persons with disabilities, enabling them to live more independently, extending their rights to control and direct their own lives and empowering them to live more producitve lives.

4210   Midland Empire Resources for Independent Living (MERIL)
4420 South 40th St
Saint Joseph, MO 64503-2157   816-279-8558
                                                 800-637-4548
                                            Fax: 816-279-1550
                                            TTY: 816-279-4943
                                            www.meril.org
Dr. Robert Bush, Chair
Jaren Pippitt, Vice Chair
Wayne Crawford, Secretary
Designed to promote independent living and to enhance the quality of life for persons with disabilities by empowering them to control and direct their lives.

4211   Northeast Independent Living Services
909 Broadway
Suite 350
Hannibal, MO 63401   573-221-8282
                                                 877-713-7900
                                            Fax: 573-221-9445
                                            www.neilscenter.org
Rose McNally, President
Dawn Davis, Vice President
Brooke Kendrick, Executive Director
To empower persons with disabilities to live as full and productive members of society.

4212   On My Own
428 E Highland Ave
Nevada, MO 64772-2609   417-667-7007
                                                 800-362-8852
                                            Fax: 417-667-6262
                                            www.omoinc.org
Jennifer Gundy, Executive Director
A non profit independent living center.

4213   Ozark Independent Living
109 Aid Ave
West Plains, MO 65775-3529   417-257-0038
                                                 888-440-7500
                                            Fax: 417-257-2380
                                            TTY: 888-440-7500
                                            info@ozarkcil.com
                                            ozarkcil.com
Michael Conner, Vice Chair
Scott Schneider, Secretary/Treasurer
Cindy Moore, Executive Director
OIL?was created to provide independent living services to persons with disabilities who reside in the following counties in Missouri: Oregon Ozark, Shannon, Wright, Howell, Texas, and Douglas. OIL is non-profit, on-residential supported by grants, donations, and volunteers

4214   Paraquad
5240 Oakland Ave
Saint Louis, MO 63110-1436   314-289-4200
                                            Fax: 314-289-4201
                                            TTY: 314-289-4252
                                            contactus@paraquad.org
                                            www.paraquad.org
Robert Funk, Executive Director
Paraquad works to empower people with disabilities to increase their independence through choice and opportunity.

4215   Places for People
4130 Lindell Blvd
Saint Louis, MO 63108-2914   314-535-5600
                                            Fax: 314-535-6037
                                            www.placesforpeople.org
Kevin Kissling, President
Robin Kolker Adkins, Vice President
Joe Yancey, Executive Director
Places for People provides individualized, high quality and effective services to adults with serious and persistent mental disorders to assist them in living, working and socializing responsibility to serve those individuals who rely on public funding.

4216   RAIL
3024 Dupont Circle
Jefferson City, MO 65109   573-526-7039
                                                877-222-8963
                                                888-667-2117
                                          Fax: 573-751-1441
                                          mo.silc@vr.dese.mo.gov
                                                www.mosilc.org

Chris Camene, Chairperson
Jessica Hatfield, Vice-Chairperson
Barrnie Cooper, Secretary/Treasurer
RAIL is an Independent Living Center, one of twenty-two in the
State of Missouri, RAIL's Mission is to assist persons with dis-
abilities to live as independently as they choose within the com-
munities of their choice. RAIL offers four core services which
are: Advocacy, Peer Support, Information & Referral, and Inde-
pendent Living Skills Training. RAIL is a Consumer Services
Directed Program vendor

4217   SEMO Alliance for Disability Independence
1913 Rusmar St
Cape Girardeau, MO 63701-7623   573-651-6464
                                                800-898-7234
                                          Fax: 573-651-6565
                                          TTY: 573-651-6464
                                                www.sadi.org

Timothy D. Woodard, President
Michelle Spooler, Vice-President
Leemon Priest, Secretary
A community based, non-profit, nonresidential center for independent living that is committed to providing services to persons
with disabilities to enable them to remain in their own home and
community, not an institution.

4218   Services for Independent Living
1401 Hathman Place
Columbia, MO 65201-5552   573-874-1646
                                                800-766-1968
                                          Fax: 573-874-3564
                                          TTY: 573-874-4121
                                                www.silcolumbia.org

Dan Dunham, President
Bonnie Gregg, Vice President
Amy Henderson, Treasurer
A non-residential, community-based center for independent living. Provides individualized and group services to persons with
severe disabilities in the Mid-Missouri area; works to help people
with disabilities achieve their highest potential in independent
living and community life.

4219   Southwest Center for Independent Living (S CIL)
2864 S Nettleton Ave
Springfield, MO 65807-5970   417-886-3619
                                                800-676-7245
                                          Fax: 417-886-3619
                                          TTY: 417-886-1188
                                                scil@swcil.org
                                                www.swcil.org

Amy C. Lewis, President
Mark Grantham, Vice President
Gary Maddox, Chief Executive Officer
Provides services, advocacy, and resources for people with any
disability in Christian, Dallas, Greene, Lawrence, Polk, Stone,
Taney and Webster Counties of Southwest Missouri.

4220   Sunnyhill, Inc.
11140 So. Towne Square
Ste. 100
Saint Louis, MO 63123   314-845-3900
                                                www.sunnyhillinc.org

Donny Mitchell, Chief Operating Officer
Amy Wheeler, Vice President, Program Services
Luke Mraz, Director, Development & Community Partnerships
Services are provided to adults and children with developmental
disabilities. Supported living arrangements are located in St.
Louis city, St. Louis county and St. Charles County. Group home
and camp services are located in Dittmer, MO. Travel program
also available.

4221   Tri-County Center for Independent Living
1420 HWY 72 East
Rolla, MO 65401   573-368-5933
                                          Fax: 573-368-5991
                                          TTY: 573-368-5933
                                                www.tricountycenter.com

Victoria Evans, Executive Director
Mission is to eliminate physical and attitudinal barriers through
the power of advocacy, enlightenment, and reformation.

4222   West Central Independent Living Solutions
610 N Ridgeview Dr
Suite B
Warrensburg, MO 64093-9323   660-422-7883
                                                800-236-5175
                                          Fax: 660-422-7895
                                          TTY: 660-422-7894
                                                info@w-ils.org
                                                www.w-ils.org

David De Frain, President
James Piatt, Vice President
Kathy Kay, Executive Director
Works to empower people with disabilities to become more inde-
pendent by providing independent living skills training, peer
support, information and referral and advocacy. West Central In-
dependent Living Solutions now has satellite offices in Sedalia,
MO and Lexington.

4223   Whole Person, The
3710 Main Street
Kansas City, MO 64111-7501   816-225-0301
                                                800-878-3037
                                          Fax: 816-931-0529
                                          TTY: 816-561-0304
                                                info@thewholeperson.org
                                                www.thewholeperson.org

Rick O'Neal, President
Jim Atwater, Vice President
Julie Dejean, CEO
The Whole Person, assists people with disabilities to live inde-
pendently and encourages change within the community to ex-
pand opportunities for independent living.

4224   Whole Person: Kansas City
3710 Main Street
Kansas City, MO 64111-7501   816-561-0304
                                                800-878-3037
                                          Fax: 816-931-0529
                                          TTY: 816-627-2202
                                                info@thewholeperson.org
                                                www.thewholeperson.org

Rick O'Neal, President
Jim Atwater, Vice President
Julie Dejean, CEO
Assists people with disabilities to live independently and encour-
ages change within the community to expand opportunities for in-
dependent living.

Montana

4225   Living Independently for Today and Tomorrow
1201 Grand Avenue
Suite 1
Billings, MT 59102-2033   406-259-5181
                                                800-669-6319
                                          Fax: 406-259-5259
                                          TTY: 406-245-1225
                                                www.liftt.org

Bobbie Becker, Executive Director
Martha Carstensen, Program Director
LIFTT's Independent living program works with people with disabilities so they can live independently and have access to the
community. LIFTT staff, most of whom have disabilities, serve as
mentors to people as they work to achieve the goals they have set
for themselves.

4226   **Montana Independent Living Project, Inc.**
825 Great Northern Blvd
Suite 105
Helena, MT 59601-4715   406-442-5755
800-735-6457
Fax: 406-442-1612
TTY: 406-442-5755
bmaffit@milp.us
www.milp.us

Bob Maffit, Executive Director
Les Clark, Independent Living Specialist
Charlene White, Financial Manager
A not-for-profit agency that provides services that promote independence for people with disabilities.

4227   **North Central Independent Living Services**
1120 25th Ave
Black Eagle, MT 59414-1037   406-452-9834
800-823-6245
Fax: 406-453-3940

Tom Osborn, Executive Director
North Central Independent Living Services is located in Great Falls and provides services from Glacier County across the Hi-Line to the North Dakota border. A satellite office is set up in Glasgow.

4228   **Summit Independent Living Center: Kalipsell**
1203 Highway 2 W.
Suite #35
Kalispell, MT 59901-6020   406-257-0048
800-995-0029
Fax: 406-257-0634
TTY: 406-257-0048
webmaster@bils.org
www.summitilc.org

Steve Hackler, President
Larry Riley, Vice President
Jenny Montgomery, Secretary
To promote community awareness, equal access, and the independence of people with disabilities through advocacy, education, and the advancement of civil rights.

4229   **Summit Independent Living Center: Hamilton**
316 North 3rd St
Suite #113
Hamilton, MT 59840-2479   406-363-5242
800-398-9013
Fax: 406-375-9035
webmaster@bils.org
www.summitilc.org

Steve Hackler, President
Larry Riley, Vice President
Jenny Montgomery, Secretary
To promote community awareness, equal access, and the independence of people with disabilities through advocacy, education, and the advancement of civil rights.

4230   **Summit Independent Living Center: Missoula**
700 SW Higgins Ave
Suite #101
Missoula, MT 59803-1489   406-728-1630
800-398-9002
Fax: 406-829-3309
missoula@summitilc.org
www.summitilc.org

Steve Hackler, President
Larry Riley, Vice President
Jenny Montgomery, Secretary
To promote community awareness, equal access, and the independence of people with disabilities through advocacy, education, and the advancement of civil rights.

4231   **Summit Independent Living Center: Ronan**
124 Main St.
Ronan, MT 59864-2718   406-215-1604
866-230-6936
Fax: 406-552-1028
ronan@summitilc.org
www.summitilc.org

Steve Hackler, President
Larry Riley, Vice President
Jenny Montgomery, Secretary
To promote community awareness, equal access, and the independence of people with disabilities through advocacy, education, and the advancement of civil rights.

Nebraska

4232   **Center for Independent Living of Central Nebraska**
3335 West Capital Street
Grand Island, NE 68803-1730   308-382-9255
877-400-1004
Fax: 308-384-7832
TTY: 308-382-9255
jthomas@cilne.org
www.cilne.org

Joni Thomas, Executive Director
Irene Britt, Western Program Manager
Lesia Gracia, Independent Living Specialist
Offers independent living skills training, peer sharing, information and referral, housing counseling and referral, accessibility and barrier removal consultation including ADA training and technical assistance, driver education and training, assistive technology services including demonstration and equipment loan, and a free lending library of adapted toys and ability switches for children with severe disabilities. Serves all disabilities and all ages.

4233   **League of Human Dignity: Lincoln**
1701 P St
Lincoln, NE 68508-1799   402-441-7871
888-508-4758
Fax: 402-441-7650
TTY: 402-441-7871
info@leagueofhumandignity.com
www.leagueofhumandignity.com

Mike Schafer, CEO
The mission of the League of Human Dignity is to actively promote the full integration of individuals with disabilities into society. To this end, we will advocate their needs and rights, and provide quality services to involve these persons in becoming and remaining independent citizens.

4234   **League of Human Dignity: Norfolk**
400 Elm Ave
Norfolk, NE 68701-4033   402-371-4475
800-843-5785
Fax: 402-371-4625
TTY: 402-371-4475
ninfo@leagueofhumandignity.com
leagueofhumandignity.com

Mike Shafer, CEO
Jean M. Kloppenborg, Norfolk CIL Director
The mission of the League of Human Dignity is to actively promote the full integration of individuals with disabilities into society. To this end, we will advocate their needs and rights, and provide quality services to involve these persons in becoming and remaining independent citizens.

4235   **League of Human Dignity: Omaha**
5513 Center St
Omaha, NE 68106-3001   402-595-1256
800-843-5784
Fax: 402-595-1410
oinfo@leagueofhumandignity.com
www.leagueofhumandignity.com

Mike Schafer, CEO
Bob Gomez, Executive Director
The mission of the League of Human Dignity is to actively promote the full integration of individuals with disabilities into soci-

ety. To this end, we will advocate their needs and rights, and provide quality services to involve these persons in becoming and remaining independent citizens.

4236   Mosaic of Axtell Bethpage Village
1044 23rd Rd.
PO Box 67
Axtell, NE 68924   308-743-2401
                                        Fax: 308-743-2659
                                   www.mosaicinfo.org/axtell

Max Miller, Chairperson
James Zils, Vice Chairperson
Linda Timmons, President/ CEO
Provides services that respect the human diginity and rights of each person. An interdisciplinary team of family, staffmembers and professional consultatns support individuals served in developing personal goals and programs, helping them to fully participate in Axtell's community life. Mosaic at Axtell offers residential and community services.

4237   Mosaic of Beatrice
722 S. 12th St.
PO Box 607
Beatrice, NE 68310-607   402-223-4066
                                        Fax: 402-223-4951
                                   www.mosaicinfo.org/beatrice

Max Miller, Chairperson
James Zils, Vice Chairperson
Linda Timmons, President/ CEO
Provides individualized services, living options, work choices, spiritual nurture and advocacy to people with disabilities in more than 250 communities across 14 states and Great Britain through the work of 4,800 employees.

4238   Mosiac: York
220 W South 21st St
York, NE 68467-9316   402-362-2180
                                        Fax: 402-362-2961
                                        www.mosaicinfo.org

Max Miller, Chairperson
James Zils, Vice Chairperson
Linda Timmons, President/ CEO
Providing a wide array of services to assist individuals and families in achieving positive life goals. Services to persons with disabilities and other special needs include community living options, training and employment options, spiritual growth and development options, training and counseling support.

Nevada

4239   Carson City Center for Independent Living
900 Mallory Way
Carson City, NV 89701   775-841-2580

Sandra Coyle, Owner
Helps consumers continue to live independently in the community through a variety of individual and community services.

4240   Northern Nevada Center for Independent Living: Fallon
1919 Grimes St
Suite B
Fallon, NV 89406-3100   775-423-4900
                                             800-885-3712
                                        Fax: 775-423-1399
                                        TTY: 775-423-4900
                                        nncilf@cccomm.net
                                             www.nncil.org

Lisa Bonie, Executive Director
Hilda Velasco, Operations Manager
Joni Inglis, Independent Living Advocate
Independent Living Center.

4241   Rural Center for Independent Living
1895 E Long St
Carson City, NV 89706-3214   775-841-2580
                                        Fax: 775-841-2580
                                        ruralcil@yahoo.com

Dee Dee Foremaster, Executive Director

Advocacy, Benefit Assistance, social security assistance, peer support, housing information and home-less day drop-in center for individuals with disabilities.

4242   Southern Nevada Center for Independent Living: North Las Vegas
3100 E Lake Mead Blvd
North Las Vegas, NV 89030-7380   702-649-3822
                                             800-398-0760
                                        Fax: 702-649-5022
                                        TTY: 702-649-3822
                                        sncilnv@aol.com
                                             www.sncil.org

Connie Kratky, President
Elliot Yug, Vice - President
Pamela Rake, Secretary
SNCIL is committed to removing barriers preventing indpendent living by providing services designed to empower people with disabilities.

4243   Southern Nevada Center for Independent Living: Las Vegas
2950 S. Rainbow Blvd.
Suite 220
Las Vegas, NV 89146-5611   702-889-4216
                                             800-870-7003
                                        Fax: 702-889-4574
                                        TTY: 702-889-4216
                                        sncil2@aol.com
                                             www.sncil.org

Connie Kratky, President
Elliot Yug, Vice - President
Pamela Rake, Secretary
SNCIL is committed to removing barriers preventing Independent Living by providing services designed to empower people with disabilities.

New Hampshire

4244   Granite State Independent Living Foundation
21 Chenell Drive
Concord, NH 3301-4079   603-228-9680
                                             800-826-3700
                                        Fax: 603-444-3128
                                        TTY: 603-228-9680
                                             info@gsil.org
                                             www.gsil.org

Ken Traum, Chair
Lorna D. Greer, Vice Chair
Clyde E. Terry, CEO
GSIL is a statewide non-profit that recognizes the fact that all of us will need some type of support in the course of the lives. GSIL offers tools and resources so that individuals can participate as fully as the choose in their lives, families and communities. Contact the Independent Living Foundation for referrals to living situations.

New Jersey

4245   Alliance Center for Independance
Alliance for Disabled in Action
629 Amboy Ave, First Floor
Edison, NJ 08837-3579   732-738-4388
                                        Fax: 732-738-4416
                                        TTY: 732-738-9644
                                        adacil@adacil.org
                                             www.adacil.org

Colleen Roche, Chair
Bernard Zuckerman, Treasurer
Carole Tonks, Executive Director
Alliance for Disabled in Action is a private, not-for-profit center for independent living serving people in Middlesex, Somerset and Union Counties of New Jersey. ADA's mission is to support and promote choice, self-direction and independent living in the lives of people with disabilities, with the right of individuals to inclusion in the community as the primary goal.

4246   Camden City Independent Living Center
2600 Mount Ephraim Ave
Camden, NJ 8104-3236   856-966-0800
                                               Fax: 856-966-0832
                                               TTY: 856-966-0830
                                          vedasmithccilc@aol.com
                                              www.camdencityilc.org

Bruce Smith, Chairperson
John Quann, Vice Chairperson
Tanya Brown, Treasurer
Provides services designed to empower people with disabilities.
To provide services to individuals with significant disabilities.
Services include information referral, advocacy, peer support,
and independent living skills training. CCILC services
individuals in Camden City

4247   Center for Independent Living: Long Branch
279 Broadway
Suite #201
Long Branch, NJ 7740-6940   732-571-4884
                                               Fax: 732-571-4003
                                               TTY: 732-571-4878
                                               www.moceanscil.org

Jennifer Sterner, Vice Chair
Maureen Poling, Secretary
Stan Soden, Director IL Services
Offers peer support, disability education and personal assistant
services. Serving Monmouth and Ocean Counties with information and referrals, advocacy, peer support and independent living
instructions.

4248   Center for Independent Living: South Jersey
1150 Delsea Drive
Suite #1
Westville, NJ 8093-2251   856-853-6490
                                                   800-413-3791
                                               Fax: 856-853-1466
                                               TTY: 856-853-7602

Hazel Lee-Briggs, Executive Director
Danuta Debicki, Program Manager
Terryama Davis, Independent Living Specialist
Dedicated to providing people with disabilities in Gloucester and
Camden counties the opportunity to actively participate in society, to provide freedom of choice, to work, to own a home, raise a
family and in general, to participate to the fullest extent in
day-to-day activities. The center provides information and referrals, advocacy, peer support, and independent living skills
training.

4249   DAWN Center for Independent Living
66 Ford Road
Suite 121
Denville, NJ 7834-1235   973-625-1940
                                                   888-383-3296
                                               Fax: 973-625-1942
                                               TTY: 973-625-1932
                                               info@dawncil.org
                                               www.dawncil.org

Elizabeth Lehmann, President
Gabrielle Waldman, Vice President
Carmela Slivinski, Executive Director
DAWN is the Center for Independent Living serving Morris, Sussex and Warren counties. DAWN empowers people with disabilities to strive for equality and to take control of their own lives by
providing the tools that encourage independence and self-advocacy, promoting public awareness of the needs, desires and rights
to individuals living with disabilities, and offering community
activities that create new experiences and opportunities.

4250   Dial: Disabled Information Awareness & Living
2 Prospect Village Plaza
Floor 1
Clifton, NJ 7013-1918   973-470-8090
                                                   866-277-1733
                                               Fax: 973-470-8171
                                               TTY: 973-470-2521
                                               info@dial-cil.org
                                               www.dial-cil.org

Cynthia DeSouza, President
Anthony Gianduso, Vice President
John Petix, Executive Director

Promotes the full inclusion of all people living with disabilities
into society and encourage the consumers and the community at
large to seek involvement in this self-governing organization to
the fullest extent.

4251   Disability Rights New Jersey
New Jersey Protection and Advocacy
210 S. Broad Street
Floor 3
Trenton, NJ 08608-2407   609-292-9742
                                                   800-922-7233
                                               Fax: 609-777-0187
                                               TTY: 609-633-7106
                                               advocate@drnj.org
                                               www.drnj.org

Walter Anthony Woodberry, Chair
Andrew McGeady, Vice Chair
Linda K. Soley, Treasurer
Assistive Technology Advocacy Center provides assistance to
personswith disabilities in helping them to obtain assistive tech-
nology devices and/or services.

4252   Family Resource Associates
35 Haddon Ave
Shrewsbury, NJ 7702-4007   732-747-5310
                                               Fax: 732-747-1896
                                               info@frainc.org
                                               www.frainc.org

Allan Proske, President
Bill Sheeser, Vice President
John Feeney, Treasurer
FRA is dedicated to helping children, adolescents and people of
all ages with disabilities to reach their fullest potential. FRA also
connects individuals to independence through modern therapies
and advanced technology. FRA provides direct services to those
in the greater Nonmouth/Ocean County area.

4253   Heightened Independence and Progress: Hackensack
131 Main St
Suite #120
Hackensack, NJ 7601-7182   201-996-9100
                                               Fax: 201-996-9422
                                               TTY: 201-966-9424
                                               www.hipcil.org

Eileen Goff, President/CEO
Trish Carney, Finance and Development Director
Empowers people with disabilities to achieve independent living
through outreach, advocacy and education.

4254   Heightened Independence and Progress: Jersey City
35 Journal Square
Suite #703
Jersey City, NJ 7306-4105   201-533-4407
                                               Fax: 201-533-4421
                                               TTY: 201-533-4409
                                               www.hipcil.org

Jean Csaposs, Board Chair
Lottie Esteban, First Vice Chair
Eileen Goff, President/CEO
Empowering People with Disabilities to Achieve Independent
Living through Outreach, Advocacy, and Education.

4255   Progressive Center for Independent Living
3525 Quakerbridge Rd.
Suite 904
Hamilton, NJ 8619-3710   609-581-4500
                                                   877-917-4500
                                               Fax: 609-581-4555
                                               TTY: 609-581-4550
                                               info@pcil.org
                                               www.pcil.org

Norman Smith, President
John Witman, Vice President
Scott Elliott, Executive Director
Advocates for the rights of people with disabilities to achieve and
maintain independent lifestyles. The Center has programs to assist with employment, transition from school to adult life, and
emergency preparedness.

4256 Progressive Center for Independent Living: Flemington
4 Walter E Foran Blvd
Suite 410
Flemington, NJ 8822-4669
908-782-1055
877-376-9174
Fax: 908-782-6025
TTY: 908-782-1081
info@pcil.org
pcil.org

Norman Smith, President
John Witman, Vice President
Scott Elliott, Executive Director
Advocates for the rights of people with disabilities to achieve and maintain independent lifestyles.

4257 Project Freedom
223 Hutchinson Rd
Robbinsville, NJ 8691-3457
609-448-2998
Fax: 609-448-7293
ProjectFreedom1@aol.com
www.projectfreedom.org

Tim Doherty, Executive Director
Norman A. Smith, Assoc Ex Director
Elizabeth Maxwell, Office Manager
Dedicated to developing, supporting, and advocating opportunities for independent living persons with disabilities.

4258 Project Freedom: Hamilton
715 Kuser Rd
Hamilton, NJ 8619-3924
609-588-9919
Fax: 609-588-8831
cfunk@projectfreedom.org
www.projectfreedom.org

Cecilia Funk, Social Service Coordinator
Judy Wilkinson, Office Manager
Paul Campanella, Property Manager
Dedicated to developing, supporting, and advocating opportunities for independent living persons with disabilities.

4259 Project Freedom: Lawrence
1 Freedom Blvd
Lawrence, NJ 8648-4531
609-278-0075
Fax: 609-278-1250
jelsowiny@projectfreedom.org
www.projectfreedom.org

Jacklene Elsowiny, Social Serv Coordinator
Tim Doherty, Executive Director
Stephen Schaefer, CFO
Dedicated to developing, supporting, and advocating opportunities for independent living persons with disabilities.

4260 Total Living Center
6712 Washington Ave
Egg Harbor Township, NJ 8234-1999
609-645-9547
Fax: 609-813-2318
TTY: 609-645-9593

Jo Hudson, President
Cliff Anderson, Vice President
Cathy Shaner, Secretary
Total Living Center is a non-profit organization whose mission is to empower individuals with significant disabilities to maximize their potential for independence and productivity, to live as fully as possible within the community, taking responsibility for themselves, and sharing this commitment with others.

New Mexico

4261 Ability Center
715 E Idaho Ave.
Suite 3E
Las Cruces, NM 88001
575-526-5016
800-376-4372
Fax: 575-526-1202
TTY: 575-210-5272
freedom@theabilitycenter.org
www.theabilitycenter.org
The Ability Center is a private, nonresidential, nonprofit, New Mexico corporation. As a center for independent living (CIL)

TACIL provides a variety of support services for individuals with disabilities.

4262 CASA Inc.
116 West Baltimore Street
Hagerstown, MD 21740
301-739-4990
Fax: 301-790-0064
casa4@myactv.net
www.casaabq.com

Sherry Donovan, President
Linda Davis, Vice-President
Melinda Marsden, Treasurer
Offers peer counseling and information and referral services.

4263 CHOICES Center for Independent Living
200 E 4th St.
Suite #200
Roswell, NM 88201-6237
575-627-6727
800-387-4572
Fax: 575-627-6754
TTY: 505-627-6727

Julia Calvert, Executive Director
Offers many core services including independent living skills training, peer support, information and referral, advocacy and transition.

4264 New Mexico Technology Assistance Program
625 Silver Ave SW
Ste. 100 B
Albuquerque, NM 87102
505-841-4464
877-696-1470
Fax: 505-841-4467
Tracy.Agiovlasitis@state.nm.us
www.tap.gcd.state.nm.us

Tracy Agiovlasitis, Program Manager
Examines and works to eliminate barriers to obtaining assistive technology in New Mexico. Has established a statewide program for coordinating assistive technology services; is designed to assist people with disabilities to locate, secure, and maintain assistive technology.

4265 New Vistas
1205 Parkway Dr.
Suite A
Santa Fe, NM 87501-2483
505-471-1001
Fax: 505-471-4427
info@newvistas.org
www.newvistas.org

Victor Ortega, President
Libby Gonzales, Vice-President
Gay Romero, Secretary/Treasurer
Partners with and supports people with disabilities and families of children with special needs to enrich their quality of life in New Mexico.

4266 San Juan Center for Independence
1204 San Juan Blvd
Farmington, NM 87401
505-566-5827
877-484-4500
Fax: 505-566-5842
TTY: 505-566-5827
sjci@sjci.org
www.sjci.org

Patricia Ziegler, Executive Director
Tim Carver, CFO
SJCI is a New Mexico private non residential, nonprofit corporation that serves people with disabilities. The purpose of SJCI is to provide a variety of community based, consumer driven service to people with disablities to promote independence, self-residence and intergration into the community.

New York

4267 AIM Independent Living Center: Corning
271 E 1st St
Corning, NY 14830-2924
607-962-8225
Fax: 607-937-5125
TTY: 607-962-8225
troche@aimcil.com
www.aimcil.com

Rene Snyder, Executive Director
Sabrina Mineo-O'Connell, President
George Spisack, Vice President
AIM is a non-profit organization dedicated to people with disabilities, their families, friends, the businesses that serve them and those with an interest in disabilities. The mission of AIM is to support the individuals ability to make independent, self-directing choices through education, advocacy, information and referral.

4268 AIM Independent Living Center: Elmira
650 Baldwin St.
Elmira, NY 14901-2216
607-733-3718
Fax: 607-733-0180
TTY: 607-733-7764
troche@aimcil.com
www.aimcil.com

Rene Snyder, Executive Director
Sabrina Mineo-O'Connell, President
George Spisack, Vice President
AIM's goal is to enable the consumer to live an independent and comfortable lifestyle in the security of their home environment so they may feel dignity and pride in their achievements while controling their own care.

4269 ARISE
635 James St
Syracuse, NY 13203-2661
315-472-3171
Fax: 315-472-9252
TTY: 315-479-6363
info@ariseinc.org
www.ariseinc.org

Tania Anderson, President
Sue Judge, Vice President
Michael Cook, Treasurer
Founded in 1979, ARISE's mission is to work with people of all abilities to create a fair and just community in which everyone can fully participate. As a center for independent living, ARISE is a non-profit organization run by and for individuals with disabilities. ARISE serves over 3,000 children and adults with disabilities each year through our programs and services in several broad areas including advocacy, employment, independent living/integrated recreation programs, and much more.

4270 ARISE: Oneida
131 Main St
Suite #107
Oneida, NY 13421-1644
315-363-4672
Fax: 315-363-4675
TTY: 315-363-2364
info@ariseinc.org
www.ariseinc.org

Tania Anderson, President
Sue Judge, Vice President
Michael Cook, Treasurer
A consumer controlled, non-profit Independent Living Center that promotes the full inclusion of people with disabilities in the community.

4271 ARISE: Oswego
9 Fourth Avenue
Oswego, NY 13126-1803
315-342-4088
Fax: 315-342-4107
TTY: 315-342-8696
info@ariseinc.org
www.ariseinc.org

Tania Anderson, President
Sue Judge, Vice President
Michael Cook, Treasurer

A consumer controlled, non-profit Independent Living Center that promotes the full inclusion of people with disabilities in the community.

4272 ARISE: Pulaski
2 Broad St
Pulaski, NY 13142-4446
315-298-5726
Fax: 315-298-5729
info@ariseinc.org
www.ariseinc.org

Tania Anderson, President
Sue Judge, Vice President
Michael Cook, Treasurer
A consumer controlled, non-profit Independent Living Center that promotes the full inclusion of people with disabilities in the community.

4273 Access to Independence of Cortland County, Inc.
26 N Main St
Cortland, NY 13045-2198
607-753-7363
Fax: 607-756-4884
info@aticortland.org
www.aticortland.org

Judy Bentley, Chair
Peter Morse-Ackley, Vice Chair
Chad W. Underwood, CEO
Access to Independence is Cortland County's foremost disability resource. It empowers people to lead independent lives in their community and strives to open doors to full participation and access for all.

4274 Action Toward Independence: Middletown
130 Dolson Avenue
Suite 35
Middletown, NY 10940-6563
845-343-4284
Fax: 845-342-5269

Stephen McLaughlin, Executive Director
Joann Hargabus, Services Director, Orange Cnty.
Gilles Malkine, Services Director, Sullivan Cnty
Independent living center that serves Orange & Sullivan counties. Provides programs and services to individuals who have disabilities and to their families. These services include peer counseling, individual & systems advocacy, independent living, skills training, information and referral, benefits advisement, recreation and a drop in center. We are designed to enable people with disabilities to achieve independence, inclusion and participation in their communities.

4275 Action Toward Independence: Monticello
309 E Broadway
Suite A
Monticello, NY 12701-8810
845-794-4228
Fax: 845-794-4475
TTY: 845-794-4228
www.atitoday.org

Steve McLaughlin, Executive Director
Joann Hargabus, Director of Services
A not-for-profit, non residential, peer run, referral and advocacy agency for persons with disaiblities in Orange and Sullivan counties. Our services are aimed at promoting accessibility, community integration, and equal opportunity in all aspects of society for persons with all types of disabilities.

4276 BRiDGES
873 Route 45
Suite 108
New City, NY 10956
845-624-1366
Fax: 845-624-1369
info@bridgesrc.org
www.bridgesrc.org

Patricia Ranieri, President
David Jacobsen, Ph.D, Psy.D, Executive Director
Michael Coleman, Director of Finance & Controller
BRiDGES is a community-based non-profit organization that serves people with disabilities. Services provided by them include personal assistance self-employers, independent living services, volunteer opportunities, advocacy and more.

4277 Bronx Independent Living Services
4419 Thrid Avenue
Suite 2C
Bronx, NY 10457

718-515-2800
Fax: 718-515-2844
TTY: 718-515-2803
webmaster@bils.org
www.bils.org

Barbara Linn, President
Anita Richichi, Vice President
Sheldon Mann, Treasurer
BILS is a not-for-profit community agency serving people with all kinds of disabilities. The mission is to empower people with disabilities toward living independent lives. BILS assists individuals by providing advocacy, peer counseling, housing information, and independent living training/counseling.

4278 Brooklyn Center for Independence of the Disabled
27 Smith Street
Suite #200
Brooklyn, NY 11201

718-998-3000
Fax: 718-998-3743
TTY: 718-998-7406
advocate@bcid.org
www.bcid.org

Joan Peters, Executive Director
Sandrina Kingston, Program Director
Princess Davis, Office Manager
Operated by a majority of people with disabilities, BCID is dedicated to guaranteeing the civil rights of people with disabilities. BCID exists to improve the quality of life of brooklyn residents with disabilities thgouh programs that empower them to gain greater control of their lives and achieve full and equal integration into society.

4279 Capital District Center for Independence
845 Central Ave
South 3
Albany, NY 12206-1342

518-459-6422
Fax: 518-459-7847
TTY: 518-459-6422
info@cdciweb.com
www.cdciweb.com

Laurel Kelley, Executive Director
Dawn Werner, Deputy Director
Judy Zuchero, Program Director
One of 37 Independent Living Centers in New York State, the Center is a non-residential, community based organization, which primarily serves Albany and Schenetady Counties. The Center's mission is to assist people with disabilities to acquire self-advocacy skills and by teaching through example, consumers achieve greater control over the direction of their lives.

4280 Catskill Center for Independence
6104 State Highway 23
Oneonta, NY 13820

607-432-8000
Fax: 607-432-6907
TTY: 607-432-8000
ccfi@ccfi.us
www.ccfi.us

Chris Zachmeyer, Executive Director
Christine Worden, Assistant Director
One of 37 community-based independent living centers located throughout the state of New York. As an advocacy agency, we provide a vareity of services to people with disabilities, their friends and family members. In addition, we provide advocacy, training, and technical assistance to our community members, organizations, businesses and state and local governments in a variety of disability related areas. Serves Otsego, Delaware and Schoharie counties.

4281 Center for Community Alternatives
115 E Jefferson St
Suite #300
Syracuse, NY 13202-2018

315-422-5638
Fax: 315-471-4924
cca@communityalternatives.org
www.communityalternatives.org

Kwame Johnson, President
Susan R. Horn, Esq., Vice-President
Carole A. Eady, Secretary

Promotes reintegrative justice and a reduced reliance on incarceration through advocacy, services and public policy development in pursuit of civil and human rights.

4282 Center for Independence of the Disabled of New York
841 Broadway
Suite 301
New York, NY 10003-4708

212-674-2300
Fax: 212-254-5953
TTY: 212-674-5619
info@cidny.org
www.cidny.org

Martin Eichel, President
Anne M. Davis, Vice President
John O'Neill, Vice President
To ensure full integration, independence and equal opportunity for all people with disabilities by removing barriers to the social, economic, cultural and civic life of the community.

4283 Center for Independence of the Disabled of New York
841 Broadway
Suite 301
New York, NY 10003-4708

212-674-2300
Fax: 212-254-5953
TTY: 212-674-5619
info@cidny.org
www.cidny.org

Martin Eichel, President
Anne M. Davis, Vice President
John O'Neill, Vice President
To ensure full integration, independence and equal opportunity for all people with disabilities by removing barriers to the social, economic, cultural and civic life of the community.

4284 DD Center/St Lukes: Roosevelt Hospital Center
St Lukes Roosevelt
1000 10th Ave
New York, NY 10019-1192

212-473-2045
Fax: 212-473-0501

Charles Raimondo, VP
Farooq Chaudry, MD
Independent living center that advocates for people with disabilities by assisting with the application process of housing, benefits, etc.

4285 Finger Lakes Independence Center
215 5th St
Ithaca, NY 14850-3403

607-272-2433
Fax: 607-272-0902
TTY: 607-272-2433
flic@clarityconnect.com
www.fliconline.org

Lenore Schwager, Executive Director
FLIC assists all people with disabilities, their families and friends to promote independence and make informed decisions in pursuit of their goals. The servides provided are free of charge, and services are primarily served to residents of Tompkins, Schyler counties.

4286 Harlem Independent Living Center
289 St. Nicholas Avenue
Suite #21
New York, NY 10027- 4805

212-222-7122
800-673-2371
Fax: 212-222-7199
harlemilc@aol.com
www.hilc.org

Christina Curry, Executive Director
Edward Randolph, Resource Specialist
Dr. Herbert Thornhill, Emeritus
A non-profit agency that advocates for people with disabilities by assisting with the application process of housing, benefits, etc. Our services are free of charge.
Monthly

4287   Independent Living
5 Washington Terrace
Newburgh, NY 12550   845-565-1162
                                         Fax: 845-565-0567
                                         TTY: 845-565-0337
                                    info@myindependentliving.org
                                    www.myindependentliving.org

Doug J Hovey, President & CEO
Shannon Zawiski, Chief Operating Officer
Emily Robisch, Chief Financial Officer
A non-profit agency run by people with disabilities for others
with disabilities. The agency offers programs and services to enhance quality of life, including benefits advising, personal assistance services, advocacy, employment and mental health
services, recovery center, supportive housing and more.

4288   Long Island Center for Independent Living
3601 Hempstead Tpke
Suites 208 & 500
Levittown, NY 11756-1331   516-796-0144
                                         Fax: 516-520-1247
                                         TTY: 516-796-0135
                                             licil@aol.com
                                             www.licil.net

Joan Lynch, Executive Director
LICIL is committed to the empowerment of consumers with disabilities. LICIL staff functions as ambassadors to the belief that
individuals with disabilities have a responsibility to take an active role in their own lives and self determined view of their
futures.

4289   Massena Independent Living Center
156 Center St.
Massena, NY 13662-1495   315-764-9442
                                             877-397-9613
                                         Fax: 315-764-9464
                                         mindepli@twcny.rr.com
                                             www.milcinc.org

Jeff Reifensnyder, Executive Director
Provides a variety of non-residential direct services as well as educating the public through community awareness campaigns.
Also seeks to address the current appropriate unmet needs of persons experiencing a disability.

4290   NYS Independent Living Council
111 Washington Ave
Suite #101
Albany, NY 12210-2280   518-427-1060
                                             877-397-4126
                                         Fax: 518-427-1139
                                             bradw@nysilc.org
                                             www.nysilc.org

Brad Williams, Executive Director
Patty Black, Administrative Assistant
Provides support and technical assistance to 37 independent living centers-community-based organizations directed by and for
people with disabilities.

4291   Nassau County Office for the Physically Challenged
60 Charles Lindberg Blvd
Uniondale, NY 11553-4812   516-227-7399
                                          www.nassaucountyny.gov

Edward P. Mangano, County Executive
This agency serves as the ADA compliance coordinating office
for all Nassau County governmental facilities, programs and services. It also serves in an advisory capacity to local, regional and
national policy-making organizations, planning committees and
legislative bodies and conducts advocacy as well as direct programs and services to enhance inclusion by people with disabilities to employment, consumerism and transportation.

4292   North Country Center for Independent Living
80 Sharron Avenue
Plattsburgh, NY 12901-3827   518-563-9058
                                         Fax: 518-563-0292
                                         TTY: 518-563-9058
                                         andrew@ncci-online.com
                                             www.ncci-online.com

Ted Graser, President
Kathy Latinville, Vice President
Robert Poulin, Executive Director

To empower people with disabilities to live more independent
and productive lives, and to promote beneficial policies and community understanding of disability issues.

**4293   Northern Regional Center for Independent Living:
Watertown**
210 Court St
Suite #107
Watertown, NY 13601-4546   315-785-8703
                                             800-585-8703
                                         Fax: 315-785-8612
                                         TTY: 315-785-8704
                                             nrcil@nrcil.net
                                             www.nrcil.net

Ronald Griffin, Chair
Michael Simmons, Vice Chair
Melanie Adkins, Secretary
A disability rights and resource center that promotes community
efforts to end discrimination, segregation, and prejudice against
people with disabilities.

**4294   Northern Regional Center for Independent Living:
Lowville**
7632 N State St
Lowville, NY 13367-1318   315-376-8696
                                         Fax: 315-376-3404
                                         TTY: 315-376-8696
                                             karenb@nrcil.net
                                             www.nrcil.net

Ronald Griffin, Chair
Michael Simmons, Vice Chair
Melanie Adkins, Secretary
A disability rights and resource center that promotes community
efforts to end discrimination, segregation, and prejudice against
people with disabilities.

4295   Options for Independence: Auburn
75 Genesee St
Auburn, NY 13021-3667   315-255-3447
                                         Fax: 315-255-0836
                                             www.ariseinc.org

Tania Anderson, President
Sue Judge, Vice President
Michael Cook, Treasurer
Options for Independence is an Independent Living Center which
assists people with disabilities to gain opportunities, make their
own decisions, pursue activities and become part of comunity
life. Options provides a variety of services to all people with disabilities, their families, friends, and service providers in Cayuga
and Seneca Counties.

4296   Putnam Independent Living Services
1961 Route 6
2nd Floor
Carmel, NY 10512-2324   845-228-7457
                                         Fax: 845-228-7460
                                         TTY: 866-933-5390
                                             info@wilc.org
                                             www.putnamils.org

Joe Bravo, Executive Director
Mildred Caballero-Ho, Deputy Executive Director
Margaret Valenzuela, Program Director, IL Services
A non-profit, community-based advocacy and resource center
that serves people with all types of disabilities.

4297   Regional Center for Independent Living
497 State St
Rochester, NY 14608-1642   585-442-6470
                                         Fax: 585-271-8558
                                         TTY: 585-442-6470
                                             bdarling@rcil.org
                                             www.rcil.org

Shelly Perrin, Chairperson
Bobbi Wallach, Vice Chairperson
Bruce E Darling, Executive Director
To empower people with disabilities to self-advocate, to live in-
dependently and to enhance the quality of community life.

4298   **Resource Center for Accessible Living**
727 Ulster Ave
Kingston, NY 12401-1709   845-331-0541
Fax: 845-331-2076
TTY: 845-331-4527
office@rcal.org
www.rcal.org

Paul Scarpati, President
Paula Kindos-Carberry, Co-Vice President
Bernadette Mueller, Co-Vice President
RCAL is a non-profit, community based service and advocacy
run by and for people with any type of disability. RCAL is dedicated to assisting and empowering individuals, of all ages, to live
independently and participate in all aspects of community life.

4299   **Resource Center for Independent Living**
347 W Main St
Amsterdam, NY 12010-2225   518-842-3561
Fax: 518-842-0905
TTY: 518-842-3593

Shelly Perrin, Chairperson
Bobbi Wallach, Vice Chairperson
Bruce E Darling, Executive Director
Peer counseling, advocacy, independent living skills training, information and referral services, self-advocacy training, ADA
consultation, home and community based services, community
education, benefits advisement and more. All programs and services are available in English and Spanish.

4300   **Southern Adirondack Independent Living**
418 Geyser Rd
Country Club Plaza
Ballston Spa, NY 12020-6002   518-584-8202
Fax: 518-584-1195
www.sail-center.org

Karen Thayer, Executive Director
Anna Livingston, Assistant Director
Barbara Potvin, Executive Assistant
To assist individuals with disabilities to become independent em-
powered self-advocates.

4301   **Southern Adirondack Independent Living Center**
71 Glenwood Ave
Queensbury, NY 12804-1728   518-792-3537
Fax: 518-792-0979
TTY: 518-792-0505

Karen Thayer, Executive Director
Anna Livingston, Assistant Director
Shirley Dumont, Director of Advocacy
To assist individuals with disabilities to become independent em-
powered self-advocates.

4302   **Southern Tier Independence Center**
135 E Frederick St
Binghamton, NY 13904-1224   607-724-2111
Fax: 607-772-3600
TTY: 607-724-2111
stic@stic-cil.org
www.stic-cil.org

Maria Dibble, Executive Director
Frank Pennisi, Accessibility Services
STIC provides assistance and services to all people with disabilities of all ages to increase their independence in all aspects of integrated community life. STIC also serves their families and
friends, and businesses, agencies, and goverments to enable them
to better meet the needs of people with disabilities, and finally
STIC educates and influences the community in pursuit of full inclusion of people with disabilities.

4303   **Southwestern Independent Living Center**
843 N Main St
Jamestown, NY 14701-3546   716-661-3010
Fax: 716-661-3011
TTY: 716-661-3012
info@ilc-jamestown-ny.org

Marie T Carrubba, Executive Director
Linda Rumbaugh, Independent Living Specialist
Christine Ahlstrom, Independent Living Specialist
A non-residential, private, nonprofit agency established to pro-
vide services throughout Chautauqua County that will assist indi-

viduals with disabilities in reaching maximum independence and
an enriched quality of life.

4304   **Staten Island Center for Independent Living, Inc.**
470 Castleton Ave
Staten Island, NY 10301   718-720-9016
Fax: 718-720-9664
TTY: 718-720-9870
ldesantis@siciliving.org
www.siciliving.org

Lorraine DeSantis, Executive Director
Claudia J. Stanton, Office Manager
Michelle Sabatino, Independent Living Specialist
Mission is to provide all individuals with disabilities the information, life skills training, and facilitative assistance which contributes to independence, individuality, and integration in the
community and provides the skills and knowledge necessary to
function in the least restrictive, personally fulfilling, most self
reliant and productive manner.

4305   **Suffolk Independent Living Organization(SILO)**
2111 Lakeland Ave.
Suite A
Ronkonkoma, NY 11779   631-880-7929
Fax: 631-946-6377
TTY: 631-946-6585
www.siloinc.org/?

Edward Ahern, Manager
Glenn Campbell, Co-Executive Director
A not-for-profit organization that helps the disabled become
more independent and more involved in the community by providing them with information on referrals on Housing, Education, Employment and Benefits.

4306   **Taconic Resources for Independence**
82 Washington St
Suite #214
Poughkeepsie, NY 12601-2305   845-452-3913
866-948-1094
Fax: 845-485-3196
tri@taconicresources.org
www.taconicresources.org

Cynthia L. Fiore, Executive Director
Patrick Muller, Program Director
Diane Barkstrom, Program Director/Staff Interpret
A center for independent living, benefits advisement informa-
tion, and referral, advocacy, independent living skills, peer coun-
seling, parent advocacy, sign language interpreters.

4307   **Westchester Disabled on the Move**
984 N. Broadway
Suite LL-10
Yonkers, NY 10701-1320   914-968-4717
Fax: 914-968-6137
info@wdom.org
www.wdom.org

Gail Cartenuto Cohn, President
Mattie Trupia, Vice President
Sandra Dolman, Secretary
WDOM empowers people with disabilities to control their own
lives; advocates for civil rights and a barrier free society; encourages people with disabilities to participate in the political process; educates government, business, other entities, and a society
as a whole to understand, accept, and accommodate people with
disabilities; creates an environment that inspires self-respect

4308   **Westchester Independent Living Center**
200 Hamilton Avenue
2nd Floor
White Plains, NY 10601- 1809   914-682-3926
Fax: 914-682-8518
TTY: 866-933-5390
Contact@wilc.org
www.wilc.org

Joseph Bravo, Executive Director
A not-for-profit, community-based advocacy and resource center
that serves people with all types of disabilities.

North Carolina

4309 Disability Awareness Network
609 Country Club Dr.
Suite C
Greenville, NC 27834-6210
252-353-5522
Fax: 252-353-5160
DAWNpittco@aol.com
Jackie Hansley, Owner
Information and referral for diabled persons; peer counseling for
diabled persons; advocacy on ADA issues; independent living
skills and training.

4310 Disability Rights & Resources
5801 Executive Center Dr.
Suite #101
Charlotte, NC 28212-8870
704-537-0550
800-755-5749
Fax: 704-566-0507
TTY: 704-537-0550
mailto@disability-rights.org
www.disability-rights.org
Maura Chavez, President
Marta Fales, Vice President
Holly Howell, Secretary
To guard the civil rights of people wtih disabilities by empower-
ing ourselves and others to live as we choose.

4311 Joy: A Shabazz Center for Independent Living
235 N Greene St
Greensboro, NC 27401-2410
336-272-0501
Fax: 336-272-0575
TTY: 336-272-0501
Aaron Shabazz, Executive Director
James Wells, President
Stephen Simpson, Vice-President
A non-profit, consumer oriented, Center for Independent Living
(CIL) providing advocacy, peer counseling and peer support, in-
dependent living skills, training, information and referrals, with
other related services for persons with disabilites.

4312 Live Independently Networking Center
P.O.Box 1135
Newton, NC 28658-1135
828-464-0331
Fax: 828-464-7375
TTY: 828-464-2838
Donavon Kirby, Deputy Director
Private, nonprofit, federally funded center for independent living
located in Western North Carolina.

4313 Live Independently Networking Center: Hickory
2830 16th St NE
Apt. 17
Hickory, NC 28601-8606
828-464-0331
Fax: 828-464-7375
Private, non-profit, federally funded center for independent liv-
ing

4314 Pathways for the Future Center for Independent Living
525 Mineral Springs Dr
Sylva, NC 28779-9077
828-631-1167
Fax: 828-631-1169
TTY: 828-631-1167
Barbara Davis, Executive Director
Dedicated to increasing independence, changing attitudes, promoting equal access and building a peer support network in western North Carolina through the use of community education,
independent living services and advocacy.

4315 Western Alliance Center for Independent Living
30b London Rd
Asheville, NC 28803-2706
828-274-0444
Fax: 828-274-4461
westernalliance.org
Katy Hollingsworth, Manager
Jerry Brewton, Independent Living Specialist

4316 Western Alliance for Independent Living
108 New Leicester Highway
Asheville, NC 28806
828-298-1977
Fax: 828-298-0875
khollingsworth@disabilitypartners.org
www.disabilitypartners.org
Kathy Hollingsworth, Associate Director
Rosemary Weaver, Independent Living Specialist
Mechelle Holt, Volunteer/Program Coordinator

North Dakota

4317 Dakota Center for Independent Living: Dickinson
26-1st street East
Suite 103
Dickinson, ND 58601-5103
701- 48- 436
800-489-5013
Fax: 701- 48- 436
TTY: 800489501363
dcil@ndsupernet.com
www.dakotacil.org
Robin Were, President
Claudia Ziegler, Vice president
Carol Mihulka, Secretary/Treasurer
Believes in self-determination for people with disabilities and
creates the environment in which it is achieved.

4318 Dakota Center for Independent Living: Bismarck
3111 E Broadway Ave
Bismarck, ND 58501-5085
701-222-3636
800-489-5013
Fax: 701-222-0511
TTY: 701-222-3636
maryr@dakotacil.org
www.dakotacil.org
Robin Were, President
Claudia Ziegler, Vice president
Carol Mihulka, Secretary/Treasurer
Believes in self-determination for people with disabilities and
creates the environment in which it is achieved.

4319 Fraser
2902 University Drive South
Fargo, ND 58103-6053
701-232-3301
Fax: 701-237-5775
fraser@fraserltd.org
fraserltd.org
Sandra Leyland, Executive Director
Mark Brodshaug, President
Michael Kirk, Vice President
Private non-profit, federally funded center for independent liv-
ing

4320 Freedom Resource Center for Independent Living: Fargo
2701 9th Ave S
Suite H
Fargo, ND 58103-8712
701-478-0459
800-450-0459
Fax: 701-478-0510
TTY: 701-478-0459
freedom@freedomrc.org
www.freedomrc.org
Nate Aalgaard, Executive Director
Angie Bosch, Office Coordinator
Mark Mark Bourdon Bourdon, Program Director
To work toward equality and inclusion for people with disabili-
ties through programs of empowerment, community education,
and systems change.

4321   Resource Center for Independent Living: Minot
300 3rd Ave SW
Suite F
Minot, ND 58701-4346   701-839-4724
                                                 800-377-5114
                                            Fax: 701-838-1677
                                            TTY: 701-839-4724
                       independencecil@independencecil.org
                                 www.independencecil.org/?

Susan Ogurek, Chair
Scott Burlingame, Executive Director
Dee Tischer, Senior Independent Living Specia
A resource center for independent living. Mission is to advocate
for the freedom of choice for individuals with disabilities to live
independently through the removal of all barriers.

Ohio

4322   Ability Center of Greater Toledo
5605 Monroe St.
Sylvania, OH 43560   419-885-5733
                                            Fax: 419-882-4813
                                              www.abilitycenter.org

Tim Harrington, Executive Director
Ash Lemons, Associate Director
Debbie Andriette, Director, Human Resources
To assist people with disabilities to live, work and socialize
within a fully accessible community.

4323   Ability Center of Greater Toledo: Bryan
1425 East High St.
Suite 108
Bryan, OH 43506   419-633-1400
                                                 855-633-1400
                                            Fax: 419-633-1410
                                              www.abilitycenter.org

Tim Harrington, Executive Director
Angie Burton, Manager, Youth Programs
To assist people with disabilities to live, work and socialize
within a fully accessible community. The Bryan office serves residents in Defiance, Fulton, Henry, and Williams Counties.

4324   Access Center for Independent Living
901 S Ludlow St
Dayton, OH 45402-2614   937-341-5202
                                            Fax: 937-341-5217
                                            TTY: 937-341-5218
                                                info@acils.com
                                                www.acils.com/?

Darrell Price, IL Team Co-Leader
Tonya Banther, IL Team Co-Leader
Melody Burba, Information & Referral Specialis
Offers peer counseling, disability education and other services to
the community.

4325   Center for Independent Living Options
2031 Auburn Avenue
Cincinnati, OH 45219-2436   513-241-2600
                                            Fax: 513-241-1707
                                            TTY: 513-241-7170
                                                      cilo.net

Lin Laing, Executive Director
Justin Bifro, President
Brian Frazier, Vice-President
The oldest center for independent living in Ohio serving individ-
uals with disabilities in the Greater Cincinnati/Northern Ken-
tucky region.

4326   Fairfield Center for Disabilities and Cerebral Palsy
681 E 6th Ave
Lancaster, OH 43130-2602   740-653-5501
                                            Fax: 740-653-6046
                                          fcdcp@sbcglobal.net
                                                 www.fcdcp.org

David Macioci, President
David Welsh, Vice-President
Mary Snider, Treasurer
Adult Day Program and Transportation. The mission of the
Fairfield Center for disabilities and Cerebral Palsy, Inc, is to cre-
ate a better future for people with a disability by increasing and
enhancing their lifestyle opportunities.

4327   Linking Employment, Abilities and Potential
2545 Lorain Ave.
Cleveland, OH 44113-3102   216-696-2716
                                            Fax: 216-687-1453
                                                 www.leapinfo.org

Charles Heindrichs, President
Brian Roof, Vice President
Vincent Shemo, Treasurer
Consumer-directed to ensure a society of equal opportunity for
all persons, regardless of disability.

**4328   Mid-Ohio Board for an Independent Living
          Environment (MOBILE)**
690 S High St
Columbus, OH 43206-1016   614-443-5936
                                            Fax: 614-443-5954
                                            TTY: 614-443-5957
                                          info@mobileonline.org
                                            www.mobileonline.org

Darry Moore, President
Thomas Shapaka, Vice-President
Mark Morton, Treasurer
A non-profit Center for Independent Living directed by persons
with disabilities. MOBILE was founded on principles that affirm
the right of persons with disabilities to live their lives with a full
measure of liberty and human dignity.

4329   Ohio Statewide Independent Living Council
670 Morrison Road
Suite 200
Gahanna, OH 43230-5324   614-892-0390
                                                 800-566-7788
                                            Fax: 614-861-0392
                                                 www.ohiosilc.org

Kay Grier, Executive Director
Eugene Iacovetta, Special Projects Coordinator
Mary Butler, Systems Change Coordinator
Committed to promoting a philosophy of consumer control, peer
support, self-help, self-determination, equal acess, and individual and systems advocacy, in order to maximize leadership, empowerment, independence, productivity and to support full
inclusion and integration of individuals with disabilities into the
mainstream of American society.

4330   Rehabilitation Service of North Central Ohio
270 Sterkel Blvd
Mansfield, OH 44907-1508   419-756-1133
                                                 800-589-1133
                                            Fax: 419-756-6544
                                          info@therehabcenter.org
                                            www.therehabcenter.org

Veronica L. Groff, President/CEO
Susan Baker, Chairman
Dan Wiegand, Vice-Chairman
Private nonprofit organization providing coordinated, team-ori-
ented comprehensive outpatient rehabilitation services to children and adults of all ages. Serves 8 counties in N/C Ohio. Four
umbrella areas of service include medical rehabilitation services,
vocational rehabilitation services, behavioral health service and
drug and alcohol addiction services. Medical rehabilitation services include physical therapy, occupational therapy, speech
therapy and audiology.

4331   Samuel W Bell Home for Sightless
3775 Muddy Creek Rd
Cincinnati, OH 45238-2055   513-241-0720
                                            Fax: 513-241-1481
                                          swbellhome@fuse.net
                                              www.samuelbell.org

Timothy Lighthal, President
Kevin Kappa, Vice-President
Miles L.Hoff, Treasurer
Offers a residential, independent living environment for blind
and legally blind adults.

4332 **Services for Independent Living**
25100 Euclid Ave
Suite #105
Cleveland, OH 44117-2663   216-731-1529
                                       Fax: 216-731-3083
                                       TTY: 216-731-1529
                                       www.sil-oh.org

Lynn Hildebrand, Executive Director
Offers support ADA, consultation and education, advocacy, transitional education services, independent living skills training, information and referrals.

4333 **Society for Equal Access: Independent Living Center**
1458 5th St NW
New Philadelphia, OH 44663-1224   330-343-9292
                                            888-213-4452
                                       Fax: 330-602-7425
                                       TTY: 330-602-2557
                                       www.seailc.org

Scott Huston, President
Edna Fillinger, Vice-President
Victoria Eichel, Secretary
The Society works with individuals to become more independent. Our agency assists with peer support, advocacy, information and referral, independent living skills and transportation. Our goal is to move those with challenges in the direction ofn independence.

Oklahoma

4334 **Ability Resources**
823 S Detroit Ave
Suite #110
Tulsa, OK 74120-4223   918-592-1235
                                            800-722-0886
                                       Fax: 918-592-5651
                                       www.ability-resources.org

Carla Lawson, Executive Director
To assist people with disabilities in attaining and maintaining their personal independence.

4335 **Green County Independent Living Resource Center**
4100 S.E. Adams Rd
Suite C-106
Bartlesville, OK 74006- 8409   918-335-1314
                                            800-559-0567
                                       Fax: 918-333-1814
                                       TTY: 918-335-1314

Vicki Haws, Executive Director
Independent living skills training, information and referrals, advocacy, a loan library of adaptive equipment and books. Services available to all individuals with disabilities and their family members who reside in Northeastern Oklahoma.

4336 **Oklahomans for Independent Living**
601 East Carl Albert Parkway
McAlester, OK 74501-5410   918-426-6220
                                             800-568-6821
                                       Fax: 918-426-3245
                                       TTY: 918-426-6263
                                       www.oilok.org

Pam Pulchny, Executive Director/ADASpecialist
Terry Yates, Administrative Assistant/Bookke
Leanna Amos, Service Management Specialist
OIL encourages individuals of all ages, with all types of disabilities to increase: personal dependence; empowerment and self determiation; and ful integration and participation in their work, community, school and home activities.

4337 **Progressive Independence**
121 N Porter Avenue
Norman, OK 73071-5834   405-321-3203
                                             800-801-3203
                                       Fax: 405-321-7601
                                       TTY: 405-321-2942
                                       www.progind.org

Scott Spray, Chairperson
Teresa Tisdell, Vice Chair
Mark Newman, Treasurer

Preovides four cores services of Information & Referral, Individaul& Systems Advocacy, Peer Counseling, and Skills Training; in addition, offers accessible computer lab, short term DME loans, ande benefits counseling for SSI/SSDI.

Oregon

4338 **Abilitree**
2680 NE Twin Knolls Dr.
Suite 3
Bend, OR 97701   541-388-8103
                                       Fax: 541-389-2337
                                       TTY: 541-388-8103
                                       www.abilitree.org

Tim Johnson, Executive Director
Greg Sublett, Director of Operations
April O'Meara, Marketing Director
CORIL empowers people with disabilities to maximize their independence, productivity and inclusio in community life. CORIL envisions a society where all people have the opportunity to develop their full capabilities with independence, productivity and more meaningful involvment in local community events and activities.

4339 **Eastern Oregon Center for Independent Living**
1021 SW 5th Ave
Ontario, OR 97914-3301   541-889-3119
                                             866-248-8369
                                       Fax: 541-889-4647
                                       eocil@eocil.org
                                       www.eocil.org

Kirt Toombs, Executive Director
EOCIL is a nonprofit community based resource and advocacy center that promotes independent living and equal access for all persons with disabilities. EOCIL serves consumers in the counties of: Baker, Gilliam, Grant, harney, Malheur, Morrow, Umatilla, Union, Wallowa and Wheeler.

4340 **HASL Independent Abilities Center**
305 NE 'E' Street
Grants Pass, OR 97526   541-479-4275
                                             800-758-4275
                                       Fax: 541-479-7261
                                       TTY: 541-479-3588
                                       haslstaff@yahoo.com
                                       www.haslonline.org

Randy Samuelson, Executive Director
To promote public awareness of the special needs and legal rights of individuals with cross-disabilities; to facilitate their integration into society and provide support through advocacy, peer counseling, skills training and information and referral to encourage independence.

4341 **Independent Living Resources**
1839 NE Couch St.
Portland, OR 97232   503-232-7411
                                       Fax: 503-232-7480
                                       TTY: 503-232-8404
                                       info@ilr.org
                                       www.ilr.org/?

Barry Fox-Quamme, Executive Director
May Altman, LCSW, Associate Director
Barbara Norris, Office Manager/Executive Assistant
ILR looks to promote the philosophy of Independent Living by creating opportunities, encouraging choices, advancing equal access, and furthering the level of independence for all people with disabilities

4342 **Laurel Hill Center**
2145 Centennial Plaza
Eugene, OR 97401-2474   541-485-6340
                                       Fax: 541-984-3124
                                       TTY: 541-684-6822
                                       info@laurel.org
                                       www.laurel.org

Tom Fauria, President
DAVE Burtner, Vice-President
EDUARDO Sifuentez, Secretary

Provides natoinall-recognized, recovery-focused rehabilitation services in Lane County, Oregon, for people with severe and persistent mental illnesses

4343 Progressive Options
611 S.W. Hurbert Street
Suite A
Newport, OR 97365-9678

541-265-4674
Fax: 541-574-4313
TTY: 541-574-1927
progop541@yahoo.com
www.progressive-options.org

Rhonda Walker, Executive Director
Progressive Options seeks to provide free services and support to people with disabilities of all kinds to help them achieve and maintain maximum independence and self-sufficiency in Lincoln County and surrounding areas in Oregon.

4344 SPOKES Unlimited
1006 Main St
Klamath Falls, OR 97601-6029

541-883-7547
Fax: 541-885-2469
TTY: 541-883-7547
www.spokesunlimited.org

Wendy Howard, Executive Director
Mission is to enhance the ability of people with disabilities to live more independently.

4345 Umpqua Valley Disabilities Network
736 SE Jackson Street
Roseburg, OR 97470-110

541-672-6336
Fax: 541-672-8606
TTY: 541-440-2882
uvdn@uvdn.org
www.uvdn.org

David Fricke, Executive Director
Heather Vialpando, Executive Assistant
UVDN's mission is to promote independent living and community inclusion for people with disabilities.

Pennsylvania

4346 Abilities in Motion
210 N 5th St
Reading, PA 19601-3304

610-376-0010
888-376-0120
Fax: 610-376-0021
TTY: 610-228-2301
www.abilitiesinmotion.org

Terry Graul, Board President
David Lerch, Vice-President
Bonnie Milke, Treasurer
Dedicated to advancing the rights of persons with disabilities in orer to promote a full life in the community through the prevention and elimination of physical, psychological, social and attitudinal barriers which serve to deny them the rights and privileges common to the general public.

4347 Anthracite Region Center for Independent Living
Pennsylvania Council on Independent Living
8 West Broad St
Suite 228
Hazleton, PA 18201-6418

570-455-9800
800-777-9906
Fax: 570-455-1731
TTY: 570-455-9800
dcorcoran@anthracitecil.org

Irene Mordosky, President
Margo Madden, Vice-President
Rand Martin, Treasurer
Enables individuals with disabilities to attain their highest possible level of independence.

4348 Brian's House
757 Springdale Dr.
Exton, PA 19341-8531

610-399-1175
ekihara@brianshouse.org
brianshouse.org

Diana L. Ramsay, MPP, OTR, FAOT, Resident and Chief Executive Off
Peter M. Shubiak, MA, Executive Vice President and Chi
Lori Plunkettt, Executive Director
A non-profit organization that provides residential, vocational and recreational/respite programs for children and adults with intellectual and developmental disabilities.

4349 Community Resources for Independence
3410 W 12th St
Erie, PA 16505-3649

814-838-7222
800-530-5541
Fax: 814-838-8491
TTY: 814-838-8115
www.crinet.org

Timothy Finegan, Executive Director
William Essigmann, Administrative Program Manager
Carl Berry, Human Resources Director
A community based, nonprofit, nonresidential organization that offers services and assistance to enable people with disabilities to expand their options, pursue their goals, and achieve and maintain self-sufficient and producitve lives in the community.

4350 Community Resources for Independence, Inc., Bradford
3410 West 12th Street
Erie, PA 16505

814-838-7222
800-530-5541
Fax: 814-838-8491
TTY: 814-838-8115
crinet.org

Timothy J. Finegan, Executive Director
William Essigmann, Administrative Program Manager
Carl Berry, Human Resources Director
Community Resources for Independence, Inc is committed to preserve, enhance and enrich the quality of life for all people with disabilities.

4351 Community Resources for Independence: Lewistown
33 East Hale Street
Suite L
Lewistown, PA 17044-2160

717-248-8011
800-309-0989
Fax: 717-248-8029
www.crinet.org

Timothy Finegan, Executive Director
William Essigmann, Administrative Program Manager
Carl Berry, Human Resources Director
A community based, nonprofit, nonresidential organization that offers services and assistance to enable people with disabilities to expand their options, pursue their goals, and achieve and maintain self-sufficient and producitve lives in the community.

4352 Community Resources for Independence: Altoona
1331 Twelth Ave
Suite #103
Altoona, PA 16601

814-994-2645
866-944-2645
Fax: 814-944-2683
www.crinet.org

Timothy Finegan, Executive Director
William Essigmann, Administrative Program Manager
Carl Berry, Human Resources Director
A community based, nonprofit, nonresidential organization that offers services and assistance to enable people with disabilities to expand their options, pursue their goals, and achieve and maintain self-sufficient and producitve lives in the community.

4353   Community Resources for Independence: Clarion
1200 Eastwood Drive
Suite #1
Clarion, PA 16214-8824   814-297-7141
                                           800-372-0140
                                      Fax: 814-297-7161
                                          www.crinet.org

Timothy J. Finegan, Executive Director
William Essigmann, Administrative Program Manager
Carl Berry, Human Resources Director
A community based, nonprofit, nonresidential organization that
offers services and assistance to enable people with disabilities to
expand their options, pursue their goals, and achieve and maintain self-sufficient and producitve lives in the community.

4354   Community Resources for Independence: Clearfield
209 E Locust St
Clearfield, PA 16830-2422   814-765-6405
                                           866-619-6405
                                      Fax: 814-765-1269
                                          www.crinet.org

Timothy Finegan, Executive Director
William Essigmann, Administrative Program Manager
Carl Berry, Human Resources Director
A community based, nonprofit, nonresidential organization that
offers services and assistance to enable people with disabilities to
expand their options, pursue their goals, and achieve and maintain self-sufficient and producitve lives in the community.

4355   Community Resources for Independence: Hermitage
3875 East State St
Suite B
Hermitage, PA 16148-3415   724-347-4121
                                      Fax: 724-347-5966
                                          www.crinet.org

Timothy J. Finegan, Executive Director
William Essigmann, Administrative Program Manager
Carl Berry, Human Resources Director
A community based, nonprofit, nonresidential organization that
offers services and assistance to enable people with disabilities to
expand their options, pursue their goals, and achieve and maintain self-sufficient and producitve lives in the community.

4356   Community Resources for Independence: Lewisburg
11 Reitz Blvd
Suite #105
Lewisburg, PA 17837-1493   570-524-4314
                                           800-332-4135
                                      Fax: 570-524-9236
                                          www.crinet.org

Timothy J. Finegan, Executive Director
William Essigmann, Administrative Program Manager
Carl Berry, Human Resources Director
A community based, nonprofit, nonresidential organization that
offers services and assistance to enable people with disabilities to
expand their options, pursue their goals, and achieve and maintain self-sufficient and producitve lives in the community.

4357   Community Resources for Independence: Oil City
250 Elm St
Oil City, PA 16301-1413   814-677-4655
                                           866-209-3882
                                      Fax: 814-677-4915
                                          www.crinet.org

Tim Finegan, Executive Director
William Essigmann, Administrative Program Manager
Carl Berry, Human Resources Director
A community based, nonprofit, nonresidential organization that
offers services and assistance to enable people with disabilities to
expand their options, pursue their goals, and achieve and maintain self-sufficient and producitve lives in the community.

4358   Community Resources for Independence: Warren
1003 Pennsylvania Ave W
Warren, PA 16365-1837   814-726-3404
                                           866-579-3404
                                      Fax: 814-726-3428
                                          www.crinet.org

Timothy Finegan, Executive Director
William Essigmann, Administrative Program Manager
Carl Berry, Human Resources Director

A community based, nonprofit, nonresidential organization that
offers services and assistance to enable people with disabilities to
expand their options, pursue their goals, and achieve and maintain self-sufficient and producitve lives in the community.

4359   Community Resources for Independence: Wellsboro
38 Plaza Ln
Wellsboro, PA 16901-1766   570-724-5852
                                           866-401-7911
                                      Fax: 570-724-3945
                                          www.crinet.org

Timothy Finegan, Executive Director
William Essigmann, Administrative Program Manager
Carl Berry, Human Resources Director
A community based, nonprofit, nonresidential organization that
offers services and assistance to enable people with disabilities to
expand their options, pursue their goals, and achieve and maintain self-sufficient and producitve lives in the community.

4360   Freedom Valley Disability Center
3607 Chapel Road
Suite B
Newtown Square, PA 19073-3602   610-353-6640
                                           800-427-4754
                                      Fax: 610-353-6753
                                      TTY: 610-353-8900

Ann Cope, Executive Director
Assists persons with disabilities in the achievement of independ-
ent living goals. Also promotes individual and community op-
tions to maximize independence for persons with disabilities.
Serves people with disabilities in Chester, Delaware, and
Montgomery Counties.

4361   Institute on Disabilities At Temple Univ.
Temple University
1755 N. 13th St
Student Center, Rm. 4115
Philadelphia, PA 19122-6099   215-204-1356
                                      Fax: 215-204-6336
                                          iod@temple.edu
                                   www.disabilities.temple.edu

James Earl Davis, Phd, Interim Executive Director
Celia Feinstein, Co-Executive- Director
Amy Goldman, Co-Executive- Director
Leads by example, creating connections and promoting networks
within and among communitites so that people with disabilities
are recognized as integral to the fabric of community life.

4362   Lehigh Valley Center for Independent Living
713 North 13th Street
Allentown, PA 18102-9121   610-770-9781
                                           800-495-8245
                                      Fax: 610-770-9801
                                      TTY: 610-770-9789
                                          info@lvcil.org
                                          www.lvcil.org

Scott Berman, President
Michelle Mitchell, Vice President
Amy Beck, Executive Director
Serves persons in Lehigh and Northampton Counties with any
type of disability and/or his/her family.

4363   Liberty Resources
714 Market St
Suite #100
Philadelphia, PA 19106-2337   215-634-2000
                                           888-634-2155
                                      Fax: 215-634-6628
                                      TTY: 215-634-6630
                                   lrinc@libertyresources.org
                                   www.libertyresources.org

Edwin Bomba, Chairman
Mary Ellen Caffrey, Chairman
Estelle B. Richman, Vice-Chairman
A non-profit, consumer driven organization that advocates and
promotes Independent Living for persons with disabilities.

4364 Life and Independence for Today
503 E Arch St
Saint Marys, PA 15857-1779
814-781-3050
800-341-5438
Fax: 814-781-1917
TTY: 814-781-3050
lift@liftcil.org
www.liftcil.org

Stephen DePrater, President
Linda McKinstry, Vice-President
Larry Caggeso, Treasurer
Offers services to enable people with disabilities to achieve new goals and broaden their horizons. It enables them to achieve and maintain self-sufficient and productive lives.

4365 Northeastern Pennsylvania Center for Independent Living
1142 Sanderson Ave
Suite #1
Scranton, PA 18509
570-344-7211
800-344-7211
Fax: 570-344-7218
TTY: 570-344-5275
nepacilinfo@nepacil.org

Robert Treptow, President
Michael Sporer, Secretary
Chris Armone,Esq, Treasurer
Established to assist in removing barriers and expanding independent living options available to people with disabilities.

4366 South Central Pennsylvania Center for Independence Living
1019 Logan Blvd
Altoona, PA 16602-2434
814-949-1905
800-237-9009
Fax: 814-949-1909
TTY: 814-949-1912
www.cilscpa.org

Susan Estep, Executive Director
The missio of the Center for Independent Living of South Central PA is to empower people with disabilities to lead independent lives in their commnuitites. The Center covers Bedford, Blair, cambria, Fulton, Huntingdon, Indiana and Somerset counties.

4367 Three Rivers Center for Independent Living: New Castle
900 Rebecca Ave
Pittsburgh, PA 15221-9383
412-371-7700
800-633-4588
Fax: 412-371-9430
TTY: 412-371-6230
www.trcil.myfastsite.net/

Kourtney T. Diaz, Chairperson
Shanicka Kennedy, Esq, Vice-Chairperson
Stanley A Holbrook, President
To empower people with disabilities to enjoy self-directed, personally meaningful lives by providing outstanding consumer controlled services and by advocating for effective community college.

4368 Three Rivers Center for Independent Livi ng: Washington
900 Rebecca Ave
Pittsburgh, PA 15221-4425
412-371-7700
800-633-4588
Fax: 412-371-9430
TTY: 412-371-6230
www.trcil.myfastsite.net/

Stanley A Holbrook, President
Kourtney T. Diaz, Chairperson
Shanicka Kennedy, Esq, Vice-Chairperson
To empower people with disabilities to enjoy self-directed, personally meaningful lives by providing outstanding consumer controlled services and by advocating for effective community college.

4369 Three Rivers Center for Independent Living
900 Rebecca Ave
Pittsburgh, PA 15221-2938
412-371-7700
800-633-4588
Fax: 412-371-9430
TTY: 412-371-6230
www.trcil.myfastsite.net/

Stanley A Holbrook, President
Kourtney T. Diaz, Chairperson
Shanicka Kennedy, Esq, Vice-Chairperson
To empower people with disabilities to enjoy self-directed, personally meaningful lives by providing outstanding consumer controlled services and by advocating for effective community college.

4370 Tri-County Patriots for Independent Living
69 East Beau St
Washington, PA 15301-4711
724-223-5115
877-889-0965
Fax: 724-223-5119
TTY: 724-228-4028
www.tripil.com

Kathleen Kleinmann, Chief Executive Officer
Maxine Berton, Administrative Assistant
Jeffry D. Woods, Chief Information Officer
Brings together individuals who share common problems in equal access, education, housing, employment, attendant care, transportation, and access to technology.

4371 Voices for Independence
1107 Payne Ave
Erie, PA 16503-1741
814-874-0064
866-407-0064
Fax: 814-874-3497
TTY: 814-874-0064
web@vficil.org
www.vficil.org

Shona Eakin, Executive Director
Edna Anabui, Executive Administrative Assista
Doug McClintock, Director of Finances
To empower people with disabilities and promote independent living.

Rhode Island

4372 Arc of Blackstone
500 Prospect St.
Wing B, Suite 203
Pawtucket, RI 2860- 4396
401-727-0150
800-257-6092
Fax: 401-727-1545
contact@bvcriarc.org
www.bvcriarc.org

Kathleen O'Neill, President
Thomas E. Hodge, Vice-President
Joseph F. McEnness, Treasurer
Committed to supporting people with developmental disabilities secure the opportunity to choose and realize their goals of where and how they live, learn, work and play

4373 Franklin Court Assisted Living
180 Franklin St
Bristol, RI 2809-3352
401-253-3679
Fax: 401-253-5855

Michelle Belmore Cabana, Chief Financial Officer
Brenda Marshall, Administrator
Lynn A. Marshall, Property Manager
Offers local seniors an affordable assisted living option with first-rate services and gracious accommodations.

4374 IN-SIGHT Independent Living
43 Jefferson Blvd
Warwick, RI 2888-1078
401-941-3322
Fax: 401-941-3356
cbutler@in-sight.org
www.in-sight.org

Jean Saylor, Chairman
Robert Tyler, Vice-Chairman
James Hahn, Treasurer

Creating opportunities and choices for people who are blind and visually impaired

4375   Ocean State Center for Independent Living
1944 Warwick Avenue
Warwick, RI 2889-2448
                                        401-738-1013
                                        866-857-1161
                                        Fax: 401-738-1083
                                        TTY: 401-738-1015
                                        info@oscil.org
                                        www.oscil.org

Lorna Ricci, Executive Director
OSCIL is a consumer controlled, community based, nonprofit organization established to provide a range of independent living services to enhance, through self direction, the quality of life of Rhode Islander with significant disability and to promote integration into the community.

4376   Office of Rehabilitation Services
40 Fountain Street
Providence, RI 02903-1898
                                        401-421-7005
                                        TTY: 401-421-7016
                                        www.ors.ri.gov

Ron Racine, Associate Director
Beth Rioles, Administrator, DDS
Laurie DiOrio, Administrator, SBVI
Goal is to help individuals with physical and mental disabilities prepare for and obtain appropriate employment.

4377   PARI Independent Living Center
500 Prospect St
Pawtucket, RI 2860-6259
                                        401-725-1966
                                        Fax: 401-725-2104
                                        TTY: 401-725-1966
                                        www.pari-ilc.org

Leo Canuel, Executive Director
Sue Bilodau, Program Director
Offers information and referral services, personal care attendant services, home modifications, advocacy services and peer counseling, independent living skills training, and recycled equipment.

South Carolina

4378   Columbia Disability Action Center
136 Stonemark Lane
Suite #100
Columbia, SC 29210
                                        800-681-6805
                                        Fax: 803-779-5114
                                        TTY: 803-779-0949
                                        www.able-sc.org/

David Dawson, President
Rochelle Gadson, Vice President
Joe Butler, Treasurer
A non-profit consumer governed Center for Independent Living. Programs and services support persons with disaibilities in taking full advantage of community resources, enhancing personal opportunities, and determining the direction of their lives.

4379   Disability Action Center
330B Pelham Rd
Suite 100 A
Greenville, SC 29615-3116
                                        864-235-1421
                                        800-681-7715
                                        Fax: 864-235-2056
                                        TTY: 864-235-8798
                                        amayne@dacsc.org
                                        www.able-sc.org/

David Dawson, President
Rochelle Gadson, Vice President
Joe Butler, Treasurer
Empowering people with disabilities to reach their highest level of independence.

4380   Graham Street Community Resources
306 Graham St
Florence, SC 29501-4735
                                        843-665-6674
                                        Fax: 843-665-6674

Faye Thompson, Manager

Promotes independent living and empowers people with disabilities to reach their highest level of independence.

4381   South Carolina Independent Living Council
136 Stonemark Lane
Suite #100
Columbia, SC 29210-7318
                                        803-217-3209
                                        800-994-4322
                                        Fax: 803-731-1439
                                        TTY: 803-217-3209
                                        scilc@scilconline.org
                                        www.scsilc.com

Mike Le Fever, President
Committed to equal opportunity, equal access, self determination, independence, and choice for all people with disabilities and pursues these goals by the means available.

4382   Walton Options for Independent Living: North Augusta
325 Georgia Ave
North Augusta, SC 29841-3848
                                        803-279-9611
                                        Fax: 803-279-9135
                                        tjohnston@waltonoptions.org
                                        www.waltonoptions.org

Cynthia Anzek, Executive Director
Empowers persons of all ages with all types of disabilities to reach their highest level of independence, community inclusion and employment.

South Dakota

4383   Adjustment Training Center
607 N 4th St
Aberdeen, SD 57401-2733
                                        605-229-0263
                                        Fax: 605-225-3455
                                        www.aspiresd.org

Jennifer Gray, Executive Director
Arlette Keller, Director of Service Coordination
Angela Huffman, Director of Nursing
Offers peer counseling, attendant care registry and referrals.

4384   Black Hills Workshop & Training Center
Black Hills Workshop
3650 Range Road
PO Box 2104
Rapid City, SD 57709-2104
                                        605-343-4550
                                        Fax: 605-343-0879
                                        TTY: 800-877-1113
                                        drosby@bhws.com
                                        www.blackhillsworks.org

Brad Saathoff, Chief Executive Officer
Janet Niehaus, VP of Finance
Michelle Aman, VP of Residential Services
Offers job placement, housing options, case coordination, supported employment and supported living for all disability groups, as well as specialized services for brian injury victims.

4385   Communication Service for the Deaf: Rapid City
200 W Cesar Chavez St
Suite 650
Austin, TX 78701-694
                                        844-222-0002
                                        800-642-6410
                                        Fax: 605-394-6609
                                        TTY: 866-273-3323
                                        csd@csd.org
                                        www.c-s-d.org

Dr. Benjamin Soukup, Founder, Chairman & CEO
Christopher Soukup, President
Brad Hermes, Chief Financial Officer
A private, nonprofit organization dedicated to providing broad-based services, ensuring public accessibility and increasing public awareness of issues affecting deaf and hard of hearing inividuals.

4386 Native American Advocacy Program for Persons with Disabilities
P.O.Box 527
Winner, SD 57580-527   605-842-3977
                                        800-303-3975
                                    Fax: 605-842-3983
                                    TTY: 605-842-3977

Marla Bull Bear, Executive Director
Charles Bull Bear, Specialist
Betty Farr, Il Specialist
The mission is to encourage a healthy organization that assists Native Americans with disabilities, by providing prevention, education and training, advocacy, support, independent living skills and referrals.

4387 Prairie Freedom Center for Independent Living: Sioux Falls
4107 S Carnegie Cr
Suite #9
Sioux Falls, SD 57106-3100   605-362-3550
                                    Fax: 605-367-5639
                                    i-l-c@ilcchoices.org
                                    www.ilcchoices.org

Steve Tripp, President
Cheri Raymond, Vice President
Matt Cain, Executive Director
Established to provide basic skills so many of us take for granted: to take care of our own needs and to make our own decisions to be independent.

4388 Prairie Freedom Center for Independent Li ving: Madison
4107 S Carnegie Cr
411 SE 10th St
Sioux Falls, SD 57106-3570   605-362-3550
                                    Fax: 605-256-5071
                                    i-l-c@ilcchoices.org
                                    www.ilcchoices.org

Steve Tripp, President
Cheri Raymond, Vice President
Matt Cain, Executive Director
Established to provide basic skills so many of us take for granted: to take care of our own needs and to make our own decisions to be independent.

4389 Prairie Freedom Center for Independent Living: Yankton
4107 S Carnegie Cr
Suite #107
Sioux Falls, SD 57106-2800   605-362-3550
                                    Fax: 605-668-3060
                                    TTY: 605-668-3060
                                    www.ilcchoices.org

Steve Tripp, President
Cheri Raymond, Vice President
Matt Cain, Executive Director
Established to provide basic skills so many of us take for granted: to take care of our own needs and to make our own decisions to be independent.

4390 South Dakota Assistive Technology Project: DakotaLink
1161 Deadwood Ave N
Suite #5
Rapid City, SD 57702-382   605-394-6742
                                    800-645-0673
                                    Fax: 605-394-6744
                                    TTY: 605-394-6742
                                    atinfo@dakotalink.net

Pat Czerny, Manager
Patrick Czerny, Technical Services Coordinator
David Scherer, Program Coordinator
DakotaLink, the South Dakota Assistive Technology Program, provides resources and supports to individuals of all ages to ensure greater access to and acquisition of assistive technology devices and services.

4391 Western Resources for dis-ABLED Independence
405 East Omaha St
Suite D
Rapid City, SD 57701-2974   605-718-1930
                                    888-434-4943
                                    Fax: 605-718-1933
                                    TTY: 605-718-1930
                                    chad@wril.org
                                    www.wril.org

Jeff Wangen, President
Dennis Coull, Vice-President
Linda Lockner, Secretary
WRDI advocates for the rights of equal inclusion of people with disabilities in all aspects of community life. WRDI also strives to identify and promote access to existing resources and to advocate for the development of new resources, which may enable people with disabilities to live more independently.

Tennessee

4392 Center for Independent Living of Middle Tennessee
955 Woodland St
Nashville, TN 37206-3753   615-292-5803
                                    866-992-4568
                                    Fax: 615-383-1176
                                    TTY: 615-292-7790

Tom Hopton, Executive Director
Tria Bridgeman, Benefits Analyst-Jackson
Dylan Brown, Benefits Analyst-Nashville
CILMT provides persons with disabilities opportunities to be self advocates and make their own decisions regarding living arrangements, means of transportation, employment, social and recreational activities, as well as other aspects of everyday life. Serves Davidson, Cheatham, Wilson, Robertson, Rutherford, Sumner and Williamson Counties.

4393 DisAbility Resource Center: Knoxville
900 E Hill Ave
Suite 205
Knoxville, TN 37915-2567   865-637-3666
                                    Fax: 865-637-5616
                                    TTY: 865-637-6976

Lillian Burch, Executive Director
Nicole Craig, Programme Director
Katherine Moore, Independent Living Specialist
DRCTN mission is to empower people with disabilities to fully integrate and participate in the community. DRC is a community-based non-residential program of services designed to assist people with disabilities to gain independence and to assist the community in eliminating barriers of independence.

4394 Jackson Center for Independent Living
1981 Hollywood Drive
Jackson, TN 38305-4388   731-668-2211
                                    Fax: 731-668-0406
                                    TTY: 731-664-3970
                                    www.j-cil.com

Glen Barr, Executive Director
JCIL works with people with significant disabilities and the Deaf Community in achieving their Independent Living Goals while assisting the community in eliminating barriers to Independent Living.

4395 Memphis Center for Independent Living
1633 Madison Ave
Memphis, TN 38104-2506   901-726-6404
                                    800-848-0298
                                    Fax: 901-726-6521
                                    TTY: 901-726-6404
                                    info@mcil.org
                                    www.mcil.org

Kevin Lofton, Chairman
Marvin Glenn Bailey, Vice-Chairman
Charles M. Weirich, Jr., Board Counsel
MCIL is a community based non-profit organization whose primary mission is to facilitate the full integration of persons with disabilities into all aspects of community life.

4396 Tennessee Technology Access Program (TTAP)
400 Deaderick St
14th Fl
Nashville, TN 37243-1403   615-313-5183
800-732-5059
Fax: 615-532-4685
TTY: 615-313-5695

Kevin Wright, Director
TTAP's mission is to maintain a statewide program of technology-rated assistance that is timely, comprehensive and consumer driven to ensure that all Tennesseans with disabilities have the information, services and deices that they need to make choices about where and how they spend their time as independently as possible.

4397 Tri-State Resource and Advocacy Corporation
6925 Shallowford Rd
#300
Chattanooga, TN 37421   423-892-4774
800-868-8724
Fax: 423-892-9866
TTY: 423-892-4774
www.1trac.org

Mark Woofall, Executive Director
Pam Jackson, Independent Living Facilitator
TRAC is dedicated to improving opportunities for individuals wuth disabilities.

Texas

4398 ABLE Center for Independent Living
1931 E 37th
St # 1
Odessa, TX 79762-6906   432-580-3439
info@ablecenterpb.org

Marilyn Hancock, Executive Director
Kathleen Story MA, Independent Living Specialist
Britni Veretto, HR Manager
To promote independent living for people with disabilities.

4399 Austin Resource Center for Independent Living
825 E. Rundberg Ln
Suite E6
Austin, TX 78753-4813   512-832-6349
800-414-6327
Fax: 512-832-1869
arcil@arcil.com
www.arcil.com

Ross Davis, Chair
Linda Loach, Vice-Chair
Sylvia Davis, Secretary/Treasurer
Serving people with disabilities, their families and communities throughout Travis and surrounding counties.

4400 Austin Resource Center: Round Rock
525 Round Rock West
Suite A120
Round Rock, TX 78681-5020   512-828-4624
Fax: 512-828-4625
sally@arcil.com
www.arcil.com

Ross Davis, Chair
Linda Loach, Vice-Chair
Sylvia Davis, Secretary/Treasurer
Serving peole with disabilities, their families and communities throughout Travis and surrounding counties.

4401 Austin Resource Center: San Marcos
618 South Guadalupe St
Suite #103
San Marcos, TX 78666- 6977   512-396-5790
800-572-2973
Fax: 512-396-5794
sanmarcos@arcil.com
www.arcil.com

Ross Davis, Chair
Linda Loach, Vice-Chair
Sylvia Davis, Secretary/Treasurer
Serving people with disabilities, their families and communities throughout Travis and surounding counties.

4402 Brazoria County Center For Independent Living
1104D East Mullberry Street
Suite D
Angleton, TX 77515- 3952   979-849-7060
888-872-7957
Fax: 979-849-8465
TTY: 979-849-7060
bccil@neosoft.com
www.hcil.cc

Chamane Barrow, Manager
To promote the full inclusion, equal opportunity and participation of persons with disabilities in every aspect of community life. We believe that people with disabilities have the right to make choices affecting their lives, a right to take risks, a right to fail, and a right to succeed.

4403 Centre, The
3550 West Dallas Rd
Houston, TX 77019   713-525-8400
Fax: 713-525-8444
thecenterhouston.org

Bill Coorsh, President
Richard Rosenberg, Vice-President
Lisa F. Schott, Secretary
Provides services for more than 600 children and adults with mental developmental disabilities. The Center also offers a wide array of programs including education, vocational training and job placement services, three different residential options representing both urban and rural living environments, special programs designed to meet the needs of older adults, and a variety of therapeutic support services.

4404 Crockett Resource Center for Independent Living
1020 Loop 304 East
Crockett, TX 75835-1806   936-544-2811
Fax: 936-544-7315
TTY: 936-544-2811
crcil@windstream.net
www.crockettresourcecenter.org

Sara Minton, Executive Director
Mary Killough, Chief Financial Officer
Cathy Newsome, Information/Outreach Coordinator
Provides independent living services to cross-disability groups to increase their personal self-determination and minimize dependence on others. Maintain comprehensive information on availability of resources and provides referrals to such resources. Provides instruction to assist people with disabilities to gain skills that would empower them to live independently. Peer counseling, advocacy - both individual and community by assisting to obtain support services to make changes in society.

4405 Houston Center for Independent Living (HCIL)
6201 Bonhomme Rd.
Suite 150-South
Houston, TX 77036   713-974-4621
Fax: 713-974-6927
hcil@neosoft.com

Sandra Bookman, Executive Director
Advocacy organization created by and for people with disabilities (PWD) to empower and protect their rights. Services include but not limited to: peer to peer support, individual and systems advocacy, independent living skills training, information and referral, disability cultural awareness, ASL and Braille classes, ADA technical assistance, Relocation/Transition to Community Services, computer technology training, SSA Work Incentives Technical Assistance, equipment loan program.

4406 Independent Life Styles
215 North Benton Drive
Sauk Rapids, MN 56379-1874   320-529-9000
888-529-0743
Fax: 320-529-0747
ilicil@independentlifestyles.org
www.independentlifestyles.org

Karen Ahles, Chair
Jay Keller, Educator
Cara Ruff, Executive Director

Offers peer counseling, advocacy and other services to the community.

4407 Independent Living Research Utilization Project
Institute For Rehabilitation & Research
1333 Moursund
Houston, TX 77030

713-520-0232
Fax: 713-520-5785
TTY: 713-520-0232
ilru@ilru.org
www.ilru.org

Lex Frieden, Director
ILRU is a national center for information, training, research and technical assistance in independent living. Its goal is to expand the body of knowledge in independent living and to improve utilization of results of research programs and demonstration projects in this field. ILRU is a program of The Institute for Rehabilitation and Research, a nationally recognized medical rehabilitation facility for persons with disabilities. TTY phone number: (713) 520-5136.

4408 LIFE/ Run Centers for Independent Living
8240 Boston Avenue
Lubbock, TX 79423-2342

806-795-5433
Fax: 806-795-5607
TTY: 806-795-5433
wilmacrain@yahoo.com
www.liferun.org

Michelle Crain, Executive Director
Committed to providing individuals with disabilities the information and skills necessary to become independent and to achieve full inclusion in every aspect of their life.

4409 Office for Students with Disabilities, University of Texas at Arlington
701 South Nedderman Drive
Arlington, TX 76019-1

817-272-3364
800-735-2989
Fax: 817-272-1447
TTY: 800-735-2989
helpdesk@uta.edu
www.uta.edu/disability

Penny Acrey, Director
Demarice Ferguson, MS, CRC, Associate Director
Scott Holmes, Assistant Director for Testing
Offers disability counseling and academic accomodation to UT Arlington community.

4410 Palestine Resource Center for Independent Living
421 Avenue a St
Palestine, TX 75801-2903

903-729-7505
888-326-5166
Fax: 903-729-7540
TTY: 903-729-7505
prcil@embarqmail.com
www.palestineresourcecenter.org/?

Sara Minton, Executive Director
Mary Killough, Chief Financial Officer
Cathy Newsome, Information/Outreach Coordinator
Provides independent living services to cross-disability groups to increase their personal self-determination and minimize dependence on others. Maintain comprehensive information on availability of resources and provides referrals to such resources. Provides instruction to assist people with disabilities to gain skills that would empower them to live independently. Peer counseling, advocacy - both individual and community by assisting to obtain support services to make changes in society.

4411 Panhandle Action Center for Independent Living Skills
417 W. 10th Avenue
Amarillo, TX 79101-4316

806-374-1400
Fax: 806-374-4550
TTY: 806-374-2774
www.panhandleilc.org

Joe Rogers, Executive Director
Alma Benavides, Employment Director
Chris White, Development Director
PILC is a non profit organization dedicated to the advancement of full participation in all aspects of life. PILC services are developed, directed, delivered, and governed primarily by individuals with disabilities.

4412 REACH of Dallas Resource Center on Independent Living
8625 King George
Suite 210
Dallas, TX 75235-2286

214-630-4796
Fax: 214-630-6390
TTY: 214-630-5995
reachdallas@reachcils.org
www.reachcils.org

Charlotte A. Stewart, Executive Director
Information and referral, peer support/peer counseling, independent living skills training and advocacy assistance.

4413 REACH of Denton Resource Center on Independent Living
405 S. Elm St
Suite 202
Denton, TX 76201-6068

940-383-1062
Fax: 940-383-2742
reachden@reachcils.org
www.reachcils.org

Charlotte A. Stewart, Executive Director
To provide for people with disabilities so that they are enabled to lead self-directed lives and to educate the general public about disability-related topics in order to promote a barrier free community.

4414 REACH of Fort Worth Resource Center on Independent Living
1000 Macon Street
Suite 200
Fort Worth, TX 76102-4527

817-870-9082
Fax: 817-877-1622
reachftw@reachcils.org
www.reachcils.org

Charlotte A. Stewart, Executive Director
To provide services for people with disabilities so that they are enabled to lead self-directed lives and to educate the general public about disability-related topics in order to promote a barrier free community.

4415 RISE-Resource: Information, Support and Empowerment
755 11th Street
Suite 101
Beaumont, TX 77701-3723

409-832-2599
Fax: 409-838-4499
TTY: 409-832-2599
www.risecil.org

Jim Brocato, Executive Director
Amanda Powe, Relocation Services Specialist
Cheryl Bass, Program Director
A non-profit center for independent living.

4416 SAILS
1028 S Alamo St
San Antonio, TX 78210-1170

210-281-1878
800-474-0295
Fax: 210-281-1759
TTY: 210-281-1878
kbrietzke@sailstx.org
www.sailstx.org

Patricia Byrd, Chair
Dennis Wolf, Vice Chair
Jerry D. King, Treasurer
SAILS advocates for the rights and empowerment of people with disabilities in San Antonio; as well as surrounding areas. Services are provided to people with disabilities in the following counties: Atacosa, Bandera, Bexar, Calhoun, Comal, DeWitt, Dimmit, Edwards, Frio, Gillespie, Goliad, Gonzalez, Guadalupe, Jackson, Karnes, La Salle, Kendall, Kerr, Kinney, Lavaca, Maverick, Medina, Real, Uvalde, Val Verde, Victoria, Wilson and Zavala.

4417 Texas Department of Assistive and Rehabilitative Services
4800 N. Lamar Blvd
Austin, TX 78756
512-472-4138
800-628-5115
Fax: 512-472-0603
TTY: 866-581-9328
dars.inquiries@dars.state.tx.us
www.dars.state.tx.us

Bill West, Manager
Daniel Bravo, Chief Operating Officer
Rebecca Trevino, Chief Financial Officer
Provides technical assistance and other support services to the state's Independent Living Council, Independent Living Centers and Independent Living Counseling programs.

4418 VOLAR Center for Independent Living
1220 Golden Key Circle
El Paso, TX 79925-5825
915-591-0800
800-591-0800
Fax: 915-591-3506
TTY: 915-591-0800
volar@volarcil.org
www.volarcil.org

Luis Chew, Executive Director
Danny Monroe, Chief Financial Officer
Nena Garcia, Records Manager/ Bookkeeper
VOLAR is committed to providing independent living ervices and information and referral, and to developing community options for persons with cross disabilities to empower them to live the kind of lives they choose. VOLAR is an organization of and for people with disabilities, advocating human and civil rights, community options and empowering people to live the lives they choose. Newsletter available.

4419 Valley Association for Independent Living (VAIL)
3012 N McColl Road
McAllen, TX 78501
956-668-8245
866-400-8245
Fax: 956-878-1601
info@vailrgv.org
vailrgv.org

Woodie Johnston, Executive Director
Offers information and referral, peer couseling, MS supprt group, independent living skills training, and advocacy, work incentives planning and assistance, transitioning people with disabilities from the nursing home into the community.

4420 Valley Association for Independent Living: Harlingen
1824 W. Jefferson Ave
Suite B
Harlingen, TX 78550-5247
956-428-1126
866-400-8245
Fax: 956-428-4339

Soledad Myers, Manager
Provides information and referral, peer counseling, support groups, independent living skills training, community rehab program and advocacy

Utah

4421 Active Re-Entry
10 S Fairgrounds Rd
Price, UT 84501
435-637-4950
Fax: 435-637-4952
TTY: 435-637-4950
active@arecil.org
www.arecil.org

Nancy Bentley, Executive Director
Active Re-Entry is a community based program which assists individuals with disabilities to acheive or maintain self-sufficient and productive live in their own communities. Active Re-Entry is committed to promoting the rights, dignity, and quality of life for all persons with disabilities.

4422 Active Re-Entry: Vernal
10 S Fairgrounds Rd
Price, UT 84501-9727
435-637-4950
Fax: 435-789-6090
TTY: 435-789-4021
active@arecil.org
www.arecil.org

Heather Moore, President
Active Re-Entry is a community based program which assists individuals with disabilities to achieve or maintain self-sufficient and productive lives in their own communities. We are committed to promoting the rights, dignity, and quality of life for all persons with disabilities.

4423 Central Utah Independent Living Center
3445 S Main St
Salt Lake City, UT 84115-2824
801-466-5565
877-421-4500
Fax: 801-466-2363
TTY: 801-373-5044
uilc@uilc.org
www.uilc.org

Debra Mair, Executive Director
Kim Meichle, Assistant Director
Patty Trent, Fiscal Manager
Empowers people with disabilities to reach their full potential in community settings through peer support, advocacy, and education.

4424 OPTIONS for Independence
Northern Utah Center for Independent Living
106 East 1120 N
Logan, UT 84341-2215
435-753-5353
Fax: 435-753-5390
TTY: 435-753-5353
www.optionsind.org

Cheryl Atwood, Executive Director
OPTIONS for Independence, the Northern Utah Center for Independent Living serves people of all ages with all types of disabilities. OPTIONS is a nonresidential Center that provides services to individuals with disabilities to facilitate their full participation in the community and raise the understanding of disability issues and access to the community. The Independent Living philosophy is strictly adhered to: consumer control and choice being the focus.

4425 OPTIONS for Independence: Brigham Satellite
106 East 1120 N
Logan, UT 84341-3379
435-753-5353
Fax: 435-753-5390
TTY: 435-723-2171
dcrockett@qwestoffice.net
www.optionsind.org

Cheryl Atwood, Executive Director
Deanna Crockett, Manager
OPTIONS is a nonresidential Independent Living Center where people with disabilities can learn skills to gain more control and independence over their lives. OPTIONS raises the vision and capability of the community at large to the point where people of all abilities will have equal access.

4426 Red Rock Center for Independence
515 W 300 N
Suite A
Saint George, UT 84770-4578
435-673-7501
800-649-2340
Fax: 435-673-8808
rrci@rrci.org
www.rrci.org

Barbara Lefler, Executive Director
Jerry Salkowe, President
Celeste Sorensen, Secretary
Red Rock Center for Independence assists people with disabilities to live and participate independently.

4427 **Tri-County Independent Living Center**
P.O.Box 428
Ogden, UT 84402-428
801-612-3215
866-734-5678
Fax: 801-612-3732
TTY: 801-612-3215
www.uilc.org

Richard Fox, Chairperson
Kim Price, Vice-Chairperson
Greg Killpack, Secretary/Treasurer
The mission of the Tri-County ILC is to enhance independence for all people with disabilities. Serves Davis, Weber and Morgan Counties.

4428 **Utah Assistive Technology Program (UTAP) Utah State University**
6855 Old Main Hill
Logan, UT 84322-6855
435-797-3811
800-524-5152
Fax: 435-797-2355
www.uatpat.org

Sachin Pavithran, UATP Program Director
Marilyn Hammond, Utah Assistive Technology Founda
Lois Summers, UATP Staff Assistant/UATF Busine
Provides expertise, resources, and a structure to enhance and expand AT services provided by private and public agencies in Utah. Occurs through monitoring, coordination, information dissemination, empowering individuals, the identification and removal of barriers, and expanding state resources.

4429 **Utah Independent Living Center**
3445 S Main St
Salt Lake City, UT 84115-4453
801-466-5565
800-355-2195
Fax: 801-466-2363
TTY: 801-466-5565
uilc@uilc.org
www.uilc.org

Debra Mair, Executive Director
Kim Meichle, Assistant Director
Julie Beckstead, Program Coordinator
Offers information and referral services. To assist persons with disabilities achieve independence by providing services and activities which enhance independent living skillspromote the public's understanding, accomodation, and acceptance of their rights, needs and abilities.

4430 **Utah Independent Living Center: Minersville**
P.O.Box 168
Minersville, UT 84752-168
435-691-7724
rrci@rrci.org
www.rrci.org

Barbara Lefler, Executive Director
Jerry Salkowe, President
Celeste Sorensen, Secretary
To enhance independence for all people with disaibilities.

4431 **Utah Independent Living Center: Tooele**
42 S Main St
Tooele, UT 84074-2132
435-843-7353
Fax: 435-843-7359
TTY: 435-843-7353
www.uilc.org

Debra Mair, Executive Director
Kim Meichle, Assistant Director
Julie Beckstead, Program Coordinator
Mission is to assist persons with disabilities achieve greater independence by providing services and activities which enhance independent living skills and promote the public's understanding, accomodation, and acceptance of their rights, needs and abilities.

Vermont

4432 **Vermont Assistive Technology Program**
Department of Aging and Independent Living
100 State Street
Montpelier, VT 05602-2305
802-871-3353
800-750-6355
Fax: 802-871-3048
TTY: 802-241-1464
www.atp.vermont.gov/tryout-centers

Julie Tucker, Program Director
David Punia ATP, Information/Education Specialist
Encompasses a state coordinating council for assistive technology issues, regional centers for demonstration, trial and technical support with computer and augmentative communication equipment and regional seating and positioning centers.

4433 **Vermont Center for Independent Living: Bennington**
601 Main St
Bennington, VT 5201-2875
802-447-0574
800-639-1522
info@vcil.org
www.vcil.org

Colleen Arcodia, Peer Advocate Counselor
Michelle Grubb, Finance & Operations Officer
Sarah Launderville, Executive Director
Believes that individuals with disabilities have the right to live with dignity and with appropriate support in their own homes, fully participate in their communities, and to control and make decisions about their lives.

4434 **Vermont Center for Independent Living: Chittenden**
11 East State Street
Montpelier, VT 05602
802-229-0501
800-639-1522
Fax: 802-229-0503
TTY: 802-229-0501
info@vcil.org
www.vcil.org

Colleen Arcodia, Peer Advocate Counselor
Nathan Besio, Peer Advocate Counselor
Chanda Beun, Receptionist/Admin Specialist
Believes that individuals with disabilities have the right to live with dignity and with appropriate support in their own homes, fully participate in their communities, and to control and make decisions about their lives.

4435 **Vermont Center for Independent Living: Montpelier**
11 E State St
Montpelier, VT 05602-3008
802-229-0501
800-639-1522
Fax: 802-229-0503
info@vcil.org
vcil.org

Colleen Arcodia, Peer Advocate Counselor
Denise Bailey, Direct Services Coordinator
Dhiresha Blose, Development Officer
Believes that individuals with disabilities have the right to live with dignity and with appropriate support in their own homes, fully participate in their communities, and to control and make decisions about their lives.

Virginia

4436 **Access Independence**
324 Hope Dr
Winchester, VA 22601-6800
540-662-4452
Fax: 540-662-4474
TTY: 540-662-5556
askai@accessindependence.org
www.accessindependence.org

Donald Price, Executive Director
Brenda Ernst, Independent Living Specialist
Joan Davis, Manager Operations/Rep Payee
Offers support services to persons with disabilities to assist in maintaining or increasing their independence and self-determination. Includes housing assistance, independent living skills

training, information, referral services, assistance and representative payee and advocacy.

4437 Appalachian Independence Center
230 Charwood Dr
Abingdon, VA 24210-2566

276-628-2979
Fax: 276-628-4931
TTY: 276-676-0920
aicadmin@ntelos.net
aicadvocates.org

Greg Morrell, Executive Director
Donna Buckland, Development Director
Scarlett Cox, Operations Director
Mission is to advocate for and with people with disabilities to promote full participation in society

4438 Blue Ridge Independent Living Center
Ste B
1502 Williamson Rd NE
Roanoke, VA 24012-5100

540-342-1231
Fax: 540-342-9505
TTY: 540-342-1231
brilc@brilc.org
brilc.org

Karen Michalski-Karn, Executive Director
Dana Jackson, Program Services Director
Lottie Diomedi, Independent Living Coordinator
BRILC assists people with disabilities to live independently. The Center also serves the community at large by helping to create and environment that is accessible to all. BRILC offers a variety of services ranging from referrals to community resources, support services, and direct services. These include peer counseling, support groups, training and seminars, advocacy, education, support services, awareness, aid in obtaining specialized equipment, and much more.

4439 Blue Ridge Independent Living Center: Christianburg
210 Pepper Street S
Christiansburg, VA 24073-3571

540-381-8829
Fax: 540-381-8833
TTY: 540-381-9149
brilc@brilc.org
brilc.org

Karen Michalski-Karney, Executive Director
Dana Jackson, Program Services Director
Lottie Diomedi, Independent Living Coordinator
Assists people with disabilities to live independently. The center also serves the community at large by helping to create an environment that is accessible to all.

4440 Blue Ridge Independent Living Center: Low Moor
P.O.Box 7
Low Moor, VA 24457-7

540-862-0252
Fax: 540-862-0252
TTY: 540-862-0252
brilc.org

Karen Michalski-Karney, Executive Director
Dana Jackson, Program Services Director
Lottie Diomedi, Independent Living Coordinator
Assists to help people with disabilities to live independently. The center also serves the community at large by helping to create an environment that is accessible to all.

4441 Clinch Independent Living Services
1139C Plaza Drive
Grundy, VA 24614-6780

276-935-6088
800-597-2322
Fax: 276-935-6342
TTY: 276-935-6088

Betty Bevins, Executive Director
Nonprofit organization providing information and referral, peer counseling, advocacy and independent living skills training to persons with disabilities.

4442 Disability Resource Center
409 Progress St
Fredericksburg, VA 22401-3337

540-373-2559
800-648-6324
Fax: 540-373-8126
TTY: 540-373-5890
drc@cildrc.org

Debe Fults, Executive Director
Eric Barnes, Equipment Connection Assistant
Grace Marshall, Community Integration Coor.
Mission is to assist people with disabilities, those who support them, and the community, through information, education and resources, to achieve the highest potential and benefit of independent living.

4443 ENDependence Center of Northern Virginia
2300 Claredon Blvd.
Suite 3305
Arlington, VA 22201-3367

703-525-3268
866-849-3852
Fax: 703-525-3585
TTY: 703-525-3553
info@ecnv.org
www.ecnv.org

Cynthia Evans, Director of Community Services
Layo Oyewole, Director of Medicaid Programs
Doris Ray, Director of Advocacy and Outreac
ECNV is a community-based resource and advocacy enter which is managed by and for people with disabilities. ENCV promotes independent living philosophy and equal access for all persons with disabilities and, like the nearly 400 centers for independent living across the country, ECNV grew from local disability rights and self-help movements.

4444 Equal Access Center for Independence
4031 University Drive
Suite #301
Fairfax, VA 22030-3409

703-934-2020
TTY: 703-277-7730

David Sharp, Executive Director
Provides information and referral, peer counseling, advocacy and independent living skills training to persons with disabilities.

4445 Independence Empowerment Center
8409 Dorsey Circle
Suite 101
Manassas, VA 20110-4414

703-257-5400
Fax: 703-257-5043
TTY: 703-257-5400
info@ieccil.org
www.ieccil.org

Mary D Lopez, Executive Director
Roberta McEachern, Program Director
Sheree Thomas, Grants Coordinator
A non-profit Center for Independent Living. One of over 500 centers in the United States with roots in civil rights models of the 1960's.

4446 Independence Resource Center
815 Cherry Ave
Charlottesville, VA 22903-3448

434-971-9629
Fax: 434-971-8242
TTY: 434-971-9629
tvandever@ntelos.net
www.charlottesvilleirc.org

Tom Vandever, Executive Director
Brenda Gianniny, Administrator
Carolyn Berry, Participant Services Coordinator
Information and referral services.

4447 Independent Living Center Network: Department of the Visually Handicapped
Ste 300
1809 Staples Mill Rd
Richmond, VA 23230-3515

Fax: 804-355-9297

Robert W Partin, Director
Robert Kastenbaum, Partner
Information and referral services.

4448 Junction Center for Independent Living
P.O.Box 1210
Norton, VA 24273-913
276-679-5988
Fax: 276-679-6569
TTY: 276-679-5988
jcil1@junctioncenter.org
junctioncenter.org

Dennis Horton, Executive Director
Cindy Mefford, Assistant to the Executive Direc
Joe Brady, Deaf and Hard of Hearing Coordin
To assist those who have significant disabilities so that they migh live independently in the least restrictive and most integrated environment possible.

4449 Junction Center for Independent Living: Duffield
P.O.Box 408
Duffield, VA 24244-408
276-431-1195
Fax: 276-431-1196
TTY: 276-431-1195
jcil1@junctioncenter.org

Dennis Horton, Executive Director
Cindy Mefford, Assistant to the Executive Direc
Joe Brady, Deaf and Hard of Hearing Coordin
To assist those who have significant disabilities so that they might live independently in the least restrictive and most integrated environment possbile.

4450 Lynchburg Area Center for Independent Living
500 Alleghany Ave
Suite #520
Lynchburg, VA 24501-2610
434-528-4971
Fax: 434-528-4976
TTY: 434-528-4972
www.lacil.org

Phil Theisen, Executive Director
LACIL is a private non-profit, non-residential consumer driven organization that promotes the efforts of persons with disabilities to live independently in the community and supports the efforts of the community to be open and accessible to all citizens.

4451 Peidmont Independent Living Center
Piedmont Living Center
601 S. Belvidere Street
Richmond, VA 23220
804-782-1986
800-828-1140
Fax: 877-VHD- 123
www.vhda.com

Kit Hale, Chairman
Timothy M. Chapman, Vice Chairman
Susan Dewey, Executive Director
Empowering indiviuals with disabilities to become self-sufficient and independent within their communities.

4452 Peninsula Center for Independent Living
2021-A Cunningham Drive
Suite #2
Hampton, VA 23666-3320
757-827-0275
Fax: 757-827-0655
TTY: 757-827-8800
iepcil@hvacil.org
www.hvacil.org

Ralph Shelman, Executive Director
IEPCIL is a private non-profit non-residential Agency established to provide services to people with disabilities. The Centers Philosophy is that people with a disability should play a major role in deciding their future.The center provides services to people with disabilities in the cities of Hampton, Newport News, Poquoson, Williamsburg, and counties of James City, York, and Gloucester.

4453 Piedmont Independent Living Center
1045 Main Street
Suite #2
Danville, VA 24541-1800
434-797-2530
Fax: 434-797-2568
TTY: 434-797-2530

Clarence Dickerson, Executive Director
Jeanette King, ILS Coordinator/BPAD
Lori Penn, Office Manager
Empowering indiviuals with disabilities to become self-sufficient and independent within their communities.

4454 Resources for Independent Living
4009 Fitzhugh Ave
Richmond, VA 23230-3953
804-353-6503
Fax: 804-358-5606
TTY: 804-353-6583
info@ril-va.org
www.ril-va.org

Gerald O'Neill, Executive Director
Marcia Guardino, Program Manager
Kelly Hickok, Community Services Manager
Assisting persons who are severly disabled to live independently in the community and to encourage necessary change within the community so independent living is a possibility.

4455 Valley Associates for Independent Living (VAIL)
Shenandoah Valley Workforce Investment Board
3210 Peoples Drive
Suite 220
Harrisonburg, VA 22801-869
540-433-6513
888-242-8245
Fax: 540-433-6313
vail@govail.org
www.govail.org

Marcia Du Bois, Executive Director
Bob Satterwhite, Executive Director
VAIL is a not-for-profit, private Center for Independent Living providing advocacy, information and referral, independent living skills training, supported employment, and peer counseling to individuals with disabilities in our planning district.

4456 Valley Associates for Independent Living: Lexington
205-B South Liberty St
Harrisonburg, VA 22801-3638
540-433-6513
888-242-8245
Fax: 540-433-6313
TTY: 540-438-9265
vail@govail.org
www.govail.org

Marcia Du Bois, Executive Director
Promoting self-direction among people with disabilities and removing barriers to independence in the community.

4457 Woodrow Wilson Rehabilitation Center Training Program
243 Woodrow Wilson Avenue
Fishersville, VA 22939-1500
540-332-7000
800-345-9972
Fax: 540-332-7132
TTY: 800-811-7893
www.wwrc.net

Rick Sizemore, Executive Director
Information & referral services. Six week Virginia residential programs and evaluation services.

Washington

4458 Alliance for People with Disabilities: Seattle
1120 E. Terrace St
Suite 100
Seattle, WA 98122
206-545-7055
866-545-7055
Fax: 206-545-7059
TTY: 206-632-3456
info@disabilitypride.org
www.disabilitypride.org

Kimberly Heymann, Executive Director
Elizabeth Kennedy, Executive Assistant
Bhelle Ollero, IL Specialist
The Alliance promotes equality and choice for people with disabilities. They provide advocacy, peer support, idependent living skills training, information and referral, transition assistance for youth, civil rights legal aid, assistive technology, training and nursing home transition back into the community.

4459 Alliance of People with Disabilities: Redmond
East King County Office
1150 140th Ave NE
Suite 101
Bellevue, WA 98005-3537

425-558-0993
800-216-3335
Fax: 425-558-4773
TTY: 425-861-4773
info@disabilitypride.org
www.disabilitypride.org

Kimberly Heymann, Executive Director
Elizabeth Kennedy, Executive Assistant
Bhelle Ollero, IL Specialist
Services include: information and referral, independent living skills training, peer groups, disAbility law project (DLP), access reviews, health insurance advising, and systems advocacy.

4460 Community Services for the Blind and Partially Sighted Store: Sight Connection
9709 Third Ave NE
Suite #100
Seattle, WA 98115-2027

206-525-5556
800-458-4888
Fax: 206-525-0422
www.sightconnection.org

Mary Lewis, Secretary
Shannon Grady Martsolf, President/CEO
Miles Otoupal, Chair
Over 300 practical products for living with vision loss selected by certified vision rehabilitation specialists from Community Services for the Blind and Partially Sighted. Easy-to-use online store features large print, large photos, secure transactions, and links to other vision-related resources.

4461 DisAbility Resource Connection: Everett
607 SE Everett Mall Way
Suite 6C
Everett, WA 98208-3210

425-347-5768
800-315-3583
Fax: 425-710-0767
TTY: 425-347-5768

Charley Lane, Executive Director
disAbility Resource Connection is all about living your life as you choose. The staff is committed to assisting every individual to connect to resources, connect to skills, connect to life.

4462 Kitsap Community Resources
845 8th St
Bremerton, WA 98337-1517

360-478-2301
Fax: 360-415-2706
info@kcr.org
www.kcr.org

Larry Eyer, Executive Director
Irmgard Davis, Fiscal Officer
Rudy Taylor, Board President
Kitsap Community Resources is a local, non-profit organization dedicated to helping people in need. KCR creates hope and opportunity for low-income Kitsap County Residents by providing resources that promote self-sufficiency.

4463 Spokane Center for Independent Living
8817 E. Mission Ave.
Suite 106
Spokane Valley, WA 99212

509-326-6355
Fax: 509-327-2420
info@scilwa.org

William Kane, Executive Director
To improve the self-determination and self-reliance of people with disabilities through systems and individual advocacy, education and independent living services.

4464 Tacoma Area Coalition of Individuals with Disabilities
6315 S 19th St
Tacoma, WA 98466-6217

253-565-9000
877-538-2243
Fax: 253-565-5578
TTY: 253-565-3486
www.tacid.org

Ken Gibson, Executive Director
Steve Pierce, CFO
Jo Ann Maxwell, Deputy Executive Director - Phil

Promotes the independence of individuals with disabilities.

West Virginia

4465 Appalachian Center for Independent Living
4710 Chimney Drive
Suite # C
Charleston, WV 25302-4841

304-965-0376
800-642-3003
Fax: 304-965-0377
TTY: 800-642-3003
acil@yahoo.com
www.mtstcil.org

Ann Weeks, President and CEO
Adam Elmer, Chief Financial Officer
Georgetta Stevens, VP, Corporate Operations
A resource center for persons with disabilities and their communities. Serves Kanawha, Clay, Boone and Putnam counties.

4466 Appalachian Center for Independent Living: Spencer
811 Madison Avenue
Suite #106
Spencer, WV 25276-1900

304-927-4080
Fax: 304-927-4330
TTY: 800-642-3003
susanacil@yahoo.com
www.mtstcil.org

Ann Weeks, President and CEO
Adam Elmer, Chief Financial Officer
Georgetta Stevens, VP, Corporate Operations
A resource center for persons with disabilities and their communities. Serves Jackson, Roane, and Calhoun counties.

4467 Mountain State Center for Independent Living
329 Prince St
Beckley, WV 25801-4515

304-255-0122
Fax: 304-255-0157
TTY: 304-255-0122
aoweeks@mtstcil.org
www.mtstcil.org

Ann Weeks, President and CEO
Adam Elmer, Chief Financial Officer
Georgetta Stevens, VP, Corporate Operations
This office provides individual and systems advocacy, independent living skills development, information and referral, peer support, personal assistance services, housing referral and training, transportation. Serves Raleigh counties.

4468 Mountain State Center for Independent Living
821 Fourth Avenue
Huntington, WV 25701-1406

304-525-3324
866-687-8245
Fax: 304-525-3360
TTY: 304-525-3324
aoweeks@mtstcil.org
www.mtstcil.org

Ann Weeks, President and CEO
Adam Elmer, Chief Financial Officer
Georgetta Stevens, VP, Corporate Operations
Services provided are: individual and systems advocacy, independent living skills development, information and referral, peer support, personal assistance services, supported employment, community integration program, housing referral and training, transportation. Serves Cabell and Wayne counties.

4469 Northern West Virginia Center for Independent Living
601-603 East Brockway
Suite A & B
Morgantown, WV 26501

304-296-6091
800-834-6408
Fax: 304-292-5217
TTY: 304-296-6091
nwvcil@nwvcil.org
www.mtstcil.org

Ann Weeks, President and CEO
Adam Elmer, Chief Financial Officer
Georgetta Stevens, VP, Corporate Operations
NWVCIL is committed to the philosophy that all persons have equal access and unconditional value, that all individuals shall be

respected for their uniqueness and shall have the right to live within the community of their choice, having equal access to participate in and contribute to that community.

Wisconsin

4470 Center for Independent Living of Western Wisconsin
2920 Schneider Avenue East
Menomonie, WI 54751-2331
715-233-1070
800-228-3287
Fax: 715-233-1083
TTY: 800-228-3287
www.cilww.com

Tim Sheehan, Executive Director
Kay Sommerfeld, Assistant Director
Tammy Grage, Fiscal & HR Manager
Advocates for the full participation in society of all persons with disabilities. Our goal is empowering individuals to exercise choices to maintain or increase their indpendence. Our strategy is providing consumer-driven services at no cost to persons with disiabilities in Western Wisconsin

4471 Independence First
540 South 1st Street
Milwaukee, WI 53204-1516
414-291-7520
Fax: 414-291-7525
TTY: 414-297-7520
lschulz@independencefirst.org
www.independencefirst.org

Lee Schulz, President and CEO
John Schmid, Chair
Judy Murphy, Vice Chair
A non-profit agency directed by, and for the benefit of, persons with disabilities, primarily serving the four county metropolitan Milwaukee area.

4472 Independence First: West Bend
735 S Main St
West Bend, WI 53095-3965
262-306-6717
lschulz@independencefirst.org
www.independencefirst.org

Lee Schulz, President and CEO
John Schmid, Chair
Judy Murphy, Vice Chair
A non-profit agency directed by, and for the benefit of, persons with disabilities, primarily serving the four county Metropolitan Milwaukee area.

4473 Inspiration Ministries
N2270 State Road 67
Walworth, WI 53184-948
262-275-6131
Fax: 262-275-3355
inspirationministries.org

Robin Knoll, President
Richard Hall, Executive Vice President
Craig Pape, VP Ministry Services
Formerly known as Christian League for the Handicapped, Inspiration Ministries is a vibrant community of adults with disabilities engaged in living, working, leisure and faith activities designed to provide a complete living experience. The campus consists of a modern residential facility offering a range of living accomodations; a work center and resale shop; and Inspiration Center, a retreat/camping center designed to be 100% wheelchair accessible.

4474 Mid-State Independent Living Consultants: Wausau
3262 Church Street
Suite #1
Stevens Point, WI 54481-5321
715-344-4210
800-382-8484
Fax: 715-344-4414
TTY: 800-382-8484
milc@milc-inc.org
www.milc-inc.org

Tom Vandehey, President
Becky Paulson, Independent Living Consultant
Working for persons with disabilities towards empowerment to make informed choices.

4475 Mid-state Independent Living Consultants: Stevens Point
3262 Church Street
Suite #1
Stevens Point, WI 54481-5321
715-344-4210
800-382-8484
Fax: 715-344-4414
TTY: 800-382-8484
milc@milc-inc.org
www.milc-inc.org

Jenny Fasula, Executive Director
Karalyn Peterson, Resource Director
Committed to enhancing personal and community relationships, providing opportunities for growth, and helping people with varying abilities achieve their personal goals.

4476 North Country Independent Living
69 N 28th St.
Suite 28
Superior, WI 54880-5138
715-392-9118
800-924-1220
Fax: 715-392-4636
northcountryil.com

John Nousaine, Executive Director
Gloria Hakkila-Johnson, Assistant Director
Jim Glaeser, Accountant
Empowers people with disabilities.

4477 North Country Independent Living: Ashland
422 3rd St. W.
Suite #114
Ashland, WI 54806-1553
715-682-5676
800-499-5676
Fax: 715-682-3144
TTY: 715-682-5676
northcountryil.com

John Nousaine, Director
Empowers people with disabilities.

4478 Options for Independent Living
555 Country Club Road
Green Bay, WI 54307-1967
920-490-0500
888-465-1515
Fax: 920-490-0700
TTY: 920-490-0600
www.optionsil.com

Thomas Diedrick, Executive Director
Kathryn C. Barry, Assistant Director
Sandra L. Popp, Independent Living Coordinator
A non-profit organization committed to empowering people with disabilities to lead independent and productive lives in their community through advocacy, the provision of information, education, technology and related services.

4479 Options for Independent Living: Fox Valley
820 West College Ave
Suite #5
Appleton, WI 54914
920-997-9999
888-465-1515
Fax: 920-997-9381
TTY: 920-490-0600
www.optionsil.com

Thomas Diedrick, Executive Director
Kathryn C. Barry, Assistant Director
Sandra L. Popp, Independent Living Coordinator
A non-profit organization committed to empowering people with disabilities to lead independent and productive lives in their community through advocacy, the provision of information, education, technology and related services.

4480 Society's Assets: Elkhorn
615 E Geneva St
Elkhorn, WI 53121-2301
262-723-8181
800-261-8181
Fax: 262-723-8184
TTY: 866-840-9763
info@societysassets.org
www.societysassets.org

Bruce Nelson, Director
Jill Vigueres, Manager
To ensure the rights of all persons with disabilities to live and function as independently as possible in the community of their

choice, through supporting individual's efforts to achieve control over their lives and become integrated into community life.

4481 Society's Assets: Kenosha
5455 Sheridan Road
Suite 101
Kenosha, WI 53140-4103
262-657-3999
800-317-3999
Fax: 262-657-1672
TTY: 866-840-9762
info@societysassets.org
www.societysassets.org

Sue Liu, Manager
Bruce Nelsen, Executive Director
To ensure the rights of all persons with disabilities to live and function as independently as possible in the community of their choice, through supporting individuals efforts to achieve controll over their lives and become integrated into community life. Offers home care and independent living services.

4482 Society's Assets: Racine
5200 Washinton Ave
Suite #225
Racine, WI 53406-4238
262-637-9128
800-378-9128
Fax: 262-637-8646
TTY: 886-840-9761
info@societysassets.org
www.societysassets.org

Deb Pitsch, Administrator
Karen Olufs, Director Independent Living
Jean Rumachik, Director Home Care Services
Society's Assets assists people with disabilities to live as independently as possible. A non-profit human services agency, Society's Assets provides information and referal, independent living skills training, peer support, advocacy, and supportive home care. Home health care is provided by SAI Home Health Care. The agency serves 5 counties in southeastern Wisconsin and also provides information about interpreters, employment, benefits, home modifications, assistive equipment and accessibility.
Fees vary

Wyoming

4483 RENEW: Gillette
35 Fairgrounds Road
Newcastle, WY 82701
307-746-4733
888-253-4653
Fax: 307-746-9701
www.renew-wyo.com

Donna Bombeck, Chairwoman
Carolyn Holso, Vice Chairwoman
Renee Nack, Secretary
Empowering persons with disabilities to enrich their lives.

4484 RENEW: Rehabilitation Enterprises of North Eastern Wyoming
1969 S Sheridan Ave
Sheridan, WY 82801-6108
307-672-7481
888-309-2020
Fax: 307-674-5117
pr@renew-wyo.com
www.renew-wyo.com

Donna Bombeck, Chairwoman
Carolyn Holso, Vice Chairwoman
Renee Nack, Secretary
Multi-disciplinary organization dedicated to the highest possible economic and social independence for persons with disabilities. Extensive referral service, specialized employment placement, occupational therapy, psychological services, evaluation services, and coordination of external services as needed to meet client plans and objectives.

4485 Rehabilitation Enterprises of North Eastern Wyoming: Newcastle
35 Fairgrounds Rd
Newcastle, WY 82701-2625
307-746-4733
888-693-9245
Fax: 307-746-9701
www.renew-wyo.com

Donna Bombeck, Chairwoman
Carolyn Holso, Vice Chairwoman
Renee Nack, Secretary
Empowering persons with disabilities to enrich their lives.

4486 Wyoming Services for Independent Living
1156 South 2nd
Lander, WY 82520-3905
307-332-4889
800-266-3061
Fax: 307-332-2491
TTY: 307-332-7582
www.wysil.org

Susan Hoesel, Business Manager
Donna Langelier, Program Manager
Marcia Henthorn, Program Manager
Committed to enhancing personal and community relationships, providing opportunities for growth, and helping people with varying abilities achieve thier personal goals.

Law

Associations & Referral Agencies

4487   Center for Disability and Elder Law, Inc.
205 W. Randolph
Suite 1610
Chicago, IL 60606   312-376-1880
Fax: 312-376-1885
info@cdelaw.org
www.cdelaw.org

Caroline Manley, Executive Director
Stephanie Ridella Vittands, Staff Attorney

A not-for-profit legal services organization which provids legal
services to low income persons residing in Chicago and Cook
County, Il., who are either elderly and/or persons with disabilities. CDEL provides legal services by matching qualified candidates with volunteer attorneys who represent them, pro-bono, in a
wide range of civil legal matters; and through special initiatives
including the Senior Center Initiative (SCI) and the Senior Tax
Opportunity program.

4488   Center for Workplace Compliance
1501 M Street NW
Suite 400
Washington, DC 20005   202-629-5650
Fax: 202-629-5651
info@cwc.org
cwc.org

Joseph S. Lakis, President
Michael Eastman, Senior Vice President, Policy
Danny Patrella, Vice President, Compliance

Formerly known as the Equal Employment Advisory Council, it
is a nonprofit employer association providing guidance to its
member companies on understanding and complying with their
affirmative action obligations.
1976

**4489   Chicago Lawyers' Committee for Civil Rights Under
Law**
100 N LaSalle Street
Suite 600
Chicago, IL 60602-2400   312-630-9744
Fax: 312-630-1127
info@clccrul.org
www.clccrul.org

Bonnie Allen, Executive Director
Timna Axel, Director, Communications
Aneel Chablani, Chief Counsel

Promotes and protects civil rights of low-income, minority and
disadvantaged people in the social, economic, and political systems of the nation.

4490   CrescentCare Legal Services
1631 Elysian Fields Ave.
New Orleans, LA 70117   504-323-2642
www.aidslaw.org

J. Lind, Attorney
J. Johnson, Attorney
J. Holmes, Attorney

The mission of CrescentCare Legal Services (formerly
AIDSLAW Louisiana) is to provide excellent, specialized legal
services for people living with HIV/AIDS in Louisiana, to improve their quality of life and access to health care, related to their
HIV/AIDS status.

4491   DNA People's Legal Services
PO Box 306
Window Rock, AZ 86515   928-871-4151
Fax: 928-871-5036
www.dnalegalservices.org

Kathy Gallagher, Development Director

A nonprofit legal aid organization working to protect civil rights,
promote tribal sovereignty and alleviate civil legal problems for
people who live in poverty in the Southwestern United States.
1967

4492   Disability Law Colorado
455 Sherman St.
Suite 130
Denver, CO 80203   303-722-3619
800-288-1376
Fax: 303-722-0720
disabilitylawco.org

Mary Anne Harvey, Executive Director
Alison L. Butler, Esq., Director, Legal Services
Mark Ivandick, Managing Attorney/Program Coordinator

Protects and promotes the rights of people with disabilities and
older people in Colorado through direct legal representation, advocacy, education and legislative analysis.

4493   Disability Rights Advocates
2001 Center St
4th Floor
Berkeley, CA 94704-1204   510-665-8644
Fax: 510-665-8511
frontdesk@dralegal.org
dralegal.org

Michelle Caiola, Managing Director, Litigation
Kate Hamilton, Managing Director, Development & Operations
Stuart Seaborn, Managing Director, Litigation

Disability Rights Advocates is a non-profit legal center representing people with disabilities, advocating for them when their
civil rights have been violated. Their clients include those with
mobility, sensory, cognitive, and psychiatric disabilities.

4494   Disability Rights Education and Defense Fund
3075 Adeline Street
Suite 210
Berkeley, CA 94703   510-644-2555
Fax: 510-841-8645
info@dredf.org
dredf.org

Susan Henderson, Executive Director
Claudia Center, Legal Director
Silvia Yee, Senior Staff Attorney

Nonprofit organization dedicated to advancing the civil rights of
individuals with disabilities through legislation, litigation, informal and formal advocacy and education and training of lawyers,
advocates and clients with respect to disability issues. DREDF
also provides training, advocacy, technical assistance and
referrals for parents of disabled children.

4495   Disability Rights Texas
2222 West Braker Lane
Austin, TX 78758-1024   512-454-4816
866-362-2851
www.disabilityrightstx.org

Mary Faithfull, Executive Director
Patty Anderson, Deputy Director

A federally designated legal protection and advocacy agency
(P&A) for people with disabilities in Texas. Helps people with
disabilities understand and exercise their rights under the law, ensuring their full and equal participation in society.

4496   Guardianship Services Associates
41A South Blvd
Oak Park, IL 60302-2777   708-386-5398
Fax: 708-386-5970

Robert R. Wohlgemuth, Executive Director

Information and counseling on guardianship and its alternatives.
Can provide direct assistance in obtaining guardianship for disabled adults in Cook County. Also provides information and direct assistance on durable powers of attorney.

4497   Independence Economic Development
210 W Truman Road
Independence, MO 64050   816-252-5777
Fax: 816-254-1641
info@inedc.biz
www.iced.org

J.D. Kehrman, President
Jodi Krantz, Vice President
Xander Winkel, Executive Director, Ennovation Center

A non-profit, public/private partnership established for the purpose of supporting and enhancing the economic growth of independence.

4498 Independent Living Research Utilization
1333 Moursund
Houston, TX 77030-7031   713-520-0232
                                 Fax: 713-520-5785
                                 TTY: 713-520-0232
                                      ilru@ilru.org
                                      ilru.org

Lex Frieden, Director
Richard Petty, Co-Director
Brooke Curtis, Program Coordinator
The ILRU is a national center for information, training, research, and technical assistance in independent living. Its goal is to expand the body of knowledge in independent living and to improve utilization of results of research programs and demonstration projects in this field.

4499 Judge David L Bazelon Center for Mental Health Law
1090 Vermont Avenue NW
Suite 220
Washington, DC 20005   202-467-5730
                      communications@bazelon.org
                                 www.bazelon.org

Holly O'Donnell, CEO
Ira Burnim, Director, Legal
Jennifer Mathis, Director, Policy & Legal Advocacy
A nonprofit organization devoted to improving the lives of people with mental illnesses through changes in policy and law.

4500 Legal Action Center
810 1st Street
Suite 200
Washington, DC 20002   202-544-5478
                                 Fax: 202-544-5712
                                      lacinfo@lac.org
                                      www.lac.org

Paul N. Samuels, Director & President
Anita R. Marton, Senior Vice President
Ellen Weber, Vice President, Health Initiatives
The only non-profit law and policy organization in the United States whose sole mission is to fight discrimination against people with histories of addiction, HIV/AIDS, or criminal records, and to advocate for sound public policies in these areas.

4501 Legal Counsel for Health Jusice
17 North State Street
Suite 900
Chicago, IL 60602   312-427-8990
                                 Fax: 312-427-8419
                                      legalcouncil.org

Tom Yates, Executive Director
Ellyce Anapolsky, Senior Staff Attorney
Julie Brennan, Program Director
Formerly known as the AIDS Legal Council of Chicago, the group provides legal assistance for people with illness and/or disability.

4502 National Health Law Program (NHeLP)
3701 Wilshire Blvd
Suite 750
Los Angeles, CA 90010   310-204-6010
                                      www.healthlaw.org

Amy Chen, Senior Attorney
Abigail Coursolle, Senior Attorney
Elizabeth G. Taylor, Executive Director
A national public interest law firm that seeks to improve health care for America's working and unemployed poor, minorities, the elderly and people with disabilities. NHeLP serves legal services programs, community-based organizations, the private bar, providers and individuals who work to preserve a health care safety net for the millions of uninsured or underinsured low-income people.
1970

4503 National Right to Work Legal Defense Foundation
8001 Braddock Rd.
Springfield, VA 22160   703-321-8510
                                 800-336-3600
                                 Fax: 703-321-9319
                                      nrtw.org

Raymond LaJeunesse, Vice President & Legal Director
Byron S. Andrus, Staff Attorney
Matthew B. Gilliam, Staff Attorney
The National Right to Work Legal Defense Foundation is a non-profit, charitable organization. Its mission is to eliminate coercive union power and compulsory unionism abuses through strategic litigation, public information, and education programs.
1968

4504 Ohio Civil Rights Commission (OCRC)
Rhodes State Office Tower
30 East Broad Street, 5th Floor
Columbus, OH 43215   614-466-2785
                                 888-278-7101
                                 Fax: 614-644-8776
                                      crc.ohio.gov

G. Michael Payton, Executive Director
Darlene Sweeney-Newbern, Director, Regional Operations
Stephanie Bostos-Demers, Chief Legal Counsel
Primary function is to enforce state laws against discrimination.

4505 REACH/Resource Centers on Independent Living
8625 King George
Suite 210
Dallas, TX 75235-2286   214-630-4796
                                 Fax: 214-630-6390
                                 TTY: 214-630-5995
                      reachdallas@reachcils.org
                                 www.reachcils.org

Sylvia Hodgins, President
Charlotte A. Stewart, Executive Director
Penny Acrey, Secretary
Providing services for people with disabilities so that they are empowered to lead self-directed lives and educating the general public on disability-related topics in order to promote a barrier-free community.

Resources for the Disabled

4506 ADA In Details: Interpreting the 2010 Americans with Disabilities Act Stands
Wiley Publishing
111 River St
Hoboken, NJ 07030-5774   201-748-6000
                                 Fax: 201-748-6088
                                      info@wiley.com
                                      www.wiley.com

Matthe S. Kissner, Chief Executive Officer
Christopher Caridi, Senior Vice President
Helps readers understand the facilities requirements of the Americans with Disabilities Act Accessibility Guidelines. Presents the technical requirements for accessible elements and spaces in new construction, alterations and additions. $40.00
304 pages Paperback 1917
ISBN 9-781119-27-7

4507 Americans With Disabilities Act Annotated: Legislative History, Regulations & Commentary
Disability Rights Education and Defense Fund
3075 Adeline Street
Suite 210
Berkeley, CA 94703   510-644-2555
                                 Fax: 510-841-8645
                                      info@dredf.org
                                      dredf.org

Arlene B. Mayerson, Author
Also known as the Blue Book, written in narrative form for both professionals and lay people, this work offers detailed, thorough analysis of all of the law's provisions, encompassing ADA legislative history, the statute and regulations. Available in alternative formats.

4508 **Americans with Disabilities Act Manual**
US Department of Justice
950 Pennsylvania Ave. NW
9th Floor
Washington, DC 20530   202-307-0663
                              800-514-0301
                              Fax: 202-307-1197
                              TTY: 800-514-0383
                              www.ada.gov

Rebecca B. Bond, Chief
Anne Raish, Principal Deputy Chief
Christina Galindo-Walsh, Deputy Chief
An in-depth analysis of the legal and practical implications of the ADA using non-technical language. *$20.00*

4509 **Americans with Disabilities Act: Selected Resources for Deaf**
Gallaudet University Bookstore
800 Florida Avenue NE
Washington, DC 20002-3695   202-651-5000
                                 800-621-2736
                                 Fax: 202-651-5508
                                 clerc.center@gallaudet.edu
                                 www.gallaudet.edu

Priscilla O'Donnell, Bookstore Manager
Iva Williams, Bookstore Secretary
Elaine Vance, Human Resources Director
This resource identifies programs and publications specific to the ADA and deafness and also lists ADA materials and programs for people with any disability.

4510 **Approaching Equality**
T J Publishers
Ste 108
2544 Tarpley Rd
Carrollton, TX 75006-2288   972-416-0800
                                 800-999-1168
                                 Fax: 301-585-5930
                                 TJPubinc@aol.com

Frank Bowe, Author
Public education laws guarantee special education for all deaf children, but may find the special education system confusing, or are unsure of their rights under current laws. For anyone with an interest in education, advocacy and the deaf community, this book reviews dramatic developments in education of deaf children, youth and adults since COED's 1988 report, Toward Equality.. *$12.95*
112 pages
ISBN 0-93266-39-6

4511 **Assessment of the Feasibility of Contracting with a Nominee Agency**
Mississippi State University
PO Drawer 6189
Mississippi State, MS 39762   662-325-2001
                                 Fax: 662-325-8989
                                 rrtc@colled.msstate.edu
                                 www.blind.msstate.edu

Michelle Capella McDonnall, Interim Director
Stephanie Hall, Business Manager
Douglas Bedsaul, Research and Training Coordinator
Only five State Licensing Agencies currently utilize nominee agreements. This study compared the Pennsylvania BE program with four states that utilize nominee agencies and four states that do not. *$20.00*
152 pages Paperback

4512 **Can America Afford to Grow Old?**
Brookings Institution
1775 Massachusetts Ave NW
Washington, DC 20036-2103   202-797-6000
                                 Fax: 202-797-6004
                                 www.brookings.edu

William Antholis, Managing Director
Steven Bennett, Vice President and Chief Operating Officer
Kimberly Churches, Vice President for Development
Social security laws and regulations. *$8.95*
144 pages Paperback
ISBN 0-815700-43-1

4513 **Childcare and the ADA**
Eastern Washington University
Rm 223
705 W 1st Ave
Spokane, WA 99201-3909   509-623-4200
                                 Fax: 509-623-4230
                                 susan.vanmeter@mail.ewu.edu
Nancy Ashworth, Director Child Development
Allen Barrom, Manager
Provides information on how childcare providers must comply with the ADA. Eight videotapes plus an instructional manual with examples of situations and problems.. *$85.00*
Set

4514 **Common ADA Errors and Omissions in New Construction and Alterations**
US Department of Justice
950 Pennsylvania Ave. NW
9th Floor
Washington, DC 20530   202-307-0663
                                 800-514-0301
                                 Fax: 202-307-1197
                                 TTY: 800-514-0383
                                 www.ada.gov

Rebecca B. Bond, Chief
Anne Raish, Principal Deputy Chief
Christina Galindo-Walsh, Deputy Chief
Lists a sampling of common accessibility errors or omissions that have been identified through the Department of Justice's ongoing enforcement efforts.
13 pages

4515 **Commonly Asked Questions About Child Care Centers and the Americans with Disabilities Act**
US Department of Justice
950 Pennsylvania Ave. NW
9th Floor
Washington, DC 20530   202-307-0663
                                 800-514-0301
                                 Fax: 202-307-1197
                                 TTY: 800-514-0383
                                 www.ada.gov

Rebecca B. Bond, Chief
Anne Raish, Principal Deputy Chief
Christina Galindo-Walsh, Deputy Chief
Explains how the requirements of the ADA apply to Child Care Centers. Also describes some of the Department of justice's ongoing enformcement efforts in the child care area and it provides a resource list on sources of information on the ADA.
13 pages

4516 **Commonly Asked Questions About Title III of the ADA**
US Department of Justice
950 Pennsylvania Ave. NW
9th Floor
Washington, DC 20530   202-307-0663
                                 800-514-0301
                                 Fax: 202-307-1197
                                 TTY: 800-514-0383
                                 www.ada.gov

Rebecca B. Bond, Chief
Anne Raish, Principal Deputy Chief
Christina Galindo-Walsh, Deputy Chief
A 6-page publication providing information for state and local governments about ADA requirements for ensuring that people with disabilities receive the same services and benefits as provided to others.
on-line

4517 **Commonly Asked Questions About the ADA and Law Enforcement**
US Department of Justice
950 Pennsylvania Ave. NW
9th Floor
Washington, DC 20530   202-307-0663
                              800-514-0301
                              Fax: 202-307-1197
                              TTY: 800-514-0383
                              www.ada.gov

Rebecca B. Bond, Chief
Anne Raish, Principal Deputy Chief
Christina Galindo-Walsh, Deputy Chief
A publication explaining ADA requirements for ensuring that people with disabilities receive the same law enforcement services and protections as provided to others.
13 pages on-line

4518 **Complying with the Americans with Disabilis Act**
Greenwood Publishing Group
130 Cremona Drive
Santa Barbara, CA 93117   805-968-1911
                                 800-368-6868
                                 Fax: 866-270-3856
                                 CustomerService@abc-clio.com
                                 www.greenwood.com

Don Fresh, Author
Peter W Thomas, Co-Author
John Gosden, Library Resource Consultants
A guidebook for management and people with disabilities. This unique guidebook presents a comprehensive analysis of the new Americans with Disabilities Act (ADA), the most significant federal civil rights law in almost 30 years, and its impact on over four million American businesses, state and local governments, nonprofit associations, 87 percent of American's private sector jobs, and 22.7 million working-age people with disabilities. *$117.95*
280 pages Hardcover
ISBN 0-899307-14-0

4519 **Court-Related Needs of the Elderly and Persons with Disabilities**
Mental Health Commission
2700 Martin Luther King Jr Ave SE
Washington, DC 20032- 2601   202-282-0027
                                    Fax: 202-373-7982
This book features the ground-breaking recommendations from the national Conference on the Court-Related Needs of the Elderly and Persons with Disabilities, funded by the States Justice Institute and co-sponsored by the American Bar Association and National Judicial College. Accompanying the recommendations are detailed commentaries and extensive background research papers organized around issues.. *$20.00*
276 pages

4520 **Criminal Law Handbook on Psychiatric & Psychological Evidence & Testimony**
New York City Bar
42 West 44th Street
New York, NY 10036-6604   212-382-6600
                                 Fax: 212-768-8116
                                 phynes@nycbar.org
                                 www.nycbar.org

Bret Parker, Executive Director
Debra Raskin, President
Alan Rothstein, General Counsel
The Criminal Law Handbook provides lawyers, judges and forensic experts with comprehensive, in-depth treatment of admissibility (and limitations on admissibility) of psychiatric and psychological evidence and testimony pertaining to key criminal mental health law standards. *$47.00*

4521 **Department of Justice ADA Mediation Program**
US Department of Justice
950 Pennsylvania Ave. NW
9th Floor
Washington, DC 20530   202-307-0663
                              800-514-0301
                              Fax: 202-307-1197
                              TTY: 800-514-0383
                              www.ada.gov

Rebecca B. Bond, Chief
Anne Raish, Principal Deputy Chief
Christina Galindo-Walsh, Deputy Chief
Provides an overview of the Department's Mediation Program and examples of successfully mediated cases.
6 pages

4522 **Dimensions of State Mental Health Policy**
Greenwood Publishing Group
130 Cremona Drive
Santa Barbara, CA 93117   805-968-1911
                                 800-368-6868
                                 Fax: 866-270-3856
                                 CustomerService@abc-clio.com
                                 www.greenwood.com

Christopher Hudson, Author
Arthur J Cox, Co-Author
John Gosden, Library Resource Consultants
Introduces students to the emerging field of state mental health policy, its history, current policies, organizational models and required programming knowledge. *$86.95*
320 pages Hardcover
ISBN 0-275932-52-7

4523 **Disability Compliance for Higher Education**
LRP Publications
360 Hiatt Dr
Palm Beach Gardens, FL 33418   561-622-6520
                                      800-341-7874
                                      Fax: 561-622-0757
                                      lrpitvp@lrp.com
                                      www.lrp.com

Kenneth Kahn, CEO
Gives guidance on the most difficult issues faced, such as supporting students with psychological disabilities, ensuring accessibility, understanding OCR rulings, and more. *$57.29*
300 pages

4524 **Disability Discrimination Law, Evidence and Testimony**
ABA Commission on Mental & Physical Disability Law
1050 Connecticut Ave. N.W.
Suite 400
Washington, DC 20036   202-662-1000
                              800-285-2221
                              Fax: 202-442-3439
                              cmpdl@americanbar.org
                              www.americanbar.org

John W Parry JD, Author
Explains and analyzes key aspects of disability discriminiation law from several different perspectives to guide you through the myriad federal and state statutes, court cases, and regulations. *$105.00*
694 pages Paperback
ISBN 1-604420-12-8

4525 **Disability Law in the United States**
William Hein & Company
2350 North Forest Rd.
Getzville, NY 14068-1296   716-882-2600
                                  800-828-7571
                                  Fax: 716-883-8100
                                  mail@wshein.com
                                  www.wshein.com

Dr Bernard D Reams Jr, Author
Peter J McGovern, Co-Author
Jon S Schultz, Co-Author
Offers thousands of pages of information on the laws and legislation affecting the disabled in the United States. Its purpose is to provide a clear and comprehensive mandate to end discrimination against individuals with disabilities and to bring disabled persons

into the economic and social midstream of American Life.
$675.00
5750 pages
ISBN 0-899417-97-3

4526 **Disability Under the Fair Employment & Housing Act: What You Should Know About the Law**
California Department of Fair Employment & Housing
2218 Kausen Drive
Suite 100
Elk Grove, CA 95758   916-478-7251
                                                         800-884-1684
                                                    Fax: 916-227-2870
                                             contact.center@dfeh.ca.gov
                                                       www.dfeh.ca.gov

Phyllis W Cheng, Director
Intended to highlight and summarize workplace disability laws enforced by the California Department of Fair Employment and Housing. It will familiarize people with the content of these laws, including recent changes and amendments to state statutes and attendent accommodation responsibilities.

4527 **Discrimination is Against the Law**
California Department of Fair Employment & Housing
2218 Kausen Drive
Suite 100
Elk Grove, CA 95758   916-478-7251
                                                         800-884-1684
                                                    Fax: 916-227-2870
                                             contact.center@dfeh.ca.gov
                                                       www.dfeh.ca.gov

Phyllis Cheng, Director
Enforces California state laws that prohibit harassment and discrimination in employment, housing, and public accomodations and that provide for pregnancy leave and family and personal leave.

4528 **Education of the Handicapped: Laws, Legislative Histories and Administrative Document**
William S Hein & Co Inc
2350 North Forest Rd.
Getzville, NY 14068-1296   716-882-2600
                                                         800-828-7571
                                                    Fax: 716-883-8100
                                                      mail@wshein.com
                                                       www.wshein.com

Bernard D Reams Jr, Editor
Focuses upon Elementary and Secondary Education Act of 1965 and its amendment, Education For All Handicapped Children Act of 1975 and its amendments and acts providing services for the blind, deaf, developmentally disabled, etc. *$2950.00*
55 volumes
ISBN 0-899411-57-6

4529 **ElderLawAnswers.com**
150 Chestnut Street
4th Floor, Box 15
Providence, RI 02903   617-267-9700
                                                         866-267-0947
                                            support@elderlawanswers.com
                                                  www.elderlawanswers.com

Harry S Margolis, Founder/President
Mark Miller, Director of Product and Business Development
Ken Coughlin, Managing Editor
Supports seniors, their families and their attorneys in achieving their goals by providing

4530 **Employment Discrimination Based on Disability**
California Department of Fair Employment & Housing
2218 Kausen Drive
Suite 100
Elk Grove, CA 95758   916-478-7251
                                                         800-884-1684
                                                    Fax: 916-227-2870
                                             contact.center@dfeh.ca.gov
                                                       www.dfeh.ca.gov

Phyllis W Cheng, Director
Prohibits employment discrimination and harassment based on a person's disability or perceived disability. Also requires employers to reasonably accommodate individuals with mental or physi-

cal disabilities unless the employer can show that to do so would cause an undue hardship.

4531 **Employment Standards Administration Department of Labor (ESA)**
200 Constitution Ave NW
Washington, DC 20210-1   800-321-6742
                                                   TTY: 877-889-5627
                                                             osha.gov

David Michaels, Assistant Secretary
Jordan Barab, Deputy Assistant Secretary
Richard Fairfax, Deputy Assistant Secretary
Monitors compliance with sub-minimum wage requirements for handicapped workers in sheltered workshops, competitive industry and hospitals and institutions under Section 14 of the Fair Labor Standards Act of 1938.

4532 **Enforcing the ADA: A Status Report from the Department of Justice**
US Department of Justice
950 Pennsylvania Ave. NW
9th Floor
Washington, DC 20530   202-307-0663
                                                         800-514-0301
                                                    Fax: 202-307-1197
                                                   TTY: 800-514-0383
                                                         www.ada.gov

Rebecca B. Bond, Chief
Anne Raish, Principal Deputy Chief
Christina Galindo-Walsh, Deputy Chief
A brief report issued by the Justice Department each quarter providing timely information about ADA cases and settlements, building codes that meet ADA accessibility standards, and ADA technical assistance activities.

4533 **Federal Laws of the Mentally Handicapped: Laws, Legislative Histories and Admin. Documents**
William Hein & Company
2350 North Forest Rd.
Getzville, NY 14068-1296   716-882-2600
                                                         800-828-7571
                                                    Fax: 716-883-8100
                                                      mail@wshein.com
                                                       www.wshein.com

Bernard D Reams Jr, Editor
Chronological compilation of all relevant federal laws dealing with the mentally handicapped along with supporting documentation necessary to create a complete legislative history. *$3500.00*
42 Volume/Set
ISBN 0-899411-06-1

4534 **Formed Families: Adoption of Children with Handicaps**
Haworth Press
711 Third Avenue
New York, NY 10017   212-216-7800
                                                         800-354-1420
                                                    Fax: 212-244-1563
                                               subscriptions@tandf.co.uk
                                                    www.haworthpress.com

William Cohen, Owner
Provides broad coverage of the issues relating to the adoption of children with handicaps. Concerned professionals can find here all the answers about clinical programs, legal issues, estimates of frequency, and important factors related to positive and negative outcomes of these adoptions. *$74.95*
242 pages Hardcover
ISBN 0-866569-14-6

4535 Free Appropriate Public Education: The Law and Children with Disabilities
Love Publishing Company
9101 E Kenyon Avenue
Suite 2200
Denver, CO 80237
303-221-7333
Fax: 303-221-7444
lpc@lovepublishing.com
www.lovepublishing.com
H Rutherford Turnbull III, Author
Matthew J Stowe, Co-Author
Nancy E Huerta, Co-Author
Includes the 2004 IDEA reauthorization and the proposed regulations. This up-to-the-minute resource brings you the most recent developments in legislation, case law techniques, due process, parent participation and much, much more. *$78.00*
448 pages Hardcover
ISBN 0-891083-25-2

4536 Health Care Quality Improvement Act of 1986
William Hein & Company
2350 North Forest Rd.
Getzville, NY 14068-1296
716-882-2600
800-828-7571
Fax: 716-883-8100
mail@wshein.com
www.wshein.com
Bernard D Reams Jr, Editor
In order to encourage more stringent peer review by doctors and hospitals, and to protect reporting physicians and institutions from retaliatory lawsuits, Congress enacted The Health Care Quality Improvement Act. The Act was also intended to address the increasing incidence of medical malpractice and to prevent the ease with which incompetent practitioners moved from state to state. Hardcover. *$125.00*
721 pages
ISBN 0-899416-93-4

4537 Housing and Transportation of the Handicapped
William Hein & Company
2350 North Forest Rd.
Getzville, NY 14068-1296
716-882-2600
800-828-7571
Fax: 716-883-8100
mail@wshein.com
www.wshein.com
Bernard D Reams Jr, Editor
National laws, recognizing the problems encountered by the handicapped in the areas of Housing and Transportation and providing assistance in an effort to surmount those problems, span more than half a century. *$1552.50*
30000 pages 250 documents
ISBN 0-899412-47-5

4538 Human Resource Management and the Americans with Disabilities Act
Greenwood Publishing Group
130 Cremona Drive
Santa Barbara, CA 93117
805-968-1911
800-368-6868
Fax: 866-270-3856
CustomerService@abc-clio.com
www.greenwood.com
John G Veres, Author
Ronald R Sims, Co-Author
John Gosden, Library Resource Consultants
Concrete advice for human resource professionals on how to cope with the vague, often obscure provisions of the Americans with Disabilities Act. *$107.95*
232 pages Hardcover
ISBN 0-899308-57-9

4539 International Handbook on Mental Health Policy
Greenwood Publishing Group
130 Cremona Drive
Santa Barbara, CA 93117
805-968-1911
800-368-6868
Fax: 866-270-3856
CustomerService@abc-clio.com
www.greenwood.com
John Gosden, Library Resource Consultants
Lina Gosden, Library Resource Consultants
Steve Pearson, Library Resource Consultants
The first major reference book for academics and practitioners that provides a systematic survey and analysis of mental health policies in twenty representative countries. *$179.95*
512 pages Hardcover
ISBN 0-313275-67-8

4540 Knowing Your Rights
A AR P Fulfillment
601 E St NW
Washington, DC 20049-1
202-434-3525
800-687-2277
Fax: 202-434-3443
TTY: 877-434-7598
member@aarp.org
www.aarp.org
William D. Novelli, CEO
Lynn Smith, Director of Human Resources
Describes how changes in Medicare's reimbursement policies are designed to reduce health care costs and suggests steps that Medicare beneficiaries, their families and friends can take to assure that they continue to receive quality care under the Prospective Payment System.
19 pages

4541 Law Center Newsletter
Public Interest Law Center of Philadelphia
1709 Benjamin Franklin Parkway
United Way Building
Philadelphia, PA 19103
215-627-7100
Fax: 215-627-3183
www.pilcop.org
Eric J Rothschild, Chair
Brian T Feeney, Vice Chair
Jennifer R. Clarke, Executive Director
Information on mental health, foster care and public education. Provides all updates concerning the law in these areas.

4542 Legal Center for People with Disabilities& Older People
455 Sherman St
Suite 130
Denver, CO 80203
303-722-0300
800-288-1376
Fax: 303-722-0720
TTY: 303-722-3619
Mary Anne Harvey, Executive Director
John R. Posthumus, President
Stephen P. Rickles, Vice President
Uses the legal system to protect and promote the rights of people with disabilities and older people in Colorado through direct legal representation, advocacy, education and legislative analysis. The Legal Center is Colorado's Protection and Advocacy System. We are also the State Ombudsman for nursing homes and assisted living facilities. Call for a free publications and products list.

4543 Legal Right: The Guide for Deaf and Hard of Hearing People
National Association of the Deaf
8630 Fenton Street
Suite 820
Silver Spring, MD 20910- 3819
301-587-1789
Fax: 301-587-1791
TTY: 301-587-1789
www.nad.org
Christopher Wagner, Board Chair
Howard A. Rosenblum, Chief Executive Officer
Marc P. Charmatz, Staff Attorney
This revised fifth edition is in easy-to-understand language, offering the latest state and federal statues and administrative pro-

cedures that prohibit discrimination against the deaf, hard of hearing and other physically challenged people. *$32.50*
264 pages Paperback
ISBN 1-563680-00-9

4544   Legal Rights of Persons with Disabilities
LRP Publications
360 Hiatt Dr
Palm Beach Gardens, FL 33418-7106   561-622-6520
800-341-7874
Fax: 561-622-0757
lrpitvp@lrp.com
www.lrp.com
Kenneth Kahn, CEO
Shows what is required, permitted and guaranteed by federal disability laws-including the ADA, Section 504 of the Rehabilitation Act and the IDEA. Explores the boundaries of accceptable behavior under disability laws and provides guidelines to help clients fulfill their legal obligations. *$365.00*
2722 pages

4545   Legislative Handbook for Parents
NAPVI
250 W 64th St
New York, NY 10023   800-284-4422
napvi@lighthouseguild.org
www.napvi.org
Alan R. Morse, President/CEO
Mark G. Ackermann, Executive Vice President
James M. Dubin, Chairman
A publication for parents who make direct contact with public officials on behalf of their children. Sample letters, do's-and-dont's, and a glossary of legislative terms are some of the topics that are contained in this manual. *$5.50*
24 pages Paperback

4546   Legislative Network for Nurses
Business Publishers
2222 Sedwick Drive
Durham, NC 27713   800-223-8720
Fax: 800-508-2592
www.bpinews.com
Provides up-to-date information on the nursing shortage, nurse training programs, AIDS and Hepatitis B, unionization, registered care technologies, compensation, child care, home health care staffing and much more. *$286.00*
8 pages Newsl./BiMonthly

4547   Loving Justice
Exceptional Parent Library
P.O.Box 1807
Englewood Cliffs, NJ 7632-1207   201-947-6000
800-535-1910
Fax: 201-947-9376
eplibrary@aol.com
www.eplibrary.com
How the Americans with Disabilities Act affects religious institutions, including congregations, hospitals, nursing homes, seminaries, universities and more. *$10.95*

4548   Making News: How to Get News Coverage of Disability Rights Issues
Advocado Press
PO Box 406781
Louisville, KY 40204   888-739-1920
Fax: 502-899-9562
www.advocadopress.org
Tari Susan Hartman, Author
Mary Johnson, Co-Author
This book gives examples and tips on how to fight back and get on the front pages, lead the newscasts and influence public debate. *$10.95*
165 pages Paperback
ISBN 0-962706-43-4

4549   Medicare and Medicaid Patient and Program Protection Act of 1987
William Hein & Company
2350 North Forest Rd.
Getzville, NY 14068-1296   716-882-2600
800-828-7571
Fax: 716-883-8100
mail@wshein.com
www.wshein.com
Bernard D Reams Jr, Editor
Enables the HHS to protect patients and federal health care programs from censured practitioners. The Act broadens the authority of HHS to exclude practitioners from Medicare and Medicaid programs; strengthens the monetary penalities HHS may impose on violators; provides for criminal penalties in certain cases; and requires states to inform HHS regarding sanctions against health care providers. *$195.00*
3 Volumes
ISBN 0-899416-95-0

4550   Mental & Physical Disability Law Reporter
American Bar Association
1050 Connecticut Ave. N.W.
Suite 400
Washington, DC 20036-1019   202-662-1570
800-285-2221
Fax: 202-442-3439
cmpdl@abanet.org
www.abanet.org
Robert M Carlson, Chair
James R Silkenat, President
Jack L Rives, Executive Director
Contains over 2,000 summaries per year of federal and state court decisions and legislation that affect persons with mental and physical disabilities. Includes bylined articles by experts in the field regarding disability law developments and trends. *$384.00*
350+ pages BiMonthly

4551   Mental Disabilities and the Americans with Disabilities Act
Greenwood Publishing Group
130 Cremona Drive
Santa Barbara, CA 93117   805-968-1911
800-368-6868
Fax: 866-270-3856
CustomerService@abc-clio.com
www.greenwood.com
John Gosden, Library Resource Consultants
Lina Gosden, Library Resource Consultants
Steve Pearson, Library Resource Consultants
A clear, practical compliance guide, written by a psychologist, to help organizations conform to provisions on mental disabilities in the Americans with Disabilities Act. Hardcover. *$91.95*
216 pages Hardcover
ISBN 0-899308-26-5

4552   Mental Disability Law, Evidence and Testimony
ABA Commission on Mental & Physical Disability Law
1050 Connecticut Ave. N.W.
Suite 400
Washington, DC 20036-1019   202-662-1000
800-285-2221
www.abanet.org
Robert M Carlson, Chair
James R Silkenat, President
Jack L Rives, Executive Director
Provides a comprehensive analysis of federal and state statues and case law with a disability discrimination focus. *$95.00*
491 pages Paperback
ISBN 1-590318-32-3

4553   Mental Health Law Reporter
Business Publishers
2222 Sedwick Drive
Durham, NC 27713   240-514-0600
800-223-8720
Fax: 800-508-2592
Leonard A Eiserer, Publisher
Jeremy Bond, Editor MHLR
Bob Grupe, Editor MHLR

MHLR brings you the most timely, focused and thorough information on the legal issues that concern mental health practitioners in mental health litigation. Topics include: malpractice litigation, patient-therapist confidentiality, sexual victimization of patients, the insanity defense, social security administrative case law and much more.. *$286.00*
8 pages Monthly

4554   Mental and Physical Disability Law Reporter
American Bar Association
1050 Connecticut Ave. N.W.
Suite 400
Washington, DC 20036-1019   202-662-1000
                                         800-285-2221
                                 service@americanbar.org
                                     www.americanbar.org

Wm T Robinson III, President
The only periodical that comprehensively covers civil and criminal mental disability law and disability discrimination law. *$ 324.00*
150+ pages Bimonthly

4555   Mentally Disabled and the Law
William S Hein & Company
2350 North Forest Rd.
Getzville, NY 14068-1296   716-882-2600
                                          800-828-7571
                                    Fax: 716-883-8100
                                       mail@wshein.com
                                        www.wshein.com

Samuel Brakel, Author
John Parry, Co-Author
Barbara A Weiner, Co-Author
Chapters retained from 1961 and 1971 editions have been substantially rewritten. Two subjects-sterilization and sexual psychopathy-have been integrated into chapters on family law. Three new chapters on treatment rights, provider-patient relationship and rights of mentally disabled persons in the community. Sixteen new tables supplement the existing revised 41. *$92.00*
845 pages
ISBN 0-910059-05-5

4556   Myths and Facts
US Department of Justice
950 Pennsylvania Ave. NW
9th Floor
Washington, DC 20530   202-307-0663
                                          800-514-0301
                                    Fax: 202-307-1197
                                    TTY: 800-514-0383
                                             www.ada.gov

Rebecca B. Bond, Chief
Anne Raish, Principal Deputy Chief
Christina Galindo-Walsh, Deputy Chief
A 3-page publication dispelling some common misconceptions about the ADA's requirements and implementation.

4557   NAD Broadcaster
National Association of the Deaf
8630 Fenton Street
Suite 820
Silver Spring, MD 20910- 3819   301-587-1789
                                    Fax: 301-587-1791
                                    TTY: 301-587-1789
                                       nad.info@nad.org
                                           www.nad.org

Christopher Wagner, Board Chair
Howard A. Rosenblum, Chief Executive Officer
Marc P. Charmatz, Staff Attorney
National newspaper published 11 times a year by the nation's largest organization safeguarding the accessbility and civil rights of 28 million deaf and hard of hearing Americans in education, employment, health care, and telecommunications. Membership: individual $30 per year. *$7.00*

4558   No Longer Disabled: the Federal Courts & the Politics of Social Security Disability
Greenwood Publishing Group
130 Cremona Drive
Santa Barbara, CA 93117   805-968-1911
                                          800-368-6868
                                    Fax: 866-270-3856
                          CustomerService@abc-clio.com
                                     www.greenwood.com

John Gosden, Library Resource Consultants
Lina Gosden, Library Resource Consultants
Steve Pearson, Library Resource Consultants
This book is a case study of judicial policy making. It focuses on the role of adjudication in the making and refining of federal policy. *$107.95*
208 pages Hardcover
ISBN 0-313254-24-9

4559   Nolo's Guide to Social Security Disability Getting and Keeping Your Benefits
NOLO
950 Parker St
Berkeley, CA 94710-2524   800-955-4775
                                    Fax: 800-645-0895
                                           www.nolo.com

David Morton, Author
This guide demystifies the program and tells you everything you need to know about qualifying and applying for benefits, maintaining your benefits, and appealing the denial of a claim. *$25.49*
512 pages paperback
ISBN 1-413311-04-4

4560   Opening the Courthouse Door: An ADA Access Guide for State Courts
American Bar Association
1050 Connecticut Ave. N.W.
Suite 400
Washington, DC 20036-1019   202-662-1000
                                         800-285-2221
                                 service@americanbar.org
                                     www.americanbar.org

Wm T Robinson III, President
Practical step-by-step guide walks the reader through the courthouse and court process, presenting a menu of straightforawrd access ideas to enhance communications in court, make the facility more accessbile, and nodify rules and procedures. *$12.00*
78 pages

4561   PPAL In Print
Parent Professional Advocacy League
77 Rumford Ave.
Waltham, MA 02453   866-815-8122
                                    Fax: 617-542-7832
                                           info@ppal.net
                                           www.ppal.net

Lisa Lambert, Executive Director
Meri Viano, Associate Director
Joel Khattar, Program Manager
The Parent Professional Advocacy League (PPAL) is a statewide organization focusing on the interests of families with children with mental health needs. PPAL advocates for improved and better access to mental health services for children and their families.

4562   Power of Attorney for Health Care
Center for Public Representation
P.O.Box 260049
Madison, WI 53726-49   608-251-4008
                                          800-369-0388
                                    Fax: 606-251-1263

Discusses Wisconsin law regarding medical decisions, the Cruzan case and ethical considerations in addition to legal implications and advantages of this document. Book tells how to create a personalized Power of Attorney document, including language for the special provisions portion. *$49.95*
132 pages
ISBN 0-93262 -38-0

4563 **Special EDitions**
Disability Rights Education and Defense Fund
3075 Adeline Street
Suite 210
Berkeley, CA 94703   510-644-2555
                                       Fax: 510-841-8645
                                         info@dredf.org
                                              dredf.org

Susan Henderson, Executive Director
Special news releases by the Disability Rights Education and De-
fense Fund, available electronically online.
Quarterly

4564 **Summaries of Legal Precedents & Law Review**
Through the Looking Glass
3075 Adeline St
Suite 120
Berkeley, CA 94703   510-848-1112
                                            800-644-2666
                                       Fax: 510-848-4445
                                    TLG@lookingglass.org
                                     www.lookingglass.org

Megan Kirshbaum, Executive Director
Summarizes legal precedents and law review articles relevant to
marital custody and child protection situations of parents with diverse disabilities. *$25.00*
24 pages

4565 **TASH Connections**
TASH
1101 15th St. NW
Suite 206
Washington, DC 20005   202-817-3264
                                       Fax: 202-999-4722
                                          info@tash.org
                                            www.tash.org

Julia M. White, Editor
Connections is the online magazine written exclusively for, and
by, TASH members, containing articles on new developments in
the disability field, while challenging readers to consider issues
affecting people with disabilities, their families and advocates.
Quarterly

4566 **Title II & III Regulation Amendment Regarding
Detectable Warnings**
US Department of Justice
950 Pennsylvania Ave. NW
9th Floor
Washington, DC 20530   202-307-0663
                                            800-514-0301
                                       Fax: 202-307-1197
                                       TTY: 800-514-0383
                                             www.ada.gov

Rebecca B. Bond, Chief
Anne Raish, Principal Deputy Chief
Christina Galindo-Walsh, Deputy Chief
This document suspends the requirements for detectable warn-
ings at curb ramps, hazardous vehicular areas, and reflecting
pools.

4567 **Title II Complaint Form**
US Department of Justice
950 Pennsylvania Ave. NW
9th Floor
Washington, DC 20530   202-307-0663
                                            800-514-0301
                                       Fax: 202-307-1197
                                       TTY: 800-514-0383
                                             www.ada.gov

Rebecca B. Bond, Chief
Anne Raish, Principal Deputy Chief
Christina Galindo-Walsh, Deputy Chief
Standard form for filing a complaint under title II of the ADA or
section 504 of the Rehabilitation Act of 1973, which prohibit discrimination on the basis of disability by State and local governments and by recipients of federal financial assistance.

4568 **Title II Highlights**
US Department of Justice
950 Pennsylvania Ave. NW
9th Floor
Washington, DC 20530   202-307-0663
                                            800-514-0301
                                       Fax: 202-307-1197
                                       TTY: 800-514-0383
                                             www.ada.gov

Rebecca B. Bond, Chief
Anne Raish, Principal Deputy Chief
Christina Galindo-Walsh, Deputy Chief
Outline of the key requirements of the ADA for State and local
governments. Provides detailed information in bullet format for
quick reference.
8 pages

4569 **Title III Technical Assistance Manual and Supplement**
US Department of Justice
950 Pennsylvania Ave. NW
9th Floor
Washington, DC 20530   202-307-0663
                                            800-514-0301
                                       Fax: 202-307-1197
                                       TTY: 800-514-0383
                                             www.ada.gov

Rebecca B. Bond, Chief
Anne Raish, Principal Deputy Chief
Christina Galindo-Walsh, Deputy Chief
Explains in lay terms what businesses and non-profit agencies
must do to ensure access to their goods, services, and facilities.
83 pages

4570 **Toward Independence**
National Council on Disability
81 E. Main Street
Xenia, OH 45385   937-376-3996
                                       Fax: 937-376-2046
                                           info@ti-inc.org

Mary Rose Zink, Chair
Paul Osterfeld, Vice Chair
Mark Schlater, Executive Director
A 1986 report to the U.S. Congress on the federal laws and pro-
grams serving people with disabilities, and recommendations for
legislation.

4571 **UCP Washington Wire**
United Cerebral Palsy
1825 K Street NW
Suite 600
Washington, DC 20006-1601   202-776-0406
                                            800-872-5827
                                       Fax: 202-776-0414
                                            info@ucp.org
                                             www.ucp.org

Stephen Bennett, President/CEO
Publication that provides a comprehensive source of information
on federal legislation, agency regulations, court decisions and
other issues of interest to the disability community.
weekly

4572 **US Department of Health and Human Services Office for
Civil Rights**
200 Independence Ave SW
Room 509F, HHH Building
Washington, DC 20201   202-619-0403
                                            800-368-1019
                                       TTY: 800-537-7697
                                          ocrmail@hhs.gov
                                             www.hhs.gov

Georgina Verdugo, Director
The Department's civil rights and health privacy law enforcement agency, OCR investigates complaints, enforces rights, and
promulgates regulations, develops policy and provides technical
assistance and public education to ensure understanding of and
compliance with non-discrimination and health information
privacy laws.

4573 US Department of Labor
200 Constitution Ave NW
Washington, DC 20210
866-487-2365
www.dol.gov

Hilda L Solis, Secretary of Labor
Seth D Harris, Deputy Secretary
To foster, promote, and develop the welfare of the wage earners, job seekers, and retirees of the United States; improve working conditions, advance opportunities for profitable employment; and assure work-related benefits and rights.

4574 US Department of Labor Office of Federal Contract Compliance Programs
200 Constitution Ave NW
Washington, DC 20210
312-596-7010
866-487-2365
Fax: 312-596-7044
OFCCP-MW-PreAward@dol.gov
www.dol.gov

Melissa L Speer, Interim Regional Director
To enforce, for the benefit of job seekers and wage earners, the contractual promise of affirmative action and equal employment opportunity required of those who do business with the Federal government.

4575 University Legal Services AT Program
Ste 130
220 i St NE
Washington, DC 20002-4364
202-547-4747
877-221-4638
Fax: 202-547-2083
TTY: 202-547-2657
atpdc@uls-dc.org

Jane Brown, Executive Director
Designed to empower individuals with disabilities; to promote consumer involvement and advocacy, and provide information, referral and training as they relate to accessing assistive technology services and devices; and to identify and improve access to funding resources..

4576 William S Hein & Company
2350 North Forest Rd.
Getzville, NY 14068-1296
716-882-2600
800-828-7571
Fax: 716-883-8100
mail@wshein.com
www.wshein.com

Kevin Marmion, President
Offers a catalog of periodicals, publications and reprints, microforms and government publications on medical, handicapped and health law.

Libraries & Research Centers

Alabama

4577 Alabama Institute for Deaf and Blind Library and Resource Center
205 E South Street
P.O. Box 698
Talladega, AL 35160   256-761-3206
                                                Fax: 256-761-3352
                                                         aidb.org

Dr. John Mascia, President
Teresa Lacy, Director, Library & Resource Center
Book collection includes discs, cassettes, braille and large print. Also closed-circuit TV and magnifiers. Offers braille production and binding.

4578 Alabama Radio Reading Service Network(ARRS)
Public Radio WBHM 90.3 FM
650 11th St S
Birmingham, AL 35233-1   205-934-2606
                                                    800-444-9246
                                                Fax: 205-934-5075
                                                        wbhm.org

Audrey Atkins, Marketing Manager
Scott E Hanley, General Manager
Theresa Kidd, Office Manager
Services and readings are broadcast over a subcarrier service of public radio WBHM. This is a statewide service devoted to Alabama's blind and handicapped community.

4579 Alabama Regional Library for the Blind and Physically Handicapped
Alabama Public Library Service
6030 Monticello Dr
Montgomery, AL 36130-1   334-213-3906
                                                    800-392-5671
                                                Fax: 334-213-3993
                                            revans@apls.state.al.us

Mike Coleman, Blind & Physically Handicapped Division
Tim Emmons, Blind & Physically Handicapped Division
Nancy Pack, Director
Recreational reading in special format for persons unable to use standard print. Reference materials offered include materials on blindness and other handicaps, films, local subjects and authors.

4580 Dothan Houston County Library System
Formerly Houston-Love Memorial Library
445 N Oates St
Dothan, AL 36303   334-793-9767
                                                  dhcls@dhcls.org
                                                     www.dhcls.org

Jason DeLuc, Library Director
Charlotte Mitchell, Main Library Manager
Offers magnifiers, summer reading programs and more for the blind and physically handicapped. Scanner, software, jaws for Windows.

4581 Huntsville Subregional Library for the Blind & Physically Handicapped
Huntsville-Madison County Public Library
915 Monroe St SW
Huntsville, AL 35804-0000   256-532-5980
                                                Fax: 256-532-5994
                                               bphdept@hmcpl.org
                                                      www.hmcpl.org

Laurel Best, Executive Director
Talking books for people who are blind or disabled offering reference materials on the blind and other disabilities, large-print photocopier, thermaform duplicator and more.

4582 Public Library Of Anniston-Calhoun County
108 E 10th St
Anniston, AL 36201   256-237-8501
                                           library@publiclibrary.cc
                                                     publiclibrary.cc

Reference materials on blindness, cassettes, large print books and discs.

4583 Technology Assistance for Special Consumers
UCP Huntsville
1856 Keats Drive
Huntsville, AL 35810   256-859-8300
                                                Fax: 256-859-4332
                                                   ucphuntsville.org

Cheryl Smith, Chief Executive Officer
Provide individuals with disabilities, their families and/or advocates, and associated professionals access to assistive technology devices and services to increase independence at home, school, and work.

Alaska

4584 Alaska State Library Talking Book Center
State of Alaska
344 W 3rd Ave
Ste 125
Anchorage, AK 99501-2338   907-465-1304
                                                    888-820-4525
                                                Fax: 907-269-6580
                                                   tbc@alaska.gov
                                             talkingbooks.alaska.gov

Patience Frederiksen, Director, Division of Libraries, Archives & Museums
Freya Anderson, Requisitions Librarian
Ginny Jacobs, Library Assistant
The Alaska State Library Talking Book Center is a cooperative effort between the Library of Congress National Library Service for the Blind and Physically Handicapped and the Alaska State Library to provide print handicapped Alaskans with talking book and Braille service. The Talking Book Center has 55,000 audiobooks that can be checked out to eligible Alaskans whose visual or physical handicap prevents them from reading standard print materials.

Arizona

4585 Arizona Braille and Talking Book Library
Arizona State Library
1030 N 32nd St
Phoenix, AZ 85008-5108   602-255-5578
                                                    800-255-5578
                                                Fax: 602-286-0444
                                                 www.azlibrary.gov

Linda Montgomery, Director
Audio and braille books and magazines, summer reading program, volunteer-produced audio books, audo described, films and more.

4586 Books for the Blind of Arizona
Unit A107
6120 E 5th St
Tucson, AZ 85711-2536   602-792-9153
                                                Fax: 520-886-9839

Betty Evans, Chairperson
Offers large print photocopier, textbooks, recreational, career, vocational, braille books, talking books, cassettes, large print books and more for the visually impaired K-12, college students and adults..

4587 Children's Center for Neurodevelopmental Studies
5430 W Glenn Dr
Glendale, AZ 85301-2628   623-915-0345
                                                Fax: 623-937-5425
                                                  admin@ccnsaz.org
                                          www.thechildrenscenteraz.org

Kent Rideout, Executive Director
Dawna Sterner, Preschool & Education Informatio
Catherine Orsak, Therapy Information
The Center is a non-profit school and therapy center for children with autism and other developmental delays specializing in the use of sensory integration.

4588   Flagstaff City-Coconino County Public Library
300 W Aspen Ave
Flagstaff, AZ 86001-5304   928-779-7670
                                          TTY: 928-214-2417
                                   www.flagstaffpubliclibrary.org
Reference materials on blindness and other handicaps, braille
writer, magnifiers and large-print photocopier. Large-type
books, closed captioned videos, adapters and books on tape.

4589   Fountain Hills Lioness Braille Service
P.O.Box 18332
Fountain Hills, AZ 85269-8332   480-837-3961

Jean Hauck, Chairperson
Braille and large print books on the subjects of recreation, career
and vocations, religion, novels and cookbooks for the visually
impaired..

4590   Prescott Public Library
215 E Goodwin St
Prescott, AZ 86303-3911   928-777-1500
                                      Fax: 928-771-5829
                                        prescottlibrary.info
Roger Saft, Director
Martha Baden, Public Services Manager
Teresa Vonk, Support Services Manager
Large print, braille and audio books; magnifiers; text to voice
scanner; talking book machine application; toy library for chil-
dren with special needs; special needs product catalogs; home
book delivery; descriptive videos; 43 point PC monitor..

4591   Special Needs Center/Phoenix Public Library
1221 N Central Ave
Phoenix, AZ 85004-1867   602-262-4636
                                       TTY: 602-254-8205
                                    www.phoenixpubliclibrary.org
Offers large print books and magazines, print/braille books, amd
braille magazines, Descriptive video services videotapes, several
video print enlargers and computer workplace for persons with
disabilities.

4592   World Research Foundation
P.O. Box 20828
Sedona, AZ 86341-8804   928-284-3300
                                      Fax: 928-284-3530
                                          info@wrf.org
                                             wrf.org
Steven A Ross, President
LaVerne Boeckmann, Co-Founder
Large research library of alternative medicine; offers a computer
search and printout of specific health issues for a nominal fee.

Arkansas

**4593   Arkansas Regional Library for the Blind and Physically
         Handicapped**
900 West Capitol Avenue
Suite 100
Little Rock, AR 72201-3108   501-682-2053
                                   www.library.arkansas.gov
J D Hall, Manager of BPH Services
Dwain Gordon, Deputy Director
Danny Koonce, Public Information Specialist
Public library books in recorded or braille format. Popular fiction
and nonfiction books for all ages, books and players are on free
loan, sent to patrons by mail and may be returned postage free.
Anyone who cannot see well enough to read regular print with
glasses on or who has a disability that makes it difficult to hold a
book or turn the pages is eligible.

4594   Arkansas School for the Blind
P.O.Box 668
Little Rock, AR 72203-668   501-296-1810
                                          800-362-4451
                                      Fax: 501-296-1831
                              www.arkansasschoolfortheblind.org
Khayyam Eddings, Chairperson
Jennifer Benedetti, Elementary Principal
Teresa Doan, Special Education Supervisor

Students at the ASB receive a quality education from specially
trained instructors of the Visually Impaired in all academic areas.
ASB features a comprehensive Music and Art program, as well as
extensive extra-curricular activities. ASB is a proud member of
the Arkansas Activities Association and The North Central
Association of Schools for the Blind.

4595   Educational Services for the Visually Impaired
2402 Wildwood Avenue
Suite 112
Sherwood, AR 72120-5085   501-835-5448
                                      Fax: 501-835-6840
                                 Angyln.Young@arkansas.gov
                                          www.esvi.org
Angyln Young, State Coordinator
Cindy Lester, Data Management Specialist
Cynthia Kelly, ESVI Office Manager
Offers textbooks, braille books and more to the visually impaired
grades K-12 in the Arizona area.

**4596   Library for the Blind and Physically Handicapped SW
         Region of Arkansas**
P.O.Box 668
2057 North Jackson St
Magnolia, AR 71754-668   870-234-1991
                                      Fax: 870-234-5077
                                     library@cocolib.org
Rhonda Rolen, Director
Dana Thornton, Assistant Director
Becky Verschage, Processing Clerk
A free library service that serves adults and children who meet the
eligiblity requirements, offers free loan of cassette machine and
recorded books, which meet the reading preferences of a highly
diverse clientele.

**4597   Northwest Ozarks Regional Library for the Blind and
         Handicapped**
Fayetteville, AR 72701   479-575-2000
                                          www.uark.edu
Offers a summer reading program, closed-circuit TV, magnifiers,
braille writers and large print books.

California

4598   Braille Institute Library
741 N Vermont Ave
Los Angeles, CA 90029-3594   323-663-1111
                                          800-808-2555
                                      Fax: 323-663-0867
                                     la@brailleinstitute.org
                                        brailleinstitute.org
Leslie E. Stocker, President
Sally H. Jameson, Vice President of Programs and S
Peter A. Mindnich, Executive Vice President
Braille Institute provides an environment of hope and encourage-
ment for people who are blind and visually impaired through inte-
grated educational, social and recreational programs and
services.

4599   Braille Institute Santa Barbara Center
2031 De La Vina St
Santa Barbara, CA 93105-3895   805-682-6222
                                          800-272-4553
                                      Fax: 805-687-6141
                                     sb@brailleinstitute.org
                                        brailleinstitute.org
Leslie E. Stocker, President
Sally H. Jameson, Vice President of Programs and S
Peter A. Mindnich, Executive Vice President
Offers programs, services and information for persons with vi-
sual impairments.

4600   Braille Institute Sight Center
741 N Vermont Ave
Los Angeles, CA 90029-3594
323-663-1111
800-808-2555
Fax: 323-663-0867
la@brailleinstitute.org
brailleinstitute.org
Sally H. Jameson, Vice President of Programs and S
Leslie E Stocker, President
Peter A. Mindnich, Executive Vice President
Offers help, programs, services and information to the blind and visually impaired children and adults.

4601   Braille and Talking Book Library: California
P.O. Box 942837
Sacramento, CA 94237-0001
916-654-0640
800-952-5666
www.library.ca.gov/services/btbl.html
Stacey A. Aldrich, State Librarian
Debbie Newton, Bureau Chief, Administrative Ser
Phyllis Smith, Manager, Human Resources and Bus
Free service for eligible Northern California residents.

4602   California State Library Braille and Talking Book Library
PO Box 942837
Sacramento, CA 94237-0001
916-654-0640
800-952-5666
btbl@library.ca.gov
www.btbl.ca.gov
A division of the California State Library, the Braille and Talking Book Library (BTBL) is a free service offering braille and audiobook to readers in Northern California who cannot read due to a visual or physical disability. The BTBL is an affiliate of the National Service for the Blind and Physically Handicapped.

4603   Clearinghouse for Specialized Media and Translations
1430 N St
Ste 3207
Sacramento, CA 95814-5901
916-319-0800
Fax: 916-323-9732
www.cde.ca.gov/re/pn/sm
Jonn Paris-Salb, Manager
Provides materials in accessible formats; aural media, braille, large print, digital talking books and electronic media access technology.

4604   Dental Amalgam Syndrome (DAMS) Newsletter
725-9 Tramway Ln NE
Albuquerque, NM 87122-1672
505-291-8239
Fax: 505-294-3339
Dedicated to informing the public about the potential risks of mercury in dental amalgam fillings..

4605   Fresno County Free Library Blind and Handicapped Services
2420 Mariposa Street
Fresno, CA 93721-3640
559-600-7323
800-742-1011
wendy.eisenberg@fresnolibrary.org
www.fresnolibrary.org/tblb
Wendy Eisenberg, Manager
Laurel Prysiazny, County Librarian
Magnifiers, home visits, volunteer-produced cassette books, discs and cassettes.

4606   Glaucoma Research Foundation
251 Post St
Ste 600
San Francisco, CA 94108-5017
415-986-3162
800-826-6693
Fax: 415-986-3763
question@glaucoma.org
glaucoma.org
Tom Brunner, President and CEO
Nancy Graydon, Executive Director of Development
Andrew L. Jackson, Director of Communications
Clinical and laboratory studies of glaucoma. We work to prevent vision loss from glaucoma by investing in innovative research, education and support with the ultimate goal of finding a cure..

4607   Herrick Health Sciences Library
Alta Bates Medical Center
2001 Dwight Way
Berkeley, CA 94704-2608
510-869-6777
Fax: 510-204-4091
www.altabatessummit.org
Laurie Bagley, Librarian
Carol Hirsch-Butler, Administrator
Carolyn Kemp, Regional Manager of Public Relations
Information on rehabilitation, psychiatry and psychoanalysis.

4608   Kuzell Institute for Arthritis and Infectious Diseases
Medical Research Institute Of San Francisco
2200 Webster St.
San Francisco, CA 94115-1821
415-561-1734
Edward Byrd, Owner
One of seven units comprising the Medical Research Institute of San Francisco that offers basic and applied research in arthritis and related diseases.

4609   New Beginnings: The Blind Children's Center
4120 Marathon St
Los Angeles, CA 90029-3584
323-664-2153
info@blindchildrenscenter.org
blindchildrenscenter.org/document-library
Sarah E. Orth, CEO
Fernanda Armenta-Schmitt, Director, Education & Family Services
The purpose of the Center is to turn initial fears into hope. Helps children and their families become independent by creating a climate of safety and trust. Children learn to develop self confidence and to master a wide range of skills. Services include an infant stimulation program, educational preschool, interdisciplinary assessment services, family services, correspondence program, toll free national hotline and a publication and research service.

4610   Research & Training Center on Mental Health for Hard of Hearing Persons
California School of Professional Psychology
Ste 140
6215 Ferris Sq
San Diego, CA 92121-3279
619-282-4443
800-HEA-R619
Fax: 800-642-0266
Raymond J Trybus, Director
Thomas J Goulder, Associate Director
Funded by the National Institute on Disability and Rehabilitation Research, this training center aims to address issues of psychological relevance to persons who are hard of hearing or late deafened (as distinct from prelingually, culturally deaf persons). Also serves as information clearinghouse on this topic.

4611   Rosalind Russell Medical Research Center for Arthritis
Suite 600
350 Parnassus Ave
San Francisco, CA 94117
415-476-1141
Fax: 415-476-3526
rrac@medicine.ucsf.edu
Ephraim P Engleman, MD, Center Director
David Wofsy, MD, Associate Director
Paula R. Gambs, Chair
Arthritis research and its probable causes.

4612   San Francisco Public Library for the Blindand Print Handicapped
100 Larkin St
San Francisco, CA 94102-4705
415-557-4400
Fax: 415-557-4252
TTY: 415-557-4433
webmail@sfpl.org
www.sfpl.org
Toni Cordova, Chief of Communications, Program
Toni Bernardi, Special Projects Manager
Laura Lent, Chief of Collections & Technical
Foreign-language books on cassette, children's books on cassettes and more.

4613 San Jose State University Library
150 E San Fernando St
San Jose, CA 95112-3580   408-808-2000
                                            Fax: 408-924-1118
                                               www.sjlibrary.org

Don W Kassing, President
Jane Light, Library/Executive Director
Jeff Barber, Security Officer
Information on physical disabilities, accessibility and learning
disabilities.

Colorado

4614 AMC Cancer Research Center
3401 Quebec Street
Suite 3200
Denver, CO 80207   303-233-6501
                                                 800-321-1557
                                            Fax: 303-239-3400
                                                      amc.org

Gary Kortz, Chairman
Steven D. Toltz, Treasurer
Cheryl Kisling, Secretary
Provides trained counselors who provide understanding and sup-
port for cancer patients; information and referral services; and
screening programs.

4615 Boulder Public Library
1001 Arapahoe Ave
Boulder, CO 80302-6015   303-441-3100
                                             www.boulderlibrary.org

Melinda Mattling, Manager
Priscilla Hudson, Manager
Offers braille books, cassettes, talking books, large print photo-
copier, large print books and more for the visually impaired.

4616 Colorado Talking Book Library
180 Sheridan Blvd
Denver, CO 80226-8101   303-727-9277
                                                 800-685-2136
                                            Fax: 303-727-9281
                                          ctbl.info@cde.state.co.us

Debbie Macleod, Executive Director
Provides free library service to Coloradans of all ages who are unable to read standard print due to visual, physical or learning disabilities whether permanent or temporary. Provides audio, braille
and large-print books and magazines.

4617 National Jewish Medical & Research Center
1400 Jackson St
Denver, CO 80206-2762   303-388-4461
                                                 877-225-5654
                                           www.nationaljewish.org

Michael Salem, MD, President and CEO
Richard A. Schierburg, Chair
Robin Chotin, Vice Chair
The only medical center in the country whose research and pa-
tient care resources are dedicated to respiratory and immunologic
diseases.

Connecticut

4618 Connecticut Braille Association
107 Vanderbilt Ave
West Hartford, CT 6110-1514   860-953-4445
                                            Fax: 860-378-0205

Nick Martino, Owner
Offers textbooks, cassettes, large print books, braille books and
more.

**4619 Connecticut Library for the Blind and Physically
Handicapped**
231 Capitol Avenue
Hartford, CT 06106-1569   860-757-6500
                                                 860-866-4478
                                            Fax: 860-721-2056
                                              ctaylor@cslib.org

Kendall Wiggin, State Librarian
Ursula Hunt, Administrative Assistant
Shelley Delisle, IT Manager
Network library of the National Library Service for the Blind and
Physically Handicapped, Library of Congress. Lends books and
magazines in Braille or recorded formats along with the necessary playback equipment, free, for any Connecticut adult or child
who is unable to read regular print due to a visual or physical disability. All materials are mailed to and from library patrons by
postage-free mail

4620 Connecticut State Library
Connecticut State Government
231 Capitol Ave
Hartford, CT 06106-1569   860-757-6500
                                                 866-866-4478
                                            Fax: 860-721-2056
                                               isref@cslib.org

Kendall Wiggin, State Librarian
Ursula Hunt, Administrative Assistant
Shelley Delisle, IT Manager
Discs, cassettes, braille, reference materials on blindness and
other handicaps, closed-circuit TV and large-print photocopier.

**4621 Connecticut Tech Act Project: Connecticut Department
of Social Services**
Bureau of Rehabilitations Services
25 Sigourney St
11th Floor
Hartford, CT 06106-5041   860-424-4881
                                                 800-537-2549
                                            Fax: 860-424-4850
                                            TTY: 860-424-4839
                                              arlene.lugo@ct.gov
                                             www.cttechact.com

Arlene Lugo, Program Director
Single point of entry, advocacy, information and referral, peer
counseling, and access to objective expert advice and consultation for people with disabilities.

4622 Prevent Blindness Connecticut
101 Whitney Avenue
New Haven, CT 06510   203-722-4653
                                                 800-850-2020
                                            Fax: 203-722-4691

Kathryn Garre-Ayars, President and CEO
Tahesha Bryan, Administrative Assistant
Naomi Hayner, Connecticut Program Manager
The mission of Prevent Blindness Connecticut is to save sight and
prevent blindness through eye screenings, education, safety ac-
tivities and research.

4623 Yale University: Vision Research Center
310 Cedar St, LH 108
PO Box 208023
New Haven, CT 06520- 8023   203-785-2759
                                                 800-395-7949
                                            Fax: 203-785-7303
                                         pamela.berkheiser@yale.edu
                                          medicine.yale.edu/pathology

George Shafranov, Chairman
Pam Burkheiser, Manager
Robert J. Alpern, Dean
Vision including studies on growth and development.

Delaware

4624 Delaware Assistive Technology Initiative (DATI)
Alfred I. duPont Hospital for Children
461 Wyoming Road
Newark, DE 19716-0269

302-831-0354
800-870-3284
Fax: 302-831-4690
TTY: 302-651-6794
dati@asel.udel.edu
www.dati.org

Beth Mineo Mollica, Director
Sonja Rathel, Project Coordinator
The Delaware Assistive Technology Initiative (DATI) connects Delawareans who have disabilities with the tools they need in order to learn, work, play and participate in community life safely and independently. DATI services include: Equipment demonstration centers in eah county; no-cost, short-term equipment loans that let you try before you buy; Equipment Exchange Program; AT workshops and other training sessions; advocacy for improved AT access policies and funding and several more.

4625 Delaware Library for the Blind and Physically Handicapped
Government
121 Duke of York Street
Dover, DE 19901-7430

302-739-4748
800-282-8676
Fax: 302-739-6787
debph@lib.de.us
libraries.delaware.gov

Dr. Annie E. Norman, Director
Sonja Brown, Administrative Specialist
Beth-Ann Ryan, Deputy Director
Books on cassette and playback equipment are provided to patrons who are unable to read regular printed books.

4626 Elwyn Delaware
321 E 11th St.
Wilmington, DE 19801-3417

302-658-8860
info@elwyn.org
elwyn.org

Charles S. McLister, President & CEO, Elwyn
Provides work training, job placement and supported employment, and elder care services.

District of Columbia

4627 District of Columbia Public Library: Services for the Deaf Community
District of Columbia Public Library
901 G St NW, Room 215
Washington, DC 20001-4531

202-727-0321
Fax: 202-727-0321
TTY: 202-559-5368
library_deaf_dc@yahoo.com
dclibrary.org

Venetia Demson, Chief Adaptive Services
Janice Roseu, Library for the Deaf Community
Offers reference services through videophone, signers for library programs, sign language classes, information about deafness, print and non-print materials for persons who have hearing disabilities. Book talks on deaf culture and American Sign Language story hours for kids, and Saturday sessions on employment-related skills are offered. Videophones for public use are available at the MLK Library.

4628 District of Columbia Regional Library for the Blind and Physically Handicapped
901 G St NW
Washington, DC 20001-4531

202-727-0321
Fax: 202-727-1129
TTY: 202-727-2145
lbphb_2000@yahoo.com
www.dclibrary.org

Richard Reyes-Gavilan, Executive Director
Jonathan Butler, Director of Business Services
Barbara Kirven, Director of Human Resources
Regional library/RPH is network library in the Library of Congress, National Library Services for the Blind and Physically Handicapped.

4629 Georgetown University Center for Child and Human Development
P.O. Box 571485
Washington, DC 20057

202-687-5000
Fax: 202-687-8899
TTY: 202-687-5000
gucdc@georgetown.edu
gucchd.georgetown.edu

Phyllis R. Magrab, PhD, Director
John J. DeGioia, President
The Georgetown University Center for Child and Human Development (GUCCHD) was established over 50 years ago to improve the quality of life for all children and youth and their families, especially those with special health care needs, behavioral health challenges, or disabilities. Located in the nation's capital, this center both directly serves vulnerable children and their families, as well as influences local, state, national, and international programs and policy.

4630 National Institute on Disability, Independent Living, and Rehabilitation Research (NIDILRR)
Administration for Community Living
330 C St. SW
Washington, DC 20201

202-401-4634
acl.gov

Anjali Forber-Pratt, Director
Alison Barkoff, Principal Deputy Administrator
Vicki Gottlich, Director, Center for Policy & Evaluation
NIDILRR is the US government's primary disability research agency.

Florida

4631 Brevard County Talking Books Library
Brevard County Libraries
2725 Judge Fran Jamieson Way
Viera, FL 32940

321-633-2000
Fax: 321-633-1964
TTY: 321-633-1838
kbriley@brev.org
www.brevardcounty.us/PublicLibraries

Camille Johnson, Manager
Catherine J Schweinsburg, Library Services Director
Subregional library for the blind and physically handicapped, assistive reading devices collection, reference materials on blindness and other handicaps, descriptive videos, CCTV, phonic ear, reading edge and LOUD-R assistive listening devices available.

4632 Broward County Talking Book Library
100 S Andrews Ave
Fort Lauderdale, FL 33301-1830

954-357-7444
Fax: 954-357-5548
www.broward.org

Robert E. Cannon, Director
Carolyn Kayne, Manager
Reference materials on blindness and other handicaps, films, closed-circuit TV, discs, cassettes and a book discussion group is offered.

4633 Dade County Talking Book Library
Miami Dade Public Library System
101 West Flagler Street
Miami, FL 33130   305-375-2665
                                    800-451-9544
                              Fax: 305-757-8401
                        talkingbooks@mdpls.org
                                  www.mdpls.org

Raymond Sanpiago, Executive Director
Lainey Brooks, Development Officer
Sylvia Mora Oria, Assistant Director
A free Outreach Service of the Miami-Dade Public Library System. A network library, or subregional, of the National Library Service for the Blind and Physically Handicapped, Library of Congress, and of the Florida Bureau of Braille and Talking Books Library Service.

4634 Florida Division of Blind Services
Regional Library
325 West Gaines Street
Turlington Building, Suite 1114
Tallahassee, FL 32399-0400   850-245-0300
                                    800-342-1828
                              Fax: 850-245-0363
                             dbs.myflorida.com

Mike Gunde, Manager
Susan Roberts, Bureau Chief
Robert Doyle, Director
Discs, cassettes, closed-circuit TV, large-print photocopier, films, children's books on cassettes and more.

4635 Florida Instructional Materials Center for the Visually Impaired (FIMC-VI)
4210 W Bay Villa Ave
Tampa, FL 33611-1206   813-837-7826
                                    800-282-9193
                              Fax: 813-837-7979
                FloridaBrailleChallenge@gmail.com
                                   www.fimcvi.org

Mary Stoltz, Database Manager
Jeffrey Fitterman, Technology Specialist
Teresa Gutierrez, Administrative Secretary
Operates a clearinghouse depository and production center for braille, large print and digital texts. Provides assistance in assessment of materials and specialized apparatus, organizes and trains volunteers for material production for the visually impaired, and provides professional development for teachers of the visually impaired. Provides electronic texts to NIMAS-eligible students in Florida.

4636 Hillsborough County Talking Book Library
Tampa-Hillsborough County Public Library
900 N Ashley Dr
Tampa, FL 33602-3704   813-273-3652
                              Fax: 813-273-3707
                              TTY: 813-273-3610
                                   www.hcplc.org

Joe Stines, Director of Libraries
Marcee Challener, Assitant Director
David Wullschleger, Chief of Operations
Serves as the reference hub and resource center for all citzens of Hillsborough County and as the flagship library of the Tampa-Hillsborough County Public Library System.

4637 Jacksonville Public Library: Talking Books/Special Needs
303 N Laura St
Jacksonville, FL 32202-3505   904-630-2665
                              Fax: 904-630-0604
                www.jpl.coj.net/lib/talkingbooks.html
Barbara Gubbin, Executive Director
Offers cassettes and digital books, reference materials on blindness and ADA issues, newsline, descriptive videos, and some assistive devices.

4638 Lee County Library System: Talking Books Library
2001 N. Tamiami Trail N.E.
North Fort Myers, FL 33903-4855   239-533-4320
                                    800-854-8195
                              Fax: 239-485-1146
                              TTY: 239-995-2665
                       talkingbooks@leegov.com
                         www.lee-county.com/library

Cynthia N Cobb, Director
Terri Crawford, Deputy Director
Debbie Parrott, Manager
Provides free books and magazines to Lee County residents of all ages who have any disability that prevents them from reading printed material. Books are played on special players provided free by the National Library Service. Circulates low tech assistive aids and devices for temporary loan to Lee County Library card holders. Directs people to assistive technology and disability related resources.

4639 Louis de la Parte Florida Mental Health Institute Research Library
University of South Florida
4202 E. Fowler Ave. LIB122
Tampa, FL 33620   813-974-2729
                              Fax: 813-974-7242
                                lib.usf.edu/fmhi

William A. Garrison, Dean
Florence Jandreau, CAP, Senior Assistant to the Dean
Claudia Dold, Assistant University Librarian
Information offered on mental illness, autism and pervasive development disabilities mental health research and archives management.

4640 Orange County Library System: Audio-Visual Department
101 E Central Blvd
Orlando, FL 32801-2429   407-835-7323
                              Fax: 407-835-7649
                              TTY: 407-835-7641
                          comments@ocls.info
                                   www.ocls.info

Ted Maines, President
Lisa Franchina, Vice President
Bob Tessier, Comptroller
Serves the residents of the Orange County Library District, with headquarters in downtown Orlando.

4641 Pearlman Biomedical Research Institute
Mt Sinai Medical Center
1600 NW 10th Ave
Miami Beach, FL 33140   305-674-2121
                              Fax: 305-674-2198
                     william-abraham@msmc.com

William Abraham, Director
A 32,000 square feet facility located on the main campus of Mount Sinai. The institute consists of laboratory space, research and administrative offices. The studies conducted within the facility are primarily pre-clinical research.

4642 Pinellas Talking Book Library for the Blind and Physically Handicapped
1330 Cleveland St
Clearwater, FL 33755-5103   727-441-8408
                              Fax: 727-441-8398
                              TTY: 727-441-3168
                           contactus@pplc.us
                                     www.pplc.us

William Horne, Chair
Cheryl Morales, Executive Director
David Saari, Facilities Manager
The Pinellas Public Library Cooperative serves Pinellas County residents in member cities and the unincorporated county. The Cooperative Office provides cooridination of activities and funding as well as marketing services for the the member counties. The Talking Book Library servces Pinellas, Manatee, and Sarasota counties.

4643   **Talking Book Service: Mantatee County Central Library**
1112 Manatee Avenue West
Bradenton, FL 34206-1000   941-748-4501
Fax: 941-751-7098
www.mymanatee.org

Patricia Schubert, Manager
Offers children's books on disc and cassette and more reference materials for the blind and physically handicapped.

4644   **Talking Books Library for the Blind and Physically Handicapped**
Palm Beach County Library
3650 Summit Blvd
West Palm Beach, FL 33406-4114   561-233-2600
888-780-4962
Fax: 561-233-2627
webmaster@pbclibrary.org
www.pbclibrary.org

John Callahan, Executive Director
Bill Rautenberg, Chair
Harriet Helfman, Vice Chair
Established in 1967, today the County Library system serves Palm Beach County through the Main Library, 2 Regional Libraries, 11 Branch Libraries, a Bookmobile and a library annex. It continues to expand through our involvement with library networks, the Internet, and the World Wide Web.

4645   **Talking Books/Homebound Services**
Brevard County Library System
2725 Judge Fran Jamieson Way
Viera, FL 32940   321-633-2000
Fax: 321-633-1838
kbriley@brev.org
www.brevardcounty.us/PublicLibraries

Kay Briley, Librarian
Camille Johnson, Executive Director
Offers reference materials on blindness and other handicaps. Subregional library for the blind and physically handicapped, assistive reading devices collection, reference materials on blindness and other handicaps; CCTV, phonic ear, reading edge and LOUD-R assistive listening devices available.

4646   **University of Miami: Bascom Palmer Eye Institute**
Department Of Ophthalmalogy
900 NW 17th St
Miami, FL 33136-1119   305-243-2020
888-845-0002
Fax: 305-326-7000
www.bascompalmer.org

Michael Gittelman, CEO
Teresa Spaulding, Manager
Eduardo C. Alfonso, M.D., Professor and Chairman
Clinical and basic research into blindness and visual impairments.

4647   **University of Miami: Mailman Center for Child Development**
1601 NW 12th Ave
Miami, FL 33136-1005   305-243-6395
Fax: 305-326-7594
pedsinformation@med.miami.edu
pediatrics.med.miami.edu

William Donelan, Vice President for Medical Admin
William W. O'Neill, M.D., Executive Dean, Chief Medical Of
Pascal J. Goldschmidt, M.D., SVP, Dean, CEO
Focuses on birth defects and children's illnesses.

4648   **West Florida Regional Library**
200 W Gregory St
Pensacola, FL 32502-4822   850-436-5060
Fax: 850-436-5039
TTY: 850-436-5063
hhudson@ci.pensacola.fl.us

Eugene Fischer, Executive Director
Helen Hudson, Outreach Librarian
Offers children's print/braille books.

Georgia

4649   **Athens Talking Book Center-Athens-Clarke County Regional Library**
2025 Baxter St
Athens, GA 30606-6331   706-613-3655
800-531-2063
Fax: 706-613-3660

Stacey Chandler, Manager
Discs, cassettes, large print books, reference materials on blindness, descriptive videos, films, closed-circuit TV, magnifiers, braille writer, summer reading programs, cassette books and magazines and more.

4650   **Augusta Talking Book Center**
823 Telfair Street
Augusta, GA 30901-2232   706-821-2600
Fax: 706-724-6762
TTY: 706-722-1639
www.ecgrl.org

Lillie Hamilton, Board Of Trustee
Audrey Bell, Manager
Loran Gray, Board Of Trustee
Discs, cassettes, braille writer, films, large print books, summer reading program, magnifiers and reference materials on blindness and other handicaps.

4651   **Bainbridge Subregional Library for the Blind & Physically Handicapped**
S W Georgia Regional Library
301 S Monroe St
Bainbridge, GA 39819-4029   229-248-2665
800-795-2680
Fax: 229-248-2670
lbph@swgrl.org
www.swgrl.org

Susans Wittle, Manager
Kathy Hutchins, Supervisor
The library houses a large collection of recorded materials as well as reference materials. For recorded and Braille materials that are provided by the National Library Service (NLS) but not currently in stock at the Bainbridge Library, the Regional Library in Atlanta can be contacted to Interlibrary Loan the requested materials.

4652   **Columbus Subregional Library For The Blind And Physically Handicapped**
1120 Bradley Dr
Columbus, GA 31906-2813   706-649-0780
800-652-0782
Fax: 706-649-1914
TTY: 706-649-0974

Dorothy Bowen, Librarian
Braille writer, magnifiers, closed-circuit TV, large-print photocopier, cassette books and magazines, children's books on cassette, home visits and other reference materials on blindness and other handicaps.

4653   **Emory Autism Resource Center**
Emory University
1551 Shoup Ct
Decatur, GA 30033   404-727-8350
Fax: 404-727-3969
tohannon@emory.edu
www.emory.edu/HOUSING/CLAIRMONT/autism.html

James W. Wagner, President
Larry Hagan, IT Manager
Paul B. Pruett, MD, Director of Residency Education
Offers on-line bulletin boards which are relevant to autism.

4654   **Emory University Laboratory for Ophthalmic Research**
1365b Clifton Rd NE
Atlanta, GA 30322-1013   404-778-4530
Fax: 404-778-4002
pbennet@emory.edu
www.eyecenter.emory.edu

James W. Wagner, President
Larry Hagan, IT Manager
Paul B. Pruett, MD, Director of Residency Education

Various studies into the aspects of blindness.

4655 **Georgia Library for the Blind and Physically Handicapped**
Georgia Public Library
1800 Century Place
Suite 150
Atlanta, GA 30345-4304
404-235-7200
800-248-6701
Fax: 404-756-4618
georgialibraries.org

Stella Cone, Director
Deborah Scott, Business Manager
Dr. Lamar Veatch, Librarian
Discs, cassettes, braille, films, closed-circuit TV, braille writer, large-print photocopier, cassette books and magazines.

4656 **Hall County Library: East Hall Branch and Special Needs Library**
127 Main St NW
Gainesville, GA 30501-3614
770-532-3311
Fax: 770-532-4305
TTY: 770-531-2520
info@hallcountylibrary.org
www.hallcountylibrary.org

Adrian Mixson, Manager
Summer reading programs, braille writer, magnifiers, scanners and readers, audio described videos, closed captioned videos, closed-circuit TV, large-print photocopier, cassette books and magazines, large print books, children's books on cassette, home visits and other reference materials on blindness and other handicaps.

4657 **Macon Library for the Blind and Physically Handicapped**
Washington Memorial Library
1180 Washington Ave
Macon, GA 31201-1762
478-744-0800
Fax: 478-742-3161
www.co.bibb.ga.us/library

Thomas Jones, Director
Leila Brittain, Finance Officer
Hannah Warren, Office Manager
Summer reading programs, braille writer, magnifiers, closed-circuit TV, large-print photocopier, cassette books and magazines, children's books on cassette, home visits and other reference materials on blindness and other handicaps.

4658 **National Center on Birth Defects and Developmental Disabilities**
Centers for Disease Control and Prevention
1600 Clifton Rd NE
MS E-87
Atlanta, GA 30333
404-639-3311
800-232-4636
Fax: 404-498-3070
TTY: 888-232-6348
cdcinfo@cdc.gov
www.cdc.gov/ncbddd/

Coleen A. Boyle, PhD, MSHyg, Director
Stephanie Dulin, MBA, Deputy Director
Vicki Kipreos, PMP, Management Officer
Promotes child development, prevents birth defects and developmental disabilities.

4659 **North Georgia Talking Book Center**
LaFayette-Walker Public Library
305 S Duke St
La Fayette, GA 30728-2936
706-638-8312
888-506-0509
888-506-0509
Fax: 706-638-4028
www.chrl.org

Tim York, Manager
June DeLong, Library Assistant
Martha McKeehan, Library Assistant
We offer books on cassette for the visual and physically disabled induvidual, books in braille, magazines on cassette, zoom text screen magnifier, computer voice program, large-print photocopier, summer reading program, home visits na dother reference materials on blindness and other disabilities.

4660 **Oconee Regional Library**
801 Bellevue Ave
Dublin, GA 31021-4847
478-272-5710
Fax: 478-275-5381
georgialibraries.org

Stella Cone, Director
Deborah Scott, Business Manager
Dr. Lamar Veatch, Librarian
Summer reading programs, braille writer, magnifiers, closed-circuit TV, large-print photocopier, cassette books and magazines, children's books on cassette, home visits and other reference materials on blindness and other handicaps.

4661 **Rome Subregional Library for the Blind and Physically Handicapped**
205 Riverside Pkwy
Rome, GA 30161-2922
706-236-4611
888-263-0769
Fax: 706-236-4631
TTY: 706-236-4618

Diana Mills, Librarian
Delana Hickman, Manager
The regional library system serves Floyd and Polk counties. System headquarters are located in Rome, Georgia, within the Rome/Floyd County Library Branch.

4662 **South Georgia Regional Library-Valdosta Talking Book Center**
300 Woodrow Wilson Dr
Valdosta, GA 31602-2532
229-333-0086
Fax: 229-333-0364
commissioner@lowndescounty.com
sgrl.org

Chuck Gibson, Manager
Summer reading programs, Braille writer, magnifiers, closed-circuit TV, large print photocopier, cassette books and magazines, children's books on cassette, home visits and other reference materials on blindness and other handicaps.

4663 **Talking Book Center Brunswick-Glynn County Regional Library**
208 Gloucester St
Brunswick, GA 31520-7007
912-267-1212
Fax: 912-267-9597
www.trrl.org

Betty Ransom, Librarian
Joe Shinnick, Executive Director
The Three Rivers Regional Library system is named for 3 rivers that flow through all 7 counties of the library system. The Three Rivers Regional Library system serves patrons in Brantley, Camden, Charlton, Glynn, Long, McIntosh, and Wayne counties in southeast Georgia.

Hawaii

4664 **Assistive Technology Resource Centers of Hawaii (ATRC)**
200 North Vineyard Boulevard
Suite 430
Honolulu, HI 96817-5362
808-532-7110
800-645-3007
Fax: 808-532-7120
TTY: 808-532-7110
atrc-info@atrc.org
www.atrc.org

Barbara Fischlowitz-Leong, Executive Director
Jeff Ah Sam, Technical Assisstant
Jodi Asato, Deputy Director
Provides information and training on assistive technology devices, services, and funding resources. Conducts presentations and demonstrations in the community to increase AT awareness and promote self-advocacy among people with disabilities.

4665 **Hawaii State Library for the Blind and Physically Handicapped**
874 Dillingham Blvd
Honolulu, HI 96817-4505
808-845-9221
800-559-4096
Fax: 808-733-8449
honcclib@hawaii.edu
www2.honolulu.hawaii.edu/library

Fusako Miyashiro, Manager
Supported by the Hawaii State Public Library System and the National Library Service for the Blind and Physically Handicapped, Library of Congress. Staff with knowledge of sign language; Special interest periodicals; Books on deafness and sign language; captioned media; Special Services: Radio Reading Service, Talking Books Reader's Club, educational and cultural programs, machine lending agency. Braille, cassette and large type. Regional and National service, quarterly newsletter.

Idaho

4666 **Idaho Assistive Technology Project**
University of Idaho
121 West Sweet Ave
Moscow, ID 83843-2268
208-885-3557
800-432-8324
Fax: 208-885-6145
idahoat@uidaho.edu
www.idahoat.org

Janice Carson, Project Director
Irene Lunsford, Loan Program Manager
Julie Magelky, Loan Program Coordinator
A federally funded program managed by the Center on Disabilities and Human Development at the University of Idaho. The goal of the IATP is to increase the availability of assistive technology devices and services for Idahoans with disabilities. The IATP offers free trainings and technical assistance, a low-interest loan program, assistive technology assessments for children and agriculture workers, and free informational materials.

4667 **Idaho Commission for Libraries: Talking Book Service**
325 W State St
Boise, ID 83702-6055
208-334-2150
800-458-3271
Fax: 208-334-4016
talkingbooks@libraries.idaho.gov
www.libraries.idaho.gov/tbs

Ann Joslin, Manager
Irene Lunsford, Library Consultant
David Harrell, IT & Telecommunications Resources Manager
Offers audio and braille books and magazines, equipment, and accessories. All materials are mailed free to users' homes. Service is available free to all Idaho residents with a disability which limits their ability to use print materials.

Illinois

4668 **Chicago Public Library Talking Book Center**
400 S State St
Chicago, IL 60605-1216
312-747-4300
800-757-4654
Fax: 312-747-4962
www.chipublib.org

Linda Johnson Rice, President
Christopher Valenti, Vice President
Cristina Benitez, Secretary
Summer reading programs, braille writer, closed-circuit TV, large print photocopier, cassette books and magazines, children's books on cassette, home visits and other reference materials on blindness and other handicaps. Three assistive technology centers designed and equipped for the blind and visually impaired, funded by the National Library Service for the Blind and Handicapped, a division of the Library of Congress. All services FREE!

4669 **Department of Ophthalmology and Visual Science**
1855 W Taylor St
Chicago, IL 60612-7242
312-996-7000
800-625-2013
Fax: 312-996-7770
TTY: 312-413-0123
www.uic.edu

Paula Allen-Meares, Chancellor
Lon S. Kaufman, Vice Chancellor for Academic Aff
Mitra Dutta, Vice Chancellor for Research
Offers help, support, information and research for persons with vision problems, including Retinitis Pigmentosa.

4670 **Guild for the Blind**
65 E. Wacker Place
Suite 1010
Chicago, IL 60601-7463
312-236-8569
Fax: 312-236-8128
www.second-sense.org

Brett Christenson, President
Laura Rounce, Vice President
Michael P. Wagner, Treasurer
provides worship on vision rehabilitation, training on computers and other adaptive technology, career counseling, and professional development workshops and offers assistive devices for sale.

4671 **Horizons for the Blind**
125 Erick St.
A103
Crystal Lake, IL 60014
815-444-8800
800-318-2000
Fax: 815-444-8830
mail@horizons-blind.org
www.horizons-blind.org

Camille Caffarelli, Executive Director
Jeff T. Thorsen, First Vice President & Treasurer
Keith Myers, Second Vice President
Horizons for the Blind is a nonprofit organization working to improve the quality of life for people who are blind or visually impaired by increasing access to consumer products, services, culture, arts, education, and recreation.

4672 **Illinois Early Childhood Intervention Clearinghouse**
51 Gerty Drive
Champaign, IL 61820-7469
217-333-1386
877-275-3227
Fax: 217-244-7732
Illinois-eic@illinois.edu
www.eiclearinghouse.org

Charlton Brandt, Manager
Patricia Traylor, Project Associate
Free lending library of materials related to early childhood and disability. Books, audiovisuals and articles available. Computerized database with more than 31,000 items available to Illinois residents.

4673 **Illinois Machine Sub-Lending Agency**
607 S Greenbriar Rd
Carterville, IL 62918-1602
618-985-8375
800-455-2665
Fax: 618-985-4211
imsastaff@imsa.lib.il.us

Loretta Broomfield, Director
The Illinois Machine Sublending Agency (IMSA) is a division of the Illinois Network of Talking Book and Braille Libraries. The primary responsibility of IMSA is to maintain Talking Book equipment and accessories and to issue Talking Book equipment and accessories to Illinois residents who are registered for the service. IMSA is also the support center for patrons in need of assistance with the Braille and Audio Reading Download (BARD) service.

4674 **Illinois Regional Library for the Blind and Physically Handicapped**
1055 W Roosevelt Rd
Chicago, IL 60608-1559
312-746-9210
800-331-2351
Fax: 312-746-9192

Shawn Thomas, Reference Librarian
Barbara Perkins, Acting Director

Summer reading programs, braille writer, magnifiers, closed-circuit TV, large-print photocopier, cassette books and magazines, descriptive videos, children's books on cassette, home visits and other reference materials on blindness and other handicaps.

4675   Mid-Illinois Talking Book Center
600 High Point Ln
East Peoria, IL 61611-9396   309-694-9200
                                      800-426-0709
Rose Chenoweth, Director
Michelle Moran, Assistant
Rebecca Rollings, Assistant
Providing a free library service to anyone unable to read regular print because of a visual or physical disability. There are books and magazines on tape and playback equipment; and also in Braille. Books and magazines are mailed free to and from library patrons, wherever they reside.

4676   National Eye Research Foundation (NERF)
Ste 207a
910 Skokie Blvd
Northbrook, IL 60062-4033   847-564-4652
                                     800-621-2258
                                Fax: 847-564-0807
                                     info@nerf.org
                                     www.nerf.org
Joel Tenner, Manager
Dedicated to improving eye care for the public and meeting the professional nees of eye care practitioners; sponsors eye research projects on contact lens applications and eye care problems. Special study sections in such fields as orthokertology, primary eyecare, pediatrics, and through continuing education programs. Provides eye care information for the public and professionals. Educational materials including pamphlets. Program activities include education and referrals.

4677   National Lekotek Center
2001 N. Clybourn
Chicago, IL 60614   773-528-5766
                                     800-366-7529
                                Fax: 773-537-2992
                                     www.lekotek.org
Elaine D. Cottey, Chair
Joanna Horsnail, Chair Elect
Eric Gastevich, Treasurer
Toy library and play-centered programs for children with special needs and their families with branches in 17 states. Sliding fee scale. Lekotek also has a Toy Resource Helpline that provides individualized assistances in the selection of toys and play materials and general resources for families with children with disabilities.

4678   Northwestern University Multipurpose Arthritis & Musculoskeletal Center
420 East Superior Street
Chicago, IL 60611-4296   312-503-8194
                                Fax: 312-503-1204
                         www.feinberg.northwestern.edu
Cynthia Barnard, MBA, Director, Quality Strategies
John Vozenilek, MD, Assistant Professor
Eric G. Neilson, MD, Vice President for Medical Affairs
Conducts biomedical, educational and health services research into musculoskeletal diseases.

4679   Skokie Accessible Library Services
Skokie Public Library
5215 Oakton St
Skokie, IL 60077-3680   847-673-7774
                                Fax: 847-673-7797
                                TTY: 847-673-8926
                                     www.skokie.lib.il.us
Carolyn A. Anthony, Director
John J. Graham, President
Diana Hunter, Vice President/President Emerita
Library services for people with disabilities, including electronic aids, materials in special formats, programs and special services.

4680   University of Illinois at Chicago: Lions of Illinois Eye Research Institute
University of Illinois at Chicago
1855 West Taylor Street, m/c 648
Room 3.138
Chicago, IL 60612   312-996-6591
                                Fax: 312-996-7770
                                     eyeweb@uic.edu
                                     www.uic.edu
Rolanda Geddis, Manager
Paula Alen Meares, Chancellor
Jerry Bauman, Vice President for Health Affairs
Visual impairments and blindness research, including glaucoma studies.

4681   Voices of Vision Talking Book Center at DuPage Library System
125 Tower Drive
Burr Ridge, IL 60527-2771   630-734-5055
                                     800-426-0709
                                Fax: 630-208-0399
                                     info@illinoistalkingbooks.org
                                     www.illinoistalkingbooks.org
Karen L. Odean, Director
Provides library service to persons who are unable to use standard printed material because of visual or physical disabilities. Part of the Illinois network of Talking Book Libraries. The service is free to those who are eligable. Provides books and magazines on audio-cassettes. Special playback equipment needed to use the books is also loaned. Braille books and magazines are also available. The collection includes popular books, classics and children's literature.

Indiana

4682   Allen County Public Library
900 Library Plaza
Fort Wayne, IN 46802-3699   260-421-1200
                                Fax: 260-421-1386
                                TTY: 260-421-1302
                                     Genealogy@ACPL.Info
                                     www.acpl.lib.in.us
Jeffrey R. Krull, Director
Martin E. Seifert, President
Alan McMahan, Vice President
Summer reading programs, braille writer, magnifiers, closed-circuit TV, large-print photocopier, cassette books and magazines, children's books on cassette, home visits and other reference materials on blindness and other handicaps.

4683   Bartholomew County Public Library
536 5th St
Columbus, IN 47201-6225   812-379-1255
                                Fax: 812-379-1275
                                     library@barth.lib.in.us
                                     barth.lib.in.us
Beth Poor, Executive Director
Summer reading programs, braille writer, magnifiers, closed-circuit TV, large-print photocopier, cassette books and magazines, children's books on cassette, home visits and other reference materials on blindness and other handicaps.

4684   Elkhart Public Library for the Blind and Physically Handicapped
300 S 2nd St
Elkhart, IN 46516-3109   574-522-2223
                                     800-622-4970
                                Fax: 574-522-2174
                                     www.myepl.org/epl
Connie Jo Ozinga, Executive Director
Barbara G. Anderson, President
Janice E. Dean, Vice-President
Summer reading programs, braille writer, magnifiers, closed-circuit TV, large-print photocopier, cassette books and magazines, children's books on cassette, home visits and other reference materials on blindness and other handicaps.

4685 Indiana Resource Center for Autism
2853 E 10th St
Bloomington, IN 47408-2696
812-855-6508
800-825-4733
Fax: 812-855-9630
TTY: 812-855-9396
iidc@indiana.edu
www.iidc.indiana.edu/irca
Dr Cathy Pratt Ph.D., BCBA, Director
Donna Beasley, Administrative Program Secretary
Pamela Anderson, Outreach/Resource Specialist
The Indiana Resource Center for Autism staff conduct outreach training and consultations, engage in research and develop and disseminate information focused on building the capicity of local communities, organizations, agencies and families to support children and adults across the autism spectrum in typical work, school, home and community settings. Please check our website for a complete list of publications.

4686 Indiana University: Multipurpose Arthritis Center
School Of Medicine, Rheumatology Division
509 E. 3rd Street
Bloomington, IN 47401-3654
812-855-0516
Fax: 812-855-9943
research.iu.edu
Dr. Kenneth Brandt MD, Director
Carmichael Center, Vice President for Research
Steven A Martin, Associate Vice President for Research
The mission of the center is to pursue major biomedical research interests relevant to the rheumatic diseases. Current areas of emphasis include; articular cartilage biology, pathogenesis of articular cartilage breakdown in osteoarthritis, causes of pain and disability in QA, the pathogenesis and treatment of various forms of amyloidosis, the pathogenesis of dermatomyositis, and immunologic and biochemical markers of cartilage breakdown and repair.

4687 Lake County Public Library Talking Books Service
1919 W 81st Ave
Merrillville, IN 46410-5488
219-769-3541
Fax: 219-769-0690
www.lcplin.org
Larry Acheff, Manager
Large-print books, descriptive videos, braille writer, magnifiers, closed-circuit TV, large-print photocopier, cassette books and magazines, children's books on cassette, and other reference materials on blindness and other handicaps.

4688 Special Services Division: Indiana State Library
140 N Senate Ave
Indianapolis, IN 46204-2207
317-232-3675
800-622-4970
Fax: 317-253-3209
TTY: 317-232-7763
www.in.gov/isloutage
Roberta Brooker, Manager
Barbara Maxwell, State Librarian
C Ewick, Manager
Circulates a collection of braille, recorded, and large print books and magazines and the special equipment needed to play the recorded materials to anyone in Indiana who cannot read regular print due to a visual or physical disability.

4689 St. Joseph Hospital Rehabilitation Center
700 Broadway
Fort Wayne, IN 46802-1402
260-425-3000
Fax: 260-425-3741
www.stjoehospital.com
Kirk Ray, CEO
Bob Hailes, Vice President
Information offered on rehabilitation.

4690 Talking Books Service Evansville Vanderburgh County Public Library
200 SE Martin Luther King Jr Blvd
Evansville, IN 47713- 1802
812-428-8200
866-645-2536
Fax: 812-428-8397
tbs@evpl.org
www.evpl.org
Marcia Learned Au, COO
Connie Davis, Vice President
Marcia Au, Executive Director
The Talking Book Service of the Evansville Vanderburgh Public Library is part of a nationwide network of cooperating libraries headed by the National Library Service & a division of the Library of Congress. This free program provides library services and materials in alternative formats to person who are unable to use standard print material due to a visual or physical handicap.

Iowa

4691 Iowa Department for the Blind Library
State Of Iowa
524 4th Street
Des Moines, IA 50309-2364
515-281-1333
800-362-2587
Fax: 515-281-1263
TTY: 515-281-1355
contact@blind.state.ia.us
www.IDBonline.org
Richard Sorey, Director
Mike Hoenig, Chair
Steve Hagemoser, Commision Board Member
Summer reading programs, large print, disc, Braille and cassette books and magazines, descriptive videos and reference materials on blindness and other handicaps.

4692 Iowa Registry for Congenital and Inherited Disorders
University of Iowa
Department of Epidemiology, Univers
100 BVC, Room W260
Iowa City, IA 52242-5000
319-335-4107
866-274-4237
Fax: 319-335-4030
ircid@uiowa.edu
www.public-health.uiowa.edu/ircid/
Paul Romitti, Ph.D, Director
Kim Keppler-Noreuil, M.D, Clinical Director for Birth Defects
Katherine. Mathews, M.D, Clinical Director for Neuromuscular Disorders
The mission of the Iowa Registry for Congenital and Inherited Disorders is; maintain statewide surveillance for collecting information on selected congenital and inherited disorders in Iowa, monitor annual trends in occurrence and mortality of these disorders, provide data for research studies and educational activities for the prevention and treatment of these disorders.

4693 Library Commission for the Blind
State Of Iowa
524 4th Street
Des Moines, IA 50309-2364
515-281-1333
800-362-2587
Fax: 515-281-1263
TTY: 515-281-1355
contact@blind.state.ia.us
Karen A Keninger, Director
Aldini Jodi, Library Support Staff
Barber Kim, Independent Living Supervisor
Summer reading programs, Braille writer, magnifiers, closed-circuit TV, large print photocopier, cassette books and magazines, children's books on cassette and other reference materials on blindness and other handicaps.

Kansas

4694 Center for the Improvement of Human Functioning
3100 N Hillside St
Wichita, KS 67219-3904
316-682-3100
Fax: 316-682-5054
information@riordanclinic.org
www.riordanclinic.org

Hugh D Riordan, President
Ron Hunninghake MD, Chief Medical Officer
Brian Riordan, Chief Executive Officer
Medical, research, and educational facility specializing in the treatment of chronic illness.

4695 Central Kansas Library Systems Headquarters (CSLS)
1409 Williams St
Great Bend, KS 67530-4020
620-792-4865
800-362-2642
Fax: 620-793-7270
www.ckls.org

Harry Williams, Administrator
Vickie Herl, Adminstrative Manager
Marquita Boehnke, Department Head
Summer reading programs, braille writer, magnifiers, closed-circuit TV, large-print photocopier, cassette books and magazines, children's books on cassette, home visits and other reference materials on blindness and other handicaps. Assistive technology available. Serving 17 counties in Central Kansas.

4696 Manhattan Public Library
629 Poyntz Ave
Manhattan, KS 66502-6131
785-776-4741
800-432-2796
Fax: 785-776-1545
refstaff@mhklibrary.org
manhattan.lib.ks.us

Linda Knupp, Director
John Pecoraro, Assistant Director
Brice Hobrock, President
Summer reading programs, Braille writer, magnifiers, closed-circuit TV, large-print photocopier, cassette books and magazines, children's books on cassette, home visits and other reference materials on blindness and other disabilities.

4697 Northwest Kansas Library System Talking Books
2 Washington Square
Norton, KS 67654-1615
785-877-5148
800-432-2858
Fax: 785-877-5697
www.nwkls.org

George Seamon, Director
Alice Evans, Business Manager & Acquisitions
David Fischer, Technology Consultant
Offers books on disc and cassette. Library of Congress talking book and program for qualified individuals. Also offers descriptive videos to eligible persons.

4698 South Central Kansas Library System
321 North Main Street
South Hutchinson, KS 67505-1145
620-663-3211
800-234-0529
Fax: 620-663-9797
sckls.info

Paul Hawkins, Director
Sharon Barnes, Technology Consultant
Larry Papenfuss, Director of Information Technology
Serving public, school, academic and special libraries in 12 counties since 1968, the South Central Kansas Library System (SCKLS) is the "go to" resource for innovative services, quality member awareness and assistance.

4699 State Library of Kansas
Esu Memorial Union
300 SW 10th Ave.
Room 312-N
Topeka, KS 66612-1593
620-341-6280
800-362-0699
KTB@ks.gov
kslib.info/talking-books

Cindy Roupe, State Librarian
Michael Lang, Director
Kansas Talking Books provides personalized library support and materials in a specialized format to eligible Kansas residents to ensure that all may read. Features: Audiobooks, magazines and audio equipment mailed directly to your house and returned postage free; special equipment lent to you at no charge; downloadable books from the Braille and Audio Reading Download (BARD) website or by using the new BARD app.

4700 Topeka & Shawnee County Public Library Talking Books Service
1515 SW 10th Ave
Topeka, KS 66604-1374
785-580-4400
800-432-2925
Fax: 785-580-4496
TTY: 785-580-4544
www.tscpl.org

Stephanie Hall, Manager
Gina Millsap, Chief Executive Officer
Robert Banks, Chief Operating Officer
Talking books is a free service that provides cassette and digital books and equipment to people who are unable to read or use standard print materials because of a visual or physical impairment. There are no fees. To apply for Talking Books you must fill out and submit an application, have it certified by the appropriate authority and return it to the library. You can find an application on our website or have one mailed out to you by contacting our office.

4701 Wichita Public Library/Talking Book Service
Wichita Public Library
223 S Main St
Wichita, KS 67202-3795
316-261-8500
Fax: 316-262-4540
TTY: 316-262-3972
admin@wichita.lib.ks.us

Cynthia Berner-Harris, Executive Director
Eric J. Larson, Member of the Board
Furnish recorded reading material (books and magazines) for visually and physically challenged citizens.

4702 Wichita Public Library/Talking Book Service
223 S Main St
Wichita, KS 67202-3795
316-261-8500
Fax: 316-262-4540
TTY: 316-262-3972
admin@wichita.lib.ks.us

Cynthia Berner-Harris, Executive Director
Eric J. Larson, Member of the Board
Furnish recorded reading material (books and magazines) for visually and physically challenged citizens.

Kentucky

4703 EnTech: Enabling Technologies of Kentuckiana
Spaulding University
851 South 3rd Street
Louisville, KY 40203-2115
502-585-9911
800-896-8941
Fax: 502-585-7103
www.spalding.edu

Laura Strickland, Manager
Mary Kaye Steinmietz, Outreach Coordinator
Tori Murden McClure, President
Assistive technology resource and demonstration center, serving persons of all ages and disabilities in Kentucky and Southern Indiana. Services include: assistive technology information, demonstration, evaluation, training, technical support and short-term loan of equipment.

4704 Kentucky Talking Book Library - Kentucky Dept. for Libraries and Archives
300 Coffee Tree Road
PO Box 537
Frankfort, KY 40602-0537

502-564-8300
800-372-2968
Fax: 502-564-5773
ktbl.mail@ky.gov
www.kdla.ky.gov

Barbara Penegor, Regional Librarian
Lauren Abner, Field Services
Katherine K. Adelberg, E-Rate Coordinator
Provides library service to those who are physically unable to read print. Audio and braille books and magazines are available via mail or download.

4705 Louisville Free Public Library
301 York Street
Louisville, KY 40203-2257

502-574-1611
Fax: 502-574-1666
lfpl.org

Craig Buthod, Manager
Summer reading programs, braille writer, magnifiers, closed-circuit TV, large-print photocopier, cassette books and magazines, children's books on cassette, home visits and other reference materials on blindness and other handicaps.

Louisiana

4706 Central Louisiana State Hospital Medical and Professional Library
P.O.Box 5031
Pineville, LA 71361-5031

318-484-6200
Fax: 318-484-6501
www.doa.la.gov

Patrick Kelly, CEO
Carol Gee, Manager
Information offered on psychiatry, psychology and mental health.

4707 Louisiana State Library
701 North 4th St
Baton Rouge, LA 70802-5345

225-342-4913
800-543-4702
Fax: 225-219-4804
admin@state.lib.la.us
www.state.lib.la.us

Rebecca Hamilton, Assistant Secretary, State Libra
Diane Brown, Deputy State Librarian
Beverly Dugas, Business Manager
Summer reading programs, braille writer, magnifiers, closed-circuit TV, large-print photocopier, cassette books and magazines, children's books on cassette. Descriptive videoss and other reference materials on blindness and other handicaps.

4708 Louisiana State University Genetics Section of Pediatrics
533 Bolivar St
New Orleans, LA 70112-1349

504-568-6151
Fax: 504-568-8500
postmaster@lsuhsc.edu
www.medschool.lsuhsc.edu

Steve Nelson, MD, Dean
Janis Letourneau, MD, Associate Dean for Faculty & Ins
Cathi Fontenot, MD, Associate Dean for Alumni Affair
Our goal is to continue building a strong department in which all of the faculty are successful in attracting funding, and committed to establishing productive programs that bring credit to the Department and to the Health Sciences Center as a whole.

4709 State Library of Louisiana: Services for the Blind and Physically Handicapped
701 North 4th St
Baton Rouge, LA 70802-5345

225-342-4913
800-543-4702
Fax: 225-219-4804
www.state.lib.la.us

Rebecca Hamilton, Assistant Secretary, State Libra
Diane Brown, Deputy State Librarian
Beverly Dugas, Business Manager
Summer reading programs, braille publications, cassette books and magazines, children's books on cassette and other reference materials on blindness and other handicaps. Louisiana Hotlines - quarterly newsletter. Affiliated with National Library Service for the Blind and Physically Handicapped, Washington, DC. Louisiana Voices recording program uses volunteers to record books for the blind.

Maine

4710 Bangor Public Library
145 Harlow St
Bangor, ME 04401-4900

207-947-8336
Fax: 207-945-6694
www.bpl.lib.me.us

Barbara Mc Dade, Executive Director
Norman Minsky, President
Franklin E. Bragg II, MD, Vice President
Summer reading programs, braille writer, magnifiers, closed-circuit TV, large-print photocopier, cassette books and magazines, children's books on cassette, home visits and other reference materials on blindness and other handicaps.

4711 Cary Library
107 Main Street
Houlton, ME 04730-2196

207-532-1302
Fax: 207-532-4350
www.cary.lib.me.us

Iva Sussman, Chair
Forrest Barnes, Treasurer
Gary Hagan, Secretary
Summer reading programs, braille writer, magnifiers, closed-circuit TV, large-print photocopier, cassette books and magazines, children's books on cassette, home visits and other reference materials on blindness and other handicaps.

4712 Lewiston Public Library
200 Lisbon St
Lewiston, ME 04240-7234

207-513-3004
Fax: 207-784-3011
TTY: 207-200-1511
LPLReference@LewistonMaine.gov
lplonline.org

Rick Speer, Library Director
Marcela Peres, Adult Services Librarian
David Moorhead, Children's Librarian
Summer reading programs, braille writer, magnifiers, closed-circuit T.V., large-print photocopier, cassette books and magazines, children's books on cassette, home visits and other reference materials on blindness and other handicaps.

4713 Maine State Library
Maine State
64 State House Sta
Augusta, ME 04333-64

207-287-5650
800-762-7106
Fax: 207-287-5624
TTY: 888-577-6690
benitad@ursus3.ursus.maine.edu
maine.gov

Chris Boynton, Manager
J Gary Nichols, State Librarian
Melora Norman, Manager
Summer reading programs, cassette books and magazines, children's books on cassette, home visits and other reference materials on blindness and other handicaps.
Newsl./BiAnnual

4714   New England Regional Genetics Group
P.O.Box 920288
Needham, MA 02492-4   781-444-0126
                                           Fax: 781-444-0127
                                          mfgnergg@verizon.net
                                              www.nergg.org

Marinell Newtown, President
Jennifer Walsh, Secretary
Merrill Henderson, Treasurer
New Englands primary network for collaborative exchange of ge-
netic health information and education.

4715   Portland Public Library
5 Monument Sq
Portland, ME 04101-4072   207-871-1700
                                           Fax: 207-871-1703
                                       reference@portland.lib.me.us
                                            portlandlibrary.com

Stephen J. Podgajny, Executive Director
Clare E. Hannan, Head of Finance and Operations
Linda Albert, Head of Human Resources
Summer reading programs, magnifiers, closed-circuit T.V.,
large-print photocopier, cassette books and magazines, children's books on cassette, home visits and other reference materials on blindness and other handicaps.

4716   Waterville Public Library
73 Elm Street
Waterville, ME 04901-6078   207-872-5433
                                           Fax: 207-873-4779
                                      wplhelpdesk@waterville.lib.me.us
                                          www.watervillelibrary.org

Sarah Sugden, Executive Director
Marnie Terhune, President
William Grant, Treasurer
Summer reading programs, braille writer, magnifiers, closed-circuit T.V., large-print photocopier, cassette books and magazines,
children's books on cassette, home visits and other reference materials on blindness and other handicaps.

Maryland

**4717   Johns Hopkins University Dana Center for Preventive
Ophthalmology**
Wilmer Ophthalmology Institute
600 N Wolfe St
Wilmer Suite 122
Baltimore, MD 21287-9019   410-955-2777
                                           Fax: 410-955-2542
                                              boland@jhu.edu

Harry Quigley, Director
Emily W. Gower, Ph.D, Director
Joanne. Katz, Sc.D, Director/Professor and Associate Chair
Established in 1979, the Dana Center for Preventive Ophthalmology is dedicated to improving knowlege of risk factors for ocular
disease and public health approaches to the prevention of these
diseases and their ensuing visual impairment and blindness
worldwide.

4718   Johns Hopkins University: Asthma and Allergy Center
5501 Hopkins Bayview Cir
Baltimore, MD 21224-6821   410-550-0545
                                           Fax: 410-550-1733
                                           jhuallergy@jhmi.edu
                                           hopkins-arthritis.org

Lawrence Lichtenstein, Director
Studies of allergic diseases and individuals with allergic disease,
pulmonary diseases and diseases involving inflammation and im-
munological processes.

**4719   Maryland State Library for the Blind and Physically
Handicapped**
Maryland State Department of Education
415 Park Avenue
Baltimore, MD 21201-3603   410-230-2424
                                                800-964-9209
                                           Fax: 410-333-2095
                                          TTY: 800-934-2541
                                          referenc@lbph.lib.md.us

Jill Lewis, Manager
Diana Jarvis, Administrative Specialist
LaTarsha Wilson, Secretary
Provide comprehensive library services to the eligible blind and
physically handicapped residents of the State of Maryland. The
vision is to provide innovative and quality services to meet the
needs and expectations of the patrons of Maryland.

**4720   Montgomery County Department of Public
Libraries/Special Needs Library**
6400 Democracy Blvd
Bethesda, MD 20817-1638   240-777-0922
                                          TTY: 301-897-2203
                                         montgomerycountymd.gov

Susan F Cohen, Assistant Head Librarian
James Montgomery, Owner
Joseph Eagan, Branch Manager
Serves the library information and reading needs of people with
disabilities, family members, students and service providers.
Some of its services include books, periodicals, and videos on
disability issues, adaptive technology, community information;
the National Library for the Blind and Physically Handicapped
Talking Book program; large print books; and computer room
with adaptive technology.

4721   National Epilepsy Library (NEL)
Epilepsy Foundation
8301 Professional Pl
Landover, MD 20785-7223   866-330-2718
                                                800-332-1000
                                           Fax: 877-687-4878
                                           ContactUs@efa.org
                                        www.epilepsyfoundation.org

Marl A Finucane, Executive Vice President
Patty Dukes, Vice President Operations/Human
Mimi Browne, Director, HRSA programs
Contains information about epilepsy and seizure disorders and
serves physicians and other health professionals. Provides
in-house bibliographic database (ESDI), searches and documents
delivery and interlibrary loans. Maintains the Albert and Ellen
Grass Archives.

4722   National Federation of the Blind Jernigan Institute
200 E. Wells St.
at Jernigan Place
Baltimore, MD 21230   410-659-9314
                                           Fax: 410-685-5653
                                              nfb@nfb.org
                                         nfb.org/programs-services

Anil Lewis, Executive Director, Blindness Initiatives
Cutting-edge research and training is conducted through the NFB
Jernigan Institute to address the real problems of blindness, such
as model education and rehabilitation methods to empower the
blind or improved instruction in Braille. The Jacobus tenBroek
Library is also hosted at the NFB headquarters.

4723   National Institute on Aging
31 Center Dr., MSC 2292
Building 31, Room 5C27
Bethesda, MD 20892   800-222-2225
                                          TTY: 800-222-4225
                                            niaic@nia.nih.gov
                                             www.nia.nih.gov

Richard J. Hodes, Director
Lisa Mascone, Deputy Director, Management
Luigi Ferrucci, Scientific Director
The National Institute on Aging (NIA) is the primary Federal
agency engaged in researching Alzheimer's disease.

4724   National Rehabilitation Information Center (NARIC)
8400 Corporate Drive
Suite 500
Landover, MD 20785-2245   301-459-5984
                                       800-346-2742
                                  Fax: 301-459-4263
                                  TTY: 301-459-5984
                           naricinfo@heitechservices.com
                                       www.naric.com

Mark X. Odum, Project Director
Natalie J. Collier, Library & Acquisitions Manager
Tamara J. Pyle, Library & Information Services Coordinator
NARIC is a federally-funded library and information center that
focuses on disability and rehabilitation information.

4725   Red Notebook
Friends of Libraries for Deaf Action
2930 Craiglawn Rd
Silver Spring, MD 20904-1816   301-572-5168
                                  Fax: 301-572-5168
                                  TTY: 301-572-5168
                                     folda86@aol.com

Alice L Hagemeyer, MLS, Founder/President
Merrie A. Davidson, Associate
Ricardo Lopez, MS, Associate
A binder containing fact sheets, library reprints, announcements
and other printed informational materials that are related to both
deaf and library issues. It is designed to help build communication among individuals and groups within the deaf community.
The focus is on assisting libraries in providing cost-effective and
efficient library and information services to these consumers in a
unbiased fashion.

4726   Social Security Library
U S Social Security Administration
6401 Security Blvd
Baltimore, MD 21235-6401   800-772-1213
                                  TTY: 800-325-0778
                                  www.socialsecurity.gov

Bill Vitek, Manager
Jo B Barnhart, Chief Executive Officer
Information on social security and disability insurance.

4727   Trace Research and Development Center
Univ. of Maryland, College of Information Studies
4130 Campus Dr.
College Park, MD 20742   301-405-2043
                                    trace-info@umd.edu
                                       trace.umd.edu

Kate Vanderheiden, Program Manager
Research focused on how standard information and communication technology products may be designed so that more people
with disabilities can use them.

4728   Warren Grant Magnuson Clinical Center
National Institue Health
9000 Rockville Pike
Bethesda, MD 20892-1   301-496-2563
                                       800-411-1222
                                  Fax: 301-480-2984
                                  TTY: 866-411-1010
                               prpl@mail.cc.nih.gov
                                       www.cc.nih.gov

John I Gallin, MD, Clinical Center Director
Clare Hastings, PhD, RN, FAA, Chief Nurse Officer
Maureen E. Gormley, MPH, MA, RN, Chief Operating Officer
Established in 1953 as the research hospital of the National Institutes of Health. Designed so that patient care facilities are close to
research laboratories so new findings of basic and clinical scientists can be quickly applied to the treatment of patients. Upon referral by physicians, patients are admitted to NIH clinical studies.

Massachusetts

4729   Boston University Arthritis Center
Boston University
715 Albany St
Boston, MA 02118-2526   617-638-4640
                                  Fax: 617-638-5226
                                       www.bumc.bu.edu

Karen Antman, Dean & Provost, Medical School
Meg Aranow, Director
Barbara A. Cole, Associate VP for Research Admin
The Arthritis Center focuses its educational, research and patient
care efforts on the diagnosis and treatment of rheumatic diseases.
These include the many forms of arthritis; the auto-immune dis-
eases such as Scleroderma, Systemic Lupus, Erythematosus,
Rheumatoid Arthritis; localized pain syndromes such as
tendonitis, bursitis, and carpal tunnel syndrome; and metabolic
bone disorders such as osteoporosis.

4730   Boston University Center for Human Genetics
840 Memorial Drive
Suite 101
Cambridge, MA 02139   617-638-7083
                                  Fax: 617-638-7092
                                     amilunsk@bu.edu
                                       www.chginc.org

Aubrey Milunsky, Co-Director
Jeff Milunsky, M.D., F.A.C., Director of Clinical Genetics
Research and molecular diagnosis.

**4731   Boston University Robert Dawson Evans Memorial Dept.
of Clinical Research**
75 East Newton St
Boston, MA 02118-2657   617-247-5019
                                  Fax: 617-638-8728

Norman G Levinsky, Director
Jack Ansel, MD
Integral unit of the University Hospital specializing in arthritis
and connective tissue studies.

**4732   Braille and Talking Book Library, Perkins School for the
Blind**
175 North Beacon Street
Watertown, MA 02472-2751   617-972-3434
                                       800-852-3133
                                  Fax: 617-926-2027
                                     Info@Perkins.org
                                       www.perkins.org

Frederic M. Clifford, Chairman
Philip L. Ladd, Vice Chairman
Dave Power, CEO & President
The Braille and Talking Book Library loans braille and recorded
reading materials and the playback equipment necessary to use
them. You are eligible for services if you are unable to read print
due to a disability.

**4733   Brigham and Women's Hospital: Asthma and Allergic
Disease Research Center**
75 Francis St
Boston, MA 02115-6110   617-732-5500
                                       855-278-8010
                                  Fax: 617-730-2858
                                     arc@partners.org

Matthew H Liang, Director
Elizabeth G Nabel, President
Arthur Mombourquette, Vice President of Support Servic
Integral unit of the hospital focusing research attention on asthma
and allergy related disorders.

4734 **Brigham and Women's Hospital: Robert B Brigham Multipurpose Arthritis Center**
Brigham and Women s Hospital
75 Francis St
Boston, MA 02115-6110
617-732-5500
855-278-8010
Fax: 617-432-0979
www.brighamandwomens.org
Matthew H Liang, Director
Elizabeth G Nabel, President
Arthur Mombourquette, Vice President of Support Servic
Research studies into arthritis and rheumatic diseases.

4735 **Caption Center**
Media Access Group at WGBH
One Guest St.
Boston, MA 02135
617-300-3600
Fax: 617-300-1020
access@wgbh.org
www.wgbh.org/caption
Pat McDonald, Director
The Caption Center was the world's first captioning agency providing access to television for viewers who are visually impaired and/or hard of hearing. The Center develops new solutions and uses closed captioning and descriptive video to promote access to technology.

4736 **Center for Interdisciplinary Research on Immunologic Diseases**
Childrens Hospital Medical Center
300 Longwood Avenue
Boston, MA 02115-5724
617-355-6000
800-355-7944
Fax: 617-355-0443
TTY: 617-730-0152
webteam@tch.harvard.edu
www.childrenshospital.org
Sandra L. Fenwick, President and Chief Executive Officer
Kevin Churchwell, MD, Executive Vice President
Dick Argys, Senior Vice President and Chief Administrative Officer
Organizational research unit of the Children's Hospital that focuses on the causes, prevention and treatments of asthma, infections and allergies.

4737 **Harvard University Howe Laboratory of Ophthalmology**
Massachusetts Eye & Ear Infirmary
243 Charles Street
Boston, MA 02114-3002
617-523-7900
Fax: 617-573-4380
TTY: 617-573-5498
richard.godfrey@schepens.harvard.edu
www.masseyeandear.org/
Wycliffe Grousbeck, Chairman
John Fernandez, President and CEO
Jonathan Uhrig, Treasurer
Development ophthalmology and eye research.

4738 **Laboure College Library**
303 Adams Street
Dorchester Center, MA 02124-5698
617-296-8300
Fax: 617-296-7947
admissions@laboure.edu
laboure.edu
Andrew Callo, Manager
Maureen A. Smith, President
Offers information on physical disabilities, independent living, peer counseling and advocacy.

4739 **Massachusetts Rehabilitation Commission**
600 Washington Street
Boston, MA 02111
617-204-3603
800-245-6543
Fax: 617-727-1354
TTY: 800-245-6543
www.mass.gov/mrc
Elmer C Bartels, Commissioner
Deval L. Patrick, Governor
Timothy P. Murray, Lieutenant Governor
Vacational Rehabilitation and Independent Living for people with disabilities.

4740 **Schepens Eye Research Institute**
20 Staniford Street
Boston, MA 02114-2508
617-912-0100
Fax: 617-912-0118
geninfo@vision.eri.harvard.edu
John Fernandez, President and CEO
Debra Rogers, Vice President for Ophthalmology
Alan A Ryan, Director Research Finance
Prominent center for research on eye, vision, and blinding diseases; dedicated to research that improves the understanding, management, and prevention of eye diseases and visual deficiencies; fosters collaboration among its faculty members; trains young scientists and clinicians from around the world; promotes communication with scientists in allied fields; leader in the worldwide dispersion of basic scientific knowledge of vision.

4741 **Talking Book Library at Worcester Public Library**
3 Salem Sq
Worcester, MA 01608-2015
508-799-1730
800-762-0085
Fax: 508-799-1676
www.worcpublib.org
James Izatt, Dept Head
Braille embosser, magnifiers, closed-circuit TV, adapted computers, cassette books and magazines, children's books on cassette, reference materials on blindness and other disabilities.

Michigan

4742 **Artificial Language Laboratory**
Michigan State University
220 Trowbridge Rd
East Lansing, MI 48824-1042
517-353-5940
Fax: 517-353-4766
finaid@msu.edu
www.msu.edu
Dr. John B Eulenberg, Phd, Director
Stephen R. Blosser, BSME, Technical Director
Shawn A. Miller, Laboratory Manager
Multidisciplinary research center in the Audiology & Speech Science department, Michigan State University. Its basic research program includes speech analysis and synthesis. Applied research is carried out on computer-based systems for persons who are blind and for persons with cerebral palsy and head injury. The laboratory develops physical, cognitive and linguistic assessment technology.

4743 **Burger School for the Autistic**
31735 Maplewood St.
Garden City, MI 48135-1993
734-793-1830
Fax: 734-762-8533
garden-city.lib.mi.us
James B Lenze, Library Director
Dan Lodge, Adult Librarian
Lindsay Fricke, Youth Librarian
Burger school for students with autism is the largest public school in the United States that specializes in the education of students with autism.

4744 **Chi Medical Library**
Ingham Regional Medical Center
401 West Greenlawn
Lansing, MI 48910-2819
517-975-6000
irmc.org
Judy Barnes, Manager
Consumer health and patient education collection in books, videotapes, pamphlets. Open to the public.

4745 **Glaucoma Laser Trial**
Sinai Hospital of Detroit: Dept. of Opthalmology
31 Center Drive
Bethesda, MI 20892-2510
301-496-5248
kcl@nei.nih.gov
www.nei.nih.gov
Paul A. Sieving, M.D., Ph.D., Director
The purpose of the trial is to compare the safety and long-term efficacy of argon laser treatment of the trabecular meshwork with standard medical treatment for primary open-angle glaucoma.

4746 **Grand Traverse Area Library for the Blind and Physically Handicapped**
610 Woodmere Ave
Traverse City, MI 49686-3103

231-932-8500
877-931-8558
Fax: 231-932-8578
webmaster@tadl.tcnet.org
www.tadl.org

Metta Lansdale, Library Director
Thomas Kachadurian, President
Jason Gillman, Vice President
The LBPH was established as a sub-regional library in 1972 and currently provides services for 783 registered individuals in 16 counties, 171 of these registrants are Grand Traverse County residents. Anyone unable to read regular printed materials because of visual or physical limitations may be eligible.

4747 **Kent District Library for the Blind and Physically Handicapped**
814 West River Center Dr. NE
Comstock Park, MI 49321-3420

616-784-2007
877-243-2466
Fax: 616-336-3256
WyomingYouthStaff@kdl.org
www.kdl.org

Charles R Myers, Chair
Vickie Hoekstra, Vice Chair
Carol Simpson, Secretary
Summer reading programs, braille writer, magnifiers, large-print photocopier, cassette books and magazines, children's books on cassette, and other reference materials on blindness and other handicaps.

4748 **Macomb Library for the Blind & Physically Handicapped**
40900 Romeo Plank
Clinton Township, MI 48038-1132

586-226-5020
800-203-5274
Fax: 586-286-0634
mlbph@cmpl.org
www.cmpl.org

Larry Neal, Library Director
Fred L. Gibson, Jr., President
Peter M. Ruggirello,, Vice Chairman
Braille writer, closed-circuit T.V., large-print books, cassette books and magazines, children's books on cassette, other reference materials on blindness and other handicaps, descriptive videos and bifokal kits. Assistive technology including JAWS, Zoomtext, OpenBook, and Duxbury.

4749 **Michigan Braille and Talking Book Library**
P.O.Box 30007
702 W. Kalamazoo St
Lansing, MI 48909-7507

517-373-5614
800-992-9012
Fax: 517-373-5865
btbl@michigan.gov
www.michigan.gov/btbl

Sue Chinault, Manager
Provides library service to people with visual or physical disabilities that are unable to utilize standard print materials. Digital book cartridges (audio books) and/or braille books are sent directly to the patron's home, completely free of charge. This program is available to all Michigan residents.

4750 **Michigan Library for the Blind and Physically Handicapped**
Genesee District Library
G-4195 Pasadena Rd.
Flint, MI 48504

810-732-1120
866-732-1120
fun@thegdl.org
www.thegdl.org/services/talking-book-center

William Delaney, Chair
David Conklin, Director
Amy Goldyn, Finance Manager
Offers Genesee County residents with visual or physical impairments a service allowing them to borrow talking books application through the Talking Book Center.

4751 **Michigan's Assistive Technology Resource**
Physically Impaired Association of Michigan
1023 S Us Highway 27
Saint Johns, MI 48879-2423

989-224-0333
800-274-7426
Fax: 989-224-0330
www.cenmi.org

Jeff Diedrich, Manager
Maryann Jones, Coordinator
Barbara Warren, Information Specialist
Provides information services, support materials, technical assistance, and training to local and intermediate school districts in michigan to increase their capacity to address the needs of students with disabilities for assistive technology.

4752 **Mideastern Michigan Library Co-op**
503 S Saginaw St
Suite 711
Flint, MI 48502

810-232-7119
800-641-6639
Fax: 810-232-6639
dhooks@mmlc.info
www.mmlc.info

Denise Hooks, Director
Irene Bancroft, Administrative Specialist
Provides resources and supports for member libraries in the areas of funding, advocacy, educational opportunities for librarians and networking with other libraries. Its members include Library for the Blind and Physically Handicapped, and Braille and Talking Book Library.

4753 **Muskegon Area District Library for the Blind and Physically Handicapped**
4845 Airline Rd
Unit 5
Muskegon, MI 49444-4503

231-737-6248
877-569-4801
Fax: 231-737-6307
TTY: 231-722-4103
madl.org

Stephen Dix, Director
Richard Schneider, Assistant Director
Brenda Hall, Business Manager
Braille typewriter, magnifiers, closed-circuit TV, large-print photocopier, cassette books and magazines, children's books on cassette, home visits and other reference materials on blindness and other handicaps, The Reading Edge, and large print books.

4754 **Northland Library Cooperative**
Library Cooperative/ Library for the blind
220 W. Clinton St.
Charlevoix, MI 49720

231-855-2206
www.nlc.lib.mi.us

Jennifer Dean, Director
Christine Johnston, Executive Director
Roger Mendel, Director
Summer reading programs, Braille writer, magnifiers, closed-circuit TV, large-print photocopier, cassette books and magazines, children's books on cassette and other reference materials on blindness and other handicaps.

4755 **Oakland County Library for the Visually & Physically Impaired**
1200 N Telegraph Rd
Pontiac, MI 48341-1032

248-858-5050
800-774-4542
Fax: 248-858-1153
TTY: 248-452-2247
www.oakgov.com/lvpi

Dave Conklin, Manager
The Oakland County Library for the Visually and Physically Impaired was established in 1974 to provide access to free library service for County residents who are unable to read standard printed material because of a visual impairment or physical limitation.

4756 St. Clair County Library Special Technologies Alternative Resources (S.T.A.R.)
210 McMorran Blvd
Port Huron, MI 48060-4014   810-982-3600
       800-272-8570
       Fax: 810-982-3600
       TTY: 810-455-0200
       www.sccl.lib.mi.us/LBPH.aspx

Arnold H. Larson, Chairperson
Arlene M. Marcetti, Trustee
Kathleen J. Wheelihan, Trustee
Offers library services to the blind, deaf and blind, visually disabled, phsyically disabled, and reading disabled.

4757 University of Michigan: Orthopaedic Research Laboratories
1500 E. Medical Center Drive
Ann Arbor, MI 48109   734-936-6641
       800-211-8181
       Fax: 734-647-0003
       www.med.umich.edu

Steve Goldstein, Lab Director
Paul Castillo, C.P.A., Chief Financial Officer
Michael ME Johns, M.D., Interim Executive Vice President for Medical Affairs
Develops and studies the causes and treatments for arthritis including new devices and assistive aids.

4758 Upper Peninsula Library for the Blind
1615 Presque Isle Ave
Marquette, MI 49855-2811   906-228-7697
       800-562-8985
       Fax: 906-228-5627
       TTY: 906-228-7697
       webmaster@uproc.lib.mi.us
       www.uplibraries.org

Suzanne Dees, Executive Director
Summer reading programs, braille writer, magnifiers, closed-circuit T.V., large-print photocopier, cassette books and magazines, children's books on cassette, home visits and other reference materials on blindness and other handicaps.

4759 Washtenaw County Library for the Blind & Physically Handicapped
P.O.Box 8645
Ann Arbor, MI 48107-8645   734-222-6860
       Fax: 734-222-6803
       ewashtenaw.org

Mary Udoji, Manager
Michigan Subregional Library, Library of Congress National Library Service network. General library service for persons unable to use standard print materials for various physical reasons. Lends audio books and listening equipment, large type books, descriptive videos. Provides reference information and programs. Kurzweil scanner with components which convert standard print to Braille, large type or audio and closed circuit TV magnifier on site.

4760 Wayne County Regional Library for the Blind
30555 Michigan Ave
Westland, MI 48186-5310   734-727-7300
       888-968-2737
       Fax: 734-727-7333
       TTY: 734-727-7330

Vanessa Morris, Regional Librarian
Sue Steiger, Librarian
Rebecca Farmer, Student Intern
Summer reading programs, braille writer, magnifiers, closed-circuit T.V., large-print photocopier, cassette books and magazines, children's books on cassette, and other reference materials on blindness and other handicaps.

4761 Wayne State University: CS Mott Center for Human Genetics and Development
42. W. Warren Avenue
Detroit, MI 48202-1405   313-577-1485
       Fax: 313-577-8554
       rsokol@med.wayne.edu
       www.media.wayne.edu

Robert Sokol, Director
Matthew Lockwood, Director of Communications
Tom Reynolds, Associate Director of Public Relations
Human growth and development disorders.

Minnesota

4762 Century College
3300 Century Ave North
White Bear Lake, MN 55110-1252   651-779-3300
       800-228-1978
       Fax: 651-779-3417
       TTY: 651-773-1715
       century.edu

Dr. Ron Anderson, President
Steven Ritt, Vice President
Harold M. Johnson, Treasurer
Programs of study - Orthotic Practitioner, Orthotic Technician, Prosethetic Practitioner, Prosthetic Technician. In addition, Century College offers more than 50 other programs in liberal arts, career and occupational programs.

4763 Communication Center/Minnesota State Services for the Blind
Services for the Blind
332 Minnesota Street
Suite 200
Saint Paul, MN 55101-1351   651-642-0500
       800-652-9000
       Fax: 651-649-5927
       DEED.CustomerService@state.mn.us
       www.mnssb.org

Katie Clark Sieben, Commissioner
Brian Allie, Chief Information Officer
Kim Babine, Director Government Affairs
Special library service for the blind and physically handicapped providing tape and Braille transcription of textbooks and vocational materials; Minnesota Radio Talking Book providing current newspaper, magazines and best selling books; Dial-in-News, a touch tone phone accessed newspaper service; Library of Congress cassette and phonograph talking book equipment; repair services for special audio reading equipment, with most services free to Minnesota Residents.

4764 Duluth Public Library
520 W Superior St
Duluth, MN 55802-1578   218-730-4200
       Fax: 218-723-3822
       www.duluth.lib.mn.us

Carla Powers, Library Manager
Renee Zurn, Digital & Outreach Manager
Davis Ouse, Public Services Manager
Main library computer lab contains one Sorenson Relay and accessibility computer with zoom text JAWS software.

4765 Minnesota Library for the Blind and Physically Handicapped
Department of Education
1500 Highway 36 West
Roseville, MN 55113   651-582-8200
       800-722-0550
       Fax: 507-333-4832
       charlene.briner@state.mn.us
       education.state.mn.us

Catherine A. Durivage, Manager
Rene Perrance, Librarian
Charlene Briner, Chief of Staff
Provides books and magazines in Braille, large print, records, and cassettes to qualified residents of Minnesota who have a visual or physical impairment, including reading disabilities due to an organic cause certified by a medical doctor, that prevents residents

from reading standard print or physically handling a book. Equipment for in-house use include magnifiers, braillers, listening equipment, and CCTV. Reference collection for in-house use only on visual impairment topics.

4766 Special U
University of Minnesota
P.O.Box 721-Umhc
Minneapolis, MN 55455
612-625-3846
800-276-8642
Fax: 612-624-0997
kdwb-var@umn.edu

Brings together comprehensive sources of information related to youth with chronic or disabling conditions and their families. Topics include psychosocial issues, disability awareness, developmental processes, family, sexuality, education, employment, independent living, cultural issues, gender issues, service delivery, professional issues, advocacy and legal issues, and health issues. Special focus on transition from childhood to adolesecence to adulthood.

Mississippi

4767 Blind and Physically Handicapped Library Services
Mississippi Library Commission
3881 Eastwood Dr
Jackson, MS 39211-6473
601-432-4492
877-594-5733
Fax: 601-432-4478
mlcref@mlc.lib.ms.us
www.mlc.lib.ms.us

Shellie Zeigler, BPHLS Director
Christy Williams, Director of Administrative Services Bureau
Gloria Washington, Public Relations Director

BPHLS serves as the MS Regional Library for the Library of Congress, NLS for the Blind and Physically Handicapped. Book collections include audio cassette, CDs, digital books, Braille, large print, children's 18-20 point large print, and standard print reference collection. Descriptive videos, magazines in Braille or on cassette are available, as well as equipment: adaptive workstation, Braille embosser, closed-circuit TV, magnifier, speech input/output, and more. Check for eligibility.

4768 Mississippi Library Commission
3881 Eastwood Dr
Jackson, MS 39211-6473
601-432-4111
800-647-7542
Fax: 601-354-4181
TTY: 601-354-6411
mslib@mlc.lib.ms.us
www.mlc.lib.ms.us/index.html

Susan Cassagne, Executive Director
Katherine Buntin, Senior Library Consultant
Tracy Carr, Library Services Bureau Director

Summer reading programs, braille writer, magnifiers, closed-circuit T.V., large-print photocopier, cassette books and magazines, children's books on cassette, home visits and other reference materials on blindness and other handicaps.

4769 Mississippi Library Commission\Talking Book and Braille Services
3881 Eastwood Dr
Jackson, MS 39211-6473
601-432-4111
800-446-0892
Fax: 601-354-4181
mslib@mlc.lib.ms.us

Susan Cassagne, Executive Director
Katherine Buntin, Senior Library Consultant
Tracy Carr, Library Services Bureau Director

Library service for the print handicapped braille, cassette and disc materials (books & periodicals) for children and adults. Large print RG production (copier & printer), braille embosser and other handicaps.

Missouri

4770 Assemblies of God Center for the Blind
1445 N Boonville Ave
Springfield, MO 65802-1894
417-862-2781
855-642-2011
Fax: 417-863-6614
www.blind.ag.org

Paul Weingartner, Director
Caryl Weingartner, Office Administrator
Sarah Sykes, Certified Braille Transcriber

Offers braille and electronic text lending library, Sunday School materials for all ages, braille and audio periodicals, resource assistance, and resources for blind children and children of blind parents. Children's braille books with tactile graphics are also avaiable for purchase or loan, as well as books in digital media for adaptive reading services.

4771 Church of the Nazarene
Nazarene Publishing House
P.O. Box 843116
Kansas City, MO 64184-3116
816-333-7000
800-877-0700
Fax: 800-849-9827
it@nazarene.org
www.nazarene.org

Dr.Eugenio R Duarte, Board of General Superintendents
Dr.Jerry D. Porter, Board of General Superintendents
Dr. David A Busic, Board of General Superintendents

Offers braille and large print books. Also offers a lending library and cassettes for the blind.

4772 Judevine Center for Autism
1333 W Lockwood Avenue
Saint Louis, MO 63132-3252
314-432-6200
800-780-6545
Fax: 888-507-4453
judevine@judevine.org
www.judevine.org

Becky Blackwell, President

Evaluations and assessments, parent and professional training programs, consultations, workshops, seminars, family support, clinical therapies, adult programs and support, residential services.

4773 Lutheran Blind Mission
7550 Watson Rd
Saint Louis, MO 63119-4409
314-918-0415
888-215-2455
Fax: 314-963-0738
blind.mission@blindmission.org

Sherry Lambing, Manager
Dave Andrus, Executive Director
Nancy Crawford, Manager

Offers Christian books in braille and large print books and cassettes for the blind and visually impaired, on loan, as well as Christian periodicals in braille, large print and cassette tape.

4774 University of Missouri: Columbia Arthritis Center
University of Missouri
1 Hospital Dr
Columbia, MO 65212-1
573-882-4141
Fax: 573-884-3996
www.muhealth.org

James Ross, Chief Executive Officer
Mitch Wasden, Chief Operating Officer
Anita Larsen, Chief Nurse Executive

Research into arthritis and rheumatic diseases. One of the most comprehensive health-care networks in Missouri, our 5 hospitals and numerous clinics, all staffed by University Physicians, offer the finest primary, secondary, and tertiary health-care services. We also provide education for future health-care providers and participate in important research.

4775 Wolfner Talking Book & Braille Library
Secretary State Office
600 West Main Street
PO Box 387
Jefferson City, MO 65101-387   573-751-4936
                                      800-392-2614
                                      Fax: 573-526-2985
                                      TTY: 800-347-1379
                                      wolfner@sos.mo.gov
                                      www.sos.mo.gov/wolfner/

Richard J Smith, Division Director
Paul Mathews, Reader Advisor, A-CO
Brandon Kempf, Reader Advisor, CP-G & Wi-Z
Wolfner Library provides reading material for Missouri State residents unable to read standard print due to a visual or physical disability. Book formats are recorded books on digital cartridge and cassette, braille and some childrens books in large print. Wolfner Library also lends out descriptive videos, playback equipment for the cartridges and cassettes are also on loan.

Montana

4776 MonTECH
029 McGill Hall
University of Montana
Missoula, MT 59803   406-243-5751
                                       877-243-5511
                                       montech@ruralinstitute.umt.edu
                                       montech.ruralinstitute.umt.edu

Kathy Laurin PhD, Project Director
Chris Clasby MSW MATP, Project Coordinator
James Poelstra MA, Info Technology Specialist
Specializing in Assistive Technology and oversee a variety of AT related grants and contracts. The overall goal is to develop a comprehensive, statewide system of assistive technology related assistance. Striving to ensure that all people in Montana with disabilities have equitable access to assistive technology devices and services in order to enhance their independence, productivity and quality of life.

4777 Montana State Library-Talking Book Library
1515 East 6th Ave
P.O. Box 201800
Helena, MT 59620-1800   406-444-2064
                                      800-332-5087
                                      Fax: 406-444-0266
                                      TTY: 406-444-4799
                                      mtbl@mt.gov
                                      msl.mt.gov/talking_book_library
Christie Briggs, Regional Librarian/Supervisor
Erin Harris, Director Recording and Volunteer Programs
Carolyn Meier, Library Clerk/Circulation
The Library offers FREE alternative audio and Braille reading materials for Montana citizens who cannot read standard print materials because of a visual, physical or reading handicap. Over 50,000 titles on 4-track cassette, WebBraille, Web0pac, WebBlud, summer reading programs, braille writer, magnifiers, closed-circuit T.V., large-print photocopier, cassette books and magazines, children's books on cassette, home visits and other reference materials on blindness and other handicaps.

Nebraska

4778 Nebraska Assistive Technology Partnership Nebraska Department of Education
Ste C
5143 S 48th St
Lincoln, NE 68516-2261   402-471-0734
                                      888-806-6287
                                      888-806-6287
                                      Fax: 402-471-6052
                                      TTY: 402-471-0734
                                      nlc.nebraska.gov/tbbs/

Steve Miller, Manager
Lilly Blase, Program Coordinator

Provides statewide assistive technology and home modification services for Nebraskans of all ages and disabilities.

4779 Nebraska Library Commission: Talking Book and Braille Service (TBBS)
Talking Book and Braille Service
1200 N St
Suite 120
Lincoln, NE 68508-2023   402-471-4038
                                      800-742-7691
                                      Fax: 402-471-6244
                                      nlc.readadv@nebraska.gov
                                      nlc.nebraska.gov/tbbs

David Oertli, Executive Director
Kay Goehring, Reader Services Coordinator
Bill Ainsley, Audio Production Studio Manager
Provides eligible users with free audio books, audio magazines and Braille via the mail. Also features in-house studios for audiobook production.

Nevada

4780 Las Vegas-Clark County Library District
7060 W. Windmill Lane
Las Vegas, NV 89113   702-734-7323
                                      Fax: 702-507-6187
                                      www.lvccld.org

Keiba Crear, Chair
Michael Saunders, Vice Chair
Randy Ence, Secretary
Summer reading programs, braille writer, magnifiers, closed-circuit T.V., large-print photocopier, cassette books and magazines, children's books on cassette, home visits and other reference materials on blindness and other handicaps.

4781 Nevada State Library and Archives
100 North Stewart Street
Carson City, NV 89701-4285   775-684-3313
                                      800-922-2880
                                      Fax: 775-684-3330

Michael Fischer, Director
Ann Brinkmeyer, Head of Government Publications
Kathy Edwards, Government Publications Libraria
Summer reading programs, braille writer, magnifiers, closed-circuit T.V., large-print photocopier, cassette books and magazines, children's books on cassette, home visits and other reference materials on blindness and other handicaps.

New Hampshire

4782 New Hampshire State Library: Talking Book Services
117 Pleasant St
Concord, NH 03301-3852   603-271-3429
                                      800-491-4200
                                      Fax: 603-271-8370
                                      TTY: 800-735-2964
                                      michael.york@dcr.nh.gov
                                      www.nh.gov/nhsl/talking_books

Michael York, State Librarian
Janet Eklund, Administrator of Library Operations
Donna Gilbreth, Supervisor
Regional Library for National Library Service for the Blind & Physically Handicapped offers digital and cassette books, magazines on cassette, children's books on digital and on cassette, descriptive videos, playaways, and downloadable digital audio books, and Braille services.

New Jersey

4783 Autism New Jersey
500 Horizon Dr.
Suite 530
Robbinsville, NJ 08691   609-588-8200
                                       800-4AU-TISM
                                  Fax: 609-588-8858
                          information@autismnj.org
                                   www.autismnj.org

Suzanne Buchanan, Executive Director
Ellen Schisler, Associate Executive Director
Elena Graziosi, Manager of Information Services
Autism New Jersey is the largest statewide network of parents
and professionals dedicated to improving lives of individuals
with autism spectrum disorders. Self-advocates, families, the
professionals who work with them, government officials, the media, and concerned state residents all turn to Autism New Jersey
for information, compassionate support, and training.

**4784 Children's Specialized Hospital Medical Library - Parent
Resource Center**
200 Somerset St.
New Brunswick, NJ 08901   888-244-5373
                          www.childrens-specialized.org

Warren E. Moore, President & CEO
Charles Chianese, Vice President & Chief Operating Officer
Joseph J. Dobosh Jr., Vice President & Chief Financial Officer
Contains some 3,000 books, and journals specializing in nursing,
pediatrics, child neurology, and rehabilitation. Also provides a
Parent Resource Center, a special collection of books, videos and
pamphlets designed to meet the information needs of parents and
families, as well as the local community.

4785 Christopher & Dana Reeve Foundation
636 Morris Turnpike
Suite 3A
Short Hills, NJ 07078   973-379-2690
                                       800-225-0292
                                  Fax: 973-912-9433
             infospecialist@christopherreeve.org
                          www.christopherreeve.org

John M Hughes, Chairman
John E McConnell, Vice Chairman
Peter Wilderotter, President & CEO
A national clearinghouse for information, referral and educational materials on paralysis. The foundation also offers a free
book titled 'Paralysis Resource Guide' in English or Spanish, as
well as a free library.

4786 Eye Institute of New Jersey
New Jersey Medical School
Suite 6100
PO Box 1709
Newark, NJ 07101-1709   973-972-2065
                                  Fax: 973-972-2068

Jacinta Ogbonna, Administrative director
Department A
Ophthamology, including research into cornea, retina and
neuro-ophthamalogy.

4787 Mycoclonus Research Foundation
Apt 17d
200 Old Palisade Rd
Fort Lee, NJ 7024-7060   201-585-0770
                                  Fax: 201-585-0770
             http://www.pspinformation.com/index.html
Mark Seiden, VP
Supports clinical and basic research into the cause and treatment
of myoclonus; four international workshops facilitated the sharing of information by physicians, scientists, and investigators active in the field, resulted in three publications; supports
promising research projects, clinical neurological fellows, with
special emphasis on posthypoxic myoclonus and encourages all
who are interested in futhering the understanding, treatment, and
cure of myoclonus.

4788 New Jersey Library for the Blind and Handicapped
2300 Stuyvesant Ave
Trenton, NJ 8618-3226   609-530-4000
                                       800-792-8322
                                  Fax: 609-406-7181
                                  TTY: 609-530-4000
                          tbbc@njstatelib.org
                                        njlbh.org

Adam Szczepaniak, Director
Maria Baratta, Assistant Director
Summer reading programs, braille writer, magnifiers, closed-circuit T.V., large-print, cassette, braille books and magazines, children's books on cassette, and other reference materials on
blindness and other handicaps. Provides reading material on audio, cassette, large print and braille to eligible NJ residents.

New Mexico

**4789 New Mexico State Library for the Blind and Physically
Handicapped**
1209 Camino Carlos Rey
Santa Fe, NM 87507-4400   505-476-9700
                                       1 -0 -6 5
                                  Fax: 505-476-9776
                                  TTY: 800-659-4915
                          lbph@state.nm.us
                          www.nmstatelibrary.org

David L. Caffey, Chairperson
Norice Lee, Vice Chairperson
Eugene Gant, Public Education Department Appointee
Summer reading programs, braille writer, magnifiers, closed-circuit T.V., large-print photocopier, cassette books and magazines,
children's books on cassette, home visits and other reference materials on blindness and other handicaps.

New York

4790 Andrew Heiskell Braille and Talking Book Library
New York Public Library
40 W 20th St
New York, NY 10011-4211   212-206-5400
                                  Fax: 212-206-5418
                                  TTY: 212-206-5458
                          ahlbph@nypl.org
                          www.nypl.org/locations/heiskell

Tony Marx, President and CEO
Mary Lee Kennedy, Chief Library Officer
Anne L. Coriston, Vice President for Public Service
The library provides talking books and talking book players to the
five boroughs of New York City, and braille books to New York
City and Long Island. These items may be circulated in person or
through the mail without charge to the borrower. Deposit collections may be arranged with agencies that provide service to people with visual impairments. The library also circulates large
print books and materials in other formats.

4791 Center on Human Policy: School of Education
Syracuse University
302 Huntington Hall
Syracuse, NY 13244   315-443-3851
                                       800-894-0826
                                  Fax: 315-443-4338
                          thechp@syr.edu
                          thechp.syr.edu

Alan Foley, Director
The Center on Human Policy is an organization that works to ensure the rights of people with disabilities. This is accomplished
through research, teaching, and advocacy in policy.

4792 DREAMMS for Kids
190 Whispering Oaks Dr
Longs, SC 29568-6973   607-539-3027
                                  Fax: 607-539-9930
                          janet@dreamms.org
                          www.dreamms.org

Janet Hosmer, Executive Director

DREAMMS is committed to increasing the use of computers, high quality instructional technology, and assistive technologies for students with special needs in schools, homes and the workplace.

4793 Ehrman Medical Library
New York University Medical Center
577 First Avenue
Room 117
New York, NY 10016-6402   212-263-5394
                                      Fax: 212-263-6534
                                 HSL_admin@nyumc.org
                                      hsl.med.nyu.edu

N. Rambo, Chair/Director
D. Peters, Executive Assistant
N. Romanosky, Department Administrator
Our mission of the Fredrick L. Ehrman Library is to enhance learning, research and patient care and New York University Medical Center by effectively managing knowledge-based resources, providing client-centered information services and education, and extending access through new initiatives in information technology.

4794 Finger Lakes Developmental Disabilities Service Office
44 Holland Avenue
Albany, NY 12229-0001   518-474-3625
                                          866-946-9733
                                      Fax: 585-461-8764
                                         opwdd.ny.gov/

Mike Feeney, Director
Carolyn Bassett, Manager
Andrew M Cuomo, Governor
Information on developmental disabilities.

4795 Helen Keller International
Fl 12
352 Park Ave S
New York, NY 10010-1723   212-532-0544
                                          877-535-5374
                                      Fax: 212-532-6014
                                          info@hki.org
                                              hki.org

Henry C. Barkhorn III, Chairman
Desmond G. FitzGerald, Vice Chairman
Mary Crawford, Secretary
Nonprofit international organization whose mission is to combat the causes and consequences of blindness and malnutrition.

4796 Helen Keller National Center for Deaf - Blind Youths And Adults
141 Middle Neck Rd
Sands Point, NY 11050-1218   516-944-8900
                                      Fax: 516-944-7302
                                      TTY: 516-944-8637
                                      hkncinfo@hknc.org
                                          www.hknc.org

Joseph McNulty, Executive Director
HKNC is the only national vocational and rehabilitation program providing services exclusively to youth and adults who are deaf-blind.

4797 Institute for Basic Research in Developmental Disabilities
1050 Forest Hill Rd
Staten Island, NY 10314-6399   718-494-0600
                                      Fax: 718-698-3803
                                       ibr@opwdd.ny.gov
                                          opwdd.ny.gov

Khalid Iqbal, Department Chairman
Joseph J Maturi, Acting Director
Wojciech Kaczmarski, Research Scientist
The Institute for Basic Research in Developmental Disabilities offers services to New Yorkers with developmental disabilities. Services include research, clinical studies, education, publications, employment supports and more.

4798 Institute for Visual Sciences
221 E 71st St
New York, NY 10021-4139   212-517-0400
                                      Fax: 212-472-0295
                                          www.mmm.edu/

Judson R. Shaver, Ph.D., President
Paul Ciraulo, Executive Vice President for Administration and Finance
Carol L Jackson, Vice President for Student Affairs and Dean of Students
Ophthalmology with emphasis on the development of care for the eye.

4799 JGB Cassette Library International
15 W 65th St
New York, NY 10023-6601   212-769-6200
                                          800-284-4422
                                      Fax: 212-769-6266
                                      www.guildhealth.org

Jerry Bechhofer, President
Summer reading programs, braille writer, magnifiers, closed-circuit T.V., large-print photocopier, cassette books and magazines, children's books on cassette, home visits and other reference materials on blindness and other handicaps.

4800 Nassau Library System
900 Jerusalem Ave
Uniondale, NY 11553-3097   516-292-8920
                                      Fax: 516-565-0950
                                 outreach@nassaulibrary.org
                                        nassaulibrary.org

Ken Ulric, President
Barbara Behrens, Vice President
Kathy Seyfried, Treasurer
Information about public library services in Nassau County, including services for people with disabilities and the Senior Connections volunteer project (information and referral for seniors and their families).

4801 National Braille Association
95 Allens Creek Road
95 Allens creek road
Suite 202
Rochester, NY 14618   585-427-8260
                                      Fax: 585-427-0263
                                 nbaoffice@nationalbraille.org
                                      www.nationalbraille.org

David Shaffer, Executive Director
Jan Carroll, President
Cindi Laurent, Vice President
Only national organization dedicated to the professional development of individuals who prepare and produce braille materials.

4802 New York State Talking Book & Braille Library
New York State Library and Education
Cultural Education Center
222 Madison Avenue
Albany, NY 12230-1   518-474-5930
                                          800-342-3688
                                      Fax: 518-474-5786
                                      tbbl@mail.nysed.gov

Loretta Ebert, Research library director
Lends audio and braille books and specialized playback equipment to eligible borrowers with print disabilities. Service is completely free. Serves 55 counties of upstate NY (Westchester and above). Also provides service to schools, nursing homes, and other facilities.

4803 Postgraduate Center for Mental Health
124 E 28th St
New York, NY 10016-8402   212-576-4150
                                      Fax: 212-696-1679
                             www.dvguide.com/newyork/postgrad.html

Marge Slobetz, Assistant Director
Marie Serrano, Manager
Evaluations and psychotherapy by social workers psychologists for children, adolescents, families and couples. Neuropsychological testing and remedation for learning disabilities.

4804 **Rehabilitation Research Library**
Human Resources Center
Albertson, NY 11507
516-741-2010
Fax: 516-746-3298

Amnon Tishler, Research Librarian
Susan Feifer, Manager
Information on rehabilitation and occupational rehabilitation.

4805 **State University of New York Health Sciences Center**
450 Clarkson Avenue
Brooklyn, NY 11203-2098
718-270-1000
Fax: 718-778-5397
www.downstate.edu

Meg O'Sullivan, Assistant Vice President
Jennifer Hayes, Staff Assistant
Child psychiatry research programs.

4806 **Suffolk Cooperative Library System: Long Island Talking Book Library**
Long Island Talking Book Library System
2 Penn Plaza
Suite 1102
New York, NY 10121
212-502-7600
888-545-8331
Fax: 631-286-1647
TTY: 631-286-4546
communications@afb.net
www.afb.org

Carl R Augusto, President & CEO
Kelly Bleach, Chief Administrative Officer
Rick Bozeman, Chief Financial Officer
Offers a variety of support services to its 55 member libraries and other patrons including, an extensive talking book program, assistive technology and other services for people with disabilities.

4807 **United Spinal Association**
75-20 Astoria Blvd
Suite 120
East Elmhurst, NY 11370
718-803-3782
800-444-0120
Fax: 718-803-0414
mkurtz@unitedspinal.org
www.unitedspinal.org

James Weisman, President & CEO
Abby Ross, COO
Information on spinal cord injury and laws and regulations concerning people with disabilities, including veterans.

4808 **Wallace Memorial Library**
Rochester Institute Of Technology
90 Lomb Memorial Dr
Rochester, NY 14623-5603
585-475-2551
Fax: 585-475-7220
TTY: 585-475-2760
twc@rit.edu
wallacecenter.rit.edu

Lynn Wild, Associate Provost for Faculty Development
Shirley Bower, Director RIT Libraries
Julia Lisuzzo, Director of TWC Administration
Information on physical disabilities and deafness.

4809 **Xavier Society for the Blind**
Two Penn Plaza,
Suite 1102
New York, NY 10121-4595
212-473-7800
800-637-9193
Fax: 212-473-7801
info@xaviersocietyfortheblind.org
www.xaviersocietyfortheblind.org
Fr. John Sheehan, SJ, Chairman of the Board / CEO
Fr. Claudio Burgaleta, SJ, Vice-President
Mr. Victor Gainor, Secretary
Provides spiritual and inspirational reading material to visually impaired persons in suitable format: braille, large print and cassette, throughout U.S. and Canada. Services are provided both by way of regular periodical publications sent through the mail and non-returnable; and by means of a lending library where books are returned. All services are provided free.

North Carolina

4810 **Genova Diagnostics**
63 Zillicoa St.
Asheville, NC 28801
828-253-0621
800-522-4762
info@gdx.net
www.gdx.net

Jeffrey Ledford, Chief Executive Officer
Craig Thiel, Chief Financial Officer
Jeff Ellis, Chief Commercial Officer
Genova Diagnostics specializes in nutritional, metabolic, and toxicant analyses. Genova is committed to helping health care professionals identify nutritional influences on health and disease, and laboratory procedures in nutritional and biochemical testing.
1984

4811 **North Carolina Library for the Blind and Physically Handicapped**
109 East Jones Street
Raleigh, NC 27635-1
919-807-7450
888-388-2460
Fax: 919-733-6910
TTY: 919-733-1462
nclbph@ncdcr.gov

Francine Martin, Manager
Carl Ginger Rush, Secretary
James Benton, President
Free loan of large print, braille, and cassette tape books and magazines and specialized playback equipment to registered eligible North Carolinians. Call for an application form. Collection contains general fiction and nonfiction titles. Registered borrowers may subscribe to receive descriptive videos for a one time fee.

4812 **Pediatric Rheumatology Clinic**
Duke Medical Center
P.O.Box 3212
Durham, NC 27708-3212
919-684-8111
Fax: 919-684-6616
rabin001@mc.duke.edu
www.duke.edu

Rebecca H. Buckley, Medical Director
Michael Duke, Owner
Clinical and laboratory pediatric rheumatoid studies.

4813 **University of North Carolina at Chapel Hill: Neuroscience Research Building**
115 Mason Farm Road
Chapel Hill, NC 27599-7250
919-843-8536
Fax: 919-966-9605
www.med.unc.edu/ophth/
Ricky D. Bass, MBA, MHA, Associate Chair for Administration
Sandy Scarlett, Development Director
Cassandra J. Barnhart, MPH, Manager of Research Administration
An interdepartmental research center on the campus of the UNC-Chapel Hill School of Medicine. Mission is to promote neuroscience research with specific emphasis on developmental, cellular, and disease-related processes.

North Dakota

4814 **North Dakota State Library Talking Book Services**
604 E Boulevard Ave
Bismarck, ND 58505-0800
701-328-4622
800-472-2104
Fax: 701-328-2040
TTY: 800-892-8622
ndsl.lib.state.nd.us

Doris Ott, Manager
Hullen E. Bivins, State Lbirarian
Susan Hammer-Schneider, Head Disability Serves
The Talking Books Program provides patrons with free access to cassette books and magazines. The Talking Books Program is administered by the National Library Service for the Blind and Physically Handicapped.

Ohio

4815 Case Western Reserve University
10900 Euclid Ave
Cleveland, OH 44106-4901

216-368-2000
president@case.edu
www.case.edu

Barbara R. Snyder, President
Stanton L. Gerson, MD
W.A. Bud Baeslack, Provost and Executive Vice President
Programs which encompass the arts and sciences, engineering, health sciences, law, management, and social work.

4816 Case Western Reserve University Northeast Ohio Multipurpose Arthritis Center
11100 Euclid Ave
Cleveland, OH 44106-1716

216-844-3969
888-844-8447

Fred Rothstein, Executive Director
Basic and clinical research into the causes, diagnosis and treatment of arthritis.

4817 Cincinnati Children's Hospital Medical Center
University Of Cincinnati Uap
3333 Burnet Ave
Cincinnati, OH 45229-3026

513-636-4200
800-344-2462
Fax: 513-636-2837
TTY: 513-636-4900
www.cincinnatichildrens.org

James Anderson, CEO
James M Anderson, Chief Executive Officer
David Schonfeld, Executive Director
Dedicated to providing the highest level of pediatric care. As Greater Cincinnati's only pediatric hospital, Cincinnati Children's is committed to bringing the very best medical care to children in our community.

4818 Cleveland FES Center
11000 Cedar Ave
Suite 230
Cleveland, OH 44106-3056

216-231-3257
Fax: 216-231-3258
TTY: 216-231-3257
fescenter.case.edu

Robert Kirsch, Executive Director
Peckham P Hunter, Director
Research and development center on functional electrical stimulation. Houses the FES Information Center, a resource center with a library. Publications, newsletters and videotapes for persons with disabilities and others interested in electrical stimulation are offered.

4819 Cleveland Public Library
325 Superior Ave E
Cleveland, OH 44114-1271

216-623-2800
Fax: 216-623-2800
cpl.org

Felton Thomas, Executive Director
Thomas D. Corrigan, President
Maritza Rodriguez, Vice President
Summer reading programs, braille writer, magnifiers, closed-circuit T.V., large-print photocopier, cassette books and magazines, children's books on cassette, and other reference materials on blindness and other handicaps.

4820 Ohio Regional Library for the Blind and Physically Handicapped
National Library Office
800 Vine St
Cincinnati, OH 45202-2009

513-369-6900
800-582-0335
Fax: 513-369-3111
TTY: 516-665-3384
www.cincinnatilibrary.org

Kimber L. Fender, Director
Ross A Wright, President
Paul G Sittenfeld, Vice President
Summer reading programs, braille writer, magnifiers, closed-circuit T.V., large-print photocopier, cassette books and magazines, children's books on cassette, and other reference materials on blindness and other handicaps.

4821 State Library of Ohio: Talking Book Program
National Library Service in Washington
Ste 100
274 E 1st Ave
Columbus, OH 43201-3692

614-644-7061
800-686-1531
Fax: 614-466-3584
library.ohio.gov

Jo Budler, Manager
Jim Buchman, Dir Patron & Catalog Services
Peter Bates, Deputy Director
A machine-lending agency for the visually impaired. Provides free recorded books, and magazines to approximately 26,000 eligible blind, visually impaired, physically handicapped, and reading disabled Ohio residents.

Oklahoma

4822 Oklahoma Library for the Blind & Physically Handicapped
300 NE 18th St
Oklahoma City, OK 73105-3296

405-521-3514
800-523-0288
Fax: 405-521-4582
TTY: 405-521-4672
library@drs.state.ok.us
www.library.state.ok.us

Paul Adams, Library Director
Vicky Golightly, Public Information Officer
Braille writer, magnifiers, closed-circuit T.V., large-print photocopier, cassette books and magazines, children's books on cassette, home visits and other reference materials on blindness and other handicaps.

4823 Oklahoma Medical Research Foundation
825 NE 13th St
Oklahoma City, OK 73104-5097

405-271-6673
800-522-0211
Fax: 405-271-7510
contact@omrf.org
www.omrf.org

Dr. Stephen Prescott, President
Mike D. 'Chip' Morgan, Executive VP and COO
Adam Cohen, Senior VP and General Counsel
Focuses on arthritis and muscoloskeletal disease research.

4824 Tulsa City-County Library System: Outreach Services
Tulsa City: County Library System
400 Civic Centre
Tulsa, OK 74103-3857

918-549-7323
os@tulsalibrary.org
www.tulsalibrary.org

Tracy Warren, Director
Tulsa City-County Library's Outreach Services Department provides library services to individuals that are unable to regularly visit a library, including monthly bookmobile visits and deliveries to residents of senior sites, along with mailing materials to homebound individuals/caretakers residing in their own homes.

Oregon

4825 Oregon Health Sciences University, Elks' Children's Eye Clinic
Casey Eye Institute
3181 S.W. Sam Jackson Park Rd.
Portland, OR 97239-3098

503-494-3000
888-222-8311
Fax: 503-494-4286
www.ohsucasey.com

Earl A Palmer, Director
Eleen Reyster, Clinic Manager
James Rosenbaum, Manager

The elks children's eye clinic is the major charitable project of the Oregon State Elks association. The clinic would not be possible without the organization's dedication and commitment to providing eye care for babies and children.

4826 Oregon Talking Book & Braille Services
250 Winter St NE
Salem, OR 97301-3950   503-378-5389
                              800-452-0292
                         Fax: 503-585-8059
                         TTY: 503-378-4334
www.oregon.gov/OSL/TBABS/Pages/index.aspx
Mary Kay Dahlgreen, Interim State Librarian
Robin Speer, Fund Development Officer
Susan Westin, Program Manager
We serve the blind and physically disabled. Cassette books and magazines, Braille books-magazines, for children and adults. Descriptive videos. Audiocassette machines are provided free of charge. Call us for an application.

4827 Talking Book & Braille Services Oregon State Library
250 Winter St NE
Salem, OR 97301-3950   503-378-5389
                              800-452-0292
                         Fax: 503-585-8059
                         TTY: 503-378-4334
www.oregon.gov/OSL/TBABS/Pages/index.aspx
Mary Kay Dahlgreen, Interim State Librarian
Robin Speer, Fund Development Officer
Susan Westin, Program Manager
Braille writer, magnifiers, large-print photocopier, cassette books and magazines, children's books on cassette and braille books.

Pennsylvania

4828 Associated Services for the Blind and Visually Impaired
ASB
919 Walnut Street
Philadelphia, PA 19107-5237   215-627-0600
                         Fax: 215-922-0692
                         asbinfo@asb.org
                         www.asb.org
Karla S. McCaney, President & CEO
Beth Deering, Chief Program Officer
Sylvia Purnell, Director of Learning & Development
Associated Services for the Blind and Visually Impaired (ASB), is a private, nonprofit organization working to provide services, education, training, and resources to promote self-esteem, independence, and self determination in people who are blind or visually impaired. In addition, ASB advocates for the rights of blind and visually impaired persons through community actions and public education.

4829 Carnegie Library of Pittsburgh Library for the Blind & Physically Handicapped
4400 Forbes Ave
Pittsburgh, PA 15213-4007   412-622-3114
                              800-242-0586
                         Fax: 412-687-2442
                         info@carnegielibrary.org
                         carnegielibrary.org
Cathy Chaparro, Manager
Sue Murdock, Manager
Jane Dayton, Assistant Director
Loans recorded books/magazines and playback equipment, large print books and described videos to western PA residents unable to use standard printed materials due to a visual, physical, or physically-based reading disability.

4830 Free Library of Philadelphia: Library for the Blind and Physically Handicapped
1901 Vine Street
Philadelphia, PA 19103   215-686-5322
                         reardons@freelibrary.org
                         www.library.phila.gov
Tobey Gordon Dichter, Chair
Richard A. Greenawalt, First Vice Chair
Miriam Spector, Vice Chair

Summer reading programs for children and teens. Closed-circuit T.V.for enlarging print for low vision; computers with screen readers and large print; cassette books and magazines; braille books and magazines; and descriptive videos for the blind and visually impaired. Unique and acclaimed adult education program for all disabilities. State of the art book recording facilities.

4831 Pennsylvania College of Optometry Eye Institute
8360 Old York Rd
Elkins Park, PA 19027-1598   215-780-1400
                         Fax: 215-780-1336
Since 1919 the college has led the field in education, in research, and in new approaches to vision diagnosis and correction.

4832 Reading Rehabilitation Hospital
Box 250
Rr 1
Reading, PA 19607   610-796-6297
                         Fax: 610-796-6353
Richard Kruczek, CEO
Doug Mehrkam, Owner
Information on physical disabilities, stroke, head injuries, aging and spinal cord injuries.

Rhode Island

4833 Office Of Library & Information Services for the Blind and Physically Handicapped
1 Capitol Hill
4th Floor
Providence, RI 02908-5803   401-574-9300
                         Fax: 401-574-9320
                         olis.webmaster@olis.ri.gov
                         www.olis.ri.gov
Howard Boksenbaum, Chief Library Officer
Chaichin Chen, Library Program Specialist: LORI
Debbie Cullerton, Information Services Technician:
Offers information and services for the visually impaired including reference materials, braille printers, braille writers, large-print books and more.

4834 Talking Books Plus
Library for the Blind & Physically Handicapped
1 Capitol Hill
4th Floor
Providence, RI 02908-5803   401-574-9300
                         Fax: 401-574-9320
                         olis.webmaster@olis.ri.gov
                         www.olis.ri.gov
Howard Boksenbaum, Chief Library Officer
Chaichin Chen, Library Program Specialist: LORI
Debbie Cullerton, Information Services Technician:
Offers talking book services for the blind and physically handicapped. Collection includes reference materials, braille printer, braille writer, large-print books, adaptive computer workstations and referrals to appropriate agencies/programs for other services.

South Carolina

4835 Medical University of South Carolina Arthritis Clinical/Research Center
171 Ashley Avenue
Charleston, SC 29425-100   843-792-1414
                              800-424-MUSC
                         Fax: 843-792-7121
                         academicdepartments.musc.edu/musc/
Jennie Ariail, Director
Tom Gasque Smith, Associate Director
Dr. David Cole, President
Offers patient care services and basic and clinical research on various types of arthritis and connective tissue diseases.

4836 South Carolina State Library
1500 Senate Street
P.O.Box 11469
Columbia, SC 29211-1469   803-734-8026
Fax: 803-734-4757
reference@statelibrary.sc.gov
statelibrary.sc.gov

Debbie Anderson,, Administrative Coordinator
Flora A. DuBose, Administrative Specialist
Leesa Benggio, Acting Director
Summer reading programs, braille writer, magnifiers, closed-circuit T.V., large-print photocopier, cassette books and magazines, children's books on cassette, home visits and other reference materials on blindness and other handicaps.

South Dakota

4837 South Dakota State Library
800 Governors Dr
Pierre, SD 57501-2294   605-773-3131
800-423-6665
Fax: 605-773-6962
TTY: 605-773-4950
library@state.sd.us
library.sd.gov

Dr. Lesta V. Turchen, President
Monte Loos, Vice President
Sarah Easter, Secretary
Summer reading programs, braille writer, magnifiers, closed-circuit T.V., large-print photocopier, cassette books and magazines, children's books on cassette, home visits and other reference materials on blindness and other handicaps.

Tennessee

4838 Tennessee Library for the Blind and Physically Handicapped
Tennessee State Library Archives
403 7th Ave N
Nashville, TN 37243-1409   615-741-3915
800-342-3308
Fax: 615-532-8856
tlbph.tsla@tn.gov
www.tennessee.gov/tsla/lbph/

Ruth Hemphill, Director
Ed Byrne, Assistant Director
Blake Fontenay, Communications Director
Provides free public library service to residents of Tennessee who are unable to read standard print due to a physical disability. Cooperating library with national network of libraries serving people with print disabilities, operating under the auspices

Texas

4839 Baylor College of Medicine Birth Defects Center
One Baylor Plaza
Houston, TX 77030-2348   713-798-4951
Fax: 832-825-3141
www.bcm.edu/obgyn/tcfs

Frank Greenberg, Director
Dr. Paul Klotman, President
One of the few centers in the world that performs fetal surgery. Provides integrated, multidisciplinary care for mothers, carrying babies with genetic or anatomic birth defects requiring therapy before or immediately after birth. This collaboration enable.

4840 Baylor College of Medicine: Cullen Eye Institute
Baylor College of Medicine
One Baylor Plaza
Houston, TX 77030-2743   713-798-4951
888-562-3937
Fax: 713-798-1521
http://www.bcm.edu/eye/index.cfm?pmid=0

Dan B. Jones, Professor and Chair
Al Vaughan, Manager
Michael Cassidy, Plant Manager
Research activities focus on restoring vision and preventing blindness through a better understanding of the disease.

4841 Brown-Heatly Library
4800 N Lamar Blvd
P O Box 149198
Austin, TX 78756-2316   800-252-5204
800-628-5115
www.dars.state.tx.us

Veronda L. Durden, Commissioner
Glenn Neal, Deputy Commissioner
Daniel Bravo, Chief Operating Officer
Houses a collection of books, audio and video tapes and periodicals focusing on rehabilitation, disabilities, employment skills and practices and management for the Texas Rehabilitation Commission. Houses materials on developmental and other disabilities.

4842 Center for Research on Women with Disabilities
Baylor College of Medicine
One Baylor Plaza
Houston, TX 77030-3411   713-798-5782
800-443-7693
Fax: 713-798-4688
crowd@bcm.tmc.edu
www.bcm.edu/crowd

Kathy Fire, Administrator
Margaret A. Nosek, Executive Director
Martha Mendez, Secretary
Research organization dedicated to conducting research and promoting, developeing, and disseminating information to expand the life choices of women with disabilities. Conducts research and training activities on issues related to the health, independence

4843 Christian Education for the Blind
Suite 702
4200 S Freeway Dr
Fort Worth, TX 76115   817-920-0044
Fax: 817-920-0777
bceb@evl.net

Rodger Dyer, Executive Director
Offers braille and large print books and cassettes for the visually impaired.

4844 Houston Public Library: Access Center
500 McKinney St
Houston, TX 77002-5000   832-393-1313
Fax: 832-393-1474
TTY: 832-393-1539
website@hpl.lib.tx.us
houstonlibrary.org

Rhea Brown Lawson, Director
Roosevelt Weeks, Deputy Director
Greg Simpson, Assistant Director
Offers full library services to the visually and hearing impaired in Houston, TX at no charge. Houses unique and critical services for its users including online access to the Internet in a private and secure area.

4845 Talking Book Program/Texas State Library
Talking Book Program
1201 Brazos St.
PO Box 12927
Austin, TX 78711-2927   512-463-5458
800-252-9605
Fax: 512-936-0685
tbp.services@tsl.state.tx.us
www.texastalkingbooks.org

Ava M Smith, Director

Providing free library service to Texans of all ages who are unable to read standard print material due to visual, physical, or reading disabilities-whether permanent or temporary. The program offers more than 80,000 titles in fiction and nonfiction, plus 80 national magazines for adults and children.

4846 University of Texas Southwestern Medical Center/Allergy & Immunology
5323 Harry Hines Blvd
Dallas, TX 75390-7208   214-648-3111
                                        www.utsouthwestern.edu

Diane Jeffries, Director
Priscilla Alderman, Executive Assistant
Daniel K Podolsky, President
Mission is to improve the health care in our community, Texas, our nation, and the world through innovation and education. To educate the next generation of leaders in patient care, biomedical science and disease prevention. To conduct high-impact, intern

4847 University of Texas at Austin Library
101 E 21st St
Austin, TX 78712-900   512-495-4350
                                        Fax: 512-495-4347
                                        webform@lib.utexas.edu
                                        www.lib.utexas.edu

Douglas Dempster, Manager
Sheldon Ekland-Olson, Chief Executive Officer
Dr. Fred Heath, Vice Provost and Director
Provides access to information for all users, including those with disabilities, in accordance with the overall mission of the General Libraries of the University of Texas at Austin.

Utah

4848 Utah State Library Division: Program for the Blind and Disabled
250 North 1950 West
Suite A
Salt Lake City, UT 84116- 7901   801-715-6789
                                        800-662-5540
                                        Fax: 801-715-6767
                                        TTY: 801-715-6721
                                        blind@utah.gov
                                        www.blindlibrary.utah.gov

Donna Morris, Director
Lisa Nelson, Program Manager
Michael Sweeney, Readers Advisor Librarian
The Program for the Blind and Disabled provides the kinds of materials found in public libraries in formats accessible to the blind and disabled. Books and magazines are available in braille, in large print, on audio cassettes, and on audio digital books. Services are provided by the Utah State Library Division in cooperation with the Library of Congress, National Library Service for the Blind and Physically Handicapped. Services are provided free of charge to eligible readers.

Vermont

4849 National Center for PTSD
VA Medical Center (116D)
215 N Main St
White River Junction, VT 05009   802-296-5132
                                        802-296-6300
                                        Fax: 802-296-5135
                                        ncptsd@va.gov
                                        www.ptsd.va.gov

Paula P Schnurr, PhD, Executive Director
Cybele Merrick, MA, MS, Associate Director for Education
Nancy Bernardy, PhD, Associate Director of Clinical Networking
The National Center for PTSD works to improve care for America's Veterans and others who suffer from trauma or PTSD. The center engages in researchand provides education and training for diagnosis and treatment of the disorder.

4850 Vermont Department of Libraries - Special Services Unit
578 Paine Tpke N
Berlin, VT 05602   802-828-3273
                                        800-479-1711
                                        Fax: 802-828-3109
                                        libraries.vermont.gov/library_for_the_blind
Teresa Faust, Special Services Librarian
Sara Blow, Library Assistant
Jennifer Hart, Librarian
Regional network library pf the National Library Service for the Blind & Physically Handicapped. The SSU makes available reading material in large print and NLS talking book formats, including these special collections: children's print braille books, audio described videos and DVDs.

4851 Vermont Department of Libraries -Special Services Unit
578 Paine Tpke N
Berlin, VT 05602-9139   802-828-3273
                                        800-479-1711
                                        Fax: 802-828-3109
                                        www.libraries.vermont.gov/ssu
Teresa Faust, Special Services Librarian
Sara Blow, Library Assistant
Jennifer Hart, Librarian

Virginia

4852 Access Services
Fairfax County Public Library
12000 Government Center Pkwy
Suite 123
Fairfax, VA 22035-1   703-324-7329
                                        Fax: 703-222-3193
                                        TTY: 703-324-8365
                                        access@fairfaxcounty.gov
                                        fairfaxcounty.gov
Janice Kuch, Branch Manager
Beena Pandey, Volunteer Coordinator
Ken Plummer, Outreach Manager
Offers talking books, TDD access, assistive devices such as decoders for three-week loans, support groups for people who are visually impaired, adapted computer work station with braille printer and assistive listening devices.

4853 Alexandria Library Talking Book Service
5005 Duke St
Alexandria, VA 22304-2903   703-746-1702
                                        Fax: 703-519-5917
                                        TTY: 703-519-5911
                                        www.alexandria.lib.va.us
Rose T. Dawson, Director
Renee DiPilato, Deputy Director
Linda Wesson, Communications Officer
Summer reading programs, braille writer, magnifiers, closed-circuit T.V., large-print photocopier, cassette books and magazines, children's books on cassette, home visits and other reference materials on blindness and other handicaps.

4854 Arlington County Department of Libraries
Arlington County Library
1015 N Quincy St
Arlington, VA 22201-4603   703-228-5990
                                        Fax: 703-228-7720
                                        TTY: 703-228-6320
                                        libraries@arlingtonva.us
                                        arlingtonva.us
Diane Kresh, Director
Margaret Brown, Chief
Anne Gable, Administrative Services/Technology Division Chief
Summer reading programs, braille writer, magnifiers, closed-circuit T.V., large-print photocopier, cassette books and magazines, children's books on cassette, home visits and other reference materials on blindness and other handicaps.

4855 Braille Circulating Library for the Blind
2700 Stuart Ave
Richmond, VA 23220-3305   804-359-3743
                                  Fax: 804-359-4777
                                      bclministries.org

Rev. Brian J Barton, Sr., Executive Director
Offers library materials for the blind and visually impaired on a
free-loan basis. Serves the entire USA and 41 foreign countries
with cassette tapes, reel to reel tapes, braille books, large print
books along with talking book records.

4856 Central Rappahannock Regional Library
1201 Caroline St
Fredericksburg, VA 22401-3701   540-372-1144
                                  Fax: 540-899-9867
                                  TTY: 540-371-9165
                                      webmaster@crrl.org
                                      www.librarypoint.org

Donna Cote, Executive Director
Alison Heartwell, Librarian
Offers reference materials on blindness and other disabilities.

4857 Council for Exceptional Children (CEC)
Council for Exceptional Children
3100 Clarendon Blvd.
Suite 600
Arlington, VA 22201-5332   888-232-7733
                                  TTY: 866-915-5000
                              service@exceptionalchildren.org
                                  www.exceptionalchildren.org

Chad Rummel, Executive Director
Laurie VanderPloeg, Associate Executive Director, Professional Affairs
Craig Evans, Chief Financial Officer
The Council for Exceptional Children aims to improve the educational success of individuals with disabilities and/or gifts and talents by advocating for appropriate policies, setting professional
standards, and providing resources and professional development for special educators.

4858 James Branch Cabell Library
Virginia Commonwealth University
901 Park Avenue
PO Box 842033
Richmond, VA 23284-2033   804-828-1110
                                       866-828-2665
                                       866-828-2665
                                  Fax: 804-828-0151
                                      library@vcu.edu
                                      www.library.vcu.edu

John Birch, Media Specialist II
Wesley Chenault, Head
Yuki Hibben, Assistant Head
Provides individualized orientations and assistance with library
research and equipment.

4859 Newport News Public Library System
2400 Washington Ave
3rd Floor
Newport News, VA 23607- 4301   757-926-8000
                                  Fax: 757-926-1365
                              icieszyn@ci.newport-news.va.us
                                      newportnewsva.com

Thomas P. Herbert, P.E., Chair
Wendy C. Drucker, Vice Chair
Sam Workman, Assistant Director of Development
Summer reading programs, braille writer, magnifiers, closed-circuit T.V., large-print photocopier, cassette books and magazines,
children's books on cassette, home visits and other reference materials on blindness and other handicaps.

**4860 Northern Virginia Resource Center for Deafand Hard of
Hearing Persons**
3951 Pender Dr
Suite 130
Fairfax, VA 22030-6035   703-352-9056
                                  Fax: 703-352-9058
                                  TTY: 703-352-9056
                                      info@nvrc.org
                                      nvrc.org

William Boyd, Chair
Jim Faughnan, Vice Chair
Steve Williams, Treasurer
Empowering deaf and hard of hearing individuals and their fami-
lies through education, advocacy and community involvement.

4861 Roanoke City Public Library System
706 S Jefferson St
Roanoke, VA 24016-5191   540-853-2473
                                  Fax: 540-853-1781
                              main.library@roanokeva.gov
                                  www.roanokegov.com/library

Michael L. Ramsey, President
Barbara Lemon, Vice President
Summer reading programs, braille writer, magnifiers, closed-circuit T.V., large-print photocopier, cassette books and magazines,
children's books on cassette, home visits and other reference materials on blindness and other handicaps.

4862 Staunton Public Library Talking Book Center
1 Churchville Ave
Staunton, VA 24401-3229   540-885-6215
                                       800-995-6215
                                  Fax: 540-332-3906
                                      www.talkingbookcenter.org

Lisa Eye, Reader Advisor
Lynn Harris, President
Daniel Swift, Treasurer
Offers free library service by circulating recorded books, maga-
zines, and playback equipment to individuals unable to use stan-
dard print materials because of visual or physical impairment.

**4863 University of Virginia Health System General Clinical
Research Group**
P.O.Box 800787
Charlottesville, VA 22908-0787   434-924-2394
                                  Fax: 434-924-9960
                                      gcrc.med.virginia.edu

Pamela Sprouse, Administrator
Eugene J. Barrett, Program Director
Mary Lee Vance, Associate Director
Provides investigators with the specialized resources necessary
to conduct advanced clinical research. The facility includes ten
inpatient beds, skilled research nurses, a core assay laboratory, a
metabolic kitchen, outpatient facilities, computing and st

4864 Virginia Autism Resource Center
4100 Price Club Blvd
PO Box 842020
Richmond, Virginia, VA 23284-2020   804-674-8888
                                       877-667-7771
                                          877- -
                                  Fax: 804-276-3970
                                      www.varc.org

Carol Schall, Ph.D., Director
Florence McLeod, Administrative Assistant
Dawn Hendricks, Ph.D., Faculty/instructor
VARC promotes and facilitates best practices for those diagnosed
within the autism spectrum. Information, resources, and education and training help parents, educators, service providers and
medical professionals provide effective support from early
childhood through adulthood.

4865 Virginia Beach Public Library Special Services Library
936 Independence Blvd
Virginia Beach, VA 23455-6006   757-385-2680
                                  Fax: 757-464-6741
                                      spaddock@vbgov.com
                                      www.vbgov.com/dept/library

Marcy Sims, Library Director
David Palmer, Public Services Manager
Susan Paddock, Library Manager

A public library for people with visual and physical disabilities, braille writer, magnifiers, closed-circuit T.V., large-print photocopier, cassette books and magazines, children's books on cassette, and other reference materials on blindness and other d

4866 Virginia Chapter of the Arthtitis Foundation
2201 W. Broad St
Suite 100
Richmond, VA 23220-3937
800-365-3811
800-456-4687
Fax: 804-359-4900
cmogel@arthritis.org
www.arthritis.org/virginia

Gail Norman, Interim President/CEO
Terri Harris, Chief Financial Officer
Nick Turvas, Senior VP of Health/Wellness
Provides free information, services and counseling to the public. Services include assistance in locating and accessing government and other health care programs for persons with arthritis, referral to doctors specializing in the treatment of arthritis,

4867 Virginia State Library for the Visually and Physically Handicapped
395 Azalea Ave
Richmond, VA 23227-3623
804-266-2477
800-552-7015
Fax: 804-266-2478
virginiavoice.org

Paula I. Otto, President
Susan C. Rucker, Secretary/Treasurer
Nicholas B Morgan, Executive Director
Summer reading programs, braille writer, magnifiers, closed-circuit T.V., large-print photocopier, cassette books and magazines, children's books on cassette, home visits and other reference materials on blindness and other handicaps.

Washington

4868 Meridian Valley Clinical Laboratory
801 SW 16th St
Suite 126
Renton, WA 98057-2632
425-271-8689
855-405-8378
Fax: 425-271-8674
meridian@meridianvalleylab.com
www.meridianvalleylab.com
Dr. Jonathan Wright, Medical Director
A clinical test facility dedicated to providing the most accurate and informative data for patient diagnosis and therapeutic monitoring. With our current research and up-to-date information and various aspects of clinical nutritional medicine, our methodo

4869 Ophthalmic Research Laboratory Eye Institute/First Hill Campus
747 Broadway
Seattle, WA 98122-4307
206-386-6000
800-833-8879
TTY: 206-386-2022
www.swedish.org

Bryan Mueller, CEO
Dan Harris, CFO
Heidi Aylsworth, Chief Strategy Officer
Color vision physiology, vision disorders and blindness research.

4870 Washington Talking Book and Braille Library
2021 9th Ave
Seattle, WA 98121-2783
206-615-0400
800-542-0866
Fax: 206-615-0437
TTY: 206-615-0418
wtbbl@sos.wa.gov
wtbbl.org

Danielle Miller, Director and Regional Librarian
Amy Ravenholt, Assistant Program Manager
Mandy Gonnsen, Youth Services Librarian
Summer reading programs, braille writer, magnifiers, closed-circuit T.V., large-print photocopier, cassette books and magazines,

children's books, and other reference materials on blindness and other handicaps, online catalog, reference station with assis

West Virginia

4871 Cabell County Public Library/Talking Book Department/Subregional Library for the Blind
455 9th St
Huntington, WV 25701-1417
304-528-5700
Fax: 304-528-5739
cabell.lib.wv.us

Judy K. Rule, Director
Angela Straight, Assistant Director
Mary Lou Pratt, Adult Services Coordinator
Summer reading programs, Braille writer, magnifiers, closed-circuit TV, cassette books and magazines, children's books on cassette reference materials on blindness and other handicaps, enlargers and Arkenstone Reader.

4872 Division of Rehabilitation Services: Staff Library
107 Capitol St
Charleston, WV 25301-2609
304-356-2060
800-642-8207
Fax: 304-766-4913
wvdrs.org

Carol Johnson, Manager
Specialized library with information on disabilities and the rehabilitation there of special collections: deaf and hard of hearing, visually impaired/blind, wellness center, literacy and career. The library has assistive devices such as CCTV, scanner and

4873 Kanawha County Public Library
123 Capitol St
Charleston, WV 25301-2686
304-343-4646
Fax: 304-348-6530
kanawha.lib.wv.us

Cheryl Morgan, President
Jennifer Pauer, First Vice President
Elizabeth O. Lord, Second Vice President
Summer reading programs, large print PC option, magnifiers, large type books, cassette books, and magazines, children's books on cassette, home visits and other reference materials on blindness and other handicaps

4874 Ohio County Public Library Services for the Blind and Physically Handicapped
52 16th St
Wheeling, WV 26003-3671
304-232-0244
Fax: 304-232-6848
wheeling.weirton.lib.wv.us

Jimmie McCamic, Chairman
Michael Baker, Secretary-Treasurer
Greg Marquart, Trustee
The Ohio Public Library exists to provide books and related materials that will assist the residents of the community in the pursuit of knowledge, information, education, research, and recreation in order to promote an enlightned citizenry and to enrich t

4875 Talking Book Department, Parkersburg and Wood County Public Library
3100 Emerson Ave
Parkersburg, WV 26104-2414
304-420-4587
Fax: 304-420-4589
Lindsay Place, Talking Books Dept. Coordinator
Brian Raitz, Director
Free program loaning recorded books and magazines, braille books and magazines to people who are unable to read or use standard print due to a visual or physical impairment.

4876 **West Virginia Autism Training Center**
Marshall University College Of Educational & Human
Old Main 316
1 John Marshall Drive
Huntington, WV 25755-1   304-696-2332
                                                       800-344-5115
                                                  Fax: 304-696-2846
                                                  www.marshall.edu/atc/
Amanda Plumley, Executive Office Manager
Ginny Painter, Communications Director
Joe Ciccarello, Associate Executive Director
Provides education, training, and treatment programs for W Virginians who have autism, pervasive devolopmental disorders or Asperger's disease and have formally been registered with the center.

4877 **West Virginia Library Commission**
1900 Kanawha Blvd E
Charleston, WV 25305-9   304-558-2041
                                                       800-642-9021
                                                  Fax: 304-558-2044
                                                  www.librarycommission.wv.gov
Karen Goff, Secretary
Deborah McNeal, Personnel Officer
Steve Tyler, Supervisor
Summer reading programs, braille writer, magnifiers, closed-circuit T.V., large-print photocopier, cassette books and magazines, children's books on cassette, home visits and other reference materials on blindness and other handicaps.

4878 **West Virginia School for the Blind Library**
301 E Main St
Romney, WV 26757-1828   304-822-4840
                                                  Fax: 304-822-3370
                                                  cjohn@access.mountain.net
                                                  wvde.state.wv.us
Patsy Shank, Administrator
Cynthia Johnson, Librarian
Summer reading programs, braille writer, magnifiers, closed-circuit T.V., large-print photocopier, cassette books and magazines, children's books on cassette, home visits and other reference materials on blindness and other handicaps.

Wisconsin

4879 **Brown County Library**
Central Library Downtown
515 Pine Street
Green Bay, WI 54301-3743   920-448-4400
                                                  Fax: 920-448-4376
                                                  TTY: 920-448-4400
                                                  bc_library@co.brown.wi.us
                                                  www.co.brown.wi.us/library
Terry Watermelon, President
Kathy Pletcher, Vice President
Carla Buboltz, Secretary
Summer reading programs, braille writer, magnifiers, closed-circuit TV, large-print photocopier, cassette books and magazines, children's books on cassette, home visits and other reference materials on blindness and other handicaps.

4880 **Eye Institute of the Medical College of Wisconsin and Froedtert Clinic**
925 N 87th St
Milwaukee, WI 53226-4812   414-456-2020
                                                  Fax: 414-456-6300
                                                  eyecare@mcw.edu
                                                  doctor.mcw.edu
Jane D Kivlin, Director
Richard Schultz, MD, Director
A national leader as a full-service academic opthalmology program. Dedicated to the highest quality patient care, education, and vision research, the faculty and staff strive to provide state-of-the-art clinical and surgical patient care in a compassionat

4881 **Wisconsin Regional Library for the Blind& Physically Handicapped**
813 W Wells St
Milwaukee, WI 53233-1436   414-286-3045
                                                       800-242-8822
                                                  Fax: 414-286-3102
                                                  TTY: 414-286-3548
                                                  lbph@mpl.org
Marsha J Valance, Manager
Meredith Wittmann, Regional Librarian
Circulates recorded materials, playback equipment and braille materials to print-handicapped Wisconsin residents.

Wyoming

4882 **Wyoming Services for the Visually Impaired**
Wyoming Department of Education
2300 Capitol Ave
Cheyenne, WY 82002-0050   307-777-7690
                                                  Fax: 307-777-6234
                                                  jackie.miller@wyo.gov
                                                  edu.wyoming.gov/in-the-classroom/special-prog
Ron Micheli, Chairman
Scotty Ratliff, Vice-Chair
Pete Ratliff, Treasurer
Services for the Visually Impaired assists people of all ages who have low vision or are blind. The goal is to provide information, education, and support to individuals with low vision in order that they may lead enjoyable and productive lives with maxim

4883 **Wyoming's New Options in Technology(WYNOT) - University of Wyoming**
1000 E University Ave
Laramie, WY 82071-2000   307-766-2761
                                                       888-989-9463
                                                  Fax: 307-766-2763
                                                  TTY: 800-908-7011
                                                  wind.uw@uwyo.edu
                                                  wind.uwyo.edu/wynot
William MacLean Jr., Ph.D., Executive Director
Designed to develop and implement a consumer oriented statewide system of technology-related assistance for people with disabilities of all ages.

Media, Print

Children & Young Adults

4884 Assistive Technology for Infants and Toddlers with Disabilities Handbook
Idaho Assistive Technology Project
University of Idaho
1187 Alturas Dr.
Moscow, ID 83843- 2268

800-432-8324
Fax: 208-885-6102
idahoat@uidaho.edu
www.idahoat.org

LaRae Rhoads, Author
Ron Seiler, Author
This handbook is designed as a guide for parents and families in Idaho who have infants and toddlers with developmental delays or disabilities.

4885 Assistive Technology for School-Age Children with Disabilities - Handbook
Idaho Assistive Technology Project
University of Idaho
1187 Alturas Dr.
Moscow, ID 83843- 2268

208-885-3557
800-432-8324
Fax: 208-885-6102
idahoat@uidaho.edu
www.idahoat.org

LaRae Rhoads, Author
Ron Seiler, Author
Michelle Doty, Author
A handbook designed to provide guidance and information for parentswho have school-aged children with disabilities, focusing on resources for assistive technologies available for their children.

4886 Children's Understanding of Disability
Routledge (Taylor & Francis Group)
711 Third Ave.
New York, NY 10017

212-216-7800
800-634-7064
Fax: 202-564-7854
enquiries@taylorandfrancis.com
www.routledge.com

Ann Lewis, Author
Children's Understanding of Disability is a valuable addition to the debate surrounding the integration of children with special needs into ordinary schools. Taking the viewpoint of the children themselves, it explores how pupils with severe learning difficulties and their non-disabled classmates interact.Ann Lewis examines what happens when non-disabled children and pupils with severe learning difficulties work together regularly over the course of a year.
Hardcover

4887 Complete IEP Guide: How to Advocate for Your Special Ed Child (8th Edition)
NOLO (Internet Brands)
909 N. Sepulveda Blvd
11th Fl.
El Segundo, CA 90245

310-280-4000
www.nolo.com

Lawrence Siegel, Attorney/Author
This all-in-one guide will help you understand special education law, identify your child's needs, prepare for meetings, develop the IEP and resolve disputes.
384 pages

4888 Don't Call Me Special: A First Look at Disability
Barron's Educational Series
250 Wireless Blvd
Hauppauge, NY 11788

800-645-3476
Fax: 631-494-3723
barrons@barronseduc.com
www.barronseduc.com

Pat Thomas, Author
This picture book explores questions and concerns about physical disabilities in a simple and reassuring way. Youger children can find out about individual disabilities, special equipment that is available to help the disabled, and how people of all ages can deal with disabilities and live happy and full lives.
Paperback

4889 Everything Parent's Guide to Special Education
Adams Media
4868 Innovation Dr
Bldg 2
Fort Collins, CO 80525

855-278-0402
www.adamsmediastore.com

Amanda Morin, Author
This handbook offers parents assistance, advice, and aid on navigating special education for their child, with information on assessment, evaluation, specific needs for specific disabilities, current law, and dealing with parent-school conflict. It includes worksheets, forms, and sample documents to help parents be effective advocates for their child's learning.

4890 It isn't Fair!: Siblings of Children with Disabilities
Praeger - ABC-CLIO
130 Cremona Dr
Santa Barbara, CA 93117

805-968-1911
800-368-6868
Fax: 866-270-3856
CustomerService@abc-clio.com
www.abc-clio.com/praeger

Stanley D. Klein, Editor
Maxwell J. Schleifer, Editor
This book presents a wide range of perspectives on the relationship of siblings to children with disabilities. These perspectives are written in the first person by parents, young adult siblings, younger siblings, and professionals.
200 pages

4891 Life Beyond the Classroom: Transition Strategies for Young People with Disabilities
Brookes Publishing
P.O.Box 10624
Baltimore, MD 21285-0624

410-337-9580
800-638-3775
Fax: 410-337-8539
custserv@brookespublishing.com
www.brookespublishing.com

Paul Wehman, Author
This textbook is an essential guide to planning, designing, and implementing successful transition programs for students with disabilities.
616 pages

4892 Mayor of the West Side
Fanlight Productions
32 Court St
21st Fl.
Brooklyn, NY 11201

718-488-8900
800-876-1710
Fax: 718-488-8642
info@fanlight.com
www.fanlight.com

Judd Ehrlich, Director
What happens when love gets in the way of letting go? As a teenager with multiple disabilities prepares for his Bar Mitzvah, his family and community consider what Mark's life will be like when they are no longer able to protect him.

4893 New Horizons Independent Living Center
8085 E Manley Dr
Prescott Valley, AZ 86314-6154

928-772-1266
800-406-2377
Fax: 928-772-3808
TTY: 928-772-1266
www.nhilc.org

Gale Dean, Executive Director
Alan Loosley, President
Sharon Geddes, Vice President
The mission of New Horizons Independent Living Center is to provide programs and services in Northern Arizona which encourage and empower people with disabilities to self-determine the goals and activities of their lives.

4894 Rolling Along with Goldilocks and the Three Bears
Woodbine House
6510 Bells Mill Rd
Bethesda, MD 20817   800-843-7323
                                    info@woodbinehouse.com
                                    www.woodbinehouse.com
Cindy Meyers, Author
Carol Morgan, Illustrator
The familiar fairytale with a special needs twist. Ages 3-7.
28 pages

4895 Shriner's Hospitals for Children Newsletter
3101 SW Sam Jackson Park Rd
Portland, OR 97201   503-241-5090
                                    Fax: 503-221-3498
                        www.shrinershospitalforchildren.org
Bi-annual publication from the Shriners Hospital for Children in
Portland, Oregon. Free. Produced by the medical staff.

4896 Sibling Forum: A FRA Newsletter
Family Resource Associates
35 Haddon Ave
Shrewsbury, NJ 07702-4007   732-747-5310
                                    Fax: 732-747-1896
                                    info@frainc.org
                                    www.frainc.org
A newsletter for brothers and sisters, aged 10 through teen, whose
sibling has a disablilty. Includes input from readers, library re-
sources and discussion of feelings. $12/year for families,
$20/year for professionals.
Quarterly

**4897 Sibshops: Workshops for Siblings of Children with
Special Needs**
Sibling Supporting Project
322-6512 23rd Ave NW
Seattle, WA 98117   206-297-6368
                                    info@siblingsupport.org
                                    www.siblingsupport.org
Don Meyer, Author
Patricia Vadasy, Author
Sibshops is a program that brings together 8-to 13-year-old broth-
ers and sisters of children with special needs. The siblings receive
support and information in a recreational setting, so they have fun
while they learn.
264 pages

4898 Special Education Report
LRP Publications
360 Hiatt Dr
Dept. 150F
Palm Beach Gardens, FL 33418   800-341-7874
                                    Fax: 561-622-2423
                                    custserv@lrp.com
                                    www.lrp.com
Published monthly, Special Education Report is the independent
news service on law, policy and funding of programs for disabled
children.
Monthly Newsletter

4899 Special Format Books for Children and Youth Ages 3-19
New York State Talking Book and Braille Library
Cultural Education Center
222 Madison Ave
Albany, NY 12230-0001   518-474-5935
                                    800-342-3688
                                    Fax: 518-474-7041
                                    tbbl@nysed.gov
                        www.nysl.nysed.gov/tbbl/index.html
The New York State Talking Book and Braille Library (TBBL)
lends audio and braille books and magazines to eligible residents
of upstate New York who have a qualifying print disability.

**4900 The Sibling Slam Book: What It's Really Like To Have a
Brother or Sister with Special Needs**
Sibling Support Project
6512 23rd Ave NW
Ste 322
Seattle, WA 98117   206-297-6368
                                    info@siblingsupport.org
                                    www.siblingsupport.org
Don Meyer, Author
A brutally honest, non-PC look at the lives, experiences, and
opinions of siblings without disabilities who have siblings with
disabilities. Formatted like the slam books passed around in many
junior high and high schools, this one poses a series of 50 personal questions, with responses drawn from the author's interviews with over 80 teens from across the United States. It reflects
experiences that range from positive to negative.

4901 The Sibling Survival Guide
Sibling Support Project
6512 23rd Ave. NW
Ste 322
Seattle, WA 98117   206-297-6368
                                    info@siblingsupport.org
                                    www.siblingsupport.org
Don Meyer, Author
Emily Holl, Author
Edited by experts in the field of disabilities and sibling relation-
ships, The Sibling Survival Guide focuses on the topmost con-
cerns identified in a survey of hundreds of siblings.

4902 Views from Our Shoes
Sibling Support Project
6512 23rd Ave NW
Ste 322
Seattle, WA 98117   206-297-6368
                                    www.siblingsupport.org
Don Meyer, Author
Siblings share what it is like to have a brother or sister with a dis-
ability. Age 9 and up.
106 pages Paperback

**4903 What About Me? Growing Up with a Developmentally
Disabled Sibling**
Da Capo Press/ Perseus Books Group
Order Department
210 American Dr
Jackson, TN 38301   800-343-4499
                                    Fax: 800-351-5073
                        www.perseusbooksgroup.com
Bryna Siegel, Author
Stuart Silverstein, Author
A compassionate and accessible guide on living with and caring
for a developmentally disabled sibling.
316 pages Paperback

4904 What It's Like to be Me
Friendship Press
P.O.Box 37844
Cincinnati, OH 45222-844   513-948-8733
                                    Fax: 513-761-3722
This was written and illustrated entirely by children with handicapped conditions. These contributions invite the reader to set
aside any pity or prejudices and listen. Black and white, and color
drawings and photographs make this book visually appealing, enjoyable for all ages.

Community

4905 'Cultural Life,' Disability, Inclusion, and Citizenship: Moving Beyond Leisure in Isolation
Routledge (Taylor & Francis Group)
711 Third Ave
New York, NY 10017
212-216-7800
800-634-7064
Fax: 202-564-7854
enquiries@taylorandfrancis.com
www.routledge.com

Simon Darcy, Editor
Jerome Singleton, Editor
This book concentrates on disability citizenship in leisure.
90 pages Hardback

4906 Active Citizenship and Disability: Implementing the Personalization of Support
Cambridge University Press
Shaftesbury Rd
Cambridge, UK CB2-8BS
information@cambridge.org
www.cambridge.org

Andrew Power, Author
Janet E. Lord, Author
Allison S. DeFranco, Author
This book provides an international comparative study of the implementation of disability rights law and policy focused on the emerging principles of self-determination and personalisation. The case studies examine how different jurisdictions have reformed disability law and policy and reconfigured how support is administered and funded to ensure maximum choice and independence is accorded to people with disabilities.
518 pages Paperback; Hardcover

4907 California Community Care News
Community Residential Care Association of CA
1924 Alhambra Blvd
P.O. Box 163270
Sacramento, CA 95816-9270
916-455-0723
Fax: 916-455-7201
www.crcac.com

Charles W Skoien Jr, Director/Lobbyist
Denise Johnson, Consultant
Forum for the exchange of ideas, information and opinions among clients, families and service providers. Information regarding services and assisted living programs for the elderly, mentally ill and disabled.
Monthly

4908 Community Disability Services: An Evidence-Based Approach to Practice
Purdue University Press
Stewart Center 190
504 W State St
West Lafayette, IN 47907-2058
265-494-2038
pupress@purdue.edu
www.thepress.purdue.edu

Ian Dempsey, Editor
Karen Nankervis, Editor
Articles by an array of international experts provide as an excellent resource for professionals and students involved in the area of disability studies. The book is divided into three parts: (1) disability and modern society; (2) working with people who are challenged; and (3) working within a disability-services environment. This approach mirrors the contemporary debate within a practice framework reflecting how individuals, organizations, and communities deal with the problem and solutions.
304 pages Paperback

4909 Comprehensive Care Coordination for Chronically Ill Adults
Wiley-Blackwell
111 River St
Hoboken, NJ 07030-5774
201-748-6000
877-762-2974
Fax: 201-748-6088
info@wiley.com
www.wiley.com

Cheryl Schraeder, Editor
Paul S. Shelton, Editor
A combination of theory and case studies, this book presents the growing demographic of chronically ill adults in the U.S., offering models for change and improvement in quality of care; recommendations on relevant and current literature; and descriptions of successful care outcomes.
440 pages Paperback

4910 Hallmarks and Features of High-Quality Community-Based Services
Independent Living Research Utilization (ILRU)
1333 Moursund
Houston, TX 77030
713-520-0232
Fax: 713-520-5785
ilru@ilru.org
ilru.org

This brief paper describes and expands on five hallmarks that are felt to greatly impact the quality of community-based services. While this list of qualities is neither exhaustive nor comprehensive, it does draw from the findings and insights of professionals in community building, and aims to inform readers of those areas that are considered to be of vital importance to high-quality experience of community services.

4911 Human Exceptionality: School, Community, and Family (12th Edition)
Cengage Learning
20 Channel Center St
Boston, MA 02210
617-289-7700
Fax: 617-289-7844
www.cengage.com/us

Michael L. Hardman, Author
M. Winston Egan, Author
Clifford J. Drew, Author
An evidence-based testament to the critical role of cross-professional collaboration in enhancing the lives of exceptional individuals and their families. This text's unique lifespan approach combines powerful research, evidence-based practices, and inspiring stories, engendering passion and empathy and enhancing the lives of individuals with exceptionalities.
544 pages Hardcover

4912 Inclusive Leisure Services (3rd Edition)
Venture Publishing Inc.
1999 Cato Ave
State College, PA 16801
814-234-4561
Fax: 814-234-1651
www.venturepublish.com

John Dattilo, Author
This text will educate future and current leisure services professionals about attitude development and actions that promote positive attitudes about people who have experienced discrimination and segregation. It provides strategies that will facilitate meaningful leisure participation by all participants, while respecting their rights.
560 pages Hardcover

4913 Independent Living for Persons with Disabilities and Elderly People
IOS Press
6751 Tepper Dr
Clifton, VA 20124
703-830-6300
Fax: 703-830-2300
sales@iospress.com
www.iospress.nl

Mounir Mokhtari, Editor
Discusses the need for assistive technology in making homes more accessible for the elderly and people with disabilities. Goes on to suggest the application of these technologies in other areas of the community, such as hospitals and schools, which allow

those with disabilities and the elderly to live their lives with some independence and autonomy.
216 pages Softcover

4914   Independent Living for Physically Disabled People
People With Disabilities Press (iUniverse)
1663 Liberty Dr
Bloomington, IN 47403   812-330-2909
                                             800-288-4677
                                             Fax: 812-355-4085
                                             media@iuniverse.com
                                             www.iuniverse.com

Nancy M. Crewe, Author
Irving Kenneth Zola, Author
This book describes the philosophy of independent living, from legislative strides to community centres, as well as future trends.
436 pages

4915   Pathways To Inclusion (2nd Edition)
Captus Press
1600 Steeles Ave W
Concord, ON, Canada L4K-4M2   416-736-5537
                                             Fax: 416-736-5793
                                             info@captus.com
                                             www.captus.com

John Lord, Author
Peggy Hutchison, Author
Pathways to Inclusion 2nd edition addresses the organizational strategies that have been used in the past and highlights areas for change. Human service organizations are examined, pinpointing common characteristics that have led to improved quality of life for people with disabilities and other vulnerable citizens.
328 pages Paperback

Employment

4916   A Supported Employment Workbook: Individual Profiling and Job Matching
Jessica Kingsley Publishers
73 Collier St
London, UK N19BE   hello@jkp.com
                                             www.jkp.com

Steve Leach, Author
Created with the goal of helping job developers, this guide offers practical tools and strategies to help job development professionals assist their clients. The workbook includes vocational forms, job analysis forms, and support review charts, and offers aid to professionals in assisting disabled persons to find and secure stable jobs in their communities.
224 pages Paperback

4917   Career Success for Disabled High-Flyers
Jessica Kingsley Publishers
73 Collier St
London, UK N19BE   hello@jkp.com
                                             www.jkp.com

Sonali Shah, Author
Drawing on case studies of 31 disabled adults, this book suggests that individual traits and patterns of behaviour are key factors in career success, and shows that it is often society rather than impairment that hinders professional progression. It will provide role models and valuable insights for young career-minded disabled people.
208 pages Paperback

4918   Job Success for Persons with Developmental Disabilities
Jessica Kingsley Publishers
73 Collier St
London, UK N19BE   hello@jkp.com
                                             www.jkp.com

David B. Wiegan, Author
This book provides a comprehensive approach to developing a successful jobs program for persons with developmental disabilities, drawn from the author's extensive experience and real success.
160 pages Paperback

4919   Making News: How to Get News Coverage of Disability Rights Issues
The Advocado Press
                                             contact145@advocadopress.org
                                             www.advocadopress.org
Book gives how-to information on influencing media coverage of disability issues.
165 pages

4920   Making Self-Employment Work for People with Disabilities
Brookes Publishing
P.O.Box 10624
Baltimore, MD 21285-0624   410-337-9580
                                             800-638-3775
                                             Fax: 410-337-8539
                                             custserv@brookespublishing.com
                                             www.brookespublishing.com

Cary Griffin, Author
David Hammis, Author
Beth Keeton, Author
Practical support for individuals with significant disabilities in starting and maintaining a small business. Covers building a business plan; pinpointing interests, strengths, and goals; and finding helpful information and support
288 pages

4921   Road Ahead: Transition to Adult Life for Persons with Disabilities (3rd Edition)
IOS Press
6751 Tepper Dr
Clifton, VA 20124   703-830-6300
                                             Fax: 703-830-2300
                                             sales@iospress.com
                                             www.iospress.nl

Keith Storey, Editor
Dawn Hunter, Editor
Explores transition planning, assessment, instructional strategies, career development and support, social life, quality of life, supported living, and post-secondary education for people with disabilities.
318 pages

4922   The Job Developer's Handbook: Practical Tactics for Customized Employment
Brookes Publishing
P.O. Box 10624
Baltimore, MD 21285-0624   410-337-9580
                                             800-638-3775
                                             Fax: 410-337-8539
                                             custserv@brookespublishing.com
                                             www.brookespublishing.com

Cary Griffin, Author
David Hammis, Author
Tammara Geary, Author
One of the most practical employment books available, this forward-thinking guide walks employment specialists step by step through customized job development for people with disabilities, revealing the best ways to build a satisfying, meaningful job around a person's preferences, skills, and goals.
264 pages

General Disabilities

4923   A Guide to Disability Rights Laws
US Department of Justice
950 Pennsylvania Ave. NW
9th Floor
Washington, DC 20530   202-307-0663
                                             800-514-0301
                                             Fax: 202-307-1197
                                             TTY: 800-514-0383
                                             www.ada.gov

Rebecca B. Bond, Chief
Anne Raish, Principal Deputy Chief
Christina Galindo-Walsh, Deputy Chief

A 21-page booklet providing a brief description of the ADA, the Telecommunications Act, Fair Housing Act, Air Carrier Access Act, Voting Accessibility for the Elderly and Handicapped Act, National Voter Registration Act, Civil Rights of Institutionalized Persons Act, Individuals with Disabilities in Education Act, Rehabilitation Act, Architectural Barriers Act, and the federal agencies to contact for more information.
Available in Large Print & Braille

4924   A Practical Guide to Art Therapy Groups
Routledge (Taylor & Francis Group)
711 Third Ave
New York, NY 10017
212-216-7800
800-634-7064
Fax: 202-564-7854
enquiries@taylorandfrancis.com
www.routledge.com

Diane Fausek, Author
Unique approaches, materials, and device will inspire you to tap into your own well of creativity to design your own treatment plans. It lays out the ingredients and the skills to get the results you want. Includes strategies that have been used for people with Alzheimer's, geri-psychiatric conditions and developmental disabilities.
124 pages Hardcover; Paperback

4925   A World Awaits You
Mobility International USA
132 E Broadway
Suite 343
Eugene, OR 97401
541-343-1284
Fax: 541-343-6812
TTY: 541-343-1284
clearinghouse@miusa.org
www.miusa.org/away

Susan Sygall, Chief Executive Officer
Cindy Lewis, Director, Programs
Publication from Mobility International USA featuring stories from people with disabilities who have participated in international exchange experiences.
Annually

4926   ADA Guide for Small Businesses
US Department of Justice, Civil Rights Division
950 Pennsylvania Ave. NW
9th Floor
Washington, DC 20530
202-307-0663
800-514-0301
Fax: 202-307-1197
TTY: 800-514-0383
www.ada.gov

Rebecca B. Bond, Chief
Anne Raish, Principal Deputy Chief
Christina Galindo-Walsh, Deputy Chief
A 15-page booklet for businesses that provide goods and services to the public. This publication explains basic ADA requirements, illustrates ways to make facilities accessible, and provides information about tax credits and deductions.

4927   ADA Information Services
US Department of Justice, Civil Rights Division
950 Pennsylvania Ave. NW
9th Floor
Washington, DC 20530
202-307-0663
800-514-0301
Fax: 202-307-1197
TTY: 800-514-0383
www.ada.gov

Rebecca B. Bond, Chief
Anne Raish, Principal Deputy Chief
Christina Galindo-Walsh, Deputy Chief
A 2-page list with the telephone numbers and internet addresses of federal agencies and other organizations that provide information and technical assistance to the public about the ADA.

4928   ADA Pipeline
DRTAC: Southeast ADA Center
1419 Mayson Street NE
Atlanta, GA 30324
404-385-0636
800-949-4232
Fax: 404-385-0641
www.sedbtac.org

Cyndi Smith, B.S., Office Assistant
Mary Morder, Information Technology Support
Sally Z. Weiss, B.A., Director
16 pages Quarterly

4929   ADA Questions and Answers
US Department of Justice, Civil Rights Division
950 Pennsylvania Ave. NW
9th Floor
Washington, DC 20530
202-307-0663
800-514-0301
Fax: 202-307-1197
TTY: 800-514-0383
www.ada.gov

Rebecca B. Bond, Chief
Anne Raish, Principal Deputy Chief
Christina Galindo-Walsh, Deputy Chief
A 31-page booklet giving an overview of the ADA's requirements affecting employers, businesses, nonprofit service agencies, and state and local governments programs, including public transportation.

4930   ADA Tax Incentive Packet for Business
US Department of Justice
950 Pennsylvania Ave. NW
9th Floor
Washington, DC 20530
202-307-0663
800-514-0301
Fax: 202-307-1197
TTY: 800-514-0383
www.ada.gov

Rebecca B. Bond, Chief
Anne Raish, Principal Deputy Chief
Christina Galindo-Walsh, Deputy Chief
A 13-page packet of information to help businesses understand and take advantage of the tax credit and deduction available for complying with the ADA.

4931   ADA and City Governments: Common Problems
US Department of Justice
950 Pennsylvania Ave. NW
9th Floor
Washington, DC 20530
202-307-0663
800-514-0301
Fax: 202-307-1197
TTY: 800-514-0383
www.ada.gov

Rebecca B. Bond, Chief
Anne Raish, Principal Deputy Chief
Christina Galindo-Walsh, Deputy Chief
A 9-page document that contains a sampling of common problems shared by city governments of all sizes, provides examples of common deficiencies and explains how these problems affect persons with disabilities.

4932   ADA-TA: A Technical Assistance Update from the Department of Justice
US Department of Justice
950 Pennsylvania Ave. NW
9th Floor
Washington, DC 20530
202-307-0663
800-514-0301
Fax: 202-307-1197
TTY: 800-514-0383
www.ada.gov

Rebecca B. Bond, Chief
Anne Raish, Principal Deputy Chief
Christina Galindo-Walsh, Deputy Chief
A serial publication that answers Common Questions about ADA requirements and provides Design Details illustrating particular design requirements. The first edition addresses Readily Achievable Barrier Removal and Van Accessible Packing Spaces.

4933   AEPS Family Report: For Children Ages Birth to Three
Brookes Publishing
P.O.Box 10624
Baltimore, MD 21285-0624   410-337-9580
                                   800-638-3775
                              Fax: 410-337-8539
                      custserv@brookespublishing.com
                          www.brookespublishing.com
Diane Bricker, Author
Betty Capt, Author
JoAnn Johnson, Author
This is a 64-item questionnaire that asks parents to rank their child's abilities on specific skills. In packages of 10.
28 pages Saddle-stiched

4934   ARC's Government Report
Arc of the District of Columbia
817 Varnum St NE
Washington, DC 20017-2144   202-636-2950
                              Fax: 202-636-2996
                                   www.arcdc.net
Mary Lou Meccariello, Executive Director
Ed Cabatic, Director of Finance
Randy Shingler, Chief Operating Officer
Reports on government activities related to individuals with disabilities with a focus on persons with developmental disabilities.
$50.00

4935   ARCA Newsletter
ARCA - Dakota County Technical College
1300 145th St E
Rosemount, MN 55068-2932   651-423-8301
                                   877-937-3282
                              Fax: 651-423-7028
                                   dctc.edu
Ron Thomas, President
Offers information on support groups, conventions, books, manuscripts and programs for the rehabilitation professional and the disabled.
Monthly

4936   Accent on Living Magazine
Cheever Publishing
P.O.Box 700
Bloomington, IL 61702-700   309-378-2961
                                   800-787-8444
                              Fax: 309-378-4420
Julie Cheever, Marketing Manager
A magazine published for forty four years, serves physically disabled people, with general interest, travel, and home modification features. *$12.00*
112 pages Quarterly

4937   Access Design Services: CILs as Experts
Independent Living Research Utilization ILRU
1333 Moursund
Houston, TX 77030   713-520-0232
                      Fax: 713-520-5785
                          ilru@ilru.org
                              ilru.org
Lex Frieden, Director, ILRU
Richard Petty, Co-Director
Featuring the Access Design Services of Alpha One in Maine, this month's Readings is another of the winners of the recent competition for innovative CIL programs.
10 pages

4938   Access To Independence Inc.
Access to Independence
3810 Milwaukee Street
Madison, WI 53714   608-242-8484
                              800-362-9877
                         Fax: 608-242-0383
                         TTY: 608-242-8485
                          info@accesstoind.org
                          www.accesstoind.org
Dee Truhn, Executive Director
Jason Belaungy, Assistant Director
Geri, Finances/HR

Independent Living Center serving people of any age and all types of disabilities in south-central Wisconsin. Empower people with disabilities, through advocacy, education, and support.
24 pages Semi-Annual

4939   Access for 911 and Telephone Emergency Services
US Department of Justice
950 Pennsylvania Ave. NW
9th Floor
Washington, DC 20530   202-307-0663
                                   800-514-0301
                              Fax: 202-307-1197
                              TTY: 800-514-0383
                                   www.ada.gov
Rebecca B. Bond, Chief
Anne Raish, Principal Deputy Chief
Christina Galindo-Walsh, Deputy Chief
A 10-page publication explaining the requirements for direct, equal access to 911 for persons who use teletypewritters (TTYs).

4940   Achieving Diversity and Independence
Independent Living Research Utilization ILRU
1333 Moursund
Houston, TX 77030   713-520-0232
                      Fax: 713-520-5785
                          ilru@ilru.org
                              ilru.org
Lex Frieden, Director, ILRU
Richard Petty, Co-Director
10 pages

4941   Activity-Based Intervention: 2nd Edition
Brookes Publishing
P.O.Box 10624
Baltimore, MD 21285-0624   410-337-9580
                                   800-638-3775
                              Fax: 410-337-8539
                      custserv@brookespublishing.com
                          readplaylearn.com
Paul H. Brooks, Chairman
Jeffrey D. Brookes, President
Melissa A. Behm, Executive Vice President
This 14 minute video illustrates how activity-based intervention can be used to turn everyday events and natural interactions into opportunities to promote learning in young children who are considered at risk for developmental delays or who have mild to significant disabilities. *$39.00*
ISBN 1-55766-86-3

4942   Ad Lib Drop-In Center: Consumer Management, Ownership and Empowerment
Independent Living Research Utilization ILRU
1333 Moursund
Houston, TX 77030   713-520-0232
                      Fax: 713-520-5785
                          ilru@ilru.org
                              ilru.org
Lex Frieden, Director, ILRU
Richard Petty, Co-Director
Joe describes how Ad Lib ensured consumer control in their Drop-In Center: the DIC came about because of consumer input, and consumers are involved in planning the program; members can choose to become volunteers or paid staff members. All of the staff at the DIC are consumers; and active consumer advisory board helps develop policies and programs and provides input to the Ad Lib board.
10 pages

4943   Adobe News
Santa Barbara Foundation
15 E Carrillo St
Santa Barbara, CA 93101-2706   805-963-1873
                                        805-966-2345
                                   Fax: 805-966-2345
Ron Gallo, CEO
8 pages Bi-Annually

4944   Advocate
Arc Massachusetts
217 South St
Waltham, MA 02453-2710   781-891-6270
                                     Fax: 781-891-6271
                                   arcmass@arcmass.org
                                      www.arcmass.org

Leo V. Sarkissian, Executive Director
Judy Zacek, Associate Editor
Beth Rutledge, Production Coordinator/Ad
Advocate is The Arc of Massachusetts' quarterly newsletter. This
is one of the ways in which we inform and educate people about
current topics in the field of developmental disabilities. *$ 20.00*
8-12 pages Quarterly

4945   American Herb Association Newsletter
P.O.Box 353
Nevada City, CA 95959-353   530-265-9552
                                     Fax: 530-274-3140
                                      www.ahaherb.com
Information on many different herbs and herb usues. *$ 20.00*

**4946   Americans with Disabilities Act Checklist for New
Lodging Facilities**
US Department of Justice
950 Pennsylvania Ave. NW
9th Floor
Washington, DC 20530   202-307-0663
                                           800-514-0301
                                     Fax: 202-307-1197
                                     TTY: 800-514-0383
                                         www.ada.gov

Rebecca B. Bond, Chief
Anne Raish, Principal Deputy Chief
Christina Galindo-Walsh, Deputy Chief
This 34-page checklist is a self-help survey that owners,
franchisors, and managers of lodging facilities can use to identify
ADA mistakes at their facilities.

4947   Americans with Disabilities Act Handbook
Aspen Publishers
76 9th Ave
7th Floor
New York, NY 10011-4962   212-790-2000
                                     Fax: 212-771-0885
                                  www.aspenpublishers.com

Henry H Perritt Jr Esq, Author
Bob Lemmond, President and CEO
Gustavo Dobles, Vice President & Chief Content Officer
The Americans With Disabilities Act (ADA) Handbook provides
comprehensive coverage of the ADA's employment, commercial
facilities, and public accommodations provisions as well as coverage of the transportation, communication, and federal, local,
and state government requirements. *$599.00*
1671 pages 2X per year
ISBN 0-735531-48-X

**4948   An Interdisciplinary Journal for the Social Study of
Health, Illness and Medicine**
Sage Publications
2455 Teller Rd
Thousand Oaks, CA 91320-2218   805-499-0721
                                           800-818-7243
                                     Fax: 805-499-0871
                                       hea.sagepub.com

Alan Radley, Editor
Blaise Simqu, Chief Executive Officer
Quarterly

4949   Annual Report Sarkeys Foundation
530 E Main St
Norman, OK 73071-5823   405-364-3703
                                     Fax: 405-364-8191
                                    susan@sarkeys.org
                                         sarkeys.org

Kim Henry, Executive Director
Lorri Sutton, Executive Assistant
Susan C. Frantz, Senior Program Officer
Yearly

**4950   Applied Kinesiology: Muscle Response in Diagnosis,
Therapy and Preventive Medicine**
Inner Traditions
P.O.Box 388
Rochester, VT 05767-388   802-767-3174
                                           800-246-8648
                                     Fax: 802-767-3726
                               orders@innertraditions.com
                                 www.InnerTraditions.com

Jessica Arsenault, Sales Associate
Rob Meadows, VP Sales & Marketing
$12.95
144 pages
ISBN 0-892813-28-8

4951   Arc Connection Newsletter
Arc of Tennessee
151 Athens Way
Suite 100
Nashville, TN 37228-1367   615-248-5878
                                           800-835-7077
                                     Fax: 615-248-5879
                                   pcooper@thearctn.org
                                         thearctn.org

Carrie Hobbs Guiden, Executive Director
*Peggy Cooper, Membership, Chapter and Communications Man-
ager*
Nicole Davidson, Business Manager
The Arc of Tennessee is a nonprofit organization that offers advocacy, information, referral and support to people with intellectual
or developmental disabilities and their families. This is their publication. It is free to members. *$10.00*
12 pages Quarterly

4952   Aromatherapy Book: Applications and Inhalations
2526 Martin Luther King Jr. Way
Berkeley, CA 94704   510-549-4270
                                     Fax: 510-549-4276
                              info@northatlanticbooks.com
                               www.northatlanticbooks.com
Minda Armstrong, Print Production Manager
Richard Grossinger, Founding Publisher
Janet Levin, Director of Sales & Distribution
A book of practical and researched information about
aromatherapy. *$18.95*
400 pages
ISBN 1-556430-73-6

4953   Aromatherapy for Common Ailments
Simon & Schuster
100 Front St
Delran, NJ 8075-1181   856-461-6500
                                           800-323-7445
                                     Fax: 856-824-2402
                                     www.simonsays.com

David Schaeffer, VP
Explains aromatherapy with emphasis on medicinal uses.
96 pages
ISBN 0-671731-34-3

4954   As I Am
Fanlight Productions
32 Court Street
21st Floor
Brooklyn, NY 11201   718-488-8900
                                           800-876-1710
                                     Fax: 718-488-8642
                                      info@fanlight.com
                                       www.fanlight.com

Ben Achtenberg, Owner
Anthony Sweeney, Marketing Director
Three young people with developmental disabilities speak for
themselves about their lives, the problems they face and their
hopes and expectations for the future. *$99.00*
ISBN 1-572950-58-7

4955 Attitudes Toward Persons with Disabilities
Springer Publishing Company
11 West 42nd Street
15th Floor
New York, NY 10036   212-431-4370
                                      877-687-7476
                               Fax: 212-941-7842
                    marketing@springerpub.com
                            www.springerpub.com
James C. Costello, Vice President, Journal Publishing
Diana Osborne, Production Manager
Megan Larkin, Managing Editor, Journals
This volume examines what is known of people's complex and
multifaceted attitudes toward persons with disabilities. Divided
into five areas of concern: theory, origin of attitudes, attitude
measurement, attitudes of specific groups and attitude change.
$38.95
352 pages Hardcover
ISBN 0-82616 -90-1

**4956 Authoritative Guide to Self- Help Resourcein Mental
Health**
Guilford Press
72 Spring St
New York, NY 10012-4019   212-431-9800
                                      800-365-7006
                               Fax: 212-966-6708
                                   info@guilford.com
                                   www.guilford.com
Linda F Campbell PhD, Author
Thomas P Smith PsyD, Author
Robert Sommer PhD, Author
Reviews and rates 600+ self-help books, autobiographies, and
popular films, and evaluates hundreds of Internet sites. Addresses 28 of the most prevalent clinical disorders and life chal-
lenges- from ADHD, Alzheimer's, and anxiety disorders, to
marital problems, mood disorders and weight management. Also
in cloth at $45.00 (ISBN# 1-57230-506-1) *$25.00*
377 pages Paperback
ISBN 1-572305-80-0

4957 AwareNews
Services for Independent Living
26250 Euclid Ave
Suite 801
Euclid, OH 44132   216-731-1529
                               Fax: 216-731-3083
                                     sil@stratos.net
                                       www.sil-oh.org
Molly Foos, Executive Director
Katherine Foley, Director of Advocacy
Lisa Marn, Assistant Director
12 pages Quarterly

4958 Bach Flower Therapy: Theory and Practice
Inner Traditions
1 Park St
Rochester, VT 05767   802-767-3174
                               Fax: 802-767-3726
                 customerservice@InnerTraditions.com
                            www.innertraditions.com
Ehud Sperling, Owner
Contemporary study of Bach's techniques, intended for practitio-
ners and lay readers alike. Includes lists of symptoms to facilitate
diagnosis, ans aims to provide an understanding of psychoso-
matic elements in relation to physical complaints.
ISBN 0-892812-39-7

**4959 Barrier Free Travel: A Nuts and Bolts Guide for
Wheelers and Slow Walkers (3rd Edition)**
Demos Health Publishing
11 W 42nd St
15th Fl
New York, NY 10036   212-683-0072
                               barrierfreetravel.net
Candy Harrington, Author

Billed as the definitive guide to accessible travel, this indispensable resource contains detailed information about the logistics of
planning accessible travel by plane, train, bus and ship. *$19.95*
200 pages Paperback
ISBN 1-932603-83-2

4960 Beliefs, Values, and Principles of Self Advocacy
Brookline Books
34 University Rd
Brookline, MA 02445-4533   800-666-2665
                               Fax: 617-734-3952
                                 brbooks@yahoo.com
                              www.brooklinebooks.com
Written by self-advocates around the world, they tell about the
beliefs, values, and principles important to them, and the empowerment and personal growth they experience through self-advocacy. *$7.00*
48 pages Paperback
ISBN 0-57129 -22-2

4961 Beliefs: Pathways to Health and Well Being
Metamorphous Press
P.O.Box 10616
Portland, OR 97296-616   503-228-4972
                               Fax: 503-223-9117
David Balding, Publisher
Explores behavioral technologies and belief change strategies
that can alter beliefs that support unhealthy habbits such as smoking, overeating, and drug use. Also covers the changing of thinking processes that create phobias and unreasonable fears,
retraining the immune system to eliminate allergies and to deal
optinally with cancer, AIDS, and other diseases. Includes strategies to transform unhealthy beliefs into lifelong constructs of
wellness.

4962 Bench Marks
Govennor's Council on Developmental Disabilities
1717 W Jefferson St
Phoenix, AZ 85007-3202   602-542-4049
                                      800-889-5893
                               Fax: 602-542-5320
Micheal Ward, Executive Director
Susan Madison, Manager
Quarterly

4963 Bodie, Dolina, Smith & Hobbs, P.C.
21 W Susquehanna Ave
Suite 110
Towson, MD 21204-5218   410-823-1250
                                      877-739-1013
                               Fax: 443-901-0802
                               chobbs@bodie-law.com
                                   www.bodie-law.com
Chester Hobbs, Esquire
Thomas G. Bodie, Lawyer
Wallace Dann, Lawyer
Law firm; provides estates, trusts and guardianship administra-
tion, estate planning, elder law, tax issues, bankruptcy, foreclo-
sures, and real estate issues. *$25.00*
Quarterly

4964 Body Reflexology: Healing at Your Fingertips
Parker Publishing Company
Ste 2605
1501 Broadway
New York, NY 10036-5600   212-869-6350
Hy Dubin, President
Features step-by-step instructions of how to send healing flows
of energy through the body to relieve back pain, headaches, ar-
thritis, and other afflictions. Illustrated.
343 pages Hardcover
ISBN 0-132997-36-3

4965 Body Silent: The Different World of the Disabled
WW Norton & Company
324 State Street
Suite H
Santa Barbara, CA 93101-2364   818-718-9900
                                      800-333-6867
                              Fax: 818-349-2027
                              editor@specialneeds.com
                              www.specialneeds.com
The author's personal account of his progressive and terminal
loss of muscle function caused by a spinal tumor, resulting in
quadripilegia. Includes society's fears, myths, and misunder-
standings about disability and the damage they inflict. *$9.95*
256 pages
ISBN 0-393320-42-1

4966 Body of Knowledge/Hellerwork
406 Berry St
Mount Shasta, CA 96067-2548   530-926-2500
                              theheller@aol.com
                              www.josephheller.com
Joseph Heller, Owner
Information, referral directory, training and certification.

4967 Bridge Newsletter
Arizona Bridge to Independent Living
1229 E Washington St
Phoenix, AZ 85034-1101   602-256-2245
                                      800-280-2245
                              Fax: 602-254-6407
                              abil.org
Phil Pangrazio, President & CEO
Regina Mitzel, V. P. & Chief Administrative Officer
Amina Kruck, V.P. of Advocacy
12 pages Monthly

**4968 Bridging the Gap: A National Directory of Services for
Women & Girls with Disabilities**
Educational Equity Concepts
71 Fifth Avenue
New York, NY 10016-5506   212-725-1803
                              Fax: 212-725-0947
                              TTY: 212-725-1803
                              www.edequity.org
Ellen Rubin, Coordinator Disability Programs
Merle Froschl, Editor
Contains a resource section of publications and videos geared
specifically to women and girls with disabilities. Available in
print, on cassette, and also in braille. *$24.95*
ISBN 0-931629-16-0

4969 Bulletin of the Association on the Handicapped
Assoc. on Handicapped Student Service Program
P.O.Box 21192
Columbus, OH 43221-0192   614-365-5216
                              Fax: 614-365-6718
Membership journal including Association news, articles and
sections such as Literature in Review and Speak Out. *$16.00*

4970 CDR Reports
Council for Disability Rights
Ste 1540
20 N Wacker Dr
Chicago, IL 60606-2903   312-201-4800
                              Fax: 312-444-1977
                              www.disabilityrights.org
Jo Holzer, Executive Director/Editor
Bruce Moore, Employment Specialist
$15.00
8 pages Monthly

4971 California Financial Power of Attorney
NOLO
950 Parker St
Berkeley, CA 94710-2524   510-549-1976
                                      800-955-4775
                              Fax: 510-548-5902
                              www.nolo.com
Maira Dizgalvis, Trade Customer Service Manager
Susan McConnell, Director Sales
Natasha Kaluza, Sales Assistant

A plain-English book packed with forms and instructions to give
a trusted person the legal authority to handle your financial
affairs.
Paperback

4972 Caring for America's Heroes
Oklahoma City VA Medical Center
921 NE 13th St
Oklahoma City, OK 73104-5007   405-270-0501
                              Fax: 405-270-1560
                              www.oklahoma.va.gov
Steven Gentlin, Director
Kathleen Fogarty, Associate Director
D Robert McCaffree MD, Chief of Staff

**4973 Center for Health Research: Eastern Washington
University**
Showalter 209a
Cheney, WA 99004   509-359-2279
                                      800-221-9369
                              Fax: 509-359-2778
                              sharon.wilson@mail.ewu.edu
Produces eight videotapes, accompanying printed materials, and
a videotaped public services announcement to serve as training
and resource materials for use by daycare centers.

4974 Center for Libraries and Educational Improvement
400 Maryland Ave SW
Washington, DC 20202-1   202-260-2226
                                      800-872-5327
                              Fax: 202-401-0689
                              TTY: 800-437-0833
                              www.ed.gov
Administers the Library Services Construction Act, which authorizes grants to the states for library services to the physically
handicapped.

4975 Centering Corporation Grief Resources
7230 Maple Street
Omaha, NE 68134   402-553-1200
                                      866-218-0101
                              Fax: 402-533-0507
                              j1200@aol.com
                              www.centering.org
Joy Johnson, Founder
Dr. Marvin Johnson, Founder
Janet Roberts, Executive Director
A full catalog of all our available bereavement resources. We are a
small, non-profit organization providing help to families in crisis
situations.
32 pages BiAnnually

4976 Centers for Disease Control and Prevention
US Department of Health and Human Services
1600 Clifton Rd NE
Atlanta, GA 30329-4018   404-639-3311
                                      800-232-4636
                              Fax: 404-498-1177
                              www.cdc.gov
Robert Delaney, Plant Manager
Publishes an annually updated list of infectious and communica-
ble diseases transmitted through the handling of food in accor-
dance with Section 103 of Title I.

**4977 Child With Special Needs: Encouraging Intellectual and
Emotional Growth**
Addison-Wesley Publishing Company
Ste 300
75 Arlington St
Boston, MA 02116-3988   617-848-7500
                                      800-238-9682
                              Fax: 617-944-7273
                              www.awprofessional.com
Bill Barke, CEO
Covering all kinds of disabilities — including cerebral palsy, au-
tism, developmental, ADD, and language problems — this guide
offers parents specific ways of helping all special needs chidren
reach their full intellectual and emotional potential. *$32.00*
496 pages
ISBN 0-201407-26-4

4978   Chinese Herbal Medicine
Shambhala Publications
300 Massachusetts Avenue
Boston, MA 02115   617-424-0030
                                         Fax: 617-236-1563
                                    editors@shambhala.com
                                          shambhala.com

Richard Reoch, President
Gives an in-depth look into herbal medicine.
176 pages
ISBN 0-877733-98-8

**4979   Christian Approach to Overcoming Disability: A
          Doctor's Story**
Haworth Press
10 Alice St
Binghamton, NY 13904-1503   607-722-5857
                                             800-429-6784
                                         Fax: 607-722-6362
                                   orders@haworthpress.com
                                      www.haworthpress.com

William Cohen, Owner
$29.95
128 pages
ISBN 0-789022-57-5

4980   Closing the Gap
P.O. Box 68
Henderson, MN 56044   507-248-3294
                                         Fax: 507-248-3810
                                      www.closingthegap.com

Dolores Hagen, Co-Founder
Budd Hagen, Co-Founder
Explores use of microcomputers as personal and educational
tools for persons with disabilities.
36+ pages BiMonthly

**4981   Conference of the Association on Higher Education &
          Disability (AHEAD)**
8015 West Kenton Circle
Suite 230
Huntersville, NC 28078   704-947-7779
                                         Fax: 704-948-7779
                                             www.ahead.org

Stephan Smith, Executive Director
Carol Funckes, Chief Operations Officer
Howard Kramer, Conference Director
An annual conference focused on aiding and meeting the needs of
persons with disabilities attending higher education institutions.

4982   Constellations
Minnesota STAR Program
Ste 309
50 Sherburne Ave
Saint Paul, MN 55155-1402   651-296-2771
                                             800-657-3862
                                         Fax: 651-282-6671
                                    star.program@state.mn.us

Chuck Rassbach, Executive Director
Free quarterly publication from the Minnesota STAR Program.
8 pages Quarterly

4983   Coping+Plus: Dimensions of Disability
Greenwood Publishing Group
130 Cremona Drive
Santa Barbara, CA 93117   805-968-1911
                                             800-368-6868
                                         Fax: 866-270-3856
                               CustomerService@abc-clio.com
                                          www.abc-clio.com

Matt Laddin, Vice President of Marketing
Mike Saltzman, Director-Eastern Territories & National Accounts
James Lingle, International Sales & Marketing
Everyone can learn new or more effective coping skills and strat-
egies to deal with times of loss, crisis and disability. $55-$59.95
280 pages Hardcover
ISBN 0-275945-44-8

4984   Council News
Northern Nevada Center for Independent Living
999 Pyramid Way
Sparks, NV 89431-4471   775-353-3599
                                         Fax: 775-353-3588
                                             www.nncil.org

Lisa Bonie, Executive Director
Hilda Velasco, Operations Manager
Joni Inglis, Independent Living Advocate
NNCIL was founded in 1982 by a small group of people with disabilities, who believe that each person, regardless of the severity
of his or her disability, has the potential to grow, develop and
share fully the joys and responsibilities of our society.
12 pages Quarterly

4985   Counseling in Terminal Care & Bereavement
Brookes Publishing
P.O.Box 10624
Baltimore, MD 21285-0624   410-337-9580
                                             800-638-3775
                                         Fax: 410-337-8539
                             custserv@brookespublishing.com
                                          readplaylearn.com

Paul H. Brooks, Chairman
Jeffrey D. Brookes, President
Melissa A. Behm, Executive Vice President
Provides practical suggestions for addressing the needs of patients and family members who are anticipating or currently dealing with grief and bereavement, such as hospice care, hospitals,
or at home care. *$34.00*
210 pages Paperback
ISBN 1-85433 -78-7

**4986   Creating Wholeness: Self-Healing Workbook Using
          Dynamic Relaxation, Images and Thoughts**
Plenum Publishing Corporation
233 Spring St
7th Floor
New York, NY 10013-1522   212-620-8000
                                             800-644-4831
                                         Fax: 212-460-1575
                                         ainy@aveda.com
                                          www.aveda.edu

232 pages
ISBN 0-306441-72-1

4987   DRS Connection
Disabled Resource Services
Ste 101
424 Pine St
Fort Collins, CO 80524-2421   970-482-2700
                                         Fax: 970-407-7072

Nancy Jackson, Executive Director
4 pages Quaterly

4988   Demand Response Transportation Through a Rural ILC
Independent Living Research Utilization ILRU
1333 Moursund
Houston, TX 77030   713-520-0232
                                         Fax: 713-520-5785
                                             ilru@ilru.org
                                             ilru.org

Lex Frieden, Director, ILRU
Richard Petty, Co-Director
Oklahomans for Independent Living's transportation program
was selected as exemplary becuase they marketed it by emphasizing people with disabilities as economic constituency.
10 pages

4989   Developing Organized Coalitions and Strategic Plans
Independent Living Research Utilization ILRU
1333 Moursund
Houston, TX 77030   713-520-0232
                                         Fax: 713-520-5785
                                             ilru@ilru.org
                                             ilru.org

Lex Frieden, Director, ILRU
Richard Petty, Co-Director
10 pages

4990 **Dictionary of Congenital Malformations& Disorders**
Informa Healthcare
Fl 16
52 Vanderbilt Ave
New York, NY 10017-3846   212-520-2777
                                      Fax: 212-661-5052
                                      orders@crcpress.com
                                      www.tandfonline.com

$55.00
193 pages
ISBN 0-850705-77-1

4991 **Dictionary of Developmental Disabilities Terminology**
Brookes Publishing
P.O.Box 10624
Baltimore, MD 21285-0624   410-337-9580
                                          800-638-3775
                                      Fax: 410-337-8539
                              custserv@brookespublishing.com
                              www.brookespublishing.com

Paul H. Brooks, Chairman
Jeffrey D. Brookes, President
Melissa A. Behm, Executive Vice President
With more than 3,000 easy-to-understand entries, this dictionary
provides thorough explanations of terms associated with devel-
opmental disabilities and disorders. *$55.95*
368 pages Hardcover
ISBN 1-557662-45-2

4992 **Directory of Members**
American Network of Community Options & Resources
1101 King St
Suite 380
Alexandria, VA 22314-2962   703-535-7850
                                      Fax: 703-535-7860
                                      ancor@ancor.org
                                      ancor.org

Dave Toeniskoetter, President
Chris Sparks, Vice President
Julie Manworren, Secretary/Treasurer
The Directory lists over 600 agencies that provide residential services and supports in 48 states and the District of Columbia. The
listings include the name of the Executive Directors, the name,
address, and phone number of the agency, describe the types of
services that are provided and how many individuals receive services from that agency. *$25.00*
189 pages

4993 **Disability Awareness Guide**
Central Iowa Center for Independent Living
655 Walnut St
Suite 131
Des Moines, IA 50309-3930   515-243-1742
                                      Fax: 515-243-5385

Bob Jeppesen, Executive Director
Frank Strong, Assistant Director Programs
Bob Jepson, Manager
The Disability Awareness Guide contains information about our
center; who we are and what we do. It also contains the telephone
numbers of local and national agencies and resources available
for people with disabilities.

4994 **Disability Rights Movement**
Children's Press
Sherman Tpke
Danbury, CT 6813   800-621-1115
                                      Fax: 800-374-4329

Elena Rockman, Marketing Manager
Author Deborah Kent illuminates both the history of the National
Disability Rights Movement and the inspiring personal stories of
individuals with various disabilities. *$18.00*
32 pages Hardcover
ISBN 0-53106-32-3

4995 **Disabled People's International Fifth World Assembly as
Reported by Two US Participants**
Independent Living Research Utilization ILRU
1333 Moursund
Houston, TX 77030   713-520-0232
                                      Fax: 713-520-5785
                                      ilru@ilru.org
                                      ilru.org

Lex Frieden, Director, ILRU
Richard Petty, Co-Director
This report describes the international conference on independent living held in Mexico City in December 1998 as experienced
by staff members from two U.S. centers. Kaye Beneke interviewed Luis Chew and Marco Antonio Coronado for this edition
of Readings in Independent Living.
10 pages

4996 **Disabled We Stand**
Brookline Books
34 University Rd
Brookline, MA 02445-4533   800-666-2665
                                      Fax: 617-734-3952
                                      brbooks@yahoo.com
                                      www.brooklinebooks.com

This book is impassioned, often angry, but also hopeful and practical, suggesting a series of actions that will lead to constructive
change. It is imbued with spirit and energy of disabled people
who are determined to take their lives into their own hands. *$
10.95*
Paperback
ISBN 0-25331-80-0

4997 **Disabled, the Media, and the Information Age**
Greenwood Publishing Group
130 Cremona Drive
Santa Barbara, CA 93117   805-968-1911
                                          800-368-6868
                                      Fax: 866-270-3856
                              CustomerService@abc-clio.com
                              www.abc-clio.com

Matt Laddin, Vice President of Marketing
Mike Saltzman, Director-Eastern Territories & National Accounts
James Lingle, International Sales & Marketing
A short and easy-to-read overview of how disabled Americans
have been portrayed by the media and how images and the role of
the handicapped are changing. *$55.00*
264 pages Hardcover
ISBN 0-313284-72-5

4998 **Discovery Newsletter**
North Dakota State Library Talking Book Services
Dept 250
604 E Boulevard Ave
Bismarck, ND 58505-605   701-328-2000
                                          800-843-9948
                                      Fax: 701-328-2040
                                      sbschneider@nd.gov
                              ndsl.lib.state.nd.us/DisabilityServices.html

Doris Ott, Manager
The North Dakota State Library Disability Services produces the
Doscovery Newsletter containing information on services,
books, catalogs and of interest to the patron.
6 pages Bi-Annually

4999 **EP Resource Guide**
Exceptional Parent Library
P.O.Box 1807
Englewood Cliffs, NJ 7632-1207   201-947-6000
                                          800-535-1910
                                      Fax: 201-947-9376
                                      eplibrary@aol.com
                                      www.eplibrary.com

Lists directories of national organizations, associations, products and services. *$9.95*

5000 **ESCIL Update Newsletter**
Eastern Shore Center for Independent Living
9 Sunburst Ctr
Cambridge, MD 21613-2057
410-221-7701
800-705-7944
Fax: 410-221-7714

Shirley Tarbox, Executive Director
Jean Reed, Administrative Assistant
Lisa Morgan, Director IL Services
6 pages Quarterly

5001 **Easy Things to Make Things Simple: Do It Yourself Modifications for Disabled Persons**
Brookline Books
34 University Rd
Brookline, MA 02445-4533
800-666-2665
Fax: 617-734-3952
brbooks@yahoo.com
www.brooklinebooks.com

This book aims at older adults and others with physical limitations who require adaptations for safer and easier living in the kitchen, bathroom, bedroom, yard, and garden. The adaptations can be done inexpensively, from common materials. Large print format and detailed diagrams, plus special sections with advice caregivers. *$15.95*
160 pages Paperback
ISBN 1-571290-24-9

5002 **Enabling Romance: A Guide to Love, Sex & Relationships for the Disabled**

Ken Kroll, Author
Erica Levy Klein, Author
An uncensored, illustrated guide to intimacy and sexual expression for persons with physical disabilities.

5003 **Encyclopedia of Disability**
Sage Publications
2455 Teller Rd
Thousand Oaks, CA 91320-2218
805-499-0721
info@sagepub.com
www.sagepub.com

Gary L Albrecht, Editor
Blaise Simqu, Chief Executive Officer
A five volume set that covers disabilities A-Z *$850.00*
2500 pages
ISBN 0-761925-65-1

5004 **EveryBody's Different: Understanding and Changing Our Reactions to Disabilities**
Brookes Publishing
P.O.Box 10624
Baltimore, MD 21285-0624
410-337-9580
800-638-3775
Fax: 410-337-8539
custserv@brookespublishing.com
readplaylearn.com
Paul H. Brooks, Chairman
Jeffrey D. Brookes, President
Melissa A. Behm, Executive Vice President
This book discusses the emotions, questions, fears, and stereotypes that people without disabilities sometimes experience when they interact with people who do have disabilities. The author teaches readers to become more at ease with the concept of disability and to communicate more effectively with each other. Features activities and exercises that encourage self-examination, helping people to create more enriching personal relationships and work toward a fully inclusive society.
Paperback
ISBN 1-55766 -59-9

5005 **Everybody's Guide to Homeopathic Medicines**
Jeremy P Tarcher
375 Hudson St
New York, NY 10014-3658
212-366-2000
academic@penguin.com
www.us.penguingroup.com

John Makinson, Chairman and CEO
Coram Williams, CFO

Covers alternative treatments in homeopathic medicines.
375 pages
ISBN 0-874778-43-3

5006 **Everyday Social Interaction: A Program for People with Disabilities**
Brookes Publishing
P.O.Box 10624
Baltimore, MD 21285-0624
410-337-9580
800-638-3775
Fax: 410-337-8539
custserv@brookespublishing.com
readplaylearn.com

Paul H. Brooks, Chairman
Jeffrey D. Brookes, President
Melissa A. Behm, Executive Vice President
This source guides teachers and human services professionals in helping people with disabilities acquire social interaction skills and develop satisfying relationships. Included is a checklist and task analyses that shows how complex skills can be broken down into major components for easy performance monitoring accompanied by tips on social courtesies, rewards, praise, and criticism. *$41.95*
342 pages Paperback
ISBN 1-55766 -58-4

5007 **Family Challenges: Parenting with a Disability**
Aquarius Health Care Videos
P.O.Box 1159
Sherborn, MA 01770-7159
508-650-1616
888-440-2963
Fax: 508-650-4216
aqvideos@tiac.net
www.aquariusproductions.com

Lesile Kussmann, Owner
When a parent has a disability, everyone in the family is affected. For children, these experiences may profoundly influence their lives and views of the world. In this sensitive film, you will hear about different roles that all the family members take on at varying times. *$195.00*

5008 **Force A Miracle**
Writer's Showcase Press

A testament to the inner human strength to overcome extreme adversity, to triumph and continue a worthwhile and self-rewarding life. *$14.95*
244 pages
ISBN 0-595226-88-4

5009 **Forum**
Coalition for the Education of Disabled Children
165 W Center St
Marion, OH 43302-3742
740-382-7362
800-374-2806
Fax: 740-382-3428

Tracie Wilson, Manager
Leeann Derugen, Manager
Forum is a newsletter reporting on legislative and other developments affecting persons with disabilities.
Quarterly

5010 **Foundation Fundamentals for Nonprofit Organizations**
Foundation Center
Department Ze
79 5th Ave
New York, NY 10003-3034
212-620-4230
800-424-9836
Fax: 212-807-3677
order@foundationcenter.org
www.fdncenter.org

Bradford K. Smith, President
Lisa Philip, Vice President for Strategic Philanthropy
Lawrence T. McGill, Vice President for Research
This video is designed to give fundraisers a general overview of the foundation funding process and to introduce them to the many resources available through our libraries and cooperating collec-

tions. The video gives clear, step-by-step instructions on how to build a fundraising program. *$24.00*
Video

5011 Four-Ingredient Cookbook
Laurel Designs
Apt A
1805 Mar West St
Belvedere Tiburon, CA 94920-1962   Fax: 415-435-1451
Janet Sawyer, Owner
Lynn Montoya, Owner
Simple, easy to follow recipes, each containing four ingredients. Particularly suited to persons with limited physical ability. Includes 400 recipes, appetizers to desserts. *$9.00*

5012 Frequently Asked Questions About Multiple Chemical Sensitivity
Independent Living Research Utilization ILRU
1333 Moursund
Houston, TX 77030   713-520-0232
          Fax: 713-520-5785
          ilru@ilru.org
          ilru.org
Lex Frieden, Director, ILRU
Richard Petty, Co-Director
This FAQ covers important information about multiple chemical sensitivity and environmental illness. The FAQ describes the conditions, recommends strategies for improving access, and lists resources for CILs and other organizations. As the fact sheet states, centers must set an example in assuring that all people can enter their offices.
10 pages

5013 Genetic Disorders Sourcebook
Omnigraphics
615 Griswold Street
Suite 520
Detroit, MI 48226   610-461-3548
          800-234-1340
          Fax: 800-875-1340
          contact@omnigraphics.com
          www.omnigraphics.com
Peter Ruffner, Co-Founder
Fred Ruffner, Co-Founder
Provides information on hereditary diseases and disorders. *$7800.00*
650 pages
ISBN 0-789892-41-1

5014 Genetic Nutritioneering
McGraw-Hill Company
2460 Kerper Blvd
Dubuque, IA 52001-2224   563-588-1451
          800-338-3987
          Fax: 614-755-5654
Kurt Strand, VP
Describes how to modify the expression of genetic traits, potentially preventing heart disease, cancer, arthritis, and hormone-related problems. Features how to slow biological aging and reduce the risk of age-related diseases. *$16.95*
288 pages
ISBN 0-879839-21-X

5015 Going to School with Facilitated Communication
Syracuse University, School of Education
230 Huntington Hall
Syracuse, NY 13244-1   315-443-4752
          Fax: 315-443-2258
          jhrusso@syr.edu
          www.soe.syr.edu
Shirley Adamczyk, Administrative Assistant
Rachael Gazdick, Executive Director
Isabelle M. Glod, Administrative Assistant
A video in which students with autism and/or severe disabilities illustrate the use of facilitated communication focusing on basic principles fostering facilitated communication.
Video

5016 Grief: What it is and What You Can Do
Centering Corporation
7230 Maple Street
Omaha, NE 68134   402-553-1200
          866-218-0101
          Fax: 402-533-0507
          j1200@aol.com
          www.centering.org
Joy Johnson, Founder
Dr. Marvin Johnson, Founder
Janet Roberts, Executive Director
General grief information for all grief issues. *$3.50*
32 pages Paperback

5017 Guidelines on Disability
US Department of Housing & Urban Development
451 7th St SW
Washington, DC 20410-1   202-708-1112
          TTY: 202-708-1455
          portal.hud.gov/hudportal/HUD
Shaun Donovan, Secretary
Helen R. Kanovsky, Acting Deputy Secretary
Jennifer Ho, Senior Advisor to the Secretary
Contains information on housing and accessibility for persons with disabilities.

5018 Handbook of Services for the Handicapped
Greenwood Publishing Group
130 Cremona Drive
Santa Barbara, CA 93117   805-968-1911
          800-368-6868
          Fax: 866-270-3856
          CustomerService@abc-clio.com
          www.abc-clio.com
Matt Laddin, Vice President of Marketing
Mike Saltzman, Director-Eastern Territories & National Accounts
James Lingle, International Sales & Marketing
A handy reference book offering information and services for disabled individuals. *$59.95-$65.00.*
291 pages Hardcover
ISBN 0-313213-85-2

5019 Healing Herbs
Rodale Press
33 E Minor St
Emmaus, PA 18098-1   610-967-5171
          Fax: 610-967-8963
Maria Rodale, Chairman/Chief Executive Officer
Scott D. Schulman, President
Heather Rodale, Board Member/Vice President/ Leadership Development
Covers everything from growing the herbs to home remedies.

5020 Helen Keller National Center for Deaf- Blind Youths And Adults
141 Middle Neck Rd
Sands Point, NY 11050-1218   516-944-8900
          Fax: 516-944-7302
          hkncinfo@hknc.org
          www.hknc.org
Joseph McNulty, Executive Director
HKNC is the only national vacational and rehabilitation program providing services exclusively to youth and adults who are deaf-blind.

5021 Hospice Alternative
Harper Collins Publishers/Basic Books
10 E 53rd St
New York, NY 10022-5244   212-207-7000
          800-242-7737
          Fax: 212-207-7203
Jane Friedman, CEO
An account of the hospice experience. An innovative and humane way of caring for the terminally ill. *$8.95*
256 pages
ISBN 0-46503 -61-0

5022 How to File a Title III Complaint
US Department of Justice
950 Pennsylvania Ave. NW
9th Floor
Washington, DC 20530　　　　202-307-0663
　　　　　　　　　　　　　　800-514-0301
　　　　　　　　　　　　Fax: 202-307-1197
　　　　　　　　　　　　TTY: 800-514-0383
　　　　　　　　　　　　www.ada.gov

Rebecca B. Bond, Chief
Anne Raish, Principal Deputy Chief
Christina Galindo-Walsh, Deputy Chief
This publication details the procedure for filing a complaint under Title III of the ADA.

5023 How to Live Longer with a Disability
Accent Books & Products
PO Box 700
Bloomington, IL 61702-700　　　309-378-2961
　　　　　　　　　　　　　　800-787-8444
　　　　　　　　　　　　Fax: 309-378-4420
　　　　　　　　　　　　acmtlvng@aol.com

Raymond C Cheever, Publisher
Betty Garee, Editor
Eleven chapters to help you enjoy every aspect of your life, and live easier and happier. Includes sexuality and disability, getting more from the medical community and benefit programs. Co-authored by Robert Mauro, sociologist and Elle Becker, counselor and psychologist, both disabled. *$11.50*
266 pages Paperback
ISBN 0-19570 -38-8

5024 Ideas for Kids on the Go
Accent Books & Products
PO Box 700
Bloomington, IL 61702-700　　　309-378-2961
　　　　　　　　　　　　　　800-787-8444
　　　　　　　　　　　　Fax: 309-378-4420
　　　　　　　　　　　　acmtlvng@aol.com

Raymond C Cheever, Publisher
Betty Garee, Editor
This guide shows kids with physical disabilities how to go for it! Lists products and where to get them, and includes tips from others for having fun and getting ahead. Ages 1-18. *$6.95*
69 pages Paperback
ISBN 0-91570 -17-5

5025 If I Only Knew What to Say or Do
AARP Fulfillment
601 E St NW
Washington, DC 20049-1　　　202-434-2277
　　　　　　　　　　　　　　800-424-3410
　　　　　　　　　　　　Fax: 202-434-3443
　　　　　　　　　　　　TTY: 877-434-7598
　　　　　　　　　　　　member@aarp.org
　　　　　　　　　　　　www.aarp.org

Carol Raphael, Chair
Ronald E. Daly, Sr., Board Vice Chair
Jeannine English, President
Provides a concise discussion of how to help a friend in crisis. Learn what to say and what not to say.

5026 If it Weren't for the Honor: I'd Rather Have Walked
Accent Books & Products
PO Box 700
Bloomington, IL 61702-700　　　309-378-2961
　　　　　　　　　　　　　　800-787-8444
　　　　　　　　　　　　Fax: 309-378-4420
　　　　　　　　　　　　acmtlvng@aol.com

Raymond C Cheever, Publisher
Betty Garee, Editor
Revealing, often humorous, highly interesting and important reading. This book offers an account told by the author who was on the scene and actually saw and participated in many events that paved the way for progress for all those with disabilities. *$14.50*
262 pages Paperback
ISBN 0-91570 -41-8

5027 Imagery in Healing Shamanism and Modern Medicine
Shambhala Publications
300 Massachusetts Avenue
Horticultural Hall
Boston, MA 02115　　　　617-424-0030
　　　　　　　　　　　　888-424-2329
　　　　　　　　　　　　Fax: 617-236-1563
　　　　　　　　　　　editors@shambhala.com
　　　　　　　　　　　www.shambhala.com

Richard Reoch, President
Patients use self imagery to fight sickness and pain throughout their lives. *$15.95*
272 pages
ISBN 1-570629-34-x

5028 Independence
Easterseals
1219 Dunn Ave
Daytona Beach, FL 32114-2405　　386-255-4568
　　　　　　　　　　　　　　877-255-4568
　　　　　　　　　　　　Fax: 386-258-7677

Jeff Blass, Chairman
Austin Brownlee, Chair-Elect
Becky Rutland, Vice Chair
4-6 pages Quarterly

5029 Independent Living Centers and Managed Care: Results of an ILRU Study on Involvement
Independent Living Research Utilization ILRU
1333 Moursund
TIRR Memorial Hermann Research Cent
Houston, TX 77030-7031　　　713-520-0232
　　　　　　　　　　　　Fax: 713-520-5785
　　　　　　　　　　　　ilru@ilru.org
　　　　　　　　　　　　www.ilru.org

Lex Frieden, Director, ILRU
Richard Petty, Co-Director
Vinh Nguyen, Program Director
This month's Readings presents findings from an ILRU study of roles centers are taking vis-a-vis managed care. Initiated in spring 1998, we asked Drew Batavia to take the lead in conducting this study for us. We were interested in collecting data on frequency with which centers are contacted by consumers with managed care problems. This is a study that will need to be repeated periodically as our experiences with managed care evolves. Meanwhile, here are the initial findings.
10 pages

5030 Independent Living Challenges the Blues
Independent Living Research Utilization ILRU
1333 Moursund
TIRR Memorial Hermann Research Cent
Houston, TX 77030-7031　　　713-520-0232
　　　　　　　　　　　　Fax: 713-520-5785
　　　　　　　　　　　　ilru@ilru.org
　　　　　　　　　　　　www.ilru.org

Lex Frieden, Director, ILRU
Richard Petty, Co-Director
Vinh Nguyen, Program Director
Patricia's article highlights the Georgia SILC's health care advocacy efforts: the Georgia legislature passed a bill enabling Georgia Bleu to convert to for-profit status without a distribution of assets to similar nonprofit corporations; the Georgia SILC joined other health care advocates in filing a class action law suit to challenge the legality of the conversion; the Georgia SILC continues advocacy efforts to involve people with disabilities in developing and monitoring health care policy.
10 pages

5031 Independent Living Office
Department of Housing & Urban Development (HUD)
451 7th St SW
Washington, DC 20410-1　　　202-863-2800

Ted Tozer, President
Rafael Diaz, Chief Information Officer/Chief Information Officer
Mike Anderson, Chief Human Capital Officer
This office within HUD is charged with encouraging the construction of housing that is accessible to handicapped persons. The Office of Independent Living encourages modifications of

apartments and other dwellings so that handicapped persons can enter without assistance.

5032 Information Services for People with Developmental Disabilities
Greenwood Publishing Group
130 Cremona Drive
Santa Barbara, CA 93117
805-968-1911
800-368-6868
Fax: 866-270-3856
CustomerService@abc-clio.com
www.abc-clio.com

Matt Laddin, Vice President of Marketing
Mike Saltzman, Director - Eastern Territories
James Lingle, International Sales & Marketing
Overviews the information needs of people with developmental disabilities and tells librarians how to meet them. $65.oo-$75.00.
368 pages Hardcover
ISBN 0-313287-80-5

5033 Innovative Programs: An Example of How CILs Can Put Their Work in Context
Culture
1333 Moursund
TIRR Memorial Hermann Research Cent
Houston, TX 77030-7031
713-520-0232
Fax: 713-520-5785
ilru@ilru.org
www.ilru.org

Lex Frieden, Director, ILRU
Richard Petty, Co-Director
Vinh Nguyen, Program Director
Another winner in the innovative CIL competition- Steve Brown describes the Talking Books Program of Southeast Alaska Independent Living, discussing their efforts to record the oral history and life experiences of people with disabilities in the larger context of disability culture.
10 pages

5034 Insurance Solutions: Plan Well, Live Better
Demos Medical Publishing
11 West 42nd Street
15th Floor
New York, NY 10036
212-683-0072
800-532-8663
Fax: 212-683-0118
support@demosmedical.com
www.demosmedpub.com

Paul Choi, Vice-President of Finance and Operations
Matt Conmy, Sr. Director of Sales
Thomas Hastings, Marketing Manager
Learn how to look at various insurance options from a new perspective — including life, disability, health, and long-term care. Concrete information for dealing with potential problems in your coverage, to secure your financial future. *$24.95*
192 pages 2002
ISBN 1-888799-55-2

5035 International Directory of Libraries for the Disabled
KG Saur/Division of RR Bowker
121 Chanlon Rd
New Providence, NJ 7974-1541
908-286-1090
800-521-8110

Michael Cairns, CEO
An essential resource for improving the quality and quantity of materials available to the print-handicapped audience. Featuring talking books, braille books, large print books as well as production centers for these materials. *$46.00*
257 pages
ISBN 3-59821 -81-1

5036 Issues in Independent Living
Independent Living Research Utilization
1333 Moursund
TIRR Memorial Hermann Research Cent
Houston, TX 77030-7031
713-520-0232
Fax: 713-520-5785
ilru@ilru.org
www.ilru.org

Lex Frieden, Executive Director
Vinh Nguyen, Program Director
This booklet is a report of the National Study Group on the Implications of Health Care Reform for Americans with Disabilities and Chronic Health Conditions.
30 pages

5037 JAMA: The Journal of the American Medical Association
American Medical Association
PO Box 10946
Chicago, IL 60654-4820
312-670-7827
800-262-2350
Fax: 312-464-5909
subscriptions@jamanetwork.com
jama.jamanetwork.com

Howard Bauchner, MD, Editor-in-Chief
Articles cover all aspects of medical research and clinical medicine. *$66.00*

5038 JCIL Advocate Times
Jackson Center for Independent Living
409 Linden Ave
Jackson, MI 49203-4065
517-782-6054
Fax: 517-782-3118

Lesia Pikaart, Executive Director
JoAnn Lucas, Associate Director
Quarterly

5039 Jason & Nordic Publishers, Inc.
PO Box 441
Hollidaysburg, PA 16648-441
814-696-2929
Fax: 814-696-4250

Norma Mc Phee, Owner/CEO
Norma Phee
Turtle Books for children with disabilities present heroes who look like them, have problems like theirs, have similar doubts and feelings in non-threatening, fun stories. They are motivational, bridge the gap and promote understanding among peers and siblings. 22 children's books (grades preK-3) plus Sensitivity and Awareness Guide containing lesson plans, activities, background information keyed to the series. Disabilities include: Down syndrome, cerebral palsy, blindness, deafness and more.

5040 Journal of Social Work in Disabilty & Rehabilitation
Haworth Press
10 Alice St
Binghamton, NY 13904-1503
607-722-5857
800-429-6784
Fax: 607-722-6362
orders@haworthpress.com
www.haworthpress.com

William Cohen, Owner
John T Oardeck PhD, Editor
S Harrington-Miller, Advertising
Presents and explores issues related to disabilities and social policy, practice, research, and theory. Reflecting the broad scope of social work in disabilty practice, this interdisciplinary journal examines vital issues aspects of the field — from innovative practice methods, legal issues, and literature reviews to program descriptions and cuttinf-edge practice research.
Quarterly

5041 Just Like Everyone Else
World Institute on Disability
3075 Adeline St.
Suite 155
Berkeley, CA 94703   510-225-6400
                              Fax: 510-225-0477
                                   wid@wid.org
                                   www.wid.org
Marcie Roth, Executive Director & Chief Executive Officer
Katherine Zigmont, Senior Director, Operations & Deputy Director
Reggie Johnson, Senior Director, Marketing & Communications
Intended for general audiences, the publication provides perspective, inspiration and information about the Independent Living Movement and the Americans with Disabilities Act.

5042 Keep the Promise: Managed Care and People with Disabilities
American Network of Community Options & Resource
1101 King St
Ste 380
Alexandria, VA 22314-2962   703-535-7850
                              Fax: 703-535-7860
                                   ancor@ancor.org
                                   www.ancor.org
Dave Toeniskoetter, President
Chris Sparks, Vice President
Julie Manworren, Secretary/Treasurer
This publication presents a detailed review of the process and the lessons learned. Details a way for all stake holders to work together for a state or local system.
119 pages $18 - $22

5043 Keeping Our Families Together
Through the Looking Glass
3075 Adeline St.
Ste. 120
Berkeley, CA 94703-2212   510-848-1112
                                   800-644-2666
                              Fax: 510-848-4445
                              TTY: 510-848-1005
                                   tlg@lookingglass.org
                                   www.lookingglass.org
Maureen Block, J.D., Board President
Thomas Spalding, Board Treasurer
Alice Nemon, D.S.W.,, Board Secretary
Report of the National Task Force on parents with disabilities and their families. Available in braille, large print or cassette. *$2.00*
12 pages

5044 Learn About the ADA in Your Local Library
US Department of Justice
950 Pennsylvania Ave. NW
9th Floor
Washington, DC 20530   202-307-0663
                                   800-514-0301
                              Fax: 202-307-1197
                              TTY: 800-514-0383
                                   www.ada.gov
Rebecca B. Bond, Chief
Anne Raish, Principal Deputy Chief
Christina Galindo-Walsh, Deputy Chief
A 10-page annotated list of 95 ADA publications and one videotape that are available in 15,000 public libraries throughout the country.

5045 LifeLines
Disabled & Alone/Life Services for the Handicapped
1441 Broadway
23rd Floor
New York, NY 10018-2326   212-532-6740
                                   800-995-0066
                              Fax: 212-532-6740
                                   info@disabledandalone.org
                         www.disabledandalone.org/lifelines.html
Leslie D. Park, Chair
Rex L. Davidson, Vice President
Lee Alan Ackerman, Executive Director

Newsletter providing current and valuable information about lifetime care and planning for persons with disabilities and their families and the organizations serving them. Free upon request.
4-10 pages Biannual

5046 Lifelong Leisure Skills and Lifestyles for Persons with Developmental Disabilities
Brookes Publishing
PO Box 10624
Baltimore, MD 21285-0624   410-337-9580
                                   800-638-3775
                              Fax: 410-337-8539
                              custserv@brookespublishing.com
                                   www.readplaylearn.com
Paul H. Brooks, Chairman
Jeffrey D. Brookes, President
Melissa A. Behm, Executive Vice President
This instructional manual offers ideas and detailed examples that describe how to guide individuals of all ages through popular activities using adaptations that foster skill acquisition and inclusion. Some of the concepts explored are home-school-community collaboration, choice making and the dignity of risk, and leisure skill acquisition for the life span. *$35.00*
352 pages Paperback
ISBN 1-55766 -47-2

5047 Livin'
Lehigh Valley Center for Independent Living
435 Allentown Dr
Allentown, PA 18109-9121   610-770-9781
                              Fax: 610-770-9801
                                   info@lvcil.org
                                   www.lvcil.org
Amy Beck, Executive Director
Cara Steidel, Director of Finance
Greg Bott, Director of Development
4 pages Quarterly

5048 Living in a State of Stuck
Brookline Books
8 Trumbull Rd
Suite B-001
Northampton, MA 01060   413-584-0184
                                   800-666-2665
                              Fax: 413-584-6184
                                   brbooks@yahoo.com
                                   www.brooklinebooks.com
Offers explanations on how adaptive technologies affect the lives of people with disabilities. *$24.95*
3rd ed., paper
ISBN 1-571290-27-3

5049 Living in the Community
Independent Living Research Utilization ILRU
1333 Moursund
TIRR Memorial Hermann Research Cent
Houston, TX 77030-7031   713-520-0232
                              Fax: 713-520-5785
                                   ilru@ilru.org
                                   www.ilru.org
Lex Frieden, Director, ILRU
Richard Petty, Co-Director
Vinh Nguyen, Program Director
James, Lori, and Jamey describe the elements of their successful program to move people out of nursing homes and into the community: providing funding for deposits, first month's rent and other neccessities, including assistive technology; providing training and the other core services before and after consumers leave the nursing home; developing relationships with housing and other service providers.
10 pages

5050 Loud, Proud and Passionate
Mobility International USA
132 E Broadway
Suite 343
Eugene, OR 97401

541-343-1284
Fax: 541-343-6812
TTY: 541-343-1284
clearinghouse@miusa.org
www.miusa.org

Susan Sygall, Chief Executive Officer
Cindy Lewis, Director, Programs
A resource book for international development and women's organization about including women with disabilities in projects in the community. Informs women with disabilities about the efforts and successes of their peers worldwide.

5051 Love: Where to Find It, How to Keep It
Accent Books & Products
PO Box 700
Bloomington, IL 61702-700

309-378-2961
800-787-8444
Fax: 309-378-4420
acmtlvng@aol.com

Raymond C Cheever, Publisher
Betty Garee, Editor
Offers ideas such as how to meet other single people, avoid the wrong type; communications skills and much more for the disabled person wanting to date. *$6.95*
104 pages Paperback
ISBN 0-91570-31-0

5052 MOOSE: A Very Special Person
Brookline Books
8 Trumbull Rd
Suite B-001
Northampton, MA 01060

413-584-0184
800-666-2665
Fax: 413-584-6184
brbooks@yahoo.com
www.brooklinebooks.com

Moose, which in very human terms, teaches us that each of us is different and that we have our own unique capacity for loving, sharing, enjoying and learning. *$10.95*
Paperback
ISBN 0-91479-73-5

5053 Mainstream Magazine
2973 Beech St
San Diego, CA 92102-1529

619-232-2727
Fax: 619-234-3155
www.mainstream-mag.com

Cyndi Jones, Executive Director
The authoritative, national voice of people with disabilities, publishes in-depth reports on employment, education, new products and technology, legislation and disability rights advocacy, recreation and travel, disability arts and culture, plus personality profiles and challenging commentary. *$24.00*
Monthly

5054 Making Changes: Family Voices on Living Disabilities
Brookline Books
8 Trumbull Rd
Suite B-001
Northampton, MA 01060

413-584-0184
800-666-2665
Fax: 413-584-6184
brbooks@yahoo.com
www.brooklinebooks.com

What are the day to day impacts on the family when a disabled child is born? Or when a child who grows up without a disability becomes disabled through accident or disease? This provocative set of reports illuminates the conditions of those peoples lives, and the way they and those around them adjust to the disabilities. *$16.95*
216 pages Paperback
ISBN 0-91479-93-

5055 Making Informed Medical Decisions: Where to Look and How to Use What You Find
Patient-Centered Guides
1005 Gravenstein Highway North
Sebastopol, CA 95472

707-827-7000
Fax: 707-829-0104
support@oreilly.com
www.oreilly.com

Nancy Oster, Author
Making Informed Medical Decisions acts like a friendly reference librarian, explaining: tips for researching for someone else; medical journal articles; statistics and risk; standard treatment options; clinical trial; making an ally of your doctor; and determining your own best course. *$17.95*
381 pages Paperback
ISBN 1-565924-59-2

5056 Making Wise Decisions for Long-Term Care
AARP Fulfillment
601 E St NW
Washington, DC 20049-1

202-434-2277
800-424-3410
Fax: 202-434-3443
TTY: 877-434-7598
member@aarp.org
www.aarp.org

Carol Raphael, Chair
Ronald E. Daly, Sr., Board Vice Chair
Jeannine English, President
Here's a comprehensive consumer education effort in the area of long-term care.
28 pages

5057 Making a Difference
Georgia Council On Developmental Disabilities
2 Peachtree St N.W.
Suite 26-246
Atlanta, GA 30303-3141

404-657-2126
888-275-4233
Fax: 404-657-2132
TTY: 404-657-2133
eejacobson@dhr.state.ga.us
www.gcdd.org

Eric E Jacobson, Executive Director
Pat Nobbie, Deputy Director
Dottie Adams, Family/Individual Support Dir.
The Georgia Council on Developmental Disabilities collaborates with Georgia's citizens, public and private advocacy organizations and policymakers to positively influence public policies that enhance the quality of life for people with disabilities and their families. GCDD provides this through education and advocacy activities, program implementation, funding and public policy analysis and research.

5058 Making a Difference: A Wise Approach
Easterseals
141 W Jackson Blvd.
Suite 1400A
Chicago, IL 60604

312-726-6200
800-221-6827
Fax: 312-726-1494
info@easterseals.com
www.easterseals.com

Angela F. Williams, President & CEO
Glenda Oakley, Chief Financial Officer
Marcy Traxler, Senior Vice President, Network Advancement
The town of Wise, Virginia, and its leading citizen, Virgil Craft, personify what Making a Difference is all about when a community supports implementing the provisions of the Americans with Disabilities Act. Craft, a person with a disability, has spent his life giving back to the community. The community, in turn, has supported Craft's efforts to improve the environment, education, healthcare and access for disabled persons. A 16-minute video.

5059   Managing Your Activities
Arthritis Foundation
PO Box 78423
Atlanta, GA 30357-0669
                                  404-237-8771
                                  800-933-7023
                              Fax: 404-872-0457
                              help@arthritis.org
                              www.arthritis.org

John H Klippel, CEO/ President

5060   Managing Your Health Care
Arthritis Foundation
PO Box 78423
Atlanta, GA 30357-0669
                                  404-237-8771
                                  800-933-7023
                              Fax: 404-872-0457
                              help@arthritis.org
                              www.arthritis.org

John H Klippel, CEO/ President

**5061   Medical Aspects of Disability: A Handbook For The
Rehabilitation Professional**
Springer Publishing Company
11 West 42nd Street
15th Floor
New York, NY 10036
                                  212-431-4370
                                  877-687-7476
                              Fax: 212-941-7842
                              cs@springerpub.com
                              www.springerpub.com

Ursula Springer, President
Theodore C. Nardin, CEO/Publisher
Jason Roth, VP/Marketing Director
$62.92
744 pages
ISBN 0-826179-71-1

5062   Meeting the Needs of Employees with Disabilities
Resources for Rehabilitation
22 Bonad Road
Ste 19a
Winchester, MA 01890-4330
                                  781-368-9080
                              Fax: 781-368-9096
                              orders@rfr.org
                              www.rfr.org

Susan Greenblatt, Editor
Provides information to help people with disabilities retain or obtain employment. Information on government programs and laws, supported employment, training programs, environmental adaptations and the transition from school to work are included. Chapters on mobility impairment, vision impairment and hearing and speech impairments. *$ 47.95*
167 pages Biennial
ISBN 0-92971 -13-5

5063   NCD Bulletin
National Council on Disability
1331 F Street Northwest
Suite 850
Washington, DC 20004- 1138
                                  202-272-2004
                              Fax: 202-272-2022
                              ncd@ncd.gov
                              www.ncd.gov

Jeff Rosen, Chairperson
Kamilah Oni Martin-Proctor, Co-Vice Chair
Lynnae Ruttledge, Co-Vice Chair
Reports on the latest issues and news affecting people with disabilities.
2 pages Monthly

**5064   NCDE Survival Strategies for Overseas Living for People
with Disabilities**
Mobility International USA
132 E Broadway
Suite 343
Eugene, OR 97401
                                  541-343-1284
                              Fax: 541-343-6812
                              TTY: 541-343-1284
                              clearinghouse@miusa.org
                              www.miusa.org

Susan Sygall, Chief Executive Officer
Cindy Lewis, Director, Programs
This book will provide individuals with disablilities information, resources and guidance on pursuing international exchange opportunities. It addresses disability-related aspects of the international exchange process such as choosing a program, applying, preparing for the trip, adjusting to a new country and returning home.

5065   National Hookup
ISC
16 Liberty St
Larkspur, CA 94939-1520
                                  415-924-3549
                              Fax: 415-927-9556

Russ Bohlke, Manager
Newsletter published by ISC, a national organization of people with physical disabilities. *$6.00*
12-16 pages Quarterly

5066   New Horizons in Sexuality
Accent Books & Products
PO Box 700
Bloomington, IL 61702-700
                                  309-378-2961
                                  800-787-8444
                              Fax: 309-378-4420
                              acmtlvng@aol.com

Raymond C Cheever, Publisher
Betty Garee, Editor
This manual helps both males and females progress toward a satisfying post-injury relationship. *$7.95*
50 pages Paperback
ISBN 0-91570 -42-6

5067   New Voices: Self Advocacy By People with Disabilities
Brookline Books
8 Trumbull Rd
Suite B-001
Northampton, MA 01060
                                  413-584-0184
                                  800-666-2665
                              Fax: 413-584-6184
                              brbooks@yahoo.com
                              www.brooklinebooks.com

A collection of original papers, many by self advocates, that vividly illustrate the dynamic, ever-growing self-advocacy movement — persons with disabilities speaking out and seeking better non-institutional living situations, social and political equality and decent jobs at reasonable pay. *$29.95*
274 pages Paperback
ISBN 1-57129 -04-4

5068   North Star Community Services
3420 University Ave
Waterloo, IA 50701-2050
                                  319-236-0901
                                  888-879-1365
                              Fax: 319-236-3701
                              jmuller@northstarcs.org
                              www.northstarcs.org

Mark Witmer, Executive Director
Matt Hinders, Director of Operations & Safety
Bridget Hartmann, Director of Human Resources
North Star Community Services is a rehabilitative services organization with home office in Waterloo, IA and several branch offices in Northeast, Northern and Central Iowa. North Star helps indiviuals with disabilities live and work in their communities. Services include: adult day services, supported community living services, employment services, and case management/service coordination.

5069   Nothing is Impossible: Reflections on a New Life
Ballantine Books
1745 Broadway
10th Floor
New York, NY 10019   212-782-9000
                    rhkidspublicity@randomhouse.com
                    www.atrandom.com
Edward Warren, Owner
Reeve offers a uniquely powerful message of hope on topics ranging from the controversial stem cell debate to the mind-body connection he credits with his recent physical improvements. *$6.99*
224 pages
ISBN 0-345470-73-7

5070   Nutritional Desk Reference
Keats Publishing
P.O.Box 876
New Canaan, CT 06840   203-966-8721
                    800-323-4900

5071   Nutritional Influences on Illness:
Third Line Press
4751 Viviana Dr
Tarzana, CA 91356-5038   818-996-0076
                    third-line.com
Melvyn R Werbach, Owner
A comprehensive summary of the world's knowledge concerning the relationship between dietary and nutrtional factors and illness. This book does not try to promote any particular school of thought. Instead of the author telling readers his opinion as to what research says, he makes it easy for them to see data for themselves and then form their own opinions.
504 pages
ISBN 0-879835-31-1

5072   Oregon Perspectives
Oregon Council on Developmental Disabilities
540 24th Pl NE
Salem, OR 97301-4517   503-945-9941
                    800-292-4154
                    Fax: 503-945-9947
                    www.ocdd.org
Laura Bronson, Office Manager
Beth Kessler, Planning & Communications Coordi
A quarterly publication from the Oregon Council on Developmental Disabilities.

5073   Organ Transplants: Making the Most of Your Gift of Life
Patient-Centered Guides
1005 Gravenstein Highway North
Sebastopol, CA 95472   707-827-7000
                    Fax: 707-829-0104
                    support@oreilly.com
                    www.oreilly.com
Robert Finn, Author
Over 64,000 people in the US are awaiting an organ transplant. Although transplant surgeries are now fairly routine and can give their recipients the gift of new life, the road to getting a transplant can be long and harrowing. Living with immunosuppressive drugs and strong emotional responses can also be more challenging than families imagine. Medical journalist Robert Finn answers the concerns of these families, with the latest facts about transplantation - as well as the stories behind them. *$5.99*
326 pages Paperback
ISBN 1-565926-34-X

5074   PEAK Parent Center
917 East Moreno Ave.
Suite 140
Colorado Springs, CO 80903   719-531-9400
                    Fax: 719-531-9452
                    info@peakparent.org
                    www.peakparent.org
Michele Williers, Executive Director
Pam Christy, Director, Parent Training & Information
PEAK Parent Center is Colorado's federally-designated Parent Training and Information Center (PTI). As a PTI, PEAK supports and empowers parents, providing them with information and strategies to use when advocating for their children with disabili-

ties. PEAK works one-on-one with families and educators helping them realize new possibilities for children with disabilities by expanding knowledge of special education and offering new strategies for success.
1986

5075   Parallels in Time
MN Governor's Council on Development Disabilities
658 Cedar St
Saint Paul, MN 55155-1603   651-296-4018
                    877-348-0505
                    Fax: 651-297-7200
                    admin.dd@state.mn.us
                    www.mncdd.org
Colleen Wieck PhD, Executive Director
Parallels in Time traces present attitudes and the treatment of people with disabilities, and supplements the first weekend seesion of Partners in Policymaking. This CD-ROM includes the History of the Parent Movement and the History of the Independent Living Movement, as well as personal stories of self advocates, leaders in the self advocacy movement.

5076   Part of the Team
Easterseals
Ste 1800
230 W Monroe St
Chicago, IL 60606-4851   312-726-6800
                    Fax: 312-726-1494
Janet D Jamieson, Communications Manager
James Williams Jr, Chief Executive Officer
Designed for employers of all sizes, rehabilitation organizations and all others concerned with the employment of people with disabilities. It addresses managers' concerns and questions about supervising persons with disabilities and can be used as a discussion/team-building tool for employees with and without disabilities. The video recognizes people with disabilities as strong contenders for almost any job. *$15.00*

5077   Partnering with Public Health: Funding& Advocacy Opportunities for CILs and SILCs
Independent Living Research Utilization ILRU
1333 Moursund
Houston, TX 77030-7031   713-520-0232
                    Fax: 713-520-5785
                    ilru@ilru.org
                    ilru.org
Lex Frieden, Director, ILRU
Richard Petty, Co-Director
Laura Rauscher discusses how CILs and SCILs can use funding from the Centers for Disease Control and partnerships with public health agencies to provide innovative programs promoting the health of people with disabilities.
10 pages

5078   Peer Counseling: Roles, Functions, Boundaries
Independent Living Research Utilization ILRU
1333 Moursund
Houston, TX 77030-7031   713-520-0232
                    Fax: 713-520-5785
                    ilru@ilru.org
                    ilru.org
Lex Frieden, Director, ILRU
Richard Petty, Co-Cirector
In this article, the following points were discussed: describing peer support as counseling suggests safeguards and expectations which cannot be provided by nonprofessionals; the purpose of peer counseling is to promote the independent living philosophy and encourage consumers to embrace it; peer counseling cannot and is not intended to help individuals deal with intense emotional stress, whether it is related to their disability or to something else.
10 pages

5079   Peer Mentor Volunteers: Empowering People for Change
Independent Living Research Utilization ILRU
1333 Moursund
Houston, TX 77030-7031   713-520-0232
                                              Fax: 713-520-5785
                                                   ilru@ilru.org
                                                      ilru.org

Lex Frieden, Director, ILRU
Richard Petty, Co-Director
Arizona Bridge to Independent Living (ABIL) in Phoenix, featured in this issue, is another winner in the innovative CIL program competition.
10 pages

5080   People and Families
New Jersey Council on Developmental Disabilities
20 West State Street, 6th Floor
P.O.Box 700
Trenton, NJ 08625-0700   609-292-3745
                                                   800-792-8858
                                              Fax: 609-292-7114
                                              TTY: 609-777-3238
                                                  njcdd@njcdd.org
                                                   www.njcdd.org

Elaine Buchsbaum, Chairman
Christopher Miller, Vice Chair
Alison M. Lozano, Ph.D, Executive Director
A free magazine for people with disabilities, their families and the public about disability topics such as personal assistance, deinstitutionalization, health care and community living. Published by the New Jersey council on Developmental Disabilities, a federally funded advocacy and policy advisory body. The council has 25 members - 15 consumer/product volunteers and 10 professionals.
48 pages Quarterly

5081   People with Disabilities & Abuse: Implications for
Center for Independent Living
Independent Living Research Utilization ILRU
1333 Moursund
P.O.Box 700
Houston, TX 77030-7031   713-520-0232
                                              Fax: 713-520-5785
                                                   ilru@ilru.org
                                                      ilru.org

Lex Frieden, Director, ILRU
Richard Petty, Co-Director
10 pages

5082   People with Disabilities Who Challenge the System
Brookes Publishing
P.O.Box 10624
Baltimore, MD 21285-0624   410-337-9580
                                                   800-638-3775
                                              Fax: 410-337-8539
                                    custserv@brookespublishing.com
                                                 readplaylearn.com

Paul H. Brooks, Chairman
Jeffrey D. Brookes, President
Melissa A. Behm, Executive Vice President
Helpful forms, tables, and case studies plus an emphasis on self-determination point the way to the development of supports so that people who are deaf-blind, have severe to profound physical and cognitive disabilities, or have serious behavior problems can be fully included in the classroom, workplace, and community. *$34.00*
464 pages Paperback
ISBN 1-55766 -29-0

5083   People's Voice
Independence CIL
300 3rd Ave SW
Suite F
Minot, ND 58701-4346   701-839-4724
                                                   800-377-5114
                                              Fax: 701-838-1677
                          independencecil@independencecil.org
                                              independencecil.org

Susan Ogurek, Chair
Heather Wittliff, Vice Chair
Scott Burlingame, Executive Director
8 pages Quarterly

5084   Personal Perspectives on Personal Assistance Services
World Institute on Disability
3075 Adeline St.
Suite 155
Berkeley, CA 94703   510-225-6400
                                              Fax: 510-225-0477
                                                   wid@wid.org
                                                   www.wid.org

Marcie Roth, Executive Director & Chief Executive Officer
Katherine Zigmont, Senior Director, Operations & Deputy Director
Reggie Johnson, Senior Director, Marketing & Communications
A collection of personal essays that explores a range of perspectives on Personal Assistance Services. Family issues and PAS concerns for people with various different disabilities, of different ages and as members of minority groups are addressed.

5085   Perspectives
National Assoc of State Directors of DD Services
113 Oronoco St
Alexandria, VA 22314-2015   703-683-4202
                                              Fax: 703-684-1395
                                              dberland@nasddds.org

Nancy Thaler, Executive Director
Provides a concise summary of national policy developments and initiatives affecting persons with devlopmental disabilities and the programs that serve them. From bills pending before Congress, to the growth in Medicaid-funded services, to changes in federal-state Medicaid policies and the shift of responsibility from Washington to the states, keeps readers in tune with the latest national issues shaping publically funded disability services.
$95.00
Monthly

5086   Place to Live
Accent Books & Products
P.O.Box 700
Bloomington, IL 61702-700   309-378-2961
                                                   800-787-8444
                                              Fax: 309-378-4420
                                                  acmtlvng@aol.com

Raymond C Cheever, Publisher
Betty Garee, Editor
Many disabled people have found that group housing or accessible apartments are the best alternative to living in a nursing home. These articles tell about some of the alternatives people have found so they can live independently. Just one idea might be the answer for better living for you. *$4.95*
64 pages Paperback
ISBN 0-91570 -30-2

5087   Psychological & Social Impact of Disability
Springer Publishing Company
11 West 42nd Street
15th Floor
New York, NY 10036   212-431-4370
                                                   877-687-7476
                                              Fax: 212-941-7842
                                              cs@springerpub.com
                                                www.springerpub.com

James C. Costello, Vice President, Journal Publishing
Diana Osborne, Production Manager
Megan Larkin, Managing Editor, Journals
$49.95
488 pages
ISBN 0-826122-13-2

5088 **Psychology and Health**
Springer Publishing Company
11 West 42nd Street
15th Floor
New York, NY 10036 212-431-4370
877-687-7476
Fax: 212-941-7842
cs@springerpub.com
www.springerpub.com
James C. Costello, Vice President, Journal Publishing
Diana Osborne, Production Manager
Megan Larkin, Managing Editor, Journals
Content of this book spans a wide range of clinical conditions, including somatization disorders, chronic pain, migraine, anxiety and cancer. *$29.95*
256 pages

5089 **Psychology of Disability**
Springer Publishing Company
11 West 42nd Street,
15th Floor
New York, NY 10036-3915 212-431-4370
877-687-7476
Fax: 212-941-7842
cs@springerpub.com
www.springerpub.com
James C. Costello, Vice President, Journal Publishing
Diana Osborne, Production Manager
Megan Larkin, Managing Editor, Journals
Reactions to the disabled. *$27.95*
288 pages
ISBN 0-82613 -40-1

5090 **Quality of Life for Persons with Disabilities**
Brookline Books
8 Trumbull Road
Suite B-001
Northampton, MA 01060 413-584-0184
800-666-2665
Fax: 413-584-6184
brbooks@yahoo.com
www.brooklinebooks.com
James C. Costello, Vice President, Journal Publishing
Quality of life generally refers to a person's subjective experience of his or her life and focuses attention on how the individual with a disabling condition experiences the world. This book presents a comprehensive and international view of this concept as applied to a broad range of settings in which persons with disabilities live, work and play. *$35.00*
Paperback
ISBN 0-91479 -92-1

5091 **REACHing Out Newsletter**
REACH of Dallas Resource on Independent Living
8625 King George
Suite 210
Dallas, TX 75235-2286 214-630-4796
Fax: 214-630-6390
TTY: 214-630-5995
reachdallas@reachcils.org
reachcils.org
Charlotte A. Stewart, Executive Director
Quarterly newsletter from REACH of Dallas Resource Center on Independent Living.
16 pages Quarterly

5092 **RTC Connection**
Research and Training Center
University of Wisconsin Stou
Menomonie, WI 54751 715-232-2236
Fax: 715-232-2251
menz@uwstout.edu
Julie Larson, Program Assistant
Bi-annual reports on disability and rehabilitation research and policy topics.
Newsletter

5093 **Relaxation: A Comprehensive Manual for Adults and Children with Special Needs**
Research Press
2612 N. Mattis Ave.
P.O.Box 7886
Champaign, IL 61822- 9177 217-352-3273
800-519-2707
Fax: 217-352-1221
orders@researchpress.com
www.researchpress.com
This unique contribution to the field of relaxation training presents: self relaxation techniques designed for adults, methods for teaching relaxation to adults and older children, and procedures for teaching relaxation to young children and children with developmental disabilities. The clear, concise text is supplemented by over 100 helpful illustrations. *$19.95*
Paperback
ISBN 0-878221-86-8

5094 **Resources for People with Disabilities and Chronic Conditions**
Resources for Rehabilitation
Ste 19a
33 Bedford St
Lexington, MA 02420-4330 781-890-6371
Fax: 781-861-7517
Susan Greenblatt
A comprehensive resource directory that helps people with disabilities and chronic conditions achieve their maximum level of independence. Chapters on spinal cord injuries, low back pain, diabetes, hearing and speech impairments, epilepsy, multiple sclerosis. Describes organizations, products and publications. *$49.95*
215 pages Biennial
ISBN 0-92971 -12-7

5095 **Role Portrayal and Stereotyping on Television**
Greenwood Publishing Group
130 Cremona Drive
P O Box 1911
Santa Barbara, CA 93117- 4208 203-226-3571
800-368-6868
805-968-1911
Fax: 866-270-3856
customerservice@abc-clio.com
www.abc-clio.com
An annotated bibliography of studies relating to women, minorities, aging, health and handicaps.
214 pages $55 - $59.95
ISBN 0-313248-55-9

5096 **Screening in Chronic Disease**
Oxford University Press
2001 Evans Rd
Cary, NC 27513-2009 800-445-9714
877-773-4325
Fax: 919-677-1303
custserv.us@oup.com
global.oup.com
Thomas Carty, Senior Vice President
Early detection, or screening, is a common strategy for controlling chronic disease, but little information has been available to help determine which screening procedures are worthwhile, until this textbook. *$42.50*
256 pages

5097 **Sexual Adjustment**
Accent Books & Products
P.O.Box 700
Bloomington, IL 61702-700 309-378-2961
800-787-8444
Fax: 309-378-4420
acmtlvng@aol.com
Raymond C Cheever, Publisher
Betty Garee, Editor
Essential information concerning sexual adjustment for the paraplegic male. *$4.95*
73 pages Paperback
ISBN 0-19570 -00-0

5098 Sexuality and Disabilities: A Guide for Human Service Practitioners
Haworth Press
2&4 Park Square
Abingdon, FL 33487-1503
561-994-0555
Fax: 561-241-7856
orders@taylorandfrancis.com
This book addresses persons with physical, sensory, intellectual and cognitive disabilities and their concerns in the areas of intimacy, family issues, sexuality and sexual functioning. $74.95
159 pages Hardcover
ISBN 1-560243-75-9

5099 Sickened: The Memoir of a Muchausen by Proxy Childhood
Bantam Books
1745 Broadway
10th Floor
New York, NY 10019-4039
212-782-9000
Fax: 212-572-6066
crownpublicity@randomhouse.com
www.randomhouse.com
From early childhood, Julie Gregory was continually X-rayed, medicated, and operated on — in the vain pursuit of an illness that was created in her mother's mind. Munchausen by proxy (MBP) in which the caretaker — almost always the mother — invents or induces symptoms in her child because she craves the attention of medical professionals. $24.95
256 pages Hardcover
ISBN 0-553803-07-7

5100 Socialization Games for Persons with Disabilities
Charles C. Thomas
2600 S First St
Springfield, IL 62704-4730
217-789-8980
800-258-8980
Fax: 217-789-9130
books@ccthomas.com
www.ccthomas.com
Michael P. Thomas, President
This text will assist those who want to teach severely multiple disabled students by providing information on: general principles of intervention and classroom organization; managing the behavior of students; physically managing students and using adaptive equipment; teaching eating skills; teaching toileting, dressing, and hygiene skills; teaching cognition, communication, and socialization skills; teaching independent living skills; and teaching infants and preschool students. $38.95
176 pages Paperback
ISBN 0-398067-46-5

5101 Sometimes You Just Want to Feel Like a Human Being
Brookes Publishing
P.O.Box 10624
Baltimore, MD 21285-0624
410-337-9580
800-638-3775
Fax: 410-337-8539
custserv@brookespublishing.com
readplaylearn.com
Paul Brooks, Owner
Case studies of empowering psychotherapy with people with disabilities. This text reveals how counseling can be beneficial to individuals with disabilities of all kinds, including autism, developmental disabilities, sensory impairment, cerebral palsy, or HIV infection. $26.95
272 pages Paperback
ISBN 1-55766 -96-0

5102 South Carolina Assistive Technology Program
8301 Farrow Road
University Center for Excellence
Columbia, SC 29203-2920
803-935-5263
800-915-4522
Fax: 803-935-5342
carol.page@uscmed.sc.edu
www.sc.edu/scatp/
Carol Page, Ph.D, Program Director
Mary r Alice Bechtle, Program Coordinator
Janet Jendron, Program Coordinator

The South Carolina Assistive Technology Program (SCATP) is a federally funded program concerned with getting technology into the hands of people with disabilities so that they might live, work, learn and be a more independent part of the community. We provide an equipment loan and demonstration program, an on-line equipment exchange program, training, technical assistance, publications, an interactive CDROM (SC Curriculum Access through AT), an information listserv and work with various state com
7-8 pages Bi-annually

5103 Space Coast CIL News
Space Coast Center for Independent Living
571 Haverty Court,
Suite W
Rockledge, FL 32955-2566
321-633-6011
Fax: 321-633-6472
TTY: 321-784-9008
www.sccil.net
Michael Lavoie, President
Howard Fetes, Vice-President
Non-profit organization that provides services which enable people with disabilities to live as independently as possible.
12 pages Quarterly

5104 Special Needs Trust Handbook
Aspen Publishers
7th Fl
76 9th Ave
New York, NY 10011-4962
301-644-3599
800-638-8437
www.aspenpublishers.com
Bob Lemmond, President and CEO
Gustavo Dobles, Vice President and Chief Content Officer
Susan Pikitch, Vice President and Chief Financial Officer
The Special Needs Trusts Handbook is the single-volume, comprehensive resource that provides information on how to handle the complex requirements of drafting and administering trusts for clients who are mentally or physically disabled, or who wish to provide for others with disabilities. $245.00
900 pages
ISBN 0-735572-88-7

5105 Special Siblings: Growing Up With Someone with A Disability
Brookes Publishing
P.O.Box 10624
Baltimore, MD 21285-0624
410-337-9580
800-638-3775
Fax: 410-337-8539
custserv@brookespublishing.com
readplaylearn.com
Paul Brooks, Owner
The author reveals what she experienced as the sister of a man with cerebral palsy and developmental disability — and shares what others have learned about being and having a special sibling. Weaving a lifetime of memories and reflections with relevant research and interviews with more than 100 other siblings and experts, McHugh explores a spectrum of feelings — from anger and guilt to love and pride — and helps readers understand the issues siblings may encounter. $21.95
256 pages Paperback
ISBN 1-557666-07-5

5106 TERI
251 Airport Rd
Oceanside, CA 92058-1321
760-721-1706
teriinc.org
Cheryl Kilmer, CEO & Founder
William E. Mara, Chief Operating Officer
Krysti DeZonia, Ed.D, Director of Education & Research
A private, nonprofit corporation which has been developing and operating programs for individuals with developmental disabilities since 1980. Offers staff training videos, staff training tools and technique manuals.

5107   That All May Worship: An Interfaith Welcome to People with Disabilities
American Association of People with Disabilities
2013 H St. NW
5th Floor
Washington, DC 20006   202-521-4316
                                    800-840-8844
                            communications@aapd.com
                            www.aapd.com/publications
Maria Town, President & Chief Executive Officer
Jasmin Bailey, Manager, Business Operations
Christine Liao, Programs Director
An interfaith handbook to assist congregations in welcoming people with disabilities to promote acceptance and full participation.

5108   The Ultimate Guide to Sex and Disability
Read How You Want Large Print Books

                                    800-797-9277
                            support@readhowyouwant.com
                            www.readhowyouwant.com
Miriam Kaufman, Author
For everyone, men and women of all ages and sexual identities, The Ultimate Guide to Sex and Disability covers the span of disabilities - from chronic fatigue and back pain to spinal cord injury, multiple sclerosis, cystic fibrosis, cerebral palsy, and many others.

5109   To Live with Grace and Dignity
LRP Publications

Lydia Gans, Author
This book combines photographs and essays to allow the reader to enter some of the real day to day relationships that develop between individuals with disabilities and their personal assistants. The individuals included in this book represent a wide range of ages, disabilities and cultural backgrounds.
72 pages Paperback
ISBN 0-934753-85-7

5110   Touch/Ability Connects People with Disabilities & Alternative Health Care Pract.
Independent Living Research Utilization ILRU
1333 Moursund
Houston, TX 77030-7031   713-520-0232
                            Fax: 713-520-5785
                                    ilru@ilru.org
                                    ilru.org
Lex Frieden, Director, ILRU
Richard Petty, Co-Director
The people at DIRECT center for Independence and Touch/Ability in Tuscon, Arizona, have collaborated to develop a wellness program that makes alternative health care choices available to people with disabilities. The Touch/Ability Wellness program was selected as one of last year's winners in the Innovative CILs competition because of this outcome of increased options open to people with disabilities.
10 pages

5111   US Role in International Disability Activities: A History
World Institute on Disability
3075 Adeline St.
Suite 155
Berkeley, CA 94703   510-225-6400
                            Fax: 510-225-0477
                                    wid@wid.org
                                    www.wid.org
Marcie Roth, Executive Director & Chief Executive Officer
Katherine Zigmont, Senior Director, Operations & Deputy Director
Reggie Johnson, Senior Director, Marketing & Communications
This study serves as an introduction to US involvement in the field of international rehabilitation and disability.

5112   Understanding and Accommodating Physical Disabilities: Desk Reference
Greenwood Publishing Group
130 Cremona Drive
P O Box 1911
Santa Barbara, CA 93117- 4208   203-226-3571
                                    800-368-6868
                                    805-968-1911
                            Fax: 866-270-3856
                            customerservice@abc-clio.com
                                    www.abc-clio.com
Medical conditions that qualify as disabilities under the American's with Disabilities Act are explained in non-medical terminology. Hardcover.
200 pages $52.95 - $55
ISBN 0-899308-14-7

5113   Vestibular Disorders Association
Vestibular Disorders Association
5018 NE 15th Ave.
P.O. Box 13305
Portland, OR 97211   503-229-7705
                                    800-837-8428
                            Fax: 503-229-8064
                                    info@vestibular.org
                                    www.vestibular.org
Cynthia Ryan, MBA, Executive Director
Tony Staser, Development Director
Kerrie Denner, Outreach Coordinator
The mission of the Vestibular Disorders Association is to serve people with vestibular disorders by providing access to information, offering a support network, and elevating awareness of the challenges associated with these disorders. They also aim to support and empower vestibular patients on their journey back to balance. *$15.00*
ISBN 0-963261-15-0

5114   Visions & Values
Idaho Council on Developmental Disabilities
650 W. State St., Room 100
P. O. Box 83720
Boise, ID 83720-5840   208-332-1824
                                    800-544-2433
                            Fax: 208-334-2307
C. L. Butch Otter, Governor
A quarterly publication from the Idaho Council on Developmental Disabilities.

5115   Weiner's Herbal
Quantum Books
355 Middlesex Avenue
Wilmington, MA 01887-1406   978-988-2470
                            Fax: 617-577-7282
                                    www.quantumbooks.com
William Szabo, Owner
A-Z index covering all aspects of herbs.
Paperback
ISBN 0-812825-86-1

5116   When the Brain Goes Wrong
Fanlight Productions
32 Court Street,
21st Floor
Brooklyn, NY 11201-1731   718-488-8900
                                    800-876-1710
                            Fax: 718-488-8642
                                    info@fanlight.com
                                    www.fanlight.com
Ben Achtenberg, Owner
Nicole Johnson, Publicity Coordinator
Anthony Sweeney, Marketing Director
An extraordinary and provocative series of seven short films which profile individuals with a range of brian dysfunctions. The seven brief segments focus on schizophrenia, manic depression, epilepsy, head injury, headaches and addiction. In addition to the personal stories, the segments include interviews with physicians who speak briefly about what is known about the disorders and treatment. #131 *$245.00*
ISBN 1-572951-31-1

5117 Women with Physical Disabilities: Achieving & Maintaining Health & Well-Being
Spina Bifida Association of America
1600 Wilson Blvd.
Suite 800
Arlington, VA 22209-4226
202-944-3285
800-621-3141
Fax: 202-944-3295
sbaa@sbaa.org
www.spinabifidaassociation.org
Ana Ximenes, Chair
Sara Struwe, President & CEO
Cindy Brownstein, CEO
Introduces the critical concept of womens health in the context of physical disabilities. *$42.00*

5118 Work in the Context of Disability Culture
Independent Living Research Utilization ILRU
1333 Moursund
Houston, TX 77030-7031
713-520-0232
Fax: 713-520-5785
ilru@ilru.org
ilru.org
Lex Frieden, Director, ILRU
Richard Petty, Co-Director
Another winner in the innovative CIL competition-Steve Brown describes the Talking Books Program of Southeast Alaska Independent Living, discussing their efforts to record the oral history and life experiences of people with disabilities in the larger context of the disability culture.
10 pages

5119 Your Role in Inclusion Theatre
Houston, TX
713-202-8840
Inclusiontheater@gmail.com
Deborah E. Nowinski, Author/Inclusion Specialist
A guidebook for educators who wish to create a successful theatre environment for individuals of all abilities. The book also includes stories, tips, and games. *$19.95*
192 pages
ISBN 1-517357-49-8

Parenting: General

5120 AEPS Family Report: Birth to Three Years
Brookes Publishing
P.O. Box 10624
Baltimore, MD 21285-0624
410-337-9580
800-638-3775
Fax: 410-337-8539
custserv@brookespublishing.com
www.brookespublishing.com
Diane Bricker, Author
Betty Capt, Author
JoAnn Johnson, Author
This Family Report was developed for use in conjunction with the AEPSr for children birth to 3 years to obtain information from parents and other caregivers about their children's skills and abilities across major areas of development. Available in packages of 10.
28 pages Saddle-stitched

5121 AEPS Family Report: For Children Ages Three to Six
Brookes Publishing
P.O.Box 10624
Baltimore, MD 21285-0624
410-337-9580
800-638-3775
Fax: 410-337-8539
custserv@brookespublishing.com
www.brookespublishing.com
Diane Bricker, Author
Betty Capt, Author
JoAnn Johnson, Author
This is a 64-item questionnaire that asks parents to rank their child's abilities on specific skills. In packages of 10 paperback.
28 pages Saddle-stiched

5122 Adapted Physical Activity
Human Kinetics
1607 N Market St
P.O.Box 5076
Champaign, IL 61820-5076
800-747-4457
Fax: 217-351-1549
info@hkusa.com
www.humankinetics.com
Human Kinetics produces a variety of resources for adapted physical education practitioners, including books on activities, a research journal and higher education references.

5123 Assistive Technology for Parents with Disabilities Handbook
Idaho Assistive Technology Project
University of Idaho
1187 Alturas Dr.
Moscow, ID 83843- 2268
208-885-3557
800-432-8324
Fax: 208-885-6102
idahoat@uidaho.edu
www.idahoat.org
handbook providing resources and information on assistive technology for parents with disabilities.

5124 Babyface: A Story of Heart and Bones
Penguin Books USA
375 Hudson St
New York, NY 10014
212-366-2000
consumerservices@penguinrandomhouse.com
www.penguin.com
Jeanne McDermott, Author
A must read for families that seek insight into coping with a chronic condition. Many useful resources provided.
288 pages Paperback

5125 Backyards and Butterflies: Ways to Include Children with Disabilities in Outdoor Activities
Brookline Books
8 Trumbull Rd
Ste B-001
Northampton, MA 01060
413-584-0184
800-666-2665
Fax: 413-584-6184
brbooks@yahoo.com
www.brooklinebks.com
Doreen Greenstein, Author
Suzanne Bloom, Author
An illustrated book with dozens of imaginative ways parents can include children with physical disabilities in outdoor activities. Offers clear concise, how-to directions for constructing homemade toys, utensils, and other items that can be enjoyed outside safely and comfortably.
72 pages Paperback

5126 Beyond Tears: Living After Losing a Child
St. Martin's Griffin (Macmillan Publishers)
75 Varick St
New York, NY 10013
212-226-7521
press.inquiries@macmillan.com
us.macmillan.com/smp
Ellen Mitchell, Author
Meant to comfort and give direction to bereaved parents, Beyond Tears is written by nine mothers who have each lost a child. This revised edition includes a new chapter written from the perspective of surviving siblings. The death of a child is that unimaginable loss no parent ever expects to face. In this book, nine mothers share their individual stories of how to survive in the darkest hour.

5127 Broken Dolls: Gathering the Pieces: Caringfor Chronically Ill Children
St. Paul Press

Jennifer Travis Cox, Author
Told from the point of view of the author, this book tracks the challenges faced by parents and caregivers of chronically ill-children - both in terms of medical care and emotional impact. It offers advice based on the author's own experiences caring for her

child, as well as insights from other families who have gone through the same experience.
164 pages Paperback

5128 Building the Healing Partnership: Parents, Professionals and Children
Brookline Books
8 Trumbull Road
Suite B-001
Northampton, MA 01060
413-584-0184
800-666-2665
Fax: 413-584-6184
brbooks@yahoo.com
www.brooklinebooks.com
Successful programs understand that the disabled child's needs must be considered in the context of a family. This book was specifically written for practitioner's who must work with families but who have insufficient training in family systems assessment and intervention. It is a valuable blend of theory and practice with pointers for applying the principles. *$24.95*
Paperback
ISBN 0-91479 -63-8

5129 Children with Disabilities
Brookes Publishing
P.O.Box 10624
Baltimore, MD 21285-0624
410-337-9580
800-638-3775
Fax: 410-337-8539
custserv@brookespublishing.com
www.brookespublishing.com
Mark L Batshaw MD, Editor
Paul Brooks, Owner
Lauren Rohe, Regional Sales Consultant
Extensive coverage of genetics, heredity, pre- and postnatal development, specific disabilities, family roles, and intervention. Features chapters on substance abuse, HIV and AIDS, Down syndrome, fragile X syndrome, behavior management, transitions to adulthood, and health care in the 21st century. Also reveals the causes of many conditions that can lead to developmental disabilities. *$69.95*
912 pages Hardcover
ISBN 1-557665-81-8

5130 Conditional Love: Parents' Attitudes Toward Handicapped Children
Greenwood Publishing Group
130 Cremona Drive
P O Box 1911
Santa Barbara, CA 93117- 4208
203-226-3571
800-368-6868
805-968-1911
Fax: 866-270-3856
customerservice@abc-clio.com
www.abc-clio.com
Offers parents information on understanding disabled children and mainstreaming them into their normal family life. *$49.95*
312 pages
ISBN 0-89789 -24-7

5131 Coordinacion De Servicios Centrado En La Familia
Brookline Books
8 Trumbull Road
Suite B-001
Northampton, MA 01060
413-584-0184
800-666-2665
Fax: 413-584-6184
brbooks@yahoo.com
www.brooklinebooks.com
This book, translated into Spanish from the English original, is designed to orient and educate parents about issues of service coordination, to assist families in caring for an infant or toddler with developmental delays or disabilities. *$7.00*
34 pages Paperback
ISBN 0-91479 -90-5

5132 Developing Personal Safety Skills in Children with Disabilities
Brookes Publishing
P.O.Box 10624
Baltimore, MD 21285-0624
410-337-9580
800-638-3775
Fax: 410-337-8539
custserv@brookespublishing.com
readplaylearn.com
Paul Brooks, Owner
A guide for teachers, parents, and caregivers, this volume explores the issue of personal safety for children with disabilities and offers strategies for empowering and protecting them at home and in school. Recognizing that children with disabilities are vulnerable to abuse, this work explores why children with disabilities need personal safety skills, offers, curriculum ideas and exercises, and advocates the development of self-esteem and assertiveness so that children can protect themselves. *$34.00*
220 pages Paperback
ISBN 1-557661-84-7

5133 Developmental Disabilities in Infancy and Childhood
Brookes Publishing
P.O.Box 10624
Baltimore, MD 21285-0624
410-767-6100
800-638-3775
Fax: 410-767-5850
custserv@brookespublishing.com
readplaylearn.com
Paul Brooks, Owner
This two volume set explores advances in assessment and treatment, retains a clinical focus, and incorporates recent developments in research and theory. Can be purchased individually or as a set (Vol. 1: Neurodevelopmental Diagnosis and Treatment Vol. 2: The Spectrum of Developmental Disabilities). *$210.00*
Hardcover
ISBN 1-55766O-CA-P

5134 Dictionary of Developmental Disabilities Terminology
Brookes Publishing
P.O.Box 10624
Baltimore, MD 21285-0624
410-337-9580
800-638-3775
Fax: 410-337-8539
custserv@brookespublishing.com
readplaylearn.com
Paul Brooks, Owner
Answers thousands of questions for medical or human services professionals, parents or advocates of children with disabilities, or students preparing for their careers. Provides thorough explanations of the most common terms associated with disabilities. *$55.95*
368 pages Hardcover
ISBN 1-557662-45-2

5135 Encyclopedia of Genetic Disorders & Birth Defects
Facts on File
132 W 31st St
17th Floor
New York, NY 10001-3406
800-322-8755
Fax: 800-678-3633
custserv@factsonfile.com
www.infobasepublishing.com/
Mark Donnell, President
Layperson-accessible entries on genetic terminology and genetically-influenced conditions. *$71.50*
474 pages
ISBN 0-816038-09-0

5136 Exceptional Parent Magazine
Psy-Ed Corporation
416 Main Street
Johnstown, PA 15901-2032
814-361-3860
877-372-7368
Fax: 814-361-3861
www.eparent.com
Vanessa B Ira, Contributing Writer / Editor
Joseph M. Valenzano, Jr., President, CEO & Publisher
Rick Rader, MD, Editor-in-Chief

Magazine that provides information, support, ideas, encouragement, and outreach for parents and families of children with disabilities and the professionals who work with them. *$39.95*
85 pages Monthly

5137   Face of Inclusion
Special Needs Project
Ste H
324 State St
Santa Barbara, CA 93101-2364   805-962-8087
                                      800-333-6867
                                      Fax: 805-962-5087
                                      eplibrary@aol.com
                                      www.eplibrary.com
Hod Gray, Owner
A unique and moving parents' perspective of inclusion for administrators, teachers, and parents of children with disabilities. *$99.00*

5138   Families Magazine
New Jersey Developmental Disabilities Council
20 West State Street, 6th Floor
P.O.Box 700
Trenton, NJ 08625-0700   609-292-3745
                                     800-792-8858
                                     Fax: 609-292-7114
                                     TTY: 609-777-3238
                                     njcdd@njcdd.org
                                     www.njddc.org
Elaine Buchsbaum, Chairman
Christopher Miller, Vice Chair
Alison M. Lozano, Ph.D, Executive Director
Quarterly magazine for people with disabilities, their families and the public, features family profiles, news, columns and the New Jersey Family support councils newsletter.
Quarterly

5139   Families, Illness & Disability
Through the Looking Glass
3075 Adeline St
Ste. 120
Berkeley, CA 94703-2212   510-848-1112
                                     800-644-2666
                                     Fax: 510-848-4445
                                     TTY: 510-848-1005
                                     tlg@lookingglass.org
                                     www.lookingglass.org
Maureen Block, J.D., Co-Founder
Karen Fessel, Ph.D., Executive Director
$35.00
320 pages

5140   Family Interventions Throughout Disability
Springer Publishing Company
11 West 42nd Street,
15th Floor
New York, NY 10036-3915   212-431-4370
                                     877-687-7476
                                     Fax: 212-941-7842
                                     cs@springerpub.com
                                     www.springerpub.com
Theodore C Nardin, Chief Executive Officer
James C. Costello, Vice President, Journal Publishing
Diana Osborne, Production Manager
Family attitudes throughout chronic illness and disability. *$31.95*
320 pages
ISBN 0-82615-80-4

5141   Family-Centered Service Coordination: A Manual for Parents
Brookline Books
8 Trumbull Road
Suite B-001
Northampton, MA 01060   413-584-0184
                                     800-666-2665
                                     Fax: 413-584-6184
                                     brbooks@yahoo.com
                                     www.brooklinebooks.com

A manual designed to orient and educate parents about issues of service coordination, to assist families in caring for an infant or toddler with developmental delays or disabilities. *$7.00*
34 pages Paperback
ISBN 0-91479-90-5

5142   Handbook About Care in the Home
AARP Fulfillment
601 E St NW
Washington, DC 20049-1   202-434-2277
                                     888-687-2277
                                     TTY: 877-434-7598
                                     member@aarp.org
                                     www.aarp.org
Offers valuable information for the disabled.
24 pages

5143   LifeLines
Disabled & Alone/Life Services for the Handicapped
1441 Broadway
23rd Floor
New York, NY 10018-2326   212-532-6740
                                     800-995-0066
                                     Fax: 212-532-6740
                                     info@disabledandalone.org
                                     www.disabledandalone.org/lifelines.html
Leslie D. Park, Chair
Rex L. Davidson, Vice President
Lee Alan Ackerman, Executive Director
Newsletter providing current and valuable information about lifetime care and planning for persons with disabilities and their families and the organizations serving them. Free upon request.
4-10 pages Biannual

5144   Living with a Brother or Sister with Special Needs: A Book for Sibs
Sibling Support Project
6512 23rd Ave NW
Ste 322
Seattle, WA 98117   206-297-6368
                                     info@siblingsupport.org
                                     www.siblingsupport.org
Don Meyer, Author
Patricia Vadasy, Author
Living with a Brother or Sister with Special Needs focuses on the intensity of emotions that brothers and sisters experience when they have a sibling with special needs, and the hard questions they ask. It talks about the good and not-so-good parts of having a brother or sister who has special needs, and offers suggestions for how to make life easier for everyone in the family.
144 pages Paperback

5145   Loving & Letting Go
Centering Corporation
7230 Maple Street
Omaha, NE 68134-5064   402-553-1200
                                     866-218-0101
                                     Fax: 402-533-0507
                                     j1200@aol.com
                                     www.centering.org
Joy Johnson, Founder
Dr. Marvin Johnson, co-Founder
For parents who decide to turn away from aggressive medical intervention for their critically ill newborn. *$5.95*
48 pages Paperback

5146   Mobility Training for People with Disabilities
Charles C. Thomas
2600 S First St
Springfield, IL 62704-4730   217-789-8980
                                     800-258-8980
                                     Fax: 217-789-9130
                                     books@ccthomas.com
                                     www.ccthomas.com
Michael P. Thomas, President

5147   Mother to Be
Through the Looking Glass
3075 Adeline St
Ste. 120
Berkeley, CA 94703-2212   510-848-1112
                                        800-644-2666
                                        Fax: 510-848-4445
                                        TTY: 510-848-1005
                                        tlg@lookingglass.org
                                        www.lookingglass.org
Maureen Block, J.D., Co-Founder
Karen Fessel, Ph.D., Executive Director
Guide to pregnancy and birth for women with disabilities. *$34.00*
410 pages

**5148   New Language of Toys: Teaching Communication Skills
to Children with Special Needs**
Spina Bifida Association of America
1600 Wilson Blvd.
Suite 800
Arlington, VA 22209-4226   202-944-3285
                                        800-621-3141
                                        Fax: 202-944-3295
                                        sbaa@sbaa.org
                                        www.spinabifidaassociation.org
Ana Ximenes, Chair
Sara Struwe, President & CEO
Cindy Brownstein, CEO
A guide for parents and teachers and a reader-friendly resource
guide that provides a wealth of information on how play activities
affect a child's language development and where to get the toys
and materials to use in these activities. *$19.00*

5149   Newsline
Federation for Children with Special Needs
529 Main St.
Suite 1M3
Boston, MA 02129   617-236-7210
                                        800-331-0688
                                        Fax: 617-241-0330
                                        fcsninfo@fcsn.org
                                        www.fcsn.org
Pam Nourse, Executive Director
Offers information and resources for families of children with
disabilities, as well as event announcements, project updates,
news and more.
Quarterly

**5150   On the Road to Autonomy: Promoting Self- Competence
in Children & Youth with Disabilities**
Brookes Publishing
P.O.Box 10624
Baltimore, MD 21285-0624   410-337-9580
                                       800-638-3775
                                       Fax: 410-337-8539
                                       custserv@brookespublishing.com
                                       readplaylearn.com
Paul Brooks, Owner
This book provides detailed conceptual, practical, and personal
information regarding the promotion of self-esteem, self-deter-
mination, and coping skills among children and youth with and
without disabilities. *$48.00*
432 pages Paperback
ISBN 1-55766 -35-5

5151   Pain Erasure
M Evans and Company
216 E 49th St
New York, NY 10017-1546   212-979-0880
                                       Fax: 212-486-4544
Mary Evans, Owner
This book explains Bonnie Prudden's method for pain relief us-
ing myotherapy, a method hailed by doctors and patients.
ISBN 0-345331-02-8

**5152   Parent Centers and Independent Living Centers:
Collectively We're Stronger**
Independent Living Research Utilization ILRU
1333 Moursund
Houston, TX 77030-7031   713-520-0232
                                       Fax: 713-520-5785
                                       ilru@ilru.org
                                       ilru.org
Lex Frieden, Director, ILRU
Richard Petty, Co-Director
This article describes several examples of effective working relationships of PTIs and CILs. The examples highlight how parent
and consumer organizations have identified complimentary
strengths and formed partnerships to better support children with
disabilities and their families. These partnerships can also be a
very important way of involving youth in the disability movement so they may become leaders of tomorrow.
10 pages

5153   Parent-Child Interaction and Developmental Disabilities
Greenwood Publishing Group
130 Cremona Drive
P O Box 1911
Santa Barbara, CA 93117   800-368-6868
                                       805-968-1911
                                       Fax: 866-270-3856
                                       customerservice@abc-clio.com
                                       www.abc-clio.com
This volume brings together the original papers by international
scholars and practitioners on the question of the effects of parent
interaction with developmentally disabled children.
$65.00-$69.50.
395 pages Hardcover
ISBN 0-275928-35-7

5154   Parenting
Accent Books & Products
P.O.Box 700
Bloomington, IL 61702-700   309-378-2961
                                       800-787-8444
                                       Fax: 309-378-4420
                                       acmtlvng@aol.com
Raymond C Cheever, Publisher
Betty Garee, Editor
Experienced parents (who are disabled) discuss: raising children
from infant to teens, balancing career and motherhood, discipline
methods and more when both parents are disabled. *$7.95*
83 pages
ISBN 0-91570 -26-4

5155   Parenting with a Disability
Through the Looking Glass
3075 Adeline St
Ste. 120
Berkeley, CA 94703-2212   510-848-1112
                                       800-644-2666
                                       Fax: 510-848-4445
                                       TTY: 510-848-1005
                                       tlg@lookingglass.org
                                       www.lookingglass.org
Maureen Block, J.D., Board President
Rusty Hendlin, M.A., LMFT, Director of Medi-Cal Services
Thomas Spalding, Board Treasurer
International newsletter. Available in braille, large print or cas-
sette.
3 per year

5156   Perspectives on a Parent Movement
Brookline Books
8 Trumbull Rd
Suite B-001
Northampton, MA 1060-4533   413-584-0184
                                       800-666-2665
                                       Fax: 413-584-6184
                                       brbooks@yahoo.com
                                       www.brooklinebooks.com

This book captures Rosemary Dybwad's truly innovative wisdom and pioneering for people with intellectual limitations in these previously unpublished essays and speeches. *$17.95*
Paperback
ISBN 0-91479 -74-3

5157 Sexuality and the Developmentally Handicapped
Edwin Mellen Press
P.O.Box 450
Lewiston, NY 14092-450   716-754-2266
                                Fax: 716-754-4056
                             jrupnow@mellenpress.com
                                   mellenpress.com

Herbert Richardson, Owner
Presents the knowledge, attitudes, and skills pertinent to responding to the sexual problems of developmentally handicapped persons, their families and communities. Details fully documented cases, issues concerning the law, and resource materials available. *$89.95*
245 pages Hardcover
ISBN 0-88946 -32-5

5158 Shattered Dreams-Lonely Choices: Birth Parents of Babies with Disabilities
Greenwood Publishing Group
130 Cremona Drive
Santa Barbara, CA 93117-4208   203-226-3571
                                  800-368-6868
                                  805-968-1911
                                Fax: 866-270-3856
                           customerservice@abc-clio.com
                                 www.abc-clio.com
Written by a mother who, without warning, gave birth to a boy with Down Syndrome, this book is meant to help parents through the initial shock and the realization that they are not able to care for their child. $29.95-$35.00. *$29.95*
208 pages Hardcover
ISBN 0-897892-86-0

5159 Since Owen, A Parent-to-Parent Guide for Care of the Disabled Child
Special Needs Project
324 State Street
Suite H
Santa Barbara, CA 93101-2364   818-718-9900
                                 800-333-6867
                               Fax: 818-349-2027
                            editor@specialneeds.com
                              www.specialneeds.com
Hod Gray, Owner
Against the background of his experience as the parent of a severely disabled young man, Callahan writes conscientiously to other parents. *$16.95*
486 pages

5160 Sleep Better! A Guide to Improving Sleep for Children with Special Needs
Brookes Publishing
P.O.Box 10624
Baltimore, MD 21285-624   410-337-9580
                                 800-638-3775
                               Fax: 410-337-8539
                          custserv@brookespublishing.com
                               readplaylearn.com
Paul Brooks, Owner
This book offers step-by-step, how to instructions for helping children with disabilities get the rest they need. For problems ranging from bedtime tantrums to night waking, parents and caregivers will find a variety of widely tested and easy-to-implement techniques that have already helped hundreds of children with special needs. *$21.95*
288 pages Paperback
ISBN 1-55766 -15-7

5161 Something's Wrong with My Child!
Charles C. Thomas
2600 S First St
Springfield, IL 62704-4730   217-789-8980
                                 800-258-8980
                               Fax: 217-789-9130
                             books@ccthomas.com
                                www.ccthomas.com
Michael P. Thomas, President
This text provides professionals and parents with the opportunity to gain insights into a family that has benefited positively and constructively from the presence of a member with a disability. The author presents a compilation of easy-to-read material that's based on real-life experiences. *$39.95*
234 pages Paperback 1998
ISBN 0-398068-99-8

5162 Sometimes I Get All Scribbly
Exceptional Parent Library
P.O.Box 1807
Englewood Cliffs, NJ 7632-1207   201-947-6000
                                 800-535-1910
                               Fax: 201-947-9376
                              eplibrary@aol.com
                               www.eplibrary.com
Clinical, educational and emotional information from the point of view of a parent. *$16.00*

5163 Son-Rise: The Miracle Continues
2080 South Undermountain Road
Sheffield, MA 01257-9643   413-229-2100
                                 877-766-7473
                               Fax: 413-229-3202
                             sonrise@option.org
                               www.son-rise.org
Barry Neil Kaufman, Co-Founder/ Co-Originator/Senior Teacher/Trainer
Samahria Lyte Kaufman, Co-Founder/ Co-Originator/Senior Teacher/Trainer
Bryn Hogan, ATCA Senior Staff
Documents Raun Kaufman's astonishing development from a lifeless, autistic child into a highly verbal, lovable youngster with no traces of his former condition. Details Raun's extraordinary progress from the age of four into young adulthood, also shares moving accounts of five families that successfully used the Son-Rise Program to reach their own special children.
372 pages
ISBN 0-915811-53-7

5164 Special Kids Need Special Parents: A Resource for Parents of Children With Special Needs
Berkley Publishing Group
375 Hudson Street
New York, NY 10014-3657   212-366-2372
                               Fax: 212-366-2933
                         ecommerce@us.penguingroup.com
                             www.us.penguingroup.com
The author, herself the parent of a child with special needs, draws on interviews with health care professionals, nationally recognized authorities, and other partens to give readers the answers, advice, and comfort they crave. *$13.95*
319 pages Paperback
ISBN 0-425176-62-2

5165 Special Parent, Special Child
Exceptional Parent Library
P.O.Box 1807
Englewood Cliffs, NJ 7632-1207   201-947-6000
                                 800-535-1910
                               Fax: 201-947-9376
                              eplibrary@aol.com
                               www.eplibrary.com
Offers information for facing the challenges of being a special parent. *$21.95*
Hardcover

5166 **Strategies for Working with Families of Young Children with Disabilities**
Brookes Publishing
P.O. Box 10624
Baltimore, MD 21285-624
410-337-9580
800-638-3775
Fax: 410-337-8539
custserv@brookespublishing.com
readplaylearn.com

Paul Brooks, Owner
This text offers useful techniques for collaborating with and supporting families whose youngest members either have a disability or are at risk for developing a disability. The authors address specific issues such as cultural diversity, transitions to new programs, and disagreements between families and professionals. *$33.00*
272 pages Paperback
ISBN 1-55766 -57-6

5167 **That's My Child**
Exceptional Parent Library
P.O. Box 1807
Englewood Cliffs, NJ 7632-1207
201-947-6000
800-535-1910
Fax: 201-947-9376
eplibrary@aol.com
www.eplibrary.com
Offers information to help parent successfully navigate the maze of resources and services available for children with special needs. *$12.95*

5168 **The Complete Guide to Creating a Special Needs Life Plan**
Jessica Kingsley Publishers
73 Collier St
London, UK N19BE
hello@jkp.com
www.jkp.com

Hal Wright, Author
The purpose of special needs planning is to create the best possible life for an adult with a disability. This book provides comprehensive guidance on creating a life plan to transition a special needs child to independence or to ensure they are well cared for in the future.
360 pages

5169 **They Don't Come with Manuals**
Fanlight Productions
32 Court Street, 21st Floor
Brooklyn, NY 11201-1731
718-488-8900
800-876-1710
Fax: 718-488-8642
orders@fanlight.com
www.fanlight.com

Ben Achtenberg, Owner
Anthony Sweeney, Marketing Director
Nicole Johnson, Publicity Coordinator
The parents and adoptive parents in this video speak candidly of their day to day experiences caring for children with physical and mental disabilities. *$145.00*

5170 **They're Just Kids**
Aquarius Health Care Videos
30 Forest Road
P.O. Box 249
Millis, MA 02054-7159
508-376-1244
Fax: 508-376-1245
aqvideos@tiac.net
www.aquariusproductions.com

Lesile Kussmann, President
Joyce Farmer, Assistant Director
The importance and value of inclusion, excellent for anyone working with kids with disabilities. The documentary explores the advantages of the inclusion of disabled children in the classroom, cub scouts and other extracurricular activities. *$99.00*
Video

5171 **To a Different Drumbeat**
Alliance for Parental Involvement in Education
P.O. Box 59
East Chatham, NY 12060-59
518-392-6900
Fax: 518-392-6900
Parents of special needs children contributed to this book. *$16.95*

5172 **Uncommon Fathers**
Woodbine House
6510 Bells Mill Rd
Bethesda, MD 20817-1636
301-897-3570
800-843-7323
info@woodbinehouse.com
woodbinehouse.com

Irv Shapell, Owner
Nineteen fathers talk about the life-altering experience of having a child with special needs and offer a welcome, seldom-heard perspective on raising kids with disabilities, including autism, cerebral palsy, and Down syndrome. Uncommon Fathers is the first book for fathers by fathers, but it is also helpful to partners, family, friends, and service providers. *$14.95*
206 pages Paperback
ISBN 0-933149-68-9

5173 **We Can Speak for Ourselves: Self Advocacy by Mentally Handicapped People**
Brookline Books
8 Trumbull Rd
Suite B-001
Northampton, MA 1060-4533
413-584-0184
800-666-2665
Fax: 413-584-6184
brbooks@yahoo.com
www.brooklinebooks.com
Practical advice and support for parents, group resident workers, and others interested in fostering self-advocacy for people with developmental disabilities. *$10.00*
246 pages Paperback
ISBN 0-25336 -65-9

5174 **You May Be Able to Adopt**
Through the Looking Glass
3075 Adeline St
Ste. 120
Berkeley, CA 94703-2212
510-848-1112
800-644-2666
Fax: 510-848-4445
TTY: 510-848-1005
tlg@lookingglass.org
www.lookingglass.org

Maureen Block, J.D., Board President
Rusty Hendlin, M.A., LMFT, Director of Medi-Cal Services
Thomas Spalding, Board Treasurer
A guide to the adoption process for prospective mothers with disabilities and their partners. Available in braille, large print or cassette. *$10.00*
112 pages

5175 **You Will Dream New Dreams**
Kensington Publishing
119 West 40th Street
New York, NY 10018
800-221-2647
www.kensingtonbooks.com
Steven Zacharius, Chairman, President & CEO
A parent's support group in print. The shared narratives come from those with newly diagnosed children, adult disabled children, and everything in between. *$13.00*
278 pages Paperback
ISBN 1-575665-60-3

5176 **Your Child Has a Disability: A Complete Sourcebook of Daily and Medical Care**
Brookes Publishing
P.O. Box 10624
Baltimore, MD 21285-624
410-337-9580
800-638-3775
Fax: 410-337-8539
custserv@brookespublishing.com
readplaylearn.com

Paul Brooks, Owner

Offers expert advice on a wide range of issues-from finding the right doctor and investigating the medical aspects of a child's condition to learning care techniques and fulfilling education requirements. *$24.95*
368 pages Paperback
ISBN 1-557663-74-2

Parenting: Specific Disabilities

5177   Cancer Clinical Trials: A Commonsense Guide to Experimental Cancer Therapies and Trials
DiaMedica Inc.
2 Carlson Pkwy N
Ste 165
Minneapolis, MN 55447   763-270-0603
                                               Fax: 763-710-4456
                                               www.diamedica.com
Tomasz M. Beer, Author
Larry W. Axmaker, Author
Cancer Clinical Trials is a comprehensive, no-nonsense, and readable guide for anyone who is considering therapeutic options in addition to standard cancer therapy. The book seeks to share knowledge about cancer clinical trials with people living with cancer, their families and loved ones. It will help readers decide if a clinical trial is a good option for them, to choose an appropriate trial, and to navigate through the clinical trial process.
192 pages

5178   Different Dream Parenting: A Practical Guide to Raising a Child with Special Needs
Discovery House Publishers
3000 Kraft Ave SE
P.O. Box 3566
Grand Rapids, MI 49512   800-653-8333
                                               support@dhp.org
                                               dhp.org
Jolene Philo, Author
In Different Dream Parenting, author Jolene Philo offers guidance and encouragement through biblical insights and her own personal experiences. Find spiritual wisdom, practical resources, and tools that can help you become an extraordinary advocate for your child. Discover how you can move beyond the challenges and experience the joy of being your childs biggest and best supporter.
336 pages

5179   Essential First Steps for Parents of Children with Autism
Woodbine House
6510 Bells Mill Rd
Bethesda, MD 20817   301-897-3570
                                               800-843-7323
                                               info@woodbinehouse.com
                                               www.woodbinehouse.com
Lara Delmolino, Author
Sandra L. Harris, Author
When autism is diagnosed or suspected in young children, overwhelmed parents wonder where to turn and how to begin helping their child. Drs. Delmolino and Harris, experienced clinicians and ABA therapists, eliminate the confusion and guesswork by outlining the pivotal steps parents can take now to optimize learning and functioning for children ages 5 and younger.
154 pages Paperback

5180   Final Report: Challenges and Strategies of Disabled Parents: Findings from a Survey (1997)
Through the Looking Glass
3075 Adeline St
Ste. 120
Berkeley, CA 94703-2212   510-848-1112
                                               800-644-2666
                                               Fax: 510-848-4445
                                               TTY: 510-848-1005
                                               tlg@lookingglass.org
                                               www.lookingglass.org
Linda Toms Barker, Author
Vida Maralani, Author

This milestone TLG-directed report presents findings from the first national survey of parents with disabilities. The report includes a description of parents with disabilities, barriers to parenting among adults with disabilities, transportation issues, personal assistance, adaptive parenting equipment, housing, as well as recommendations for legal and service system changes.

5181   Pervasive Developmental Disorders: Findinga Diagnosis and Getting Help
Patient-Centered Guides/O'Reilly Media
1005 Gravenstein Highway North
Sebastopol, CA 95472   707-827-7000
                                               Fax: 707-829-0104
                                               support@oreilly.com
                                               www.oreilly.com
Mitzi Waltz, Author
This book encompasess both the practical aspects and the personal stories and emotional facets of living with PDD-NOS, the most common pervasive developmental disorder. Parents of an undiagnosed child may suspect many things, from autism to servere allergies. Pervasive Developmental Disorders is for parents (or newly diagnosed adults) who struggle with this neurological condition that profoundly impacts the life of child and family.
580 pages Paperback 1999

5182   Teaching Children with Down Syndrome about Their Bodies, Boundaries, and Sexuality
Woodbine House
6510 Bell Mills Rd
Bethesda, MD 20817   800-843-7323
                                               info@woodbinehouse.com
                                               www.woodbinehouse.com
Terri Couwenhoven, Author
Drawing on her unique background as both a sexual educator and mother of a child with Down syndrome, the author blends factual information and practical ideas for teaching children with Down syndrome about their bodies, puberty, and sexuality. This book gives parents the confidence to speak comfortably about these sometimes difficult subjects.
332 pages Paperback

5183   Thinking Differently: An Inspiring Guidefor Parents of Children with Learning Disabilities
William Morrow Paperbacks (HarperCollins)
195 Broadway
New York, NY 10007   212-207-7000
                                               orders@harpercollins.com
                                               www.harpercollins.com
David Flink, Author
An innovative, comprehensive guide—the first of its kind—to help parents understand and accept learning disabilities in their children, offering tips and strategies for successfully advocating on their behalf and helping them become their own best advocates.

5184   Your Child in the Hospital: A Practical Guide for Parents (3rd Edition)
Childhood Cancer Guides/O'Reilly Media
1005 Gravenstein Hwy N
Sebastopol, CA 95472   707-827-7019
                                               800-889-8969
                                               Fax: 707-824-8268
                                               orders@oreilly.com
                                               shop.oreilly.com
Nancy Keene, Author
This book offers advice from dozens of veteran parents on how to cope with a child's hospitalization, relieving anxious parents so they can help dispel their child's fears and concerns. Parents will find easy-to-read tips on preparing their child, handling procedures without trauma, and preventing insurance snafus. The second edition features a journal to help open communication and give the child a measure of control over the experience.
176 pages Paperback

Parenting: School

5185 Allergy & Asthma Today
Allergy & Asthma Network
8229 Boone Blvd
Ste 260
Vienna, VA 22182 800-878-4403
Fax: 703-288-5271
canderson@allergyasthmanetwork.org
www.allergyasthmanetwork.org
Tonya Winders, President
Charmayne Anderson, Director, Advocacy
Gary Fitzgerald, Managing Editor
Practical, medical,information for school patients, physicians, caregivers and families.

5186 Carolina Curriculum for Infants and Toddlers with Special Needs (3rd Edition)
Brookes Publishing
P.O.Box 10624
Baltimore, MD 21285-0624 410-337-9580
800-638-3775
Fax: 410-337-8539
custserv@brookespublishing.com
www.brookespublishing.com
Nancy M. Johnson-Martin, Author
Susan M. Attermeier, Author
Bonnie J. Hacker, Author
This book includes detailed assessment and intervention sequences, daily routine integration strategies, sensorimotor adaptations, and a sample 24-page Assessment Log that shows readers how to chart a child's individual progress.
504 pages Spiral-bound

5187 Choosing Outcomes and Accommodations for Children (COACH) (2nd Edition)
Brookes Publishing
P.O.Box 10624
Baltimore, MD 21285-0624 410-337-9580
800-638-3775
Fax: 410-337-8539
custserv@brookespublishing.com
www.brookespublishing.com
Michael F. Giangreco, Author
Chigee J. Cloninger, Author
Virginia Salce Iverson, Author
A guide to educational planning for students with disabilities, second edition. Focuses on life outcomes such as social relationships and participation in typical home, school, and community activities.
232 pages Spiral bound

5188 Complete IEP Guide: How to Advocate for Your Special Ed Child (8th Edition)
NOLO (Internet Brands)
909 N. Sepulveda Blvd
11th Fl.
El Segundo, CA 90245 310-280-4000
www.nolo.com
Lawrence Siegel, Author/Attorney
This all-in-one guide will help you understand special education law, identify your child's needs, prepare for meetings, develop the IEP and resolve disputes.
384 pages

5189 Exceptional Student in the Regular Classroom (6th Edition)
Pearson
330 Hudson St
New York, NY 10013 212-641-2400
www.pearsoned.com
Bill R. Gearheart, Author
Mel W. Weishan, Author
Carol J. Gearheart, Author
Offers good, solid information through a practical understandable presentation unencumbered by specialized jargon. Covers topics associated with special learners.
517 pages

5190 Study Power Workbook: Exercises in Study - Skills to Improve Your Learning and Your Grades
Brookline Books
8 Trumbull Rd
Ste B-001
Northampton, MA 1060-4533 413-584-0184
800-666-2665
Fax: 413-584-6184
brbooks@yahoo.com
www.brooklinebks.com
Sara Beth Huntley, Author
William Luckie, Author
Wood Smethurst, Author
The techniques in the easy-to-use, self-teaching manual have yielded remarkable success for students from elementary to medical school, at all levels of intelligence and achievement. Key skills covered include: listening, note taking, concentration, summarizing, reading comprehension, memorization, test taking, preparing papers and reports, time management, and more. These abilities are vital to success throughout every stage of learning; the benefits will last a lifetime.

Parenting: Spiritual

5191 A Good and Perfect Gift: Faith, Expectations, and a Little Girl Named Penny
Bethany House Publishers (Baker Publishing Group)
6030 E Fulton Rd
Ada, MI 49301 616-676-9185
800-877-2665
Fax: 616-676-9573
bakerpublishinggroup.com
Amy Julia Becker, Author
When her first baby, Penny, is given a frightening diagnosis, Amy Julia's world comes crashing down. Could she continue to trust God's goodness through what felt like personal tragedy? But challenging surprises often lead to unforeseen joy, and disappointments can turn into blessings. This wise and beautiful book is more than a courageous story of raising a child against the odds—it is a journey through the unexpected ups and downs of life and the discoveries that come along the way.
240 pages

5192 Before and After Zachariah
Chicago Review Press
814 N Franklin St
Chicago, IL 60610 312-337-0747
800-888-4741
Fax: 312-337-5110
www.chicagoreviewpress.com
Fern Kupfer, Author
This intimate chronicle of one family's life with a severely brain damaged child is recently back in print.
247 pages 1982

5193 Bethy and the Mouse: A Father Remembers His Children with Disabilities
Brookline Books
8 Trumbull Rd
Ste B-001
Northampton, MA 1060-4533 413-584-0184
800-666-2665
Fax: 413-584-6184
brbooks@yahoo.com
www.brooklinebks.com
Donald C. Bakely, Author
A moving collection of poetry, photographs, and prose following a father's experiences with two disabled children—one with Down Syndrome and one with an underdeveloped brain.
184 pages Paperback 1999

5194 Disabled God: Toward a Liberatory Theology of Disability
Abingdon Press
2222 Rosa L. Parks Blvd
Nashville, TN 37288   615-749-6615
                                       800-251-3320
                          orders@abingdonpress.com
                          www.abingdonpress.com
Nancy L. Eisland, Author
Draws on themes of the disability rights movement to identify people with disabilities as members of a socially disadvantaged minority group rather than as individuals who need to adjust. Highlights the history of people with disabilities in the church and society.
139 pages Paperback 1994

5195 Farewell, My Forever Child
CreateSpace, an Amazon Company
4900 Lacross Rd
North Charleston, SC 29406   843-760-8000
                          www.createspace.com
Kalila Smith, Author
Based on her own experiences following the loss of her 29-year-old daughter, Kalila Smith discusses the complex grief felt by parents who have lost a developmentally disabled child, and offers strategies to help families achieve peace and deal with the loss.
134 pages

5196 In Time and with Love: Caring for the Special Needs Infant and Toddler
William Morrow Paperbacks (HarperCollins)
195 Broadway
New York, NY 10007   212-207-7000
                          orders@harpercollins.com
                          www.harpercollins.com
Marilyn Segal, Author
Roni Leiderman, Author
Wendy S. Masi, Author
For families and caregivers of preteen and handicapped children in their first three years - more than one hundred tips for adjusting and coping. Part of the Your Child At Play series.
240 pages

5197 Journal of Disability & Religion
Routledge (Taylor & Francis Group)
711 Third Ave
New York, NY 10017   212-216-7800
                                       800-354-1420
                          Fax: 202-564-7854
                          orders@taylorandfrancis.com
                          www.tandfonline.com
This journal aims to inform religious professionals about developments in the field of disability and rehabilitation in order to facilitate greater contributions on the part of pastors, religious educators and pastoral counselors.
Quarterly

5198 Spiritually Able: A Parents Guide to Teaching Faith To Children with Special Needs
Loyola Press
3441 N Ashland Ave
Chicago, IL 60657   800-621-1008
                          Fax: 773-281-0555
                          customerservice@loyolapress.com
                          www.loyolapress.com
David Rizzo, Author
Both memoir and manual, Spiritually Able: A Parent's Guide to Teaching the Faith to Children with Special Needs is a life-preserver to parents who are seeking ways to grow and nourish a deeper relationship to God and their faith for their child with special needs. Full of tips, advice, and personal accounts, Spiritually Able helps bridge the gap and invites all into the welcoming embrace of the Church.
140 pages

5199 The Spiritual Art of Raising Children with Disabilities
Judson Press
P.O. Box 851
Valley Forge, PA 19482   800-458-3766
                          www.judsonpress.com
Kathleen Deyer Bolduc, Author
In The Spiritual Art of Raising Children with Disabilities, Bolduc uses the metaphor of the mosaic to life as parents of children with disabilities. Readers are walked through the process using the spiritual disciplines to help you recognize God's presence in your life and regain the balance we all need. this book offers readers the unique perspective of a parent raising a child with disabilities and dealing with it through faith and spiritual direction.
192 pages Paperback

5200 Worst Loss: How Families Heal from the Death of a Child
Holt Paperbacks (Macmillan Publishers)
75 Varick St
New York, NY 10013   212-226-7521
                          press.inquiries@macmillan.com
                          us.macmillan.com/henryholt
Barbara D. Rosof, Author
Combines anecdotal case histories and the latest research to help bereaved parents cope with the loss of a child, offering practical and comforting advice on how to overcome the disabling symptoms of grief.
304 pages 1995

Professional

5201 American Journal of Physical Medicine & Rehabilitation
Lippincott, Williams & Wilkins
2001 Market St
Ste 5
Philadelphia, PA 19103-1551   215-521-8300
                                       800-638-3030
                          Fax: 215-521-8902
                          orders@lww.com
                          www.lww.com
Walter R. Frontera, MD, PHD, Editor-in-Chief
Journal of the Association of Academic Psychiatrists. Articles covering research and clinical studies and applications of new equipment, procedures and therapeutic advances.
Monthly

5202 American Journal of Psychiatry
American Psychiatric Association
1000 Wilson Blvd
Ste 1825
Arlington, VA 22209-3924   703-907-7322
                                       800-368-5777
                          Fax: 703-907-1091
                          ajp@psych.org
                          ajp.psychiatryonline.org
Robert Freedman, Editor
Peer-reviewed articles focus on developments in biological psychiatry as well as on treatment innovations and forensic, ethical, economic, and social topics.
Monthly

5203 American Journal of Public Health (AJPH)
American Public Health Association
800 I St. NW
Washington, DC 20001   202-777-2742
                          Fax: 202-777-2534
                          TTY: 202-777-2500
                          www.apha.org
Georges C. Benjamin, Executive Director
Alfredo Morabia, Editor-in-Chief
Association journal containing editorials, commentary, and analyses on public health.
Monthly

5204 Art Therapy
American Art Therapy Association
4875 Eisenhower Ave.
Suite 240
Alexandria, VA 22304   703-548-5860
                                    888-290-0878
                               Fax: 703-548-5860
                               info@arttherapy.org
                                    arttherapy.org

Jordan Potash, Editor-in-Chief
Publishes articles on news, developments, ideas and research relating to the field of art therapy.
Quarterly

5205 CAREERS & the disABLED Magazine
Equal Opportunity Publications
445 Broad Hollow Rd
Ste 425
Melville, NY 11747-3615   631-421-9421
                               Fax: 631-421-1352
                                    info@eop.com
                                    www.eop.com

Barbara Capella Loehr, Editor
A career magazine for professional career seekers who have disabilities. Profiles disabled people who have achieved successful careers. Features a career section in Braille, career guide.

**5206 Clinician's Practical Guide to
Attention-Deficit/Hyperactivity Disorder**
Brookes Publishing
P.O.Box 10624
Baltimore, MD 21285-0624   410-337-9580
                                    800-638-3775
                               Fax: 410-337-8539
                          custserv@brookespublishing.com
                               www.brookespublishing.com

Marianne Mercugliano, Author
Quick reference volume with comprehensive data on psychoeducational and neuropsychological assessment, related symptoms, drug and counseling therapies and critical issues.
368 pages

**5207 Counseling Parents of Children with Chronic Illness or
Disability**
Wiley
111 River St
Hoboken, NJ 07030-5774   201-748-6000
                                    877-762-2974
                               Fax: 201-748-6088
                                    info@wiley.com
                                    www.wiley.com

Hilton Davis, Author
This book aims to help medical staff and carers relate to parents in ways that facilitate their adaptation to their child's illness. The key to this is in effective communication.
148 pages Paperback

**5208 Creating Options for Family Recovery: A Provider's
Guide to Promoting Parental Mental Health**
Employment Options Inc.
82 Brigham St
Marlboro, MA 01752-3137   508-485-5051
                               Fax: 508-485-8807
                          options@employmentoptions.org
                               www.employmentoptions.com

Joanne Nicholson, Author
Toni Wolf, Author
Chip Wilder, Author
This book seeks to advise professionals and providers on strategies to use when working with families who are dealing with mental illness, assisting them with the promotion of a healthy recovery. The resources in this guide are drawn from over 20 years of research and practice, and the lived experiences of parents, children and family members.
120 pages Paperback

5209 Cystic Fibrosis: Medical Care
Lippincott, Williams & Wilkins
16522 Hunters Green Pkwy
Hagerstown, MD 21740   301-223-2300
                                    800-638-3030
                               Fax: 301-223-2400
                                    orders@lww.com
                                    www.lww.com

David M. Orenstein, Author
Beryl J. Rosenstein, Author
Robert C. Stern, Author
A guide to the medical community to the principles and practices of cystic fibrosis care. After chapters on the molecular and cellular bases of CF and its diagnosis, they cover the major organ systems affected by CF and deal with surgery for CF patients, transplantation (lung and liver), hospitalization, and terminal care. Also included are chapters on special populations, exercise, and laboratory testing.
365 pages

5210 Disability & Rehabilitation Journal
Taylor & Francis Online
6000 Broken Sound Pkwy NW
Ste 300
Boca Raton, FL 33487   212-216-7800
                                    800-634-7064
                               Fax: 212-564-7854
                     enquiries@taylorandfrancis.com
                               www.taylorandfrancis.com

Dave Muller, Editor-in-Chief
Peer-reviewed journal offering the latest news, research, and insights on disability and rehabilitation medicine.
Bi-weekly

**5211 Disability Analysis Handbook: Tools for Independent
Practice**
American Board of Disability Analysts
1483 N. Mt. Juliet Rd.
Suite 175
Nashville, TN 37122   629-255-0870
                               Fax: 615-296-9980
                               office@eventsm3.com
                               www.americandisability.org

Handbook providing information on physical and mental disabilities, including diabetes, substance abuse, aging, nonverbal learning, chronic pain, etc.
396 pages

**5212 Enhancing Everyday Communication for Children with
Disabilities**
Brookes Publishing
P.O.Box 10624
Baltimore, MD 21285-0624   410-337-9580
                                    800-638-3775
                               Fax: 410-337-8539
                          custserv@brookespublishing.com
                               www.brookespublishing.com

Jeff Sigafoos, Author & Editor
Michael Arthur-Kelly, Author
Nancy Butterfield, Author
Practical and concise, this introductory guide is filled with real-world tips and strategies for anyone working to improve the communication of children with moderate, severe, and multiple disabilities. Emphasizing the link between behavior and communication, three respected researchers transform up-to-date research and proven best practices into instructional procedures and interventions ready for use at home or in school.
176 pages Paperback

5213 Ethical Issues In Home Health Care (2nd Edition)
Charles C. Thomas
2600 S First St
Springfield, IL 62704-4730   217-789-8980
                                    800-258-8980
                               Fax: 217-789-9130
                               books@ccthomas.com
                               www.ccthomas.com

Sheri Smith, Author
Rosalind Ekman Ladd, Author
Lynn Pasquerella, Author

This book will help to answer some of the growing number of ethical questions and more complex issues that home health care nurses face. The cases presented in each chapter of the book are fictionalized situations based on interviews conducted with home health care nurses in both hospital-sponsored and private agencies, in hospices, and in urban and rural settings. Each chapter of the book is devoted to one of the main areas of concern for home health care nurses.
258 pages

5214   Journal of Public Health
Oxford Journals, Oxford University Press
2001 Evans Rd
Cary, NC 27513   919-677-0977
                                       800-852-7323
                                  Fax: 919-677-1714
                            www.oxfordjournals.org
Eugene Milne, Editor
Ted Schrecker, Editor
Scholarly articles on issues that relate to public health and the healthcare system.

5215   PM&R Journal
American Academy of Physical Medicine & Rehab
9700 W Bryn Mawr Ave
Ste 200
Rosemont, IL 60018-5701   847-737-6000
                                       877-227-6799
                                  Fax: 847-737-6001
                                  TTY: 800-437-0833
                                     info@aapmr.org
                                  www.pmrjournal.org
Stuart M. Weinstein, Editor-in-Chief
Cathy Mendelsohn, Managing Editor
Covers medical, social and employment aspects of vocational rehabilitation. The content of PM&R includes articles that are contemporary and important to both research and clinical practice. The various sections of the journal include original research such as clinical trials, outcomes studies, and clinically relevant translational science; reviews (narrative and analytical); case presentations; point/counterpoint debates; ethical/legal topics; practice management updates; and statistical themes.
Monthly

5216   Provider Magazine
American Health Care Association
1201 L St NW
Washington, DC 20005-4024   202-842-4444
                                       888-656-6669
                                  Fax: 202-842-3860
                                     sales@ahca.org
Joanne Erickson, Editor-in-Chief
Amy Mendoza, Managing Editor
Magazine for long-term healthcare professionals.
Monthly

5217   Public Health Reports
Association of Schools & Programs of Public Health
1900 M St NW
Ste 710
Washington, DC 20036   202-296-1099
                                  Fax: 202-296-1252
                           www.publichealthreports.org
Frederic E. Shaw, Editorn-in-Chief
Sasha M. Ruiz, Acting Managing Editor
PHR is a peer-reviewed journal published on a bi-monthly basis. Each issue offers recurring guest columns such as Local Acts, Global Health Matters, ASPPH From the Schools and Programs of Public Health, Law and the Public's Health, Public Health Chronicles, NCHS Dataline, and the Surgeon General's Perspectives.
Bi-monthly

5218   Sociopolitical Aspects of Disabilities(2nd Edition)
Charles C. Thomas
2600 S First St
Springfield, IL 62704-4730   217-789-8980
                                       800-258-8980
                                  Fax: 217-789-9130
                               books@ccthomas.com
                                  www.ccthomas.com
Willie V. Bryan, Author
Provides understanding of the social and political histories of people with disabilities in the United States. This understanding is pivotal in working with persons with disabilities, to provide background and perspective on current policies and attitudes.
284 pages

5219   Starting and Sustaining Genetic Support Groups
Johns Hopkins University Press
2715 N Charles St
Baltimore, MD 21218-4363   410-516-6900
                                  Fax: 410-516-6968
                          webmaster@jhupress.jhu.edu
                                  www.press.jhu.edu
Joan O. Weiss, Author
Jayne S. Mackta, Author
Guide to the establishment and maintenance of genetic support groups for individuals with genetic disorders and their families. For therapists and group leaders. Discusses practical matters including finding a leader, fund-raising, organizing peer support training programs.
152 pages

5220   The Essential Brain Injury Guide (5th Edition)
Brain Injury Association of America
3057 Nutley St.
Suite 805
Fairfax, VA 22031-1931   703-761-0750
                                  Fax: 703-761-0755
                                     info@biausa.org
                                    shop.biausa.org
Susan H. Connors, President & Chief Executive Officer
Shana De Caro, Chairowman
Page Melton Ivie, Vice Chairwoman
The expanded and updated Essential Brain Injury Guide 5.0 is a hard cover, 25 chapter, 500-page text that provides information about brain injury, as well as brain injury treatment and rehabilitation. *$135.00*

5221   What Psychotherapists Should Know about Disabilty
Guilford Press
370 Seventh Ave
Ste 1200
New York, NY 10001-1020   800-365-7006
                                  Fax: 212-966-6708
                                    info@guilford.com
                                   www.guilford.com
Rhoda Olkin, Author
This comprehensive volume provides the knowledge and skills that mental health professionals need for more effective, informed work with clients with disabilities. Topics addressed include etiquette with clients with disabilities; special concerns in assessment, evaluation, and diagnosis. Filled with clinical examples and observations, the volume also discusses strategies for enhancing teaching, training, and research.
368 pages

5222   Women with Visible & Invisible Disabilitiees: Multiple Intersections, Issues, Therapies
Routledge (Taylor & Francis Group)
711 Third Ave
New York, NY 10017   212-216-7800
                                       800-634-7064
                                  Fax: 202-564-7854
                        enquiries@taylorandfrancis.com
                                   www.routledge.com
Martha E. Banks, Editor
Ellyn Kaschak, Editor
Addresses the issues faced by women with disabilities, examines the social construction of disability, and makes suggestions for

the development and modification of culturally relevant therapy to meet the needs of disabled women.
414 pages Hardcover; Paperback

Specific Disabilities

5223 **inMotion Magazine**
Amputee Coalition
601 Pennsylvania Ave. NW
Suite 600, South Bldg.
Washington, DC 20004   888-267-5669
                                www.amputee-coalition.org
Mary Richards, President & Chief Executive Officer
inMotion Magazine is published bimonthly for amputees, caregivers and health care professionals, offering timely and comprehensive information. Offered both in print and online, free subscription.

Vocations

5224 **Ability Magazine**
P.O. Box 10878
Costa Mesa, CA 92627   www.abilitymagazine.com
Features articles on living, working, playing and entertainment for the disabled.
Bi-monthly

5225 **Chemists with Disabilities Committee - American Chemical Society**
American Chemical Society
1155 16th St NW
Washington, DC 20036   202-872-4600
                                         800-227-5558
                                    Fax: 202-872-4574
                                         cwd@acs.org
                                         www.acs.org

John Johnston, Ph.D, MBA, Chair
James Schiller, Chair Elect
Paula Christopher, Staff Liaison
Promotes the full involvement of individuals with physical and learning disabilities in educational and career opportunities in the chemical and allied sciences. CWD members help individuals with disabilities to connect with employers and educators of persons with disabilities.

5226 **Demystifying Job Development: Field-Based Approaches to Job Development for the Disabled**
Training Resource Network
266 Roaring Dr.
St. Augustine, FL 32084   Fax: 904-823-3554
                                         www.trn-store.com

David Hoff, Author
Cecilia Gandolfo, Author
Marty Gold, Author
A guide to successful placement of individuals with severe disabilities in quality jobs in the community.
105 pages

5227 **Hiring Idahoans with Disabilities**
Idaho Assistive Technology Project
University of Idaho
1187 Alturas Dr.
Moscow, ID 83843- 8331   208-885-3557
                                         800-432-8324
                                    Fax: 208-885-6102
                                    idahoat@uidaho.edu

Jane Frederickson, Author
Kristen Hagen, Author
The purpose of this handbook is to inform employers in Idaho business and industry about the promise of hiring Idahoans with disabilities.

5228 **Life Beyond the Classroom: Transition Strategies for Young People with Disabilities**
Brookes Publishing
P.O.Box 10624
Baltimore, MD 21285-0624   410-337-9580
                                         800-638-3775
                                    Fax: 410-337-8539
                                www.brookespublishing.com
Paul Wehman, Author
Specialists in a variety of disciplines use creative and practical techniques to ensure careful transition planning, to build young people's confidence and competence in work skills, and to foster support from businesses and community organizations for training and employment programs.
616 pages

5229 **More Than a Job: Securing Satisfying Careers for People with Disabilities**
Brookes Publishing
P.O. Box 10624
Baltimore, MD 21285-0624   800-638-3775
                                    Fax: 410-337-8539
                            custserv@brookespublishing.com
                                www.brookespublishing.com
Paul Wehman, Editor
John Kregel, Editor
This book transforms job placement into career counseling for people with physical and developmental disabilities. It presents step-by-step guidelines for helping people with disabilities to identify their own interests.
384 pages 1998

5230 **OT Practice Magazine**
American Occupational Therapy Association
6116 Executive Blvd.
Suite 200
North Bethesda, MD 20852-4929   301-652-6611
                                         800-729-2682
                                    otpractice@aota.org
                        www.aota.org/Publications-News/otp.aspx
Sherry Keramidas, Executive Director
Neil Harvison, Chief Officer, Knowledge Division
Matthew Clark, Chief Officer, Innovation & Engagement
OT Practice covers professional information on all aspects of occupational therapy practice today. Features include hands-on techniques, continuing education, legislative issues, career advice, job opportunities, and the latest professional news. Also available online.

5231 **Occupational Therapy and Vocational Rehabilitation**
Wiley
111 River St
Hoboken, NJ 07030-5774   201-748-6000
                                         877-762-2974
                                    Fax: 201-748-6088
                                         info@wiley.com
                                         www.wiley.com

Joanne Ross
This book introduces the occupational therapist to the practice of vocational rehabilitation. As rehabilitation specialists, Occupational Therapists work in a range of diverse settings with clients who have a variety of physical, emotional and psychological conditions. This book highlights the contribution, which can be made by occupational therapists in assisting disabled, ill or injured workers to access, remain in and return to work.
280 pages Paperback

5232 **Work and Disability: Contexts, Issues & Strategies for Enhancing Employment Outcomes**
PRO-ED Inc.
8700 Shoal Creek Blvd
Austin, TX 78757-6897   512-451-3246
                                         800-897-3202
                                    Fax: 800-397-7633
                                    general@proedinc.com
                                         www.proedinc.com

Edna Mora Szymanski, Editor
Randall M. Parker, Editor
492 pages

Media, Electronic

Audio/Visual

5233 A Place for Me
Educational Productions
9000 SW Gemini Dr
Beaverton, OR 97008-7151

503-644-7000
800-950-4949
Fax: 503-350-7000
custserve@edpro.com
www.teachingstrategies.com

Diane Trister Dodge, Founder/President/Lead Author
Arnitra Duckett, VP, Sales & Strategic Marketing

In this video, parents discuss the issues they face in planning for their child's future. This program is designed to stimulate discussion of these issues and help increase awareness of the options available in your local community.

5234 Able to Laugh
Fanlight Productions
32 Court St.
21st Floor
Brooklyn, NY 11201-4421

718-488-8900
800-876-1710
Fax: 718-488-8642
info@fanlight.com
www.fanlight.com

Jonathan Miller, President
Patricio Guzman, Director
Meredith Miller, Sales Manager

An exploration of the world of disability as interpreted by six professional comedians who happen to be disabled. It is also about the awkward ways disabled and able-bodied people relate to one another. *$199.00*
ISBN 1-572951-05-2

5235 Acting Blind
Fanlight Productions
32 Court St.
21st Floor
Brooklyn, NY 11201-4421

718-488-8900
800-876-1710
Fax: 718-488-8642
info@fanlight.com
www.fanlight.com

Jonathan Miller, President
Patricio Guzman, Director
Meredith Miller, Sales Manager

Takes audiences behind the scenes as a company of non-professional actors rehearse a play about life without sight. The performers have no problem imagining themselves in these roles: they are blind themselves. *$229.00*

5236 Adaptive Baby Care
Through the Looking Glass
3075 Adeline St
Suite 120
Berkeley, CA 94703-2577

510-848-1112
800-644-2666
Fax: 510-848-4445
TTY: 510-848-1005
tlg@lookingglass.org
www.lookingglass.org

Megan Kirshbaum, Executive Director
Paul Preston, Assoc. Dir

This publication is presented as a catalyst for problem-solving regarding the development of adaptive baby care equipment. This newest publication is designed for parents, family members and professionals. It includes: guidelines for problem-solving baby care barriers; photographs and descriptions of prototypes and resources for adaptive baby care equipment; adaptive baby care techniques; adaptive baby care equipment checklist; commercial product safety commission guidelines; and local and natio
$250.00

5237 Adaptive Baby Care Equipment Video and Book
Through the Looking Glass
Through the Looking Glass
3075 Adeline St
Suite 120
Berkeley, CA 94703-2577

510-848-1112
800-644-2666
Fax: 510-848-4445
TTY: 510-848-1005
tlg@lookingglass.org
www.lookingglass.org

Stephanie Miyashiro, Board President
Thomas Spalding, Board Treasurer
Alice Nemon, D.S.W., Board Secretary

Includes Adaptive Baby care Equipment: Guide Lines; Prototypes and Resources, plus a twelve minute video. Available in braille, large print or cassette. *$79.00*

5238 All About Attention Deficit Disorders, Revised
Parent Magic
800 Roosevelt Rd
B-309
Glen Ellyn, IL 60137-5839

630-208-0031
800-442-4453
Fax: 630-208-7366
www.parentmagic.com

Nancy Roe, Administrator/Exec Admin
Thomas Phelan, Owner/President/CEO

A psychologist and expert on ADD outlines the symptoms, diagnosis and treatment of this neurological disorder. Video ($49.95 - 2 parts) and audio cassette ($24.95). Also in DVD format (1 disk-$39.93).

5239 Autism
Aquarius Health Care Media
30 Forest Rd
PO Box 249
Millis, MA 2054-1511

508-376-1244
Fax: 508-376-1245
www.nmm.net

Lesile Kussmann, Owner/President/Producer
Kathy Newkirk, Director
Jane Hutchinson, Assoc. Director

This video takes you into the lives of autistic people and their families to understand more about autism. What defines autism and how can we help those living with the disability? Children, teens, and adults are also profiled and we begin to see the varying levels of development and new technology to help these people communicate. Preview Available. *$149.00*
Video

5240 Basic Course in American Sign Language(B100) Harris Communications, Inc.
Harris Communications
15155 Technology Dr
Eden Prairie, MN 55344

800-825-6758
Fax: 952-906-1099
TTY: 952-388-2152
info@harriscomm.com
www.harriscomm.com

Ray Harris, CEO

This series of four one-hour tapes is designed to illustrate the various exercises and dialogues in the text. *$39.95*
Video

5241 Beginning ASL Video Course
Harris Communications
15155 Technology Dr
Eden Prairie, MN 55344

800-825-6758
Fax: 952-906-1099
TTY: 952-388-2152
info@harriscomm.com
www.harriscomm.com

Ray Harris, CEO

You'll watch a family teach you to learn American Sign Language during funny and touching family situations. A total of 15 tapes in the course.
Video

5242 Blindness
Landmark Media
3450 Slade Run Dr
Falls Church, VA 22042-3940   703-241-2030
                                           800-342-4336
                                      Fax: 703-536-9540
                                 info@landmarkmedia.com
Michael Hartogs, President/Owner
Joan Hartogs, Owner/Vice President
Peter Hartogs, Vice President
Landmark Media is an independent family-owned company currently celebrating our 28th anniversary. We have been fortunate to be able to offer the finest quality educational DVDs available. *$250.00*
Video

5243 Boy Inside, The
Fanlight Productions
32 Court St.
21st Floor
Brooklyn, NY 11201-4421   718-488-8900
                                           800-876-1710
                                      Fax: 718-488-8642
                                       info@fanlight.com
                                       www.fanlight.com
Jonathan Miller, President
Patricio Guzman, Director
Meredith Miller, Sales Manager
Filmmaker Marianne Kaplan tells the personal and often distressing story of her son Adam, a 12-year-old with Asperger Syndrome, during a tumultuous year in the life of their family.

5244 Braille Documents
Metrolina Association for the Blind
704 Louise Ave
Charlotte, NC 28204-2128   704-887-5118
                                           800-926-5466
                                      Fax: 704-372-3872
                                      bschmiel@mabnc.org
                                          www.mabnc.org
Robert Scheffel, President
Richard Hartness, Vice President, Product Design & Development
Barbara Schmiel, Vice President, Accessible Braille Services
This production shop creates Braille and large-print documents. We work with our clients to find the most cost effective solutions for their needs. Unlike other modified statement service providers, we accept your existing style of statement or allow you to design your own statement.Documents may be received in electronic data files as encrypted data sent over public networks, data sent to a file transfer protocol drop box, or data sent over a dedicated data line. ABS also accepts paper hardcopi

5245 Bringing Out the Best
PO Box 9177
Dept. 11W
Champaign, IL 61826-9177   217-352-3273
                                           800-519-2707
                                      Fax: 217-352-1221
                                 orders@researchpress.com
                                    www.researchpress.com
David Parkinson, Chairman
Russell Pence, President
Gail Salyards, Dir. Of Marketing/President

5246 Business as Usual
Fanlight Productions
32 Court St.
21st Floor
Brooklyn, NY 11201-4421   718-488-8900
                                           800-876-1710
                                      Fax: 718-488-8642
                                       info@fanlight.com
                                       www.fanlight.com
Jonathan Miller, President
Patricio Guzman, Director
Meredith Miller, Sales Manager
An enlightening documentary, brings a unique international perspective to this struggle. This film examines five innovative programs which create opportunities for people with mental and physical disabilities to own and operate their own businesses. *$145.00*

5247 Buying Time: The Media Role in Health Care
Fanlight Productions
32 Court St.
21st Floor
Brooklyn, NY 11201-4421   718-488-8900
                                           800-876-1710
                                      Fax: 718-488-8642
                                       info@fanlight.com
                                       www.fanlight.com
Jonathan Miller, President
Patricio Guzman, Director
Meredith Miller, Sales Manager
This video program is a thoughtful and disturbing examination in the role of the media in determining the allocation of health care resources. This program is a powerful tool on ethics, policy, journalism, sociology, medicine and nursing as well as for professional workshops, and continuing education programs. *$99.00*

5248 Caring for Persons with Developmental Disabilities
PO Box 9177
Dept. 11W
Champaign, IL 61826-9177   217-352-3273
                                           800-519-2707
                                      Fax: 217-352-1221
                                    www.researchpress.com
David Parkinson, Chairman
Russell Pence, President
Gail Salyards, Dir. Of Marketing/President

5249 Clockworks
Learning Corporation of America
6493 Kaiser Dr
Fremont, CA 94555-3610   510-490-7311
Oonchia Chia, Owner
Scotty, who has Down Syndrome, is fascinated by clocks. This film follows him on his adventures of employment in the clock shop.
Film

5250 Close Encounters of the Disabling Kind
Mainstream
6930 Carroll Ave
Suite 204
Takoma Park, MD 20912-4468   301-891-8777
                                      Fax: 301-891-8778
Lillie Harrison, Information Programs Clerk
Fritz Rumpel, Editor
A training video that provides a hiring manager with information on how to learn the basics of disability etiquette and, by the end of the video, seems much better prepared and willing to interview qualified individuals with disabilities. Includes trainer and trainee guides. *$99.95*
Video

5251 Deaf Children Signers
Harris Communications
15155 Technology Dr
Eden Prairie, MN 55344   800-825-6758
                                      Fax: 952-906-1099
                                      TTY: 952-388-2152
                                   info@harriscomm.com
                                    www.harriscomm.com
Ray Harris, CEO
Graduate to voicing for Deaf children ages 5-11. This unique tape lets eleven young children demonstrate their abilities by signing about what is important to them. *$49.95*
Video

5252 Deaf Culture Series
Harris Communications
15155 Technology Dr
Eden Prairie, MN 55344   800-825-6758
                                      Fax: 952-906-1099
                                      TTY: 952-388-2152
                                   info@harriscomm.com
                                    www.harriscomm.com
Ray Harris, CEO
Each video in this five-part series features a topic dealing with the unique culture of deaf people. It is an excellent resource for deaf

studies programs, Interpreter Preparation programs and Sign Language programs. *$49.95*
Video

5253   Do You Hear That?
Alexander Graham Bell Association
3417 Volta Pl. NW
Washington, DC 20007   202-337-5220
                                        Fax: 202-337-8314
                                        TTY: 202-337-5221
                                        info@agbell.org
                                        www.agbell.org
Emilio Alonso-Mendoza, Chief Executive Officer
This video shows auditory-verbal therapy sessions of a therapist working individually with 11 children who range in age from 7 months to 7 years old and have hearing aids or cochlear implants.
Video

5254   Doing Things Together
Britannica Film Company
345 4th St
San Francisco, CA 94107-1206   415-928-8466
                                        Fax: 415-928-5027
Dave Bekowich, Owner
Steve went with his parents to an amusement park. He met another boy named Martin who at first was shocked by Steve's prosthetic hand.
Film

5255   Emerging Leaders
Mobility International USA
132 E Broadway
Suite 343
Eugene, OR 97401   541-343-1284
                                        Fax: 541-343-6812
                                        TTY: 541-343-1284
                                        clearinghouse@miusa.org
                                        www.miusa.org
Susan Sygall, Chief Executive Officer
Cindy Lewis, Director, Programs
Pioneering short-term international disability leadership programs in the U.S. and abroad with 2,000 youth, young adults and professionals from over 100 countries.
Video

5256   Face First
Fanlight Productions
32 Court St.
21st Floor
Brooklyn, NY 11201-4421   718-488-8900
                                        800-876-1710
                                        Fax: 718-488-8642
                                        info@fanlight.com
                                        www.fanlight.com
Jonathan Miller, President
Patricio Guzman, Director
Meredith Miller, Sales Manager
In this documentary, the stories told reflect the reality faced by all those who are seen as different. Despite their difficult experiences, the survival of the profiled individuals affords comic relief &, by adulthood, they possess unusual strengths that shape their careers in pediatrics, disability care, public speaking, and journalism. *$195.00*

5257   Family-Guided Activity-Based Intervention for Toddlers & Infants
Brookes Publishing
PO Box 10624
Baltimore, MD 21285-0624   410-337-9580
                                        800-638-3775
                                        Fax: 410-337-8539
                                        custserv@brookespublishing.com
Paul Brooks, Owner
This 20-minute video was created to assist early childhood professionals to incorporate therapeutic intervention into daily living. It includes a discussion and demonstration of how intervention professionals actively may involve caregivers in the

planning and implementation of activities aimed at encouraging development of a child's target skills *$37.00*
20 Minutes
ISBN 1-55766-19-3

5258   Filmakers Library
124 E 40th St
Suite 901
New York, NY 10016-1798   212-808-4980
                                        Fax: 212-808-4983
                                        www.filmakers.com
Sue Oscar, Co-President
Linda Gottesman, Co-President
Andrea Traubner, Dir., Broadcast Sales
Filmakers Library has been a leading source of outstanding films for the education, library, and non-theatrical markets. Now, as an imprint of award-winning online publisher Alexander Street Press, Filmakers Library is able to offer online streaming access to most of our titles, ensuring that our films receive the greatest possible exposure and accessibility through the most flexible delivery platforms. We market and promote our films throughout the world by direct mail, print advertising, exhib

5259   Filmakers Library: An Imprint Of Alexander Street Press
124 E 40th St
Suite 901
New York, NY 10016-1798   212-808-4980
                                        Fax: 212-808-4983
                                        www.filmakers.com
Sue Oscar, Co-President
Linda Gottesman, Co-President
Andrea Traubner, Dir., Broadcast Sales
Filmakers Library has been a leading source of outstanding films for the education, library, and non-theatrical markets. Now, as an imprint of award-winning online publisher Alexander Street Press, Filmakers Library is able to offer online streaming access to most of our titles, ensuring that our films receive the greatest possible exposure and accessibility through the most flexible delivery platforms. We market and promote our films throughout the world by direct mail, print advertising, exhib
$100 - $300

5260   Films & Videos on Aging and Sensory Change
Lighthouse International
111 E 59th St
New York, NY 10022-1202   212-821-9200
                                        800-829-0500
                                        Fax: 212-821-9706
                                        info@lighthouse.org
Joanna Mellor, VP Information Services
Tara Cortes, President
An annotated list of over 80 films and videos dealing with age-related sensory change, divided into sections on vision impairment, hearing impairment, and multiple sensory impairments. *$5.00*

5262   Heart to Heart
Blind Children's Center
4120 Marathon St
Los Angeles, CA 90029-3584   323-664-2153
                                        info@blindchildrenscenter.org
                                        www.blindchildrenscenter.org
Nancy Chernus-Mansfield, Co-Author
Dori Hayashi, Co-Author
Parents of blind and partially sighted children talk about their feelings. *$35.00*
VHS/DVD

5263   Helping Hands
Fanlight Productions
32 Court St.
21st Floor
Brooklyn, NY 11201-4421   718-488-8900
                                        800-876-1710
                                        Fax: 718-488-8642
                                        info@fanlight.com
                                        www.fanlight.com
Jonathan Miller, President
Patricio Guzman, Director
Meredith Miller, Sales Manager

The ADA mandates equal access and opportunity for the 43 million people with disabilities in the United States. These individuals may have limited speech, sight or mobility; a developmental disability; or a medical condition which limits some life activities. Many, however, are ready, willing and very able to join the workforce. This video demonstrates that many modifications or adaptations can be made simply by using ingenuity or common sense — such as keeping the aisles clear, etc. *$145.00*
37 Minutes

5264   Home is in the Heart: Accommodating Peoplewith Disabilities in the Homestay Experience
Mobility International USA
132 E Broadway
Suite 343
Eugene, OR 97401   541-343-1284
                                     Fax: 541-343-6812
                                     TTY: 541-343-1284
                              clearinghouse@miusa.org
                                          www.miusa.org

Susan Sygall, Chief Executive Officer
Cindy Lewis, Director, Programs
Provides information and ideas for exchange organizations. Discusses how to recruit homestay families, meet accessibility needs and accommodate international participants with disabilities.
Video

5265   How Difficult Can This Be ? (Fat City) - Rick Lavoie
CACLD
PO Box 210
Barnstable, MA 02630-210   508-362-1052
                              scheduling@ricklavoie.com
                                       www.ricklavoie.com

Rick Lavoie, Film Maker
This unique program allows viewers to experience the same frustration, anxiety and tension that children with learning disabilities face in their daily lives. Teachers, social workers, psychologists, parents and friends who have participated in Richard Lavoie's workshop reflect upon their experience and the way it changed their approach to L.D. children. 1989.

5266   How We Play
Fanlight Productions
32 Court St.
21st Floor
Brooklyn, NY 11201-4421   718-488-8900
                                          800-876-1710
                                     Fax: 718-488-8642
                                       info@fanlight.com
                                         www.fanlight.com

Jonathan Miller, President
Patricio Guzman, Director
Meredith Miller, Sales Manager
Though most of the people in this new, short documentary are in wheelchairs, and one is blind, they are anything but handicapped. Playing tennis, snorkeling, whitewater canoeing, practicing karate - they are living proof that a disability can be a challenge, not an obstacle. *$99.00*

5267   I'm Not Disabled
Landmark Media
3450 Slade Run Dr
Falls Church, VA 22042-3940   703-241-2030
                                          800-342-4336
                                     Fax: 703-536-9540
                              info@landmarkmedia.com

Michael Hartogs, President
Joan Hartogs, Vice President
Peter Hartogs, Vice President
Young people talk about their disabilities and the importance of sports in their lives. The afflictions range from blindness and missing limbs to paralysis. Through physical education and therapy they enjoy freedom of movement and participate in sports such as tennis, basketball, kayaking, skiing, and swimming. *$195.00*
Video

5268   Imagery Procedures for People with Special Needs
Research Press
PO Box 9177
Dept. 11W
Champaign, IL 61826-9177   217-352-3273
                                          800-519-2707
                                     Fax: 217-352-1221
                                    rp@researchpress.com
                                   www.researchpress.com

David Parkinson, Chairman
Russell Pence, President
Gail Salyards, Dir. Of Marketing/President
This video was developed at the Groden Center and illustrates imagery based procedures including the use of positive reinforcement, covert modeling, and a self-control triad to assists individuals to self-regulate their behaviors in stressful situations or under conditions that may evoke extreme fear. Recommended for professionals and family members interested in teaching self-control strategies that individuals with autism spectrum disorders can use in community settings. *$195.00*
32 Minutes

5269   In the Middle
Fanlight Productions
c/o Icarus Films
32 Court Street, 21st Floor
Brooklyn, NY 11201   718-488-8900
                                          800-876-1710
                                     Fax: 718-488-8642
                                       info@fanlight.com
                                         www.fanlight.com

Ben Achtenberg, Founder, Owner
Documents the problems and joys shared by Ryanna, who has Spina Bifida, and her parents, teachers and classmates during her first year of being mainstreamed in a Head Start Program. *$99.00*

5270   Include Us
Exceptional Parent Library
PO Box 1807
Englewood Cliffs, NJ 7632-1207   201-947-6000
                                          800-535-1910
                                     Fax: 201-947-9376
                                       eplibrary@aol.com

First children's video to feature a proportionate number of children with disabilities. Inclusion works via eight songs. *$19.95*

5271   Intensive Early Intervention and Beyond
PO Box 9177
Dept. 11W
Champaign, IL 61826-9177   217-352-3273
                                          800-519-2707
                                     Fax: 217-352-1221
                                   www.researchpress.com

David Parkinson, Chairman
Russell Pence, President
Gail Salyards, Dir. Of Marketing/President

5272   Invisible Children
Learning Corporation of America
6493 Kaiser Dr
Fremont, CA 94555-3610   510-490-7311

Oonchia Chia, Owner
Renaldo was blind, Mandy was deaf, and Mark had Cerebral Palsy and used a wheelchair. These child-size puppet characters interacted with non-handicapped puppets.
Film

5274   Let's Eat Video
Blind Children's Center
4120 Marathon Street
Los Angeles, CA 90029-3584   323-664-2153
                              info@blindchildrenscenter.org
                                 blindchildrenscenter.org

Jill Brody, Co-Author
Lynne Webber, Co-Author
Babies and toddlers with visual impairments lack one major avenue of exploration, and this significantly infulences their awareness, perceptions, and anticipation of the food which is presented to them. *$35.00*
VHS/DVD

5275 Look Who's Laughing
Aquarius Health Care Videos
30 Forest Rd
PO Box 249
Millis, MA 2054-1511   508-376-1244
Fax: 508-376-1245
aqvideos@tiac.net
www.aquariusproductions.com
Lesile Kussmann, Owner/President/Producer
Kathy Newkirk, Director
Jane Hutchinson, Assoc. Director
This video is packed with laugh-out-loud comedic moments, but is also full of intelligent and inspiring messages. Look Who's Laughing introduces viewers to some of today's funniest comedians - who just happen to be physically disabled. We hear them talk openly and honestly about their limitations as well as their abilities and talents. Helpful for those who work with the disabled and motivational to both the disabled and able-bodied. Preview option available. *$95.00*
Video

5276 My Body is Not Who I Am
Aquarius Health Care Videos
30 Forest Rd
PO Box 249
Millis, MA 2054-1511   508-376-1244
Fax: 508-376-1245
aqvideos@tiac.net
www.aquariusproductions.com
Lesile Kussmann, Owner/President/Producer
Kathy Newkirk, Director
Jane Hutchinson, Assoc. Director
This thought-provoking video introduces viewers to people who openly discuss the struggles and triumphs they have experienced living in a body that is physically disabled. They talk honestly about the social stigma of their disability and the problems they face in terms of mobility, health care and family relationships, as well as the challenges of emotional and sexual intimacy. Preview option available. *$195.00*
Video

5277 My Country
Aquarius Health Care Videos
30 Forest Rd
PO Box 249
Millis, MA 2054-1511   508-376-1244
Fax: 508-376-1245
aqvideos@tiac.net
www.aquariusproductions.com
Lesile Kussmann, Owner/President/Producer
Kathy Newkirk, Director
Jane Hutchinson, Assoc. Director
By telling the stories of three people with disabilities and their struggle for equal rights under the law, this film draws a powerful parallel between the efforts of disability rights activists and the civil rights struggle of the 1960s. Great for disability awareness programs, and for discussions of disability rights issues. Should be part of every college curriculum on disabilities. Awarded Best of Show Superfest 98. Preview option available. *$195.00*
Video

5278 Narcolepsy
Fanlight Productions
c/o Icarus Films
32 Court Street, 21st Floor
Brooklyn, NY 11201   718-488-8900
800-876-1710
Fax: 718-488-8642
info@fanlight.com
www.fanlight.com
Ben Achtenberg, Founder, Owner
Jason Margolis, Producer
Presents the experiences of three individuals who lives and relationships have been disrupted by narcolepsy. Rental $50/day. *$199.00*
VHS/25 Minutes

5279 No Barriers
Aquarius Health Care Videos
30 Forest Rd
PO Box 249
Millis, MA 2054-1511   508-376-1244
Fax: 508-376-1245
aqvideos@tiac.net
www.aquariusproductions.com
Lesile Kussmann, Owner/President/Producer
Kathy Newkirk, Director
Jane Hutchinson, Assoc. Director
Everyone faces the world with different abilities and disabilities. But everyone has at least one goal in common...to break through their own barriers says Mark Wellman. Mark, a paraplegic, knows this well. No Barriers takes us into Mark's world where he defies the odds for most able bodied individuals by climbing Yosemite's Half Dome and El Capitan. This video is more than inspiring and fun to watch...it helps one make that paradigm shift from can't do to can do! Preview option available *$90.00*
Video

5280 On The Spectrum
Fanlight Productions
32 Court St.
21st Floor
Brooklyn, NY 11201-4421   718-488-8900
800-876-1710
Fax: 718-488-8642
info@fanlight.com
www.fanlight.com
Jonathan Miller, President
Patricio Guzman, Director
Meredith Miller, Sales Manager
Adults living with Asperger syndrome describe the ways AS has affected their lives, their work and their relationships. They discuss learning to cope with the disorder and the comfort and reinforcement of participating with others 'like them' in an Asperger's support group. 53 min. *$199.00*

5281 Open for Business
Disability Rights Education and Defense Fund
3075 Adeline Street
Suite 210
Berkeley, CA 94703-2219   510-644-2555
800-841-8645
Fax: 510-841-8645
info@dredf.org
www.dredf.org
Sue Henderson, Executive Director
Jenny. Kern, Esq, President/Chair
Claudia Center, Esq, Treasurer
Documentary video captures the drama and emotions of the historic civil rights demonstration of people with disabilities in 1977, resulting in the signing of the 504 Regulations, the first Federal Civil Rights Law protecting people with disabilities. Includes contemporary news footage and news interviews with participants and demonstration leaders. *$179.00*

5282 Open to the Public
Aquarius Health Care Videos
30 Forest Rd
PO Box 249
Millis, MA 2054-1511   508-376-1244
Fax: 508-376-1245
aqvideos@tiac.net
www.aquariusproductions.com
Lesile Kussmann, Owner/President/Producer
Kathy Newkirk, Director
Jane Hutchinson, Assoc. Director
Provides an overview of the Americans with Disabilities Act as it applies to state and local governments. The ADA doesn't provide recommendations for solving common problems, but this film could provide enough information for governments to solve some common problems without turning to high-priced consultants. Preview option available. *$125.00*
Video

5283 Our Own Road
Aquarius Health Care Videos
30 Forest Rd
PO Box 249
Millis, MA 2054-1511

508-376-1244
Fax: 508-376-1245
aqvideos@tiac.net
www.aquariusproductions.com

Lesile Kussmann, Owner/President/Producer
Kathy Newkirk, Director
Jane Hutchinson, Assoc. Director
This video shows the disabled helping other people who are disabled and portrays the sense of pride they get from helping others. This multicultural program features many different healing techniques, and teaches the importance of helping those who are disabled become independent and productive. *$99.00*

5284 Outsider: The Life and Art of Judith Scott
Fanlight Productions
32 Court St.
21st Floor
Brooklyn, NY 11201-4421

718-488-8900
800-876-1710
Fax: 718-488-8642
info@fanlight.com
www.fanlight.com

Jonathan Miller, President
Patricio Guzman, Director
Meredith Miller, Sales Manager
Judith Scoot has Down Syndrome, is deaf, and does not speak. Yet after 35 years of institutionalization, with the help of a sister who never gave up on her, she emerged to create a series of sculptures that have fascinated and mystified art experts and collectors around the world. 26 minutes. *$199.00*

5285 Passion for Justice
Fanlight Productions
32 Court St.
21st Floor
Brooklyn, NY 11201-4421

718-488-8900
800-876-1710
Fax: 718-488-8642
info@fanlight.com
www.fanlight.com

Jonathan Miller, President
Patricio Guzman, Director
Meredith Miller, Sales Manager
An unusually penetrating examination of the question of inclusion, this is an engaging portrait of Bob Perske, the author of Unequal Justice, and a crusader for the legal rights of people with developmental disabilities. A Passion for Justice asks challenging questions about society's responsibility to this population, and about ways to protect everyone's rights to equality and justice. *$99.00*
29 Minutes

5286 Phoenix Dance
Fanlight Productions
32 Court St.
21st Floor
Brooklyn, NY 11201-4421

718-488-8900
800-876-1710
Fax: 718-488-8642
info@fanlight.com
www.fanlight.com

Jonathan Miller, President
Patricio Guzman, Director
Meredith Miller, Sales Manager
A heroic journey of transformation and healing, Phoenix Dance challenges our expectations of what it means to be disabled. In March, 2001, renowned dancer Homer Avila discovered that the pain in his hip was cancer. A month later, his right leg and most of his hip were amputated. *$199.00*

5287 Pool Exercise Program - Arthritis Water Exercise / Arthritis Foundation
Arthritis Foundation Distribution Center
PO Box 932915
Atlanta, GA 31193-2915

440-872-7100
800-283-7800
Fax: 404-872-0457
aforders@arthritis.org
www.arthritis.org

John Klippel, President/CEO
This video features water exercises that will help you increase and maintain joint flexibility, strengthen and tone muscles, and increase endurance. All exercises are performed in water at chest level. No swimming skills are necessary. *$19.50*

5288 Potty Learning for Children who Experience Delay
Exceptional Parent Library
PO Box 1807
Englewood Cliffs, NJ 7632-1207

201-947-6000
800-535-1910
Fax: 201-947-9376
eplibrary@aol.com

This video presents a unique developmental approach to supporting the child in learning independence in the management of bathroom skills. *$39.95*

5289 Pushin' Forward
Fanlight Productions
32 Court St.
21st Floor
Brooklyn, NY 11201-4421

718-488-8900
800-876-1710
Fax: 718-488-8642
info@fanlight.com
www.fanlight.com

Jonathan Miller, President
Patricio Guzman, Director
Meredith Miller, Sales Manager
Growing up poor and Latino, James Lilly was a gang member and drug dealer until, at fifteen, he was shot in the back and paralyzed. Today, he shares his story with inner city kids, and tells them about one thing that helped him move on; wheelchair racing. In Pushin' Forward he takes on the world's longest wheelchair race, from Fairbanks to Anchorage, Alaska, in six days! 39 minutes. *$229.00*

5290 Recognizing Children with Special Needs
Films Media Group
132 W. 31st St
16th Fl.
New York, NY 10001

800-322-8755
Fax: 800-678-3633
custserv@films.com
www.films.com

A great overview for caregivers of children on how to recognize special needs. Often-times it is the little things children do everyday to compensate for, or express, a disability that can be observed by their caregiver. All types of disabilities are addressed: emotional, physical, psychological, and chronic illness. A wonderful tool for teachers, childcare staff, and students on how to play a vital role in our children's development. Preview option available.
DVD/Video

5291 Relaxation Techniques for People with Special Needs
Research Press
PO Box 9177
Dept. 11W
Champaign, IL 61826-9177

217-352-3273
800-519-2707
Fax: 217-352-1221
rp@researchpress.com
www.researchpress.com

David Parkinson, Chairman
Russell Pence, President
Gail Salyards, Dir. Of Marketing/President
The developers discuss and demonstrate how to use special relaxation procedures with children and adolescents who have developmental disabilities. They emphasize the need for students to learn relaxation as a means of coping with stress and developing

self-control. During the scenes of Dr June Groden conducting relaxation training, viewers will see how to correctly use the training procedures, how to use reinforcement during training and how to use guided imagery. 23 minutes. Includes book. *$195.00*
Video

5292 Right at Home
Aquarius Health Care Videos
30 Forest Rd
PO Box 249
Millis, MA 2054
508-376-1244
Fax: 508-376-1245
aqvideos@tiac.net
www.aquariusproductions.com
Lesile Kussmann, Owner/President/Producer
Kathy Newkirk, Director
Jane Hutchinson, Assoc. Director
Shows simple solutions for complying with the Fair Hoiusing Act amendments. Emphasizes low-cost, practical solutions, and working with people with disabilities to find the best applicable solution. Ideal for people with disabilities and their families, as well as housing providers, university courses, and disability awareness organizations. Preview option is available. *$99.00*
Video

5293 Seat-A-Robics
PO Box 630064
Little Neck, NY 11363-64
718-631-4007

Daria Alinovi, President
Offers a variety of safe, affordable and medically approved video exercise programs that are listed in our video chapter. In addition the company offers two resources. The first Healthy Eating & Facts For Kids is geared specifically to health professionals and educators that work with disabled children ($39.95). The second is a recreational resource guide that stimulates children to be creative and get involved. It keeps them actively engaged while having fun and getting fit ($29.95).

5294 Shining Bright: Head Start Inclusion
Brookes Publishing
PO Box 10624
Baltimore, MD 21285-624
410-337-9580
800-638-3775
Fax: 410-337-8539
custserv@brookespublishing.com
Paul Brooks, Owner
This documentary depicts the collaborative efforts of a Head Start and a local education agency to include children with severe disabilities in a Head Start program. This video addresses issues such as support for children with severe health impairments, benefits of participating in Head Start, ability of teachers with a general education background to serve children with severe disabilities, and staff relations. Includes a 28-page saddle-stitched booklet. *$45.00*
23 Minutes
ISBN 1-55766-95-9

5295 Small Differences
Aquarius Health Care Videos
30 Forest Rd
PO Box 249
Millis, MA 2054-1511
508-376-1244
Fax: 508-376-1245
aqvideos@tiac.net
www.aquariusproductions.com
Lesile Kussmann, Owner/President/Producer
Kathy Newkirk, Director
Jane Hutchinson, Assoc. Director
What happens when you give children with and without disabilities a camera and ask them to produce a video about disabilities? The result is an uplifting, award-winning disability video that both children and adults can relate to. The kids interviewed adults and children with physical and sensory disabilities. A top-quality production that increases understanding and awareness. Winner, Columbus International Film & Video Festival. Winner, National Education Media Network. Preview option availabe *$110.00*
Video

5296 Someday's Child
Educational Productions
9000 SW Gemini Dr
Beaverton, OR 97008-7151
503-644-7000
800-950-4949
Fax: 503-350-7000
custserv@edpro.com
www.edpro.com
Diane Trister Dodge, Founder/President/Lead Author
Arnitra Duckett, VP, Sales & Strategic Marketing
This video focuses on three families' search for help and information for their children with disabilities.

5297 Sound & Fury
Aquarius Health Care Videos
30 Forest Rd
PO Box 249
Millis, MA 2054-1511
508-376-1244
Fax: 508-376-1245
aqvideos@tiac.net
www.aquariusproductions.com
Lesile Kussmann, Owner/President/Producer
Kathy Newkirk, Director
Jane Hutchinson, Assoc. Director
This film takes viewers inside the seldom seen world of the deaf to witness a painful family struggle over a controversial medical technology called the cochlear implant. Some of the family members celebrate the implant as a long overdue cure for deafness while others fear it will destroy their language and way of life. This documentary explores this seemingly irreconcilable conflict as it illuminates the ongoing struggle for identity among deaf people today. *$195.00*
Video

5298 Special Children/Special Solutions
Option Indigo Press
2080 S Undermountain Rd
Sheffield, MA 1257-9643
413-229-8727
800-714-2779
Fax: 413-229-8727
indigo@option.org
Barry Kaufmans, Owner/Founder/Author
Samahria Kaufmans, Owner/Founder
This four-tape audio series presents concrete, down-to-earth, no-nonsense alternatives which are full of love and acceptance for the special child while being wholly supportive of parents, professionals and helpers who want to reach out. The accepting (nonjudgmental) attitude presented is the basis of all Samahria's work and is the foundation for the nurturing teaching process that has encouraged and helped parents, children and others to accomplish more than most would have believed. *$55.00*
Audio

5299 Technology for the Disabled
Landmark Media
3450 Slade Run Dr
Falls Church, VA 22042-3940
703-241-2030
800-342-4336
Fax: 703-536-9540
info@landmarkmedia.com
landmarkmedia.com
Michael Hartogs, President
Joan Hartogs, Vice President
Peter Hartogs, Vice President
Physically disabled people cope with the frustrations of a body they cannot control. The computer age has made many disabled more self-reliant; armless feed themselves, the blind read newspapers and the voiceless speak through marvelous technological breakthroughs. *$195.00*
Video

5300   Three R's for Special Education: Rights, Resources, Results
Brookes Publishing
PO Box 10624
Baltimore
MD, 21 0624-624   410-337-9580
                                                   800-638-3775
                                              Fax: 410-337-8539
                                 custserv@brookespublishing.com
Paul Brooks, Owner
This is a guide for parents, and a tool for educators. Through this video parents learn how to work through the steps of the special education system and work toward securing the best education and services for their children. Reviews the laws to protect children with disabilities in easy to understand language. Also provides a list of national organizations that can offer resources, information and advice to parents. *$49.95*
50 Minutes
ISBN 0-96461-80-7

5301   Tools for Students
Aquarius Health Care Videos
30 Forest Rd
PO Box 249
Millis, MA 2054-1511   508-376-1244
                                               Fax: 508-376-1245
                                              aqvideos@tiac.net
                                        www.aquariusproductions.com
Lesile Kussmann, Owner/President/Producer
Kathy Newkirk, Director
Jane Hutchinson, Assoc. Director
Provides a series of 26 fun occupational therapy sensory processing activities. Designed as an in-home, in-workshop, and in-class exercise leader with students. Activities include: Strenghten the muscles necessary for normal activities, provide the muscles necessary to enhance alertness and concentration, increase the ability to use good posture, help social skills and fitting in and increase coordination; concludes with emphasis on team collaboration between the student, teacher, and parents. *$99.00*
Video

5302   Twitch and Shout
Fanlight Productions
c/o Icarus Films
32 Court Street, 21st Floor
Brooklyn, NY 11201   718-488-8900
                                                   800-876-1710
                                              Fax: 718-488-8642
                                               info@fanlight.com
                                                www.fanlight.com
Ben Achtenberg, Founder, Owner
Laurel Chitden, Producer
This documentary provides an intimate journey into the startling world of Tourette Syndrome (TS), a genetic disorder that can cause a bizarre range of involuntary movements, vocalizations, and compulsions. Through the eyes of a photojournalist with TS, the film introduces viewers to others who have this puzzling disorder. This is an emotionally absorbing, sometimes, unsettling, and finally uplifting program about people who must contend with a society that often sees them as crazy or bad. *$225.00*

5303   Video Guide to Disability Awareness
Aquarius Health Care Videos
30 Forest Rd
PO Box 249
Millis, MA 2054-1511   508-376-1244
                                               Fax: 508-376-1245
                                              aqvideos@tiac.net
                                        www.aquariusproductions.com
Lesile Kussmann, Owner/President/Producer
Kathy Newkirk, Director
Jane Hutchinson, Assoc. Director
President Clinton opens and concludes this informative video about disability awareness. A series of candid interviews with people who have a wide range of disabilities provide personal insights into the issues surrounding visual, hearing, physical and mental disabilities. Video comes with written reference guide and is also available with open or closed captioning. Preview option available. *$195.00*
Video

5304   Video Intensive Parenting
Systems Unlimited/LIFE Skills
1556 S 1st Ave
Iowa City, IA 52240-6007   319-356-5412

Geoffrey Lauer, Program Director
Bill Gorman, President
Ginny Kirschling, Public Information Specialist
Parents who have children with special needs share their reactions to their child's diagnosis and how they have learned to cope with their feelings. *$69.95*

5305   Vital Signs: Crip Culture Talks Back
Fanlight Productions
32 Court St.
21st Floor
Brooklyn, NY 11201-4421   718-488-8900
                                                   800-876-1710
                                              Fax: 718-488-8642
                                               info@fanlight.com
                                                www.fanlight.com
Jonathan Miller, President
Patricio Guzman, Director
Meredith Miller, Sales Manager
This edgy, raw video documentary explores the politics of disability through the performances, debates and late-night conversations of artists at a recent national conference of disabilities and the art's. Vital Signs conveys the intensity, variety and vitality of disability culture today. *$225.00*
Video

5306   What About Me?
Educational Productions
9000 SW Gemini Dr
Beaverton, OR 97008-7151   503-644-7000
                                                   800-950-4949
                                              Fax: 503-350-7000
                                              custserve@edpro.com
                                        www.teachingstrategies.com
Diane Trister Dodge, Founder/President/Lead Author
Arnitra Duckett, VP, Sales & Strategic Marketing
This video focuses on two siblings of children with disabilities. The siblings (Brian and Julie) share their perspectives, their worries, concerns and victories about living with a sibling with a disability.

5307   When Billy Broke His Head...and Other
Fanlight Productions
32 Court St.
21st Floor
Brooklyn, NY 11201-4421   718-488-8900
                                                   800-876-1710
                                              Fax: 718-488-8642
                                               info@fanlight.com
                                                www.fanlight.com
Jonathan Miller, President
Patricio Guzman, Director
Meredith Miller, Sales Manager
When Billy Golfus, an award-winning journalist, became brain damaged as the result of a motor scooter accident, he joined the ranks of the 43 million Americans with disabilities, this country's largest and most invisible minority. He helped create this video, which blends humor with politics and individual experience with a chorus of voices, to explain what it is really like to live with a disability in America. #136 *$195.00*
ISBN 1-57295-36-2

5308   When I Grow Up
Britannica Film Company
345 4th St
San Francisco, CA 94107-1206   415-928-8466
                                              Fax: 415-928-5027
Dave Bekowich, Owner
At a costume party each child was to come as what they wanted to be when they grew up. Some of the children had handicaps, and they talked about why their handicaps would not prevent them from fulfilling their desires.
Film

5309   When Parents Can't Fix It
Fanlight Productions
32 Court St.
21st Floor
Brooklyn, NY 11201-4421   718-488-8900
                                            800-876-1710
                                        Fax: 718-488-8642
                                        info@fanlight.com
                                        www.fanlight.com

Jonathan Miller, President
Patricio Guzman, Director
Meredith Miller, Sales Manager
This documentary looks at the lives of five families who are raising children with disabilities - the problems they face, how they have learned to cope, and the rewards and stresses of adapting to their child's condition. It explores the medical complexities and financial pressures families encounter, the emotional and physical toll on parents and siblings, and the dangers of child abuse in this population. It offers a very realistic look at different family strengths and coping styles.
58 Min. DVD/VHS
ISBN 1-572958-76-6

5310   White Cane and Wheels
Fanlight Productions
32 Court St.
21st Floor
Brooklyn, NY 11201-4421   718-488-8900
                                            800-876-1710
                                        Fax: 718-488-8642
                                        info@fanlight.com
                                        www.fanlight.com

Jonathan Miller, President
Patricio Guzman, Director
Meredith Miller, Sales Manager
Carmen and Steve once dreamed of lives on stage and screen, but their plans were cut short by her blindness and his muscular dystrophy. This program is a funny and touching exploration of a relationship filled with frustration, but held together with patience, stubborness, forgiveness, and love. 26 minutes. *$169.00*

Web Sites

5311   ADA Questions and Answers
US Department of Justice, Civil Rights Division
950 Pennsylvania Ave. NW
9th Floor
Washington, DC 20530   202-307-0663
                                            800-514-0301
                                        Fax: 202-307-1197
                                        TTY: 800-514-0383
                                             www.ada.gov
Rebecca B. Bond, Chief
Anne Raish, Principal Deputy Chief
Christina Galindo-Walsh, Deputy Chief
A 31-page booklet giving an overview of the ADA's requirements affecting employers, businesses, nonprofit service agencies, and state and local governments programs, including public transportation. Available in electronic format only.

5312   Ability Jobs
Ability Magazine
P.O. Box 10878
Costa Mesa, CA 92627   www.abilityjobs.com
Provides an electronic classified system which allows employers to recruit qualified individuals with disabilities, and people with disabilities to locate employment opportunities.

5313   AbleApparel - Affordable Adaptive Clothing and Accessories
2121 Hillside Ave
New Hyde Park, NY 11040-2712   516-873-6552
                                        Fax: 516-248-7308
                                        www.ableapparel.com
Mary Ann Tenaglia, Partner
Marie Harmon, Partner
Donna Lo Monica, Partner/Designer

AbleApparel is always designing and creating new products that will make Matty's life and others with disabilities a little easier. Most of the people spoken to regardless of age want to be able to wear clothes that are functional, affordable and, above all, fashionable.

5314   AbleData
103 W Broad St
Suite 400
Falls Church, VA 22046   301-608-8998
                                            800-227-0216
                                        Fax: 301-608-8958
                                        TTY: 301-608-8912
                                        www.abledata.com
Katherine Belknap, Director
David Johnson, Publications Director
AbleData provides objective information on assistive technology and rehabilitation equipment available from domestic and international sources to consumers, organizations, professionals, and caregivers within the United States. AbleData serves the nation's disability, rehabilitation and senior communities.

5315   Access Unlimited
570 Hance Rd
Binghamton, NY 13903-5700   607-669-4822
                                            800-849-2143
                                        Fax: 607-669-4595
                                        www.accessunlimited.com
Thomas Egan, President/Owner
Tom 'TC' Cole, National Sales Manager
Adaptive transportation and mobility equipment for people with disabilities. ccess Unlimited products empower people with disabilities to regain control of their mobility.

5316   Ai Squared
130 Taconic Business Park
Manchester Center, VT 05255-9752   802-362-3612
                                            800-859-0270
                                        Fax: 802-362-1670
                                        sales@aisquared.com
                                        www.aisquared.com
David Wu, CEO
Jost Eckhardt, VP of Engineering
Doug Hacker, VP of Business Development
Ai Squared has been a leader in the assistive technology field for over 20 years. Our flagship product, ZoomText, is the world's best magnification and reading software for the vision impaired. We pride ourselves on delivering the highest quality software products and superior technical support.

5317   Alternatives in Education for the Hearing Impaired (AEHI)
9300 Capitol Drive
Wheeling, IL 60090-7207   847-850-5490
                                        Fax: 847-850-5493
                                        info@agbms.org
                                        www.agbms.org
Sandra L. Mosetick, Board President Emeritus
Bridget Chevez, Board President
Daniel Konopacki, Treasurer
AEHI is a program of the Alexander Graham Bell Montessori School in Mt. Prospect, IL, that fosters literacy and empowers people with hearing impairments to achieve their full potential through unique educational options. AEHI provides Cued Speech workshops, individualized parental training and support, educational consulting, professional development opportunities, and access to a wide variety of information on Cued Speech and its benefits.

5318   American Academy of Audiology (AAA)
11480 Commerce Park Dr.
Suite 220
Reston, VA 20191   703-790-8466
                                        Fax: 703-790-8631
                                        infoaud@audiology.org
                                        www.audiology.org
Patrick E. Gallagher, Executive Director
Kathryn Werner, Vice President, Public Affairs
Amy Miedema, Vice President, Communications & Membership
The American Academy of Audiology is the world's largest professional organization for audiologists. The Academy is dedi-

cated to providing quality hearing care services through professional development, education, research, and increased public awareness of hearing and balance disorders.

5319   American Association of People with Disabilities (AAPD)
2013 H St. NW
5th Floor
Washington, DC 20006   202-521-4316
                                         800-840-8844
                             communications@aapd.com
                                         www.aapd.com

Maria Town, President & Chief Executive Officer
Jasmin Bailey, Manager, Business Operations
Christine Liao, Programs Director
Nonprofit cross-disability member organization dedicated to ensuring economic self-sufficiency and political empowerment for Americans with disabilities. AAPD works in coalition with other disability organizations for the full implementation and enforcement of disability nondiscrimination laws, particularly the Americans With Disabilities Act (ADA) of 1990 and the Rehabilitation Act of 1973.

5320   American College of Rheumatology, Researchand Education Foundation
2200 Lake Boulevard NE
Atlanta, GA 30319-5310   404-633-3777
                                    Fax: 404-633-1870
                                 acr@rheumatology.org
                                 www.rheumatology.org

Audrey B. Uknis, MD, President
David I. Daikh, MD, PhD, Foundation President
Jan K. Richardson, PT, PhD, O, ARHP President
The American College of Rheumatology's mission is advancing rheumatology.The organization represents over 8,500 rheumatologists and rheumatology health professionals around the world. The ACR offers its members the support they need to ensure that they are able to continue their innovative work by providing programs of education, research, advocacy, and practice support.

5321   American Liver Foundation
39 Broadway
Suite 2700
New York, NY 10006-3054   212-668-1000
                                    Fax: 212-483-8179
                                www.liverfoundation.org

Ryan Reczek, National Director, Field Development
Rolf Taylor, National Director, Corporate Relations
Pritha Kuchaculla, National Director, Programs
Is the only national voluntary health organization dedicated to preventing, treating, and curing hepatitis and other liver and gall bladder diseases through research and education.

5322   American Mobility: Personal Mobility Solutions
60 Island St
Lawrence, MA 1840-1835   978-794-3030
                             www.americanmobility.com

David Lacroix, President
Source of Pride Scooters, Jazzy Power Chairs, personal mobility vehicles, and lift and recline chairs.

5323   American Speech-Language and Hearing Association
2200 Research Blvd
Rockville, MD 20850-3289   301-296-5700
                                         800-638-8255
                                    Fax: 301-296-8580
                                    TTY: 301-296-5650
                                 actioncenter@asha.org
                                         www.asha.org

Wayne A. Foster, PhD, CCC-SLP/A, Chair, Audiology Advisory Council
Patricia A. Prelock, PhD, CCC-SLP, President
Carolyn W. Higdon, EdD, CCC-SLP, Vice President for Finance
Exhibits by companies specializing in alternative and augmentative communications products, publishers, software and hardware compinies, and hearing aid testing equipment manufacturers.

5324   Americans with Disabilities Act: ADA Home Page
                                         800-514-0301
                                    TTY: 800-514-0383
                                 webmaster@usdoj.gov
                                         www.ada.gov
Provides facts on the Americans with Disabilities Act and other information relating to disability rights.

5325   Aspies For Freedom (AFF)
                             www.aspiesforfreedom.com
Gwen Nelson, Co-Founder
Amy Nelson, Co-Founder
Seeks to change the discourse on autism, including negative treatment in the media. Runs an online chatroom and promotes Autistic Pride Day.

5326   Association for the Cure of Cancer of the Prostate (CaP CURE)-Prostate Cancer Foundation
1250 Fourth St
Suite 360
Santa Monica, CA 90401-1444   310-570-4700
                                         800-757-2873
                                    Fax: 310-570-4701
                                         info@pcf.org
                                         www.pcf.org

Mike Milken, Founder/Chairman
Jonathon Simons, MD, President/CEO
Ralph Finerman, Chief Financial Officer/Treasurer/Secretary
CURE is a nonprofit public charity that is dedicated to supporting prostate cancer research and hastening the conversion of research into cures or controls.

5327   Asthma and Allergy Foundation of America
8201 Corporate Drive
Suite 1000
Landover, MD 20785-2266   800-727-8462
                                         info@aafa.org
                                         www.aafa.org

Lynn Hanessian, Chair
Michele Abu Carrick, LICSW, Co-Chair, Governance
Judi McAuliffe, RN, Co-Chair, Programs & Services
AAFA is dedicated to improving the quality of life for people with asthma and allergic diseases through education, advocacy and research.

5328   AudiologyOnline
12333 Sowden Rd.
Ste. B. #79931
Houston, TX 77080-2059   800-753-2160
                                    Fax: 210-579-7010
                                www.audiologyonline.com

Ted A. Meyer, Chair
Catharine McNally, Chair-Elect
Susan Lenihan, Secretary
Online continuing education resources for audiology professionals.

5329   BDRC Newsletter
Birth Defect Research for Children
976 Lake Baldwin Lane
Suite 104
Orlando, FL 32814   407-895-0802
                                 staff@birthdefects.org
                                 www.birthdefects.org

Betty Mekdeci, Executive Director
A monthly electronic newsletter offering the latest news, research, and updates on birth defects.
Monthly

5330   Braille and Audio Reading Download (BARD)
National Library Service
1291 Taylor St NW
Washington, DC 20542   202-707-5100
                                         800-424-8567
                                         888-657-7323
                                    Fax: 202-707-0712
                                 NLSDownload@loc.gov
                                         nlsbard.loc.gov

501

A program of the National Library Service, where eligible users may download Braille and audiobooks.

5331   Cancer Research Institute
29 Broadway
4th Floor
New York, NY 10006   212-688-7515
                                      800-992-2623
                                      Fax: 212-832-9376
                                      info@cancerresearch.org
                                      www.cancerresearch.org
Jill O'Donnell-Tormey, CEO & Director of Scientific Affairs
Lynne Harmer, Director of Grants Administration and Special Events
Alfred R. Massidas, Chief Financial Officer and Director of Human Resources
Nonprofit organization dedicated to cancer immunotherapy.

5332   Center on the Social & Emotional Foundations for Early Learning (CSEFEL)
Vanderbilt University 110 Magnolia
Box 328 GPC
Nashville, TN 37203   615-322-8150
                                      Fax: 615-343-1570
                                      ml.hemmeter@vanderbilt.edu
                                      csefel.vanderbilt.edu
Mary-Louise Hemmeter, Principal Investigator
Rob Corso, Project Coordinator
Tweety Yates, Project Coordinator
The center will: focus on promoting the social and emotional developmental of children as a means of preventing challenging behaviors; collaborate with existing T/TA providers for the purpose of ensuring the implementation and sustainability of practices at the local level; provide ongoing identification of training needs and preferred delivery formats of local programs and T/TA providers; disseminate evidence-based practices.

5333   Damon Runyon Cancer Research Foundation
Walter Winchell Foundation
One Exchange Plaza, 55 Broadway
Suite 302
New York, NY 10006-3720   212-455-0500
                                     877-722-6237
                                     info@damonrunyon.org
                                     www.damonrunyon.org
Lorraine Egan, President/Chief Executive Officer
Elizabeth Portland, Director of Development
Marialice C. Pagnotta, Director of the Damon Runyon Broadway Tickets Service
The Damon Runyon Cancer Research Foundation funds early career cancer researchers who have the energy, drive and creativity to become leading innovators in their fields. We identify the best young scientists in the nation and support them through four award programs: our Fellowship, Pediatric Cancer Fellowship, Clinical Investigator and Innovation Awards.

5334   DisAbility Information and Resources
                                     jlubin@eskimo.com
                                     www.makoa.org
Jim Lubin, Creator/Owner
Offers dozens of links to sites with information, services and products for the disabled.

5335   Disability Rights Activist
                                     www.disrights.org
Provides information to enable anyone intersted in the rights of disabled people to work for those rights.

5336   DisabilityAdvisor.com
37 North Orange Ave.
Suite 500
Orlando, FL 32801   321-332-7800
                                      888-393-1010
                                      Fax: 888-985-6060
                                      www.disabilityadvisor.com
Joseph E. Ram, Publisher
Kay Derochie, Editor
Jackie Booth, Ph.D., Editor

DisabilityAdvisor.com provides free information on federal and state disability benefits programs and other resources for readers and their families. This includes disabled children and students, military veterans, injured workers and disabled seniors. Readers are encouraged to submit their questions and comments online. The website also offers information on managing finances, education, parenting, relationships and other issues of interest to the disabled and their friends and families.

5337   DisabilityResources.org
Four Glatter Lane
Dept. IN
Centereach, NY 11720-1032   631-585-0290
                                     Fax: 631-585-0290
Julie Klauber, Co-founder/Managing Editor
Avery Klauber, Co-Founder/Executive Director
Sally Rosenthal, Contributing Editor
Disability Resources, inc. is a nonprofit 501(c)(3) organization established to promote and improve awareness, availability and accessibility of information that can help people with disabilities live, learn, love, work and play independently.

5338   Discover Technology
Houston, TX   713-885-1519
                                     dtinc8888@hotmail.com
                                     www.discovertechnology.com
Amantha Cole, Founder
The primary mission of Discover Technology, Inc.is to create and administer computer labs for persons with disabilities, to encourage communication between persons with and without disabilities and to educate the general population about the disabled population.

5339   Dynamic Living
125 Old Iron Ore Road
Bloomfield, CT 06002-1315   860-683-4442
                                     888-940-0605
                                     Fax: 860-243-1910
                                     www.dynamic-living.com
Andrea Tannenbaum, Owner
Kitchen products, bathroom helpers, and unique daily living products that provide a convienient, comfortable, and safe environment for people with disabilities.

5340   ERIC Clearinghouse on Disabilities and Gifted Education
                                     www.hoagiesgifted.org/eric
The ERIC Clearinghouse was disbanded by the government in 2003. This website acts as an archive of ERIC material.

5341   ElderLawAnswers.com
150 Chesnut St
4th Floor, Box #15
Providence, RI 02903   866-267-0947
                                     support@elderlawanswers.com
                                     www.elderlawanswers.com
Harry S. Margolis, Founder/President
Ken Coughlin, Editor
Mark Miller, Director of Product and Business Development
Provides information about legal issues facing senior citizens and a searchable directory of attorneys.

5342   Exploring Autism: A Look at the Genetics of Autism
Box 3445 DUMC
Durham, NC 27710   Fax: 919-684-0952
Chantelle Wolpert, Project Director
Dedicated to helping families who are living with the challenges of autism stay informed about the exciting breakthroughs involving the genetics of autism. Report and explain new genetic research findings. Explain genetic principles as they relate to autism, provide the latest research news, and seek your imput.

5343 FHI 360
1825 Connecticut Ave., NW
Suite 800
Washington, DC 20009-5721   202-884-8000
                                   Fax: 202-884-8400
                        CareerCenterSupport@fhi360.org
                                   www.fhi360.org
Willard Cates Jr, MD, MPH, President Emeritus
Albert J. Siemens, PhD, Chief Executive Officer
Patrick C. Fine, MS, Chief Operating Officer
FHI 360 is a nonprofit human development organization dedicated to improving lives in lasting ways by advancing integrated, locally driven solutions.

5344 Foundation Fighting Blindness
7168 Columbia Gateway Dr.
Suite 100
Columbia, MD 21046   410-423-0600
                                   800-683-5555
                                   TTY: 410363713951
                            info@FightBlindness.org
                                   www.blindness.org
William T. Schmidt, Chief Executive Officer
Valerie Navy-Daniels, Chief Development Officer
Stephen M. Rose, PhD, Chief Research Officer
The Foundation Fighting Blindness (FFB) works to promote research in order to prevent, treat and restore vision. FFB is currently the world's leading private funder of retinal disease research, funding over 100 research grants and 150 researchers.

5345 Freedom Scientific
11830 31st Court North
St. Petersburg, FL 33716-1805   727-803-8000
                                   800-444-4443
                                   Fax: 727-803-8001
                            info@freedomscientific.com
                                   www.freedomscientific.com
Lee Hamilton, President/CEO/Chairman
Mike Self, Sales Representative
Joseph McDaniel, Sales Representative
Assistive technology for blind and visually impaired computer users.

5346 Gallaudet University Press
800 Florida Ave, NE
Washington, DC 20002-3695   202-651-5488
                                   Fax: 202-651-5489
                            gupress@gallaudet.edu
                                   www.gupress.gallaudet.edu
Gallaudet University Press is a vital, self-supporting member of the Gallaudet educational and scholarly community. The mission of the Press is to disseminate knowledge about deaf and hard of hearing people, their languages, their communities, their history, and their education through print and electronic media.

5347 Glaucoma Research Foundation
251 Post Street
Suite 600
San Francisco, CA 94108-5017   415-986-3162
                                   800-826-6693
                            question@glaucoma.org
                                   www.glaucoma.org
Andrew Iwach, MD, Board Chair/Executive Director
Thomas r M. Brunne, President/CEO
H. Allen Bouch, Vice Chair
Our mission is to prevent vision loss from glaucoma by investing in innovative research, education, and support with the ultimate goal of finding a cure.

5348 HealthyWomen
P.O. Box 430
Red Bank, NJ 07701   732-530-3425
                                   877-986-9472
                                   Fax: 732-865-7225
                            info@healthywomen.org
                                   www.healthywomen.org
Oxana K Pickeral, Ph.D, MBA, Chair
Beth Battaglino, CEO
Phyllis E Greenberger, MSW, Senior Vice President, Science & Health Policy

Website providing information for women with disabilities, health professionals, researchers, and caretakers.

5349 Herb Research Foundation
5589 Arapahoe Ave
Suite 205
Boulder, CO 80303-8115   303-449-2265
                                   www.herbs.org
Rob McCaleb, President
John Lowe, Director of Research
Research and public education on the health benefits of medicinal plants. Dedicated to world health through the informed use of herbs.

5350 Hypokalemic Periodic Paralysis Resource Page
155 West 68th St
Suite 1732
New York, NY 10023-5830   407-339-9499
                                   lfeld@cfl.rr.com
                                   www.periodicparalysis.org
Jacob Levitt, President/Medical Director
Linda Feld, Vice President
Provides understandable information on HKPP, dynamia linkage to several additional sources of helpful information on the Internet, and offers several online networking opportunities.

5351 INCLUDEnyc
Formerly Resources for Children with Special Needs
116 E. 16th St.
5th Fl.
New York, NY 10003   212-677-4650
                                   Fax: 202-254-4070
                            info@includenyc.org
                                   www.includenyc.org
Barbara Glassman, Executive Director
Todd Dorman, Senior Director of Communications and Outreach
Mariko Sakita, Director of Parent & Family Services
Provides free services and resources for youth and families with disabilities in all five state boroughs. Organizational services include: Parenting & Advocacy; School and Community Activities; Parent counseling and Training for students with Autism; Medicaid Waiver services; Transition and Adult Services; and Social skills and building relationships.

5352 Innovation Management Group
179 Niblick Road
Suite 454
Paso Robles, CA 93446-4845   818-701-1579
                                   800-889-0987
                                   Fax: 818-936-0200
                            sales@imgpresents.com
                                   www.imgpresents.com
US and international onscreen keyboards, Word Prediction, Switch Scanning, Hover and Dwell, Joystick emulation, and Magnification software programs.

5353 Interstitial Cystitis Association
1760 Old Meadow Road
Suite 500
McLean, VA 22102-2651   703-442-2070
                                   800-435-7422
                                   Fax: 703-506-3266
                            icamail@ichelp.org
                                   www.ichelp.org
Barbara Gordon, Co-Chair/Executive Director
Eric Zarnikow, MBA, Co-Chair
Marilynn Schreibstein, CFO
The Interstitial Cystitis Association (ICA) advocates for interstitial cystitis (IC) research dedicated to discovery of a cure and better treatments, raises awareness, and serves as a central hub for the healthcare providers, researchers and millions of patients who suffer with constant urinary urgency and frequency and extreme bladder pain called IC. (IC is also referred to as painful bladder syndrome, bladder pain syndrome, and chronic pelvic pain.)

5354 JoanBorysenko.Com
PO Box 1300
Tesuque, NM 87574   www.joanborysenko.com
Joan Borysenko, Founder

503

Publishes resources for credible information about the intersection of mind-body health, positive psychology, and spiritual exploration.

5355 LD OnLine - WETA Public Television
2775 S. Quincy Street
Arlington, VA 22206-2269   Fax: 703-998-2060
                                        ldonline@weta.org
                                        www.ldonline.org

Noel Gunther, Executive Director
Christian Lindstrom, Director, Learning Media
Tina Chovanec, Director, Reading Rockets
LD OnLine seeks to help children and adults reach their full potential by providing accurate and up-to-date information and advice about learning disabilities and ADHD. The site features hundreds of helpful articles, multimedia, monthly columns by noted experts, first person essays, children's writing and artwork, a comprehensive resource guide, very active forums, and a Yellow Pages referral directory of professionals, schools, and products.

5356 Lighthouse Guild
250 West 64th Street
New York, NY 10023   800-284-4422
                                        www.lighthouseguild.org

Calvin W. Roberts, President & CEO
James M. Dubin, Chairman
Lawrence E. Goldschmidt, Vice Chairman & Treasurer
Lighthouse Guild is a not-for-profit vision & healthcare organization, addressing the needs of people who are blind or visually impaired, including those with multiple disabilities or chronic medical conditions.

5357 Lyme Disease Foundation
PO Box 332
Tolland, CT 6084-332   860-870-0070
                                        Fax: 860-870-0080
                                        www.lyme.org

Karen Forschuer, Chairman
Thomas Forschuer, Executive Director
Provides critical information about tick-borne disease prevention, improves healthcare and funds research for solutions. 500,000 children, adults, and professionals assisted 25 countries.

5358 Mainstream Living
333 SW 9th St
Des Moines, IA 50309   515-243-8115
                                        Fax: 515-243-5017
                                        www.mainstreamliving.org
Provides a full range of community-based residential and non-residential supports to people with disabilities, including community housing, therapy, and employment services.

5359 Mainstream Online Magazine of the Able-Disabled

                                        www.mainstream-mag.com

Cyndi Jones, Publisher
William G. Stothers, Editor
The leading news, advocacy and lifestyle magazine for people with disabilities.

5360 Microsoft Accessibility Technology for Everyone
One Microsoft Way
Redmond, WA 98052-6399   425-882-8080
                                        800-642-7676
                                        Fax: 425-936-7329
                                        TTY: 800-892-5234
                                        www.microsoft.com/enable

William Gates III, Chairman
Steven Ballmer, CEO/Director
Information about accessibility features and options included in Microsoft products.

5361 MossRehab ResourceNet
1200 West Tabor Road
Philadelphia, PA 19141-3099   215-456-9900
                                        800-225-5567
                                        www.mossresourcenet.org

John Whyte, Owner
Ruth Lefton, COO
Anthony Allonardo, Director of Technology

MossRehab, a modern, 147-bed facility, offers comprehensive care to people with a broad range of conditions—including stroke, brain injury, orthopaedic and musculoskeletal disabilities, spinal cord dysfunction, pulmonary disorders, amputations, and other forms of disability.

5362 Multiple Sclerosis National Research Institute
11350 SW Village Parkway
Port St. Lucie, FL 34987-2352   858-597-3872
                                        866-676-7400
                                        Fax: 858-597-3804
                                        www.ms-research.org

Robin Offord, Chairman
Richard Houghten, President/CEO
Donald B. Cooper, C.F.O
Multiple Sclerosis National Research Institute is a division of Torrey Pines Institute for Molecular Studies, a not-for-profit basic research center dedicated to the discovery and development of innovative research methods that lead to treatments for major medical conditions, including multiple sclerosis, AIDS, Alzheimer's disease, pain, heart disease, many types of cancer, and more.

5363 National Alliance of the Disabled(NAOTD)

Walton Dutcher, Executive Director/Operations
Fred Temple, Director
Spike Spikberg, Director
The National Alliance OF The DisAbled is an online informational and advocacy organization dedicated to working towards gaining equal rights for the disAbled in all areas of life.

5364 National Birth Defect Registry
Birth Defect Research for Children
976 Lake Baldwin Lane
Suite 104
Orlando, FL 32814   407-895-0802
                                        staff@birthdefects.org
                                        www.birthdefects.org

Betty Mekdeci, Executive Director
Data collection project by Birth Defect Research for Children to answer parents' questions about birth defects.

5365 National Brain Tumor Foundation - National Brain Tumor Society
55 Chapel Street
Suite 200
Newton, MA 02458-2599   617-924-9997
                                        800-770-8287
                                        Fax: 617-928-9998
                                        info@braintumor.org
                                        www.braintumor.org

Jeffrey Kolodin, Chair
Michael Nathanson, Vice Chair
N. Paul TonThat, Executive Director
An organization serving people whose lives are affected by brain tumors. The organization is dedicated to promoting a cure for brain tumors, improving the quality of life and giving hope to the brain tumor community by funding meaningful research and providing patient resources, timely information and education.

5366 National Business & Disability Council
201 I.U. Willets Road
Albertson, NY 11507-1516   516-465-1516
                                        lfrancis@viscardicenter.org
                                        www.business-disability.com

Michael C. Pascucci, Executive Leadership Team Chairman
Laura Francis, Executive Director
John D. Kemp, President
The NBDC is the leading resource for employers seeking to integrate people with disabilities into the workplace and companies seeking to reach them in the consumer marketplace.

5367   National Organization on Disability (NOD)
77 Water St.
13th Floor
New York, NY 10005   646-505-1191
                                  Fax: 646-505-1184
                                       info@nod.org
                                       www.nod.org
Carol Glazer, President
Moeena Das, Chief Operating Officer
Priyanka Ghosh, Director, External Affairs
The National Organization on Disability is a private, nonprofit organization that promotes the full and equal participation of men, women, and children with disabilities in all aspects of American life.
1982

5368   National Rehabilitation Information Center (NARIC)
8400 Corporate Drive
Suite 500
Landover, MD 20785-2266   301-459-5984
                                       800-346-2742
                                  Fax: 301-459-4263
                                  TTY: 301-459-5984
                                       www.naric.com
Mark X. Odum, Project Director
Serves both professionals and the general public intersted in disability and rehabilitation.

5369   National Youth Leadership Network Youth Leader Blog (NYLN)

                                          nyln.org
Articles and documentaries about youth leadership, including overcoming disabilities.

5370   Nebraska Library Commission: Talking Book and Braille Service (TBBS)
Talking Book and Braille Service
1200 N St
Suite 120
Lincoln, NE 68508-2023   402-471-4038
                                       800-742-7691
                                  Fax: 402-471-6244
                            nlc.readadv@nebraska.gov
                                  nlc.nebraska.gov/tbbs
David Oertli, Executive Director
Kay Goehring, Reader Services Coordinator
Bill Ainsley, Audio Production Studio Manager
Provides eligible users with free audio books, audio magazines and Braille via the mail. Also features in-house studios for audiobook production.

5371   NeuroControl Corporation
8333 Rockside Rd
Valley View, OH 44125-6134   216-912-0101
                                       800-378-6955
                                  Fax: 216-912-0129
Helps people with spinal cord injuries lead more independent lives.

5372   Newsletter of PA's AT Lending Library
Temple University Institute on Disabilities
1755 N 13th Street
Student Center, Room 411S
Philadelphia, PA 19122-6024   215-204-1356
                                       800-204-PIAT
                                  Fax: 215-204-6336
                                  TTY: 215-204-1805
                                       iod@temple.edu
                        www.disabilities.temple.edu/atlend
Celia Feinstein, Co-Executive Director of the Institute on Disabilities
Amy Goldman, Co-Executive Director of the Institute on Disabilities
Ann Marie, Deputy Director
Newsletter from the Assistive Technology Lending Library in Pennsylvania. It is produced quarterly, is free of charge, and is available online only.
4-8 pages Quarterly

5373   Office of Juvenile Justice and Delinquency Prevention
810 Seventh St NW
Washington, DC 20531-3718   202-307-5911
                                       800-851-3420
                                  Fax: 301-519-5600
                                       www.ojjdp.gov
Kathi Grasso, Director, Concentration of Federal Efforts Program
Robert Listenbee, Jr., Administrator
Melodee Hanes, Principal Deputy Administrator
The Office of Juvenile Justice and Delinquency Prevention (OJJDP) provides national leadership, coordination, and resources to prevent and respond to juvenile delinquency and victimization. OJJDP supports states and communities in their efforts to develop and implement effective and coordinated prevention and intervention programs and to improve the juvenile justice system so that it protects public safety, holds offenders accountable, and provides treatment and rehabilitative services tailored

5374   Osteogenesis Imperfecta Foundation
804 W. Diamond Ave.
Suite 210
Gaithersburg, MD 20878- 1414   301-947-0083
                                       800-981-2663
                                  Fax: 301-947-0456
                                       bonelink@oif.org
                                       www.oif.org
Mary Beth Huber, Director of Program Services
Tom Costanzo, Director of Finance & Administration
Erika r Ruebensaal Carte, Director of Communications & Development
Strives to improve the quality of life for indivduals with this brittle bone disorder through research, education, awareness, and mutual support.

5375   Quantum Technologies
25242 Arctic Ocean Drive
Lake Forest, CA 92630-6217   949-930-3400
                                  Fax: 949-399-4600
                                       www.qtww.com
Dale Rasmussen, Chairman
Alan Niedzwieck, President/Director
W. Brian Olson, Chief Executive Officer
Provides access to information and tools for independence to serve the visually impaired and those with a learning disability.

5376   Regional Resource Centers Program
1 Quality Street
Suite 721
Lexington, KY 40507   859-257-4921
                                  Fax: 859-257-4353
                                  TTY: 859-257-2903
                                       mike.abell@uky.edu
                                       www.rrcprogram.org
Shauna Crane, RRCP Coordinator
Perry Williams, OSEP, Team Member
Mike Abell, Team Member
The Regional Resource Centers Program provides service to all states as well as the Pacific jurisdictions, the Virgin Islands, and Puerto Rico. The six regional program centers are funded by the federal Office of Special Education Programs (OSEP) to assist state education agencies in the systemic improvement of education programs, practices, and policies that affect children and youth with disabilities.

5377   Research!America
1101 King Street
Suite 520
Alexandria, VA 22314-2960   703-739-2577
                                       800-366-2873
                                  Fax: 703-739-2372
                                  info@researchamerica.org
                                       www.researchamerica.org
Hon. John Edward Porter, Chair
Hon. Michael Castle, Vice Chair
Mary Woolley, President/CEO
Builds active public support for more government and private-industry research to find treatments and cures for both physical and mental disorders.

5378   Social Security Online
5 Park Centre Court
Suite 100
Owings Mills, MD 21117-1   800-772-1213
                                        TTY: 800-325-0778
                                            www.ssa.gov
Carolyn W. Colvin, Commissioner
James A. Kissko, Chief of Staff
Katherine A. Thornton, Deputy Chief of Staff
Official website of the Social Security Administration.

5379   Special Clothes for Children
PO Box 333
E. Harwich, MA 02645-333   508-430-2410
                                       Fax: 508-430-2410
                                       TTY: 508-430-2410
                                         lou@lnrmusic.com
A catalog of adaptive clothing for children with disabilities -
helping boys and girls with special needs meet the world with
pride and confidence since 1987.

5380   The Arc of the United States
1825 K St NW
Suite 1200
Washington, DC 20006   202-534-3700
                                            800-433-5255
                                       Fax: 202-534-3731
                                          info@thearc.org
                                            www.thearc.org
Peter Berns, Chief Executive Officer
Ruben Rodriguez, Chief Operating Officer
Julie Ward, Senior Executive Officer, Public Policy
The Arc promotes and protects the rights of people with intellectual and developmental disabilities and actively supports their inclusion and participation in the community throughout their
lifetimes. The Arc's clients include people with autism, Down
syndrome, Fragile X syndrome, and various other developmental
disabilities. Some services offered by The Arc include public policy advocacy, education and vocational services.

5381   V Foundation for Cancer Research
106 Towerview Court
Cary, NC 27513-3595   919-380-9505
                                            800-454-6698
                                         info@jimmyv.org
                                            www.jimmyv.org
Sherrie Mazur, Director of Marketing & Communication
Danielle Smith, Director of Corporate and Market Development
*Mark Steudel, Associate Director of Development for Prospect
Research*
Named after basketball coach and broadcaster, Jim Valvano. The
V Foundation funds critical stage research conducted by young
researchers at NCI approved cancer research facilities.

5382   ValueOptions
240 Corporate Blvd.
Norfolk, VA 23502-4900   757-459-5100
                                       Fax: 501-707-0940
                                       TTY: 877-334-0077
                                         www.valueoptions.com
Heyward R. Donigan, President/CEO
Scott Tabakin, Chief Financial Officer
*Kyle A. Raffaniello, Executive Vice President and Chief Strategy
Officer*
Serves over 22 million people in behavioral healthcare through
publicaly funded, federal, and commercial contracts.

5383   Wardrobe Wagon: The Special Needs Clothing Store
258B Route 46 E
Fairfield, NJ 7004-2324   973-244-2414
                                            800-992-2737
                                       wardrobew@aol.com
                                         www.wardrobewagon.com
E Oppenberg, President
Bonnie Oppenberg
Jerome Oppenberg, Owner
Wearing apparel for individuals with special clothing needs.

5384   We Magazine
130 William St
New York, NY 10038   646-769-2722
                                       Fax: 212-375-6266
                                       TTY: 212-375-6235
                                         sales@wemedia.com
Lifestyle magazine for people with disabilities.

5385   We Media
1801 Reston Parkway
Suite 300
Reston, VA 20190-4303   703-880-2659
                                         help@wemedia.com
                                            www.wemedia.com
Andrew Nachison, Founder
Dale Peskin, Founder
Online network for people with disabilities.

5386   WebABLE
                             www.hisoftware.com/press/webable.html
Provides disability-related internet resources.

5387   WheelchairNet
6425 Penn Ave
Suite 401 BAKSQ, Department of Reha
Philadelphia, PA 15206   412-624-6279
                                          ruffing@pitt.edu
                                            www.wheelchairnet.org
Joseph Ruffing, Communications Specialist
A virtual community of people who care about wheelchairs.

5388   World Association of Persons with Disabilities
2441 N Sterling Ave
302W
Oklahoma, OK 73127-2009   405-672-4440
                                            www.wapd.org
Byron R. Kerford, Founder/Leader
Thomas J. Mecke, Executive Director
Sierra Hebron, Director of Human Resources
Dedicated to improving the quality of life for those with disabili-
ties.

Toys & Games

General

5389 Age Appropriate Puzzles
7756 Winding Way
Fair Oaks, CA 95628-5735
916-961-3507
Fax: 916-961-0765

Cheryl Meyers, President
These unique puzzles teach numerous concepts: picture, name, color and shape recognition. Each of the two themes (holidays, and clothing) comes with self-adhesive stickers that name each picture in English, Hmong, Russian, Spanish and Vietnamese. A notch at each puzzle piece makes grasping and lifting the pieces easy to use., They are designed for children from 18 months and up. Special needs children, preschool through high school would also benefit. *$9.95*

5390 All-Turn-It Spinner
AbleNet, Inc.
2625 Patton Road
Roseville, MN 55113-1137
651-294-2200
800-322-0956
Fax: 651-294-2259
customerservice@ablenetinc.com
www.ablenetinc.com

Jennifer Thalhuber, President & CEO
Paul Sugden, CFO & Trustee
The All-Turn-It Spinner is a random spinner that comes with a dice overlay allowing users to participate in any commercially-available game that require dice. Activate the spinner with its built-in switch or connect an external switch. Overlays are interchangeable with AbleNet designed spinner games or users can create their own overlay. *$145.00*

5391 Anthony Brothers Manufacturing
Convert-O-Bike
9 Capper Drive
Dailey Industrial Park,
Pacific, MO 63069-5196
636-257-0533
800-346-6313
Fax: 636-257-5473
www.angelesstore.com

Tim Lynch, Director of Sales
David Curry, General Manager
Michelle Vondera, Customer Service Manager
Manufacture wheeled toys and goods for disabled children.

5392 Automatic Card Shuffler
Maxi Aids
42 Executive Blvd.
Farmingdale, NY 11735-4710
631-752-0521
800-522-6294
Fax: 631-752-0689
TTY: 631-752-0738
sales@maxiaids.com
www.maxiaids.com

Elliot Zaretsky, Founder, President & CEO
Allows for hands-free card shuffling. Holds up to two decks at a time. Designed for those with limited hand dexterity. *$ 13.95*

5393 Backgammon Set: Deluxe
Maxi Aids
42 Executive Blvd.
Farmingdale, NY 11735-4710
631-752-0521
800-522-6294
Fax: 631-752-0689
TTY: 631-752-0738
sales@maxiaids.com
www.maxiaids.com

Elliot Zaretsky, Founder, President & CEO
Backgammon game board set featuring raised white dividers and color contrast for players with low vision. *$59.95*

5394 Board Games: Peg Solitaire
Maxi Aids
42 Executive Blvd.
Farmingdale, NY 11735-4710
631-752-0521
800-522-6294
Fax: 631-752-0689
TTY: 631-752-0738
sales@maxiaids.com
www.maxiaids.com

Elliot Zaretsky, Founder, President & CEO
This version of the solo board game uses wood marbles and a wood game board with 33 indentations. *$12.95*

5395 Board Games: Snakes and Ladders
Maxi Aids
42 Executive Blvd.
Farmingdale, NY 11735-4710
631-752-0521
800-522-6294
Fax: 631-752-0689
TTY: 631-752-0738
sales@maxiaids.com
www.maxiaids.com

Elliot Zaretsky, Founder, President & CEO
A board game for two to four players. Comes with a raised board and wood die braille spinner. *$72.59*

5396 Braille Playing Cards
Maxi Aids
42 Executive Blvd.
Farmingdale, NY 11735-4710
631-752-0521
800-522-6294
Fax: 631-752-0689
TTY: 631-752-0738
sales@maxiaids.com
www.maxiaids.com

Elliot Zaretsky, Founder, President & CEO
Playing cards that offer regular print and braille on plastic cards for the blind or visually impaired player.

5397 Braille: Bingo Cards, Boards and Call Numbers
Maxi Aids
42 Executive Blvd.
Farmingdale, NY 11735-4710
631-752-0521
800-522-6294
Fax: 631-752-0689
TTY: 631-752-0738
sales@maxiaids.com
www.maxiaids.com

Elliot Zaretsky, Founder, President & CEO
Bingo products for the visually impaired. Cards, boards and call numbers in regular print and braille.

5398 Braille: Rook Cards
Maxi Aids
42 Executive Blvd.
Farmingdale, NY 11735-4710
631-752-0521
800-522-6294
Fax: 631-752-0689
TTY: 631-752-0738
sales@maxiaids.com
www.maxiaids.com

Elliot Zaretsky, Founder, President & CEO
This set of cards for Rook, the popular bidding card game with 23 variations, has regular size print and braille print for the blind/visually impaired player. *$18.95*

5399 Cards: Musical
ASB
919 Walnut Street
Philadelphia, PA 19107-5237
215-627-0600
Fax: 215-922-0692
asbinfo@asb.org
www.asb.org

Karla S. McCaney, President & CEO
Beth Deering, Chief Program Officer
Sylvia Purnell, Director of Learning & Development
These cards, for all occasions, play music when they are opened for the visually impaired and blind persons.. *$2.50*

5400 **Cards: UNO**
Maxi Aids
42 Executive Blvd.
Farmingdale, NY 11735-4710
631-752-0521
800-522-6294
Fax: 631-752-0689
TTY: 631-752-0738
sales@maxiaids.com
www.maxiaids.com

Elliot Zaretsky, Founder, President & CEO
Traditional card game in braille for blind or visually impaired players. *$14.50*

5401 **Chess Set: Deluxe**
Maxi Aids
42 Executive Blvd.
Farmingdale, NY 11735-4710
631-752-0521
800-522-6294
Fax: 631-752-0689
TTY: 631-752-0738
sales@maxiaids.com
www.maxiaids.com

Elliot Zaretsky, Founder, President & CEO
Wooden board contains holes for inserting pieces. Black pieces contain a metal tip to distinguish them from white pieces. *$46.95*

5402 **Dice: Jumbo Size**
ASB
919 Walnut Street
Philadelphia, PA 19107-5237
215-627-0600
Fax: 215-922-0692
asbinfo@asb.org
www.asb.org

Karla S. McCaney, President & CEO
Beth Deering, Chief Program Officer
Sylvia Purnell, Director of Learning & Development
The large white and black dice are over-sized and have grooved dots to indicate the numbers, for easy reading for the visually handicapped. *$4.95*

5403 **Dominoes with Raised Dots**
Maxi Aids
42 Executive Blvd.
Farmingdale, NY 11735-4710
631-752-0521
800-522-6294
Fax: 631-752-0689
TTY: 631-752-0738
sales@maxiaids.com
www.maxiaids.com

Elliot Zaretsky, Founder, President & CEO
Standard set with tactile pieces for easier identification. *$14.95*

5404 **Dual Switch Latch and Timer**
AbleNet, Inc.
2625 Patton Road
Roseville, MN 55113-1137
651-294-2200
800-322-0956
Fax: 651-294-2259
customerservice@ablenetinc.com
www.ablenetinc.com

Jennifer Thalhuber, President & CEO
Paul Sugden, CFO & Trustee
Dual Switch Latch and Timer allows a user to activate a battery-operated toy or appliance in the latch, timed seconds and timed minutes modes of control. Choose for one user and one device at a time. *$235.00*

5405 **Early Learning 1**
MarbleSoft
12301 Central Ave NE
Suite 205
Blaine, MN 55434-4902
763-755-1402
888-755-1402
Fax: 763-862-2920
sales@marblesoft.com
www.marblesoft.com

Vicki Larson, Manager
Early learning 2.1 includes four activities that teach prereading skills. Single and dual-switch scanning are built in and special prompts allow blind students to use all levels of difficulty. Includes Matching Colors, Learning Shapes, Counting Numbers and Letter Match. Runs on Windows 98 or later and MAC OS 9 or OSX (classic not required). *$70.00*

5406 **Enabling Devices**
50 Broadway
Hawthorne, NY 10532
914-747-3070
800-832-8697
Fax: 914-747-3480
sales@enablingdevices.com
www.enablingdevices.com

Seth Kanor, President & CEO
Enabling Devices is a company dedicated to developing affordable learning and assistive devices to help people of all ages with disabling conditions. Founded by Steven E. Kanor, Ph.D. and orginally known as Toys for Special Children, the company has been creating innovative communicators, adapted toys and switches for the physically challenged for more than 35 years.

5407 **Four in a Row Game: Tactile**
Maxi Aids
42 Executive Blvd.
Farmingdale, NY 11735-4710
631-752-0521
800-522-6294
Fax: 631-752-0689
TTY: 631-752-0738
sales@maxiaids.com
www.maxiaids.com

Elliot Zaretsky, Founder, President & CEO
Comes with game console, 23 red disks, and 23 yellow disks. Red disks are drilled for tactile identification. *$22.95*

5408 **Hands-Free Controller**
Nintendo
PO Box 957
Redmond, WA 98073-957
800-255-3700
www.nintendo.com

Yoshio Tsuboike, Editor-in-Chief
Nintendo controller for the physically disabled.

5409 **National Lekotek Center**
2001 N. Clybourn Av.
1st Floor
Chicago, IL 60614-3716
773-528-5766
800-366-PLAY
Fax: 773-537-2992
TTY: 773-973-2180
www.lekotek.org

Elaine D. Cottey, Chair
Joanna Horsnail, Chair
Eric Gastevich, Treasurer
Maximizes the development of children with special needs through play. Supports families through nationwide family play centers, toy lending libraries and computer play programs. Publishes six-page newsletter three times per year.

5410 **New Language of Toys: Teaching Communication Skills to Children with Special Needs**
Spina Bifida Association of America
4590 MacArthur Blvd,NW,
Suite 250
Washington, DC 20007- 4226
202-944-3285
800-621-314
Fax: 202-944-3295
sbaa@sbaa.org
www.spinabifidaassociation.org

Lisa Raman, Director-National Resource Center
Mary Nethercutt, National Walk Director
Christopher Vance, Director of Development
A guide for parents and teachers and a reader-friendly resource guide that provides a wealth of information on how play activities affect a child's language development and where to get the toys and materials to use in these activities. *$19.00*

5411 Playing Card Holders
Maxi Aids
42 Executive Blvd.
Farmingdale, NY 11735-4710
631-752-0521
800-522-6294
Fax: 631-752-0689
TTY: 631-752-0738
sales@maxiaids.com
www.maxiaids.com

Elliot Zaretsky, Founder, President & CEO
A playing card holder for those with arthritis, dexterity issues or visual impairments. Holds up to 15 cards. *$8.95*

5412 Puzzle Games: Cooking, Eating, Community and Grooming
PCI
PO Box 34270
San Antonio, TX 78265-4270
210-670-3866
800-594-4263
Fax: 218-210-3771

Janie Haugen, Program Director
Jeff McLane, President/CEO
Rebecca Phillips, Executive Director
Each game has 63 pieces which are 2 inches in size. The completed full color puzzle is 19 inch x 15 inch. Step 1 - Work the puzzle. Step 2 - Match picture or word cards to the correct space on the puzzle. These puzzles teach basic life skills. *$19.95*

5413 Single Switch Games
MarbleSoft
12301 Central Ave NE
Suite 205
Blaine, MN 55434-4902
763-755-1402
888-755-1402
888-755-1402
Fax: 763-862-2920
sales@marblesoft.com
www.marblesoft.com

Vicki Larson, Manager
Mark Larson
Theres alot of educational software for single switch users, but how about something that's just fun? We've taken some games similar to the ones you enjoyed as a kid and made them work just right for single switch users. Includes Single Switch Maze, A Frog's Life, Switching Lanes, Switch Invaders, Slingshot Gallery and Scurry. Runs on Windows 98 or later and MAC OS9 or OSX (classic not required) *$60.00*

5414 Socialization Games for Persons with Disabilities
Charles C. Thomas
2600 S First St
Springfield, IL 62704-4730
217-789-8980
800-258-8980
Fax: 217-789-9130
books@ccthomas.com
www.ccthomas.com

Michael P. Thomas, President
Nevalyn Nevil, Author
Marna Beatty, Author
This text will assist those who want to teach severely multiple disabled students by providing information on: general principles of intervention and classroom organization; managing the behavior of students; physically managing students and using adaptive equipment; teaching eating skills; teaching toileting, dressing, and hygiene skills; teaching cognition, communication, and socialization skills; teaching independent living skills; and teaching infants and preschool students. *$38.95*
176 pages Paperback
ISBN 0-398067-46-5

5415 Tactile Checkers Set
Maxi Aids
42 Executive Blvd.
Farmingdale, NY 11735-4710
631-752-0521
800-522-6294
Fax: 631-752-0689
TTY: 631-752-0738
sales@maxiaids.com
www.maxiaids.com

Elliot Zaretsky, Founder, President & CEO
A wooden board with peg holes and high-contrast tactile squares. Game pieces are tactile wooden discs with pegs. *$33.92*

5416 Take a Chance
Speech Bin
1965 25th Ave
Vero Beach, FL 32960-3062
772-770-0007
800-477-3324
Fax: 772-770-0006
info@speechbin.com

Jan J Binney, Senior Editor
Card game for practice of commonly misarticulated speech sounds. *$18.75*
16 pages Book & Cards
ISBN 0-93785 -46-7

5417 Tic Tac Toe
Maxi Aids
42 Executive Blvd.
Farmingdale, NY 11735-4710
631-752-0521
800-522-6294
Fax: 631-752-0689
TTY: 631-752-0738
sales@maxiaids.com
www.maxiaids.com

Elliot Zaretsky, Founder, President & CEO
Comes with wooden board with peg holes/grooves and three-dimensional tactile game pieces. *$8.95*

Travel & Transportation

Newsletters & Books

5418   A World Awaits You
Mobility International USA
132 E Broadway
Suite 343
Eugene, OR 97401   541-343-1284
                                            Fax: 541-343-6812
                                            TTY: 541-343-1284
                                        clearinghouse@miusa.org
                                            www.miusa.org/away
Susan Sygall, Chief Executive Officer
Cindy Lewis, Director, Programs
A journal of success stories and tips of people with disabilities
participating in international exchange programs.
Annually

5419   Hostelling North America
Hostelling International
8455 Colesville Rd.
Suite 1225
Silver Spring, MD 20910   240-650-2100
                                            Fax: 240-650-2094
                                               www.hiusa.org
Charles Hokanson, Chair
Violet Apple, Vice Chair
Eric Oetjen, Vice Chair
HI-USA has hostels in major cities, in national and state parks,
near beaches, and in the mountains. Hostelling North America is
a directory of hostels in U.S. and Canada, including hostels that
are accessible.
400 pages

5420   Sports 'N Spokes Magazine
Paralyzed Veterans of America
801 18th St. NW
Washington, DC 20006-3517   800-424-8200
                                                    888-888-2201
                                            TTY: 800-795-4327
                                                 info@pva.org
                                        www.sportsnspokes.com
Tom Fjerstad, Editor
Andy Nemann, Assistant Editor
John Groth, Editorial Coordinator
Publication of the PVA, a congressionally chartered veterans ser-
vice organization. Sports 'N Spokes serves as a source for wheel-
chair sports and recreation.

**5421   United States Department of the Interior National Park
Service**
1849 C St. NW
Washington, DC 20240   202-208-6843
                                               www.nps.gov
Shawn Benge, Deputy Director, Operations
Lena McDowall, Deputy Director, Management & Administration
Susan Farinelli, Acting Chief of Staff
Offers an informational packet containing books, guides and
tours for the disabled and elderly.

5422   Wheelin Around e-Guide
Wheelers Accessible Van Rentals
6614 W Sweetwater Ave.
Glendale, AZ 85304   623-776-8830
                                                    800-456-1371
                                            Fax: 623-900-2708
                                        corporate@wheelersavr.com
                                        www.wheelersvanrentals.com
Wheelers' objective is to make the world more accessible by providing solutions to transportation challenges. The Wheelin
Around e-Guide provides information on the accessible transportation options offered by Wheelers.
1987

Associations & Programs

5423   American Airlines
                                                    800-433-7300
                                               www.aa.com
Robert Isom, Chief Executive Officer
Derek Kerr, Vice Chair & Chief Financial Officer
*Maya Leibman, Executive Vice President & Chief Information
Officer*
This airline trains employees to make sure that passengers with
disabilities enjoy convenient, safe, and comfortable travel.

5424   American Hotel and Lodging Association
1250 Eye St. NW
Suite 1100
Washington, DC 20005   202-289-3100
                                            Fax: 202-289-3199
                                        membership@ahla.com
                                               www.ahla.com
Chip Rogers, President & Chief Executive Officer
Kevin Carey, Executive Vice President & Chief Operating Officer
Brian Crawford, Executive Vice President, Government Affairs
Disseminates information, develops and conducts a series of
seminars for the hotel and motel industry at state-level associa-
tion conferences, and develops and distributes an ADA Compli-
ance handbook for use by the lodging industry.

5425   Amtrak
1 Massachusetts Ave. NW
Washington, DC 20001   215-856-7924
                                                    800-872-7245
                                            TTY: 800-523-6590
                                               www.amtrak.com
Stephen J. Gardner, President & Chief Executive Officer
Eleanor D. Acheson, Executive Vice President & General Counsel
Roger Harris, Executive Vice President, Marketing & Revenue
Amtrak provides services for passengers with disabilities and
works to make facilities more accessible. Contact Amtrak's Special Services Desk at 1-800-USA-RAIL at least 24 hours in advance to arrange for special assistance. The type of equipment
and accessibility vary from train to train and station to station.

5426   Easterseals Project Action Consulting
1101 Vermont Ave. NW
Suite 510
Washington, DC 20005   202-347-3066
                                                    844-227-3772
                                            TTY: 202-347-7385
                                        espaconsulting@easterseals.com
                                            www.projectaction.com
*Carol Wright Kenderdine, Assistant Vice President, Mobility &
Transportation*
Grozda Tisma, Procurement & Special Project Coordinator
Kristi McLaughlin, Consultant
A national technical assistance program designed to improve ac-
cess to transportation services for people with disabilities and as-
sist transit providers in implementing the Americans with
Disabilities Act.

**5427   General Motors Mobility Program for Persons with
Disabilities**
GM Mobility Program
PO Box 33170
Detroit, MI 48232   800-323-9935
                                            Fax: 866-234-3036
                                            TTY: 800-833-9935
                                               mobility@gm.com
                                               www.gmmobility.com
GM Mobility Program provides up to $1000 reimbursement to-
ward mobility adaptations for drivers or passengers and/or vehi-
cle alerting devices for drivers who are deaf or hard of hearing.
Provided on eligible new Chevrolet, Buick, Cadillac and GMC
vehicles. Complete GMC financing available. GM Mobility also
offers free resource information, including list of area adaptive
equipment installers, plus free resource video.

5428 **Marriott International**
10400 Fernwood Rd.
Bethesda, MA 20817   301-380-3000
                                  800-228-9290
                                  www.marriott.com

J.W. Marriott Jr., Executive Chairman
Anthony Capuano, Chief Executive Officer
Stephanie Linnartz, President
Marriott International operates 30 brands and 7000+ properties
across 131 countries and territories, with an emphasis on diver-
sity, inclusion, sustainability and social impact.

5429 **MedEscort International**
PO Box 8766
Allentown, PA 18105   800-255-7182
                                 service@medescort.com
                                 www.medescort.com

Craig Poliner, President
MedEscort International serves the health care community
throughout the world. They specialize in the long-distance transportation of patients by air ambulance, commercial airline, or
other forms of transportation. Other services include pre-trip
preparations, bedside to bedside service, ground transportation
service, and worldwide travel coordination.

5430 **MossRehab Travel Resources**
Moss Rehabilitation Hospital
60 Township Line Rd.
Elkins Park, PA 19027   215-663-6000
                                 800-225-5667
                                 Fax: 215-663-8891
                                 www.mossrehab.com

Thomas Smith, Chief Operating Officer
Alberto Esquenazi, Chief Medical Officer
Eileen Hartranft, Program Director
Offers information and resources for persons with special travel-
ing/accessibility needs.

5431 **Nantahala Outdoor Center**
13077 Hwy. 19 W
Bryson City, NC 28713   828-785-4851
                                 reservations@noc.com
                                 www.noc.com

Colin McBeath, President
Nantahala Outdoor Center offers whitewater rafting adventures
on six rivers in the Southeast for all skill levels, as well as kayak
and canoe adaptive instruction. NOC can tailor whitewater programs to a variety of skills and ability levels, modify gear, and
pace instruction.

5432 **Paralyzed Veterans of America**
801 18th St. NW
Washington, DC 20006-3517   800-424-8200
                                 TTY: 800-795-4327
                                 info@pva.org
                                 www.pva.org

Charles Brown, National President
Marcus Murray, National Secretary
Carl Blake, Executive Director
A national organization serving veterans and individuals with
spinal cord injury/disorder (SCI/D), as well as their family mem-
bers and caregivers.

5433 **Rehabiliation Engineering Research Center on
Accessible Public Transportation**
SUNY Buffalo, School of Architecture & Planning
3435 Main St.
Buffalo, NY 14214-3087   716-829-5899
                                 www.rercapt.org

Aaron Steinfeld, Co-Director
Jordana Maisel, Co-Director
A partnership between the Robotics Institute at Carnegie Mellon
University and the Center for Inclusive Design and Environmental Access at University at Buffalo, the RERC on Accessible Public Transportation conducts research and develops methods to
further advance accessible transportation systems and
equipment.

5434 **Shilo Inns & Resorts**
11707 NE Airport Way
Portland, OR 97220   503-641-6565
                                 800-222-2244
                                 guestservices@shiloinns.com
                                 www.shiloinns.com

Mark S. Hemstreet, Founder & Owner
Shilo Inns offers special assist rooms at many locations throughout the Western United States. These rooms include larger sized
bathrooms equipped with assistance railings and wheelchair access. Special assist dogs are welcome at most Shilo Inns.

5435 **Travelers Aid International**
110 Maryland Ave. NE
Suite 508
Washington, DC 20002   202-546-1127
                                 www.travelersaid.org

Kathleen Baldwin, President & Chief Executive Officer
Edward Powers, Membership Director
Ellen Horton, Communications Director
Provides crisis intervention and casework services, limited fi-
nancial assistance, protective travel assistance and information
and referrals for travelers, transients, and newcomers.

5436 **US Servas**
PO Box 3419
Berkeley, CA 94703-0419   800-509-1450
                                 info@usservas.org
                                 www.usservas.org

Marguerite Hills, Chair
Joanne Ferguson Cavanaugh, Secretary
Steve Kanters, Treasurer
International network that links travelers with hosts in 120+
countries with the hope of building world peace through under-
standing and friendship.

5437 **Wheelers Accessible Van Rentals**
6614 W Sweetwater Ave.
Glendale, AZ 85304   623-776-8830
                                 800-456-1371
                                 Fax: 623-900-2708
                                 corporate@wheelersavr.com
                                 www.wheelersvanrentals.com

Rental wheelchairs and scooter accessible vans. Technically advanced engineering features bring a world of independence to the
user. Locations throughout the U.S.
1987

5438 **Wilderness Inquiry**
1611 County Rd. B West
Suite 315
St. Paul, MN 55113   612-676-9400
                                 Fax: 612-676-9401
                                 info@wildernessinquiry.org
                                 www.wildernessinquiry.org

Kim Keprios, Executive Director
Julie K. Edmiston, Associate Executive Director
Jeff Hanson, Operations Manager
Allows people of all ages and abilities to share the adventure of
wilderness travel.
1978

Tours

5439 **Able Trek Tours**
510 K St.
PO Box 384
Reedsburg, WI 53959   608-524-3021
                                 800-205-6713
                                 Fax: 608-524-8302
                                 staff@abletrektours.com
                                 abletrektours.com

Don Douglas, Owner & President
Able Trek Tours offers vacation programs and charter bus services for individuals with special needs.

5440 Access Pass
National Park Service
1849 C St. NW
Washington, DC 20240   202-208-6843
                                      www.nps.gov

Shawn Benge, Deputy Director, Operations
Lena McDowall, Deputy Director, Management & Administration
Susan Farinelli, Acting Chief of Staff
A free passport to federally operated parks, monuments, historic sites, recreation areas, and wildlife refuges for persons who are permanently disabled.

5441 Accessible Journeys
35 W Sellers Ave.
Ridley Park, PA 19078   610-521-0339
                                      800-846-4537
                                      Fax: 610-521-6959
Howard McCoy, President & Chief Executive Officer
Accessible Journeys is a vacation planner and tour operator for wheelchair travelers and people with disabilities.

5442 Anglo California Travel Service
10620 Creston Dr.
Los Altos, CA 94024   408-257-2257
                                      800-339-4484
                                      Fax: 408-257-2664
                                      anglocalifornia@yahoo.com
                                      www.anglocalifornia.com
Audrey Cooper, Contact
Tony Cooper, Contact
Provides plans for one and two week accessible tours.
1968

5443 Courier Travel
532 Duane St.
Glen Ellyn, IL 60137   630-469-0511
                                      info@couriertravelinc.com
                                      www.couriertravelinc.com
Fred Mueller, Owner
Offers specialized assistance for independent travel or tours for persons with disabilities. Vacations include cruises and travel in the USA and abroad.

5444 Cunard Line
24303 Town Center Dr.
Suite 200
Valencia, CA 91355   800-728-6273
                                      www.cunard.com
Simon Palethorpe, President
The Cunard Line is a British cruise line providing luxury cruise vacations and ocean travel experiences. The fleet consists of Queen Elizabeth, the Queen Mary 2, and the Queen Victoria. The Cunard Line accommodates guests with disabilities and reduced mobility.

5445 Dialysis at Sea Cruises
5230 Land O' Lakes Blvd.
PO Box 1158
Land O' Lakes, FL 34639-9998   813-775-4040
                                      800-544-7604
                                      Fax: 727-372-7490
                                      info@dialysisatsea.com
                                      www.dialysisatsea.com
Steve Debroux, Owner
Provides travel opportunities for persons on hemodialysis and CAPD. Handles all aspects of their travel and medical requirements. Not sold through travel agents. Makes all reservations and coordinates the total set-up and operation of an onboard ship mobile dialysis clinic. Cruises run from seven days to three weeks and have departures from cities around the world on a variety of cruise lines.
1977

5446 Dvorak Raft Kayak & Fishing Expeditions
17921 US Hwy. 285
Nathrop, CO 81236   719-539-6851
                                      800-824-3795
                                      info@dvorakexpeditions.com
                                      www.dvorakexpeditions.com
Bill Dvorak, Co-Owner
Jaci Dvorak, Co-Owner

Dvorak offers a wide range of whitewater rafting trips on the Arkansas, Colorado, Dolores, Gunnison, Green, North Platte, Rio Grande, and San Miguel rivers ranging from half-day to multi-day excursions. Provides river trips for people who are deaf, visually impaired, and physically or mentally disabled. Colorado's first Licensed Outfitter.
1969

5447 Easy Access Travel
1716 Morning Glory
Carrollton, TX 75007   951-202-2208
                                      debra@easyaccesstravel.com
                                      www.easyaccesstravel.com
Debra Kerper, Owner
Specializes in accessible cruise vacations and land tours for individuals with disabilities.

5448 Environmental Traveling Companions
Fort Mason Center
2 Marina Blvd.
Suite C385
San Francisco, CA 94123   415-474-7662
                                      Fax: 415-474-3919
                                      info@etctrips.org
                                      www.etctrips.org
Diane Poslosky, Executive Director
Magen Kuzma, Administrative Director
Jenny Jedeikin, Communications Manager
Provides accessible outdoor experiences for people with disabilities and under-resourced youth.

5449 Guide Service of Washington
1400 Eye St. NW
Washington, DC 20005-2259   202-628-2842
                                      Fax: 202-638-2812
                                      sales@dctourguides.com
                                      www.dctourguides.com
A guide service offering tours of Washington DC and vicinity.
1964

5450 New Directions For People With Disabilities
5276 Hollister Ave.
Suite 207
Santa Barbara, CA 93111   805-967-2841
                                      888-967-2841
                                      Fax: 805-964-7344
                                      hello@newdirectionstravel.org
                                      www.newdirectionstravel.org
Dee Duncan, Executive Director
A nonprofit organization providing local, national, and international travel vacations and holiday programs for people with mild to moderate developmental disabilities.
1985

5451 Norwegian Cruise Line
7665 Corporate Center Dr.
Miami, FL 33126   866-234-7350
                                      www.ncl.com
Harry Sommer, President & Chief Executive Officer
Christine Da Silva, Senior Vice President, Branding & Communications
Todd Hamilton, Senior Vice President, Sales
Accommodates guests with disabilities and special needs, but advance notice is required. Cruise fares vary.

5452 ROW Adventures
PO Box 579
Coeur d'Alene, ID 83816   208-765-0841
                                      800-451-6034
                                      Fax: 208-667-6506
                                      info@rowadventures.com
                                      www.rowadventures.com
Peter Grubb, Co-Founder
Betsy Bowen, Co-Founder
Jonah Grubb, Operations Manager
Offers one to six day rafting trips to physically disadvantaged people. Designs custom itineraries, or trips with a special focus for small groups. For those with special dietary needs, they prepare special meals. They also offer canoe trips along the trail of Lewis and Clark on Montana's upper Missouri River.
1979

5453 Sundial Special Vacations
750 Marine Dr.
Suite 100
Astoria, OR 97103   503-325-4484
                                 800-547-9198
                            Fax: 503-325-4536
                      info@sundial-travel.com
                          www.sundialtour.com

Bruce Conner, Owner
Provides special vacations for developmentally disabled persons. Tour ratio is 1 to 4 depending on capabilities.
1968

5454 The Guided Tour, Inc.
7900 Old York Rd.
Suite 111-B
Elkins Park, PA 19027   215-782-1370
                            Fax: 215-635-2637
                      director@guidedtour.com
                          www.guidedtour.com

Ari Segal, Director
Jon Fash, Administrator
Lynsey Trohoske, Administrator
The Guided Tour is a program that offers supervised vacations for adults with developmental disabilities.
1965

5455 Trips Inc.
PO Box 10885
Eugene, OR 97440   541-686-1013
                            trips@tripsinc.com
                          www.tripsinc.com

Jim Peterson, Founder & President
Leslie Peterson, Executive Director
Rhonda Reed, Accounting & Travel Manager
Trips Inc. Special Adventures provides travel outings to adults with intellectual and developmental disabilities.

5456 Ventures Travel
3600 Holly Lane N
Suite 95
Plymouth, MN 55447   952-852-0107

Jayleen Pfitzer, Manager
Seeks to enhance independence and self-esteem and provide necessary support to facilitate safe and memorable travel experiences for people with developmental disabilities.

5457 Wilderness Inquiry
1611 County Rd. B West
Suite 315
St. Paul, MN 55113   612-676-9400
                            Fax: 612-676-9401
                      info@wildernessinquiry.org
                          www.wildernessinquiry.org

Kim Keprios, Executive Director
Julie K. Edmiston, Associate Executive Director
Jeff Hanson, Operations Manager
Allows people of all ages and abilities to share the adventure of wilderness travel.

Vehicle Rentals

5458 Accessible Vans of America

                                 866-224-1750
                          www.accessiblevans.com
David Adams, Executive Director
Accessible Vans of America (AVA) is dedicated to providing wheelchair accessible vehicles to people with disabilities.

5459 Avis Rent A Car System, LLC
6 Sylvan Way
Parsippany, NJ 07054   973-496-3500
                                 800-352-7900
                            TTY: 800-331-2323
                                 www.avis.com

Joe Ferraro, President & Chief Executive Officer
Brian Choi, Chief Financial Officer
Izzy Martins, Executive Vice President, Americas
Avis Access is a program of Avis Rent A Car that provides a full range of complementary products and services to drivers and passengers with physical disabilities. Products or services include transfer boards, hand controls, swivel seats, and more.

5460 National Car Rental System
600 Corporate Park Dr.
St. Louis, MO 63105   844-393-9989
                                 888-273-5262
                          www.nationalcar.com

Chrissy Taylor, President & Chief Executive Officer
Andrew C. Taylor, Executive Chairman
Accommodates special requests subject to availability. Offers hand controls, bench seats, extra mirrors and vans with lifts at many major locations.
1947

5461 Northwest Limousine Service
Yonkers, NY 10710   914-294-0777
                      northwestlimony@gmail.com
                          northwestlimoinc.com
Offers wheelchair accessible transportation.

5462 The Creative Mobility Group, LLC
32217 Stephenson Hwy.
Madison Heights, MI 48071   248-577-5430
                                 888-940-8337
                            Fax: 248-577-5450
                      info@creativemobilitygroup.com
                          www.creativemobilitygroup.com

Christina Duggan, Contact
Provides wheelchair accessible van rentals, as well as mobility scooter rentals, stairlift rentals, ramp rentals, and wheelchair rentals. Locations in Madison Heights, Michigan; Wayne, Michigan; and Byron Center, Michigan.
Founded in 2009. 1909

5463 Wheelchair Getaways
PO Box 1098
Mukilteo, WA 98275   425-353-8213
                                 866-224-1750
                                 888-433-6970
                            Fax: 425-355-6159
                          www.wheelchairgetaways.com

Wheelchair Getaways is a wheelchair/scooter accessible van rental company with over 30 franchise locations serving major cities and airports throughout the continental US and Hawaii. Rentals by the day, week, month or longer. Delivery/pickup available. Now owned by Accessible Vans of America.
1988

5464 Wheelers Accessible Van Rentals
6614 W Sweetwater Ave.
Glendale, AZ 85304   623-776-8830
                                 800-456-1371
                            Fax: 623-900-2708
                      corporate@wheelersavr.com
                          www.wheelersvanrentals.com

Wheelers provides accessible rental services through many locations across the United States.
1987

Veteran Services

National Administrations

5465 Department of Medicine and Surgery Veterans Administration
810 Vermont Ave NW
Washington, DC 20420
202-273-8504
800-827-1000
www.va.gov

David J. Shulkin, Secretary
Vivieca Wright, Chief of Staff
Provides hospital and outpatient treatment as well as nursing home care for eligible veterans in Veterans Administration facilities. Services elsewhere provided on a contract basis in the United States and its territories. Provides non-vocational inpatient residential rehabilitation services to eligible legally blinded veterans of the armed forces of the United States.

5466 Department of Veterans Affairs Regional Office - Vocational Rehab Division
810 Vermont Ave NW
Washington, DC 20420
202-273-8504
800-827-1000
www.va.gov

David J. Shulkin, Secretary
Vivieca Wright, Chief of Staff
Vocational rehabilitation is a program of services administered by the Department of Veterans Affairs for service members and veterans with service-connected physical or mental disabilities. If persons are compensibly disabled and are found in need of rehabilitation services because they have an employment handicap, this program can prepare them for a suitable job; get and keep that job; assist persons to become fully productive and independent.

5467 Department of Veterans Benefits
810 Vermont Ave NW
Washington, DC 20420
202-461-6913
800-827-1000
www.va.gov

David J. Shulkin, Secretary
Vivieca Wright, Chief of Staff
Furnishes compensation and pensions for disability and death to veterans and their dependents. Provides vocational rehabilitation services, including counseling, training, assistance and more towards employment, to blinded veterans disabled as a result of service in the armed forces during World War II, Korea and the Vietnam era; also provides rehabilitation services to certain peace-time veterans.

5468 Disabled American Veterans Headquarters
3725 Alexandria Pike
Cold Spring, KY 41076
877-426-2838
feedback@davmail.org
www.dav.org

David W Riley, Chairman
Barry Jesinoski, Executive Director
James Killen, Associate National Communications Director
Serves America's disabled veterans and their families. Direct services include legislative advocacy; professional counseling about compensation, pension, educational and job training programs and VA health care; and assistance in applying for those entitlements.

5469 Federal Benefits for Veterans and Dependents
810 Vermont Ave NW
Washington, DC 20420
202-273-6763
800-827-1000
www.benefits.va.gov

David J. Shulkin, Secretary
Viveca Wright, Chief of Staff
Offers information on benefits for veterans and their families.
93 pages
ISBN 0-16048 -58-

5470 US Department of Veterans Affairs National Headquarters
810 Vermont Ave NW
Washington, DC 20420
202-273-5400
800-827-1000
www.va.gov

David J. Shulkin, Secretary
Vivieca Wright, Chief of Staff
A federal agency that provides healthcare services to military veterans at VA medical centers and outpatient clinics located throughout the country; several non-healthcare benefits including disability compensation, vocational rehabilitation, education assistance, home loans, and life insurance; and provides burial and memorial benefits to veterans and family members at 135 national cemeteries.
80 pages

5471 Veteran's Voices Writing Project
406 W 34th St
Suite 103
Kansas City, MO 64111-3043
816-701-6844
veteransvoices@sbcglobal.net
www.veteransvoices.com

Deann Mitchell, President
Sheryl Liddle, Vice President
Marianne Watson, Treasurer
Individuals and organizations united to encourage veterans to write for pleasure and rehabilitation. The organization also maintains speakers' bureau and audio tape versions for the blind. Also offered are numerous monetary awards, articles, book reviews, cartoons and drawings, light verse, poetry and short stories.
$15.00
64 pages Magazine
ISSN 0504-07 9

Alabama

5472 Alabama VA Benefits Regional Office - Montgomery
U.S. Department of Veteran Affairs
345 Perry Hill Rd
Montgomery, AL 36109
800-827-1000
Fax: 334-213-3565
montgomery.query@vba.va.gov
www.va.gov

Cory A. Hawthorne, Director
Erica P. Worthington, Assistant Director
Jamie Bozeman, Vocational Rehabilitation & Employment Officer
The Veterans Benefits Administration (VBA) provides a variety of benefits and services to Servicemembers, Veterans, and their families.

5473 Alabama VA Medical Center - Birmingham
Veterans Health Administration U.S. Dept. of VA
700 S. 19th St
Birmingham, AL 35233
205-933-8101
www.birmingham.va.gov

Thomas Smith, Director
Veterans medical clinic offering disabled veterans medical treatments.

5474 Central Alabama Veterans Healthcare System
Veterans Health Administration, U.S. Dept. of VA
215 Perry Hill Rd
Montgomery, AL 36109-3798
334-272-4670
800-214-8387
www.centralalabama.va.gov

Paul Bockelman, Interim Director
Thomas Huettemann, Associate Director for Resources
Linda Townsend-Green, Acting Associate Director, Operations
CAVHCS exists to provide excellent services to veterans across the continuum of healthcare. We take pride in providing delivery of timely quality care by staff who demonstrate outstanding customer service, the advancement of health care through research, and the education of tomorrow's health care providers.

5475   Tuscaloosa VA Medical Center
Veterans Health Administration, U S Dept. of V A
3701 Loop Rd E
Tuscaloosa, AL 35404-5015   205-554-2000
                                              888-269-3045
                                         Fax: 205-554-2845
                                         www.tuscaloosa.va.gov

John F. Merkle, Medical Center Director
David L. Carden, Associate Director, Nursing & Patient Care Services
Carlos Berry, Chief of Staff
To serve America's Heroes by improving their health and well-being through Veteran and Family Centered Care.

Alaska

5476   Alaska VA Healthcare System - Anchorage
1201 North Muldoon Road
Ste 115
Anchorage, AK 99504-5914   907-257-4700
                                              888-353-7574
                                         Fax: 907-561-7183
                                         www.alaska.va.gov

Linda L. Boyle, Interim Director
Shawn Bransky, Associate Director
Veterans medical clinic offering disabled veterans medical treatments.

5477   DAV Department of Alaska
2925 Debarr Rd
Room 3101
Anchorage, AK 99508-2983   907-257-4803
                                         Fax: 907-258-9828
                                         www.davmembersportal.org

Pamela F. Beale, Alaska Commander
Robert W. Bingham, Membership Chairman

5478   Veteran Benefits Administration - Anchorage Regional Office
U.S. Department of Veteran Affairs
1201 Muldoon Rd
Anchorage, AK 99504   907-257-4803
                                              800-827-1000
                                         anchorage.query@vba.va.gov
                                         www.benefits.va.gov/anchorage

Robert A. McDonald, Secretary of Veterans
Robert D. Snyder, Chief of Staff
The Anchorage Regional Office is remotely managed by the Salt Lake City Regional Office. The VBA operation includes a one-stop Veterans Service Center made up of the merged Adjudication and Veterans Service Divisions. There is also a one person Loan Guaranty Division and a Vocational Rehabilitation and Employment Division.

Arizona

5479   Carl T Hayden VA Medical Center
Veterans Health Administration, U S Dept. of V A
650 E Indian School Rd
Phoenix, AZ 85012-1839   602-277-5551
                                              800-554-7174
                                         Fax: 602-222-6472
                                         g.vhacss@forum.va.gov
                                         www.phoenix.va.gov

D Gregg Gordon, President
Marva Greene, Vice President
John Fears, CEO

5480   Northern Arizona VA Health Care System
Veterans Health Administration, US Dept. of VA
500 Hwy 89N
Prescott, AZ 86313-5001   928-445-4860
                                              800-949-1005
                                         Fax: 928-768-6076
                                         g.vhacss@forum.va.gov
                                         www.prescott.va.gov

Deborah Thompson, Manager

5481   Southern Arizona VA Healthcare System
Veterans Health Administration, U S Dept. of V A
3601 S 6th Ave
Tucson, AZ 85723   520-792-1450
                                              800-470-8262
                                         Fax: 520-629-1818
                                         g.vhacss@forum.va.gov
                                         www.tucson.va.gov

Jonathan H. Gardner, MPA, FACHE, Director
Jennifer S Gutowski, MHA, FACHE, Associate Director
Katie A. Landwehr, MBA, Assistant Director
The Southern Arizona VA Health Care System (SAVAHCS) located in Tucson AZ serves over 170,000 Veterans located in eight counties in Southern Arizona and one county in Western New Mexico.

Arkansas

5482   Eugene J Towbin Healthcare Center
Veterans Health Administration, U S Dept. of V A
2200 Fort Roots Dr
North Little Rock, AR 72114-1706   501-257-1000
                                              800-827-1000
                                         Fax: 501-257-1779
                                         g.vhacss@forum.va.gov
                                         www.littlerock.va.gov

Michael R. Winn, Director
Toby T. Mathew, MHA/MBA, Deputy Director
Cyril O. Ekeh, MHA, Associate Director
CAVHS is reaching out to veterans through its community-based outpatient clinics in Mountain Home, El Dorado, Hot Springs, Mena, Pine Bluff, Searcy, Conway, Russellville, its Home Health Care Service Center in Hot Springs, and a VA Drop-In Day Treatment Center for homeless veterans in downtown Little Rock.

5483   Fayetteville VA Medical Center
Veterans Health Administration, US Dept. of VA
1100 N College Ave
Fayetteville, AR 72703-1944   479-443-4301
                                              800-691-8387
                                         g.vhacss@forum.va.gov
                                         www.fayettevillear.va.gov

W. Todd Grams, Chief Financial Officer
Glenn D. Haggstrom, Principal Executive Director
Stephen W. Warren, Principal Deputy Assistant Secretary
Honor America's Veterans by providing exceptional health care that improves their health and well-being.

5484   John L McClellan Memorial Hospital
Veterans Health Administration, US Dept. of VA
4300 W 7th St
Little Rock, AR 72205-5446   501-257-1000
                                              800-827-1000
                                         g.vhacss@forum.va.gov
                                         www.littlerock.va.gov

Michael R. Winn, Director
Toby T. Mathew, MHA/MBA, Deputy Director
Cyril O. Ekeh, MHA, Associate Director
CAVHS is reaching out to veterans through its community-based outpatient clinics in Mountain Home, El Dorado, Hot Springs, Mena, Pine Bluff, Searcy, Conway, Russellville, its Home Health Care Service Center in Hot Springs, and a VA Drop-In Day Treatment Center for homeless veterans in downtown Little Rock. Throughout its rich 90 year history, CAVHS has been widely recognized for excellence in education, research, and emergency preparedness, and -first and foremost -for a tradition of quality an

5485 **North Little Rock Regional Office**
Veterans Benefits Administration, U S Dept. of V A
2200 Fort Roots Drive
Building 65
N Little Rock, AR 72114-1756   501-370-3820
                                       800-827-1000
                                 Fax: 501-370-3829
                         littlerock.query@vba.va.gov
                                          www.va.gov

Eric K. Shinseki, Secretary
Stephen W. Warren, Principal Deputy Assistant Secretary
W. Todd Grams, Chief Financial Officer
The Little Rock VA Regional Office offers services to veterans in
the State of Arkansas and the city of Texarkana in Bowie County,
Texas. Based on 2004 information provided by the Office of Policy, Planning, and Preparedness, the veteran population of Arkansas is 268,000 and the city of Texarkana, Texas, has a veteran
population of 3,545. With a staff of approximately 124 employees, the Regional Office determines entitlement to disability
compensation and pension, survivors' benefits, vocational

California

5486 **Jerry L Pettis Memorial VA Medical Center**
Veterans Health Administration, U S Dept. of V A
11201 Benton St
Loma Linda, CA 92357-1000   909-825-7084
                                       800-741-8387
                           g.vhacss@forum.va.gov
                            www.lomalinda.va.gov
Barbara Fallen, RD, MPA, FACHE, Acting Director
Prachi V. Asher, FACHE, Assistant Director
Dwight C. Evans, M.D., Chief of Staff
Since 1977, VA Loma Linda Healthcare System has been improv-
ing the health of the men and women who have so proudly served
our nation. We consider it our privilege to serve your health care
needs in any way we can.

5487 **Long Beach VA Medical Center**
Veterans Health Administration, U S Dept. of V A
5901 E 7th St
Long Beach, CA 90822-5201   562-826-8000
                                       800-827-1000
                                       888-769-8387
                           g.vhacss@forum.va.gov
                             www.longbeach.va.gov
Isabel Duff, Medical Center Director
John M. Tryboski, MSN, Associate Director
Anthony DeFrancesco, FACHE, Associate Director

5488 **Los Angeles Regional Office**
Veterans Benefits Administration, U S Dept. of V A
11000 Wilshire Blvd
Los Angeles, CA 90024-3602   800-827-1000
                          losangeles.query@vba.va.gov
                                          www.va.gov
Eric K. Shinseki, Secretary
Stephen W. Warren, Principal Deputy Assistant Secretary
W. Todd Grams, Chief Financial Officer
The Los Angeles Regional Office (RO) provides benefits and ser-
vices to approximately 706,000 veterans residing in the Southern
California counties of Los Angeles, San Bernardino, Riverside,
Ventura, Santa Barbara, San Luis Obispo, and Kern. VA benefits
expenditures for veterans residing within the jurisdiction of the
RO exceed $800 million annually. All Loan Guaranty activities
for the six counties are under jurisdiction of the Phoenix Regional
Office.

5489 **Martinez Outpatient Clinic**
Veterans Health Administration, U S Dept. of V A
150 Muir Rd
Martinez, CA 94553-4668   925-372-2000
                                       800-382-8387
                           g.vhacss@forum.va.gov
                                          www.va.gov
John H Simms, Director
Brian E. Schuman, Chief of Police

The Martinez Outpatient Clinic offers a full range of medical,
surgical, mental health, and diagnostic outpatient services, including nuclear medicine, ultrasound, CT and MRI. The Center
for Rehabilitation and Extended Care is located adjacent to the
outpatient clinic.

5490 **Oakland VA Regional Office**
Veterans Benefits Administration U S Dept. of V A
1301 Clay Street
12th Floor
Oakland, CA 94612-5217   800-827-1000
                            oakland.query@vba.va.gov
                          www.benefits.va.gov/oakland
Geri Spearman, Director
The jurisdiction includes all Northern California, except for
Modoc, Lassen, Alpine and Mono counties, which are assigned to
the Reno Regional Office. All Loan Guaranty activities are under
the jurisdiction of the Phoenix Regional Office. Seven service organizations are collocated on the eleventh floor of the Federal Office building occupied by the regional office.

5491 **Rehabilitation Research and Development Center**
Department of Veteran s Affairs
810 Vermont Avenue, NW
Washington, DC 94304-1207   202-443-0575
                                 Fax: 202-495-6153
                             tiffany.asqueri@va.gov
Patricia A. Dorn, Ph.D., Acting Director, Rehab R&D Service
Ricardo Gonzalez, Administrative Officer
Gloria Winford, Staff Assistant
The VA Center of Excellence on Mobility in Palo Alto, CA is dedicated to developing innovative clinical treatments and assistive
devices for veterans with physical disabilities to increase their independence and improve their quality of life. The clinical emphasis of the center is to improve mobility, either ambulation or
manipulation, in individuals with neurologic impairments or orthopaedic impairments. We do not publish any printed books,
journals or periodicals.

5492 **Sacramento Medical Center**
Veterans Health Administration U S Department of V
10535 Hospital Way
Mather, CA 95655-4200   916-843-7000
                                       800-382-8387
                           g.vhacss@forum.va.gov
                       www.northerncalifornia.va.gov
David G. Mastalski, Interim Director
Donna Iatarola, RN, MSN, Associate Director
William T. Cahill, MD, Chief of Staff
It is an integrated health care delivery system, offering a comprehensive array of medical, surgical, rehabilitative, mental health
and extended care to veterans in Northern California. The health
system is comprised of a medical center in Sacramento; a rehabilitation and extended care facility in Martinez, and seven
outpatient clinics.

5493 **San Diego VA Regional Office**
Veterans Benefits Administration, U S Dept. of V A
8810 Rio San Diego Dr
San Diego, CA 92108-1698   858-552-8585
                                       800-827-1000
                                 Fax: 858-552-7436
                            oakland.query@vba.va.gov
                         www.benefits.va.gov/sandiego
Janet M Peyton, Administrative Officer
The San Diego VA Regional Office provides benefit services for
over 600,000 Veterans and their dependents in the Southern California Counties of Imperial, Orange, Riverside and San Diego.
Since the Regional Office shares occupancy of the building with
a VA Outpatient Clinic and the Employment Development Department of the State of California, it truly offers a one stop
Service Center.

5494 VA Central California Health Care System
Veterans Health Administration, U S Dept. of V A
2615 E Clinton Ave
Fresno, CA 93703-2223
559-225-6100
888-826-2838
Fax: 559-268-6911
g.vhacss@forum.va.gov
www.fresno.va.gov

Joanne Krumberger, Director
Susan Shyshka, Associate Director
Patricia Richardson Ed.D, RN, N, Nursing Executive
VA Central California Health Care System (VACCHCS) has been improving the health of the men and women who have so proudly served our nation. We consider it our privilege to serve your health care needs in any way we can.

5495 VA Greater Los Angeles Healthcare System
Veterans Health Administration U S Deptartment of
11301 Wilshire Blvd
Los Angeles, CA 90073-1003
310-478-3711
800-827-1000
Fax: 310-268-4848
g.vhacss@forum.va.gov
www.losangeles.va.gov

Donna M. Beiter, RN, MSN, Director
Christopher Sandles, Assistant Director
Marlene Brewster, RN, MSN, Acting Associate Director, Nursing and Patient Care Services
The VA Greater Los Angeles Healthcare System is the largest, most complex healthcare system within the Department of Veterans Affairs.GLA consists of three ambulatory care centers, a tertiary care facility and 10 community based outpatient clinics. GLA serves veterans residing throughout five counties: Los Angeles, Ventura, Kern, Santa Barbara, and San Luis Obispo. There are 1.4 million veterans in the GLA service area. GLA is affiliated with both UCLA School of Medicine and USC School of Medici

5496 VA Northern California Healthcare System
Veterans Health Administration, U S Dept. of V A
150 Muir Rd
Martinez, CA 94553-4668
925-372-2000
800-382-8387
g.vhacss@forum.va.gov
www.northerncalifornia.va.gov

David G. Mastalski, Interim Director
Donna Iatarola, RN, MSN, Associate Director
William T. Cahill, MD, Chief of Staff
VA Northern California Health Care System (VANCHCS) is an integrated health care delivery system, offering a comprehensive array of medical, surgical, rehabilitative, mental health and extended care to veterans in Northern California. The health system is comprised of a medical center in Sacramento; a rehabilitation and extended care facility in Martinez, and seven outpatient clinics.

5497 VA San Diego Healthcare System
Veterans Health Administration, U S Dept. of V A
3350 La Jolla Village Dr
San Diego, CA 92161
858-552-8585
800-331-8387
g.vhacss@forum.va.gov
www.sandiego.va.gov

Jeffrey T. Gering, FACHE, Director
Cynthia Abair, MHA, Associate Director
Robert M. Smith, MD, Chief of Staff/Medical Director
We provide medical, surgical, mental health, geriatric, spinal cord injury, and advanced rehabilitation services. VASDHS has 296 authorized beds, including skilled nursing beds and operates several regional referral programs including cardiovascular surgery and spinal cord injury. The facility also supports three Vet Centers at the following locations: Chula Vista, San Diego, and San Marcos.

Colorado

5498 Boulder Vet Center
4999 Pearl East Circle
Suite 106
Boulder, CO 80301
303-440-7306
877-927-8387
Fax: 303-449-3907
www.va.gov

Gail N Bennett, Office Manager
Michael J Pantaleo, Team Leader
Annette Matlock, Counselor
Offers trauma and readjustment from military and civilian life counseling and assistance with disability claims, military benefits and employment are provided.

5499 Colorado/Wyoming VA Medical Center
Veterans Benefits Administration U S Dept. of V A
155 Van Gordon St
Suite 395
Lakewood, CO 80225
303-914-2680
800-827-1000
denver.query@vba.va.gov
www.denver.va.gov

Forest Farley Jr, Medical Center Director
Thomas E Bowen, Chief of Staff

5500 Denver VA Medical Center
Veterans Health Administration, U S Dept. of V A
1055 Clermont St
Suite 6A138
Denver, CO 80220-3808
303-393-2869
888-336-8262
www.denver.va.gov

Lynnette Roth, Executive Director
Peggy Kearns MS, RD, FACHE, Associate Director
Judith Burke RN, MS, NEA-BC, Associate Director, Patient Care Services
Construction of our 1.1m sq foot, $800m replacement facility is well under way! Concrete is being poured, steel is being put in, and we're working hard to open in 2015.

5501 Grand Junction VA Medical Center
Veterans Health Administration
2121 North Ave
Grand Junction, CO 81501-6428
970-242-0731
866-206-6415
Fax: 970-244-1300
g.vhacss@forum.va.gov
www.grandjunction.va.gov

Patricia A. Hitt, MS, Acting Director
Michael Murphy, Manager
Randal France, M.D., Chief Psychiatry Service/ Int. Chf. of Staff
The VAMC operates 53 beds comprised of 23 acute care and 30 Transitional Care Unit beds. The VAMC provides primary and secondary care including acute medical, surgical, and psychiatric inpatient services, as well as a full range of outpatient services.

Connecticut

5502 Hartford Regional Office
Veterans Benefits Administration
555 Willard Ave
Building 2E
Newington, CT 6111-2631
860-666-6951
800-827-1000
hartford.query@vba.va.gov

Jeanette A Chirico Post, Network Director
The Hartford Regional Office now provides one-stop service to veterans and their families seeking assistance in compensation, pension, and vocational rehabilitation and employment in an accessible campus environment.

5503   **Hartford Vet Center**
25 Elm St
Suite A
Rocky Hill, CT 06067-2305   860-563-8800
                                             877-927-8387
                                        Fax: 860-563-8805
                                             www.va.gov

Donna Hryb LCSW, Team Leader
Pedro Ortiz, Counselor
Amy Otzel, Counselor
A U.S. Department of Veterans Affairs counseling center offering counseling to Vietnam era and combat veterans. Sexual trauma/harassment counseling, medical screening and benefit referral is available to all veterans.

5504   **VA Connecticut Healthcare System: Newington Division**
Veterans Health Administration U S Department. of
555 Willard Ave
Newington, CT 6111-2631   860-666-6951
                                             800-827-1000
                                        Fax: 860-667-6764
                                     g.vhacss@forum.va.gov
                                     www.connecticut.va.gov

Janice M. Boss, MS, Director
Margaret Veazey, RN, MSN, Associate Director for Patient Care Services
John Callahan, Associate Director
The mission of VA Connecticut Healthcare Systems is to fulfill a nation's commitment to its veterans by providing quality healthcare, promoting health through prevention and maintaining excellence in teaching and research. Provides primary, secondary and tertiary care in medicine, geriatrics, neurology, psychiatry and surgery with an operating capacity of 211 hospital beds.

5505   **VA Connecticut Healthcare System: West Haven**
Veterans Health Administration, U S Dept. of V A
950 Campbell Ave
West Haven, CT 06516-2770   203-932-5711
                                             800-827-1000
                                        Fax: 203-937-3868
                                     g.vhacss@forum.va.gov
                                     www.connecticut.va.gov

Janice M. Boss, MS, Director
Margaret Veazey, RN, MSN, Associate Director for Patient Care Services
John Callahan, Associate Director
The mission of VA Connecticut Healthcare Systems is to fulfill a nation's commitment to its veterans by providing quality healthcare, promoting health through prevention and maintaining excellence in teaching and research. Provides primary, secondary and tertiary care in medicine, geriatrics, neurology, psychiatry and surgery with an operating capacity of 211 hospital beds.

Delaware

5506   **Delaware VA Regional Office**
Veterans Benefits Administration U S Dept. of V A
1601 Kirkwood Hwy
Wilmington, DE 19805-4917   302-994-2511
                                             800-461-8262
                                        Fax: 302-633-5516
                                  wilmington.query@vba.va.gov
                                     www.wilmington.va.gov

Daniel D. Hendee, FACHE, MHA, Director
Mary Alice Johnson, MS, RN, Associate Director for Patient Care Services
William E. England, Associate Director for Finance and Operations
We offer comprehensive services ranging from preventive screenings to long-term care. Wilmington VAMC proudly serves Veterans in multiple locations for convenient access to the services we provide.

5507   **Wilmington VA Medical Center**
Veterans Health Administration, US Dept. of VA
1601 Kirkwood Hwy
Wilmington, DE 19805-4917   302-994-2511
                                             800-461-8262
                                        Fax: 302-633-5516
                                     g.vhacss@forum.va.gov
                                     www.wilmington.va.gov

Daniel D. Hendee, FACHE, MHA, Director
Mary Alice Johnson, MS, RN, Associate Director for Patient Care Services
William E. England, Associate Director for Finance and Operations
We offer comprehensive services ranging from preventive screenings to long-term care. Wilmington VAMC proudly serves Veterans in multiple locations for convenient access to the services we provide.

5508   **Wilmington Vet Center**
2710 Centerville Road
Suite 103
Wilmington, DE 19808- 4917   302-994-1660
                                             877-927-8387
                                        Fax: 302-994-8361
                                             www.va.gov

Joan Spencer, Team Leader
Patricia Elwood, Office Manager
Valerie Feeley, Counselor
Veterans counseling program offering individual counseling services, advocacy services and group counseling. The focus is the counseling of all veterans coping with the aftermath of war, sexual abuse/harassment in the military and all veterans of the Vietnam era. The center also has an active outreach program to seek veterans needing services. Hours of operation are between 8:00 AM - 4:30 PM, Monday - Friday and other times by appointment only. Services are free.

District of Columbia

5509   **Disabled American Veterans**
Legislative HQ
807 Maine Ave SW
Washington, DC 20024   202-554-3501
                                        Fax: 202-554-3581
                                     feedback@davmail.org
                                             www.dav.org

David W Riley, Chairman
Delphine Metcalf-Foster, National Commander
J. Marc Burgess, National Adjutant
Serves America's disabled veterans and their families. Direct services include legislative advocacy; professional counseling about compensation, pension, educational and job training programs and VA health care; and assistance in applying for those entitlements.

5510   **PVA Adaptive Sports**
Paralyzed Veterans of America
801 18th St. NW
Washington, DC 20006-3517   800-424-8200
                                        TTY: 800-795-4327
                                             info@pva.org
                                  www.pva.org/adaptive-sports

Charles Brown, National President
Marcus Murray, National Secretary
Carl Blake, Executive Director
Sports include air guns, bass fishing, billiards, boccia, bowling, golf, handcycling, quad rugby, and trapshooting.

5511   **VA Medical Center, Washington DC**
50 Irving St NW
Washington, DC 20422-1   202-745-8000
                                             800-827-1000
                                             877-328-2621
                                     g.vhacss@forum.va.gov
                                     www.washingtondc.va.gov

Brian A. Hawkins, MHA, Medical Center Director
Bryan C. Matthews, MBA, Associate Medical Center Director
Natalie Merckens, Assistant Medical Center Director

Acute general and specialized services in medicine, surgery, neurology, and psychiatry.

5512 Washington DC VA Medical Center
Veterans Health Administration, U S Dept. of V A
50 Irving St NW
Washington, DC 20422-1
202-745-8000
800-827-1000
877-328-2621
Fax: 202-754-8530
g.vhacss@forum.va.gov
www.washingtondc.va.gov
Brian A. Hawkins, MHA, Medical Center Director
Bryan C. Matthews, MBA, Associate Medical Center Director
Natalie Merckens, Assistant Medical Center Director
Acute general and specialized services in medicine, surgery, neurology, and psychiatry.

Florida

5513 Bay Pines VA Medical Center
Veterans Health Administration, U S Dept. of V A
10000 Bay Pines Blvd
PO Box 5005
Bay Pines, FL 33744
727-398-6661
800-827-1000
888-820-0230
g.vhacss@forum.va.gov
www.baypines.va.gov
Suzanne M. Klinker, Medical Center Director
Kristine Brown, MPH, Associate Director
Teresa Kumar, RN, MSN, CPHQ,, Associate Director for Patient / Nursing Services
Since 1933, Bay Pines VA Healthcare System has been improving the health of the men and women who have so proudly served our nation. We consider it our privilege to serve your health care needs in any way we can. Our services are available to Veterans living in a ten county catchment area in west central Florida.

5514 Gainesville Division, North Florida/South Georgia Veterans Healthcare System
Veterans Health Administration, U S Dept. of V A
1601 SW Archer Rd
Gainesville, FL 32608-1611
352-376-1611
800-324-8387
Fax: 352-379-7445
g.vhacss@forum.va.gov
www.northflorida.va.gov/northflorida
Thomas Wisnieski, MPA, FACHE, Director
Nancy Reissener, Deputy Director
Maureen Wilkes, Associate Director
In addition to our medical centers in Gainesville and Lake City, we offer services in three satellite outpatient clinics and several community-based outpatient clinics across North Florida and South Georgia.

5515 James A Haley VA Medical Center
Veterans Health Administration, U S Dept. of V A
13000 Bruce B Downs Blvd
Suite T72
Tampa, FL 33612-4745
813-972-2000
800-827-1000
888-811-0107
g.vhacss@forum.va.gov
www.tampa.va.gov
Kathleen R. Fogarty, Director
Roy L. Hawkins Jr., Deputy Director
David J. VanMeter, Associate Director
Comprehensive health care is provided through primary care, tertiary care, and long-term care in areas of medicine, surgery, psychiatry, physical medicine and rehabilitation, spinal cord injury, neurology, oncology, dentistry, geriatrics, and extended care.

5516 Miami VA Medical Center
Veterans Health Administration, U S Dept. of V A
1201 NW 16th St
Suite B822
Miami, FL 33125-1693
305-575-7000
800-827-1000
888-276-1785
Fax: 305-575-3266
g.vhacss@forum.va.gov
www.miami.va.gov
Paul M. Russo, Director
Mark E. Morgan, Associate Director
Marcia Lysaght, Associate Director, Patient Care Services
The Miami VA is an accredited comprehensive medical provider, providing general medical, surgical, inpatient and outpatient mental health services, the Miami VA Healthcare System includes an AIDS/HIV center, a prosthetic treatment center, spinal cord injury rehabilitative center, and Geriatric Research, Education, and Clinical Center (GRECC).

5517 St. Petersburg Regional Office
Veterans Benefits Administration, U S Dept. of V A
9500 Bay Pines Blvd
St Petersburg, FL 33708
727-319-7492
800-827-1000
stpete.query@vba.va.gov
www.va.gov
Warren McPherson, Executive Director

5518 West Palm Beach VA Medical Center
Veterans Health Administration, U S Dept. of V A
7305 N Military Trl
West Palm Beach, FL 33410-7417
561-422-8262
800-972-8262
Fax: 561-882-6707
g.vhacss@forum.va.gov
www.westpalmbeach.va.gov
Charleen R. Szabo, FACHE, Medical Center Director
Cristy McKillop, FACHE, MHA, Medical Center Associate Director
Gloria A. Bays, MSN, ARNP, NE-BC, Associate Director for Patient Care Services
The medical center is a general medical, psychiatric and surgical facility. It is a teaching hospital, providing a full range of patient care services, with state-of-the-art technology as well as education and limited research. Comprehensive healthcare is provided through primary care and long-term care in the areas of dentistry, extended care, medicine, neurology, oncology, pharmacy, physical medicine, psychiatry, rehabilitation and surgery. The West Palm Beach VA Medical Center operates a Blin

Georgia

5519 Atlanta Regional Office
Veterans Benefits Administration, U S Dept. of V A
1700 Clairmont Road
Decatur, GA 30033-1210
404-463-3100
800-827-1000
Fax: 404-929-5819
atlanta.query@vba.va.gov
www.va.gov
Chick Krautler, Executive Director
The Atlanta VA Regional Office is responsible for delivering non-medical VA benefits and services to Georgia Veterans and their dependent family members. This is accomplished through the administration of comprehensive and diverse benefit programs established by Congress. Our goal is to deliver these benefits and services in a timely, accurate, and compassionate manner.

5520 Atlanta VA Medical Center
Veterans Health Administration, U S Dept. of V A
1670 Clairmont Rd
Decatur, GA 30033-4004
404-321-6111
800-827-1000
Fax: 404-728-7734
g.vhacss@forum.va.gov
www.atlanta.va.gov
Leslie B. Wiggins, Director
Tom Grace, MBA/MHA, Associate Director
Sheila Meuse, PhD, Assistant Director

The Atlanta VA Medical Center (VAMC), located on 26 acres in Decatur, is one of eight medical centers in the VA Southeast Network. It is a teaching hospital, providing a full range of patient care services complete with state-of-the-art technology, education, and research.

5521 Augusta VA Medical Center
Veterans Health Administration, U S Dept. of V A
950 15th Street Downtown/1 Freedom
Augusta, GA 30904-6258
706-733-0188
800-827-1000
Fax: 706-731-7227
g.vhacss@forum.va.gov
Robert U. Hamilton, MHA, FACHE, Medical Center Director
Richard Rose, Associate Director
Michelle Cox-Henley, MS, RN, Associate Director for Nursing/Patient Services
The Charlie Norwood VA Medical Center is a two-division Medical Center that provides tertiary care in medicine, surgery, neurology, psychiatry, rehabilitation medicine, and spinal cord injury. The Downtown Division is authorized 155 beds (58 medicine, 37 surgery, and 60 spinal cord injury). The Uptown Division, located approximately three miles away, is authorized 315 beds (68 psychiatry, 15 blind rehabilitation and 40 medical rehabilitation. In addition, a 132-bed Restorative/Nursing Home C

5522 Carl Vinson VA Medical Center
Veterans Health Administration, U S Dept. of V A
1826 Veterans Blvd
Dublin, GA 31021-3699
478-272-1210
Fax: 478-277-2717
www.dublin.va.gov
John S. Goldman, Director
Gerald M. DeWorth, Associate Director
Sue Preston, RN, Associate Director for Patient and Nursing Services
Since 1948, Carl Vinson VA Medical Center has been improving the health of the men and women who have so proudly served our nation. We consider it our privilege to serve your health care needs in any way we can. Services are available to veterans living in the Middle Georgia area.

5523 Southeastern Paralyzed Veterans of America
4010 Deans Bridge Rd.
Hephzibah, GA 30815
706-796-6301
800-292-9335
Fax: 706-796-0363
paravet@comcast.net
www.southeasternpva.org
Carl Morgan, President
Kurt Glass, Vice President
Lonnie Burnett, Treasurer
Works to maximize the quality of life for its members and all people with SCI/D as a leading advocate for healthcare, SCI/D research and education, veteran's benefits, and rights, accessibility and the removal of architectural barriers, sports programs, and disability rights.
1946

Hawaii

5524 Hilo Vet Center
70 Lanihuli St
Suite 102
Hilo, HI 96720-2067
808-969-3833
877-927-8387
Fax: 808-969-2025
www.va.gov
Felipe Sales, Team Leader
Samuelito Labasan, Office Manager
Peter Ehlich, Counselor
Veterans medical clinic offering disabled veterans medical treatments, readjustment and PTSD counseling to combat veterans

5525 Honolulu VBA Regional Office
Veterans Benefits Administration, U S Dept. of V A
459 Patterson Road, E-Wing
Honolulu, HI 96819-1522
808-566-1412
800-827-1000
Fax: 808-433-0478
honolulu.query@vba.va.gov
www.vba.va.gov/ro/honolulu
Claude M Kicklighter, Chief of Staff
Alan Furuno, Manager
Alvin Kalawe, Elderly Program Coordinator
The Honolulu Regional Office is responsible for administering VA's benefit programs under the leadership and direction of the Under Secretary for Benefits for the Veterans Benefits Administration. Formerly part of the Honolulu VA Medical & Regional Office Center (VAMROC), the Honolulu Regional Office (RO) was renamed as a stand alone RO on June 2, 2003. The office is co-located with the Spark M. Matsunaga Pacific Islands Health Care System medical center, on the grounds of the Tripler Army Medic

5526 Pacific Islands Health Care System
Veterans Health Administration, US Dept. of VA
459 Patterson Rd
Honolulu, HI 96819-1522
808-433-0600
800-214-1306
Fax: 808-433-0390
g.vhacss@forum.va.gov
www.hawaii.va.gov
William F. Dubbs, M.D., Acting Director
Brandon K. Yamamoto, Acting Associate Director
Jane Wellman, APRN, Associate Director of Patient Care Services
The VA Pacific Islands Health Care System (VAPIHCS) Honolulu provides a broad range of medical care services, serving an estimated 127,600 veterans throughout Hawaii and the Pacific Islands. The VAPIHCS provides outpatient medical and mental health care through a main Ambulatory Care Clinic on Oahu (Honolulu) and through five Community Based Outpatient Clinics (CBOCs) on the neighboring islands including: Hawaii (Hilo and Kona), Maui, Kauai, and Guam. Traveling clinicians also provide episodi

Idaho

5527 Boise Regional Office
Veterans Benefits Administration, U S Dept. of V A
444 W. Fort Street
Boise, ID 83702-4531
800-827-1000
boise.query@vba.va.gov
www.va.gov
Jim Vance, Director
Pat Teague, Service Officer
Tom Ressler, Manager
The Boise Regional Office administers monetary benefits to 17,283 veterans in Idaho, Utah, and Oregon. The Regional Office issued monthly disability and death benefit payments of over $15 million in January 2007. VBA's annual compensation and pension benefits for veterans residing within the RO's jurisdiction now exceed $185 million

5528 Boise VA Medical Center
Veterans Health Administration, U S Dept. of V A
500 W Fort St
Boise, ID 83702-4531
208-422-1000
800-827-1000
Fax: 208-422-1326
g.vhacss@forum.va.gov
www.boise.va.gov
Jennifer T Shalz, Chief of Staff
We truly hope to improve your health and well-being and will make your visit or stay as pleasant as possible. We are committed to veterans and the nation and strive to continually enhance the care we provide. We also train future healthcare professionals, conduct research and support our nation in times of emergency. In all of these activities, our employees will respect and support your rights as a patient.

Illinois

5529 Edward Hines Jr Hospital
Veterans Health Administration, U S Dept. of V A
5000 South 5th Avenue
Hines, IL 60141
708-202-8387
800-827-1000
Fax: 708-202-2684
g.vhacss@forum.va.gov
www.hines.va.gov

Joan Ricard, FACHE, Hospital Director
Dr. Daniel Zomchek, Associate Director
Carol A. Gouty, RN, MSN, PhD, Associate Director of Patient Care
Specialized clinical programs include Blind Rehabilitation, Spinal Cord Injury, Neurosurgery, Radiation Therapy and Cardiovascular Surgery. The hospital also serves as the VISN 12 southern tier hub for pathology, radiology, radiation therapy, human resource management and fiscal services. Hines VAH currently operates 471 beds and six community based outpatient clinics in Elgin, Kankakee, Oak Lawn, Aurora, LaSalle, and Joliet.

5530 Marion VA Medical Center
Veterans Health Administration U S Department of V
2401 W Main St
Marion, IL 62959-1188
618-997-5311
800-827-1000
www.marion.va.gov

Paul Bockelman, Medical Center Director
Frank Kehus, Associate Director
The VA Medical Center in Marion, Illinois, is a general medical and surgical facility that operates 55 acute care beds and a 60 bed Community Living Center. Ten Outpatient Clinics that provide primary care and behavioral medicine services are located in Harrisburg; Carbondale; Effingham; and Mt. Vernon, IL; Paducah; Hanson; Owensboro; and Mayfield, Kentucky; Vincennes and Evansville, IN.

5531 North Chicago VA Medical Center
Veterans Health Administration, U S Dept. of V A
3001 North Green Bay Rd
North Chicago, IL 60064-3048
847-688-1900
800-393-0865
g.vhacss@forum.va.gov
www.lovell.fhcc.va.gov

Patrick L. Sullivan, Director
Captain Jos, A. Acosta, MC, US, Commanding Officer/Deputy Director
Captain Jami Kersten, Associate Director
The arrangement incorporates facilities, services and resources from the North Chicago VA Medical Center (VAMC) and the Naval Health Clinic Great Lakes (NHCGL). A combined mission of the health care center means active duty military, their family members, military retirees and veterans are all cared for at the facility.

5532 VA Illiana Health Care System
Veterans Health Administration, U S Dept. of V A
1900 E Main St
Danville, IL 61832-5198
217-554-3000
800-320-8387
Fax: 217-554-4552
g.vhacss@forum.va.gov
www.danville.va.gov

Emma Metcalf, MSN, RN,, Director
Diana Carranza, Associate Director
Alesia Coe, MSN, RN,, Associate Director for Patient Care Services
Since 1898, our buildings, facilities, patients, and missions have changed, but remaining constant is VA Illiana Health Care System's endeavor in improving the health of the men and women who have so proudly served our nation. Being the 8th oldest VA facility, we consider it our privilege to serve your health care needs in any way we can.

Indiana

5533 Indianapolis Regional Office
Veterans Benefits Administration
575 N Pennsylvania St
Indianapolis, IN 46204-1563
317-226-7860
800-827-1000
TTY: 800-829-4833
indianapolis.query@vba.va.gov
www.benefits.va.gov/indianapolis
The Department of Veterans Affairs provides a variety of services and benefits to honorably discharged veterans of the U. S. Military and their dependents. The purpose of this Web page is to assist Indiana's veterans, their dependents and survivors, in contacting the nearest VA facility to inquire about their veterans benefits or health care services. The State of Indiana maintains a Web page for veterans that explains many of the programs that are available to them.

5534 Richard L Roudebush VA Medical Center
Veterans Health Administration, U S Dept. of V A
1481 W 10th St
Indianapolis, IN 46202-2803
317-554-0000
800-827-1000
Fax: 317-554-0127
g.vhacss@forum.va.gov
www.indianapolis.va.gov

Thomas Mattice, Director
Jeff Nechanicky, Associate Director
Kimberly Radant, Associate Director for Patient Care Services
Since 1932, Richard L. Roudebush VA Medical Center has been improving the health of the men and women who have so proudly served our nation. We consider it our privilege to serve your health care needs in any way we can. Services are available to more than 196,000 veterans living in a 45-county area of Indiana and Illinois.

5535 VA North Indiana Health Care System: Fort Wayne Campus
Veterans Health Administration, U S Dept. of V A
2121 Lake Ave
Fort Wayne, IN 46805-5100
260-426-5431
800-360-8387
g.vhacss@forum.va.gov
www.northernindiana.va.gov

Denise M. Deitzen, Medical Center Director
Audrey L. Frison, MHA, RN, Associate Director
Helen Rhodes MPA, RN, Associate Director for Operations
The Fort Wayne Campus offers primary and secondary medical and surgical services. Primary care clinics are available at both medical center campuses and at Community Based Outpatient Clinics (CBOCs) located in South Bend, Goshen, Peru and Muncie Indiana. Recently completed renovations and construction, and continuous maintenance, ensure an attractive, state-of-the-art healthcare environment.

5536 VA Northern Indiana Health Care System: Marion Campus
Veterans Health Administration, U S Dept. of V A
1700 E 38th St
Marion, IN 46953-4568
765-674-3321
800-360-8387
g.vhacss@forum.va.gov
www.northernindiana.va.gov

Denise M. Deitzen, Medical Center Director
Audrey L. Frison, MHA, RN, Associate Director
Helen Rhodes MPA, RN, Associate Director for Operations
The Marion Campus offers a full range of mental health, nursing home care, and extended care services. Primary care clinics are available at both medical center campuses and at Community Based Outpatient Clinics (CBOCs) located in South Bend, Goshen, Peru and Muncie Indiana.

Iowa

5537 Des Moines VA Medical Center
Veterans Health Administration, U S Dept. of V A
3600 30th St
Des Moines, IA 50310-5753

515-699-5999
800-294-8387
Fax: 515-699-5862
g.vhacss@forum.va.gov
www.centraliowa.va.gov

Donald Cooper, Director
Susan Martin, Associate Director for Resources and Operations
Tammy Neff, RN, MBA, MSN, M, Acting Associate Director for Patient Services/Nurse Executi
The VA Central Iowa Health Care System (VACIHCS) operates a Veterans Health Administration (VHA) medical facility in Des Moines, with Community Based Outpatient Clinics (CBOCs) in Mason City, Fort Dodge, Knoxville, Marshalltown and Carroll. The medical center provides acute and specialized medical and surgical services, residential outpatient treatment programs in substance abuse and post-traumatic stress and a full range of mental health and long-term care services, as well as sub-acute and r

5538 Des Moines VA Regional Office
Veterans Benefits Administration, U S Dept. of V A
210 Walnut Street
Des Moines, IA 50309-2115

515-323-7580
800-827-1000
Fax: 515-323-7580
leander@vba.va.gov
www.va.gov

Rich Anderson, Service Director
The Des Moines VA Regional Office provides Compensation, Pension and Vocational Rehabilitation and Counseling services for all military veterans in the State of Iowa. The Des Moines VA Regional Office currently provides approximately $260 million in benefits to the approximately 270,000 veterans in Iowa.

5539 Iowa City VA Medical Center
Veterans Health Administration, U S Dept. of V A
601 Highway 6 West
Iowa City, IA 52240-2202

319-338-0581
800-637-0128
866-687-7382
Fax: 319-339-7171
g.vhacss@forum.va.gov
www.iowacity.va.gov

Barry Sharp, Director
Timothy McMurry, Associate Director for Operations
Dawn Oxley, RN, Associate Director Patient Care Services/Nurse Executive
Tertiary care facility, affiliated teaching hospital, and research center seving an aging veteran populatiaon in eastern Iowa and western Illinois. Satellite clinics are located in Bettendorf, Dubuque, and Waterloo, Iowa and in Quincy and Galesburg, Illinois.

5540 Knoxville VA Medical Center
Veterans Health Administration, U S Dept. of V A
1515 W Pleasant St
Knoxville, IA 50138-3399

641-842-3101
800-816-8878
Fax: 641-828-5124
g.vhacss@forum.va.gov
www.centraliowa.va.gov

Claudia M Kicklighter

5541 VA Central Iowa Health Care System
3600 30th St
Des Moines, IA 50310-5753

515-699-5999
800-294-8387
Fax: 515-699-5862
www.centraliowa.va.gov

Donald Cooper, Director
Susan Martin, Associate Director for Resources and Operations
Tammy Neff, RN, MBA, MSN, M, Acting Associate Director for Patient Services/Nurse Executi
The VA Central Iowa Health Care System (VACIHCS) operates a Veterans Health Administration (VHA) medical facility in Des Moines, with Community Based Outpatient Clinics (CBOCs) in

Mason City, Fort Dodge, Knoxville, Marshalltown and Carroll. The medical center provides acute and specialized medical and surgical services, residential outpatient treatment programs in substance abuse and post-traumatic stress and a full range of mental health and long-term care services, as well as sub-acute and r

Kansas

5542 Colmery-O'Neil VA Medical Center
Veterans Health Administration, U S Dept. of V A
2200 SW Gage Blvd
Topeka, KS 66622

785-350-3111
800-574-8387
g.vhacss@forum.va.gov
www.topeka.va.gov

A. Rudy Klopfer, FACHE, Director
John Moon, Associate Director
Nelson L. Dean, RN, BSN, MA, Associate Director for Patient Care Services
Since 1946, the staff of the Colmery-O'Neil VA Medical Center has been serving veterans. Today, we proudly serve our nation's veterans with excellent health care as part of the VA Eastern Kansas Health Care System (VAEKHCS). We consider it our privilege to serve your health care needs in any way we can.

5543 Dwight D Eisenhower VA Medical Center
Veterans Health Administration, U S Dept. of V A
4101 4th Street Trafficway
Leavenworth, KS 66048-5014

913-682-2000
800-952-8387
g.vhacss@forum.va.gov
www.leavenworth.va.gov

A. Rudy Klopfer, FACHE, Director
John Moon, Associate Director
Nelson L. Dean, RN, BSN, MA, Associate Director for Patient Care Services
Since 1886, the staff of the Dwight D. Eisenhower VA Medical Center has been serving veterans. Today, we proudly serve our nation's veterans with excellent health care as part of the VA Eastern Kansas Health Care System (VAEKHCS). We consider it our privilege to serve your health care needs in any way we can.

5544 Kansas VA Regional Office
Veterans Benefits Administration, U S Dept. of V A
5500 E Kellogg Dr
Wichita, KS 67218-1607

800-827-1000
wichita.query@vba.va.gov
www.benefits.va.gov/wichita

Edgar L Tucker, Medical Center Director

5545 Robert J Dole VA Medical Center
Veterans Health Administration, U S Dept. of V A
5500 E Kellogg Dr
Wichita, KS 67218-1607

316-685-2221
800-827-1000
888-827-6881
Fax: 316-651-3666
g.vhacss@forum.va.gov
www.wichita.va.gov

Kevin Inkley, MA, Director
Vicki Bondie, MBA, Associate Director
Carol A. Kaster, MA, RN, Associate Director of Patient Care/Nurse Executive
For over 70 years, the Dole VA Medical and Regional office center has been honored to serve Kansas area veterans. The center provides a full range of primary and specialty acute and extended care services to veterans in 59 counties of Kansas. Special emphasis programs include substance abuse, post traumatic stress disorder (PTSD), women's health, spinal cord injury, visual impairment, prosthetic and sensory aids, and homeless services.

Kentucky

5546 **Lexington VA Medical Center**
Veterans Health Administration, U S Dept. of V A
1101 Veterans Dr
Lexington, KY 40502-2235 859-281-4900
800-352-4000
g.vhacss@forum.va.gov
www.lexington.va.gov
Martin J. Traxler, Acting Medical Center Director
Patricia Breeden, MD, Acting Chief of Staff
Laura Faulkner, Acting Associate Medical Center Director
The Lexington Veterans Affairs Medical Center is a fully accredited, two-division, tertiary care medical center with an operating bed complement of 199 hospital beds. Acute medical, neurological, surgical and psychiatric inpatient services are provided at the Cooper Division, located adjacent to the University of Kentucky Medical Center. Other available services include: emergency care, medical-surgical units, acute psychiatry, ICU, progressive care unit, (includes Cardiac Cath Lab) ambulatory s

5547 **Louisville VA Medical Center**
Veterans Health Administration, U S Dept. of V A
800 Zorn Ave
Louisville, KY 40206-1433 502-287-4000
800-376-8387
g.vhacss@forum.va.gov
www.louisville.va.gov
Wayne L. Pfeffer, MHSA, FACHE, Medical Center Director
Douglas V Paxton, Sr, Associate Director / Operations
Pamala Thompson, RN, MSA, MSN, Associate Director for Patient Care Services
Since 1952, Robley Rex VAMC has been improving the health of the men and women who have so proudly served our nation. We consider it our privilege to serve your health care needs in any way we can. Services are available to more than 166,000 veterans living in a 35-county area of the Kentuckiana area.

5548 **Louisville VA Regional Office**
Veterans Benefits Administration, U S Dept. of V A
800 Zorn Avenue
Louisville, KY 40206-1433 502-287-4000
800-376-8387
louisville.query@vba.va.gov
www.louisville.va.gov
Wayne L. Pfeffer, MHSA, FACHE, Medical Center Director
Douglas V Paxton, Sr, Associate Director / Operations
Pamala Thompson, RN, MSA, MSN, Associate Director for Patient Care Services
Since 1952, Robley Rex VAMC has been improving the health of the men and women who have so proudly served our nation. We consider it our privilege to serve your health care needs in any way we can. Services are available to more than 166,000 veterans living in a 35-county area of the Kentuckiana area.

Louisiana

5549 **Alexandria VA Medical Center**
Department of Veterans Affairs
2495 Shreveport Highway
Pineville, LA 71360-9004 318-466-4000
800-375-8387
Fax: 318-483-5029
richard.wright2@va.gov
www.alexandria.va.gov
Martin J. Traxler, Medical Center Director
Yolanda Sanders-Jackson, Associate Director
Jose N Rivera, MD, Acting Chief of Staff
The VAMC Alexandria is categorized as a primary and secondary care facility. It is a teaching hospital, providing a full range of primary care services with state-of-the-art technology and education. Comprehensive acute and extended health care is provided on a primary and secondary basis in areas of medicine, surgery, psychiatry, physical medicine and rehabilitation, neurology, oncology, dentistry, geriatrics, and extended care. The Medical Center serves a potential veteran population of over 1

5550 **New Orleans VA Medical Center**
Veterans Health Administration, U S Dept. of V A
1601 Perdido St
New Orleans, LA 70112-1262 504-412-3700
800-935-8387
Fax: 504-589-5210
Stacie.Rivera@med.va.gov
www.neworleans.va.gov
John D Church Jr, Medical Director/President
Fernando Rivera, Association Medical Center Direc
Sam Lucero, Special Assistant to Director
A teaching hospital, providing a full range of patient care services, with state-of-the-art technology as well as education and research. Comprehensive health care is provided through primary care, tetiary care, and long-term care in areas of medicine, surgery, psychiatry, physical medicine and rehabilitation, neurology, oncology, dentistry, geriatrics, and extended care.

5551 **Shreveport VA Medical Center**
Veterans Health Administration, U S Dept. of V A
510 E Stoner Ave
Shreveport, LA 71101-4295 318-221-8411
800-827-1000
www.shreveport.va.gov
Shirley M. Bealer, Medical Center Director
Todd M. Moore, Assistant Medical Center Director
Erik J. Glover, Associate Medical Center Director

Maine

5552 **Maine VA Regional Office**
Veterans Benefits Administration, U S Dept. of V A
1 VA Center
Augusta, ME 4330-6719 207-623-8411
877-421-8263
togus.query@vba.va.gov
www.va.gov
Dale Demers, Director
Scott Karczewski, Manager

5553 **Togus VA Medical Center**
Veterans Health Administration, U S Dept. of V A
1 VA Center
Augusta, ME 04330-6795 207-623-8411
877-421-8263
Fax: 207-623-5792
g.vhacss@forum.va.gov
Scott Karczewski, Regional Office Director
Denise Benson, Veterans Sevice Center Manager
Gregg Morin, Assistant Veterans Service Center Manager

Maryland

5554 **Baltimore Regional Office**
Veterans Benefits Administration, U S Dept. of V A
31 Hopkins Plz
Baltimore, MD 21201-2825 800-827-1000
baltimore.query@vba.va.gov
www.va.gov
Jerry L Calhoun
The Baltimore Regional Office serves 484,013 veterans living in the State of Maryland, 2% of the national veteran population. The Regional Office's jurisdiction includes all counties in the State of Maryland. The Baltimore Regional Office has an assigned staffing of 218. We provide services at the VA Medical Center in Baltimore and Transition Assistance throughout the State. We actively participate in a homeless veterans outreach program based at the Maryland Center for the Veterans Educatio

5555 Baltimore VA Medical Center
Veterans Health Administration, U S Dept. of V A
10 N Greene St
Baltimore, MD 21201-1524   410-605-7000
                                  800-463-6295
                                  Fax: 410-605-7901
                                  g.vhacss@forum.va.gov
                                  www.maryland.va.gov

Dennis H. Smith, Director
Nancy Quailey-Giannopoulis, Associate Director for Operations
Frederick P. Soetje, Associate Director for Finance
The Baltimore Medical Center is nationally recognized for its outstanding patient safety and state-of-the-art technology, the VA Maryland Health Care System is proud of its reputation as a leader in veterans' health care, research and education.

5556 Fort Howard VA Medical Center
Veterans Health Administration, U S Dept. of V A
9600 N Point Rd
Fort Howard, MD 21052-3050   410-477-1800
                                    800-351-8387
                                    Fax: 410-477-7177
                                    www.mdva.state.md.us

Thomas Hutchins, Secretary

5557 Maryland Veterans Centers
10 N Greene St
Baltimore, MD 21201-1524   410-605-7000
                                  800-463-6295
                                  Fax: 410-605-7901
                                  www.maryland.va.gov

J Y Jacks, Manager
Dennis H Smith, Executive Director
Veterans medical clinic offering disabled veterans medical treatments.

5558 Perry Point VA Medical Center
Veterans Health Administration, U S Dept. of V A
Circle Drive
Perry Point, MD 21902   410-642-2411
                               800-949-1003
                               Fax: 410-642-1165
                               g.vhacss@forum.va.gov
                               www.maryland.va.gov

Dennis H. Smith, Director
Nancy Quailey-Giannopoulis, Associate Director for Operations
Frederick P. Soetje, Associate Director for Finance
It is nationally recognized for its outstanding patient safety and state-of-the-art technology, the VA Maryland Health Care System is proud of its reputation as a leader in veterans' health care, research and education.

5559 VA Maryland Health Care System
10 N Greene St
Baltimore, MD 21201-1524   410-605-7000
                                  800-463-6295
                                  Fax: 410-605-7900
                                  www.maryland.va.gov

Dennis H. Smith, Director
Nancy Quailey-Giannopoulis, Associate Director for Operations
Frederick P. Soetje, Associate Director for Finance
A dynamic and exciting health care organization that is dedicated to providing quality, compassionate and accessible care and service to Maryland's veterans. As a part of one of the largest health care systems in the United States, the VAMHCS has a reputation as a leader in veterans' health care, reserch and education. Provides comprehensive service to veterans including medical, surgical, rehabilitative, nurological and mental health care on both an inpatient and outpatient basis.

5560 Boston VA Regional Office
Veterans Benefits Administration, U S Dept. of V A
15 New Sudbury Street
JFK Bldg
Boston, MA 2203-9928   617-232-9500
                              800-827-1000
                              boston.query@vba.va.gov
                              www.boston.va.gov

Liza Catucci, Administrative Officer
Michael Lawson, President

5561 Edith Nourse Rogers Memorial Veterans Hospital
Veterans Health Administration U S Deptartment of
200 Springs Rd Bldg #23
Bedford, MA 1730-1114   781-687-2000
                               800-827-1000
                               Fax: 781-687-3536
                               g.vhacss@forum.va.gov
                               www.bedford.va.gov

Michael Mayo-Smith, Manager

5562 Northampton VA Medical Center
Veterans Health Administration, U S Dept. of V A
421 N Main St
Leeds, MA 1062   413-584-4040
                        800-827-1000
                        g.vhacss@forum.va.gov

Richard Woloss, Manager

5563 VA Boston Healthcare System: Brockton Division
Veterans Health Administration, U S Dept. of V A
940 Belmont St
Brockton, MA 02301-5596   508-583-4500
                                 800-865-3384
                                 Fax: 617-323-7700
                                 g.vhacss@forum.va.gov
                                 www.boston.va.gov

Vincent Ng, Acting Director
Susan A. MacKenzie, PhD, Associate Director
Cecilia McVey, BSN, MHA, CAN, Associate Director Nursing & Patient Care Services
VA Boston Healthcare System's consolidated facility consists of the Jamaica Plain campus, located in the heart of Boston's Longwood Medical Community; the West Roxbury campus, located on the Dedham line; and the Brockton campus, located 20 miles south of Boston in the City of Brockton.

5564 VA Boston Healthcare System: Jamaica Plain Campus
Veterans Health Administration, U S Dept. of V A
150 S Huntington Ave
Boston, MA 2130-4817   617-232-9500
                              800-865-3384
                              Fax: 617-278-4549
                              g.vhacss@forum.va.gov
                              www.boston.va.gov

Vincent Ng, Acting Director
Susan A. MacKenzie, PhD, Associate Director
Cecilia McVey, BSN, MHA, CAN, Associate Director Nursing & Patient Care Services
VA Boston Healthcare System's consolidated facility consists of the Jamaica Plain campus, located in the heart of Boston's Longwood Medical Community; the West Roxbury campus, located on the Dedham line; and the Brockton campus, located 20 miles south of Boston in the City of Brockton.

5565 VA Boston Healthcare System: West Roxbury Division
Veterans Health Administration, U S Dept. of V A
1400 VFW Pkwy
West Roxbury, MA 2132-4927   617-323-7700
                                    800-865-3384
                                    g.vhacss@forum.va.gov
                                    www.boston.va.gov

Susan A Mac Kenzie, Associate Director
VA Boston Healthcare System's consolidated facility consists of the Jamaica Plain campus, located in the heart of Boston's Longwood Medical Community; the West Roxbury campus, located on the Dedham line; and the Brockton campus, located 20 miles south of Boston in the City of Brockton.

Michigan

5566 Aleda E Lutz VA Medical Center
Veterans Health Administration, U S Dept. of V A
1500 Weiss St
Saginaw, MI 48602-5251   989-497-2500
800-827-1000
Fax: 989-791-2428
g.vhacss@forum.va.gov
www.saginaw.va.gov

Jeff Nechanicky, Acting Medical Center Director
Stephanie Young, Associate Director
Penny Holland, R.N., MSN, Associate Director for Patient Care Svcs
Since 1950, the Aleda E. Lutz VA Medical Center has been improving the health of the men and women who have so proudly served our nation. We consider it our privilege to serve your health care needs in any way we can. Services are available to more than 31,000 veterans living in the Central and Northern 35 counties of Michigan's Lower Peninsula.

5567 Battle Creek VA Medical Center
Veterans Health Administration, U S Dept. of V A
5500 Armstrong Rd
Battle Creek, MI 49037-7314   269-966-5600
888-214-1247
888-214-1247
Fax: 269-966-5483
g.vhacss@forum.va.gov
www.battlecreek.va.gov

Mary Beth Skupien, Director
Edward Dornoff, Associate Director
Kay Bower, Associate Director for Patient Care Services
Since 1924, the Battle Creek, Michigan VA Medical Center has been improving the health of the men and women who have so proudly served our nation. The Battle Creek VA Medical Center consists of 104 medical and psychiatric beds, 32 residential rehabilitation beds, and 103 nursing home care unit beds. In addition, specialized services offered include a Palliative Care Unit, a Substance Abuse Clinic, a Post Traumatic Stress Disorder Program and a Domicilliary.

5568 Iron Mountain VA Medical Center
Veterans Health Administration, U S Dept. of V A
325 East H Street
Iron Mountain, MI 49801-4760   906-774-3300
800-827-1000
Fax: 906-779-3114
g.vhacss@forum.va.gov
www.ironmountain.va.gov

James W. Rice, Medical Center Director
William Caron, FACHE, Associate Medical Center Director
Andrea Collins, RN, MSN, Associate Director for Nursing and Patient Care Service
OGJVAMC is a primary and secondary level care facility with 17 acute care beds, 13 in the medical/surgical ward and 4 in the intensive care unit (ICU). The main facility provides limited emergency and acute inpatient care, and collaborates with larger VA Medical Centers in Milwaukee and Madison, WI, to provide higher-level emergency and specialty care services. OGJVAMC also provides rehabilitation and extended care, including palliative and hospice care, in its 40-bed Community Living Center.

5569 John D Dingell VA Medical Center
Veterans Health Administration, U S Dept. of V A
4646 John R St
Detroit, MI 48201-1916   313-576-1000
800-827-1000
Fax: 313-576-1112
g.vhacss@forum.va.gov
www.detroit.va.gov

Pamela J. Reeves, M.D., Director
Annette Walker, M.S.H.A., B.S., Associate Director
Ann M. Herm, R.N., B.S.N., M., Associate Director, Patient Care Services
Our mission is to provide timely, compassionate and high quality care to those we serve by encouraging teamwork, education, research, innovation, and continuous improvement.

5570 Michigan VA Regional Office
Veterans Benefits Administration, U S Dept. of V A
477 Michigan Ave
Patrick V McNamara Federal Building
Detroit, MI 48226-1217   800-827-1000
detroit.query@vba.va.gov
www.benefits.va.gov/detroit

David Leonard, Director
Dennis W Paradowski, Assistant Director
The Regional Office Staff are dedicated to providing responsive and timely service to the veterans of Michigan and their families. Their duties include processing and making decisions on claims for disability compensation, and assisting with applications for a wide range of VA benefits.

5571 VA Ann Arbor Healthcare System
Veterans Health Administration, U S Dept. of V A
2215 Fuller Rd
Ann Arbor, MI 48105-2303   734-769-7100
800-361-8387
Fax: 734-761-7870
g.vhacss@forum.va.gov
www.annarbor.va.gov

Robert P. McDivitt, FACHE, Director
Randall E. Ritter, Associate Director
Stacey Breedveld, R.N., Associate Director Patient Care
Since 1953, the VA Ann Arbor Healthcare System (VAAAHS) has provided state-of-the-art healthcare services to the men and women who have so proudly served our nation. We consider it our privilege to serve your healthcare needs in any way we can.

5572 Vet Center Readjustment Counseling Service
1940 Eastern Ave SE
Grand Rapids, MI 49507-2771   616-285-5795
800-905-4675
Fax: 616-285-5898
www.va.gov

William Busby, Executive Director
Branden K Lyon, Counselor
Lynn Hall, Clinical Coordinator
Providing a broad range of counseling outreach and referral services to eligible veterans in order to help make readjustments to cilvilian life.

Minnesota

5573 Minneapolis VA Medical Center
Veterans Health Administration, U S Dept. of V A
1 Veterans Dr
Minneapolis, MN 55417-2399   612-725-2000
866-414-5058
Fax: 612-725-2049
g.vhacss@forum.va.gov
www.minneapolis.va.gov

Judy Johnson-Mekota, Director
Erik J. Stalhandske, Associate Director
Kent Crossley, Chief of Staff
Minneapolis VA Health Care System (VAHCS) is a teaching hospital providing a full range of patient care services with state-of-the-art technology, as well as education and research. Comprehensive health care is provided through primary care, tertiary care and long-term care in areas of medicine, surgery, psychiatry, physical medicine and rehabilitation, neurology, oncology, dentistry, geriatrics and extended care.

5574 St. Cloud VA Medical Center
Veterans Health Administration, U S Dept. of V A
4801 Veterans Dr
Saint Cloud, MN 56303-2015   320-252-1670
800-247-1739
Fax: 320-255-6472
g.vhacss@forum.va.gov
www.stcloud.va.gov

Barry I. Bahl, Director
Cheryl Thieschafer, Associate Director
Meri Hauge, BSN, MSN Nurse, Executive/Associate Director for Patient Care Services

Specialty care services include audiology, cardiology, dentistry, hematology, oncology, optometry, orthopedics, podiatry, pulmonology, urology and rheumatology. A new Ambulatory Surgery (same-day) Center opened in the fall of 2011 and will provide access to additional outpatient surgical procedures. The medical center offers extensive mental health programming, including acute psychiatric care, Residential Rehabilitation Treatment programs and an outpatient mental health clinic. The programs u

5575 St. Paul Regional Office
Veterans Benefits Administration, U S Dept. of V A
1 Federal Dr
Fort Snelling, MN 55111-4080   800-827-1000
                                                stpaul.query@vba.va.gov
                                                www.benefits.va.gov/stpaul

Vincent Crawford, Director

5576 Vet Center
405 E Superior St
Ste 160
Duluth, MN 55802-2240   218-722-8654
                                                877-927-8387
                                                Fax: 218-723-8212
                                                www.vetcenter.va.gov

Cynthia Macaulay MEd, Counselor
Rob Evanson, Counselor
Debbie Burt, Office Manager
Counseling, social services and benefits assistance for combat veterans and those sexually traumatized in the military.

Mississippi

5577 Biloxi/Gulfport VA Medical Center
Veterans Health Administration, U S Dept. of V A
400 Veterans Ave
Biloxi, MS 39531-2410   228-523-5000
                                                800-296-8872
                                                Fax: 228-563-2898
                                                g.vhacss@forum.va.gov
                                                www.biloxi.va.gov

Anthony L. Dawson, Director
Nancy Weaver, Associate Director
Kenneth Shimon, Chief of Staff

5578 Jackson Regional Office
Veterans Benefits Administration, U S Dept. of V A
1600 E Woodrow Wilson Ave
Jackson, MS 39216-5100   601-364-7000
                                                800-827-1000
                                                Fax: 601-364-7007
                                                jackson.query@vba.va.gov
                                                www.benefits.va.gov/jackson

Neil Anthony Mcphie, Chairman
Barbara Sapin, Vice Chairman

Missouri

5579 Harry S Truman Memorial Veterans' Hospital
Veterans Health Administration, U S Dept. of V A
800 Hospital Dr
Columbia, MO 65201-5275   573-814-6000
                                                800-827-1000
                                                Fax: 573-814-6551
                                                g.vhacss@forum.va.gov
                                                www.columbiamo.va.gov

Sallie Houser-Hanfelder, Director
Robert Ritter, Associate Director
Lana Zerrer, Chief of Staff

5580 John J Pershing VA Medical Center
Veterans Health Administration, U S Dept. of V A
1500 N Westwood Blvd
Poplar Bluff, MO 63901-3318   573-686-4151
                                                888-557-8262
                                                Fax: 573-778-4156
                                                g.vhacss@forum.va.gov
                                                www.poplarbluff.va.gov

Merk Hedstrom, Medical Center Director
Linda Haga, Research Contact

5581 Kansas City VA Medical Center
Veterans Health Administration, U S Dept. of V A
4801 E Linwood Blvd
Kansas City, MO 64128-2226   816-861-4700
                                                800-827-1000
                                                g.vhacss@forum.va.gov
                                                www.kansascity.va.gov

Kenneth Grasing, Research/Development
Ram Sharma, Administrative Officer
Kent Hill, Executive Director
The Kansas City VA Medical Center is a modern, well-equipped teriary care inpatient and outpatient center. As the third largest teaching hospital in the metropolitan area, it maintains educational affiliations with the University of Kansas School of Medicine.

5582 St. Louis Regional Office
Veterans Benefits Administration, U S Dept. of V A
400 S 18th St
Saint Louis, MO 63103-2265   800-827-1000
                                                stlouis.query@vba.va.gov
                                                www.stlouis.va.gov

5583 St. Louis VA Medical Center
Veterans Health Administration, U S Dept. of V A
915 N Grand Blvd
Saint Louis, MO 63106-1621   314-652-4100
                                                800-228-5459
                                                Fax: 314-289-7009
                                                g.vhacss@forum.va.gov
                                                www.stlouis.va.gov

Dolores Minor, Administrative Officer

Montana

5584 Montana VA Regional Office
3633 Veterans Drive
Fort Harrison, MT 59636-188   406-442-7310
                                                800-827-1000
                                                www.va.gov

5585 V A Montana Healthcare System
U S Dept. of V A
3687 Veterans Drive
PO Box 1500
Fort Harrison, MT 59636-1500   406-442-6410
                                                877-468-8387
                                                Fax: 406-447-7916
                                                ftharrison.query@vba.va.gov
                                                www.montana.va.gov

Christine Gregory, Director
Vicki Thennis, Interim Associate Director
Trena Bonde, Chief of Staff
This is a complete, medically reliable dictionary of congenital malformations and disorders. As the authors explain, 'Down syndrome is the only common congenital disorder, the other defects and disorders are rare or very rare, some having been reported fewer than 20 times worlwide.' This dictionary covers them all. Examples: Aagenaes syndrome, Acrocallosal syndrome, and Acrodysostosis

5586   VA Montana Healthcare System
Veterans Health Administration, U S Dept. of V A
1892 William St
Fort Harrison, MT 59636   406-447-7945
                                           800-827-1000
                                      Fax: 406-447-7965
                                    g.vhacss@forum.va.gov
                                       www.montana.va.gov

Joseph Underkofel, Executive Director
Gregory Johnson, MD

5587   Vet Center
Readjusment Counciling Service Western Mountain Re
2795 Enterprise Ave.
Suite 1
Billings, MT 59102-3238   406-657-6071
                                      Fax: 406-657-6603
                                            www.va.gov

Bob Phillips, Manager
Luanne Anderson, Office Manager
Barry Osgard MS, Counselor
Readjustment counseling service for counseling veterans who
are having difficulty adjusting from military service especially
those diagnosed with PTSD.

Nebraska

5588   Grand Island VA Medical System
Veterans Health Administration, U S Dept. of V A
2201 N Broadwell Ave
Grand Island, NE 68803-2153   308-382-3660
                                          866-580-1810
                                    g.vhacss@forum.va.gov

John Hilbert, Executive Director
Daniel L Parker, Deputy Director

5589   Lincoln Regional Office
Veterans Benefits Administration, U S Dept. of V A
3800 Village Dr.
Lincoln, NE 68501-4103   402-471-4444
                                           800-827-1000
                                      Fax: 402-479-5124
                                   lincoln.query@vba.va.gov
                                   www.veteranprograms.com

Bill Gibson, CEO
Daniel Parker, Deputy Director

5590   Lincoln VA Medical Center
Veterans Health Administration, U S Dept. of V A
600 S 70th St
Lincoln, NE 68510-2451   402-489-3802
                                           800-827-1000
                                      Fax: 402-486-7860
                                    g.vhacss@forum.va.gov

Ryon L Adams, Research/Development Coordinator

5591   VA Nebraska-Western Iowa Health Care System
Veterans Health Administration, U S Dept. of V A
4101 Woolworth Ave
Omaha, NE 68105-1850   402-449-0610
                                           800-451-5796
                                      Fax: 402-449-0684
                                      www.nebraska.va.gov

Marci Mylan, Director
Rowen Zetterman, Chief of Staff

Nevada

5592   Las Vegas Veterans Center
1919 S. Jones, Suite A
Las Vegas, NV 89146-905   702-251-7873
                                      Fax: 702-388-6664
                                      www.lasvegas.va.gov

Daryl Harding, Resident Counselor LCSW
Matt Watson, Team Leader MSW
Veterans clinical counseling center for veterans and their dependent individual and group counseling, marital and family counseling, alcohol and drug assessment referral or treatment. Community education and consultation, employment counseling.

5593   Reno Regional Office
Veterans Benefits Administration
1000 Locust St
Reno, NV 89502-2597   775-328-1486
                                           800-827-1000
                                      Fax: 775-328-1447
                                     reno.query@vba.va.gov
                                         www.reno.va.gov

Joseph E Dardillo, Administrative Officer

5594   VA Sierra Nevada Healthcare System
Veterans Health Administration, U S Dept. of V A
957 Kirman Ave
Reno, NV 89502-2597   775-786-7200
                                           888-838-6256
                                      Fax: 775-328-1816
                                         www.reno.va.gov

Kurt W. Schlegelmich, Director
Michael C. Tadych, Associate Director
Rachel Crossley, Associate Director

5595   VA Southern Nevada Healthcare System
Veterans Health Administration, U S Dept. of V A
6900 North Pecos Rd
Las Vegas, NV 89086   702-791-9000
                                           800-827-1000
                                      Fax: 707-636-3027
                                    g.vhacss@forum.va.gov
                                       www.lasvegas.va.gov

Isabel M. Duff, Acting Director
Ramu Komanduri, Chief of Staff
Sandra L. Solem, Acting Nurse Executive

New Hampshire

5596   Manchester Regional Office
Veterans Benefits Administration, U S Dept. of V A
275 Chestnut St
Manchester, NH 3101-2411   800-827-1000
                                  manchester.query@vba.va.gov
                                            www.va.gov

Jerry Beale, Director

5597   Manchester VA Medical Center
Veterans Health Administration, U S Dept. of V A
718 Smyth Rd
Manchester, NH 03104-7007   603-624-4366
                                           800-892-8384
                                    g.vhacss@forum.va.gov
                                     www.manchester.va.gov

Susan MacKenzie, Acting Med Center Director
Tammy A. Krueger, Associate Director
Andrew J. Breuder, Chief of Staff

5598   New Hampshire Veterans Centers
103 Liberty St
Manchester, NH 3104-3118   603-668-7060
                                           800-562-3127
                                      Fax: 603-666-7404
                                            www.va.gov

Caryl Ahern, Manager
Paulette Landry, Office Manager
Veterans clinic offering combat veterans outpatient counseling

New Jersey

5599   Disabled American Veterans: Ocean County
P.O.Box 1806
Toms River, NJ 8754-1806   732-929-0907

Mary Bencivenga, Contact

5600 **East Orange Campus of the VA New Jersey Healthcare System**
385 Tremont Ave
East Orange, NJ 07018-1023 973-676-1000
Fax: 973-676-4226
www.newjersey.va.gov

Kenneth Mizrach, Director
Glen Giaquinto, Associate Director
John A. Griffith, Associate Director

5601 **Lyons Campus of the VA New Jersey Healthcare System**
Veterans Health Administration, U S Dept. of V A
151 Knollcroft Rd
Lyons, NJ 7939-5001 908-647-0180
800-827-1000
Fax: 908-647-3452
g.vhacss@forum.va.gov
www.newjersey.va.gov

James J Farsetta, Director
Donna Henderson, Coordinator

5602 **Newark Regional Office**
Veterans Benefits Administration, U S Dept. of V A
20 Washington Pl
Newark, NJ 07102-3174 973-645-1441
800-827-1000
newark.query@vba.va.gov
www.newjersey.va.gov

Stephen G Abel, Deputy Commissioner for Veterans

New Mexico

5603 **New Mexico State Veterans' Home**
992 South Broadway
Truth or Consequences, NM 87901-927 575-894-4200
800-964-3976
Fax: 575-894-4270

Lori S Montgomery, Administrator
Carol B Wilson, Admission Coordinator
Veterans medical clinic offering disabled veterans medical treatments.

5604 **New Mexico VA Healthcare System**
Veterans Health Administration, US Dept. of VA
1501 San Pedro Dr SE
Albuquerque, NM 87108-5154 505-265-1711
800-465-8262
Fax: 505-256-2855
g.vhacss@forum.va.gov
www.albuquerque.va.gov

George Marnell, Executive Director
Pamela Crowell, Acting Associate Director
Peter Woodbridge, Chief of Staff

New York

5605 **Albany VA Medical Center: Samuel S Stratton**
Veterans Health Administration, U S Dept. of V A
113 Holland Ave
Albany, NY 12208-3410 518-626-5000
800-233-4810
888-838-7890
Fax: 518-626-5500
g.vhacss@forum.va.gov
www.albany.va.gov

Donald W Stuart, Associate Director (Interim)
Linda W Weiss, Director
Laurdes Irzarry, Chief of Staff

5606 **Albany Vet Center**
Ste 2
17 Computer Dr W
Albany, NY 12205-1618 518-458-7998
Fax: 518-458-8613

Lloyd Mc Omber, Owner
Melodie Krahula, Team Leader

Provides readjustment counseling for combat veterans and also provides benefits and job counseling for all veterans.

5607 **Bath VA Medical Center**
Veterans Health Administration U S Deptartment of
76 Veterans Avenue
Bath, NY 14810 607-664-4000
877-845-3247
888-823-9659
Fax: 607-664-4000
g.vhacss@forum.va.gov
www.bath.va.gov

Michael Swartz, Medical Center Director
David B. Krueger, Associate Director
Felipe Diaz, Chief of Staff

5608 **Bronx VA Medical Center**
Veterans Health Administration, U S Dept. of V A
130 W Kingsbridge Rd
Bronx, NY 10468-9938 718-584-9000
800-877-6976
Fax: 718-733-1223
g.vhacss@forum.va.gov
www.bronx.va.gov

Eric Langhoff, Director
Vincent F Immiti, Associate Director
Kathleen M. Capitulo, Chief of Staff

5609 **Brooklyn Campus of the VA NY Harbor Healthcare System**
Veterans Health Administration, U S Dept. of V A
800 Poly Place
Brooklyn, NY 11209-7104 718-836-6600
800-827-1000
g.vhacss@forum.va.gov
www.nyharbor.va.gov

Martina A Parauda, Director
Veronica J Foy, Associate Director, Facilities &
Michael S Simberkoff, Executive Chief of Staff

5610 **Buffalo Regional Office - Department of Veterans Affairs**
Veterans Benefits Administration
130 South Elmwood Avenue
Buffalo, NY 14202-2465 716-852-3028
800-827-1000
www.va.gov

5611 **Canandiagua VA Medical Center**
Veterans Health Administration, U S Dept. of V A
400 Fort Hill Ave
Canandaigua, NY 14424-1159 585-394-2000
800-204-9917
g.vhacss@forum.va.gov
www.canandaigua.va.gov

Craig S Howard, Medical Center Director
Margaret Owens, Associate Director
Dr. Robert B Babcock, Chief of Staff

5612 **Castle Point Campus of the VA Hudson Valley Healthcare System**
Veterans Health Administration, U S Dept. of V A
Route 9D
Castle Point, NY 12511 845-831-2000
800-827-1000
Fax: 845-838-5193
g.vhacss@forum.va.gov
www.hudsonvalley.va.gov

Gerald F Culliton, Director
John M. Gary, Associate Director
Patricia A. Burke, Associate Director

5613 **New York City Campus of the VA NY Harbor Healthcare System**
Veterans Health Administration, U S Dept. of V A
423 E 23rd St
New York, NY 10010-5011 212-686-7500
800-827-1000
Fax: 718-567-4082
g.vhacss@forum.va.gov
www.nyharbor.va.gov

Camille R Varacchi, Administrative Officer

5614   New York Regional Office
Veterans Benefits Administration, U S Dept. of V A
245 W Houston St
New York, NY 10014-4805   212-714-0699
                                           800-827-1000
                                       Fax: 212-807-4042
                              newyork.query@vba.va.gov
                                              www.va.gov

Ronna Brown, President

5615   Northport VA Medical Center
Veterans Health Administration, U S Dept. of V A
79 Middleville Rd
Northport, NY 11768-2296   631-261-4400
                                           800-827-1000
                                       Fax: 631-266-6710
                               g.vhacss@forum.va.gov
                                     www.northport.va.gov

Philip C Moschitta, Medical Center Director
Rosie A Chatman, Associate Director for Patient &
Maria Favale, Associate Director

5616   Syracuse VA Medical Center
Veterans Health Administration, U S Dept. of V A
800 Irving Ave
Syracuse, NY 13210-2716   315-425-4400
                                           800-792-4334
                                           888-838-7890
                               g.vhacss@forum.va.gov
                                     www.syracuse.va.gov

James Cody, VA Medical Center Director
Judy Hayman, Associate Medical Center Director
William H Marx, Chief of Staff

5617   Torah Alliance of Families of Kids with Disabilities
T AF KI D
1433 Coney Island Ave
Brooklyn, NY 11230-4119   718-252-2236
                                       Fax: 718-252-2216
Juby Shapiro, Manager
Serves over 1k families whose children have a variety of disabilities and special needs. Many of these families are large families in
the low socioeconomic level. Offers monthly meetings, guest lectures, parent matching, information of new developments in software, technology and techniques, sibling support groups, pen pal
lists, audio and video library, alternative medicine and nutrition
information and education on legal awareness and rights of
disabled citizens.

5618   VA Hudson Valley Health Care System
Veterans Health Administration, U S Department of
2094 Albany Post Road
Montrose, NY 10548-1454   914-737-4400
                                       Fax: 845-788-4244
                                  www.hudsonvalley.va.gov

James J Farsette, Network Director
Michael Sabo, Executive Director

5619   VA Western NY Healthcare System, Batavia
Veterans Health Administration, U S Dept. of V A
222 Richmond Ave
Batavia, NY 14020-1227   585-297-1000
                                           800-827-1000
                                       Fax: 585-786-1258
                               g.vhacss@forum.va.gov
                                              www.va.gov

William F Feeley, Medical Center Director
Miguel Rainstein, Chief of Staff
Jason C Petti, Associate Medical Center Directo

5620   VA Western NY Healthcare System, Buffalo
Veterans Health Administration, U S Dept. of V A
3495 Bailey Ave
Buffalo, NY 14215-1129   716-834-9200
                                           800-532-8387
                                        www.buffalo.va.gov

Brian Stiller, Medical Center Director
Jason C. Petti, Chief of Staff
Royce Calhoun, Associate Medical Center Directo

North Carolina

5621   Asheville VA Medical Center
Veterans Health Administration, U S Dept. of V A
1100 Tunnel Rd
Asheville, NC 28805-2043   828-298-7911
                                           800-932-6408
                                       Fax: 828-299-2502
                               g.vhacss@forum.va.gov
                                     www.asheville.va.gov

Cynthia Beyfogle, Executive Director
David A. Pattillo, Assistant Medical Director
James Wells, Chief of Staff

5622   Charlotte Vet Center
2114 Ben Craig Drive
Charlotte, NC 28262-2350   704-549-8025
                                       Fax: 704-549-8261
                                              www.va.gov

Loretta Deaton, Team Leader
Cynthia Algra, Office Manager
Billy Moore, Counselor
Preadjustment Counseling for Combat Veterans with Post Trau-
matic Stress Disorder (PTSD).

5623   Durham VA Medical Center
Veterans Health Administration, U S Dept. of V A
508 Fulton St
Durham, NC 27705-3875   919-286-0411
                                           800-827-1000
                                           888-878-6890
                                       Fax: 919-286-5944
                                     www.durham.va.gov

Deanne M Seekins, Director
Rudy A Klopfer, Associate Director
John D Shelburne, Chief of Staff
Since 1953, Durham Veterans Affairs Medical Cetner has been
improving the health of the men and women who have so proudly
served our nation. We consider it our privilege to serve your
health care needs in any way we can. Services are available to
more than 200,000 veterans living in a 26-county area of central
and eastern North Carolina.

5624   Fayetteville VA Medical Center
Veterans Health Administration, U S Dept. of V A
2300 Ramsey St
Fayetteville, NC 28301-3856   910-488-2120
                                           800-771-6106
                                       Fax: 910-822-7926
                               g.vhacss@forum.va.gov
                                              www.va.gov

Elizabeth Goolsby, Director
James Galkowski, Associate Director, Operations
Jesse Howard III, Acting Chief of Staff
Since 1940, the Fayetteville VA Medical Center (VAMC)
hasimproved the health of the men and women who have so
proudly served our nation. We consider it our privilege to serve
your health care needs in any way we can. Medical, mental health,
women's health careand specialty servicesare available to more
than 157,000 veterans living in a 21-county area of North
Carolina and South Carolina.

5625   WG Hefner VA Medical Center - Salisbury
Vet Health Administration U S Department of VA
1601 Brenner Ave
Salisbury, NC 28144-2515   704-638-9000
                                           800-469-8252
                                       Fax: 704-638-3395
                               g.vhacss@forum.va.gov
                                     www.salisbury.va.gov

Kaye Green, Director
Linette Barker, Associate Medical Center Directo
Subbarao Pemmaraju, Chief of Staff (Interim)
Since 1953, Hefner VAMC has been improving the health of the
men and women who have so proudly served our nation. We consider it our privilege to serve your health care needs in any way we
can. Primary and secondary inpatient health care are available to
more than 287,000 veterans living in a 24-county area of the Central Piedmont Region of North Carolina. This includes the Char-

lotte area with over 100,000 veterans, and the Winston-Salem area with 65,000 veterans.

5626 Winston-Salem Regional Office
Veterans Benefits Administration, U S Dept. of V A
251 N Main St
Winston-Salem, NC 27155-2 336-768-5560
800-827-1000
Fax: 336-768-7295
TTY: 800-829-4833
winsalem.query@vba.va.gov
www.va.gov

Glenn Cobb, Executive VP

North Dakota

5627 Fargo VA Medical Center
Veterans Health Administration, U S Dept. of V A
2101 North Elm
Fargo, ND 58102-2417 701-232-3241
800-410-9723
Fax: 701-239-7166
g.vhacss@forum.va.gov
www.va.gov

Michael J Murphy, Healthcare Center Director
Dale DeKrey, Associate Director for Operation
J Brian Hancock, Chief of Staff

5628 North Dakota VA Regional Office - Fargo Regional Office
Veterans Benefits Administration, U S Dept. of V A
2101 Elm St N
Fargo, ND 58102-2417 701-451-4690
800-410-9723
Fax: 701-451-4690
fargo.query@vba.va.gov
www.fargo.va.gov

Thomas Santoro, Director Research Department

Ohio

5629 Chillicothe VA Medical Center
Veterans Health Administration, U S Dept. of V A
17273 State Route 104
Chillicothe, OH 45601-9718 740-773-1141
800-358-8262
888-838-6446
Fax: 740-772-7023
g.vhacss@forum.va.gov
www.chillicothe.va.gov

Wendy J. Hepker, Medical Center Director
Keith Sullivan, Associate Medical Center Directo
Deborah M Meesig, Chief of Staff
The Chillicothe VA Medical Center provides acute and chronic mental health services, primary and secondary medical services, a wide range of nursing home care services, specialty medical services as well as specialized women Veterans health clinics. The facility is an active ambulatory care setting and serves as a chronic mental health referral center for VA Medical Center in southern Ohio and parts of West Virginia and Kentucky

5630 Cincinnati VA Medical Center
Veterans Health Administration, U S Dept. of V A
3200 Vine St
Cincinnati, OH 45220-2213 513-861-3100
800-827-1000
888-267-7873
Fax: 513-475-6500
g.vhacss@forum.va.gov
www.cincinnati.va.gov

Linda Smith, Director
David Ninneman, Associate Director
Robert Falcone, Chief of Staff

5631 Cleveland Regional Office
Veterans Benefits Administration, U S Dept. of V A
1240 E 9th St
Cleveland, OH 44199-2068 800-827-1000
Fax: 216-522-8262
cleveland.query@vba.va.gov
www.va.gov

P Hunter Peckham, Director
Robert Ruff, Assistant Director
William Bunkley, Minority Veterans Program Coordi

5632 Dayton VA Medical Center
Veterans Health Administration U S Department of V
4100 W 3rd St
Dayton, OH 45428-9000 937-268-6511
800-368-8262
888-838-6446
Fax: 937-262-2170
g.vhacss@forum.va.gov
www.dayton.va.gov

Glenn Costie, Acting Director
Mark Murdock, Associate Director
James T. Hardy, Chief of Staff
The Dayton VAMC is a state of the art teaching facility that has been serving Veterans for 146 years, having accepted its first patient in 1867. The Dayton VA Medical Center provides a full range of health care through medical, surgical, mental health (inpatient and outpatient), home and community health programs, geriatric (nursing home), physical medicine and therapy services, neurology, oncology, dentistry, and hospice.

5633 Louis Stokes VA Medical Center - Wade Park Campus
Veterans Health Administration, U S Dept. of V A
10701 East Blvd
Cleveland, OH 44106-1702 216-791-3800
877-838-8262
888-838-6446
Fax: 440-838-6017
g.vhacss@forum.va.gov
www.cleveland.va.gov

Susan M Fuehrer, Medical Center Director
Darwin Goodspeed, Associate Medical Center Director
Murray D. Altose, Chief of Staff

Oklahoma

5634 Jack C. Montgomery VA Medical Center
Veterans Benefits Administration, U S Dept. of V A
1011 Honor Heights Dr
Muskogee, OK 74401-1318 918-577-3000
800-827-1000
muskogee.query@vba.va.gov
www.muskogee.va.gov

Alef Nancy Graham, Manager

5635 Jack C. Montomery VA Medical Center
1011 Honor Heights Dr
Muskogee, OK 74401-1318 918-577-3000
800-827-1000
muskogee.query@vba.va.gov
www.muskogee.va.gov

James R. Floyd, Medical Director
Inez Reitz, Acting Associate Director
Thomas D. Schneider, Chief of Staff

5636 Oklahoma City VA Medical Center
Veterans Health Administration, U S Dept. of V A
921 NE 13th St
Oklahoma City, OK 73104-5007 405-456-1000
800-827-1000
Fax: 405-270-1560
www.oklahoma.va.gov

Jimmy A. Murphy, Director
Debra A. Colombe, Associate Director
Mark Huycke, Chief of Staff

5637 Oklahoma Veterans Centers Vet Center
3033 N Walnut Ave
Ste W101
Oklahoma City, OK 73105-2833   405-270-5184
                                     Fax: 405-270-5125

Peter Sharp, Manager
Steve Kenzie, Owner
PTSP counseling for all combat Veterans and victims of sexual
trauma/sexual harassment.

Oregon

5638 Oregon Health Sciences University
3181 SW Sam Jackson Park Rd
Portland, OR 97239-3098   503-494-8311
                                        ohsu.edu

Joe Robertson, President
James Morgan, Executive Director

5639 Portland Regional Office
Veterans Benefits Administration, U S Dept. of V A
100 SW Main St, Floor 2
Portland, OR 97204-2802   503-373-2388
                                     800-827-1000
                           portland.query@vba.va.gov
                                       www.va.gov

5640 Portland VA Medical Center
Veterans Health Administration, U S Dept. of V A
3710 SW U.S. Veterans Hospital Rd.
Portland, OR 97239-2964   503-220-8262
                                     800-949-1004
                                Fax: 503-273-5319
                             g.vhacss@forum.va.gov
                                 www.portland.va.gov

John E Patrick, Director
David Stockwell, Deputy Director of Administratio
Tom Anderson, Chief of Staff
The Portland VA Medical Center (PVAMC) is a 303-bed consolidated facility with two main divisions. The medical center serves
as the quaternary referral center for Oregon, Southern Washington, and parts of Idaho for the U.S. Department of Veterans Affairs. The Portland VAMC is located atop Marquam Hill on 28.5
acres overlooking the city of Portland. In addition to comprehensive medical and mental health services, the Portland VAMC supports ongoing research and medical education, including nati

5641 Roseburg VA Medical Center
Veterans Health Administration, U S Dept. of V A
913 NW Garden Valley Blvd
Roseburg, OR 97471-6523   541-440-1000
                                     800-549-8387
                                Fax: 541-440-1225
                             g.vhacss@forum.va.gov
                                 www.roseburg.va.gov

Jim Willis, Director
Mark Traines, MD

5642 Southern Oregon Rehabilitation Center & Clinics
Veterans Health Administration, U S Dept. of V A
8495 Crater Lake Hwy
White City, OR 97503   541-826-2111
                                     800-809-8725
                                Fax: 541-830-3500
                             g.vhacss@forum.va.gov
                              www.southernoregon.va.gov

George Andries, Executive Director

Pennsylvania

5643 Butler VA Medical Center
Veterans Health Administration, U S Dept. of V A
325 New Castle Rd
Butler, PA 16001-2418   724-282-7171
                                     800-362-8262
                                Fax: 724-282-7640
                             g.vhacss@forum.va.gov
                                 www.butler.va.gov

John Gennaro, Director
Rebecca Hubscher, Associate Director
Sharon Parson, Nurse Executive
VA Butler Healthcare is located in the heart of Butler County, on
the bus line, and convenient to community support services for
Western Pennsylvania and Eastern Ohio-area Veterans. We have
been attending to Veterans' total care since 1947 and are the
health care choice for over 18,000 Veterans - providing comprehensive Veteran care including primary, specialty, and mental
health care - as well as health maintenance plans, management of
chronic conditions and preventative medicine needs.

5644 Coatesville VA Medical Center
Veterans Health Administration, U S Dept. of V A
1400 Blackhorse Hill Rd
Coatesville, PA 19320-2040   610-384-7711
                                     800-290-6172
                                     888-558-3812
                             g.vhacss@forum.va.gov
                                 www.coatesville.va.gov

Gary Devansky, Director
Sheila Chelleppa, Chief of Staff
Nancy Schmid, Associate Director Patient Care

5645 Erie VA Medical Center
Veterans Health Administration, U S Dept. of V A
135 E 38th Street Blvd
Erie, PA 16504-1559   814-868-8661
                                     800-274-8387
                                     888-860-2124
                                Fax: 814-860-2425
                             g.vhacss@forum.va.gov
                                 www.erie.va.gov

Michael Adelman, Medical Center Director
Melissa Sundin, Associate Medical Center Directo
Dr. Anthony Behm, Chief of Staff

5646 James E Van Zandt VA Medical Center
Veterans Health Administration, U S Dept. of V A
2907 Pleasant Valley Blvd
Altoona, PA 16602-4377   814-943-8164
                                     800-827-1000
                                Fax: 814-940-7898
                             g.vhacss@forum.va.gov
                                       www.va.gov

Cecil B Hengeveld, Director
Gerald Williams, Executive Director

5647 Lebanon VA Medical Center
Veterans Health Administration, U S Dept. of V A
1700 S Lincoln Ave
Lebanon, PA 17042-7597   717-272-6621
                                     800-409-8771
                                Fax: 717-228-5907
                             g.vhacss@forum.va.gov
                                 www.lebanon.va.gov

Robert (Bob) Callahan Jr., Director
Robin C. Aube-Warren, Associate Director
Kanan Chatterjee, Chief of Staff

5648 Pennsylvania Veterans Centers
Veterans Health Administration, U S Department of
135 E 38th St
Erie, PA 16504   814-868-8661
                                     800-274-8387
                                Fax: 717-861-8589
                                 www.erie.va.gov

Michael Aldeman, medical Center Director
Melissa Sundin, Associate Director
Anthony Behm, Chief of Staff

Veterans medical clinic offering disabled veterans medical treatments.

5649 Philadelphia Regional Office and Insurance Center
Veterans Benefits Administration, U S Dept. of V A
5000 Wissahickon Ave
Philadelphia, PA 19144-4867
215-336-3003
800-827-1000
Fax: 215-336-5542
phillyro.query@vba.va.gov
www.va.gov

Sonny Dicrecchio, Executive Director

5650 Philadelphia VA Medical Center
Veterans Health Administration, U S Dept. of V A
3900 Woodland Avenue
Philadelphia, PA 19104
215-823-5800
800-949-1001
g.vhacss@forum.va.gov
www.philadelphia.va.gov

Joseph M Dalpiaz, Director
Ralph Schapira, Chief of Staff
Margaret O'Shea Caplan, Associate Director for Finance

5651 Pittsburgh Regional Office
Veterans Benefits Administration
1000 Liberty Avenue
Pittsburgh, PA 15222
412-688-6100
800-827-1000
Fax: 412-688-6121
pittsburgh.query@vba.va.gov
www.pittsburgh.va.gov

Micahel E Moreland

5652 VA Pittsburgh Healthcare System, University Drive Division
Veterans Health Administration, U S Dept. of V A
University Dr
Pittsburgh, PA 15240-2400
412-688-6000
866-482-7488
Fax: 412-688-6901
g.vhacss@forum.va.gov
www.pittsburgh.va.gov

Timothy Mar Carlos, CEO

5653 VA Pittsburgh Healthcare System, Highland Drive Division
Veterans Health Administration, U S Dept. of V A
7180 Highland Dr
Pittsburgh, PA 15206-1206
412-688-6000
800-827-1000
Fax: 412-365-4213
g.vhacss@forum.va.gov
www.pittsburgh.va.gov

Kristin Best, Deputy Adjutant General
Roger Sutton, MD

5654 Wilkes-Barre VA Medical Center
Veterans Health Administration, U S Dept. of V A
1111 E End Blvd
Wilkes Barre, PA 18711-30
570-824-3521
877-928-2621
Fax: 570-821-7278
g.vhacss@forum.va.gov
www.wilkes-barre.va.gov

William H Mills, Director (Interim)
Douglas V Paxton Sr., Associate Director
Mirza Z Ali, Chief of Staff

Rhode Island

5655 Providence Regional Office
Veterans Benefits Administration, U S Dept. of V A
380 Westminster St
Providence, RI 2903-3246
401-462-0324
800-827-1000
Fax: 401-254-2320
providence.query@vba.va.gov
www.va.gov

Daniel Evangelista, Acting Associate Director

5656 Providence VA Medical Center
Veterans Health Administration, U S Dept. of V A
830 Chalkstone Ave
Providence, RI 02908-4799
401-273-7100
866-363-4486
Fax: 401-457-3360
g.vhacss@forum.va.gov
www.providence.va.gov

Vincent W Ng, Medical Center Director
William J Burney, Medical Center Associate Directo
Gregory M Gillette, Medical Center Chief of Staff
To fulfill President Lincoln's promise To care for him who shall have borne the battle, and for his widow, and his orphan by serving and honoring the men and women who are America's veterans.

South Carolina

5657 Columbia Regional Office
Veterans Benefits Administration, U S Dept. of V A
6437 Garners Ferry Rd
Columbia, SC 29209-2401
803-401-1094
800-827-1000
columbia.query@vba.va.gov
www.va.gov

Jimmie Ruff, Executive Director

5658 Ralph H Johnson VA Medical Center
Veterans Health Administration, U S Dept. of V A
109 Bee St
Charleston, SC 29401-5703
843-577-5011
800-827-1000
888-878-6884
Fax: 843-876-5384
g.vhacss@forum.va.gov
www.charleston.va.gov

Carolyn L Adams, Director
Scott Isaacks, Associate Director
Florence N Hutchinson, Chief of Staff

5659 William Jennings Bryan Dorn VA Medical Center
Veterans Health Administration U S Department of V
6439 Garners Ferry Rd
Columbia, SC 29209-1638
803-776-4000
800-293-8262
Fax: 803-695-6739
www.columbiasc.va.gov

Carolyn L Adams, Director
Barbara Temeck, Chief of Staff
David L. Omura, Chief of Staff

South Dakota

5660 Royal C Johnson Veterans Memorial Medical Center
Veterans Health Administration, U S Dept. of VA
2501 W. 22nd St
Sioux Falls, SD 57105-5046
605-336-3230
800-316-8387
Fax: 605-333-6878
g.vhacss@forum.va.gov
www.siouxfalls.va.gov

Patrick J Kelly, Director
Sara Ackert, Associate Director
Victor Waters, Chief of Staff

5661 Sioux Falls Regional Office
Veterans Benefits Administration, U S Dept. of V A
2501 W. 22nd St
Sioux Falls, SD 57105-5046
605-336-3230
800-827-1000
Fax: 605-333-5316
siouxfalls.query@vba.va.gov
www.siouxfalls.va.gov

Tennessee

5662 Alvin C York VA Medical Center
Veterans Health Administration, U S Dept. of V A
3400 Lebanon Pike
Murfreesboro, TN 37129-1237   615-867-6000
800-876-7093
Fax: 615-867-5768
g.vhacss@forum.va.gov
www.tennesseevalley.va.gov

Juan Morales, Medical System Director
Janice Cobb, Associate Director, Nursing Serv
Emma Metcalf, Chief Operating Officer

5663 Memphis VA Medical Center
Veterans Health Administration, U S Dept. of V A
1030 Jefferson Ave
Memphis, TN 38104-2127   901-523-8990
800-636-8262
g.vhacss@forum.va.gov
www.memphis.va.gov

Jay Robinson III, Associate Medical Center Directo
Douglas D Southall, Assistant Medical Center Directo
Margarethe Hagemann, Chief of Staff

5664 Mountain Home VA Medical Center - James H Quillen VA Medical Center
Veterans Health Administration, US Dept. of VA
Corner of Lamont & Veterans Way
Mountain Home, TN 37684   423-926-1171
877-573-3529
g.vhacss@forum.va.gov
www.mountainhome.va.gov

Charlene S Ehret, Medical Center Director
Jimmy H McGlawn, Associate Director
David R Reagan, Chief of Staff

5665 Nasheville Regional Office
Veterans Benefits Administration, U S Dept. of V A
110 9th Ave S
Nashville, TN 37203-3817   800-827-1000
nashville.query@vba.va.gov
www.va.gov

Michael R Walsh, Administrative Officer
Donald H Rubin, Research/Development Coordinator

5666 Nashville VA Medical Center
Veterans Health Administration, US Dept. of VA
1310 24th Ave S
Nashville, TN 37212-2637   615-327-4751
800-228-4973
Fax: 615-321-6350
g.vhacss@forum.va.gov
www.tennesseevalley.va.gov

Juan Morales, Medical System Director
Michael A Doukas, Chief of Staff
Gary D Trende, Associate Director, Nursing Serv

Texas

5667 Amarillo VA Healthcare System
Veterans Health Administration, U S Dept. of V A
6010 Amarillo Blvd West
Amarillo, TX 79106-1991   806-355-9703
800-687-8262
Fax: 806-354-7869
g.vhacss@forum.va.gov
www.amarillo.va.gov

David Welch, Director
Lance Robinson, Associate Director
Grace Stringfelow, Chief of Staff

5668 Amarillo Vet Center
Department of Veterans Affairs
3414 Olsen Blvd
Suite E
Amarillo, TX 79109-3072   806-351-1104
Fax: 806-351-1104
www.va.gov

Pedro Garcia Jr., Team Leader
Simon Camarillo, Counsilor
William C Santer, Family Therapist
Provides individual, group and family counseling to veterans who served in combat theaters of World War II and Korea, veterans of the Vietnam Era, and veterans of conflicts zones in Lebanon, Grenada, Panama, the Persian Guld and Somalia.

5669 El Paso VA Healthcare Center
Veterans Health Administration, U S Dept. of V A
5001 N Piedras
El Paso, TX 79930-4210   915-564-6100
800-672-3782
Fax: 915-564-7920
g.vhacss@forum.va.gov
www.elpaso.va.gov

John A. Mendoza, Director
Elizabeth Lowery, Associate Director
Homer LeMar, Interim Chief of Staff

5670 Houston Regional Office
Veterans Benefits Administration, U S Dept. of V A
6900 Almeda Rd
Houston, TX 77030-4200   713-791-1414
800-827-1000
houston.query@vba.va.gov
www.va.gov

Cecil Aultman, Executive Director
Edgar Tucker, Chief Executive Officer

5671 Michael E. Debakey VA Medical Center
Veterans Health Administration, U S Dept. of V A
2002 Holcombe Blvd
Houston, TX 77030-4211   713-791-1414
800-553-2278
g.vhacss@forum.va.gov
www.houston.va.gov

Adam C Walmus, Director
J Kalavar, Chief of Staff
Francisco Vazquez, Associate Director

5672 South Texas Veterans Healthcare System
Veterans Health Administration, U S Dept. of V A
7400 Merton Minter
San Antonio, TX 78229-4404   210-617-5300
877-469-5300
888-686-6350
g.vhacss@forum.va.gov
www.southtexas.va.gov

Marie L. Wedon, Director
Wade Vlosich, Associate Director
Joe A. Perez, Assistant Director

5673 VA North Texas Health Veterans Affairs Care System: Dallas VA Medical Center
Veterans Health Administration, U S Dept. of V A
4500 S Lancaster Rd
Dallas, TX 75216-7167   214-742-8387
800-849-3597
Fax: 214-857-1171
www.northtexas.va.gov/index.asp

Jeffrey Milligan, Director
Peter Dancy, Associate Director
Clark R. Gregg, Chief of Staff
Health care system which serves veterans with medical care and rehabilitation services including spinal cord injury center. For VA benefit inquiries contact 1-800-827-1000. This system has locations in Bonham, Dallas, and Fort Worth.

5674 Waco Regional Office
Veterans Benefits Administration, U S Dept. of V A
4800 Memorial Dr
Waco, TX 76711-1   254-752-6581
                                   800-423-1111
                                   TTY: 800-829-4833
                                   waco.query@vba.va.gov
                                   www.centraltexas.va.gov

William F. Harper, Chief of Staff
Russell E. Lloyd, Associate Director of Resources
Karen Spada, Associate Director for Patients
Mission is to honor America's Veterans by providing exceptional
health care that improves their health and well being.

5675 West Texas VA Healthcare System
Veterans Health Administration, U S Dept. of V A
300 Veterans Blvd
Big Spring, TX 79720-5566   432-263-7361
                                   800-472-1365
                                   Fax: 915-264-4834
                                   g.vhacss@forum.va.gov
                                   www.bigspring.va.gov

Andrew M. Welch, Interim Director
Kenneth Allensworth, Associate Director
Raul Zambrano, Chief of Staff
The West Texas VA Health Care System (WTVAHCS) proudly
serves Veterans in 33 counties across 53,000 square miles of rural
geography in West Texas and Eastern New Mexico. The George
H. O'Brien, Jr. VA Medical Center is located in Big Spring, Texas
and the six Community Based Outpatient Clinics (CBOC's) that
comprise the remainder of the health care system are located in
Abilene, TX, Stamford, TX, San Angelo, TX, Odessa, TX, Fort
Stockton, TX, and Hobbs, NM.

Utah

5676 Utah Division of Veterans Affairs
Utah Division of Veterans Affairs
550 Foothill Blvd
Ste 202
Salt Lake City, UT 84113-1106   801-582-1565
                                   800-894-9497
                                   Fax: 801-326-2369
                                   www.saltlakecity.va.gov

David J Peifer, Director
Todd Andrews, Assistant to the Director
Karen H. Gribbin, Manager
Our mission is to serve the veteran who served us. The VA Salt
Lake City Health Care System is committed to providing our pa-
tients with the highest Quality of Care in an environment that is
safe. We do this by focusing on Continuous Process Improvement
and by supporting a Culture of Safety

5677 VA Salt Lake City Healthcare System
Veterans Health Administration, U S Dept. of V A
500 Foothill Drive
Salt Lake City, UT 84148-1   801-582-1565
                                   800-613-4012
                                   Fax: 801-584-1289
                                   www.saltlakecity.va.gov

Steven W Young, Director
Warren E Hill, Associate Director
Karen H. Gribbin, Chief of Staff
Our mission is to serve the veteran who served us. The VA Salt
Lake City Health Care System is committed to providing our pa-
tients with the highest Quality of Care in an environment that is
safe. We do this by focusing on Continuous Process Improvement
and by supporting a Culture of Safety

Vermont

5678 Vermont VA Regional Office Center
Veterans Benefits Administration
215 N Main St
White River Junction, VT 05009-1   802-295-9363
                                   866-687-8387
                                   Fax: 802-290-6354
                                   whiteriver.query@vba.va.gov
                                   www.whiteriver.va.gov

Deborah Amdur, Executive Director
Danielle S. Ocker, Associate Director
Melanie Thompson, Acting Chief of Staff
The White River Junction VA Medical Center (WRJ VAMC) is re-
sponsible for the delivery of health care services to eligible Veter-
ans in Vermont and the 4 contiguous counties of New Hampshire.
These services are delivered at the Medical Center's main campus
located in White River Junction, Vermont, and at its seven Outpa-
tient Clinics (Bennington, Brattleboro, Colchester, Newport, and
Rutland, Vermont; Keene and Littleton, New Hampshire). The
White River Junction VA is closely affiliated with the Ge

5679 Vermont Veterans Centers
359 Dorset St
South Burlington, VT 05403-6210   802-862-1806
                                   877-927-8387
                                   Fax: 802-865-3319
                                   www.va.gov

Fred Forehand, Team Leader
William Newkirk, Counsilor
George Troutman, Counsilor
Veterans medical clinic offering disabled veterans medical treat-
ments.

Virginia

5680 Hampton VA Medical Center
Veterans Health Administration, U S Dept. of V A
100 Emancipation Dr
Hampton, VA 23667-1   757-722-9961
                                   800-827-1000
                                   Fax: 757-728-3135
                                   mike.eisenberg@med.va.gov
                                   www.hampton.va.gov

Deanne M Seekins, Medical Center Director
Benita K Stoddard, Associate Director for Operation
G. Arul, Chief of Staff

5681 Hunter Holmes McGuire VA Medical Center
Veterans Health Administration, U S Dept. of V A
1201 Broad Rock Blvd
Richmond, VA 23249-1   804-675-5000
                                   800-784-8381
                                   Fax: 804-675-5236
                                   g.vhacss@forum.va.gov
                                   www.richmond.va.gov

Charles E Sepich, Director
David P Budinger, Associate Director
Julie Beales, Interim Chief of Staff

5682 Roanoke Regional Office
Veterans Benefits Administration, U S Dept. of V A
116 North Jefferson St
Roanoke, VA 24016-1906   540-362-1999
                                   800-827-1000
                                   Fax: 540-563-4838
                                   www.va.gov

Roger Bohm, Executive
Bert Boyd, COO/Executive Director

5683 **Salem VA Medical Center**
Veterans Health Administration, U S Dept. of V A
1970 Roanoke Blvd
Salem, VA 24153-6478 540-982-2463
800-827-1000
888-982-2463
Fax: 540-983-1096
g.vhacss@forum.va.gov
www.salem.va.gov

Miguel H LaPuz, Director
Carol S Bogedain, Associate Director
Maureen McCarthy, Chief of Staff

5684 **Virginia Department of Veterans Services**
270 Franklin Rd SW
Roanoke, VA 24011-2204 540-857-7102
Fax: 540-857-6437

Colbert Boyd, Manager

Washington

5685 **Jonathan M Wainwright Memorial VA Medical Center**
Veterans Health Administration, U S Dept. of V A
77 Wainwright Dr
Walla Walla, WA 99362-3975 509-525-5200
888-687-8863
Fax: 509-946-3062
www.va.gov

Michael W Parnicky, R and D Coordinator

5686 **Seattle Regional Office**
Veterans Benefits Administration
915 2nd Ave
Seattle, WA 98174-1060 206-762-1010
800-827-1000
seattle.query@vba.va.gov
www.va.gov

Va Ad Harabanim, Executive Director
Timothy Williams, Chief Executive Officer

5687 **Spokane VA Medical Center**
Veterans Health Administration, U S Dept. of V A
4815 N Assembly St
Spokane, WA 99205-6185 509-434-7000
800-325-7940
Fax: 509-434-7119
g.vhacss@forum.va.gov
www.spokane.va.gov

Alan Prentiss, Chief of Staff
Dirk Minatre, Coordinator
Joseph Manley, Executive Director

5688 **VA Puget Sound Health Care System**
Veterans Health Administration, U S Dept. of V A
1660 S Columbian Way
Seattle, WA 98108-1532 206-762-1010
800-329-8387
g.vhacss@forum.va.gov
www.pugetsound.va.gov

Michael Fisher, Director
Michael Tadych, Deputy Director
Walt Dannenberg, Assistant Director

West Virginia

5689 **Huntington Regional Office**
Veterans Benefits Administration, U S Dept. of V A
640 4th Ave
Huntington, WV 25701-1340 304-525-5131
800-827-1000
Fax: 304-399-9344
huntington.query@vba.va.gov
www.va.gov

Mark Bugher, President

5690 **Huntington VA Medical Center**
Veterans Health Administration, U S Dept. of V A
1540 Spring Valley Dr
Huntington, WV 25704-9300 304-429-6741
800-827-8244
Fax: 304-429-6713
www.huntington.va.gov

Edward H Seiler, Director
Suzanne Jene, Associate Director
Jeffery B Breaux, Chief of Staff

5691 **Louis A Johnson VA Medical Center**
Veterans Health Administration, U S Dept. of V A
1 Medical Center Drive
Clarksburg, WV 26301-4155 304-623-3461
800-733-0512
Fax: 304-626-7048
g.vhacss@forum.va.gov
www.clarksburg.va.gov

William E Cox, Director
Jeffrey A Beiler II, Associate Director
Glenn R Snider, Chief of Staff

5692 **Martinsburg VA Medical Center**
Veterans Health Administration, U S Dept. of V A
510 Butler Avenue
Martinsburg, WV 25405-9990 304-263-0811
800-817-3807
Fax: 304-262-7433
www.martinsburg.va.gov

Ann R Brown, Director
Timothy J Cooke, Associate Medical Center Directo
Jonathan E Fierer, Chief of Staff

5693 **US Department Veterans Affairs Beckley Vet Center**
200 Veterans Ave
Beckley, WV 25801-4301 304-255-2121
877-902-5142
Fax: 304-254-8711
www.beckley.va.gov

Karin L. McGraw, Director
Vet Center services includes individual and group readjustment counseling, referral for benefits assistance, liason with community agencies, marital and family counseling, substance abuse counseling, job counseling and referral, sexual trauma counseling, and community education.

Wisconsin

5694 **Clement J Zablocki VA Medical Center**
Veterans Health Administration U S Department of V
5000 W National Ave
Milwaukee, WI 53295-1 414-384-2000
888-827-1000
888-469-6614
Fax: 414-382-5319
www.milwaukee.va.gov

Robert H Beller, Director
Michael D Erdmann, Chief of Staff
Judith A Murphy, Associate Director for Patient/N
In an effort to improve access to veterans in Milwaukee County, the VAMC has deployed a mobile clinic that provides primary care four days a week to veterans. The Medical Center also assists the Vet Center located in the City of Milwaukee. In addition, this Medical Center participates in a four-way partnership with the WDVA, the Center for Veterans Issues, Ltd., and the Social Development Commission, to operate Vets Place Central, a 72-bed transitional housing program.

5695 **Tomah VA Medical Center**
Veterans Health Administration, U S Dept. of V A
500 E Veterans St
Tomah, WI 54660-3105 608-372-3971
800-872-8662
Fax: 608-372-1224
www.tomah.va.gov

Mario V. DeSanctis, Medical Center Director
David Huffman, Associate Director
David J. Houlihan, Chief of Staff

VAMCTomah has been improving the health of the men and women who have so proudly served our nation. We consider it our privelege to serve your health care needs in any way we can. Services are available to veterans living in a Western/Central area of Wisconsin.

5696   William S Middleton Memorial VA Hospital Center
Veterans Health Administration, U S Dept. of V A
2500 Overlook Ter
Madison, WI 53705-2254   608-256-1901
                                                   888-478-8321
                                                   888-256-1901
                                              Fax: 608-280-7244
                                                www.madison.va.gov

Judy McKee, Director
John Rohrer, Associate Director
Alan J. Bridges, Chief of Staff

5697   Wisconsin VA Regional Office
Veterans Benefits Administration, U S Dept. of V A
5000 W National Ave
Milwaukee, WI 53295-1   414-384-2000
                                                   800-827-1000
                                              Fax: 414-382-5374
                                          milwaukee.query@vba.va.gov
                                                www.milwaukee.va.gov

Philip L Cook, Executive Director
Neil S Mandel, Research/Development Coordinator
Glen Grippen, CEO
In an effort to improve access to veterans in Milwaukee County, the VAMC has deployed a mobile clinic that provides primary care four days a week to veterans. The Medical Center also assists the Vet Center located in the City of Milwaukee. In addition, this Medical Center participates in a four-way partnership with the WDVA, the Center for Veterans Issues, Ltd., and the Social Development Commission, to operate Vets Place Central, a 72-bed transitional housing program.

Wyoming

5698   Casper Vet Center
1030 N. Poplar Suite B
Casper, WY 82601-2665   307-261-5355
                                              Fax: 307-261-5439
                                                www.vetcenter.va.gov

James Whipps, Office Manager
Vet Center offering re-adjustment counseling for combat veterans.

5699   Cheyenne VA Medical Center
Veterans Health Administration, U S Dept. of V A
2360 E Pershing Blvd
Cheyenne, WY 82001-5356   307-778-7370
                                                   877-927-8387
                                                   888-483-9127
                                              Fax: 307-638-8923
                                                       www.va.gov

Cynthia McCormack, Medical Center Director
Elizabeth Lowery, Associate Director
Jerry Zang, Chief of Staff

5700   Sheridan VA Medical Center
Veterans Health Administration, U S Dept. of V A
1898 Fort Rd
Sheridan, WY 82801-8320   307-672-3473
                                                   800-827-1000
                                                   866-822-6714
                                              Fax: 307-672-1639
                                          www.sheridan.va.gov/index.asp

Debra L Hirschman, Director
Michele Beach, Director
Wendell Robison, Chief of Staff

5701   Wyoming/Colorado VA Regional Office
Veterans Benefits Administration, U S Dept. of V A
155 Van Gordon St
Lakewood, CO 80228-1709   303-894-7474
                                                   800-827-1000
                                              Fax: 303-894-7442
                                          denver.query@vba.va.gov
                                                       www.va.gov

E William Belz, Director

Vocational & Employment

Alabama

5702   ADRS Lakeshore
Alabama Department Of Rehabilitation Services
602 S. Lawrence St.
Montgomery, AL 36104   334-293-7500
                                     800-441-7609
                                     Fax: 334-293-7383
                                     TTY: 800-499-1816
                                     www.rehab.alabama.gov

Michelle K. Glaze, District 1, Mobile
Jimmy Varnado, District 2, Montgomery
Eddie Williams, District 5, Huntsville
Rehabilitation offering employment services to severely disabled persons. Programs include Adaptive Driving Training, Assistive Technology; Employability Development, and Vocational Evaluation.

5703   Alabama Goodwill Industries
2350 Green Springs Highway S
Birmingham, AL 35205   205-323-6331
                                     alabamagoodwill.org
                                     www.alabamagoodwill.org
David Wells, President & Chief Executive Officer
Amanda Ford, Vice President, Organizational Development
Doug Prescott, Vice President, Operations
The mission of Goodwill is to provide rehabilitation services, training, employment, and opportunities for personal growth to the disabled/disadvantaged.

5704   Arc of Central Alabama
6001 Crestwood Blvd
Birmingham, AL 35212   205-323-6383
                                     Fax: 205-323-0085
                                     www.arcofcentralalabama.org
Chris B. Stewart, President & Chief Executive Officer
Mike Mitchell, Chief Operating Officer
N. Brooks Greene, Chief Financial Officer
The Arc of Central Alabama provides the following services to people with intellectual and developmental disabilities: day programs; residential services; employment services; early intervention; and advocacy.

5705   Butler Adult Training Center
South Central Alabama Mental Health
680 Hardscramble Rd.
Greenville, AL 36037   334-382-2353
                                     Fax: 334-382-9518
                                     www.scamhc.org
Clients receive training in Independent Living Skills, Self-Care, Language Skills, Learning, Self Direction and Economic Self-Sufficiency. The clients also participate in Special Olympics activities.

5706   Coffee County Training Center
South Central Alabama Mental Health
801 Aviation Blvd.
Enterprise, AL 36330   334-393-1732
                                     Fax: 334-347-0252
                                     www.scamhc.org
Clients 21 years and up receive training in Independent Living Skills, Self-Care, Language Skills, Learning, Self-Direction and Economic Self-Sufficiency. Transportation is also provided to clients of the center.

5707   Easterseals: Achievement Center
Easterseals of Alabama
510 W Thomason Circle
Opelika, AL 36801-5499   334-745-3501
                                     866-239-2237
                                     Fax: 334-749-5808
                                     info@achievement-center.org
                                     www.achievement-center.org
Star Wray, Executive Director
Randy Burke, Director, Industrial Operations
Joni House, Director, Business & Finance
Provides vocational development and extended employment programs for physically, mentally, and developmentally disabled individuals and to non-disabled persons who are culturally, socially, or economically disadvantaged.
1961

5708   Easterseals: Opportunity Center
6300 McClellan Blvd
Anniston, AL 36206   256-820-9960
                                     Fax: 256-820-9592
                                     smiles@opportunity-center.com
                                     www.opportunity-center.com
A nationally accredited non-profit organization providing vocational evaluation/assessment, paid work training, and employment services for people with disabilities in Calhoun, Cleburne, Clay, Talladega, Coosa and Randolph counties.

5709   Montgomery Comprehensive Career Center
1060 East South Blvd.
Montgomery, AL 36116   334-286-1746
                                     Fax: 334-288-7286
                                     montgomery@alcc.alabama.gov
                                     joblink.alabama.gov

5710   Vocational Rehabilitation Service (VRS)
Alabama Department Of Rehabilitation Services
602 S. Lawrence St.
Montgomery, AL 36104   334-293-7500
                                     800-441-7609
                                     Fax: 334-293-7383
                                     TTY: 800-499-1816
                                     www.rehab.alabama.gov
Availiable through any of the 20 VRS offices statewide, services can include educational services, vocational assesment, evaluation and counseling, job training, assistive technology, orientation and mobility training and job placement.

5711   Vocational Rehabilitation Service - Opelika
Alabama Department Of Rehabilitation Services
520 W Thomason Circle
Opelika, AL 36801   334-749-1259
                                     800-671-6835
                                     Fax: 334-749-8753
                                     TTY: 800-499-1816
                                     www.rehab.alabama.gov

5712   Vocational Rehabilitation Service - Dothan
Alabama Department Of Rehabilitation Services
795 Ross Clark Circle NE
Ste 2
Dothan, AL 36303   334-699-8600
                                     800-275-0132
                                     Fax: 334-792-1783
                                     TTY: 800-499-1816
                                     www.rehab.alabama.gov

5713   Vocational Rehabilitation Service - Gadsden
Alabama Department of Rehabilitation Services
1100 George Wallace Dr.
Gadsden, AL 35903-6501   256-547-6974
                                     800-671-6839
                                     Fax: 256-543-1784
                                     TTY: 800-499-1816
                                     www.rehab.alabama.gov

5714 Vocational Rehabilitation Service - Homewood
Alabama Department Of Rehabilitation Services
236 Goodwin Crest Dr.
Birmingham, AL 35209
205-290-4400
800-671-6837
Fax: 205-290-0486
TTY: 800-499-1816
www.rehab.alabama.gov

5715 Vocational Rehabilitation Service - Huntsville
Alabama Department Of Rehabilitation Services
3000 Johnson Rd. SW
Huntsville, AL 35805-5847
256-650-1700
800-671-6840
Fax: 256-650-1795
TTY: 800-499-1816
www.rehab.alabama.gov

Eddie C. Williams, Manager

5716 Vocational Rehabilitation Service - Jackson
Alabama Department Of Rehabilitation Services
1401 Forest Ave.
PO Box 1005
Jackson, AL 36545
251-246-5708
800-671-6836
Fax: 251-246-5224
TTY: 800-499-1816
www.rehab.alabama.gov

5717 Vocational Rehabilitation Service - Jasper
Alabama Department Of Rehabilitation Services
4505 Hwy 78 E
Suite 300
Jasper, AL 35501
205-221-7840
800-671-6841
Fax: 205-221-1062
TTY: 800-499-1816
www.rehab.alabama.gov

5718 Vocational Rehabilitation Service - Mobile
Alabama Department Of Rehabilitation Services
3101 International Drive
Bldg. 7
Mobile, AL 36606
251-479-8611
800-671-6842
Fax: 251-478-2197
TTY: 800-499-1816
www.rehab.alabama.gov

Stephen G. Kayes, Manger

5719 Vocational Rehabilitation Service - Muscle Shoals
Alabama Department Of Rehabilitation Services
1615 Trojan Dr
Suite 2
Muscle Shoals, AL 35661
256-381-3184
800-275-0166
Fax: 256-389-3149
TTY: 800-499-1816
www.rehab.alabama.gov

5720 Vocational Rehabilitation Service - Selma
Alabama Department Of Rehabilitation Services
722 Alabama Ave.
Selma, AL 36701
334-877-2927
888-761-5995
Fax: 334-877-3796
TTY: 800-499-1816
www.rehab.alabama.gov

5721 Vocational Rehabilitation Service - Talladega
Alabama Department Of Rehabilitation Services
31 Arnold St.
Talladega, AL 35160
256-362-1300
800-441-7592
Fax: 256-362-6387
TTY: 800-499-1816
www.rehab.alabama.gov

5722 Vocational Rehabilitation Service - Troy
Alabama Department of Rehabilitation Services
1109 Troy Plaza St.
Troy, AL 36081
334-566-2491
800-441-7608
Fax: 334-566-9415
TTY: 800-499-1816
www.rehab.alabama.gov

5723 Vocational Rehabilitation Service - Tuscaloosa
Alabama Department of Rehabilitation Services
1400 James I Harrison Jr Parkway E
Suite 300
Tuscaloosa, AL 35405
205-554-1300
800-331-5562
Fax: 205-554-1369
TTY: 800-499-1816
www.rehab.alabama.gov

William Strickland, Manager

5724 Vocational Rehabilitation Services - Andalusia
Alabama Department of Rehabilitation Services
1082 Village Square Dr.
Suite 1
Andalusia, AL 36420
334-222-4114
800-671-6833
Fax: 334-427-1216
TTY: 800-499-1816
www.rehab.alabama.gov

5725 Vocational Rehabilitation Services - Anniston
Alabama Department of Rehabilitation Services
1910 Coleman Rd.
Anniston, AL 36207
256-240-8800
800-671-6834
Fax: 256-240-6580
TTY: 800-499-1816
www.rehab.alabama.gov

5726 Vocational and Rehabilitation Service - Decatur
Alabama Department of Rehabilitation Services
621 Cherry St. NE
Decatur, AL 35602
256-353-2754
800-671-6838
Fax: 256-351-2476
TTY: 800-499-1816
www.rehab.alabama.gov

5727 Wiregrass Rehabilitation Center, Inc.
795 Ross Clark Circle
Suitr 1
Dothan, AL 36303
334-792-0022
Fax: 334-712-7632
www.wrcjobs.com

John Brown, Chair
Tom West, Vice-Chairman
Ryan Hendrix, Treasurer
Trains individuals to become employable and assists them in finding jobs withing their communities. Also assists individuals who have difficulty maintaining employment, those who are on forms of public assistance such as welfare and those who are employable and underemployed.
1958

5728 Workshops Empowerment, Inc.
4244 3rd Ave. S
Birmingham, AL 35222
205-592-9683
800-368-5688
info@weincal.org
www.weincal.org

Susan Crow, Executive Director
Nathalie Brasher, Director, Programs
Kathy Dunn, Director, Operations
Provides vocational training, sheltered employment and other support services to people with disabilities in central Alabama.

Alaska

5729 Alaska Division of Vocational Rehabilitation
Department of Labor & Workforce Development
P.O. Box 115516
Juneau, AK 99811-5516
907-465-2814
800-478-2815
Fax: 907-465-2856
dol.dvr.info@alaska.gov
www.labor.state.ak.us/dvr

Duane Mayes, Director
Assists individuals with disabilities to obtain and maintain employment.

5730 Alaska Job Center Network
Alaska Department of Labor & Workforce Development
P.O. Box 115514
Juneau, AK 99811-5514
907-465-4562
Fax: 907-465-2984
TTY: 907-465-4562
juneau.jobcenter@alaska.gov
www.jobs.alaska.gov

5731 Alaska State Commission for Human Rights
800 A St
Suite 204
Anchorage, AK 99501-3669
907-274-4692
800-478-4692
Fax: 907-278-8588
hrc@alaska.gov
humanrights.alaska.gov

Arizona

5732 Arizona Developmental Disabilities Planning Council (ADDPC)
3839 North 3rd St.
Suite 306
Phoenix, AZ 85012
602-542-8970
877-665-3176
Fax: 602-542-8978
addpc@azdes.gov
addpc.az.gov

Jon Meyers, Executive Director
Marcella Crane, Grants Manager
Lani St. Cyr, Fiscal Manager
A successor of the Governor's Council on Developmental Disabilities, the ADDPC serves Arizona residents with developmental disabilities and their families through research, education, advocacy, and financial support. The council aims to improve employment, self-advocacy, and community inclusion.

5733 Beacon Group
308 W Glenn St.
Tucson, AZ 85705
520-622-4874
Fax: 520-620-6620
www.beacongroup.org

Provides employment and rehabilitation opportunities for people with disabilities.

5734 Business Enterprise Program (BEP)
Arizona Department of Economic Security
3425 East Van Buren
Suite 102
Phoenix, AZ 85008
602-774-9100
Fax: 602-250-8548
des.az.gov

Michael Wisehart, Director
Provides employment opportunties for legally blind individuals to own merchandising businesses.

5735 Division of Developmental Disabilities
Arizona Department of Economic Security
1789 West Jefferson St.
Phoenix, AZ 85007
844-770-9500
Fax: 602-542-6870
DDDCustomerServiceCenter@azdes.gov
des.az.gov

Michael Wisehart, Director
Provides supports and serivces that help empower individuals with developmental disabilities to exercise their rights, lead independent lives, and be involved in their communities.

5736 Fair Employment Practice Agency: Arizona
Arizona Civil Rights Division
2005 N Central Ave.
Phoenix, AZ 85004-2926
602-542-5025
Fax: 602-542-8885
TTY: 877-624-8090
www.azag.gov

Joseph Sciarrotta, Division Chief
Provides legal advice to most state agencies. The office also investigates and prosecutes consumer fraud, white collar crime, organized crime, public corruption, and civil rights.

5737 Temporary Assistance for Needy Families (TANF)
1717 W Jefferson St.
Phoenix, AZ 85007
602-542-9935
www.tanf.us/arizona.html
Assist applicants and recipients of temporary assistance to needy families to obtain job training and employment that will lead to economic independence.

5738 Vocational Rehabilitation
Department of Economic Security
1789 W. Jefferson St.
Phoenix, AZ 85007
844-770-9500
Fax: 602-542-6870
des.az.gov

Michael Wisehart, Director
This program serves individuals with disabilities seeking jobs and job training by providing them with services that prepare them for entry or rentry into the workforce.

5739 Yavapai Regional Medical Center-West
1003 Willow Creek Rd.
Prescott, AZ 86301
928-445-2700
877-843-9762
yrmc.org

Mike Beatty, Chair
Tony Ferrulli, Vice Chair
Daniel Storvick, Secretary
Widely recognized for the quality and success of the physical, occupational, and speech therapy programs it offers. Provides a wide range of programs and services that enable patients to reach their maximum level of function and independence and enjoy the highest possible quality of life.

Arkansas

5740 Arkansas Department of Workforce Services
P.O. Box 2981
Little Rock, AR 72203
501-682-2121
844-908-2178
Fax: 501-682-8845
ADWS.Info@arkansas.gov
www.dws.arkansas.gov

Charisse Childers, Director
Jay Bassett, Deputy Director
Courtney Traylor, Deputy Director
Provides a wide range of services, including unemployment insurance, employment assistance, and Temporary Assistance for Needy Families.

5741   Arkansas Rehabilitation Services (ARS)
1 Commerce Way
Little Rock, AR 72202   501-296-1600
                                    Fax: 501-296-1141
                        ACECommunications@arkansas.gov
                                  arcareereducation.org
Charisse Childers, Director
Joseph Baxter, Commissioner
Trenia Miles, Director, Adult Education
The Arkansas Rehabilitation Services prepares people with disabilities to work and lead productive, independent lives.

5742   Easterseals Arkansas
3920 Woodland Heights Rd.
Little Rock, AR 72212   501-227-3600
                                 info@eastersealsar.com
                            www.easterseals.com/arkansas
Ron Ekstrand, President & Chief Executive Officer
Stephanie Smith, Chief Program Officer
Stacy Ferguson, Chief Administration & Financial Officer
Mission is to provide exceptional services to ensure that all people with disabilities or special needs have equal opportunities to live, learn, work, and play in their communities.
1944

5743   Vocational Rehabilitation Services
Arkansas Division of Services for the Blind
P.O. Box 1437
Little Rock, AR 72203   501-682-1001
                                    TTY: 501-682-8820
                        humanservices.arkansas.gov/about-dhs/dsb
Cindy Gillespie, Secretary
Keesa M. Smith, Deputy Director, Youth & Families
Dawn Stehle, Deputy Director, Health & State Medicaid Director
A comprehensive state program designed to assess the needs of blind or visually impaired individuals, and to plan, develop, and provide them with employment services.

California

5744   ABLE Industries, Inc.
8929 W. Goshen Ave.
Visalia, CA 93291   559-651-8150
                               kstump@ableindustries.org
                                  www.ableindustries.org
Keith R. Stump, Executive Director
Tracy Hart, President
Michael Stafford, Vice President
Committed to improving the lives of people with disabilities by creating opportunities to maximize their independence through job training, employment, life skills education, and community support services.
1962

5745   AbilityFirst

                                          626-396-1010
                                          877-768-4600
                                   info@abilityfirst.org
                                     www.abilityfirst.org
Lori Gangemi, President & Chief Executive Officer
Kashif Khan, Chief Financial Officer
Keri Castaneda, Chief Program Officer
Provides programs and services to help children and adults with physical and developmental disabilities reach their full potential throughout their lives. Offers a broad range of employment, recreational, and socialization programs.

5746   Achievement House & NCI Affiliates
3003 Cuesta College Rd.
San Luis Obispo, CA 93405   805-543-9383
                                info@achievementhouse.org
                                 www.achievementhouse.org
Provides vocational opportunities for individuals with special needs that respect personal choice and diversity, and reflect individualized goals that support enhanced independence, personal responsibility, and self-esteem.

5747   Anthesis
1063 W. 6th Street
Ontario, CA 91762   909-624-3555
                                             anthesis.us
Mitch Gariador, Executive Director
Kitty DuBois, Director of Human Resources
Terri Perkins, Director of Employment Programs
Anthesis seeks to assist adults with disabilities to reach their full potential through services such as vocational training, employment preparation, and placement services.

5748   Bakersfield ARC
4500 California Ave
Bakersfield, CA 93309   661-834-2272
                                        www.barc-inc.org
A nonprofit organization that provides essential job training, employment, and support services for the developmentally disabled and their families.
1949

5749   California Department of Fair Employment& Housing
2218 Kausen Dr.
Suite 100
Elk Grove, CA 95758   800-884-1684
                                     TTY: 800-700-2320
                             contact.center@dfeh.ca.gov
                                         www.dfeh.ca.gov
Kevin Kish, Director
Mary Wheat, Chief Deputy Director
Jannette Wipper, Chief Counsel
The Department of Fair Employment and Housing protects Californians from employment, housing, and public accomodation discrimination, as well as hate violence.

5750   Colton-Redlands-Yucaipa Regional Occupational Program (CRY-ROP)
1214 Indiana Ct.
Redlands, CA 92374   909-793-3115
                                    Fax: 909-793-6901
                                         www.cryrop.org
Provides hands-on training programs in over 40 high-demand career fields to assist high school students and adults in acquiring marketable job skills. Works in cooperation with local high schools, adult education colleges, and employers to ensure a coordinated integration of academic and career preparation. Support services, career guidance, and services are provided to disabled people.

5751   Community Employment Services
Hope Services
30 Las Colinas Ln.
San Jose, CA 95119-1212   408-284-2850
                                     www.hopeservices.org
Charles "Chip" Huggins, President & Chief Executive Officer
Clayton Ng, Chief Financial Officer
Sujan Vatturi, Chief Information Officer
Hope Services provides a comprehensive and integrated employment service that provides job training, job placement, and on-the-job training for individuals with developmental disabilities.

5752   Continuing Education & Employment Development Program
The Arc San Francisco
1500 Howard St.
San Francisco, CA 94103   415-255-7200
                                    Fax: 415-255-9488
                                      info@thearcsf.org
                                        www.thearcsf.org
Kristen Pedersen, Director
Jennifer Dresen, Senior Director, Programs
Nina Asay, Senior Director, Administration & Operations
Preparing individuals with disabilities for employment through real-world experiences, trainings, and internships.

5753   Desert Haven Enterprises
43437 Copeland Circle
P.O. Box 2110
Lancaster, CA 93535   661-948-8402
                                    Fax: 661-948-1080
                                      www.deserthaven.org

A private, nonprofit organization dedicated to developing, enhancing, and promoting the capabilities of persons with developmental disabilities.

5754 Employment Development Department
P.O. Box 826880
MIC 83
Sacramento, CA 94280-0001
916-654-7799
800-758-0398
www.edd.ca.gov

Nancy Farias, Director
Provides job and unemployment listings, disability insurance, and other information for job seekers and employers.

5755 Fresno City College: Disabled Students Programs and Services
Fresno City College
1101 E. University Ave.
Fresno, CA 93741
559-442-8237
Fax: 559-499-6038
TTY: 559-442-8237
susan.arriola@fresnocitycollege.edu
www.fresnocitycollege.edu

Susan Arriola, Director
The Disabled Students Programs & Services (DSPS) at Fresno City College provides services for students with physical, learning and/or psychological disabilities to successfully pursue their individual educational, vocational, and personal goals. Some programs offered include basic computer training, adaptive software training, independent living and consumer skills training, note-taking assistance, special classes, and more.

5756 Heartland Opportunity Center
323 N.E. St.
Madera, CA 93638
559-674-8828
Fax: 559-674-8857

Provides employment, job placement, vocational, and life skills training to adults with mental, physical and/or emotional disabilities in order to help them reach their personal and vocational goals.

5757 INALLIANCE Inc.
6950 21st Ave.
Sacramento, CA 95820
916-381-1300
Fax: 916-381-9026
acroom@inallianceinc.com
inallianceinc.com

Andrea Croom, Executive Director
Auriel Taurone, Intake Coordinator
Committed to providing services that contribute to the independence of adults with developmental disabilities and acquired brain injury. Services focus on job placement, employment training, and the facilitation of supports necessary for integrated employment and community living.

5758 Kings Rehabilitation Center
490 E. Hanford Armona Rd.
Hanford, CA 93230
559-582-9234
www.kingsrehab.com

Steve Mendoza, Executive Director
Kings Rehabilitation Center provides day program services, vocational training, and employment opportunities for individuals with disabilities.

5759 Mother Lode Rehabilitation Enterprises, Inc. (MORE)
399 Placerville Dr.
Placerville, CA 95667
530-622-4848
www.morerehab.org

Susie Davies, Chief Executive Officer
Nancy Cramer, Chair
Steve Shortes, Vice Chair
A private, nonprofit organization dedicated to supporting persons with disabilities. Established by parents, educators, rehabilitation professionals, and concerned citizens in 1973, MORE now offers training for social, living, and vocational skills.
1973

5760 Napa Valley PSI Inc.
651 Trabajo Ln.
P.O. Box 600
Napa, CA 94559-600
707-255-0177
lea@napavalleypsi.org
www.napavalleypsi.org

Carol Gonsalves, President
Raymond Ingersoll, Vice President
Eleanor Cullum, Secretary
Provides work training, work opportunities, and job placement services for developmentally disabled adults. Emphasis is on manufacture of quality wood products, primarily wooden office furniture.

5761 PRIDE Industries
10030 Foothills Blvd.
Roseville, CA 95747-7102
916-788-2100
800-550-6005
Fax: 800-888-0447
info@prideindustries.com
www.prideindustries.com

Jeff Dern, President & Chief Executive Officer
Casey Blake, Chief Operating Officer
Everett Crane, Chief Financial Officer
Provides vocational and employment services that create jobs for people with disabilites; services include career counseling, vocational assessment, work adjustment, work services, job seeking skills, job development, job placement, on-the-job support (coaching), mentoring, independent living skills, transition services, and case management.

5762 Parents and Friends, Inc
306 E. Redwood Ave.
P.O. Box 656
Fort Bragg, CA 95437
707-964-4940
Fax: 707-964-8536
rmoon@parentsandfriends.org
www.parentsandfriends.org

Rick Moon, Chief Executive Director
Sage Statham, President
Jacqueline Bazor, Vice President
Serves people with developmental disabilities by providing them with oppotunities to participate in their community.

5763 PathPoint
315 W. Haley St.
Suite 202
Santa Barbara, CA 93101
805-966-3310
Fax: 805-966-5582
jeannie.barbieri-low@pathpoint.org
www.pathpoint.org

Henry Bruell, President & Chief Executive Officer
Mark Maynard, Chief People Officer
Stephanie Eubanks, Treasurer
Dedicated to providing comprehensive training and support services that empower people with disabilities or disadvantages to live and work as valued members of the community.

5764 People Services, Inc
4195 Lakeshore Blvd.
Lakeport, CA 95453
707-263-3810
Fax: 707-263-0552
info@peopleservices.org
www.peopleservices.org

Dana Lewis, Executive Director
Cindy Ustrud, President
Kathy Windrem, Vice President
Dedicated to serving as the local community agency, providing the delivery of quality services for people with disabilities.

5765 Porterville Sheltered Workshop
194 W. Poplar Ave.
Porterville, CA 93257
559-784-1399
pswcares.org

Don Sowers, Executive Director
Carol Ledbetter, Director of Program Services
Elizabeth Tellez, Director of Finance
Provides work adjustment and remunerative work programs. Their mission is to assist disabled individuals achieve a more independent and productive life.
1956

5766   Project Independence
3505 Cadillac Ave.
Suite O-103
Costa Mesa, CA 92626   714-549-3464
                                    877-444-0144
                               Fax: 714-549-3559
                       www.proindependence.org
Robert Watson, President & Chief Executive Officer
Dorothy M. Blubaugh, Chief Operations Officer
Meka Green, Director of Human Resources
Promotes civil rights for people with developmental disabilities
through services which expand independence and choice.

5767   Projects with Industry (PWI) Program
Whittier Union High School District
9401 S. Painter Ave.
Whittier, CA 90605   562-698-8121
                                    www.wuhsd.org
The Transitional and Vocational Services Department runs the
PWI program, which focuses on career planning, employment
preparation, job placement, and career advancement for individu-
als with mild to significant disabilities.

5768   Shasta County Opportunity Center
1265 Redwood Blvd.
Redding, CA 96003   530-225-5781
                               Fax: 530-225-5751
                 oppcenter_info@co.shasta.ca.us
                          www.co.shasta.ca.us
Donnell Ewert, Director, Health and Human Services Agency
An employment training program for people with disabilities in
Shasta County. These individuals perform paid work in a number
of different work environments and at the same time learn the
skills necessary to obtain competetive employment in the local
community.

5769   Social Vocational Services
3555 Torrance Blvd.
Torrance, CA 90503   310-944-3303
                               Fax: 310-944-3304
                   www.socialvocationalservices.org
The leading provider of services for people with developmental
disabilities in the state of California. Social Vocational Services
provides a paid work program for adults with developmental
disabilities.

5770   South Bay Vocational Center
20706 Main St.
Carson, CA 90745   310-817-5116
                               Info@SBVC1.com
                               www.sbvc1.com
A not-for-profit organization that has been providing excellent
vocational programs and services for individuals with
disabilities.

5771   The Arc Los Angeles and Orange Counties
12049 Woodruff Ave.
Downey, CA 90241   562-803-4606
                               Fax: 562-803-6550
                               www.thearclaoc.org
Dedicated to improving the lives of children and adults with intellectual and developmental disabilities and their families through
educational and employment opportunities.
1956

5772   Tri-County Independent Living Center
139 5th St.
Eureka, CA 95501   707-445-8404
                                    833-866-8444
                               aa@tilinet.org
                               www.tilinet.org
Eddie Morgan, Executive Director
Kevin O'Brien, President
Devva Kasnitz, Vice President
Aims to provide programs, services, and information for people
with disabilities living in Humboldt, Del Norte, and Trinity
Counties in northern California in an effort to allow choices for
individuals to optimize their independence.

5773   Unyeway
11657 Riverside Dr.
Suite 165
Lakside, CA 92040   619-334-6502
                               Fax: 619-334-6504
                               www.unyeway.com
Kimberly Kelley, Executive Director
A California nonprofit that provides employment opportunities
for adults with developmental disabilities such as job placement
programs, remunerative work services, and work adjustment
training programs.

5774   Valley Light Industries
5360 N. Irwindale Ave.
Baldwin Park, CA 91706   626-337-6200
                          admin@valleylightind.org
                          www.valleylightctr.org
Sage Newman, Chief Executive Officer
Ivan Campos, Director of Operations
Aims to recognize the unique capacities of individuals with dis-
abilities, and provide them with the same opportunities of
employment.

5775   Work Training Center
80 Independence Circle
Chico, CA 95973   530-343-7994
                               info@ewtc.org
                               www.wtcinc.org
Brett Barker, Chief Executive Director
Laura Carter, Chief Financial Officer
Julie Ellen, Director, Facilities & Maintenance
A nonprofit organization providing work and leisure services to
people with disabilities.

Colorado

5776   Blue Peaks Developmental Services
703 Fourth St.
Alamosa, CO 81101-2638   719-589-5135
                               Fax: 719-589-0680
                               www.bluepeaks.org
Cindy Espinoza, Executive Director
Loren Velasquez, Operations Diretor
Brock Gallegos, Finance Director
Provides remunerative work for persons with intellectual and de-
velopmental disabilities in the San Luis Valley.

5777   Cheyenne Village
6275 Lehman Dr.
Colorado Springs, CO 80918   719-592-0200
                               Fax: 719-548-9947
                               TTY: 719-592-0224
                          www.cheyennevillage.org
Tim Cunningham, Chief Executive Officer
Mary Dice, Chief Financial Officer
Travers Hyde, Director of Operations
Serves adults with developmental disabilities and intellectual
disabilities in El Paso, Teller, and Park Counties.

5778   Colorado Civil Rights Divsion
1560 Broadway
Suite 110
Denver, CO 80202   303-894-2997
                                    800-262-4845
                                    TTY: 711
                          dora_ccrd@state.co.us
                          www.ccrd.colorado.gov
Aubrey Elenis, Director
Embraces the Department's mission of consumer protection and
works to protect individuals from discrimination in employment,
housing, and at places of public accommodation through enforce-
ment and outreach consistent with the Colorado Civil Rights
Laws.

5779   Developmental Disabilities Resource Center (DDRC)
11177 West 8th Ave.
Lakewood, CO 80215   303-233-3363
                                    contact@ddrcco.com
                                              ddrcco.com

C. David Pemberton, President
Joanne Elliott, Vice President
Susan Hartley, Treasurer
Residental and employment programs for adults with developmental and intellectual disabilities.

5780   Division of Vocational Rehabilitation
Department of Labor and Employment
633 17th St.
Suite 1501
Denver, CO 80202   303-318-8571
                              CDLE_voc.rehab@state.co.us
                                      www.colorado.gov/dvr
Assists people with disabilities to succeed at work and living independently.

5781   Dynamic Dimensions
567 18th St.
Burlington, CO 80807   719-346-5367
                                      Fax: 719-346-6010
                              exdir@dynamicdimensions.org
                                    dynamicdimensions.org

Ginny Hallagin, Executive Director
Shawn Calhoon, Finance Manager
Debbie Lamm, Assistant Executive Director & Program Manager
An organization that provides training, advocacy, job placement, and community involvement for individuals with disabilities.

5782   Eastern Colorado Services for the Developmentally Disabled (ECSDD)
617 S. 10th Ave.
Sterling, CO 80751   970-522-7121
                                      Fax: 970-522-1173
                                              www.ecsdd.org

Rhonda Roth, Executive Director
Kasha Sheets, Finance Director
Lori Araujo, Case Management Director
Assists developmentally disabled individuals by providing vocational opportunities within their communities.

5783   Hope Center
3400 Elizabeth St.
Denver, CO 80205-4801   303-388-4801
                                      Fax: 303-388-0249
                                      gghope@comcast.net
                                    www.hopecenterinc.org

Gerie Grimes, President & Chief Executive Officer
Janell Lindsey, Acting Chair
Mary A. Davis, Secretary & Treasurer
Provides educational and vocational opportunities for special-needs and at-risk children and adults from 2-1/2 to adulthood.

5784   Imagine!
1400 Dixon Ave.
Lafayette, CO 80026-2790   303-665-7789
                                    www.imaginecolorado.org

Rebecca Novinger, Executive Director
Jeff Tucker, Director of Human Resources
Jenna Corder, Director of Client Relations
Provides support services to people of all ages with developmental delays and cognitive disabilities including Autism Spectrum Disorder, Cerebral Palsy, and Down Syndrome.

5785   Las Animas County Rehabilitation Center
1205 Congress Dr.
P.O. Box 781
Trinidad, CO 81082-781   719-846-3388
                                      Fax: 719-846-4543
                                          info@scdds.com
                                              www.scdds.com

Duane Roy, Executive Director
Mari Mason, Case Management Director
David Moore, Chief Financial Officer
Provides job placement programs, remunerative work services, and work adjustment training programs.

Connecticut

5786   Abilities Without Boundaries
615 W. Johnson Ave.
Cheshire, CT 06410   203-272-5607
                                      Fax: 203-272-4284
                              www.abilitieswithoutboundaries.org
Amanda Barnes, Executive Director
Lloyd R. Saberksi, President
Clay Yalof, Vice President
Formerly known as Cheshire Occupational & Career Opportunities (COCO), Abilities Without Boundaries provides opportunities in the community through employment and social experiences for people with developmental disabilities.

5787   Allied Community Services
3 Pearson Way
Enfield, CT 06082   860-741-3701
                                      Fax: 860-741-6870
                                      www.alliedgroup.org
Carol Bohnet, President & Chief Executive Officer
Provides individuals with disabilities or other challenges the opportunity to live and enjoy a productive, independent, and fulfilling life.

5788   Area Cooperative Educational Services(ACES)
350 State St.
North Haven, CT 06473   203-498-6800
                                      Fax: 203-498-6890
                                              www.aces.org
Thomas M. Danehy, Executive Director
Timothy Howes, Deputy Executive Director
Steve Cook, Director, Human Resources
Offers adult and vocational programs for persons with disabilities.

5789   Bureau of Rehabilitation Services
Department of Rehabilitation Services
55 Farmington Ave.
12th Fl.
Hartford, CT 06105   860-424-5055
                                      Fax: 860-424-4850
                                      TTY: 860-247-0775
                              kathleen.sullivan@ct.gov
                                          www.ct.gov/brs
A program which aids disabled persons with preparing for, finding, and keeping employment.

5790   CCARC, Inc.
950 Slater Rd.
New Britain, CT 06053-1658   860-229-6665
                                          ccarc@ccarc.com
                                              www.ccarc.com
Lind Iovanna, Chief Executive Officer
Stacey Vonrichthofen, Chief Operating Officer
Julie Erickson, Senior Vice President
Provides support to people with a variety of disabilities by offering day, residential, recreational, and advocacy services.

5791   CW Resources
200 Myrtle St.
New Britain, CT 06053   860-229-7700
                                      Fax: 860-229-6847
                                      info@cwresources.org
                                    www.cwresources.org
Offers integrated vocational training and employment opportunities for individuals with a variety of different disabilities.

5792   Connecticut Governor's Committee on Employment of People with Disabilities
Connecticut Department of Labor
200 Folly Brook Blvd.
Wethersfield, CT 06109   860-263-6007
                                      dol.webhelp@ct.gov
                                    www.ctdol.state.ct.us
The Committee promotes the employment of people with disabilities by developing programs and initiatives to increase statewide employment opportunities for disabled individuals.

5793 Fotheringhay Farms
The Caring Community of CT
84 Waterhole Rd.
Colchester, CT 06415   860-267-4463
Fax: 860-267-7628
info@caringcommunityct.org
caringcommunityct.org
The Caring Community offers an agri-based vocational skill development through Fotheringhay Farms in green house, barnyard, and garden settings.
1984

5794 George Hegyi Industrial Training Center
5 Coon Hollow Rd.
Derby, CT 06418   203-735-8727

A private, nonprofit agency that offers work programs to individuals with special needs.

5795 Goodwill of Southern New England
432 Washington Ave.
North Haven, CT 06473   203-777-2000
888-909-8188
www.goodwillsne.org
H. Richard Borer, President
Robert Burns, Chief Operations Officer
Marcus O. Notz, Chief Information Officer & Marketing/Public Relations
Provides training, education and other services which result in employment and expanded opportunities for people with disabilities and other barriers to employment in order to enhance their capacity for independent living, increased quality of life and work.

5796 Kennedy Center
2440 Reservoir Ave.
Trumbull, CT 06611   203-365-8522
Fax: 203-365-8533
info@kennedyctr.org
www.thekennedycenterinc.org
Richard E. Sebastian, Jr., President & Chief Executive Officer
Stuart Gordon, Vice President of Finance
Greg Pierson, Facilities Manager
Provides vocational rehabilitation, job training, and job placement services to adults with disabilities.

Delaware

5797 Delaware Division of Vocational Rehabilitation
Delaware Department of Labor
4425 North Market St.
Wilmington, DE 19802   302-761-8275
TTY: 302-761-8275
www.delawareworks.com
The state's public program that helps people with physical and mental disabilities obtain or retain employment. DVR's commitment is to help people with disabilities increase independence through employment.

5798 Service Source
13 Reads Way
Suite 101
New Castle, DE 19802   302-762-0300
DRIVE@servicesource.org
www.servicesource.org
Mark Hall, President
Bruce Patterson, Chief Executive Officer
Nate Hoover, Chief Financial Officer
ServiceSource is a leading nonprofit disability resource organization with regional offices and programs located in eight states and the District of Columbia. They offer a range of innovative employment, training, habilitation, housing, and other support services. ServiceSource directly employs more than 1,500 individuals on government and commercial affirmative employment contracts.

District of Columbia

5799 District of Columbia Department of Employment Services
4058 Minnesota Ave. NE
Washington, DC 20019   202-724-7000
Fax: 202-673-6993
TTY: 202-698-4817
does@dc.gov
does.dc.gov
Unique Morris-Hughes, Director
Jason Washington, Chief of Staff
Ramon Perez-Goizueta, Chief Compliance Officer
Their mission is to foster economic development and growth in the District of Columbia by providing workforce training, bringing together job seekers and employers, compensating unemployed and injured workers, and promoting safe and healthy workplaces.

5800 Goodwill of Greater Washington
2200 South Dakota Ave. NE
Washington, DC 20018   202-636-4225
888-817-4323
Fax: 202-526-3994
info@dcgoodwill.org
dcgoodwill.org
Catherine Meloy, President & Chief Executive Officer
Colleen Paletta, Chief Integration Officer
Rosa Proctor, Chief Financial Officer
Offers vocational training, job training, sheltered employment, and work experience.

5801 Palladium
1331 Pennsylvania Ave. NW
Suite 600
Washington, DC 20004   202-775-9680
thepalladiumgroup.com
Kim Bredhauer, Chairman
Christopher Hirst, Managing Director & Chief Executive Officer
Residential and employment programs for adults with developmental disabilities.

5802 Rehabilitation Services Administration
400 Maryland Ave. SW
Washington, DC 20202   202-401-2000
800-872-5327
TTY: 800-730-8913
www2.ed.gov
State Rehabilitation Agency providing services to eligible persons with disabilities.

5803 The District of Columbia Office of Human Rights (OHR)
441 4th St. NW
Suite 570 North
Washington, DC 20001   202-727-4559
Fax: 202-727-9589
TTY: 711
ohr@dc.gov
ohr.dc.gov
Hnin Khaing, Interim Director
Upholds local and federal human rights laws, and aims to eradicate discrimination and increase equal opportunity for residents of the District of Columbia.

Florida

5804 Abilities of Florida: An Affiliate of Service Source
2735 Whitney Rd.
Clearwater, FL 33760   727-538-7370
servicesource.org/florida
Provides a full range of employment services including work evaluation, training, job coaching, job placement, advocacy, and education. Also provides housing assistance and specialized to adults with cystic fibrosis.

5805 Able Trust, The
3320 Thomasville Rd.
Suite 200
Tallahassee, FL 32308   850-224-4493
                              Fax: 850-224-4496
                              info@abletrust.org
                              www.abletrust.org
Allison Chase, President & Chief Executive Officer
Joey D'Souza, Vice President, External Engagement
Donna Wright, Vice President, Development & Marketing
Provides grant funds for employment-related programs for non-profit agencies in Florida. Assists families, individuals, and agencies through educational conferences and youth training programs. Provides businesses free resources for hiring people with disabilities.

5806 Florida Division of Blind Services
325 West Gaines St.
Turlington Building, Suite 1114
Tallahassee, FL 32399-0400   850-245-0300
                               800-342-1828
                               Fax: 850-245-0363
                               dbs.myflorida.com
Robert Doyle, Director
An organization that aims to help blind and visually impaired individuals have access to tools, support, and oppotunities in order to live independent lives. Offers a Vocational Rehabilitation program for adults, and a Transition Services program for young adults.

5807 Florida Division of Vocational Rehabilitation
4070 Esplanade Way
Tallahassee, FL 32399-7016   800-451-4327
                               Fax: 850-245-3399
                               rehabworks.org
A federal-state program that helps people with physical or mental disabilities get a job.

5808 Florida Fair Employment Practice Agency
Florida Commission on Human Relations
4075 Esplanade Way
Room 110
Tallahassee, FL 32399   850-488-7082
                               800-342-8170
                               Fax: 850-487-1007
                               fchrinfo@fchr.myflorida.com
                               fchr.state.fl.us
Michelle Wilson, Executive Director
The Commission is the state agency charged with enforcing the state's civil rights laws and serves as a resource on human relations for the people of Florida.

5809 Goodwill Life Skills Development Program
Goodwill Industries-Suncoast, Inc.
10596 Gandy Blvd.
St. Petersburg, FL 33702   727-523-1512
                               888-279-1988
                               Fax: 727-579-0850
                               TTY: 727-579-1068
                               goodwill-suncoast.org
Deborah A. Passerini, President & Chief Executive Officer
Tracey Boucher, Corporate Treasurer & Chief Financial Officer
Kris Rawson, Vice President for Mission Services & Chief Mission Officer
A training program that enables people with developmental disabilities to gain independence by practicing job skills.

5810 Goodwill Temporary Staffing
Goodwill Industries-Suncoast, Inc.
10596 Gandy Blvd.
St. Petersburg, FL 33702   727-523-1512
                               888-279-1988
                               Fax: 727-579-0850
                               TTY: 727-579-1068
                               goodwill-suncoast.org
Deborah A. Passerini, President & Chief Executive Officer
Tracey Boucher, Corporate Treasurer & Chief Financial Officer
Kris Rawson, Vice President for Mission Services & Chief Mission Officer
Provides employment links from potential employees, both disabled and non-disabled alike to employers with immediate em-

ployment opportunities seeking qualified candidates. Pre-screening on all applicants includes employment history, personal references, law enforcement background checks, and substance screening.

5811 Goodwill's Community Employment Services
Goodwill Industries-Suncoast, Inc.
10596 Gandy Blvd.
St. Petersburg, FL 33702   727-523-1512
                               888-279-1988
                               Fax: 727-579-0850
                               TTY: 727-579-1068
                               goodwill-suncoast.org
Deborah A. Passerini, President & Chief Executive Officer
Tracey Boucher, Corporate Treasurer & Chief Financial Officer
Kris Rawson, Vice President for Mission Services & Chief Mission Officer
Provides employment opportunities for people with developmental disabilities. Community Employment Services offer on-the-job training and check ups from a support facilitator.

5812 Goodwill's Job Connection Center
Goodwill Industries-Suncoast, Inc.
10596 Gandy Blvd.
St. Petersburg, FL 33702   727-523-1512
                               888-279-1988
                               Fax: 727-579-0850
                               TTY: 727-579-1068
                               www.goodwill-suncoast.org
Deborah A. Passerini, President & Chief Executive Officer
Tracey Boucher, Corporate Treasurer & Chief Financial Officer
Kris Rawson, Vice President for Mission Services & Chief Mission Officer
A local, community-based space where people can search for employment. The center offers carrer planning and exploration, employability workshops, and training.

5813 Goodwill's JobWorks
Goodwill Industries-Suncoast, Inc.
10596 Gandy Blvd.
St. Petersburg, FL 33702   727-523-1512
                               888-279-1988
                               Fax: 727-579-0850
                               TTY: 727-579-1068
                               www.goodwill-suncoast.org
Deborah A. Passerini, President & Chief Executive Officer
Tracey Boucher, Corporate Treasurer & Chief Financial Officer
Kris Rawson, Vice President for Mission Services & Chief Mission Officer
A program that provides employment for people with disabilities at MacDill Air Force Base in dining or postal services.

5814 Lighthouse Central Florida
215 East New Hampshire St.
Orlando, FL 32804   407-898-2483
                               Fax: 407-898-0236
                               lighthousecentralflorida.com
Kyle Johnson, President & Chief Executive Officer
Kaleb Stunkard, Executive Vice President & Chief Operations Officer
Ryan Brown, Vice President, Operations
Lighthouse Central Florida (LCF) is the only nonprofit organization offering comprehensive, professional, vision rehabilitation services to Central Floridians of all ages with low vision or blindness.

5815 One-Stop Service Center
Goodwill Industries-Suncoast, Inc.
10596 Gandy Blvd.
St. Petersburg, FL 33702   727-523-1512
                               888-279-1988
                               Fax: 727-579-0850
                               TTY: 727-579-1068
                               goodwill-suncoast.org
Deborah A. Passerini, President & Chief Executive Officer
Tracey Boucher, Corporate Treasurer & Chief Financial Officer
Kris Rawson, Vice President for Mission Services & Chief Mission Officer
Provides universal job search and placement related services to any person entering the service center. Each One-Stop Services Center provides on-site representation from a variety of employ-

ment-related service providers. All Centers host and/or facilitate local employment fairs and provides access to computerized job postings.

5816 Palm Beach Habilitation Center
4522 South Congress Ave.
Palm Springs, FL 33461 561-965-8500
Fax: 561-433-2073
pbhab.com

Patty Isola, Interim Chief Executive Officer
Cara Webster, Controller
Danielle Hanson, Chief Development Officer
Providing work evaluation, work adjustment, job placement, employment, residential, and retirement services for mentally, emotionally, and physically disabled adults.

5817 Primrose Center
2733 South Ferncreek Ave.
Orlando, FL 32806 407-898-7201
www.primrosecenter.org

Bill McCormac, Chief Executive Officer
Karen Schlachter, Chief Financial Officer
Leslie North, President & Chair
A nonprofit organization that aims to transform the lives of people with developmental disabilities by providing opportunities to achieve their fullest potential. Primrose Center offers an Adult Day Program and an Employment Services Program, which provide opportunities for individuals with intellectual and developmental disabilities to gain employment.

5818 Project SEARCH
Goodwill Industries-Suncoast, Inc.
10596 Gandy Blvd.
St. Petersburg, FL 33702 727-523-1512
888-279-1988
Fax: 727-579-0850
TTY: 727-579-1068
www.goodwill-suncoast.org
Deborah A. Passerini, President & Chief Executive Officer
Tracey Boucher, Corporate Treasurer & Chief Financial Officer
Kris Rawson, Vice President for Mission Services & Chief Mission Officer
A program for students with disabilities that provides work experience.

5819 Quest, Inc.
PO Box 531125
Orlando, FL 32853 407-218-4300
888-807-8378
Fax: 407-218-4301
contact@questinc.org
www.questinc.org
John Gill, President & Chief Executive Officer
Brooke Eakins, Chief Operating Officer
Todd Thrasher, Chief Financial Officer
Quest helps individuals with developmental disabilities in Central Florida achieve their goals by providing services that increase their capabilities and quality of life. Quest serves more than 1,000 individuals each day in the Orlando and Tampa areas.

5820 Quest, Inc. - Tampa Area
3910 US Hwy. 301 N
Tampa, FL 33619 813-423-7700
888-807-8378
Fax: 813-423-7701
contact@questinc.org
www.questinc.org
John Gill, President & Chief Executive Officer
Brooke Eakins, Chief Operating Officer
Todd Thrasher, Chief Financial Officer
Quest helps individuals with developmental disabilities in Central Florida achieve their goals by providing services that increase their capabilities and quality of life. Quest serves more than 1,000 individuals each day in the Orlando and Tampa areas.

5821 SCARC, Inc.

973-383-7442

A nonprofit organization that provides a training and employment program for adults with disabilities. SCARC offers voca-

tional evaluation, training, work services, transportation, supported independent living, and community based training.

5822 Seagull Industries for the Disabled
3879 Byron Dr.
West Palm Beach, FL 33404 561-842-5814
Info@Seagull.org
www.seagull.org
Laura Fowler, Chair
Judy Dynia, Vice Chair
Jim Weber, Secretary
Dedicated to improving the quality of life of mentally, physically, and emotionally challenged adults in Palm Beach County, Florida through advocacy and the provision of a variety of social service, vocational training, and residential programs designed to encourage self reliance and independence.

Georgia

5823 Fair Housing and Equal Employment
Georgia Commission on Equal Opportunity
205 Jesse Hill Jr. Dr. SE
14th Floor-1470B East Tower
Atlanta, GA 30334 404-656-1736
800-473-6736
Fax: 404-656-4399
gceo@gceo.state.ga.us
www.gceo.state.ga.us
Allona Lane Cross, Executive Director & Administrator
Jonathan Paul Harris, Deputy Director
Caprisa T. Clowney, Equal Employment Division Director
The mission of the Commission on Equal Opportunity is to investigate housing and employment discrimination in the state of Georgia.

5824 Goodwill Career Centers
Goodwill of North Georgia
2201 Lawrenceville Hwy.
Suite 300
Decatur, GA 30033 404-420-9900
goodwillng.org
Keith T. Parker, President & Chief Executive Officer
Jenny Taylor, Vice President of Career Services
Employment training, assessment, and job placement for people who have disabilities and/or are disadvantaged. The center also provides access to computers and phones to aid in acquiring employment.

5825 Griffin Area Resource Center
931 Hamilton Blvd.
Griffin, GA 30224 770-228-9919
Fax: 770-228-9920
griffinarearesourcecenter.com
Lisa Sassaman, Executive Director
Connie Moody, Director of Support Services
Kim Byrom, Day Support Supervisor
A CARF (The Rehabilitation Accreditation Commission) accredited Employment and Community Support organization providing daily services to participants with disabilities from 16 years of age and up in a 5 county area.
1955

5826 New Ventures
306 Fort Dr.
LaGrange, GA 30240 706-882-7723
dhigh@newventures.org
newventures.org
J.M. Rawlinson, Chair
David Kegel, Vice Chair
Kathleen Ernest, Secretary
A rehabilitation and work training facility for individuals with barriers to employability. The program utilizes community based industrial work of varying levels of difficulty. A return to work conditioning program for the industrially injured is offered which features first-day contact, workers compensation rehabilitation team management, and light-duty work conditioning. A training stipend is paid to defray costs associated with training.

5827 Vocational and Rehabilitation Agency
1718 Peachtree St. NW
Suite 376 S.
Atlanta, GA 30309
844-367-4872
gvs.georgia.gov

Chris Wells, Executive Director
Thomas W. Wilson, Chair
Faye Perdue, Vice Chair
Purpose is to assist eligible individuals with disabilities to become productive members of the Georgia workforce and to live independently.

Hawaii

5828 Assets School
One Ohana Nui Way
Honolulu, HI 96818
808-423-1356
Fax: 808-422-1920
info@assets-school.net
assets-school.net

Kitty Yannone, Chair
Assets School serves gifted and capable students, specializing in those with dyslexia and other language-based learning differences. They provide a strength-based program, complemented by outreach and training, that empowers students to become effective learners and confident self-advocates.

5829 Hawaii Fair Employment Practice Agency
Hawaii Civil Rights Commission
830 Punchbowl St.
Room 411
Honolulu, HI 96813
808-586-8636
Fax: 808-586-8655
TTY: 808-586-8692
DLIR.HCRC.INFOR@hawaii.gov
labor.hawaii.gov/hcrc

William Hoshijo, Executive Director
HCRC enforces state laws prohibiting discrimination in employment.

5830 Hawaii Vocational Rehabilitation Division
P.O. Box 339
Honolulu, HI 96809-0339
808-586-9741
Fax: 808-586-9755
dhs@dhs.hawaii.gov
humanservices.hawaii.gov/vocationalrehab/

Cathy Betts, Director
Joseph Campos, Deputy Director
Amanda Stevens, Public Information & Communications Officer
Provides services to Hawaiian residents who experience barriers to employment due to physical or cognitive disabilities.

5831 Lanakila Rehabilitation Center
1809 Bachelot St.
Honolulu, HI 96817
808-531-0555
TTY: 808-531-0555
hello@lanakilapacific.org
www.lanakilapacific.org

Rona Yagi Fukumoto, President & Chief Executive Officer
Karen Wong, Vice President of Administration
Dwayne Masutani, Director of Finance
Lanakila is a private nonprofit organization whose mission is to provide services and supports that assist individuals with physical, mental, or age-related challenges to live as independently as possible within their community. A broad range of services are offered which include meal/senior services, community based adult day programming for individuals with disabilities, work training opportunities, and extended/supported employment for individuals with special needs.

5832 Services for the Blind Branch
Division of Vocational Rehabilitation
1390 Miller Street
Room 209
Honolulu, HI 96813
808-586-5679
Fax: 808-586-5700
dhs@dhs.hawaii.gov
humanservices.hawaii.gov/vocationalrehab/

Daisy Hartsfield, Administrator

Provides employment services to Hawaiian residents who are blind or have visual impairments.

Idaho

5833 Idaho Commission for the Blind & Visually Impaired
341 W. Washington St.
P.O. Box 83720
Boise, ID 83720- 0012
208-334-3220
800-542-8688
Fax: 208-334-2963
bcunningham@icbvi.idaho.gov
www.icbvi.state.id.us

Beth Cunningham, Administrator
Steve Achabal, Independent Living Coordinator
Mike Walsh, Rehabilitation Services Chief
A state agency that provides vocational rehabilitation, independent living training, medical intervention, adaptive technology and devices, and employer advocacy.

5834 Idaho Department of Labor
317 W. Main St.
Boise, ID 83735
208-332-8942
Fax: 208-639-3256
www@labor.idaho.gov
labor.idaho.gov

Jani Revier, Director
Provides workforce services and connects job seekers with employers.

5835 Idaho Division of Vocational Rehabilitation
650 W. State St.
Room 150
Boise, ID 83720
208-334-3390
Fax: 208-334-5305
vr.idaho.gov

Jane Donnellan, Administrator
Vocational Rehabilitation assists many individuals with disabilities to go to work. With VR assistance, these individuals have overcome numerous obstacles and disability related barriers to achieve employment.

5836 Idaho Governor's Committee on Employment of People with Disabilities
317 W. Main St.
Boise, ID 83735
208-332-3750
Fax: 208-327-7331
www.dol.gov

Purpose is to promote greater independece for people with disabilities through employment.

5837 Idaho Human Rights Commission
317 W. Main St.
Boise, ID 83735-0660
208-334-2873
888-249-7025
Fax: 208-334-2664
HRC.inquiry@labor.idaho.gov
humanrights.idaho.gov

Jani Revier, Director
Administers state and federal anti-discrimination laws in Idaho in a manner that is fair, accurate, and timely. Works towards ensuring that all people within the state are treated with dignity and respect in their places of employment, housing, education, and public accomodations.

Illinois

5838 Ada S. McKinley Community Services, Inc.
1359 W. Washington Blvd.
Chicago, IL 60607
312-554-0600
Fax: 312-554-0292
info@adasmckinley.org
adasmckinley.org

Jamal Malone, Chief Executive Officer
Peter Greetis, Director of Information Technology
Valerie R. Mercer, Senior Director of Human Resources

Mission is to serve those who, because of disabilities or other limiting conditions, need help in finding and pursuing paths leading to healthy, productive, and fulfilling lives.

5839   Anixter Center
6610 N. Clark St.
Chicago, IL 60626   773-973-7900
                                    AskAnixter@anixter.org
                                            anixter.org

Rebecca Clark, President & Chief Executive Officer
Jonathan Linas, Chair
Tanya Curtis, Secretary
A Chicago-based human services agency that assists people with disabilities to live and work successfully in the community. Anixter Center provides vocational training, employment services, residences, special education, prevention programs, community services, and health care. In addition, Anixter Center offers Illinois' only substance abuse treatment programs specifically for people with disabilities including Addiction Recovery of the Deaf.

5840   C-4 Work Center
4740 North Clark St.
Chicago, IL 60640   773-769-0205
                                           888-968-7282
                                    infoc4@c4chicago.org
                                       www.c4chicago.org

Kerri Brown, Chief Executive Officer
Doug Myers, Interim Chief Financial Officer
Patrick Dombrowski, Chief Clinical Officer
A social service provider that offers aftercare, case finding, information and referrals, vocational training, and work activities offered to mentally ill persons.

5841   Clearbrook
1835 W. Central Rd.
Arlington Heights, IL 60005   847-870-7711
                                      Fax: 847-870-7741
                                      TTY: 847-870-2239
                                     info@clearbrook.org
                                       www.clearbrook.org

Anthony Di Vittorio, President
Kevin Anderko, Vice President of Human Resources
Don Frick, Vice President of Operations
A nonprofit organization that offers educational, employment, and residential services to the developmentally disabled children and adults.

5842   Cornerstone Services
777 Joyce Rd.
Joliet, IL 60436   815-741-7600
                                           877-444-0304
                                      Fax: 815-723-1177
                                   cornerstoneservices.org

Ben Stortz, President & Chief Executive Officer
Kim Hudgens, Vice President & Chief Operating Officer
Ken Mihelich, Vice President & Chief Financial Officer
Cornerstone Services provides progressive, comprehensive services for people with disabilities, promoting choice, dignity, and the opportunity to live and work in the community. Established in 1969, the agency provides developmental, vocational, employment, residential, and behavioral health services at various community-based locations. The nonprofit social service agency helps approximately 750 people each day.
1969

5843   Fulton County Rehab Center
500 N. Main St.
Canton, IL 61520   309-647-6510

Residential rehab center with health care incidental. Manufactures wood pallets and skids and offers job training and vocational rehabilitation services.

5844   Glenkirk
3504 Commercial Ave.
Northbrook, IL 60062   847-272-5111
                                             glenkirk.org
                                           , glenkirk.org

Nicole Zanon, Director, Community & Family Supports

A nonprofit organization serving people in north and northwest Chicago that helps infants, children, and adults with developmental disabilities reach higher levels of independence. Glenkirk's residential, vocational, educational, and support programs include services which provide individual evaluation, therapeutic treatment, and training.

5845   Illinois Life Span Program
The Arc of Illinois
20901 LaGrange Rd.
Suite 209
Frankfort, IL 60423   800-588-7002
                                    www.illinoislifespan.org

Amie Lulinski, Executive Director
Becca Schroeder, Director of Development
Deb Fornoff, Life Span Director
A program of The Arc of Illinois that provides resources, advocacy, and services to individuals of all ages with developmental or intellectual disabilities. The program aims to help individuals with disabilities participate fully in their community.

5846   Jewish Vocational Services
216 West Jackson Blvd.
Suite 700
Chicago, IL 60606   855-275-5237
                                           ask@jcfs.org
                                      www.jvschicago.org

Stacey Shor, President & Chief Executive Officer
Karen Corken, Vice President & Chief Operating Officer
Vincent Everson, Vice President & Chief Financial Officer
Occupational training and job placement for handicapped persons of all religions.

5847   Kennedy Job Training Center
St. Coletta's of Illinois, Inc.
18350 Crossing Dr.
Tinley Park, IL 60487   708-342-5200
                                      Fax: 708-342-2579
                                 information@stcolettail.org
                                            www.stcil.org

Michael Kahne, Board Chair
William A. Brennan, Secretary & Treasurer
St. Coletta's of Illinois offers vocational evaluation, vocational training work adjustment training, and job placement services for developmentally disabled and hearing impaired persons.

5848   Knox County Board of Developmental Disabilities
11700 Upper Gilchrist Rd.
Mount Vernon, OH 43050   740-397-4656
                                              kccdd.com

Robert Drews, President
Tonya Boucher, Vice President
Korey Kidwell, Recording Secretary
Offers developmental training, vocational evaluation, work adjustment training, extended training, placement, and supported employment.

5849   Kreider Services
500 Anchor Rd.
Dixon, IL 61021-0366   815-288-6691
                                      Fax: 815-288-1636
                                      TTY: 815-288-5931
                                       kreiderservices.org

Mike Hickey, President
Dr. Richard L. Piller, Vice President
Don Vock, Secretary & Treasurer
A private nonprofit organization that offers day service programs, vocational training programs, job placement, supported employment, respite care, residential and family support for children ages 0-3.

5850   Lambs Farm
14245 W. Rockland Rd.
Libertyville, IL 60048   847-362-4636
                                      info@lambsfarm.org
                                           lambsfarm.org

Person-centered, comprehensive program of residential, vocational, and social support service for adults with developmental disabilities.

5851 Land of Lincoln Goodwill Industries
1220 Outer Park Dr.
Springfield, IL 62704   217-789-0400
info@llgi.org
www.llgi.org

Ron Culves, President & Chief Executive Officer
Jason Goodman, Vice President of Finance
Wally Proenza, Vice President of Retail Operations
Empowers people with special needs to become self-sufficient through the power of work.

5852 Orchard Village
7660 Gross Point Rd.
Skokie, IL 60077   847-967-1800
Fax: 847-967-1801
ov@orchardvillage.org
www.orchardvillage.org

Susan Kaufman, President & Chief Executive Officer
Marlene Hodges, Executive Vice President & Chief Financial Officer
Vocational program and counseling, respite services and community living group homes for the disabled and cognitively impaired. Orchard village also operates a private school especially devoted to teaching young adults independent living and skills necessary to flourish in the community.

5853 Sertoma Centre
4343 W. 123rd St.
Alsip, IL 60803   708-371-9700
Fax: 708-371-9747
sertomacentre.org

Gus van den Brink, Executive Director
Sarah Wiemeyer, Assistant Executive Director
Debra Marillo, Director of Advancement & Communications
A nationally accredited, not-for-profit agency that provides services to students and adults with developmental disabilities and mental illness. MIssion is to provide opportunities that empower individuals with disabilities to achieve success.

5854 Shore Training Center
Shore Community Services
8350 Laramie Ave.
Skokie, IL 60077   847-982-2030
info@shoreservices.org
shoreservices.org

Alexis India Alm, Chief Executive Officer
Mission is to improve the quality of life for citizens with developmental disabilities through community based services providing education/training.

5855 The Workshop
706 West St.
P.O. Box 6087
Galena, IL 61036   815-777-2211
Fax: 815-777-3386
theworkshopgalena@theworkshopgalena.org
theworkshopgalena.org

Alyssa Havens, Executive Director
Courtney Busch, Program Director
Laura Moyer, Creative Director
An organization that provides services to individuals with disabilities in Jo Daviess County such as intake and referral, early intervention for children, vocational evaluation, and work adjustment training services.

5856 Thresholds
4101 N Ravenswood Ave.
Chicago, IL 60613   773-572-5500
thresholds@thresholds.org
www.thresholds.org

Mark Ishaug, Chief Executive Officer
Mark Furlong, Chief Operating Officer
Brent Peterson, Chief Development Officer
Provider of recovery services for persons with mental illnesses and substance abuse disorders in Illinois. It offers 30 programs at more than 75 locations throughout Chicago and surrounding suburbs and counties. Services include case management, housing, employment, education, psychiatry, primary care, substance use treatment, and research.

5857 Vocational Rehabilitation Services
Illinois Department of Human Services
100 South Grand Ave. East
Springfield, IL 62762   800-843-6154
TTY: 866-324-5553
www.dhs.state.il.us
Provides support for individuals who are looking for employment. Specialized services for individuals who are blind, visually impaired, deaf, or hard of hearing.

5858 Washington County Vocational Workshop
781 E. Holzhauer Dr.
Nashville, IL 62263   618-327-3348

Provides job training and related services and vocational rehabilitation services.

Indiana

5859 ADEC Resources for Independence
19670 State Rd. 120
P.O. Box 398
Bristol, IN 46507   574-848-7451
Fax: 574-848-5917
info@adecinc.com
adecinc.com

Donna Belusar, President & Chief Executive Officer
Timothy Donlin, Chief Financial Officer
Lisa Kendall, Vice President, Human Resources
Serves individuals of all ages with developmental disabilities and delays, as well as visual or physical impairments.

5860 Arc Northwest Indiana
4315 E. Michigan Blvd.
Michigan City, IN 46360   219-510-3888
btrowbridge@ArcNWI.com
thearc.org/chapter/the-arc-northwest-indiana/

Peter Berns, Chief Executive Officer
Ruben Rodriguez, Chief Operating Officer
The Arc Northwest Indiana serves people with intellectual and developmental disabilities and their families by providing programs that aren't adressed by governmental agencies or local providers.

5861 BI-County Services
425 East Harrison St.
Bluffton, IN 46714   260-824-1253
Fax: 260-824-1892
bi-countyservices.com
A nonprofit organization that serves individuals with disabilities in Wells and Adam Counties. Provides infant services, Medicaid waivers, music therapy, ICF, MR, group homes, sheltered employment, pay program, and supported employment services.

5862 Carey Services
2724 S. Carey St.
Marion, IN 46953   765-668-8961
Fax: 765-664-6747
info@careyservices.com
www.careyservices.com

James Allbaugh, President & Chief Executive Officer
Yolanda Kincaid, Chief Operations Officer
David Smith, Director of Finance
The mission of Carey Services is to create pathways towards self-sufficiency with personal satisfaction. Carey Services offers employment training and job coaching services.

5863 Evansville Association for the Blind
500 North 2nd Ave.
Evansville, IN 47710   812-422-1181
www.evansvilleblind.org

Karla L. Horrell, Executive Director
Prince Samuel, President
Fred Dormeier, Vice President
A nonprofit ogranization that offers employment services to people who are visually impaired.

5864 Four Rivers Resource Services
P.O. Box 249
Hwy. 59 South
Linton, IN 47441   812-847-2231
fourrivers@frrs.org
frrs.org
Shane Burton, Chief Executive Officer
Mel Fields, Chief Operating Officer
Employment; community living; connections; follow-along;
early intervention; preschool; healthy families; child care re-
source, referral, and child care voucher program; impact; and
transpotation services.

5865 Gateway Services/JCARC
3500 North Morton St.
P.O. Box 216
Franklin, IN 46131   317-738-5500
www.gatewayarc.com
A nonprofit organization that offers employment services to
individduals with disabilities. Economic advisors aid disabled
individuals throughout the entire process of finding a job, and
continue to check in on them after employment.

5866 Goodwill of Central & Southern Indiana
1635 W. Michigan St.
Indianapolis, IN 46222   317-524-4313
goodwill@goodwillindy.org
www.goodwillindy.org
Kent A. Kramer, President & Chief Executive Officer
Daniel J. Riley, Senior Vice President & Chief Financial Officer
Eric Schlegel, Senior Vice President & Chief Operating Officer
Offers employment services such as vocational rehabilitation,
employer support, and job coaches for individuals with
disabilities.

5867 Indiana Civil Rights Commission
100 North Senate Ave.
Room N300
Indianapolis, IN 46204   317-232-2600
800-628-2909
Fax: 317-232-6580
TTY: 800-743-3333
info@icrc.in.gov
www.in.gov/icrc
Gregory L. Wilson, Sr., Executive Director
Doneisha Posey, Deputy Director & General Counsel
Pamella Cook, Chief Financial Officer
Works to develop public policies that ensure equal opportunity in
education to all and enforces the civil rights laws of the State of
Indiana.

5868 Indiana Disability Employment Initiative
Indiana Department of Workforce Development
10 North Senate Ave.
Indianapolis, IN 46204   800-891-6499
www.in.gov/dwd/2416.htm
Jointly funded by the US Department of Labor's Employment and
Training Administration, DEI aims to improve education, train-
ing, and employment opportunities for adults with disabilities.

5869 New Hope Services
725 Wall St.
Jeffersonville, IN 47130   812-288-8248
info@newhopeservices.org
newhopeservices.org
James A. Bosley, Chief Executive Officer
Jody Reschar Heazlitt, President
John Broady, Senior Vice President & Chief Financial Officer
Mission is to provide hope through services which are responsive
to individual needs. New Hope Services offers a vocational training program for individuals with intellectual or physical
disabilities.

5870 New Horizons Rehabilitation
237 Six Pine Ranch Rd.
Batesville, IN 47006   812-934-4528
contact@nhrinc.org
www.nhrinc.org
Provides training and services to children and adults with men-
tal/physical disabilities. The Community Employment services
helps individuals ages 14 and up acquire employment.

5871 Noble of Indiana
Noble, Inc.
7701 East 21st St.
Indianapolis, IN 46219   317-375-2700
Fax: 317-375-2719
www.mynoblelife.org
Julia Huffman, President & Chief Executive Officer
Judy Tidwell, Chief Financial Officer
Erin Hardwick, Director of Pre-Vocational Services
Since 1953, Noble of Indiana has been dedicated to its mission: to
create opportunities for people with developmental disabilities to
live meaningful lives.

5872 Paladin
4315 East Michigan Blvd.
Michigan City, IN 46360   219-874-4288
Fax: 219-874-2689
Paladin@paladin.care
www.paladin.care
Steve Hobby, President & Chief Executive Officer
Evelyn Marvel, Chief Financial & Operations Officer
Alanna Konieczka, Human Resources Manager
A nonprofit organization that offers pre-vocational and employ-
ment services to individuals with disabilities.

5873 Putnam County Comprehensive Services
630 Tennessee St.
Greencastle, IN 46135   765-653-9763
Fax: 765-653-3646
aranck_pccs@yahoo.com
www.pccsinc.org
Andrew Ranck, Executive Director
Ken Heeke, President
Sue McCune, Treasurer
A not-for-profit organization serving individuals with disabilities and similar characteristics in Indiana. Their mission is to provide services to individuals with disabilities in order for them to
reach their optimum potential in attitudes, habits, and skills
through training and integration, making them contributing members of their community, and to promote community awareness
and acceptance of people with different abilities.
1968

5874 Southern Indiana Resource Solutions
1579 S. Folsomville Rd.
Boonville, IN 47601   812-897-4840
Fax: 812-897-0123
www.sirs.org
Cheryl Mullis, President & Chief Executive Officer
Adult services including jobs, community connections, and residential and childrens services, including service coordination
and all therapies.

5875 Sycamore Rehabilitation Services
1001 Sycamore Ln.
P.O. Box 369
Danville, IN 46122-1474   317-745-4715
866-573-0817
Fax: 317-745-8271
info@sycamoreservices.com
sycamoreservices.com
Terry Kessinger, President
Steve Patterson, Vice President
Carol Thralls, Treasurer
Provides training and services for persons with disabilities that
enhance independence in all areas of life.

Iowa

5876 Access, Inc.
20 5th St. NW
Hampton, IA 50441   641-456-2532
info@accessincorporated.org
www.accessincorporated.org
Dale Schirmer, Executive Director
A nonprofit organization providing residential and vocational
services in Franklin, Butler, and Hardin counties in the state of
Iowa. Residential Services include RCF/MR services, Supported

Community Living Services, and Community Supervised Apartment Living Arrangement Services. Vocational Services include Work Services and Supported Employment Services. Accredited by the Commission on Accreditation of Rehabilitation Facilities since 1984, and serves individuals with a wide range of needs.

5877 Iowa Career Connection
3408 Woodland Ave.
Suite 201
West Des Moines, IA 50266   515-282-5823
contact@iowacareerconnection.com
www.iowacareerconnection.com
Specializes in accounting and human resources talent acquisition in the Upper-Midwest.

5878 Iowa Civil Rights Commission
400 E. 14th St.
Des Moines, IA 50319-0201   515-281-4121
800-457-4416
Fax: 515-242-5840
www.state.ia.us/government/crc
Stan Thompson, Executive Director
A neutral, fact-finding administrative agency that enforces the 'Iowa Civi Rights Act of 1965,' Iowa's anti-discrimination law. The commission doesn not provide legal representation. The commission's vision is a state free of discrimination.

5879 Iowa Economic Development Authority
1963 Bell Avenue
Suite 200
Des Moines, IA 50315   515-348-6200
info@iowaeda.com
www.iowaeconomicdevelopment.com
Debi Durham, Director
To engender and promote economic development policies and practices which stimulate and sustain Iowa's economic growth and climate and that integrate efforts across public and private sectors.

5880 Iowa Valley Community College
3702 S. Center St.
Marshalltown, IA 50158   641-752-4643
800-284-4823
Fax: 641-752-5909
ivinfo@iavalley.edu
www.iavalley.edu
Kristie Fisher, Chancellor
Julie Eastridge, Director of Marketing
Mike Mosher, Chief Information Officer
Offers two levels of specialized vocational preparatory programming for adults with disabilities. The Career Development Center serves dependent adults. The goal of the program is to maintain or improve skills to enable persons served to enter sheltered or supported employment. The IRP/CBVT programs are non-credit specialized vocational programs for independent adults served by Vocational Rehabilitation and our programs. The goals are for competitive placements in jobs. CARF accredited.

5881 Iowa Vocational Rehabilitation Services
510 East 12th St.
Jessie Parker Building
Des Moines, IA 50319-0240   800-532-1486
www.ivrs.iowa.gov/index.html
Iowa Vocational Rehabilitation Services aims to help individuals with disabilities achieve their employment, independence, and economic goals.

5882 New Focus
102 W. Washington St.
Centerville, IA 52544   641-437-1722

Provides vocational services for adults with disabilities. Includes work activity, supported employment, and supported community living.

Kansas

5883 Kansas Human Rights Commission
900 SW Jackson St.
Suite 568-S
Topeka, KS 66612-1258   785-296-3206
Fax: 785-296-0589
khrc@ks.gov
www.khrc.net
Ruth Glover, Executive Director
Mission is to assure equal opportunities in employment, public accommodations, and housing, as well as to prevent discrimination.

5884 Kansas Vocational Rehabilitation Agency
Department for Children & Families
555 S. Kansas
3rd Fl.
Topeka, KS 66603   785-368-7471
www.dcf.ks.gov
Helps people with disabilities achieve employment and self-sufficiency. Also links employers with qualified and productive individuals to meet thier work force needs.

Kentucky

5885 Kentucky Commission on Human Rights
332 West Broadway
Suite 1400
Louisville, KY 40202   502-595-4024
Fax: 502-696-5230
kchr.mail@ky.gov
kchr.ky.gov/Pages/default.aspx
Terrance A. Sullivan, Executive Director
Samar Syeda, Executive Administrator
The state government authority that enforces the Kentucky Civil Rights Act, making it unlawful to discriminate in the areas of employment, financial transactions, housing, and public accommodations.

5886 Kentucky Office for the Blind
500 Mero Street 4th Floor NE
Frankfort, KY 40601   502-564-4440
800-372-7172
TTY: 800-372-7172
cora.mcnabb@ky.gov
blind.ky.gov
Cora McNabb, Acting Executive Director
Tiffany Smither, Fiscal Administrator
The Office for the Blind offers a wide variety of employment services aimed at providing the skills and opportunities for independence to individuals with visual disabilities.

5887 Kentucky Vocational Rehabilitation Agency
500 Mero Street
4th Floor NE
Frankfort, KY 40621   502-564-4440
800-372-7172
TTY: 800-372-7172
WFD.VOCREHAB@ky.gov
kcc.ky.gov/Vocational-Rehabilitation/
Assists eligible individuals with disabilities achieve their employment goals.

5888 Pioneer Vocational/Industrial Services
150 Corporate Dr.
P.O. Box 1396
Danville, KY 40422   859-236-8413
800-527-4198
Fax: 859-238-7115
TTY: 859-236-1251
pioneer@pioneerservices.org
www.pioneerservices.org
Mike Pittman, Executive Director
Steve Lovell, Director of Marketing and Production

Mission is to provide vocational development and extended employment programs to people who are disabled and/or disadvantaged, and to assist them in maximizing independent living skills.
1967

Louisiana

5889 **Blind Services**
Louisiana Rehabilitation Services
1001 North 23rd St.
P.O. Box 94094
Baton Rouge, LA 70804-9094   225-342-3111
Fax: 225-342-7960
owd@lwc.la.gov
www.laworks.net

Ava Cates, Secretary
A section of the Louisiana Rehabilitation Services, Blind Services offers employment opportunities to individuals who are blind or visually impaired.

5890 **COEA The Arc of East Ascension**
1122 E. Ascension Complex Blvd.
Gonzales, LA 70737-4265   225-621-2000
Fax: 225-621-2022
opportunities@eatel.net
thearc.org/chapter/the-arc-of-east-ascension/

Peter Berns, Executive Director
Ruben Rodriguez, Chief Operating Officer
Committed to affording individuals the opportunities that reflect and support their choices, dignity, individuality, self-determination, community, coherency, and common sense. The Arc of East Ascension offers educational, employment, community, housing, and recreational services.

5891 **Louisiana Rehabilitation Services**
Office of Workforce Development
1001 North 23rd St.
P.O. Box 94094
Baton Rouge, LA 70804-9094   225-342-3111
Fax: 225-342-7960
owd@lwc.la.gov
www.laworks.net/WorkforceDev/LRS/LRS_Main.asp

Melissa Bayham, Director
Provides services for job seekers and job training programs for individuals with disabilities. Programs include Blind Services and Vocational Rehabilitation.

5892 **The Arc Westbank**
401 Gretna Blvd.
Gretna, LA 70053   504-361-1131
jennifer@westbankarc.org
westbankarc.org
Provides day and employment services to individuals with disabilities.
1956

5893 **Vocational Rehabilitation Program**
Office of Workforce Development
1001 North 23rd St.
P.O. Box 94094
Baton Rouge, LA 70802-9094   225-342-3111
Fax: 225-342-7960
owd@lwc.la.gov
www.laworks.net

Offers individuals with disabilities a wide range of services designed to provide them with the skills and resources needed to compete in the interview process, get the job, keep the job, and develop a lifetime career.

Maine

5894 **Bangor Veteran Center: Veterans Outreach Center**
615 Odlin Rd.
Suite 3
Bangor, ME 04401   207-947-3391
Fax: 207-941-8195
www.maine.va.gov

Denis McDonough, Secretary of Veterans Affairs
Donald M. Remy, Deputy Secretart of Veterans Affairs
Tanya J. Brasher, Chief of Staff of Veterans Affairs
Readjustment counseling services for veterans of Vietnam, Vietnam Era, Persian Gulf, Panama, Grenada, Lebanon, Somalia, WWII and Korean conflicts, as well as Iraq, Afganistan, and military sexual trauma.

5895 **Creative Work Systems**
10 Speirs St.
Westbrook, ME 04092   207-879-1140
Fax: 207-879-1146
creativeworksystems.com

Heidi Howard, Executive Director
Jim Harrison, President
Carolyn Faulkner, Vice President
Provides residential, day habilitation, and supported employment services in Central and Southern Maine.

5896 **Division for the Blind and Visually Impaired**
Bureau of Rehabilitation Services
150 State House Station
Augusta, ME 04333-0150   207-623-7948
www.maine.gov/rehab/dbvi/index.shtml
The Division provices services to persons with severe visual impairments, including counseling and vocational assessment, job training and placement, and orientation and mobility instruction.

5897 **Maine Commission on Disability & Employment**
State Workforce Board
45 Commerce Dr.
Augusta, ME 04330   207-621-5087
SWB.DOL@maine.gov
www.maine.gov

Jennifer Kimble, Chair
Established in 1997, the Commission aims to influence policy related to employment for people with disabilities.

5898 **Maine Department of Labor**
54 State House Station
Augusta, ME 04333-0054   207-623-7900
mdol@maine.gov
www.state.me.us/labor

Laura Fortman, Commissioner
Provides a wide range of services such as employment, labor market information, rehabilitation/disability, and others.

5899 **Maine Human Rights Commission**
Maine Human Rights Commission
51 State House Station
Augusta, ME 04333   207-624-6290
Fax: 207-624-8729
TTY: 711
www.maine.gov/mhrc

Amy Sneirson, Executive Director
Barbara Archer Hirsch, Commission Counsel
Melody Piper, Operations Director
The State agency with the responsibility of enforcing Maine's anti-discrimination laws. The Commission investigates complaints of unlawful discrimination in employment, housing, education, access to public accommodations, extension of credit, and offensive names.

5900 **Northeast Occupational Exchange**
29 Franklin St.
Bangor, ME 04401   800-857-0500
Fax: 207-561-4725
TTY: 207-992-2298
www.noemaine.org

Charles O. Tingley, Executive Director
Sharon Greenleaf, Assistant Director

A fully licensed, comprehensive mental health and substance abuse treatment and rehabilitation facility.
1975

Maryland

5901 Ardmore Developmental Center
4300 Forbes Boulevard
Suite 110
Lanham, MD 20706   301-577-2575
                                Fax: 301-259-3634
                          grow@ArdmoreEnterprises.org
                          www.ardmoreenterprises.org
Lori Sedlezky, Chief Executive Officer
David Schey, Chief Financial Officer
Melissa Scholfield, Director of People & Culture
Offers supported employment programs and vocational education for persons with intellectual and developmental disabilities, as well as residential services and a Day Support program.
1963

5902 Maryland Commission on Civil Rights (FEPA)
6 Saint Paul St.
Suite 900
Baltimore, MD 21202-1631   410-767-8600
                                     800-637-6247
                                Fax: 410-333-1841
                                mccr@maryland.gov
                                www.mccr.maryland.gov
Alvin O. Gillard, Executive Director
Cleveland L. Horton II, Deputy Director
Glendora Hughes, General Counsel
The Maryland Commission on Civil Rights represents the interests of the State of Maryland in ensuring equal opportunity for all individuals in the areas of housing, public accommodations, employment, and state contracts.

5903 Maryland Department of Disabilities
217 E. Redwood St.
Suite 1300
Baltimore, MD 21202   410-767-3660
                                     800-637-4113
                                Fax: 410-333-6674
                             info.mdod@maryland.gov
                                  mdod.maryland.gov
Carol Beatty, Secretary
Christian Miele, Deputy Secretary
John Brennan, Assistant Deputy Secretary
The Maryland Department of Disabilities is charged with improving services for individuals with disabilities in the areas of housing, employment, community living, technology assistance, transportation, and more.

5904 Maryland Employment Network
Bel Air, MB   410-803-7184
                                     855-384-2844
                                Fax: 410-803-8732
                               www.ticket2workmd.org
Keirstyn Silver, Director, Self-Sufficiency & Education
Molly Hall, Program Administrator
A state-wide network of 9 partner agencies that aim to help individuals with disabilities gain quality employment.

5905 Maryland State Department of Education
Division of Rehabilitation Services (DORS)
2301 Argonne Dr.
Baltimore, MD 21218   410-554-9442
                                     888-554-0334
                                TTY: 443-798-2840
                                  dors@maryland.gov
                                  dors.maryland.gov
Scott Dennis, Assistant State Superintendent
Sandy Bowser, Executive Associate
Kimberlee Schultz, Director, Office of Public Affairs
The Division of Rehabilitation Services provides opportunities for individuals with physical and/or mental disabilities that help them gain employment. The Division is composed of the public

vocational rehabilitation program, and the Disability Determination Services.

5906 Melwood
5606 Dower House Rd.
Upper Marlboro, MD 20772   301-599-8000
                                Fax: 301-599-0180
                                services@melwood.org
                                www.melwood.org
Larysa Kautz, President & CEO
Scott Gibson, Chief Strategy Officer
Rebecca Cheraquit, Chief Program Officer
Melwood is a dynamic nonprofit that creates jobs and opportunities to improve the lives of people with disabilities. Melwood serves more than 2000 people with disabilities each year.

5907 NFB Career Mentoring
National Federation of the Blind
200 E. Wells St.
at Jernigan Place
Baltimore, MD 21230   410-659-9314
                                Fax: 410-685-5653
                                     nfb@nfb.org
                                     www.nfb.org
Mark A. Riccobono, President
A primary initiative of the NFB Jernigan Institute, the Career Mentoring program aims to increase the employment of visually impaired adults. The National Federation of the Blind also offers an employment resource page.

5908 Office of Fair Practices
Department of Labor, Licensing & Regulation
1100 North Eutaw St.
Room 613
Baltimore, MD 21202   410-230-6319
                                Fax: 410-225-3282
                               dlofp-dllr@maryland.gov
                          www.dllr.state.md.us/oeope/
Yvette Dickens, Director & ADA/504 Officer
Andrea Somerville, EEO Specialist
Aims to ensure qual opportunities for all individuals by enforcing the Equal Employment Opportunity (EEO) Program, the Americans with Disabilities Act, and other equal opportunity programs.

5909 TLC Speech-Language/Occupational TherapyCamps
2092 Gaither Rd.
Suite 100
Rockville, MD 20850   301-424-5200
                                Fax: 301-424-8063
                                     info@ttlc.org
                                     www.ttlc.org
Patricia Ritter, Executive Director
TLC provides small group summer programs for children with special needs. Offers speech-language and occupational therapy summer camps for children ages 3-7.

Massachusetts

5910 Executive Office of Labor & Workforce Development
State of Massachusetts
One Ashburton Pl.
Suite 2112
Boston, MA 02108   617-626-7122
                                Fax: 617-727-1090
                                     www.mass.gov
Charlie Baker, Governor
Karyn Polito, Lt. Governor
Manages the Commonwealth's workforce development and labor departments.

5911 Gateway Arts Center: Studio, Craft Store & Gallery
Vinsen Corporation
60-62 Harvard St.
Brookline, MA 02445   617-734-1577
                                gatewayarts@vinfen.org
                                www.gatewayarts.org
Rae Edelson, Director
Stephanie Schmidt-Ellis, Clinical Program Director
Ted Lampe, Program Director

Award-winning, nationally recognized arts-based rehabilitation service with over 100 talented adults with disabilities.

5912 Life-Skills, Inc.
44 Morris St.
Webster, MA 01570
508-943-0700
Fax: 508-949-6129
info@life-skillsinc.org
life-skillsinc.org

J. Thomas Amick, Chief Executive Officer
Kathy Nolan, Chief Financial Officer
Lisa Morgan, Director of Compliance
Accredited through the Commission on Accreditation of Rehabilitation Facilities; offers day, residential, and employment services for individuals with intellectual, developmental, physical, and emotional disabilities.

5913 Massachusetts Commission Against Discrimination (FEPA)
1 Ashburton Pl.
Suite 601
Boston, MA 02108
617-994-6000
Fax: 617-994-6024
TTY: 617-994-6196
mcad@mass.gov
www.mass.gov

Sunila Thomas-George, Chairwoman
The commission works to eliminate discrimination on a variety of bases and areas, and strives to advance the civil rights of the people of commonwealth through law enforcement, outreach, and training.

5914 Massachusetts Commission for the Blind
600 Washington St.
Boston, MA 02111
617-727-5550
800-392-6450
Fax: 617-626-7512
www.mass.gov/eohhs/gov/departments/mcb/
David D'Arcangelo, Commissioner
Provides vocational and social rehabilitation for individuals with visual impairments.

5915 Massachusetts Governor's Commission on Employment of People with Disabilities
Department of Employment & Training
19 Standford St.
3rd Fl.
Boston, MA 02114
617-262-5239
Fax: 617-727-0315
www.dol.gov/odep/contact/
Charlie Baker, Governor
State vocational rehabilitation agency.

5916 Massachusetts Rehabilitation Commission
600 Washington St.
Boston, MA 02111
617-204-3600
Fax: 617-727-1354
TTY: 800-245-6543
MRC.generalinformation@Massmail.State.MA.US
www.mass.gov
Toni Wolf, Commissioner
Helps individuals with disabilities work and live independently. The Commission runs the Vocational Rehabilitation and Community Living programs.

5917 Viability
60 Brookdale Dr.
Springfield, MA 01104
413-781-5359
viability.org

Francis Fitzgerald, Chair
Jonathon Stephen "Steve" Dean, Vice Chair
Charlene Smolkowicz, Treasurer
Viability's mission is to help individuals with disabilities achieve their full potential. Services include day programs, employment services, and job training and placements.

5918 Work Inc.
25 Beach St.
Dorchester, MA 02122
617-691-1500
info@workinc.org
workinc.org

James Cassetta, President
Sharon Smith, Chief Executive Officer
Paul Lemieux, Chief Financial Officer
A nationally recognized organization that provides supportive services need to help people with disabilities reach their career goals.

Michigan

5919 Department of Health & Human Services
333 S. Grand Ave.
P.O. Box 30195
Lansing, MI 48909
517-373-3740
TTY: 800-649-3777
www.michigan.gov/mdhhs/
Elizabeth Hertel, Director
Farah Hanley, Chief Deputy for Health
David Knezek, Chief Deputy Director for Administration
The DHHS is Michigan's public assistance, child, and family welfare agency. DHS directs the operations of public assistance and service programs through a network of over 100 county department of human service offices around the state.

5920 Division on Deaf, DeafBlind & Hard of Hearing
3054 W. Grand Blvd.
Suite 3-600
Detroit, MI 48202
313-437-7035
877-499-6232
Fax: 319-456-3721
TTY: 877-499-6232
DODDBHH@Michigan.gov
www.michigan.gov/mdcr/divisions/doddbhh
Annie Urasky, Division Director
Alayna Lail, Executive Secretary
A state office with the mission of helping to improve the lives of Michigan citizens who are deaf, deafblind and hard of hearing.

5921 Michigan Department of Civil Rights
3054 W. Grand Blvd.
Suite 3-600
Detroit, MI 48202
313-456-3700
800-482-3604
Fax: 313-456-3791
TTY: 877-878-8464
MDCR-INFO@michigan.gov
www.michigan.gov/mdcr
John E. Johnson, Jr., Executive Director
Investigates and resolves discrimination complaints and works to prevent discrimination through educational programs that promote voluntary compliance with civil rights laws.

5922 Michigan Rehabilitation Services
Department of Health & Human Services
320 S. Walnut St.
Lansing, MI 48933
800-854-9090
Fax: 517-335-0135
www.michigan.gov/mrs
Jenny Piatt, Bureau Division Director
State vocational rehabilitation agency that provides specialized employment and educational services to teens and adults with disabilities in order to help them find and retain employment.

5923 Michigan Workforce Development Agency
Department of Labor and Economic Opportunity (LEO)
201 N. Washington Square
Lansing, MI 48913
517-335-5858
Fax: 517-241-8217
TTY: 888-605-6722
www.michigan.gov/mdcd
Offers job development and placement services to dislocated workers with disabilities.

5924 Straits Area Services, Inc. (SAS)
1320 W. State St.
P.O. Box 6042
Cheboygan, MI 49721   231-627-4319
                            www.sastogether.org

Cyril Drier, President
David Johnson, Vice President
Theresa Sorenson, Treasurer
Provides community integration, supported employment, skill building, rehabilitative training, business support, work enclaves, and more to individuals with developmental disabilities.
1976

Minnesota

5925 Jewish Vocational Service of Jewish Familyand Children's Services
5905 Golden Valley Rd.
Golden Valley, MN 55422   952-546-0616
                            Fax: 952-593-1778
                            jfcs@jfcsmpls.org
                            www.jfcsmpls.org

Judy Halper, Chief Executive Officer
Lee Friedman, Chief Operating Officer
John Maloy, Chief Financial Officer
The mission of JVS is to be a recognized leader in delivering employment, training, and career development services that positively impact individuals of all backgrounds, businesses, and society. JVS offers a vocational rehabilitation program that includes job placement, work adjustment training, and extended employment.

5926 Minnesota Department of Employment & Economic Development: State Services for the Blind
2200 University Ave. W.
Suite 240
St. Paul, MN 55114   651-539-2300
                            800-722-0550
                            Fax: 651-649-5927
                            ssb.info@state.mn.us
                            mn.gov/deed/ssb/

Ed Lecher, Program Director
Offers tools, services, and training for individuals who are blind, DeafBlind, or have a visual impairment and are seeking employment or to live more indepedently.

5927 Minnesota Department of Employment and Economic Development: Vocational Rehab Services
332 Minnesota St.
1st National Bank Bldg., Suite E200
St. Paul, MN 55101   651-259-7114
                            800-657-3858
                            DEED.CustomerService@state.mn.us
                            mn.gov/deed/

Steve Grove, Commissioner
Elizabeth Frosch, Chief of Staff
Marc Majors, Deputy Commissioner of Workforce Development
Service for people with disabilities who need skills to prepare for work, or to find and keep a job.

5928 Minnesota Department of Human Rights (FEPA)
Griggs Midway Building
540 Fairview Ave North, Suite 201
St. Paul, MN 55104   651-539-1100
                            800-657-3704
                            TTY: 800-627-3529
                            Info.MDHR@state.mn.us
                            mn.gov/mdhr/

Rebecca Lucero, Commissioner
Irina Vaynerman, Deputy Commissioner
Nick Pladson, General Counsel
Mission and vision is to make Minnesota discrimination free. The Minnesota Department of Human Rights investigates charges of discrimination, and ensures that businesses comply with equal opportunity requirements.

Mississippi

5929 AbilityWorks
P.O. Box 1698
Jackson, MS 39215   601-898-7076
                            www.mdrs.ms.gov
Vocational evaluation, work adjustment, and job placement of disabled persons in a rehabilitation workshop. AbilityWorks is a division of the Mississippi Department of Rehabilitation.

5930 Mississippi Department of Rehabilitation Services
1281 Highway 51
Madison, MS 39110   800-443-1000
                            TTY: 800-443-1000
                            www.mdrs.ms.gov/

Anita Naik, Office Director, Special Disability Programs
Billy Taylor, Chief of Staff
Dorothy Young, Office Director, Vocational Rehabilitation for the Blind
Offers low vision aids and appliances, counseling, social work, educational and professional training, residential services, recreational services, computer training and employment opportunities for Mississippians with disabilities.

5931 Mississippi Employment Security Commission
1235 Echelon Prkwy.
P.O. Box 1699
Jackson, MS 39215-1699   601-321-6000
                            comments@mdes.ms.gov
                            www.mdes.ms.gov

Jackie Turner, Executive Director
A federally funded state agency. The programs of MDES, under direction of the governor of Mississippi, report to the federal government. The goal of the department is to help citizens of Mississippi get jobs.

5932 National Research and Training Center on Blindness and Low Vision
Mississippi State University
108 Herbert-South, Room 150
PO Drawer 6189
Mississippi State, MS 39762-6189   662-325-2001
                            Fax: 662-325-8989
                            nrtc@colled.msstate.edu
                            www.blind.msstate.edu

Michele McDonnall, Research Professor & Director
Kendra Farrow, Program Director
Lisa Gooden-Hunley, Program Coordinator
The NRTC focuses on enhancing the employment and independence of individuals who are blind and visually impaired.

Missouri

5933 Missouri Commission on Human Rights
421 E. Dunklin
P.O. Box 1129
Jefferson City, MO 65102- 1129   573-751-3325
                            877-781-4236
                            Fax: 573-751-2905
                            TTY: 800-735-2966
                            mchr@labor.mo.gov
                            labor.mo.gov/MOHUMANRIGHTS

Anna S. Hui, Director
The Missouri Commission on Human Rights enforces the state's anti-discrimination law that prohibits discrimination in housing, employment, and places of public accommodations. It prohibits discrimination due to race, color, religion, national origin, ancestry, sex, disability, age, and familial status. Complaints must be filed within 180 days of the alleged discrimination. If discrimination is found after investigation, the Commission can hold hearings to enforce the law.

5934 Missouri Governor's Council on Disability
301 West High St., Room 620
P.O. Box 1668
Jefferson City, MO 65102
800-877-8249
Fax: 573-526-4109
TTY: 573-751-2600
gcd@oa.mo.gov
disability.mo.gov/gcd/

Claudia Browner, Executive Director
The Council promotes the full participation of Missouri citizens
with disabilities, and provides information about the American
with Disabilities Act. They aim to protect persons with disabilities through equal access to services and employment
opportunities.

5935 Missouri Vocational Rehabilitation Agency
Department of Elementary & Secondary Education
205 Jefferson St.
Jefferson City, MO 65101
573-751-3251
info@vr.dese.mo.gov
dese.mo.gov

Margie Vandeven, Commissioner
A team of dedicated individuals working for the continuous improvement of education and services for all citizens. Vocational
Rehabilitation offers specialized employment and training services for individuals with a physical or mental impairment.

5936 Vocational Rehabilitation Services for the Blind
Missouri Department of Social Services
615 Howerton Court
P.O. Box 2320
Jefferson City, MO 65102-2320
573-751-4249
Fax: 573-751-4984
TTY: 800-735-2966
askrsb@dss.mo.gov
dss.mo.gov/fsd/rsb/vr.htm

Robert J. Knodell, Acting Director
A state organization that aims to create employment opportunities for blind and visually impaired persons.

Montana

5937 Disability Employment & Transitions
Department of Public Health & Human Services
111 North Last Chance Gulch
P.O. Box 4210
Helena, MT 59604
406-444-5622
dphhs.mt.gov/detd

Adam Meier, Director
Provides services for individuals with disabilities who want to
become employed. Focuses on transitions from high school to
post-secondary education and work.

5938 Montana Human Rights Bureau (FEPA)
P.O. Box 1728
Helena, MT 59624-1728
406-444-2884
800-542-0807
Fax: 406-443-3234
www.erd.dli.mt.gov/human-rights

Enforces state and federal laws prohibiting unlawful discrimination based on age, marital status, disability, race/nationality,
color, religion, sex, etc., in the areas of employment, housing, education, and public accommodations.

Nebraska

5939 Nebraska Department of Labor
1111 O Street
Suite 222
Lincoln, NE 68508
402-471-4474
800-833-7352
TTY: 402-471-0016
ndol.lincolnwfd@nebraska.gov
dol.nebraska.gov

John Albin, Commissioner

Services for individuals with disabilities who want to become
employed.

5940 Nebraska Equal Opportunity Commission (FEPA)
1526 K Street
Suite 310
Lincoln, NE 68508-2709
402-471-2024
800-642-6112
Fax: 402-471-4059
www.neoc.ne.gov

Patrick Borchers, Chairperson
John Arnold, Vice-Chairperson
Paula Gardner, Executive Director
The Nebraska Equal Opportunity Commission is a neutral administrative agency that enforces state policy against discrimination
in the areas of employment, housing, and public
accommodations.

5941 Nebraska VR
Department of Education
PO Box 94987
Lincoln, NE 68509
402-471-3644
877-637-3422
Fax: 402-471-0788
marketingteam.vr@nebraska.gov
www.vr.nebraska.gov

Lindy Foley, Director
An employment program for citizens of Nebraska who experience a disability and are seeking employment.

Nevada

5942 Bureau of Vocational Rehabilitation
Rehabilitation Division
500 E. Third Street
Carson City, NV 89713
702-486-5230
TTY: 702-486-1018
detr.state.nv.us

Shelley Hendren, Rehabilitation Administrator
A state and federally funded program that helps people with disabilities find employment, and helps advance the skills of disabled individuals who are already employed.

5943 Nevada Equal Rights Commission
1820 East Sahara Ave.
Suite 314
Las Vegas, NV 89104
702-486-7161
800-326-6868
Fax: 702-486-7054
detr.state.nv.us/nerc.htm

Connye Harper, Commissioner
Stewart Chang, Commissioner
Tiffany Young, Commissioner
Oversees the state's Equal Employment Opportunity program in
order to make sure that all citizens of Nebraska recieve the same
employment opportunities.

**5944 Nevada Governor's Council on Developmental
Disabilities**
808 W. Nye Ln.
Carson City, NV 89703
775-684-8619
Fax: 775-684-8626
elmarquez@dhhs.nv.gov
www.nevadaddcouncil.org

Catherine Nielsen, Executive Director
The Council provides advocacy for individuals with intellectual
or developmental disabilities, so that they may live more independent lives and be involved in the community.

New Hampshire

5945 New Hampshire Bureau of Vocational Rehabilitation
New Hampshire Department of Education
101 Pleasant St.
Concord, NH 03301 603-271-3494
Fax: 603-271-1953
info@doe.nh.gov
www.education.nh.gov

Lisa Hinson-Hatz, State Director
The Bureau of Vocational Rehabilitation assists citizens of New Hampshire with disabilities secure employment.

5946 New Hampshire Commission for Human Rights (FEPA)
2 Industrial Park Dr.
Building 1
Concord, NH 03301 603-271-2767
Fax: 603-271-6339
humanrights@nh.gov
www.nh.gov/hrc

Ahni Malachi, Executive Director
Sarah Burke Cohen, Assistant Director
Established for the purpose of eliminating discrimination in employment, public accomodations, and the sale or rental of housing or commercial property.

5947 New Hampshire Employment Security
45 South Fruit St.
Concord, NH 03301 603-224-3311
800-852-3400
TTY: 800-735-2964
webmaster@nhes.nh.gov
www.nhes.nh.gov

George N. Copadis, Commissioner
Operates a free public employment service and provides assisted and self-directed employment and career-related services and labor market information for employers and the general public.

New Jersey

5948 ARC of Hunterdon County, The
53 Frontage Road
Suite 150
Hampton, NJ 08827 908-730-7827
www.archunterdon.org

Jeff Mattison, Executive Director
Kathy Walsh, President
Jessica Lui, Vice President
Mission is to provide support, training, and opportunities to individuals with intellectual and developmental disabilities so that they can achieve the greatest degree of independence and productivity, and become contributing, responsible, and proud members of society.

5949 ARC of Mercer County
180 Ewingville Rd.
Ewing, NJ 08638 609-406-0181
Fax: 609-406-9258
familysupports@arcmercer.org
www.arcmercer.org

Steve Cook, Executive Director
Committed to securing for all people with developmental disabilities the opportunity to choose and realize their goals.

5950 ARC of Monmouth
1158 Wayside Rd.
Tinton Falls, NJ 07712 732-493-1919
Fax: 732-493-3604
info@arcofmonmouth.org
www.arcofmonmouth.org

Lauren Zalepka, President
Joyce Nunziata, First Vice President
Robert Angel, Executive Director
A nonprofit organization providing services and supports for individuals who have cognitive and developmental disabilities and their families.

5951 Abilities Center of New Jersey
1208 Delsea Dr.
Westville, NJ 08093 856-848-1025
Fax: 856-848-8429
info@abilities4work.com
abilities4work.com

Susan Perron, President & CEO
Stephanie Berridge, Secretary & Treasurer
Jack Sheppard, Chairman
A nonprofit organization dedicated to developing employment opportunities for people with disabilities or other disadvantages through education, training, and job placement.

5952 Abilities of Northwest New Jersey Inc.
264 Rt 31 North
Washington, NJ 07882 908-689-1118
info@abilitiesnw.com
abilities-nw.com

Cynthia B. Wildermuth, Chief Executive Officer
Sue Zukoski, Chief Operating Officer
Michelle Savino, Director of Training & Quality Improvement
Private not-for-profit community rehabilitation program providing vocational training and employment services since 1974 to the disabled and disadvantaged population.

5953 Alliance Center for Independence (ACI)
629 Amboy Ave.
First Floor
Edison, NJ 08837 732-738-4388
Fax: 732-738-4416
TTY: 732-738-9644
ctonks@adacil.org
www.adacil.org

Carole Tonks, Executive Director
Luke Koppisch, Deputy Director
ACI is a nonprofit Center for Independent Living that provides information and referral services and develops and implements educational programs and innovative activities that promote activism, peer support, health, wellness, employment, and independent living skills for people with disabilities.

5954 Arc of Bergen and Passaic Counties
223 Moore St.
Hackensack, NJ 07601 201-343-0322
Fax: 201-343-0401
arc@arcbp.com
arcbergenpassaic.org

Kathy Walsh, President & CEO
Catherine Pescatore, Vice President & CFO
Alice Siegel, Senior Vice President
A membership organization serving persons with disabilities and their families in Bergen and Passaic Counties, NJ.

5955 Career Opportunity Development of New Jersey
901 Atlantic Ave.
Egg Harbor City, NJ 08215-1810 609-965-6871
Fax: 609-965-3099
njcodi.org

Linda Carney, President & CEO
Karen Gardner, Chief Financial Officer
Mary Pat Braudis, Board Chairperson
A nonprofit organization that provides services to individuals with varying forms of physical, mental, and economic disabilities and disadvantages. Provides services to more than 1,500 unduplicated consumers annually.

5956 Center for Educational Advancement New Jersey
11 Minneakoning Rd.
Flemington, NJ 08822 908-782-1480
cea-nj.org

Michael Skoczek, President & CEO
Philip Ferri, Chair
Michael Collins, Treasurer
A CARF-accredited, nonprofit organization that provides opportunities for disbaled individuals to lead productive lives. Programs offered throughout Central New Jersey.

5957 **Easterseals New Jersey**
25 Kennedy Blvd.
Suite 600
East Brunswick, NJ 08816   732-257-6662
                                            Fax: 732-257-7373
                                            www.easterseals.com/nj
Brian Fitzgerald, President & CEO
Helen Drobnis, Chief Advancement Officer & Corporate Secretary
Michael Owen, Chief Human Resources Officer & General Counsel
A nonprofit organization that provides opportunities for disabled
citizens of New Jersey to be independent and participate in their
communities. Easterseals New Jersey serves over 9,000
individuals.

5958 **Eden Autism**
2 Merwick Rd.
Princeton, NJ 08540   609-987-0099
                                            edenautism.org
Michael K. Decker, President & CEO
Jennifer Bizub, Chief Operating Officer
Melinda Gorny McAleer, Chief Development Officer
A nonprofit organization that provides a variety of services for
chidlren and adults with autism. Services include individualized
education, employment training/placement, group residences,
and early intervention.

5959 **Edison Sheltered Workshop**
48 Ethel Road
Edison, NJ 08817   732-985-8834
                                            Fax: 732-985-2216
                                            info@eswnj.org
                                            www.eswnj.org
Brij Chawla, Executive Director
Rick Parker, President
Mark Viggiano, Vice President
An organization that provides vocational training and job place-
ment services for disabled individuals who are 16 years old and
living in Middlesex County.

5960 **Goodwill Industries of Southern New Jersey**
2835 Route 73
Maple Shade, NJ 08052   856-439-0200
                                            Fax: 856-439-0843
                                            juli.lundberg@goodwillnj.org
                                            goodwillnj.org
Mark Boyd, President & CEO
Michael Shaw, Chief Operating Officer
Stephen Castro, Chief Financial Officer
A nonprofit, community-based organization that empowers indi-
viduals with special needs by providing them with the opportu-
nity to develop marketable job skills.

5961 **Hudson Community Enterprises**
68-70 Tuers Ave.
Jersey City, NJ 07306   201-434-3303
                                            Fax: 201-434-3660
                                            info@hce.works
                                            hce.works
Joseph F. Brown, President
Vocational rehab, transition services and training programs are
offered.

5962 **Inroads to Opportunities**
301 Cox St.
Roselle, NJ 07203   908-241-7200
                                            Fax: 908-241-2025
                                            ocuc@inroadsto.com
                                            www.occupationalcenter.org
Michele Ford, President & CEO
Ken Rowinsky, Board Treasurer
Lynn Boyko, Recording Secretary
Formerly known as the Occupational Center of Union County, the
organization offers vocational preparation, transition from
school to work, job placement and mental health services to over
500 individuals annually.

5963 **Jersey Cape**
152 Crest Haven Road
Cape May Court House, NJ 08210-1651   609-465-4117
                                            www.jerseycape.org
Joe Sittineri, Executive Director

Offers a range of employment programs and services for people
with disabilities.

5964 **Jewish Vocational Service (JVS) - East Orange**
7 Glenwood Ave.
Lower Level
East Orange, NJ 07017   973-674-6330
                                            info@jvsnj.org
                                            jvsnj.org
Michael Andreas, Executive Director
Rebecca Shulman, Senior Program Director
Hetal Narciso, Chief Operating Officer
Offers vocational rehabilitation services, as well as education
and literacy.

5965 **Jewish Vocational Service (JVS) - Livingston**
354 Eisenhower Parkway
Plaza 1, Suite 2150
Livingston, NJ 07039   973-674-6330
                                            info@jvsnj.org
                                            jvsnj.org
Michael Andreas, Executive Director
Rebecca Shulman, Senior Program Director
Hetal Narciso, Chief Operating Officer
Houses JVS administration, as well as providing career counsel-
ing, job placement and corporate training services.

5966 **Jewish Vocational Service (JVS) - Montclair**
83 Walnut St.
Montclair, NJ 07042   973-674-6330
                                            info@jvsnj.org
                                            jvsnj.org
Michael Andreas, Executive Director
Rebecca Shulman, Senior Program Director
Hetal Narciso, Chief Operating Officer
Provides vocational rehabilitation services.

5967 **New Jersey Commission for the Blind and Visually
Impaired (CBVI)**
Department of Human Services
153 Halsey St
6th Floor, PO Box 47017
Newark, NJ 07101   973-648-3333
                                            877-685-8878
                                            askcbvi@dhs.state.nj.us
                                            www.state.nj.us/humanservices/cbvi
Bernice Davis, Executive Director
Edward Szajdecki, Chief, Fiscal Services
Eva Scott, Director of Blindness Education
The Commission for the Blind and Visually Impaired (CBVI)
promotes and provides services in the areas of education, employment, independence and eye health for persons who are blind
or visually impaired, their families and the community. It seeks to
provide or ensure access to services that will enable consumers to
obtain their fullest measure of self-reliance and quality of life and
fully integrated into their community.

5968 **New Jersey Division of Vocational Rehabilitation
Services (DVRS)**
Department of Labor and Workforce Development
1 John Fitch Plaza
Trenton, NJ 08611   www.nj.gov/labor/career-services/
Robert Asaro-Angelo, Commissioner
Julie Diaz, Chief of Staff
Caroline M. Stout, Director, Disability Determination Services
Services for individuals with disabilities who want to become
employed.

5969 **New Jersey Institute for Disabilities (NJID)**
10A Oak Dr.
Edison, NJ 08837   732-549-6187
                                            www.njid.org
Robert J. Ferrara, Acting President
Robert J. Gross, Controller
Frank A. Ursino, Director of Security
Dedicated to the provision of comprehensive, superior,
multi-faceted programs of service to individuals with develop-
mental and related disabilities.

5970 Occupational Training Center of Burlington County (OTCBC)
2 Manhattan Drive
Burlington, NJ 08016   609-267-6677
Fax: 609-265-8418
info@otcbc.org
otcbc.org

Isaac Manning, Executive Director
Mission is to assist individuals with disabilities in reaching their maximum potential.

5971 Occupational Training Center (OTC)
The Arc of Camden County
520 Market Street
Camden, NJ 08102   856-768-0845
Fax: 856-767-1378
commissioners@camdencounty.com
www.camdencounty.com

Loret McClain, Contact
Provides the following to residents of Camden County: job placement; supported employment; extended employment; vocational evaluation and assessment; work adjustment training; and contract work.

5972 Pathways to Independence, Inc.
60 Kingsland Ave.
Kearny, NJ 07032   201-997-6155
www.pathwaysnj.org

Alvin Cox, Executive Director
Tessa Farrell, Program Director
Marie Yakobofski, Finance Director
Pre-vocational and vocational programming for people with disabilities. Specializing in developmental disabilities, learning disabilities and mental health issues. Serving over 100 people in Hudson, Bergen and Essex Counties. CARF accredited.

5973 Somerset Community Action Program, Inc.
155 Pierce St.
Suite F
Somerset, NJ 08873   732-846-8888
Fax: 732-214-9754
info@somersetcap.org
www.somersetcap.org

Steven Nagel, Executive Director
Sabah Hussein, Finance Director
Abdul Jackson, Program Coordinator
Provides services for low-income individuals and those with disabilities who want to become employed.

5974 St. John of God Community Services Vocational Rehabilitation
1145 Delsea Dr.
Westville Grove, NJ 08093   856-848-4700
Communications@sjogcs.org
www.sjogcs.org

Thomas Osorio, Executive Director
Serves Gloucester and Camden Counties providing special education, vocational and habilitative services to residents of southern New Jersey since 1967.

5975 The Arc Gloucester
1555 Gateway Blvd.
West Deptford, NJ 08096   856-848-8648
www.thearcgloucester.org

Lisa Conley, Chief Executive Officer
A nonprofit organization serving people with intellectual and related developmental disabilities and their families through education, advocacy, and direct services.

5976 United Cerebral Palsy Associations of New Jersey
1005 Whitehead Rd. Extension
Suite 1
Ewing, NJ 08638   609-882-4182
888-322-1918
Fax: 609-882-4054
info@advopps.org
advopps.org

Paul Ronollo, Acting Chief Executive Officer
Charlie Morin, Acting Chief Financial Officer
Scott Kutcher, Controller

Dedicated to changing lives and bringing independence to people with all types of disabilities.

New Mexico

5977 Adelante Development Center
3900 Osuna Rd. NE
Albuquerque, NM 87109   505-341-2000
Fax: 505-341-2001
info@GoAdelante.org
www.goadelante.org

Rebecca Sanford, President & CEO
Ryan Baca, Chair
Merritt Allen, Secretary
Serves Albuquerque and Belen.

5978 Goodwill Industries of New Mexico
5000 San Mateo Blvd. NE
Albuquerque, NM 87109   505-881-6401
866-376-0182
Fax: 505-884-3157
media@goodwillnm.org
goodwillnm.org

Shauna Kastle, President & CEO
Tom Downey, Chief Financial Officer
Sara Penn, Chief Services Officer
Serves Albuquerque, Santa Fe and Rio Rancho.

5979 LifeROOTS
1111 Menaul Blvd. NE
Albuquerque, NM 87107   505-255-5501
StephanieH@LifeROOTSNM.org
www.liferootsnm.org

Matthew Molina, President & CEO
Michelle Hayden, Finance Director
Angela Ortega, Community Services Director
Albuquerque, Rio Rancho and the surrounding area. Mission is to improve the abilities, interests, and choices of children and adults with physical, developmental or behavioral challenges with the goal of achieving their highest levels of self-sufficiency.

5980 New Mexico Commission for the Blind (NMCFTB)
2905 Rodeo Park Dr E
Bldg 4, Suite 100
Santa Fe, NM 87505   505-476-4479
888-513-7968
www.cfb.state.nm.us

Arthur A. Schreiber, Chairman
Shirley Lansing, Commissioner
Robert Reidy, Commissioner
Offers services for the totally blind, legally blind, visually impaired, and more with health, counseling, educational, recreational, rehabilitation, computer training and professional training services.

5981 New Mexico Division of Vocational Rehabilitation
505-954-8500
800-224-7005
www.dvr.state.nm.us

Casey Stone-Romero, Director
Robert Alirez, Chief Information Officer
Therese "Terry" Trujillo, Admin. Services Deputy Director & Chief Financial Officer
Purpose is to help people with disabilities achieve a suitable employment outcome.

5982 New Mexico Workforce Connection
New Mexico Department of Workforce Solutions
501 Mountain Rd NE
Albuquerque, NM 87102   505-843-1900
www.dws.state.nm.us

Assists with job searches, referrals and placement. Partner of the American Job Center Network.

5983 Tohatchi Area of Opportunity & Services
PO Box 49
Tohatchi, NM 87325   505-722-9287
                                              Fax: 505-722-9189
                                                  taos-inc.org

Kimber Crowe, Chief Executive Officer
Gerald Morris, Manager, Program Service
Provides a range of programs for Native Americans with developmental disabilities.

New York

5984 Adult Career and Continuing Ed Services - Vocational Rehabilitation (ACCESS-VR)
New York State Education Department
89 Washington Ave.
Albany, NY 12234   518-474-3852
                                                  800-222-5627
                                              www.acces.nysed.gov/vr

MaryEllen Elia, Commissioner
Aims to assist people with disabilities attain and maintain employment.

5985 National Business & Disability Council
The Viscardi Center
201 I.U. Willets Rd.
Albertson, NY 11507   516-465-1400
                                              info@viscardicenter.org
                                          viscardicenter.org/services/nbdc

Dr. Chris Rosa, President & Chief Executive Officer
Sheryl P. Buchel, Executive Vice President & Chief Financial Officer
Michael Caprara, Chief Information Officer
The NBDC is a resource for employers seeking to integrate people with disabilities into the workplace and companies seeking to reach them in the consumer marketplace.

5986 New York State Department of Labor
Building 12
State Office Campus
Albany, NY 12240   518-457-9000
                                                  888-469-7365
                                                  www.labor.ny.gov

Scott Melvin, Executive Deputy Commissioner
The mission of the New York State Department of Labor is to help New York work by preparing individuals for jobs. Provides direct job search and counseling services to job seekers, and can refer people who have disabilities for training opportunities. Provides unemployment insurance for those out of work through no fault of their own.

North Carolina

5987 Division of Vocational Rehabilitation Services (DVRS)
Western Regional Office
2801 Mail Service Center
Raleigh, NC 27699-2801   919-579-5100
                                                  800-689-9090
                                              TTY: 919-855-3579
                                                  www.ncdhhs.gov

Kody Kinsley, Secretary of Health & Human Services
Services include vocational evaluation, work adjustment, job placement, and an on-site work services program.

5988 Division of Vocational Rehabilitation Services (DVRS)
NC Department of Health and Human Services
2801 Mail Service Center
Raleigh, NC 27699-2801   919-579-5100
                                                  800-689-9090
                                              TTY: 919-855-3579
                                              www.ncdhhs.gov/divisions/dvrs

Kody Kinsley, Secretary of Health & Human Services
Seeks to promote employment and independence for people with disabilities through customer partnership and community leadership.

5989 Division of Workforce Solutions
NC Department of Commerce
301 North Wilmington St.
Raleigh, NC 27601-1058   919-814-4600
                                              info@nccommerce.com
                                          www.nccommerce.com/jobs-training

Machelle Baker Sanders, Secretary of Commerce
Jordan Whichard, Chief Deputy Secretary
Marqueta Welton, Chief of Staff
Offers vocational assessment, training, and adult developmental activities.

5990 LIFESPAN Incorporated
1511 Shopton Rd.
Suite A
Charlotte, NC 28217   704-944-5100
                                              www.lifespanservices.org

Ken D. Fuquay, President & Chief Ambassador, Empowerment
Christopher White, Chief Operating Officer
Robin Devore, Chief Compliance Officer
Aims to transform the lives of children and adults with developmental disabilities by providing education, employment, and enrichment programs that promote inclusion, choice, family supports, and other best practices.

5991 NCWorks Commission
NC Department of Commerce
301 North Wilmington St.
Raleigh, NC 27601-1058   919-814-4600
                                          NCWorksCommission@nccommerce.com
                                              www.nccommerce.com

Machelle Baker Sanders, Secretary of Commerce
Jordan Whichard, Chief Deputy Secretary
Marqueta Welton, Chief of Staff
North Carolina's workforce development board. Seeks to prepare workers in the state for the future by increasing access to education and skills training, among other initiatives.

5992 North Carolina Division of Services for the Blind
Department of Health and Human Services
2601 Mail Service Center
Raleigh, NC 27699-2601   919-527-6700
                                                  800-222-1546
                                              www.ncdhhs.gov/divisions/dsb

Kody Kinsley, Secretary of Health & Human Services
Since 1935, the mission of the North Carolina Division of Services for the Blind has been to enable people who are blind or visually impaired to reach their goals of independence and employment.

5993 Rowan Vocational Opportunities, Inc. (RVO)
2728 Old Concord Rd.
Salisbury, NC 28146   704-633-6223
                                              www.rowanvocopp.org

Gary Yelton, Executive Director
Skip Kraft, Director, Operations
Glenn McDonald, Director, Sales & Marketing
Offers vocational assessment, training, and adult developmental activities.

5994 Rutherford Vocational Workshop
230 Fairground Rd.
Spindale, NC 28160   828-286-4352
                                          rutherfordlifeservices@gmail.com
                                              rutherfordlifeservices.com

Amanda Freeman, Executive Director
T.J. Francis, Director, Finance
John Jarrett, Director, Human Resources
Offers vocational assessment, training, and adult developmental activities.

5995 Transylvania Vocational Services (TVS)
11 Mountain Industrial Drive
PO Box 1115
Brevard, NC 28712   828-884-3195
                                                  info@tvsinc.org
                                                  www.tvsinc.org

Jamie Brandenburg, Chief Executive Officer
A private nonprofit corporation with the mission to provide skills development, career opportunities and related services in a supportive environment for people with barriers to employment.

5996 **WestBridge Vocational**
140 Little Savannah Rd.
Sylvia, NC 28779 828-586-8981
jrigdon@westbridgevoc.org
www.westbridgevoc.org

Joe Rigdon, Product Information
A community-based employment and training program for people with disabilities. Their full-service program includes a transitional youth program for life beyond high school, job coaching, vocational assessment and job placement.

North Dakota

5997 **Job Service North Dakota**
Job Service North Dakota
P.O. Box 5507
Bismarck, ND 58506-5507 701-328-2825
Fax: 701-328-4000
TTY: 800-366-6888
www.jobsnd.com

Doug Burgum, Executive Director
Offers vocational assessment, training, and adult developmental activities.

5998 **North Dakota Department of Labor, and Human Rights**
Dept 406
600 East Boulevard Avenue
Bismarck, ND 58505- 0340 701-328-2660
800-582-8032
800-366-6888
Fax: 701-328-2031
TTY: 800-366-6888
labor@nd.gov
www.nd.gov/labor

Erica Thunder, Labor Commissioner
Through a work-sharing agreement with the Equal Employment Opportunity Commission (EEOC), the North Dakota Department of Labor's Human Rights Division enforces the Americans with Disabilities Act (ADA) as related to employment discrimination.

5999 **North Dakota Vocational Rehabilitation Agency**
100 E Divide Avenue
Bismarck, ND 58501 701-328-8950
800-755-2745
Fax: 701-328-8969
dhsvr@nd.gov
www.nd.gov/dhs/dvr/

Damian Schlinger, State Director
Alicia Halle, Assistant Director
Patty Wanner, Operations Administrator
The North Dakota Vocational Rehabilitation Agency offers services for blind and visually impaired people such as health, counseling, educational, recreational, rehabilitation, computer training and professional training services.

Ohio

6000 **Bureau of Vocational Rehabilitation (BVR)**
400 East Campus View Blvd.
Columbus, OH 43235 614-438-1200
800-282-4536
susan.pugh@ood.ohio.gov
ood.ohio.gov

Susan Pugh, Deputy Director
State agency that provides vocational rehabilitation services to help people with disabilities become employed and independent.

6001 **Greater Cincinnati Behavioral Health Services - Employment Services**
1501 Madison Rd.
Cincinnati, OH 45206 513-354-5200
gcbhs.com

Jeff O'Neil, President & CEO
Jeff Kirschner, Chief Operations Officer
Tracey Skale, Chief Medical Officer
Offers the following services: job exploration; job development; job coaching and employment supports; and specialized programs.

Oklahoma

6002 **Office of Disability Concerns**
1112 N May Ave.
Suite 103A
Oklahoma City, OK 73103 405-521-3756
odc@odc.ok.gov
www.odc.ok.gov

Doug MacMillan, Director
William Ginn, Disability Program Specialist, Client Assistance Program
Mission is to promote the employment of people with disabilities. The vision of the committee is to facilitate partnerships with commitment to full, high-quality employment of people with disabilities.

6003 **Oklahoma Department of Rehabilitation Services**
3535 NW 58th St.
Suite 500
Oklahoma City, OK 73112-4824 405-951-3400
800-845-8476
Fax: 405-951-3529
www.oklahoma.gov/okdrs.html

Melinda Fruendt, Executive Director
The Oklahoma Department of Rehabilitation Services (DRS) provides assistance to Oklahomans with disabilities through vocational rehabilitation, employment, independent living, residential and outreach programs, and the determination of medical eligibility for disability benefits.

6004 **Oklahoma Employment Security Commission (OESC)**
PO Box 52003
Oklahoma City, OK 73152-2003 405-557-7100
888-980-9675
TTY: 800-722-0353
OESCHelps@oesc.state.ok.us
www.ok.gov/oesc

Shelley Zumwalt, Executive Director
Michelle Britten, Chief Operations Officer
Taylor Adams, Director of Communications
Connects Ohioans with work, as well as enhancing skills and providing unemployment compensation.

Oregon

6005 **Bureau of Labor and Industries (BOLI)**
800 NE Oregon St
Suite 1045
Portland, OR 97232 971-673-0761
BOLI_help@boli.oregon.gov
www.oregon.gov/boli

Val Hoyle, Commissioner
Protects Oregonians from unlawful discrimination, defends workers' rights, and provides training to employees and employers.

6006 **Opportunities Foundation of Central Oregon**
P.O. Box 430
835 E. Hwy 126
Redmond, OR 97756 541-548-2611
Fax: 541-548-9573
info@opportunityfound.org
www.opportunityfound.org

Margee O'Brien, President
Shelly Hudspeth, Vice President
Marci Campbell, Secretary
Offers supported employment, residential support and behavior consultation services, including employment at three thirft stores.

6007   Oregon Commission for the Blind
535 SE 12th Avenue
Portland, OR 97214   971-673-1588
                                         888-202-5463
                                    Fax: 503-234-7468
                                    ocb.mail@state.or.us
                                    www.oregon.gov/Blind
Dacia Johnson, Executive Director
Angel Hale, Director, Rehabilitation Services
Malinda Carlson, Director, Independent Living Services
A resource for visually impaired Oregonians, as well as their families, friends, and employers. Nationally recognized programs and staff that make a difference in people's lives every day.

**6008   Oregon Department of Human Services Vocational
         Rehabilitation (DHS VR)**
500 Summer St. NE
Suite E-15
Salem, OR 97301   503-945-5600
                                    Fax: 503-581-6198
                                    TTY: 503-945-6214
                                    odhs.directorsoffice@dhsoha.state.or.us
                                    www.oregon.gov/dhs/employment/VR
Fariborz Pakseresht, Director
Ashley Carson Cottingham, Director, Aging & People With Disabilities
Lilia Teninty, Director, Office of Developmental Disabilities Services
Offers vocational assessments and training, adult developmental activities, and helps remove disability related barriers to employment.

Pennsylvania

6009   Office of Vocational Rehabilitation (OVR)
Pennsylvania Department of Labor & Industry
1521 North Sixth St.
Harrisburg, PA 17102   dli.pa.gov/Individuals/Disability-Services
Helps individuals with disabilities prepare for, obtain, and manage employment, with services provided both directly and through a network of vendors.

6010   Pennsylvania Department of Labor and Industry (DLI)
1700 Labor & Industry Building
Harrisburg, PA 17102   717-787-5729
                                    www.dli.state.pa.us
Administers benefits to unemployed individuals, oversees the administration of worker's compensation benefits to individuals with job related injuries, and provides vocational rehabilitation to individuals with disabilities.

**6011   Pennsylvania Governor's Cabinet Committee for People
         With Disabilities**
Department of Human Services
234 Health and Welfare Bldg.
Harrisburg, PA 17105-2675   717-787-3422
                                         800-692-7462
                                    Fax: 717-772-2490
                                    www.dhs.pa.gov
Teresa Miller, Chair
Mission is to assist with disabilities to secure and maintain employment and independence.

6012   Pennsylvania Human Relations Commission Agency
Executive Offices
333 Market St.
8th Fl.
Harrisburg, PA 17101-2210   717-787-4410
                                    TTY: 717-787-7279
                                    phrc@pa.gov
                                    phrc.state.pa.us
Jennifer Berrier, Secretary of Labor & Industry
Mission is to administer and enforce the PHRAct and the PFEOA of the Commonwealth of Pennsylvania for the identification and elimination of discrimination and the providing of equal opportunity for all persons.

Rhode Island

6013   Groden Network
610 Manton Ave.
Providence, RI 02909   401-274-6310
                                    grodennetwork.org
Michael Pearis, Chief Executive Officer
Grace Toe, Chief Financial Officer
Cooper Woodard, Chief Clinical Officer
The Groden Network aims to support children & adults with autism, as well as other developmental disailities, by providing educational, therapeutic and other services. The Network also engages in research, and educates families as well. The Network consists of The Groden Center, The Cover Center, and The Halcyon Center.

6014   Office of Rehabilitation Services
40 Fountain Street
Providence, RI 02903-1898   401-421-7005
                                    TTY: 401-421-7016
                                    www.ors.ri.gov
Joseph Murphy, Associate Director
Beth Rioles, Administrator, DDS
Laurie DiOrio, Administrator, SBVI
Goal is to help individuals with physical and mental disabilities prepare for and obtain appropriate employment.

**6015   Rhode Island Services for the Blind and Visually
         Impaired**
40 Fountain Street
Providence, RI 02903-1898   401-421-7005
                                    TTY: 401-421-7016
                                    www.ors.ri.gov/SBVI.html
Ron Racine, Associate Director
Beth Rioles, Administrator, DDS
Laurie DiOrio, Administrator, SBVI
Provides qualifying people with visual impairments opportunities to become self-sustaining members of the community.

South Carolina

6016   South Carolina Commission for the Blind (SCCB)
1430 Confederate Ave.
Columbia, SC 29201-79   803-898-8731
                                    publicinfo@sccb.sc.gov
                                    www.sccb.state.sc.us
Goal is to help individuals with visual impairments prepare for and obtain appropriate employment.

**6017   South Carolina Department of Employment and
         Workforce (DEW)**
1550 Gadsden St.
P.O. Box 995
Columbia, SC 29202   803-737-2400
                                         866-831-1724
D. Ellzey, Executive Director
T. Timmons, Chief Legal Officer
J. Michaelson, Chief Financial Officer
Public agency that offers job search assistance, unemployment benefits and a WIA program. Also offered are services for individuals with disabilities.

**6018   South Carolina Governor's Committee on Employment
         of the Handicapped**
S.C. Vocational Rehabilitation Department
1410 Boston Ave.
West Columbia, SC 29171   803-896-6500
                                         800-832-7526
                                    TTY: 806-896-6553
                                    communications@scvrd.net
                                    www.scvrd.net
Felicia W. Johnson, Commissioner
Goal is to help individuals with physical and mental disabilities prepare for and obtain appropriate employment.

6019 **South Carolina Vocational Rehabilitation Department (SCVRD)**
1410 Boston Ave.
West Columbia, SC 29171   803-896-6500
800-832-7526
TTY: 806-896-6553
communications@scvrd.net
www.scvrd.net

Felicia W. Johnson, Commissioner
The SCVRD's mission is to enable eligible South Carolinians with disabilities to prepare for, achieve and maintain competitive employment.

South Dakota

6020 **South Dakota Department of Human Services**
Hillsview Plaza
3800 E Hwy 34
Pierre, SD 57501   605-773-5990
Fax: 605-773-5483
infodhs@state.sd.us
dhs.sd.gov

Shawnie Rechtenbaugh, Secretary
Provides resources for individuals with developmental disabilities, including rehabilitation services, services for the blind and visually impaired, and long-term services and supports.

6021 **South Dakota Department of Human Services: Div. of Service to the Blind & Visually Impaired**
Hillview Plaza
3800 E Highway 34
Pierre, SD 57501   605-773-3195
Fax: 605-773-5483
dhs.sd.gov/servicetotheblind

Shawnie Rechtenbaugh, Secretary
To provide individualized rehabilitation services that result in optimal employment and independent living outcomes for people with visual impairments.

6022 **South Dakota State Vocational Rehabilitation**
Department of Human Services
3800 E Hwy 34
Hillview Plaza
Pierre, SD 57501   605-773-3195
Fax: 605-773-5483
dhs.sd.gov/rehabservices/vr.aspx

Shawnie Rechtenbaugh, Secretary
Provides employment services to people with significant disabilities.

6023 **South Dakota Workforce Investment Act Training Programs**
123 W Missouri Ave.
Pierre, SD 57501-0405   605-773-3101
Fax: 605-773-6184
dlr.sd.gov/workforce_services/wioa

Marcia Hultman, Department Secretary
Dawn Dovre, Deputy Secretary
Andrew Szilvasi, Technology Development
Mission is to enhance the South Dakota workforce by providing business with employment-related solutions and helping people with job placement and career transition services

Tennessee

6024 **Tennessee Department Human Services: Vocational Rehabilitation Services**
505 Deaderick St.
Nashville, TN 37243-1403   615-313-4891
Fax: 615-741-6508
TTY: 800-270-1349
www.tn.gov/humanservices

Clarence H. Carter, Commissioner, Human Services
Determines eligibility and nature/scope of required VR services, and provides those employment-focused rehabilitation services for individuals with disabilities.

6025 **Tennessee Department of Labor and Workforce Development**
220 French Landing Dr.
Nashville, TN 37243   844-224-5818
www.tn.gov/workforce

Jeff McCord, Commissioner
Dewayne Scott, Deputy Commissioner
Deniece Thomas, Deputy Commissioner
Offers services to employees and employers, including job training and adult education.

6026 **Tennessee Human Rights Commission**
312 Rosa L Parks Ave.
23rd Fl.
Nashville, TN 37243   615-741-5825
800-251-3589
Fax: 615-253-1886
ask.thrc@tn.gov
www.tn.gov/humanrights

Muriel Malone, Interim Executive Director
Tanya Webster, Title VI Compliance Director
Dawn Cummings, General Counsel
An independent state agency charged with preventing and eradicating discrimination in employment, public accomodations, and housing.

Texas

6027 **Ability Connection**
8802 Harry Hines Blvd.
Dallas, TX 75235   214-351-2500
info@abilityconnection.org
abilityconnection.org

Jim Hanophy, President & CEO
Laura Mahaley, Chief Financial Officer
Brian Petty, Chief Operating Officer
Provides training and support services to children and adults with both physical and intellectual disabilities.

6028 **Concentra**
5080 Spectrum Dr.
Suite 1200W
Addison, TX 75001   866-944-6046
www.concentra.com

Keith Newton, President & CEO
John Anderson, Executive VP & Chief Medical Officer
John deLorimier, Executive VP, Customer Growth & Experience
Offers employers comprehensive occupational health services and state-of-the-art physical and occupational therapy. Staff works as a team to produce the best possible patient care while delivering cost savings through workers compensation disability management programs.

6029 **Texas Workforce Commission (TWC)**
101 E 15th St.
Austin, TX 78778-0001   800-628-5115
customers@twc.state.tx.us
www.twc.state.tx.us

Ed Serna, Interim Executive Director
Courtney Arbour, Division Director, Workforce Development
Cheryl Fuller, Division Director, Vocational Rehabilitation Services
State government agency charged with overseeing and providing workforce development services to employers and job seekers of Texas. Offers career development information, job search resources, training programs, and, as appropriate, unemployment benefits.

6030 **Texas Workforce Commission: Vocational Rehabilitation Services**
101 E 15th St.
Austin, TX 78778-0001   800-628-5115
customers@twc.state.tx.us
twc.texas.gov

Ed Serna, Interim Executive Director
Cheryl Fuller, Division Director, Vocational Rehabilitation Services

Helps people with disabilities prepare for, find and keep jobs. Work related services are individualized and may include counseling, training, medical treatment, assistive devices, job placement assistance and other services.

Utah

6031   Utah Department of Human Services: Division of Services for People with Disabilities
195 North 1950 West
Salt Lake City, UT 84116   801-538-4171
                                             844-275-3773
                                         dhsinfo@utah.gov
                                             dspd.utah.gov
Information and referral services for people with disabilities, including DD/MR, brain injury and physical disabilities throughout the state of Utah.

6032   Utah Employment Services
2292 South Redwood Rd.
Salt Lake City, UT 84119   801-978-0378
                                      info@utahemploy.com
                                      www.utahemploy.com
To help individuals prepare and obtain appropriate employment.

6033   Utah Governor's Committee on Employment for People with Disabilities (GCEPD)
Utah State Office of Rehabilitation
P.O. Box 45249
Salt Lake City, UT 84145-0249   801-526-9675
                                     dwscontactus@utah.gov
                                         jobs.utah.gov/usor
Casey Cameron, Executive Director
Greg Paras, Deputy Director
Nate McDonald, Deputy Director
Promotes opportunities and provide support for persons with disabilities to lead self-determined lives.

6034   Utah State Office for Rehabilitation (USOR)
P.O. Box 45249
Salt Lake City, UT 84145-0249   801-526-9675
                                     dwscontactus@utah.gov
                                         jobs.utah.gov/usor
Casey Cameron, Executive Director
Greg Paras, Deputy Director
Nate McDonald, Deputy Director
Provides services for individuals who are blind or visually impaired, deaf or hard of hearing, and those with other disabilities, including vocational rehabilitation.

6035   Utah State Office of Rehabilition: Vocational Rehabilitation
P.O. Box 45249
Salt Lake City, UT 84145-0249   801-526-9675
                                         jobs.utah.gov/usor/vr
Casey Cameron, Executive Director
Greg Paras, Deputy Director
Nate McDonald, Deputy Director
Vocational Rehabilitation Services for individuals with disabilities. To assist individuals with disabilities to prepare for and obtain employment and increase their independence.

6036   Utah State Office of Rehabilition: Services for the Blind and Visually Impaired
P.O. Box 45249
Salt Lake City, UT 84145-0249   801-526-9675
                                     dwscontactus@utah.gov
                                         jobs.utah.gov/usor/vr
Casey Cameron, Executive Director
Greg Paras, Deputy Director
Nate McDonald, Deputy Director
Individuals who are blind or visually impaired receive training, adjustment services, and other assistive aids.

6037   Veterans Support Center (VSC)
Union Building
Room 418
Salt Lake City, UT 84112   801-587-7722
                                       vetcenter@sa.utah.edu
                                     veteranscenter.utah.edu
Paul Morgan, Director
Matt Root, Veterans Program Coordinator
Angela Brink, Office Manager
Readjustment counseling services to veterans.

Vermont

6038   Vermont Department of Disabilities, Aging and Independent Living (DAIL)
280 State Dr.
HC2 South
Waterbury, VT 05671-2020   802-241-2401
                                        Fax: 802-241-0386
                                          dail.vermont.gov
Monica White, Interim Commissioner
Provides programs and services for people with physical and developmental disabilities, as well as those with visual impairments, and those over 60 years of age. Employment services for people with disabilities are also provided.

6039   Vermont Department of Labor
5 Green Mountain Dr.
PO Box 488
Montpelier, VT 05601- 0488   802-828-4000
                               labor.commissioner@vermont.gov
                                         labor.vermont.gov
Michael A. Harrington, Commissioner
Dustin Degree, Deputy Commissioner
The primary focus is to help support the efforts to make Vermont a more competitive place to do business and create good jobs.

6040   Vermont Division of Vocational Rehabilitation
280 State Dr.
HC2 South
Waterbury, VT 05671-2040   866-879-6757
                                        Fax: 803-241-0341
                                        vocrehab.vermont.gov
Diane Dalmasse, Division Director
Provides employment services to individuals with physical or developmental disabilities.

Virginia

6041   Campagna Center
418 S Washington St.
Alexandria, VA 22314   703-549-0111
                                        Fax: 703-549-2097
                                     www.campagnacenter.org
Janice Abraham, Board Chair, President & CEO
Don Lubreski, Chief Financial Officer
Edith Hawkins, Chief Program Officer
Offers social services, on-the-job-training for parents, play therapy, physical therapy, speech therapy and other specialized services.

6042   Didlake
8641 Breeden Ave.
Manassas, VA 20110-8431   703-361-4195
                                             866-361-4195
                                        Fax: 703-369-7141
                                           ask@didlake.org
                                          www.didlake.com
Donna Hollis, Chief Executive Officer
Den,e Fortune McKnight, Vice President, Finance & Administration/CFO
Offers situational assessments, work training, employment and job placement services to people with disabilities.

6043 Richmond Research Training Center (RRTC)
PO Box 842011
1314 West Main St.
Richmond, VA 23284-2011
804-828-1851
Fax: 804-828-2193
TTY: 804-828-2494
RRTC@vcu.edu
vcurrtc.org

Paul Wehman, Professor & Director
John Kregel, Associate Director
Katherine Inge, Director, Employment
Research and training center report on the supported employment of persons with developmental and other disabilities.

6044 ServiceSource Disability Resource Center
10467 White Granite Dr.
Oakton, VA 22124
703-461-6000
www.servicesource.org

Bruce Patterson, Chief Executive Officer
Mark Hall, President
Nate Hoover, Chief Financial Officer
Provides training, job placement and employment services in private sector and government contract employment.

6045 SourceAmerica
8401 Old Courthouse Rd.
Vienna, VA 22182
888-411-8424
www.sourceamerica.org

Richard Belden, President & CEO
Jeffrey McCaw, Chief Financial Officer
Wes Tyler, Executive Vice President & Chief Operating Officer
SourceAmerica facilitates the Federal AbilityOne Program, which provides employment opportunities for people with disabilities. Provides products and services to government, corporate and nonprofit clients, as well as advocating on behalf of the disabled.

6046 Virginia Department for the Blind and Vision Impaired (DBVI)
397 Azalea Ave.
Richmond, VA 23227
804-371-3140
800-622-2155
www.vdbvi.org

Raymond E. Hopkins, Commissioner
Rick L. Mitchell, Deputy Commissioner, Services
Matt Koch, Deputy Commissioner, Enterprises
Offers services for the totally blind, legally blind, visually impaired, and more with health, counseling, educational, recreational, rehabilitation, computer training and professional training services.

Washington

6047 Business Enterprise Program (BEP)
Department of Services for the Blind
PO Box 40959
4565 7th Ave. SE
Olympia, WA 98504-0959
206-906-5500
800-552-7103
info@dsb.wa.gov
dsb.wa.gov

Michael MacKillop, Acting Executive Director
The Program allows qualified legally-blind individuals to operate food service businesses in government buildings.

6048 Department of Services for the Blind (DSB)
PO Box 40959
4565 7th Ave. SE
Olympia, WA 98504-0959
206-906-5500
800-552-7103
info@dsb.wa.gov
dsb.wa.gov

Michael MacKillop, Acting Executive Director
Offers a range of services for citizens with viosual impairments, including employment services.

6049 Department of Social & Health Services: Division of Vocational Rehabilitation
Customer Service Center
P.O. Box 11699
Tacoma, WA 98411-6699
877-501-2233
TTY: 800-833-6384
www1.dshs.wa.gov/dvr

Jilma Meneses, Secretary
Lisa Yanagida, Chief of Staff
Terry Redmon, Director
Mission is to empower individuals with disabilities to achieve a greater quality of life by obtaining and maintaining employment.

6050 Department of Social & Health Services: Developmental Disabilities Administration (DDA)
Customer Service Center
P.O. Box 11699
Tacoma, WA 98411-6699
877-501-2233
TTY: 800-833-6384
askdshs@dshs.wa.gov
www.dshs.wa.gov/dda

Jilma Meneses, Secretary
Lisa Yanagida, Chief of Staff
Terry Redmon, Director
Offers persons with developmental disabilities quality supports and services that are individual/family driven, stable and flexible, satisfying to the person and their family, and able to meet individual needs.

6051 SL Start Washington
909 SE Everett Mall Way
Everett, WA 98208
206-365-0809
www.lsrserviceswa.com

Kendra Ellis, Executive Director
LaceyJay Switzer, Area Director Snohomish & King County
Enola Stark, Program Manager
A diversified and innovative human and health services company focused on a wide range of social, employment and long-term services.

West Virginia

6052 West Virginia Division of Rehabilitation Services (DRS)
P.O. Box 50890
Charleston, WV 25305-0890
304-356-2060
800-642-8207
TTY: 304-766-4809
www.wvdrs.org

DRS specializes in helping people with disabilities who want to find a job or maintain current employment. Rehabilitation counselors at more than 30 field offices help with applications. Once eligibility is determined, counselors & clients work as a team to develop a plan to meet the individuals employment goal. Services may include work-related counseling/guidance, evaluation/assessment, job development & placement assistance, vocational training, college assistance & assistive technology.

6053 WorkForce West Virginia
P.O. Box 2753
1321 Plaza East Shopping Ctr.
Charleston, WV 25330-2753
800-252-5627
Fax: 304-558-1979
workforcelmi@wv.gov
workforcewv.org

Workforce West Virginia is funded through the U.S. Department of Labor, and oversees the state unemployment insurance program as well as workforce development services across the state.

Wisconsin

6054 Department of Workforce Development: Vocational Rehabilitation
P.O. Box 7852
201 East Washington Avenue
Madison, WI 53707
608-261-0050
800-442-3477
Fax: 608-266-1133
dvr@dwd.wisconsin.gov
dwd.wisconsin.gov/dvr

Delora Newton, Administrator
Meredith Dressel, Deputy Administrator
Assists eligible individuals with disabilities with finding employment.

Wyoming

6055 Department of Workforce Services: Vocational Rehabilitation
Disability Determination Services
5221 Yellowstone Road
Cheyenne, WY 82002
307-777-8650
Fax: 307-777-5857
wyomingworkforce.org/workers/vr

Robin Sessions Cooley, Director
Provides services to disabled individuals to enable them to reach vocational goals.

6056 Wyoming Department of Workforce Services: Unemployment Insurance Division
5221 Yellowstone Road
Cheyenne, WY 82002
307-777-8650
Fax: 307-777-5857
wyomingworkforce.org/workers/ui

Robin Sessions Cooley, Director
The Department is responsible for unemployment claims and payments, unemployment adjudication, employer protests and charging, and benefit payment control.

6057 Wyoming State Rehabilitation Council (SRC)
Disability Determination Services
5221 Yellowstone Road
Cheyenne, WY 82002
307-777-8650
Fax: 307-777-5307
wyomingworkforce.org/workers/vr/src

Robin Sessions Cooley, Director
Assists, empowers and supports people with disabilities to achieve employment, independence and intergration in the workplace and community.

Rehabilitation Facilities, Acute

Alabama

6058 **HealthSouth Lakeshore Rehabilitation Hospital**
3800 Ridgeway Dr
Birmingham, AL 35209-5599
205-868-2000
Fax: 205-868-2029
www.healthsouthlakeshorerehab.com
Vickie Demers, Chief Executive Officer
April Cobb, Chief Nursing Officer
Al Rayburn, Director, Therapy Operations
A 100 bed facility whos key services is physical rehabilitation. Also specialized services (inpatient) infection isolation room. In addition, also has outpatient physical rehabilitation and sports medicine. Patient family support services include patient representative, transportation for elderly/handicapped and patient support groups. Imaging services(diagnostic & theraputic) include ct scanner, diagnostic diagnostic radioisotope facility, MRI, and ultrasound.

6059 **HealthSouth Rehabilitation Hospital of North Alabama**
107 Governors Dr
Huntsville, AL 35801
256-535-2300
Fax: 256-428-2608
www.healthsouthhuntsville.com
Douglas H. Beverly, Chief Executive Officer
Susan Creekmore, Director, Therapy Operations
Risha Hoover, Director, Marketing Operations
A comprehensive 50 bed rehabilitation hospital serving the need of patients in the North Alabama area. Guides patients with physically disabling conditions along an individualized treatment pathway so they can reach their highest level of physical, social and emotional well-being. A wide range of medical and theraputic services are delivered by qualified and experienced professionals.

6060 **J.L. Bedsole/Rotary Rehabilitation Hospital**
Infirmary Health
5 Mobile Infirmary Circle
Mobile, AL 36607-3513
251-435-3417
www.infirmaryhealth.org
D. Mark Nix, President & CEO
Kenneth C. Brewington, Chief Medical Office, Mobile Infirmary
Jennifer Eslinger, President, Mobile Infirmary
Provides rehabilitation for patients affected by stroke, spinal cord injury, brain injury or other neurological illnesses.

6061 **More Than Just a Job**
Institute On Disability/UCED
60 5th Avenue
Suite 101
New York, NY 10011
212-366-8900
Fax: 603-862-0555
www.forbes.com
Narrative case studies and interviews with persons with disabilities, their employers, families and experts in the field. *$ 20.00*

6062 **Rocky Mountain Resource & Training Institute**
3630 Sinton Road
Suite 103
Colorado Springs, CO 80907- 5072
719-444-0268
800-949-4262
Fax: 719-444-0269
TTY: 800-949-4232
www.adainformation.org
Jana Copeland, Principal Investigator
Patrick Going, Senior Advisor
Serves people with disabilities and provides training to the agencies that assist them. Facilitates disabled individuals' transition from school to adult life; provides information and resources concerning assistive technology, devices, and services; promotes and ensures compliance with the federal Americans with Disabilities Act (ADA) and other legislation promoting the rights and inclusion of people with disabilities; promotes supported employment, strategic planning and development.

Arkansas

6063 **Central Arkansas Rehab Hospital**
2201 Wildwood Ave
Sherwood, AR 72120-5074
501-834-1800
Fax: 501-834-2227
www.stvincentrehabhospital.com
Lee Frazier, MPH, Dr, CEO
Dr. Sean Foley, Medical Director
Debbie Taylor, Director of Marketing Operations
A nonprofit hospital licensed for 69 acute care beds with all private rooms. Opened in 1999the hospital offers a full range of outpatient diagnostic services, including MRI,CT,PET along with surgical procedures, cardiology, neurology, neurosurgery, othopedic, rehab and a 24 hour emergency department staffed with board certified emergency room physicians. Includes an outpatient surgery center, rehabilitation hospital, senior health program, diabetic program and physician offices.

6064 **HealthSouth Rehabilitation Hospital**
1401 South J St
Fort Smith, AR 72901-5158
479-785-3300
Fax: 479-785-8599
www.healthsouth.com
Juli Stec, CEO
Provides physical rehabilitation as its key services. Also provides other services such as end-of-life services, pain management and an infection isolation room.

6065 **Northwest Arkansas Rehabilitation Hospital**
153 E Monte Painter Dr
Fayetteville, AR 72703-4002
479-444-2233
Fax: 479-444-2390
www.healthsouthfayetteville.com
Marty Hurlbut, Medical Director
Denise Wilson, Director Of Clinical Services
A 60-bed acute medical rehabilitation hospital that offers comprehensive inpatient and outpatient rehabilitation services.

6066 **Rebsamen Rehabilitation Center**
P.O.Box 159
Jacksonville, AR 72078-159
501-985-7000
Fax: 501-985-7384
www.rebsamenmedicalcenter.com
Mack McAlister, Chairperson
Murice Green, Vice Chairman
Tommy Swaim, Secretary
Mission is to provide personal healthcare for your family. Vision is to develop a family of caregivers to become your community hospital. A 113 bed acute care facility operated by a volunteer Board of Directors made up of community leaders. Rebsamen Medical Center is accredited by the Joint Commission on Accreditation of Healthcare Organizations as well as the Arkansas Department of Health. Through JCAHO we voluntary sumbit to evaluations of our compliance with nationwide hospital standards.

Arizona

6067 **Barrow Neurological Institute Rehab Center**
350 W Thomas Rd
Phoenix, AZ 85013-4409
602-406-3000
Fax: 602-406-4104
www.stjosephs-phx.org
Jackie Aragon, VP Care Management
Linda Hunt, President
Dedicated resources to delivering compassionate, high-quality, affordable health services; serving and advocating for our sisters and brothers who are poor and disenfranchised; and partnering with others in the community to improve the quality of life. Our vision:a growing and diversified health care ministry distinguished by excellent quality and committed to expanding access to those in need.

6068 HealthSouth Sports Medicine Center
5111 N Scottsdale Rd
Ste 100
Scottsdale, AZ 85250-7076   480-990-1379
                                  Fax: 480-423-8458
                                  www.healthsouth.com

Troy Meiners, Manager
An out patient facility specialising in sports medicine and treatment of sports injuries.

6069 Healthsouth Rehab Institute of Tucson
2650 N Wyatt Dr
Tucson, AZ 85712-6108   520-325-1300
                                  800-333-8628
                                  Fax: 520-327-4045
                                  www.rehabinstituteoftucson.com

Lee Sanford, Plant Manager
Jon Larson, Medical Director
An accredited member of the Joint Commission On Accreditation of Health Care Organizaions (JCAHO) An 80 bed facility specializing in rehabilitation

6070 Scottsdale Healthcare
9630 E Shea Blvd
Scottsdale, AZ 85260-6285   480-551-5400
                                  Fax: 480-551-5401
                                  preiley@shc.org

Thomas Sadvary, CEO
Pegg Reiley, Chief Nursing Officer
Kathy Zarubi, Associate VP of Nursing Practice
A 343 bed full-service hospital providing medical/surgical, critical care, obstetrics, pediatrics, surgery, cardiovascular, and oncology services, as well as the Sleep Disorder Center. All patient rooms are private. Emergency department is a level II Trauma Center. The Radiology Department offers state-of-the-art diagnostic equipment, including MRI, PET/CT scanning, nuclear medicine and ultrasound. Also located are the Piper Surgery Center, Cancer Center, and several medical office plazas.

6071 St. Joseph Hospital and Medical Center
350 W Thomas Rd
Phoenix, AZ 85013-4496   602-406-3000
                                  Fax: 602-406-4190
                       http://hospitals.dignityhealth.org/stjosephs/
Linda Hunt, President
Rehabilitation programs offered by the clinic assists clients with rehabilitation health needs in the comfort of their own home. The home care rehabilitation team of professionals focuses on correcting deficiencies in self-care, mobility skills and communication. Services offered include physical therapy, occupational therapy, speech pathology, rehabilitative nursing and restorative nursing assistants.

California

6072 Bakersfield Regional Rehabilitation Hospital
5001 Commerce Dr
Bakersfield, CA 93309-648   661-323-5500
                                  800-288-9829
                                  Fax: 661-633-5254
                                  www.healthsouthbakersfield.com

Chris Yoon, Medical Director
Sandra Hegland, Chief Executive Officer
A specialty hospital that treats an array of physical disabilities. It has 60 beds and offers physical rehabilitation services including support groups and education classes on illnesses such as arthritis, asthma and strokes. No surgery facilities on site.

6073 Brotman Medical Center: RehabCare Unit
3828 Delmas Ter
Culver City, CA 90232-6806   310-836-7001
                                  Fax: 310-202-4141

Howard Levine, CEO
The mission of Brotman Medical Center is to deliver innovative, quality health care to our patients and their families in an environment of compassion, respect, patient saftey, education, and fiscal responsibility.

6074 Casa Colinas Centers for Rehabilitation
255 E Bonita Ave
Pomona, CA 91767-1923   909-596-7733
                                  866-724-4127
                                  Fax: 909-593-0153
                                  TTY: 909-596-3646
                                  rehab@casacolina.org
                                  www.casacolina.org

Felice Loverso, CEO/President
Steve Norin, Chairman
Stephen W. Graeber, Vice Chairman
Casa Colina will provide individuals the opportunity to maximize their medical recovery and rehabilitation potential efficiently in an environment that recognizes their uniqueness, dignity and self esteem. The vision is to strategically reposition themselves at the forefront of the post-acute continuum by becoming the center of excellence in the provision of services to persons who can benefit from rehabilitation care.

6075 Community Hospital of Los Gatos Rehabilitation Services
815 Pollard Rd
Los Gatos, CA 95032-1400   408-378-6131
                                  Fax: 408-866-4003

Ned Borgstrom, CEO
Rehabilitation Services provide individualized treatment programs for inpatient/outpatient care. The team is supervised by a Physiatrist and may include Nurses, Physical Therapists, Occupational Therapists, Speech/Language Therapists, Psychologists, Case Managers, Dietitians, Respiratory Therapists, Recreation Therapists and/or Prosthetists/Orthotists.

6076 Garfield Medical Center
525 N Garfield Ave
Monterey Park, CA 91754-1205   626-573-2222
                                  Fax: 626-571-8972
                                  www.garfieldmedicalcenter.com

Philip Cohen, CEO
Provides quality care to all citizens of all ages. We are forward looking to meet the changing health care needs of Forsyth and the surrounding area. At the same time, we are a stable organization that is financially sound. We involve all of our medical staff through good communication. We support them by trying to meet their professional needs in training, equipment and services. We emphasize good communication with all county citizens who support us financially and through the use of services

6077 Grossmont Hospital Rehabilition Center
5555 Grossmont Center
La Mesa, CA 91942   619-740-6000
                                  800-827-4277
                                  Fax: 619-644-4159
                                  www.sharp.com

Michael Murphy, President/CEO
Daniel Gross, EVP
It is our mission to improve the health of those we serve with a commitment to excellence in all that we do. Our goal is to offer quality care and programs that set community standards, exceed patients' expectations and are provided in a caring, convenient, cost-effective and accessible manner.

6078 Health South Tustin Rehabilitation Hospita
14851 Yorba St
Tustin, CA 92780-2925   714-832-9200
                                  Fax: 714-508-4550
                                  www.healthsouth.com

Sandra Yule, CEO

6079 Holy Cross Comprehensive Rehabilitation Center
15031 Rinaldi St
Mission Hills, CA 91345-1207   818-365-8051
                                  888-432-5464
                                  Fax: 818-898-4472
                                  www.providence.org

Larry Bowe, CEO
Derek Berz, COO
Known for providing exceptional treatment through its Cancer Centers, Heart Center, Orthopedics, Neurosciences and Rehabilitation Services, as well as Woman's and Children's Services. As a 254-bed, not-for-profit facility, Providence offers a full continuum of health services, from outpatient to inpatient to home

health care. Providence operates one of the only round-the-clock trauma centers in the San Fernando Valley and surrounding communities.

6080 Job Hunting Tips for the So-Called Handicapped
Special Needs Project
324 State Street
Suite H
Santa Barbara, CA 93101-2364

818-718-9900
800-333-6867
Fax: 818-349-2027
editor@specialneeds.com
www.specialneeds.com

Hod Gray, Owner
This nifty booklet from the guru of job hunting himself is sincere, useful and brief. *$4.95*

6081 Kentfield Rehabilitation Hospital & Outpatient Center
1125 Sir Francis Drake Blvd
Kentfield, CA 94904-1418

415-456-9680
Fax: 415-485-3563
info@kentfieldrehab.com
www.kentfieldrehab.com

Deborah Doherty, MD
Provides specialized inpatient and outpatient programs. We provide quality services that are patient centered and family-oriented. Under the medical direction of board-certified hospitalists and other physician specialists, our dedicated interdisciplinary teams provide a coordinated, comprehensive treatment approach to a wide range of neurological, orthopedic, pulmonary and complex medical problems.

6082 Laurel Grove Hospital: Rehab Care Unit
20103 Lake Chabot Rd
Castro Valley, CA 94546-4093

510-537-1234
Fax: 510-727-2778
nissims@sutterhealth.org
www.edenmedcenter.org

George Bischalaney, CEO & President
Kent Myers, Treasurer
Jeffrey Randall, Secretary
The mission of Eden Medical Center is carried out by our Board of Directors, employees, physicians and volunteers who are committed to providing our patients and their families with the highest quality medical care and customer service. Creating standards of excellence to ensure quality and value for our patients. Maintaining a financially sound organization through effective clinical and administrative support. Encouraging a culture that supports employees and physicians in development.

6083 Lodi Memorial Hospital West
Lodi Memorial Hospital
975 S Fairmont Ave
Lodi, CA 95240

209-334-3411
800-323-3360
Fax: 209-333-7131

Joseph Harrington, President
Ron Kreutner, Vice President And CFO
Judy Begley RN, MSN, Chief Nursing Officer
Our vision is to provide a system of health-care services which is clinically effective, quality driven and community focused in an environment that supports and encourages excellence. In partnership with our medical staff, we will assume accountability for the health of our community, be responsible for illness and injury prevention and provide care for the ill and injured. We will measure our success on quality outcomes and customer satisfaction.

6084 Long Beach Memorial Medical Center Memorial Rehabilitation Hospital
2801 Atlantic Ave
Long Beach, CA 90806-1701

562-933-2000
Fax: 562-933-9018
www.memorialcare.org

Nissar Syed, Administrator
Barry Arbuckle, President
The hospital offers rehabilitation after catastrophic injury of disabling disease to give patients the opportunity for maximum recovery. The Hospital offers many of the area's finest rehabilitation specialists and most advanced technology, making it one of Southern California's most respected rehabilitation centers.

6085 North Coast Rehabilitation Center
1165 Montgomery Drive
Santa Rosa, CA 95405-4869

707-546-3210
Fax: 707-525-8413

Joyce Cavagnaro, Admissions
Combines state-of-the-art medicine, compassionate care, and the widest array of resources to enhance your health and promote healthy communities. Dedicated to continually introducing new programs and services that help you live life to the fullest.

6086 Northridge Hospital Medical Center
18300 Roscoe Blvd
Northridge, CA 91328

818-885-8500
Fax: 818-885-5435
www.northridgehospital.org

Mike Wall, CEO
dedicating resources to delivering compassionate, high-quality, affordable health services; serving and advocating for our sisters and brothers who are poor and disinfranchised; and partnering with others in the community to improve the quality of life.

6087 PEERS Program
8912 W Olympic Blvd
Beverly Hills, CA 90211-3514

310-553-4833
Fax: 310-553-4833

Paul Berns, Medical Director
Offers a new approach for wheelchair users. PEERS uses a combination of modern physical therapy, the DOUGLAS Reciprocating Gait System and when necessary, functional electrical stimulation to assist selected individuals to walk with recently patented specially made lightweight braces.

6088 PIRS Hotsheet
Placer Independent Resource Services
11768 Atwood Rd
Ste 29
Auburn, CA 95603

530-885-6100
800-833-8453
Fax: 530-885-3032
TTY: 530-885-0326
lbrewer@pirs.org
pirs.org

Susan Miller, Executive Director
Harry Powell, President
Paul Opper, Vice President
Monthly newletter to customers and other constituents.
6 pages Monthly

6089 Providence Holy Cross Medical Center
Providence Health System
15031 Rinaldi St
Mission Hills, CA 91345-1285

818-365-8051
818-898-4603
Fax: 818-365-4472
www.providence.org

Kerry Carmody, CEO
Physicains and nurses are among the best and are reconginzed nationally for clinical excellence. We are committed to improving your health and wellness as you journey through life. Our services span beyond the latest advancements in medical procedures, equipment and medication to also include education and wellness services-all provided with compassion and respect. We help our patients understand and use some of the healthiest tools at their disposal, including nutrition & excercise.

6090 Queen of Angels/Hollywood Presbyterian Medical Center
1300 N Vermont Ave
Los Angeles, CA 90027-6005

213-413-3000
Fax: 213-413-3500
www.hollywoodpresbyterian.com

Kathy Wong, Manager
A 434 bed acute-care facility that has been caring for the Hollywood community and surrounding areas since 1924. The hospital is committed to serving local multicultural communities with quality medical and nursing care. With more then 500 physicians representing virtually every speciality. Ready to serve your medical needs and those of your loved ones and strive to distinguish itself as a leading healthcare provider, recognized for providing quality, innovative care in a compassionate manner.

6091 Queen of the Valley Hospital
1000 Trancas St
Napa, CA 94558-2941   707-252-4411
                                        Fax: 707-257-4032
                                        www.thequeen.org

Walt Mickens, President
Vincent Morgese, Vice President
For more then 40 years, Queen of the Valley Hospital has been the premiere medical facility in the Napa Valley. Our long history of providing high quality and caring service is founded on 4 core values:Dignity, Service, Excellence and Justice. These central principals inspire us to reach out to those in need and to help heal the whole person-mind, body and spirit.They are the driving force behind our mission to improve the health and quality of life of people in the community we serve.

6092 Rancho Los Amigos National Rehabilitation Center
7601 E Imperial Hwy
Downey, CA 90242-3496   562-401-7111
                                             877-726-2461
                                           888-RAN-CHO1
                                        Fax: 562-401-6690
                                        TTY: 562-401-8450
                        dhs.lacounty.gov/wps/portal/dhs/rancho

Jorge Orozco, CEO
Mindy Lipson Aisen, Chief Medical Officer
Michelle Sterling, Interim Chief Nursing Officer
Internationally renowned in the field of medical rehabilitation, consistently ranked in the top Rehabilitation Hospitals in the United States by U.S. News and World Report. It is one of the largest comprehensive rehabilitaion centers in the United States. Licensed for 395 beds, providing service through over 20 centers of excellence.

6093 San Joaquin Valley Rehabilitation Hospital
7173 N Sharon Ave
Fresno, CA 93720-3329   559-436-3600
                                        Fax: 559-436-3606
                                        sjvrehab.com

Edward Palacios, CEO
Complete comprehensive rehabilitation services from acute rehab, outpatient and community fitness services.

6094 Santa Clara Valley Medical Center
County of Santa Clara
751 S Bascom Ave
San Jose, CA 95128-2699   408-885-5000
                                        www.scvmed.org

Paul E. Lorenz, CEO
Jeffrey Arnold, Medical Officer
Trudy Johnson, Director of Patient Care Services & Nursing
The mission of the medical center is to provide high-quality, cost-effective medical care to all residence of Santa Clara County regardless of their ability to pay. Make availiable a wide range of inpatient, outpatient, emergency services within resource constraints. Maintain an environment within which the needs of our patients are paramount and where patients, their families and all our visitors are treated in a compassionate, supportive, friendly, and dignified manner.

6095 Scripps Memorial Hospital at La Jolla
9888 Genesee Ave
La Jolla, CA 92037-1205   858-626-4123
                                             800-727-4777
                                        Fax: 858-626-6122
                                        www.scripps.org

Sean A Deitch, President/CEO
Gary Fybel, Executive Director/Administrator
One of the county's 6 designated trauma centers, offers a wide range of clinical and surgical services including 24-hour emergency services; intensive care; interventional cardiology and radiology; radiation oncology; cardiothoracic and orthopedic services; neurology; ophthalmology; and mental health and psychology services.

6096 South Coast Medical Center
12 Mason
Ste A
Irvine, CA 92618-2733   714-669-4446
                                        Fax: 714-669-4448
                                        info@southcoastmedcenter.com

Leigh Erin Connealy, Manager
Bruce Christian, President
A 208 bed acute care hospital. Services include maternity, surgical, subacute care, psychiatric program, eating disorder treatment, chemical dependency treatment, radiology, ICU/CCU, comprehensive rehabilitation services, bariatric surgery and movement disorders program..

6097 St. Joseph Rehabilitation Center
St. Joseph Health System
2200 Harrison Ave
Eureka, CA 95501-3215   707-441-4414
                                        Fax: 707-441-4429
                                        www.stjosepheureka.org

Mission is to provide physical rehabilitation services in a positive patient-centered environment. This promotes restoration of maximum functional abilities and allows for a dignified quality of life experience. As a staff we are guided by our core values of Dignity, Excellence, Service, and Justice.

6098 St. Jude Brain Injury Network
St. Jude Hospital
130 W Bastanchury Rd
Fullerton, CA 92835-1058   714-446-5626
                                             866-785-8332
                                        Fax: 714-446-5979
                                        ocrcuser@stjoc.org
                                        www.tbioc.org

Jana Gable, Program Coordinator
David Bogdan, Service Coordinator
Lina Marroquin, Servicer Coordinator
Provides comprehensive planning, program referral, assists with funding possibilities, and interagency coordination of services. Areas of emphasis include day treatment, vocational and housing options, and the requirements are adults who have suffered a brain injury from an external force.

6099 St. Jude Medical Center
101 E Valencia Mesa Dr
Fullerton, CA 92835-3809   714-871-3280
                                             800-627-8106
                                        Fax: 714-992-3029
                                        stjudemedicalcenter.org

Robert Fraschetti, President
We are one of Southern California's most respected and technologically advanced hospitals, and our four core values: dignity, excellence, service and justice are the guiding principles for everything we do. St. Jude is synonymous with exceptional care that extends beyond good medicine to a commitment to caring for you - mind, body and spirit.

6100 St. Mary Medical Center
1050 Linden Ave
Long Beach, CA 90813-3393   562-491-9000
                                        Fax: 562-491-9053
                                        www.stmarymedicalcenter.org

Chris Desicco, CEO

6101 Sunnyside Nursing Center
22617 S Vermont Ave
Torrance, CA 90502-2595   310-320-4130
                                        Fax: 310-212-3232
                                        www.sunnysidenursing.com

Shane Dahl, Administrator
Manny Cordero, Director of Nursing
El Sayad, Medical Director
Skilled nursing care facility; residential care facility; intermediate care facility; specialty hospital.

6102 UCLA Medical Center: Department of Anesthesiology, Acute Pain Services
U CL A Medical Center
1245 16th Street Medical Plz
Ste 225
Santa Monica, CA 90404

310-794-1841
Fax: 310-794-1511
access@mednet.ucla.edu

Michael Ferrante, Clinical Director
A 337-bed acute-care medical center, has been serving the healthcare needs of West Los Angeles and Santa Monica since 1926. Highly regarded for its primary and specialty care, the medical center features many outstanding clinical programs, including its women's and children's services, emergency services, and family medicine programs.

Colorado

6103 Children's Hospital Rehabilitation Center
University of Colorado Health Sciences Center
1056 E 19th Ave
Denver, CO 80218-1007

303-861-8888
800-624-6553
chipteam.org

Lou Blankenship, CEO
Michael J Farrell, Chief Operating Officer
Helen Martinez, Manager
Private not-for-profit pediatric healthcare network, the hospital is 100 percent dedicated to caring for kids of all ages and stages of growth. That dedication is evident in more then 1000 pediatric specialists and more then 2400 employees. It is also our continual dedication that has placed us at the forefront of research in childhood disease with several nationally and internationally recognized medical programs.

6104 Craig Hospital
3425 S Clarkson St
Englewood, CO 80113-2899

303-789-8000
Fax: 303-789-8214
khosack@craighospital.org
www.craighospital.org

Michael Fordyce, President
Thomas Balazy, Medical Director
Julie Keegan, VP of Finance
A 93-bed, private, not-for-profit, free-standing, acute care and rehabilitation hospital that provides a comprehensive system of inpatient and outpatient medical care, rehabilitation, neurosurgical rehabilitative care, an equipment company, and long-term follow up services.

6105 HealthSouth Rehabilitation Hospital of Colorado Springs
HealthSouth Corporation
325 S Parkside Dr
Colorado Springs, CO 80910-3134

719-630-8000
Fax: 719-520-0387
www.healthsouthcoloradosprings.com

Steve Schaefer, CEO
A 56 bed rehabilitation hospital, its key services are: cardiology department, physical rehabilitation, and orthopedics department. Accredidted to the Joint Commission on Accreditation of Health Care Organizations (JCAHO)

6106 Mapleton Center
North Broadway & Balsam
Boulder, CO 80301-9130

303-440-2273
Fax: 303-441-0536
pr@bch.org
www.bch.org

David Gehant, President/CEO
Comprehensive inpatient and outpatient rehabilitation services for all age groups. Treatment provided by interdisciplinary teams and staff physicians. CARF accredited in brain injury rehabilitation, pediatric rehabilitation, pain management, work hardening and inpatient rehabilitation.

6107 Mediplex Rehab: Denver
Vibra Health Care
8451 Pearl St
Thornton, CO 80229-4804

303-288-3000
Fax: 303-496-1120
info@vhdenver.com
www.northvalleyrehab.com

Walter Sacckett, CEO
Encompasses the broadest mix of professional talent, the finest technology and a total commitment by our people to deliver the highest quality care today, and well into the future. The services can be divided into 4 main categories: long term Acute Care and rehab. Skilled nursing facility and residential ventilator program. Outpatient services and pain management. Adult and Geriatric inpatient psychiatric services.

Connecticut

6108 Mariner Health Care: Connecticut
23 Liberty Way
Niantic, CT 06357

860-739-4007
Fax: 860-701-2202

District of Columbia

6109 National Rehabilitation Hospital
102 Irving St NW
Washington, DC 20010-2949

202-877-1760
Fax: 202-829-2789
www.nrhrehab.org

Edward Healton, Medical Director
Robert Bunning, Associate Medical Director
A private facility dedicated solely to medical rehabilitation. The hospital offers intensive inpatient programs and full-service outpatient programs.

Florida

6110 Florida Hospital Rehabilitation Center
601 E Rollins St
Orlando, FL 32803-1248

407-303-1527
855-303-3627
Fax: 407-303-7566
fh.web@flhosp.org

Rex Alleyne, President
Florida Hospital Orlando uses the latest technology to treat over 32,000 inpatients and 53,600 outpatients annually. This 881-bed, acute-carecommunity hospital also serves as a major tertiary facility for much of the Southeast, the Caribbean and South America

6111 HealthSouth Regional Rehab Center/Florida
20601 Old Cutler Rd
Miami, FL 33189-2441

305-251-3800
Fax: 305-259-0498
www.healthsouth.com

Murray Rolnick, Medical Director
Elizabeth Izquierdo, Chief Executive Officer
HealthSouth Rehabilitation Hospital of Miami is a member of the HealthSouth Corporation, the nation's largest healthcare services provider. The hospital is accredited by the Joint Commission on Accreditation of Healthcare Organizations (JCAHO) and Commission on Accreditaion of Rehabilitation Facilities (CARF). Services offered include dietary services, occupational therapy, and respitory care.

6112 HealthSouth Rehab Hospital: Largo
901 Clearwater Largo Rd N
Largo, FL 33770-4121

727-586-2999
Fax: 727-588-3404
www.healthsouthlargo.com

Elaine Ebaugh, CEO
Linda Russo, Director, Therapies

A specialty hospital devoted to providing comprehensive medical rehabilitation services. The hospital is licensed as a Comprehensive Medical Rehabilitation Hospital by the state of Florida, and accredited by the Joint Commission on Accreditation of Healthcare Organizations (JCAHO). HealthSouth of Largo is the only free standing Rehabilitation Hospital in the Tampa Bay region, and serves patients of all ages. Provides inpatient medical rehabilitation services as well as outpatient programs.

6113 HealthSouth Sports Medicine & Rehabilitation Center
3280 Ponce De Leon Blvd
Coral Gables, FL 33134-7252 305-444-0909
Fax: 305-444-5760
www.healthsouth.com

Jay Greeney, President
Ray Jaffet, Administrator
Provides specialized medical and therapeutic services designated to help physically disabled individuals reach their optimum level of independence and function by providing inpatient and outpatient comprehensive medical rehabilitation services.

6114 HealthSouth Sports Medicine and Rehabilitation Center
2141 South Highway A1A Alt
Jupiter, FL 33477 561-743-8890
Fax: 561-743-8795

Diane Reiley, Manager
Outpatient orthopedic and sports medicine/physical therapy.

6115 HealthSouth Treasure Coast Rehabilitation Hospital
Health South Corporation of Alabama
1600 37th St
Vero Beach, FL 32960-4863 772-778-2100
Fax: 772-567-7041
www.healthsouthtreasurecoast.com
Jimmy Lockhart, Medical Director
HealthSouth Treasure Coast Rehabilitation Hospital is a 90-bed inpatient comprehensive rehabilitation hospital serving Indian River, St. Lucie, Martin and Okeechobee counties. Outpatient services are available at the hospital and at four other clinics. Therapies include physical, occupational, speech and psychology services.

6116 Manatee Springs Care & Rehabilitation Center
5627 9th St E
Bradenton, FL 34203-6105 941-753-8941
Fax: 941-739-4409
www.manateespringsrehab.com
Donna Steiermann, Administrator
Skilled rehabilitation facility specializing in PT, OT, speech therapy, aquatic therapy and an indoor pool. Piped oxygen bed for specialized respiratory care. Compassionate end of life care. Some Medicare, private insurance, and Medicaid.

6117 Perry Health Facility
207 Marshall Dr
Perry, FL 32347-1897 850-584-6334
Fax: 850-838-1801
Rebkah Hatch, Administrator
Full rehabilitation team available, Physiatrist, DOR, Psychiatrist, Psychologist, RD, Geriatric Nursing, PT/OT/ST/RT, Orthotiet/Prosthetist. Provider for PPO's & HMO's as well as medicare, private insurance and medicare/medicaid.

6118 Pinecrest Rehabilitation Hospital and Outpatient Centers
Tenet South Florida
5352 Linton Blvd
Delray Beach, FL 33484-6514 561-498-4440
800-283-8326
Fax: 561-495-3103
www.pinecrestrehab.com
Mark Bryan, CEO
Pinecrest Rehabilitation Hospital is a 90 bed, accredited hospital and is comprised of a Specialty Unit, a Neuro Trauma Unit and Joint Replacement Unit. Additional services at Pincrest include six outpatient rehab centers throughout Palm Beach County. The Outpatient Centers each focus on various specialties such as orthopedic and neurological rehab, pain management, cardiac and pulmonary rehab, occupational medicine, Hearing Institute, dizziness and balance and wellness.

6119 Rehabilitation Institute of Sarasota
3251 Proctor Rd
Sarasota, FL 34231-8538 941-921-8796
Fax: 941-922-6228
Stacy Shepherd, Director Clinical Services
a 75-bed hospital that offers individualized medical and theraputic services tailored to patients and clinics for those affected with stroke, multiple sclerosis, Parkinson's, muscular dystrophy and Lou Gehrig's disease (ALS)

6120 Sea Pines Rehabilitation Hospital
101 E Florida Ave
Melbourne, FL 32901-8398 321-984-4600
Fax: 321-727-7440
ellen.lyons-olski@healthsouth.com
www.healthsouthseapines.com
Stuart Miller, Medical Director
Donna Bohdal, Director of Therapy Operations
Denise McGrath, Administrator
A 90-bed facility specializing in rehabilitation of brain and spinal injuries.

6121 Shriners Hospitals for Children: Tampa
12502 USF Pine Dr
Tampa, FL 33612-9411 813-972-2250
813-281-0300
Fax: 813-975-7125
aargiz-lyons@shrinenet.org
www.shrinershq.org/hospitals/tampa
David Ferrell, FACHE
Maureen Maciel, Chief of Staff
Alicia Argis-Lyons, Develpoment Officer
Recognizing that the family plays a vital role in a child's ability to overcome an illness or injury, Shriners Hospitals helps the family provide the support the child needs by involving the family in all aspects of the child's care and recovery. The purpose of all Shriners Hospitals for Children is to provide care to children with orthopedic problems and burn injuries to help them lead fuller, more productive lives.

6122 South Miami Hospital
6200 SW 73rd St
South Miami, FL 33143-4679 786-662-4000
Fax: 786-662-5302
www.baptisthealth.net
Brian E. Keely, CEO
The mission is to improve the health and well-being of individuals, and to promote the sanctity and preservation of life, in the communities we serve. We are committed to maintaining the highest standards of clinical and service excellence, rooted in utmost integrity and moral practice.

6123 St. Anne's Nursing Center
11855 Quail Roost Dr
Miami, FL 33177-3956 305-252-4000
Fax: 305-969-6752
www.catholichealthservices.org
Tony Farinella, Executive Director
Francisco Cruz, Medical Director
Julia Shillingford, Director of Nursing
Provides spacious, comfortable accommodations with ample recreational areas in a beautifully landscaped setting.

6124 St. Anthony's Hospital
1200 7th Ave N
St Petersburg, FL 33705-1388 727-825-1100
www.stanthonys.com
William Ulbricht, President
James McClint, VP
Ron Colaguori, VP Operations
A not-for-profit, 395-bed hospital established in 1931. St. Anthony's is dedicated to improving the health of the community through community-owned health care that sets the standard for high-quality, compassionate care.

6125 **St. Anthony's Rehabilitation Hospital**
3487 NW 35th Ave
Lauderdale Lakes, FL 33311-1107   954-485-4023
                                         954-739-6233
                              www.catholichealthservices.org
Linda Motte, Hospital Administrator
Kathy Torbertsonn, Dir. Rehab.
Provides spacious, comfortable accommodations with ample recreational areas in a beautifully landscaped setting.

6126 **St. Catherine's Rehabilitation Hospital and Villa Maria Nursing Center**
1050 NE 125th St
North Miami, FL 33161-5805   305-357-1735
                                         305-891-3361
                              www.catholichealthservices.org
Virginia Irving, Hospital Administrator
Jim Reiss, Executive Director
Greg Hartley, Director Rehab
St. Catherine's Rehabilitation Hospital is a CARF accredited, 60 bed facility offering inpatient and outpatient rehabilitation and medical clinics; including physical, occupational, and speech therapy, neurology, neurodiagnostics, wound care, and hyperbaric medicine. Villa Maria Nursing center is a JCAHO accredited, 212 bed skilled nursing center providing short term nursing and rehabilitation, as well as long term care.

6127 **St. John's Nursing Center**
3075 NW 35th Ave
Lauderdale Lakes, FL 33311-1107   954-739-6233
                                    Fax: 954-733-9579
                              www.catholichealthservices.org
Ralph E. Lawson, Chairman
Elizabeth Worley, Vice Chairman
Thomas Marin, Assistant Secretary
Provides spacious, comfortable accommodations with ample recreational areas in a beautifully landscaped setting.

6128 **Successful Job Accommodation Strategies**
LRP Publications
36- Hiatt Dr
Palm Beach Gardens, FL 33418   561-622-6520
                                         800-341-7874
                                    Fax: 561-622-0757
                                   webmaster@lrp.com
                                         www.lrp.com
Honora McDowell, Product Group Manager
Kenneth Kahn, Chief Executive Officer
This monthly newsletter provides you with quick tips, new accommodation ideas and innovative workplace solutions. You learn the outcomes of the latest cases involving workplace accommodations. *$ 140.00*
12 pages Monthly

6129 **Tampa General Rehabilitation Center**
1 Tampa General Circle
Tampa, FL 33601-1289   813-844-7000
                                    Fax: 813-844-1477
                                         tgh.org
Ron Hytoff, President/CEO
Devanand Mangar MD, Vice Chief of Staff
Thomas L. Bernasek MD, Chief of Staff
Offers a full range of inpatient and outpatient programs all aimed at helping patients achieve their full potentials. JCAHO and CARF accredited and V.R. designated center. A wide range of inpatient and outpatient programs are available such as Brain and Spinal Cord Injury Programs, Comprehensive Medical Rehabilitation, Pain Management, Cardiac Rehab, Pediatric Therapy Service, Sleep Disorders, Epilepsy, and Wheelchair Seating. Hosts the Florida Alliance for Assistive Services and Technolgy.

6130 **University of Miami: Jackson Memorial Rehabilitation Center**
University of Miami
1611 NW 12th Ave
Miami, FL 33136-1005   305-585-6970
                                    Fax: 305-585-6092
                                    info@jhsmiami.org
                                    www.jhsmiami.org
Michael Butler, Chief Medical Officer

An accredited, non-profit, tertiary care hospital and the major teaching facility for the University of Miami School of Medicine. With more then 1,550 beds, Jackson Memorial is a referral center, a magnet for medical research, and home to the Ryder Trauma Center- the only adult and pediatric level 1 trauma center in Miami-Dade County.

6131 **Winter Park Memorial Hospital**
Florida Hospital
200 N Lakemont Ave
Winter Park, FL 32792-3273   407-646-7000
                                    Fax: 407-646-7639
                              healthcare@winterparkhospital.com
                                   www.winterparkhospital.com
Ken Bradley, CEO
Offers Acute Rehabilitation.

Georgia

6132 **Candler General Hospital: Rehabilitation Unit**
5353 Reynolds St
Savannah, GA 31405-6015   912-819-6000
                                    Fax: 912-819-8829
                              www.sjchs.org/body.cfm?id=383
Paul Hinchey, President/CEO
Special Physical Therapy Services at Candler Outpatient Center: Aquatic therapy, pediatric services, outpaitient neurological rehabilitation program, woman's health therapy, orthotics, and spine specialty

6133 **Children's Healthcare of Atlanta at Egleston**
1405 Clifton Rd. NE
Atlanta, GA 30322   www.choa.org
Donna Hyland, President & CEO
Ruth Fowler, Chief Financial Officer
Stephanie M. Jernigan, Campus Director, Egleston
Rehabilitation Center at Egleston accepts children from birth to age 18 with acute or chronic problems. The length of rehab stay varies for each child according to the determined program of care. The center offers inpatient, outpatient and day rehab programs for comprehensive evaluation and treatment.

6134 **Cobb Hospital and Medical Center: Rehab Care Center**
3950 Austell Rd
Austell, GA 30106-1121   770-732-5126
                                         www.wellstar.org
David Anderson, Executive VP
Michael Andrews, Chief Cancer Network Officer
Avril Beckford, Chief Pediatrics Officer
To deliver world class healthcare we equip our healthcare facilities and employees with the best technology, resources and education aviailable. To deliver world class healthcare we keep seeking ways to improve the way we deliver care knowing each day holds more miracles, more life, more chances, more compassion, and more opportunities.

6135 **HealthSouth Central Georgia Rehabilitation Hospital**
3351 Northside Dr
Macon, GA 31210-2587   478-201-6500
                                    Fax: 478-471-6536
                                   www.centralgarehab.com
HealthSouth Central Georgia rehabilitation hospital is a 55 bed comprehensive medical rehabilitation hospital meeting the medical patients and famloity members in Central Georgia.

6136 **Specialty Hospital**
Floyd Healthcare Resources
304 Turner McCall Blvd SW
Rome, GA 30165-5621   706-509-5000
                                    Fax: 706-802-4175
                                   contactus@floyd.org
                                         www.floyd.org
Kurt Stuenkel, CEO
Dee Russell, Chief Medical Officer
Our mission is to be responsive to the communities we serve with a comprehensive and technologically advanced heal care system commited to the delivery of care that is characterized by continually improving quality, accessability, affordability and personal dignity.

Hawaii

6137   Shriners Hospital for Children: Honolulu
1310 Punahou St
Honolulu, HI 96826-1099   808-941-4466
                                          888-888-6314
                                          Fax: 808-942-8573
                                          jburda@shrinenet.org
                                          www.shrinershospitalsforchildren.org
Kenneth Guidera, Chief Medical Officer
Eugene D'Amore, Vice President
Kathy A. Dean, Vice President Human Resources
One of 22 hospitals across North America that provide excellent,
no-cost medical care to children with orthopedic problems and
burn industries.

Idaho

6138   Pocatello Regional Medical Center
777 Hospital Way
Pocatello, ID 83201-2797   208-234-6154
                                          Fax: 208-239-3719
                                          robbieo@portmed.org
                                          www.portmed.org

Mark Bukalew, Chairman
John Abreu, VP Finance
Stephen Weeg, Vice-Chairman
Pocatello Regional Medical Center offers 24-hour emergency
care, specialized heart services, a dialysis center, a full service rehabilitation unit including transition care, and the Woman's Center For Health including obstetrics.

Illinois

6139   Builders of Skills
515 Busse Hwy
Park Ridge, IL 60068-3154   847-318-0870
                                          Fax: 847-292-0873
                                          www.avenuestoindependence.org
Jacqueline Kinmel, Chair
Peg O'herron, Vice Chair
Eric Johnson, Treasurer
Residential setting for hearing-impaired, developmentally dis-
abled adults who are assisted with daily living skills.

6140   Center for Learning
National-Louis University
2840 Sheridan Rd
Evanston, IL 60201-1730   847-256-5150
                                          Fax: 845-256-1057

Jerry Dachs, Manager
Psycho-educational evaluations for children, adolescents, and
adults. Individualized remedial academic programs, individual
counseling

6141   DBTAC-Great Lakes ADA Center
1640 W Roosevelt Road
Room 405
Chicago, IL 60608-1316   312-413-1407
                                          800-949-4232
                                          Fax: 312-413-1856
                                          www.adagreatlakes.org
Robin Jones, Project Director
Glenn Fujiura, PhD, Director of Research and Co-Inve
Claudia Diaz, Associate Project Director
Provides training, technical assistance and consultation on the
rights and resposibilities of indiviualsand entities covered by the
ADA. Toll free number for technical assistance and materials pro-
vided electronically or via mail at no cost.

6142   Institute of Physical Medicine and Rehabilitation
6501 N Sheridan Rd
Peoria, IL 61614-2932   309-692-8110
                                          800-957-4767
                                          Fax: 309-692-8673
Lisa Snyder, Medical Director
Comprehensive CARF accredited programs in outpatient medical rehabilitation services. Eight outpatient locations, specialty
programs include adult day services, driving evaluations, balance and visual rehabilitation board certified physiatrists.

6143   LaRabida Children's Hospital and Research Center
E 65th At Lake Michigan
Chicago, IL 60649   773-363-6700
                                          Fax: 773-363-9554
                                          pr@larabida.org
                                          www.larabida.org
Brenda Wolf, President/CEO
Dedicated to excellence in caring for children with chronic ill-
ness, disabilitiesm or who have been abused, allowing them to
achieve their fullest potential through expertise and innovation
within the health care and academic communities.

6144   Marianjoy Rehabilitation Hospital and Clinics
26W171 Roosevelt Rd
Wheaton, IL 60187-6078   630-909-8000
                                          800-462-2366
                                          Fax: 630-909-8001
                                          www.marianjoy.org
Maureen Beal, Chairperson
John Oliverio, Vice Chairman
Kathleen Dvorakk, Treasurer
Goal at Marianjoy Rehabilitation Hospital is to help you and your
family return to the lifestyle you enjoyed before your illness or in-
jury. To meet this goal, we provide you with a dedicated team of
experienced professionals to assist you every step of the way.

6145   Rush Copley Medical Center-Rehab Neuro Physical Unit
2040 Ogden Ave
Ste 303
Aurora, IL 60504-7222   630-898-3700
                                          866-426-7539
                                          Fax: 630-898-3681
                                          clord@rsh.net
                                          www.rushcopley.com
Barry Finn, CEO
Mary Shilkaitis, VP, Patient Care Services
The mission of the medical center and the medical staff is to work
together to serve your healthcare needs through excellence in ed-
ucation, technology and a caring touch. Rush-Copley Medical
Center will be the leading healthcare provider of the greater Fox
Valley area. At Rush-Copley we pride ourselves on providing ev-
eryone with extrodinary service.

Indiana

6146   ATTAIN
U S Department of Education/ NI DR R
32 E Washington St
Ste 1400
Indianapolis, IN 46204-3552   317-534-0236
                                          800-528-8246
Gary Hand, Executive Director
The mission of Attain is to create solutions that enable people
with functional limitations to live, learn, work and play in the
community of their choice. All will have access to assistive devices. We will do this in partnership with people with functional
limitations, families and members of the community through
training, system change, services and support, research, dissemination and consumer advocacy.

6147 **About Special Kids**
7172 Graham Rd
Suite 100
Indianapolis, IN 46250-2879   317-257-8683
                                     800-964-4746
                                     Fax: 317-251-7488
                          FamilyNetw@aboutspecialkids.org
                               www.aboutspecialkids.org

Joe Brubaker, Executive Director
Jane Scott, Director Of Information
Nancy Stone, Project Director

A Parent to Parent organization that works throughout the state of Indiana to answer questions and provide support, information and resources. We are parents and family members of children with special needs and we help other families and professionals understand the various systems that are encountered related to special needs. Our central office is where parents from the entire state can access information, resources and support.

6148 **ArtMix**
1505 N. Delaware St.
Indianapolis, IN 46202   317-974-4123
                                Fax: 317-974-4124
                          info@artmixindiana.org
                               www.artmixindiana.org

Gayle Holtman, President/CEO
Linda Wisler, Vice President of Programs
Kathy Pataluch, Vice President of Development

Since 1982, ArtMix has been a statewide leader in its mission to transform the lives of people with disabilities through the creation of art. ArtMix programs serve over 6,000 people of all abilities each year, creating opportunities for learning, self-expression, and socialization, as well as increasing community understanding of people with disabilities. ArtMix strives to create a welcoming environment that breaks down barriers, providing an inclusive space for people of all ages and abilities.

6149 **Clark Memorial Hospital: RehabCare Unit**
1220 Missouri Ave
Jeffersonville, IN 47130-3743   812-282-6631
                                       Fax: 812-283-2656
                                       clarkmemorial.org

Martin Padgett, CEO

The mission of Clark Memorial Hospital is to provide superior health services to the people and communities we serve. The vision of Clark Memorial Hospital is to be the best community healh care provider in the United States. We value each individual and work together to explore new ways to improve the quality of life of all. We persue excellence in all we do. We treat all individuals with the same compassion, dignity, and privacy that we want in ourselves.

6150 **Developmental Disabilities Planning Council**
402 W Washington St
Indianapolis, IN 46204-2855   317-232-7770
                                     Fax: 317-233-3712
                                     www.state.in.us/gpcpd

Suellen Jackson-Boner, Executive Director
Christine Dahlberg, Associate Director
Jim Geswein, CFO

The mission of the Indiana Governor's Council is to promote public policy which leads to the independence, productivity and inclusion of people with disabilities in all aspects of society. This mission is accomplished through planning, evaluation, collaboration, education, research and advocacy. The Council is consumer-driven and is charged with determining how the service delivery system in both the public and private sectors can be most responsible to the people with disabilities.

6151 **Easterseals Crossroads**
4740 Kingsway Dr.
Indianapolis, IN 46205   317-466-1000
                                Fax: 317-466-2000
                          www.eastersealscrossroads.org

Harold Tenbarge, Chair
Darlisa E. Davis, Treasurer
John Seever, Secretary

Provides services for people with disabilities in central Indiana.

6152 **IN-SOURCE**
Indiana Resource Center for Families with Special
1703 S Ironwood Dr
South Bend, IN 46613-3414   574-234-7101
                                   800-332-4433
                                   Fax: 574-234-7279
                          insource@insource.org
                               insource.org

Richard Burden, Executive Director
Scott Carson, Assistant Director
Dory Lawrence, Project Director

The mission of IN*SOURCE is to provide parents, families and service providers in Indiana the information and training necessary to assure effective educational programs and appropriate services for children and young adults with disabilities.

6153 **Indiana Congress of Parent and Teachers**
2525 N Shadeland Ave
Ste D4
Indianapolis, IN 46219-1770   317-357-5881
                                     Fax: 317-357-3751
                                     www.indianapta.org

Sharon Wise, President
Theresa Distelrath, VP
Job Wise, Secretary

The mission of the Indiana PTA is three-fold: to support and speak on behalf of children and youth in the schools, community and before governmental agencies and other organizations that make decisions affecting children; to assist parents in developing the skills they need to raise and protect their children; and, to encorage parent and community involvement in the public schools of this state and nation.

6154 **Indiana Protection and Advocacy Services Commission**
4701 N Keystone Ave
Ste 222
Indianapolis, IN 46205-1561   317-722-5555
                                     800-838-1131
                                     Fax: 317-722-5564
                                     dward@ipas.IN.gov
                                     www.in.gov/ipas

Karen Pedevilla, Education and Training Director

IPAS was created in 1977 by state law to protect and advocate the rights of people with disabilities and its Indiana's federally designated Protection (P&A) system and client assist program. It is an independent state agency, with receives no state funding and is independent from all service providers, as required by federal and state law.

6155 **Kokomo Rehabilitation Hospital**
829 N Dixon Rd
Kokomo, IN 46901-7709   765-452-6700
                               Fax: 765-452-7470

Brenda Harry, Admissions Director

a 60 bed facility specializing in rehabilitation services to the people of Indiana.

6156 **Memorial Regional Rehabilitation Center**
615 N Michigan St
South Bend, IN 46601-1033   574-647-1000

20-bed CARF accredited inpatient rehabilitation, outpatient orthopedic clinic and work performance program, head injury clinic. Outpatient neuro rehab and a driver education and training program are provided.

6157 **Methodist Hospital Rehabilitation Institute**
8701 Broadway
Merrillville, IN 46410-7035   219-738-5500
                                     Fax: 219-755-0448
                                     methodisthospitals.org

Ian McFadden, President/CEO
Matthew Doyle, VP & CFO
Wright Alcorn, VP Operations

Methodist Hospitals, of all the hospitals in Northwest Indiana, attracts the most complex cases across a range of specialties, including stroke, brain tumor, cancer, trauma and high-risk pregnancy. This is the result of our commitment to providing the expertise and technology needed to offer the most advanced clinical care.

6158 **NAMI Indiana**
P.O.Box 22697
Indianapolis, IN 46222-697   317-925-9399
                                               800-677-6442
                                               Fax: 317-925-9398
                                               info@namiindiana.org
                                               www.namiindiana.org

Marilynn Walker, President
Joshua Sprunger, Executive Director
Linda Williams, Program Coooridnator
NAMI Indiana is a non-profit grassroots organization dedicated
to improving the lives of people afflicted by serious and
persistant mental illness. We are dedicated to helping families
through a network of support, education, advocacy, and promotion of research. NAMI's goal is to help establish a system of care
that provides community based services for persons with serious
mental illness, as well as support for them and their families.

6159 **Parkview Regional Rehabilitation Center**
2200 Randallia Dr
Fort Wayne, IN 46805-4638   260-373-4000
                                               888-480-5151
                                               Fax: 260-373-4288
                                               www.parkview.com

Mike Packnett, President & CEO
Mike Browning, CFO
Rick Henvey, Chief Administrative Officer
Provides a full range of inpatient, theraputic services and pro-
grams for patients as young as 3 years of age to the very elderly.
Our accute care rehabilitation center, is well equipped to care for
patients with neurological and orthopedic injuries and diseases.

6160 **Programs for Children with Disabilities: Ages 3 through
5**
Indiana Department of Education
151 W Ohio St
Indianapolis, IN 46204-1905   317-232-0570
                                               877-851-4106
                                               Fax: 317-232-0589
                                               specialed@doe.in.gov
                                               www.doe.in.gov

Heather Neal, Chief of Staff
The division provides leadership and state-level support for public school gifted and talented (grades K-12) programs and for students with disabilities from ages 3-21. The division ensures that
Indiana, in its compliance with the federal Individuals With Disabilities Education Act, through monitoring of special education
programs, oversight of community and residential programs, provision of mediation and due process rights, and sound fiscal
management.

6161 **Programs for Children with Special Health Care Needs**
Indiana State Department of Health
2 N Meridian St
Indianapolis, IN 46204-3021   317-233-1325
                                               www.in.gov/isdh/

Sean Keefer, Chief of Staff
The Children's Special Health Care Services (CSHCS) program
provides financial assistance for needed medical treatment to
children with serious and chronic medical conditions to reduce
complications and promote maximum quality of life.

6162 **Programs for Infants and Toddlers with Disabilities:
Ages Birth through 2**
402 W Washington St
Indianapolis, IN 46204-2773   317-232-1144
                                               800-441-7837
A family-centered, locally-based, coordinated system that provides early intervention services to infants and young children
with disabilities or who are developmentally vulnerable. First
Steps brings together families and professionals from education,
health and social service agencies. By coordinating locally
availiable services, First Steps is working to give Indiana's children and their families the widest possible array of early
intervention resources.

6163 **Riley Child Development Center**
705 Riley Hospital Drive
Rm 5837
Indianapolis, IN 46202-5128   317-274-7819
                                               Fax: 317-944-9760
                                               info@child-dev.com

Cristy James, Communication Coordinator
Riley Hospital for Children is Indiana's only comprehensive children's hospital, with pediatric specialists in evry field of medicine and surgery. Riley is committed to providing the highest
quality health care to children in a compassionate, family-centered environment. Riley is a national leader in cutting edge research and medical education, ensuring health care excellence for
children for generations to come. Riley provides medical care to
all children, regardless of family's ability to pay.

6164 **St. Anthony Memorial Hospital: Rehab Unit**
301 W Homer St
Michigan City, IN 46360-4358   219-879-8511
                                               Fax: 219-877-1409
                                               www.saintanthonymemorial.org

Joseph Allegreti, Board of Directors
Calvin Bellamy, Board of Directors
Saint Anthony Memorial is an acute care hospital located in
Michigan City, primary serving La Porte and Porter Counties in
Indiana as well as Berrien County Michigan.

6165 **State Division of Vocational Rehabilitation**
402 W Washington St
P O Box 7083
Indianapolis, IN 46207-7083   317-233-4475
                                               800-545-7763
                                               Fax: 317-232-6478
                                               vrcommission@fssa.in.gov
                                               www.state.in.us/fssa

Megan Ornellas, Chief of Staff
Susie Howard, Deputy Chief of Staff

Iowa

6166 **Younker Rehabilitation Center of Iowa Methodist
Medical Center**
1776 W Lakes Pkwy
Des Moines, IA 50266   515-241-6161
                                               888-584-6311
                                               Fax: 515-241-5137
                                               www.ihs.org

Bill Leaver, President
Kevin Vermeer, EVP
Danny Drake, VP
Iowa Health System is the state's first and largest integrated
healthcare system. We are physicians, hospitals, civic leaders and
local volunteers committed to providing the highest possible
quality and the lowest possible cost. We serve over 70 communities in Iowa, Western Illinois, and Eastern Nebraska.

Kansas

6167 **Kansas Rehabilitation Hospital**
1504 SW 8th Ave
Topeka, KS 66606-2714   785-235-6600
                                               Fax: 785-232-8545
                                               www.kansasrehabhospital.com

Mark LeNeave, CEO
Mindy Mitchell, Chief Nursing Officer
A free standing physical rehabilitation hospital located in Topeka
Kansas. Designated to provide a barrier-free access to all treatment and patient service areas. This 79-bed facility offers a total
rehabilitation environment in a warm, caring setting that encourages patient, family and staff interaction.

6168 Mid-America Rehabilitation Hospital HealthSouth
Health South Corporation
5701 W 110th St
Overland Park, KS 66211-2503   913-491-2400
                                    Fax: 913-491-1097
                                    tiffany.kiehl@healthsouth.com
                                    www.midamericarehabhospital.com

Kristen De Hart, CEO
Tiffany Kiehl, Director Marketing/Operations
Paul Matlack, Director Therapy Operations
97 bed Acute Rehab hospital offering full continuum from in-patient, day treatment and outpatient services for individuals with physical limitations due to CVA, TBI, SCI, other traumas, joint replacement, etc.

Kentucky

6169 Cardinal Hill Rehabilitation Hospital
2050 Versailles Rd
Lexington, KY 40504-1499   859-254-5701
                                800-233-3260
                                Fax: 859-231-1365
                                webmaster@cardinalhill.org
                                www.cardinalhill.org

Kerry Gillihan, CEO
William J. Lester, Medical Director
Russell Travis, Assistant Medical Director
CARF-accredited rehab center provides comprehensive inpatient and outpatient services in two locations to people with physical and cognitive disabilities. We provide diagnosis-specific programs to 100 inpatients, outpatient clinics, outpatient therapies, pain management and therapeutic pool services. The Pediatric Center serves children from birth to age 18 years of age.

6170 HealthSouth Rehabilitation of Louisville
1227 Goss Ave
Louisville, KY 40217-1287   270-769-3100
                                 Fax: 502-636-0351
                                 www.healthsouth.com

Tim Nichol, Manager
Regina Durbin, Administrator
HealthSouth Rehabilitation Hospitals lead the way, consistently outperforming peers with a unique, intensive approach to rehabilitative care, partnering with every patient to find a treatment plan that works for them. We offer a wide range of comprehensive rehabilitation programsfor a wide variety of diagnoses. At HealthSouth, we provide access to independent private practice physicians, specializing in physical medicine and rehabilitation, who work in conjunction with HealthSouth's highly qual

6171 Lakeview Rehabilitation Hospital
134 Heartland Dr
Elizabethtown, KY 42701-2778   270-769-3100
                                    Fax: 270-769-6870
                                    www.healthsouthlakeview.com

Lori Jarboes, CEO
Chris Koford, Medical Director
HealthSouth Rehabilitation Hospitals lead the way, consistently outperforming peers with a unique, intensive approach to rehabilitative care, partnering with every patient to find a treatment plan that works for them. We offer a wide range of comprehensive rehabilitation programsfor a wide variety of diagnoses. At HealthSouth, we provide access to independent private practice physicians, specializing in physical medicine and rehabilitation, who work in conjunction with HealthSouth's highly qual

6172 Shriners Hospitals for Children, Lexington
1900 Richmond Rd
Lexington, KY 40502-1204   859-266-2101
                                800-444-8314
                                Fax: 859-268-5636
                                Dwallenius@shrinenet.org
                                www.shrinershq.org/hospitals/lexington

Warren E. Hopkins, Chairman
Kirk E. Carter, Vice Chairman
Ken R. Dougherty, Treasurer
Shriners Hospitals for Childrenr - Lexington, is a 50-bed pediatric orthopaedic hospital. Our family-centered approach to care is designed to support the whole family during the acute and reconstructive phases of a child's injury. Located in Lexington, Ky., our hospital treats children from all over the country and around the world, and has unique relationships with some of the top hospitals and universities in the world.

Louisiana

6173 HealthSouth Specialty Hospital Of North Louisiana
1401 Ezelle St
Ruston, LA 71270-7218   318-251-3126
                             800-548-9157
                             Fax: 318-251-1594
                             mark.rice@lifecare-hospitals.com
                             www.healthsouth.com

Mark Rice, CEO
A 90-bed specialty hospital offering both inpatient and outpatient services. Acute long term care.

6174 Our Lady of Lourdes Rehabilitation Center
4801 Ambassador Caffery Pkwy
Lafayette, LA 70508   337-470-2000
                           Fax: 318-289-2681
                           info@lourdesrmc.com
                           www.lourdesrmc.com

William Barrow, CEO
Gerald R. Boudreaux, Chairman of the Board
D. Wayne Elmore, Secretary
Our Lady of Lourdes outpatient physical medicine and rehabilitation department is compprised of a multi-disciplinary team of physical therapists, oppcuptational therapists and speech languare pathologists.

6175 Rehabilitation Center of Lake Charles Memorial Hospital
1701 Oak Park Boulevard
Lake Charles, LA 70601-8911   337-494-3000
                                   Fax: 337-494-2656
                                   webmaster@lcmh.com
                                   www.lcmh.com

Dale Shearer, Director
Larry Graham, President/CEO
Ben F. Thompson, MD, Medical Staff President
Rehabilitation center offering intensive physical, occupational, speech, neuropsychology, recreational therapies along with rehabilitation nursing.

6176 Shriners Hospital for Children-Shreveport
3100 Samford Ave
Shreveport, LA 71103-4239   318-222-5704
                                 Fax: 318-424-7610
                                 jburda@shrinenet.org
                                 www.shrinershospitalsforchildren.org

Richard McCall, Chief of Staff
Phillip Gates, Assistant Chief
An interdisciplinary approach is used in patient care programs to ensure comprehensive care for each patient. The staff includes orthopaedists, pediatricians, nurses, therapists, social workers, child life specialists, and more. The Shreveport Hospital is equipped and staffed to provide care for virtually all pediatric orthopaedic problems, with the exception of acute trauma.

6177 South Louisiana Rehabilitation Hospital
715 W Worthy Rd
Gonzales, LA 70737-3844   225-647-8277
                               Fax: 225-647-2446
                               sober@powerhouseprograms.com
                               www.powerhouseprograms.com

Cody Gautreux, Executive Director
Tonja Randolph, President
Power House Programs is a male only facility for the treatment of Chemical Dependency/Dual Diagnosis, located in Gonzales, Louisiana. Applicants must have participated in a primary treatment program for substance abuse prior to acceptance. Our program is divided into 3 phases and is staffed by Board Certified Social Workers and Board Certified Substance Abuse Counselors. We provide individual, group and family therapy; plus 12 step meetings in a community setting.

6178   St. Frances Cabrini Hospital: Rehab Unit
St Frances Cabrini Hospital
3330 Masonic Dr
Alexandria, LA 71301-3899   318-487-1122
                                  Fax: 318-448-6822
                        www.christusstfrancescabrini.org
Curman Gaines, Chairperson
Dallas Hixson, Vice Chairperson
CHRISTUS St. Frances Cabrini Hospital is a 265-bed facility located in Alexandria, Louisiana. Employing approximately 1,400 Associates and with a staff of neary 320 physicians, CHRISTUS St. Frances Cabrini Hospital offers a comprehensive array of services providing the highest quality patient care in a compassionate setting.

6179   St. Patrick Hospital: Rehab Unit
524 Doctor Michael Debakey Dr
Lake Charles, LA 70601-5725   337-491-7577
                                     888-722-9355
                                 Fax: 337-430-4284
                           www.christusstpatrick.org
Ellen Jones, CEO
Committed to providing care and service of the highest quality for children and adults, and to ensuring that the basic human rights of expression, decision making and personal dignity are preseved. We are also committed to treating our patients with respect, understanding and Christian love. We realize that this committment involves much more then attending to your medical needs.

6180   Thibodaux Regional Medical Center
602 N Acadia Rd
PO Box 1118
Thibodaux, LA 70301-4847   985-447-5500
                                  800-822-8442
                              Fax: 985-449-4600
                              info@thibodaux.com
                              www.thibodaux.com
Greg Stock, CEO
Jacob Giardina, Chairman
Andrew Hoffman, Chief of Staff
Mission is to provide the highest quality, most cost effective health care services possible to the people of Thibodaux and surrounding areas. The vision is to be the regional medical center of choice for health care services in the southeast Louisiana by recognizing the value of physicians and employees, committing to quality improvement, partnering with other health care providers, and remaining financially viable in a competitive environment.

Maine

6181   Brewer Rehab and Living Center
74 Parkway S
Brewer, ME 04412-1628   207-989-7300
                               800-359-7412
                           Fax: 207-989-4240
Janet Hope, Executive Director
Brewer Rehab and Living Center accomodates 106 residents. We are located in Brewer, Maine. We have a 24-hour nursing staff and experienced dedicated on-site physical therapists, occupational therapists and speech language pathologists. We have a specialized inpatient program for individuals with brain injury resulting from a traumatic injury or neurological event such as a stroke. We also have a specialized care unit for individuals with Alzheimer's disease and other dementias.

6182   New England Rehabilitation Hospital of Portland
335 Brighton Ave
Portland, ME 04102-2363   207-662-8000
                             Fax: 207-879-8168
                             www.nerhp.org
Elissa Charbonneau, Medical Director
Amy Morse, CEO
Mission is to provide individuals with guidance, education, support, and motivation while helping them achieve maximum independence and function. Our professionals work with the patient and family through a team approach, to establish and implement an individualized rehabilitation plan designed to meet specific patient goals.

Maryland

6183   Mt. Washington Pediatric Hospital
1708 W Rogers Ave
Baltimore, MD 21209-4596   410-578-8600
                              Fax: 410-466-1715
                              www.mwph.org
Sheldon Stein, President
Richard Katz, VP, Medical Affairs
Provides inpatient, outpatient and day programs for infants and children with rehabilitation and/or complex medical needs. We are dedicated to maximizing the rehabilitation and development of our patients through the delivery of interdisciplinary services and programs and providing every resource availiable to enable our patients to attain the highest quality of life within their families and their communities.

Massachusetts

6184   New Bedford Rehabilitation Hospital
4499 Acushnet Ave
New Bedford, MA 02745-4707   508-995-6900
                                Fax: 508-998-8131
New Bedford Rehabilitation Hospital provides safe, high-quality, cost-effective medical and rehabilitation care to our patients and their families with the goal of improving quality of life and maximizing function.

6185   New England Rehabilitation Hospital: Massachusetts
2 Rehabilitation Way
Woburn, MA 01801-6098   781-939-5050
                               Fax: 781-933-9257
                           www.newenglandrehab.com
Deniz Ozel, Medical Director
A 168-bed comprehensive inpatient rehabilitation hospital, which includes 2 off-campus satellite units. Offers an array of area outpatient rehabilitation centers. New England Rehabilitation Hospital remains committed to a personal caring approach. The vision is to provide the communities with a complete continuum of acute rehabilitative programs and services.

6186   Shriners Burns Hospital: Boston
51 Blossom St
Boston, MA 02114-2623   617-722-3000
                               800-255-1916
                           Fax: 617-523-1684
                    www.shrinershospitalsforchildren.org
Thomas D'Esmond, Administrator
Matthias Donelan, Chief of Staff
Provides treatment for children to their 18th birthday with acute, fresh burns, plastic reconstructive surgery for patients with healed burns, severe scarring and facial deformity. Some non-burn conditions such as Scalded Skin Syndrome, Cleft Lip, Cleft Palate and purpura fulminians are also treated. Call the Hospital for information. All medical treatment is without cost to the patient, parents, or any third party.

6187   Shriners Hospital Springfield Unit Springfield Unit for Crippled Children
516 Carew St
Springfield, MA 01104-2330   413-787-2000
                                    800-237-5055
                                Fax: 413-787-2009
                    www.shrinershospitalsforchildren.org
Kenneth Guidera, Chief Medical Officer
Eugene D'Amore, Vice President
Kathy A. Dean, Vice President Human Resources
Shriners Hospital for Children is fully equipped and staffed to provide care for pediatric orthopaedic conditions and disorders.

Michigan

6188 Covenant Healthcare Rehabilitation Program
1447 N Harrison
Saginaw, MI 48602-4316
989-583-2930
Fax: 989-583-0000
www.covenanthealthcare.com

Spence Maidlow, President
Juli Martin, Program Director
Offers a broad spectrum of programs and services ranging from obstetrics, neonatal and pediatric care, to acute care including cardiology, oncology, surgery and many other services on the leading edge of medicine. All our programs and services exemplify our commitment to providing quality, compassionate care. As a medical facility with more then 700 beds, and a complete range of medical services, Covenant stands ready to meet the healthcare needs of the 15 counties in Michigan we serve.

6189 Farmington Health Care Center
34225 Grand River Ave
Farmington, MI 48335-3440
248-477-7373
Fax: 248-477-2888

Brian Garavaglia, Administrator
Skilled nursing facility specializing in ventilator dependent residents.

6190 Flint Osteopathic Hospital: RehabCare Unit
3921 Beecher Rd
Flint, MI 48532-3602
810-606-5000
Fax: 810-762-2153
TTY: 888-633-2368
www.genesys.org

Susan Malone, Program Manager
Joy Finkenbiner, Executive Director
Genesys Health System takes great pride in the fact that we strive to deliver the highest quality health care, in a model healing environment, for the entire continuum of care needed throughout one's life. From birth to the twilight years, and everywhere in between, Genesys is there to get you back to the things you love to do.

6191 Integrated Health Services of Michigan at Clarkston
4800 Clintonville Rd
Clarkston, MI 48346-4297
248-674-0903
Fax: 248-674-3359
donna.cook@fundltc.com

Carol Doll, Admissions Director
Margaret Canny, Administrator
At Clarkston Specialty Healthcare Center, our mission is to deliver personalized care to the members of our community at a time when our support is most needed. We strive to maximize and enhance the quality of life in a compassionate and professional environment.

6192 St. John Hospital: North Shore
Ascension Health
26755 Ballard St
Harrison Township, MI 48045-2419
586-465-5501
866-501-3627
Fax: 586-466-5352
webcenter@stjohn.org
www.stjohnprovidence.org

David Sessions, CEO
A 96-bed specialty hospital that provides comprehensive physical medicine and rehabilitation, along with a wide range of medical and surgical services. St. John North Shores Hospital also provides emergency and urgent care, extensive outpatient rehabilitation services, and most ancillary diagnostic services.

Minnesota

6193 Alinna Health
800 E 28th St
Minneapolis, MN 55407-3798
612-863-4200
866-880-3550
Fax: 612-863-5698
sisterkenny@allina.com
www.allinahealth.org/ahs/ski.nsf/

Helen Kettner, Nurse-Liaison
Courage Kenny Rehabilitation Institute provides a continuum of rehabilitation services for people with short- and long-term conditions and disabilities in communities throughout Minnesota and western Wisconsin. Our goal is to improve health outcomes, make it easier for clients and families to get the right services for their needs, and reduce costs by preventing complications.

Missouri

6194 Columbia Regional Hospital: RehabCare Unit
404 N Keene St
Columbia, MO 65201-6698
573-882-2501
Fax: 573-449-7588
www.muhealth.org

James Ross, CEO
Anita Larsen, COO
A medical and physical rehabilitation program serving patients throughout Mid-Missouri with functional deficits due to neurologic, orthopaedic or other medical conditions.

6195 Jewish Hospital of St. Louis: Department of Rehabilitation
1 Barnes Jewish Hospital Plz
Saint Louis, MO 63110-1003
314-747-3000
855-925-0631
Fax: 314-454-5277
www.barnesjewish.org

Richard Liedweg, President
Mark Krieger, VP/CFO
John Lynch, Chief Medical Officer
We take exceptional care of people by providing world-class healthcare, delivering care in a compassionate, respectful and responsive way. By advancing medical knowledge and continously improving our practices. By educating current and future generations of healthcare professionals.

6196 St. Mary's Regional Rehabilitation Center
201 NW R D Mize Rd
Blue Springs, MO 64014-2513
816-228-5900
Fax: 816-655-5348

Fleury Yelvington, President/CEO
Amy McKay, Executive Director of Nursing
A 143-bed inpatient physical rehabilitation unit offering PT, OT, ST, recreational therapy, psychiatry and all other ancillary services of a full-service hospital. Specialize in orthopedic and neurologic disabilities.

6197 Three Rivers Health Care
2620 N Westwood Blvd
Poplar Bluff, MO 63901-3396
573-785-7721
800-582-9533
Fax: 573-686-5388
info@pbrmc.hma-corp.com
www.poplarbluffregional.com

Charles Stewart, Market CEO
Gerald Faircloth, Administrator
Melissa Samuelson, Chief Nursing Officer
Poplar Bluff Regional Medical Center is a regional medical center with 2 hospital campuses and more then 100 active physicians. The 423-bed facility is the largest medical center in Southeast Missouri and is located in ButlerCounty. With outreach clinics in Bloomfield, Dexter, Malden, Piedmont, and Puxico, Poplar Bluff Regional Medical Center is committed to serving its 6 county region.

Montana

6198   St. Vincent Hospital and Health Center
1233 N 30th St
Billings, MT 59101-165
603-657-7000
Fax: 406-657-8817
www.svhhc.org

Jason Barker, CEO
Steve Loveless, COO
Joan Thullberry, Chief Nursing Officer
Vision is to be recognized for our vitality, best in class performance and providing easy access to compassionate and trust-worthy healthcare. The healthcare we offer is based on community need. We strive to improve the health status of the community, with a special concern for the poor and those who have limited access to healthcare.

Nebraska

6199   Madonna Rehabilitation Hospital
5401 South St
Lincoln, NE 68506-2150
402-489-7102
800-676-5448
Fax: 402-483-9406
info@madonna.org
www.madonna.org

Marsha Lommel, CEO
Provides a complete range of inpatient and outpatient rehabilitation for patients of all ages and abilities. Through highly specialized programs and services, Madona offers individualized treatment and support to help every patient.

Nevada

6200   University Medical Center
1800 W Charleston Blvd
Las Vegas, NV 89102-2386
702-383-2000
Fax: 702-383-2536
feedback@umcsn.com
www.umcsn.com

Brian Brannman, CEO
Lawrence Barnard, Chief Operating Officer
Joan Brookhyser, Chief Medical Officer
University Medical Center is dedicated to providing the highest level of health care possible by maintaining its ongoing commitment to personal, individualized care for each patient.Through the latest treatment techniques, comfortable surroundings and a dedicated staff, that commitment is expressed every day, in every area of the hospital.

New Hampshire

6201   Head Injury Treatment Program at Dover
307 Plaza Dr
Dover, NH 03820-2455
603-742-2676
Fax: 603-749-5375
www.doverrehab.com

Sue Mills, Program Rep
Jill Bosa, Administrator
A provider of postacute services in the greater New Hampshire Seacost area. We accomodate 112 residents and are licensed by the state of New Hampshire. We employ nearly 150 licensed nurses, therapists, and other healthcare professionals, who strive to provide quality care. The goal of our patient service model is to bridge the gap between hospitalization and home so that recovery and physical functioning are maximized and hospital re-admission is minimized.

6202   Lakeview NeuroRehabilitation Center
244 Highwatch Road
Effingham, NH 03882
603-539-7451
800-473-4221
Fax: 603-539-8815
www.lakeviewsystem.com

Anton Merka, Chairman
Carolyn McDermott, President
Christopher Slover,, Chief Executive Officer
Residential treatment center serving individuals with neurologic/behavioral disorders. Lakeview serves both children and adults in functionally based program environment. Transistional programs in various group homes also available to clients as they progress in their treatment.

6203   Northeast Rehabilitation Hospital
70 Butler St
Salem, NH 03079-3974
603-893-2900
800-825-7292
Fax: 603-893-1638
TTY: 800-439-2370
www.northeastrehab.com

John Prochilo, CEO
NRHN is an organization characterized by the positive and proactive commitment to the delivery of customer centered care. Our employees exemplify our organizational commitment to providing quality rehabilitation services throughout the continuum. NRHN will be prudent with all resources and will take individual and collective responsibility for fiscal health. NRHN will remain a model by which other rehabilitation and post acute networks seek to emulate.

6204   St. Joseph Hospital Rehabilitation
172 Kinsley St
Nashua, NH 03060-3688
603-595-3076
800-210-9000
Fax: 603-595-3635
www.stjosephhospital.com

Judy Grilli, Medical Staff Officer
A comprehensive healthcare system that serves the Greater Nashua area, western New Hampshire and Northern Massachusetts. Our hospital is licensed for 208 beds and includes a Level 2 Trauma Center. In addition to the hospital, St. Joseph Healthcare system also includes a satellite emergency center in Milford, 5 family medical centers, a large network of primary care and specialty physician practices.

New Jersey

6205   Betty Bacharach Rehabilitation Hospital
61 W Jimmie Leeds Rd
Pomona, NJ 08240-9102
609-652-7000
Fax: 609-652-7487
www.bacharach.org

Philip J. Perskie, Esq., Chairman
Roy Goldberg, Vice Chairman
Craig Anmuth, Medical Director
Therapists, nurses and other specialists, led by physiatrists - doctors specially trained in the medical practice of physical medicine and rehabilitation.

6206   Children's Specialized Hospital
200 Somerset St.
New Brunswick, NJ 08901
888-244-5373
www.childrens-specialized.org

Warren E. Moore, President & CEO
Charles Chianese, Vice President & Chief Operating Officer
Joseph J. Dobosh Jr., Vice President & Chief Financial Officer
New Jersey's largest comprehensive pediatric rehabilitation hospital, treats children and adolescents from birth through 21 years of age. Programs include spinal dysfunction, brain injury, respiratory, burn, Day Hospital, early intervention, preschool, and cognitive rehabilitation.

6207 HealthSouth Rehabilitation Hospital
14 Hospital Dr
Toms River, NJ 08755-6402   732-244-3100
                                   Fax: 732-244-7790
                                   www.rehabnj.com/tomsriver/

Patty Ostaszewski, CEO
Joseph Stillo, Medical Director
A comprehensive 131-bed medical rehabilitation hospital dedicated to treating individuals with a variety of physical disabilities
resulting from injury and illness. We serve all of New Jersey,
Manhattan, and Philiadelphia. Accredited by the Joint Commission on Accreditation of Healthcare Organizations (JCAHO).
The mission of the hospital is to get people back to work, to play,
to living.

6208 JFK Johnson Rehab Institute
65 James St
Edison, NJ 08820-3947   732-321-7070
                               Fax: 732-321-0994
                               www.njrehab.org

Krishna Urs, Physician
David Brown, Physician
JRI has developed programs in such specialties as stroke rehabilitation, orthopedic programs, fitness, cardiac rehabilitation,
women's health, pediatrics and brain injury rehabilitation. We
also offer the most sophisticated diagnostic services available.

6209 Kessler Institute for Rehabilitation
1199 Pleasant Valley Way
West Orange, NJ 07052   973-731-3600
                               877-322-2580
                               Fax: 973-243-6819
                               www.kessler-rehab.com

Sue Kida, President
Provides physical medicine and rehabilitation through the integration of highly specialized care, treatment, technology, education, research, and advocacy.

6210 Mediplex Rehab: Camden
1 Cooper Plz
Camden, NJ 08103-1461   856-342-2300
                               Fax: 856-342-7979
                               www.cooperhealth.org

John P. Sheridan, Jr. President/CEO
Adrienne Kirby, Phd, President/CEO
Raymond L. Baraldi, Interim Chief Medical Officer
Cooper University Hospital is the leading provider of comprehensive health services, medical education and clinical research
in Southern New Jersey and the Delaware Valley. With over 550
physicians in over 75 specialties, Cooper is uniquely equipped to
provide an almost unlimited number of medical services. The
hospital is committed to excellence in medical education, patient
care, and research. Offers training programs to medical students,
residents, and nurses in a variety of specialties.

6211 Universal Institute Rehabilitation & Fitness Center
15 Microlab Rd
Ste 101
Livingston, NJ 07039   973-992-8181
                              800-468-5440
                              Fax: 973-992-7178
                              www.uirehab.com

Adam Steinberg, President
Lisa Lasso, Vice President, Chief Financial Officer
Universal institute is a 15,000 square foot, state of the art rehabilitation facility that specializes in neurological disorders such as
brain injuries, spinal cord injury, strokes, etc. Services include
PT, OT, speech patholgy, cognitive remediation, aqua therapy
and EMG biofeedback.

New Mexico

6212 HealthSouth Rehabilitation Center: New Mexico
7000 Jefferson St NE
Albuquerque, NM 87109-4357   505-344-9478
                                    800-293-7226
                                    Fax: 505-345-6722
                                    www.healthsouthnewmexico.com

Sylvia Kelly, CEO
Rocky BigCrane, Director of Plant Operations
Lisa Brower, Director of Therapy Operations
Our hospital offers highly specialized inpatient rehabilitation
services. From hip fractures to joint replacements and stroke to
Parkinson's disease - our hospital has the experts, technology and
experience to meet your rehabilitation needs.

6213 St. Joseph Rehabilitation Hospital and Outpatient Center
Ardence
505 Elm St NE
Albuquerque, NM 87102-2500   505-727-4700
                                    Fax: 505-727-4793

Janelle Raborn, Administrator/CEO
Sherrie Peterson, Director
A member of the four hospital, St. Joseph healthcare system, this
facility provides inpatient and outpatient care for those requiring
physical medicine and rehabilitation. Specialty programs include
brain injury, stroke, spinal cord, orthopedics, occupational and
physical therapies, clinical psychology, speech/language pathology, hand clinic and functional capacity evaluations. The only facility in New Mexico accredited in four areas by the commission
on accreditation of rehab facilities.

New York

6214 Burke Rehabilitation Hospital
785 Mamaroneck Ave
White Plains, NY 10605-2523   914-597-2500
                                     888-99 -URKE
                                     Fax: 914-946-0866
                                     web@burke.org
                                     www.burke.org

John Ryan, Executive Director
Mary Beth Walsh, M.D., Executive Medical Director/CEO
Brett Langley, Physician.
We provide inpatient and outpatient care for a broad range of neurological, musculoskeletal, cardiac, and pulmonary disabilities
caused by disease or injury. Burke treats patients who have suffered a stroke, spinal cord injury, brain injury, amputation, joint
replacement, complicated fracture, arthritis, cardiac and pulmonary disease, and neurological disorders. Patients are most frequently transferred to Burke from acute care hospitals once their
condition is stable and they are able to partici

6215 Occupational Therapy Strategies and Adaptations for Independent Daily Living
Haworth Press
10 Alice St
Binghamton, NY 13904-1503   607-722-5857
                                   800-429-6784
                                   Fax: 607-722-6362
                                   orders@haworthpress.com
                                   www.tandf.co.uk

This contains clinical expertise of some fourteen authors or author teams addressing the issue of occupational therapy to assist
in independent daily living. Also available as hardcover. *$74.95*
186 pages Softcover
ISBN 0-866563-50-4

6216 Rusk Institute of Rehabilitation Medicine
301 East 17th Street
Second Avenue (in the Hospital for
New York, NY 10016-4901   212-263-6034
                                 Fax: 212-263-8510
                                 DevelopmentOffice@nyumc.org
                                 www.med.nyu.edu/rusk

Steven Flanagan, Chairman

Operates under the auspices of the Dept. Of Rehabilitation Medicine of New York University School of Medicine, one of the nations foremost medical schools. The relationship between Rusk and other clinical and research units within the medical center contributes to an environment which provides the optimal rehabilitation setting for patients. Rusk provides patients with access to treatment across a continuum of care depending on their individual medical needs.

6217 Silvercrest Center for Nursing & Rehabilitation
144-45 87th Ave
Briarwood, NY 11435-3109   718-480-4000
                                            800-645-9806
                                      Fax: 718-658-2367
                                admissions@silvercrest.org
                                        www.silvercrest.org
Andrea Gibbon, Clinical Care Coordinator
Penny Blakely, Unit Manager
The Silvercrest Center for Nursing and Rehabilitation has earned a widespread reputatiopn for combing the best in clinical care with the best in nursing care and for making available to its communities the broadest menu of services to ease a patients' path to recovery from hospital to home. The Center is for the treatment of medically complex patients beginning their recovery, for the rehabilitation of patients who need restorative therapy before going home and much more.

6218 Vocational Rehabilitation and Employment
Books on Special Children
PO Box 305
Congers, NY 10920-305   845-638-1236
                                      Fax: 845-638-0847
                                   www.vba.va.gov/bln/vre/
Defines kinds of work, expectations, goals and programs. Contributions in general issues of supported employment, training and management and community based programs. *$47.00*
372 pages Hardcover

North Carolina

6219 Horizon Rehabilitation Center
Trans Health Incorporated
3100 Erwin Rd
Durham, NC 27705-4505   919-383-1546
                                            800-541-7750
                                      Fax: 919-383-0862
A 125-bed rehabilitation, subacute and long term care facility. HRC is JCAHO and CARF accredited with a physician-directed rehabilitation program, internal case management and a therapy department composed of physical, occupational, speech, recreational and respiratory therapists - pulmonary rehabilitation/ventilator unit.

6220 Integrated Health Services of Durham
Duke University Medical Center
3100 Erwin Rd
Durham, NC 27705-4505   919-383-1546
                                      Fax: 919-383-0862
Aaron Lony, Administrator

6221 Learning Services Corporation
Corporate Office
10 Speen St
Ste 4
Framingham, MA 01701-4661   508-626-3671
                                            888-419-9955
                                      Fax: 866-491-7396
                                   www.learningservices.com
Susan Snow, Director of Admissions
Deb. Braunling-McMorrow, Ph, President and CEO
A licensed postacute rehabilitation program for adults who have an acquired brain injury. Individuals who are enrolled in the program participate in active, intensive rehabilitation carried out by a team of neuropsychology, speech/language therapy, physical therapy, occupational therapy, vocational services, family services and life skills training. Services include residential rehabilitation, home based treatment, day treatment, subacute rehabilitation and supported living.

Ohio

6222 Columbus Rehab & Subactute
44 S Souder Ave
Columbus, OH 43222-1539   614-228-5900
                                      Fax: 614-228-3989
                           www.columbusrehabskillednursing.com
Kelly Fligor, Administrator
Columbus Rehabilitation and Subacute Institute is a leading provider of long-term skilled nursing care and short-term rehabilitation solutions. Our 120 bed facility offers a full continuum of services and care focused around each individual in today's ever-changing healthcare environment.

6223 Great Lakes Regional Rehabilitation Center
3700 Kolbe Rd
Lorain, OH 44053-1611   440-960-3470
                                      Fax: 440-960-4636
Julie Jones, Manager
Provides excellent, innovative and comprehensive rehabilitation programs to people in our community. Committed to a better quality of life for all individuals, the Rehabilitation Center has grown to become a regional resource for individuals needing all types of rehabilitation services.

6224 HCR Health Care Services
1 Seagate
Toledo, OH 43604-1541   419-321-5470
                                            800-736-4427
                                      Fax: 419-252-5543
Specialty transitional care and intensive rehabilitation services. Specialized services are focused on patients with catastrophic conditions or whose length of stay at an acute care or rehabilitation hospital can be dramatically reduced by transferring to a subacute level of care.

6225 Heather Hill Rehabilitation Hospital
Heather Hill
12340 Bass Lake Rd
Chardon, OH 44024-8327   440-285-4040
                                            800-423-2972
                                      Fax: 440-285-0946
                                   info@heatherhill.org
Ed Davis, Operations
Donald Goddard, Chief Medical Officer
Individualized treatment programs for adults and adolescents can participate in and benefit from three-plus hours a day of active therapy.

6226 Parma Community General Hospital Acute Rehabilitation Center
7007 Powers Blvd
Parma, OH 44129-5437   440-743-3000
                                      Fax: 440-843-4387
                                   www.parmahospital.org
David Nedrich, Chairman
Thomas P. O'Donnell, First Vice Chairman
Nancy E. Hatgas, Second Assistant Treasurer
Parma Hospital offers acute and subacute inpatient care including specialty centers for heart, cancer, robotic surgery, orthopedics, pain management, acute rehabilitation and bariatric care.

6227 Rehabilitation Institute of Ohio at Miami Valley Hospital
1 Wyoming St
Dayton, OH 45409-2793   937-208-8000
                                      TTY: 937-208-2006
                                   www.miamivalleyhospital.com
Vanessa Sandarusi, Executive Director
Anita Marie Greer, Program Manager, Acute Therapy Services
Jessica Hallum, Nurse Manager of the Inpatient Rehabilitation Unit
The Miami Valley Hospital Rehabilitation Institute of Ohio (RIO) is one of the largest and most comprehensive rehabilitation services providers in the United States. RIO offers a full spectrum of specialized rehabilitation programs delivered by the region's most experienced rehabilitation experts.

6228 Shriners Burn Institute: Cincinnati Unit
Shriners Hospitals for Children Cincinnati
3229 Burnet Ave
Cincinnati, OH 45229-3095   513-872-6000
                                   800-875-8580
                              Fax: 513-872-6999
                www.shrinershospitalsforchildren.org

Richard Kagan, Chief of Staff
Petra Warner, Assistant Chief of Staff
Tony Lewgood, Interim Administrator
All the attention and resources are focused on just one kind of patient-the burn-injured child. Shriners combine excellent clinical skill, compassionate care, and innovative research, providing comprehensive pediatric burn care and reconstructive rehabilitation to achieve the best possible outcome for a child that has suffered a burn injury. There is never a charge to the patient or family for any of the medical care or services provided by the Shriners Hospitals throughout North America.

6229 St. Francis Health Care Centre
401 N Broadway St
Green Springs, OH 44836-9653   419-639-2626
                                    800-248-2552
                               Fax: 419-639-6225

Kim Eicher, CEO
Jane Holmer, Admissions Coordinator
Provides compassionate care for the elderly and physically challenged. We are a healthcare ministry under the sponsorship of the Franciscan Sisters of Our Lady of Perpetual Help. As a Catholic facility. we respectfully offer those we serve, care hope and dignity in a joyful and compassionate manner.

6230 St. Rita's Medical Center Rehabilitation Services
730 W Market St
Lima, OH 45801-4602   419-227-3361
                                    800-232-7762
                               Fax: 419-226-9750

James Reber, CEO
The St. Rita's Inpatient Acute Care Rehabilitation service provides individualized service to you or your family member 7 days a week, wherever you might stay in the hospital. Acute rehabilitation care includes physical, occupational, and speech therapy services. Our goal is to make you as independent as possible before your discarge to home or, when necessary to extended services in other parts of the hospital.

6231 University of Cincinnati Hospital
Health Alliance
234 Goodman St
Cincinnati, OH 45219-2316   513-584-1000
                               Fax: 513-584-7712
                       universityhospital.uchealth.com/

James Kingsbury, President/CEO
University Hospital has an international reputation, bringing thousands of people, from the region and around the world to Cincinnati to receive care from world renowned physicians in state-of-the-art medical facilities.

6232 Upper Valley Medical/Rehab Services
3130 N County Road
25-A
Troy, OH 45373-1309   937-440-4000
                               Fax: 937-440-7337
                                    info@uvmc.com
                                    www.uvmc.com

Rafay Atiq, Director Rehab Services
A not-for-profit health care system serving the health care needs of Miami County and the surrounding area. The health care system features a state-of-the-art acute care hospital which opened in 1998. Comprehensive inpatient and outpatient services are provided with a full compliment of diagnostic and treatment services and behavioral health care programs.

Oklahoma

6233 Hilcrest Medical Center: Kaiser Rehab Center
1125 S Trenton Ave
Tulsa, OK 74120-5498   918-579-7100
                               Fax: 918-579-7110
                                    www.hillcrest.com

Perri Craven, Medical Director
Kaiser Rehabilitation Center offers a wide range of services to help people regain functionality and independence after a debilitating injury or illness. Our approach to rehabilitation is a team approach, bringing the expertise of physicians, therapists, nurses and other health professionals together with patient family to achieve the best possible outcome. Each patient is given an individualized treatment plan that stimulates and challenges them to achieve their maximum potential.

6234 Jane Phillips Medical Center
Jane Phillips Medical Center
3500 E Frank Phillips Blvd
Bartlesville, OK 74006-2464   918-333-7200
                               Fax: 918-331-1360
                                    www.jpmc.org

David Stire, CEO
Mike Moore, CFO
Jane Phillips Health System is sponsored by St. John Health System. This partnership helps our patients by ensuing access to the most sophisticated levels of care availiable in this area. It offers a wide range of services, including general medicine, surgery, cardiopulmonary care, maternal and infant care, cancer treatment, geriatric care, orthopedics, and physical medicine.

6235 Jim Thorpe Rehabilitation Center at Southwest Medical Center
Southwest Medical Center
4100 S. Douglas Ave.
Oklahoma City, OK 73109   405-644-5445
                                    800-677-1238
                               Fax: 405-644-5384

Al Moorad, Medical Director
Provides inpatient rehabilitation for people with head injuries, spinal cord injuries, orthopedic conditions, pain management, neurological diseases, strokes and a variety of diagnoses that stop individuals from being able to take care of themselves independently. Services available include medical direction, physical therapy, social work, occupational therapy, speech therapy, recreational therapy, and aftercare follow-up.

6236 Mercy Memorial Health Center-Rehab Center
1011 14th Ave NW
Ardmore, OK 73401-1828   580-223-5400
                                    800-572-1182
                               Fax: 580-220-6463
                                    www.mercy.net

Jan Shores, Manager
Lynn Britton Britton, President/CEO
Randy Combs, Executive Vice President Strategic Growth
A full service tertiary hospital with 176 licensed beds, 913 co-workers and 100 physicians. Four primary care clinics

6237 St. Anthony Hospital: Rehabilitation Unit
St. Anthony Hospital
1000 N Lee Ave
Oklahoma City, OK 73102-1036   405-272-7000
                                    800-851-0888
                               Fax: 405-272-7075
                               st_anthony@ssmhc.com
                                    www.saintsok.com

S Beaver, President
18 spacious private rooms, each with bathroom, and furnishings designed with patient safety in mind. Horticulture room where patients can work with plants and flowers as part of their rehabilitation. And a residential-style training apartment with fully equipped kitchen, bathroom, and bedroom to make the patient feel more at home.

6238   Valir Health
700 NW 7th St
Oklahoma City, OK 73102-1212

405-609-3600
888-898-2080
Fax: 405-605-8638
info@valir.com
www.valir.com

Dirk O'Hara, Principal
Tonya Purvine, Corporate Compliance Officer
Inpatient Rehab Facility including all therapy services serving people who have been injured and had an illness resulting in a decreased level of independence.

Oregon

6239   Shriners Hospitals for Children: Portland
3101 SW Sam Jackson Park Rd
Portland, OR 97239-3095

503-241-5090
800-237-5055
Fax: 503-221-3701
www.shrinershospitalsforchildren.org

Michael Aiona, Chief of Staff
Craig Patchin, Administrator
Mark Thoreson, Development Officer
Pediatric orthopedic and plastic surgery; inpatient and outpatient services. No charge for any services provided at the Hospital. Diagnosis, rehabilitation, surgery, sports and recreation for ages 0-18 for people with physical disabilities involving bones, muscles or joints or in need of plastic surgery for burn scars or cleft lip/palate.

Pennsylvania

6240   Allied Services John Heinz Institute of Rehabilitation Medicine
150 Mundy St
MAC III Building, 1st Floor
Wilkes Barre, PA 18702-6830

570-826-3900
Fax: 570-830-2027
www.allied-services.org

Gerald Franceski, Chairman
Thomas Speicher, Vice-Chairman
William Conaboy, CEO
John Heinz Rehab is one of the foremost providers of rehabilitation in the country. Under the supervision of board-certified psychiatrists, a team of highly qualified professionals provides a broad range of specialized services and therapies for inpatients, with speacialized programs in the areas of brain injury, injured worker recovery and pediatrics. John Heinz Rehab is the only CARF accredited program in northeastern Pennsylvania for treatment of brain injury rehabilitation.

6241   Allied Services Rehabilitation Hospital
475 Morgan Hwy
Scranton, PA 18508-2656

570-348-1359
Fax: 570-341-4548
www.allied-services.org

Gerald Franceski, Chairman
Thomas Speicher, Vice-Chairman
William Conaboy, CEO
Committed to help people overcome challenges and reach their greatest potential by providing quality care, people-oriented services and comfort.

6242   Brighten Place
131 North Main St
Chalfont, PA 18914-245

215-997-7746
Fax: 215-997-2517
brightenplace@enter.net

William Koffros, CEO
A residential brain injury program with the mission to encourage growth and foster independence on an individual level for each resident. We are CARF accredited and provide additional services which include a day program and respite care.

6243   Chestnut Hill Rehabilitation Hospital
8601 Stenton Ave
Wyndmoor, PA 19038-8312

215-233-6200
Fax: 215-233-6879
www.extendedcare.com

Cammi Lubking, Administrator
Chestnut Hill Rehab Hospital is dedicated to meeting patients' physical, emotional, social, and vocational goals. Through innovative programs, sophisticated equipment, and support by specially trained staff members committed to the progress of every patient, Chestnut Hill achieves results.

6244   Doylestown Hospital Rehabilitation Center
595 W State St
Doylestown, PA 18901-2597

215-345-2200
Fax: 215-345-2512
www.dh.org

James Brexler, President and Chief Executive Officer
Eleanor Wilson, RN, MSN, MHA, Vice President, Patient Services/Chief Operating Officer
Dan Upton, Vice President, Chief Financial Officer
The mission of Doylestown Hospital is to provide a responsive healing environment for patients and their families, and to improve the quality of life for all members of our community. We combine the creative energies of Medical Staff, Board, Associates and Volunteers to make Doylestown Hospital a place where each patient and family feels healed and whole, even when disease cannot be cured.

6245   Health Care Solutions
500 Abbott Dr
Ste B
Broomall, PA 19008-4301

610-544-6023
800-451-1671
Fax: 610-544-6035
www.lincare.com

John Byrnes, CEO
Shawn Schabel, President/COO
Develops unique containment programs, offers equipment set-up, patient instruction, patient assessment and equipment usage. Offers clinical services that include oxygen systems, ventilators, aerosol therapy, suction equipment, T.E.N.S. programs, compression pumps, custom orthotics, enteral feeding.

6246   HealthSouth Harmarville Rehabilitation Hospital
P.O.Box 11460
320 Guys Run Road
Pittsburgh, PA 15238-460

412-828-1300
877-937-7342
Fax: 412-828-7705
www.healthsouthharmarville.com

Ken Anthony, Chief Executive Officer
Thomas Franz, M.D., Medical Director
Catherine M. Birk, M.D., Staff Physiatrist
A 202-bed facility providing inpatient and outpatient physical medicine and rehabilitation to adults and adolescents in Pennsylvania, West Virginia, Ohio and Maryland.

6247   HealthSouth Nittany Valley Rehabilitation Hospital
Health South of Nittany Valley
550 W College Ave
Pleasant Gap, PA 16823-7401

814-359-3421
800-842-6026
Fax: 814-359-5898
www.nittanyvalleyrehab.com

Richard Allatt, Medical Director
Susan Hartman, CEO
Sara Godwin, CNO
Comprehensive inpatient and outpatient facilities. Treatment for symptoms relating to: stroke, head injury, pulmonary disease, orthopedic conditions, neurological disorders, cardiac illnesses and spinal cord injuries. Healthsouth Nittany Valley Rehabilitation Hospital is a part of Healthsouth's national network of more than 2,000 facilities in 50 states.

6248 HealthSouth Rehab Hospital Of Erie
143 E 2nd St
Erie, PA 16507-1501
814-878-1200
800-234-4574
Fax: 814-878-1399
www.healthsoutherie.com
Douglas Grisier, Medical Director
Shelly Mayes, Director of Therapy Operations
An acute inpatient rehabilitation hospital that was founded in 1986. HealthSouth Erie is one of the only rehabilitation hospitals in the country to hold a triple-certification by the Joint Commission in the areas of Brain Injury, Stroke and Parkinson's disease Rehabilitation.

6249 HealthSouth Rehabilitation Hospital of Altoona
2005 Valley View Blvd
Altoona, PA 16602-4548
814-944-3535
800-873-4220
Fax: 814-944-6160
www.healthsouthaltoona.com
Scott Filler, Chief Executive Officer
Paul Sutton, Director Of Clinical Services
Rakesh (Rock Patel, D.O., Medical Director
Inpatient and outpatient physical rehabilitation programs and services.

6250 Healthsouth Rehabilitation Hospital of Greater Pittsburgh
2380 McGinley Rd
Monroeville, PA 15146-4400
412-856-2400
Fax: 412-856-9320
www.lifecare-hospitals.com
Mary Lee Dadey, Administrator
Rehabilitation and long-term acute care hospital that treats brain injury, stroke, multiple sclerosis, Parkinson's disease, back and spinal cord injuries, cancer, pulmonary disease, cardiac disease, traumatic and work injuries.

6251 Healthsouth Rehabilitation Hospital of Mechanicsburg
175 Lancaster Blvd
Mechanicsburg, PA 17055-3562
717-691-3700
800-933-3831
Fax: 717-697-6524
www.healthsouthpa.com
Mark Freeburn, CEO
Annette Bates, Director of Marketing Operations
Jeff Brandenburg, MPT, Director of Therapy Operations
HealthSouth provides comprehensive rehabilitation and recovery services to patients with stroke, brain injury, hip fracture, medically complex, pulmonary, wound, spinal cord injury, amputation, and other neuro-muscular, and orthopedic impairments. Our primary goal is to provide individualized treatment programs to people requiring physical rehabilitation and medical recovery in order to help patients get back to work, to play, to living.

6252 Healthsouth Rehabilitation Hospital of York
1850 Normandie Dr
York, PA 17408-1552
717-767-6941
Fax: 717-767-8776
www.healthsouthyork.com
Sally Arthur, Director of Human Resources
Bruce Sicilia, Medical Director
Elaine Charest, Director of Therapy Operations
A 120-bed rehabilitation hospital dedicated to providing advanced, comprehensive services to patients who have suffered head injury, spinal cord injury, stroke, burns, amputation, chronic pain and other neurological and musculoskeletal disorders. HRH of York provides outpatient services in seven locations. Healthsouth is located in York, Pennsylvania, approximately 50 miles north of Baltimore and 25 miles south of Harrisburg.

6253 Magee Rehabilitation Hospital
1513 Race St
Philadelphia, PA 19102-1177
215-587-3000
800-966-2433
Fax: 215-568-3736
www.mageerehab.org
Jack Carroll, CEO
A not-for-profit health organization which is the home to the nation's first brain injury rehabilitation program to be accredited by the Commission on the Accreditation of Rehabilitation Facilities

(CARF) and is one of 14 federally designated Regional Spinal Cord Injury Centers. Our staff and management are committed to restoring the highest level of independence possible to individuals with disabilities.

6254 Moss Rehabilitation Hospital
1200 W Tabor Rd.
Philadelphia, PA 19141
215-456-9800
Fax: 215-456-9381
www.mossrehab.com
Thomas Smith, Chief Operating Officer
Alberto Esquenazi, Chief Medical Officer
Eileen Hartranft, Program Director
An outpatient services center providing rehabilitation services. This 152 bed facility offers comprehensive care to people with broad ranges of conditions, diagnostic laboratories and a multidisciplinary team of rehabilitation professionals.

6255 Shriners Hospitals for Children, Philadelphia
Shrinners Hospitals for Children
3551 N Broad St
Philadelphia, PA 19140-4131
215-430-4000
800-281-4051
Fax: 215-430-4126
www.shrinershq.org
Alan W. Madsen, Chairman of the Board
John A. Cinotto, 1st Vice President
Dale W. Stauss, 2nd Vice President
At Shriners Hospitals for Childrenr - Philadelphia, we provide state-of-the-art medical care for children with spinal cord injuries, as well as a host of orthopaedic and neuromusculoskeletal disorders and diseases

6256 Shriners Hospitals for Children, Erie
1645 W 8th St
Erie, PA 16505-5007
814-875-8700
Fax: 814-875-8756
www.shrinershq.org
John Lubahn, Chief of Staff
Charles Walczak, Administrator
The Shriners Hospitals for Children, Erie, is a 30-bed pediatric orthopaedic hospital providing comprehensive orthopaedic care to children at no charge. The hospital is one of 22 Shriners Hospitals throughout North America. The Erie Hospital accepts and treats children with routine and complex orthopaedic and neuromuscular problems, utilizing the latest treatments and technology available in pediatric orthopaedics, resulting in early ambulation and reduced length of stay.

6257 Shriners Hospitals, Philadelphia Unit, for Crippled Children
3551 N Broad St
Philadelphia, PA 19140-4105
215-430-4000
Fax: 215-430-4079
www.shrinershq.org/hospitals/philadelphia
Randal Betz, Chief of Staff
Ernest Perilli, Administrator
Provides comprehensive medical, surgical and rehabilitative care for children with orthopaedic conditions and spinal cord injuries. All services are provided at no charge. The hospital is one of 22 located throughout North America. In addition to treating children with routine and complex orthopaedic problems, the Philadelphia hospital provides a comprehensive and individualized rehabilitation program for children and adolescents who have sustained a traumatic injury to their spine.

South Carolina

6258 Colleton Regional Hospital: RehabCare Unit
501 Robertson Blvd
Walterboro, SC 29488-5714
843-782-2000
Fax: 843-549-7562
www.colletonmedical.com
Mitchell Mongel, CEO
Colleton Medical Center's 8-bed physical and mental rehabilitation department is the oldest in the Lowcountry and has been serving the community for nearly 20 years. Strives to provide patient-centered care in a family atmosphere. The team includes nurses, physical therapists, occupational therapists, speech ther-

apists, and nutritionists. The typical patient requires rehabilitation following a stroke, spinal injury, close head injury, and orthopedic rehabilitation.

6259 HealthSouth Rehab Hospital: South Carolina
2935 Colonial Dr
Columbia, SC 29203-6811   803-254-7777
Fax: 803-414-1414
www.healthsouthcolumbia.com
W. Anthony Jackson, CEO
Lydia Carpenter, Director of Therapy Operations
Devin Troyer, M.D., Medical Director
Offers a wide range of specialized medical and therapeutic services designed to help physically disabled individuals reach their optimum level of function and independence.

6260 Shriners Hospitals for Children, Greenville
950 W Faris Rd
Greenville, SC 29605-4255   864-271-3444
866-459-0013
Fax: 864-271-4471
www.shrinershq.org/hospitals/greenville
Randall Romberger, Administrator
Peter Stasikelis, Chief of Staff
Tracy McReynolds,, Development Officer
A 50-bed pediatric orthopaedic hospital providing comprehensive orthopaedic care to children at no charge to their families. The hospital is one of 22 Shriners Hospitals throughout North America. The hospital accepts and treats children with routine and complex orthopaedic problems, utilizing the latest tretments and technology availiable in pediatric orthopaedics, resulting in early ambulatory and reduced length of stay.

Tennessee

6261 Health South Cane Creek Rehabilitation Center
Health South Corporation
180 Mount Pelia Rd
Martin, TN 38237-3812   731-587-4231
Fax: 731-588-1454
dayle.unger@healthsouth.com
www.healthsouthcanecreek.com
Eric Garrard, CEO
William Eason, Medical Director
Lindsey Box-Rotger, BSN, RN, C, Director of Quality and Risk Management
Offers a wide variety of programs and services for patients in need of acute rehabilitation. Programs and services are availiable through inpatient and outpaitent. Thereapy services availiable are physical, occupational, speech, and respiratory.

6262 HealthSouth Chattanooga Rehabilitation Hospital
2412 McCallie Ave
Chattanooga, TN 37404-3398   423-697-9129
800-763-5189
Fax: 423-697-9124
www.healthsouthchattanooga.com
Scott Rowe, CEO
Amjad Munir, Medical Director
Karen Jonakin, Director Clinical Services
Offers orthopaedic rehabilitation, stroke rehabilitation, amputee rehabilitation, brain injury program, pain management, ventilator weaning, carpal tunnel screening, low intensity program, oncology program, aquatic therapy, day treatment, burn program and outpatient services.

6263 HealthSouth Rehabilitation Cntr/Tennessee
1282 Union Ave
Memphis, TN 38104-3414   901-722-2000
Fax: 901-729-5171
healthsouthmemphis.com
Tracy Willis, CEO
Toni Wackerfuss, Director of Therapy Operation
An 80-bed acute medical rehabilitation hospital that offers comprehensive inpatient and outpatient rehabilitation services.

6264 James H And Cecile C Quillen Rehabilitation Hospital
2511 Wesley St
Johnson City, TN 37601-1723   423-952-1700
800-235-1994
Fax: 423-283-0906
www.msha.com
Tammy Bishop, Manager
A 60-bed, freestanding comprehensive medical rehabilitation hospital. Full range of outpatient and day treatment, 14-bed traumatic brain injury unit, in ground therapeutic pool, transitional living apartment, outdoor ambulation course. All inpatient and outpatient programs utilize an interdisciplinary team approach designed to improve a patient's physical and cognitive functioning.

6265 Nashville Rehabilitation Hospital
610 Gallatin Ave
Nashville, TN 37206-3225   615-650-2600
800-227-3108
Fax: 615-650-2562
Alan Miller, CEO
Marc Miller, President
A free-standing physical rehabilitation facility offering services to patients on an inpatient and outpatient basis. Programs include CVA, orthopedic, neuromuscular, traumatic brain injury, spinal cord injury, general rehabilitation and Bridges - geriatric psychiatric unit. Intra-disciplinary team approach is utilized to assist patients in obtaining their maximum fuctional level.

6266 Patricia Neal Rehab Center : Ft. Sanders Regional Medical Center
Covenant Health
1901 W Clinch Ave
Knoxville, TN 37916-2307   865-541-1111
800-728-6325
Fax: 865-541-2247
www.patneal.org
J.E. Henry, Co-Chair
David Kugley, Co-Chair
Mary Dillon, M.D., Medical Director, Patricia Neal Rehabilitation Center
A CARF accredited 73-bed facility, it offers a comprehensive team approach to care. Physical, occupational, recreational, behavioral medicine and speech language therapists work with physiatrists to develop individual plans of care designed to return patients to a normal lifestyle as quickly as possible. In addition, rehabilitation nurses collaborate with specialists to teach self-care techniques and provide education to help patients reach optimal functionality.

6267 Rehabilitation Center Baptist Hospital
137 E Blount Ave
Suite 6-B
Knoxville, TN 37920-1643   865-632-5520

Primary focus: Mix of mental health and substance abuse services.

6268 Rehabilitation Center at McFarland Hospital
University Medical Center
500 Park Ave
Lebanon, TN 37087-3721   615-449-0500
Fax: 615-453-7405
www.universitymedicalcenter.com
Saad Ehtisham, CEO
Matt Caldwell, Chief Executive Officer
Michael Cherry, Chief Financial Officer
An Acute Inpatient Rehab, located on the hospital's second floor. The center has 26 patient rooms, three therapy treatment rooms, a patient dining area, and an 'activities of daily living' area which includes a kitchen/laundry area and a patient apartment, for those individuals who will be returning home.

6269 St. Mary's Medical Center: RehabCare Center
900 E Oak Hill Ave
Knoxville, TN 37917-4505   865-545-7962
Fax: 865-545-8133
www.tennova.com
Jeffrey Ashin, President
Committed to providing individualized and flexable treatment programs designed for individuals who have been disabled by an

injury or illness. The primary mission of the RehabCare Center is to help patients achieve basic skills that may allow independent living and working.

6270   Sumner Regional Medical Center
555 Hartsville Pike
Gallatin, TN 37066-2400   615-328-8888
                                     Fax: 615-328-3903
                              www.mysumnermedical.com

Susan Peach, BSN, MBA, CEO
Kevin Rinks, Chief Financial Officer
Michael S. Herman, Chief Operating Officer
SRMC operates as a 155-bed healthcare facility and provides quality Gallatin hospital and medical care services in numerous areas, including cancer treatment, cardiac care, same- day surgery, orthopaedics, diagnostics, women's health and rehabilitation services. As the community grows, SRMC strives to continually improve its services and programs to meet the changing needs of its service area.

Texas

6271   Bayshore Medical Center: Rehab
4000 Spencer Hwy
Pasadena, TX 77504-1202   713-359-2000
                                     Fax: 713-359-1283
                              www.bayshoremedical.com

Dr. Charles Bessire, Board
Jeanna Barnard, FACHE,, CEO
Alice Hopkins Adams, Board
A 345-bed facility, providing the award-winning care for which we have been nationally recoginzed. Members are here to care for the physical and emotional well-being of those who arrive at Bayshore Medical Center often frightned, in pain and perhaps even alone. We offer patients solace and security through constant communication and compassionate listening in the midst of their medical emergencies and surgical or diagnostic procedures. Kindness, empathy & quality are triats that patients trust.

6272   Cecil R Bomhr Rehabilitation Center of Nacogdoches Memorial Hospital
1204 N Mound St
Nacogdoches, TX 75961-4027   936-564-4611
                                     Fax: 936-564-4616
                                     info@nacmem.org
                                     www.nacmem.org

Jerry Whitaker, Chairperson
Larry Walker, M.D., Vice-Chairperson
Lisa King, Secretary
The goal of Nacogdoches Memorial Hospital's rehabilitation services is to assist patients in attaining their highest potential activity level for independent daily living, thereby reducing the number of necessary hospitalizations. Keeping folks healthy and in their homes lowers healthcare costs for all of us.

6273   Covenant Health Systems Owens White Outpatient Rehab Center
9812 Slide Rd
Lubbock, TX 79424-1116   806-725-5627
                                     Fax: 806-723-6009
                              www.covenanthealth.org

Walt Cathey, Manager
A comprehensive rehabilitation program designed to help patients attain their maximum level of independence following a debilitating stroke, illness or injury. Our fully accredited program features outpatient physical, occupational and speech language therapies, as well as certified athletic trainers and a certified strength and conditioning specialist.

6274   Gonzales Warm Springs Rehabilitation Hospital
200 Memorial Dr
Luling, TX 78648-3213   830-875-8400
                                     Fax: 830-875-5029
                              www.warmsprings.org

Anthony Misitano, President/CEO
Vonnie Cromwell, Operations Manager
Statewide not-for-profit system of inpatient and outpatient rehabilitation speciality centers. Throughout the communities we

serve, the Warm Springs Rehabilitation System offers hope and acts as a catalyst for achieving an optimal quality of life by providing comprehensive physical and/or cogenitive care. Investing resources in educational and recreational programs. Supporting research efforts.

6275   Harris Methodist Fort Worth Hospital Mabee Rehabilitation Center
1301 Pennsylvania Ave
Fort Worth, TX 76104-2122   817-250-2760
                                     866-847-7342
                                     Fax: 814-250-6846
                              www.texashealth.org

Lillie Biggins, B.S.N., M.S.N, CEO/President
Elaine Nelson, R.N., M.S.N., Chief Nursing Officer
Joseph Prosser, M.D., M.B.A., Chief Medical Officer
Professionals at the Harris Methodist Fort Worth Hospital's Mabee Rehabilitation Center work closely with each patient to develop a specialzed treatment plan for personal achievement. The center offers highly trained clinical staff members and spacious facilities An incredibly wide range of treatment programs and educational services are provided for both inpatient and outpatient needs.

6276   HealthSouth Plano Rehabilitation Hospital
6701 Oakmont Blvd.
Fort Worth, TX 76132-7526   817-370-4700
                                     Fax: 972-423-4293
                              www.healthsouth.com

Jon F. Hanson, Chairman
John W. Chidsey, Board of director
Donald L. Correll, Board of director
A 62-bed medical reahabilitation facility serving inpatient and out patient needs in the Northern Dallas area. The team coordinate all aspects of the patient's rehabilitation to maximize results. The overall effort is directed by board-certified physical medicine and rehabilitation physicians who specialize in medical rehabilitation. Whatever the cause of the disability, our services can benefit patients who have functional limitations in such areas as mobility, communication and self care.

6277   HealthSouth Rehab Hospital Of Arlington
3200 Matlock Rd
Arlington, TX 76015-2911   817-468-4000
                                     Fax: 817-468-3055
                              www.healthsouth.com

Jon F. Hanson, Chairman
John W. Chidsey, Board of director
Donald L. Correll, Board of director
A modern 65-bed hospital dedicated to providng inpatient programs in a general rehabilitation setting for persons recovering for a disabling injury or illness. As part of our continuum of care, we also offer outpatient therapy, a day program, and individual therapy services. Our goal is to help our patients resume a productive and more meaningful life through appropriate rehabilitative care and restorative nursing in a wellness-oriented environment that promotes healing and functional recovery.

6278   HealthSouth Rehab Hospital Of Austin
1215 Red River St
Austin, TX 78701-1921   512-474-5700
                                     Fax: 512-479-3765
                              www.healthsouthaustin.com

Duke Saldiver, CEO
Corey Helm Swartz, Director of Therapy Operations
Maria Arizmendez, M.D., Medical Director
A comprehensive 83 bed medical rehabilitation hospital serving the needs of patients in the Central Texas area. The mission is to promote recovery for persons with disabling conditions by providing individualized treatment so they can reach the highest level of physical, social and emotional well-being.

6279   HealthSouth Rehabilitation Center of Humble Texas
19002 McKay Blvd
Humble, TX 77338   281-446-6148
                                     Fax: 281-446-5616
                              www.healthsouthhumble.com

Angie Simmons, CEO
Mikeal Simpson, Director of Therapy Operations
Emile Mathurin, Jr., M.D., Medical Director

Offers comprehensive rehabilitation services for patients with diverse diagnoses. Rehabilitation can be defined as multidisciplinary therapy designed to increase patient's overall functioning to a level that meets or exceeds where the patient was prior to illness or injury or to maximize current level of ability. The benefits of these services to patients and their families is invaluable.

6280 HealthSouth Rehabilitation Hospital
6701 Oakmont Blvd
Fort Worth, TX 76132-2957   817-370-4700
                                   Fax: 817-370-4977
                                   www.healthsouthcityview.com
Deborah Hopps, CEO
Mark Bussell, Medical Director
Mark Bussell, M.D., Medical Director
A 62-bed acute medical rehabilitation hospital that offers comprehensive inpatient and outpatient rehabilitation services.

6281 HealthSouth Rehabilitation Hospital of Beaumont
3340 Plaza 10 Dr
Beaumont, TX 77707-2551   409-835-0835
                                  Fax: 409-835-0898
Sam Coco, Director of Therapy Operations
HJ Gaspard, CEO
Linda Smith, M.D., Medical Director
A state of the art freestanding 61-bed comprehensive physical rehabilitation hospital. The hospital is specifically designed to meet the needs of individuals and their families who have experienced a disabling injury or illness or are recovering from a surgery. An experienced team of physicians, nurses, therapists, treat conditions and other disorders.

6282 HealthSouth Rehabilitation Institute Of San Antonio (RIOSA)
9119 Cinnamon Hill
San Antonio, TX 78240-5401   210-691-0737
                                  Fax: 210-558-1297
                                  www.hsriosa.com
Scott Butcher, CEO
Richard Senelick, Medical Director
Christine Chesnut, OTR, MPH, Director of Therapy Operations
HealthSouth Rehabilitation Institute of San Antonio is the largest free-standing physical rehabilitation hospital in San Antonio and is proud to enter our 11th year of delivering quality, comprehensive medical rehabilition in a pristine environment. HealthSouth annually serves over 1,500 inpatients and more then 20,000 outpatient visits from throughout San Antonio and Mexico. 108-bed hospital has more then 300 personell on staff providing extensive experience.

6283 Hillcrest Baptist Medical Center: Rehab Care Unit
100 Hillcrest Medical Blvd
Waco, TX 76712-3239   254-202-2000
                                  Fax: 254-202-8975
Fred Walters, President
Jon Ellis, Secretary
A fully accredited 393-bed acute care facility in Waco including a Level II Trauma Center, Hillcrest Family Health Center, a network of family medicine clinics; and many key services. Hillcrest is a ministry of Texas Baptists and is one of 7 health care institutions affiliated with the Baptist General Convention of Texas.

6284 Institute for Rehabilitation & Research
1333 Moursund St
Houston, TX 77030-3405   713-942-6159
                                  800-447-3422
                                  Fax: 713-942-5289
                                  tirr.referrals@memorialhermann.org
                                  www.memorialhermann.org
Jeffrey Berliner, Physician
Michelle Pu, Physician
A national center for information, training, research, and technical assistance in independent living. The goal is to extend the body of knowledge in independent living and to improve the utilization of results of research programs and demonstration projects in this field. It has developed a variety of strategies for collecting, synthesizing, and disseminating information related to the field of independent living.

6285 Midland Memorial Hospital & Medical Center
400 Rosalind Redfern Grover Parkway
Midland, TX 79701-9980   432-685-1111
                                  800-833-2916
                                  russell.meyers@midland-memorial.com
                                  www.midland-memorial.com
J.T. Lent Jr., President
Russell Meyers, CEO
Greg Wright, Board of Directors
The Occupational and Physical Therapy Center is a specialzed outpatient clinic. The clinic provides a wide variety of rehabilitation services designed to adequately assist you in returning back to your normal duties. Our highly trained professionals are here to help you with all your rehabilitation needs.

6286 Navarro Regional Hospital: RehabCare Unit
Navarro Hospital
3201 W State Highway 22
Corsicana, TX 75110-2469   903-654-6800
                                  Fax: 903-654-6955
                                  www.navarrohospital.com
Xavier Villarreal, CEO
Glenda Teri, Chief Nursing Officer
The rehab unit is located on the 4th floor and is designed for individuals who require intense rehab for an injury or disease process where the goal would be to return home. Our team is committed to helping individuals return to the highest level of functioning. Our team consists of physicians, nurses, physical therapist, occupational therapist, speech therapist, social workers, dieticians and other professionals as needed.

6287 Rebound: Northeast Methodist Hospital
12412 Judson Rd
Live Oak, TX 78233-3255   210-757-7000
                                  Fax: 210-757-5072
Joe Hernandez, Manager
Methodist Healthcare provides quality, comprehensive rehabilitation services for children and adults. Working as a team, rehabilitation professionals help patients define and achieve individual goals in restoring function and productivity.

6288 Rio Vista Rehabilitation Hospital
1740 Curie Dr
El Paso, TX 79902-2900   915-544-8336
                                  800-999-8392
                                  Fax: 915-544-4838
Gene Miller, Administrator

6289 San Antonio Warm Springs Rehabilitation Hospital
5101 Medical Dr
San Antonio, TX 78229-4801   210-595-2380
                                  Fax: 210-614-0649
                                  www.warmsprings.org
Kurt Meyer, SVP Operations
Rick Marek, VP Post Acute Medical
A statewide not-for-profit system of inpatient and outpatient rehabilitation specialty centers. Warm Springs Rehabilitation System offers hope and acts as a catalyst for achieving an optimal quality of life by providing comprehensive physical and/or cognitive rehabilitative care. Invensting resources in educational and recreational programs. Supporting research efforts.

6290 Shannon Medical Center: RehabCare Unit
120 E Harris Ave
San Angelo, TX 76903-5904   325-653-6741
                                  Fax: 325-657-5706
                                  www.shannonhealth.com
Bryan Horner, CEO
Irv Zeitler, VP Medical Affairs
Shane Plymell, Chief financial officer
Committed to improving the health of our community, using the latest technologies available in the spirit of caring and integrity. Strives to create an environment committed to the values of accountability, service, pride, integrity, respect and excellence. We foster growth toward the highest quality care and customer service and strive for excellent financial performance. We hire and develop the best people to accomplish these tasks.

6291 Shriners Burn Institute: Galveston Unit
815 Market St
Galveston, TX 77550-2725   409-770-6600
Fax: 409-770-6919
www.totalburncare.com

David Herndon, Chief Of Staff
David Ferrell, F.A.C.H.E., Administrator
Providing expert, orthopaedic and burn care to children under 18 regardless of ability to pay.

6292 Shriners Hospitals for Children, Houston
6977 Main St
Houston, TX 77030-3701   713-797-1616
800-853-1240
Fax: 713-797-1029
www.shrinershq.org

David Ferrell, Administrator
Douglas Barnes, Chief of Staff
Melanie Lux, M.D.,, Director
Shriners Hospitals provides at no charge quality pediatric orthopedic serivces to children ages newborn to 18 years old. These services include both outpatient and inpatient needs. Specialties include cerebrel palsy, spina bifida, scoliosis, hand, hip and feet problems. An application is required and may be completed by phone.

6293 South Arlington Medical Center: Rehab Care Unit
3301 Matlock Rd
Arlington, TX 76015-2908   817-472-4849
Fax: 817-472-4946
mca@hcahealthcare.com
www.medicalcenterarlington.com
Patrice Oliver, Manaager
Above all else, we are committed to the care and improvement of human life. In recognition of this committment, we strive to deliver high-quality, cost-effective healthcare in the communities we serve.

6294 South Texas Rehabilitation Hospital
Ernest Health
425 E Alton Gloor Blvd
Brownsville, TX 78526-3361   956-554-6000
Fax: 956-350-6150
www.strh.ernesthealth.com
Christopher Wilson, Medical Director
Jessie Eason, CEO
Mary Valdez, Director of Marketing
STRH was designed for the provision of specialized rehabilitative care, in the only freestanding acute rehabilitation hospital serving Brownsville and the Rio Grande Valley. The hospital provides rehabilitative services for patients with functional deficits as a result of debilitating illnesses or injuries.

6295 St. David's Rehabilitation Center
St. David s Medical Center
621 Radam Lane
Suite 200
Austin, TX 78745-4237   512-447-1083
Fax: 512-447-1338
www.stdavids.com
Anisa Godinez, Medical Director
Everett Heinze, MD Neurology, Medical Director
Tom Hill, MD, Medical Director
Mission is to provide exceptional care to every patient every day with a spirit of warmth, friendliness and personal pride. Values are integrity, compassion, accountability, respect and excellence.

6296 Texas NeuroRehab Center
1106 W Dittmar Rd
Austin, TX 78745-6328   512-444-4835
800-252-5151
Fax: 512-462-6749
Alison Crawford Sinsky, Inpatient and Outpatient Manager
Ed Varando, Occupational Therapy Manager
Internationally recognized provider in brain injury/neurobehavioral treatment for children, adolescents, and adults with complex medical, physical and/or behavioral issues. Medical rehabilitation, neurobehavioral, and neuropsychiatric programs combine traditional therapies with education, vocational, substance abuse, and sensory integration services.

6297 Texas Specialty Hospital at Dallas
7955 Harry Hines Blvd
Dallas, TX 75235-3305   214-637-0000
Robin Burns, CEO
66 beds offering active/acute rehabilitation, brain injury day treatment, cognitive rehabilitation, complex care, extended rehabilitation and short term evaluation.

6298 Touchstone Neurorecovery Center
Nexus Health Systems
9297 Wahrenberger Rd
Conroe, TX 77304-2441   936-788-7770
800-414-4824
Fax: 936-788-7785
tncinfo@nhsltd.com
John W. Cassidy, MD, Executive Medical Director
Jude Theriot, MD, Medical Director
Ron Tintner, MD, Associate Clinical Director
Touchstone provides treatment and rehabilitation in a residential environment on a tranquil, wooded 26-acre site just north of Houston in Conroe, TX. Touchstone offers customized treatment programs designed to help individuals with known or suspected brain injury or neurological deficits progress to their highest functional level possible. Touchstone offers both on-campus and off-campus housing in home-like settings for residents based on their needs.

6299 Valley Regional Medical Center: RehabCare Unit
100A E Alton Gloor Blvd
Brownsville, TX 78526-3328   956-350-7000
Fax: 956-350-7111
www.valleyregionalmedicalcenter.com
Billy Bradford Jr.,, Chair
Francisco Javier Del Castillo, M, Vice Chair
Subramaniam Anandasivam, MD, Board
Our mission is to treat our community as family by providing quality compassionate care.

Utah

6300 HealthSouth Rehab Hospital Of Utah
8074 S 1300 E
Sandy, UT 84094-743   801-561-3400
801-565-6666
Fax: 801-565-6576
www.healthsouthutah.com
Phil Eaton, CEO
William McNutt, Director of Therapy Operations
Mark Rada, M.D., Interim Medical Director
A full spectrum of services, including inpatient, outpatient, day hospital and home health. Holistic patient care, education and community assimilation are the hallmarks of our programs, and evidence of our leadership in the field of rehabilitation. Working together as a team, we are able to tailor the needs of our patients and provide the highest quality services. We believe that education and involvement of family and friends, will assist them in maintaining independence after discharge.

6301 LDS Hospital Rehabilitation Center
8th Ave & C Street
Salt Lake City, UT 84143-0001   801-408-1100
800-527-1118
Fax: 801-408-5610
www.intermountainhealthcare.org
Lizz Daley, Administrator
Jim Sheets, Administrator
Located within a Trauma I Center, this facility provides comprehensive inpatient and outpatient rehabilitation to people with physical disabilities. CARF/JCAHO accredited. Low cost family housing is available and Medicaid/Medicare is accepted.

589

6302   Primary Children's Medical Center
100 Mario Capecchi Dr
Salt Lake City, UT 84113-1100   801-662-1000
                                       Fax: 801-588-2318
                             www.intermountainhealthcare.org
Scott Parker, President
Kevin Jones, Manager
Ore-Ofe O. Adesina, MD, Ophthalmology
Primary Children's Medical Center is the pediatric center serving
5 states in the Intermountain West Utah, Idaho, Wyoming, Nevada
and Montana. The 289-bed facility is equipped and staffed
to treat children with complex illness and injury. PCMC is owned
by Intermountain Healthcare, a non-profit health care system. In
addition, it is affiliated with the Dept. of Pediatrics, University of
Utah, integrating pediatric programs. The hospital is designed to
meet the needs of children & their families.

6303   Shriners Hospitals for Children: Intermountain
Fairfax Road at Virginia St
Salt Lake City, UT 84103   801-536-3500
                                       800-313-3745
                                       Fax: 801-536-3782
                                       www.shrinershq.org
Kevin Martin, Administrator
Jacques D'Astous, Chief of Staff
One of nineteen hospitals in North America specializing in pediatric orthopedics (plus four hospitals providing pediatric burn
treatment). This hospital serves the Intermountain region. All
services provided in the hospital are at no cost to family, insurance company, nor state/federal agency regardless of ability to
pay.

6304   Stewart Rehabilitation Center: McKay Dee Hospital
4401 Harrison Blvd
Ogden, UT 84403-3195   801-387-2080
                                       Fax: 801-387-7720
                             www.intermountainhealthcare.org
Corey Anden, Nurse Coordinator
Judy Grover, Manager
With 10 affiliated clinics, McKay-Dee serves northern Utah, and
portions of southeast Idaho and western Wyoming. A part of
Intermountain Healthcare's system of 21 hospitals, McKay-Dee
Hospital Center offers nationally ranked programs such as the
Heart & Vascular Institute, the Newborn ICU and a new Cancer
Treatment Center.

6305   University Healthcare-Rehabilitation Center
50 N Medical Dr
Salt Lake City, UT 84132-1   801-587-3422
                                       801-58 -EHAB
                                       Fax: 801-581-2111
                             www.healthcare.utah.edu/rehab/
David Entwistle, Administrator
Trish Jensen, Program Coordinator
Provides quality, comprehensive, rehabilitation services to persons with complex rehabilitation needs, including spinal cord injuries, head trauma, stroke, and other disabling conditions.
Rehabilitation Services has been serving physicians, their patients, and the community since 1965. Rehabilitation Services
has been an established leader in comprehensive inpatient, outpatient and home/community rehabilitation programs. Accredited
by CARF and JCAHO.

Vermont

6306   Vermont Achievement Center
88 Park St
Rutland, VT 05701-4715   802-775-2395
                                       Fax: 802-773-9656
                                       www.vac-rutland.com
Kiki Mc Shane, CEO
Rebecca Wisell, Administrator
Vermont Achievement Center is recognized as a catalyst in building a community where all people are capable of change. Individuals flourish because they are nutured, valued and treated with
respect. Education is empowering. The family is the primary influence in a person's life. Children belong in a family. Families

are enhanced by support of the community. Children and family
services are flexible and responsive to changing needs.

Virginia

6307   Inova Mount Vernon Hospital Rehabilitation Program
Inova Rehabilitation Center
2501 Parkers Ln
Alexandria, VA 22306-3209   703-664-7000
                                       800-554-7342
                                       Fax: 703-664-7423
                                       www.inova.com
Barbara Doyle, CEO
Inova Mount Vernon Hospital is a 237-bed hospital offering patients convenience and state-of-the-art care in a community environment. Our hospital sits on 26 acres of beautifully landscaped
open space, where patients can find moments of serenity in our
specially designed gardens..

6308   Kluge Children's Rehabilitation Center
University of Virginia
2270 Ivy Rd
Charlottesville, VA 22903-4977   434-924-5161
                                       800-627-8596
                                       Fax: 434-924-5559
                             www.healthsystem.virginia.edu
Janet Allaire, Administrator
Richard Stevenson, Research Director
The Kluge Childrens's Rehabilitation Center (KCRC) is a place
dedicated to serving children with special needs. Children be-
tween the ages of birth and 21 come to the KCRC from all over
Virginia, the United States, and even overseas for many reasons.
Some need specific therapy or rehabilitation after injuries, accidents, or surgery. Others have chronic illness such as diabetes,
and cystic fibrosis. Many families come to find out why their
child is experiencing behavior problems.

Washington

**6309   Good Samaritan Healthcare Physical Medicine and
Rehabilitation**
Good Samaritan Hospital
407 14th Ave SE
Puyallup, WA 98372-3770   253-697-4000
                                       Fax: 253-697-5157
                                       info@goodsamhealth.org
                                       www.multicare.org
Glenn Kassman, President
Vince Schmitz, CFO
Good Samaritan is part of the Multi-Care Health System, a
non-for-profit medical system serving the growing populations
of Pierce and King Counties in the greater Puget Sound region of
Washington. Our medical staff includes 1,600 of the regions most
respected primary care physicians and specialists.

6310   Northwest Hospital Center for Medical Rehabilitation
1550 N 115th St
Seattle, WA 98133-9733   206-364-0500
                                       Fax: 206-364-0500
                                       TTY: 877-694-4677
                                       www.nwhospital.org
Peter Evans, Chairman
Scott L. Hardman, Vice Chairman
James K. Anderson, Board
Provides complete medical and surgical services in both inpatient
and outpatient settings. Services across multiple specialties include: 24hr emergency services, critical care, cardiac care, stroke
program, cancer care, childbirth center, rehabilitation center, diagnostic imaging and education and wellness services. Mission is
to raise the long-term health status of our community by providing personalized, quality care with compassion dignity, and
respect.

6311 **Providence Medical Center**
500 17th Ave
Seattle, WA 98122-5711   206-000-1111
                        Fax: 206-320-3387
                        www.providence.org
Swedish offers a complete continuum of rehabilitation services, from acute inpatient care to extensive outpatient therapies, to meet virtually every rehabilitative need for patients of all ages. Nearly 7,000 patients turn to Swedish for these services every year. Through our multidisciplinary team of physical and occupational therapists and speech-language pathologists, Swedish provides the reassurance of a high level of clinical expertise in comfortable, state-of-the-art facilities.

6312 **Providence Rehabilitation Services**
Providence Rehabilitation Services
1321 Colby Ave
Everett, WA 98201-1665   425-261-3825
                        Fax: 425-261-3823
                        www.providence.org
Jim Phillips, Manager
Leslie Baumgarten, Manager
Continuum of care available: Acute Care, Inpatient Rehabilitation Unit, Transitional Care, Outpatient therapies, and In-home services.

6313 **Shriners Hospitals for Children: Spokane**
Shriners Hospitals
911 W 5th Ave
Spokane, WA 99204-2901   509-455-7844
                        Fax: 509-744-1223
                www.shrinershq.org/hospitals/spokane
Kristin Monasmith, Public Relations Director
Craig Patchin, Administrator
Paul M. Caskey, M.D., Chief of Staff
Provides pediatric orthopedic services plus burn scar revision to children birth to 18. All services at no charge to the family.

West Virginia

6314 **HealthSouth Mountain View Regional Rehab Hospital**
1160 Van Voorhis Rd
Morgantown, WV 26505-3437   304-598-1100
                        800-388-2451
                        Fax: 304-598-1103
                www.healthsouthmountainview.com/
Vicki Demers, Chief Executive Officer
Govind Patel, M.D., Medical Director
Robbin Butler, OTR/L, Director of Therapy Operations
A 96-bed inpatient acute rehabilitation hospital. Outpatient services, physical, occupational and speech therapy, and interior therapy pool. Programs include neuro/stroke, brain injury, spinal cord injury and pediatric.

6315 **HealthSouth Western Hills Regional Rehab Hospital**
3 Western Hills Dr
Parkersburg, WV 26105-8122   304-420-1392
                        Fax: 304-420-1374
                        www.healthsouthwesternhills.com
Kalapala Rao, Medical Director
Candace Ross, Director of Human Resources
Greg Holland, Director of Marketing Operations
A 40-bed medical rehabilitation hospital serving inpatient and outpatient needs in the western West Virginia area. Our hospital is accredited by the Joint Commission on Accreditation of Healthcare Organizations (JCAHO) Our mission is to guide patients whtih physically disabling conditions along an individualized treatment pathway so they can reach the highest level of physical, social and emotional well-being. We strive to provide the highest quality care for you and your family.

Wisconsin

6316 **Extendicare Health Services, Inc.**
3540 South 43rd Street
Milwaukee, WI 53220-2903   414-541-1000
                        800-395-5000
                        Fax: 414-541-1942
                        www.extendicare.com
Timothy Lukenda, CEO
Douglas Harris, SVP
David Pearce, Vice President, General Counsel
Sunrise Care Center is a leading provider of long-term skilled nursing care and short-term rehabilitation solutions. Our 99 bed facility offers a full continuum of services and care focused around each individual in today's ever-changing healthcare environment. Our facility is Medicare and Medicaid certified.

6317 **St. Catherine's Hospital**
9555 76th St
Pleasant Prairie, WI 53158   262-577-8000
                        Fax: 262-653-5795
                        www.uhsi.org
Vicki Lewis, Manager
Committed to living out the healing ministries of the Judeo-Christian faiths by providing exceptional and compassionate healthcare service that promotes the dignity and well-being of the people we serve.

6318 **St. Joseph Hospital**
611 Saint Joseph Ave
Marshfield, WI 54449-1898   715-387-1713
                        Fax: 715-389-3939
                        www.ministryhealth.org
Michael Schmidt, CEO
Catherine Olson, Director
A values-driven healthcare delivery network of aligned hospitals, clinics, long-term care facilities, home care agencies, dialysis centers and many other programs and services in Wisconsin and Minnesota.

Wyoming

6319 **Spalding Rehabilitation Hospital at Memorial Hospital of Laramie**
2301 House Ave
Suite 300
Cheyenne, WY 82001-3748   307-635-4141
                        800-374-7687
                        Fax: 307-638-2656
                        www.imgwy.com
Mitchell Schwarzbach, Executive Director
Tanya Boerkircher, Wyoming Endoscopy Center Manager
Andrea Bailey, Charge Entry Supervisor
We are a professional corporation of physicians trained in various medical specialties and subspecialties including Internal Medicine, Gastroenterology and Chest Diseases.It is our mission to provide the highest quality, cost-effective primary and subspecialty medical care, and education to the people of southern Wyoming, western Nebraska, and northern Colorado.

Rehabilitation Facilities, Post-Acute

Alabama

6320   Alabama Department of Rehabilitation Services
602 S. Lawrence St.
Montgomery, AL 36104
                                334-293-7500
                                800-441-7609
                                Fax: 334-293-7383
                                TTY: 800-499-1816
                                www.rehab.alabama.gov
Jane E. Burdeshaw, Commissioner
State agency which provides services and assistance to Alabama's children and adults with disabilities.

6321   Briarcliff Nursing Home & Rehab Facility
3201 North Ware Road
McAllen, TX 78501
                                956-631-5542
                                Fax: 956-631-5777
                                http://www.briarcliffnursingcenter.com
Postacute rehabilitation program.

6322   Centers for The Developmentally Disabled - North Central Alabama
1602 Church St SE
P.O. Box 2091
Decatur, AL 35602
                                256-350-1458
                                Fax: 256-350-1485
                                info@cddnca.org
                                www.cddnca.org
Earl Brightwell, Executive Director
CDD NCA provides services and programs for individuals who are mentally and/or physically challenged, or developmentally delayed. These services range from early intervention services for infants and toddlers to residential and employment programs for adults. All services are typically provided at no cost to the individual or their family, regardless of income. Funding sources for the CDD NCA include DMH, United Way, and ADRS.

6323   Cheaha Regional Mental Health Center
351 W 3rd St
Sylacauga, AL 35150
                                256-245-1340
                                Fax: 256-245-1343
Cynthia L. Atkinson, Executive Director
Dr. Shakil Khan, Medical Director
Karen McKinney, Clinical Director, Mental Health Services
CRMHC provides a continuum of services for persons with intellectual disabilities, serious mental illness and substance abuse in a four county area in east Alabama, which includes Clay, Coosa, Randolph, and Talladega Counties.

6324   Children's Rehabilitation Service
Alabama Department of Rehabilitation Services
602 S. Lawrence St.
Montgomery, AL 36104
                                334-293-7500
                                800-441-7609
                                Fax: 334-293-7383
                                TTY: 800-499-1816
                                www.rehab.alabama.gov
Jane E. Burdeshaw, Commissioner
CRS provides individualized services to children with special health care needs from birth to age 21 and their families at home, school, and in the community. In addition, CRS provides disability services, expertise, and adaptive technology to and for local school systems, assisting teachers, school nurses and other staff in the education of children with disabilities. The CRS Hemophilia Program serves Alabama's children and adults with this life-threatening blood disorder.

6325   Chilton-Shelby Mental Health Center
110 Medical Center Dr
Calera, AL 35045
                                205-755-8800
                                Fax: 205-668-4957
                                chiltonshelby.org
Melodie D. Crawford, Chief Executive Officer
Vicki M. Potts, Chief Financial Officer
Kathryn T. Crouthers, Chief Operations Officer

Mental health rehabilitation services and more for the recovery of mentally disabled adults. Serves Chilton and Shelby counties.
Business Office Location

6326   Darden Rehabilitation Center
1001 E Broad Street
Ste C
Gadsden, AL 35903-2400
                                256-547-5751
                                Fax: 256-547-5761
                                darden@dardenrehab.org
                                dardenrehab.org
Lynn Curry, Executive Director
Derek Coburn, Operations Manager
Dana Johnson, Program Coordinator
Work adjustment and job placement programs. Serves the counties of Etowah, Marshall, Dekalb, Clair and Cherokee.

6327   Easterseals Central Alabama
2185 Normandie Dr.
Montgomery, AL 36111
                                334-288-0240
                                Fax: 334-288-7171
                                info@eastersealsca.org
                                www.eastersealscentralalabama.org
Lynne Stokley, Chief Executive Officer
Debbie Lynn, Administrator
Serves people with disabilities and their families by providing programs and services.

6328   Easterseals Northwest Alabama
1615 Trojan Dr.
Suite 1
Muscle Shoals, AL 35661
                                256-381-1110
                                info@eastersealsnwal.org
                                www.eastersealsnwal.org
Lynne Stokley, Chief Executive Officer
Danny Prince, Administrator
Easterseals provides services for people with disabilities and their families. Services include occupational therapy, physical therapy, speech therapy, and vocational services.

6329   Easterseals West Alabama
1110 Dr. Edward Hillard Drive
Tuscaloosa, AL 35401-7446
                                205-759-1211
                                800-726-1216
                                Fax: 205-349-1162
                                eswa@eswaweb.org
                                eswaweb.org
Ronny Johnston, Executive Director
Dusty Beam, Administrative Coordinator
Holly Hillard, Director, Development
Leading organization in helping children and adults with disabilities to live with equality, dignity and independence. Rehabilitation services are provided in two divisions: outpatient rehabilitation division (physical therapy, occupational therapy, speech therapy, hearing evaluation, sell and service hearind aids) and vocational division (vocational evaualtion and vocational development). Services are rendered regardless of age, race, sex, color, creed, national origin, veteran's status.

6330   Easterseals West Central Alabama Rehabilitation Center
2906 Citizens Pkwy
P.O. Box 750
Selma, AL 36702-0750
                                334-872-8421
                                800-801-4776
                                Fax: 334-872-3907
                                www.eswcarc.us
Vocational evaluation, job development, employment development, job coaching, counseling, medical services, audiology, pre-school development programs.

6331   Geer Adult Training Center
P.O.Box 419
83 South Canaan Road
Canaan, CT 06018-419
                                860-824-7067
                                Fax: 205-367-8032
                                geercares.org/content/about-geer
Yvonne Williams, Program Coordinator

6332 Goodwill Easterseals of the Gulf Coast
2440 Gordon Smith Dr.
Mobile, AL 36617-2319
251-471-1581
info@al.easterseals.com
www.gesgc.org

Peter D'Olive, Chairman
Frank Harkins, President & CEO
Bill Dillman, Vice President, Marketing & Development
Vocational, medical, pre-school education, day care, recreation and other support services.

6333 HealthSouth Corporation
3660 Grandview Parkway
Ste 200
Birmingham, AL 35243-3332
205-967-7116
800-765-4772
Fax: 225-928-0317
healthsouth.com

Jacque Shadle, CEO
Derrick Landreneau, Director of Nursing services
Dedicated to one field of medicine - physical rehabilitation medicine - and are committed to one goal, helping patients achieve the highest level of functioning possible after a debilitating injury or illness.

6334 Indian Rivers Mental Health Center - Bibb
2439 Main St
Brent, AL 35034
205-926-4681
Fax: 205-296-6016
www.irmhc.org

6335 Indian Rivers Mental Health Center - Pickens
890 Reform St.
Carrollton, AL 35447
205-367-8032
Fax: 205-367-9291
www.irmhc.org

6336 Indian Rivers Mental Health Center - Tuscaloosa
2209 - 9th St
Tuscaloosa, AL 35401
205-391-3131
Fax: 205-391-3135
http://www.irmhc.org

Barbara Friedman, President
Elizabeth Rice, First Vice President
Services are available to adults who have serious mental illness resulting in personal, family or work-related problems. Counseling may take place in either individual or group settings, identification, evaluation and treatment services are available to persons who experience problems related to alcohol and drug abuse and counseling services are available for children and adolescents who have a severe emotional disturbance causing discipline problems at home and school.

6337 Mobile ARC
2424 Gordon Smith Dr
Mobile, AL 36617-2397
251-479-7409
Fax: 251-473-7649
jzoghby@mobilearc.org
mobilearc.org

Jeff Zoghby, Executive Director
Amy Odom, Public Relations and Development Director
Mobile Arc, Inc. (MARC) offers a wide range of services for persons with intellectual and developmental disabilities.

6338 Southeastern Blind Rehabilitation Center
U.S. Department of Veteran Affairs
700 S 19th St
Birmingham, AL 35233-1927
205-558-4706
Fax: 205-933-4484
www.rehab.va.gov/blindrehab/
The Center is a 32-bed inpatient blind rehabilitation program which serves the southeastern region. The majority of client services are for basic adjustment and management to sight loss. Basic services include: low vision, orientation and mobility, manual skills, ADL and communications. Training on electronic mobility aids and adapted computers is also available on a restricted basis. The program maintains graduate education affiliations and an active applied research program.

6339 UAB Eye Care
University Of Alabama at Birmingham
1716 University Blvd
Birmingham, AL 35233
205-975-2020
Fax: 205-934-6755
www.uab.edu/optometry/home/eyecare
Rodney W. Nowakowski, Dean
Dr. Marsha Snow, Chief, Low Vision Patient Care
Brittney Bolen, Optometric Technician
Complete eye services, including low vision services and materials.

6340 Vaughn-Blumberg Services
2715 Flynn Rd
P.O. Box 8646
Dothan, AL 36304
334-793-3102
Fax: 334-793-7740
www.vaughnblumbergservices.com
Ed Dorsey, Executive Director
Linda Cunningham, Director of Human Resources
Billy McCarthy, Director of Finance
Provides comprehensive services for people with intellectual disabilities that reside in Houston County as well as assist in facilitating their participation in society to the fullest extent of their individual capabilities. Offers early intervention services for the mentally handicapped adult including diagnosis and evaluation and physical, speech, and occupational therapies. They also offer counseling, day training,employment assistance and residental homes.

Alaska

6341 Alaska Center for the Blind and Visually Impaired
3903 Taft Drive
Anchorage, AK 99517-3069
907-248-7770
800-770-7517
Fax: 907-248-7517
info@alaskabvi.org
www.alaskabvi.org
Regan Mattingly, Executive Director
Robert Tasso, Program Manager
Caren Ailleo, Development & Communications Director
Services to help the adult residential or community-based student become independent and self-sufficient by offering independent travel, Braille reading and writing, use of assiative technology such as talking computers, manual skills and personal, as well as home management. There is a special program for those 55 years of age and older who are experiencing a vision loss and another program for rural Alaska Native youth who are visually impaired.

Arizona

6342 Arizona Center for the Blind and Visually Impaired
3100 E Roosevelt St
Phoenix, AZ 85008-5036
602-273-7411
Fax: 602-273-7410
jlamay@acbvi.org
acbvi.org
James La May, CEO
Frank Vance, Director
Christine Boisen, Chair
A private, nonprofit organization that provides comprehensive rehabilitation services and more for the blind and visually handicapped. The staff includes 20 instructional and adminstrative professionals.

6343 Arizona Industries for the Blind
Suite 130
515 N 51st Avenue
Phoenix, AZ 85043-2711
602-771-9100
Fax: 602-353-5701
DanielMartinez@azdes.gov
www.azdes.gov/aib
Richard Monaco, General Manager
Daniel Martinez, Community Services Liaison

Offers rehabilitation services, vocational/pre-vocational evaluation and training, work adjustment, job development and employment and training opportunities for individuals who are blind.

6344 Banner Good Samaritan Medical Center
1111 E McDowell Road
Phoenix, AZ 85006-2666
602-839-2000
Fax: 602-239-5868
www.bannerhealth.com

Steve Narang, MD, Chief Executive Officer
Lorraine Hudspeth, Controller
Letty Cerpa, Senior Accountant
Nearly 1,700 physicians representing more than 50 specialties work with Banner Good Samaritan staff to care for more then 36,000 inpatients a year. Houses more then 650 licensed patient care beds. A teaching hospital that trains more then 220 physicians annually and a premier medical center in Arizona and the Southwest. Provides a comprehensive foundation of major programs and an equally impressive offering of highly specialized programs not availiable in most hospitals.

6345 Beacon Group
308 W Glenn St.
Tucson, AZ 85705
520-622-4874
Fax: 520-620-6620
www.beacongroup.org
Committed to effectively assisting adults with disabilities to maximize their personal, social, vocational and educational skills in order to attain a successful and meaningful independence within the Tucson community.

6346 Carondelet Brain Injury Programs and Services (Bridges Now)
2202 N. Forbes Blvd.
Tucson, AZ 85745-2602
520-872-7324
Fax: 520-873-3743
comments@carondelet.org
carondelet.org

Daisy M Jenkins, Executive VP, Chief HR/Administr
James K Beckmann, President/Chief Executive Officer
Alan Strauss, Executive VP, Finance and Chief Financial Officer
Comprehensive outpatient rehabilitation program. PT, OT, ST, Psychology and Rehab Counseling Services.

6347 Desert Life Rehabilitation & Care Center
1919 W Medical St
Tucson, AZ 85704-1133
520-369-9620
Fax: 520-867-6612
Amad Nazifi, Executive Director
Accomodates 240 residents. Provides skilled and intermediate nursing with occupational, physical, speech and respiratory therapy services. Offers special programs including an Alzheimer's Unit and a Young Adult program

6348 Devereux Advanced Behavioral Health Arizona - Scottsdale
Scottsdale Administrative Office
2025 N 3rd St
Suite 250
Phoenix, AZ 85004
602-283-1573
Fax: 480-443-5587
azadmissions@devereux.org
www.devereuxaz.org

Lane Barker, Executive Director
Yvette Jackson, Director of Operations
Donovan S Carman, MBA, Director of Finance
Engages in the treatment of behavioral health issues through services such as residential treatment centers, day school, outpatient services, prevention programs, adult foster care, and foster care for children. Also offered are evidence-based interventions to improve lives.

6349 Devereux Arizona - Tucson
Tuscon Administrative Office
6141 E Grant Rd
Tucson, AZ 85712
520-296-5551
Fax: 520-296-8244
azadmissions@devereux.org
www.devereuxaz.org

Lane Barker, Executive Director
Yvette Jackson, Director of Operations
Donovan S Carman, MBA, Director of Finance
Organization offering culturally competent care for individuals with emotional and behavioral health disorders. Some of the programs offered include Adult Foster Care, kinship program, Therapeutic Foster Care Program, Parent Aide and more.

6350 Freestone Rehabilitation Center
10617 E Oasis Drive
Mesa, AZ 85208
480-986-1531
Fax: 480-986-1538

Randy Gray, Executive Director
Cherie Vance, Manager

6351 HealthSouth Valley Of The Sun Rehabilitation Hospital
13460 N 67th Ave
Glendale, AZ 85304-1000
623-878-8800
Fax: 623-878-5254
healthsouth.com

Beth Bacher, Manager
A 60-bed free-standing hospital that offers acute physical rehabilitation, outpatient therapy services and day hospital treatment. Works in cooperation with local, regional and national managed care organizations and other sources to maximise patient recovery while conserving financial resources.

6352 Institute for Human Development
Northern Arizona University
912 Riordan Rd. P.O.Box 5630
Flagstaff, AZ 86011-5630
928-523-4791
Fax: 928-523-9127
TTY: 928-523-1695
ihd@nau.edu
www.nau.edu/ihd

Levi Esguerra, Director
Lisa Andrew, Advisory Commitee
Lynn Black, Advisory Commitee
The Institute values and supports the independence, productivity and inclusion of Arizona's citizens with disabilities. Based on the values and beliefs, the Institute conducts training, research and services that further these goals.

6353 John C Lincoln Hospital North Mountain
250 E Dunlap Ave
Phoenix, AZ 85020-2871
602-943-2381
Fax: 602-944-8062
webmaster@jcl.com
www.jcl.com/content/northmountain/default.htm
Rhonda Forsyth, President
Bruce Pearson, FACHE, Senior Vice President
Maggi Griffin, RN, MS, Vice President & Chief Executive Officer
Mission is to assist each person entrusted to our care to enjoy the fullest gift of health possible, and work with others to build a community where a helping hand is available for our most vulnerable members.

6354 La Frontera Center
504 W 29th St
Tucson, AZ 85713-3394
520-884-9920
Fax: 520-792-0654
www.lafronteraaz.org

Kevin Heath, Board Chair
Frank Valenzuela, Vice Chair
Celestino Fernandez, Treasurer
A nonprofit community-based behavioral health agency that has been helping southern Arizona children, adults, and families since 1968.

6355 Manor Care Nursing and Rehab Center: Tucson
3705 N Swan Rd
Tucson, AZ 85718-6939   520-299-7088
                                         Fax: 520-529-0038
                                         www.hcr-manorcare.com

Clifton J. Porter II, Vice President - Government Rela
Martin Allen, Vice President
A leading provider of short-term post-acute medical care and rehabilitation and long-term skilled nursing care. High quality medical care is provided through registered (RN) and licensed practical (LPN) nurses and certified nursing assistants (CNA) in concert with physical, occupational and speech rehabilitation therapists. Our more then 275 skilled nursing centers are Medicare-and Medicaid-certified.

6356 Nova Care
Second Floor
680 American Avenue
King of Prussia, PA 19406-2607   800-331-8840
                                         Fax: 602-256-7292
                                         novacare.com

Scott Lusted, General Manager
Brian Beal, Market Manager
NovaCare Rehabilitation's highly respected clinical team provides preventative and rehabilitative services that maximize functionality and promote well-being. NovaCare Rehabilitation also provides physical therapy and athletic training services to more then 20 professional sports teams and 300 universities, colleges, and highschools thoughout the nation.

6357 Perry Rehabilitation Center
3146 E Windsor Avenue
Phoenix, AZ 85008-1199   602-956-0400
                                         Fax: 602-957-7610
                                         perrycenter@qwest.net
                                         www.azafh.com

Diana Casillas, Human Resources Director
Jim Musick, President
Provides services for people with disabilities, cognitive disabilities including residential services, day treatment, job training and job placement.

6358 Phoenix Veterans Center
Ste 100
1544 W. Grant St.
Phoenix, AZ 85004-1554   602-358-8494
                                         Fax: 602-379-4130
                                         www.azcremationcenter.com/?

Ken Benckwitz, Manager
Veterans medical clinic offering disabled veterans medical treatments.

6359 Progress Valley: Phoenix
10505 North 69th Street
Suite 1100
Paradise Valley, AZ 85253-6106   480-922-9427
                                         Fax: 602-274-5473
                                         recovery@progressvalley.org
                                         alcoholism.about.com

Susanne Lambert, Executive Director
Jennifer White, Director of Programs
Cathie Scott, Sober Housing Manager
Residential aftercare for alcoholism and chemical dependency. Certified chemical dependency counselors provide individual treatment.

6360 Rehabilitation Services Administration
Suite 102
3425 East Van Buren
Phoenix, AZ 85008-3202   602-771-9100
                                         800-563-1221
                                         Fax: 602-250-8584
                                         TTY: 855-475-8194
                                         azrsa@azdes.gov

Katharine Levandowsky, Administrator
Provides a variety of specialized services to assist in removing barriers to employment and/or independent living for individuals with physical or mental disabilities. RSA offers 3 major service programs and several specialized programs/services.

6361 Southern Arizona Association For The Visually Impaired
3767 East Grant Rd
Tucson, AZ 85716-2935   520-795-1331
                                         Fax: 520-795-1336
                                         reception@saavi.us
                                         www.saavi.us

Michael Gordon, Executive Director
Amy Murillo, Associate Director
Carol Lopez, Finance Director
Offers health services, counseling, social work, home and personal management, computer training, low vision aids and more for the visually handicapped 18 years or older.

6362 Toyei Industries
Hc 58 Box 55
Ganado, AZ 86505-55   928-736-2417
                                         888-45T-OYEI
                                         Fax: 928-736-2495

Anthony Lincoln, CEO
Serves the needs of developmentally disabled and the severely mentally impaired adult citizens of the Navajo Nation and other Indian Nations. Staff of 60+ serves the needs of all the Navajo adults. Services include day treatment programs, and residential and group home services.

6363 Yuma Center for the Visually Impaired
328 W. Spears Street
Yuma, AZ 85365-6580   928-247-8890
                                         Fax: 928-344-1863
                                         https://www.azdes.gov

Calvin Roberts, Executive Director
Kathy Lucero, Store Manager
Dana Clayton, Human Resources Specialist
A private nonprofit agency offering services for totally blind and legally blind children and adults in the Arizona area.

Arkansas

6364 Arkansas Lighthouse for the Blind
P.O.Box 192666
6818 Murray St.
Little Rock, AR 72209- 2666   501-562-2222
                                         Fax: 501-568-5275
                                         info@arkansaslighthouse.org
                                         arkansaslighthouse.org

Bill Johnson, Chief Executive Officer
Danny Novielli, COO
John McAtee, Chief Financial Officer
Manufacturer of textiles, apparel and paper products and employs blind and legally blind individuals.

6365 Beverly Enterprises Network
1 Thousand Beverly
Fort Smith, AR 72901-2629   479-201-2000
                                         800-666-9996
                                         Fax: 479-452-5131

Randy Churchey, CEO
Offers a progressive approach to subacute care. The goal of this organization is to assist injured and disabled individuals regain the level of independence to which they have been accustomed. Provides support and training programs, patient and family services and specialty programs for patients.

6366 Easterseals: Arkansas
3920 Woodland Heights Rd
Little Rock, AR 72212-2495   501-227-3600
                                         877-533-3700
                                         Fax: 501-227-4021
                                         TTY: 501-227-3686
                                         lrogers@ar.easterseals.com

Sharon Moone-Jochums, President/ CEO
Linda Rogers, VP Programs
Michael E. Stock, Treasurer
Their mission is to provide exceptional services to ensure that all people with disabilities or special needs have equal opportunities to live, learn, work and play in their communitites.

6367 **HealthSouth Rehabilitation Hospital Of Fort Smith**
1401 South J. Street
Fort Smith, AR 72901-5158 479-785-3300
Fax: 479-785-8599
healthsouth.com

Ryan Cassedy, CEO
Cygnet Schroeder, M.D., Medical Director
Donna Beallis, D.O., Director of Medical Management
A free-standing 80-bed comprehensive physical medicine and re-habilitation hospital offering inpatient and outpatient services. Provides specialized medical and therapy services, designed to assist physically challenged persons to reach their highest level of independent function.

6368 **Lions World Services for the Blind**
2811 Fair Park Blvd
Little Rock, AR 72204-5044 501-664-7100
800-248-0734
Fax: 501-664-2743
training@lwsb.org
www.wsblind.org/

Larry Dickerson, President/ CEO
Tony Woodell, President & Chief Executive Officer
Bill Smith, Director of Development
Offers services in the areas of health education, recreation, reha-bilitation, counseling, employment, computer training and more for all legally blind residents of the U.S. The staff includes 56 full time employees.

6369 **Little Rock Vet Center #0713**
Department of Veterans Affairs of Washington DC
Suite A
201 W Broadway St
North Little Rock, AR 72114- 5505 501-324-6395
877-927-8387
Fax: 501-324-6928

Elizabeth N Ruggiero, Team Leader
Ida L Fogle, Counselor
Van A Hall, Counselor
Vet Center provides PTSD counseling to veterans of a combat zone. No medical care provided.

6370 **Timber Ridge Ranch NeuroRestorative Services**
4500 W Commerce Dr
North Little Rock, AR 72116 501-758-8799
800-743-6802
Fax: 501-758-8778
neuroinfo@thementornetwork.com
www.neurorestorative.com

Bill Duffy, Chief Operating Officer
Michael E. Hofmeister, MS, MBA, Vice President of Operations
Sean Byrne, MBA, Chief Financial Officer
Comprehensive, individualized services from a transdisciplinary team of licensed professionals assist clients along a course to greater independence. A separate team is dedicated to the needs of children, adolescents, and their families. A clinical team may include professionals from the disciplines of: behavior analysis, neuropsychology, physiatry, psychology, speech-language pa-thology, occupational therapy, physical therapy, social work, couseling, education, nursing, and case management.

California

6371 **ARC Fresno-Kelso Activity Center**
4567 N Marty Ave
Fresno, CA 93722-7810 559-226-6268
Fax: 559-226-6269
arcfresno@arcfresno.org
arcfresno.org

Lori Ramirez, Executive Director
Catherine Wooliever, Director of Human Resources
Jamie Marrash, Director of Program Services
The Arc Fresno is a private, non-profit 501(c)(3) organization who was founded in 1953. They provide services and supports for over 550 individuals with developmental disabilities throughout Fresno County. They currently offer eight (8) programs, and do so with the help of 145 employees.

6372 **ARC Of San Diego-ARROW Center**
3030 Market Street
San Diego, CA 92102-3297 619-685-1175
Fax: 619-234-3759
arc-sd.com

Anthony J. DeSalis, President & CEO
The ARC of San Diego is a provider of services to persons with disabilities.

6373 **ARC Of San Diego-Rex Industries, The**
9575 Aero Dr
San Diego, CA 92123-1803 858-571-4369
800-748-5575
Fax: 858-715-3788
arc-sd.com

Dwight Stratton, Chair
Jerry Wechsler, 1st Vice Chairman
David W. Schneider, President & CEO
Offers many different programs including: North County Par-ent/Infant Program which is an educational program for children, birth to three years who are showing delays in development or who are at risk for developmental delays. The Adult Develop-ment Center is a program for adults, eighteen and over, with a de-velopmental disability in the severe to profound range. The program focuses on self-help, communication, daily living and pre-vocational skills. Other programs are available..

6374 **ARC Of San-Diego-South Bay**
1280 Nolan Avenue
Chula Vista, CA 91911-3738 619-427-7524
Fax: 619-427-4657
info@arc-sd.com
www.arc-sd.com/locations

Becky Thaller, Director
Steve Hojsan, Arc Enterprises Director
Michael Bruce, Workshop Manager
Provides remunerative work.

6375 **ARC Of Southeast Los Angeles-Southeast Industries**
9501 Washburn Rd
Downey, CA 90242-2913 562-803-1556
Fax: 562-803-4080
www.arcselac.org/

Provides an offsite extension of your production and warehouse facility. We have reliable and highly trained personnel to meet your needs, including pick-up and delivery service with prompt turn-around times. We offer assembly and packaging at competi-tive rates while maintaining the highest standards.

6376 **ARC: VC Community Connections West**
5103 Walker Street
Ventura, CA 93003-7358 805-650-8611
Fax: 805-644-7308
www.arcvc.org

Robert Hogan, President
Gene West, First Vice President
Eve Liebman, Recording Secretary
Caring and experienced staff is dedicated to serving participants with a variety of physical, mental and social disabilities who re-quire a higher level of support and supervision. Using a per-son-centered planning approach, Arc Ventura County promotes self-directed services for all clients and families served. Adult development centers serve individuals with physical and mental disabilities, as well as people with challenging behaviors, who re-quire assistance with basic skills such as self care.

6377 **ARC: VC Ventura**
5103 Walker Street
Ventura, CA 93003-7358 806-650-8611
Fax: 806-644-7308
www.arcvc.org

Robert Hogan, President
Gene West, First Vice President
Eve Liebman, Recording Secretary
Arc Ventura County is a private, nonprofit organization that pro-vides educational, vocational and residential services for people with developmental disabilities. Informed decisions, positive changes, and integration in the community are fundamental prin-cipals in all programs. As evidence of our programming excel-lence, Arc Ventura County has been accredited by CARF (The Rehabilitation Accreditation Commission.

6378   AbilityFirst

626-396-1010
877-768-4600
info@abilityfirst.org
www.abilityfirst.org

Lori Gangemi, President & Chief Executive Officer
Kashif Khan, Chief Financial Officer
Keri Castaneda, Chief Program Officer

AbilityFirst serves children and adults with special needs through 24 locations in Southern California.

6379   Accentcare
17855 North Dallas Pkwy
Dallas, TX 75287-2468

972-201-3800
800-834-3059
info@accentcare.com
accentcare.com

Mark Pacala, Chairman of the Board and CEO (i
Vincent E. Cook, EVP and Chief Financial Officer
Melvin Warriner, SVP and Chief Culture Officer

Postacute rehabilitation program: home care aides follow through with rehabilitation instructions given by physical, occupational and speech therapists. Other home care services are available, serving special needs for Alzheimer's, blind, brain injury, MS, ostomies, parkinsonism, spinal injury and stroke.

6380   Anaheim Veterans Center
859, South Harbor Blvd
Anaheim, CA 92805-4680

714-776-0161
800-225-8387
Fax: 714-776-8904
anaheimvetcenter@yahoo.com
www.longbeach.va.gov/visitors/vet_center.asp

Veterans medical clinic offering disabled veterans medical treatments.

6381   Azure Acres Recovery Center
5777 Madison Avenue
Suite 1210
Sacramento, CA 95841-9034

877-977-3755
877-762-3735
Fax: 707-823-8972
info@azureacres.com
azureacres.com

Joe Tinervin, MSW, Executive Director
Michael Roeske, Psy.D., Clinical Director
Christie Splitstone, MA, Counselor/Case Manager

Offers rehabilitation services and residential care for the person with an alcohol or drug abuse related problems.

6382   Back in the Saddle
2 BITS Trail
P.O. Box 3336
Chelmsford, MA 01824-0936

800-865-2478
877-756-5068
Fax: 800-866-3235
help@BackInTheSaddle.com
www.thesaddle.com

Richard Smith PhD, Owner
Erika Reed, Co-Director

A long term community residential facility for head injured adults. House parents live on-site; and oversee a variety of programs which are individually designed and might include classes in community college, placement in a workshop or on a workstation, volunteer positions and home skills assignments. Recreational outing range from horseback riding to weekend camping. Apartment programs available as set-up. Price: $2800-$3000 per month.

6383   Ballard Rehabilitation Hospital
1760 W 16th St
San Bernardino, CA 92411-1150

909-473-1200
800-761-1226
Fax: 909-473-1276
www.ballardrehab.com

Edward C. Palacios, RN,MPH, Administrator
Mary Hunt, Chief Operating Officer
Patty Meinhardt, Director Marketing/Admissions

Ballard Rehab Hospital is a free standing specialty hospital and provides the complete continuum of acute rehabilitation and out-patient rehabilitation, dedicated to providing rehab care to adults and children. The following inpatient and outpatient programs are available: CNA (Stroke) Rehab; Spinal Cord Injury Rehab; Brain Injury Rehab; Pain Management Rehab; Bariatric program, pulmonary program, injured Worker Programs; and Post Amputation Rehab.

6384   Bayview Nursing and Rehabilitation
516 Willow Street
Alameda, CA 94501-6132

510-521-5600
Fax: 510-865-6441
TTY: 800-735-2922
http://www.bayviewnursing.com/

Richard S Espinoza, Administrator

Offers a full range of medical services to meet the individual needs of our residents, including short-term rehabilitative services and long termed skilled care. Working with the resident's physician, our staff-including medical specialists, nurses, nutritionists, dietitians, and social workers-establishes a comprehensive treatment plan intended to restore you or your loved one to the highest practicable potential.

6385   Belden Center
606 Humboldt St
Santa Rosa, CA 95404-4219

707-579-2735
Fax: 707-579-4145

Casey Harding, Owner
Pamela Fadden, Owner

Postacute rehabilitation program.

6386   Blind Babies Foundation
Suite 300
1814 Franklin St
Oakland, CA 94612-3487

510-446-2229
Fax: 510-446-2262
blindbabies.org

Dottie Bridge, President
Aben Hill, 1st Vice President
Clare Friedman, PhD, 2nd Vice President

Mission: when an infant or pre school child is identified as blind or visually impaired, provides family-centered services to support the child's optimal development and access to the world.

6387   Brotman Medical Center: RehabCare Unit
Brotman Medical Center
3828 Delmas Terrace
Culver City, CA 90232-2713

310-836-7000
800-677-1238
Fax: 310-202-4105
phvc.com

Jennifer Cortez, Program Manager
Kevin O'Connor, CEO
Scott Leonard, CTO

Culver City is centrally located within the city of Los Angeles. These are two programs offering inpatient rehabilitation. The acute rehab program is designed for patients who need physical rehabilitation due to injury or medical disability. This program requires patients to participate in 3 hours therapy per day. The sub-acute program is designed especially for patients who need rehab but cannot tolerate the intensity of the acute rehab program..

6388   Build Rehabilitation Industries
12432 Foothill Blvd
Sylmar, CA 91342

818-898-0020
Fax: 818-898-1949
buildindustries.com

Comprehensive C.A.R.F. Accredited vocational rehabilitation services for adults with disabilities or other barriers to employment. Programs include: Sheltered Workshops, Work Evaluation, Work Hardening and Adjustment, Supported Employment, Job Placement, Independent Living Skills, Behavior Management, Adult Development Center, On-the-Job Training, and One-Stop Workforce Development Career Center.

6389 California Elwyn
18325 Mt. Baldy Circle
Fountain Valley, CA 92708-6115   714-557-6313
Fax: 714-963-2961
info@elwyn.org
elwyn.org

Charles S. McLister, President & CEO, Elwyn
Provides opportunities for people with disabilities who are 18 or older. Offers Individual Rehabilitation Plans and Supported Employment Services.

6390 California Eye Institute
1360 E Herndon Ave
Fresno, CA 93720-3326   559-449-5000
www.samc.com

Nancy Hollingsworth, President and CEO
Michael W. Martinez, EVP/Chief Operating and Financial Officer
Stephen Soldo, Chief Medical Officer
A private, nonprofit agency offering services such as health, educational, recreational, rehabilitation and employment counseling to the totally blind, legally blind and visually impaired. The staff includes two full time workers.

6391 Camp Recovery Center
3192 Glen Canyon Rd
Scotts Valley, CA 95066-4916   877-557-6237
Fax: 831-438-2789
camprecovery.com

Michael Johnson, Ph.D, Executive Director
Tim Sinnott, Clinical Director
Zoe R., Case Manager
A free-standing social model recovery center for chemical dependency located on 25 wooded acres in the Santa Cruz Mountains. The services include: medical detoxification, complete medical evaluation, psychiatric evaluation and counseling, psychological testing, individual counseling and more. Helps the recovery from chemical dependency in a easier, warm and caring environment.

6392 Campobello Chemical Dependency Recovery Center
2448 Guerneville Road
Suite 400
Santa Rosa, CA 95402- 4030   707-546-1547
800-805-1833
Fax: 707-579-1603
campobello.org

Our mission is to provide primary treatment, education, ongoing support and family services for clients seeking a more rewarding, chemically free lifestyle. Our primary goals are: to improve understanding/acceptance of the disease model of addiction. To improve self esteem. To reduce family, job and legal problems. To improve physical/emotional health. To enhance coping and problem solving strategies for recovery.

6393 Casa Colina Centers for Rehabilitation
P.O.Box 6001
255 East Bonita Avenue
Pomona, CA 91767- 6001   909-596-7733
866-724-4127
Fax: 909-593-0153
TTY: 909-596-3646
casacolina.org

Steve Norin, Chairman
Felice L Loverso, President
Chandrahas Agarwal, Medical Director
Casa Colina, has pioneered effective programs to create opportunity for health, productivity and self-esteem for persons with disability since 1936. Through medical rehabilitation, transitional living, residential, community, and prevention and wellness programs. Casa Colina serves more than 7,000 persons annually. Casa Colina, a non-profit organization, offers a unique spectrum of opportunities, achievement and results to patients and their families.

6394 Casa Colina Padua Village
P.O.Box 6001
255 East Bonita Avenue
Pomona, CA 91767- 6001   909-596-7733
866-724-4127
Fax: 909-593-0153
TTY: 909-596-3646
casacolina.org

Steve Norin, Chairman
Chandrahas Agarwal, Medical Director
Felice L Loverso, President
Long term residential services for adults with developmental disability. Residences include Malmquist House, Woodbend House, and Hillsdale House, all located in Claremont, California.

6395 Casa Colina Residential Services: Rancho Pino Verde
Casa Colina Center for Rehabilitation
P.O.Box 6001
255 East Bonita Avenue
Pomona, CA 91767- 7517   909-596-7733
866-724-4127
Fax: 909-593-0153
TTY: 909-596-3646
www.casacolina.org

Steve Norin, Chairman
Randy Blackman, Vice Chairman
Felice L. Loverso, President
Long term residential services in rural environment for adults with brain injury.

6396 Casa Colina Transitional Living Center
255 East Bonita Avenue
P.O.Box 6001
Pomona, CA 91767- 1923   909-596-7733
866-724-4127
Fax: 909-593-0153
TTY: 909-596-3646
casacolina.org

Steve Norin, Chairman
Felice L Loverso, President
Chandrahas Agarwal, Medical Director
Postacute rehabilitation program.

6397 Casa Colina Transitional Living Center: Pomona
P.O.Box 6001
255 East Bonita Avenue
Pomona, CA 91767- 6001   909-596-7733
866-724-4127
Fax: 909-593-0153
TTY: 909-596-3646
casacolina.org

Steve Norin, Chairman
Felice L Loverso, President
Chandrahas Agarwal, Medical Director
Post acute short term residential program for persons with brain injury. In a home-like setting, therapy promotes successful re-entry to home and community living.

6398 Cedars of Marin
PO Box 947
Ross, CA 94957-947   415-454-5310
Fax: 415-454-0573
thecedarsofmarin.org

Jefferson Rice, Board Chair
James Brentano, Board Vice President
Andrew Hinkelman, Board Treasurer
The Cedars of Marin has provided residential and day programs for adults with developmental disabilities for over 91 years. Our award-winning programs help our clients to live creative, productive, joyous lives.

6399 Center for Neuro Skills
5215 Ashe Rd.
Bakersfield, CA 93313-2988   661-872-3408
800-922-4994
Fax: 661-872-5150
skatomski@neuroskills.com
neuroskills.com

Mark J Ashley, President/CEO and Co-Founder
A comprehensive, post-acute, community based head-injury rehabilitation program serving over 100 clients per year. Since

1980, CNS has effectively treated the entire spectrum of head-injured clients, including those with severe behavioral disorders, cognitive/perceptual impairments, speech/language problems, physical disabilities and post-concussion syndrome.

6400   Center for the Partially Sighted
Suite 150
6101 W. Centinela Ave.
Culver City, CA 90230   310-988-1970
                                           Fax: 310-988-1980
                                                low-vision.org

La Donna S. Ringering, Ph.D, President/CEO
Pam Thompson, Director of Psychological Servic
Phyllis Amaral, Clinical Director
Services for partially sighted and legally blind people include low vision evaluations, the design and prescription of low vision devices and adaptive technology, as well as counseling and rehabilitation training (independent living skills and orientation/mobility training). Special programs include children's program, diabetes and vision loss program, Technology demonstrations. Store carries low vision aids. Catalog available.

6401   Central Coast Neurobehaviorial Center OPTIONS
P.O.Box 877
800 Quintana Road Suite 2C
Morro Bay, CA 93442-877   805-772-6066
                                           Fax: 805-772-6067

Michael Mamot, CEO
Ole von Frausing-Borch, COO
Serves adults with developmental disabilities, traumatic head injuries, or other neurological impairments. OPTIONS operates two transitional living centers, eight licensed residential facilities, two licensed community integration day programs and a licensed short term stabilization center. Services offered include: supported and independent living services, group and individual vocational services, neuropsychological assessment, occupational therapy, cognitive therapy, speech therapy and more.

6402   Cerebral Palsy: North County Center
#209
8525 Gibbs Drive
San Diego, CA 92123-1758   858-571-7803
                                           Fax: 858-571-0919
                                              info@ucpsd.org
                                              www.ucpsd.org

David Carucci, Executive Director
Mary Krieger, Associate Executive Director
Bruce Neufeld, Chief Financial Officer
The mission of UCP San Diego County is to advance the independence, productivity and full citizenship of people affected by cerebral palsy and other disabilities. By making solid steps, UCP can build a better community for all in the process.

6403   Children's Hospital Central California Rehabilitation Center
9300 Valley Childrens Place
Madera, CA 93636-8762   559-353-3000
                                        www.valleychildrens.org
Todd Suntrapak, President & Chief Executive Officer
David Christensen, MD, SVP Medical Affairs & Chief Medical Officer
Beverly Hayden-Pugh, Vice President & Chief Nursing Officer
A 297-bed pediatric medical center on a 50-acre campus. We now have more then 500 doctors practicing in over 40 pediatric subspecialties with clinics and services throughout the state.

6404   Children's Hospital Los Angeles Rehabilitation Program
4650 W Sunset Blvd
Los Angeles, CA 90027-6062   323-361-4155
                                               888-631-2452
                                           Fax: 323-361-8101
                                        webmaster@chla.usc.edu
                                      www.childrenshospitalla.org
Richard D. Cordova, President & CEO
Rodney B. Hanners, Senior Vice President and Chief
Henri R. Ford, M.D.
Designated as a Level I Pediatric Trauma Canter by the Los Angeles County EMS Agency, the hospital treats more then 1,500 pediatric trauma patients per year. Performs more then 13,900 pediatric surgeries a year, including more complex surgical procedures then any other hospital in Southern California

6405   Children's Therapy Center
Ste 120
770 Paseo Camarillo
Camarillo, CA 93010-6092   805-383-1501
                                           Fax: 805-383-1504

Beth Maulhardt, Owner
Provides individual occupational therapy, speech/language therapy, family/child consulting, education services and physical therapy consultation for children. Evaluations and treatment are on an individual basis and special emphasis is placed on a multidisciplinary approach with information sharing, and often team treatment.

6406   Clausen House
88 Vernon Street
Oakland, CA 94610-4217   510-839-0050
                                              clausenhouse.org

Deborah Levy, Interim Executive Director
Michael A. Scott, Director of Development
Stan Nicholson, Director of Human Resources
Residential, supported employment, independent and supported living, adult education, and social recreation activities. Serving the developmentally disabled since 1967.

6407   Community Gatepath
350 Twin Dolphin Dr
Suite 123
Redwood City, CA 94065   650-259-8500
                                           Fax: 650-697-5010
                                             info@gatepath.org
                                                 gatepath.org

Bryan Neider, CEO
Steve D'Eredita, Chief Financial Officer
Tracey Fecher, Vice President of Programs
Gatepath is a non-profit organization serving children, youth and adults with special needs and developmental disabilities and their families in the greater San Francisco Bay Area. The organization partners with various local non-profits, businesses, government agencies and third party providers to better serve this community.

6408   Community Hospital and Rehabilitation Center of Los Gatos-Saratoga
815 Pollard Rd
Los Gatos, CA 95032-1438   408-378-6131
                                           Fax: 408-866-4003

Gary Honts, CEO
Offers rehabilitation services, inpatient and outpatient care, physical therapy, occupational therapy and more for the physically challenged adult. We have a commitment to health care excellence. It is in this commitment that we have dedicated ourselves to provide personal and professional service to our patients. Our goal is to work closely with staff, physicians and the community to attain shared goals and positive changes, now and in the future..

6409   Contra Costa ARC
1340 Arnold Drive
Suite 127
Martinez, CA 94553-4189   925-370-1818
                                           Fax: 925-370-2048
                                        www.ContraCostaARC.com

Barbara Maizie, Executive Director
Diana Jorgensen, Program Coordinator
Andrey George, Administrative Coordinator
A private nonprofit membership-based organization dedicated to enhancing the quality of life of individuals with developmental disabilities.

6410   Corona Regional Medical Center- Rehabiltation Center
800 S. Main St.
Corona, CA 92882-3117   951-737-4343
                                           Fax: 951-736-7276
                                         www.coronaregional.com

Diane Mc Donald, Manager
Mark Uffer, Chief Executive Officer
Doreen Dann, Chief Nursing Officer
Offers inpatient and outpatient rehabilitation services. The Center consists of an acute rehab unit, a subacute rehab unit containing modules for long-term ventilator care, respiratory rehab, coma intervention and orthopedics. In addition to inpatient thera-

pies, the Center's outpatient programs include sports and industrial medicine.

6411   Critical Air Medicine
Montgomery Field
8775 Aero Drive
Suite 235
San Diego, CA 92123-1705   858-300-0224
                                  800-247-8326
                             Fax: 858-300-0228
                             www.aircharterguide.com

Frank Craven, Publisher of the Air Charter Guide

Offers emergency medical care by air medical transport carriers. These carriers are fully equipped with medical equipment and supplies for cardiovascular emergencies, respiratory supplies, orthopedic supplies and medications..

6412   Crutcher's Serenity House
P.O.Box D
50 Hillcrest Drive
Deer Park, CA 94576-504   707-963-3192
                            Fax: 707-963-2309

Robert Crutcher, Owner/CEO
Lu Crutcher, Executive Director

A privately owned and operated facility that introduces to residents a new lifestyle free of all chemicals, and a new awareness of their total being. The length of the program is four weeks and is within five minutes of an acute care hospital. The Center is licensed for 19 beds, male and female located in a home-like setting with an emphasis on maintaining a family atmosphere.

6413   Daniel Freeman Rehabilitation Centers
333 N Prairie Ave
PO Box 28990
Santa Ana, CA 92799-4501   714-230-3150
                             Fax: 714-850-0153
                        advertising@acupuncturetoday.com
                             www.acupuncturetoday.com

H Arndt, Associate Administrator
Gabrielle Lindsley, Business Development Manager
Evelyn Petersen, Human Resources / Payroll Manager

Comprehensive rehabilitation services which address needs and issues of the physically diabled and their families. We offer accute input rehabilitation, outpatient and short term skilled nursing rehabilitaion. Specialty areas include: brain injury, stroke, spinal chord injury, chronic pain, arthritis..

6414   Delano Regional Medical Center
1401 Garces Highway
Delano, CA 93215-3690   661-725-4800
                              drmc.com

Bahram Ghaffari, President
Jeremy Klemm, HealthStream Regional Director
Robert A. Frist, HealthStream CEO

Delano Regional Medical Center (DRMC) is proud to be known throughout California & beyond as an innovative regional hospital, deeply rooted in the local communities and committed to providing an exceptional patient experience. A non-profit acute-care facility serving a region of 10 rural central Californiatowns. With over 100 physicians on our active medical staff and additional courtesy or consulting physicians, patients are assured of receiving high-quality care in multiple specialties.

6415   Desert Regional Medical Center
1150 N Indian Canyon Dr
Palm Springs, CA 92262   760-323-6511
                                800-491-4990
                           www.desertmedctr.com

Carolyn Caldwell, Chief Executive Officer
Tracey Cowles, Physician Relations Manager
Jeanne Stanton, RN, Chair

Our dedicated physicians and caregivers provide a broad array of quality programs and services, including comprehensive cancer care, women's health services, heart care, surgical weight loss reduction and orthopedics.

6416   Devereux Advanced Behavioral Health California
P.O. Box 6784
Santa Barbara, CA 93160   805-968-2525
                            Fax: 805-968-3247
                            rpopke@devereux.org
                            www.devereuxca.org

Amy Evans, Executive Director
Rebecca Popke, Marketing & Admissions Manager
Wendy Cooper, Manager of External Affairs

Serves adults age 18 through 85 who have intellectual and developmental disabilities such as emotional disturbances, neurological impairments, autism, dementia and more. Devereux California currently provides a continuum of services, including on-campus residential, day programs, behavior management and supported living services in the community.

6417   Division of Physical Medicine and Rehabilitation
San Joaquin General Hospital
500 W Hospital Rd
French Camp, CA 95231-9693   209-468-6000
                               Fax: 209-468-6501

Offers rehabilitation services, inpatient and outpatient care, speech therapy, physical therapy, occupational therapy and more for the physically challenged individual.

6418   Dr. Karen H Chao Developmental Optometry Karen H. Chao. O.D.
Suite A
121 S Del Mar Ave
San Gabriel, CA 91776-1345   626-287-0401
                               Fax: 626-287-1457
                               drkhchao@yahoo.com
                               www.healthgrades.com

Karen Chao, Owner
Karen Chao OD, Owner
Roger C. Holstein, Chief Executive Officer

Developmental optometrist specializing in the testing and treatment of vision problems and the enhancement of visual performance. Performs visual perceptual testing and training for children and adults. Undetected vision problems interfere with the ability to achieve and are highly correlated with learning difficulties and developmental problems. Provides the opportunity to overcome vision and visual-perceptual dysfunctions..

6419   Early Childhood Services
Desert Area Resources and Training
201 E Ridgecrest Blvd
Ridgecrest, CA 93555-3919   760-375-9787
                               Fax: 760-375-1288
                               www.dartontarget.org/

Peter V. Berns, Chief Executive Officer
Cris Bridges, Chief of Client Services
Bob Beecroft, Chief Operations Officer

Provides early intervention services to children who have disabilities or are experiencing delays in development. Provides developmental activities to promote the attainment of developmental milestones so that each child may reach his/her maximum potential. The program also provides therapeutic and educational intervention and offers support and guidance to families.

6420   East Los Angeles Doctors Hospital
4060 Whittier Boulevard
Los Angeles, CA 90023-2526   323-268-5514
                               www.elalax.com

Hector Hernandez, Chief Executive Officer
Kamlesh Dhawan, Chief Of Staff
Michael Austerlitz, Vice-Chief Of Staff

Postacute rehabilitation program.

6421   Easterseals Northern California
2730 Shadelands Dr.
Walnut Creek, CA 94598   925-266-8400
                          customerservice@esnorcal.org
                          www.esnorcal.org

Jim Kelleher, Chief Executive Officer
Andrea Pettiford, Vice President, Operations

Creates solutions that change the lives of children and adults with disabilities and special needs, and provides support to family members.

6422 Easterseals Superior California
3205 Hurley Way
Sacramento, CA 95864 916-485-6711
Fax: 916-485-2653
info@myeasterseals.org
www.easterseals.com/superior-ca
Gary T. Kasai, President & CEO
Don Nguyen, Chief Financnial Officer
Gary Novak, Chief Marketing & Donor Relations Officer
Dedicated to empowering people with disabilities by providing services, including medical rehabilitation and employment and training services, and promoting independence.

6423 Exceed: A Division of Valley Resource Center
P.O.Box 1773
1285 N. Santa Fe
Hemet, CA 92543-1773 951-766-8659
800-423-1227
Fax: 951-929-9758
vrctwohip@aol.com
Pattie Robert, Business Development Specialist
Mary Morse, Marketing Director
Kathy Cooke, Manager
Our vision is an environment where each client is valued as an individual and is provided the opportunity to reach his/her maximum potential. Our mission is to provide service and advocacy, which creates choices and opportunities, for adults with disabilities to reach their maximum potential..

6424 Eye Medical Center of Fresno
Eye Medical Center
1360 E. Herndon Avenue
Suite 301 & 210
Fresno, CA 93720-1498 559-486-5000
emcfresno.com
A private, nonprofit agency offering services such as health, educational, recreational, rehabilitation, employment and counseling to the totally blind, legally blind and visually impaired. The staff includes hundreds of full time workers.

6425 Fontana Rehabilitation Workshop
Industrial Support Systems
8333 Almeria Ave
Fontana, CA 92335-3283 909-428-3883
800-755-4755
Fax: 909-428-3835
www.industrial-support.org
Silvia Anderson, Executive Director
U. Jones, CFO
C.Steven Bowen Plant, Operations manager
The Fontana Rehabilitation Workshop, Inc., through its business divisions is committed to maintaining a stable environment wherein people with disabilities are provided with those services and supports that enable them to overcome barriers to employment and empower them to maximize their employment potential.

6426 Foothill Vocational Opportunities
789 North Fair Oaks Avenue
Pasadena, CA 91103-3045 626-449-0218
Fax: 626-449-0218
info@foothillvoc.org
foothillvoc.org
Foothill Vocational Opportunities maximizes the personal and economic potential of disabled individuals by creating meaningful employment opportunities. Foothill provides our clients and their families with the tools they need to live fuller, richer lives, bringing a sense of inclusion and dignity to a chronically marginalized and underdeserved group of people.

6427 Fred Finch Youth Center
3800 Coolidge Ave
Oakland, CA 94602-3399 510-482-2244
Fax: 510-488-1960
receptionist@fredfinch.org
fredfinch.org
Thomas N. Alexander, President/CEO
FFYC seeks to provide a continuum of high quality programs for the care and treatment of children, youth, young adults, and their families, whose changing needs can best be met by a variety of mental health and support services. The goal is for the program participants to receive the most effective services in the least restrictive environment appropriate to their needs so that they may function at their highest potential.

6428 Gateway Center of Monterey County
850 Congress Ave
Pacific Grove, CA 93950-4898 831-372-8002
Fax: 831-372-2411
info@gatewaycenter.org
gatewaycenter.org
Stephanie Lyon, Executive Director
Mike Price, Chief Financial Officer
Desiree Boller, Accounting Assistant
Our mission is to be a caring and stimulating environment for the Developmentally Disabled where all people can achieve their individual goals safely and with dignity. Our goal is to continue our programs and to find new and innovative ways of assisting the developmentally disabled to live in our community in surroundings compatable with their ability to live and work at the highest level possible.

6429 Gateway Industries: Castroville
7055 Veterans Blvd
Unit A
Burr Ridge, IL 60527 630-321-1333
888-473-3744
Fax: 630-321-1321
www.redshift.com
Located in the Sand City Industrial Park, it provides vocational training and employment to developmentally disabled adults so they can achieve their vocational potential while also providing quality services to bussiness along the Central Coast. The sheltered work environment assists the employees by increasing their income, improving their work skills and habits, and enabling them to participate in the community.

6430 Gilroy Workshop
7471 Monterey Street
Gilroy, CA 95020-3629 408-430-2810
Fax: 408-842-6770
info@leadershipgilroy.org
www.leadershipgilroy.org/
Kristi Alarid, Manager
Sally French, Manager
Denise Martin, Executive Director
Work adjustment and remunerative work programs..

6431 Glendale Adventist Medical Center
1509 Wilson Ter
Glendale, CA 91206-4098 818-409-8000
Fax: 818-546-5609
Kevin Roberts, President/CEO
Warren Tetz, Sr. Vice President and COO
Kelly Turner, Sr. Vice President and CFO
Rehabilitative team is made up of physician specialists, as well as professional and certified staff nurses, thereapists and others who meet regularly to ensure tht each patients progress is carefully planned and closely monitored.

6432 Glendale Memorial Hospital and Health Center Rehabilitation Unit
Glendale Memorial Hospital and Health Center
1420 South Central Ave
Glendale, CA 91204-2508 818-502-1900
Fax: 818-409-7688
www.glendalememorialhospital.org
Catherine M. Pelley, President
Offers rehabilitation services, occupational therapy, physical therapy, residential services and more for the disabled.

6433 Goleta Valley Cottage Hospital
Cottage Health System
351 S Patterson Ave
Santa Barbara, CA 93111-2496 805-967-3411
Fax: 805-681-6437
cverkiak@cottagehealthsystem.org
www.sbch.org
Ronald C. Wreft, President & CEO
Rosemary Bray, Clinical Manager
Diana Gray Miller, Administrator
A 122-bed acute care hospital was founded in 1966 to serve the growing community of Goleta Valley. Today, we admit more then

2,000 patients a year, see more then 17,000 emergency visits, and welcome nearly 400 newborns to our designated 'Baby Friendly' Birth Center each year. We are also recognized for our Level IV trauma designation. We take great pride in fulfilling our goal of providing each patient with comfortable, personalized care.

6434   HealthSouth Tustin Rehabilitation Hospital
Health South Corporation
14851 Yorba St
Tustin, CA 92780-2925   714-832-9200
www.tustinrehab.com/

Diana Hanyak, Chief Executive Officer
Rodric Bell, Medical Director
Lindsey Barrett, Director of Case Management
HealthSouth Tustin Rehabilitation Hospital is part of the HealthSouth Corportation, the nation's largest provider of rehabilitative healthcare services, we are the only facility of its kind in Orange County. Fully accredited by the Joint Commission on Accreditation of Healthcare Organizations (JACHO) we provide inpatient and outpatient care designed to meet individual needs of patients and their families.

6435   Hi-Desert Medical Center
6601 White Feather Road
Joshua Tree, CA 92252-760   760-366-3711
hdmc.org

Lionel Chadwick, Chief Executive Officer
Tom Duda, Chief Financial Officer
Judy Austin, Chief Operating Officer & Chief
Postacute rehabilitation program.

6436   Home of the Guiding Hands
Suite 200
1825 Gillespie Way
El Cajon, CA 92020-0501   619-938-2850
Fax: 619-938-3055
info@guidinghands.org
guidinghands.org

Mary Miller, President
Debby McNeil, Vice President
Michael Harris, Treasurer
The mission of Home og the Guiding Hands is to provide quality services, training and advocacy for people with developmental disabilities, their families, and others who will benefit.

6437   Hospital of the Good Samaritan Acute Rehabilitation Unit
1225 Wilshire Blvd
Los Angeles, CA 90017-1901   213-977-2121
800-366-8338
Fax: 213-482-2770
info@goodsam.org
goodsam.org

Andrew B Leeka, President and CEO
Charles T. Munger, Chairman
Physicians, researchers and staff are united by a common mission: to foster growth into one of the most comprehensive medical centers in the West. Services offered include: cardiology and cardiovascular services, neurosciences, movement disorders and Parkinsons disorder, wound care center and transfusion-medicine and surgery center.

6438   Innovative Rehabilitation Services
Hacienda La Puente Unified School District
15959 E. Gale Ave
City Of Industry, CA 91745   626-933-1000
Fax: 626-934-2900
info@hlpusd.k12.ca.us
www.hlpusd.k12.ca.us

Matthew Smith, Site Administrator
George Stransky, Counselor
Crystal Ontiveros, Counselor
Provides innovative student-centered learning opportunities and support services to a diverse population that enable individuals to achieve thier goals as lifelong learners, productive workers and effective communicators.

6439   Janus of Santa Cruz
Suite 150
200 7th Ave
Santa Cruz, CA 95062-4669   831-462-1060
866-526-8772
janussc.org

Rod Libbey, Executive Director
Bill Morris, Medical Director
Margie Storms, Clinical Director
A private not-for-profit corporation, licensed by the state of California. The Janus Clinic has a 3 year accreditation by the Council on Accreditation for Health Care Facilities.

6440   John Muir Medical Center Rehabilitation Services, Therapy Center
1601 Ygnacio Valley Rd
Walnut Creek, CA 94598-3122   925-939-3000
Fax: 925-308-8944
www.johnmuirhealth.com

Calvin Knight, President and CEO
Helen Doughty, Librarian
A 324-bed acute care facility that is designated as the only trauma center for Contra Costa County and portions of Solano County. Recognized as one of the region's premier healthcare providers, areas of specialty include high-and low-risk obstetrics, orthopedics, neurosciences, cardiac care and cancer care. The campus is accredited by the Joint Commission on Accreditation of Healthcare Organizations (JCAHO), a national surveyor of quality patient care.

6441   Kindred Hospital-La Mirada
14900 E. Imperial Hwy
La Mirada, CA 90638-2172   562-944-1900
Fax: 562-906-3455
TTY: 800-735-2922
www.kindredlamirada.com

April Myers, Administrator
Adam Darvish, Executive Director
Committed to the delivery of high quality care in a cost-effective manner to enable us to become 'a model of excellence' in Long-Term Acute Care. Committed to treat our patients and families with dignity and respect, in the same manner we would want to be treated.

6442   King's View Work Experience Center- Atwater
559 East Bardsley Avenue
P. O. Box 688
Tulare, CA 93275-0688   559-688-7531
Fax: 559-688-3509
info@kingsview.org
www.kingsview.org

Leon Hoover, Chief Executive Officer
Vida Jalali, Chief Financial Officer Interim
Sue Essman, Director of Human Resources
The primary mission of the Kings View Work Experience Center (KVWEC) is to serve people who have developmental disabilities. We believe in the dignity and worth of each person and in their right to rehabilitation, education and community integration. It is Kings View's aim to provide quality services to people who need assistance in the development of social, vocational and independent living skills.

6443   LaPalma Intercommunity Hospital
7901 Walker St
La Palma, CA 90623-1764   714-670-7400
LPIHInfo@primehealthcare.com
www.lapalmaintercommunityhospital.com

Virg Narbutas, Regional CEO
Sami Shoukair, Chief Medical Officer
Linda Gonzaba, Medical Staff Office Director
Lapalma Intercommunity Hospital endeavors to provide comprehensive, quality healthcare in a convenient, compassionate and cost effective manner. Lapalma is consistently at the forefront of evolving national healthcare reform. Our organization provides an innovative and integrated healthcare delivery system. We remain ever cognizant of our patient's needs and desires for high quality affordable healthcare.

6444 Learning Services of Northern California
131 Langley Drive
Suite B
Lawrenceville, GA 30046-9315   408-848-4379
                                      888-419-9955
                                  Fax: 866-491-7396
                              www.learningservices.com
Dr. Debra Braunling-McMorrow, President and CEO
Jeanne Mack, Chief Financial Officer and Vice President of Operations
Michael Weaver, Chief Development Officer
Located on 10 acres of ranchland in rural Santa Clara Valley, our Gilroy Program offers treatment, structure, and support in a spacious, campus-based living environment. Sharing living residences are complimented by a treatment and recreation facility for individuals who require intensive support.

6445 Learning Services: Morgan Hill
131 Langley Drive
Suite B
Lawrenceville, GA 30046-9315   408-848-4379
                                      888-419-9955
                                  Fax: 866-491-7396
                              www.learningservices.com
Dr. Debra Braunling-McMorrow, President and CEO
Jeanne Mack, Chief Financial Officer and Vice President of Operations
Michael Weaver, Chief Development Officer
Located in the quaint rural town within walking distance from the old main street of Morgan Hill. Our Morgan Hill program offers the convenience and amenities of small-town living within the supportive community of Morgan Hill.

6446 Learning Services: Supported Living Programs
131 Langley Drive
Suite B
Lawrenceville, GA 30046-9315   408-848-4379
                                      888-419-9955
                                  Fax: 866-491-7396
                              www.learningservices.com
Dr. Debra Braunling-McMorrow, President and CEO
Jeanne Mack, Chief Financial Officer and Vice President of Operations
Michael Weaver, Chief Development Officer
We offer a variety of diverse and stimulating environments for people with different needs, capabilities and personal goals. Within comfortable, homelike, age-appropriate settings we provide the structure and support necessary to ensure the richest possible quality of life. Program offered in both Northern and Southern facilities of California

6447 Leon S Peters Rehabilitation Center
2823 Fresno St
Fresno, CA 93721-1324   559-459-6000
                          www.communitymedical.org
Florence Dunn, Chairwoman
John McGregor, Esquire, Secretary
Tim A. Joslin, President, Chief Executive Officer
Community's flagship hospital that offers world class specialized critical care with the area's only stroke unit with 24-hour vascular neurology and neurosurgery coverage and a team of specially trained stroke nurses. The world's first G4 CyberKnife. The table Mountain Rancheraia Level 1 Trauma Center. The Leon S. Peters burn center. The region's only perinatology program for high rish pregnancies and deliveries. The Da-Vinci robotic surgical system, and 3 helicopeter landing pads.

6448 Lion's Blind Center of Diablo Valley, Inc. Lions Center For The Visually Impaired
175 Alvarado Ave
Pittsburg, CA 94565-4862   925-432-3013
                                  800-750-3937
                              Fax: 925-432-7014
                              www.seniorvision.org
Edward Schroth, Executive Director
Barbara Cronin, President
Charles Dunham, First Vice President
A private, nonprofit agency offering services such as health, educational, recreational, rehabilitation, employment and counseling to the totally blind, legally blind and visually impaired. The staff includes two full time workers..

6449 Lion's Blind Center of Oakland
2115 Broadway
Oakland, CA 94612-2698   510-450-1580
                            Fax: 510-654-3603
Michelle Taylor Lagunas, Executive Director/ CEO
Christina Easiley, Administrative Manager
Scott Blanks, Director of Rehabilitation Servi
A private nonprofit organization offering services for the totally blind, legally blind, deaf-blind and multihandicapped blind. Services include: professional training, rehabilitation, education, counseling, social work, self help and more. The staff includes 12 full time and 1 part time worker.

6450 Living Skills Center for the Visually Impaired
2430 Road 20
#B112
San Pablo, CA 94806-5005   510-234-4984
                              Fax: 510-234-4986
                              info@hcblind.org
                              www.hcblind.org
Patricia Williams, Executive Director
Patricia Maffei, Program Director
Ronald Hideshima, Adaptive Technology Instructor
A private, nonprofit agency offering services such as independent living skills training, recreational, employment and accessible technology training to the totally blind, legally blind and visually impaired. The staff includes six full time teachers.

6451 Loma Linda University Orthopedic and Rehabilitation Institute
25333 Barton Rd
Loma Linda, CA 92354-3123   909-558-1000
                              Fax: 909-558-0308
                                  www.llu.edu
Richard H. Hart, MD, DrPH, President & Chief Executive Officer
Ronald L. Carter, PhD, Senior Vice President, Educational Affairs
Cari Dominguez, DHS, Senior Vice President, Human Resources
Offers a full range of clinical programs for both inpatients and outpatient. The specific diagnosis leading to patient admission includes stroke, spinal cord injury, traumatic or anoxic brain damage, amputation, post neurosurgery, chronic neurological disease, Guillain-Barre syndrome, arthritis, multiple trauma or other complex orthopedic problems. The facilities and professional services are comprehensive and ensure that the best care is provided to pediatric and adult patients..

6452 Manor Care Health Services- Citrus Heights
7807 Uplands Way
Citrus Heights, CA 95610-7500   916-967-2929
                                  Fax: 916-965-8439
                                  hcr-manorcare.com
Steven M. Cavanaugh, Chief Financial Officer
Paul A. Ormond, Chairman, President and Chief Ex
The nations leader in skilled nursing and rehabilitation care. Our facility has been serving the Sacramento area for more then 12 years. We are known for our beautiful decor, outstanding rehabilitation staff and loving nursing care. We offer short term rehabilitation, long term skilled nursing care, respite care and post hospital surgical care.

6453 Manor Care Health Services- Palm Desert
74-350 Country Club Dr
Palm Desert, CA 92260-1608   760-341-0261
                              Fax: 760-779-1563
                              hcr-manorcare.com
Steven M. Cavanaugh, Chief Financial Officer
Paul A. Ormond, Chairman, President and Chief Ex
Centrally located in the Coachella Valley, specializing in skilled nursing whith an emphasis on rehabilitation, post surgery recovery, hospice, alzheimer's care and long term care. In addition, we offer 2 unique service options for the discriminating consumer. Our Arcadia unit offers a specialized Alzheimer's care program in a dedicated secure wing. ManorCare offers rehabilitation services including physical, occupational and speech therapies for those recovering from illness injury or surgery.

603

6454 Manor Care Health Services-Fountain Valley
11680 Warner Ave
Fountain Valley, CA 92708-2513   714-241-9800
                                   Fax: 714-966-1654
                                   hcr-manorcare.com
Steven M. Cavanaugh, Chief Financial Officer
Paul A. Ormond, Chairman, President and Chief Ex
Provides 24-hour skilled nursing, rehabilitative therapies and
specialized Alzheimer's care. Our in-house therapists provide
physical, occupational and speech therapies in our rehabilitation
area. Our team is goal oriented and focuses on producing positive
outcomes for those recovering from illness, injury or surgery. Our
respite care program provides a full range of services for a few
days, a week or even a season.

6455 Manor Care Health Services-Hemet
1717 W Stetson Ave
Hemet, CA 92545-6882   951-925-9171
                                   Fax: 951-925-8186
                                   hcr-manorcare.com
Steven M. Cavanaugh, Chief Financial Officer
Paul A. Ormond, Chairman, President and Chief Ex
Provides skilled nursing, Rehabilitation services, and specialized Alzheimer's care. In addition we offer short term respite
stays for family caregivers that simply need a break from the
stress of daily care. Our Arcadia unit staff is specially trained in
the care of residents with Alzheimer's disease. The secured unit is
designed to provide a soothing and homelike environment while
enhancing each resident's remaining abilities.

6456 Manor Care Health Services-Sunnyvale
1150 Tilton Dr
Sunnyvale, CA 94087-2440   408-735-7200
                                   Fax: 408-736-8629
                                   hcr-manorcare.com
Steven M. Cavanaugh, Chief Financial Officer
Paul A. Ormond, Chairman, President and Chief Ex
Our in-house therapists provide physical, occupational and
speech therapies in our rehabilitation area. Our team is goal oriented and focuses on producing positive outcomes for those recovering from illness, injury or surgery. Our skilled nursing staff
works with our therapy department and dietary department to provide positive wound care programs for patients requiring skin
management care.

6457 Manor Care Health Services-Walnut Creek
1226 Rossmoor Pkwy
Walnut Creek, CA 94595-2538   925-975-5000
                                   Fax: 925-937-1132
                                   hcr-manorcare.com
Steven M. Cavanaugh, Chief Financial Officer
Paul A. Ormond, Chairman, President and Chief Ex
Provides luxurious long term care and rehabilitation services. In
house therapists provide, physical, occupational and speech therapies in our rehabilitation area. Our team is goal oriented and focuses on producing positive outcomes for those recovering from
illness, injury or surgery. Our years of combined management experience add value to our resident's quality of life.

6458 Maynord's Chemical Dependency Recovery Centers
19325 Cherokee Road
Tuolumne, CA 95379-1657   209-928-3737
                                        800-228-8208
                                   Fax: 209-928-1152
                                        maynords.com
James Berry, Director
Maynord's Recovery Centers has always been dedicated to the recovery of good people whose lives are being destroyed by alcohol
and drugs. Since 1978, Maynord's residential program has helped
thousands of people put their lives back together after addiction
has taken its toll. Today, Maynord's offers a treatment system
over much of the San Joaquin Valley and the San Francisco Bay
Area.

6459 Maynord's Ranch for Men
19325 Cherokee Road
Tuolumne, CA 95379-1657   209-928-3737
                                        800-228-8208
                                   Fax: 209-928-1152
                                        maynords.com
James Berry, Director

Provides treatment for chemical dependency problems to men.
The treatment addresses their recovery through a comprehensive
plan created for their individual needs. Also offers a program for
women called the Meadows.

6460 Meadowbrook Manor
431 West Remington Boulevard
Bolingbrook, IL 60440   630-759-1112
                                   Fax: 630-759-6925
                                   www.meadowbrookmanor.com
Postacute rehabilitation program.

6461 Meadowview Manor
41 Crestview Terrace
Bridgeport, WV 26330   304-842-7101
                                   Fax: 304-842-7104
Provides treatment designed for women that is directed at every
important facet of their lives - mentally, physically and spiritually. Clients receive a variety of treatment approaches to facilitate
their recovery and a comprehensive treatment plan is created for
their individual needs. Issues relating to the cause of addictions
are addressed in lectures, one-on-one counseling sessions, group
therapy and re entry groups. Also offers a male treatment
programs called Maynord's Ranch.

6462 Memorial Hospital of Gardenia
1145 West Redondo Beach Blvd
Gardena, CA 90247-3528   310-532-4200
                                        800-782-2288
                                   www.avantihospitals.com
Edward Mirzabegian, Corporate Chief Executive Officer
Postacute rehabilitation program.

6463 Mercy Medical Group
Mercy Hospital
3000 Q Street
Sacramento, CA 95816   916-733-3333
                                   www.mymercymedicalgroup.org
Located near the Old Rosevill Hospital. There are several pri-
mary care physicians, including Family Practice, Internal Medi-
cine and Pediatrics at this location. Specialty services include
Diagnostic Imaging, Laboratory and Mental Health Services.

6464 Napa County Mental Health Department
2344 Old Sonoma Road
Bldg. D
Napa, CA 94559-3708   707-259-8151
                                        800-648-8650
                       www.countyofnapa.org/MentalHealth/
Work hardening and disciplinary programs.

6465 Napa Valley Support Systems
1700 Second Street Suite 212
Napa, CA 94559-1344   707-253-7490
                                   Fax: 707-253-0115
                                   napavalleysupportservices.org
Beth Kahiga, Executive Director
Heather Jump, Administrative Manager
Katy Vanzant, Program Director
Work hardening and disciplinary programs.

6466 North Valley Services
1040 Washington
Red Bluff, CA 96080-4509   530-527-0407
                                   Fax: 530-527-7091
                                   www.northvalleyservices.org
Joe Brown, President
Larry Donnelley, Vice President
Lynn DeFreece, CEO
Provides vocational rehabilitation services, such as job counsel-
ing, job training, and work experience, to unemployed and under-
employed persons, persons with disabilities.

6467 Northridge Hospital Medical Center Rehabiltation Medicine
18300 Roscoe Blvd
Northridge, CA 91328-4167   818-885-8500
                                   Fax: 818-701-7367
                                   www.northridgehospital.org/index.htm
Mike L. Wall, President
Thomas L. Hedge, Medical Director
Joel S. Rosen, Associate Medical Director

A full service, comprehensive rehabilitation program suited to treat patients of all ages who have suffered catastrophic or debilitating injury or illness. The goal of the program is to deliver exceptional patient care to maximise each individual's skills and independence.

6468 Northridge Hospital Medical Center: Centerfor Rehabilitation Medicine
18300 Roscoe Blvd
Northridge, CA 91328-4167
818-885-8500
Fax: 818-701-7367
www.northridgehospital.com

Mike L. Wall, President
Thomas L. Hedge, Medical Director
Joel S. Rosen, Associate Medical Director
Committed to serving the health needs of our communities with particular attention to the needs of the poor, the disadvantaged, and vulneralbe, and the comfort of the suffering and dying. Catholic Healthcare West has a commitment to quality-quality healthcare services and the promotion of optimal quality of life for all of life.

6469 Old Adobe Developmental Services
1301A Rand Street
Suite A
Petaluma, CA 94954-5697
707-763-9807
Fax: 707-763-7708
www.oadsinc.org

Elizabeth Clary, Executive Director
Marie Padgett, Controller
The mission of Old Adobe to provide opportunities for individuals with developmental challenges to reach thier fullest potentials. Our job at OADS is to find ways for these individuals to find full expression in all parts of their lives. We have a partnership with the Adult Education Department of the Petaluma School District in providing services to persons with developmental challenges. We are funded by the Dept. of Rehabilitation and the Dept. Of Developmental services.

6470 Old Adobe Developmental Services-Rohnert Park Services (Behavioral)
5401 Snyder Ln.
Rohnert Park, CA 94928-3124
707-584-5859
Fax: 707-664-8057

Elizabeth Clary, Executive Director
Helen Gunderson, Administrative Assistant
The program services are designed to assist individuals who demonstrate basic work skills, to develop social skills and work habits necessary to succeed in supported or competitive employment. Most often individual program services involve working with the client to replace those behavioral excesses that have been a barrier to vocational placement.

6471 PRIDE Industries
10030 Foothills Blvd
Roseville, CA 95747-7102
916-788-2100
800-550-6005
Fax: 800-888-0447
info@prideindustries.com
prideindustries.com

Michael Ziegler, President & CEO
Bob Selvester, Vice Chair
Mike Snegg, Treasurer
To provide opportunities through employment, training, evaluation and placement maximizing community access, independence and quality of life for people with barriers to employment.

6472 Pacific Hospital Of Long Beach-Neuro Care Unit
2776 Pacific Ave
Long Beach, CA 90806-2613
562-997-2000
webmaster@phlb.org

Michael D. Drobot, CEO
Clark Todd, President
Teri Plemmons, Administrative Assistant
Our mission is to heal with compassion and to perform with distinction. Our vision: to improve the hospital's orthopedic and Spine Center of Excellence. Achieve exceptional financial performance to enhance hospital services. Improve the vertically integrated ancillary, outpatient and inpatient surgery system. Develop a professionally challenging work environment that reflects an agile, peak performance culture.

6473 Paradise Vally Hospital-South Bay Rehabilitation Center
2400 East 4th St
National City, CA 91950-2026
619-470-4321
paradisevalleyhospital.net

Prem Reddy, Chairman
Neerav Jadeja, Administrator
Luis Leon, President
South Bay Rehabilitation Center, offers a complete range of treatment for patients with physical disabilities. Our specialized inpatient and outpatient programs are designed to meet each person's individual needs or injuries, with the goal of restoring as much independence as possible and significantly improving their lives.

6474 Parents and Friends
350 South Main Street
Fort Bragg, CA 95437-5408
707-964-4940
parentsandfriends.org

Rick Moon, Executive Director
Jessica Dickey, Administrative Assistant
Kristy Tanguay, Manager
Parents and Friends provides opportunities for persons with developmental challenges and similar needs to participate fully in our community.

6475 People Services
4195 Lakeshore Blvd
Lakeport, CA 95453-6411
707-263-3810
peopleservices.org

Ilene Dumont, Executive Director
Martin Diesman, Director
Vicki Cole, Director
Providing an array of services for adults with developmental disabilities and other people with disabilities. Services include supported employment, work services, supported living, personal, social and community training, transportation, specialized individual services and much more.

6476 Petaluma Recycling Center
Old Adobe Developmental Services
315 2nd St
Petaluma, CA 94952-4230
707-763-4761
Fax: 707-763-4921

Elizabeth Clary, Executive Director
Began in 1974; has been one of the major employers of persons with developmental challenges for 26 years; is the primary recycling facility in the growing city of 52,000; accepts over 20 different kinds of recyclables; employs 20-25 persons a day.

6477 Pomerado Rehabilitation Outpatient Service
15615 Pomerado Rd
Poway, CA 92064-2405
858-485-6511
Fax: 858-613-4248

Bob Blake, Director Rehab Services
Jonathan Pee, Manager
A 107-bed acute care hospital. In addition to a round-the-clock Emergency Department, Pomerado offers the area's finest outpaitent surgery center and general medical/surgical services. Pomerado Hospital also is home to a world-class Birth Center and a Level II NICU. Fully JCAHO-accredidted, Pomerado is well-known for offering only private rooms, each with a scenic view of the North Countryside, which enhances the healing atmosphere..

6478 Pride Industries: Grass Valley
12451 Loma Rica Dr
Grass Valley, CA 95945-9059
530-477-1832
800-550-6005
Fax: 530-477-8038
info@prideindustries.com
www.prideindustries.com

Bob Olsen, Chairman
Bob Selvester, Vice Chairman
Walt Payne, President/CEO
Work adjustment and remunerative work programs. We offer an adult day program as well.

605

6479 Rancho Adult Day Care Center
Rancho Los Amigos Medical Center
7601 Imperial Hwy
Downey, CA 90242-3456   562-401-7111
                                     Fax: 562-401-7991
                                     TTY: 562-401-8450
                           dhs.lacounty.gov/wps/portal/dhs/rancho
Valerie Orange, CEO
Margaret L Campbell, Research Director
Provides personal care, social services and a therapeutic program
to older adults in order to improve their quality of life. Offers a
Clinical Gerontology Service, an Alzheimer's Disease Diagnos-
tic and Treatment Center and a Geriatric Assessment and
Rehabilitation Unit..

6480 Regional Center for Rehabilitation
2288 Auburn Blvd
Sacramento, CA 95821-1618   916-421-4167
                                     Fax: 916-925-1586

Postacute rehabilitation program..

6481 Rehabilitation Institute of Santa Barbara
   2415 De La Vina St
Santa Barbara, CA 93105-3819   805-569-8999
                                     Fax: 805-687-3707
Ralph Pollock, President
Scott Silic MBA, Vice President Of Operations
Cheryl Ellis MD, MHA, VP Medical Services
A regional rehabilitation system with an acute care hospital at the
center, the Institute provides specialized inpatient and outpatient
programs for brain injury, spinal cord injury, stroke, work-related
injury, chronic pain, orthopedic problems and more. Offers a
46-bed acute-care rehabilitation hospital, a free-standing outpatient center, the brain injury continuum, chronic pain program..

6482 Rehabilitation Institute of Southern California
1800 E La Veta Ave
Orange, CA 92866-2902   714-633-7400
                                     Fax: 714-633-4586
                                            riorehab.org
Praim S. Singh, Executive Director
Carol Reese, Executive Assistant
Grace Lee, Administrative Assistant
Outpatient rehabilitation serving physically and disabled children and adults. Child development programs, adult day care for
disabled seniors, child care for disabled and non-disabled children, outpatient therapy, aquatics, adult day healthcare, independent living, vocational services, social services, and housing.

6483 Rubicon Programs
2500 Bissell Avenue
Richmond, CA 94804-1815   510-235-1516
                                     Fax: 510-235-2025
                           www.rubiconprograms.org
Rob Hope, Chief Program Officer
Jane Fischberg, President and Executive Director
Roger Contreras, CFO
Rubicon Programs Inc. helps people and communities build assets to achieve greater independence. Since 1973, Rubicon has
built and operated affordable housing and provided employment,
job training, mental health, and other supportive services to individuals who have disabilities, are homeless, or are otherwise
economically disadvantaged.

6484 San Bernardino Valley Lighthouse for the Blind
762 North Sierra Way
San Bernardino, CA 92410-4438   909-884-3121
                                     Fax: 909-884-2964
                                            www.afb.org
Robert Mc Bay, Executive Director
Sandra Wood, Administrative Assistant
Provides training in independent living skills - cooking, mobility
and orientation, sewing, Braille and typing. Also, we have classes
in macrame, ceramics and basket weaving. Weekly support group
and Bible study..

6485 Santa Clara Valley Blind Center, Inc.
101 N Bascom Ave
San Jose, CA 95128-1805   408-295-4016
                                     Fax: 408-295-1398
                           info@visionbeyondsight.org
                                 visionbeyondsight.org
Arnold Chew, President
John Glass, Vice President
Arlene Holmes, Secretary
SCVBC's mission is to increase the confidence, independence,
and quality of life of the blind and visually impaired through edu-
cational, recreational, and rehabilitative programs.

6486 Scripps Memorial Hospital: Pain Center
4275 Campus Point Ct.
San Diego, CA 92121-1205   858-626-4123
                                          800-727-4777
                           clinicalresearch@scrippshealth.com
                                        www.scripps.org
Chris Van Gorder, President and CEO
Richard K Rothberger, Vice President, Chief Financial Officer
Robin B Brown, Chief Executive
Offers both inpatient and outpatient programs including: physical activity management, individual pain management, group
therapy, medication adjustment, pain control classes, occupational therapy, biofeedback training, family counseling, vocational and leisure counseling and recreational therapy.

6487 Sharp Coronado Hospital
250 Prospect Place
Coronado, CA 92118-1999   619-522-3600
                           erica.carlson@sharp.com
                                            sharp.com
Marcia Hall, CEO
Mark Tamsen, Chairman
Tom Smisek, Vice Chairman
Providing medical and surgical care, intensive care, sub-acute
and long-term care, rehabilitation therapies and emergency services in a peaceful setting is part of our live+heal+grow philosophy. We are one of the county's few community-owned hospitals
and are proud of our history of providing convenient, award-winning heath care to Coronado and San Diego.

6488 Shriners Hospitals For Children-Northern California
2425 Stockton Blvd.
Sacramento, CA 95817   916-453-2000
                           patientreferrals@shrinenet.org
                           www.shrinershospitalsforchildren.org
John McCabe, Executive Vice President
Dale W Stauss, Chairman
Jerry G Gantt, 1st Vice President
The only hospital in the Shriners system that houses facilities for
treatment of all 3 Shriner specialties -spinal cord injuries, orthopaedic, and burns. The hospital features 80 patient beds, 9 parent
apartments, 5 state-of-the-art operating rooms, a high-tech Motion Analysis lab, and an entire floor devoted to research.

6489 Shriners Hospitals for Children: Los Angeles
3160 Geneva Street
Los Angeles, CA 90020-1199   213-388-3151
                           patientreferrals@shrinenet.org
                           www.shrinershospitalsforchildren.org
John McCabe, Executive Vice President
Dale W Stauss, Chairman
Jerry G Gantt, 1st Vice President
Shriners Hospitals for Children: Los Angeles, treats children un-
der age 18 with burn scars, orthopedic conditions, cleft lip and
palate and limb deficiencies at no cost to the patient or their
families.

6490 Society for the Blind
1238 S St.
Sacramento, CA 95811-3256   916-452-8271
                                     Fax: 916-492-2483
                           info@societyfortheblind.org
                                 societyfortheblind.org
Shari Roesler, Executive Director
Shane Snyder, Director of Programs
A private, local nonprofit organization providing blind and visu-
ally impaired people with the training supplies and support they
need to live independent, productive and fulfilled lives with lim-

ited vision. Services include the Low Vision Clinic, Braille classes, computer training, support groups, living skills instruction, mobility training and the Products for Independence Store.

6491   Solutions at Santa Barbara: Transitional Living Center
1135 N Patterson Ave
Santa Barbara, CA 93111-1113   805-683-1995
Fax: 805-683-4793
sol1135@aol.com
solutionsatsantabarbara.com
Sue Hannigan, Director
Postacute rehabilitation program. Short-term transitional living program for individuals with traumatic brain injury, stroke, aneurysm and other neurological disorders.

6492   St. John's Pleasant Valley Hospital Neuro Care Unit
2309 Antonio Ave
Camarillo, CA 93010-1414   805-389-5800

Jerry Conway, President
Maureen M. Malone, Administrator
Raye Burkhardt, Vice President and Chief Nursing
Houses 82 acute-care beds, a 99-bed extended care unit, and the only hyperbaric medicine unit in Ventura County. Employ's 1,800 people and count 250 active medical staff.

6493   St. John's Regional Medica Center- Industrial Therapy Center
1600 North Rose Ave
Oxnard, CA 93030-3723   805-988-2500
www.stjohnshealth.org
Gudrun Moll, Vice President and Chief Nursing
Laurie Harting, President & CEO
Kim Wilson, Vice President
A non-profit health care facility offering multi-disciplinary programs for pain management and work hardening, as well as physical and occupational therapy.

6494   Sub-Acute Saratoga Hospital
13425 Sousa Lane
Saratoga, CA 95070-4663   408-378-8875
Fax: 408-378-7419
subacutesaratoga.com
Jack Stephens, President & CEO
Paul Quintana, Medical Director
Gary Vernon, NHA Administrator
Dedicated to the fulfillment of human needs, desires, and wishes in illness and in health. The cohesiveness of caring in a family community of staff, patients, and their loved ones. The celebration of each unique life through their therapeutic journey, while preserving their individual spirit. The achievement of advanced medical expertise, knowledge, and skill given with the human touch of caring toward the ultimate goal: enhancing the healing process from acute illness to the joy of going home.

6495   Synergos Neurological Center: Hayward
27200 Calaroga Avenue
Hayward, CA 94545-4383   510-264-4000
Fax: 510-264-4007
strosehospital.org
Richard C. Hardwig, Chair
Alan McIntosh, Vice Chair
Lex Reddy, President and CEO
Postacute rehabilitation program.

6496   Synergos Neurological Center: Mission Hills
27200 Calaroga Avenue
Hayward, CA 94545-4383   510-264-4000
Fax: 510-264-4007
www.strosehospital.org
Richard C. Hardwig, Chair
Alan McIntosh, Vice Chair
Lex Reddy, President and CEO
For over 30 years, St. Rose Hospital Rehabilitation Services Department has helped thousands of patients recover from illness and injury through the help of our specially trained therapists. These therapists have been trained in specific rehabilitative areas such as physical, occupational, and speech therapies.

6497   Temple Community Hospital
235 N Hoover St
Los Angeles, CA 90004-3672   213-382-7252
Fax: 213-382-1874
templecommunityhospital.com
The mission of Temple Community Hospital is to improve the quality of health in our community and to provide necessary hospital services for those individuals requiring such care.

6498   The Arc of the East Bay
1101 Walpert St
Hayward, CA 94541-3721   510-582-8151
arcalameda.org
Son Luter, President & CEO
Offers a variety of services and programs for adults and children with intellectual and developmental disabilities.

6499   Tunnell Center for Rehab
680 South Fourth Street
Louisville, CA 40202-4807   502-596-7300
Fax: 800-545-0749
web_administrator@kindred.com
kindredhealthcare.com
Mary R., Activities Assistant
Kristen W., Health and Rehabilitation Center
The Tunnell Center for Rehabilitation and Healthcare accomodates 178 residents. We are dedicated to short-term complex medical and rehabilitative care. Using a holistic care management approach we work with residents who have suffered debilitating injury or illness, and who need comprehensive nursing and rehabilitation services to achieve their highest practicable level of functional ability and independence.

6500   Ukiah Valley Association for Habilitation
Ukiah, CA 95482-689   707-468-8824
Fax: 707-468-9149
TTY: 800-735-2929
www.uvah.org
Pamela Jensen, Executive Director
Kris Vipond, Business Manager
Sharrae Elston, Director
Work adjustment and suppoted employment and social and community services.

6501   Valley Center for the Blind
2491 W Shaw Avenue
Suite 124
Fresno, CA 93711-3331   559-222-4088
Fax: 559-222-4844
Bud Breslin, Executive Director
Millie Marshall, Marriage Family Therapist
Saramarie Katich, Office Mngr/Program Director
A private, nonprofit organization that offers educational, health, recreational and professional training services to the totally blind, legally blind or severely visually impaired.

6502   Villa Esperanza Services
2060 East Villa Street
Pasadena, CA 91107   626-449-2919
Fax: 626-449-2850
info@villaesperanzaservices.org
www.villaesperanzaservices.org
Candice Rogers, Chairman
Richard Hubinger, President
Vicky Castillo, CFO
Serving disabled infants to seniors in a school, adult day program, adult work program and residences and adult day health care program and care management program.

6503   Village Square Nursing And Rehabilitation Center
Kindred Healthcare, Inc.
1586 West San Marcos Blvd
San Marcos, CA 92078-4019   760-471-2986

Accomodates 118 residents offering spacious private and semi-private rooms. We are Medicare and Medi-Cal certified and contracted with most managed care insurance groups.

6504   Vista Center for the Blind & Visually Impaired
2500 El Camino Real,
Suite 100
Palo Alto, CA 94306   650-858-0202
                                               800-660-2009
                                          Fax: 650-858-0214
                                          info@vistacenter.org
                                          www.vistacenter.org

Pam Brandin, Executive Director
Nacole Barth-Ellis, Co-Director of Development
Terry Kurfess, Co-Director of Development
Private nonprofit agency that serves the visually impaired in the San Mateo, Santa Clara, San Benito and Santa Cruz Counties with offices in Palo Alto and Santa Cruz. Offers Low Vision Evaluations, mobility training, daily living skills training, social services, counseling, support groups, computer training, other rehabilitation services, and a store.

6505   Winways at Orange County
7732 E Santiago Canyon Rd
Orange, CA 92869-1829   714-771-5276
                                          Fax: 714-771-1452
                                          winwaysrehab.com

Pamela Kauss, Director
The program offers clients highly personalized, comprehensive programs to meet the needs of individuals with traumatic brain injury, stroke, tumors, aneurysm, post concussive syndrome or other neurological disorders. Winways also has a special program that provides services to Spanish speaking clients, called Contigo Adelante with materials in Spanish, and Spanish speaking interpreters to assist in the therapy process.

Colorado

6506   Capron Rehabilitation Center
Penrose Hospital/ St. Francis Healthcare System
2222 N Nevada Ave
Colorado Springs, CO 80907-6819   719-776-5000
                                          penrosestfrancis.org

Margaret Sabin, President & CEO
Nate Olson, Chief Executive Officer
Jameson Smith, Senior VP & Chief Admnistrative Officer
Southern Colorado's most complete inpatient and outpatient rehabilitation center.

6507   Cerebral Palsy of Colorado
801 Yosemite Street
Denver, CO 80230   303-691-9339
                                          Fax: 303-691-0846
                                          abilityconnectioncolorado.org

Judith I Ham, CEO
James Reuter, Chairman of the Board
Penfield Tate, Vice Chairman
Provides services for children birth-5 years, employment services for adults, information and referral, donation pickup and cell phone/ink cartridge recycling services.

6508   Cherry Hills Health Care Center
Kindred
3575 S Washington St
Englewood, CO 80110-3807   303-789-2265

Accomodates 92 residents. We serve Medicare, Medicaid, managed-care and private pay clients. Our 2 story facility has a home-like environment with a dining room and a day room one each floor. Our short-term rehab unit was designed for patients who have been in the hospital and need continued intensive nursing care or rehabilitation before returning home.

6509   Community Hospital Back and Conditioning Clinic
1060 Orchard Ave
Grand Junction, CO 81501-2997   970-243-3400
                                               800-621-0926
                                          Fax: 970-856-6510

Amy Hibberd, Executive Director
David Scherman, Manager
Post-accute rehabilitation program.

6510   Devereux Advanced Behavioral Health Colorado
8405 Church Ranch Blvd.
Westminster, CO 80021   303-466-7391
                                               800-456-2536
                                          www.devereuxco.org

Lisa Gaudia, Interim Clinical Director
A non-profit partner for individuals, families, schools and communities, serving people in the areas of autism, intellectual and developmental disabilities, mental health issues, and child welfare. Programs offered include residential services, community based services, educational programs, employment supports and more.

6511   Laradon Hall Society for Exceptional Children and Adults
5100 Lincoln St
Denver, CO 80216-2056   303-296-2400
                                               866-381-2163
                                          Fax: 303-296-4012
                                          laradon.org

William Mitchell, Chair
Suzanne Bradeen, Vice Chair
Jason Adams, Treasurer
Laradon provides educational, vocational and residential services to children and adults with developmental disabilities and other special needs. Laradon was founded in 1948. It is among the largest and most comprehensive service providers in Colorado.

6512   Learning Services: Bear Creek
7201 W Hampden Ave
Lakewood, CO 80227-5305   303-989-6660
                                               888-419-9955
                                          Fax: 866-491-7396
                                          learningservices.com

Susan Snow, Director of Admissions
Dr. Debra Braunling-McMorrow, President and CEO
Jeanne Mack, Chief Financial Officer
Supported living program for persons with acquired brain injury.

6513   MOSAIC In Colorado Springs
888 W. Garden of the Gods Road
Ste 100
Colorado Springs, CO 80907-6251   719-380-0451
                                          Fax: 719-380-7055
                                          mosaic_cosprings@mosaicinfo.org
                                          www.mosaicincoloradosprings.org

Tom Maltais, Executive Director
Mosaic in Colorado Springs provides a variety of services to assist adults and families in achieving positive goals. Services to persons with intellectual disabilities include community living options, vocational training and supported employment, spiritual growth and personal development options, and day programs habilitation and community participation.

6514   Manor Care Nursing and Rehabilitation Center: Boulder
Manor Care Ohio
2800 Palo Pkwy
Boulder, CO 80301-1540   303-440-9100
                                          Fax: 303-440-9251
                                          www.hcr-manorcare.com

Steven M. Cavanaugh, Chief Financial Officer
Paul A. Ormond, Chairman, President and Chief Ex
150 bed center offers a full spectrum of nursing care and rehabilitation. This includes our Arcadia Special Care Unit for Alzheimer's patients. Specialized unit for post acute skilled nursing care. Physical and massage therapies. And a 48 bed upscale Heritage unit offering additional amenities and furnishings.

6515   Manor Care Nursing: Denver
290 S Monaco Pkwy
Denver, CO 80224-1105   303-355-2525
                                          Fax: 303-333-6960
                                          www.hcr-manorcare.com

Steven M. Cavanaugh, Chief Financial Officer
Paul A. Ormond, Chairman, President and Chief Ex
Our center has delveloped a reputation for its luxurious environment, comprehensive rehabilitation service and focus on quality care. A wide range of individual and group activities and many gracious amenities create the finest combination of elegance and professional skilled nursing care. Arcadia, our special care unit for persons with Alzheimer's disease and related memory impair-

ments, promotes independence and preserves dignity within a safe and secure environment.

6516   Mediplex of Colorado
8451 Pearl St
Thornton, CO 80229-4804   303-288-3000
                                   Fax: 303-286-5136
                                   info@vhdenver.com

Jan Eyer, Chief Executive Officer
Our programs and services help each patient along the road to recovery toward our ultimate aim; the greatest possible restoration of the individual's self-esteem, ability to set goals, and self-sufficiency. Also offer specialized acute inpatient rehabilitative services, including special programs in Trauma Rehabilitation.

6517   Platte River Industries
490 Bryant St
Denver, CO 80204-4808   303-825-0041
                                   Fax: 303-825-0564

Bob Smith, Executive Director
Postacute rehabilitation facility and program..

6518   Pueblo Diversified Industries
2828 Granada Blvd
Pueblo, CO 81005-3198   800-466-8393
                                   Fax: 719-564-3407
                                   info@pdipueblo.org
                                   www.pdipueblo.net

Karen K Lillie, President & CEO
Robin Forbes, Director Human Services
Tom Drolshagen, Chief Operating Officer
A place where people can turn limitations into opportunities. People can experience the independence, pride and self worth of securing and maintaining a job.

6519   SHALOM Denver
2498 W 2nd Ave
Denver, CO 80223-1007   303-623-0251
                                  Fax: 303-620-9584
                                  shalomdenver.com

Arnie Kover, Disability and Employment Servic
Sara Leeper, Coordinator of Client Services
Vicky Brittain, Mailing Business Manager
SHALOM Denver provides employment, training, and job placement opportunities to people with disabilities, resettled immigrants, and people moving from welfare to work.

6520   SPIN Early Childhood Care & Education Cntr
1333 Elm Ave
Canon City, CO 81212-4431   719-275-0550
                                  www.starpointco.com/spin

Diane Trujillo, Manager
SPIN center is a fully inclusive non-discriminating community early childhood program, offering a variety of schedule choices for families. The philosophy of the SPIN program is to promote each child's growth and development. Special attention is given to cognitive, physical, speech language and social-emotional growth. Staff is specifically trained to facilitate and prepare environments that promote exploration, key experiences, creativity and self-expression..

6521   Schaefer Enterprises
500 26th Street
P.O. Box 200009
Greeley, CO 80631-8427   970-353-0662
                                  Fax: 970-353-2779
                                  www.schaeferenterprises.com

Valorie Randall, Executive Director
Alex Witt, Executive Assistant
Veronica Griego, Production Director
Schaefer Enterprises, Inc., located in Greely, Colorado, is a vaulable community resource that has been fulfilling the outsourcing needs of businesses in Weld County and outlying areas since 1952.

6522   Spalding Rehab Hospital West Unit
150 Spring St
Morrison, CO 80465   303-697-4334
                                  Fax: 303-697-0570

Postacute rehabilitation program.

Connecticut

6523   ACES/ACCESS Inclusion Program
350 State Street
North Haven, CT 06473-3218   203-498-6800
                                  Fax: 203-234-1369
                                  acesinfo@aces.org
                                  www.aces.org

Thomas M Danehy, Executive Director
Erika Forte, Assistant Executive Director
Evelyn Rossetti, Manager
Provides a person centered planning approach for integrated employment, volunteer community based opportunities for adults who have developmental disabilities..

6524   Apria Healthcare
Apria Healthcare Group, Inc.
1975 Wehrle Dr
Buffalo, NY 14221   716-631-8726

Provides a broad range of high-quality and cost-effective specialty infusion therapies and related services to patients in their homes throughout the Northeastern United States. Offer home infusion antibiotic therapy, quality pharmacy services, skilled nursing services and related support services.

6525   Arc Of Meriden-Wallingford, Inc.
200 Research Parkway
Meriden, CT 06450   203-237-9975
                                  Fax: 203-639-0946
                                  www.arcmw.org

Pamela Fields, Executive Director
Joseph Palfini, Board President
Becky Blazejowski, Financial Director
A membership agency that provides comprehensive, full-service, community-based opportunities for people with disabilities. Guided by over 120 community members and an active Board of Directors, the Arc always has its focus on improving the lives of people with disabilities. The Arc of Meriden-Wallingford offers advocacy and assistance to our members along with advocating for the rights and choices of people with disabilities in our community.

6526   Connecticut Subacute Corporation
19 Tuttle Pl
Middletown, CT 06457-1881   860-347-6300
                                  Fax: 860-347-2446

Evan K Lyle, Managed Care Director
Cheri Kauset, Corporate Rep.
Specializes in subacute medical and rehabilitation programming. The strength of our system is in its' ability to service a broad range of clinical and psychosocial needs which enable each individual to attain his/her optimal potential. Programming includes neurological and orthopedic rehabilitation, post-surgical and wound care management, intravenous therapy, pulmonary rehabilitation including ventilator services, and long term care..

6527   Datahr Rehabilitation Institute
4 Berkshire Blvd
Bethel, CT 06801-1001   203-775-4700
                                  888-8DA-TAHR
                                  Fax: 203-775-4688

Thomas Fanning, CEO
Providers of comprehensive rehabilitation services with a history of nearly 5 decades of service. This institute is recognized as a leading resource in meeting the needs of those disabled by illness, injury or developmental disorders in Connecticut and New York. A team of rehabilitation and health care professionals offering career development, residential services, supported employment, volunteer services, occupational therapy, day activities and more.

6528   Eastern Blind Rehabilitation Center
810 Vermont Avenue
Washington, DC 20420   202-461-7600
                                  800-273-8255

Eric K. Shinseki, Secretary of Veterans Affairs
W. Scott Gould, Deputy Secretary of Veterans Aff
Jose D Riojas, Chief of Staff

Provides residential rehabilitation services to eligible legally blind veterans in the Northeast and Middle Atlantic portions of the country. Referral applications by Veterans Administration Medical Centers and Outpatient Clinics in the geographical area served by the Blind Rehabilitation Center.

6529 FAVRAH Senior Adult Enrichment Program
23 W Avon Rd
Avon, CT 06001
860-674-8839
Fax: 860-676-0275

Nancy Ralston, Manager
Provides remunerative work. Post acute rehabilitation programs and facility.

6530 Gaylord Hospital
Gaylord Farm Road
P.O.Box 400
Wallingford, CT 06492-7048
203-284-2800
866-429-5673
Fax: 203-284-2894
TTY: 203-284-2700
lcrispino@gaylord.org
www.gaylord.org

James Cullen, President
Works to restore ability and build courage. Offers rehabilitation care with one goal in mind: to help patients return to their homes, communities and jobs.

6531 Hockanum Greenhouse
Hockanum Industry
290 Middle Tpke
Storrs Mansfield, CT 06268-2908
860-429-6697
Fax: 860-429-7496

Christopher Campbell, Manager
Beth Chaty, Director
Betsy Treiber, Director
A non profit agency that strives to provide gainful employment, training, support and retirement services for developmentally disabled individuals through the dignity of work, community interaction and structured activities.

6532 Kuhn Employment Oppurtunities
1630 North Colony Road
P.O.Box 941
Meriden, CT 06450
203-235-2583
860-347-5843
www.kuhngroup.org

Paul O'Sullivan, Chairperson
Mark DuPuis, Vice Chairperson
John J. Ausanka III, Treasurer
Kuhn is committed to developing quality skill enhancement programs which provide meaningful employment for persons with disabilities so that they will become independentm gain self-esteem, and be accepted by the community. Our vision is that all individuals have the ability to fully participate in the community through work. Kuhn believes that all participants have a right to integrated community employment.

6533 Norwalk Hospital Section Of Physical Medicine And Rehabilitation
34 Maple Street
Norwalk, CT 06856
203-852-2000
Fax: 800-789-4584

Diane M. Allison, Chair
Edward A. Kangas, Vice Chair
Andrew J. Whittingham, Treasurer
A 25 bed inpatient Rehabilitation Unit. This CARF and JCAHO accredidted rehab unit is located on the 8th floor of Norwalk Hospital. The focus of the rehab unit is to restore lost function and assist patients in returning to the community. Who have recently experienced a life changing medical event. The progam is tailored to meet individual therapy needs and address activities of daily living. Family and caregiver participation in the program is welcomed and encouraged.

6534 Rehabilitation Associates, Inc.
1931 Black Rock Tpke
Fairfield, CT 06825-3506
203-384-8681
Fax: 203-384-0956
info@rehabassocinc.com
www.rehabilitationassociatesinc.com

Carol Landsman, Director
A comprehensive outpatient rehabilitation facility offering physical therapy, occupational therapy, speech-language pathology, clinical social work services and nutritional services to all age groups. Facility locations in Fairfield, Stratford, Milford, Shelton and Westport.

6535 Reliance House
40 Broadway
Norwich, CT 06360-5702
860-887-6536
Fax: 860-885-1970
reliancehouse.org

Jack Malone, President
Jackie Falman, Vice President
Sam Bliven, Secretary
A residential vocational and recreational support network. An active and productive clubhouse where people with mental illness can gain skills, strength and self-esteem.

6536 Yale New Haven Health System-Bridgeport Hospital
789 Howard Avenue
New Haven, CT 06519
203-384-3000
www.yalenewhavenhealth.org

Marna P. Borgstrom, President and CEO
Richard D'Aquila, Executive Vice President
Peter N. Herbert, MD, Senior VP, Medical Affairs
Medical services are provided by physicians who are specialists in physical medicine and rehabilitation. The physical therapy department provides a variety of services and utilizes sophisticated modalities to restore and reinforce physical abilities.

Delaware

6537 Alfred I DuPont Hospital for Children
Division of Rehabilitation
1600 Rockland Road,
PO Box 269
Wilmington, DE 19803-269
302-651-4000
888-533-3543
Fax: 302-651-4055
infodupont@nemours.org
www.nemours.org

William G. Mackenzie, MD, Chair
David J. Bailey, President and Chief Executive Officer
Robert D. Bridges, Executive Vice President, Enterprise Services/Chief Financia
The hospital is a division of Nemours, which operates one of the nations largest subspecialty group practices devoted to pediatric patient care, teaching, and research. A 180-bed hospital that offers all the specialties of pediatric medicine, surgery, and dentistry in a spacious, comfortable, and family focused facility.

6538 Community Systems Inc.
2 Penns Way
Suite 301
New Castle, DE 19720
302-325-1500
Fax: 302-325-1505
communitysystems.org

David Paige, Executive Director
Amy Yento, Chair
A 4 state family of non-profit, tax exempt corporations whose mission is helping persons with disabilities to find happiness in their own homes, in their personal relationships, and as contributing members of their community.

6539 DDDS/Georgetown Center
5 Academy St
Georgetown, DE 19947-1915
302-856-5366
Fax: 302-856-5305
dhss.delaware.gov/dhss

Mission is to improve the quality of life for Delaware's citizens by promoting health and well-being, fostering self-sufficiency, and protecting vulnerable operations. The vision statement is that together we provide quality services as we create a better future for the people of Delaware.

6540 **Delaware Association for the Blind**
2915 Newport Gap Pike
Landis Lodge Building
Wilmington, DE 19808
302-998-5913
888-777-3925
Fax: 302-691-5810
dabdel.org

Janet L. Berry, Executive Director
Ken Rolph, President
Jennifer Smith, Secretary
A private, nonprofit organization that offers adjustment to blindness counseling, recreation activities, summer camps and financial assistance for the legally blind. The staff includes five full time, nine part time and twelve seasonal. Operates a store selling items for the blind.

6541 **Delaware Veterans Center**
810 Vermont Avenue
Washington, DC 20420
302-994-2511
800-273-8255
Fax: 302-633-5591
Slaon D Gibson, Acting Secretary of Veterans Affairs
Jose D Riojas, Chief of Staff
Richard J Griffin, Acting Inspector General
A 60-bed hospital and 60-bed NHCU, both accredited by the Joint Commission on Accreditation of Healthcare Organizations with a VBA Regional Office and 2 Vet Centers (one on campus) offering veterans the unique opportunity to obtain heathcare, benefits services, and Readjustment Counseling at one location. The center provides a wide spectrum of primary and tertiary acute and extended care inpatient and outpatient activities an an academic setting..

6542 **Easterseals Delaware & Maryland's Eastern Shore**
61 Corporate Cir.
New Castle, DE 19720
302-324-4444
Fax: 302-324-4441
www.easterseals.com/de
Kenan J. Sklenar, President & CEO
Pamela Reuther, Chief Operating Officer
Manuel Arencibia, Vice President, Development
Provides services to ensure that all people with disabilities or special needs and their families have equal opportunities to live, learn, work and play in their communities.

6543 **Edgemoor Day Program**
500 Duncan Rd
Wilmington, DE 19809-2369
302-762-9077
Fax: 302-762-1652
www.dhss.delaware.gov/dhss/main/maps/other/ed
Scott Borino, Executive Director
Carol Koyste, Manager, Finance & Administratio
Brandon Furrowh, Director, Recreation & Youth Pro
Our mission is providing affordable and accessible services which help improve the quality of life for community members of all ages through a broad range of educational, recreational, self-enrichment, and family support services. ECC is a not-for-profit, community-based, multi-service agency located just north of Wilmington. We provide a broad range of educational, recreational, self-enrichment, and family support services.

6544 **Elwyn Delaware**
321 E 11th St.
Wilmington, DE 19801-3417
302-658-8860
info@elwyn.org
elwyn.org
Charles S. McLister, President & CEO, Elwyn
Provides work training, job placement and supported employment, and elder care services.

6545 **First State Senior Center**
291a N Rehoboth Blvd
Milford, DE 19963-1303
302-422-1510
dhss.delaware.gov/dhss/main/maps/other/dddssr
Improves the quality of life for Delaware's citizens by promoting health and well-being, fostering self-sufficiency, and protecting vulnerable populations.

6546 **Woodside Day Program**
941 Walnut Shade Rd
Dover, DE 19901-7765
302-739-4494
Fax: 302-697-4490

Connie Grace, Supervisor
Joyce Oliver, Manager

District of Columbia

6547 **Barbara Chambers Children's Center**
1470 Irving St NW
Washington, DC 20010-2804
202-387-6755
Fax: 202-319-9066
barbarachambers.org
Barbara Chambers, Founder
Mission is to provide comprehensive, quality child care services to the community at large, by offering a variety of opportunities for childrens's intellectual, emotional, social and physical development in a clean, safe, and nurturing environment. Our philosophy is to provide a supportive environment in which children can be children..allowing each child to learn at his/her pace and most of all allowing the child to learn through his/her daily play.

6548 **District of Columbia General Hospital Physical Medicine & Rehab Services**
Room 1358
19th and Mass Ave
Washington, DC 20003
202-727-6055
Fax: 202-675-7819
Dr. Maribel Bieberach, Chairperson PM&R
Dr. Raman Kapur, Staff Physiatrist
Offers comprehensive physical medicine and rehabilitation services including in and outpatient consultations and electrodiagnostic testing; in and outpatient physical and occupational therapy; inpatient recreational therapy, and a multidisciplinary prosthetic clinic which meets once a month..

6549 **George Washington University Medical Center**
George Washington University Medical Center
2150 Pennsylvania Ave NW
Washington, DC 20037-3201
202-741-3000
Fax: 202-741-3183
www.gwdocs.com
Offers an Ambulatory Physical Therapy/Sports Medicine Center, a Medical Center Prosthetics/Orthotics Clinic and a Speech and Hearing Center to persons in the District of Columbia, Virginia and Maryland.

6550 **HSC Pediatric Center, The**
1731 Bunker Hill Rd NE
Washington, DC 20017-3026
202-832-4400
800-226-4444
Fax: 202-467-0978
Debbie Zients, CEO
Dr Murry M Pollack, VP, Medical Affairs
Eva Fowler, Media Contact
Provides the highest quality rehabilitative and transitional care for infants, children, adolescents, and young adults with special health care needs and their families in a supportive environment that respects their needs, strengths, vslues and priorities..

6551 **Howard University Child Development Center**
1911 5th St NW
Washington, DC 20001-2314
202-797-8134
Fax: 202-986-6580
Connie Siler, Manager
Offers children with developmental problems diagnosis, treatment, evaluation and follow along visits..

6552 **Psychiatric Institute of Washington**
4228 Wisconsin Ave NW
Washington, DC 20016-2138
202-885-5600
800-369-2273
Fax: 202-885-5614

Ken Courage, Chairman
Carol Desjuns, Chief Operations Officer
Howard Hoffman, Executive Medical Director

611

Psychiatric intensive care, crisis intervention, adult day treatment, drug treatment and other services to children and adults who have psychiatric and chemical dependency problems.

6553 Spina Bifida Program of Children's National Medical Center
Children's National Medical Center
111 Michigan Ave. NW
Washington, DC 20010   202-476-5000
                                         888-884-2327
                                      childrensnational.org

Kurt Newman, President & CEO
Mark Batshaw, Executive Vice President & Physician-in-Chief
Denice Cora-Bramble, Chief Medical Officer
Provides care and treatment for infants, children and youth with spina bifida of all forms, including spina bifida occulta, meningocele, and myelomeningocele.

Florida

6554 Bayfront Rehabilitation Center
Bayfront Medical Center
701 6th St S
St Petersburg, FL 33701-4814   727-823-1234
                                      www.bayfrontstpete.com

Kathryn Gillette, President and CEO
Eric Smith, Chief Financial Officer
Lavah Lowe, Chief Operating Officer
Bayfront Medical Center has an Inpatient Rehabilitation Hospital and two outpatient rehabilitation clinics that each provide progressive, comprehensive, individualized treatment. Specialized care in Physiatry (physical medicine), rehab nursing, occupational therapy, speech language pathology, recreational therapy, patient/family services and psychology is tailored to each patient from admission to community and/or school reintegration.

6555 Brain Injury Rehabilitation Center Dr. P. Phillips Hospital
Brain Injury Rehabilitation Center Dr. P. Phillips
9400 Turkey Lake Rd
Orlando, FL 32819-8001   407-351-8580

Shannon Elswick, President
Linda Chapin, Chairman
Mark Swanson, Chief Quality Officer
Dedicated to restoring brain injured patients with rehabilitation potential to their highest level of functioning. This is accomplished through an interdisciplinary team demonstrating personal responsibility to the patient, their family and each other.

6556 Brooks Memorial Hospital Rehabilitation Center
3599 University Blvd. South
Jacksonville, FL 32207-6215   904-858-7600
                                   Fax: 904-858-7619
                          louise.spierre@brookshealth.org
                                      www.brookshealth.org

Douglas Baer, Chief Executive Officer/ Preside
Holly Morris, Director, Brooks Rehabilitation
Louise Spierre, Medical Director
An entire care facility featuring five day inpatient evaluation, pre-operative evaluation programs, five week pain management program, referral criteria and treatment goals, therapy services, psychological services and more to the physically challenged.

6557 Center for Pain Control and Rehabilitation
Ste 607
2780 Cleveland Ave
Fort Myers, FL 33901-5858   239-337-4332

Mary Bonnette, Owner

6558 Comprehensive Rehabilitation Center at Lee Memorial Hospital
2776 Cleveland Ave
Fort Myers, FL 33901-5864   239-343-2000
                                        leememorial.org

James R. Nathan, Chief Executive Officer System P
Larry Antonucci, Chief Operating Officer
Jon Cecil, Chief Human Resources Officer
Lee Memorial hospital has achieved national recognition as one of the top 100 hospitals for stroke, orthopedics, and Intensive Care Unit (ICU) It is a 367 bed hospital that provides 24-hour emergency and trauma care, inpatient rehabilitation, orthopedics, neuroscience, trauma, cancer, diabetes, digestive, general surgery, urology, endocrinology, gastroenterology, opthamology, and many others.

6559 Comprehensive Rehabilitation Center of Naples Community Hospital
350 7th Street North
Naples, FL 34102   239-436-5000
                                   Fax: 239-436-5250
                                        www.nchmd.org

Allen S. Weiss, CEO
Mariann MacDonald, Chairman
Thomas Gazdic, Chairman/Treasurer
Offers rehabilitation services, inpatient and outpatient care at 5 locations in the county and more for the benefit of the disabled.

6560 Conklin Center for the Blind
405 White St
Daytona Beach, FL 32114-2999   386-258-3441
                                   Fax: 386-258-1155
                              info@conklincenter.org
                                   www.conklincenter.org

Robert T Kelly, Executive Director
The Conklin Center's mission is to empower children and adults who are blind and have one or more additional disabilities to develop their potential to be able to obtain competitive employment, live independently and fully participate in community life.

6561 Davis Center for Rehabilitation Baptist Hospital of Miami
8900 N Kendall Dr
Miami, FL 33176-2118   786-596-1960
                          corporatepr@baptisthealth.net
                               www.baptisthealth.net/bhs
Brian E. Keeley, President and Chief Executive Of
Calvin Babcock, Chairman
A full-service, nonprofit community hospital providing a full range of inpatient and outpatient rehabilitation services. The overall commitment to excellence has extended to this specialized field. Access to medical expertise and services ensures that the best in medical resources are available should an unforeseen medical problem arise.

6562 Devereux Advanced Behavioral Health Florida - Titusville Campus
1850 S. Deleon Ave.
Titusville, FL 32780   407-473-5238
                                        800-338-3738
                                 referral@devereux.org
                                      www.devereuxfl.org

Gwendolyn B Skinner, Vice President of Operations
Dave Detro, Human Resource Director
Carlos F Pozzi-Montero, Psy.D, Clinical Director
The Devereux Florida Titusville Campus offers a variety of residential, foster care and community support services for youth with behavioral and intellectual/developmental disabilities. Services include a residential group home with private rooms and a therapeutic group home.

6563 Devereux Advanced Behavioral Health - Florida
Devereux Florida Corporate Office
5850 T.G. Lee Blvd.
Suite 400
Orlando, FL 32822   407-362-9210
                                     800-338-3738
                                     referral@devereux.org
                                     www.devereuxfl.org
Gwendolyn B Skinner, Vice President of Operations
Dave Detro, Human Resource Director
Carlos F Pozzi-Montero, Psy.D, Clinical Director
Offering care for children with mental health, behavioral, intellectual and developmental disabilities and challenges. Some services offered include a psychiatric program, community based group homes, foster care, counseling centers, case management, abuse and neglect prevention services, community-based care and outreach programs.

6564 Devereux Florida - Orlando Campus
Devereux Orlando Campus
6147 Christian Way
Orlando, FL 32808   407-296-5300
                                     800-338-3738
                                     referral@devereux.org
                                     www.devereuxfl.org
Gwendolyn B Skinner, Vice President of Operations
Dave Detro, Human Resource Director
Carlos F Pozzi-Montero, Psy.D, Clinical Director
The Orlando Campus provides intensive residential services for children and adolescents who suffer from emotional, behavioral and psychological problems. Programs offered include Devereux's Statewide Inpatient Psychiatric Program (SIPP), Residential Group Care and the Residential Treatment Center.

6565 Devereux Florida - Viera Campus
Devereux Viera Campus
8000 Devereux Dr.
Viera, FL 32940   321-242-9100
                                     800-338-3738
                                     Fax: 321-259-0786
                                     vischool@devereux.org
                                     www.devereuxfl.org
Gwendolyn B Skinner, Vice President of Operations
Dave Detro, Human Resource Director
Carlos F Pozzi-Montero, Psy.D, Clinical Director
The campus offers two residential programs for youth with developmental or behavioral challenges: the Intensive Residential Treatment Center (IRTC) and the Intellectual/Developmental Disabilities (I/DD) Program. The Viera Campus also offers six residential units and the Devereux School.

6566 Devereux Threshold Center for Autism
Threshold Center For Autism
3550 N Goldenrod Rd
Winter Park, FL 32792   407-671-7060
                                    800-338-3738
                                    Fax: 407-671-6005
                                    referral@devereux.org
                                    www.devereuxfl.org
Gwendolyn B Skinner, Vice President of Operations
Dave Detro, Human Resource Director
Carlos F Pozzi-Montero, Psy.D., Clinical Director
The Devereux Threshold Center for Autism includes a therapeutic residential program and an adult day treatment program for people with intellectual/developmental disabilities.

6567 Division of Blind Services
325 West Gaines Street
Suite 1114
Turlington Building, FL 32399-0400 850-245-0300
                                    800-342-1828
                                    Fax: 850-245-0386
                                    ana.saint-ford@dbs.fldoe.org
                                    dbs.myflorida.com
Aleisa McKinlay, Interim Director
Phyllis Vaughn, Bureau Chief, Administrative Services
William Findley, Bureau Chief, Business Enterprise Program
Serves the totally blind, legally blind, visually impaired, deaf-blind, learning disabled, and more by offering health, counseling, educational, recreational and computer training services.

6568 Easterseals Northeast Central Florida
1219 Dunn Ave.
Daytona Beach, FL 32114   386-255-4568
                                    877-255-4568
                                    Fax: 386-258-7677
                                    TTY: 386-310-1157
                                    www.easterseals.com/necfl
Bev Johnson, President & CEO
Melissa Chesley, Vice President, Finance & CFO
Susan B. Moor, Vice President, Philanthropy
Provides services for individuals with physical, intellectual, and other disabilities.

6569 Easterseals South Florida
1475 NW 14th Ave.
Miami, FL 33125   305-325-0470
                                    Fax: 305-325-0578
                                    www.easterseals.com/southflorida
Maurice Woods, President & CEO
Barry R. Vogel, Chief Administrative Officer
Maher Malak, Chief Financial Officer
The mission of Easterseals South Florida is to provide services to ensure that all children and adults with disabilities or special needs and their families have equal opportunities to live, learn, work and play in their communities.

6570 Easterseals Southwest Flordia
Sarasota, FL 34243-2001   941-355-7637
                                    themeadowscup.com
Easterseals Sothwest Florida creates solutions that change lives for children, adults and their families through high quality therapeutic, educational and supportive services.

6571 Easterseals Southwest Florida
350 Braden Ave.
Sarasota, FL 34243   941-355-7637
                                    Fax: 941-358-3069
                                    www.easterseals-swfl.org
Tom Waters, President & CEO
Patrick Ryan, Chief Operating Officer
George Pfeiffer, Vice President, Government Relations
Provides services to children and adults with physical, neurological and communications disabilities and their families.

6572 Florida CORF
Columbia Medical Center: Peninsula

John Feore, Executive VP
Sandra Trovato, Executive Director
Offers Medicare authorized therapy programs for seniors, disabled and others who need rehabilitation. CORF can provide coordinated and extended services in the home after a hospital stay, or when physical status changes. Patients who are treated at CORF, include amputations, arthritis, chronic/acute pain, depression/anxiety, nerve injury, sports injury, stroke and swallowing problems.

6573 Florida Institute Of Rehabilitation Education (FIRE)
3071 Highland Oaks Terrace
Tallahassee, FL 32301-4876   850-942-3658
                                    888-827-6033
                                    Fax: 850-942-4518
                                    info@lighthousebigbend.org
Barbara Ross, Executive Director
Evelyn Worley, Assistant Director
Wayne Warner, Vocational Program Director
Provides independent living and vocational rehabilitation services to Florida residents who are legally blind. Services include instruction in orientation and mobility, accessible technology, daily living skills and employability skills. Information, referral and counseling services are also offered. All services are provided without charge.

6574 Florida Institute for Neurologic Rehabilitation, Inc
1962 Vandolah Road
P O Box 1348
Wauchula, FL 33873-1348   863-773-2857
                                           800-697-5390
                                      Fax: 863-773-0867
                                               finr.net
John Richards, Administrator
Stephanie Ortiz, RN, Director of Nursing
Kevin E. O'Keefe, Program Director
A residential rehabilitation facility providing a therapeutic environment in which children, adolescents and adults who have survived head-injury can develop the independence and skills necessary to re-enter the community.

6575 Fort Lauderdale Veterans Medical Center
713 NE 3rd Ave
Fort Lauderdale, FL 33304-2619   954-356-7926
                                      Fax: 954-356-7609
                                 www.va.gov/directory/guide/
Robert White, Executive Director
Sloan D Gibson, Acting Secretary
Jose D Riojas, Chief of Staff
Veterans medical clinic offering disabled veterans medical treatments.

6576 Halifax Hospital Medical Center Eye Clinic Professional Center
308 Farmington Avenue
Farmington, CT 06032   860-658-4388
                                           888-444-3598
                                 webmaster@evariant.com
                                       www.evariant.com
Bill Moschella, CEO
Rob Grant, Executive Vice President
Michael Clark, Chief Operating Officer
Offers services for the totally blind, legally blind, visually impaired, and more with health, counseling, educational, recreational, rehabilitation, computer training and professional training services.

6577 HealthQuest Subacute and Rehabilitation Programs
Regenta Park
8700 a C Skinner Pkwy
Jacksonville, FL 32256-836   Fax: 904-641-7896
HealthQuest offers four centers within the state of Florida offering exceptional staff, comfortable surroundings and individually designed, closely monitored programs dedicated to enabling patients to achieve their goals. Each location offers a progressive and cost effective alternative to in-hospital subacute and rehabilitative care. Centers are offered in Jacksonville, Winter Park, Sarasota and Sunrise..

6578 HealthSouth Emeral Coast Sports & Rehabilitation Center
1847 Florida Avenue
Panama City, FL 32405-3730   850-784-4878
                                      Fax: 850-769-7566
                            www.healthsouthpanamacity.com
Tony Bennett, CEO
Michelle Miller, Manager
Outpatient sports medicine and rehabilitation center providing physical therapy, occupational therapy, industrial rehab, work hardening/work simulation, worksite and ergonomic analysis, FCE's, work assessment and pre-employment goals of returning the clients back to work, and returning to all recreational, sports and functional activities safely..

6579 HealthSouth Rehabilitation Hospital of Tallahassee
Healthsouth Corporation
1675 Riggins Rd
Tallahassee, FL 32308-5315   850-656-4800
                            www.healthsouthtallahassee.com
Heath Phillips, Chief Executive Officer
Robert Robert Rowland, Medical Director
Tom Abbruscato, Controller
North Florida's sole acute rehabilitation hospital between Jacksonville \, Panama City, and Gainesville. With 250 employees providing a full continuum of care form its 70 bed facility, the hospital is accredited by JCAHO, CARF and state designated and certified by Vocational Rehabilitation for traumatic brain injury,

as well as a wide variety of other diagnoses. With the addition of our outpatients, the facility has served the greater community by touching the lives of over 50,000 patients.

6580 HealthSouth Rehabilitation Hospital Of Miami
20601 Old Cutler Rd
Miami, FL 33189-2441   305-251-3800
                                 www.healthsouthmiami.com
Elizabeth Izquierdo, Chief Executive Officer
Angelo Appio, Director of Marketing Operations
Reyna M. Hernandez, Chief Financial Officer
A comprehensive source of medical rehabilitation services for Pinellas County, Florida area residents, their families and their physicians. Offers the people of Florida all the clinical, technical and professional resources of the nation's leading provider of comprehensive rehabilitation care.

6581 HealthSouth Rehabilitation Hospital of Sarasota
Health South Corporation in Burmingham Alabama
6400 Edgelake Drive
Sarasota, FL 34240-8813   941-921-8600
                                           866-330-5822
                                 www.healthsouthsarasota.com
Marcus Braz, Chief Executive Officer
Alexander DeJesus, Medical Director
Nancy Arnold, Director of Marketing Operations
HealthSouth Rehabilitation Hospital of Sarasota is a 96-bed inpatient rehabilitation hospital that offers comprehensive inpatient rehabilitation services designed to return patients to leading active and independent lives.

6582 HealthSouth Sea Pines Rehabilitation Hospital
Sea Pines Rehabilitation Hospital
101 E Florida Ave
Melbourne, FL 32901-8398   321-984-4600
                                      Fax: 321-952-6532
                                 www.healthsouthseapines.com
Stuart Miller, Medical Director
Denise McGrath, Chief Executive Officer
Donna Anderson, Director of Human Resources
Designed to return patients to leading active, independent lives, HealthSouth Sea Pines Rehabilitation Hospital is a 90-bed rehabilitation hospital that provides a higher level of comprehensive rehabilitation services.

6583 Holy Cross Hospital
Catholic Southwest
4725 North Federal Hwy
Fort Lauderdale, FL 33308-4668   954-771-8000
                                       www.holy-cross.com
Patrick Taylor, President & Chief Executive Offi
Luisa Gutman, Senior Vice President & Chief Op
Linda Wilford, Senior Vice President & Chief Fi
Holy Cross Hospital in Fort Lauderdale is a full-service, non-profit Catholic hospital, sponsored by the Sisters of Mercy. Holy Cross is a US News & World Report 'Best Hospital' and HealthGrades Distinguished Hospital for Clinical Excellence, 2004 and 2005

6584 Lee Memorial Hospital
2776 Cleveland Ave
Fort Myers, FL 33901-5855   239-343-2000
                                       www.leememorial.org
Sanford Cohen, Chairman
Chris Hansen, Vice Chairman
David Collins, Treasurer
Offers a complete inpatient program of intensive rehabilitation designed to restore a patient to a more independent level of functioning. The comprehensive care includes medical rehabilitation and training for spinal cord injury, brain injury, stroke and neurological disorders.

6585 Lighthouse for the Blind of Palm Beach
1710 Tiffany Drive East
West Palm Beach, FL 33407-3224   561-586-5600
                                      Fax: 561-84- 80
                            lighthousepalmbeaches.org
Marvin A. Tanck, President and CEO
Dont, Mickens, Chair
John R. Banister, Vice Chairman

A private, non-profit rehabilitation and education agency in its 55th year of service. Offers programs to assist persons who areblind or visually impaired, an on-site Industrial Center, a technology training center, an Aids and appliances Store, special equipment grant programs, outreach services for children and adults, Early Intervention and Preschool Services, and a variety of support groups. These programs provide services and education for blind children and their parents.

6586   Lighthouse for the Visually Impaired and Blind
8610 Galen Wilson Blvd
Port Richey, FL 34668-5974   727-815-0303
                                                   866-962-5254
                                              Fax: 727-815-0203
                                              lighthouse@lvib.org
                                                   www.lvib.org

Sylvia Stinson-Perez, Executive Director
Dr. John Mann, President
Melissa M. Suess, Orientation and Mobility Instruc
The Lighthouse offers services for visually impaired or blind adults and children ages 0-5 years old. Counseling, educational services, recreational services, rehabilitation, computer training and support groups.

6587   MacDonald Training Center
5420 W Cypress Street
Tampa, FL 33607-1706   813-870-1300
                                                   866-948-6184
                                              Fax: 813-872-6010
                                              TTY: 813-873-7631
                                              macdonaldcenter.org

Jim Freyvogel, President/CEO
Judith DeStasio, CFO
Debi Hamilton, Director of Services
A private, non-profit, community-based human services organization serving adults with disabilities (since 1953). Persons are provided the opportunity to achieve their highest potential through the Center's various programs that include day training, employment, community living and various support services.

6588   Medicenter of Tampa
4411 North Habana Avenue
Tampa, FL 33614-7211   813-872-2771
                                              Fax: 813-871-2831
                              rehabilitationandhealthcarecenteroftampa.com
Dan Davis, President
Mariluz G, Social Services Director
Brenda Pace, Secretary
Postacute rehabilitation program. A 174 bed non-profit facility with postacute reahbilitation programs..

6589   Miami Heart Institute Adams Building
4300 Alton Rd
Miami Beach, FL 33140-2997   305-674-2121
                                                   www.msmc.com
Steven D. Sonenreich, President/CEO
The mission is to provide high quality health care to our diverse community enhanced through teaching, research, charity care and financial responsibility.

6590   Miami Lighthouse for the Blind
601 SW 8th Ave
Miami, FL 33130-3200   305-856-2288
                                              Fax: 305-285-6967
                                         info@miamilighthouse.com
                                              miamilighthouse.org
Virginia A. Jacko, President & Chief Executive Officer
Sharon Caughill, Special Projects Manager
Jeannie Reinoso, Executive Assistant
Offers services for the legally blind and severely visually impaired (including those who are developmentally delayed) of all ages in the areas of counseling and educational, recreational, rehabilitation, computer and vocational training services.

6591   Mount Sinai Medical Center Rehabilitation Unit
4300 Alton Rd
Miami Beach, FL 33140-2997   305-674-2121
                                                   www.msmc.com
Steven D. Sonenreich, President/CEO
A comprehensive inpatient and outpatient rehabilitation programs have been helping patients recover for more then 20 years.

Fully customized treatment plans based on the needs of each patient is 1 reason why our services are among the best in South Florida. Our team approach takes into account the medical, physical, psychological, social, spiritual, cultural and economic needs of patients and their families.

6592   Neurobehavioral Medicine Center
Ste 1
4821 Us Highway 19
New Port Richey, FL 34652-4259   727-849-2005
                                              Fax: 727-849-2087

Otsenre Matos, Medical Director
Gerard Taylor PhD, Counseling/Stress Management
Donna Taylor RN, Manager
A multidisciplinary outpatient program for the evaluation and treatment of chronic pain. Consultation services for hospitalized patients are also provided upon request. Comprehensive treatment of individuals with closed traumatic brain injuries..

6593   North Broward Rehab Unit
North Broward Medical Center
201 E Sample Rd
Deerfield Beach, FL 33064-3596   954-941-8300
                                              www.browardhealth.org

Douglas Ford, Chiefs of Staff
Pauline Grant, Chief Executive Officer
CARF accredited, 30-bed inpatient rehabilitation unit treating adults with brain injuries, spinal cord injuries, stroke, orthopedic and neurologic injuries.

6594   Northwest Medical Center
Health Care Corporation of America
2801 North State Road 7
Margate, FL 33063-5727   954-974-0400
                                                   866-256-7720
                                              northwestmed.com

Mark Rader, CEO
Above all else, we are committed to the care and improvement of human life. In recognition of this commitment, we strive to deliver high quality, cost effective healthcare in the communities we serve. We recognize and affirm the unique and intrinsic work of each individual. We treat all those we serve with compassion and kindness. We act with absolute honesty, integrity, and fairness in the way we conduct our business and the way we live our lives.

6595   Pain Institute of Tampa
4178 N Armenia Ave
Tampa, FL 33607-6429   813-875-5913

John E Barsa, Founder & MD
Offers a comprehensive and multidisciplinary approach to pain controll and management. Most services are provided on-site but other services may require you to be referred elswhere. We will monitor and coordinate your care in a manner to provide optimal recovery potential.

6596   Pain Treatment Center, Baptist Hospital of Miami
8900 N Kendall Dr
Miami, FL 33176-2118   786-596-1960
                                         corporatepr@baptisthealth.net
                                              www.baptisthealth.net

Calvin Babcock, Chairman
Brian E. Keeley, President and Chief Executive Of
Since 1960, Baptist Hospital of Miami has been one of the most respected medical centers in South Florida. The hospitals full range of medical and technological services is the natural choice for a growing number of people throughout the world.

6597   Pine Castle
4911 Spring Park Rd
Jacksonville, FL 32207-7496   904-733-2650
                                              Fax: 904-733-2681
                                              info@pinecastle.org
                                                   pinecastle.org
Jonathan May, Executive Director
Randall Duncan, Associate Executive Director
Leigh Griffin, Director of Finance
Provides remunerative work, training, community employment and community living options for adults with developmental disabilities.

6598 Polk County Association for Handicapped Citizens
1038 Sunshine Dr E
Lakeland, FL 33801-6338   863-858-2252
                                 Fax: 863-665-2330
Kecia Howell, Owner
Anthony J. Senzamici Jr., 1st Vice Chairman
Carol N. Asbill, 2nd Vice Chairman
A private non-profit organization that provides an adult day training program to people with developmental disabilities and is under the direction of a volunteer board of directors. The primary goal for our services is to provide people with knowledge and practical experience to be independent adults so they can become contributing members of their community..

6599 Quest, Inc.
PO Box 531125
Orlando, FL 32853   407-218-4300
                                 888-807-8378
                               Fax: 407-218-4301
                            contact@questinc.org
                                 www.questinc.org
John Gill, President & Chief Executive Officer
Brooke Eakins, Chief Operating Officer
Todd Thrasher, Chief Financial Officer
Quest helps individuals with developmental disabilities in Central Florida achieve their goals by providing services that increase their capabilities and quality of life. Quest serves more than 1,000 individuals each day in the Orlando and Tampa areas.

6600 Quest, Inc. - Tampa Area
3910 US Hwy. 301 N
Tampa, FL 33619   813-423-7700
                                 888-807-8378
                               Fax: 813-423-7701
                            contact@questinc.org
                                 www.questinc.org
John Gill, President & Chief Executive Officer
Brooke Eakins, Chief Operating Officer
Todd Thrasher, Chief Financial Officer
Quest helps individuals with developmental disabilities in Central Florida achieve their goals by providing services that increase their capabilities and quality of life. Quest serves more than 1,000 individuals each day in the Orlando and Tampa areas.

6601 Rehabilitation Center for Children and Adults
300 Royal Palm Way
Palm Beach, FL 33480-4305   561-655-7266
                               Fax: 561-655-3269
                                    info@rcca.org
                                       rcca.org
John C. Whelton, Chairman
Jacob L. Lochner, Co-Chairman
Christopher Adams, MD
A private, nonprofit organization whose purpose is to improve physical function, independence and communication of people with physical disabilities. Any child or adult with a physical or speech disability is eligible for services.

6602 Renaissance Center
3599 University Blvd
Suite 604
Jacksonville, FL 32216- 9249   904-399-0905
                               Fax: 904-743-5109
                    www.obiplasticsurgery.com/index.php
Lewis Obi, MD

6603 Rosomoff Comprehensive Pain Center, The
5200 NE 2nd Avenue
Miami, FL 33137-2706   305-532-7246
                               Fax: 305-534-3974
Elsayed Abdel-Moty, Director
Hubert Rossomoff, Owner
A state-of-the-art Center of Excellence offering inpatient, outpatient, outpatient rehabilitation services and seniors programs. The Center became an internationally renowned model for the evalutation and treatment of all persons seeking pain relief.

6604 Sarasota Memorial Hospital/Comprehensive Rehabilitation Unit
1700 S Tamiami Trail
Sarasota, FL 34239-3509   941-917-9000
                               Fax: 941-917-2211
                                    www.smh.com
Marguerite G Malone, Chair
Gregory Carter, First Vice Chair
Alex Miller, Second Vice Chair
The goal of the 34-bed Comprehensive Rehabilitation Unit (CRU) is to increase patient functional independence, adjust to illness or disability and successfully return to the community. The unit is dedicated to patients who have experienced conditions such

6605 Strive Physical Therapy Centers
2620 SE Maricamp RD
Ocala, FL 34471-4517   352-732-8868
                               Fax: 352-732-8890
                               www.striverehab.com
R W Shutes, Owner
Johanna Solbato, Administrator
R.W. Shutes, President and CEO
Certified as an Outpatient Rehabilitation Agency, providing a comprehensive approach to patient evaluation and treatment. Our objective is to return our patients back to a productive life as quickly as possible and safely as possible.

6606 Sunbridge Care and Rehabilitation
101 East State Street,
Kennett Square, FL 19348-6105   610-444-6350
                               Fax: 610-925-4000
                               info@genesishcc.com
                               www.genesishcc.com
Dan Hirschfeld, President
George V Hager, Chief Executive Officer
Robert A Reitz, Executive Vice President & Chief Operating Officer
A comprehensive medical rehabilitation facility that is committed to helping individuals with disabilities improve their quality of life. This is a 120-bed facility offering a full range of acute and sub-acute inpatient programs as well as community-based

6607 Tampa Bay Academy
12012 Boyette Rd
Riverview, FL 33569-5631   813-677-6700
                                 800-678-3838
                               Fax: 813-671-3145
                            tlamb@tampahope.org
                              www.tampahope.org
Renee Scott, Chair
Amy McClure, Vice-Chair
Titania Lamb, Executive Director
A psychiatric residential treatment center and partial hospitalization program for ages 7 to 17.

6608 Tampa General Rehabilitation Center
1 Tampa General Circle
P.O.Box 1289
Tampa, FL 33606-3571   813-844-7700
                                866-844-1411
                              Fax: 813-844-1477
                                      tgh.org
James R. Burkhart, President & CEO
Bruce Zwiebel, Chief Of Staff
Deana L. Nelson, Chief Operating Officer
Offers a full range of programs all aimed at helping patients achieve their full potentials. It is one of three centers in the state that provides Driver Training and Evaluation Programs for persons with disabilities, and also an Assisted Reproduction Pro

6609 Tampa Lighthouse for the Blind
1106 West Platt Street
Tampa, FL 33606-2142   813-251-2407
                              Fax: 813-254-4305
                              tampalighthouse.org
Sheryl Brown, Executive Director
Offers services for the totally blind, legally blind, visually impaired, and more with health, counseling, educational, recreational, rehabilitation, computer training and professional training services.

6610 **The Arc Tampa Bay**
1501 N Belcher Rd.
Suite 249
Clearwater, FL 33765
727-799-3330
Fax: 727-799-4632
thearctb.org
Seeks to support and empower people with intellectual and developmental disabilities through services such as adult day training programs, employment programs, residential programs, and more.

6611 **Visually Impaired Persons of Southwest Florida**
35 W Mariana Ave
North Fort Myers, FL 33903-5515
239-997-7797
Fax: 239-997-8462
Doug Fowler, Executive Director
Margaret Ruhe Lincoln, Director of operations
Provides training in independent living skills, orientation and mobility, counseling, computer and other communication skills, family support groups, peer counseling, socialization and a low vision clinic. Second location in Charlotte County. Phone: 941-6

6612 **West Florida Hospital: The Rehabilitation Institute**
8383 North Davis Hwy
Pensacola, FL 32514-6039
850-494-4000
800-342-1123
Fax: 850-494-4881
www.westfloridahospital.com
Roman S Bautista, President/CEO
Carol Saxton, Senior VP Patient Care Services
A 58-bed comprehensive rehabilitation facility offering inpatient and outpatient services. JCAHO and CARF accredited and a State designed head and spinal cord injury center. CARF accredited programs include: comprehensive inpatient rehab, spinal cord inju

6613 **West Gables Health Care Center**
2525 SW 75th Ave
Miami, FL 33155-2800
305-262-6800
Fax: 888-453-1928
www.westgablesrehabhospital.com
Jose Vargas, Medical Director
Walter Concepcion, Chief Executive Officer
Cesar Sepulveda, Materials Manager
Services provide by West Gables Health Center: activities services are provided onsite to residents. Clinical laboratory services are provided, dental, dietary, housekeeping, mental health services, nursing services, occupational therapy, pharmacy, physic

6614 **Willough at Naples**
9001 Tamiami Trail East
Naples, FL 34113-3397
239-775-4500
800-722-0100
Fax: 239-793-0534
info@thewilloughatnaples.com
thewilloughatnaples.com
James O'Shea, President
A licensed psychiatric hospital in Southwest Florida which provides quality management and treatment for eating disorders and chemical dependency in adults.

Georgia

6615 **Annandale Village**
3500 Annandale Ln
Suwanee, GA 30024-2150
770-945-8381
Fax: 770-945-8693
annandale.org
Adam Pomeranz, Chief Executive Officer
Melissa Burton, Chief Financial Officer
Keith Fenton, Chief Development & Marketing Officer
Private nonprofit residential facility for adults with developmental disabilities. Located on 124 acres just north of Atlanta. Annandale provides full program and 24 hour residential services, pay program services, respite care and skilled nursing services.

6616 **Atlanta Institute of Medicine and Rehabilitation**
Ste E
2911 Piedmont Rd NE
Atlanta, GA 30305-2782
404-365-0160
Fax: 404-365-0751
Lawrence E Eppelbaum, Founder
Galina Vayner, MD
One of the most famous medical centers in the state of Georgia. The Institute employs more then 40 highly qualified medical professionals and fully equipped with the latest medical equipment. It has gathered recognition and respect from the people of Atla

6617 **Bobby Dodd Institute (BDI)**
2120 Marietta Blvd NW
Atlanta, GA 30318-2122
678-365-0071
Fax: 678-365-0098
TTY: 678-365-0099
bobbydodd.org
Rodney Hall, Chair
Christopher Rosselli, Vice Chair
Wayne McMillan, President & CEO
BDI annually serves approximately 400 clients in Atlanta, GA. BDI works primarily with people with developmental disabilities such as autism and down syndrome, but includes clients with physical or acquired disabilities.

6618 **Cave Spring Rehabilitation Center**
Georgia Department of Labor
7 Georgia Ave
P.O.Box 303
Cave Spring, GA 30124-2718
706-777-2341
Fax: 706-777-2366
gvra.georgia.gov/cave-spring-center-contacts-
Russell Fleming, Director
Karen Hulsey, Administrative Operations Coordinator
Renee Lambert, Rehabilitation Assistant

6619 **Center for the Visually Impaired**
739 West Peachtree St NW
Atlanta, GA 30308-1137
404-875-9011
Fax: 404-607-0062
cviga.org
Susan Hoy, Chair
Fontaine M. Huey, President
Doreen Zaksheske, Vice President of Finance & Operations
Offers services to people of all ages who are blind or visually impaired with training in orientation and mobility, computer technology, activities of daily living, communication skills and employment readiness. Aso offers two children's programs, a comm

6620 **Devereux Advanced Behavioral Health Georgia**
Devereux Georgia Treatment Network
1291 Stanley Rd.
Kennesaw, GA 30152
770-427-0147
800-342-3357
Fax: 770-427-4030
info@devereux.org
www.devereuxga.org
Gwendolyn B Skinner, Vice President of Operations
Dave Detro, Human Resource Director
Carlos F Pozzi-Montero, Psy.D, Clinical Director
Facility offering services to youth with emotional and behavioral health challenges. Services include Intensive Residential Treatment, Foster Care Program, Group Homes, and educational programs.

6621 **Easterseals East Georgia**
1500 Wrightsboro Rd.
Augusta, GA 30904
706-667-9695
Fax: 706-667-8831
www.easterseals.com/eastgeorgia
Lynn Smith, Chief Executive Officer
Easterseals East Georgia assists people with disabilities and other special needs to maximize opportunities for employment, independence and full inclusion into society.

6622   Georgia Industries for the Blind
700 Faceville Highway
Bainbridge, GA 39819-218   229-248-2666
                                        Fax: 229-248-2669
                                  gvra.georgia.gov/gib/about-us
James Hughes, Executive Director
Offers services for the totally blind, legally blind, visually impaired, and more with health, counseling, educational, recreational, rehabilitation, computer training and professional training services.

6623   Hillhaven Rehabilitation
26 Tower Rd NE
Marietta, GA 30060-6947   770-422-8913
                                             800-526-5782
                                        Fax: 770-425-2085
Leslie Ann Marie Parrish, Case Manager
Valerie Hamilton, Administrator
Routine skilled and subacute medical and rehabilitation care including physical therapy, occupational therapy, speech pathology and therapeutic recreation. Programs include stroke and head injury rehab; orthopedic rehab; complex IV therapy; woundcare; can.

6624   In-Home Medical Care
Care Master Medical Services
240 Odell Rd
P.O.Box 278
Griffin, GA 30223-4787   770-227-1264
                                             800-542-8889
                                        Fax: 770-412-0014
                                    caremastermedical.com
Nancy Frederick, VP
Eddie Grogan, Chief Executive Officer
Offers the devoted attention of a professional nurse, the use of I.V. therapies, pain management and provision of medical equipment and supplies right where the patient wants to be.

6625   Learning Services: Harris House Program
131 Langley Drive
Suite B
Lawrenceville, GA 30046-4446   404-298-0144
                                             888-419-9955
                                        Fax: 866-491-7396
                                      learningservices.com
Dr. Debra Braunling-McMorrow, President and CEO
Susan Snow, Director of Admissions
Michael Weaver, Chief Development Officer
Situated in the small, historic district of Stone Mountain, just outside of Atlanta, this 6 bed program is designed to encourage independence while providing appropriate support for each individuals needs. Community-based productive activities are customi

6626   Pain Control & Rehabilitation Institute of Georgia
Ste 120
2784 N Decatur Rd
Decatur, GA 30033-5993   404-297-1400
                                        Fax: 404-297-1427
Shulim Spektor, CEO
Anna Britman, Office Manager
Provides pain management for chronic and acute pain resulted from injuries, diseases of muscles and nerve, Reflex Sympathetic Dystrophy, perform disabilities and impairment ratings.

6627   Savannah Association for the Blind
214 Drayton Street
Savannah, GA 31401-4021   912-236-4473
                                        Fax: 912-234-9286
Gregory Hodges, President
Robert Falligant, Vice-president
Gary Sadowski, Treasurer
Offers services for the totally blind, legally blind, visually impaired, and more with health, counseling, educational, recreational, rehabilitation, computer training and professional training services.

6628   Shepherd Center for Treatment of Spinal Injuries
2020 Peachtree Rd NW
Atlanta, GA 30309-1465   404-352-2020
                                        Fax: 404-350-7479
                                    admissions@shepherd.org
                                         www.shepherd.org
Gary R. Ulicny, President & CEO
David F. Apple, Jr., M.D., Medical Director
Angela Beninga, D.O., Staff Physiatrist
Dedicated exclusively to the care of patients with spinal cord injuries and other paralyzing spinal disorders. It serves predominately residents of Georgia and neighboring states as one of the only 14 hospitals designated by the U.S. Department of Educati

6629   Transitional Hospitals Corporation
Ste 1000
7000 Central Pkwy NE
Atlanta, GA 30328-4592   770-821-5328
                                             800-683-6868
                                        Fax: 770-913-0015
                                             csins.com
Dean Kozee, Owner
Carolyn Norton, Special Projects Consultant/Broker
Amaury Rentas, Event Insurance/Broker
A national network of intensive care hospitals providing care for patients who suffer from a chronic illness and/or catastrophic accident. The mission is founded on providing quality health care to patients who require highly skilled nursing care and acce.

6630   Walton Rehabilitation Health System
1355 Independence Dr
Augusta, GA 30901-1037   706-823-8584
                                             866-492-5866
                                        Fax: 706-724-5752
                                    www.waltonfoundation.net
Robert Taylor, Chair
Dennis Skelley, President/CEO
David Dugan, Treasurer
A 58-bed comprehensive physical rehabilitation hospital offering inpatient and outpatient services. Services offered include: stroke recovery, orthopedic injury, pediatrics, head injury, pain management for chronic pain syndrome, TMJ/Craniofacial pain and

Hawaii

6631   Rehabilitation Hospital of the Pacific
226 N Kuakini St
Honolulu, HI 96817-2498   808-531-3511
                                        Fax: 808-566-3411
                                rehabfoundation@rehabhospital.org
                                     www.rehabhospital.org
John Komeiji, Chair
Glenn O. Sexton, Vice Chair
E. Lynne Madden, Secretary/Treasurer
The only acute care medical rehabilitation organization serving both Hawaii and the Pacific. For over 52 years, the hospital and its 7 outpatient clinics on Oahu, and Maui and Hawaii have been dedicated to providing comprehensive, cost effective rehabilit

Idaho

6632   Ashton Memorial Nursing Home and Chemical Dependency Center
700 N 2nd
Ashton, ID 83420   208-652-7461
                                        Fax: 208-652-7595
                                        ashtonmemorial.com
Sheila Kellogg, Administrator

6633 Idaho Elks Rehabilitation Hospital
600 N Robbins Rd
Boise, ID 83702   208-489-4444
                                              Fax: 208-344-8883
                                              info@elksrehab.org
                                              www.elksrehab.org

Joseph P. Caroselli, CEO
Doug Lewis, Chief Financial Officer
Mellisa Honsinger, Chief Operating Officer
A nonprofit hospital serving Idaho and the Pacific Northwest. All
inpatient and outpatient programs and services are supervised by
the hospital's full-time medical directors whose specialty is physical rehabilitative medicine. Services include: occupation

6634 Portneuf Medical Center Rehabilitation
777 Hospital Way
Pocatello, ID 83201-4004   208-239-1000
                                              charlesa@portmed.org
                                              www.portmed.org

Mark Buckalew, Chairman
Michael Nosacka, MD
Dan Ordyna, CEO
Provides compassionate, quality health care services needed by
the people of eastern Idaho in collaboration with other providers
and community resources.

Illinois

6635 Advocate Christ Hospital and Medical Center
4440 W 95th St
Oak Lawn, IL 60453-2600   708-684-8000
                                              Fax: 708-684-4440
                                              advocatehealth.com

Jim Skogsbergh, CEO
Bill Santulli, COO
Kate K, Director
A 665-bed, not-for-profit teaching, research and referral medical
center in Oak Lawn, Illinois. It also is home to the Advocate Hope
Childrens's Hospital, one of the most comprehensive providers
of pediatric care in the state. The medical center is a lead

**6636 Advocate Christ Medical Center & Advocate Hope
Children's Hospital**
4440 W 95th St
Oak Lawn, IL 60453-2600   708-684-8000
                                              Fax: 708-684-4440
                                              advocatehealth.com

Kenneth Lukhard, CEO
Darcie Brazel, Market Chief Nurse Executive
Jan McCrea, Rehab Services Director
The largest fully integrated not-for-profit health care delivery
system in metropolitan Chicago and is recognized as one of the
top 10 systems in the country. The mission of Advocate Health
Care is to serve the health needs of individuals, families and co

6637 Advocate Illinois Masonic Medical Center
836 W Wellington Ave
Chicago, IL 60657-5147   773-975-1600
                                              www.advocatehealth.com/immc
Jim Skogsbergh, CEO
Ajay V. Maker, MD
Consultation, education, family counseling, parent training in
behavior modification techniques offered to developmentally
disabled adults.

6638 Alexian Brothers Medical Center
800 Biesterfield Rd
Elk Grove Village, IL 60007-3396   847-437-5500
                                              www.alexian.org
Mark Frey, President/CEO
Tracy Rogers, Senior Vice President and Chief Operating Officer
Paul Belter, Senior Vice President and Chief Financial Officer
A threefold mission: Works toward maximizing physical function, enhance independent social skills and optimize communication skills consistent with an individual's ability. The Center
helps those disabled by accident or illness achieve a new personal
best

6639 Back in the Saddle Hippotherapy Program
Corcoran Physical Therapy
4200 W Peterson Ave
Chicago, IL 60646-6074   312-286-2266
                                              847-604-4145
                                              Fax: 847-673-8895
Julie Naughton, Program Coordinator
Maureen Corcoran, Physical Therapist
Tom Corcoran, Owner
A direct medical treatment used by licensed physical therapists
who have a strong treatment background in posture and move-
ment, neuromotor function and sensory processing. The benefits
of Hippotherapy are available to individuals with just about any
disab

6640 Barbara Olson Center of Hope
3206 N Central Ave
Rockford, IL 61101-1797   815-964-9275
                                              Fax: 815-964-9607
                                              info@b-olsoncenterofhope.org
                                              b-olsoncenterofhope.org
Carm Herman, Executive Director
Pam Sondell, Director of Programs and Services
Pam Carey, Director of Human Resources
We provide vocational employment, educational and social op-
portunities for adults with developmental disabilities.

6641 Bartolucci Center, The- ILC Enterprises
6415 Stanley Ave
Berwyn, IL 60402-3130   708-745-5277
                                              Fax: 708-698-5090
                                              www.pillarscommunity.org
Zada Clarke, Chairman
Ann Schreiner, President & CEO
Jennifer Hogberg, Vice Chair
A nonprofit tax exempt private social service agency serving sub-
urban Chicago offering day treatment and vocational counseling
to individuals who encountered a pattern of job loss due to
emotional problems.

6642 Baxter Healthcare Corporation
1 Baxter Pkwy
Deerfield, IL 60015-4625   224-948-2000
                                              800-422-9837
                                              224-948-1812
                                              Fax: 800-568-5020
*Phillip L. Batchelor, Corporate Vice President - Quality and Regu-
latory Affairs*
Jean-Luc Butel, Corporate Vice President - President, International
*Robert M. Davis, Corporate Vice President - President, Medical
Products*
Baxter International Inc. is a global healthcare company that,
through its subsidiaries assists healthcare professionals and their
patients with treatment of complex medical conditions including
hemophilia, immune disorders, kidney disease, cancer, trauma
and other conditions. Baxter applies its expertise in medical devices, pharmaceuticals, and biotechnology to make a meaningful
difference in patient's lives.

6643 Beacon Therapeutic Diagnostic and Treatment Center
10650 S Longwood Dr
Chicago, IL 60643-2617   773-881-1005
                                              Fax: 773-881-1164
Susan Reyha-Guerrero, President & CEO
Cheryl Thompson, Deputy CEO
Paul Morley, Chief Operating Officer
Offers community day treatment, education, diagnostic services,
family counseling, learning disabled, speech and hearing and
psychiatric services.

6644 Blind Service Association
17 N State St
Ste 1050
Chicago, IL 60602-3510   312-236-0808
                                              blindserviceassociation.org
Ann Lousin, President
Linda Schwartz, Executive Vice President
Arthur M. Shapiro, Secretary
Offers services for the totally blind, legally blind and visually im-
paired with reading and recording low vision network, social ser-
vices, referrals and support groups.

619

6645 Brentwood Subacute Healthcare Center
T HI Brentwood
5400 W 87th St
Burbank, IL 60459-2913 866-300-3257
www.savaseniorcare.com
Audrey Protrowski, Director Business Development
Jill Sattersield, Administrator
John Walton, CEO
Seeks to help patients and their families through what can be a very emotional decision-making process. We provide guidance and consultation on everything from how to properly choose the facility to providing resources that help you cope with the nature of the decision itself.

6646 Caremark Healthcare Services
2211 Sanders Rd
Northbrook, IL 60062-6128 847-559-4700
800-423-1411
Fax: 847-559-3905
www.caremark.com
Larry J. Merlo, President & CEO
Mark Cosby, Executive Vice President
An 80-service-center network providing services anywhere in the U.S. Offers 24 hour access to nursing and pharmacy services, case management resource centers, HIV/AIDS services, women's health services, transplant care services, nutrition support services

6647 Centegra Northern Illinois Medical Center
4209 West Shamrock Lane
Suite B
McHenry, IL 60050-8499 815-759-8017
877-236-8347
Fax: 815-759-8062
www.centegra.org
Michael S. Eesley, CEO
Jason Sciarro, President
David L. Tomlinson, Executive Vice President
Providing rehabilitation services in Lake and McHenry Counties, the Rehabilitation Unit is a complete living environment for up to 15 patients after a debilitating illness of trauma. Various locations offering a multitude of services: PT, OT, speech, HT,

6648 Center for Comprehensive Services
Mentor Network
P.O.Box 2825
Carbondale, IL 62902-2825 618-457-4008
800-582-4227
Fax: 618-457-5372
dayna.foreman@thementornetwork.com
mentorabi.com
Bill Duffy, Chief Operating Officer
Michael E. Hofmeister, Vice President
Sean Byrne, Chief Financial Officer
Post-acute rehabilitation services for adults and adolescents with acquired brain injuries. Residential, day-treatment and out-patient services tailored to individual needs.

6649 Center for Rehabilitation at Rush Presbyterian:
Johnston R Bowman Health Center
1653 W Congress Parkway
Chicago, IL 60612-3833 312-942-5000
Fax: 312-942-3601
TTY: 312-942-2207
teri_sommerfeld@rush.edu
www.rush.edu
Larry J. Goodman, CEO
A 613-bed hospital serving adults and children, the John R. Bowman Health Center and Rush University is home to one of the first medical colleges in the Midwest and one of the nation's top-ranked nursing colleges, as well as graduate programs in allied he

6650 Center for Spine, Sports & Occupational Rehabilitation
345 E Superior St
Chicago, IL 60611-2654 312-238-7767
800-354-7342
Fax: 312-238-7709
webmaster@ric.org
www.rehabchicago.org
Joanne C. Smith, President & CEO
Edward B. Case, Executive Vice President
M. Jude Reyes, Chair
Offers evaluation and treatment of patients with acute and sub-acute musculoskeletal and sports injuries. RIC offers different levels of care, including inpatient, day rehabilitation, and outpatients services, according to the special needs of each patient

6651 Children's Home and Aid Society of Illinois
125 South Wacker Drive
14th Floor
Chicago, IL 60606-4448 312-424-0200
www.childrenshomeandaid.org
Beverley Sibblies, Chairman
Chris Leahy, Vice-Chairman
Mark Tresnowski, Secretary
Private state-wide. Multi-service, racially integrated staff and client populations. Provides educational, placement and community services for children-at-risk and their families. Advocacy, consultation and follow-up services provided according to our ph

6652 Clinton County Rehabilitation Center
1665 North Fourth Street
P O Box 157
Breese, IL 62230- 1791 618-526-8800
Fax: 618-526-2021
info@commlink.org
commlink.org
Wesley A. Gozia, President
Judge Joseph L. Heimann, Vice President
John L. Lengerman, Treasurer
Provides Adult Day Programs (developmental training, work training, job readiness and job placements); Residentail Programs (CILA Intermittent Care, CILA 24 hour care); Infant Programs (early interventions, early head start); Community Services (specializ

6653 Continucare, A Service of the Rehab Institute of Chicago
West Suburban Hospital Medical Center
3 Erie Ct
Oak Park, IL 60302-2519 708-383-6200
800-354-7342
Fax: 312-908-1369
Heidi Asbury MD
We respond to the needs of the whole person: body, mind and spirit. We foster a climate of care, hospitality and a spirit of community. We develop systems and structures that attend to the needs of those at risk of discrimination because of age, gender, lifestyle, ethnic background, religious beliefs or socioeconomic status.

6654 Delta Center
1400 Commercial Ave
Cairo, IL 62914-1978 618-734-2665
800-471-7213
Fax: 618-734-1999
deltacenter.org
Lisa Tolbert, Executive Director
Lisa Tholbert, Assistant Executive Director
The Delta Center is a non-profit mental health center, substance abuse counseling facility, and also provides various community services to Alexander and Pulaski County, Illinois. The purpose and mission is to promote, encourage, foster and engage exclusi

6655 Division of Rehabilitation-Education Services, University of Illinois
Beckwith Hall
201 E. John Street
Champaign, IL 61820- 6901 217-333-4603
Fax: 217-333-0248
disability@uiuc.edu
Ann Fredricksen, Disability Specialist
Jon Gunderson, Coordinator
Pat Malik, Director

6656   Easterseals DuPage and Fox Valley
830 S Addison Ave.
Villa Park, IL 60181-1153   630-620-4433
                                    Fax: 630-620-1148
                                    info@eastersealsdfvr.org
                                    www.easterseals.com/dfv

Theresa Forthofer, President & CEO
Dave Gardner, Chief Financial Officer
Kathy Moreland, Vice President, Development
The mission of Easterseals DuPage and Fox Valley is to enable infants, children and adults with disabilities to achieve maximum independence and to provide support to their families. Key services provided include physical, occupational, speech-language, nutrition and assistive technology therapies and audiology services for all ages.

6657   Easterseals Gilchrist Marchman Child Development Center
1312 S Racine Ave.
Chicago, IL 60608   312-492-7402
                                    Fax: 312-492-9014
                                    www.easterseals.com

Sara Ray Stoelinga, Chief Executive Officer
Ann O'Malley, Contact
An early childhood and education program for children ages 6 weeks to 5 years. Focuses on social and intellectual development through family-centered education.

6658   Easterseals Jayne Shover Center
799 S McLean Blvd.
Elgin, IL 60123   847-742-3264
                                    Fax: 847-742-9436
                                    www.easterseals.com/dfv

Theresa Forthofer, President & CEO
Kimberly Garcia, Contact
A free-standing, comprehensive outpatient rehabilitation center serving children and adults with physical and developmental disabilities.

6659   Easterseals Joliet Region
212 Barney Dr.
Joliet, IL 60435   815-725-2194
                                    Fax: 815-725-5150
                                    www.easterseals.com/joliet

Deb Condotti, President & CEO
David Gardner, Chief Financial Officer
Vanessa Hunter, Director, Residential & Social Services
Services for children and adults with disabilities and their families. Pediatric therapy, residential programs, special home placement, inclusive child care, and early intervention.

6660   El Valor
Main Office & Developmental Training Center
1850 W 21st St
Chicago, IL 60608   312-666-4511
                                    Fax: 312-666-6677
                                    TTY: 312-666-3361
                                    info@elvalor.net
                                    elvalor.org

Rafael Malpica, Chairman
Rey B Gonzalez, President & CEO
Carmen Ziegler, Chief Financial Officer
El Valor's mission is to serve people with disabilities and their families, by offering programs in the areas of early childhood education, adult services and parental and community engagement.

6661   Elgin Training Center
Association For Individual Development Elgin Area
1135 Bowes Road
Elgin, IL 60123-1321   847-931-6200
                                    Fax: 847-888-6079
                                    www.the-association.org

Chuck Miles, Chairmen
Patrick Flaherty, Vice Chairmen
Walter Dwyer, Treasurer
Day training services to develop work habits and attitudes while providing training in small product assembly, sorting, packaging, collating, & material handling. Instruction also offered in job related knowledge & in personal, social and independent living skills. There is also an on-site specialized Autism Program. Addi-

tionally, residential programs (group homes & apartments) are also available for people with developmental disabilities.

6662   Family Counseling Center
PO Box 759
Golconda, IL 62938   618-683-2461
                                    Fax: 618-683-2066
                                    fccinconline.org

Larry Mizell, Executive Director
Connie Duncan, Director
Nora Beth Hacker, Financial Director
Provides counseling, developmental training, evaluations, assisted living services, referrals, psychosocial rehabilitation, and a variety of work services.

6663   Family Matters
A RC Community Support Systems
1901 S. 4th St
Ste 209
Effingham, IL 62401-4123   217-347-5428
                                    866-436-7842
                                    Fax: 217-347-5119
                                    deinhorn@arc-css.org
                                    www.fmptic.org

Debbie Einhorn, Executive Director
Debbie Einhorn, Director Family Support
Nancy Mader, Project Coordinator
Parent Training and Information Center and family support programs for families of children who have disabilities from the ages of birth through 21. Services include: Parent support and training, school advocacy, home visits, information and referral, pa

6664   Five Star Industries
1308 Wells Street Road
P O Box 60
Du Quoin, IL 62832-60   618-542-5421
                                    Fax: 618-542-5556
                                    5starind.com

Susan Engelhardt, Executive Director
Incorporated as a private, non-profit corporation under the laws of the State of Illinois, is an equal opportunity employer and provides equal opportunity in compliance with the Civil Rights Act of 1964 and all other appropriate laws, rules and regulation

6665   HSI Austin Center For Development
1819 S Kedzie Ave
Chicago, IL 60623-2623   773-854-1676
                                    Fax: 773-854-8300
Provides an educational program designed to enhance academic, behavioral and social performance of children 4-14 years of age experiencing emotional disorders that result in exclusion from the public school setting.

6666   Hyde Park-Woodlawn
950 E 61st St
Chicago, IL 60637-2623   773-324-0280
                                    Fax: 773-324-0285

Clarissa Williams, Manager

6667   Illinois Center for Autism
548 South Ruby Lane
Fairview Heights, IL 62208-2614   618-398-7500
                                    Fax: 618-394-9869
                                    info@illinoiscenterforautism.org
                                    illinoiscenterforautism.org

Hardy Ware, Chairperson
Thomas E. Berry, Vice Chairperson
Gary Guthrie, Secretary
A community-based mental health/educational treatment center dedicated to serving autistic clients.

6668   Julius and Betty Levinson Center
1825 K Street NW
Suite 600
Washington, DC 60304-1557   202-776-0406
                                    800-872-5827
                                    Fax: 708-383-9025
                                    www.ucp.org

Woody Connette, Chair
Ian Ridlon, Vice Chair
Mark Boles, Treasurer

621

Houses one of its three adult developmental training programs for substantially physically disabled men and women.

6669 Lake County Health Department
18 N. County Street
Waukegan, IL 60085
847-377-2000
Fax: 847-336-1517
www.lakecountyil.gov

Aaron Lawlor, Chairman
Stevenson Mountsier, Vice Chairman
Barry Burton, Administrator
Includes counseling, crisis intervention, emergency management, psychotherapy and chemotherapy management for individuals and families.

6670 Little Friends, Inc.
140 N Wright Street
Naperville, IL 60540-4799
630-355-6533
Fax: 630-355-3176
info@lilfriends.com
www.littlefriendsinc.com

Dan Casey, Chairman
Matt Johanson, Vice Chairman
Michele Calbi, Treasurer
Little Friends has been serving children and adults with autism and other developmental disabilities for over 40 years. Based in Naperville, Little Friends operates three schools, vocational training programs, community-based residential services and the

6671 MAP Training Center
7th and Mc Kinley St
Karnak, IL 62956
618-634-9401
Fax: 618-634-9090

Larry Earnhart, President
Cindy Earnhart, Community Liaison
Training, employment, residential and support services, targeted for adults with developmental disabilities.

6672 Macon Resources
2121 Hubbard Ave.
P O Box 2760
Decatur, IL 62524-2760
217-875-1910
Fax: 217-875-8899
TTY: 217-875-8898
maconresources.org

Tom Hill, President
Michael Breheny, Vice President
Barb Nadler, Secretary
The purpose is to provide a comprehensive array of habilitative/rehabilitative training programs and support services to assist individuals and/or family units of an individual with a developmental disability, mental illness, or other handicapping conditi

6673 Mary Bryant Home for the Blind
2960 Stanton
Springfield, IL 62703-4385
217-529-1611
888-529-1611
Fax: 217-529-6975
mbha@marybryanthome.org
marybryanthome.org

Jerry Curry, Executive Director
Robert E. Maxey, President
Allan J. Rupel, Vice President
Supportive living facility for blind or visually impaired adults over the age of 22. A supportive living facility remodeled to foster the move to increased independence for residents. The new apartment style housing combined with personal care and other a

6674 Northern Illinois Special Recreation Association (NISRA)
285 Memorial Drive
Crystal Lake, IL 60014-3650
815-459-0737
Fax: 815-459-0388
info@nisra.org
www.nisra.org

Brian Shahinian, Executive Director
Carol Amoroso, Manager of Finance and Personnel
Kerri Ruddy, Manager of Office Services

Leisure and recreation services to those with disabilities who are unable to participate successfully in park district and city recreation programs.

6675 Oak Forest Hospital of Cook County
15900 Cicero Ave
Oak Forest, IL 60452
708-687-7200
Fax: 708-687-7979
TTY: 708-687-4794
http://www.cchil.org

Robert Weinstein, Department Chair
Suja Mathew, Associate Chair
A 654 bed health care center devoted to the diagnosis, rehabilitation and long-term care of adults suffering from chronic illnesses, diseases and physical impairments.

6676 PARC
1913 W. Townline Road
P.O.Box 3418
Peoria, IL 61615-3418
309-691-3800
Fax: 309-689-3613
parcway.org

Pat Kawczynski, Chair
Heyl Royster, Vice Chair
Terry Waters, Treasurer
Serves all ages that are diagnosed with developmental and physical disabilities. Programs include early intervention, family support, respite care, vocational training, supported employment, adult day programs and residential.

6677 Peoria Area Blind People's Center
2905 W Garden St
Peoria, IL 61605-1316
309-637-3693
Fax: 309-637-3693
info@cicbvi.org
cicbvi.org

Carol Warren, President
Cora Quinn, Vice President
Prasad Parupalli, Treasurer
Offers services for the totally blind, legally blind, visually impaired, and more with health, counseling, educational, recreational, rehabilitation, computer training and professional training services.

6678 Pioneer Center for Human Services
4031 W Dayton St
McHenry, IL 60050
815-344-1230
Fax: 815-344-3815
TTY: 815-344-6243
gethelp@pioneercenter.org

Dan McCaleb, Chairman
Sam Tenuto, Co-CEO
Frank Samuel, Co-CEO
Pioneer Center is a non-profit agency in McHenry County delivering services to more than 4,000 people annually. Pioneer Center provides developmental disability services, youth and family behavioral health services and homeless services (McHenry County PADS).

6679 Prosthetics and Orthotics Center in Blue Island
2310 York St
Blue Island, IL 60406-2411
708-597-2611
800-354-7342
Fax: 800-908-1932
www.rehabchicago.org/about/blue_island.php
Provides orthotic and prosthetic fittings and follow-up services to adults and children in the south suburbs of Chicago.

6680 RB King Counseling Center
2300 N Edward St
Decatur, IL 62526-4163
217-877-8121
Fax: 217-875-0966

Gordon Cross MD
Offers outpatient, individual, group, divorce and meditation, family and re-adjustment counseling.

6681   REHAB Products and Services
3715 N Vermilion St
Danville, IL 61832-1130   217-446-1146
                                 Fax: 217-446-1191
                                 workse.org

Frank L. Brunacci, President/CEO
Crystal Meece, Vice President Production
Todd Seabaugh, VP Programs
janitorial, lawn care, distribution services.

6682   RIC Northshore
Rehabilitation Institute of Chicago
345 E Superior St
Chicago, IL 60611-2654   312-238-1000
                                800-354-7342
                                webmaster@ric.org
                                www.rehabchicago.org

Joanne C. Smith, President/CEO
Edward B. Case, Vice President
Provides rehabilitation for sports-related injuries,
musculoskeletal conditions, neurological conditions, stroke, arthritis, amputation, burns, and general deconditioning.

6683   RIC Prosthetics and Orthotics Center
Rehabilitation Institute of Chicago
345 E. Superior Street
Suite 101
Chicago, IL 60611-4615   312-238-1000
                                800-345-7342
                                Fax: 708-957-8353
                                webmaster@rehabchicago.org
                                ric.org

Martin Buckner, CPO, Inpatient Coordinator
Nicole T. Soltys, CP, Clinical Coordinator
Robert D. Lipschutz, CP, Director of Prosthetic and Orthotic
Education
Offers almost all the prosthetics and orthotics services provided
at RIC's main hospital in downtown Chicago, including consulta-
tions, fittings and training.

6684   RIC Windermere House
5548 S Hyde Park Blvd
Chicago, IL 60637-1909   773-256-5050
                                800-354-7342
                                Fax: 773-256-5060
                                www.rehabchicago.org

Meghan Scalise, Manager
Evaluation, therapeutic services and patient education are offered in the areas of arthritis, multiple sclerosis, musculoskeletal
conditions, orthopedics, stroke, spinal cord injury, brain injury
and sports medicine.

6685   Ray Graham Association for People with Disabilities
901 Warrenville Road
Suite 500
Lisle, IL 60532-1038   630-620-2222
                                Fax: 630-628-2350
                                TTY: 630-628-2352
                                cathyfickerterill@yahoo.com
                                ray-graham.org

Michael Komoll, Chairperson
Neville Bilimoria, Vice Chairperson
Kim zoeller, President & CEO
Provides developmental services at 15 sites to infants, children
and adults with disabilities. Services range from 1 hr/wk respite
to full-time residential.

6686   Reach Rehabilitation Program: Americana Healthcare
9401 S Kostner Ave
Oak Lawn, IL 60453-2697   708-423-1505
                                Fax: 708-423-3822

Jean M Roche, Owner
Postacute rehabilitation program.

6687   Rehabilitation Achievement Center
345 E Superior St
Chicago, IL 60611-4805   312-238-1000
                                800-354-7342
                                www.ric.org

M. Jude Reyes, Chair
Mike P. Krasny, Vice Chair
Joanne C. Smith, President & CEO
Rehabilitation Institute of Chicago (RIC) has aquired the assets
of the Rehabilitation Achievement Center (RAC).

**6688   Rehabilitation Institute of Chicago: Alexian Brothers
Medical Center**
800 Biesterfield Rd
Elk Grove Village, IL 60007-3361   847-437-5500
                                      866-253-9426
                                      Fax: 847-631-5663
                                      TTY: 847-956-5116
                                      www.alexianbrothershealth.org

Mark Frey, President and Chief Executive Officer
Tracy Rogers, Senior Vice President and Chief Operating Officer
Paul Belter, Senior Vice President and Chief Financial Officer
A 32-bed rehabilitation unit under the medical direction and su-
pervision of the Rehabilitation Institute of Chicago.

6689   Riverside Medical Center
Mental Health Unit
350 N Wall St
Kankakee, IL 60901-2991   815-933-1671
                                Fax: 815-935-8160
                                rhuber@rsh.net
                                riversidehealthcare.org

Phillip Kambic, CEO
Bill W. Douglas, Vice President
Offers recreation, parenting therapy, emergency services, psychological testing and inpatient treatment programs. Riverside is
nationally recognized for its specialty programs in heart care, obstetrics, trauma, oncology, rehabilitation, geriatrics, occupa

**6690   Robert Young Mental Health Center Division of Trinity
Regional Haelth System**
Trinity Health Foundation
2701 17th St
Rock Island, IL 61201-5351   309-779-2800
                                800-322-1431
                                Fax: 309-779-2027
                                www.unitypoint.org

Rick Seidler, President & CEO
Jim Hayes, CFO
Tamara Byram, VP, Legal/Compliance
Services include comprehensive inpatient rehabilitation, chronic
pain management programs, outpatient medical rehabilitation,
work hardening programs, vocational evaluation, alcohol and
other drug dependency rehabilitation programs, Burn Center, and
menta

6691   Sampson-Katz Center
216 West Jackson Blvd
Suite 700
Chicago, IL 60606-2104   312-673-3400
                                Fax: 312-553-5544
                                TTY: 773-761-6672
                                jvsskc@jvschicago.org
                                www.jvschicago.org

Andrew M. Glick, Chair
John L. Daniels, Vice Chair
H. Debra Levin, President

6692   Shelby County Community Services
160 North Main Street
Memphis, TN 38103-650   901-222-2300
                                Fax: 912-222-2090
                                www.shelbycountytn.gov

Dottie Jones, Director
Primary focus is substance abuse treatment.

6693   Streator Unlimited
305 N Sterling St
P O Box 706
Streator, IL 61364-2369   815-673-5574
                                      Fax: 815-673-1714
                            contact@streatorunlimited.org
                              www.streatorunlimited.org
Jeffrey Dean, Executive Director
Lynn Fukar, Director of Day Services
Julie Caestens, Director Residential Services
Vocational and personal skills training, residential services, client and family support, supported and computerized employment. Serves adults with intellectual disabilities with the goal of enabling them to reach their fullest potential, live as independ

6694   Swedish Covenant Hospital Rehabilitation Services
5145 N California Ave
Chicago, IL 60625-3661   773-878-8200
                                      Fax: 773-561-0490
Mark Newton, President & CEO
Provides acute rehabilitation services, subacute care and outpatient services for many types of disabling injuries and conditions, including amputation, arthritis, brain injury, general deconditioning, multiple sclerosis, musculoskeletal injuries, stroke,

6695   TCRC Sight Center
21310 Route 9
Tremont, IL 61568-2558   309-347-7148
                                      Fax: 309-925-4241
                                      info@tcrcorg.com
                                      www.tcrcorg.com
Jamie Durdel, President & CEO
Molly Anderson, Vice President
Offers services for persons who are totally blind, legally blind, partially sighted or visually impaired along with other disabilities. Have support group, rehabilitation classes, orientation and mobility services, counseling services, low vision clinic,

6696   Tazewell County Resource Center
Box 12
Rr 1
Tremont, IL 61568   309-347-7148
                                      Fax: 309-925-4241
                                      info@tcrcorg.com
                                      http://www.tcrcorg.com
Jamie Durdel, President & CEO
Molly Anderson, Vice President
A private, nonprofit agency providing programs for the special needs of infants, adults, children and their families residing in Tazewell County. Services offered include: birth-three infant/parent program, adult day care services, family support, residen

6697   Trumbull Park
10530 S Oglesby Ave
Chicago, IL 60617-6140   773-375-7022
                                      Fax: 773-375-5528
Gregory Terry, Director
Diana Moore, Site Supervisor
Ada McKinley, Manager
Offers consultation, education, general counseling, recreation, self-help and social services for children and adults.

6698   University of Illinois Medical Center
1740 West Taylor Street
Chicago, IL 60612-7232   312-355-4000
                                           866-600-2273
                                      Fax: 312-996-7770
                                      hospital.uillinois.edu
Rajiv Pai, Chief
Marilyn Plomann, Manager
Offers services for the totally blind, legally blind, visually impaired, and more with health, counseling, educational, recreational, rehabilitation, computer training and professional training services.

6699   VanMatre Rehabilitation Center
950 S Mulford Rd
Rockford, IL 61108-4274   815-381-8500
                                           866-754-3347
                                      Fax: 815-484-9953
                            webcontentcoordinator@rhsnet.org
                              www.vanmatrerehab.com
Gary E. Kaatz, President and Chief Executive Officer
Scott Craig, Medical Director
A CARF-accredited comprehensive rehabilitation center based within the Rockford Memorial Hospital providing inpatient and outpatient services for physically and cognitively challenged persons with debilitating illness and injuries.

6700   Warren Achievement Center
1220 E 2nd Ave
Monmouth, IL 61546-2404   309-734-3131
                                      Fax: 309-734-7114
                            info@warrenachievement.com
                              warrenachievement.com
Rick Barnhill, President
Jim Kesse, Vice President
Sherry Waite, Chief Operations Officer
For developmentally disabled children and adults. Parent-infant education programs are for parents of infants with disabilities or developmental delays; Children's Group Homes which serve children on a fulltime basis and can serve additional children on a

Indiana

6701   Ball Memorial Hospital
2401 W University Ave
Muncie, IN 47303-3499   765-747-3111
                                      Fax: 765-747-3313
                              iuhealth.org/ball-memorial
Mike Haley, CEO
Offers rehabilitation services, occupational therapy, physical therapy and more for the physically challenged child or adult.

6702   Community Health Network
1500 N Ritter Ave
Indianapolis, IN 46219-3027   317-355-4275
                                           800-775-7775
                                      Fax: 317-351-7723
                                      www.ecommunity.com
Keith Thompson, Manager
Anita Harden, President
A leading not-for-profit health system offering convenient access to expert physicians, advanced treatments and leading edge technology, all focused on getting patients well and back to their lives. With caring compassion, Community's 5 hospitals and 70 + sites of care continually strive to improve the health and well-being of those individuals in central Indiana who entrust care to us.

6703   Crossroads Industrial Services
8302 E 33rd Street
Indianapolis, IN 46226   317-897-7320
                                      Fax: 317-897-9763
                         info@crossroadsindustrialservices.com
                         www.crossroadsindustrialservices.c om
Anne Shupe, Finance Executive
Curtiss Quirin, CEO
Assisting customers with short-term, seasonal, and long-term outsourcing needs. Many consider Crossroads an extension of their company

6704   Department of Veterans Affairs Vet Center #418
302 W. Washington St
Room E120
Indianapolis, IN 46204- 2738   317-232-3910
                                           800-490-4520
                                      Fax: 317-232-7721
                              www.in.gov/veteran/sso/fac
Charles T. Applegate, Director
Provides readjustment counseling to combat veterans. Onsite assistance for employment problems, vocational rehabilitation and sexual trauma counsel.

6705 **Easterseals Rehabilitation Center**
3701 Bellemeade Ave.
Evansville, IN 47714   812-479-1411
                            www.easterseals.com/in-sw
Kelly Schneider, President
Guy Davis, Vice President, Administration
Laura Terhune, Vice President, Development
Services include therapy and medical rehabilitation, assistive
technology, early intervention, early care and education, and
community employment.

6706 **Frasier Rehabilitation Center Division of Clark**
Memorial Hospital
2201 Greentree N
Clarksville, IN 47129-8957   812-218-6590
                            Fax: 812-218-6597
            http://www.jhsmh.org/Frazier-Rehab-Institute-
Catherine Lucas Spalding, Administrator
Designed to help patients in their adjustment to a physically limiting condition, both psychologically and physically, by helping to
maximize each patient's abilities so he or she can function as independently as possible. The program treats patients whos

6707 **HealthSouth Deaconess Rehabilitation Hospital**
4100 Covert Ave
Evansville, IN 47714-5559   812-476-9983
                                  800-677-3422
                            Fax: 812-476-4270
                        www.healthsouthdeaconess.com
Barbara Butler, Chief Executive Officer
Ashok. Dhingra, M.D, Medical Director
Brett Hirt, Director, Therapy Operations
AHealthSouth Deaconess Rehabilitation Hospital is a joint venture partner with Deaconess Health System. Our hospital is an
80-bed inpatient rehabilitation hospital that offers comprehensive inpatient and outpatient rehabilitation services designed to
return patients to leading active and independent lives.

6708 **Healthwin Specialized Care**
20531 Darden Rd
South Bend, IN 46637-2999   574-272-0100
                            Fax: 574-277-3233
                              info@healthwin.org
                                  healthwin.org
Connie McCahill, President
Lauren Davis, Vice President
John Cergnul, Treasurer
No other facility in the area has a homelike environment like ours.
Its simply part of our culture. Rehabilitation therapy that includes
physical, occupational, speech, respiratory and a full time
in-house therapist. Other services include a wound special

6709 **Memorial Regional Rehabilitation Center**
615 N Michigan St
South Bend, IN 46601-1033   574-647-1000
                                  877-282-0964
Johan Kuitse, MSA, PT, Outpatient Clinical Manager
Anne Clifford, DPT, Physical Therapists
Shanti Shrestha Dalson, DPT, Physical Therapists
20-bed CARF accredited inpatient rehabilitation, outpatient orthopedic clinic and work performance program, head injury
clinic. Outpatient neuro rehab and a driver education and training
program are provided.

6710 **Saint Joseph Regional Medical Center- South Bend**
5215 Holy Cross Parkway
Mishawaka, IN 46545-2814   574-335-5000
                            Fax: 574-237-7312
                            thefoundation@sjrmc.com
                                  sjmed.com
Albert Gutierrez, President & CEO
Steven Gable, Vice President
Janice Dunn, CFO
Continuum of rehabilitation services offered. Included are: acute
rehabilitation, a 26 bed CARF accredited comprehensive inpa-
tient unit, a CARF certified inpatient brain injury program, a
CARF outpatient day treatment brain injury program,
comprehensive o

Iowa

6711 **Crossroads of Western Iowa**
1 Crossroads Pl
Missouri Valley, IA 51555-6069   712-642-4114
                            Fax: 712-642-4115
                                info@cwiowa.org
                              explorecrossroads.com
Brent Dillinger, CEO
Pat Kocour, President
Steven Van Riper, Vice President
CWI provides services in Missouri Valley, Onawa and Council
Bluffs, Iowa. An array of services for people with mental illness,
developmental disabilities and brain injury are provided in each
location.

6712 **Des Moines Division-VA Central Iowa Health Care**
System
3600 30th St
Des Moines, IA 50310-5753   515-699-5999
                                  800-294-8387
                            Fax: 515-699-5862
                              www.centraliowa.va.gov
Judith Johnson-Mekota, Director
Fredrick Bahls, Chief Of Staff
Susan A. Martin, Associate Director
VA Cental Iowa Health Care System is the result of the 1997
merger of the Des Moines and Knoxville, Iowa, VA Medical Cen-
ters. This integrated healthcare system brings 2 previously sepa-
rate organizational structures, located 40 miles apart, into one
cohesi

6713 **Easterseals Iowa**
401 NE 66th Ave.
Des Moines, IA 50313   515-289-1933
                            Fax: 515-289-1281
                            TTY: 515-289-4069
                              www.easterseals.com/ia
Sherri Nielsen, President & CEO
Kevin Small, Chief Financial Officer
Allison Piazza, Chief Development Officer
Provides services to Iowans with disabilities. Services include
vocational and employment training, camping recreation and re-
spite services, craft training and sales, home and farm adapta-
tions, and transportation.

6714 **Genesis Regional Rehabilitation Center**
Genesis Health System
1227 E.Rusholme Street
Davenport, IA 52803-3396   563-421-1000
                            Fax: 563-421-3499
                                genesishealth.com
Doug Cropper, President & CEO
Kenneth Croken, Vice President
Joseph Lohmuller, Chief Medical Officer
Serves persons of all ages experiencing a disability, whether ac-
quired at birth or following a serious interdisciplinary service.
Rehabilitation programs include acute rehabilitation; adult reha-
bilitation, pediatric rehabilitation, outpatient orthopaedics

6715 **Homelink**
Van G Miller & Associates
1101 W S Marnan Drive
Waterloo, IA 50701-2817   319-235-7173
                                  866-575-8483
                            Fax: 319-235-7822
                    homelinkprivacyofficer@vgm.com
                              www.vgmhomelink.com
Dave Kazynski, President
Rick Hibben, Coordinator
A national network of home medical equipment, respiratory ther-
apy, rehabilitation and infusion therapy service providers with
over 2,500 locations serving all fifty states.

6716 **Iowa Central Industries**
127 Avenue M
Fort Dodge, IA 50501-5797   515-576-2126
                            Fax: 515-576-2251
Tom Eckman, Executive Director

Services include evaluation and training in pre-vocational and vocational skills, personal behavior management, cognitive skills, communication skills, self-care skills and social skills. Services arranged include: independent living training, medical ser

6717 Life Skills Laundry Division
1510 Industrial Rd SW
Le Mars, IA 51031-3009
712-546-4785
Fax: 712-546-4985

Don Nore, Executive Director

6718 MIW
909 S 14th Ave
Marshalltown, IA 50158-3610
641-752-3697
Fax: 641-752-1614

Rich Byers, President/CEO
Vocational services for adults with disabilities. Includes organizational employment services, supported employment, job placement.

6719 Mercy Dubuque Physical Rehabilitation Unit
250 Mercy Drive
Dubuque, IA 52001-7320
563-589-8000
Fax: 563-589-8162
www.mercydubuque.com

Russel M. Knight, CEO
Provides services which open the door to improved communication, offering the opportunity to enrich the quality of life. Mercy offers many other branches of services including, rehabilitation services for children and a pulmonary rehabilitation program.

6720 Mercy Medical Center-Pain Services
1111 6th Ave
Des Moines, IA 50314-2611
515-247-3121
Fax: 515-248-8867
webmaster@mercydesmoines.org

Dana L. Simon, MD
Dave Vellinga, President & CEO
Laurie Conner, Vice President
An outpatient program dedicated to helping people with chronic pain live more productive, satisfying lives. The program is not designed for conditions that are surgically curable, but rather approaches the problem using a comprehensive, holistic treatment.

6721 Nishna Productions-Shenandoah Work Center
902 Day Street
Shenandoah, IA 51601-70
712-246-1242
Fax: 712-246-1243

Mary Rolf, President
Sherri Clark, Executive Director
Melissa Mueller, Program Manager
Shelter, workshop and job training for the disabled. Some of the services we provide are Work Activity, Adult Day Activity Program, Personal & Social Adjustment, Residential Services, Home & Community Based Services & Employment Resources.

6722 Northstar Community Services
3420 University Avenue
Waterloo, IA 50701-2050
319-236-0901
888-879-1365
Fax: 319-236-3701
www.northstarcs.org

Mark Witmar, Executive Director
Jeff Conrey, President
Kathy Folkerts, Vice President
Provides adult day services, employment services and supported community living so people with disabilities can live and work in the community.

6723 Options of Linn County
935 2nd street
SW
Cedar Rapids, IA 52404-3100
319-892-5000
Fax: 319-892-5849
linncounty.org

Joel D. Miller, Auditor
Sharon Gonzalez, Treasurer
Options of Linn County works with community businesses in providing employment services to adults with disabilities. Options is a publicly operated service provider within the Linn County Community Services department.

6724 RISE
106 Rainbow Dr
Elkader, IA 52043-9075
563-245-1868
Fax: 563-245-2859

Ed Josten, Manager

6725 Ragtime Industries
116 N 2nd St
Albia, IA 52531-1624
641-932-7813
Fax: 641-932-7814

Lisa Glenn, Executive Director
A work-oriented rehabilitation organization which provides training for mentally and physically disabled adults in Monroe County. A variety of programs which help to develop each person's individual potential are offered.

6726 Sunshine Services
1106 East 9th St
Spencer, IA 51301-225
712-262-7805
Fax: 712-262-8369

Ann Vandehar, Executive Director

6727 Tenco Industries
710 Gateway Dr
Ottumwa, IA 52501-2204
641-682-8114
Fax: 641-684-4223
www.tenco.org

Ben Wright, Executive Director
Dixie Merritt, Vocational Director
Brenda Miller, Marketing and Development DirectoR
To advocate and provide opportunities for people with disabilities, or conditions that limit their abilities, to develop and maintain the skills necessary for personal dignity and independence in all areas of life. Provide a wide array of services to individuals with disabilities. By looking at each person as individuals, we are able to work with them to maximize their skills. Residentials services, including HCBS and CSALA are also provided in all communities.

Kansas

6728 Arrowhead West
1100 E Wyatt Earp Blvd
Dodge City, KS 67801-5337
620-227-8803
Fax: 620-227-8812
web@arrowheadwest.org
www.arrowheadwest.org

Kelly Mason, Chairperson
Michael Stein, Vice Chairperson
Lori Pendergast, President
Services and programs offered include: developmental and therapy services for children birth to age 3; adult center-based work services and community integrated employment options; adult life skills and retirement programs; and adult residential services.

6729 Big Lakes Developmental Center
1416 Hayes Dr
Manhattan, KS 66502-5066
785-776-9201
Fax: 785-776-9830
biglakes@biglakes.org
biglakes.org

Lori Feldkamp, President
Shawn Funk, Community Education Director
A private nonprofit Community Developmental Disability Organization (CDDO) serving individuals with developmental disabilities in Riley, Geary, Clay and Pottawatome counties in Kansas. Big lakes is supported by county mill levy and federal and state fundi

6730 Developmental Services of Northwest Kansas
2703 Hall St
Suite 10
Hays, KS 67601-1964
785-625-5678
800-637-2229
Fax: 785-625-8204

Jerry Michaud, President
Ruth Lang, Administrative Assistant
A private nonprofit organization serving both children and adults with disabilities. Offers services to children ages birth to three

years, youth and adults through a network of community-based and outreach programs and inter-agency agreements with other

6731 ENVISION
2301 S Water St
Wichita, KS 67213-4819
316-267-2244
Fax: 316-267-4312
Info@envisionus.com
www.envisionus.com

Sam Williams, Chair
Jon Rosell, PhD, Vice-Chair
Michael Monteferrante, President and CEO
Provides jobs, job training and vision rehabilitation services to people who are blind or low vision. A private not-for-profit agency uniquely combining employment opportunitites with rehabilitation services and public education.

6732 Heartspring
8700 E 29th St N
Wichita, KS 67226-2169
316-634-8700
800-835-1043
Fax: 316-634-0555
kgrover@heartspring.org
www.heartspring.org

Gary W. Singleton, President and CEO
Paul Faber, Executive Vice President, Operations
Katie Grover, Director Of Marketing
Heartspring provides outpatient therapies, evaluations and consultations for children with special needs through Heartspring Pediatric Services. The Heartspring School is a residential and day school for children ages 5-21 with multiple disabilities. Children with autism and their families receive resources through the Heartspring CARE program. The Heartspring Hearing Center provides services to individuals of all ages.

6733 Indian Creek Nursing Center
6515 W 103rd St
Overland Park, KS 66212-1798
913-633-7000
Fax: 913-642-3982
www.savaseniorcare.com

Randy Sutterfield, Administrator
Postacute rehabilitation program. A 120-bed nursing home facility.

6734 Johnson County Developmental Supports
111 South Cherry Street
Olathe, KS 66061-1223
913-715-5000
Fax: 913-715-0800
info@jocogov.org
www.jocogov.org

Ed Eilert, Chairman
Michael Lally, Vice Chair
Scott Tschudy, Treasurer
JCDS is the community Developmental Disability Organization for Johnson County, Kansas. Provides supports in the form of direct services to people on a daily basis.

6735 Ketch Industries
1006 E Waterman St
Wichita, KS 67211-1525
316-383-8700
800-766-3777
Fax: 316-383-8715
webmaster@ketch.org
ketch.org

Fred Badders, Chairman
Carla Bienhoff, Chairman
Loren Anthony, Secretary
The mission of Ketch is to promote independence for persons with disabilities through innovative learning experiences that support individuals choices for working, living and playing in their community.

6736 Lakemary Center
100 Lakemary Dr
Paola, KS 66071-1855
913-557-4000
Fax: 913-557-4910
lakemaryctr.org

William Craig, President
Paul Sokoloff, Chair
Gayle Richardson, Vice Chair

A private, not-for-profit day and residential training facility which provides for the assessment, education, training, therapy and social development of children and adults, moderate and severe developmental disabilities.

6737 Northview Developmental Services
700 E 14th St
Newton, KS 67117-5702
316-283-5170
Fax: 316-283-5196
http://northviewdev.mennonite.net/

Mary Holloway, CEO
The mission is to provide quality supportive and coordinating services to persons with developmental disabilities, assisting them to grow as they integrate into the community. Further, our mission is to improve the quality of their lives by providing acce

Kentucky

6738 Cardinal Hill Rehabilitation Hospital
Cadinal Hill Medical Center
2050 Versailles Rd
Lexington, KY 40504-1499
859-254-5701
800-233-3260
Fax: 859-231-1365
www.cardinalhill.org

Gary R. Payne, CEO
Provides occupational health services, therapy services and urgent medical treatment of injured workers.

6739 Frazier Rehab Institute
220 Abraham Flexner Way
Louisville, KY 40202-1887
502-582-7400
Fax: 502-582-7477

Jamie Ochsner, Manager
Steve Ahr, VP Frazier Rehab/Neurscience
Frazier Rehab Institute is a regional healthcare system dedicated entirely to rehabilitation. Through an expansive network of inpatient and outpatient facilites in Kentucky and southern Indiana, Frazier offers a wide array of services based on one common

6740 HealthSouth Northern Kentucky Rehabilitation Hospital
201 Medical Village Dr
Edgewood, KY 41017-3407
859-341-2044
800-860-6004
Fax: 859-341-2813
www.healthsouthkentucky.com

Richard Evans, CEO
Mary Pfeffer, Director Therapy Operations
Neal Moser, M.D., Medical Director
Offers all types of inpatient and outpatient rehabilitation services such as occupational therapy, physical therapy, speech therapy. Respiratory therpay, Psychology, Aquatics, Case Managemenet/Social Work and Nutritional Services.

6741 King's Daughter's Medical Center's Rehab Unit/Work Hardening Program
2201 Lexington Ave
Ashland, KY 41101-2843
606-408-4000
888-377-5362
Fax: 606-327-7542
info@kdmc.net
www.kdmc.com

Kristie Whitlatch, President & CEO
Matt Ebaugh, VP / Chief Strategy and Information Officer
Philip Fioret, M.D., VP / Chief Medical Officer
Offers a 27-bed, inpatient rehabilitation services unit treating physical disabilities related to accident or illness. The program provides an interdisciplinary inpatient program designed to restore the individual to the highest level of independence. It

6742 LifeSkills Industries
380 Suwannee Trail St
Bowling Green, KY 42103-6499
270-901-5000
800-223-8913
Fax: 270-782-0058
sbell@lifeskills.com
lifeskills.com

Alice Simpson, CEO

LifeSkills will be the reliable advocate, dependable safety net and provider of choice, for high quality, accessible services and supports for the citizens of south-central Kentucky whos lives are affected by mental illness, developmental disablilities or

6743   Low Vision Services of Kentucky
120 N. Eagle Creek Drive
Suite 500
Lexington, KY 40509- 1827

859-263-3900
800-627-2020
Fax: 859-977-1136
jvanarsdall@retinaky.com
www.lowvisionky.com

Regina Callihan-May, O.D.
Jeanne Van Arsdall, Co-ordinator
Maryanne Inman, Practice Administrator
Offers educational, recreational and rehabilitational services and devices for the visually impaired, legally blind, totally blind.

6744   Muhlenberg County Opportunity Center
PO Box 511
Greenville, KY 42345-1416

270-754-5590
Fax: 270-338-5977
muhlon.com

Chuck Hammonds, Manager
Charles Hamonds, Director
Post-acute rehabilitation facility with programs including a workshop with hand packaging of manufactured goods.

6745   New Vision Enterprises
1900 Brownsboro Rd
Louisville, KY 40206-2102

502-893-0211
800-405-9135
Fax: 502-893-3885

Larry Sherman, Plant Manager
Offers employment training and services for the blind and legally blind.

6746   Park DuValle Community Health Center, Inc.
3015 Wilson Ave
Louisville, KY 40211-1969

502-774-4401
Fax: 502-775-6195
www.pdchc.org

Richard K Jones, President
John Howard MD, Medical Director
Dave Gerwig, CFO
Offers services for the totally blind, legally blind, visually impaired, and more with health, counseling, educational, recreational, rehabilitation, computer training and professional training services.

Louisiana

6747   Alliance House
427 S Foster Drive
Baton Rouge, LA 70806-2723

225-987-0013
Fax: 225-346-0857

A non-residential facility serving male and female chronically mentally ill. Services include: social service, vocational evaluation, pre-vocational training and job placement.

6748   Assumption Activity Center
4201 Highway 1
Napoleonville, LA 70390-8628

985-369-2907
Fax: 985-369-2657

Warren Gonzales, Manager
A community work center providing prevocational training and extended employment for adults with disabilities. Services include: social services, work activities, specialized training and supported employment.

6749   Bancroft Rehabilitation Living Centers
425 Kings Highway East
P.O. Box 20
Haddonfield, NJ 08033-0018

504-482-3075
800-774-5516
Fax: 504-483-2135
lynn.tomaio@bancroft.org
www.bancroft.org

Dr. Robert Voogt, Owner
Toni Pergolin, President & CEO
Cynthia Boyer, Executive Director
Mission is to nurture abilities and independence of people with neurological challenges by providing a broad spectrum of advanced therapeutic and educational programs and by fostering the development of best practices in the field through research and pro

6750   Deaf Action Center Of Greater New Orleans
Catholic Charities
1000 Howard Ave
Suite 200
New Orleans, LA 70113-1903

504-523-3755
866-891-2210
Fax: 504-523-2789
TTY: 504-615-4944
www.ccano.org

Tommie A. Vassel, Chairman
Sr.Marjorie Hebert, MSC, President & CEO
This community service and resource center serves deaf, deaf-blind, hard of hearing and speech-impaired persons in the greater New Orleans area regardless of age, religion, race or secondary disability. DAC provides interpreting services, equipment distri

6751   Donaldsville Area Arc
1030 Clay St
Donaldsonville, LA 70346-3518

225-473-4516
daarc@eatel.net

Provides a range of services for developmentally disabled adults and children.

6752   East Jefferson General Hospital Rehab Center
4200 Houma Blvd
Metairie, LA 70006-2996

504-454-4000
www.ejgh.org

Newell D. Normand, Chairman
Ashton J. Ryan, Jr., Vice Chairman
Mark J, Peters, President & CEO
Provides the highest quality, compassionate healthcare to the people we serve. East Jefferson General Hospital will be the region's healthcare leader providing the highest quality care through innovation and collaboration with our team members, medical st

6753   Family Service Society
2515 Canal Street
Suite 201
New Orleans, LA 70119-6489

504-822-0800
Fax: 504-822-0831
family@fsgno.org
www.fsgno.org

L. Blake Jones, Chair
Jackie Sullivan, 1st Vice Chair
Kathleen Vogt, 2nd Vice Chair
Offers services for the totally blind, legally blind, visually impaired, and more with health, counseling, educational, recreational, rehabilitation, computer training and professional training services.

6754   Foundation Industries
9995 Highway 64
Zachary, LA 70791

225-654-6288
Fax: 225-654-3988

Jim Lambert-Oswald, President
Jim Oswald, General Manager
A private, nonprofit sheltered workshop providing extended employment and work activities for the developmentally disabled. Objectives are to build work skills through supervision and develop social interaction.

6755 Handi-Works Productions
2700 Lee St
Alexandria, LA 71301-4358   318-442-3377
                                Fax: 318-473-0858
This is a nonprofit workshop for male and female clients who have vocational handicapping conditions. All types of handicapped persons are served in this non-residential workshop.

6756 Lighthouse for the Blind in New Orleans
123 State St
New Orleans, LA 70118-5793   504-899-4501
                                   888-792-0163
                                Fax: 504-895-4162
                                lighthouselouisiana.org

Curtis Eustis, Chair
Paul Masinter, Chair Elect
Tabatha George, Secretary
Offers services for the totally blind, legally blind, visually impaired, and more with health, counseling, educational, recreational, rehabilitation, computer training and professional training services.

6757 Louisiana Center for the Blind
101 South Trenton Street
Ruston, LA 71270-4431   318-251-2891
                                   800-234-4166
                                Fax: 318-251-0109
                                www.louisianacenter.org

Pam Allen, Executive Director
Neita Ghrigsby, Office Manager
Janette Woodard, Residential Manager
A new kind of orientation and training center for blind persons. The center is privately operated and provides quality instruction in the skills of blindness. Offers employment assistance, computer literacy training, summer training and employment project

6758 Louisiana State University Eye Center
Lousiana State University
433 Bolivar Street
New Orleans, LA 70112-2272   504-568-4808
                                Fax: 504-412-1315
                                www.lsuhsc.edu

Jayne S. Weiss, Director
Kelli McMichael, Manager
The LSU Eye Center is part of the LSU Medical Center complex in downtown New Orleans. It is in the LSU-Lions Building at 2020 Gravier Street between South Bolivar and South Prieur streets.

6759 New Orleans Speech and Hearing Center
1636 Toledano St
New Orleans, LA 70115-4598   504-897-2606
                                Fax: 504-891-6048

Mary Beth Green, President
Jessica Vinturella, Treasurer
Kindall James, Secretary
This non-residential facility serves male and female clients for purposes of evaluating speech and hearing problems and providing speech therapy, hearing aids and other assistive technology for speech and hearing.

6760 Port City Enterprises
836 North Seventh Street
Port Allen, LA 70767-113   225-344-1142
                                   877-344-1142
                                Fax: 225-344-1192
                                www.portcityenterprises.org

William Kleinpeter, President
Mark Graffeo, Vice President
L.J. Treuil Jr, Secretary
Offers supported employment, sheltered work and supervised programs for the developmentally disabled, ages 22 and over.

6761 Rehabilitation Center at Thibodeaux Regional
Rehab Care
602 N Acadia Rd
Thibodaux, LA 70301-4847   985-493-4731
                                   800-822-8442
                                Fax: 985-449-4600
                                www.thibodaux.com/centers-services
Jan Torres, Program Manager
Rose Pipes, Clinical Coordinator
Designed to help patients in their adjustment to a physically limiting condition, both physically and psychologically, by helping to maximize each patients abilities so he or she can function as independently as possible.

6762 St. Patrick RehabCare Unit
RehabCare
524 Doctor Michael Debakey Dr
Lake Charles, LA 70601-5725   337-491-7590
                                   888-722-9355
                                Fax: 337-491-7157
Larry A Hauskins, Manager
Ruth Thornton, Admissions
A comprehensive physical and cognitive rehabilitation program designed to help individuals who have experienced a disabling injury or illness.

6763 The Arc - Iberville
PO Box 264
Plaquemine, LA 70765-0264   225-687-4062
                                arciberville@bellsouth.net
Provides a range of services for adults and children with developmental disabilities.

6764 The Arc Caddo-Bossier
351 Jordan St.
Shreveport, LA 71101   318-221-8392

Janet Parker, Executive Director
Chris Hackler, COO, Program & Services
Nonprofit agency providing services to adults and children with developmental disabilities

6765 Touro Rehabilitation Center - LCMC (Louisiana Children's Medical Center)
1401 Foucher St
New Orleans, LA 70115-3515   504-897-8565
                                Fax: 504-897-8393
                                www.touro.com/rehab
Jeanette Ray, VP of Rehab and Post Acute Srv
Janet Clark, Director of Inpatient Rehabilitation Programs
Marylee Pontillas, Director of Outpatient Rehab Srv
Located in New Orleans' Garden District, Touro Rehabilitation is a comprehensive rehabilitation facility dedicated to the restoration of function and independence for individuals with disabilities. The scope of rehabilitation services is broad, with 3 CARF accreditations for Brain Injury, Spinal Cord Injury and General Rehabilitation. TRC opened in 1984 and offers 69 rehab beds. TRC is part of Touro Infirmary which has a proud 150 year history as a nonprofit teaching hospital.

6766 Training, Resource & Assistive-Technology
2000 Lakeshore Drive
New Orleans, LA 70148-1   504-280-6000
                                   888-514-4275
                                Fax: 504-280-5707
                                ggaglian@uno.edu
                                www.uno.edu
Ken Zangla, Director
Naomi Moore, Assistant Director
Connie Lanier, Coordinator
Provides quality services to persons with disabilities, rehabilitation professionals, educators and employers. Built a solid reputation for its innovative training programs and community outreach efforts. The Center is recognized as a valuable resource st

Maine

6767   Charlotte White Center
572 Bangor Rd
Dover Foxcroft, ME 04426-3373   207-564-2426
                                          888-440-4158
                                          Fax: 207-564-2404
                                          charlottewhitecenter.com

Richard M. Brown, CEO
Charles G. Clemons, COO
Dale Shaw, CFO
A nonprofit agency, devoted to assisting adults and children with
developmental disabilities, mental health, physical handicaps,
and elder age related issues. With headquarters in Do-
ver-Foxcroft Maine, the agency provides multiple levels of social
services.

6768   Iris Network for the Blind
189 Park Avenue
Portland, ME 04102-2909   207-774-6273
                                          Fax: 207-774-0679
                                          ashah@theiris.org
                                          theiris.org

Leonard Cole, Chairman
Katharine Ray, 1st Vice Chairman
Bruce Roullard, 2nd Vice Chairman
A statewide resource and catalyst for people who are visually im-
paired or blind so they can attain their determined level of inde-
pendence and integration into the community.

6769   Roger Randall Center
45 School St
Houlton, ME 04730-2010   207-532-4068
                                          Fax: 207-532-7334

Rob Moran, Executive Director
Tom Moakler, President
Vicki Moody, Vice President
The Roger Randall Cneter is one of five Day Habilitation Programs adminsitered by Community Living Association, a private,
non-profit agency. These programs may provide a supportive environment that allows the individual to achieve their maximum
growth po

6770   Sebasticook Farms-Great Bay Foundation
P.O.Box 65
Saint Albans, ME 04971   207-487-4399
                                          Fax: 207-938-5670

Tom Davis, Executive Director
Pam Erskin, Program Coordinator
Provides residential, educational and vocational services to
adults who are developmentally disabled in order to maximize independent living and to provide assistance in obtaining an earned
income.

6771   Social Learning Center
10 Shelton McMurphey Blvd
Eugene, OR 97401-3363   541-485-2711
                                          877-208-6134
                                          Fax: 541-485-7087
                                          www.oslc.org

Sam Vuchinich, Ph.D, Chair
Gordon Naga Hall, Ph.D., Vice President
Susan Miller, J.D., Secretary/Treasurer
Post accute rehabilitation program.

Maryland

6772   Blind Industries and Services of Maryland
3345 Washington Blvd
Baltimore, MD 21227-1602   410-737-2600
                                          888-322-4567
                                          Fax: 410-737-2665
                                          info@bism.org
                                          bism.org

Donald J. Morris, Chairperson
Walter A. Brown, Vice Chairperson
Fredrick J. Puente, President
Offers a comprehensive residential rehabilitation training program for people who are blind. Areas of instruction: braille, cane
travel, independent living, computer, adjustment and blindness
seminars.

6773   Center for Neuro-Rehabilitation
2340238 N Cary St
Annapolis, MD 21223   410-263-1704
                                          410-462-4711

Jeanne Fryer
Laurent Pierre-Philippe
Provide community-based inpatient and outpatient acute rehabilitation, vocational services and long-term care. Specializing in
treating complex neurological conditions including spinal cord
injuries, multiple sclerosis, strokes, and other brain injuries resulting from trauma, anoxia, tumors, genetic malformations and
other related conditions. Locations in Annapolis, Bethesda, Frederick, Towson, MD and Fairfax, Va. CNR is licensed, a Medicare
provider and CARF accredited.

6774   Child Find/Early Childhood Disabilities Unit
Montgomery County Public Schools
Ste A4
10731 Saint Margarets Way
Kensington, MD 20895- 2831   301-929-2224
                                          Fax: 301-929-2223

Julie Bader, Supervisor
Offers free developmental screening for children ages 3 years until eligible for kindergarten, evaluation and placement services.

6775   Greater Baltimore Medical Center
6701 N Charles St
Baltimore, MD 21204-6881   443-849-2000
                                          800-597-9142
                                          Fax: 443-849-2631
                                          www.gbmc.org

John B. Chessare MD, President & CEO
Harold J. Tucker MD, Chief Of Staff
Eric L. Melchoir, Vice President & CFO
Offers services for the visually impaired and blind with low vi-
sion exams. Rehabilitation teaching and orientation and mobility
in the home or workplace. Also offers a bimonthly newsletter for
$12/yr for Hoover patients and monthly share group.

6776   James Lawrence Kernan Hospital
2200 Kernan Drive
Baltimore, MD 21207-6697   410-285-6566
                                          888-453-7626
                                          Fax: 410-448-6854
                                          www.umrehabortho.org

Michael Jablonover MD,MBA, President & CEO
John P. Straumanis MD, FAAP, Vice President
W. Walter x Augustin, III, CPA, Vice President of Financial
Services
Kernan reigns as Maryland's origional orthopaedic hospital with
a staff which consists of a support team of orthopaedic physician
assistants and dedicated nurses in the Post Anesthesia Care Unit
and on the Medical/Surgical Unit, guaranteeing the highest q

6777   Levindale Hebrew Geriatric Center
2401 W Belvedere Ave.
Baltimore, MD 21215-5271   410-601-9355
                                          www.lifebridgehealth.org/Levindale
A 330-licensed bed facility providing post-acute services for patients affected by life-altering illness or injury.

6778   Meridan Medical Center For Subacute Care
770 York Rd
Towson, MD 21204   410-821-5500
                                          Fax: 410-821-6735

Yvette Caldwell, Administrator
Patients receive around-the-clock professional nursing care;
physical and occupational, speech and respiratory therapists also
assist patients. Each patient's individualized plan of care is reviewed and updated as patient needs change. Careful discharge p.

6779 Rehabilitation Opportunities
5100 Philadelphia Way
Lanham, MD 20706-4412 301-731-4242
Fax: 301-731-4191
roiworks.org

Tom Purcell, President
Bruce Shapiro, Vice President
David Fierst, Secretary
Organization offering day programs, evaluation, work adjustments and sheltered workshops for persons who are developmentally disabled.

6780 Rosewood Center
410-951-5000
888-300-7071
Fax: 410-581-6157
www.dhmh.state.md.us/dda/rosewood

Leslie Smith, Program Director
James Anzalone, Director
Rosewood Center is a State residential Center that supports adults with developmental disabilities from the central Maryland region.

6781 TLC Speech-Language/Occupational TherapyCamps
2092 Gaither Rd.
Suite 100
Rockville, MD 20850 301-424-5200
Fax: 301-424-8063
info@ttlc.org
www.ttlc.org

Patricia Ritter, Executive Director
TLC provides small group summer programs for children with special needs. Offers speech-language and occupational therapy summer camps for children ages 3-7.

6782 Workforce and Technology Center
Division of Rehabilitation Services
2301 Argonne Drive
Baltimore, MD 21218-1628 410-554-9442
888-554-0334
Fax: 410-554-9112
www.dors.state.md.us

Dan Frye, Chairperson
Josie Thomas, Vice Chairperson
Is one of nine state operated comprehensive rehabilitation facilities in the country providing a wide range of services to individuals with disabilities. The Maryland Division of Rehabilitation Services operates the Workforce and Technology Program. Avail

Massachusetts

6783 Baroco Corporation
136 West Street
Northampton, MA 01060-2711 413-534-9978
Fax: 413-585-9019
www.baroco.com

Rick Barnard, President/Owner
Suzanne Darby, Executive Administrator
Julia McLaughlin, Executive Administrator
Provides training and therapeutic support for its recipients with developmental disabilities in order to aid them in securing and maintaining placement in a less-restrictive setting.

6784 Berkshire Meadows
160 Gould Street
Suite 300
Needham, MA 02494-2300 781-559-4900
Fax: 413-528-0293
lkelly@jri.org
berkshiremeadows.org

Andy Pond, President
Gregory Canfield, Vice President
Deborah Reuman, CFO
Private, non profit school for children, adolescents, young adults who are severely, developmentally disabled. Approved special education learning center, work site program and foster care. Physical therapy, speech and language development, behavioral pro *$8200.00*

6785 Blueberry Hill Healthcare
75 Brimbal Ave
Beverly, MA 01915-6009 978-927-2020
Fax: 978-922-5213
admissions@BlueberryHillRehab.com
www.blueberryhillrehab.com

Ralph Epstein, Medical Director
Accomodates 146 residents. We are centrally located close to Route 128 and Route 1A in Beverly Massachusetts. We offer short-term rehab care, long term care and Alzheimer's Special Care Programs. Our interdisciplinary team designs individual care plans fo

6786 Boston University Hospital Vision Rehabilitation Services
One Boston Medical Center Place
Boston, MA 02118-2371 617-638-8000
Fax: 617-638-7769
www.bmc.org/rehab.htm

Simona Manasian, Medical Director
Karen Mattie, Director
Jenn Blake, Clinical Outpatient Supervisor
Offers services for the totally blind, legally blind, visually impaired, and more with health, counseling, educational, recreational, rehabilitation, computer training and professional training services.

6787 Burbank Rehabilitation Center
275 Nichols Rd
Fitchburg, MA 01420-1919 978-343-5000
888-840-3627
Fax: 978-343-5342
www.umassmemorialhealthcare.org

David Bennett, Chair
Eric Dickson, President & CEO
The largest community hospital and regional referral center in the area. Offers the most extensive high quality, cost-effective healthcare services in the region. The hospital provides outstanding hospital-based services such as case management of high ri

6788 Carl and Ruth Shapiro Family National Center for Accessible Media
WGBH Educational Foundation
1 Guest St.
Boston, MA 02135-2016 617-300-3400
Fax: 617-300-1035
TTY: 617-300-2489
ncam@wgbh.org
ncam.wgbh.org

Donna Danielewski, Director
Madeleine Rothberg, Senior Subject Matter Expert
Geoff Freed, Director of Technology
The Carl and Ruth Shapiro Family National Center for Accessible Media (NCAM) is a research and development facility dedicated to addressing barriers to media and emerging technologies for people with disabilities in their homes, schools, workplaces, and communities.

6789 Carroll Center for the Blind
770 Centre St
Newton, MA 02458-2597 617-969-6200
800-852-3131
Fax: 617-969-6204
www.carroll.org

Josepth Abely, President
Arthur O'Neill, Vice President
Brian Charlson, Director of Computer Training Services
Offers services for the totally blind, legally blind, visually impaired, and more with health, counseling, educational, in dependent living, tronell skills, computer traing, recreational, rehabilitation, computer training and professional training services.

6790   Center for Psychiatric Rehabilitation
Boston University
940 Commonwealth Ave
West
Boston, MA 02215-1203   617-353-3549
                                    Fax: 617-353-7700
                                    psyrehab@bu.edu
                                    cpr.bu.edu

Kim T. Mueser, Executive Director
Deborah Dolan, Director of operations
Larry Kohn, Director of Development
The mission of the Center is to increase knowledge, to train treatment personnel, to develop effective rehabilitation programs and to assist in organizing both personnel and programs into efficient and coordinated service delivery systems for people with

6791   Clark House Nursing Center At Foxhill Village
Kindred Healthcare
30 Longwood Dr
Westwood, MA 02090-1132   781-326-5652
                                    800-359-7412
                                    Fax: 781-326-4034
                                    www.clarkhousefhv.com

Chris Wasel, Administrator
Clark House At Fox Hill Village accomodates 70 residents. We are part of the Fox Hill Village Assisted Living and Retirement Center campus. Clark House Nursing center has been named a recipient of a 2005 step II quality Award from the American Health Care

6792   College Internship Program at the Berkshire Center
18 Park St
Lee, MA 01238-1702   413-243-2576
                                    Fax: 413-243-3351

Lucy Gosselin, Program Director
Laina Hubbard, Admissions Coordinator
Charles D. Houff, Head Therapist
A highly individualized postsecondary program for learning disabled young adults 18-30. Provides job placement services and follow-ups; college support; money management and social skills. Residential students share an apartment and have their own room.

6793   Devereux Advanced Behavioral Health Massachusetts & Rhode Island
Devereux School
60 Miles Rd.
P.O. Box 219
Rutland, MA 01543   508-886-4746
                                    800-338-3738
                                    Fax: 508-886-4773
                                    tbeauvai@devereux.org
                                    www.devereuxma.org
Stephen Yerdon, Executive Director
Bonnie Byer, Business Development Director
Evans Chiyombwe, Quality Management Director
Serving children and youth with emotional, behavioral, intellectual and developmental disorders. Services include residential treatment, community-based group homes, therapeutic foster care, special needs day school, substance abuse and autism spectrum programs, diagnostic services and in-home services.

6794   Eagle Pond Rehabilitation and Living Center
1 Love Lane
P.O.Box 208
South Dennis, MA 02660-3445   508-385-6034
                                    Fax: 508-385-7064
                                    www.eaglepond.com

Paul Marchwat, Executive Director
Ellen Reil, Marketing Director
Eagle Pond accomodates 142 residents. Medicare and Medicaid certified as well as being accredited by the Joint Comission (formerly (JCAHO) which enables us to contract with many insurance companies.

6795   FOR Community Services
75 Litwin Ln
Chicopee, MA 01020-4817   413-592-6142
                                    Fax: 413-598-0478
                                    ggolash1@aol.com

Gina Golash, Executive Director

Providing a world of meaning for individuals with developmental disabilities throughout Western Massachusetts since 1967.

6796   Fairlawn Rehabilitation Hospital
189 May Street
Worcester, MA 01602-4399   508-791-6351
                                    Fax: 508-831-1277
                                    www.fairlawnrehab.org

Dave Richer, CEO
Peter Bagley MD, Medical Director
Matthew Akulonis, Director Of Support Operations
Offers comprehensive rehabilitation on both an inpatient and outpatient basis. Specialty programs include: head injury, spinal cord injury, young/senior stroke, oncology, geriatrics and orthopedics.

6797   Greenery Extended Care Center: Worcester
59 Acton Street
Worcester, MA 01604-4899   508-791-3147
                                    800-633-0887
                                    Fax: 508-753-6267
                                    worcester@wingatehealthcare.com
                                    wingatehealthcare.com
Scott Schuster, Founder & President
Brian Callahan, CFO
Michael Benjamin, Vice President
173 beds offering complex care, extended rehabilitation and neurobehavioral intervention. Offering life care homes and Nursing home services. Specialties include life events and physical care, long term and home health care, and nursing homes and nursing

6798   Greenery Rehabilitation & Skilled Nursing Center
P.O.Box 1330
Middleboro, MA 02346-4330   508-947-9295
                                    Fax: 508-947-7974
201 beds offering programs of active/acute rehabilitation, cognitive rehabilitation, respiratory care and short-term evaluations.

6799   Harrington House Nursing And Rehabilitation Center
160 Main Street
Walpole, MA 02081-4037   508-660-3080
                                    Fax: 508-660-1634
                                    www.harringtonrehab.com

Joseph Haron, Medical Director
Accomodates 90 residents. Our state-of-the-art center offers post-accute services including rehabilitation and medical management. Our center also provides a long term care program including hospice services.

6800   HealthSouth Rehabilitation Hospital Of Western Massachusetts
222 State Street
Ludlow, MA 01056-3478   413-308-3300
                                    Fax: 413-547-2738
                                    www.healthsouthrehab.org

Victoria Healy, CEO
Adnan Dahdul, M.D., Medical Director
Deborah Cabanas, Chief Nursing Officer
A 53-bed acute Rehabilitation Hospital. The facility has been operating for 14 years and has provided rehabilitative care to patients and families in the greater Springfield area with an outstanding reputation for attention to detail and compassion. Becau

6801   Holiday Inn Boxborough Woods
242 Adams Pl
Boxborough, MA 01719-1735   978-263-8701
                                    800-465-4329
                                    Fax: 978-263-0518
                                    box_sales@fine-hotels.com
                                    www.ihg.com/holidayinn

Kevin Murray, Manager
Marcel Girard, Manager
Nancy Ellen Hurley, Chief Marketing Officer
Located on 35 acres of wooded countryside just off I-495 at exit #28. Minutes from the Mass Turnpike, Route 2, 290 and 9. Conference center located on main level with 30,000 square feet of meeting space. Guest rooms feature two-line telephones, voice mail
$129 - $159

6802 Lifeworks Employment Services
1400 Providence Highway
Suite 2300
Norwood, MA 02062- 4551   781-769-3298
                                  Fax: 781-551-0045
                                  www.lifeworksma.org
Dan Burke, President & CEO
Chris Page, Vice President
Brenda Calder, CFO
Providing homes, jobs, education and supportive living for people with developmental disabilities.

6803 Massachusetts Eye and Ear Infirmary & Vision Rehabilitation Center
243 Charles Street
Boston, MA 02114-3002   617-523-7900
                                Fax: 617-573-4178
                                TTY: 617-523-5498
                                www.masseyeandear.org
Wycliffe Grousbeck, Chairman
John Fernandaz, President & CEO
Lily H. Bentas, Secretary
Visual rehabilitation encompasses a low vision rehabilitation evaluation, occupational therapy evaluation (with home visit if necessary), and social service evaluation.

6804 New England Center for Children
260 Tremont Street
Boston, MA 02116-2108   617-636-4600
                                Fax: 617-636-4866
                                cwelch@necc.org
                                necc.org
Lisel Macenka, Chair
James C. Burling, Vice Chair
L.Vincent Strully, President
A comprehensive year-round program for students with autism and PDD who require a highly specialized educational and behavior management program. Students are from all over the country and receive intensive, positive, behavioral counseling and social skil

6805 New England Eye Center - Tufts Medical Center
Tufts Medical Center
260 Tremont St
Boston, MA 02116   617-636-4600
                          800-231-3316
                          Fax: 617-636-4866
                          eli_peli@meei.harvard.edu
                          www.neec.com
Jeannette Spillane, Executive Director
Shana Bellus, Director, Admitting Operations
Linnea Olsson, Special Projects Consultant
The New England Eye Center offers services for the legally blind and visually impaired, as well as for health care providers. Services include health care, counseling, education, vision research and professional training. Emphasis is on mobility related vision enhancement, including devices for driving and safe walking.

6806 New Medico Rehabilitation and Skilled Nursing Center at Lewis Bay
89 Lewis Bay Rd
Hyannis, MA 02601-5207   508-775-7601
                                Fax: 508-790-4239
Edmund Steinle, Executive Director
Post acute rehabilitation services.

6807 Protestant Guild Learning Center
411 Waverley Oaks Rd
Suite 104
Waltham, MA 02452-8449   781-893-6000
                                Fax: 781-893-1171
                                www.theguildschool.org
Eric H. Rosenberger, President
Thomas P. Corcoran, Vice President & Treasurer
Thomas Belski, Chief Executive Officer
Offers services for the diagnostically disabled children and adolescents with ages 6-22 years with health, counseling, educational, recreational, rehabilitation, computer training and professional training services.

6808 Shaughnessy-Kaplan Rehabilitation Hospital
1 Dove Ave
Salem, MA 01970   978-745-9000
                          Fax: 978-740-4730
                          skrhinfo@partners.org
                          spauldingrehab.org
Anthony Sciola, CEO
Maureen Banks, RN, MS, MBA, CN, President
Mary Beth DiFilippo, Vice President
A 160-bed private, non-profit hospital. We have been providing care for residents of greater North Shore communities since 1975. Shaughnessy has 120 long-term care hospital beds and a 40-bed transitional care unit sometimes referred to as a skilled nursin

6809 Son-Rise Program
2080 South Undermountain Road
Sheffield, MA 01257-9643   413-229-2100
                                  877-766-7473
                                  Fax: 413-229-3202
                                  correspondence@option.org
                                  www.autismtreatmentcenter.org
Barry Neil Kaufman, Co Founder
Samahria Lyte Kaufman, Co Founder
THe Son-Rise Program is a powerful, effective and totally unique treatment for children and adults challengedby Autism, Autuism Spectrum Disorders, Pervasive Developmental Disorder (PDD), Asperger's Syndrome and other developmental difficulties.

6810 Southern Worcester County Rehabilitation Inc. D/B/A Life-Skills, Inc.
44 Morris St
Webster, MA 01570-1812   508-943-0700
                                Fax: 508-949-6129
                                www.life-skillsinc.org
J Thomas Amick, Executive Director
Kristin Nelson, Board President
Barbara Butrym, Board Vice President
Life-Skills, Inc. assists mentally and developmentally challenged adults with meeting their individual needs, and empowering them to take full advantage of meaningful opportunities in their communities. We provide residential, employment, transportation, behavior, and theraputic day habilitation services to 350 adults in MA. We operate thrift & consignment stores, a small cafe, an ice cream shop, mini golf & arcade center, vending and greenhouse businesses, bank courier service, and others.

6811 Vinfen Corporation
950 Cambridge Street
Cambridge, MA 02141-1001   617-441-1800
                                  877-284-6336
                                  Fax: 617-441-1858
                                  TTY: 617-225-2000
                                  info@vinfen.org
                                  www.vinfen.org
Philip A. Mason, Ph.D., Chairperson
Bruce L. Bird, Ph.D., CEO/ President
Elizabeth K. Glaser, Chief Operations Officer
A private, nonprofit company, Vinfen Corporation is the largest human services provider in Massachusetts. Vinfen offers clinical, educational, residential and support services to individuals of all ages with mental illness and or developmental disabilities, who also may have another disability (e.g. substance abuse, homelessness, AIDS). The company also trains professionals in the mental health field and helps consumers to learn to live in community-based settings at the highest levels.

6812 Visiting Nurse Association of North Shore
5 Federal St
Danvers, MA 01923-3687   508-751-6926
                                800-728-1862
                                Fax: 978-777-0308
                                www.vnacarenetwork.org
Mary Ann O'Connor, CEO/ President
Stephanie Jackman-Havey, Chief Operating Officer/Chief Financial Officer
David Rose, Vice President of Human Resources
Home health services including nurses, physical, occupational and speech therapy, home health aides and more. Special programs include nutrition counseling, IV care, pediatric therapy, HIV/AIDS services and wound management. Provides services 7

days a week, 365 days a year and we accept Medicare, Medicaid and most HMO's and health insurers.

6813   Weldon Center for Rehabilitation
233 Carew St
Springfield, MA 01104-2377

413-748-6800
Fax: 413-748-6806
mercycares.com

Barbara Haswell, Manager
One of the most vital, necessary health resources in the region by helping thousands of people toward restored health and independence. A comprehensive, integrated, non-profit facility offering inpatient, outpatient, day rehabilitation and pediatric services on one site.

6814   Youville Hospital & Rehab Center
1575 Cambridge St
Cambridge, MA 02138-4398

617-876-4344
Fax: 617-547-5501

Meets the long and short term health care and rehabilitation needs of patients who are physically disabled and chronically ill. Strives to develop and maintain health as a human right on physical, social, vocational and spiritual levels. The ultimate goal of the hospital is to treat and assist each individual patient in reaching his or her optimal level of living. Services include: stroke, brain injury, spinal cord trauma, orthopedic disabilities and more.

Michigan

6815   Botsford Center For Rehabilitation & Health Improvement-Redford
28050 Grand River Ave.
Farmington Hills, MI 48336-5919

248-471-8000
877-442-7900
Fax: 313-387-3838
www.botsford.org

John Darin, Manager
A 20 bed inpatient physical rehabilitation unit, servicing individuals who have experienced a stroke, amputation, orthopedic fracture, or other neurological impairment.

6816   Bureau of Services for Blind Persons Training Center
1541 Oakland Dr
Kalamazoo, MI 49008

269-337-3848
800-292-4200
Fax: 269-337-3872
mossc@michigan.gov

Cheryl Heibeck, Director
Bruce Schultz, Assistant Director
Residential facility that provides instruction to legally blind adults in braille, computer operation and assistive technology, handwriting, cane travel, cooking, personal management, industrial arts and also crafts. During training students will develop career plans which may include work experience, internships, volunteer opprtunities and even part-time paid employment.

6817   Chelsea Community Hospital Rehabilitation Unit
775 South Main Street
Chelsea, MI 48118-1383

734-593-6000
800-231-2211
Fax: 734-475-4191
www.stjoeschelsea.org

Nancy K. Graebner, CEO/ President
Kathy Brubaker, RN, Vice President and Chief Nursing Officer
Randall Forsch, MD, Chief Medical Officer
A private, non-profit, acute care facility that combines the best of small town values with national standards of healthcare excellence. The hospital has a 19-bed acute care inpatient rehabilitation unit with comprehensive outpatient programs, including a coordinated brain injury program.

6818   Clare Branch
790 Industrial Dr
Clare, MI 48617-9224

989-386-7707
888-773-7664
Fax: 989-386-2199
mail@mmionline.com
www.mmionline.org

Cris Zeigler, Executive Director

MMI will strive to be the premier provider of person-centered services to people with barriers to employment. We will connect individuals with community resources that provide mutual benefit to them and to the community. MMI will be known for excellence in service provision, ethical business practices, a quality work environment, and for providing services that enhance the dignity and value of the people we serve.

6819   Clarkston Spec Healthcare Center
4800 Clintonville Rd
Clarkston, MI 48346-4297

800-454-5909

Margaret Canny, Administrator
120 beds offering active/acute rehabilitation, complex care, day treatment, extended rehabilitation, neurobehavioral intervention and short-term evaluation.

6820   DMC Health Care Center-Novi
42005 W 12 Mile Rd
Novi, MI 48377-3113

248-305-7575
Fax: 425-201-1450
novi@patch.com
novi.patch.com

Bud Rosenthal, CEO
Leigh Zareli Lewis, COO
Andreas Turanski, CTO
The Detroit Medical Center's record of service has provided medical excellence throughout the history of the Metropolitan Detroit area. From the founding of the Children's Hospital in 1886, to the creation of the first mechanical heart at Harpers Hospital 50 years ago, to our compassion for the underdeserved, our legacy of caring is unmatched.

6821   Eight CAP, Inc. Head Start
904 Oak Drive
Greenville, MI 48838-9277

616-754-9315
Fax: 616-754-9310
laurelm@8cap.org
www.8cap.org

Ralph Loeschner, Executive Director
Nancy Secor, Contact
Post accute rehabilitation programs.

6822   Greater Detroit Agency for the Blind and Visually Impaired
16625 Grand River Ave
Detroit, MI 48227-1419

313-272-3900
Fax: 313-272-6893
gdabvi.org

Frederick J Simpson, Board Chairman
Charles L. Cone, Vice Chairman
Leonard W Robinson, Board Secretary
Offers services for seniors 60 and over who are legally blind. Also provides eye health information, counseling, education and rehabilitation services.

6823   Hope Network Neuro Rehabilitation
3075 Orchard Vista Dr. SE
PO Box 890
Grand Rapids, MI 49546

616-301-8000
800-695-7273
Fax: 616-301-8010
www.hopenetworkrehab.org

Phil Weaver, President & Chief Executive Officer
Tim Becker, Chief Operating Officer
Andre Pierre, Chief Financial Officer
Neuro Rehabilitation is a service line of Hope Network, helping those with brain or spinal cord injuries or other neurological conditions recover through treatment techniques and person-centered care.

6824   Lakeland Center
26900 Franklin Rd
Southfield, MI 48033-5312

248-350-8070
Fax: 248-350-8078
peggys@thelakelandcenter.net
thelakelandcenter.net

Irving Shapiro, CEO
Santhosh Madhavan, Director Physical Medicine
Gary Yashinsky, Associate Medical Director

Subacute rehabilitation program directed toward those with severe neurologic diagnoses, ie: TBI, cerebral aneurysm, anoxic encephalopathy, CVA and cerebral hemorrhage, orthopedic injuries, and spinal cord injury. Subacute rehabilitation is provided for those who recover slowly and require individualized treatment plans. Residential program available as well.

6825   Mary Free Bed Rehabilitation Hospital
235 Wealthy St SE
Grand Rapids, MI 49503-5247
616-493-9657
800-528-8989
Fax: 616-454-3939
info@maryfreebed.com
maryfreebed.com

Kent Riddle, CEO
John Butzer, MD, Medical Director
Randy DeNeff, Vice President of Finance
Founded more than 100 years ago, Mary Free Bed Rehabilitation Hospital is and 80-bed, not-for-profit, acute rehabilitation center. Its mission is to restore hope and freedom through rehabilitation to people with disabilities. Mary Free Bed offers comprehensive inpatient and outpatient rehabilitationfor children and adults using an interdisciplinary approach. Also available are numerous specialty programs designed to increase the quality of life and independence of people with disabilities.

6826   Michigan Career And Technical Institute
11611 Pine Lake Rd
Plainwell, MI 49080-9225
269-664-4461
877-901-7360
Fax: 269-664-5850

Dennis Hart, Executive Director
A residential vocational training center for adults with physical, mental or emotional disabilities.

6827   Mid-Michigan Industries
2426 Parkway Dr
Mt Pleasant, MI 48858-4723
989-773-6918
888-773-7664
888-773-7664
Fax: 989-773-1317
mmionline.com

Alan Schilling, President
Andrea Christopher, Director Admissions
Linda Wagner, Branch Director
Providing jobs and training for persons with barriers to employment. Services include vocational evaluation, job placement, supported employment, work services, prevocational training and case management

6828   New Medico Community Re-Entry Service
216 St Marys Lake Rd
Battle Creek, MI 49017-9710
Fax: 269-962-2241
James Rekshan, Executive Director

6829   Sanilac County Community Mental Health
171 Dawson St
Sandusky, MI 48471-1062
810-648-0330
888-225-4447
888-225-4447
Fax: 810-648-0319

Roger Dean, Executive Director
Post-acute rehabilitation facility and programs.

6830   Special Tree Rehabilitation System
600 Stephenson Highway
Troy, MI 48083-1110
248-616-0950
800-648-6885
Fax: 248-616-0957
info@specialtree.com
www.specialtree.com

Joseph Richart, CEO
Special Tree exists to provide hope, encouragement, and expertise for people who have experienced life-altering changes. Our team approach to rehabilitation, custom designed for each person's needs and goals, offers these individuals the best opportunity for healing and recovery.

6831   Thumb Industries
1263 Sand Beach Rd
Bad Axe, MI 48413-8817
989-269-9229
Fax: 989-269-2587
thumbindustries@hotmail.com
www.thumbindustries.com

Rhonda Wisenbaugh, Executive Director
Provides job training and employment for disabled persons. Vocational rehabilitation agency, manufactures household furnishings, direct mail advertising service.

6832   Visually Impaired Center
1422 W Court St
Flint, MI 48503-5008
810-767-4014
Fax: 810-767-0020
www.vicflint.org

Committed to developing resources and collaborative programs as well as providing services that enable independent life for people with vision loss. Services include: Information and referals, assessments of needs, peer support groups, training by a Rehabilitation teacher of the blind and visually impaired, independent living skills, computer skills, training by an Orientation and Mobility Specialist, safe traveling skills, Diabetes management/education.
a pages

6833   Welcome Homes Retirement Community for the Visually Impaired
1953 Monroe Ave NW
Grand Rapids, MI 49505-6242
616-447-7837
888-939-9292
888-939-9292
Fax: 616-447-9891

Beth Lucksted, Manager
Offers services for the totally blind, legally blind, visually impaired, and more with health, counseling, educational, recreational, rehabilitation, computer training and professional training services.

6834   William H Honor Rehabilitation Center Henry Ford Wyanclotte Hospital
Henry Ford Health System
2333 Biddle Ave
Wyandotte, MI 48192-4668
734-246-6000
Fax: 734-246-6926
www.henryfordwyandotte.com
Denise Dailing, Administration Leader/rehabilita
James Sexton, Chief Executive Officer
Henry Ford, Owner
Henry Ford Wyandotte Hospital offers an array of educational programs, health screenings, and support groups. The hospital is CARF accredited and has a CARF certified stroke specialty unit.

Minnesota

6835   Industries: Cambridge
601 Cleveland St S
Cambridge, MN 55008-1752
763-689-5434
Fax: 763-552-1281
jspicer@industriesinc.org
www.industriesinc.org

Daryl Peterson, Board Chair
Bruce Montgomery, Vice Chair
Marilyn Bachman, Secretary
Nonprofit organization that does vocational assessment and training for people with disabilities.

6836   Industries: Mora
500 Walnut St S
Mora, MN 55051-1936
320-679-2354
Fax: 320-679-2355
jspicer@industriesinc.org
www.industriesinc.org

Daryl Peterson, Board Chair
Bruce Montgomery, Vice Chair
Marilyn Bachman, Secretary
Nonprofit organization that does vocational assessment and training for people with disabilities.

6837 Shriners Hospitals for Children: Twin Cities
2025 E River Pkwy
Minneapolis, MN 55414-3696   612-596-6100
                                 888-293-2832
                                 888-293-2832
                            Fax: 612-339-5954
www.shrinershospitalsforchildren.org
Charles C. Lobeck, Administrator
Cary Mielke, M.D, Interim Chief of Staff
Don Engel, Development Officer
Shriners Hospital for Children-Twin Cities offers quality orthopedic medical care regardless of the patients' ability to pay.
Shriners Hospitals provide inpatient and outpatient services, surgery, casts, braces, artificial limbs, x-rays and physical and occupational therapy to any child under the age of 18 who may benefit
from treatment.

6838 Vision Loss Resources
1936 Lyndale Ave S
Minneapolis, MN 55403-3101   612-871-2222
                            Fax: 612-872-0189
                            TTY: 612-382-8422
                                 info@vlrw.org
                       www.visionlossresources.org
Barry Shear, Chair
Lisa David, Vice Chair
Mary McDougall, Secretary
Offers services for the totally blind, legally blind, visually im-
paired, and more with health, counseling, educational, recre-
ational, rehabilitation, computer training and professional
training services.

Mississippi

6839 Addie McBryde Rehabilitation Center for the Blind
PO Box 5314
Jackson, MS 39296-5314   601-364-2700
                                800-443-1000
                            Fax: 601-364-2677
H. S. McMillan, Executive Director
Shelia Browning, Deputy Director Non-Vocational P
Offers services for the totally blind, legally blind, visually im-
paired, blind and more with health, counseling, educational, rec-
reational, rehabilitation, computer training services and
orientation and mobility.

6840 Mississippi Methodist Rehabilitation Center
1350 E Woodrow Wilson Ave
Jackson, MS 39216-5198   601-981-2611
                                800-223-6672
                            Fax: 601-364-3571
                       www.methodistonline.org
Mark A. Adams, President/ CEO
Matthew L. Holleman, III, Chair
Mike P. Sturdivant Jr, Vice Chairman
Rebuild lives that have been broken by disabilities and impairments from serious illness or severe injury. The challenge is to
help patients regain abilities, restore function and movement, and
renew emotionally. It features personal rehabilitation treatment
plans administered by specialized teams of health care professionals through a variety of outpatient programs, treatments and
other services.

Missouri

6841 Alpine North Nursing and Rehabilitation Center
4700 NW Cliff View Dr
Kansas City, MO 64150-1237   816-741-5105
                            Fax: 816-746-1301
Mike Stacks, Executive Director
Bob Richard, Administrator
Postacute rehabilitation program.

6842 Christian Hospital Northeast
11133 Dunn Rd
Saint Louis, MO 63136-6119   314-653-5000
                                 877-747-9355
                            Fax: 314-653-4130
                                 christianhospital.org
Ron McMullen, President
Bryan Hartwick, Vice President Human Resources
Sebastian Rueckert, MD, Vice President and Chief Medical Officer
A non-profit organization, a 493 bed acute care facility on 28
acres. Christian Hospital has more then 600 physicians on staff
and a diverse workforce of more then 2,5000 health-care professionals who are dedicated to providing the absolute best care with
the latest technology and medical advances.

6843 Easterseals Midwest
11933 Westline Industrial Dr.
St. Louis, MO 63146   800-200-2119
                            Fax: 314-394-4007
                                 info@esmw.org
                       www.easterseals.com/midwest
Wendy Sullivan, Chief Executive Officer
Jeff Arledge, Chief Financial Officer
Tom Barry, Chief Development Officer
Enhances the independence and quality of life of people with dis-
abilities through services, education, outreach and advocacy.

6844 Integrated Health Services of St. Louis at Gravois
10954 Kennerly Rd
Saint Louis, MO 63128-2018   314-843-4242
                            Fax: 314-843-4031
Lisa Niehaus, Administrator
Subacute, skilled and intermediate care; ventilator/tracheostomy
management program; wound management program and complex
rehabilitation program.

6845 Metropolitan Employment & Rehabilitation Service
M ER S Goodwill
1727 Locust St
Saint Louis, MO 63103-1703   314-241-3464
                            Fax: 314-241-9348
                       www.mersgoodwill.org
Lewis C. Chartock, Ph.D., President/ CEO
Dawayne Barnett, CFO
Mark Arens, Executive Vice President, Chief of Program Services
Vocational rehabilitation, primarily with the disabled, skills
training and placement services.

6846 Poplar Bluff RehabCare Program
Lucy Lee Hospital
2620 N Westwood Blvd
Poplar Bluff, MO 63901-3396   573-785-7721
                            Fax: 573-686-5987
Jim Martin, Program Manager
Chris Murray, Care Coordinator
Darlene Hill, Care Admissions Coordinator
Provides physical medicine and rehabilitation to individuals with
a physically limiting condition. The program is designed to help
individuals function as independently as possible by maximizing
their strength and abilities.

6847 Shriners Hospitals for Children St. Louis
2001 S Lindbergh Blvd
Saint Louis, MO 63131-3597   314-432-3600
                                 800-850-2960
                            Fax: 314-432-2930
                       www.shrinershq.org/hospitals/st.louis
John McCabe, Executive Vice President
Kenneth Guidera, M.D., Chief Medical Officer
Eugene R. D'Amore, Vice President, Hospital Operations
Medical care is provided free of charge for children 18 and under
with orthopaedic conditions.

6848 St. Louis Society for the Blind and Visually Impaired
8770 Manchester Rd
Saint Louis, MO 63144-2724   314-960-9000
                            Fax: 314-968-9003
                                 www.slsbvi.org
David Ekin, President
Chris Pickel, Chair
Ann Shapiro, Vice Chair

Offers vision rehabilitation services for the totally blind, legally blind, visually impaired, including counseling, educational, recreational, rehabilitation, computer training and professional training services. Low vision aids and appliance available through low vision clinic by appointment.

6849 Truman Medical Center Low Vision Rehabilitation Program
Eye Foundation of Kansas City
2300 Holmes St.
Kansas City, MO 64108   816-404-1780
                                     Fax: 816-404-1786

Nelson R. Sabates, M.D., Chairman
Monika Malecha, MD, Residency Program Director
Abraham Poulose, MD, Director of Clinics
Our program is designed to maximize daily tasks for a person with low vision. We are able to evaluate a person's home and provide recommendations as needed.

6850 Truman Neurological Center
12404 E. US 40 Highway
Independence, MO 64055-1354   816-373-5060
                                     Fax: 816-373-5787
                                     tnccommunity.com

James Landrum, Executive Director
Ann Johnson, Finance Director
Terri Boyce, Office Assistant
A licensed habilitation center established for the purpose of assisting persons with developmental disabilities. The minimum age is 18. Residential care is provided in four group homes in the community licensed by the DMH and CARF accredited.

Montana

6851 Benefis Healthcare
1101 26th St S
Great Falls, MT 59405-5104   406-455-5000
                                     Fax: 406-455-2110
                                     benefis@benefis.org
                                     www.benefis.org

John Goodnow, CEO
Laura Goldhahn-Konen, President
Forrest Ehlinger, Chief Financial & Treasury Officer
Benefis Healthcare is a not-for-profit community asses governed by a 15-member local board of directors. Benefis is locally owned and controlled. Benefis is a Level II trauma center- one of only 4 in the state and 107 in the country.

6852 Disability Services Division of Montana
Department of Public Health
Helena, MT 59604   406-444-7734
                                     Fax: 406-444-3465

Keith Messmer, Manager
Sandi Gory, Administrative Assistant
Janice Frisch, Chief Management Operations
Responsible for coordinating, developing and implementing comprehensive programs to assist Montanans with disabilities with activities of daily living, community base services and coordinated programs of habilitation, rehabilitation and independent living.

6853 Easterseals-Goodwill Northern Rocky Mountain
Easterseals National
425 1st Ave. N
Great Falls, MT 59401-2507   406-761-3680
                                     www.esgw.org

Michelle Belknap, President & CEO
Provides services for children and adults with disabilities and other special needs, and support to their families.

Nebraska

6854 Las Vegas Healthcare And Rehabilitation Center
680 South Fourth Street
Louisville, KY 40202   502-596-7300
                                     TTY: 800-545-0749
                     web_administrator@kindredhealthcare.com
                                     kindredhealthcare.com

Paul J. Diaz, President/ CEO
Accomodates 79 residents. Serving the community for approximately 40 years. Located in close proximity to local hospitals and surrounded by medical complexes, out center offers both short-term rehabilitation and long term.care.

6855 Sierra Pain Institute
265 Golden Ln
Reno, NV 89502-1205   775-323-7092
                                     Fax: 775-323-5259

Lyle Smith, Owner
The program consists of a medically supervised outpatient program managed by an interdisciplinary team with input from specialties of Pain Medicine, Physical Therapy and Occupational Science. The format insures that each patient receives the full range of behavioral techniques in a well-integrated, individually tailored therapeutic regimen.

New Hampshire

6856 Department of Physical Medicine and Rehabilitation
Exeter Hospital
5 Alumni Dr
Exeter, NH 03833-2128   603-778-7311
                                     Fax: 603-580-6592
                                     www.exeterhospital.com

Kevin Calahan, President
Offers patient treatment, committed to enhancing the lives of individuals with short and long term physically disabling conditions.

6857 Farnum Rehabilitation Center
580 Court St
Keene, NH 03431-1718   603-354-6630
                                     Fax: 603-355-2078

Susan Loughrey, Program Director
Judy Bell, Manager
Offers rehabilitation services, occupational therapy, physical therapy and more for the physically challenged individual.

6858 Hackett Hill Nursing Center and Integrated Care
191 Hackett Hill Rd
Manchester, NH 03102-8993   603-668-8161
                                     Fax: 603-622-2584

Daniele Peckham, Administrator
Brett Lennerton, Administrator
A 68-bed certified nursing home.Postacute rehabilitation program.

6859 Mental Health Center: Riverside Courtyard, The
3 Twelfth St
Berlin, NH 03570-3860   603-752-7404
                                     Fax: 603-752-5194

Eileen Theriault, Manager
A center to help people that have mental disabilities.

6860 New Hampshire Rehabilitation and Sports Medicine
Catholic Medical Center
Ste 201
769 S Main St
Manchester, NH 03102-5166   603-647-1899
                                     800-437-9666
                                     Fax: 603-668-5348

Stuart Draper, Owner
Victor Carbone, Manager
A specialized facility for comprehensive rehabilitation for individuals who have been injured or have a disability.

6861   New Medico, Highwatch Rehabilitation Center
Highwatch Rd
Center Ossipee, NH 03814   Fax: 603-539-8888
William Burke, Executive Director
Post-acute rehabilitation service.

6862   Northern New Hampshire Mental Health and Developmental Services
87 Washington St
Conway, NH 03818-6044   603-447-3347
                                            Fax: 603-447-8893
                                            www.northernhs.org
Dennis Mackay, CEO
Provides mental health and developmental services to northern New Hampshire, including early intervention, elderly services, residential program, outpatient services, employee assistance programs, inpatient services, etc.

New Jersey

6863   All Garden State Physical Therapy
44 Ridge Road
North Arlington, NJ 07031   201-998-6300
                                            Fax: 201-998-6344
Post-acute rehabilitation program.

6864   Bancroft
425 Kings Highway East
PO Box 20
Haddonfield, NJ 08033- 1284   856-429-0010
                                            800-774-5516
                                            Fax: 856-429-1613
                                            TTY: 856-428-2697
                                            inquiry@bancroft.org
                                            www.bancroft.org
Cynthia Boyer, PhD, Executive Director, Brain Injury Services
Toni Pergolin, President and Chief Executive
Clair Rohrer, Med, Executive Director, Programs for Adults
Private, not-for-profit organization serving people with disabilities since 1883. Based in Haddonfield, New Jersey, help more than 1000 children and adults with autism, developmental disabilities, brain injuries, and other neurological impairments. Operates more than 140 sites throughout the U.S. and abroad.

6865   Daughters of Miriam Center/The Gallen Institute
155 Hazel St
Clifton, NJ 07011-3423   973-772-3700
                                            Fax: 973-253-5389
                                            administration@daughtersofmiriamcenter.org
                                            www.daughtersofmiriamcenter.o rg
Fred Feinstein, Executive Director
Dedicated to providing the highest quality care, the Center has far exceeded a stereotypical nursing home by offering a continuum of care environment, making us a leader in Jewish eldercare.

6866   Devereux Advanced Behavioral Health New Jersey
Devereux New Jersey
286 Mantua Grove Rd.
Building 4
West Deptford, NJ 08066   856-599-6400
                                            Fax: 856-423-8916
                                            drenner@devereux.org
                                            www.devereuxnj.org
Brian Hancock, Executive Director
Christine DiGiampaolo, Human Resources Department
Kelly McGhee, Quality Improvement Department
Serves people of all ages who have special needs. Individuals with emotional, behavioral, and developmental disabilities are offered services such as community-based homes and apartments, vocational training programs, family care homes, and consulting services. Devereux New Jersey also has a residential/educational center for individuals with autism.

6867   Ladacain Network
Schroth School & Technical Education Center
1701 Kneeley Blvd
Wanamassa, NJ 07712-7622   732-493-5900
                                           Fax: 732-493-5980
                                           ladacin.org
Patricia Carlesimo, Executive Director
Provides an array of services and programs specifically for children and adults with developmental and physical disabilities. Services include approved Department of Education school programs; adult education and training; vocational training, personal care assistance services, in-home and Saturday respite; child care programs, housing opportunities, and more.

6868   Lourdes Regional Rehabilitation Center
Our Lady of Lourdes Medical Center
1600 Haddon Ave
Camden, NJ 08103-3101   856-757-3864
                                          856-757-3500
                                          Fax: 856-968-2511
                                          www.lourdesnet.org
Alexander J. Hatala, President
Kimberly D. Barnes, Vice President, Planning and Development
Michael Hammond, Chief Financial Officer
The only comprehensive rehabilitation facility located within an acute care hospital in Southern New Jersey. Patients benefit from the proximity to the full range of state of the art medical and surgical services should the need arise.

6869   Mt. Carmel Guild
1160 Raymond Blvd
Newark, NJ 07102-4168   973-596-4100
                                          Fax: 973-639-6583
Anita Holland, Manager
Offers services for the totally blind, legally blind, visually impaired, and more with health, counseling, educational, recreational, rehabilitation, computer training and professional training services.

6870   Pediatric Rehabilitation Department, JFK Medical Center
65 James St
Edison, NJ 08818-3947   732-321-7362
                                          732-321-7000
                                          Fax: 732-548-7751
                                          www.jfkmc.org
Michael A. Kleiman, DMD, Chair
Douglas A. Nordstrom, Vice Chair
John L. Kolaya, PE, Secretary
Comprehensive interdisciplinary, family focused outpatient pediatric rehabilitation services including evaluation and individual and group treatment programs for children birth-21.

6871   REACH Rehabilitation Program: Leader Nursing and Rehabilitation Center
550 Jessup Rd
West Deptford, NJ 08066-1921   856-848-9551
Karen Fattore, Case Manager
Anthony Stenson, Administrator
Postacute rehabilitation program.

6872   REACH Rehabilitation and Catastrophic Long-Term Care
1180 Us Highway 22
Mountainside, NJ 07092-2810   908-654-0020
                                        Fax: 908-654-8661
Allen Swanson, Manager
Archie Ordana, Manager
Postacute rehabilitation program.

6873 Rehabilitation Specialists
18-01 Pollitt Drive
Ste 1A
Fair Lawn, NJ 07410-2815   201-478-4200
                                         800-441-7488
                                    Fax: 201-478-4201
                          www.rehab-specialists.com
Virgilio Caraballo, President/CEO
Dustin Gordon, Director of Neuropsychological and Clinical Services
Dr. Brian Greenwald, Medical Director
Rehabilitation Specialists, founded in 1983, is a quality, cost effective community re-entry center treating individuals with acquired brain injury. A non clinical environment based in the community is utilized that offers professional services enabling participants to learn skills they need to return to a productive life. Both our Day and Residential programming emphases focus on Functional Life Skills, Work Skills and Learning Skills. Each participant's program is tailored to meet their needs.

6874 Somerset Valley Rehabilitation and Nursing Center
Care-One
11300 Cornell Park Drive
Suite 360
Cincinnati, OH 45242   513-469-7222
                                    Fax: 513-469-7230
                              info@healthbridge.org
Trudi Matthews, Director of Policy and Public Re
Subacute rehabilitation program, long term care, respite care.

6875 Summit Ridge Center
101 East State Street
Kennett Square, PA 19348   973-736-2000
                                    Fax: 973-736-2764
                                       genesishcc.com
Offers rehabilitation services, occupational therapy, physical therapy and more for the physically challenged. A 152-bed nursing home.

New Mexico

6876 SJR Rehabilitation Hospital
525 S Schwartz Ave
Farmington, NM 87401-5955   505-609-2625
                                    Fax: 505-327-6562
                                 eniemand@sjrmc.net
                                     www.sjrrh.com
Ena M Niemand, Executive Director
Sue Clay, Program Director
Jill Morgan, Nursing Director
Uses a team of professionals to provide a comprehensive rehabilitation program. Accomplishing the best possible physical and cognitive improvement is the aim of the following treatment members: nurses, physical therapists, physicians, speech and occupational therapists, therapeutic recreation specialist. Providing inpatient and out patient services.

6877 Southwest Communication Resource
P.O.Box 788
Bernalillo, NM 87004-788   505-867-3396
                                    Fax: 505-867-3398
                                 info@abrazosnm.org
                                          swcr.org
Services for infants, children and adults with developmental disabilities in Sandoval County New Mexico.

New York

6878 Aspire of Western New York
2356 N Forest Rd
Getzville, NY 14068-1224   716-838-0047
                                    Fax: 716-894-8257
                                 info@aspirewny.org
                                      aspirewny.org
Thomas A. Sy, Executive Director
Janet Hansen, Chief Operating Officer
Mary Anne Coombe, V.P. of Service Coordination & Fiscal Management Services
Provides comprehensive services to individuals with disabilities from infancy through adulthood. Also serves people with all types of developmental disabilities as well as providing clinical services to persons with other types of disabilities such as: spinal cord injury, head trauma and others. Aspire employs 1500 people.

6879 Bronx Continuing Treatment Day Program
1527 Southern Blvd
Bronx, NY 10460-5619   718-893-1414
                                    Fax: 718-893-0707
Mary Jane Purcell, Manager
Post-acute rehabilitation program.

6880 Brooklyn Bureau of Community Service
285 Schermerhorn St
Brooklyn, NY 11217-1098   718-310-5600
                                    Fax: 718-855-1517
                                 info@WeAreBCS.org
                                   www.wearebcs.org
Marla Simpson, Executive Director
Anthony B. Edwards, MBA, CCF, MFM, CFO
Janelle Farris, Chief Operating Officer
Offers independent living skills, counseling, work readiness, vocational trianing, job placement and job follow-up services to individuals with disabilities (to include individuals with psychiatric, physical, and developmental disabilities). Special programs to move disabled welfare recipients from welfare to work. Publishes a bi-annual newsletter.

6881 Buffalo Hearing and Speech Center
50 E North St
Buffalo, NY 14203-1002   716-885-8318
                                    Fax: 716-885-4229
                                       askbhsc.org
Frank J. Polino, Chairman
Dennis J. Szefel, First Vice Chairman
Kenneth J. Wilson, Treasurer
Assists individuals with speech, language and/or hearing impairments to achieve maximum communication potential.

6882 Cora Hoffman Center Day Program
2324 Forest Ave
Staten Island, NY 10303-1506   718-447-8205
                                    Fax: 718-815-2182
Kevin Kenney, Manager
Post-acute rehabilitation program specializing in Cerebral Palsy. Part of the Cerebral Palsey Association of New York State.

6883 Devereux Advanced Behavioral Health New York
Devereux New York
40 Devereux Way
Red Hook, NY 12571   845-758-1899
                                    Fax: 845-758-1817
                                   www.devereuxny.org
John Lopez, Executive Director
Arthur Roberts, Director of Human Resources
Jeffrey Obiekwe, Program Supervisor
Devereux New York provides a wide range of educational, clinical, residential, and community-based programs and services to people of all ages with intellectual disabilities, Autism Spectrum Disorder, and dual diagnoses. Some services include psychotherapy, life skills development, physical therapies, residential programs, case management, self advocacy and more.

6884   Elmhurst Hospital Center
7901 Broadway
Elmhurst, NY 11373-1368   718-334-4000
www.nyc.gov/html/hhc/ehc/html/home/home.shtml
Chris D Constantino, Executive Director
Hospital is comprised of 525 beds and is a Level I Trauma Center, and Emergency Heart Care Stattion and a 911 recieving hospital. It is the premiere health care organization for key areas such as Surgery, Cardiology, Women's health, Pediatrics, Rehabilitation Medicine, Renal and Mental Health Services.

6885   Federation Employment And Guidance Service(F-E-G-S)
315 Hudson St
New York, NY 10013-1086   212-366-8400
Fax: 212-366-8441
info@fegs.org
www.fegs.org

Gail Magaliff, CEO
Ira Machowsky, Executive Vice President
Thomas M. Higgins, CFO
The largest and most diversified private, not-for-profit health related and human service organization in the United States. With operations in over 258 facilities, residences, and off-site locations, F-E-G-S has served more then 2 million people since its inception.

6886   Flushing Hospital
4500 Parsons Blvd
Flushing, NY 11355-2205   718-670-5000
Fax: 718-670-3082
flushinghospital.org
Robert V. Levine, Executive Vice President and COO
Bruce J. Flanz, President/ CEO
Mounir Doss, Executive Vice President/CFO
Offers services for the totally blind, legally blind, visually impaired, and more with health, counseling, educational, recreational, rehabilitation, computer training and professional training services.

6887   Gateway Community Industries Inc.,
1 Amy Kay Pkwy
Kingston, NY 12401-6444   845-331-1261
800-454-9395
Fax: 845-331-4920
info@gatewayindustries.org
gatewayindustries.org
Francoise C. Gunefsky, President/ CEO
Eva Graham, CFO
Ralph Smith, Chief Information Officer
Gateway Community Industries, Inc., founded in 1957, is one of the leading independent not-for-profit vocational rehabilitation and training centers for people with mental and/or physical disabilities. The agency provides comprehensive services in vocational evaluation, job training, job placement, vocational work center employment, supported employment, psychiatric rehabilitation, continuing day treatment, and residential habilitation/rehabilitation.

6888   Henkind Eye Institute Division of Montefiore Hospital
111 East 210th Street
Bronx, NY 10467-2404   718-920-4321
www.montefiore.org
Philip O. Ozuah, MD, PhD, Executive Vice President/ COO
Steven M. Safyer, MD, President/ CEO
Joel A. Perlman, Executive Vice President, Chief Financial Officer
Offers services for the totally blind, legally blind, visually impaired, and more with health, counseling, educational, recreational, rehabilitation, computer training and professional training services. Low vision services offered.

6889   Industries for the Blind of New York State
194 Washington Ave
Ste 300
Albany, NY 12210-6314   518-456-8671
800-421-9010
Fax: 518-456-3587
customercare@nyspsp.org
www.abilityone.com
Richard Healey, CEO

Offers services for the totally blind, legally blind, visually impaired, and more with health, counseling, educational, recreational, rehabilitation, computer training and professional training services.

6890   Inpatient Pain Rehabilitation Program
550 First Avenue
New York, NY 10016   212-263-7300
Fax: 212-598-6468
www.med.nyu.edu
William Pinter Phd, Administrative Director
The Inpatient Rehabilitation Program, established in 1983 specializes in the treatment of chronic pain. Our inpatient program is one of the oldest and well established pain programs in the country. It is the only interdisciplinary inpatient pain program in the tri-state area and one of only 20 pain programs in the entire US to have CARF accreditation. Upon completion of an extensive evaluation, patients are admitted for an 18-day inpatient stay.

6891   Koicheff Health Care Center
2324 Forest Ave
Staten Island, NY 10303-1506   718-447-0200
Fax: 718-981-1431
Paul Castello, Clinic Director
Post-accute rehabilitation programs.

6892   New York-Presbyterian Hospital
622 W 168th St
New York, NY 10032-3796   212-305-4600
Fax: 212-305-1017
www.nyp.org
Steven J. Corwin, MD, CEO
Robert E. Kelly, MD, President
New York Presbyterian Hospital is internationally recognized for its outstanding comprehensive services. Its medical, surgical, and emergency care services provide each patient with the highest possible level of care. In addition, as part of the Hospital's commitment to the total well-being of each patient, it offers a range of specialized services, as well as special healthcare programs for neighboring communities.

6893   Norman Marcus Pain Institute
30 E 40th St
Ste 1100
New York, NY 10016   212-532-7999
Fax: 212-532-5957
support@nmpi.com
backpainusa.com
Norman J Marcus, Medical Director
We focus on muscles as the cause of most common pains, i.e. back, neck, shoulders, and headaches. We make specific muscle diagnoses and have specific treatments that in many cases will eliminate the need for surgery or relieve the pain. Patients diagnosed with herniated disc, spinal stenosis, rotator cuff tear, impingement syndrome, sciatica, fibromyalgia and headache will generally find relief.

6894   Pain Alleviation Center
Comprehensive Pain Management Associates
125 S Service Rd
Jericho, NY 11753-1038   516-997-7246
Fax: 516-997-7281
www.paincenter.com
Alex Weingarten, Director
Phillip Fyman, Director
Marisa French, Manager
One of the first pain clinics to gain national accreditation from the Commission on Accreditation of Rehabilitation Facilities. This is due largely to a patient-centered program based on the latest research.

6895   Pathfinder Village
3 Chenango Rd
Edmeston, NY 13335-2314   607-965-8377
Fax: 607-965-8655
info@pathfindervillage.org
www.pathfindervillage.org
Paul Landers, CEO
Caprice S. Eckert, Chief Financial Officer
Kelly A. Meyers, Director of Admissions

Pathfinder Village is a warm, friendly community in the rolling hills of Central New York. Here children and adults with Down Syndrome gain independence, build lasting friendships, become partners in the world and take in all that life has to offer.

6896 Pilot Industries: Ellenville
845-331-4300
48 Canal St
Ellenville, NY 12428-1327
845-647-7711
Fax: 845-647-7711

Peter Pierri, Executive Director
Betty Marks, Plant Manager
Post-acute rehabilitation services.

6897 Skills Unlimited
405 Locust Ave
Oakdale, NY 11769-1695
631-567-3320
Fax: 631-567-3285
info@skillsunlimited.org
skillsunlimited.org

Richard Kassnove, Executive Director
Our basic goals is to offer persons with disabilities the opportunity to explore and develop their full vocational potential. Our programs are unique in that by offering comprehensive services, individuals are able to deal with many different issues that could potentially affect their vocational success. Any individual that has an impairment that interferes with their ability to work is entitles to the services that we offer.

North Carolina

6898 Center for Vision Rehabilitation
Academy Eye Associates
3115 Academy Rd
Durham, NC 27707-2652
919-493-7456
800-942-1499
Fax: 919-493-1718
henry.greene@academyeye.com
academyeye.com

Henry A Greene, Owner
Vision rehabilitation and low-vision care for the visually impaired, post-stroke, head trauma and for neuro-oncology vision complications.

6899 Diversified Opportunities
1010 Herring Ave E
Wilson, NC 27893-3311
252-291-0378
Fax: 252-291-1402
www.diversifiedopportunitiesinc.com

Cindy Dixon, Executive Director
Carlton Goff, Business Manager
Ericka Simmons, QP Program Manager
Vocational rehabilitation agency, better outcomes, lower cost, guaranteed performance standards.

6900 Forsyth Medical Center
3333 Silas Creek Pkwy
Winston Salem, NC 27103-3090
336-718-5000
Fax: 336-718-9250
www.novanthealth.org

Jeffrey T. Lindsay, President
Denise Mihal, Chief Operating Officer
Stephen J. Motew, MD, Senior Vice President
Provides care that is state-of-the-art and second to none, both because of advanced treatments availiable through our clinical research and technology to the academic excellence-and caring nature-of our doctors and nurses.

6901 Industries of the Blind
914-920 W Lee St
Greensboro, NC 27403-2803
336-274-1591
800-909-7086
Fax: 336-544-3739
customerservice@iob-gso.com
industriesoftheblind.com

David Thompson, Chairperson
Scott Thornhill, 1st Vice Chairperson
Ashley S. James, Jr., 2nd Vice Chairperson

Offers services for the totally blind, legally blind, visually impaired, and more with health, counseling, educational, recreational, rehabilitation, computer training and professional training services.

6902 Johnston County Industries
1100 East Preston Street
Selma, NC 27576-3162
919-743-8700
Fax: 919-965-8023
jcindustries.com

John Shallcross, Jr., President
Durwood Woodall, Vice President
Lina Sanders-Johnson, Secretary/Treasurer
JCI is an entrepreneurial not-for-profit corporation dedicated to empowering people with disabilities or disadvantages to succeed through training and employment

6903 Learning Services: Carolina
707 Morehead Ave
Durham, NC 27707-1319
919-688-4444
888-419-9955
Fax: 919-419-9966
learningservices.com

Debra Braunling-McMorrow, President and CEO
Jeanne Mack, Chief Financial Officer and Vice President of Operations
Michael Weaver, Chief Development Officer
Located in an historic neighborhood in the heart of Durham, this campus-style setting offers easy access to resources at 3 outstanding facilities: Duke University, The University of North Carolina at Chapel Hill, and Research Triangle Park. This program provides a range of services and activities that draw upon the many resources availiable in the community.

6904 Lions Club Industries for the Blind
4500 Emperor Blvd.
Durham, NC 27703
919-596-8277
800-526-1562
Fax: 919-598-1179
inquire@buylci.com

Bill Hudson, President
Offers services for the totally blind, legally blind, visually impaired, and more with health, counseling, educational, recreational, rehabilitation, computer training and professional training services.

6905 Lions Services Inc.
5 Penn Plaza
New York, NY 10001
21 -62 -210
lsisale@aol.com

Jimmy R Cranford, President
Jimmy Cranford, President
Offers services for the totally blind, legally blind, visually impaired, and more with health, counseling, educational, recreational, rehabilitation, computer training and professional training services.

6906 Regional Rehabilitation Center Pitt County Memorial Hospital
2100 Stantonsburg Rd
Greenville, NC 27834-2818
252-847-4448
Fax: 252-816-7552

Martha M Dixon, VP General Services
An accredited, comprehensive rehabilitation center-part of a statewide network- and we're the largest such facility in eastern North Carolina. Our service area covers 29 counties, and we offer a complete array of rehabilitation services for patients of all ages. Because the Regional Rehabilitation Center is associated with both Pitt County Memorial Hospital And the Brody School of Medicine at East Carolina University, patients have access to a full range of state of the art medical services.

6907 Rehab Home Care
2660 Yonkers Rd
Raleigh, NC 27604-3384
800-447-8692
Fax: 919-831-2211

Alan Silver, CEO
Janis Hansen, Chief Operating Officer
A Medicare/Medicaid certified, state-licensed home health agency with emphasis on rehabilitation.

6908   Thoms Rehabilitation Hospital
Thoms Rehabilitation Hospital
68 Sweeten Creek Rd
Asheville, NC 28803-2318
828-277-4800
Fax: 828-277-4812
TTY: 800-735-2962
www.carepartners.org

Tracy Buchanan, President & CEO
Gary Bowers, COO
Freestanding physical rehabilitation hospital, founded 1938 -
100 beds, including 90 acute and 10 transitional - JCAHO
accredited.

6909   Winston-Salem Industries for the Blind
7730 N Point Blvd
Winston Salem, NC 27106-3310
336-759-0551
800-242-7726
Fax: 336-759-0990
info@wsifb.com
www.wsifb.com

Mike Faircloth, Chairman
Karen Carey, Vice Chairman, Secretary
W. Robert Newell, Treasurer
Offers services for the totally blind, legally blind, visually impaired, and more with health, counseling, educational, recreational, rehabilitation, computer training and professional
training services.

Ohio

6910   Bellefaire Jewish Children's Bureau
22001 Fairmount Blvd
Cleveland, OH 44118-4819
216-932-2800
800-879-2522
Fax: 216-932-6704
www.bellefairejcb.org

Adam Jacobs, CEO
Adam G. Jacobs PhD, Executive Vice President
Residential treatment for ages 12 to 17 1/2 at time of admission
offering individualized psychotherapy, special education, and
group living for severaly emotionally disturbed children and adolescents. Also offers a variety of other programs including specialized and therapuetic foster care, partial hospitilization,
outpatient counseling, home-based intensive counseling and
adoption services.

6911   Christ Hospital Rehabilitation Unit
2139 Auburn Ave
Cincinnati, OH 45219-2906
513-585-2737
Fax: 513-585-4353
www.thechristhospital.com

Mike Keating, President and CEO
Chris Bergman, Vice President and Chief Financial Officer
Berc Gawne, MD, Vice President and Chief Medical Officer
Patients of this 555-bed, not-for-profit acute care facility receive
personalized health care provided by trained specialists using the
most sophisticated medical technology available, including
state-of-the-art intensive care units, surgical facilities, cardiac
catheterization labs, three new electrophysiology labs, and the
tristates first positron emission tomography (PET) scanning
capabilities.

6912   Cleveland Sight Center
1909 E 101st St.
Cleveland, OH 44106
216-791-8118
Fax: 216-791-1101
TTY: 216-791-8119
info@clevelandsightcenter.org
www.clevelandsightcenter.org

Larry Benders, President & CEO
Kevin Krencisz, Chief Financial & Administrative Officer
Jassen Tawil, Director, Business Development & Customer Success
Social, rehabilitation, education and support services for blind
and visually impaired children and adults, early intervention program for children birth to age 6, low vision clinic, aid and appliance shop, Braille and taping transcription, training for
rehabilitation, orientation, mobility and computer access, employment services and job placement, recreation program, resi-

dent camping, talking books, radio reading services. Free
screening.

6913   Columbus Speech and Hearing Center
510 E North Broadway St
Columbus, OH 43214-4114
614-263-5151
Fax: 614-263-5365
columbusspeech.org

Dawn Gleason, Au.D., President/ CEO
Karen Deeter, Director of Operations
Serves persons who have speech-language and hearing challenges. Provides vocational rehabilitation services for individuals who are deaf, hard-of-hearing or deaf-blind.

**6914   CommuniCare of Clifton Nursing and Rehabilitation
Center**
Communi Care Health Services
4700 Ashwood Drive
Cincinnati, OH 45241
513-489-7100
Fax: 513-281-2559
communicarehealth.com

Stephen L. Rosedale, Founder/ CEO
A long term care facility which specializes in rehabilitation. Offers a full range of rehabilitative services including physical therapy, occupational therapy and speech therapy.

6915   Doctors Hospital
5100 W Broad St
Columbus, OH 43228-1672
614-544-1000
800-837-7555
Fax: 614-544-1844
www.ohiohealth.com/homedoctors

David Blom, President/ CEO
Michael Bernstein, Senior Vice President and Chief
We believe our first responsibility is to the patients we serve. We
respect the physical, emotional and spiritual needs of our patients
and find that compassion is essential to fostering healing and
wholeness.

6916   Dodd Hall at the Ohio State University Hospitals
410 W 10th Ave
Columbus, OH 43210-1240
614-293-3300
800-293-5123
OSUCareConnection@osumc.edu
www.medicalcenter.osu.edu

Steven G. Gabbe, MD, Senior Vice President / CEO
Larry Anstine, CEO
Gail Marsh, Chief Strategy Officer
Dodd Hall is a full service medical rehabilitation hospital offer-
ing comprehensive inpatient and outpatient rehabilitation.

**6917   Easterseals of Mahoning, Trumbull and Columbiana
Counties**
299 Edwards St.
Youngstown, OH 44502-1599
330-743-1168
Fax: 330-743-1616
www.easterseals.com/mtc

Maureen Pusch, Chief Executive Officer
Outpatient medical rehabilitation, skill development, vocational
support, and transportation services.

6918   Four Oaks Center
245 N. Valley Road
Xenia, OH 45385-2605
937-562-6500
Fax: 937-562-6520
www.greenedd.org

Todd McManus, President
Jill A. LaRock, Director
Dr. Vijay Gupta, Vice President
Starts children on the road to discovery by providing a learning
environment rich in opportunities and encouragement. The program was designed to give children with delays or disabilities, or
those at-risk the extra help needed to develop fully. Any child under the age of six who exhibits developmental delays, handicapping conditions, or is considered at risk may qualify to
participate.

6919   Genesis Healthcare System
Rehabilitation Services
800 Forest Ave
Zanesville, OH 43701-2881   740-454-5000
                                             800-322-4762
                                        Fax: 740-455-7527
                                        llynn@genesishcs.org
                                        www.genesishcs.org

Matt Perry, President/ CEO
Paul Masterson, CFO
Richard Helsper, COO
A CARF and JACHO accredited 19-bed rehabilitation facility located within Genesis Healthcare System, a 732 bed, non-profit hospital system, located in Zanesville, Ohio. Freestanding outpatient services, including work hardening, pain management, vocational services, audiology, lymphedema, vestibular rehab, off-the-road driving evals, aquatic therpay, womens health and sports enhancement.

6920   George A Martin Center
3603 Washington Ave
Cincinnati, OH 45229-2009   513-221-1017
                                        Fax: 513-221-3817

Karen Doggett, Executive Director
Offers services for the totally blind, legally blind, visually impaired, and more with health, counseling, educational, recreational, rehabilitation, computer training and professional training services.

6921   Grady Memorial Hospital
561 W Central Ave
Delaware, OH 43015-1489   740-615-1000
                                             800-487-1115
                                        Fax: 740-368-5114
                                        ohiohealth.com

Bruce Hagen, Regional Executive and President
As a progressive healthcare leader, Grady Memorial Hospital is committed to excellence while providing the Deleware community with comprehensive quality service delivered with compassionate, personal care. Our membership in Ohio's largest healthcare system, Ohio Health, enables us to improve access to a broader range of healthcare services, enhance development of new programs and services, and provide a complete continuum of care for patients in the deleware area.

6922   Hamilton Adult Center
3400 Symmes Rd
Hamilton, OH 45015-1359   513-867-5970
                                        Fax: 513-874-2977

Donald Musnuff, Executive Director

6923   Holzer Clinic
100 Jackson Pike
Gallipolis, OH 45631-1560   740-446-5000
                                        Fax: 740-446-5532
                                        info@holzer.org
                                        www.holzer.org

T. Wayne Munro, MD, CEO
Brent A. Saunders, Chair
Christopher Meyer, Chief Medical Officer
Serves medical needs of patients in an 8 county area, including counties in Ohio and West Virginia.

6924   Holzer Clinic Sycamore
Holzer Medical Center
4th Avenue & Sycamore St
Gallipolis, OH 45631-1560   740-446-5244
                                        Fax: 740-446-5448
                                        info@holzer.org
                                        www.holzer.org

T. Wayne Munro, MD, CEO
Brent A. Saunders, Chair
Christopher Meyer, Chief Medical Officer
Offers an individualized quality comprehensive rehabilitation program for people with disabilities by an interdisciplinary team including physical therapy, occupational, speech, nursing and social services to restore the patient to the highest degree of rehab outcomes attainable.

6925   IKRON Institute for Rehabilitative and Psychological Services
2347 Vine St
Cincinnati, OH 45213-1745   513-621-1117
                                        Fax: 513-621-2350
                                        ikron@ikron.org
                                        ikron.org

Randy Strunk, MA, LPCC-S, Executive Director
Ken Carbonell, BBA, Fiscal Director
Melissa Harmeling, MA, PCC-S, Program Director
An accredited mental health facility and a certified rehabilitation center. Through a variety of creative treatment and rehabilitation services, IKRON assists adults with mental health and/or substance abuse problems to attain greater independence, to lead lives of sobriety, to obtain competitive work and live more satisfying lives. IKRON places a strong emphasis on respect and support for persons with problems of adjustment. Special contracts to persons desiring job placement.

6926   Integrated Health Services at Waterford Commons
955 Garden Lake Pkwy
Toledo, OH 43614-2777   419-382-2200
                                        Fax: 419-381-8508

Nicole Giesige, Executive Director
A subacute and rehabilitation program specializing in ventilator weaning and management, I.V. therapeutics and pain management, wound management and subacute rehabilitation.

6927   Lester H Higgins Adult Center
3041 Cleveland Ave SW
Canton, OH 44707-3625   330-484-4814
                                        Fax: 330-484-9416
                                        http://www.theworkshopsinc.com/

Margalie Belazaire, Manager
Ed Allar, Manager
Post-accute rehabilitation service

6928   Live Oaks Career Development Campus
5936 Buckwheat Rd
Milford, OH 45150   513-575-1906
                                        Fax: 513-575-0805

Harold Carr MD, Superintendent
Robin White, President/CEO
Jim Dixon, Principal
Post-accute rehabilitation facility and services.

6929   Metro Health: St. Luke's Medical Center Pain Management Program
2500 Metrohealth Dr
Cleveland, OH 44109-1900   216-778-7800
                                        www.metrohealth.org

Mark Moran, President
CARF accredited comprehensive multidisciplinary pain management program.

6930   MetroHealth Medical Center
2500 Metrohealth Dr
Cleveland, OH 44109-1900   216-778-7800
                                        www.metrohealth.org

Mark Moran, President
Located on the near west side of Cleveland, is a leader in trauma, emergency, and critical care; women's and childrens's services, including high risk obstetrical care and neonatal intensive care; comprehensive medical and surgical subspecialties.

6931   Middletown Regional Hospital: Inpatient Rehabilitation Unit
105 McKnight Dr
Middletown, OH 45044-4838   513-422-1401
                                             800-338-4057
                                        Fax: 513-422-1520
                                        www.middletownhospital.org

C N Reddy, Owner
Douglas McNeill, Chief Executive Officer
Our mission is to serve and help people, improving the status of their health and the quality of thier lives. Our vision is to be the premier integrated delivery system in Southwest Ohio. Our Values are quality, respect, service and teamwork

6932 Newark Healthcare Center
680 South Fourth Street
Louisville, KY 40202
502-596-7300
TTY: 800-545-0749
web_administrator@kindred.com
kindredhealthcare.com

Paul J. Diaz, President/ CEO
Accomodates 300 residents. We are located in the heart of Newark, Ohio. Newark Healthcare is a 2004 recipient of the American Health Care Association's Quality Award.

6933 Parma Community General Hospital Acute Rehabilitation Center
7007 Powers Blvd
Parma, OH 44129-5495
440-743-3000
Fax: 440-843-4387
www.parmahospital.org

David Nedrich, Chairman
Thomas P. O'Donnell, First Vice Chairman
Alex I. Koler, First Assistant Treasurer
The mission of this CARF accredited unit is to provide the most comprehensive, cost-effective, acute rehabilitation program possible in order for every patient and family to adjust to his/her disability and to achieve the maximum potential of independent functioning when returning to community living.

6934 Peter A Towne Physical Therapy Center
Ste 10
447 Nilles Rd
Fairfield, OH 45014-2626
513-829-7726
Fax: 513-829-7726

Debbie Wilkerson, Office Manager
Outpatient, private practice physical and occupational therapy. Three other offices in Hamilton, Monroe and West Chester.

6935 Philomatheon Society of the Blind
2701 Tuscarawas St W
Canton, OH 44708-4638
330-453-9157
www.philomatheon.com

David Miller, President
Denise Dessecker, Vice President
Angela Randall, Secretary
Offers services for the totally blind, legally blind, visually impaired, and more with health, counseling, educational, recreational, rehabilitation, computer training and professional training services.

6936 Providence Hospital Work
2270 Banning Rd
Cincinnati, OH 45239-6621
513-591-5600
Fax: 513-591-5604

Kay Brogle, Executive Director
Post-acute rehabilitation services.

6937 Six County, Inc.
2845 Bell St
Zanesville, OH 43701-1794
740-454-9766
800-344-5818
Fax: 740-588-6452
www.sixcounty.org

John A Creek, President
Tim Llewellyn, Senior VP/Community Intervention
Robert Santos, Ex Vp & Coo
Six County, Inc., is a private, not-for-profit corporation under contract with the Mental Health and Recovery Services Board. Six County, Inc., provides comprehensive community mental health services to people of all ages in each of the six Southeastern Ohio counties served: Coshocton, Guernsey, Morgan, Muskingum, Noble, and Perry. SCI's counseling centers provide a full range of services including outpatient counseling; diagnostic assessment, referrals, and psychological testing.

6938 Society for Rehabilitation
9290 Lake Shore Blvd
Mentor, OH 44060-1664
440-352-8993
800-344-3159
Fax: 440-352-6632

Richard Kessler, Executive Director
Vision is to provide individuals with comprehensive services to improve their quality of life. Our mission is to meet the needs of individuals and their families by delivering a wide range of affordable accessible and personalized services, providing treatment by a team of highly qualified, caring professionals. Collaborating with other agencies to meet community needs.

6939 Southeast Ohio Sight Center
425 E. Alvarado Street
Suite E
Fallbrook, CA 92028
800-677-4180
www.charityadvantage.com
Offers services for the blind and visually impaired to include functional low vision evaluations, community rehabilitation trading, counseling, educational, recreational, rehabilitation and vocational services.

6940 St. Francis Rehabilitation Hospital
401 N Broadway St
Green Springs, OH 44836-9638
419-639-2626
800-248-2552
Fax: 419-639-6225

Kim Eicher, CEO
Dan Schwanke, Chief Executive Officer
Program offers specialized treatment for patients who have suffered a head injury, spinal cord injury, or stroke, or who have an orthopedic injury. The Head Injury Program provides a continuum of care from coma stimulation through transitional living. Their physicians, nurses, counselors and therapists are dedicated to helping our patients develop the motivation, strength and skills needed to overcome or adapt to their disability.

6941 TAC Enterprises
2160 Old Selma Rd
Springfield, OH 45505-4600
937-525-7400
Fax: 937-525-7401
info@tacind.com
www.tacind.com

Clifford Meyer, CEO
TAC Enterprises provides employment opportunities for individuals to develop marketable skills by completing contract work in partnership with other industries. Work and self-help skills, social adjustment, and a variety of daily living experiences are offered to the workers by our specialized staff.

Oklahoma

6942 Dean A McGee Eye Institute
608 Stanton L Young Blvd
Oklahoma City, OK 73104-5065
405-271-6060
800-787-9012
Fax: 405-271-4442
www.mei.org

Gregory L. Skuta, M.D., President/CEO
Matthew D. Brown, Executive Vice President
Lana G. Ivy, Vice President of Development
Offers services for the totally blind, legally blind, visually impaired, and more with health, counseling, educational, recreational, rehabilitation, computer training and professional training services.

6943 Jane Phillips Medical Center
Rehab Care
3500 E Frank Phillips Blvd
Bartlesville, OK 74006-2464
918-333-7200
Fax: 918-333-7801
webmaster@jpmc.org
jpmc.org

David Stire, President/ COO
Mike Moore, Chief Financial Officer/Vice President Fiscal Services
Susan Herron, RN, Vice President Nursing Services
Comprehensive inpatient rehabilitation services are provided to patients with orthopedic, neurologic, and other medical conditions of recent onset or regression, who have experienced a loss of function in activities of daily living, mobility, cognition and communication.

6944 McAlester Regional Health Center RehabCare Unit
1 E Clark Bass Blvd
McAlester, OK 74501-4255   918-426-1800
                                    Fax: 918-421-6832
                                    nbrinlee@mrhcok.com
                                    www.mrhcok.com

David Keith, President/ CEO
Cara Bland, Chairman
Evans McBride, Vice-Chairman
A 19-bed inpatient physical rehabilitation unit serving the Southeast Oklahoma area. Offers physical therapy, occupational therapy, social work, speech and psychological services in an interdisciplinary framework.

6945 Oklahoma League for the Blind
501 N Douglas Ave
Oklahoma City, OK 73106-5085   405-232-4644
                                        888-522-4644
                                    Fax: 405-236-5438
                                    info@newviewoklahoma.org
                                    www.newviewoklahoma.org

Lauren White, President/ CEO
Carol Campbell, Executive Assistant
John Wilson, Chief Financial Officer
Offers services for the blind and visually impaired, counseling, educational, recreational, rehabilitation, computer training and professional training services.

6946 Valley View Regional Hospital-RehabCare Unit
430 N Monte Vista St
Ada, OK 74820-4657   580-332-2323
                                    Fax: 580-421-1395

W. Kent Rogers, President/ CEO
Comprehensive physical medicine and rehabilitation services designed to help patients in their adjustment to a physically limiting condition.

Oregon

6947 Garten Services
PO Box 13970
Salem, OR 97309   503-581-1984
                                    Fax: 503-581-4497
                                    garten@garten.org
                                    garten.org

Tim Rocak, CEO
Pamela Best, CFO
Steve Babcock, Mail Services Manager
Garten's mission is to support people with disabilities in their effort to contribute to the community through employment, career, and retirement opportunities. Our actions increase society's awareness of human potential. Garten's vision is to be recognized as an organization positively demonstrating to the community that people with disabilities can be contributing and valued employees of a thriving business.

6948 Legacy Emanuel Rehabilitation Center
2801 N. Gantenbein
Portland, OR 97227-1542   503-413-2200
                                    Fax: 503-413-1501
                                    www.legacyhealth.org

Gary Guidetta, Executive Director
Gail Weisgerber, Manager
A non-profit tax-exempt corporation that includes 5 full-service hospitals and a children's hospital. The Legacy system provides an integrated network of healthcare services, including acute and critical care, inpatient and outpatient treatment, community health education and a variety of specialty services.

6949 Oakcrest Care Center
2933 Center St NE
Salem, OR 97301-4527   503-585-5850
                                    Fax: 503-585-8781

Postacute rehabilitation program.

6950 Oakhill-Senior Program
1190 Oakhill Ave SE
Salem, OR 97302-3496   503-364-9086
                                    Fax: 503-365-2879

Jan Dillon, Senior Services Manager
Garten Senior Services provides an adult day service program to seniors with and without developmental disabilities. The program will provide community opportunities, college classes and a wide variety of leisure activities in group and individual settings.

6951 Pacific Spine and Pain Center
1801 Highway 99 N
Ashland, OR 97520-9152   541-488-2255
                                        866-482-5515
                                    Fax: 541-482-2433

Janel R Guyette, Manager

6952 Vision Northwest
9225 SW Hall Blvd
Portland, OR 97223-6794   503-684-8389
                                        800-448-2232
                                    Fax: 503-684-9359
                                    visionnw.com

Evelyn Maizels, Executive Director
Offers services for the totally blind, legally blind, visually impaired, and more with health, counseling, educational, recreational, rehabilitation, computer training and professional training services.

6953 Willamette Valley Rehabilitation Center
1853 W Airway Rd
Lebanon, OR 97355-1233   541-258-8121
                                    Fax: 541-451-1762
                                    wvrc.org

Martin Baughman, Executive Director
Provides the best professional vocational services to those adults in the community who, by virtue of their physical or mental limitations, are negatively impacted by their ability to attain or maintain employment.

Pennsylvania

6954 Alpine Nursing and Rehabilitation Center of Hershey
Pennstate
405 Martin Ter
State College, PA 16803-3426   814-865-1710
                                    Fax: 814-863-9423

Melissa A Hardy, Director
Anna Shuey, Administrative Assistant
Postacute rehabilitation program.

6955 Beechwood Rehabilitation Services A Community Integrated Brain Injury Program
469 E Maple Ave
Langhorne, PA 19047-1600   215-750-4299
                                        800-782-3299
                                    Fax: 215-750-4327
                                    beechwoodrehab.com

Thomas Felicetti, President
Services include residential, day treatment and community based support services. Individuals with brain injury are served. The facility is Care Accredited.

6956 Blind & Vision Rehabilitation Services Of Pittsburgh
1800 West St
Homestead, PA 15120-2578   412-368-4400
                                        800-706-5050
                                    Fax: 412-368-4090
                                    www.bvrspittsburgh.org

Erika M. Arbogast, President
Brian Glass, Director of Information Services and Facilities
Leslie Montgomery, Director of Development and Public Relations
Offers services for the totally blind, legally blind, visually impaired, and more with health, counseling, educational, recreational, rehabilitation, computer training and professional training services.

6957 Bradford Regional Medical Center
116 Interstate Pkwy
Bradford, PA 16701-1036   814-368-4143
                                    Fax: 814-368-4130
                                        www.brmc.com

Marek Dzionara, Owner
Andrew Lehman, Executive Director
Timothy J. Finan, President and CEO
Offers rehabilitation services to individuals with an alcohol or drug related problem.

6958 Bryn Mawr Rehabilitation Hospital
414 Paoli Pike
Malvern, PA 19355-3311   610-251-5400
                                       888-734-2241
                                       888-734-2241
                                    Fax: 610-647-3648

Donna M. Phillips, President
We are dedicated to serving individuals and their families whose lives can be enhanced through physical or cognitive rehabilitation. We continually strive for excellence by providing care and services which are valued by those we serve and by contributing to the community through education, research and prevention of disability.

6959 Devereux Advanced Behavioral Health - National Office
National Headquarters
444 Devereux Dr
Villanova, PA 19085   800-345-1292
                              devereuxhr@devereux.org
                                     www.devereux.org

Samuel G Coppersmith, Esq, Chairman
Robert Q Kreider, President & CEO
Marilyn B Benoit, MD, Senior Vice President, Chief Clinical & Medical Officer
Devereux is a behavioral health organization supporting people with autism, intellectual and developmental disabilities, and specialty mental health needs. Some of the services offered by Devereux include diagnostics, special education, professional training, research and advocacy.

6960 Devereux Pennsylvania
444 Devereux Dr
Villanova, PA 19085   610-788-6565
                                       800-345-1292
                                    Fax: 610-430-0567
                                      www.devereuxpa.org

Carol Oliver, MS, State Director & Vice President of Operations
Melanie Beidler, MS, Executive Director, Intellectual/Developmental Disabilities
Stephen Bruce, M.Ed, BCBA, Executive Director, Adult Services
Devereux Pennsylvania provides educational and residential programs, therapeutic foster care, case management, customized employment and community-based behavioral health programs to children and adults with intellectual and behavioral challenges.

6961 Fox Subacute Center
2644 Bristol Rd
Warrington, PA 18976-1404   800-782-2288

James Foulke, CEO
Vic Costenko, COO
Walter Dunsmore, CFO
Fox subacute recognizes the great need for alternative programs for today's medically compromised patients. Fox has developed Models of Care and offers subacute programs fore the management of ventilator-dependent patients. We recognize that the best road to recovery for these patients is an environment with special care in an alternative setting. We believe that setting should be outside the hospital, in facilities where the focus is on the management of individual patients.

6962 Fox Subacute at Clara Burke
251 Stenton Ave
Plymouth Meeting, PA 19462-1220   610-828-2272
                                       800-424-7201
                                    Fax: 610-828-7939
                              admissions@foxsubacute.com
                                    www.foxsubacute.com

Terri Herd, Director of Marketing
Amy Swartley, RN,, Director of Admissions
Kathy Palladino, Director of Human Resources
Fox Subacute at Clara Burke in Plymouth Meeting, PA offers attentive, nurturing management of ventilator dependent, medically compromised patients in the PA, NJ, DE, Tri-State area. This sixty-bed facility, with its picturesque setting on 16 acres in historic Plymouth Meeting, is ideal for the specialized services and programs offered by Fox. With a team of highly motivated professionals, we offer the discharge alternative to prolonged lengths of stay in more costly acute care settings.

6963 Good Samaritan Health System
4th & Walnut Sts
P.O.Box 1281
Lebanon, PA 17042-1281   717-270-7500
                                        www.gshleb.org

Robin Weiler, Manager
Frederick Davis, VP Clinical Services
Offers services for the totally blind, legally blind, visually impaired, and more with health, counseling, educational, recreational, rehabilitation, computer training and professional training services.

6964 Good Samaritan Hospital-Health System Center
Good Samaritan Hospital
4th & Walnut Sts
P.O.Box 1281
Lebanon, PA 17042-1281   717-270-7500
                                        www.gshleb.org

June Nafziger-Eberl, Manager
Stuart Hartman, Medical Director
Comprehensive inpatient rehab unit for adults regarding general physical rehabilitation. Specific programs include orthopedic, neurological, stroke, amputee, etc.

6965 Pediatric Center at Plymouth Meeting Integrated Health Services
491 Allendale Rd
King of Prussia, PA 19406-1426   610-265-9290
                                       800-220-7337

Fran Currick, Manager
Subacute programs such as intensive respiratory care, stressing ventilator dependent children, pre and post transplant care, total parenteral nutrition, IV therapy, intensive/behavioral oral feeding programs. Provides extensive discharge planning including teaching or review for all the above programs with an emphasis on development and accessing community resources.

6966 Penn State Milton S. Hershey Medical Center College Of Medicine
500 University Dr
Hershey, PA 17033-2360   717-531-8521
                                       800-243-1455
                                    Fax: 717-531-4558
                                   www.pennstatehershey.org

Harold L Paz, CEO
Alan L. Brechbill, Executive Director
Wayne Zolko, Associate Vice President for Finance and Business
a non-sectarian, not-for-profit community hospital whose purpose is to provide high quality acute, rehabilitative and preventive health services for the entire community, regardless of creed, race, nationality, or ability to pay.

6967 Pennsylvania Pain Rehabilitation Center
Ste 2
252 W Swamp Rd
Doylestown, PA 18901-2465   215-230-9707
                                    Fax: 215-348-5106

Kenneth Lefkowitz, Manager
Post acute rehabilitation facility and programs.

6968 Rehabilitation & Nursing Center at Greater Pittsburgh, The
890 Weatherwood Ln
Greensburg, PA 15601-5777   724-837-8076
Fax: 724-837-7456
Nancy Flenner, Administrator
Marsha Echard, Admissions Coordinator
Subacute care, ventilator and pulmonary managment, comprehensive rehabilitation.

Rhode Island

6969 In-Sight
43 Jefferson Blvd
Warwick, RI 02888-6400   401-941-3322
Fax: 401-941-3356
cbutler@in-sight.org
in-sight.org
Chris Butler, Executive Director
Lucille Gaboriault, Director of Community Resources
Paul Hopkins, Director of First Impressions
Offers services for the totally blind, legally blind, visually impaired, and more with health, counseling, educational, recreational, rehabilitation, computer training and professional training services.

6970 Vanderbilt Rehabilitation Center
Newport Hospital
167 Point Street
Providence, RI 02903   401-444-3500
www.lifespan.org
Timothy J. Babineau, President/CEO
Kenneth E. Arnold, SVP, General Counsel
Carole M. Cotter, SVP, Chief Information Officer
The Vanderbilt Rehabilitation Center at Newport Hospital has been providing comprehensive rehabilitation sercices for more than 40 years and is known throughout the region for its unique programs and high-quality, patient focused care.

South Carolina

6971 Association for the Blind
One Carriage Lane
Building A
Charleston, SC 29407   843-723-6915
Fax: 843-577-4312
www.abvisc.org
J. Douglas Hazelton, President
Capers A. Grimball, Vice President
Lea B. Kerrison, Secretary
Offers services for people who are blind, or are visually impaired with health, counseling, educational, recreational, rehabilitation, computer training and professional training services.

6972 Hitchcock Rehabilitation Center
690 Medical Park Dr
Aiken, SC 29801-6348   803-648-8344
800-207-6924
Fax: 803-648-1631
Karen Bowlen, Administrator
Dan Hillman, Case Manager
Carrie Morgan, Finance Director
Comprehensive outpatient rehabilitation for adults, children, geriatrics, pediatric therapy, special needs preschool, sports medicine, home health and hospice.

6973 Mentor Network, The
3600 Forest Drive
Suite 100
Columbia, SC 29204-1891   803-799-9025
800-297-8043
Fax: 803-931-8959
thementornetwork.com
Edward Murphy, Executive Chairman
Bruce Nardella, President and CEO
Denis Holler, Chief Financial Officer
Mentor provides a full network of individually tailored services for people with development disabilities and their families. Individuals may be served in their homes, shared living home, or in a host home.

Tennessee

6974 Humana Hospital: Morristown RehabCare
726 McFarland St
Morristown, TN 37814-3989   423-522-6000
www.lakewayregionalhospital.com
James Perry, Program Director
Designed to help patients in their adjustment to a physically limiting condition by helping to maximize each patient's abilities so he or she can function as independently as possible.

6975 Opportunity East Rehabilitation Services for the Blind
758 W Morris Blvd
Morristown, TN 37813-2136   423-586-3922
800-278-6274
Fax: 423-586-1479
volblind.org
Fred Overbay, CEO
Vic Mende, Director Rehabilitation Services
Offers services for the totally blind, legally blind, visually impaired, and more with health, counseling, educational, recreational, rehabilitation, computer training and professional training services.

6976 Patrick Rehab Wellness Center
Lincoln County Health System
106 Medical Center Blvd
Fayetteville, TN 37334-2684   931-433-0273
Fax: 931-433-0378
Gloria Meadows, Administrator
Jim Stewart, Principal
Provides rehabilitation services of physical, occupational, and speech therapy. Also, wellness memberships are available to the public.

6977 PharmaThera
1785 Nonconnah Blvd
Memphis, TN 38132-2104   901-348-8100
800-767-6714
Fax: 901-348-8270
Offers 10 locations serving patients throughout the southern United States, each with an in-house, expertly trained staff. All locations use the latest technologies and techniques in infusion care to provide a broad range of individualized home infusion therapies.

6978 Siskin Hospital For Physical Rehabilitation
1 Siskin Plz
Chattanooga, TN 37403-1306   423-634-1200
info@siskinrehab.org
siskinrehab.org
Bob Main, CEO
Robert P. Main, President
Dedicated exclusively to physical rehabilitation and offers specialized treatment programs in brain injury, amputation, stroke, spinal cord injury, orthopedics, and major multiple trauma. The hospital also provides treatment for neurological disorders and loss of muscle strength and controll following illness or surgery.

6979 St. Mary's RehabCare Center
900 E Oak Hill Ave
Knoxville, TN 37917-4556   865-545-7962
Fax: 865-545-8133
Debbie Keeton, Director
Beth Greco, Executive Director
Provides comprehensive rehabilitation services for patients experiencing CVA, head trauma, orthopedic conditions, spinal cord injury or neurological impairment.

Texas

6980 Alpine Ridge and Brandywood
444 Devereux Drive
Victoria, TX 19085-2666
361-575-8271
800-345-1292
Fax: 361-575-6520
devereux.org

Robert Q. Kreider, President and CEO
Margaret McGill, SVP, Chief Operations Officer
Robert C. Dunne, SVP & Chief Financial Officer, Treasurer

6981 Amity Lodge
Devereux Foundation
444 Devereux Drive
Victoria, TX 19085-2666
361-575-8271
800-345-1292
Fax: 361-575-6520
devereux.org

Robert Q. Kreider, President and CEO
Margaret McGill, SVP, Chief Operations Officer
Robert C. Dunne, SVP & Chief Financial Officer, Treasurer
Offers residents a continuum of services ranging from minimal care and supervision to total physical and medical care.

6982 Baylor Institute for Rehabilitation
3500 Gaston Avenue
Dallas, TX 75246-2017
214-820-9300
800-4BA-YLOR
Fax: 214-841-2679
www.baylorhealth.com

Joel T. Allison, Chief Executive Officer
Gary Brock, President and Chief Operating Officer
LaVone Arthur, Vice President of Business Development
A 92-bed specialty hospital offering comprehensive rehabilitation services for persons with spinal cord injury, traumatic brain injury, stroke, amputation, and other orthopedic and neurological disorders.

6983 Beneto Center
Devereux Foundation
444 Devereux Drive
Victoria, TX 19085-2666
361-575-8271
800-345-1292
Fax: 361-575-6520
devereux.org

Robert Q. Kreider, President and CEO
Margaret McGill, SVP, Chief Operations Officer
Robert C. Dunne, SVP & Chief Financial Officer, Treasurer
Offers a continuum of services for residents requiring services ranging from minimal care and supervision to total physical and medical care.

6984 CORE Health Care
E&J Health Care
400 Highway 290
Bldg B, Suite. 205,
Dripping Springs, TX 78620
512-894-0801
866-683-1007
Fax: 512-858-4627

Eric Makowski, CEO
Kristi Jones, Marketing/Admissions Director
Erika Mountz, MBA, OTR/L, Director of Rehabilitation
Post acute and transitional rehabilitation, long-term care, community re-entry, for brain injury and complex psychiatric disorders.

6985 Center for Neuro Skills
1320 W Walnut Hill Ln
Irving, TX 75038-3007
972-580-8500
800-544-5448
Fax: 972-255-3162
srobinson@neuroskills.com
neuroskills.com

John Schultz, Administrator
Mark J. Ashley, President
Centre for Neuro Skills (CNS) seeks to provide medical rehabilitation programs, lifecare programs, advocacy, and research for people with brain injury in order to achieve a maximum quality of life.

6986 Dallas Services
4242 Office Pkwy
Dallas, TX 75204-3629
214-828-9900
Fax: 214-828-9901
www.dallasservices.org

Thomas. Turnage, Ph.D, Executive Director
Clark Thomas, Ph.D., Chair
Melissa Malonson, Vice-Chair
Offers four programs: 1) an early education for children(6weeks-6yrs) with and without special needs. 2) low vision clinic-provides low cost eye examsand glasses to low-income families as well as assistance to individuals who vision problems which cannot be corrected with glasses/surgery. 3) mesquite day school- an early head start program for infants and toddlers of low-income families. 4) special needs advocacy and inclusion program that offers families of special need children guidance and education.

6987 Daman Villa
Devereux Foundation
444 Devereux Drive
Victoria, TX 19085-2666
361-575-8271
800-345-1292
Fax: 361-575-6520
devereux.org

Robert Q. Kreider, President and CEO
Margaret McGill, SVP, Chief Operations Officer
Robert C. Dunne, SVP & Chief Financial Officer, Treasurer
Offers residents a continuum of services ranging from minimal care and supervision to total physical and medical care.

6988 Devereux Advanced Behavioral Health - Texas Victoria Campus
Texas Victoria Campus
120 David Wade Dr.
P.O. Box 2666
Victoria, TX 77902
361-574-7208
800-383-5000
Fax: 361-575-6250
www.devereuxtx.org

Pam Reed, Executive Director
Offering residential services for people of all ages with emotional, behavioral, developmental, and psychiatric disorders. Services include community based living and vocational programs, residential programs and foster care.

6989 Devereux Advanced Behavioral Health Texas - League City Campus
Texas League City Campus
1150 Devereux Dr
League City, TX 77573
281-335-1000
800-373-0011
Fax: 281-554-6290
www.devereuxtx.org

Gail Atkinson, Vice President of Operations & Marketing
Offering long-term hospitalization and intensive residential services for adolescents and young adults with emotional, behavioral, developmental and psychiatric disorders.

6990 El Paso Lighthouse for the Blind
200 Washington St
El Paso, TX 79905-3897
915-532-4495
Fax: 915-532-6338
www.lighthouse-elpaso.com

Craig Hays, President
Lea Cochran, Vice President
Lola Dawkins, Secretary
Enables people of all ages to embody blindness and vision impairment through training, rehabilitation, employment opportunity, advocacy and research. Provides access to opportunities and quality of life so that the blind and visually impaired can reach their fullest potential for self-sufficiency and independence.

6991 Harris Methodist Fort Worth/Mabee Rehabilitation Center
612 E. Lamar Boulevard
Arlington, TX 76011-2122
877-847-9355
Fax: 817-882-2753
www.texashealth.org

Louise Baldwin, President
Peggyo Ehrlich, Rehab Manager
Karen Mallett, Executive Director
A hospital based inpatient rehab program and outpatient day programs in chronic pain management, work hardening and brain injury transitional services.

6992 HealthSouth Hospital of Cypress
13031 Wortham Center Dr
Houston, TX 77065
832-280-2500
feedback@healthsouth.com
healthsouthcypress.com

Jerome Lengel, Executive Officer
Dewitt Hilton, Owner
Offers an individualized approach to the process of rehabilitation for severely injured or disabled individuals. The process begins with a pre-admissions assessment of each referred patient. The Center combines state-of-the-art technology and equipment with multi-disciplinary therapy and education in a cheerful, secure environment.

6993 Heights Hospital Rehab Unit
1917 Ashland St
Houston, TX 77008-3994
713-861-6161
Fax: 713-802-8660
www.selectmedical.com

Theresa Davis, CEO
Robert A. Ortenzio, Executive Chairman and Co-Founder
Rocco A. Ortenzio, Vice Chairman and Co-Founder
This program is designed to assist patients with physical disabilities achieve their maximum functional abilities.

6994 Hillcrest Baptist Medical Center
100 Hillcrest Medical Blvd
Waco, TX 76712
254-202-2000
Fax: 254-202-5105
www.sw.org

Anne Hott Kimberly, Program Director
Ann Gammel, Nurse Manager
Debbie Meurer, Manager
Designed to assist patients in adjustment to a physically limiting condition, utilizing interdisciplinary strategies to maximize each patient's ability and capability.

6995 Institute for Rehabilitation & Research
1333 Moursund St
Houston, TX 77030-3405
713-799-5000
800-447-3422
Fax: 713-797-5289
tirr.memorialhermann.org

Carl Josehart, CEO
Jean Herzog, President
Gerard E. Francisco, M.D., Chief Medical Officer
A national center for information, training, research, and technical assistance in independent living. The goal is to extend the body of knowledge in independent living and to improve the utilization of results of research programs and demonstration projects in this field. It has developed a variety of strategies for collecting, synthesizing, and disseminating information related to the field of independent living.

6996 Integrated Health Services of Amarillo
6141 Amarillo Blvd. West
Amarillo, TX 79106
806-356-0488
Fax: 806-356-8074

Mary Bearden, Chairman
Jay L. Barrett, President
Marvin Franz, Executive Director & CEO
Provides acute, post acute, residential and outpatient health care services. IHS of Amarillo is a 153-bed facility with 120 beds licensed by The Texas Department of Health and Human Services, and is accredited by JCAHO. We serve urban and rural populations of over 500,000, drawing from a 5-state region.

6997 Kanner Center
Devereax Foundation
444 Devereux Drive
Victoria, TX 19085-2666
361-575-8271
800-345-1292
Fax: 361-575-6520
devereux.org

Robert Q. Kreider, President and CEO
Margaret McGill, SVP, Chief Operations Officer
Robert C. Dunne, SVP & Chief Financial Officer, Treasurer
A private nonprofit nationwide network of treatment services for individuals of all ages with emotional and/or developmental disabilities.

6998 Lighthouse of Houston
3602 W Dallas St
Houston, TX 77019-1704
713-527-9561
Fax: 713-284-8451
custserv@houstonlighthouse.org
houstonlighthouse.org

Gibson DuTerroil, President
Shelagh Moran, VP/COO
Serves the blind, visually impaired, deaf-blind and multihandicapped blind. Provides workshops, vocational training and placement, low vision clinic, orientation and mobility, housing, Braille, volunteer services, senior center, visual aid sales, counseling and support, diabetic education and day health activity services and day summer camp, Summer Transition for Youth.

6999 Mainland Center Hospital RehabCare Unit
6801 Emmett F Lowry Expy
Texas City, TX 77591-2500
409-938-5000
Fax: 409-938-5501
www.mainlandmedical.com

Michael Ehrai, CEO
The RehabCare program is designed and staffed to assist functionally impaired patients improve to their maximum potential. The opportunities for improvement and adjustments are provided in a pleasant, supportive inpatient environment by therapists from the occupational, physical, recreational and speech therapy disciplines.

7000 North Texas Rehabilitation Center
1005 Midwestern Pkwy
Wichita Falls, TX 76302-2211
940-322-0771
Fax: 940-766-4943
ntrehab.org

Mike Castles, President/ CEO
Provides outpatient rehabilitation services to maximize independence or promote development to children and adults with disabilities. Programs include: physical, occupational, speech therapy, closed head injury, infant/child development, support groups, aquatics and wellness program and a child achievement program.

7001 South Texas Lighthouse for the Blind
PO BOX 9697
Corpus Christi, TX 78469-3321
361-883-6553
888-255-8011
Fax: 361-883-1041
Customer.service@stlb.net
www.stlb.net

Regis Barber, President
Nicky Ooi, Chief Operations Officer
Alana Manrow, Public Affairs Director
Their mission is to Employ, Educate and Empower their neighbors who are blind and visually impaired. They offer job opportunities in manufacturing, retail and administration, as well as orientation and mobility and adaptive technology training.

7002 Texas Specialty Hospital at Dallas
7955 Harry Hines Blvd
Dallas, TX 75235-3305
214-637-0000
Fax: 214-637-6512
Mary.Alexander@fundltc.com

Mary Alexander, CEO
Cathy Campbell, Chief Executive Officer
66 beds offering active/acute rehabilitation, brain injury day treatment, cognitive rehabilitation, complex care, extended rehabilitation and short term evaluation.

7003 **Transitional Learning Center at Gavelston and Lubbock**
1528 Post Office St
Galveston, TX 77550   409-762-6661
                                 Fax: 409-763-3930
                                 www.tlcrehab.org

Brent Masel, MD, President and Medical Director
Gary Seale, Ph.D., VP Clinical Programs
Jim Lovelace, MBA, VP of Operations
Specializes solely in post-acute brain injury. A nationally known pioneer in the field and a not for profit with a three fold mission: treatment, research and education. Offers 6 hours of therapy a day from licensed/certified staff, on site physician and nursing services and long-term living for brian injured adults at Tideway on Gavelston Island. Accredited by CARF.
1982

7004 **Treemont Nursing And Rehabilitation Center**
5550 Harvest Hill Rd
Dallas, TX 75230-1684   972-661-1862
                                 Fax: 972-788-1543

Bob Barker, Administrator
Postacute rehabilitation program.

7005 **West Texas Lighthouse for the Blind**
2001 Austin St
San Angelo, TX 76903-8796   325-653-4231
                                 Fax: 325-657-9367
            customerservice@lighthousefortheblind.org
                        www.lighthousefortheblind.org

David Wells, Executive Director
Stephen Horton, Operations Manager
Fonda V. Galindo, Finance & Human Resources Manager
Offers services for the totally blind, legally blind, visually impaired, and more with health, counseling, educational, recreational, rehabilitation, computer training and professional training services.

Utah

7006 **Quincy Rehabilitation Institute of Holy Cross Hospital**
1050 E South Temple
Salt Lake City, UT 84102-1507   801-350-8140
                                 Fax: 801-350-4791

Dave Jenson, President
Postacute rehabilitation program.

7007 **Wasatch Vision Clinic**
849 E 400 S
Salt Lake City, UT 84102-2928   801-328-2020
                                 Fax: 801-363-2201
                        email@wasatchvision.com
                              eyeappointment.com

Craig Cutler, Owner
Camron Bateman OD, Doctor
Postacute rehabilitation program.

Vermont

7008 **Rutland Mental Health Services**
78 S Main St
Rutland, VT 05701-4594   802-775-2381
                                 Fax: 802-775-4020
                                 rmhsccn.org

Dan Quinn, President/ CEO
Scott Dikeman, Vice Chairman
Ron Holm, Secretary
A private, non-profit comprehensive community mental health center. It provides services to individuals and families for mental health and substance abuse related problems and also to persons who are developmentally disabled.

Virginia

7009 **Bay Pine-Virginia Beach**
680 South Fourth Street
Louisville, KY 40202   502-596-7300
                                 TTY: 800-545-0749
                        web_administrator@kindred.com
                              kindredhealthcare.com

Paul J. Diaz, President/ CEO
Postacute rehabilitation program.

7010 **Carilion Rehabilitation: New River Valley**
2013 S Jefferson Street
Roanoke, VA 24014   540-981-7377
                                 Fax: 540-981-8233
                                 www.carilionclinic.org

Nancy Howell Agee, President/ CEO
James A. Hartley, Chair
Briggs W. Andrews, Corporate Secretary
CARF-accredited pain management program, work hardening program and comprehensive outpatient therapy clinic, massage therapy, outpatient programs and more. Program emphasis is on interdisiplinary behavioral rehab based pain management and functional restoration in conjunction with medical treatment. Work hardening is a transdisciplinary work simulation program taylored to the individual. Comprehensive outpatient program is multi-disciplinary with emphasis on manual treatment.

7011 **Faith Mission Home**
3540 Mission Home Ln
Free Union, VA 22940-1505   434-985-2294
                                 Fax: 434-985-7633
                                 www.beachyam.org

Paul Beiler, Manager
Reuben Yoder, Director
A Christian residential center that serves 60 developmentally disabled children, including individuals with Down Syndrome, Cerebral palsy and other similar conditions. Children may be admitted from the time they are ambulatory until they reach 15 years of age. He or she may stay as long as it is in the child's best interests. The training program stresses the following areas: self-care, social, academic, vocational, crafts, speech and physical development.

7012 **ManorCare Health Services-Arlington**
333 N. Summit St.
Toledo, OH 43604   800-366-1232
                        CareLine@hcr-manorcare.com
                              hcr-manorcare.com

Marcia K Jarrell, Administrator
Ric Birch, Marketing Director
ManorCare-Arlington offers residents a full Continuum of Care in a caring environment. ManorCare's wide range of services includes subacute medical and rehabilitation programs for short term patients transitioning from hospital to home and Skilled Nursing Care.

7013 **Pines Residential Treatment Center**
825 Crawford Pkwy
Portsmouth, VA 23704-2301   757-393-0061
                                 Fax: 757-393-1029

Lenard J Lexier, Medical Director
Judy Kemp, Admissions Director
A 310-bed residential treatment center in Portsmouth Virginia, providing a therapeutic environment for severely emotionally disturbed children and youth. Five unique programs meet behavioral, educational and emotional needs of males and females, five to twenty-two years of age. Multi-disciplinary teams devise individual service plans to enhance strengths and reverse self-defeating behavior. A highly effective positive reinforcement program with a proven track record.

7014 Roanoke Memorial Hospital
Carilion Health System
2013 S Jefferson Street
Roanoke, VA 24014 540-981-7377
Fax: 540-981-8233
www.carilionclinic.org
Nancy Howell Agee, President/ CEO
James A. Hartley, Chair
Briggs W. Andrews, Corporate Secretary
Carilion Health System exists to improve the health of the communities it serves. The vision is to assure accessible, affordable, high quality healthcare that meets the needs of the community. Motivate and educate individuals to improve their health. Champion community initiatives to reduce health risk

7015 Southside Virginia Training Center
P.O.Box 4030
Petersburg, VA 23803-30 804-524-7000
Fax: 804-524-7228
www.svtc.dbhds.virginia.gov
Bob Kaufman, Director, Administrative Service
Offers residential, vocational, occupational, physical, and speech therapies.

7016 Woodrow Wilson Rehabilitation Center
P.O.Box 1500
Fishersville, VA 22939-1500 540-332-7000
800-345-9972
Fax: 540-332-7132
www.wwrc.net
Rick Sizemore, Executive Director
Amy Blalock, Admissions and Marketing Director
Comprehensive residential rehabilitation center offering complete medical and vocational rehabilitation services including: vocation evaluation, vocational training, transition from school to work, occupational therapy, physical therapy, speech, language and audiology, assistive technology, rehabilitation engineering, counseling/case management, behavioral health services, nursing and physician services, etc.

Washington

7017 Arden Rehabilitation And Healthcare Center
680 South Fourth Street
Louisville, KY 40202 502-596-7300
TTY: 800-545-0749
web_administrator@kindred.com
kindredhealthcare.com
Paul J. Diaz, President/ CEO
Arden can accomodate 90 residents- post-acute/rehabilitation patients as well as long term residents. Medicare certified, the center also takes most managed healthcare insurance plans, as well as VA, respite and hospice patients.

7018 Bellingham Care Center
680 South Fourth Street
Louisville, KY 40202 502-596-7300
TTY: 800-545-0749
web_administrator@kindred.com
kindredhealthcare.com
Paul J. Diaz, President/ CEO
Postacute rehabilitation program.

7019 Division of Vocational Rehabilitation Department of Social and Health Services
P.O.Box 45130
Olympia, WA 98504-5130 360-704-3560
800-737-0617
Fax: 360-570-6941
krulik@dshs.wa.gov
www1.dshs.wa.gov/dvr
Patrick Raines, Manager
Lynnea Ruttledge, Manager
Information on computers, supported employment, marketing rehabilitation facilities and transition.

7020 First Hill Care Center
1334 Terry Ave
Seattle, WA 98101 206-682-2661
Fax: 206-624-0188
www.khseattlefirsthill.com
Postacute rehabilitation program.

7021 Harborview Medical Center, Low Vision Aid Clinic
Harborview Medical Center
325 9th Ave
Seattle, WA 98104-2499 206-744-3300
TTY: 206-744-3246
comment@u.washington.edu
www.uwmedicine.org
Eileen Whalen, Executive director
J. Richard Goss, M.D.,, Medical director
Darcy Jaffe, Chief nursing officer and senior associate for patient care
Harborview Medical Center is the only designated Level 1 adult and pediatric trauma and burn center in the state of Washington and serves as the regional trauma and burn referral center for Alaska, Montana and Idaho. UW Medicine physicians and staff based at Harborview provide highly specialized services for vascular, orthopedics, neurosciences, ophthalmology, behavioral health, HIV/AIDS and complex critical care.

7022 Integrated Health Services of Seattle
820 NW 95th St
Seattle, WA 98117-2207 206-783-7649
Fax: 206-781-1448
Jerry Harvey, Administrator
Marlette Basada, Director Nursing
Flavia Lagrange, Director Admissions
Postacute rehabilitation program. IHS provides 24 hour subacute and long-term care. We can handle vent/trach/hemo andritoneal dialysis and provide a full scope of rehabilitation services.

7023 Lakeside Milam Recovery Centers (LMRC)
3315 S. 23rd Street
Ste 102
Tacoma, WA 98405 253-272-2242
800-231-4303
Fax: 253-272-0171
help@lakesidemilam.com
www.lakesidemilam.com
Michael Kinder, Administrator
LMRC was established in 1983 with a single mission, to help victims and families recover from the pain of drug/alcohol addiction. Enlightned by the work of Dr. James Milam in the 1960's and 70's, the founders of LMRC created a treatment system based on a bedrock set of principals.

7024 Lakewood Health Care Center
11411 Bridgeport Way SW
Lakewood, WA 98499-3047 253-581-9002
800-359-7412
Fax: 253-581-7016
www.lakewoodhc.com
Gwynn Rucker, Executive Director
Patty Wood, Administrator
Linda Doll, Social Services
Accomodates 80 residents. We offer 24 hour skilled nursing services, long-term care and rehab services which include Physical, Occupational and Speech Therapy.

7025 Manor Care Health Services-Tacoma
5601 S Orchard St
Tacoma, WA 98409-1371 253-474-8421
Fax: 253-471-8857
www.hcr-manorcare.com
Tina Irwin, Administrator
124-bed skilled nursing and rehabilitation center provides services for those seeking long term Skilled Nursing Care, short term subacute care, hospice services, Alzheimer's and respite care. Our Acadia Wing, a specialized Alzheimer's care unit, provides specialized programming and trained staff that truly makes us the leader in Alzheimers Services.

7026 ManorCare Health Services-Lynnwood
3701 188th St SW
Lynnwood, WA 98037-7626   425-775-9222
                                                          Fax: 425-712-3685
                                                          www.hcr-manorcare.com

Liza Loyet, Administrator
Our in-house therapists provide physical, occupational and
speech therapies in our state-of-the-art therapy gym. Our team is
goal oriented and focuses on producing positive outcomes for
those recovering from illness, injury or surgery.

7027 ManorCare Health Services-Spokane
6025 N Assembly St
Spokane, WA 99205-7674   509-326-8282
                                                          Fax: 509-326-4790
                                                          www.hcrmanorcare.com

Cheri Kubu, Administrator
Sandra Hayes, Administrator
Provides skilled nursing and respite stays for those needing a
break from care giving. We specialize in Rehabilitation Services
provided by our in-house occupational, physical and speech
therapists.

7028 Northwest Continuum Care Center
Kindred Health Care
128 Old Beacon Hill Dr
Longview, WA 98632-5859   360-423-4060
                                                          Fax: 360-636-0958

Steve M. Ross, Executive Director
Tami Wilson, Director of Nursing
Mary R., Activities Assistant
Accomodates 69 residents. Employs the Angel Care Program designed to address any special needs that may arise during a resident's stay in our facility. The program focuses extra attention on
residents and, in some cases, family members. The goal is to meet
the special needs of the people we provide care to every day.

7029 Park Manor Convalescent Center
1710 Plaza Way
Walla Walla, WA 99362-4362   509-529-4218
                                                          Fax: 509-522-1729
                                                          egines@ensigngroup.net
                                                          www.parkmanorcare.com

Jed Gines, Administrator
Krista Maiuri, Directr Of Nursing
Sonya Taylor, Director of Rehabilitation
Residents of Park Manor enjoy a range of activities, developed to
meet their needs, inculding excercise programs, social and recreational activities, arts and crafts, shopping trips and other excursions. We also offer religious services.

7030 Queen Anne Health Care
Queen Anne Health Care
2717 Dexter Ave N
Seattle, WA 98109-1914   206-284-7012
                                                          Fax: 206-283-3936
                                                          www.queenannehealthcare.com

Heather Eacker, Executive Director
Mary R., Activities Assistant
Kristen W., Health and Rehabilitation Center
Our goal is to provide quality, compassionate care. Our cozy
building accomodates 120 residents. We offer semi private rooms
with space to add items from home for a special personalized
touch

7031 Rainier Vista Care Center
920 12th Ave SE
Puyallup, WA 98372-4920   253-841-3422
                                                          Fax: 253-848-3937

Linda Larson, Administrator
Nancy L. Erckenbrack, Executive Director
Kristen W., Health and Rehabilitation Center
Accomodates 120 residents. We are certified for Medicare and
Medicaid and we offer a continuum of healthcare services from
short-term or outpatient rehabilitation to long-term care. We offer
semi-private and private rooms as well as rehabilitation and hospice suites. Rainier Vista Care Center is a recipient of the American Health Care Association Quality Award.

7032 Rehabilitation Enterprises of Washington
430 E Lauridsen Blvd
Port Angeles, WA 98362-7978   360-452-9789
                                                          Fax: 360-452-9700

Brett White, President
REW is the professional trade association representing community rehabilitation programs before government and other
publics. These organizations provide a wide array of employment
and training services for people with disabilities. The goal is to
assist member organizations to provide the highest quality rehabilitative and employment services to their customers.

7033 Seattle Medical and Rehabilitation Center
Evergreen Healthcare
12040 NE 128th St
Kirkland, WA 98034-3013   425-899-3000
                                                          877-601-2271
                                                          TTY: 425-899-2007
                                                          evergreenhealthcare.org

Al DeYoung, Chair
Robert H. Malte, Chief Executive Officer
*Neil Johnson, RN, MSA, Senior Vice President & Chief Operating
Officer*
103 beds offering subacute rehabilitation, complex care, sub-
acute treatment and short-term evaluation. Pulmonary unit offering long and short term care for ventilator dependent patients.

7034 Slingerland Institute for Literacy
Educators Publishing Service
12729 Northup Way
Suite 1
Bellevue, WA 98005   425-453-1190
                                                          Fax: 425-635-7762
                                                          mail@slingerland.org
                                                          www.slingerland.org

Bonnie Meyer, Executive Director
Elyce Newton, Program Support
A nonprofit public corporation founded in 1977 to carry on the
work of Beth H. Slingerland in providing classroom teachers with
the techniques, knowledge and understanding necessary for identifying and teaching children with Specific Language Disability.
The main objective is to educate teachers in successful methods
of identifying, diagnosing and instructing children and adults
with SLD and to promote literacy through reading, writing and
oral expression.

7035 Timberland Opportunities Association
400 W Curtis St
Aberdeen, WA 98520-7698   360-533-5823
                                                          Fax: 360-533-5848

Jim Eddy, Executive Director
Provides training and employment for disabled people.

7036 Vancouver Health and Rehabilitation Center
400 E 33rd St
Vancouver, WA 98663-2238   360-696-2561
                                                          Fax: 360-696-9275
                                                          www.vancouverhealthcare.com

Jody Wigen, Human Resources
Joe Joy, Executive Director
Kristen W., Health and Rehabilitation Center
Postacute rehabilitation program.

Wisconsin

7037 Colonial Manor Medical And Rehabilitation Center
1010 E Wausau Ave
Wausau, WI 54403-3101   715-842-2028
                                                          Fax: 715-848-0510
                                                          www.colonialmanormrc.com

Ericca Ylitalo, Administrator
Shelley Solberg, Executive Director
Colonial Manor Medical and Rehabilitation Center is part of the
Kindred Community and is located in Wausau, Wisconsin. The
corporate headquarters are based in Louisville Kentucky. Our fa-
cility accomodates 150 residents.

7038   Waushers Industries
210 E Chicago Rd
Wautoma, WI 54982-6932   920-787-4696
                                          Fax: 920-787-4698

Richard King, Human Resources
Provides various programming for individuals with disabilities
in waushara county.

7039   Woodstock Health and Rehabilitation Center
3415 Sheridan Rd
Kenosha, WI 53140-1924   262-657-6175
                                          Fax: 262-657-5756

Debra Lamb, Administrator
Darlene Einerson, Executive Director
Kristen W., Health and Rehabilitation Center
Offers a full range of medical services to meet the individual
needs of our residents, including short term rehabilitative ser-
vices and long-tern skilled care.

Rehabilitation Facilities, Sub-Acute

Alabama

7040 UAB Spain Rehabilitation Center
1717 6th Ave S
Birmingham, AL 35233-7330   205-934-3450
www.uab.edu/medicine/physicalmedicine/
Tracy L Brewer, Administrative Manager
A 49-bed rehabilitation hospital featuring advanced, individualized care for adolescents and adult patients recovering from a broad variety of health problems. Patient care teams include physiatrists (doctors who specialized in rehabilitation medicine), nurses, nurse practitioners, physical therapists, occupational therapists, speech/language pathologists, psychologists, social workers, rehabilitation professionals and other health care professionals from all areas of the UAB Health System.

Alaska

7041 Fairbanks Memorial Hospital & Denali Center
1650 Cowles St
Fairbanks, AK 99701-5998   907-452-8181
Fax: 907-458-5324
www.fmhdc.com
Sheldon Stadnyk, MD, Interim Chief Executive Officer
The Denali Center offers the following rehabilitation services: Physical Therapy, Occupational Therapy, Speech Therapy, Sub-Acute Rehab.

Arizona

7042 Desert Life Rehabilitation & Care Center
Kindred Healthcare
1919 W Medical St
Tucson, AZ 85704-1133   520-297-8311
Fax: 520-544-0930
Amad Nazifi, Executive Director
Jane Olmstead, Director of Nursing
Accomodates 240 residents. We provide skilled and intermediate nursing with occupational, physical, speech and respiratory therapy services. We offer special programs including an Alzheimer's Unit and a Young Adult Program, and are located in beautiful Southern Arizona where there is plenty of sunshine, mountains and desert views. Desert Life is a 2005 recipient of the American Health Care Association Quality Award.

7043 Hacienda Rehabilitation and Care Center
660 S Coronado Dr
Sierra Vista, AZ 85635-3386   520-459-4900
Fax: 520-458-4082
www.haciendarcc.com
Monica Vandivort, Medical Director
Kristen W., Health and Rehabilitation Center Executive Director
Becky D., Activity Director
Accomodates 100 residents. We are located in Sierra Vista, near Kartchner Caverns, Fort Huachuca, Coronado National Forest and historic Tombstone. Serving the medical needs of the community since 1983, we strive to provide care with quality, compassion and integrity.

7044 Kachina Point Health Care & Rehabilitation Center
505 Jacks Canyon Rd
Sedona, AZ 86351-7856   928-284-1000
Fax: 928-284-0626
Michael Amadei, Medical Director
Accomodates 120 residents. We have met the healthcare needs of the community since 1984. Kachina Point is a 2004 recipient of the American Health Care Association's Quality Award.

7045 Mayo Clinic Scottsdale
13400 E Shea Blvd
Scottsdale, AZ 85259-5499   480-301-8000
800-446-2279
Fax: 480-301-9310
www.mayoclinic.org/arizona
Neena S. Abraham, Gastroenterology/ Hepatology
Roberta H. Adams, Hematology/Oncology
Charles H. Adler, Parkinson's Disease and Movement Disorders Center
Mayo clinic is a not-for-profit medical practice dedicated to the diagnosis and treatment of virtually every type of complex illness. Mayo clinic staff members work together to meet your needs. You will see as many doctors, specialists, and other health care professionals as needed to provide comprehensive diagnosis, understandable answers and effective treatment.

7046 Sonoran Rehabilitation and Care Center
Kindred
4202 N 20th Ave
Phoenix, AZ 85015-5101   602-264-3824
Fax: 602-279-6234
Jeffrey Barrett, Executive Director
Offers the following rehabilitation services: Respiratory Therapy, Physical Therapy, Speech Therapy, Occupational Therapy, Restorative Therapy, Sub-Acute Rehabilitation, Wound Care.

7047 Valley Health Care and Rehabilitation Center
Kindred Health Care Center
5545 E Lee St
Tucson, AZ 85712-4205   520-296-2306
Fax: 520-296-4072
Dale Pelton, Executive Director
Sandra Lewis, Administrator
Offers the following rehabilitation services: Physical Therapy, Occupational Therapy, Speech Therapy, Sub-Acute Rehab.

California

7048 Alamitos-Belmont Rehab Hospital
3901 E 4th St
Long Beach, CA 90814-1699   562-434-8421
Fax: 562-433-6732
www.alamitosbelmont.com
John L. Sorensen, Chairman of the Board of Directors.
Jonathan Sloey, Administrator
Offers the following rehabilitation services: Speech Therapy, Occupational Therapy, Physical Therapy, Sub-Acute Rehab.

7049 Bay View Nursing and Rehabilitation Center
Kindred Health Care
516 Willow St
Alameda, CA 94501-6132   510-521-5600
Fax: 510-865-9035
www.kindredhealthcare.com
Richard S Espinoza, Administrator
Say Silva, Assistant Executive Director
Accomodates 180 residents. Bay View is a 2004 recipient of the American Health Care Association's Quality Award. We provide short-term rehabilitative care, traditional long-term skilled care and Alzheimer's/dementia special care. Our combination of clinical skill and comprehensive rehabilitation services enables us to care for a variety of complex medical conditions.

7050 Foothill Nursing and Rehab Center
401 W Ada Ave
Glendora, CA 91741-4241   626-335-9810
Fax: 626-963-0720
www.foothillnursing.com
Arnie Shafer, Executive Director
Marianne Schultz, Administrator
Offers the following rehabilitation services: Physical Therapy, Occupational Therapy, Speech Therapy, In and Out Patient Rehab.

7051 Long Beach Memorial Medical Center Memorial Rehabilitation Hospital
2801 Atlantic Ave
Ground Floor
Long Beach, CA 90806-1701   562-933-9001
                                        Fax: 562-933-9019
                              www.memorialcare.org/long_beach
Barry Arbuckle, President/CEO
The goal of the MemorialCare Rehabilitation Institute is to help persons with disabilities regain independence and rebuild their lives in an environment where loved ones are involved in the rehabilitation process. We are dedicated to the pursuit of our mission, vision and values.

7052 Mercy Medical Center Mt. Shasta
914 Pine St
Mount Shasta, CA 96067-2143   530-926-6111
                                        Fax: 530-926-0517
                                      www.mercymtshasta.org
Greg Lippert, Senior Director of Support and Information Services
Scott Foster, Director of Hospital Finance
Sister Anne Chester, Director of Mission Integration
Mercy Medical Center is committed to furthering the healing ministry of Jesus, and to provide high-quality, affordable healthcare to the communities we serve.

7053 Northridge Hospital Medical Center
18300 Roscoe Blvd
Northridge, CA 91328-4167   818-885-8500
                                    www.northridgehospital.org
Michael Wall, CEO
Offers the following rehabilitation services: Physical Therapy, Occupational Therapy, Speech Therapy, Sub-Acute Rehab. As a member of the Catholic Heathcare West Northridge Hospital Medical Center is committed to serving the health needs of our communities with particular attention to the needs of the poor, the disadvantaged and vulnerable, and the comfort of the suffering and dying.

7054 Riverside Community Hospital
4445 Magnolia Ave
Riverside, CA 92501   951-788-3000
                                        Fax: 630-792-5636
                              complaint@jointcommission.org
                          www.riversidecommunityhospital.com
Jaime Wesolowski, President/CEO
Patrick Brilliant, CEO
At Riverside Community Hospital, we are able to provide the healthcare services that you and your family will need through the many stages of your life. Services like Emergency/Trauma, Labor and Delivery, Cardiac Care, Orthopedics and Transplant are among our many Centers of Excellence.

7055 Saint Jude Medical Center
101 E Valencia Mesa Dr
Fullerton, CA 92835-3809   714-871-3280
                                             800-870-7537
                                        Fax: 714-992-3029
                              www.stjudemedicalcenter.org
April De Cou, Wellness Educator
Jane Wang, Wellness Programs Supervisor
Offers the following rehabilitation services: Out-patient Rehab, Sub-Acute Rehab, Occupational Therapy, Physical Therapy, Speech and Audiology Therapy, Pain Management Program.

7056 South Coast Medical Center
12 Mason
Suite A
Irvine, CA 92618-2733   714-669-4446
                                        Fax: 714-669-4448
                              info@southcoastmedcenter.com
                                     www.mission4health.com
Leigh Erin Connealy, Manager
Bruce Christian, President
Offers the following services: physical therapy, occupational therapy, speech therapy, cardica rehabilitation, incontinence program, sub-acute rehabilitation.

7057 Valley Garden Health Care and Rehabilitation Center
1517 Knickerbocker Dr
Stockton, CA 95210-3119   209-957-4539
                                        Fax: 209-957-5831
                              www.valleygardenshealth.com
Dr. Alexande Chan, Medical Director
Accomodates 120 residents. Our center provides short-term nursing and rehabilitative care as well as traditional long-term skilled care. Our combination of clinical skill and comprehensive rehabilitation services enables us to care for a variety of complex medical conditions. Rehabilitative therapies are provided as needed by physical, occupational and speech therapists.

Colorado

7058 Boulder Community Hospital Mapleton Center
1100 Balsam
PO Box 9019
Boulder, CO 80301-9019   303-440-2273
                                             info@bch.org
                                             www.bch.org
Lou DellaCava, Chairman
Ric Porreca, Vice Chairman
Jean Dubofsky, Secretary
159-bed acute care hospital and 24-hour emergency department.

7059 Fairacres Manor
1700 18th Ave
Greeley, CO 80631-5152   970-353-3370
                                        Fax: 970-353-9347
Kathy Gardner, Admissions/Marketing Director
Marla Trujillo, Director of Nursing
Ben Gonzales, Admissions/Marketing Assistant Director
Offers the following rehabilitation services: Physical Therapy, Occupational Therapy, Speech Therapy, Restorative Therapy, Skilled Nursing, and Sub-Acute Rehabilitation.

7060 Rowan Community
4601 E Asbury Cir
Denver, CO 80222-4722   303-757-1228
                                        Fax: 303-759-3390
Tammy Gleisner, Director/Admissions/Marketing Director
Jeff Jerebker, President/CEO
Bruce Odenthal, VP Operations
Rowan is a 70-bed community, small enough to support personal relationships between residents and caregivers. Our residents vary in age, reflecting the diversity of a much larger community. Rowan's focus is on a psycho-social model of care with a dynamic activities and social service program. Our staff is specially trained in behavior management and many are certified Eden AlternativeT associates and certifid Elder Care Specialists.

Connecticut

7061 Hamilton Rehabilitation and Healthcare Center
89 Viets St
New London, CT 6320-3355   860-447-1471
                                        Fax: 860-439-0107
Steve Roizen, Executive Director
Offers the following rehabilitation services: Sub-Acute, Occupational Therapy, Speech Therapy, Physical Therapy.

7062 Hospital For Special Care (HSC)
2150 Corbin Ave
New Britain, CT 06053-2298   860-223-2761
                                        Fax: 860-827-4849
                                             www.hfsc.org
John J. Votto, President/CEO
Paul J. Scalise, M.D., F.C.C.P, Senior Vice President
HSC is a private, not-for-profit 200-bed rehabilitation long-term acute and chronic care hospital, widely-known and respected for its expertise in physical rehabilitation, respiratory care, and medically-complex pediatrics. Special programs for spinal cord injuries, pulmonary rehabilitation, acquired brain injuries, stroke, ventilator management and geriatrics, make HSC an important regional resource for patients with special healthcare needs.

7063   Masonic Healthcare Center
MasoniCare Corporation
22 Masonic Ave
PO Box 70
Wallingford, CT 06492-3048
203-679-5900
877-424-3537
Fax: 203-679-6459
info@masonicare.org
www.masonicare.org
Stephen B. McPherson, President
Arthur Santilli, President
The states leading provider of healthcare and retirement living communities for seniors. We are not-for-profit and have more then 100 years of experience behind us. We're recognized for the quality, compassionate care and steadfast support we provide to our residents and patients.

7064   Stamford Hospital
30 Shelburne Rd
Stamford, CT 06904-3628
203-276-1000
Fax: 203-325-7905
info@stamhealth.org
www.stamfordhospital.org
Brian Grissler, President/CEO
Kathleen Silard, EVP/Chief Operating Officer
Kevin Gage, Senior Vice President, Finance/Chief Financial Officer
A not-for-profit, community teaching hospital that has been serving Stamford and surrounding communities for more then 100 years. We have 305 inpatient beds in medicine, surgery, obstetrics/gynecology, psychiatry, and medical and surgical critical care units and maintain an educational partnership with Columbia University College of Physicians and Surgeons for its teaching program in the internal medicine, family practice, obstetrics/gynecology and surgery

7065   Windsor Rehabilitation and Healthcare Center
581 Poquonock Ave
Windsor, CT 06095-2202
860-688-7211
Fax: 860-688-6715
www.windsorrehab.com
Jeffrey Robbins, Medical Director
Accomodates 116 residents. We offer private and semi-private rooms with access to private telephones and cable television. Our goal is to be a comprehensive, leading care center viewed by our community as an excellent resource for patients, families, and professionals.

Delaware

7066   Arbors at New Castle
32 Buena Vista Dr
New Castle, DE 19720-4660
302-328-2580
Fax: 302-326-4132
www.extendicareus.com/newcastle
Annette Moore, Administrator
A subacute and rehabilitation center offering skilled medical services, infusion therapies, cardiac recovery services, renal disease services, cancer services and digestive disease services. Skilled rehabilitation services include physical therapy, occupational therapy and speech therapy. Also provides case management and discharge planning, general nursing and restorative care and respite care.

Florida

7067   Avon Oaks Skilled Care Nursing Facility
37800 French Creek Rd
Avon, OH 44011-1763
440-934-5204
800-589-5204
jreidy@avonoaks.net
www.avonoaks.net
Natalie McIntyre, Human Resources Director
Stephanie Auvil, RN, BC, Director of Nursing
Joan Reidy, Administrator

Oaks at Avon provides a full range of skilled nursing services including infusion therapy, enteral therapy, wound care, tracheotomy care, and portable diagnostics.

7068   Boca Raton Rehabilitation Center
755 Meadows Rd
Boca Raton, FL 33486-2384
561-391-5200
Fax: 561-391-0685
Stanley Mucinic, Administrator
Tracey Dougherty, Administrator
Offers the following rehabilitation services: Occupational Therapy, Speech Therapy, Physical Therapy, Sub-Acute Rehabilitation

7069   Cape Coral Hospital
636 Del Prado Blvd
Cape Coral, FL 33990
239-424-2000
Fax: 239-574-1935
www.leememorial.org
Richard Akin, Chairman
Sanford Cohen, MD, Vice Chairman
Marilyn Stout, Treasurer
A 291-bed acute care facility, Cape Coral Hospital features all private rooms. The hospital currently is undergoing a complete renovation, expansion and modernization of the Weigner-Taeni Center for Emergency Services, which will make the emergency department the largest in Lee County.

7070   Evergreen Woods Health and Rehabilitation Center
7045 Evergreen Woods Trl
Spring Hill, FL 34608-1306
352-596-8371
Fax: 352-596-8032
Janet Hanciles, Administrator
Offers the following rehabilitation services: Sub-Acute rehabilitation, Occupational therapy, Speech pathology therapy, Physical therapy.

7071   Healthcare and Rehabilitation Center of Sanford
950 Mellonville Avenue
Sanford, FL 32771-2237
407-322-8566
Fax: 407-322-0121
www.healthcareandrehabofsanford.com
Dr. S. Joshi, Medical Director
Kate Hilgar, Administrator
Vicky Smith, Director Admissions
We provide post-acute services, rehabilitative services, skilled nursing, short and long term care through Physical, Occupational, and Speech Therapists; Registered and Licensed Practical Nurses; and Certified Nursing Assistants. This is complemented by Social Services, Activities, Nutritional Services, Housekeeping and Laundry Services. With over 224 years of combined experience, our staff of professionals is here to meet the needs of each and every patient and resident.

7072   Highland Pines Rehabilitation Center
1111 S Highland Ave
Clearwater, FL 33756-4432
727-446-0581
Fax: 727-442-9425
Paula Anthony, Administrator
Offers the following rehabilitation services: Sub-Acute rehabilitation, Occupational Therapy, Speech Therapy, Physical Therapy.

7073   Jupiter Medical Center-Pavilion
1210 S Old Dixie Hwy
Jupiter, FL 33458-7205
561-747-2234
Fax: 561-744-4467
JCouris@jupitermed.com
www.jupitermed.com
John D. Couris, President/Chief Executive Officer
Dale Hocking, Vice President, Finance/Chief Financial Officer
Mike Fehr, Vice President, Information Services/Chief Information Offic
Offers the following rehabilitation services: Sub-Acute Rehabilitation, Occupational Therapy, Speech Therapy, Physical Therapy.

7074   North Broward Medical Center
201 E Sample Rd
Deerfield Beach, FL 33064-4441   954-941-8300
                                      Fax: 954-941-4233
                                      www.browardhealth.org
Pauline Grant, CEO
Douglas Ford, Chief of Staff
Offers the following rehabilitation services: Sub-Acute rehabili-
tation, Physical Therapy, Occupational Therapy, Speech Ther-
apy, Respiratory Therapy.

7075   Pompano Rehabilitation and Nursing Center
Senior Health Care Management
51 W Sample Rd
Pompano Beach, FL 33064-3542   954-942-5530
                                    Fax: 954-942-0941
Jeff Nusbusn, Administrator
Offers the following rehabilitation services: Sub-Acute Rehabil-
itation, Physical Therapy, Occupational Therapy, Speech
Therapy

7076   Rehabilitation Center of Palm Beach
300 Royal Palm Way
Palm Beach, FL 33480-4385   561-655-7266
                                 Fax: 561-655-3269
                                 info@rcca.org
                                 www.rcca.org
Ellen O'Bannon, Manager
Pamela Henderson, Executive Director
Our mission is to improve the physical function, communication
& independence of people with disabilities.

7077   Rehabilitation and Healthcare Center of Tampa
4411 N Habana Ave
Tampa, FL 33614-7211   813-872-2771
                            Fax: 813-871-2831
Dr. Gustavo Barrazuetta, Medical Director
We provide post-acute services, rehabilitative services, skilled
nursing, short and long term care through Physical, Occupational, and Speech Therapists; Registered and Licensed Practical
Nurses; and Certified Nursing Assistants. This is complemented
by Social Services, Activities, Nutritional Services, Housekeeping and Laundry Services. With over 60 years of combined experience, our staff of professionals is here to meet the needs of each
and every patient and resident.

7078   Shands Rehab Hospital
4101 NW 89th Blvd
Gainesville, FL 32606-3813   352-265-8938
                                  Fax: 352-265-5420
                                  www.ufhealth.org/shands-rehab-hospital
Tim Goldfarb,M.S., Chief Executive Officer
David S. Guzick, M.D., Ph.D., Senior Vice President
Ed. Jimenez, M.B.A, Senior Vice President/Chief Operating Officer
UF Health Shands Rehab Hospital is a 40-bed acute rehab hospi-
tal for patients who have suffered strokes, traumatic brain and
spinal cord injuries, amputations, burns or major joint replace-
ments.

7079   St. Anthony's Hospital
1200 7th Ave N
St Petersburg, FL 33705-1388   727-825-1100
                                    www.stanthonys.com
William Ulbricht, President
Ron Colaguori, VP Operations
James McClintic, M.D., Vice President, Medical Affairs
We offer outstanding diagnostic and treatment options of all
types of cancer. Our Susan Sheppard McGillicuddy Breast Center
is unmatched in the community in diagnostic services and helping
patients navigate their treatment options should they find a
cancer diagnosis.

7080   Winkler Court
3250 Winkler Avenue Ext
Fort Myers, FL 33916-9414   239-939-4993
                                 Fax: 239-939-1743
                                 www.winklercourt.com
Michael Collier, Medical Director
Michael Stens, Medical Director
We provide post-acute services, rehabilitative services, skilled
nursing, short and long term care through Physical, Occupa-

tional, and Speech Therapists; Registered and Licensed Practical
Nurses; and Certified Nursing Assistants. This is complemented
by Social Services, Activities, Nutritional Services, Housekeeping and Laundry Services. With over 100 years of combined experience, our staff of professionals is here to meet the needs of each
and every patient and resident.

7081   Winter Park Memorial Hospital
Florida Hospital
200 N Lakemont Ave
Winter Park, FL 32792-3273   407-646-7000
                                  Fax: 407-646-7639
                                  healthcare@winterparkhospital.com
                                  www.winterparkhospital.com
Ken Bradley, CEO
Nestled among the oak-shaded, brick-paved streets of one of the
most picturesque hometowns in the country, Winter Park Memorial Hospital has continuously served the residents of Winter Park
and its surrounding communities for more than 50 years.

Georgia

7082   Athena Rehab of Clayton
2055 Rex Rd
Lake City, GA 30260-3944   404-361-5144
                                Fax: 404-363-6366
Reginald Washington, Administrator
Offers the following rehabilitation services: Sub-Acute rehabili-
tation, Occupational therapy, Speech therapy, Physical therapy,
Restorative care.

7083   Lafayette Nursing and Rehabilitation Center
110 Brandywine Blvd
Fayetteville, GA 30214-1500   770-461-2928
                                   Fax: 770-461-8507
                                   www.lafayetterehab.com
Wendy Goza, Medical Director
Lafayette Nursing and Rehab Center accomodates 179 residents.
We are Medicare certified and our center also features a 25-bed
postacute rehab unit and a 24-bed dementia unit. We have RN's
LPN's and CNA's 24 hours a day. We also have physician services
availiable seven days a week.

7084   Savannah Rehabilitation and Nursing Center
815 E 63rd St
Savannah, GA 31405-4499   912-352-8615
                               Fax: 912-355-4642
Sandra Casper, Executive Director
At our facility, we provide quality care with modern rehabilitation and restorative nursing techniques. We aim to provide an atmosphere which encourages family involvement in the
care-planning process, with the right mix of activities addressing
the social, spiritual and intellectual needs of our residents.

7085   Specialty Hospital
PO Box 1566
Rome, GA 30162-1566   706-509-4100
                           Fax: 706-509-4159
A 34-bed acute long-term care hospital located in Rome, Georgia,
designed for those patients who require treatment for extended
periods of time. The patients of The Specialty Hospital are those
who do not need the medical resources of a general hospital but
whose conditions are too severe for a lower level of care. Patients
are admitted to TSH through physician and case manager
referrals.

7086   Walton Rehabilitation Health System
523 13th St.
Augusta, GA 30901-1037   706-823-8505
                              866-492-5866
                              Fax: 706-724-5752
Dennis Skelley, President/CEO
Has Centers of Excellence in Stroke Brain Injury, Complex Orthopedics, Spinal Cord Injury and Pain Management. 58-bed
nonprofit facility.

7087 Warner Robins Rehabilitation and Nursing Center
1601 Elberta Rd
Warner Robins, GA 31093-1393   478-922-2241
                                       Fax: 478-328-1984
                        www.warnerrobinsrehabilitation.com
Laura Fergason, Administrator
Offers the following rehabilitation services: Sub-Acute rehabilitation, Physical Therapy, Occupational Therapy, Speech Therapy.

Hawaii

7088 Aloha Nursing and Rehab Center
45-545 Kamehameha Hwy
Kaneohe, HI 96744-1943   808-247-2220
                                       Fax: 808-235-3676
                                  info@alohanursing.com
                                        alohanursing.com
Charles Harris, Executive Director
Amy Lee, Administrator
Our unique nursing care facility is nestled in the picturesque town of Kaneohe, Oahu, amid the towering Koolau Mountains and the panoramic vistas of Kaneohe Bay. In this tranquil setting, our 141-bed facility offers both long and short term care to residents who meet intermediate or skilled level of care criteria.

Idaho

7089 Boise Health And Rehabilitation Center
1001 S Hilton St
Boise, ID 83705-1925   208-345-4464
                                       Fax: 208-345-2998
Jason Ludwig, Medical Director
Aaron Moorhouse, Medical Director
Debbie Mills, Executive Director
Offers the following rehabilitation services: Sub-acute rehabilitation, occupational therapy, speech therapy, physical therapy.

7090 Eastern Idaho Regional Medical Center
3100 Channing Way
Idaho Falls, ID 83404-7533   208-529-6111
                                       Fax: 208-529-7021
                                           www.eirmc.com
Cindy Smith-Putnam, Executive Director of Business Development, Marketing & Comm
Lou Fatkin, Executive Director of Risk Management, Physician Relations,
Matt Campbell, Director of Human Resources
The largest medical facility in the region, Eastern Idaho Regional Medical Center (EIRMC) is a modern, JCAHO-accredidted, full-service hospital. EIRMC serves as the region's healthcare hub, offering specialty services including open-heart surgery, leading-edge cancer treatment, trauma, neurosurgery, intensive care for adults and infants, and a helicopeter service.

7091 Kindred Transitional Care and Rehabilitation
3315 8th St
Lewiston, ID 83501-4966   208-743-9543
                                       Fax: 208-746-8662
                                     www.lewistonrehab.com
Debbie Freeze, Administrator
Lewiston Rehabilitation and Care Center has years of experience providing diversified healthcare services. We have our own staff of physical, occupational and speech therapists. Our therapy gym and rehab kitchen are a lovely atmosphere in which to work toward your therapy goals. We are an Eden Alternative Certified facility.

7092 Mountain Valley Care and Rehabilitation Center
601 West Cameron Avenue
PO Box 689
Kellogg, ID 83837- 2004   208-784-1283
                                       Fax: 208-784-0151
                                  www.mountainvalleycare.com
Maryruth Butler, Executive Director

Mountain Valley Care and Rehabilitation Center accomodates 68 residents. We are conveniently located in the heart of Kellogg Idaho. We strive to offer quality care and superior customer service in a home-like environment. Upon admission, you or your loved one is looked after by an assigned staff member. We call this our 'Angel Care' program. Our rehabilitation program focuses on meething the individual needs of the resident so you or your loved one can see how they are going to progress.

7093 River's Edge Rehabilitation and Healthcare
Kindred Healthcare
714 N Butte Ave
Emmett, ID 83617-2799   208-365-4425
                                       Fax: 208-365-6989
                                  GDecker@ensigngroup.net
                                   www.riversedgerehab.com
Janis Shields, Executive Director
Steve Balle, MPT, Director of Rehabilitation
Margaret Williams RN, BSN, Director of Nursing
Emmett Rehab & healthcare accomodates 95 residents. We are located in Emmett, Idaho, a rural community located an easy 30 minute drive from Boise. Emmett Rehab &'healthcare has served the area for more then 40 years by providing healthcare for residents of Gem County.

Illinois

7094 Chevy Chase Nursing and Rehabilitation Center
3400 S Indiana Ave
Chicago, IL 60616-3841   312-842-5000
                                       Fax: 312-842-3790
Tony Prather, Administrator
Our approach to care is multidisciplinary; our medical staff members work together as a team in a proactive fashion, challenging residents each and every day, in order to motivate them to rehabilitate and achieve their ultimate potential.

7095 Glenview Terrace Nursing Center
1511 Greenwood Rd
Glenview, IL 60026-1513   847-729-9090
                                       Fax: 847-729-9135
                                   www.glenviewterrace.com
Ian Crook, Administrator
We're best known as the industry leader in post-hospital rehabilitation, including orthopedic rehabilitation and stroke recovery. Our highly effective rehabilitation services feature one-on-one physical, occupational, speech and respiratory therapies up to seven days a week.

7096 Halsted Terrace Nursing Center
10935 S Halsted St
Chicago, IL 60628-3189   773-928-2000
                                       Fax: 773-928-9154
Ted O'Brien, Administrator
Offers the following rehabilitation services: Sub-acute rehabilitation, physical therapy, occupational therapy, speech therapy, cardiac rehabilitation.

7097 Harmony Nursing and Rehabilitation Center
3919 W Foster Ave
Chicago, IL 60625-6056   773-588-9500
                                       Fax: 773-588-9533
                                  www.harmonychicago.com
John Sianghio, Administrator
Offers a friendly healthcare experience. You'll find compassionate experts who provide short-term rehabilitation and therapy, wound care, Alzheimer's and memory loss care, long-term nursing care and more.

7098 Imperial
1366 W Fullerton Ave
Chicago, IL 60614-2199   773-248-9300
                                       Fax: 773-935-0036
                                   www.imperialpavilion.com
David Hartman, Administrator
Mary Bangayan, M.D., Pulmonary Care Programme
Sanjay Gill, M.D., Cardiac Management Program
We offer a comprehensive approach to post acute care. One that takes into consideration our guests' unique needs, and utilizes a

progressive healthcare model to provide them with a personalized rehabilitation program designed to offer them the fullest possible recovery.

7099 Jackson Square Nursing and Rehabilitation Center
5130 W Jackson Blvd
Chicago, IL 60644-4332   773-921-8000
                                Fax: 773-287-9302
                    www.jacksonsquarecare.com

Rick Walworth, Administrator
At Jackson Square, there is one primary goal: to help guests regain maximum independence and functioning so that they can safely, comfortably, and happily get their life back. Our physicians, therapists, and nurses use their experience, compassion, and skill-combined with the latest and best technology-to provide comprehensive rehabilitation for a wide range of physical disabilities and medical conditions.

7100 Renaissance at 87th Street
2940 W 87th St
Chicago, IL 60652-3832   773-434-8787
                                Fax: 773-434-8717
                      www.renaissanceat87.com

Juli Foy, Administrator
At Renaissance at 87th, there is one primary goal: to help guests regain maximum independence and functioning so that they can safely, comfortably, and happily get their life back. Our physicians, therapists, and nurses use their experience, compassion, and skill-combined with the latest and best technology-to provide comprehensive rehabilitation for a wide range of physical disabilities and medical conditions.

7101 Renaissance at Hillside
4600 N. Frontage Rd.
Hillside, IL 60162-1761   708-544-9933
                                Fax: 708-544-9966
                       www.ariapostacute.com

John Stare, Administrator
Utilizing a progressive healthcare model that takes into account each patient's individual needs, Aria Post Acute Care designs a personalized rehabilitation program offering guests the best chance at the fullest possible recovery.

7102 Renaissance at Midway
4437 S Cicero Ave
Chicago, IL 60632-4333   773-884-0484
                                Fax: 773-884-0485
                   www.renaissanceatmidway.com

Jeff Baker, Executive Director
At Renaissance at Midway, there is one primary goal: to help guests regain maximum independence and functioning so that they can safely, comfortably, and happily get their life back. Our physicians, therapists, and nurses use their experience, compassion, and skill-combined with the latest and best technology-to provide comprehensive rehabilitation for a wide range of physical disabilities and medical conditions.

7103 Renaissance at South Shore
2425 E 71st St
Chicago, IL 60649-2612   773-721-5000
                                Fax: 773-721-6850
                       www.rensouthshore.com

Dave Schechter, Administrator
The Renaissance at South Shore is a 248 bed skilled nursing facility with multiple services that include short-term rehabilitation, specialized dementia care and long-term care and hospice care. Our highly trained nursing professionals provide loving care in a home-like atmosphere.

7104 Schwab Rehabilitation Hospital
Mt. Sinai
1401 S California Ave
Chicago, IL 60608-1858   773-522-2010
                       www.schwabrehab.org

Suzan Rayner, Medical Director
Lisa Thornton, Medical Staff President
Alan Channing, President/ Chief Executive Officer
Schwab Rehabilitation Hospital is a freestanding, not-for-profit, 102-bed rehabilitation hospital located on Chicago's west side. It offers a therapeutic environment of comprehensive inpatient and outpatient rehabilitation, both for adults and children.

Indiana

7105 Angel River Health and Rehabilitation
5233 Rosebud Ln
Newburgh, IN 47630-9283   812-473-4761
                                Fax: 812-473-5190

Kay Congleton, Executive Director
Our wide array of services enables our patients and residents to receive the medical care they need, the restorative therapy they require, and the support they and their families deserve. We serve many types of patient and resident needs - from short-term rehabilitation to traditional long-term care. Our resident council meets regularly to ensure that our residents' needs are being met to their satisfaction.

7106 Chalet Village Health and Rehabilitation Center
Magnolia Health Systems
1065 Parkway St
Berne, IN 46711-2366   260-589-2127
                                Fax: 260-589-3521
                        www.chalet-village.net

Vicki Shepherd, Administrator
We provide dedicated, community-centered healthcare which was founded in Indiana, operates in Indiana, for people who live in Indiana.

7107 Columbus Health and Rehabilitation Center
2100 Midway St
Columbus, IN 47201-3722   812-372-8447
                                Fax: 812-375-5117
                          www.columbushrc.com

Sherry Harrison, Executive Director
William Lustig, Medical Director
Accomodates 235 residents. We offer a continuum of healthcare services. Our center also provides a Special Care Alzheimer's Unit. We are licensed by the Stat of Indiana and are Medicare and Medicaid approved provider. We are proud to offer a friendly home-like atmosphere while providing comprehensive healthcare services. These services include short-term medical and rehabilitation treatment, which is designed to address the individual needs of our residents and patients.

7108 Harrison Health and Rehabilitation Centre
150 Beechmont Drive
Corydon, IN 47112-1717   812-738-0550
                                Fax: 812-738-6273
                          www.harrisonrehab.com

Sheila Bieker, Executive Director
Bruce Burton, Medical Director
We serve many types of patient and resident needs - from short-term rehabilitation to traditional long-term care. Working with your physician, our staff - including medical specialists, nurses, nutritionists, therapists, dietitians and social workers - establishes a comprehensive treatment plan intended to restore you or your loved one to the fullest practicable potential.

7109 Indian Creek Health and Rehabilitation Center
240 Beechmont Dr
Corydon, IN 47112-1718   812-738-8127
                                877-380-7211
                                Fax: 812-738-2917
                          www.indiancreekhrc.com

Bonnie Fallin, Executive Director
Bruce Burton, Medical Director
140 bed facility offering the following rehabilitation services: Sub-Acute rehabilitation, Physical therapy, Occupational Therapy, Speech Therapy, pain management, Wound rehabilitation. Short and long term skilled nursing care certified for Medicare, Medicaid, Private Pay and Private Insurance. Hospice and respite care rated #1 in clinical care in southern Indiana district for 2002.

7110 Meadowvale Health and Rehabilitation Center
Kindred Health Care
1529 Lancaster St
Bluffton, IN 46714-1507   260-824-4320
                                800-743-3333
                                Fax: 260-824-4689

Todd Beaulieu, Executive Director
Yadagiri Jonna, Medical Director

Working with your physician, our staff - including medical specialists, nurses, nutritionists, therapists, dietitians and social workers - establishes a comprehensive treatment plan intended to restore you or your loved one to the fullest practicable potential.

7111   Muncie Health Care and Rehabilitation
680 South Fourth Street
Louisville, KY 40202   502-596-7300
                                              800-545-0749
                                web_administrator@kindred.com
                                     www.kindredhealthcare.com

Dee Harrold, Executive Director
Dr. Jeffery Hiltz, Medical Director
Offers the following rehabilitation services: Sub-Acute rehabilitation, physical therapy, occupational therapy, speech therapy.

7112   Rehabilitation Hospital of Indiana
4141 Shore Dr
Indianapolis, IN 46254-2607   317-329-2000
                                         Fax: 317-329-2104
                                              www.rhin.com

Ian Worden, MHA, MBA, CPA, RHI Board Chair
James G. Terwilliger, MPH, Vice Chair/Secretary
Kyle Netter, MBA, PT, Executive Director of Corporate and Affiliate Relations
We approach every patient understanding that every diagnosis, every illness, and every injury are different. It's the collective effort of trained and compassionate team members who value the quality of life of every patient and their caregivers. It's the right kind of treatment- inpatient, outpatient, and follow-up services-provided under the same roof. It's one step closer to home. It's a continuum of care

7113   Sellersburg Health and Rehabilitation Centre
7823 Old State Road 60
Sellersburg, IN 47172-1858   812-246-4272
                                         Fax: 812-246-8160
                                    www.sellersburgrehab.com

Dave Powell, Administrator
Chris Hansen, Executive Director
Sellersburg is a modern healthcare center conveniently located on the edge of the community. Our center accomodates 110 residents and includes a rehabilitative program with a goal of returning residents home as quickly as possible. Sellersburg is a 2006 recipient of the American Health Care Association Quality Award.

7114   Westpark Rehabilitation Center
1316 N Tibbs Ave
Indianapolis, IN 46222-3024   317-634-8330
                                         Fax: 317-263-9442
                                    www.westparkhealthcare.com
Dave Mc Carroll, Owner
Offers the following rehabilitation services: Sub-acute rehabilitation, occupational therapy, physical therapy, speech therapy, respiratory therapy.

7115   Westview Nursing and Rehabilitation Center
1510 Clinic Dr
Bedford, IN 47421-3530   812-279-4494
                                         Fax: 812-275-8313
                          www.ascseniorcare.com/westview-nursing—rehab
Sholin Montgomery, Executive Director
Mike Spencer, Executive Director
Offers the following rehabilitation services: Sub-acute rehabilitation, physical therapy, occupational therapy, speech therapy.

7116   Windsor Estates Health and Rehab Center
429 W Lincoln Rd
Kokomo, IN 46902-3508   765-453-5600
                                         Fax: 765-455-0110
                                        www.kindredkokomo.com
Brenda Alfrey, Administrator
Monica Martin, Executive Director
Our wide array of services enables our patients and residents to receive the medical care they need, the restorative therapy they require, and the support they and their families deserve. We serve many types of patient and resident needs - from short-term rehabilitation to traditional long-term care.

Iowa

7117   Madison County Rehab Services
Madison County Hospital
300 W Hutchings St
Winterset, IA 50273-2109   515-462-2373
                                         Fax: 515-462-4492
Marcia Harris, CEO
Panndee Stebbins, Director
Offers the following rehabilitation services: Sub-acute rehabilitation, occupational therapy, physical therapy, speech therapy, home health rehab, wellness programs.

7118   Mercy Subacute Care
603 E 12th St
Des Moines, IA 50309-5515   515-247-4400
                                         Fax: 515-643-0945
Bonnie Mc Coy, Manager
Pam Nelson, Intake Coordinator
Offers the following rehabilitation services: Sub-acute rehabilitation, physical therapy, speech therapy, occupational therapy.

Kentucky

7119   Danville Centre for Health and Rehabilitation
642 N 3rd St
Danville, KY 40422-1125   859-236-3972
                                         Fax: 859-236-0703
                                      www.danvillecentre.com
Debbie Gibson, Executive Director
We offer short-term rehabilitative care as well as long-term care. Our emphasis is on service excellence - providing quality care in a home-like environment to allow for independence and to enable our patients and residents to receive the medical care they need, the restorative therapy they require, and the support they and their families deserve.

7120   Fountain Circle Health & Rehabilitation
Kindred Healthcare
200 Glenway Rd
Winchester, KY 40391   859-744-1800
                                         Fax: 859-744-0285
William Whited, Executive Director
Kathryn Jones, Medical Director
Offers the following rehabilitation services: Sub-acute rehabilitation, speech therapy, physical therapy, occupational therapy.

7121   Lexington Center for Health and Rehabilitation
353 Waller Ave
Lexington, KY 40504-2974   859-252-3558
                                         Fax: 859-233-0192
Karole Ward, Administrator
Offers the following rehabilitation services: Sub-acute rehabilitation, speech therapy, occupational therapy, physical therapy.

7122   Paducah Centre For Health and Rehabilitation
Wellsouth Health Systems
501 N 3rd St
Paducah, KY 42001-0749   270-444-9661
                                         Fax: 270-443-9407
Jean Glisson, RN, Director of Nursing
Elizabeth Kay Chilton, Admissions Director
Tracy Summers, Rehab/Specialty Program Director
Paducah Center is an 86-bed skilled and long-term care facility with a 28-bed Alzheimer's secure unit. This unit has a private courtyard and structured activities throughout the day, and is the only true Alzheimer's secure unit in the area.

7123   Pathways Brain Injury Program
4200 Browns Ln
Louisville, KY 40220-1523   502-459-8900
                                         Fax: 502-459-5026
                                      www.hcr-manorcare.com
Pam Pearson, Manager
Offers the following rehabilitation services: Sub-acute rehabilitation, speech therapy, occupational therapy, physical therapy, recreational therapy.

Louisiana

7124   **Guest House of Slidell Sub-Acute and Rehab Center**
1051 Robert Blvd
Slidell, LA 70458-2011   985-643-5630
800-303-9872
Fax: 985-649-6065

Brandy Wheat, Administrator
116 bed healthcare center offering the following subacute services within the skilled nursing setting: physical, occupational, and speech therapies, infusion therapy, respiratory care, wound care, neurological rehabilitation, cardiac reconditioning, pain management, post surgical recovery, orthopedic rehabilitation.

7125   **Irving Place Rehabilitation and Nursing Center**
1736 Irving Pl
Shreveport, LA 71101-4606   318-631-9121
Fax: 318-222-2095

Webster Johnson, Administrator
Offers the following rehabilitation services: sub-acute rehabilitation, speech therapy, occupational therapy, physical therapy

Maine

7126   **Augusta Rehabilitation Center**
188 Eastern Ave
Augusta, ME 04330-5928   207-622-3121
800-457-1220
Fax: 207-623-7666
www.augustarehabcenter.com

Malcolm Dean, Executive Director
Cathleen O'Connor
From intensive short term rehabilitation therapy to longer-term restorative care, our Nursing and Rehabilitation Centers provide a full range of nursing care and social services to treat and support each of our patients and residents. Our clinical capabilities allow us to accept patients with greater medical complexity than a traditional nursing home. This is increasingly important as many patients require transitional care before they are ready to return home.

7127   **Brentwood Rehabilitation and Nursing Center**
370 Portland St
Yarmouth, ME 04096-8101   207-846-9021
800-457-1220
Fax: 207-846-1497

Malcolm Dean, Executive Director
Daniel M. Pierce, Medical Director
Brentwood accomodates 82 residents. We are located at 370 Portland Street in Yarmouth, Maine. We strive to meet the healthcare needs of the greater Yarmouth community, including Portland and Brunswick, which are located within 10 miles of the center. In addition to Brentwood's rehabilitation and skilled nursing services, we also offer Alzheimer's specialty care in a comfortable setting.

7128   **Den-Mar Rehabilitation and Nursing Center**
44 South St
Rockport, MA 01966-1800   978-546-6311
800-439-2370
Fax: 978-546-9185

Christine Marek, Executive Director
Den-Mar nursing and Rehab center accomodates 80 residents. We provide skilled nursing and rehabilitation services as well as long term care. We are certified for Medicare and Medicaid as well as many insurance carriers. We offer semi-private and private rooms, with many common areas for socializing.

7129   **Eastside Rehabilitation and Living Center**
516 Mount Hope Ave
Bangor, ME 04401-4215   207-947-6131
800-457-1220
Fax: 207-942-0884
www.eastsiderehab.com

Ryan Kelley, Executive Director
From intensive short term rehabilitation therapy to longer-term restorative care, our Nursing and Rehabilitation Centers provide a full range of nursing care and social services to treat and support each of our patients and residents. Our clinical capabilities allow us to accept patients with greater medical complexity than a traditional nursing home. This is increasingly important as many patients require transitional care before they are ready to return home.

7130   **Kennebunk Nursing & Rehabilitation Center**
158 Ross Rd
Kennebunk, ME 04043-6532   207-985-7141
800-457-1220
Fax: 207-985-0961

Stephen Alaimo, Executive Director
We treat a variety of conditions and provide an array of services including, but not limited to:Respiratory conditions such as pneumonia and post-acute COPD episodes Cardiac conditions and post surgical care (grafts, valves, stints) Wound Stroke Orthopedic Neurological illnesses Diabetes

7131   **Norway Rehabilitation and Living Center**
29 Marion Ave
Norway, ME 04268-5601   207-743-7075
800-457-1220
Fax: 207-743-9269

Carolyn Farley, Administrator
Norway Rehabilitation and Living Center has been a fixture in the Norway community since 1976. We are a 70-bed facility offering short-term rehabilitation, skilled nursing services, long term care and residential care services. Utilizing an interdisciplinary team led by a physician and consisting of qualified health care specialists, we develop individualized plans of care for each patient that are designed to restore maximum health and optimize functional abilities and independence

7132   **Shore Village Rehabilitation & Nursing Center**
201 Camden St
\, ME 04841-2534   207-596-6423
800-457-1220
Fax: 207-596-7235

Phyllis Nickerson, Administrator
Shore Village accomodates 60 residents and is located in the mid-coast region of the state of Maine. We have a cozy size and a primary goal for the staff is to ensure a home-like atmosphere for all the residents. Shore Village provides skilled nursing and rehabilitation, respite care, and long term care. The facility is dually certified for Medicare and Medicaid and accepts many commercial insurance plans.

Maryland

7133   **Greater Baltimore Medical Center**
6701 N Charles St
Baltimore, MD 21204-6881   443-849-2000
Fax: 443-849-3024
TTY: 800-735-2258
www.gbmc.org

John B. Chessare, M.D., President/Chief Executive Officer
Eric L. Melchior, Executive Vice President/Chief Financial Officer
Keith Poisson, Executive Vice President/Chief Operating Officer
The 281-bed medical center (acute and sub-acute care) is located on a beautiful suburban campus and handles more than 26,700 inpatient cases and approximately 60,000 emergency room visits annually.

Massachusetts

7134   **Bolton Manor Nursing Home**
400 Bolton St
Marlborough, MA 01752-3912   508-481-6123
800-439-2370
Fax: 508-481-6130

Michele Ricard, Medical Director
Thomas Sullivan, Executive Director
Bolton Manor accomodates 157 residents. We are located in Marlboro, Massachusetts. We provide medical management and long-term care through comprehensive skilled and post-acute

nursing services. We also provide physical, occupational, and speech therapy services from an onsite dedicated staff of therapists. The facility is Joint Commission (formerly JCAHO) accredited and has an excellent survey history with the State Department of Public Health.

7135   Brigham Manor Nursing and Rehabilitation Center
77 High St
Newburyport, MA 01950-3071   978-462-4221
                                                        800-439-2370
                                                   Fax: 978-463-3297

Stephen Cynewski, Executive Director
Brigham Manor accomodates 64 residents. We are a Medicare-certified facility offering private, semi-private and multi-bed suites. Our bright, formal dining room, with French doors that open to a shaded courtyard, provides a warm atmosphere for entertaining family and friends. Each resident's personal tastes and medical needs are considered in the planning of our weekly menus.

7136   Country Gardens Skilled Nursing and Rehabilitation Center
2045 Grand Army Hwy
Swansea, MA 02777-3932   508-379-9700
                                                        800-439-2370
                                                   Fax: 508-379-0723

Sandy Sarza, Executive Director
Country Gardens Skilled Nursing and Rehabilitation Center accomodates 86 residents. We are located in a beautiful rural setting conveniently located about 15 minutes east of Providence and 10 minutes west of Fall River. We have provided healthcare service to the greater Swansea area for over 34 years.

7137   Country Manor Rehabilitation and Nursing Center
180 Low St
Newburyport, MA 01950-3519   978-465-5361
                                                        800-439-2370
                                                   Fax: 978-463-9366
                                                 www.countryrehab.com

Stephen Doyle, Executive Director
Country Rehabilitation and Nursing Center accomodates 123 residents. We are located in the quaint seaport town of Newburyport, Massachusetts. We provide medical management and long-term care through comprehensive skilled and intermediate nursing services. We also provide physical, occupational, and speech therapy services from an onsite dedicated staff of therapists. The center offers an Alzheimer's special care unit with staff trained in dimentia care and dementia specific programs.

7138   Franklin Skilled Nursing and Rehabilitation Center
130 Chestnut St
Franklin, MA 02038-3903   508-528-4600
                                                        800-439-2370
                                                   Fax: 508-528-7976

Paula Topijan, Executive Director
We treat a variety of conditions and provide an array of services including, but not limited to :Respiratory conditions such as pneumonia and post-acute COPD episodes,Cardiac conditions and post surgical care (grafts, valves, stints),Wound,Stroke,Orthopedic,Neurological illnesses,Diabetes

7139   Great Barrington Rehabilitation and Nursing Center
148 Maple Ave
Great Barrington, MA 01230-1906   413-528-3320
                                                        800-439-2370
                                                   Fax: 413-528-2302
                                           www.greatbarringtonrnc.com

William Kittler, Executive Director
Andrew Potler, Medical Director
Great Barrington Rehabilitation and Nursing Center accomodates 106 residents. As part of a national network of long-term healthcare centers, we have the expertise and resources to provide care appropriate to the individual needs of each and every one of our residents. We provide personal care with minimal daily living assistance to the most skilled treatment for medically complex patients.

7140   Ledgewood Rehabilitation and Skilled Nursing Center
87 Herrick St
Beverly, MA 01915-2773   978-921-1392
                                                        800-439-2370
                                                   Fax: 978-927-8627
                                              www.ledgewoodrehab.com

Frank Silvia, Executive Director
Ledgewood Rehabilitation and Skilled Nursing Center is a unique provider of healthcare services. We are part of a continuum of services that includes acute care services at Beverly Hospital, subacute care at Ledgewood, and care after discharge through Northeast Homecare. We believe this partnership offers the highest quality post-acute services north of Boston.

7141   Leo P La Chance Center for Rehabilitation and Nursing
59 Eastwood Cir
Gardner, MA 01440-3901   978-632-8776
                                                   Fax: 978-632-5048

Mark Alinger, Administrator
Leo P. LaChance, Founder
A privately owned facility, combines the best of medical technology with the ultimate in healing, compassionate rehabilitation and nursing care. Our goal is to help each client reach that ultimate goal of living life to the fullest.

7142   Oakwood Rehabilitation and Nursing Center
11 Pontiac Ave
Webster, MA 01570-1629   508-943-3889
                                                        800-439-2370
                                                   Fax: 508-949-6125
                                              www.oakwoodrehab.com

Thomas Sullivan, Executive Director
Oakwood Rehabilitation and Nursing Center accomodates 81 residents. We offer 24-hour skilled nursing, inpatient rehabilitation, respite care, and hospice services. Our center has been successfully serving the greater Webster, Massachusetts, community for 35 years. We have a dedicated and caring staff and our common goal is to promote recovery and enhance quality of live whether your needs are short or long term.

7143   Walden Rehabilitation and Nursing Center
785 Main St
Concord, MA 01742-3310   978-369-6889
                                                        800-439-2370
                                                   Fax: 978-369-8392

Ladan Azarm, Executive Director
Walden Rehabilitation and Nursing Center accomodates 123 residents. We are located in the quaint town of Concord, Massachusetts, across the street from Emerson Hospital and a short drive from the town center. Walden provides medical management and long-term care through comprehensive skilled and intermediate nursing services. We also provide physical, occupational, and speech therapy services from an onsite dedicated staff of therapists.

Michigan

7144   Boulder Park Terrace
14676 W Upright St
Charlevoix, MI 49720-1201   231-547-1005
                                                   Fax: 231-547-1039

Reezie DeVet, President/CEO
Mary-Anne Ponti, COO
A partnership formed with Charlevoix Area Hospital, Boulder Park Terrace is a long-term care facility and Sub-acute Rehabilitation Center located in Chalrevoix near the shores of Lake Michigan. The Sub-acute Rehabilitation Center was created as a transition between an acute care hospital and home. Patients enter into the program to increase their strength, endurance and over-all functioning before returning home.

Minnesota

7145 Park Health And Rehabilitation Center
4415 W 36 1/2 St
St Louis Park, MN 55416-4890
952-927-9717
Fax: 952-927-7687
www.extendicare.com

Jennifer Kuhn, Administrator
Park Health & Rehabilitation Center is a leading provider of long-term skilled nursing care and short-term rehabilitation solutions. Our 93 bed facility offers a full continuum of services and care focused around each individual in today's ever-changing healthcare environment.

Missouri

7146 Barnes-Jewish Hospital Washington University Medical Center
1 Barnes Jewish Hospital Plz
Saint Louis, MO 63110-1003
314-747-3000
866-867-3627
Fax: 314-362-8877
www.barnesjewish.org

Richard Liekweg, President
John Beatty, Vice President of Human Resources
John Lynch, MD, Chief Medical Officer
Barnes-Jewish Hospital at Washington University Medical Center is the largest hospital in Missouri and the largest private employer in the St. Louis region. An affiliated teaching hospital of Washington University School of Medicine, Barnes-Jewish Hospital has a 1,700 member medical staff with many who are recognized in the 'Best Doctors in America.'

Montana

7147 Parkview Acres Care and Rehabilitation Center
200 N Oregon St
Dillon, MT 59725-3624
406-683-5105
866-253-4090
Fax: 406-683-6388

Claire Miller, Executive Director
We are Medicare and Medicaid certified skilled nursing facility which accomodates 108 residents serving scenic Dillon and surrounding Montana communities.

Nebraska

7148 Homestead Healthcare and Rehabilitation Center
4735 S 54th St
Lincoln, NE 68516-1335
402-488-0977
800-833-0920
Fax: 402-488-4507
www.homesteadrehab.com

Matt Romshek, Executive Director
Gay Bate, RN, Director of Nursing
James Murray, Administrator
Homestead Healthcare and Rehabilitation Center is one of the area's oldest providers of skilled nursing and rehabilitation services. We are a 163-bed skilled nursing and rehabilitation center nestled in a lovely, quiet established neighborhood in South Lincoln.

7149 Madonna Rehabilitation Hospital
5401 South St
Lincoln, NE 68506-2150
402-413-3000
800-676-5448
Fax: 402-486-5448
info@madonna.org
www.madonna.org

Marsha Lommel, CEO
Tom Stalder, VP Medical Affairs

Madonna provides intensive rehabilitation and expertise for a wide variety of conditions, such as: orthopedic injuries, work injuries, arthritis, amputation, neuromuscular diseases, cardiac conditions, pulmonary disease and conditions including those dependent upon a ventilator, cancer, lymphedema, osteoporosis, wounds, renal disorders, burns, fibromyalgia, multiple sclerosis, parkinson's disease and degenerative diseases.

7150 Mary Lanning Memorial Hospital
715 N Saint Joseph Ave
Hastings, NE 68901-4497
402-463-4521
866-460-5884
tanderson@mlmh.org
www.mlmh.org

Beth Schlichtman, Compensation/Benefit Services - Director
Lisa Brandt, Public Relations & Marketing Services - Director
Carrie Edwards, Home Care Services - Director
Mary Lanning Healthcare is in its 95th year of providing quality healthcare for residents of the central Nebraska area. We continue to grow and expand, working to provide patient-centered care in a positive environment, while implementing some of the newest technologies available.

Nevada

7151 Las Vegas Healthcare and Rehabilitation Center
2832 S Maryland Pkwy
Las Vegas, NV 89109-1502
702-735-5848
800-326-6888
Fax: 702-735-6218
www.lasvegaskindred.com

Randall Fuller, Executive Director
Las Vegas Healthcare accomodates 79 residents. We have been serving the community for approximately 40 years. Located in close proximity to local hospitals and surrounded by medical complexes, our center offers both short-term rehabilitation and long-term care.

New Hampshire

7152 Dover Rehabilitation and Living Center
307 Plaza Dr
Dover, NH 03820-2455
603-742-2676
800-735-2964
Fax: 603-749-5375
www.doverrehab.com

Daniel Estee, Executive Director
Dover Rehab is a provider of postacute services in the greater New Hampshire Seacost area. We accomodate 112 residents and are licensed by the state of New Hampshire. We employ nearly 150 licensed nurses, therapists and other healthcare professionals, who strive to provide quality care. The goal of our patient service model is to bridge the gap between hospitalization and home so that recovery and physical functioning are maximized and hospital readmission is minimized.

7153 Northeast Rehabilitation Clinic
70 Butler St
Salem, NH 03079-3925
603-893-2900
800-825-7292
Fax: 603-893-1638
TTY: 800-439-2370
www.northeastrehab.com

John Prochilo, CEO/Administrator
Subacute rehabilitation at NRH was designed for people who have experienced an acutely disabling orthopedic, medical, or neurologic condition but who either do not require or are unable to participate in a full acute inpatient program. Impairment groups pertinent to this level of care include brain injury, spinal cord injury (traumatic/non-traumatic), stroke, orthopedic injury, amputation, and neurologic disorder.

New Jersey

7154 Atlantic Coast Rehabilitation & Healthcare Center
485 River Ave
Lakewood, NJ 08701-4720
732-364-7100
Fax: 732-364-2442
abby@atlanticcoastrehab.com
www.atlanticcoastrehab.com

Simon Shain, Administrator
Sharon Sckbower, Director of Nursing
Atlantic Coast is family owned and operated. It's a warm, friendly place where caregivers and patients know each other by first name. But it's also an innovative and energetic place, where the most advanced therapies and cutting edge techniques are offered. It's a comprehensive health care center that provides three distinct areas of care:Rehabilitative Therapy & Sub Acute Care, Long Term Care,Alzheimer's/Memory Impaired Care.

7155 Crestwood Nursing & Rehabilitation Center
101 Whippany Rd
Whippany, NJ 7981-1407
973-887-0311
Fax: 973-887-8355

Carol Shepard, Administrator
Sub-acute rehabilitation facility.

7156 Lakeview Subacute Care Center
130 Terhune Dr
Wayne, NJ 7470-7104
973-839-4500
87 -UBA-UTE
Fax: 973-839-2729
www.lakeviewsubacute.com

Richard Grosso, Jr, Director
Sue Ahlers, Director of Admission
Kerry Iamurri, Director of Rehab
Our comprehensive medical, nursing and rehabilitation services cater to a diverse patient population. In addition to long-term care, we offer exceptional inpatient subacute programs. We're proud to report that our average length of stay for subacute patients is a brief 14 days.

7157 Merwick Rehabilitation and Sub-Acute Care
79 Bayard Ln
Princeton, NJ 8540-3045
609-497-3000
Fax: 609-497-3024
Ryan Wismer, Administrator
76-bed skilled nursing and residential center as well as a separate 17-bed comprehensive rehabilitation center. Offers rehabilitation, physiatry, occupational therapy, respite care, speech/hearing therapy, sub-acute care.

7158 Seacrest Village Nursing Center
1001 Center St
Little Egg Harbor Twp, NJ 8087-1364
609-296-9292
Fax: 609-296-0508
info@seacrestvillagenj.com
seacrestvillagenj.com

Brian T Holloway, Administrator
Seacrest Village Nursing and Rehabilitation Center has specialized in quality rehabilitation, transitional and restorative care for more then a decade and is a perfect alternative for bridging the gap between hospital and home.

7159 St. Lawrence Rehabilitation Center
2381 Lawrenceville Rd
Lawrenceville, NJ 08648-2098
609-896-9500
Fax: 609-895-0242
epiechota@slrc.org
www.slrc.org

Kevin McGuigan, MD, Medical Director
Robyn F. Agri, MD, Doctor
Dr. Madhu Jain, Doctor
St. Lawrence Rehabilitation Center, a non-profit facility sponsored by the Roman Catholic Diocese of Trenton, is committed to maximizing the quality of human life by providing comprehensive physical rehabilitation and related programs to meet the healthcare needs of our communities.

7160 Summit Ridge Center Genesis Eldercare
20 Summit St
West Orange, NJ 07052-1501
973-736-2000
800-699-1520
Fax: 973-736-2764
info@genesishcc.com
www.genesishcc.com

Michele Cartagena, Director of Admissions
Elizabeth (L Orlando, Rehabilitation Program Director
Tsega Asefaha, LNHA, BS, MHA, Administrator
Summit Ridge Center provides skilled nursing, medical and rehabilitative care for patients requiring post-hospital, short stay rehabilitation and for longer term residents. Our Clinical Care Teams are focused on implementing your personalized care program to facilitate your recovery and improve your well-being.

New York

7161 Beth Abraham Health Services
612 Allerton Ave
Bronx, NY 10467-7495
718-519-4037
888-238-4223
Fax: 718-547-1366
info@bethabe.org
www.bethabrahamhealthservices.org

Maria Provenzano, Program Director
Yolanda Lester, Director of Admissions
Rosalie Bernard, Director of Nursing Services
Offers the following rehabilitation services: Sub-Acute rehabilitation, brain injury rehabilitation, pain management, post-operative recovery. Home visits and a network of community-based programs help patients and their families with a successful transition home.

7162 Central Island Healthcare
825 Old Country Rd
Plainview, NY 11803-4913
516-433-0600
Fax: 516-868-7251

Michael Ostreicher, Administrator
Serving the community for over 33 years, Central Island Healthcare is Long Island's largest and most active sub-acute care provider. We offer comprehensive programs focused on restoring our patients to their maximum potential and returning home. Central Island's 202-bed facility provides top notch professionals and the latest in rehabilitation and therapeutic equipment in a beautiful and comfortable setting.

7163 Clove Lakes Health Care and Rehabilitation Center
25 Fanning St
Staten Island, NY 10314-5307
718-289-7900
Fax: 718-761-8701
info@clovelakes.com
www.clovelakes.com

Helene Demisay, CEO
Clove Lakes seeks to rehabilitate those who have sustained injury or illness to the highest level of independence possible and support those with disabling conditions to live meaningful and productive lives.

7164 Dr. William O Benenson Rehabilitation Pavilion
36-17 Parsons Blvd
Flushing, NY 11354-5931
718-961-4300
Fax: 718-939-5032

Esther Benenson, Executive Director
Liza Marie Dowd, Director of Nursing
Erika Rossi, Director of Social Services
The Dr. William O Benson Reahbilitation Pavilion is a subacute short-term rehabilitation center committed to the excellence of elevated health care for our patients. Through the use of the most comprehensive and specialized services available, our staff of dedicated professionals are devoted to putting patients back to the road to full recovery 24 hours a day.

7165 Flushing Manor Nursing and Rehab
35-15 Parsons Blvd
Flushing, NY 11354-4297   718-961-3500
                                 Fax: 718-461-1784

Esther Benenson, Executive Director
Dr. Ion Oltean, Medical Director
Myung Chung, Director of Nursing
At the Flusing Manor Nursing and Rehabilitation, we stress the importance of family involvement because it is the true source of strength and stability in ones life...a tie that brings us all together as a team, enhancing the quality of life of the patients in our care.

7166 Glengariff Health Care Center
141 Dosoris Ln
Glen Cove, NY 11542   516-676-1100
                             Fax: 516-759-0216
                             www.glenhaven.org

Jean Campo, Director Admissions
Michael Miness, President
Licensed skilled nursing and subacute medical and rehabilitation facility.

7167 Haym Salomon Home for The Aged
2340 Cropsey Ave
Brooklyn, NY 11214-5706   718-266-4063
                                 Fax: 718-372-4781

Chain Lipschitz, Administrator
Religious nonmedical health care institution.

7168 Kings Harbor Multicare Center
2000 E Gun Hill Rd
Bronx, NY 10469-6016   718-320-0400
                              Fax: 718-671-5022
                              info@kingsharbor.com
                              www.kingsharbor.com

Morris Tenenbaum, Owner
Octavio Marin, Vice President
Kings Harbor Multicare Center provides long-term and short-term skilled nursing care for more then 700 residents. Kings Harbor is located in the Pelham Gardens neighborhood of Northeast Bronx, easily accessible to major highways and near public transportation. A 3 building campus facility with surrounding gardens ensures that residents with similar capabilities are grouped together.

7169 Northwoods of Cortland
28 Kellogg Rd
Cortland, NY 13045-3155   607-753-9631
                                 Fax: 607-756-2968

Lawrence Mennig, Administrator
Subacute rehabilitation facility.

7170 Port Jefferson Health Care Facility
141 Dosoris Lane
Glen Cove, NY 11542   631-676-1100
                             Fax: 631-759-0216
                             www.glengariffcare.com

Ellen Harte, Administrator
Subacute medical and rehabilitative care and long term residential skilled nursing care.

7171 Rehab Institute at Florence Nightingale Health Center
1760 3rd Ave
New York, NY 10029-6810   212-410-8760
                                 800-786-8968
                                 Fax: 212-410-8792
Sub-acute rehabilitation facility.

7172 Schnurmacher Center for Rehabilitation and Nursing
Beth Abraham of Family Health Services
12 Tibbits Ave
White Plains, NY 10606-2438   914-287-7200
                                     888-238-4223
                                     Fax: 914-428-1824
                                     info@schnurmacher.org
                                     www.schnurmacher.org

Linda Murray, Executive Director
Thomas Camisa, Medical Director
Iryn Obaldo Fontanosa, Director of Rehabilitation
The environment at Schnurmacher is tailored to the needs of patients who require medical and nursing services but who do not need the complexity of services associated with an acute-care hospital. And Schnurmacher Subacute Medical patients are out of bed more quickly and as often as possible, which helps them maintain functional status while recovery progresses.

7173 South Shore Healthcare
275 W Merrick Rd
Freeport, NY 11520-3346   516-623-4000
                                 Fax: 516-223-4599

Winnie Mack, RN, BSN, MPA, Regional Executive Director
Gene Tangney, Senior Vice President/ Regional Executive Director
Michael J. Dowling, President/ CEO
North Shore-LIJ Health System includes 16 award-winning hospitals and nearly 400 physician practice locations throughout New York, including Long Island, Manhattan, Queens and Staten Island. Proudly serving an area of seven million people, North Shore-LIJ delivers world-class services designed for every step of your health and wellness journey.

7174 St. Camillus Health and Rehabilitation Center
813 Fay Rd
Syracuse, NY 13219-3009   315-488-2951
                                 Fax: 315-488-3255
                                 info@st-camillus.org
                                 www.st-camillus.org

Aileen Balitz, President
Patrick VanBeveren, PT, DPT, M, Supervisor of Physical Therapy
Nancy, Pirro, RN, Case Manager
Since our founding in 1969, St. Camillus' mission has been to provide high-quality services and facilities emphasizing the rehabilitation of individuals to their maximum potential. The importance of the human spirit drives all we do. We are dedicated to caring for life and helping individuals achieve their highest possible level of independence.

North Carolina

7175 Chapel Hill Rehabilitation and Healthcare Center
1602 E Franklin St
Chapel Hill, NC 27514-2892   919-967-1418
                                    800-735-8262
                                    Fax: 919-918-3811

Turner Prichett, Executive Director
Chapel Hill Rehabilitation and Healthcare Center accomodates 120 residents. We are located in downtown Chapel Hill on Franklin Street and we provide roud the clock nursing care 365 days a year. Intensive rehabilitation services are administered by our licensed speech, occupational and physical therapists. Our staff is trained to care for medically complex patients such as those requiring intensive wound care, dialysis, and artificial nutrition.

7176 Cypress Pointe Rehabilitation and Healthcare Center
2006 S 16th St
Wilmington, NC 28401-6613   910-763-6271
                                   800-735-8262
                                   Fax: 910-251-9803

Sara Deiter, Executive Director
Dr. Jose Gonzalez, Medical Director
Cypress Pointe offers comprehensive physical, occupational, speech and respiratory therapy services. Following a physician's referral, patients are evaluated to determine their needs. Recommendations are then made for the appropriate interventions and rehabilitation. If therapy is required, a personalized care plan is developed.

7177 Pettigrew Rehabilitation and Healthcare Center
1551 W Pettigrew St
Durham, NC 27705-4821   919-286-0751
                               800-735-8262
                               Fax: 919-286-5992

La'Ticia Beatty, Executive Director
Pettigrew Rehabilitation and Healthcare Center accomodates 107 residents. Our healthcare center is certified by Medicare and Medicaid. We have experienced staff members who care for our residents. We strive to improve the quality of life our residents experience as a result of the services they receive from our nursing and therapy departments.

7178 Raleigh Rehabilitation and Healthcare Center
616 Wade Ave
Raleigh, NC 27605-1237   919-828-6251
800-735-8262
Fax: 919-828-3294
www.raleighrehabhc.com
Steven Jones, Executive Director
Raleigh Rehabilitation and Healthcare Center accomodates 172 residents. We provide short-term rehabilitation-including, physical, occupational, and speech therapies-as well as long-term nursing services. We specialize in neurological disorders, complex diabetes treatment, amputation recovery and pain management. We welcome short stays (respite care). Transportation services are availiable for physician appointments and dialysis treatments.

7179 Rehabilitation and Healthcare Center of Monroe
1212 E Sunset Dr
Monroe, NC 28112-4318   704-283-8548
800-735-8262
Fax: 704-283-4664
Judy Olson, Executive Director
We accomodate 159 residents and are certified for Medicare and Medicaid. We specialize in short-term rehabilitation as well as long-term care. Our therapists, wound nurse and dietician work closely to administer wound care. We hav 2 dialysis centers within a 10-block radius and gladly accpet their patients. We have an on-staff medical director as well as a psychiatrist.

7180 Winston-Salem Rehabilitation and Healthcare Center
1900 W 1st St
Winston Salem, NC 27104-4220   336-724-2821
800-735-8262
Fax: 336-725-8314
Tom Bauer, Administrator
We accommodate 230 residents and we have approximately 250 employees. Our staffing ratio averages 1 licensed nurse for every 20 residents and 1 Certified Nursing Assistant for every 10 residents. We offer a wide range of services including but not limited to respiratory care, tracheotomy care and gastric tube feeding and we also feature an in house licensed therapy program.

Ohio

7181 Arbors East Subacute and Rehabilitation Center
5500 E Broad St
Columbus, OH 43213-1476   614-575-9003
Fax: 614-575-9101
Arbors East is a leading provider of long-term skilled nursing care and short-term rehabilitation solutions. Our 100 bed facility offers a full continuum of services and care focused around each individual in today's ever-changing healthcare environment.

7182 Arbors at Canton Subacute And Rehabilitation Center
2714 13th St NW
Canton, OH 44708-3121   330-456-2842
Fax: 330-456-5343
www.laurelsofcanton.com
Amy McDermand, Director of Marketing
Beth Jones, PT, DPT, Rehabilitation Services Director
Cindy Shingler, RN,, Director of Nursing
We provide individualized, quality care to guests staying short-term for rehabilitation services or long-term for extended care services. The highest level of independence for our guests is the creed of The Laurels of Canton.

7183 Arbors at Dayton
320 Albany St
Dayton, OH 45408-1402   937-496-6200
Fax: 937-496-1990
www.extendicareus.com/dayton
Dave Maxwell, Administrator
Carlisa Pedalino, Administrator
Arbors at Dayton is a leading provider of long-term skilled nursing care and short-term rehabilitation solutions. Our 106 bed facility offers a full continuum of services and care focused around each individual in today's ever-changing healthcare environment.

7184 Arbors at Marietta
400 N 7th St
Marietta, OH 45750-2024   740-373-3597
Fax: 740-376-0004
www.extendicareus.com/marietta
Joan Florence, Director of Nursing
Kenneth Leopold, Medical Director
Arbors at Marietta is a leading provider of long-term skilled nursing care and short-term rehabilitation solutions. Our 150 bed facility offers a full continuum of services and care focused around each individual in today's ever-changing healthcare environment.

7185 Arbors at Milford
5900 Meadow Creek Dr
Milford, OH 45150-5641   513-248-1655
Fax: 513-248-7340
www.extendicareus.com/milford
Bruce Yarwood, President/CEO
Mark Ostendorf, Administrator
Arbors at Milford is a leading provider of long-term skilled nursing care and short-term rehabilitation solutions. Our 139 bed facility offers a full continuum of services and care focused around each individual in today's ever-changing healthcare environment.

7186 Arbors at Sylvania
7120 Port Sylvania Dr
Toledo, OH 43617-1158   419-841-2200
Fax: 419-841-2822
www.extendicareus.com/sylvania
Sheril Flowers, Administrator
Graig Hopple, Medical Director
Arbors at Sylvania is a leading provider of long-term skilled nursing care and short-term rehabilitation solutions. Our 79 bed facility offers a full continuum of services and care focused around each individual in today's ever-changing healthcare environment.

7187 Arbors at Toledo Subacute and Rehab Centre
2920 Cherry St
Toledo, OH 43608-1716   419-242-7458
Fax: 419-242-6514
www.extendicare.com
Jill Schlievert, Administrator
Subacute rehabilitation services and facility.

7188 Bridgepark Center for Rehabilitation and Nursing Services
145 Olive St
Akron, OH 44310-3236   330-762-0901
800-750-0750
Fax: 330-762-0905
Joseph Burick, Medical Director
A skilled nursing and rehabilitation center located in Akron, Ohio, across the street from St. Thomas Hospital with a beautiful view of the Akron skyline. Access to Interstate 77 and State Route 8 is just minutes away. Our entire staff is committed to providing caring, customer-focused skilled nursing and rehabilitation. For your convenience, we accept Medicare, Medicaid and most managed care and private insurance.

7189 Broadview Multi-Care Center
5520 Broadview Rd
Parma, OH 44134-1605   216-749-4010
Fax: 216-749-0141
www.broadviewmulticare.com
Harold Shachter, Owner
Mike Flank, VP
Broadview Multi-Care Center is a family run business with more than 40 years of experience providing quality care to the community. We are committed to meeting your needs and providing you with a warm, home-like environment. Our family is on-site and our doors are always open for your suggestions or to drop in and say hello. We always try to take and honor requests, whether it's a favorite food, an exciting activity or a particular room.

7190 Caprice Care Center
9184 Market St
North Lima, OH 44452-9558   330-965-9200
                                    Fax: 330-726-6097
                                    www.chcccompanies.com

Lori Crowl, Owner
Becky Berger, Director of Nursin
Stacey Howell, Administrator
A 106-bed skilled nursing, subacute and rehabilitation facility.
Our goal is to provide comfortable living to all who are in our
care. Caprice Health Care Center is a contemporary Medicare and
Medicaid approved facility specializing in short-term rehabilitation services. The inpatient/outpatient rehab department includes
physical, occupational, speech therapies, indoor aquatic therapy
pool, as well as complimentary van transportation for outpatient
services.

7191 Cleveland Clinic
9500 Euclid Ave
Cleveland, OH 44195-2   216-444-2200
                                         800-801-2273
                                    Fax: 216-444-7021
                                    my.clevelandclinic.org/default.aspx
Gene Altus, Executive Director
Delos M. Cosgrove, MD, Chief Executive Officer, Preside
Joseph F. Hahn, MD, Chief of Staff, Vice Chairman of
A not-for-profit, multispecialty academic medical center that in-
tegrates clinical and hospital care with research and education.
Cleveland clinic was founded in 1921 by 4 renowned physicians
with a vision of providing outstanding patient care based upon
the principals of cooperation, compassion and innovation. Today,
Cleveland Clinic is one of the largest and most respected
hospitals in the country.

7192 Columbus Rehabilitation And Subacute Institute
111 West Michigan Street
Milwaukee, WI 53203-2903   800-395-5000
                                    kschaewe@extendicare.com
                                    www.extendicareus.com
Kelly Fligor, Administrator
Jillian Fountain, Secretary
Subacute rehabilitation programs and facility.

7193 LakeMed Nursing and Rehabilitation Center
70 Normandy Dr
Painesville, OH 44077-1616   440-357-1311
                                         800-750-0750
                                    Fax: 440-352-9977
                                    www.lakemednursing.com
Connie Eyman, Administrator
Vesta Jones, Executive Director
Our goal is to provide you with quality care and we are known for
our successful short-term rehab and care of the clinically complex. We also offer respite services to give caregivers a rest, and
hospice services through our local hospice care provider. Our interdisciplinary team works together as they strive to deliver quality care and responsive service to our residents.

7194 Oregon Nursing And Rehabilitation Center
904 Isaac Streets Dr
Oregon, OH 43616-3204   419-691-2483
                                    Fax: 419-697-5401
                                    www.extendicareus.com/oregon
Mark Rogers, Administrator
Subacute rehabilitation facility and services.

**7195 Sunset View Castle Nursing Homes Castle Nursing
Homes**
434 N Washington St
Millersburg, OH 44654-1188   330-674-0015
                                    Fax: 330-763-2238
Becky Snyder, Admissions Coordinator
Kathy Edwards, Admissions And Marketing
310 licensed, certified beds. Subacute rehabilitation facility and
programs.

Oregon

7196 Care Center East Health & Specialty Care Center
Expendicare
11325 NE Weidler St
Portland, OR 97220-1950   503-253-1181
                                    Fax: 503-253-1871
                                    www.extendicareus.com
Glydon Kimbrough, Administrator
Subacute rehabilitation facility and programs

7197 Medford Rehabilitation and Healthcare Center
Kindred Healthcare
625 Stevens St
Medford, OR 97504-6719   541-779-3551
                                         800-735-1232
                                    Fax: 541-779-3658
Grant Gloor, Administrator
Dane Reeves, Executive Director
Kristen W., Health and Rehabilitation Center
We strive to provide quality, compassionate care. Our cozy build-
ing accomodates 110 residents. Our smaller size creates an invit-
ing and homelike environment. We offer semi-private rooms with
space to add items from home for a special personalized touch.

Pennsylvania

7198 Dresher Hill Health and Rehabilitation Center
1390 Camp Hill Rd
Dresher, PA 19034-2805   215-643-0600
                                    Fax: 215-641-0628
Earl Kimble, Administrator
Subacute rehabilitation facility and programs: physical/speech.

7199 Good Shepherd Rehabilitation
850 S 5th St
Allentown, PA 18103-3295   610-776-3586
                                         888-447-3422
                                    Fax: 610-776-8336
                                    goodshepherdrehab.org
John Kristel, MBA, MPT, President & CEO
Mike Bonner, MBA, Vice President, Neurosciences
*Ronald J. Petula, CPA, Senior Vice President, Finance and Chief
Financial Officer*
A world class rehabilitation network, Good Shepherd provides
comprehensive inpatient and outpatient services throughout
Pennsylvania's Lehigh Valley. Founded in 1908, Good Shepherd
has steadily expanded over last 95 years. Good Shepherd is one of
the most comprehensive rehabilitation institutes in the world.

7200 Statesman Health and Rehabilitation Center
2629 Trenton Rd
Levittown, PA 19056-1428   215-943-7777
                                    Fax: 215-943-1240
                                    www.statesmanskillednursing.com
Jamie Tanner, Administrator
Subacute rehabilitation facility and programs.

7201 UPMC Braddock
200 Lothrop St.
Pittsburgh, PA 15213-2582   412-647-8762
                                         800-533-8762
                                    Fax: 412-636-5398
                                    hospitalbill@upmc.edu
                                    upmc.com
Mark Sevco, Administrator
Rodney Jones, Vice President
With a team of more then 43,000 employees, UPMC serves the
health needs of more then 4 million people each year, improving
lives in western Pennsylvania-and beyond-through redefined
models of health care delivery and superb clinical outcomes.

7202 UPMC McKeesport
Presby
1500 5th Ave
McKeesport, PA 15132-2422

412-664-2000
Fax: 412-664-2309
fisherpj@upmc.edu
upmc.com

Ronald H Ott, CEO
Offers 56 beds for patients who need skilled nursing care. Offers ongoing rehabilitation and educational programs to patients with cardiac, neurologic, and orthopaedic diagnosis.

7203 UPMC Passavant
9100 Babcock Blvd
Pittsburgh, PA 15237-5842

412-367-6700
800-533-8762
gloordc@ph.upmc.edu
upmc.com

William Kristan, Dir Inpatient Physical Therapy
Teresa Petrick, Chief Executive Officer
Patients who have had an acute illness, injury, or exacerbation of a disease and no longer need the intensity of services in the acute care setting, but still require some complex medical care or supervision and rehabilitation services, may be appropriate to be transferred into the Subacute Unit.

Rhode Island

7204 Kindred Heights Nursing & Rehabilitation Center
Kindred Healthcare
680 South Fourth Street
Louisville, KY 40202

502-596-7300
800-545-0749
web_administrator@kindred.com
www.kindredheights.com

Sandra Sarza, Manager
Jean Aubin, Director
Kindred Heights Nursing and Rehabilitation Center accomodates 58 residents and serves the needs of elders in the greater East Bay and Providence area. We are conveniently located on Wampanoag Trail in East Providence. Kindred Heights provides skilled nursing, short-term rehab and long-term care in a family environment, but we are large enough to manage the complex nursing and rehab care needs our residents may have.

7205 Oak Hill Nursing and Rehabilitation Center
Kindered Health Care
544 Pleasant St
Pawtucket, RI 02860-5776

401-725-8888
800-745-6575
Fax: 401-723-5720
www.oakhillrehab.com

Scott M. Sandborn, Executive Director
Heidi Capela, Director Nursing
Amybeth Almeida, Director Admissions
Accomodates 143 residents. Throughout our 40 year history, Oak Hill has developed a reputation as one of the finest healthcare centers in Rhode Island. Our center consists of 3 separate units. A 34-bed post-acute unit provides care to the medically complex and those in need of extensive rehabilitative services. A 20-bed Alzheimer's Special Care Unit provides a unique style of care utilizing habilitative therapy in comfortable, home-like surroundings.

7206 Southern New England Rehab Center
200 High Service Avenue
North Providence, RI 02904

401-456-3801
888-456-4501
Fax: 401-456-3784
www.snerc.com

Vivian Hagstrom, Manager
The Center's skilled staff of over 100 professionals provides a full range of coordinated rehabilitative care. Our clinical expertise and compassion make a big difference as we develop first-rate plans of care for the unique needs of each patient. Our medical staff is comprised of physicians board-certified in rehabilitation medicine and internal medicine.

South Carolina

7207 Tuomey Healthcare System
129 N Washington St
Sumter, SC 29150-4949

803-774-9000
Fax: 803-774-8737
www.tuomey.com

R Jay Cox, CEO
Here to anticipte the needs of the communities we serve, responding with proactive healthcare initiatives, providing expert rehabilitative services and delivering life-saving acute care.

Tennessee

7208 Camden Healthcare and Rehabilitation Center
680 South Fourth Street
Louisville, KY 40202

502-596-7300
800-545-0749
web_administrator@kindred.com
kindredhealthcare.com

Mark Walker, Administrator
Subacute rehabilitation products and services, nursing and life care homes.

7209 Centennial Medical Center Tri Star Health System
2300 Patterson St
Nashville, TN 37203-1538

615-342-1000
800-242-5662
Fax: 615-342-1045
Laurel.Haskamp@HCAHealthcare.com
tristarcentennial.com

Thomas L Herron, President/Chief Executive Office
Above all else we are committed to the care and improvement of human life by caring for those we serve with integrity, compassion, a positive attitude, respect and exceptional quality.

7210 Cordova Rehabilitation and Nursing Center
955 N Germantown Pkwy
Cordova, TN 38018-6215

901-754-1393
800-848-0299
Fax: 901-754-3332
cdadmi@gracehc.com
www.gracehccordova.com

John Palmer, Administrator
Renee Tutor, Executive Director
Our professional staff can help you make an informed decision. Upon admission, our interdisciplinary team develops a comprehensive care plan to meet not only physical and rehabilitative goals, but also social and emotional needs. We understand the importance of family and resident involvement and encourage participation in the development of a personalized plan of care.

7211 Erlanger Medical Center Baronness Campus
975 E 3rd St
Chattanooga, TN 37403-2147

423-778-7000
Fax: 423-778-7615
guestrelations@erlanger.org
www.erlanger.org

Kevin M. Spiegel, FACHE, President and CEO
James Creel, MD, Chief Medical Officer
Gregg T. Gentry, Chief Administrative Officer
Our mission is to improve the health of the people we touch. Our vision is to be recognized locally, regionally, and and nationally, as a premiere healthcare system.

7212 Huntington Health and Rehabilitation Center
635 High St
Huntingdon, TN 38344-1703

731-986-8943
Fax: 731-986-3188
huntingdonhealth.com

Heidi Hawkins, Administrator
Windi Summers, Admissions Director
Subacute rehabilitation facility and programs.

7213 Madison Healthcare and Rehabilitation Center
431 Larkin Springs Rd
Madison, TN 37115-5005   615-865-8520
                                           800-848-0299
                                           Fax: 615-868-4455

Phyllis Cherry, Executive Director
At our facility, we provide quality care with modern rehabilitation and restorative nursing techniques. We aim to provide an atmosphere which encourages family involvement in the
care-planning process, with the right mix of activities addressing
the social, spiritual and intellectual needs of our residents.

7214 Mariner Health of Nashville
3939 Hillsboro Cir
Nashville, TN 37215-2708   615-297-2100
                                           Fax: 615-297-2197

David Reeves, Administrator
Amy Artrip, Director of Nursing
Religious nonmedical health care institution. 150-bed subacute
rehabilitation facility

7215 Pine Meadows Healthcare and Rehabilitation Center
700 Nuckolls Rd
Bolivar, TN 38008-1531   731-658-4707
                                           Fax: 731-658-4769
                                           www.pinemeadowshc.com

Larry Shrader, Administrator
Sharon McKeen, Admissions Director
Our goal is to take care of your loved ones. Our professional team
works with skilled hands, is directed by creative minds and is
guided by compassionate hearts. Upon your admission, our interdisciplinary team develops a comprehensive care plan designed
with a goal of meeting not only physical and rehabilitative objectives, but also social and emotional needs. We understand the importance of family and resident involvement and encourage
participation in the development of a plan of care.

7216 Primacy Healthcare and Rehabilitation Center
Kindred Health Care
6025 Primacy Pkwy
Memphis, TN 38119-5763   901-767-1040
                                           800-848-0299
                                           Fax: 901-685-7362

Donnie Dubert, Executive Director
Dr. Mark Hammond, Medical Director
Kristen W., Health and Rehabilitation Center
Upon a resident's admission, our interdisciplinary team develops
a comprehensive care plan with a goal of meeting not only physical and rehabilitative objectives but also social and emotional
needs. We understand the importance of family and resident involvement and encourage participation in the development of a
personalized plan of care.

7217 Ripley Healthcare and Rehabilitation Center
118 Halliburton St
Ripley, TN 38063-2011   731-635-5180
                                           Fax: 731-635-0663
                                           www.ripleyhc.com

Johnny Rea, Executive Director
Brandon Whiteside, Executive Director
Jan Hodge, Admissions Directo
Upon admission, our interdisciplinary team develops a comprehensive care plan to meet not only physical and rehabilitative
goals, but also social and emotional needs. We understand the importance of family and resident involvement and encourage participation in the development of a personalized care plan. Our
goal is to take care of your loved ones.

7218 Shelby Pines Rehabilitation and Healthcare Center
3909 Covington Pike
Memphis, TN 38135-2281   901-377-1011
                                           Fax: 901-377-0032

Rene Tutor, Executive Director
Subacute rehabiltation facility and programs.

7219 Siskin Hospital for Physical Rehabilitation
1 Siskin Plz
Chattanooga, TN 37403-1306   423-634-1200
                                           Fax: 423-634-4538
                                           TTY: 423-634-1201
                                           info@siskinrehab.org
                                           siskinrehab.org

Robert Main, CEO
Lindsay Wyatt, Media Coordinator, Marketing Co
Dedicated exclusively to physical rehabilitation and offers specialized treatment programs in brain injury, amputation, stroke,
spinal cord injury, orthopeadics, and major multiple trauma.

Texas

7220 North Hills Hospital
4401 Booth Calloway Rd
North Richland Hills, TX 76180-7399   817-255-1000
                                           Fax: 817-255-1991
                                           northhillshospital.com

Randy Moresi, CEO
North Hills Hospital's services include a wide range of cardiovascular services, surgical services, emergency services, radiology,
a rehabilitation unit, a senior health center, therapy services, and
women's services.

7221 Valley Regional Medical Center
100 E Alton Gloor Blvd
Brownsville, TX 78526-3328   956-350-7000
                                           Fax: 956-350-7111
                                           valleyregionalmedicalcenter.com

Susan Andrews, CEO
Francisco Javier Del Castillo, MD
Subramaniam Anandasivam, MD
Above all else, we are committed to the care and improvement of
human life. In recognition of this committment, we strive to deliver high quality, cost effective healthcare in the communities
we serve. In persuit of our mission, we recognize and affirm the
unique and intrinsic worth of each individual. We treat all those
we serve with compassion and kindness. We act with absolute
honesty and integrity and fairness in the way we conduct our business and the way we live our lives.

Utah

7222 Crosslands Rehabilitation and Healthcare Center
680 South Fourth Street
Louisville, KY 40202   502-596-7300
                                           800-545-0749
                                           web_administrator@kindred.com
                                           www.kindredhealthcare.com

John Williams, Executive Director
Lyle Black, Manager
Crossroads Rehabilitation and Healthcare accomodates 120 residents. We are fully Medicare and Medicaid certified. We are
proud of our reputation for providing quality, compassionate
care. Services availiable include in-house physical, occupational
and speech therapies, as well as 24-hour licensed nursing staff
coverage. We offer therapeutic recreation, in-house social services and registered dietician services, among many other
professional services.

7223 Federal Heights Rehabilitation and Nursing Center
Kindred Health Care
680 South Fourth Street
Louisville, KY 40202   502-596-7300
                                           800-545-0749
                                           web_administrator@kindred.com
                                           www.kindredhealthcare.com

Pete Zeigler, Executive Director
Dr. Charles Canfield, Medical Director
Federal Heights accomodates 120 residents. We are located near
three major hospitals in the Salt Lake Valley. We specialize in
providing nursing services for complex medical and rehabilitation conditions. Our discharge planning works jointly with the

669

family and resident in determining the future needs and goals upon discharge.

7224   St. George Care and Rehabilitation Center
Kindred Health Care Publications
1032 E 100 S
Saint George, UT 84770-3005   435-628-0488
                                                800-346-4128
                                            Fax: 435-628-7362
                                            www.stgeorgecare.com

John Larson, Plant Manager
Erin Hammon, Director of Nursing
Derrick Glum, Executive Director
St. George Care and Rehabilitation accomodates 95 residents. We offer a 4,000 square foot rehabilitation gym with an indoor therapy pool for inpatient and outpatient services. Therapy is provided to meet specific needs seven days a week. There is a dietitian on staff for individualized nutritional needs. We offer an Alzheimer's unit with specialized staff. We provide compassionate health services including physicians, nurses, physical therapists, and occupational therapist and licensed aides.

7225   St. Mark's Hospital
1200 E 3900 S
Salt Lake City, UT 84124-1390   801-268-7111
                                            Fax: 801-270-3489
                                            www.stmarkshospital.com

Steve B. Bateman, CEO
Above all else we are committed to the care and improvement of human life. In recognition of this commitment, we strive to deliver high quality, cost effective healthcare in the communities we serve. We define quality as 'caring people with the commitment to a continuous process of improvement in the services provided, that will better enable the hospital to meet or exceed our customer's needs and expectations.

7226   Wasatch Valley Rehabilitation
Kindred Healthcare
680 South Fourth Street
Louisville, KY 40202   502-596-7300
                                                800-545-0749
                                    web_administrator@kindred.com
                                            www.kindredhealthcare.com

Alex Stevenson, Executive Director
Ric Toomer, Executive Director
Wasatch Valley accomodates 110 residents. We are licensed for Medicare and Medicaid and we are conveniently located in the heart of Salt Lake City with easy access from I-15 and I-215. We are known by the area hospitals as a specialist in wound care and for the care we provide to those with complex medical conditions.

Virginia

7227   Nansemond Pointe Rehabilitation and Healthcare Center
200 Constance Rd
Suffolk, VA 23434-4960   757-539-8744
                                                800-828-1140
                                            Fax: 757-539-6128
                                            www.nansemondhc.com

Mel Epelle, Executive Director
Mary R, Activities Assistant
Kristen W., Health and Rehabilitation Center
Nansemond Pointe Rehabilitation and Healthcare Center accomodates 160 residents in private and semi-private rooms. We have been serving the needs of Suffolk, Virginia and the surrounding areas for over 38 years. We offer an entire continuum of care from assisted living apartments to skilled nursing to long-term care. Our licensed therapists, working with our dedicated nursing staff, share a common goal- to help our residents improve their level of recovery and independence.

7228   Rehabilitation and Research Center Virginia Commonwealth University
1250 East Marshall Street
Richmond, VA 23298   804-828-9000
                                            Fax: 804-828-5074
                                            www.vcuhealth.org

Michael Rao, Ph.D., VCU President & VCUHS President,
Sheldon M. Retchin, M.D., VP Health Sciences & CEO, VCUHS
John Duval, Chief Executive Officer MCV Hosp
The Rehabilitation and Research Center is a collaborative effort between the Department of Physical Medicine and Rehabilitation and the Medical College of Virginia Hospitals. The goals of the Rehabilitation and Research Center at the Medical College of Virginia Hospitals (MCVH) are to provide highly-skilled, interdisciplinary, inpatient rehabilitative care to adults with complex needs; to be an advocate and educator for patients and people with disabilities.

7229   Warren Memorial Hospital
1000 N Shenandoah Ave
Front Royal, VA 22630-3598   540-636-0300
                                                800-994-6610
                                            Fax: 540-636-0258
                                    complaint@jointcommission.org
                                            www.valleyhealthlink.com

Mark H. Merrill, President & Chief Executive Officer
Tonya Smith, Vice President of Operations
Pete Gallagher, Senior Vice President & CFO
A nonprofit organization of health care providers, Valley Health offers a full spectrum of services in acute care, rehabilitation and extended care facilities, and outpatient and community settings to help the people of the region manage their health and enjoy a high quality of life. Valley Health has the resources to diagnose, treat and help patients manage virtually any medical problem that may be encountered.

7230   Winchester Rehabilitation Center
333 W Cork St
Suite 230
Winchester, VA 22601-3870   540-536-5114
                                                800-994-6610
                                            Fax: 540-536-1122
                                    complaint@jointcommission.org
                                            www.valleyhealthlink.com

Mark H. Merrill, President & Chief Executive Officer
Tonya Smith, Vice President of Operations
Pete Gallagher, Senior Vice President & CFO
Offers the following rehabilitation services: Sub-Acute inpatient rehabilitation, Speech therapy, Physical therapy, Occupational therapy, Disability evaluations. 30-bed inpatient center.

Washington

7231   Aldercrest Health and Rehabilitation Center
21400 72nd Ave W
Edmonds, WA 98026-7702   425-775-1961
                                            Fax: 425-771-0116
                                            www.aldercrestskillednursing.com

Rick Milsow, Administrator
Aldercrest Health & Rehabilitation Center is a leading provider of long-term skilled nursing care and short-term rehabilitation solutions. Our 124 bed facility offers a full continuum of services and care focused around each individual in today's ever-changing healthcare environment.

7232   Arden Rehabilitation and Healthcare Center
16357 Aurora Ave N
Seattle, WA 98133-5651   206-542-3103
                                                800-833-6384
                                            Fax: 206-542-7192
                                            www.ardenrehab.com

Matthew Preston, Administrator
Ann Zell, Executive Director
Kristen W., Health and Rehabilitation Center
Arden Rehabilitation has been an integral part of the Shoreline community since 1953. It is a one-level building set on mature grounds with several beautiful courtyards for the residents to enjoy. Arden can accomodate 90 residents-post acute/rehabilitation

patients as well as long-term residents. Medicare certified, the center also takes most managed healthcare insurance plans, as well as VA, respite and hospice patients.

7233   Bellingham Health Care and Rehabilitation Services
1200 Birchwood Ave
Bellingham, WA 98225-1302   360-734-9295
                                     800-833-6384
                                Fax: 360-671-4368
                        www.avamererehabofbellingham.com
Melissa Nelson, Executive Director
Dr. Richard McClenahan, Medical Director
Kristen W., Health and Rehabilitation Center
At Bellingham Health Care and Rehab, we strive to provide quality, compassionate care. Our cozy building accomodates 84 residents. Our smaller size creates an inviting and homelike environment for your loved one. We offer semi-private rooms with space to add items from home for a special personalized touch. Provides meals served restaurant style in our dinning room overlooking our beautiful grounds.

7234   Bremerton Convalescent and Rehabilitation Center
2701 Clare Ave
Bremerton, WA 98310-3313   360-377-3951
                                Fax: 360-377-5443
                        bremertonskillednursing.com
Stephanie Bonanzino, Administrator
Subacute rehabilitation facility and programs.

7235   Edmonds Rehabilitation & Healthcare Centerer
Kindred Healthcare
21008 76th Ave W
Edmonds, WA 98026-7104   425-778-0107
                                     800-833-6384
                                Fax: 425-776-9532
Jane Davis, Executive Director
At Edmonds Rehabilitation and Healthcare, we strive to provide quality, compassionate care. Our center accomodates 91 residents. Our smaller size creates an inviting and homelike environment. We offer semi-private rooms with space to add items from home for a special personalized touch. Edmonds Rehabilitation and Healthcare provides delicious meals served restaurant style in our dinning room.

7236   Heritage Health and Rehabilitation Center
Kindred Health Care
3605 Y St
Vancouver, WA 98663-2647   360-693-5839
                                     800-833-6384
                                Fax: 360-693-3991
                        www.heritagerehab.com
Michael Moses, Executive Director
Su Patchett, Director of Nursing
Heritage Health & Rehabilitation Center is the smallest free-standing healthcare center in southwest Washington with accomodations of 49, enabling more personal care and a more home-like environment. Heritage has licensed nursing staff, restorative aides, and certified nurses assistants, trained and experienced in providing Alzheimer's care, end of life/hospice care, psychiatric care, rehabilitative care, and respite care.

7237   North Auburn Rehabilitation And Health Center
111 West Michigan Street
Milwaukee, WI 53203-2903   800-395-5000
                                extendicare.com
Allyson Jenkins, Administrator
Subacute rehabilitation facility and programs.

7238   Northwoods Lodge
2321 NW Schold Pl
Silverdale, WA 98383-9504   360-698-3930
                                Fax: 360-692-2169
                        www.encorecommunities.com
Leslie Krueger, Owner
Debbie Griffin, Director of Rehab Services
Silverdale Campus, Executive Director
Provides you with a full-range of services from weekly housekeeping and laudry services, to grounds keeping and maintenance. Our monthy fee inculdes utilities and hot, delicious, nutritious meals served table side every day. We offer transporta-

tion services, full-time activities directors, and numerous amenities to add to your comfort and enjoyment.

7239   Pacific Specialty & Rehabilitation Center r
1015 N Garrison Rd
Vancouver, WA 98664-1313   360-694-7501
                                Fax: 360-694-8148
Rebecca Pruett, Administrator
Subacute rehabilitation facility and programs.

7240   Puget Sound Healthcare Center
4001 Capitol Mall Dr SW
Olympia, WA 98502-8657   360-754-9792
                                Fax: 360-754-2455
                        www.pugetsoundskillednursing.com
Sheila Oberg, Administrator
Our goal is to provide excellence in patient care, veteran's benefits and customer satisfaction. We have reformed our department internally and are striving for high quality, prompt and seamless service to veterans. Our department employees continue to offer their dedication and commitment to help veterans get the services they have earned.

7241   Vancouver Health & Rhabilitation Center
400 E 33rd St
Vancouver, WA 98663-2238   360-696-2561
                                     800-833-6384
                                Fax: 360-696-9275
                        www.vancouverhealthcare.com
Jody Wigen, Human Resources
Joe Joy, Executive Director
Kristen W., Health and Rehabilitation Center
At Vancouver Health and Rehab Center we strive to provide quality, compassionate care. Our cozy building accomodates 98 residents. Our smaller size creates an inviting and homelike environment. We offer semi-private rooms with space to add items from home for a special personalized touch. Provides delicious meals served restaurant style in our dining room.

West Virginia

7242   War Memorial Hospital
1 Healthy Way
Berkeley Springs, WV 25411-1743   304-258-1234
                                Fax: 304-258-5618
                        complaint@jointcommission.org
                        www.valleyhealthlink.com
Mark H. Merrill, President & Chief Executive Officer
Tonya Smith, Vice President of Operations
Pete Gallagher, Senior Vice President & Chief Financial Officer
Offers physical therapy, occupational therapy, speech therapy, social services, and patient/family education for individuals who have experienced a recent physical disability due to disease, dysfunction, or general debilitation. Helps patients to maximize their abilities through activities of daily living, mobility, self-medication, and self-care and restore their ability to return to their previous lifestyle.

Wisconsin

7243   Cedar Spring Health and Rehabilitation Center
N27w5707 Lincoln Blvd
Cedarburg, WI 53012-2852   262-376-7676
                                Fax: 262-376-7808
Mary Wirth, Executive Director
Subacute rehabilitation facility and programs.

7244   Clearview-Brain Injury Center
198 Home Rd
Juneau, WI 53039-1401   920-386-3400
                                     877-386-3400
                                Fax: 920-386-3800
Jane E. Hooper, Administrator
Jacqueline Kuhl, Household Coordinator
Laura Bertagnoli
A 30-bed, state certified, subacute neuro-rehabilitation program in Juneau, WI. We are located just 45 minutes northeast of Madi-

son WI and 10 minutes east of Beaver Dam, WI. We are the first and longest standing of only 2 community re-entry programs in the state of Wisconsin providing subacute neuro-rehabilitation to teens and adults who have experienced a brain injury.

7245 Colonial Manor Medical and Rehabilitation Center
1010 E Wausau Ave
Wausau, WI 54403-3101　　　　715-842-2028
　　　　　　　　　　　　　　800-947-6644
　　　　　　　　　　　　　Fax: 715-848-0510

Ericca Ylitalo, Administrator
Shelley Solberg, Executive Director
Kristen W., Health and Rehabilitation Center
Colonial Manor Medical and Rehabilitation Center is part of the Kindred Community and is located in Wausau, Wisconsin. The corporate headquarters are based in Louisville Kentucky. Our facility accomodates 150 residents.

7246 Eastview Medical and Rehabilitation Center
729 Park St
Antigo, WI 54409-2745　　　　715-623-2356
　　　　　　　　　　　　　　800-947-6644
　　　　　　　　　　　　　Fax: 715-623-6345

Wanda Hose, Administrator
Wanda Hose, Executive Director
Kristen W., Health and Rehabilitation Center
Eastview Medical Center and Rehabilitation Center accomodates 165 residents. We are Medicare and Medicaid certified, as well as being Joint Commission accredited. Our 'TEAM' approach means specially trained staff work around the clock to assist in meeting rehabilitative goals established by our team of professionals. We encourage family involvement in our rehabilitative process. The support of loved ones is a major key to a speedy recovery.

7247 Hospitality Nursing Rehabilitation Center
8633 32nd Ave
Kenosha, WI 53142-5187　　　　262-694-8300
　　　　　　　　　　　　　Fax: 262-694-3622

Marla Benson, Administrator
LaRae Nelson, President
Lisa Behling, Secretary
Subacute rehabilitation facility and programs.

7248 Kennedy Park Medical Rehabilitation Center
Kindred Healthcare
6001 Alderson St
Schofield, WI 54476-3614　　　　715-359-4257
　　　　　　　　　　　　　　800-947-6644
　　　　　　　　　　　　　Fax: 715-355-4867

Judy Kowalski, Manager
Jim Torgerson, Executive Director
Kristen W., Health and Rehabilitation Center
Kennedy Park Medical & Rehabilitation Center accomodates 154 residents. We are located in Schofield, WI. At Kennedy Park, we specialize in dementia care, with our Reflections and Passages Units. Short-term rehabilitation and sub-acute care are provided in a setting conducive to meeting the individual needs of our residents and patients. We also provide general nursing care for persons with long-term care needs.

7249 Middleton Village Nursing & Rehabilitation
Kindred
6201 Elmwood Ave
Middleton, WI 53562-3319　　　　608-831-8300
　　　　　　　　　　　　　　800-947-6644
　　　　　　　　　　　　　Fax: 608-831-4253
　　　　　　　　　　　www.middletonvillage.com

Nicholas Stamatas, Manager
Ashley Ostrowski, Executive Director
Kristen W., Health and Rehabilitation Center
Middleton Village accomodates 97 residents. We specialize in post-surgical and post-acute rehabilitation and long-term care services.

7250 Mount Carmel Health & Rehabilitation Center
5700 W Layton Ave
Milwaukee, WI 53220-4099　　　　414-281-7200
　　　　　　　　　　　　　Fax: 414-281-4620

Mike Berry, Administrator
Darrin Hull, Executive Director
Kristen W., Health and Rehabilitation Center
Subacute rehabilitation facility and programs.

7251 Mount Carmel Medical and Rehabilitation Center
680 South Fourth Street
Louisville, KY 40202　　　　502-596-7300
　　　　　　　　　　　　　800-545-0749
　　　　　　　　web_administrator@kindred.com
　　　　　　　　　　　kindredhealthcare.com

Randy Nitschke, Administrator
Jeanne Piccioni, Executive Director
Mount Carmel Medical and Rehabilitation Center accomodates 155 residents. We are located in Burlington Wisconsin. Mount Carmel Medical and Rehabilitation center is a recipient of the American Health Care Association Quality Award.

7252 North Ridge Medical and Rehabilitation Center
1445 N 7th St
Manitowoc, WI 54220-2011　　　　920-682-0314
　　　　　　　　　　　　　　800-947-6644
　　　　　　　　　　　　　Fax: 920-682-0553

Jane Conway, Interim ED
Mary Ann Hamer, Executive Director
North Ridge Medical and Rehabilation Center accomodates 110 residents. We have been serving the Manitowoc, Wisconsin area for over 25 years. Our goal is to provide services in a warm, homey environment. Many of our staff in all departments have a long history with North Ridge and have worked here for more then 20 years. We also take pride in the fact that we have all in-house staff. Our therapy team is availiable to provide physical, occupational and speech therapy 7 days a week.

7253 Oshkosh Medical and Rehabilitation Center
1580 Bowen St
Oshkosh, WI 54901　　　　920-233-4011
　　　　　　　　　　　Fax: 920-233-5177

Tom Wagner, President
Subacute rehabilitation facility and programs.

7254 San Luis Medical and Rehabilitation Center
680 South Fourth Street
Louisville, KY 40202　　　　502-596-7300
　　　　　　　　　　　　　800-545-0749
　　　　　　　　web_administrator@kindred.com
　　　　　　　　　www.kindredhealthcare.com

Heather Dreier, Administrator
Tim Dietzen, Executive Director
Dr. John T. Warren, Medical Director
San Luis Medical and Rehabilitation Center accomodates 126 residents. We are located in Green bay, WI. At San Luis, we strive to meet the needs of our residents and we specialize in dementia care, with our Reflections Unit. Our goal is to provide short-term rehabilitation and sub-acute care in a setting conducive to assisting the needs of our residents.

7255 Strawberry Lane Nursing & Rehabilitation Center
130 Strawberry Lane
Wisconsin Rapids, WI 54494-2156　　　715-424-1600
　　　　　　　　　　　　　Fax: 715-424-4817

Cyndi Glodoski, Admissions Director
Carrie Russert, Administrator
Skilled nursing facility that provides both long term and short term care. Offer Alzheimer's and Dementia care units, as well as Hospice Care. Medicare and Medicaid certified.

Wyoming

7256 **Mountain Towers Healthcare & Rehabilitation Center**
3128 Boxelder Dr
Cheyenne, WY 82001-5808   307-634-7901
                                           800-877-9975
                                           Fax: 307-634-7910

Dan Stackis, Administrator
Toni Wyenn, Director of Nursing
Daniel G. Stackis, Executive Director
Mountain Towers Healthcare and Rehabilitation Center accomodates 170 residents, including a 16-bed acute secure unit. We offer a full range of nursing and medical care to meet individual needs. We have a full staff to meet the needs of our residents.

7257 **South Central Wyoming Healthcare and Rehabilitation**
Kindred Healthcare
542 16th St
Rawlins, WY 82301-5241   307-324-2759
                                           800-877-9975
                                           Fax: 307-324-7579

Chris Tanner, Executive Director
Anthony Janusz, Administrator
Kristen W., Health and Rehabilitation Center
South Central Wyoming Healthcare and Rehabilitation accomodates 52 residents. We are located in Rawlings, in south central Wyoming. We are Medicare and Medicaid certified by the State of Wyoming. We strive to provide quality personal services, long-term care or short-term rehabilitation to our residents in a comfortable home-like environment.

7258 **Wind River Healthcare and Rehabilitation Center**
Kindred Health Care
1002 Forest Dr
Riverton, WY 82501-2918   307-856-9471
                                           800-877-9975
                                           Fax: 307-856-1665

Jo Ann Aldrich, Executive Director
Amelia Asay, Business Office Manager
Kristen W., Health and Rehabilitation Center
Offers a full range of medical services to meet the individual needs of our residents, including short-term rehabilitative services and long-term skilled care. Working with the residents physician, our staff-including medical specialists, nurses, nutritionists, dietitians and social workers-establishes a comprehensive treatment plan intended to restore you or your loved one to the highest practicable potential.

Aging

Associations

7259 AARP
601 E Street NW
Washington, DC 20049 202-434-3525
888-687-2277
member@aarp.org
www.aarp.org

Jo Ann Jenkins, CEO
Formerly the American Association of Retired Persons. AARP is a collection of diverse individuals and ideas working as one to influence positive change and improve the lives of those 50 and over. AARP reflects a wide range of attitudes, cultures, lifestyles, and beliefs.
1919

7260 AARP Alabama
400 South Union Street
Suite 100
Montgomery, AL 36104 866-542-8167
alaarp@aarp.org
states.aarp.org/region/alabama

Candi Williams, State Director
Lisa Billingsley, Senior Operations Administrator
Provides information, events, news, and resources to Alabamians over 50 years of age, and to a membership of over 430,000.
1920

7261 AARP Alaska
3601 C Street
Suite 1420
Anchorage, AK 99503 866-227-7447
Fax: 907-341-2270
ak@aarp.org
states.aarp.org/region/alaska

Ken Helander, Advocacy Director
Ann Secrest, Media Contact
Serves 95,000 members in Alaska, providing information, resources, news, and advocacy on matters relevant to individuals aged 50 years and older.

7262 AARP Arizona
7250 N 16th Street
Suite 302
Phoenix, AZ 85020 866-389-5649
aarpaz@aarp.org
states.aarp.org/region/arizona
David Parra, Director, Community Outreach
Alex Suarez, Communications Contact
The chapter seeks to enhance the quality of life for all Arizonans, with an emphasis on individuals 50 years and older.

7263 AARP Arkansas
1701 Centerview Drive
Suite 205
Little Rock, AR 72211 866-544-5379
Fax: 501-227-7710
araarp@aarp.org
states.aarp.org/region/arkansas
Charlie Wagener, State President
Seeks to redefine and improve life for Arkansans over the age of 50.

7264 AARP California: Pasadena
200 S Los Robles Avenue
Suite 400
Pasadena, CA 91101- 2422 866-448-3614
Fax: 626-583-8500
caaarp@aarp.org
states.aarp.org/region/california
Nancy McPherson, State Director
Joy Hepp, Media Contact, Southern California
Provides news, tools, resources, and research to Californians 50 years and older.

7265 AARP California: Sacramento
1415 L Street
Suite 960
Sacramento, CA 95814 866-448-3614
Fax: 916-446-2223
caaarp@aarp.org
states.aarp.org/region/california
Nancy McPherson, State President
Mark Beach, Media Contact, Northern California
Provides news, tools, resources, and research to Californians 50 years and older.

7266 AARP Colorado
303 E 17th Avenue
Denver, CO 80203-5012 866-554-5376
Fax: 303-764-5999
coaarp@aarp.org
states.aarp.org/region/colorado
Bob Murphy, State Director
Angela Cortez, Media Contact
The Colorado chapter seeks to keep Coloradans 50 years and older informed, engaged, and active.

7267 AARP Connecticut
21 Oak Street
Suite 104
Hartford, CT 06106 866-295-7279
ctaarp@aarp.org
states.aarp.org/region/connecticut
Nora Duncan, State Director
Anna Doroghazi, Assoc. State Dir., Advocacy & Outreach
With nearly 600,000 members, the chapter provides recent news, information, and events for residents of Connecticut who are 50 years and older, as well as advocating for positive social change.

7268 AARP Delaware
222 Delaware Avenue
Suite 1630
Wilmington, DE 19801 866-227-7441
kiapalucci@aarp.org
states.aarp.org/region/delaware
Lucretia Young, State Director
Kimberly Iapalucci, Media Contact
Provides news, advocacy, education, and lifestyle information for residents of Delaware who are 50 years and older.

7269 AARP Florida: Doral
3750 Nw 87th Avenue
Suite 650
Doral, FL 33178 866-595-7678
Fax: 786-804-4544
flaarp@aarp.org
states.aarp.org/region/florida
Donna L. Ginn, State President
Jeff Johnson, State Director
The chapter provides information, research, and events to 2.7 million members, and Floridians 50 years and older.

7270 AARP Florida: St. Petersburg
360 Central Avenue
Suite 1750
St. Petersburg, FL 33701 866-595-7678
Fax: 727-369-5191
flaarp@aarp.org
states.aarp.org/region/florida
Donna L. Ginn, State President
Jeff Johnson, State Director
The chapter provides information, research, and events to 2.7 million members, and Floridians 50 years and older.

7271 AARP Florida: Tallahassee
200 West College Avenue
Suite 304
Tallahassee, FL 32301 866-595-7678
Fax: 850-222-8968
flaarp@aarp.org
states.aarp.org/region/florida
Donna L. Ginn, State President
Jeff Johnson, State Director
The chapter provides information, research, and events to 2.7 million members, and Floridians 50 years and older.

7272 AARP Georgia
999 Peachtree Street NE
Suite 1110
Atlanta, GA 30309 866-295-7281
Fax: 404-815-7940
gaaarp@aarp.org
states.aarp.org/region/georgia
Debra Tyler-Horton, State Director
Alisa Jackson, Media Contact
The chapter strives to help Georgians 50 years and older.

7273 AARP Hawaii
1132 Bishop Street
Suite 1920
Honolulu, HI 96813 866-295-7282
Fax: 808-537-2288
hiaarp@aarp.org
states.aarp.org/region/hawaii
Jessica Wooley, Director, Advocacy
With 150,000 members, the chapter advocates at the state level,
and provides information, resources, and volunteer opportunities.

7274 AARP Idaho
250 S 5th Street
Suite 800
Boise, ID 83702 866-295-7284
Fax: 208-288-4424
aarpid@aarp.org
states.aarp.org/region/idaho
Lupe Wissel, Idaho AARP State Media Relations
Randy Simon, Media Contact
The chapter advocates for and seeks to improve the lives of resi-
dents aged 50 years and older.

7275 AARP Illinois: Chicago
222 N LaSalle Street
Suite 710
Chicago, IL 60601 866-448-3613
Fax: 312-372-2204
aarpil@aarp.org
states.aarp.org/region/illinois
Bob Gallo, State Director
Dina Anderson, Media Contact
Advocates for and provides recent news, events, and lifestyle tips
to Illinois residents aged 50 years and older.

7276 AARP Illinois: Springfield
300 W Edwards Street
3rd Floor
Springfield, IL 62704 866-448-3613
Fax: 217-522-7803
aarpil@aarp.org
states.aarp.org/region/illinois
Bob Gallo, State Director
Dina Anderson, Media Contact
Legislative office of the Illinois chapter.

7277 AARP Indiana
One N Capitol Avenue
Suite 1275
Indianapolis, IN 46204- 2025 866-448-3618
Fax: 317-423-2211
inaarp@aarp.org
states.aarp.org/region/indiana
Sarah Waddle, State Director
Jason Tomcsi, Media Contact
The chapter seeks to improve life for residents of Indiana aged 50
years and older.

7278 AARP Iowa
600 E Court Avenue
Suite 100
Des Moines, IA 50309 866-554-5378
Fax: 515-244-7767
ia@aarp.org
states.aarp.org/region/iowa
Brad Anderson, State Director
Jeremy Barewin, Media Contact
Provides news, information, and resources to Iowans aged 50
years and older.

7279 AARP Kansas
6220 SW 29th Street
Suite 300
Topeka, KS 66614 866-448-3619
Fax: 785-232-1465
ksaarp@aarp.org
states.aarp.org/region/kansas
Maren Turner, Kansas AARP State Media Relations
Mary Tritsch, Media Contact
The chapter provides news, events, and more to Kansans aged 50
years and older.

7280 AARP Kentucky
10401 Linn Station Road
Suite 121
Louisville, KY 40223 866-295-7275
kyaarp@aarp.org
states.aarp.org/region/kentucky
Scott Wagenast, Associate State Director
Provides news and resources for Kentuckians over the age of 50.

7281 AARP Louisiana: Baton Rouge
301 Main Street
Suite 1012
Baton Rouge, LA 70825 866-448-3620
la@aarp.org
states.aarp.org/region/louisiana
Denise Bottcher, State Director
Andrew Muhl, Director, Advocacy
The office seeks to advocate for and provide resources to resi-
dents of Louisiana aged 50 and over.

7282 AARP Louisiana: New Orleans
3502 S Carrollton Avenue
Suite C
New Orleans, LA 70118 866-448-3620
la@aarp.org
states.aarp.org/region/louisiana
Denise Bottcher, State Director
Andrew Muhl, Director, Advocacy
AARP Louisiana's Community Resource Center.

7283 AARP Maine
53 Baxter Boulevard
Suite 202
Portland, ME 04101 866-554-5380
me@aarp.org
states.aarp.org/region/maine
Lori Parham, State Director
Amy Gallant, Director, Advocacy and Outreach
Seeks to enhance the lives of Mainers aged 50 years and over
through advocacy, information sharing, volunteer opportunities,
and service. The chapter counts 230,000 members.

7284 AARP Maryland
200 St. Paul Place
Suite 2510
Baltimore, MD 21202 866-542-8163
Fax: 410-837-0269
md@aarp.org
states.aarp.org/region/maryland
Jim Campbell, State President
Nancy Carr, Assoc. State Director, Communications
The chapter seeks to enhance the lives of Maryland residents aged
50 and over, as well as caregivers, through resources and a variety
of social opportunities.

7285 AARP Massachusetts
1 Beacon Street
Suite 2301
Boston, MA 02108 866-448-3621
Fax: 617-723-4224
ma@aarp.org
states.aarp.org/region/massachusetts
Mike Festa, State Director
Cindy Campbell, Director, Communications
Provides news, events, and resources to Massachusetts residents
aged 50 and over.

7286 AARP Michigan
309 N Washington Square
Suite 110
Lansing, MI 48933   866-227-7448
Fax: 517-482-2794
miaarp@aarp.org
states.aarp.org/region/michigan
Paula D. Cunningham, State Director
The chapter seeks to enhance the quality of life for aging residents of Michigan through information, advocacy, and services.

7287 AARP Minnesota
1919 University Avenue
Suite 500
St. Paul, MN 55104   866-554-5381
aarpmn@aarp.org
states.aarp.org/region/minnesota
Will Phillips, State Director
Maro Jo George, Associate State Director, Advocacy
Aims to connect aging residents of Minnesota with financial and other resources to enhance quality of life.

7288 AARP Mississippi
141 Township Avenue
Suite 302
Ridgeland, MS 39157   866-554-5382
Fax: 601-898-5429
msaarp@aarp.org
states.aarp.org/region/mississippi
John McDonald, AARP Missouri State Director
Ronda Gooden, Media Contact
Seeks to improve the lives of Mississippians, particularly those over 50 years of age, through events, news, resources, and advocacy.

7289 AARP Missouri
9200 Ward Parkway
Suite 350
Kansas City, MO 64114   866-389-5627
Fax: 816-561-3107
aarpmo@aarp.org
states.aarp.org/region/missouri
Craig Eichelman, State Director
Jamayla Long, Media Contact
Provides information to Missourians aged 50 and over on health, finances, and lifestyle, as well as providing advocacy.

7290 AARP Montana
30 W 14th Street
Suite 301
Helena, MT 59601   866-295-7278
mtaarp@aarp.org
states.aarp.org/region/montana
Tim Summers, State Director
Stacia Dahl, Media Contact
With 150,000 members, the chapter provides advocacy, education, information, resources, and collaborative projects for Montana residents aged 50 and over.

7291 AARP Nebraska: Lincoln
301 S 13th Street
Suite 201
Lincoln, NE 68508   866-389-5651
Fax: 402-323-6908
neaarp@aarp.org
states.aarp.org/region/nebraska
Connie Benjamin, AARP Nebraska State President
Devorah Lanner, Media Contact
Works on behalf of over 200,000 members and their families to provide news, services, information, resources, and advocacy for individuals 50 years and older.

7292 AARP Nebraska: Omaha
1941 S 42nd Street
Suite 220
Omaha, NE 68105   402-398-9568
omnebraska@aol.com
states.aarp.org/region/nebraska
Connie Benjamin, AARP Nebraska State President
Devorah Lanner, Media Contact
AARP Nebraska's Information Center.

7293 AARP Nevada
5820 S Eastern Avenue
Suite 190
Las Vegas, NV 89119   866-389-5652
aarpnv@aarp.org
states.aarp.org/region/nevada
Maria Dent, State Director
Scott Gulbransen, Media Contact
Provides news, information, and resources to 320,000 members, on matters affecting the lives of individuals aged 50 and over.

7294 AARP New Hampshire
45 South Main Street
Suite 202
Concord, NH 03301   866-542-8168
Fax: 603-224-6211
nh@aarp.org
states.aarp.org/region/new-hampshire
Todd Fahey, State Director
Doug McNutt, Associate State Director, Advocacy
Provides information, resources, and advocacy services to 228,000 members, on matters relevant to individuals aged 50 years and older.

7295 AARP New Jersey
303 George Street
Suite 505
New Brunswick, NJ 08901   866-542-8165
Fax: 609-987-4634
aarpnJ@aarp.org
states.aarp.org/region/new-jersey
Stephanie Hunsinger, State Director
Jeff Abramo, Media Contact
The chapter seeks to educate and advocate for New Jersey residents aged 50 and over, and their families.

7296 AARP New Mexico
535 Cerrillos Road
Suite A
Santa Fe, NM 87501   866-389-5636
Fax: 505-820-2889
aarpnm@aarp.org
states.aarp.org/region/new-mexico
Jennifer Baier, Interim State Director
DeAnza Valencia, Associate State Director, Advocacy
The chapter advocates on behalf of individuals 50 years and older, monitoring seniors' services, utility rates, transportation services, as well as providing financial planning services to members.

7297 AARP New York: Albany
1 Commerce Plaza
Suite 706
Albany, NY 12260   866-227-7442
nyaarp@aarp.org
states.aarp.org/region/new-york
Beth Finkel, State President
Erik Kriss, Media Contact
Provides information, resources, news, and advocacy services to residents of New York who are 50 years and older.

7298 AARP New York: New York City
750 Third Avenue
31st Floor
New York, NY 10017   866-227-7442
nyaarp@aarp.org
states.aarp.org/region/new-york
Beth Finkel, State President
Erik Kriss, Media Contact
Provides information, resources, news, and advocacy services to residents of New York who are 50 years and older.

7299 AARP New York: Rochester
435 E Henrietta Road
Rochester, NY 14620   866-227-7442
nyaarp@aarp.org
states.aarp.org/region/new-york
Beth Finkel, State President
Erik Kriss, Media Contact
Provides information, resources, news, and advocacy services to residents of New York who are 50 years and older.

7300 AARP North Carolina
5511 Capital Center Drive
Suite 400
Raleigh, NC 27606 866-389-5650
ddickerson@aarp.org
states.aarp.org/region/north-carolina
Doug Dickerson, State Director
Michael Oldender, Manager, Outreach and Advocacy
Advocates for community issues such as health care, employment/income security, retirement planning, utilities, and protection from financial abuse, on behalf of a membership 1.1 million strong.

7301 AARP North Dakota
107 W Main Avenue
Suite 125
Bismarck, ND 58501 866-554-5383
Fax: 701-255-2242
aarpnd@aarp.org
states.aarp.org/region/north-dakota
Josh Askvig, State Director
Doreen Redman, Assoc. State Dir., Community Outreach
Provides news, information, resources, events, advocacy, and more to North Dakotans aged 50 and over.

7302 AARP Ohio
17 S High Street
Suite 800
Columbus, OH 43215 866-389-5653
Fax: 614-224-9801
ohaarp@aarp.org
states.aarp.org/region/ohio
Barbara Sykes, State Director
The chapter shares information, advocates, and performs community services for 1.5 million members, 50 years and older, across the state.

7303 AARP Oklahoma
126 N Bryant Avenue
Edmond, OK 73034 866-295-7277
Fax: 405-844-7772
ok@aarp.org
states.aarp.org/region/oklahoma
Sean Voskuhl, State Director
Chad Mullen, Associate State Director, Advocacy
Assists individuals aged 50 and over through advocacy, news, information, resources, and more.

7304 AARP Oregon
9200 SE Sunnybrook Boulevard
Suite 410
Clackamas, OR 97015 866-554-5360
oraarp@aarp.org
states.aarp.org/region/oregon
Ruby Haughton-Pitts, State Director
Joyce DeMonnin, Media Contact
Strives for social change for its 500,000 members, and all individuals 50 years and over, through advocacy and community services.

7305 AARP Pennsylvania: Harrisburg
30 N 3rd Street
Suite 750
Harrisburg, PA 17101 866-389-5654
Fax: 717-236-4078
aarpa@aarp.org
states.aarp.org/region/pennsylvania
Bill Johnston-Walsh, State Director
Steve Gardner, Media Contact
Seeks to enhance the quality of life for 1.8 million members across the state.
1919

7306 AARP Pennsylvania: Philadelphia
1650 Market Street
Suite 675
Philadelphia, PA 19103 866-389-5654
Fax: 215-665-8529
aarpa@aarp.org
states.aarp.org/region/pennsylvania
Bill Johnston-Walsh, State Director
Steve Gardner, Media Contact
Seeks to enhance the quality of life for 1.8 million members across the state.

7307 AARP Rhode Island
10 Orms Street
Suite 200
Providence, RI 02904 866-542-8170
Fax: 401-272-0596
ri@aarp.org
states.aarp.org/region/rhode-island
Kathleen Connell, State Director
John Martin, Director, Communications
Provides news, information, resources, advocacy, and community services to those aged 50 and older in the state.

7308 AARP South Carolina
1201 Main Street
Suite 1720
Columbia, SC 29201 803-765-7381
866-389-5655
scaarp@aarp.org
states.aarp.org/region/south-carolina
Teresa Arnold, State Director
Nikki Hutchison, Associate State Director, Advocacy
Seeks to enhance the quality of life for members and individuals aged 50 and older, through information, resources, education, advocacy, and more.

7309 AARP South Dakota
5101 S Nevada Avenue
Suite 150
Sioux Falls, SD 57108 866-542-8172
sdaarp@aarp.org
states.aarp.org/region/south-dakota
Erik Gaikowski, State Director
Provides news, information, resources, advocacy, and community services to 110,000 members and those aged 50 and older in the state.

7310 AARP Tennessee
150 4th Avenue N
Suite 1350
Nashville, TN 37219 866-295-7274
tnaarp@aarp.org
states.aarp.org/region/tennessee
Rebecca Kelly, State Director
Rob Naylor, Director, Communications
Strives for positive social change for 660,000 members and individuals aged 50 and over.

7311 AARP Texas: Austin
1905 Aldrich Street
Suite 210
Austin, TX 78723 866-227-7443
states.aarp.org/region/texas
Bob Jackson, State Director
Junita Jiminez-Soto, Associate State Director, Communications
The chapter offers news, information, research, and events for individuals aged 50 and over, as well as conducting advocacy on their behalf.

7312 AARP Texas: Dallas
8140 Walnut Hill Lane
Suite 108
Dallas, TX 75231 866-227-7443
states.aarp.org/region/texas
Bob Jackson, State Director
Junita Jiminez-Soto, Associate State Director, Communications
The chapter offers news, information, research, and events for individuals aged 50 and over, as well as conducting advocacy on their behalf.

7313 AARP Texas: Houston
2323 S Shepherd Drive
Suite 1100
Houston, TX 77019 866-227-7443
states.aarp.org/region/texas

Bob Jackson, State Director
Junita Jiminez-Soto, Associate State Director, Communications
The chapter offers news, information, research, and events for individuals aged 50 and over, as well as conducting advocacy on their behalf.

7314 AARP Texas: San Antonio
1314 Guadalupe Street
Suite 209
San Antonio, TX 78207 866-227-7443
states.aarp.org/region/texas

Bob Jackson, State Director
Junita Jiminez-Soto, Associate State Director, Communications
The chapter offers news, information, research, and events for individuals aged 50 and over, as well as conducting advocacy on their behalf.

7315 AARP Utah
6975 Union Park Center
Suite 320
Midvale, UT 84047 866-448-3616
Fax: 801-561-2209
utaarp@aarp.org
states.aarp.org/region/utah

Alan Ormsby, State Director
Danny Harris, Director, Advocacy
Serves 211,000 members in 10 regions across the state, with advocacy, communications, programming, and outreach.

7316 AARP Vermont
199 Main Street
Suite 225
Burlington, VT 05401 866-227-7451
Fax: 802-651-9805
vtaarp@aarp.org
states.aarp.org/region/vermont

Greg Marchildon, State Director
Seeks to represent the concerns and interests of Vermonters aged 50 and over.

7317 AARP Virginia
707 E Main Street
Suite 910
Richmond, VA 23219 866-542-8164
Fax: 804-819-1923
vaaarp@aarp.org
states.aarp.org/region/virginia

Jim Dau, State Director
Serves Virginians aged 50 and older, and their families, through advocacy, information, resources, and outreach.

7318 AARP Washington
18000 International Blvd.
Suite 1020
SeaTac, WA 98188 866-227-7457
Fax: 206-517-9350
waaarp@aarp.org
states.aarp.org/region/washington

Doug Shadel, State Director
Serves 950,000 members through information, advocacy, and a variety of services.

7319 AARP Washington DC
100 M Street SE
Suite 650
Washington, DC 20003 866-554-5384
Fax: 202-434-7946
dcaarp@aarp.org
states.aarp.org/region/washington-dc

Louis Davis, Jr., State Director
Peter Rankin, Associate State Director, Advocacy
Provides information, advocacy, and a variety of services to 87,000 members aged 50 and over.

7320 AARP West Virginia
300 Summers Street
Suite 400
Charleston, WV 25301 866-227-7458
Fax: 304-344-4633
wvaarp@aarp.org
states.aarp.org/region/west-virginia

Gaylene Miller, State Director
Tom Hunter, Associate State Director, Communications
Provides information, resources, advocacy, and more to individuals aged 50 and over in West Virginia.

7321 AARP Wisconsin
222 W Washington Avenue
Suite 600
Madison, WI 53703 866-448-3611
Fax: 608-251-7612
wistate@aarp.org
states.aarp.org/region/wisconsin

Sam Wilson, State Director
Jim Flaherty, Media Contact
The chapter advocates for, and provides a variety of services to, its 840,000 members, aged 50 years and over.

7322 AARP Wyoming
2020 Carey Avenue
Mezzanine
Cheyenne, WY 82009 866-663-3290
wyaarp@aarp.org
states.aarp.org/region/wyoming

Sam Shumway, State Director
Tom Lacock, Assoc. State Dir., Advocacy & Comm.
Provides resources, information, and advocates for indviduals in Wyoming aged 50 and older, with an emphasis on health care, retirement, and utility issues.

7323 ABA Commission on Law and Aging
1050 Connecticut Avenue
Suite 400
Washington, DC 20003 202-662-8690
Fax: 202-662-8698
aging@americanbar.org
www.americanbar.org/aging

Charles P. Sabatino, JD, Director
Erica F. Wood, JD, Assistant Director
The Commission examines the issues that affect the elderly as victims of abuse, dispute resolution, international rights, medicare, voting, health care decision-making and other issues arising from the aging prisons populations.

7324 ACL Regional Support Center: Region I
Administration for Community Living
John F. Kennedy Building
Room 2075
Boston, MA 02203 617-565-1158
Fax: 617-565-4511
www.acl.gov

Jennifer Throwe, Regional Administrator
Region I includes CT, MA, ME, NH, RI, and VT.

7325 ACL Regional Support Center: Region II
Administration for Community Living
26 Federal Plaza
Room 38-102
New York, NY 10278 212-264-2976
Fax: 212-264-0114
www.acl.gov

Rhonda Schwartz, Regional Administrator
Region II includes NY, NJ, PR, and VI.

7326 ACL Regional Support Center: Region III
Administration for Community Living
801 Market St.
Philadelphia, PA 19107 267-831-2329
www.acl.gov

Laura House, Regional Administrator
Region III includes DC, DE, MD, PA, VA, and WV.

7327   **ACL Regional Support Center: Region IV**
Administration for Community Living
Atlanta Federal Center
61 Forsyth St. SW, Suite 5M69
Atlanta, GA 30303-8909   404-562-7600
                                     Fax: 404-562-7598
                                          www.acl.gov

Costas Miskis, Regional Administrator
Region IV includes AL, FL, GA, KY, MS, NC, SC, and TN.

7328   **ACL Regional Support Center: Region IX**
Administration for Community Living
90 7th St.
T-1800
San Francisco, CA 94103   415-437-8780
                                     Fax: 415-437-8782
                                          www.acl.gov

Fay Gordon, Regional Administrator
Region IX includes CA, NV, AZ, HI, GU, CNMI, and AS.

7329   **ACL Regional Support Center: Region V**
Administration for Community Living
233 N Michigan Ave.
Suite 790
Chicago, IL 60601-5527   312-938-9858
                                     Fax: 312-886-8533
                                          www.acl.gov

Amy Wiatr-Rodriguez, Regional Administrator
Region V includes IL, IN, MI, MN, OH, and WI.

7330   **ACL Regional Support Center: Region VI**
Administration for Community Living
1301 Young St.
Suite 106-850
Dallas, TX 75201   214-767-1865
                                     Fax: 214-767-2951
                                          www.acl.gov

Derek Lee, Regional Administrator
Region VI includes AR, LA, OK, NM, and TX.

7331   **ACL Regional Support Center: Region VII**
Administration for Community Living
601 E 12th St.
Suite S-1801
Kansas City, MO 64106   816-702-4180
                                          www.acl.gov

Lacey Boven, Regional Administrator
Region VII includes IA, KS, MO, and NE.

7332   **ACL Regional Support Center: Region VIII**
Administration for Community Living
1961 Stout St.
Denver, CO 80294-3638   303-844-2951
                                     Fax: 303-844-2943
                                          www.acl.gov

Percy Devine, Regional Administrator
Region VIII includes CO, MT, UT, WY, ND, and SD.

7333   **ACL Regional Support Center: Region X**
Administration for Community Living
701 Fifth Ave., M/S RX-33
Suite 1600
Seattle, WA 98104   206-615-2299
                                     Fax: 206-615-2305
                                          www.acl.gov

Louise Ryan, Regional Administrator
Region X includes AK, ID, OR, and WA.

7334   **AMDA - The Society for Post-Acute andLong-Term Care Medicine**
10500 Little Patuxent Parkway
Suite 210
Columbia, MD 21044   410-740-9743
                                          800-876-2632
                                     Fax: 410-740-4572
                                          info@paltc.org

Arif Nazir, MD, FACP, CMD, President
Karl Steinberg, MD, HMCD, Vice President
The only medical specialty society representing the community of over 50,000 medical directors, physicians, nurse practitioners, physician assistants, and other practitioners working in the various post-acute and long-term care (PA/LTC) settings.
1919

7335   **Academy for Gerontology in HigherEducation**
1220 L Street NW
Suite 901
Washington, DC 20005   202-289-9806
                                   membership@geron.org
                                          www.aghe.org

Judith L. Howe, President
Lisa Hollis-Sawyer, Treasurer
Membership organization comprised of more than 130 colleges and universities that offer education and research program in the field of aging. Affiliated with the Gerontological Society of America.
1919

7336   **Aging Life Care Association**
3275 W Ina Road
Suite 130
Tucson, AZ 85741-2198   520-881-8008
                                     Fax: 520-325-7925
                                  info@aginglifecare.org
                                   www.aginglifecare.org

Julie Wagner, Interim CEO
Amanda Mizell, Member Relations
Julie Wagner, Director of Administration
A nonprofit association providing geriatric care for aging individuals through sharing of knowledge in 8 areas: health and disability, financial matters, housing, planning, local resources, advocacy, legal and crisis intervention.

7337   **Aging Services of Michigan**
201 North Washington Square
Suite 920
Lansing, MI 48933   517-323-3687
                                     Fax: 517-323-4569
                                    www.leadingagemi.org

David Herbel, President & CEO
Deanna Mitchell, Senior Vice President for Performance & Education
Aging Services of Michigan represents and supports organizations that provide services to the elderly and disabled adults. Types of supports offered by Aging Services include advocacy, education and other programs that enhance an organization's ability to serve their constituencies.

7338   **Aging Services of South Carolina**
2711 Middleburg Dr
Suite 309-A
Columbia, SC 29204   803-988-0005
                                     Fax: 803-988-1017
                                    www.leadingagesc.org

Frazier Jackson, Chair
Vickie Moody, President
Aging Services of South Carolina represents non-profit organizations dedicated to providing high-quality health care, housing and services to the seniors of South Carolina. Supports include public policy initiatives and education.

7339   **Aging Services of Washington**
1102 Broadway
Suite 201
Tacoma, WA 98402   253-964-8870
                                     Fax: 253-964-8876
                                  info@leadingagewa.org
                                      leadingagewa.org

Jay Woolford, Chair
Deb Murphy, CEO
Laura Hofmann, Director, Clinical & Nursing Facility Services
LeadingAge Washington is a state association supporting non-profit organizations that specialize in housing and long term care for the elderly. Supports offered include advocacy, education and more.

7340 Aging and Disability Services
2100 Washington Blvd
4th Floor
Arlington, VA 22204
703-228-1700
TTY: 703-228-1788
arlaaa@arlingtonva.us
aging-disability.arlingtonva.us
Anita Friedman, Director, Department of Human Services
The Aging and Disability Services Division offers care coordination, home care, and supportive services to the aging residents of Arlington. Services are provided to adults over 60, adults with developmental disabilities and their caregivers.

7341 Aging in America
2975 Westchester Ave
Suite 301
Purchase, NY 10577
914-205-5030
Fax: 718-824-4242
contact@aginginamerica.org
aginginamerica.org
Katharine Weiss, Chair
William T Smith, President & CEO
Dina Nejman, Service Coordinator
Non-profit organization providing services for individuals and caregivers to assist them with the challenges of aging. One strategy employed towards this goal is collaboration with other organizations with experience in senior housing and community based services.

7342 AgingCare

www.agingcare.com
An online resource for aiding family caregivers. AgingCare.com covers questions on assisted living, long-term and home care, veterans benefits, Alzheimer's disease, financial aid, funeral planning, and more.

7343 Alliance for Aging Research
1700 K Street NW
Suite 740
Washington, DC 20006
202-293-2856
info@agingresearch.org
www.agingresearch.org
Sue Peschin, President & CEO
Sue Peschin, President & CEO
Non-profit organization dedicated to supporting and accelerating the pace of medical discoveries to vastly improve the universal human experience of aging and health.

7344 Alliance for Retired Americans
815 16th Street NW
4th Floor
Washington, DC 20006
202-637-5399
retiredamericans.org
Robert Roach, Jr., President
Joseph Peters, Jr., Secretary & Treasurer
Joe Etta Brown, Executive Vice President
National grassroots organization advocates for a progressive political and social agenda that improves the lives of retirees and older Americans.
1920

7345 American Aging Association
2885 Sanford Ave SW
Suite 39542
Grandville, MI 49418
contact@americanagingassociation.org
www.americanagingassociation.org
Janko Nikolich-Zugich, Chair & CEO
Christian Sell, President
Dudley Lamming, Secretary
A group of experts dedicated to understanding the basic mechanisms of aging and the development of interventions in age-related diseases to increase human lifespans. This is accomplished through biomedical aging studies and public education.

7346 American Association for GeriatricPsychiatry
6728 Old McLean Village Drive
McLean, VA 22101
703-556-9222
Fax: 703-556-8729
main@aagponline.org
www.aagponline.org
Christopher Wood, Executive Director
Information and resources for physician members and affiliates on improving quality of life for older persons with mental disorders. Provides news, facts, tools and expert information for adults coping with mental health issues and aging.
1919

7347 American Association of Retired Persons
601 E Street NW
Washington, DC 20049
202-434-3525
888-687-2277
888-687-2277
member@aarp.org
www.aarp.org
Jo Ann Jenkins, Chief Executive Officer
Scott Frisch, Executive Vice-President and COO
Cindy Lewin, Executive Vice President & General Counsel
AARP is the nation's leading organization for people age 50 and older. It serves their needs and interests through information and education, advocacy and community services provided by a network of local chapters and experienced volunteers.

7348 American Disabled for Attendant Programs Today (ADAPT)
4513 Tyson Ave.
Philadelphia, PA 19135
adapt.org
National organization fighting for the rights of disabled people through non-violent activism tactics and advocacy.

7349 American Geriatrics Society
40 Fulton Street
18th Floor
New York, NY 10038
212-308-1414
Fax: 212-832-8646
info.amger@americangeriatrics.org
www.americangeriatrics.org
Nancy E. Lundebjerg, CEO
Elvy Ickowicz, Senior Vice President of Operations
The premier professional organization of healthcare providers dedicated to improving the health and well-being of older adults. With an active membership of over 6,000 health care professionals, the AGS has a long history of affecting change in the provision of healthcare in older adults. The AGS Foundation for Health in Aging (FHA) aims to build a bridge between the research and practice of geriatrics health care professionals and the public.
1919

7350 American Planning Association
205 N Michigan Ave
Suite 1200
Chicago, IL 60601
312-431-9100
Fax: 312-786-6700
foundation@planning.org
www.planning.org/ontheradar/aging/
Mary Kay Peck, FAICP, Chair
James Drinan, CEO
Ann Simms, Chief Operating Officer
An association supporting planners to develop communities that would be more livable for aging people. The association offers membership, a knowledge center, publications, conferences and meetings, certification, policy and advocacy services, community outreach and more.

7351 American Public Health Association
800 I St. NW
Washington, DC 20001
202-777-2742
Fax: 202-777-2534
TTY: 202-777-2500
www.apha.org
Georges C. Benjamin, Executive Director
James Carbo, Chief of Staff
Regina Davis Moss, Associate Executive Director
The association works to protect all Americans and their communities from preventable, serious health threats.

7352 American Society for Neurochemistry
9037 Ron Den Lane
Windermere, FL 34786
407-909-9064
Fax: 407-876-0750
asnmanager@asneurochem.org
asneurochem.org

Sheilah Jewart, Executive Director
Karen Gottlieb, Conference Coordinator
The Society aims to advance and promote cellular and molecular neuroscience knowledge, and to facilitate communication and the dissemination of information within the field and with related disciplines.

7353 American Society on Aging
575 Market Street
Suite 2100
San Francisco, CA 94105
415-974-9600
800-537-9728
Fax: 415-974-0300
info@asaging.org
www.asaging.org

Peter Kaldes, President & CEO
Robert R. Lowe, COO
Robert R Lowe, Chief Operating Officer
Health care and social service professionals, educators, researchers, administrators, businesspersons, students, and senior citizens. Works to enhance the well-being of older individuals and to foster unity among those working with and for the elderly. Offers 25 continuing education programs for professionals in aging-related fields. Publishes 'Aging Today,' a bi-monthly newspaper, and 'Generations, a quarterly journal.
1919

7354 American Urogynecologic Society
1100 Wayne Avenue
Suite 825
Silver Spring, MD 20910
301-273-0570
Fax: 301-273-0778
info@augs.org
www.augs.org

Michelle Zinnert, CEO
Colleen Hughes, COO
The leader in female pelvic medicine and reconstructive surgery.
1919

7355 Argentum
1650 King Street
Suite 602
Alexandria, VA 22314
703-894-1805
www.alfa.org

James Balda, President & CEO
Maribeth Bersani, COO
Argentum is the leading national association exclusively dedicated to supporting companies operating professionally managed, resident-centered senior living communities and the older adults and families they serve.
1919

7356 Arizona Center on Aging
1501 N Campbell
PO Box 245027
Tucson, AZ 85724
520-626-5800
Fax: 520-626-5801
info@aging.arizona.edu
www.aging.arizona.edu

Mindy Fain, MD, Co-Director
Janko Nikolich-Zugish, MD, Co-Director
The mission at Arizona Center of Aging (ACOA) is to promote healthy and functional lives for older adults through comprehensive programs in research, education and training, and clinical care.

7357 Association for Adult Development and Aging
5999 Stevenson Avenue
Alexandria, VA 22304
www.aadaweb.org
Amber Randolph, President
A division of the American Counseling Association. Individuals holding a master's degree or its equivalent in adult counseling or a related field. Seeks to: improve the competence and skills of ACA and AADA members; expand professional work opportunities in adult development and aging counseling; promote the development of guidelines for professional preparation of counselors. Provides leadership and information to families, legislators, and communities.
1919

7358 Association for Gerontology in Higher Education
1220 L St NW
Suite 901
Washington, DC 20005
202-289-9806
Fax: 202-289-9824
geron@geron.org
www.aghe.org

Nina M Silverstein, President
Judith L Howe, President-Elect
Dana B Bradley, Treasurer
Membership association of colleges and universities offering gerontology education, training, and research programs on the subject of aging. The association seeks to enhance the knowledge and skills of those who work with older adults and their families.

7359 Association of Jewish Aging Services
2519 Connecticut Ave NW
Washington, DC 20008
202-543-7500
Fax: 202-543-4090
info@ajas.org
www.ajas.org

Daniel Reingold, Chair
Don Shulman, President & CEO
Rachel Stevens, Director of Operations
The Association of Jewish Aging Services is a non-profit community-based organization offering support services for the aging population. Inspired by Jewish values, the organization offers resources, conferences, education, professional development and advocacy to its members so they could better serve their communities.

7360 Association on Aging with Developmental Disabilities
2385 Hampton Ave.
St. Louis, MO 63139
314-647-8100
Fax: 314-647-8105
agingwithdd@msn.com
agingwithdd.org

Pamela Merkle, Executive Director
Michelle Darden, Program Development Coordinator
Erika Donaldson, Department Director
The organization offers services to accommodate the complex needs of older adults with developmental disabilities such as cerebral palsy, epilepsy, autism, severe learning disabilities and head injuries.

7361 BrightFocus Foundation
22512 Gateway Center Drive
Clarksburg, MD 20871
800-437-2423
Fax: 301-258-9454
info@brightfocus.org
www.brightfocus.org

Stacy Pagos Haller, President & CEO
Offers updated and trustworthy information on research, treatments, and resources. Free publications and newsletters.
1919

7362 Brookdale Center for Healthy Aging
2180 Third Avenue
8th Floor
New York, NY 10035
212-396-7835
Fax: 212-396-7852
info@brookdale.org
www.brookdale.org

Ruth K. Finkelstein, Executive Director
Jerry Antonatos, Director, Finance/Administration
Brookdale Center for Healthy Aging is one of the country's first university-based gerontology centers. The Center is dedicated to improving the lives of older adults through research, professional development, and advancements in policy and practice. Brookdale works to ensure that aging is framed not as a disease, but as another stage in the life course.
1919

7363 CARF International
6951 East Southpoint Rd.
Tucson, AZ 85756-9407   520-325-1044
                              888-281-6531
                         Fax: 520-318-1129
                         TTY: 520-495-7077
                              info@carf.org
                              carf.org

Brian J. Boon, President & Chief Executive Officer
Leslie Ellis-Lang, Managing Director, Child & Youth Services
Darren M. Lehrfeld, Chief Accreditation Officer
An independent, nonprofit accreditor of human service providers in the areas of aging services, behavioral health, child and youth services, DMEPOS, employment and community services, medical rehabilitation, and opioid treatment programs.
1966

7364 Center for Benefits Access
National Council on Aging
251 18th Street S
Suite 500
Arlington, VA 22202   571-527-3900
                    centerforbenefits@ncoa.org
                    www.ncoa.org/centerforbenefits

Leslie Fried, Director
Benefits outreach and enrollment for seniors and younger adults with disabilities.
1919

7365 Center for Healthy Aging
National Council on Aging
251 18th Street S
Suite 500
Arlington, VA 22202   571-527-3900
                              cha@ncoa.org
                              www.ncoa.org

Binod Suwal, Senior Program Manager
Helping older adults live longer and healthier lives through evidence-based health promotion and disease prevention programs.
1919

7366 Center for Medicare Advocacy
PO Box 350
Willimantic, CT 06226   860-456-7790
                          Fax: 860-456-2614
               mshepard@medicareadvocacy.org
                    www.medicareadvocacy.org

Judith A. Stein, Executive Director
Matthew Shepard, Media Contact
Offers consultation, training, presentation, and materials on an array of topics pertaining to aging.
1919

7367 Center for Positive Aging
1440 Dutch Valley Place NE
Suite 120
Atlanta, GA 30324   404-872-9191
                       Fax: 404-872-1737
               www.centerforpositiveaging.org

Ginny Helms, President & CEO
Jacque Thornton, SVP
Jacque Thornton, Sr. Vice President
The Center for Positive Aging is a partnership of individuals, community organizations and congregations working together to provide health, educational and recreational opportunities for older persons and their families. Through our programs, services, and affiliations, we educate people of all ages and walks of life about living independent and creative lives.
1919

7368 Children of Aging Parents
PO Box 167
Richboro, PA 18954-0167   800-227-7294
                             Fax: 215-945-8720

Louise Fradkin, Co-Founder
Mirca Liberti, Co-Founder
A non-profit clearinghouse for caregivers of the elderly, providing information, referral, educational programs and materials to caregivers.

7369 Colorado Association of Homes and Services for the Aging
1888 Sherman St
Suite 610
Denver, CO 80203   303-837-8834
                      Fax: 303-837-8836
                      Karen@CAHSA.org
                      www.cahsa.org

Maureen Hewitt, President
Lynn O'Connor, President-Elect
Laura Landwirth, Executive Director
The association represents nonprofit organizations dedicated to providing health care and housing services to Colorado's elderly. Some services provided by the association include information and education to assist in developing programs for long term care.

7370 Easter Seals
40 Holly St.
Suite 401
Toronto, ON, Canada M4S-3C3   416-932-8382
                                     877-376-6362
                                Fax: 416-932-9844
                                info@easterseals.ca
                                www.easterseals.ca

Dave Starrett, President & CEO
Frank Williamson, Director, Finance
Casey Sabawi, Senior Manager, National Corporate Partnerships
Provides services to those with disabilities to help them achieve greater independence, accessibility, and integration.
1919

7371 Experience Works
4401 Wilson Boulevard
Suite 220
Arlington, VA 22203   703-522-7272
                             866-397-9757
                         www.experienceworks.org

Sally A. Boofer, President & CEO
Rosemary Schmidt, CFO
Helps low income seniors with multiple barriers to employment, get the training they need to find good jobs in their local community.
1919

7372 Family Caregiver Alliance/National Centeron Caregiving
101 Montgomery Street
Suite 2150
San Francisco, CA 94104   415-434-3388
                                 800-445-8106
                              www.caregiver.org

Jacquelyn Kung, PhD, Chief Executive Officer
Wyatt Ritchie, MBA, Managing Director
Caregiver information and assistance via phone or e-mail; fact sheets and publications describing and documenting caregiver needs and services.

7373 Gerontological Society of America
1220 L Street NW
Suite 901
Washington, DC 20005   202-842-1275
                          Fax: 202-842-1150
                              geron@geron.org
                              www.geron.org

James Appleby, Chief Executive Officer
Karen Tracy, VP, Strategic Alliances & Communications
Nonprofit professional organization with more than 5,500 members in the field of aging. Provides researchers, educators, practitioners and policy makers with opportunities to understand, advance, integrate and use basic and applied research on aging populations. Also runs the National Adult Vaccination Program (www.navp.org).

7374 Goodwill Industries International, Inc.
15810 Indianola Dr.
Rockville, MD 20855   contactus@goodwill.org
                            www.goodwill.org

Steven C. Preston, President & Chief Executive Officer
Goodwill strives to achieve the full participation in society of disabled persons and other individuals with special needs by expanding their opportunities and occupational capabilities

through a network of autonomous, nonprofit, community-based organizations providing services throughout the world in response to local needs.

7375 Goodwill Industries-Suncoast
10596 Gandy Boulevard
St. Petersburg, FL 33702   727-523-1512
                                  888-279-1988
                             Fax: 727-579-0850
                             TTY: 727-579-1068
                          www.goodwill-suncoast.org
Deborah A. Passerini, President & Chief Executive Officer
Tracey Boucher, Corporate Treasurer & Chief Financial Officer
Kris Rawson, Vice President for Mission Services & Chief Mission Officer
A nonprofit, community-based organization whose mission is to help people achieve self-sufficiency through the dignity and power of work, serving people who are disadvantaged, disabled or elderly. The mission is accomplished through providing independent living skills, affordable housing, and training and placement in community employment.
1919

7376 Harvey A. Friedman Center for Aging
Washington University
St. Louis, Campus Box 8217
660 S Euclid
St. Louis, MO 63110   314-747-9212
                          centerforaging@wustl.edu
                          publichealth.wustl.edu/aging
Nancy Morrow-Howell, PhD, Director
Natalie Galucia, Center Manager
The Center promotes research, education, policy and service initiatives that enable older adults to remain healthy, active, empowered, contributing and independent for as long as possible.
1919

7377 Healthy Aging Association
3500 Coffee Rd
Suite 19
Modesto, CA 95355   209-523-2800
                      Fax: 209-523-2800
                    healthy.aging2000@gmail.com
                    www.healthyagingassociation.org
Mike Mallory, Board President
Dianna L Olsen, Executive Director
Samantha Borba, MA, Fitness Program Manager
A non-profit organization whose mission is to help older Americans live longer, healthier, more independent lives by promoting increased physical activity through fitness programs.

7378 Heart Touch Project™
3400 Airport Avenue
Suite 42
Santa Monica, CA 90405   310-391-2558
                           Fax: 310-391-2168
                           www.hearttouch.org
Shawnee Isaac Smith, Co-Founder
Rene Russo, Co-Founder
Non-profit, educational and service organization devoted to the delivery of compassionate and healing touch to home or hospital-bound men, women, and children.
1919

7379 Institute for Life Course and Aging
246 Bloor Street W.
Room 238
Toronto, Ontario, Canada M5S-1V4   416-978-0377
                                      Fax: 416-978-4771
                                      aging@utoronto.ca
                                    www.grandparentfamily.com
Esme Fuller-Thomson, Director
Susan Murphy, Administration
The Institute is a research center under the auspices of the Faculty of Social Work at the University of Toronto.

7380 International Federation on Aging
1 Bridgepoint Drive
Toronto, Ontario, Canada M4M-2B5   416-342-1655
                                      Fax: 416-639-2165
                                      jbarratt@ifa-fiv.org
                                      www.ifa-fiv.org
Greg Shaw, Director, Int'l & Corporate Relations
Dr. Jane Barratt, Secretary General
The IFA seeks to inform, educate and promote policies and practice to improve the quality of life of older persons around the world.
1919

7381 International Network for the Preventionof Elder Abuse
The Somers Law Firm
PO Box 368
Nassau, NY 12123   518-281-2777
                      contactus@inpea.net
                      www.inpea.net
Susan B. Somers, President
Amanda Phelan, Secretary
Organization for the prevention of elder abuse.
1919

7382 Jewish Council for the Aging
12320 Parklawn Drive
Rockville, MD 20852   301-255-4200
                        senior.helpline@accessjca.org
                        www.accessjca.org
Norman Goldstein, President
Seeks to assist the elderly of all faiths lead independent lives. Provides transportation, job search assistance, fitness training, computer training and information and referrals. Conducts educational programs and presents an annual productive aging award. Maintains speakers' bureau.
1919

7383 Jewish Council for the Aging of Greater Washington
12320 Parklawn Drive
Rockville, MD 20852   301-255-4200
                        senior.helpline@accessjca.org
                        www.accessjca.org
Norman Goldstein, President
Seeks to assist the elderly of all faiths lead independent lives. Provides transportation, job search assistance, fitness training, computer training and information and referrals. Conducts educational programs and presents an annual productive aging award. Maintains speakers' bureau.
1919

7384 Justice in Aging
1444 Eye St NW
Suite 1100
Washington, DC 20005   202-289-6976
                          Fax: 202-289-7224
                          info@justiceinaging.org
                          www.justiceinaging.org
Phyllis J Holmen, Esq., Chair
Kevin Prindiville, Executive Director
Jennifer Goldberg, Directing Attorney
Justice in Aging is a non-profit legal organization whose principal mission is to protect the rights of low-income older adults and vulnerable groups in society. Through advocacy, litigation, and training of local advocates, Justice in Aging seeks to ensure the health and economic security of those they serve.

7385 Leadership Council of Aging Organizations
                          lcao@aarp.org
                          www.lcao.org
Coalition of national non-profit organizations concerned with the well-being of older Americans.

7386 Leading Age
2519 Connecticut Avenue NW
Washington, DC 20008-1520   202-783-2242
                              info@LeadingAge.org
                              www.leadingage.org
Katie Smith Sloan, President & CEO
Nicole Fallon, Vice President, Health Policy

National association of more than 6,000 nonprofit nursing homes, continuing care retirement communities, independent living centers and community service providers serving more than 60,000 older Americans each year.

7387 LeadingAge
2519 Connecticut Avenue NW
Washington, DC 20008   202-783-2242
info@leadingage.org
www.leadingage.org
Lea Chambers-Johnson, Executive Team Administrator
Robyn I Stone, Senior Vice President, Research
The work of LeadingAge is focused on advocacy, leadership development, and applied research and promotion of effective services, home health, hospice, community services, senior housing, continuing care communities, nursing homes, as well as technology solutions to seniors and thers with special needs.
1919

7388 LeadingAge Arizona
3877 N 7th St
Suite 240
Phoenix, AZ 85014   602-230-0026
Fax: 602-230-0563
pkoester@leadingageaz.org
www.arizonaleadingage.org
Steven Kolnacki, President
Pam Koester, CEO
Donald G Isaacson, Lobbyist
LeadingAge Arizona is a non-profit association representing organizations that provide health care, housing and services to the elderly citizens of Arizona. The association supports these organizations by offering them leadership, education and advocacy services.

7389 LeadingAge California
1315 I Street
Suite 100
Sacramento, CA 95814   916-392-5111
Fax: 916-428-4250
info@leadingageca.org
Kathryn Roberts, Chair
Jeannee Parker Martin, President & CEO
Jan Guiliano, Vice President of Education
LeadingAge California advocates for non-profit organizations that provide health care, housing and community services to older adults. Services offered by LeadingAge include advocacy, public education and advertising.

7390 LeadingAge Connecticut
110 Barnes Rd
Wallingford, CT 06492   203-678-4477
Fax: 203-678-4650
leadingagect@leadingagect.org
www.leadingagect.org
William Fiocchetta, Chair
Mag Morelli, President
Nurka Carrero, Office Manager
LeadingAge Connecticut is a provider of support services to non-profit organizations serving elderly and chronically ill individuals. Supports include advocacy and information provided to members of skilled nursing facilities, intermediate care facilities, residential care homes, chronic disease hospitals, adult day centers, senior housing communities and more.

7391 LeadingAge Gulf States
P.O. Box 1748
Marrero, LA 70073   504-442-0483
Fax: 504-689-3982
kcontrenchis@leadingagegulfstates.org
www.leadingagegulfstates.org
Dennis Adams, Chair
Karen Contrenchis, NFA, CASP, President
Scott Crabtree, Vice Chair
Organization offering educational and advocacy supports to long term care organizations working in the areas of senior housing, nursing homes, adult day care, assisted living, retirement communities, Alzheimer programs and home and community based services.

7392 LeadingAge Illinois
1001 Warrenville Rd
Suite 150
Lisle, IL 60532   630-325-6170
Fax: 630-325-0749
info@leadingageil.org
Deb Reardanz, Chair
Karen Messer, President & CEO
Angela Schnepf, Executive Vice President
LeadingAge Illinois represents organizations specializing in the field of senior care services, offering them advocacy, networking, public policy and employment resources to help them thrive in their missions.

7393 LeadingAge Indiana
PO Box 68829
Indianapolis, IN 46268-0829   317-733-2380
Fax: 317-733-2385
mrinebold@leadingageindiana.org
www.leadingageindiana.org
Mike Rinebold, President
Susan Darwent, Vice President of Operations
Kathy Johnson, RN, WCC, Vice President of Clinical & Regulatory Services
LeadingAge Indiana is an association representing non-profit organizations that provide health care, services and housing for seniors throughout Indiana. LeadingAge offers education, advocacy and networking opportunities to their members.

7394 LeadingAge Iowa
4200 University Ave
Suite 305
West Des Moines, IA 50266   515-440-4630
888-440-4630
Fax: 515-440-4631
info@leadingageiowa.org
www.leadingageiowa.org
Bert Vigen, Chair
Shannon Strickler, President & CEO
Matt Blake, Director, Government Relations & Member Services
LeadingAge Iowa serves non-profit and missiondriven organizations dedicated to providing quality housing, health, community, and related services to Iowa's seniors. Supports provided include advocacy, education and collaboration.

7395 LeadingAge Kentucky
2501 Nelson Miller Pkwy
Suite 101
Louisville, KY 40223   502-992-4380
Fax: 502-992-4390
info@leadingageky.org
leadingageky.org
Timothy Veno, President & CEO
LeadingAge Kentucky represents non-profit organizations that offer services for the elderly and the disabled. LeadingAge offers advocacy and educational services and resources to their members.

7396 LeadingAge Maine & New Hampshire
55 Main St
Suite 316
Newmarket, NH 03857   603-292-6441
lhenderson@leadingagemenh.org
www.leadingagemenh.org
Rebecca Smith, Chair
Deb Riddell, Vice Chair
Lisa Henderson, Executive Director
LeadingAge Maine & New Hampshire aims to promote the interests of its non-profit members which provide healthy, affordable and ethical long-term care to the older citizens of Maine and New Hampshire. LeadingAge offers this support through education, advocacy, representation and collaboration.

7397 LeadingAge Massachusetts
246 Walnut St
Suite 203
Newton, MA 02460   617-244-2999
                                     Fax: 617-244-2995
                                     www.leadingagema.org

Jered Stewart, Chairperson
Elissa Sherman, President
Lynn Monaghan, Events & Education Manager
LeadingAge Massachusetts represents non-profit providers of
health care, housing, and services for seniors in Massachusetts.
Some services offered by LeadingAge include education and
events, webinars, networking opportunities, technology re-
sources, advocacy and consumer resources.

7398 LeadingAge Missouri
3412 Knipp Dr
Suite 102
Jefferson City, MO 65109   573-635-6244
                                     Fax: 573-635-6618
                         debbiecheshire@leadingagemissouri.org
                                 www.leadingagemissouri.org

Chris Crouch, Chair
Bill Bates, CEO
Nancie McAnaugh, Chief Operating Officer
LeadingAge Missouri's work is dedicated to assisting its members to be leaders in the delivery of quality long-term health care,
housing, and services for older adults in Missouri. Some services
provided by LeadingAge include advocacy, public education,
consumer resources and more.

7399 LeadingAge Nebraska
900 N 90th St
Suite 940
Omaha, NE 68114   402-326-2790
                                     www.leadingagene.org

Julie Sebastian, Board Chair
Jeremy Hohlen, CEO
Cheryl Wichman, Director of Professional Development
LeadingAge Nebraska represents the full continuum of mis-
sion-driven, non-profit providers of health care, housing and ser-
vices for older adults in Nebraska. Some supports offered by
LeadingAge include educational conferences, webinars, work-
shops and advocacy.

7400 LeadingAge New Jersey
3705 Quakerbridge Rd
Suite 102
Hamilton, NJ 08619   609-452-1161
                                     Fax: 609-452-2907
                                     www.leadingagenj.org

Toni Lynn Davis, Chairperson
Michele M Kent, President & CEO
Diane Borgstrom, Finance Coordinator
LeadingAge New Jersey represents non-profit nursing homes, assisted living residences, residential health care centers, independent senior housing, and continuing care retirement
communities throughout New Jersey. Members are supported
through advocacy, education, and fellowship.

7401 LeadingAge New York
13 British American Blvd
Suite 2
Latham, NY 12110-1431   518-867-8383
                                     Fax: 518-867-8384
                                     info@leadingageny.org
                                     www.leadingageny.org

James W Clyne, President & CEO
Daniel J Heim, Executive Vice President
Ellen Quinn, SPHR, Vice President of Human Resources
LeadingAge New York represents non-profit, mission-driven and
public continuing care providers, including nursing homes, senior housing, adult care facilities, continuing care retirement
communities, assisted living and community service providers.
LeadingAge provides its members with education, publications,
conferences and consultation services to help them better serve
their communities.

7402 LeadingAge North Carolina
222 N Person St
Raleigh, NC 27601   919-571-8333
                                     Fax: 919-571-1297
                                     info@leadingagenc.org
                                     www.leadingagenc.org

Robert Wernet, Chair
Tom Akins, President & CEO
Leslie Roseboro, Vice President
LeadingAge North Carolina represents non-profit providers of
care, housing, health, community and related services to the elderly. One of its primary goals is to advance policies, practices
and research to empower the aging population.

7403 LeadingAge Ohio
2233 N Bank Dr
Columbus, OH 43220   614-444-2882
                                     Fax: 614-444-2974
                                     info@leadingageohio.org
                                     www.leadingageohio.org

Judy Budi, Chair
Kenneth Daniel, Vice Chair
Kathryn Brod, President & CEO
LeadingAge Ohio represents long-term care organizations. Service providers supported include those working in the fields of
senior housing, adult day care, home- and community-based services, assisted living and nursing. Some supports offered by
LeadingAge Ohio include policy advocacy, education, employment support and resources for families.

7404 LeadingAge Oklahoma
P.O. Box 1383
El Reno, OK 73036   405-640-8040
                                     inquiry@leadingageok.org
                                     leadingageok.org

Lindsay Fick, President
Mary Brinkley, Executive Director
Mark Gray, Public Policy Congress
LeadingAge Oklahoma represents non-profit organizations that
serve the aging people of Oklahoma. LeadingAge assists these organizations through advocacy, consumer services, directories,
education, a job bank and more.

7405 LeadingAge Oregon
7340 SW Hunziker
Suite 104
Tigard, OR 97223   503-684-3788
                                     Fax: 503-624-0870
                                     info@leadingageoregon.org
                                     www.leadingageoregon.org

Greg Franks, President
Ruth Gulyas, MHA, CEO
Margaret Cervenka, Deputy Director
LeadingAge Oregon represents non-profits that provide housing,
health care, community and related services to the elderly and
disabled of Oregon. LeadingAge offers its members advocacy,
networking events and education to help them succeed in their
missions.

7406 LeadingAge PA
1100 Bent Creek Blvd
Mechanicsburg, PA 17050   717-763-5724
                                         800-545-2270
                                     Fax: 717-763-1057
                                     info@leadingagepa.org
                                     www.leadingagepa.org

Susan Drabic, Chair
Ronald Barth, President & CEO
Heidie Dolan, Office Manager & Executive Assistant
LeadingAge PA's mission is to promote the interests of its members through education, advocacy, community forums and
events. Member organizations include adult day care services, assisted living residences, home care services, skilled nursing facilities and other non-profits that serve the aging population of
Pennsylvania.

7407 LeadingAge RI
1 Virginia Ave
Providence, RI 02905 401-490-7612
Fax: 401-490-7614
TTY: 401-383-6578
info@leadingageri.org
www.leadingageri.org

Sandra Cullen, President
Stephanie Igoe, Vice President
James Nyberg, MPA, Director
LeadingAge RI seeks to advance excellence in the field of aging services by fostering innovation, collaboration, and ethical leadership through advocacy for public policy, education and professional development.

7408 LeadingAge Texas
2205 Hancock Dr
Austin, TX 78756 512-467-2242
Fax: 512-467-2275
info@leadingagetexas.org
www.leadingagetexas.org

Roque Christensen, Chair
George Linial, President & CEO
Melanie Harrison, Director of Education
LeadingAge Texas provides leadership, advocacy, and education for non-profit retirement housing and nursing home communities that serve the needs of Texas retirees.

7409 LeadingAge Wisconsin
204 S Hamilton St
Madison, WI 53703 608-255-7060
Fax: 608-255-7064
info@leadingagewi.org
www.leadingagewi.org

Fran Petrick, Chair
John Sauer, President & CEO
Jim Williams, Director of Member Enrichment
LeadingAge Wisconsin is committed to advancing the fields of long-term care, assisted living and retirement living. Towards this purpose, LeadingAge offers advocacy, education and collaborative strategies to its members so they could better serve aging people.

7410 LeadingAge Wyoming
2005 Warren Ave
Cheyenne, WY 82001 307-632-9344
Fax: 307-632-9347
eric@wyohospitals.com
www.leadingagewyoming.org
LeadingAge Wyoming represents non-profit organizations dedicated to providing long-term care and assisted living services to Wyoming's elderly. LeadingAge works to develop policies and practices and offer education so their members can thrive in their missions.

7411 Legal Council for Health Justice
17 N State Street
Suite 900
Chicago, IL 60602 312-427-8990
Fax: 312-427-8419
legalcouncil.org

Tom Yates, Executive Director
Ruth Edwards, Senior Director, Program Services
Provides legal advice and services for persons who are HIV positive or have AIDS, as well as their families. Also serves individuals with disabilities and chronic illnesses, senior citizens, and the homeless.
1919

7412 LifeSpan Network
10280 Old Columbia Rd
Suite 220
Columbia, MD 21044 410-381-1176
Fax: 410-381-0240
www.lifespan-network.org

Dennis Hunter, Chair
Kevin Heffner, President
Danna Kauffman, Public Policy Consultant
Senior care provider representing more than 330 senior care provider organizations in Maryland and the District of Columbia. Lifespan members include non-profit and proprietary independent living, assisted living, continuing care retirement communities, nursing facilities, subsidized senior housing and community and hospital based services. LifeSpan provides education, advocacy, products and services to its members.

7413 Medicare Rights Center: New York
266 W 37th Street
3rd Floor
New York, NY 10018 212-869-3850
Fax: 212-869-3532
info@medicarerights.org
www.medicarerights.org

Frederic Riccardi, President
Seeks to ensure the rights of senior citizens and people with disabilities to quality, affordable health care. Provides counseling services to Medicare beneficiaries with health insurance problems and questions; compiles information on inquiries to detect issues and systemic problems in Medicare claims administration. Educates beneficiaries, advocates, providers, and social workers about developments in Medicare law and how to handle problems.
1919

7414 Medicare Rights Center: Washington, DC
1444 I Street NW
Suite 1105
Washington, DC 20005 202-637-0961
Fax: 202-637-0962
info@medicarerights.org
www.medicarerights.org

Frederic Riccardi, President
A consumer service organization that works to ensure access to affordable health care for older adults and peoplw tih disabilities through counseling and advocacy, educational programs, and public policy intiatives.
1919

7415 National Adult Day Services Association
11350 Random Hills Road
Suite 800
Fairfax, VA 22030 877-745-1440
info@nadsa.org
www.nadsa.org

Donna Hale, Executive Director
Lance Roberts, Associate Director, Membership
Aims to be the leading voice of the Adult Day Services industry, representing providers, associations of providers, corporations, educators, students, and retired workers.

7416 National Alliance for Caregiving
1730 Rhode Island Avenue NW
Suite 812
Washington, DC 20036 202-918-1013
Fax: 202-918-1014
info@caregiving.org
www.caregiving.org

C. Grace Whiting, President & CEO
Coalition of organizations focused on improving the lives of family caregivers.
1919

7417 National Asian Pacific Center on Aging
1511 3rd Avenue
Suite 914
Seattle, WA 98101 206-624-1221
Fax: 206-624-1023
napca.org

Joon Bang, President & CEO
Tina Masuda-Draughon, CFO
Advocating for the specific needs of aging Asian Americans and Pacific Islanders.
1919

7418 National Association for Home Care and Hospice
228 Seventh St, SE
Washington, DC 20003 202-547-7424
Fax: 202-547-3540
www.nahc.org

Denise Schrader, Chair
Val J Halamandaris, President
Lucy Andrews, Vice Chair

Professional association representing the interests of chronically ill, disabled, and dying Americans and their caregivers. The association offers advocacy services on policy, resources related to hospice and home care, research sponsorships, education for the public on hospice services and more.

7419 National Association of Area Agencies on Aging
1730 Rhode Island Ave, NW
Suite 1200
Washington, DC 20036
202-872-0888
Fax: 202-872-0057
info@n4a.org
www.n4a.org

Kathryn Boles, President
Doug McKenzie, Chief, Finance & Administration
Martin Kleffner, Director of Operations
The National Association of Area Agencies on Aging (n4a) is the leading voice on aging issues for Area Agencies on Aging and a champion for Title VI Native American aging programs. n4a provides advocacy, training and technical assistance, employment support and information resources to these agencies.

7420 National Association of Counties
660 N Capitol St NW
Suite 400
Washington, DC 20001
202-393-6226
888-407-6226
Fax: 202-393-2630
nacomeetings@naco.org
www.naco.org

Bryan Desloge, President
Matthew Chase, Executive Director
Deborah Stoutamire, Director of Operations
NACO brings together elected officials and aging administrators who are interested in providing quality programs and better policies for their older constituents. NACO members work with Congress, the Administration on Aging, and other federal agencies to ensure that the nation maintains an effective and efficient safety net of services for the elderly and their families.

7421 National Association of Nutrition and Aging Services Programs (NANASP)
1612 K St NW
Suite 200
Washington, DC 20006
202-682-6899
Fax: 202-223-2099
pcarlson@nanasp.org
www.nanasp.org

Tony Sarmiento, Chair
Robert Blancato, Executive Director
Pam Carlson, Membership & Education
A national membership organization supporting those working to provide older adults with healthy food and nutrition through community-based services. NANASP engages in advocacy on issues such as nutrition, Medicare and Medicaid, elder justice, social security and other retirement security, transportation, and older workers' issues.

7422 National Association of States United for Aging and Disabilities
1201 15th St NW
Suite 350
Washington, DC 20005
202-898-2578
Fax: 202-898-2583
info@nasuad.org
www.nasuad.org

Gary Jessee, President
Martha Roherty, Executive Director
Camille Dobson, Deputy Executive Director
The National Association of States United for Aging and Disabilities (NASUAD) represents the nation's agencies serving in the areas of aging and disabilitie. NASUAD supports state leadership as well as national policies that support home and community based services for seniors and individuals with disabilities.

7423 National Center on Elder Abuse
Administration for Community Living
c/o USC Keck School of Medicine
1000 South Fremont Ave., Unit 22
Alhambra, CA 91803
855-500-3537
Fax: 626-470-9978
ncea-info@aoa.hhs.gov
www.ncea.acl.gov
The NCEA is a national resource center providing up-to-date information on elder abuse, neglect and exploitation to policy makers and the public.
1919

7424 National Clearinghouse on Abuse in Later Life
1400 E Washington Avenue
Suite 227
Madison, WI 53703
608-255-0539
Fax: 608-255-3560
ncall@wcadv.org
www.ncall.us

Bonnie Brandl, Director
Working to end abuse in later life.
1919

7425 National Committee to Preserve SocialSecurity & Medicare
111 K Street NE
Suite 700
Washington, DC 20002
202-216-0420
800-966-1935
Fax: 202-216-0446
webmaster@ncpssm.org
www.ncpssm.org

Max Richtman, President & CEO
An advocacy and education membership organization, works to protect and enhance Federal programs vital to senior's health and economic well-being.
1919

7426 National Council for Aging Care
1200 G Street NW
Washington, DC 20005
877-664-6140
www.aging.com
Seeks to provide older adults with information and resources on health & well-being, caregiving, money and financial planning, and lifestyle, through their Aging.com website.

7427 National Council on Aging
251 18th Street S
Suite 500
Arlington, VA 22202
571-527-3900
membership@ncoa.org
www.ncoa.org

James Knickman, Interim President & CEO
Kristin Kiefer, Cheif Administrative Officer
Donna Whitt, Senior Vice President & Chief Financial Officer
Emphasizes the needs for in-home and community-based health care and social services designed to help older persons remain in or return to their homes and live independently, works to educate and assist voluntary organizations to help develop such services.
1919

7428 National Falls Prevention Resource Center
Center for Healthy Aging
251 18th Street S
Suite 500
Arlington, VA 22202
571-527-3900
www.ncoa.org
Supporting the implementation and dissemination of evidence-based falls prevention programs and strategies across the nation.

7429 National Gerontological Nursing Association
121 W State St
Geneva, IL 60134
630-748-4616
ngna@affinity-strategies.com
www.ngna.org

Joanne Alderman, President
Sandra Kuebler, Treasurer
Elizabeth Tanner, Secretary

An association providing clinical care for older adults. Their member organizations include clinicians, educators, and researchers specializing in different areas of senior care services.

7430   National Hispanic Council on Aging
734 15th St NW
Suite 1050
Washington, DC 20005

202-347-9733
Fax: 202-347-9735
nhcoa@nhcoa.org
www.nhcoa.org

Octavio Martinez, Ph.D, Chair
Yanira Cruz, Ph.D, President & CEO
Maria Eugenia Hernandez-Lane, Vice President
The National Hispanic Council on Aging (NHCOA) works to improve quality of life for Hispanic seniors. With a Hispanic Aging Network of community-based organizations across the U.S., the District of Columbia and Puerto Rico, NHCOA aims to provide public education and adovocacy in areas such as economic security, health, and housing.

7431   National Hospice & Palliative CareOrganization (NHPCO)
1731 King Street
Suite 100
Alexandria, VA 22314

703-837-1500
800-646-6460
Fax: 703-837-1233
www.nhpco.org

Edo Banach, JD, President & CEO
Hannah Yang Moore, MPH, Chief Advocacy Officer
The organization seeks to improve end-of-life care, widen access to hospice care, and improve quality of life for the dying and their loved ones.
1919

7432   National Indian Council on Aging, Inc.
8500 Menaul Blvd. NE
Suite B470
Albuquerque, NM 87112

505-292-2001
Fax: 505-292-1922
info@nicoa.org
www.nicoa.org

Randella Bluehoose, Executive Director
A non-profit organization was founded by members of the National Tribal Chairmen's Association that called for a national organization to advocate for improved, comprehensive health and social services to American Indian and Alaska Native Elders.

7433   National Institute of Senior Centers
National Council on Aging
251 18th Street S
Suite 500
Arlington, VA 22202

571-527-3900
www.ncoa.org

Supporting the nation's senior centers.
1919

7434   National Institute on Aging
31 Center Dr., MSC 2292
Building 31, Room 5C27
Bethesda, MD 20892

800-222-2225
TTY: 800-222-4225
niaic@nia.nih.gov
www.nia.nih.gov

Richard J. Hodes, Director
Lisa Mascone, Deputy Director, Management
Luigi Ferrucci, Scientific Director
Seeks to understand the nature of aging, and to extend healthy, active years of life. Free resources are available on topics such as Alzheimer's & dementia, caregiving, cognitive heath, end of life care, and more.

7435   National Institutes of Health
9000 Rockville Pike
Bethesda, MD 20892

301-496-4000
nihinfo@od.nih.gov
www.nih.gov

Francis S. Collins, Director
The nation's medical research agency.
1918

7436   National Older Worker Career Center
3811 N Fairfax Drive
Suite 900
Arlington, VA 22203

703-558-4200
www.nowcc.org

Cito Vanegas, President & CEO
National non-profit promoting experienced workers as staffing options to government agencies.
1919

7437   National Resource Center on Nutrition & Aging
Meals on Wheels America
1550 Crystal Drive
Suite 1004
Arlington, VA 22202

703-548-5558
Fax: 703-548-8024
nutritionandaging.org

Ucheoma Akobundu, Director, Nutrition Strategy
Sharron Corle, Director, Learning & Development
Promoting better nutrition and active healthy aging.
1920

7438   National Senior Citizens Law Center:Oakland
1330 Broadway
Suite 525
Oakland, CA 94612

510-663-1055
www.justiceinaging.org

Kevin Prindiville, Executive Director
Advocates nationwide to promote the independence and well-being of low-income elderly individuals, as well as persons with disabilities, with particular emphais on women and racial and ethnic minorities. Advocates through litigation and agency representation and assistance to attotneys and paralegals in field programs.

7439   National Senior Citizens Law Center: Los Angeles
3660 Wilshire Boulevard
Suite 718
Los Angeles, CA 90010

213-639-0930
www.justiceinaging.org

Kevin Prindiville, Executive Director
Legal services support center specializing in the legal problems of the elderly poor. Acts as advocate on behalf of elderly, poor clients in litigation and administrative affairs. Sponsors conferences and workshops on areas of the law affecting the elderly. See Legal Resources chapter for specific state resorces.

7440   National Senior Corps Association
PO Box 360
Farmington, UT 84025

928-523-6585
sgrove@jfsmetrowest.org
www.nscatogether.org

Erin Kruse, President
Stephanie Grove, Membership Director
Provides service for aging adults.
1919

7441   National Seniors Council
1100 North Glebe Road
Suite 1010
Arlington, VA 22201

571-425-4153
nationalseniorscouncil.org

Carole Rhodes, National Director
The council seeks to serve the needs of the new generation of retirees, as an alternative to organizations such as the AARP.

7442   Office for American Indian, Alaskan Native and Native Hawaiian Elders
Administration for Community Living
330 C St. SW
Washington, DC 20201

202-401-4634
800-677-1116
olderindians@acl.hhs.gov
olderindians.acl.gov/about

Cynthia LaCounte, Director
Administers the Title VI program by overseeing Title VI funding to programs that provide nutrition, support, and caregiver support services for Native Americans. The Office operates a website that provides technical assistance resources to Title VI directors and serves as a forum for communication between Title VI programs.

7443 Points of Light: Atlanta
600 Means Street
Suite 210
Atlanta, GA 30318
404-979-2900
Fax: 404-979-2901
info@pointsoflight.org
www.pointsoflight.org

Natalye Paquin, President & CEO
Robert E. Herrera, CFO
Mobilizing people to take action on the causes they care about.

7444 Points of Light: Washington, DC
1400 G Street NW
Washington, DC 20005
404-979-2900
Fax: 404-979-2901
info@pointsoflight.org
www.pointsoflight.org

Natalye Paquin, President & CEO
Robert E. Herrera, CFO
Mobilizing people to take action on the causes they care about.

7445 Quality Improvement Organizations
qioprogram.org

Coalition of 28 organizations working to make nursing homes better places to live, work and visit.
1920

7446 Senior Resource LLC
questions@seniorresource.com
www.seniorresource.com
The company operates Seniorresource.com, which provides information to older adults on needed facilities and services, including through internet directories and an archive of E-zines.
1995 pages

7447 Senior Service America
8403 Colesville Rd
Suite 200
Silver Spring, MD 20910
301-578-8900
Fax: 301-578-8947
contact@ssa-i.org
www.seniorserviceamerica.org

Spence Limbocker, Chair
Gary A Officer, Executive Director
Donna Satterthwaite, Director, Workforce Development
Senior Service America offers employment programs for seniors in America.

7448 Society for Neuroscience
1121 14th Street NW
Suite 1010
Washginton, DC 20005
202-962-4000
marty@sfn.org
sfn.org

Marty Saggese, Executive Director
Melissa Garcia, Associate Executive Director
Large international organization of scientists and physicians devoted to the study of the brain and the nervous system.
1919

7449 Tennessee Hospital Association
5201 Virginia Way
Brentwood, TN 37027
615-256-8240
Fax: 615-242-4803
yjames@tha.com
tha.com

Alan Watson, Chairman
Craig Becker, President & CEO
Mary Layne Van Cleave, Executive Vice President & Chief Operating Officer
The Tennessee Hospital Association provides education and information to its members in the health care field so that organizations may serve their constituencies more effectively. The association also offers professional development programs in the areas of insurance, administration and operations, project management, financial services and human resources.

7450 The Gerontological Society of America
1220 L St NW
Suite 901
Washington, DC 20005
202-842-1275
geron@geron.org
www.geron.org

Barbara Resnick, PhD, CRNP, President
James Appleby, Executive Director & CEO
Patricia M D'Antonio, Senior Director, Professional Affairs & Membership
The organization seeks to advance the study of aging by supporting gerontology research. This is accomplished through encouraging communication among professionals, promoting research publications, expanding gerontology education programs and more.

7451 US Administration on Aging
330 C St. SW
Washington, DC 20201
202-401-4634
aclinfo@acl.hhs.gov
acl.gov/about-acl/administration-aging
Edwin Walker, Deputy Assistant Secretary for Aging
The Administration on Aging, an agency in the US Department of Health and Human Services, and under the Administration for Community Living, provides home and community-based care for older persons and their caregivers.

7452 Unbound
1 Elmwood Avenue
Kansas City, KS 66103
913-384-6500
800-875-6564
mail@unbound.org
www.unbound.org

Scott Wasserman, President & CEO
Seeks to advance the physical, mental, spiritual, and social welfare of the economically disadvantaged, especially children and aging persons in developing countries. US sponsors provide financial support and correspond with individuals in need; volunteers help provide social services, including medical, educational, and nutritional programs.
1919

7453 Virginia Center on Aging
Virginia Commonwealth University
Box 980229
Richmond, VA 23298
804-828-1525
vcoa@vcu.edu
vcoa.chp.vcu.edu

Edward F. Ansello, PhD, Director
Leland Waters, PhD, Associate Director
The Virginia Center on Aging is a statewide agency created by the Virginia General Assembly, with our home at Virginia Commonwealth University. Since 1978, VCoA has worked diligently to protect and improve the quality of life of older Virginians, so that they may remain independent and contributing members in their communities. Our four program areas include: abuse in later life, dementia research, geriatrics education, and lifelong learning.

Books

7454 Activities in Action
Routledge (Taylor & Francis Group)
270 Madison Ave
Fl 4 #4
New York, NY 10016-0601
212-695-6599
800-634-7064
Fax: 212-563-2269
www.routledgementalhealth.com

Jeffrey Lim, Director
Francis Chua, Manager
Tamaryn Anderson, Marketing Manager
An invaluable resource which serves as a catalyst for professional and personal growth and provides a national forum on geriatric and activity issues. *$30.00*
116 pages Hardcover
ISBN 1-560241-32-4

7455 Activities with Developmentally Disabled Elderly and Older Adults
Routledge (Taylor & Francis Group)
270 Madison Ave
Fl 4 #4
New York, NY 10016-601

212-695-6599
800-637-7064
Fax: 212-563-2269
www.routledgementalhealth.com

Jeffrey Lim, Director
Francis Chua, Manager
Tamaryn Anderson, Marketing Manager
Learn how to effectively plan and deliver activities for a growing number of older people with developmental disabilities. It aims to stimulate interest and continued support for recreation program development and implementation among developmental disability and aging service systems. *$42.00*
164 pages Hardcover
ISBN 1-560241-74-4

7456 Aging and Developmental Disability: Current Research, Programming, and Practice
Routledge (Taylor & Francis Group)
270 Madison Ave
Fl 4 #4
New York, NY 10016-601

212-695-6599
800-634-7064
Fax: 212-563-2269
www.routledgementalhealth.com

Joy Hammel, Author
Susan Nochajski, Co-Author
Explores research findings and their implications for practice in relation to normative and disability-related aging experiences and issues. It discusses the effectiveness of specific intervention targeted toward aging adults with developmental disabilities such as Down's Syndrome, cerebral palsy, autism, and epilepsy, and offers suggestions for practice and future research in this area. *$48.00*
112 pages Hardcover
ISBN 0-789010-39-1

7457 Aging and Family Therapy: Practitioner Perspectives on Golden Pond
Routledge (Taylor & Francis Group)
270 Madison Ave
Fl 4 #4
New York, NY 10016-601

212-695-6599
800-634-7064
Fax: 212-563-2269
www.routledgementalhealth.com

George Hughston, Author
Victor Christopherson, Co-Author
Marilyn Bojean, Co-Author
Here are creative strategies for use in therapy with older adults and their families. This significant new book provides practitioners with information, insight, reference tools, and other sources that will contribute to more effective intervention with the elderly and their families. *$48.00*
260 pages Hardcover
ISBN 0-866567-78-7

7458 Aging in Stride
IlluminAge Communications Partners
2200 1st Ave South
Suite 400
Seattle, WA 98134-1408

206-269-6363
888-620-8816
Fax: 206-269-6350

Dennis Kenny, Owner
Elizabeth N Oettinger, Co-Author
Dennis E Kenny JD, Co-Author
Guide to aging, the special needs of older adults, and the demands of providing care and support. Experts explain potential conflicts, planning opportunities and strategies for success. Six guides. *$24.95*
Paperback

7459 Aging in the Designed Environment
Routledge (Taylor & Francis Group)
270 Madison Ave
Fl 4 #4
New York, NY 10016-601

212-216-7800
800-634-7064
Fax: 212-563-2269
www.routledgementalhealth.com

Margaret Christenson, Author
Ellen D Taira, Co-Author
The key sourcebook for physical and occupational therapists developing and implementing environmental designs for the aging. *$30.00*
146 pages Hardcover
ISBN 1-560240-31-0

7460 Aging with a Disability
Special Needs Project
324 State Street
Suite H
Santa Barbara, CA 93101-2364

818-718-9900
800-333-6867
Fax: 818-349-2027
editor@specialneeds.com
www.specialneeds.com

Hod Gray, Owner
Laura Mosqueda, Co-Author
Aging with a Disability provides clinicians with a complete guide to the care and treatment of persons aging with a disability. Divided into five parts, this book first addresses the perspective of the person with a disability and his or her family. *$ 24.95*
328 pages Paperback

7461 Assistive Technology for Older Persons: A Handbook
Idaho Assistive Technology Project
University of Idaho
1187 Altiras Dr.
Moscow, ID 83843

208-885-3557
800-432-8324
Fax: 208-885-6102
idahoat@uidaho.edu
www.idahoat.org

Ron Seiler, Project Director
This handbook is designed as a guide for Idaho's older citizens who, as they age, wish to preserve their independence, autonomy, productivity, and dignity. It is intended to provide information about assistive technology, home modifications, and the many service options available to older people in the mcomunities across the state.

7462 Caring for Those You Love: A Guide to Compassionate Care for the Aged
Horizon Publishers & Distributors
191 N 650 E
Bountiful, UT 84010-3628

801-295-9451
866-818-6277
Fax: 801-298-1305
www.duanescrowther.com

Duane S. Crowther, Author/President
Jean Crowther, Vice President/Sec
David Crowther, Vice President
This book is a practical guide to coping with special problems of the aged and infirm, and examines the many challenges of caring for the elderly on a personal and family level. *$12.98*
108 pages
ISBN 0-882902-70-9

7463 Chronically Disabled Elderly in Society
Greenwood Publishing Group
88 Post Rd W
Westport, CT 06880-4208

203-226-3571
800-225-5800
Fax: 877-231-6980
www.greenwood.com

Merna J Alpert, Author
Lisa Scott, President
Herman Bruggink, CEO
This timely work increases awareness of and knowledge about problems of societal living among the chronically disabled el-

derly, with implications for policy makers, educational institutions, advocacy groups, families and individuals. *$76.95*
160 pages Hardcover
ISBN 0-313291-09-8

7464 Coping and Caring: Living with Alzheimer's Disease
AARP Fulfillment
601 E St NW
Washington, DC 20049
800-687-2277
TTY: 877-434-7589
member@aarp.org
www.aarp.org

Charles Leroux, Author
Steve Cone, Executive Vice President of Inte
Addresses the questions: What is Alzheimer's? How does the disease progress? How long does it last? How can families cope?
24 pages

7465 Elder Abuse and Mistreatment
Routledge (Taylor & Francis Group)
270 Madison Ave
Fl 4 #4
New York, NY 10016-601
212-695-6599
800-634-7064
Fax: 212-563-2269
www.routledgementalhealth.com

Joanna Mellor, Author
Patricia Brownell, Co-Author
Elder Abuse and Mistreatment is a comprehensive overview of current policy issues, new practice models, and up-to-date research on elder abuse and neglect. Experts in the field provide insight into elder abuse with newly examined populations to create an understanding of how to design service plans for victims of abuse and family mistreatment. The book addresses all forms of abuse and neglect, examining the value issues and ethical dilemmas that social workers face in providing service to elderl *$120.00*
284 pages Paperback
ISBN 0-789030-22-1

7466 Explore Your Options
Kansas Department on Aging
503 S Kansas Ave
New England Building
Topeka, KS 66603- 3404
785-296-4986
800-432-3535
Fax: 785-296-0256
TTY: 785-291-3167
wwwmail@kdads.ks.gov
www.agingKansas.org

Maria Russo, President
This book will help you through the maze of services available to Kansas seniors. It is designed to help you take an active role in making decisions that affect your health care and living situation.

7467 Falling in Old Age
Springer Publishing Company
11 W 42nd St
Fl 15 #15
New York, NY 10036-8002
212-431-4370
877-687-7476
Fax: 212-941-7842
cs@springerpub.com
www.springerjournals.com

Ursula Springer, President
Ted Nardin, CEO
Edie Lambiase, CFO
Presented are practical techniques for the prevention of falls and for determining and correcting the causes. *$60.00*
412 pages Hardcover
ISBN 0-826152-91-6

7468 Family Intervention Guide to Mental Illness
New Harbinger Publications
5674 Shattuck Ave
Oakland, CA 94609-1662
510-652-0215
800-748-6273
Fax: 800-652-1613
customerservice@newharbinger.com
www.newharbinger.com

Matthew McKay, Owner
Kim T Mueser, Co-Author
Kirk Johnson, CFO
The Family Intervention Guide to Mental Illness outlines the nine fundamental steps to recognizing, managing, and recovering from mental illness. It provides both diagnostic information and details about therapy options and useful medications. With the right advice, determined effort, and a lot of love, you can make a difference. *$17.95*
240 pages
ISBN 1-572245-06-8

7469 Handbook of Assistive Devices for the Handicapped Elderly
Routledge (Taylor & Francis Group)
270 Madison Ave
Fl 4 #4
New York, NY 10016-601
212-695-6599
800-634-7064
Fax: 212-563-2269
www.routledgementalhealth.com

Joseph A Breuer, Author
Jeffrey Lin, Director
Francis Chua, Manager
Concise yet comprehensive reference of assistive devices for handicapped elders. *$42.00*
77 pages Hardcover
ISBN 0-866561-52-5

7470 Handbook on Ethnicity, Aging and Mental Health
Greenwood Publishing Group
88 Post Rd W
Westport, CT 6880-4208
203-226-3571
800-225-5800
Fax: 877-231-6980
www.greenwood.com

Deborah K Padgett, Author
Lisa Scott, President
Herman Bruggink, CEO
State-of-the-art reference by leading experts and first book-length appraisal of research, practices and policies concerning mental health needs of the ethnic elderly in America. *$141.95*
376 pages Hardcover
ISBN 0-313282-04-8

7471 Health Care of the Aged: Needs, Policies, and Services
Routledge (Taylor & Francis Group)
270 Madison Ave
Fl 4 #4
New York, NY 10016-601
212-695-6599
800-634-7064
Fax: 212-563-2269
www.routledgementalhealth.com

Abraham Monk, Author
Jeffrey Lim, Director
Francis Chua, Manager
Focusing on the need for developing new service delivery models for the aged, this book examines fiscal, political, and social criteria influencing this challenge of the 1990's. The aged are caught in the sweeping changes currently occurring in the financing, organizing and delivery of human health care services. *$36.00*
800 pages Hardcover
ISBN 1-560240-65-5

7472 Health Promotion and Disease Prevention in Clinical Practice
Lippincott, Williams & Wilkins
2001 Market Street
Two Commerce Square
Philadelphia, PA 19103-3603   215-521-8300
                                           800-638-3030
                                           Fax: 215-521-8902
                                           customerservice@lww.com
                                           www.lww.com

Steven H Woolf MD, Co-Author
Steven Jonas MD, Co-Author
Evonne Kaplan-Liss, Co-Author
Incorporating the latest guidelines from major organizations, including the U.S. Preventive Services Task Force, this book offers the clinician a complete overview of how to help patients adopt healthy behaviors and to deliver recommended screening tests and immunizations. *$52.95*
218 pages Softcover
ISBN 0-781775-99-1

7473 Life Planning for Adults with Developmental Disabilities
New Harbinger Publications
5674 Shattuck Ave
Oakland, CA 94609-1662   510-652-0215
                                           800-748-6273
                                           Fax: 800-652-1613
                                           customerservice@newharbinger.com
                                           www.newharbinger.com

Matthew McKay, Publisher
Kirk Johnson, CFO
Judith Greenbaum PhD, Author
The book begins by assessing the quality of life of the adult with a disability. It offers a wealth of suggestions for making that person's life even better. The book then focuses on long-term planning for the individual with a disability and helps answer the question, Who will take care of my child after I'm gone? *$19.95*
208 pages
ISBN 1-572244-51-1

7474 Long-Term Care: How to Plan and Pay for It
NOLO
950 Parker St
Berkeley, CA 94710-2524   510-549-1976
                                           800-728-3555
                                           Fax: 800-645-0895
                                           www.nolo.com

Joseph L Matthews, Author
Ralph Warner, Chariman/CEO
Ann Heron, COO
This book helps you choose a nursing home, or find a viable alternative. Covers how to get the most out of Medicare and other benefit programs.
384 pages Paperback
ISBN 1-413305-21-0

7475 Mentally Impaired Elderly: Strategies and Interventions to Maintain Function
Routledge (Taylor & Francis Group)
270 Madison Ave
Fl 4 #4
New York, NY 10016-601   212-695-6599
                                           800-634-7064
                                           Fax: 212-653-2269
                                           www.routledgementalhealth.com

Ellen D Taira, Author
Jeffrey Lim, Director
Francis Chua, Manager
Provides effective support and sensitive care for the most vulnerable segment of the elderly population, those with mental impairment. *$34.00*
171 pages Hardcover
ISBN 1-560241-68-3

7476 Mirrored Lives: Aging Children and Elderly Parents
Praeger Publishers
88 Post Rd W
Westport, CT 06880-4208   203-226-3571
                                           800-225-5800
                                           Fax: 877-231-6980
                                           www.greenwood.com

Tom Koch, Author
Lisa Scott, President
Herman Bruggink, CEO
Discusses geriatric decline connected to nonterminal illness in old age. Koch takes a sensitive but thorough look at the declining years of his father. *$117.95*
240 pages Hardcover
ISBN 0-275936-71-6

7477 Physical & Mental Issues in Aging Sourcebook
Omnigraphics
615 Griswold Street
Suite 520
Detroit, MI 48226-3261   610-461-3548
                                           800-234-1340
                                           Fax: 800-875-1340
                                           contact@omnigraphics.com
                                           www.omnigraphics.com

Peter Ruffner, Co-Founder
Fred Ruffner, Co-Founder
Basic information about maintaining health through the post-reproductive years. Includes stats, recommendations for lifestyle modifications, a glossary and resrouce information *$84.00*
660 pages Hard cover
ISBN 0-780802-33-9

7478 Prescriptions for Independence: Working with Older People Who are Visually Impaired
American Foundation for the Blind/AFB Press
11 Penn Plz
Suite 300
New York, NY 10001-2006   212-502-7600
                                           800-232-3044
                                           Fax: 212-502-7777
                                           www.afb.org

Carl Augusto, President
Gerda Groff, Co-Author
Richard Obnen, Chairman of the Board
Easy-to-read manual on how older visually impaired persons can pursue their interests and activities in community residences, senior centers, long-term care facilities and other community settings. Paperback.
99 pages Paperback
ISBN 0-891282-44-0

7479 Sharing the Burden
Brookings Institution
1775 Massachusetts Ave NW
Washington, DC 20036-2188   202-797-6000
                                           Fax: 202-797-6004
                                           www.brookings.edu

Joshua N Weiner, Author
Laurel Hixon Illston, Co-Author
Raymond J Hanley, Co-Author
The authors examine the cost of public and private initiatives and who would pay for them. Their answers emerge from a large computer simulation model that the authors developed. *$42.95*
342 pages Cloth
ISBN 0-815793-78-2

7480 Social Security, Medicare, and Government Pensions
NOLO
950 Parker St
Berkeley, CA 94710-2524   510-549-1976
                                           800-728-3555
                                           Fax: 800-645-0895
                                           www.nolo.com

Joseph L Matthews, Author
Dorothy Matthews Berman, Co-Author
Ralph Warner, Chairman/CEO

Social Security, Medicare, SSI and more explained in this all-in-one resource that gets you the most out of your retirement benefits. *$24.95*
480 pages Paperback
ISBN 1-413307-53-5

7481 Successful Models of Community Long Term Care Services for the Elderly
Routledge (Taylor & Francis Group)
270 Madison Ave
Fl 4 #4
New York, NY 10016-601
212-695-6599
800-637-7064
Fax: 212-563-2269
www.routledgementalhealth.com

Eloise Killeffer, Author
Ruth Bennett, Co-Author
Jeffrey Lim, Director
Experienced practitioners provide examples of successful community-based long term care service programs for the elderly. *$ 72.00*
174 pages Hardcover
ISBN 0-866569-87-3

7482 Therapeutic Activities with Persons Disabled by Alzheimer's Disease
Sage Publications
804 Anacapa Stree
Sanat Barbara, CA 93101-2212
805-899-8620
info@sagepub.com
www.sagepub.com

Sara Miller McCune, Founder, Publisher, Chairperson
Blaise Simqu, CEO
Tracey Ozmina, COO
A program of functional skills for activities of daily living. Hardcover. *$86.00*
432 pages
ISBN 0-834211-62-9

7483 Visually Impaired Seniors as Senior Companions: A Reference Guide
American Foundation for the Blind/AFB Press
11 Penn Plz
Suite 300
New York, NY 10001-2006
212-502-7600
800-232-3044
Fax: 212-502-7777
www.afb.org

Carl Augusto, President
Alan Lindroth, Principal
Richard Obnen, Chairman of the Board
This useful guide describes the Senior Companion Program that is intended to broaden opportunities for older persons with disabilities. Appendix includes training materials, evaluation forms, recruitment and public relations information. *$15.00*
108 pages Paperback
ISBN 0-891282-38-6

7484 Work, Health and Income Among the Elderly
Brookings Institution
1775 Massachusetts Ave NW
Washington, DC 20036-2188
202-797-6000
Fax: 202-797-6004
www.brookings.edu

Gary Burtless, Author
Strobe Talbott, President
Steven Bennett, Vice President/COO
Employment, health and financial information for the elderly. *$26.95*
276 pages Cloth
ISBN 0-815711-76-6

Journals

7485 ATS Journals
25 Broadway
New York, NY 10004
212-315-8600
atsjournals.org

Marc Moss, President
Polly E. Parsons, President Elect
Juan C. Celedón, Secretary/Treasurer
The American Thoracic Society publishes medical research journals with a focus on respiratory issues. Publications include: Respiratory and Critical Care Medicine, Respiratory Cell and Molecular Biology, and Annals of the American Thoracic Society.

7486 Gerontology: Abstracts in Social Gerontology
National Council on the Aging
1901 L St NW
4th Floor
Washington, DC 20036-3506
202-479-1200
Fax: 202-479-0735
TTY: 202-479-6674
info@ncoa.org
www.ncoa.org

James Knickman, Interim President & CEO
Detailed abstracts are provided for recent major journal articles, books, reports and other materials on many facets of aging, including: adult education, demography, family relations, institutional care and work attitudes. Item No. AB100; Journals $114.00; Member Discount: $94.00.
Quarterly

7487 Inclusive Practices
TASH
1101 15th St. NW
Suite 206
Washington, DC 20005
202-817-3264
Fax: 202-999-4722
info@tash.org
www.tash.org

Andrea Ruppar, Co-Editor-in-Chief
Jennifer Kurth, Co-Editor-in-Chief
Quarterly online journal featuring articles on special topics in the disability field.
Quarterly

7488 Journal of the American Academy of Audiology (JAAA)
American Academy of Audiology
11480 Commerce Park Dr.
Suite 220
Reston, VA 20191
703-790-8466
Fax: 703-790-8631
infoaud@audiology.org
www.audiology.org

Gary P. Jacobson, Editor-in-Chief
Devin McCaslin, Deputy Editor-in-Chief
James Jerger, Emeritus Editor-in-Chief
The scholarly peer-reviewed journal of the American Academy of Audiology. Publishes articles and clinical reports in all areas of audiology.

7489 Physical & Occupational Therapy in Geriatrics
Taylor & Francis Group, LLC
325 Chestnut Street
Suite 800 #800
Philadelphia, PA 19106-2608
215-625-8900
800-354-1420
Fax: 215-625-2940
haworthpress@taylorandfrancis.com
www.tandf.co.uk

Ellen Dunleavey Taira, Editor
Barbara Pucher, CFO
Focuses on current practices and emerging issues in the care of the older client, including long-term care in institutional and community settings, crisis intervention, and innovative programming; the entire range of problems experienced by the elderly; and the current skills needed for working with older clients. *$99.00*
Quarterly

7490 **Research, Advocacy, and Practice for Complex and Chronic Conditions**
Council for Exceptional Children
3100 Clarendon Blvd.
Suite 600
Arlington, VA 22201-5332
888-232-7733
TTY: 866-915-5000
service@exceptionalchildren.org
www.exceptionalchildren.org

Dusty Columbia Embury, Editor
Peer-reviewed journal covering research, issues, and programs relating to the needs of people with physical, health, or multiple disabilities.

Magazines

7491 **A Better Tomorrow**
Thomas Nelson
5301 Wisconsin Avenue NW
Suite 620
Washington, DC 20015
202-364-8000
Fax: 202-364-8910
www.thomasnelson.com/

Bruce Barbour, Publisher
Dale Hanson, Editor
Magazine focusing on issues and concerns of senior citizens.

7492 **AARP Bulletin**
AARP
601 E Street NW
Washington, DC 20049
888-687-2277
www.aarp.org
Resources for online classes, training and more. Topics include Computers/Technology, Health/Wellbeing, Personal Finance. AARP Membership open to individuals age 50+, benefits include access to insurance services, travel discounts, advice on healthy living, financial planning, consumer protection. AARP represents members on issues like Medicare, Social Security, and consumer safety. Publications include the AARP Magazine and AARP Bulletin.

7493 **AARP Magazine**
American Association of Retired Persons
601 East Street NW
Washington, DC 20049
202-434-3525
888-687-2277
member@aarp.org
www.aarp.org

A Barry Rand, CEO
Steve Cone, Executive Vice President of Integrated Value
Celebrity interviews. Features on health and finance. Movie reviews and more. All with an eye toward the topics and issues you care about most.

7494 **ACE Fitness Matters**
American Council on Exercise (ACE)
4851 Paramount Drive
San Diego, CA 92123
858-576-6500
888-825-3636
Fax: 858-576-6564
support@acefitness.org
www.acefitness.org/

Herb Flentye, Chair
Scott Murdoch, PhD., RD, Vice Chair
Consumer magazine covering health and fitness news. *$ 25.00*

7495 **AER Report**
Association for Education & Rehabilitation
5680 King Centre Dr.
Suite 600
Alexandria, VA 22315
703-671-4500
Fax: 703-671-6391
www.aerbvi.org

Neva Fairchild, President
Contains organizational news, conference dates and information concerning services to visually impaired people.

7496 **ASN NEURO**
Sage Journals
2455 Teller Road
Thousand Oaks, CA 91320
805-499-9774
journals@sagepub.com
journals.sagepub.com/home/asn

Douglas L. Feinstein, Editor-in-Chief
Sandra J. Hewitt, Deputy Editor-in-Chief
Peer-reviewed open access journal focusing on recent advances in the cellular and molecular neurosciences. It is the official publication of the American Society for Neurochemistry.

7497 **Abstracts in Social Gerontology**
National Council on Aging
1901 L Street NW
4th Floor
Washington, DC 20036
202-479-1200
800-677-1116
Fax: 202-479-0735
TTY: 202-479-6674
info@ncoa.org
www.ncoa.org

James Knickman, Interim President & CEO
Detailed abstracts are provided for recent major journal articles, books, reports and other materials on many facets of aging, including adult education, demography, family relations, institutional care and work attitudes. *$114.00*

7498 **Adapted Physical Activity Quarterly**
Human Kinetics
PO Box 5076
1607 N Market Street
Champaign, IL 61820
217-351-5076
800-747-4457
Fax: 217-351-1549
info@hkusa.com
www.humankinetics.com

Brian Holding, CEO
Rainer Martens, Founder
Journal on the study of physical activity for special populations.

7499 **Aging International**
Transaction Publishers
35 Berrue
New Brunswick, NJ 08901
732-445-1245
888-999-6778
Fax: 732-445-3138
orders@transactionpub.com
www.transactionpub.com/

Mary E. Curtis, Chair
Irving Louis Horowitz, Co-Founder
Journal dedicated to the well-being of older persons worldwide. Explores productive aging, empowerment, life-long learning, health promotion, and services for the elderly, with an emphasis on sharing both common concerns and practical applications. Focuses on social and economic issues, public policies, and use of resources. Published in cooperation with the International Federation on Aging.

7500 **Aging News Alert**
CD Publications
2222 Sedwick Drive
Durham, NC 27713
301-588-6380
855-237-1396
Fax: 800-508-2592
www.cdpublications.com

Michael Gerecht, President
Twice-monthly newsletter reporting on senior programs, funding opportunities and federal actions affecting the elderly.

7501 **Aging Research & Training News**
Business Publishers, Inc.
2222 Sedwick Drive
Durham, NC 27713
800-223-8720
Fax: 800-508-2592
www.bpinews.com

Kimberly Gilbert, Managing Editor
Alexa Chew, Contributing Editor

Compilation of studies of aging populations; reports on innovative programs with aging community; federal funding and laws. *$ 267.00*
8 pages

7502   Aging and Society
Cambridge University Press
32 Avenue of the Americas
New York, NY 10013   212-924-3900
                                      800-221-4512
                                 Fax: 212-691-3239
              www.cambridge.org/us/information/contact
Ken Blakemore, Editor
Bill Bythwway, Editor
International journal publishing on topics which further the understanding of human aging. The journal of the Centre for policy on aging and the British Socie for Gerontology.

7503   American Journal of Geriatric Psychiatry
Elsevier
1600 John F Kennedy Boulevard
Philadelphia, PA 19103   www.journals.elsevier.com
Charles F. Reynolds III, MD, Editor-in-Chief
Peer-reviewed articles on the rapidly developing field of geriatric psychiatry, including areas such as the diagnosis and classification of psychiatric disorders, epidemiological and biological correlates of mental health of older adults, and psychopharmacology and other somatic treatments. *$582.00*

7504   American Journal of Speech-LanguagePathology
American Speech-Language-Hearing Association (ASHA
2200 Research Boulevard
Rockville, MD 20850   301-296-5700
                                      800-638-8255
                                 Fax: 301-296-8580
                                      www.asha.org/
Elizabeth S. McCrea, PhD, CCC-SLP, President
Barbara K. Cone, PhD, CCC-A, Vice President for Academic Affa

7505   American Legion Magazine
American Legion National Headquarters
PO Box 1055
700 N. Pennsylvania St.
Indianapolis, IN 46206   317-630-1200
                                      800-433-3318
                                 Fax: 317-630-1223
                                      www.legion.org/
Daniel S. Wheeler, National Adjutant
Philip B. Onderdonk Jr., National Judge Advocate
General interest magazine for veterans. *$152.50*

7506   American Rehabilitation ServicesAdministration (RSA)
American Rehabilitation Services Administration (R
400 Maryland Avenue, SW
Washington, DC 20202   202-205-8296
                                      800-USA-LEAR
                                 Fax: 202-205-9874
                 www2.ed.gov/about/offices/list/osers/rsa
Arne Duncan, Secretary of Education
Jim Shelton, Acting Deputy Secretary
Magazine on rehabilitation of the handicapped. *$9.50*

7507   Assistive Technology
RESNA
2001 K Street NW
3rd Floor North
Washington, DC 20006   202-367-1121
                                 Fax: 202-367-2121
                                      info@resna.org
                                      www.resna.org
Maureen Linden, President
Andrea Van Hook, Interim Executive Director
Journal focusing on assistive technology for persons with disabilities. *$35.00*

7508   Audecibel
International Hearing Society
16880 Middlebelt Road
Suite 4
Livonia, MI 48154   734-522-7200
                                      800-521-5247
                                 Fax: 734-522-0200
                                      www.ihsinfo.org/
Kathleen Mennillo, Executive Director
Magazine publishing technical articles and product announcements on hearing aids and hearing. *$25.00*

7509   Buena Vida
Casiano Communications
1700 Fern ndez Juncos Avenue
San Juan, PR 00909   787-728-3000
                                      800-468-8167
                                 Fax: 787-268-1001
                                      www.casiano.com/
Manuel A. Casiano, Chairman & CEO
Carlos Rom, Executive Vice President
Health and fitness magazine. *$23.95*

7510   Challenge Magazine
Disabled Sports, USA
451 Hungerford Drive
Suite 100
Rockville, MD 20850   301-217-0960
                                 Fax: 301-217-0968
                                      dsusa@dsusa.org
                                www.disabledsportsusa.org/
Robert Meserve, President
Steven Goodwin, Vice President
Magazine providing information on sports for people with physical disabilities.

7511   Closing the Gap
P.O. Box 68
Henderson, MN 56044   507-248-3294
                                 Fax: 507-248-3810
                                      www.closingthegap.com
Dolores Hagen, Co-Founder
Budd Hagen, Co-Founder
Online membership that includes access to the Solutions on-line magazine and archives, archived webinars and the Resource Directory, a guide to over 2,000 products for children and adults with disabilities

7512   Communication Outlook: Artificial LanguageLaboratory
Artificial Language Laboratory
405 Computer Center
Michigan State University
Lansing, MI 48824   517-353-0870
                                 Fax: 517-353-4766
                    www.msu.edu/~artlang/CommOut.html
Dr. John B. Eulenberg, Ph.D., Director
Stephen R. Blosser, B.S.M.E., Technical Director
Magazine reporting on the newest developments in the application of technology for neurologically impaired persons. *$18.00*

7513   Conscious Choice
Conscious Communications
920 N Franklin Street
Suite 202
Chicago, IL 60610   312-440-4373
                                 Fax: 312-751-3973
                                      www.consciouscomms.com/
Ross Thompson, Managing Editor
Jim Slama, Publisher
Consumer magazine covering health, nutrition and environmental issues. *$184.00*

7514 Contemporary Gerontology
Springer Publishing Company
11 West 42nd Street
15th Floor
New York, NY 10036   212-431-4370
                                      877-687-7476
                                 Fax: 212-941-7842
         cs@springerpub.com, journals@springerpub
                                 www.springerpub.com
James C. Costello, Vice President, Journal Publishi
Theodore C. Nardin, Chief Executive Officer & Publis
Scholarly journal covering gerontology.

7515 Dementia and Geriatric Cognitive Disorders
S. Karger Publishers, Inc.
26 W Avon Road
P.O. Box 529
Unionville, CT 06085   860-675-7834
                                      800-828-5479
                                 Fax: 860-675-7302
                                 www.karger.com/DEM
Victoria Chan-Pilay, Editor-in-Chief
Open-access journal devoted to the study of cognitive dysfunc-
tion in preclinical and clinical studies, concentrating on Alzhei-
mer's and Parkinson's disease, Huntington's chorea and other
neurodegenerative diseases.

7516 Disability Rag's Ragged Edge Magazine
Advocado Press
PO Box 145
Louisville, KY 40201   502-894-9492
                                 Fax: 502-899-9562
                                 www.advocadopress.org/
Mary Johnson, Mailing Contact/Editor
Magazine of debate on disability rights issues. ISSN# 1095-3949
$17.50
35 pages

7517 Disability Rights Now
Disability Rights Education and Defense Fund
3075 Adeline Street
Suite 210
Berkeley, CA 94703   510-644-2555
                                      800-466-4232
                                 Fax: 510-841-8645
                                 info@dredf.org
                                 dredf.org/
Claudia Center, President and Chair
Susan Henderson, Executive Director
Free quarterly publication describing the activities of the Dis-
ability Rights Education and Defense Fund, available in alterna-
tive formats.

7518 Disability Statistics Report
Institute for Health & Aging
2 Koret Way, #N-319X
UCSF Box 0602
San Francisco, CA 94143   415-476-1435
                                 Fax: 415-476-9707
                                 info@nursing.ucsf.edu
                                 nursing.ucsf.edu/iha
David Vlahov, RN, PhD, Dean and Professor
Yolanda Abrea, Fiscal Analyst
Magazine providing statistical data on disability in the US as col-
lected by the Disability Statistics Program.

7519 Disability Studies Quarterly
University of Hawaii at Manoa
2500 Campus Road
Honolulu, HI 96822   808-956-8111
                                 Fax: 808-956-3162
                                 manoa.hawaii.edu/
M.R.C. Greenwood, President
Tom Apple, Chief Executive Officer
Scholarly journal containing articles on all aspects of disability.
$3545.00

7520 Disabled American Veterans Magazines
Disabled American Veterans National Headquarters
PO Box 14301
Cincinnati, OH 45250   859-441-7300
                                 Fax: 859-441-8056
                                 www.dav.org/
Thomas K Keller, Editor
James Chaney, Mailing Contact
Veterans magazine on disability issues. *$15.00*

7521 Disabled People as Second Class Citizens
Springer Publishing Company
11 West 42nd Street
15th Floor
New York, NY 10036   212-431-4370
                                      877-687-7476
                                 Fax: 212-941-7842
         cs@springerpub.com, journals@springerpub
                                 www.springerpub.com
James C. Costello, Vice President, Publisher
Theodore C. Nardin, Chief Executive Officer
Disability and legal practice. *$26.95*
320 pages

**7522 Domestic Mistreatment of the Elderly:Towards
Prevention**
AARP
601 E Street NW
Washington, DC 20049   202-434-3525
                                      888-687-2277
                                 Fax: 202-434-3443
                                 member@aarp.org
                                 www.aarp.org
Gail E. Aldrich, Board Chair
Robert G. Romasco, President
This comprehensive publication addresses the problem of mis-
treatment or neglect in the home.
39 pages

7523 Duplex Planet
Duplex Planet
PO Box 1230
Saratoga Springs, NY 12866   518-692-7410
                                 Fax: 518-692-8208
                                 www.duplexplanet.com/
David Greenberger, Editor/ Founder
Consumer journal covering issues of aging and popular culture.
$122.50

7524 Eating Well Magazine
Eating Well
6221 Shelburne Road
Suite 100
Charlotte, VT 05482   802-985-4500
                                      800-344-3350
                                 Fax: 802-425-3675
                                 www.eatingwell.com
Thomas Witschi, President
Brierley Wright, Managing Editor
Food magazine with emphasis on delicious low-fat cooking and
sensible nutrition. *$19.94*

7525 Educational Gerontology
Taylor & Francis
711 3rd Avenue
8th Floor
New York, NY 10017   212-216-7800
                                      800-634-7064
                                 Fax: 212-564-7854
                                 www.taylorandfrancis.com/
D Barry Lumsden, Editor
Kevin Bradley, CEO
Journal publishing original research in the fields of gerontology,
adult education, and the social and behavioral sciences.

7526 Elderly Health Services Letter
Health Resources Online
P.O. Box 456
Allenwood, NJ 08720   800-516-4343
                                 Fax: 732-292-1111
Robert K Jenkins, Publisher

An essential tool for senior services professionals. Stays on top of the most current challenges facing senior services professionals, including financing and funding senior services, marketing, positioning senior services for managed care, getting administrative support and more.

7527 Experimental Aging Research
Taylor & Francis
711 3rd Avenue
8th Floor
New York, NY 10017
212-216-7800
800-634-7064
Fax: 212-564-7854
www.taylorandfrancis.com/
Jeffrey Elias, Editor
Kevin Bradley, CEO
International journal devoted to the scientific study of the aging process.

7528 Fitness Diet and Exercise Guide
Family Circle
110 5th Avenue
New York, NY 10011
212-463-1673
800-627-4444
Fax: 212-463-1906
fcfeedback@familycircle.com
www.familycircle.com/
Darcy Jacobs, Executive Editor
Linda Fears, Vice President/Editor in Chief
Magazine suggesting ways to eat healthier and exercise better.

7529 Focus on Geriatric Care and Rehabilitation
Aspen Publishers
7201 McKinney Circle
Frederick, MD 21704
301-644-3599
800-234-1660
Fax: 800-901-9075
www.aspenpublishers.com/
Bob Lemmond, President & CEO
Gustavo Dobles, Vice President & CCO
Monthly journal written for nurses, occupational therapists and administrators in geriatric settings. *$95.00*

7530 Generations
American Society on Aging
575 Market Street
Suite 2100
San Francisco, CA 94105
415-974-9600
800-537-9728
Fax: 415-974-0300
info@asaging.org
www.asaging.org
Peter Kaldest, President & CEO
Robert R. Lowe, COO
Peer-review quarterly journal featuring guest editor. *$30.00*

7531 Geriatrics
ModernMedicine
7500 Old Oak Boulevard
Cleveland, OH 44130
440-891-2769
Fax: 440-891-2635
Don Berman, Director, Business Development
Terry Tetzlaff, Digital Traffic Coordinator
Peer-reviewed, clinical journal for physicians and laypersons relating to medical care of middle-aged and older adults.

7532 Gerontologist
Gerontological Society of America
1220 L Street North West
Washington, DC 20005
202-842-1275
Fax: 202-842-1150
geron@geron.org
www.geron.org
James Appleby, Executive Director and CEO
Linda Krogh Harootyan, Deputy Executive Director
Multidisciplinary peer-reviewed journal presenting new concepts, clinical ideas, and applied research in gerontology. Includes book and audiovisual reviews.

7533 Gerontology
S. Karger Publishers, Inc.
PO Box 529
26 West Avon Road
Unionville, CT 06085
860-675-7834
800-828-5479
Fax: 860-675-7302
karger@snet.net
www.karger.com/
W Meier-Rage, Managing Editor
Monica Brendel, President
Medical journal. *$276.00*

7534 Get Up and Go
Liberty Media Corporation
11551 Forest Central Drive
Suite 305
Dallas, TX 75243
214-341-9429
877-772-1518
Fax: 214-341-9779
www.libertymedia.com/
John C. Malone, Chairman
Gregory B. Maffei, President & CEO
Magazine (tabloid) for people age 50 and over.

7535 Independent Living Provider
Equal Opportunity Publications
1160 E Jericho Turnpike
Suite 200
Huntington, NY 11743
516-421-9421
Fax: 516-421-0359
info@eop.com
www.eop.com/
Tamara Flaum-Dreyfuss, President and Publisher
Maureen Gladstone, Account Executive
Business magazine for home health care.

7536 Informer
The Simon Foundation for Continence
PO Box 815
Wilmette, IL 60091
847-864-3913
800-23S-mon
Fax: 847-864-9758
info@simonfoundation.org
www.simonfoundation.org
Cheryle Gartley, President and Founder
Elizabeth Tr LaGro, Vice President, Communications a
Magazine for persons with bladder or bowel incontinence.

7537 Innovations
National Council on Aging
1901 L Street NW
4th Floor
Washington, DC 20036
202-479-1200
800-677-1116
Fax: 202-479-0735
TTY: 2024796674
info@ncoa.org
www.ncoa.org
James Knickman, Interim President & CEO
Explores significant developments in the field of aging through opinion articles, profiles and research summaries. Features articles on social trends, articles on specific aging programs and information on NCOA's activities. *$50.00*

7538 Inside MS
National Multiple Sclerosis Society
733 3rd Avenue
3rd Floor
New York, NY 10017
212-986-3240
800-FIG-HTMS
Fax: 212-986-7981
editor@nmss.org
www.nationalmssociety.org/
Eli Rubenstein, Chairman of the Board
Cynthia Zagieboylo, President & CEO
Magazine for people with multiple sclerosis, their families, attending professionals, and interested donors. Provides information on coping, research, legislation, medical advances and disability rights advocacy. *$2027.00*
80 pages

7539 International Journal of Aging and Human Development
Baywood Publishing Company, Inc.
PO Box 337
26 Austin Avenue
Amityville, NY 11701   631-691-1270
800-638-7819
Fax: 631-691-1770
www.baywood.com/
Adult development and aging featuring original research theory, critial reviews.

7540 International Journal of Technology and Aging
Human Sciences Press
233 Spring Street
New York, NY 10013-1522   212-620-8000
800-221-9369
Fax: 212-463-0742
www.springer.com
Designed to serve health-care professionals, researchers, academicians and industries concerned with the convergence of two recent trends, the dramatic advances in technology and the rapidly growing elderly population. $60.00

7541 International Psychogeriatrics
Springer Publishing Company
11 West 42nd Street
15th Floor
New York, NY 10036   212-431-4370
877-687-7476
Fax: 212-941-7842
cs@springerpub.com, journals@springerpub
www.springerpub.com
James C. Costello, Vice President
Theodore C. Nardin, Chief Executive Officer
Scholarly journal covering psychogeriatric practice, research, and education worldwide.

7542 International Rehabilitation Review
Rehabilitation International
866 United Nations Plaza
Office 422
New York, NY 10017   212-420-1500
Fax: 212-505-0871
info@riglobal.org
www.riglobal.org
Teuta Rexhepi, Secretary General
Zhang Haidi, President

7543 JNeurosci
Society for Neuroscience
1121 14th Street NW
Suite 1010
Washginton, DC 20005   202-962-4000
jn@sfn.org
www.jneurosci.org
Marina R. Picciotto, Editor-in-Chief
Teresa Esch, Features Editor
Official peer-reviewed journal of the Society for Neuroscience, publishing research on a broad range of topics of interest to those working on the nervous system.

7544 Journal of Aging and Ethnicity
Springer Publishing Company
11 West 42nd Street
15th Floor
New York, NY 10036   212-431-4370
877-687-7476
Fax: 212-941-7842
www.springerpub.com
James C. Costello, Vice President
Theodore C. Nardin, Chief Executive Officer
Scholarly journal for researchers and professionals in gerontology and geriatrics, emphasizing the ethnic population of North America.

7545 Journal of Aging and Health
Sage Publications
2455 Teller Road
Thousand Oaks, CA 91320   805-499-0721
Fax: 805-499-0871
www.sagepub.in/
Kyriakos S Markides, Editor
C Anderson, Circulation Manager
Journal presenting research relative to the social and behavioral factors related to aging and health.

7546 Journal of Aging and Physical Activity
Human Kinetics
PO Box 5076
1607 N Market Street
Champaign, IL 61820   217-351-5076
800-747-4457
Fax: 217-351-1549
info@hkusa.com
www.humankinetics.com
Brian Holding, CEO
Rainer Martens, Founder
Journal examining the relationship between physical activity and the aging process.

7547 Journal of American Aging Association
American Aging Association
52373 Tyndall Falls Drive
Olmstead Falls, OH 44138   440-793-6565
Fax: 440-793-6598
ameraging@gmail.com
www.americanaging.org
Mitch Harman, Chairperson
LaDora Thompson, President

7548 Journal of Developmental and Physical Disabilities
Kluwer Academic Publishers
101 Philip Drive
Norwell, MA 02061   212-620-8000
Fax: 212-463-0742
vlib.ustu.ru/storon/kluwer/
Vincent B Hassett, Editor
V Hersen, Advertising Manager
Professional journal.

7549 Journal of Ethics, Law, and Aging
Springer Publishing Company
11 West 42nd Street
15th Floor
New York, NY 10036   212-431-4370
877-687-7476
Fax: 212-941-7842
www.springerpub.com
James C. Costello, Vice President, Journal Publishing
Theodore C. Nardin, Chief Executive Officer & Publisher
Scholarly journal covering ethical and legal issues regarding aging for professionals who plan, administer, and provide and finance services to the elderly.

7550 Journal of Mental Health and Aging
Springer Publishing Company
11 West 42nd Street
15th Floor
New York, NY 10036   212-431-4370
877-687-7476
Fax: 212-941-7842
www.springerpub.com
James C. Costello, Vice President
Theodore C. Nardin, Chief Executive Officer
Scholarly journal covering aging population for mental health professionals.

7551   Journal of Nuclear Medicine
Society of Nuclear Medicine and Molecular Imaging
1850 Samuel Morse Drive
Reston, VA 20190   703-708-9000
                                         800-513-6853
                                    Fax: 703-708-9015
                              subscriptions@snm.org
                                  jnm.snmjournals.org
Johannes Czernin, MD, Editor-in-Chief
Susan Alexander, Associate Director, Publications
Peer-reviewed journal with clinical investigations, science reports, articles benefitting continuing education, book reviews, employment opportunities, and updates on practice and research. *$58.00*

7552   Journal of Nuclear Medicine Technology
Society of Nuclear Medicine and Molecular Imaging
1850 Samuel Morse Drive
Reston, VA 20190   703-708-9000
                                         800-513-6853
                                    Fax: 703-708-9015
                              subscriptions@snm.org
                                  tech.snmjournals.org
Kathy S. Thomas, MHA, CNMT, PET, Editor-in-Chief
Susan Alexander, Associate Director, Publications
Peer-reviewed journal dedicated to nuclear medicine technology, with information on credentialing, continuing education and licensure requirements, as well as current news and updates on the field. *$58.00*

7553   Journal of Rehabilitation
National Rehabilitation Association
PO Box 150235
Alexandria, VA 22315   703-836-0850
                                         888-258-4295
                  journalofrehab@email.arizona.edu
                  nationalrehab.org/journal-of-rehabilitation
Wendy Parent-Johnson, Editor
Official journal of the National Rehabilitation Association.
Quarterly

7554   Journal of Religion, Spirituality & Aging

                                    www.tandfonline.com
James W. Ellor, Editor
Features articles, research reports and reviews of new books and audiovisual resources on religion and aging.

7555   Journal of Therapeutic Horticulture
American Horticultural Therapy Association
610 Freedom Business Center
Suite 110
King of Prussia, PA 19406   610-992-0020
                                    Fax: 301-869-2397
                                            ahta.org/
MaryAnne Millan, HTR, President
Leigh Anne Starling, MS, CRC, HTR, Vice President
Journal containing articles on the therapeutic aspects of gardening and agriculture for persons with disabilities. *$15.00*

7556   Kaleidoscope: Exploring the Expirence of Disability through Literature/Fine Arts
United Disability Services
701 S Main Street
Akron, OH 44311   330-762-9755
                                    Fax: 330-762-0912
                                    www.udsakron.org
Karen A. Bozzelli, Chairperson
Bill Choler, Vice Chairperson
Magazine featuring articles on literature and the arts. Disabilitiy related. *$9.00*
64 pages

7557   Macrobiotics Today
George Ohsawa Macrobiotic Foundation
PO Box 3998
Chico, CA 95927   530-566-9765
                                         800-232-2372
                                    Fax: 530-566-9768
                              www.ohsawamacrobiotics.com/
Carl Ferr,, President
Peter Milbury, Director
Magazine covering macrobiotics, health, and nutrition. *$20.00*

7558   Magazines in Special Media for theHandicapped
National Library Service for the Blind and Physic
1291 Taylor Street NW
Washington, DC 20011   202-707-5100
                                         800-424-8567
                                    Fax: 202-707-0712
                                    TTY: 202-707-0744
                                    www.loc.gov/nls
Karen Keninger, Director
Isabella Marqu,s de Castilla, Deputy Director
Publication includes: List of over 100 public and private organizations that publish magazines in Braille, on cassette, on disc and computer diskette, or in large print or moon type for visually impaired and physically disabled individuals. Entries include: Name of publisher, address, price. Principal content is a bibliography of periodicals, with brief description, frequency, format, and price of each.

7559   Massage Therapy Journal
American Massage Therapy Association
500 Davis St.
Suite 900
Evanston, IL 60201   877-905-2700
                                    info@amtamassage.org
                                    www.amtamassage.org
Michaele M. Colizza, President
Publication focusing on massage therapy research, techniques, and practices. *$20.00*

7560   Mature Health
New York - Haymarket
114 West 26th Street
4th Floor
New York, NY 10001   646-638-6000

Michael Heseltine, Chairman
Kevin Costello, Chief Group Executive
Magazine featuring articles on health aspects of aging, as well as articles on recreation and leisure. *$7.00*

7561   Mature Years
United Methodist Publishing House
201 8th Avenue S
PO Box 801
Nashville, TN 37202   615-749-6000
                                    Fax: 615-749-6079
                                            umph.org/
Neil Alexander, President/Publisher
Jeff Barnes, Executive Director
Magazine promoting the physical and spiritual well-being of older adults.

7562   Men's Health
Rodale Inc
400 South 10th Street
Emmaus, PA 18098   610-967-5171
                                         800-848-4735
                                    Fax: 610-967-7725
                        RodaleBooks@cdsfulfillment.com
Maria Rodale, CEO and Chairman
Scott D. Schulman, President
Magazine offering health advice for men.

7563   Mental Health Report
Business Publishers, Inc.
2222 Sedwick Drive
Durham, NC 27713   301-495-5570
                                            800-223-8720
                                       Fax: 800-508-2592
                                        www.bpinews.com
Kimberly Gilbert, Managing Editor
Alexa Chew, Contributing Editor
Magazine reporting on legislation affecting the mentally ill and
their families. *$325.00*

7564   Modern Maturity
AARP
601 E Street NW
Washington, DC 20049-0003   202-434-2277
                                            202-434-3525
                                       Fax: 888-687-2277
                                         member@aarp.org
                                            www.aarp.org
Gail E. Aldrich, Board Chair
Robert G. Romasco, President
Offers news and information of concern to those 50 and older.
Features articles on current events, health, recreation, housing,
family life, legislation and other issues.

7565   Molecular Imaging
Sage Journals
2455 Teller Road
Thousand Oaks, CA 91320   805-499-9774
                                      journals@sagepub.com
                              journals.sagepub.com/home/mix
Henry F. VanBrocklin, PhD, Editor-in-Chief
Peer-reviewed open access journal focusing on molecular imag-
ing research, including basic science, preclinical studies and hu-
man applications. Published in association with the Society of
Nuclear Medicine and Molecular Imaging.

7566   New Living
New Living Magazine
PO Box 1001
Patchogue, NY 11772   631-751-8819
                                             800-NEW-LIVI
                                       Fax: 631-751-8910
                                        www.newliving.com
Christine Ly Harvey, Publisher and Editor-in-Chief
Features and articles about holistic health and fitness;herbal rem-
edies, preventive medicine, nutrition, mind/body health, spiritu-
ality, fitness, recipes, book reviews and more!

7567   PN
PVA Publications
2111 E Highland Avenue
Suite 180
Phoenix, AZ 85016   602-224-0500
                                            888-888-2201
                                       Fax: 602-224-0507
                                      www.pn-magazine.com
Richard Hoover, Editor
Sherri Shea, Marketing & Circulation Director
Magazine spotlighting independent living for paraplegics and
quadriplegics. *$23.00*

7568   Prevention
Rodale Inc
400 South 10th Street
Emmaus, PA 18098   610-967-5171
                                            800-848-4735
                                       Fax: 910-967-8963
                         RodaleBooks@cdsfulfillment.com
                                             rodaleinc.com/
Maria Rodale, CEO and Chairman
Scott D. Schulman, President
Magazine containing articles on wellness, preventive medicine,
self-care, and fitness. *$21.97*

7569   Remedy
Rx Remedies
500 Highway 51 North
Suite Q
Ridgeland, MS 39157   601-981-0070
                                            800-826-1197
                                       Fax: 800-729-0167
                                    www.rxremediesms.com/
Joan Montgomery, Publisher
Consumer magazine covering health and wellness for individuals
over 50 years in the US. *$183.00*

7570   Research on Aging
Sage Publications
2455 Teller Road
Thousand Oaks, CA 91320   805-499-0721
                                       Fax: 805-499-0871
                                         info@sagepub.com
                                           www.sagepub.in/
Angela M O'Rand, Editor
Blaise R Simqu, CEO
Social gerontology journal.

7571   SELF Magazine
Cond, Nast
4 Times Square
New York, NY 10036   212-286-2860
                                            800-223-0780
                                       Fax: 212-880-8248
                          communications@condenast.com
                                        www.condenast.com/
Rochelle Udell, Editor-in-Chief
Larry Burstein, Publisher
Magazine serving as a health sourcebook for contemporary
women.

**7572   Secure Retirement, The Newsmagazine for Mature
Americans**
The National Committee to Preserve Social Security
111 K Street NE
Suite 700
Washington, DC 20002   202-216-0420
                                            800-966-1935
                                       Fax: 202-216-0446
                                     webmaster@ncpssm.org
                                           www.ncpssm.org
Max Richtman, President & CEO
Magazine for senior citizens and others interested in politics and
government and how they affect senior concerns and issues.

7573   Senior Times Magazine
Senior Times Magazine
4400 NW 36th Avenue
Gainesville, FL 32601   352-372-5468
                                       Fax: 352-373-9178
                              www.seniortimesmagazine.com/
Charlie Delatorre, Publisher
Albert Issac, Editor-in-Chief
Magazine devoted to educating senior citizens on recreational,
political, health and financial issues. *$15.00*

7574   Serenity
Little Sisters of The Poor
601 Maiden Choice Lane
Baltimore, MD 21228   410-744-9367
                                       Fax: 410-788-5614
                          serenitys@littlesistersofthepoor.org
                             www.littlesistersofthepoor.org/
S R Marguerite, Publications Coordinator
Saint Jeanne Jugan, Founder
Magazine making known the apostolate of Little Sisters of the
Poor and providing a positive view of the elderly and the respect
due them.
32 pages

7575 Society of Nuclear Medicine and MolecularImaging
1850 Samuel Morse Drive
Reston, VA 20190 703-708-9000
Fax: 703-708-9015
feedback@snmmi.org
www.snmmi.org
Virginia Pappas, CEO
Rebecca Maxey, Director, Communications
The mission of this nonprofit scientific and professional organization is to promote the science, technology and application of nuclear medicine and molecular imaging. Molecular imaging techniques are used to diagnose and manage the treatment of brain disorders such as Alzheimer's and Parkinson's disease, among other conditions.

7576 Spirit of Change Magazine
Spirit of Change Magazine
PO Box 405
Uxbridge, MA 01569 508-278-9640
Fax: 508-278-9641
info@spiritofchange.org
www.spiritofchange.org/
Carol Bedrosian, Publisher/Editor
Michella Bedrosian, Advertising Director
Consumer magazine covering holistic health and New Age issues. *$255.00*

7577 The American Wanderer
American Volkssport Association (AVA)
1001 Pat Booker Road
Suite 101
Universal City, TX 78148 210-659-2112
Fax: 210-659-1212
AVAHQ@ava.org
www.ava.org
Henry Rosales, Executive Director, AVA
Consumer magazine covering sports and health news. *$ 20.00*

7578 Ultrasonic Imaging
Sage Journals
2455 Teller Road
Thousand Oaks, CA 91320 805-499-9774
journals@sagepub.com
journals.sagepub.com/home/uix
Ernest J. Feleppa, Editor-in-Chief
Roslyn Raskin, Managing Editor
The journal focuses on the rapid publication of original papers on the development and application of ultrasonic techniques, with emphasis on medical diagnosis. Also published are research notes, comments on papers appearing in the journal, book reviews, and occasional review articles.

7579 VANTAGE
Signature Group Inc.
15-598 Falconbridge Rd.
Sudbury, ON P3A 5 877-688-1989
Fax: 877-688-0808
www.signaturegroupinc.com/
Paul Misniak, Publisher
Joanie Davies, Mailing Contact
Magazine for active consumers over 55 years of age.

7580 VFW Auxiliary
Ladies Auxiliary to the VFW
406 W 34th Street
10th Floor
Kansas City, MO 64111 816-561-8655
Fax: 816-931-4753
info@ladiesauxvfw.org
www.ladiesauxvfw.org/
Armithea "Si Borel, National President
Marilyn Ebersole, Mailing Contact/Editor
VFW auxiliary patriotic services magazine.

7581 Vegetarian Voice
North American Vegetarian Society
PO Box 72
Dolgeville, NY 13329 518-568-7970
Fax: 518-568-7979
navs@telenet.net
www.navs-online.org
Maribeth Abrams, Managing Editor
Brian Graff, Executive Manager
Consumer magazine covering vegetarianism, health, cooking, environmental and animal protection issues. *$203.00*
40 pages

7582 Veggie Life
EGW.com
4075 Papazian Way
208
Fremont, CA 94538 925-671-9852
Fax: 925-671-0692
www.egw.com/
Shanna Masters, Editor
Rickie Wilson, Advertising Manager
Consumer magazine covering health, nutrition, and vegetarian cooking. *$23.70*
68 pages

7583 Vim & Vigor Magazine
McMurry
1010 E. Missouri Ave.
Phoenix, AZ 85014 602-395-5850
800-282-5850
Fax: 602-395-5853
mcmurrytmg.com/
Matthew Peterson, CEO
Fred Petrovsky, COO
Magazine offering articles on health, fitness, and medical research. *$7.00*

7584 WebMD Magazine
WebMD, LLC
395 Hudson Street
New York, NY 10014 www.webmd.com/magazine
Vanessa Cognard, Publisher
Kristy Hammam, Editor in Chief

7585 eNeuro
Society for Neuroscience
1121 14th Street NW
Suite 1010
Washginton, DC 20005 202-312-7305
eNeuro@sfn.org
www.eneuro.org
Christophe Bernard, Editor-in-Chief
Kelly Newton, Director, Scientific Publications
Open-access journal of the Society for Neuroscience.

Newsletters

7586 AGRAM
Assoc of Ohio Philanthropic Homes, Housing/Service
855 S Wall St
Columbus, OH 43206-1921 614-444-2882
Fax: 614-444-2974
www.aopha.org
John Alfano, CEO
Tim White, Executive Director
P Alfano, President/CEO
Weekly

7587 Aging & Vision News
Lighthouse International
111 E 59th St
New York, NY 10022-1202 212-821-9216
800-829-0500
Fax: 212-821-9707
info@lighthouse.org
www.lightfair.com
Laurie A Silbersweig, Editorial Director

Intended for professionals engaged in research, education or service delivery in the field of vision and aging.
6-12 pages Newsletter

7588 Aging News Alert
C D Publications
8204 Fenton St
Silver Spring, MD 20910-4502   301-588-6380
                                             800-666-6380
                                             Fax: 301-588-6385
Michael Gerecht, President
Ash Gerecht, Co-Owner
Reports on successful senior programs, funding opportunities, and federal actions that effect the elderly. Available in 6, 12 or 24 month subscriptions online and online/print combinations. *$192.00*
8 pages Monthly

7589 CAHSA Connecting
Colorado Assoc of Homes and Services for the Aging
1888 Sherman St
Suite 610
Denver, CO 80203-1160   303-837-8834
                                             Fax: 303-837-8836
                                             info@cahsa.org
                                             www.leadingagecolorado.org
Laura Landwirth, Executive Director
Elisabeth Borden, Director
Maureen Hewitt, President
CAHSA Connecting is published monthly by the Colorado Association of Homes and Services for the Aging (CAHSA)

7590 CANPFA-Line
CT Assoc of Not-for-Profit Providers of the Aging
1340 Wilmington Rdg
Berlin, CT 6037   860-828-2903
                                             Fax: 860-828-8694
                                             leadingagect@leadingagect.org
                                             www.leadingagect.org
Mag Morelli, President
Nurka Carrero, Office Manager
Andrea Bellofiore, Director of Member Programs & Se
LeadingAge Connecticut promotes and advocates for a vision of the world in which every community offers an integrated and co-ordinated continuum of high quality, affordable health care, housing and community based services.
Bi-Monthly

7591 Capitol Focus
Colorado Assoc of Homes and Services for the Aging
1888 Sherman St
Suite 610
Denver, CO 80203-1160   303-837-8834
                                             Fax: 303-837-8836
                                             info@cahsa.org
                                             www.leadingagecolorado.org
Laura Landwirth, Executive Director
Elisabeth Borden, Director
Maureen Hewitt, President
Capitol Focus is a weekly activities summary of the Colorado Legislature for CAHSA members, provided by staff of the Colorado Association of Homes and Services for the Aging.

7592 Capsule
Children of Aging Parents
P.O.Box 167
Richboro, PA 18954-167   215-945-6900
                                             800-227-7294
                                             Fax: 215-945-8720
                                             www.caps4caregivers.org
Karen Rosenberg, Director
An informative newsletter for caregivers.
Quarterly

7593 Elder Visions Newsletter
National Indian Council on Aging
8500 Menaul Blvd. NE
Suite B470
Albuquerque, NM 87112   505-292-2001
                                             Fax: 505-292-1922
                                             info@nicoa.org
                                             www.nicoa.org
Randella Bluehouse, Executive Director
Provides information on issues affecting American Indian and Alaska Native Elders.
Quarterly

7594 Enabling News
Access II Independent Living Centers
101 Industrial Parkway
Gallatin, MO 64640-1280   660-663-2423
                                             888-663-2423
                                             Fax: 660-663-2517
                                             TTY: 660-663-2663
                                             access@accessii.org
                                             www.accessii.org
Debra Hawman, Executive Director
Gary Matticks, Owner
Debra Hawman, Executive Director
It is a newsletter published by Access II.
8 pages Quarterly

7595 Independence
Easterseals
141 W Jackson Blvd.
Suite 1400A
Chicago, IL 60604   312-726-6200
                                             800-221-6827
                                             Fax: 312-726-1494
                                             info@easterseals.com
                                             www.easterseals.com
Angela F. Williams, President & CEO
Glenda Oakley, Chief Financial Officer
Marcy Traxler, Senior Vice President, Network Advancement
Newsletter featuring information on Easterseals services, stories and news from the Office of Public Affairs.
Quarterly

7596 Innovations
National Council on Aging
1901 L Street NW
4th Floor
Washington, DC 20036-3506   202-479-1200
                                             Fax: 202-479-0735
                                             TTY: 202-479-6674
                                             info@ncoa.org
                                             www.ncoa.org
James Knickman, Interim President & CEO
Explores significant developments in the field of aging, keeping individuals informed on a broad range of topics.
Quarterly

7597 Legacy
Easterseals
141 W Jackson Blvd.
Suite 1400A
Chicago, IL 60604   312-726-6200
                                             800-221-6827
                                             Fax: 312-726-1494
                                             info@easterseals.com
                                             www.easterseals.com
Angela F. Williams, President & CEO
Glenda Oakley, Chief Financial Officer
Marcy Traxler, Senior Vice President, Network Advancement
Newsletter focusing on planned giving and charitable gift annuities for Easterseals.

7598   NASUA News
National Association of State Units on Aging
1201 15th Street NW
Suite 350
Washington, DC 20005-2842   202-898-2578
                                       Fax: 202-898-2583
                                       www.nasuad.org

Martha Roherty, Executive Director
Peggie Rice, Director of Policy and Legislative Affairs
Eric Risteen, Chief Operating Officer
It is the newsletter of the National Association of State Units on Aging
Monthly

7599   NCOA Week
National Council on Aging
1901 L Street NW
4th Floor
Washington, DC 20036-3540   202-479-1200
                                       Fax: 202-479-0735
                                       TTY: 202-479-6674
                                       info@ncoa.org
                                       www.ncoa.org

James Knickman, Interim President/CEO
Donna Whitt, SVP/CFO
A concise e-newsletters focused on the issues you care about, including policies that affect funding, grants and awards you can apply for, and best practices you can adapt for your center.
Weekly

7600   NNEAHSA
Northn New England Assoc of Homes & Svcs for Aging
PO Box 1428
Standish, ME 04084-1428   207-773-4822
                                       Fax: 207-773-0101
                                       www.agingservicesmenh.org

Sheila Deringis, Editor
Providing healthy, affordable and ethical long-term care to older citizens throughout Maine, New Hampshire and Vermont.

7601   NSCLC Washington Weekly
National Senior Citizens Law Center
1444 Eye St NW
Suite 1100
Washington, DC 20005-6547   202-289-6976
                                       Fax: 202-289-7224
                                       www.nsclc.org

Paul Nathanson, Executive Director
Edward King, Executive Director
Edward Spurgeon, Executive Director
Provides the latest case information, administration and congressional developments of importance for the elderly.

7602   Part B News
DecisionHealth
9737 Washingtonian Blvd
Two Washingtonian Center, Suite. 20
Gaithersburg, MD 20878-7364   301-287-2682
                                          855-225-5341
                                       Fax: 301-287-2535
                                       customer@decisionhealth.com
                                       www.decisionhealth.com

Scott Kraft, Editor
Scott Kraft, Director, Content Management
Steve Greenberg, President
Each week Part B News brings you comprehensive Medicare Part B regulatory coverage, plain-English interpretive guidance, Fee Schedule updates, claims filing strategies, coding, documentation and payment best practices, and the latest on Congressional health care deliberations and how they affect your practice.
$519.00
Yearly

7603   Post-Polio Health
Post-Polio Health International
50 Crestwood Executive Ctr.
Suite 440
St. Louis, MO 63126   314-534-0475
                                       Fax: 314-534-5070
                                       editor@post-polio.org
                                       www.post-polio.org

Brian M. Tiburzi, Editor
Post-Polio Health supports Post-Polio Health International's educational, research, and advocacy efforts. Offers information about relevant events. Published in February, May, August and November.
12 pages Quarterly

7604   Quality First
American Assoc of Homes and Services for the Aging
2519 Connecticut Ave NW
Washington, DC 20008-1520   202-783-2242
                                       Fax: 202-783-2255
                                       www.leadingage.org

William L Minnix Jr, President
Features helpful tips for marketing services and earning the public's trust through the web site.
Quarterly

7605   Senior Focus
National Council on Aging
1901 L Street
4th Floor
Washington, DC 20036-3540   202-479-1200
                                       Fax: 202-479-0735
                                       TTY: 202-479-6674
                                       info@ncoa.org
                                       www.ncoa.org

James Knickman, Interim President & CEO
Contains health, financial, lifestyle tips written for seniors
Quarterly

7606   Social Security Bulletin
US Social Security Administration

                                          800-772-1213
                                       TTY: 800-325-0778
                                       www.ssa.gov/policy
Stephen G. Evangelista, Acting Deputy Commissioner
Dawn S. Wiggins, Associate Commissioner
Natalie T. Lu, Associate Commissioner
Reports on results of research and analysis pertinent to the Social Security and SSI programs. *$16.00*
Monthly

Support Groups

7607   Area Agency on Aging of Southwest Arkansas
600 Columbia Road 11 East
PO Box 1863
Magnolia, AR 71753   870-234-7410
                                          800-272-2127
                                       Fax: 870-234-6804
                                       www.agewithdignity.com

Janet Morrison, Executive Director
The Area Agency on Aging of Southwest Arkansas, Inc. is a non-profit organization serving adults age 60 or older, family caregivers, agencies and organizations working with seniors. It is part of a national network of more than 650 Area Agencies on Aging throughout the United States.

7608   Area Agency on Aging: Region One
1366 E Thomas Rd
Suite 108
Phoenix, AZ 85014-5739   602-264-2255
                                          888-783-7500
                                       Fax: 602-230-9132
                                       www.aaaphx.org

Mary Lynn Kasunic, President
Jeannine Berg, Vice Chairman
Bobbie Garland, Vice Chairman

We have a vast variety of programs and services to enhance the quality of life for residents of Maricopa County, Arizona. If you would like more information about services mentioned within the website please call.

7609 High Country Council of Governments Area Agency on Aging
468 New Market Blvd
Boone, NC 28607-1820
828-265-5434
Fax: 828-265-5439
breece@regiond.org
www.regiond.org

Robert L. Johnson, Chairman
Gary D. Blevins, Vice Chair
Brenda Lyerly, Secretary
High Country Council of Governments is the multi-county planning and development agency for the seven northwestern North Carolina counties of Alleghany, Ashe, Avery, Mitchell, Watauga, Wilkes, and Yancey. The High Country region is a voluntary association of towns and counties located in the northern mountains of North Carolina.

7610 Institute on Aging
3575 Geary Blvd
San Francisco, CA 94118-3212
415-750-4111
877-750-4111
Fax: 415-750-5337
info@ioaging.org
www.ioaging.org

J. Thomas Briody, MHSc, President
Dustin Harper, Vice President, Community Living Services
Cindy Kauffman, MS, COO
Support Services for Elders (SSE) provides care coordination, household management, personal support, bookkeeping, and other assistance to help protect your financial affairs.

7611 Land-of-Sky Regional Council Area Agency on Aging
339 New Leicester Hwy
Suite 140
Asheville, NC 28806-2087
828-251-6622
Fax: 828-251-6353
info@landofsky.org
www.landofsky.org

LeeAnne Tucker, Aging & Volunteer Services Director
Terry Albrecht, Program Director
Joan Tuttle, Director
Is the designated regional organization to meet the needs of persons over 60 in Buncombe, Henderson, Madison, and Transylvania counties, by the North Carolina Division of Aging and Adult Services.

7612 Lumber River Council of Governments Area Agency on Aging
30 Cj Walker Rd
COMtech Park
Pembroke, NC 28372-7340
910-618-5533
Fax: 910-521-7556
lrcog@mail.lrcog.dst.nc.us
www.lumberrivercog.org

Michelle Gaitley, Nutrition Program Director
Renee Cooper, Nutrition Program Assistant
Kristen Elk Maynor, Aging Program Coordinator
The Family Caregiver Support Program was created to assist family members, neighbors, and friends who help care for a person over the age of 60, or minor grandchildren being reared by a grandparent over 60.

7613 Mid-America Regional Council - Aging and Adult Services
600 Broadway
Suite 200
Kansas City, MO 64105-1659
816-474-4240
Fax: 816-421-7758
marcinfo@marc.org
www.marc.org/Community/Aging/

James Stowe, Director of Aging & Adult Services
Bob Hogan, Manager of Aging Administrative Services
Shannon Halvorsen, Information & Referral Coordinator
The Department of Aging and Adult Services offers community-based services to aging people in the Cass, Clay, Jackson,

Platte and Ray counties. Services include home care, transportation, legal aid, breaks for caregivers and meal delivery.

7614 Mid-Carolina Area Agency on Aging
130 Gillespie Street
3rd Floor, Post Office Drawer 1510
Fayetteville, NC 28301-1510
910-323-4191
Fax: 910-323-9330
gdye@mccog.org
www.mccog.org

James Caldwell, COG Executive Director
Glenda Dye, Aging Director
Lynda Barnett, Aging Care Manager
The Mid-Carolina Area Agency on Aging is designated for planning, administration, and advocacy of services for persons aged 60 and older and their spouses who need assistance in order to remain as independent as possible.

7615 Piedmont Triad Council of Governments Area Agency on Aging
2216 W Meadowview Rd
Suite 201
Greensboro, NC 27407-3480
336-294-4950
Fax: 336-632-0457
www.ptcog.org

Blair Barton-Percival, Director
Adrienne Calhoun, Assistant Director
Bob Cleveland, Aging Program Planner
Responsible for planning, developing, implementing, and coordinating aging services for seven counties in the Piedmont Triad (Alamance, Caswell, Davidson, Guilford, Montgomery, Randolph, and Rockingham) and their 185,00 residents age 60 and older.

7616 Southwestern Commission Area Agency on Aging
125 Bonnie Ln
Sylva, NC 28779-8552
828-586-1962
Fax: 828-586-1968
www.regiona.org

Ryan Sherby, Executive Director
Beth Cook, Workforce Development Director
Janne Mathews, Aging Program Coordinator
The Area Agency on Aging (AAA) works on behalf of older adults and their caregivers in the seven southwestern counties of North Carolina. The Southwestern Commission Area Agency on Aging was established in 1980 as mandated by the 1977 Amendments of the Older Americans Act in order for a Planning and Service Area (PSA) to receive funds from the Act.

7617 Tompkins County Office for the Aging
214 W. Martin Luther King Jr./State
Ithaca, NY 14850-4299
607-274-5482
Fax: 607-274-5495
lholmes@tompkins-co.org

Lisa Holmes, Director
Lisa Lunas, Aging Services Planner
Katrina Schickel, Aging Services Specialist
We provide objective and unbiased information regarding the array of services available for older adults and their caregivers. Established in 1975, our mission is to assist the senior population of Tompkins County to remain independent in their homes as long as is possible and appropriate, and with a decent quality of life and human dignity.

7618 Triangle J Council of Governments Area Agency on Aging
4307 Emperor Blvd
Suite 110
Durham, NC 27703
919-549-0551
Fax: 919-549-9390
ejones@tjcog.org
www.tjaaa.org

Kristen Jackson, Aging Program Coordinator
Mary Warren, Director
Ashley Price, Program Specialist
The Triangle J Council of Governments serves to facilitate and support the development of programs addressing the needs of older adults and to support investment in their talents and interests.

7619 University of California Memory and Aging Center
675 Nelson Rising Lane
Suite 190
San Francisco, CA 94143-1207   415-353-2057
                                     Fax: 415-476-5591

Bruce L Miller, Director
Mary Koestler, Project Administrator
Carrie Cheung, Clinic Coordinator
Provides support for patients and families affected by
neurodegenerative diseases. In addition to our established sup-
port groups, we continue to develop new support groups.

**7620 Upper Coastal Plain Council of Governments Area
Agency on Aging**
PO Box 9
Wilson, NC 27894-9   252-234-5952
                                     Fax: 252-234-5971
                                     www.ucpcog.org

Greg Godard, Executive Director
Jody Riddle, AAA Program Director
Helen Page, Aging Programs Specialist
The Upper Coastal Plain Area Agency On Aging is one of 16 Area
Agencies on Aging across the state of NC, serving Region L.
Counties include Edgecombe, Halifax, Nash, Northampton, and
Wilson. The mission of the Area Agency on Aging is to empower
senior adults, family caregivers, and individuals with disabilities
residing in Edgecombe, Halifax, Nash, Northampton, and Wilson
Counties to live independent, meaningful, healthy, and dignified
lives.

Blind & Deaf

Audio/Visual

5261 Getting in Touch
2612 N Mattis Ave
PO Box 7886
Champaign, IL 61826-1053

217-352-3273
800-519-2707
Fax: 217-352-1221
orders@researchpress.com
www.researchpress.com

Russell Pence, President
David Parkinson, Chairman
Cynthia Martin, Principal

5273 Journey
Landmark Media
3450 Slade Run Dr
Falls Church, VA 22042-3940

703-241-2030
800-342-4336
Fax: 703-536-9540
info@landmarkmedia.com
landmarkmedia.com

Michael Hartogs, President
Richard Hartogs, VP Acquisitions
Peter Hartogs, VP New Business & Development
A moving portrayal of the extraordinary journey to Japan of 74-year-old Billie Sinclair, who is deaf, blind and mute. He funds his travels by weaving and selling baskets. In Japan he rides a roller coaster, tries judo and visits a deaf and blind acupuncturist. He demonstrates how it is possible to communicate by touch alone. *$195.00*
Video

Associations

7621 American Association of the Deaf-Blind
248 Rainbow Drive
Suite 14864
Livingston, TX 77399-2048

aadb-info@aadb.org
www.aadb.org

Rene Pellerin, President
Mindy Dill, Vice President
Tara Invidiato, Secretary
The American Association of the Deaf-Blind (AADB) is a non-profit national consumer organization run by and for deaf-blind Americans and their supporters. Deaf-Blind includes all types and degrees of dual vision and hearing loss. The association offers an information clearinghouse, service provider summit, deaf-blind technology summit, research projects, interpretation services, conferences and more.

7622 American Society for Deaf Children
PO Box 23
Woodbine, MD 21797

800-942-2732
info@deafchildren.org
deafchildren.org

Alisha Joslyn-Swob, President
Mark Drolsbaugh, Vice President
Rachel Berman, Secretary
The American Society for Deaf Children provides information for the caretakers of deaf children so children can have full communication access in their home, school and community. The society covers areas such as visual language, audiologists, healthcare providers, assistive technology and more.

7623 Arena Stage
The Mead Center for American Theater
1101 Sixth St. SW
Washington, DC 20024

202-554-9066
Fax: 202-488-4056
TTY: 202-484-0247
info@arenastage.org
arenastage.org

Edgar Dobie, Executive Director
Molly Smith, Artistic Director
Joseph Berardelli, CFO
Arena Stage has played a pioneering role in providing access to all productions for people with disabilities. Access services and programs include wheelchair accessible seating; infrared assistive listening devices; Braille, large print, audio description and sign interpretation at designated performances.

7624 Association of Late-Deafened Adults
8038 Macintosh Ln
Suite 2
Rockford, IL 61107-5336

815-332-1515
TTY: 815-332-1515
www.alda.org

Rick Brown, President
Cynthia Moynihan, Vice President
Matt Ferrara, Treasurer
The Association of Late-Deafened Adults supports the empowerment of late-deafened people by offering programs and information resources on a variety of topics: technology, disability laws, airline travel and more.

7625 Canadian Deafblind Association
1860 Appleby Line
Unit 14
Burlington, ON, Canada L7L-7H7

905-331-6279
866-229-5832
Fax: 905-319-2027
info@cdbanational.com
www.cdbanational.com

Carolyn Monaco, President
Tom McFadden, National Executive Director
The mission of the Canadian Deafblind Association is to promote and enhance the well-being of people who are deafblind by offering them advocacy, developing and dissemination information, and supporting members and community partners who also serve deafblind people.

7626 Foundation Fighting Blindness
7168 Columbia Gateway Dr.
Suite 100
Columbia, MD 21046

410-423-0600
800-683-5555
TTY: 410-363-7139
info@FightBlindness.org
www.blindness.org

Benjamin R. Yerxa, Chief Executive Officer
Jason Menzo, Chief Operating Officer
Todd Durham, VP, Clinical & Outcomes Research
The Foundation Fighting Blindness (FFB) works to promote research in order to prevent, treat and restore vision. FFB is currently the world's leading private funder of retinal disease research, funding over 100 research grants and 150 researchers.

7627 Future Reflections
Deaf-Blind Division of the Ntn'l Fed of the Blind
200 E. Wells St.
at Jernigan Place
Baltimore, MD 21230

410-659-9314
Fax: 410-685-5653
nfbpublications@nfb.org
www.nfb.org

Deborah Kent Stein, Editor
A quarterly magazine for parents and teachers of blind children.

7628 Hearing Loss Association of America
7910 Woodmont Ave
Suite 1200
Bethesda, MD 20814
301-657-2248
Fax: 301-913-9413
inquiry@hearingloss.org
www.hearingloss.org

Barbara Kelley, Executive Director
Lise Hamlin, Director of Public Policy
Carla Beyer-Smolin, National Chapter & Membership Coordinator
The mission of the Hearing Loss Association of America is to open the world of communication to people with hearing loss by offering information, education, resources, advocacy and training.

7629 Helen Keller National Center for Deaf- Blind Youths and Adults
141 Middle Neck Rd
Sands Point, NY 11050
516-944-8900
TTY: 516-570-3246
hkncinfo@hknc.org
www.helenkeller.org

Kim Zimmer, President & CEO
Marc Feldman, CPA, Chief Financial Officer
Mary Fu, Chief Development Officer
The center serves deafblind people by offering them assistive technology, vocational services, education, case management, interpretation, medical and mental health services, professional training and other supports that would empower them to work and live independently within their communities.

7630 Idaho Commission for the Blind and Visually Impaired
341 W. Washington St
PO Box 83720
Boise, ID 83720-0012
208-334-3220
800-542-8688
Fax: 208-334-2963
bcunningham@icbvi.idaho.gov
www.icbvi.state.id.us

Britt Raubenheimer, Chair
Beth Cunningham, Administrator
Bailie Welton, Management Assistant
The Idaho Commission for the Blind and Visually Impaired works to empower persons who are blind or visually impaired by providing vocational rehabilitation training, skills training and educational opportunities to achieve self fulfillment ang gain employment. The Commission also strives to serve as a resource to families and employers and to expand public awareness regarding the potential of all persons who are blind or visually impaired.

7631 International Hearing Society
16880 Middlebelt Rd
Suite 4
Livonia, MI 48154
734-522-7200
Fax: 734-522-0200
interact@ihsinfo.org
ihsinfo.org

Annette Cross, BC-HIS, President
Kathleen Mennillo, MBA, Executive Director
Fran Vincent, Director, Membership & Marketing
The International Hearing Society (IHS) represents hearing healthcare professionals worldwide. Members include professionals engaged in the practice of testing human hearing and selecting, fitting and dispensing hearing instruments. IHS offers accreditation programs, advocacy, education and training in support of these services.

7632 Lilac Services for the Blind
1212 N Howard St
Spokane, WA 99201
509-328-9116
800-422-7893
Fax: 509-328-8965
contact@lilacblind.org
lilacblind.org

Eddie Eugenio, President
Cheryl L Martin, Executive Director
Robin Waller, Development Director
Lilac Services for the Blind provides independent living instruction, adaptive aids, counseling, low-vision evaluations, support groups, Braille transcription services and more for 14 counties in the inland Northwest.

7633 National Center on Deaf-Blindness (NCDB)
Hellen Keller National Center
141 Middle Neck Rd.
Sands Point, NY 11050
541-800-0412
support@nationaldb.org
www.nationaldb.org

Sam Morgan, Director
Julie Durando, Evaluation Coordinator
Peggy Malloy, Information Services & Technology Coordinator
Funded by the federal Department of Education, the Center seeks to improve quality of life for children who are deaf-blind and their families.

7634 National Family Association for Deaf-Blind
PO Box 1667
Sands Point, NY 11050
800-255-0411
Fax: 516-883-9060
nfadb.org

Patti McGowan, President
Diana Griffen, Vice President
Jacqueline Izaguirre, Treasurer
The National Family Association for Deaf-Blind (NFADB) is a nonprofit, volunteer-based family association. The association offers advocacy, education and family supports to help create empowerment opportunities for deaf-blind people.

7635 National Federation of the Blind
200 E. Wells St.
at Jernigan Place
Baltimore, MD 21230
410-659-9314
Fax: 410-685-5653
nfb@nfb.org
www.nfb.org

Mark A. Riccobono, President
John Berggren, Executive Director, Operations
Anil Lewis, Executive Director, Blindness Initiatives
The National Federation of the Blind (NFB) works to help blind people achieve self-confidence, self-respect and self-determination and to achieve complete integration into society on a basis of equality. The Federation provides public educations, information and referral services, scholarships, literature and publications, adaptive equipment, advocacy services, legal services, employment assistance and more.

Camps

7636 Florida Lions Camp
Lions of Multiple District 35
2819 Tiger Lake Road
Lake Wales, FL 33898-9582
863-696-1948
Fax: 863-696-2398
bjcage@hotmail.com
www.lionscampfl.org

Barbara Cage, Executive Director
Liz Cage, Program Director
Carissa Moen, Bookkeeping/Registrar
One-week sessions June-August for youths and adults with visual impairments and other challenging disabilities. Coed, ages 5 and up. A variety of traditional summer camp activities which include: swimming, canoeing, fishing, hiking, camping out and cooking over a fire, games, arts & crafts, singing & dancing, hay-wagon rides, challenge course and much more. Activities are adapted to the age and ability of each camper to ensure maximum participation, safety and fun.

7637 Florida School for the Deaf and Blind
207 San Marco Ave
St Augustine, FL 32084-2799
904-827-2200
800-344-3732
Fax: 904-827-2325
www.fsdb.k12.fl.us

Dr. Jeanne Glidden Prickett, EdD, Shelter Administrator
Debbie Schuler, Administrator of Instructional S
Cindy Day, Executive Director of Parent Ser

Statewide public boarding school for eligible students who are deaf/hard-of-hearing or blind/visually impaired. FSDB serves children who are pre-k through high school.

Books

7638 A Handbook for Writing Effective Psychoeducational Reports (2nd Edition)
PRO-ED Inc.
8700 Shoal Creek Blvd.
Austin, TX 78757-6897
512-451-3246
800-897-3202
Fax: 800-397-7633
general@proedinc.com
www.proedinc.com

Sharon Bradley-Johnson, Author
C. Merle Johnson, Author
This comprehensive book shows how to write useful reports once assessment information has been attained. It is a valuable resource for professionals working in school systems, as well as for those graduate students who are just learning to write reports. *$32.00*
134 pages Paperback
ISBN 1-416401-40-7

7639 Communicating with People Who Have Trouble Hearing & Seeing: A Primer
National Association for Visually Handicapped
22 W 21st St
Fl 6
New York, NY 10010-6943
212-255-2804
Fax: 212-727-2931
info@lighthouse.org
www.lighthouse.org

Roger O Goldman, Chairman Of The Board
Line drawings that depict problems for those with both deficiencies. *$2.00*

7640 Helen and Teacher: The Story of Helen & Anne Sullivan Macy
American Foundation for the Blind/AFB Press
11 Penn Plz
Suite 300
New York, NY 10001-2006
212-502-7600
800-232-5463
Fax: 212-502-7777
afbinf@afb.net
www.afb.org

Carl Augusto, President
Richard Obnen, Chairman Of The Board
Michael Gilliam, Vice Chairman
A pictorial biography emphasizing Hellen Keller's accomplishments in public life over a period of more than 60 years. Traces Anne Sullivan's early years and her meeting with Helen Keller, and goes on to recount the joint events of their lives. A definitive biography. $29.95.
Paperback
ISBN 0-891282-89-0

7641 Independence Without Sight and Sound: Suggestions for Practitioners
American Foundation for the Blind/AFB Press
11 Penn Plz
Suite 300
New York, NY 10001-2006
212-502-7600
800-232-8463
Fax: 212-502-7777
afbinfo@afb.net
www.afb.org

Carl Augusto, President
Richard Obnen, Chairman Of The Board
Michael Gilliam, Vice Chairman
This practical guidebook covers the essential aspects of communicating and working with deaf-blind persons. Includes useful information on how to talk with deaf-blind people, and adapt orientation and mobility techniques for deaf-blind travelers. *$39.95*
193 pages Paperback
ISBN 0-891282-46-7

7642 Reclaiming Independence: Staying in the Drivers Seat When You Are no Longer Drive.
American Printing House for the Blind
1839 Frankfort Ave
Louisville, KY 40206-3148
502-895-2405
800-223-1839
Fax: 502-899-2274
info@aph.org
www.aph.org

Tuck Tinsley, President
Joseph Paradis, Chairman
Kathleen Huebner, Vice Chairman
Useful for both individuals and professionals, this video/resource guide will help you successfuly use rehabilitation and transportation resources. *$60.00*

7643 Verbal View of the Web & Net
American Printing House for the Blind
1839 Frankfort Ave
Louisville, KY 40206-3148
502-895-2405
800-223-1839
Fax: 502-899-2274
info@aph.org
www.aph.org

Tuck Tinsley, President
Joseph Paradis, Chairman
Kathleen Huebner, Vice Chairman
One of a series of Verbal View titles, Verbal View of the Net & Web explains how to access information on the internet and teaches accessability features of Internet Explorer. *$50.00*

Magazines

7644 Braille Montior
National Federation of the Blind
200 E. Wells St.
at Jernigan Place
Baltimore, MD 21230
410-659-9314
Fax: 410-685-5653
nfbpublications@nfb.org
www.nfb.org

Gary Wunder, Editor
The Braille Monitor is the leading publication of the National Federation of the Blind. It covers the events and activities of the NFB and addresses the many issues and concerns of the blind. *$40.00*
11 times a year

7645 Deaf-Blind American
American Association of the Deaf-Blind
248 Rainbow Drive
Suite 14864
Livingston, TX 77399-2048
aadb-info@aadb.org
www.aadb.org

Rene Pellerin, President
The official magazine of the American Association of the Deaf-Blind (AADB).
Quartlery

7646 Hearing Life Magazine
Hearing Loss Association of America
7910 Woodmont Ave
Ste 1200
Bethesda, MD 20814-7022
301-657-2248
Fax: 301-913-9413
inquiry@hearingloss.org
www.hearingloss.org

Barbara Kelley, Executive Director
Formerly known as Hearing Loss Magazine, this official publication of the Hearing Loss Association of America helps individuals with hearing loss live a better life.
Bi-Monthly

7647 Hearing Professional Magazine
International Hearing Society
Ste 4
16880 Middlebelt Rd
Livonia, MI 48154-3374   734-522-7200
                                  Fax: 734-522-0200
                             knacarato@ihsinfo.org
                                    www.ihsinfo.org

Kathleen Mennillo, Executive Director
The Hearing Professional magazine is the official publication of
the International Hearing Society. This quarterly publication includes industry news, membership highlights and best practices,
hearing healthcare legislation, and other information and tools
for hearing healthcare professionals.

Newsletters

7648 AADB E-News
American Association of the Deaf-Blind
248 Rainbow Drive
Suite 14864
Livingston, TX 77399-2048   aadb-info@aadb.org
                                       www.aadb.org
Rene Pellerin, President
Contains information about the latest events occurring within
AADB and in the deaf-blind community.

7649 ALDA Newsletter
ALDA
8038 Macintosh Ln
Suite 2
Rockford, IL 61107-5336   815-332-1515
                                  TTY: 815-332-1515
                                       www.alda.org
Rick Brown, President
Articles, stories and poems by and about late-deafened adults.

7650 Beam
1850 W Roosevelt Rd
Chicago, IL 60608-1298   312-666-1331
                                  Fax: 312-243-8539
                                  TTY: 312-666-8874
                             www.chicagolighthouse.org
James Kesteloot, President
Terrence Longo, Assistant Director
Quarterly newsletter of the organization offering progressive
programs for the blind, visually impaired, deaf-blind and
multi-disabled children and adults, including vocational programs, computer and office skills training, job placement, independent living skills, orientation and mobility training,
counseling and a low vision clinic.

7651 Deaf-Blind Perspective
National Consortium on Deaf-Blindness
345 Monmouth Ave
Monmouth, OR 97361   503-838-8391
                                       800-438-9376
                                  Fax: 503-838-8150
                                  TTY: 800-854-7013
                                       dbp@wou.edu
John Reiman PhD, Director
Peggy Malloy, Managing Editor
A free publication with articles, essays, and announcements
about topics related to people who are deaf-blind. The primary fo-
cus is on the education of children and youth with deaf-blindness.
Published two times a year (Spring and Fall) by the national con-
sortium on Deaf-blindness at the Teaching Research Institute at
Western Oregon University.

7652 Endeavor Magazine
American Society for Deaf Children
PO Box 23
Woodbine, MD 21797   800-942-2732
                             info@deafchildren.org
                                  www.deafchildren.org
Tami Dominguez, Editor

ASDC's qurterly publication featuring committee reports, stories, and fun.
Quarterly

7653 HKNC Newsletter
Helen Keller National Center
141 Middle Neck Rd
Sands Point, NY 11050-1218   516-944-8900
                                  Fax: 516-944-7302
                                  TTY: 516-944-8637
                                  hkncinfo@hknc.org
                                       www.hknc.org
Joseph McNulty, Executive Director
Highlights recent activities at the national center.

7654 InFocus
7168 Columbia Gateway Dr.
Suite 100
Columbia, MD 21046   410-423-0600
                                       800-683-5555
                                  TTY: 410-363-7139
                             info@FightBlindness.org
                                    www.blindness.org
Benjamin R. Yerxa, Chief Executive Officer
Presents articles on coping, research updates, and Foundation
news.
3x/year

7655 NAT-CENT
Helen Keller National Center
141 Middle Neck Rd
Sands Point, NY 11050-1218   516-944-8900
                                  Fax: 516-944-7302
                                  TTY: 516-944-8637
                                  hkncinfo@hknc.org
                                       www.hknc.org
Joseph McNulty, Executive Director
Contains articles on legislation, services, aids and devices, hu-
man interest and issues related to deaf-blindness.

7656 News from Advocates for Deaf-Blind
National Family Association for Deaf-Blind
PO Box 1667
Sands Point, NY 11050   800-225-0411
                                  Fax: 516-883-9060
                                     www.NFADB.org
Patti McGowan, President
A membership organization which provide resources, education,
advocacy, referrals and support for families with children who
are deaf-blind; professionals in the field; and individuals who are
deaf-blind.
20 pages TriAnnual

Software

7657 Braille + Mobile Manager
American Printing House for the Blind
1839 Frankfort Ave
Louisville, KY 40206-0085   502-895-2405
                                       800-223-1839
                                  Fax: 502-899-2284
                                      info@aph.org
                                           aph.org
Tuck Tinsley, President
Joseph Paradis, Chairman
Kathleen Huebner, Vice Chairman
Use it like a hand-held PDA or like a laptop. *$1395.00*

7658 MaximEyes
American Printing House for the Blind
1839 Frankfort Ave
Louisville, KY 40206-0085   502-895-2405
                                       800-223-1839
                                  Fax: 502-899-2284
                                      info@aph.org
                                           aph.org
Tuck Tinsley, President
Joseph Paradis, Chairman
Kathleen Huebner, Vice Chairman

MaximEyes is a plug-in for Internet Explorer that adds a toolbar that allows you to controll the size of website text and images.
$59.95

Sports

7659 ASD Athletics
Alabama Institute for Deaf and Blind
205 South St E
Talladega, AL 35160-2411   256-761-3222
                                         Fax: 256-761-3278
                              Ripley.Walter@aidb.state.al.us
John Jernigan, Director, Student Development (ASD)
Walter Ripley, Director, Athletics & After-School Programs
Offers students opportunities to participate in a number of organizzed sports including basketball, volleyball, baseball, football, and cheerleading. Student athletes compete at national and international levels.

Support Groups

7660 Aurora of Central New York
518 James Street
Suite 100
Syracuse, NY 13203-2282   315-422-7263
                                       Fax: 315-422-4792
                                       TTY: 315-422-9746
                                       auroraofcny.org
John Scala, President
John McCormick, President
Ryan Emery, Treasurer
Professional counseling services to assist individuals and their families deal with the trauma of hearing or vision loss.

7661 Wendell Johnson Speech And Hearing Clinic
University Of Iowa
250 Hawkins Dr
Iowa City, IA 52242-1025   319-335-8736
                                       Fax: 319-335-8851
                                       kathy-miller@uiowa.edu
                    www.clas.uiowa.edu/comsci/clinical-services
Linda Souke, Clinic Director
Kathy Miller, Clinic Assistant
The clinic offers assessment and remediation for communication disorders in adults and children. The clinic also offers services during the Summer for school age children needing intervention services because of speech, language, hearing and/or reading problems.

Cognitive

Associations

7662 Academy of Cognitive Therapy
245 N. 15th St
Suite 403
Philadelphia, PA 19102
Fax: 215-537-1789
info@academyofct.org
www.academyofct.org

Lata K McGinn, Ph.D, President
Troy Thompson, Executive Director
Allen Miller, Ph.D, MBA, Treasurer
The Academy of Cognitive Therapy is a non-profit organization that supports continuing education and research in cognitive therapy, provides resources for professionals and the public, and offers certification for those skilled in the field.

7663 Adults & Children with Learning & Developmental Disabilities (ACLD)
807 S Oyster Bay Rd.
Bethpage, NY 11714
516-822-0028
www.acld.org

Robert C. Goldsmith, Executive Director
Robert Ciatto, Chief Operating Officer
Aimee C. Keegan, Director, Development & Community Relations
Nonprofit serving Long Island by supporting individuals with developmental disabilities and their families.

7664 Albert Ellis Institute
145 East 32nd St.
9th Fl.
New York, NY 10016
212-535-0822
Fax: 212-249-3582
info@albertellis.org
albertellis.org

Kristene A. Doyle, Director
Psychotherapy training Institute focused on the teachings of Albert Ellis, primarily the therapeutic approach known as Rational Emotive Behavior Therapy (REBT).

7665 American Academy of Child & Adolescent Psychiatry
3615 Wisconsin Ave NW
Washington, DC 20016-3007
202-966-7300
Fax: 202-464-0131
communications@aacap.org
www.aacap.org

Gregory K Fritz, MD, President
Heidi B Fordi, CAE, Executive Director
Karen Ferguson, Deputy Director of Clinical Practice
The American Academy of Child & Adolescent Psychiatry is a non-profit organization engaged in research, education and advocacy specific to child and adolescent psychiatry. The academy's mission is to provide resources and knowledge beneficial to patients, their families and psychiatric professionals.

7666 American Delirium Society
1183 University Dr
Suite 105 - 106
Burlington, NC 27215
410-955-2343
info@americandeliriumsociety.org
www.americandeliriumsociety.org

Rakesh C Arora MD, Ph.D, Director
Noll Campbell, PharmD, MS, Director
John W Devlin, PharmD, Director
The American Delirium Society fosters research, education, quality improvement, advocacy and science to minimize the impact of delirium on short- and long-term health and well being and the effects of delirium on the health care system as a whole. The organization offers educational resources including videos and publications on the subject.

7667 American Psychiatric Association
1000 Wilson Blvd
Suite 1825
Arlington, VA 22209-3901
703-907-7300
703-907-7300
888-357-7924
Fax: 703-907-1085
apa@psych.org
www.psychiatry.org

Anita Everett, MD, President
Saul M Levin, MD, MPA, CEO & Medical Director
Mark Myers, Director, Administrative Services
The American Psychiatric Association is a medical specialty society with over 37,000 member physicians engaged in the field of psychiatric practice, research, and academia. The association's mission is to ensure humane care and effective treatment of all persons with mental disorders, including substance use disorders. Services offered by them include collegial support, advocacy, publications and more.

7668 Anxiety and Depression Association of America (ADAA)
8701 Georgia Ave.
Suite 412
Silver Spring, MD 20910
240-485-1001
Fax: 240-485-1035
information@adaa.org
adaa.org

Susan K. Gurley, Executive Director
Lise Bram, Deputy Executive Director
Vickie Spielman, Associate Director, Membership & Education
The Anxiety and Depression Association of America is an international nonprofit organization and a leader in education, training, and research for anxiety, OCD, PTSD, depression, and related disorders. ADAA encourages the advancement of scientific knowledge about the causes and treatment for mental health issues.

7669 Association for Behavioral and Cognitive Therapies (ABCT)
305 7th Ave
16th Floor
New York, NY 10001
212-647-1890
Fax: 212-647-1865
www.abct.org

Gail Steketee, Ph.D, President
Barbara Kamholz, Ph.D, Convention & Continuing Education Issues
Shireen Rizvi, Ph.D, Academic & Professional Issues
The ABCT is an organization committed to the advancement of scientific approaches to address the issues of soldiers with PTSD. The association offeres information in a number of areas: combat related stress, military posttraumatic stress disorder, military suicide and veterans' health.

7670 Association for Contextual Behavioral Science
1880 Pinegrove Dr
P.O. Box 655
Jenison, MI 49429
225-302-8688
staff@contextualscience.org
contextualscience.org

Emily Rodrigues, Executive Director
Courtney Zirkle, CMP, Administrative & Social Media Manager
The Association for Contextual Behavioral Science specializes in helping people through research and practice based in contextual behavioral science (including RFT and CBS). The association offers learning resources, training, internships, events, consultations, conferences, continuing education opportunities and more.

7671 Autism National Committee (AUTCOM)
3 Bedford Green
South Burlington, VT 05403
info@autcom.org
www.autcom.org

Anne Bakeman, Membership Coordinator
Seeks to protect and advnce the rights of all individuals with autism, Pervasive Developmental Disorder, and related conditions.

7672 Autism Network International (ANI)
PO Box 35448
Syracuse, NY 13235-5448   www.autismnetworkinternational.org
Jim Sinclair, Coordinator

Autistic-run organization offering advocacy and self-help services for autistic people.

7673 Autism Research Institute
4182 Adams Ave.
San Diego, CA 92116-2599   866-366-3361
                                            www.autism.com
Stephen Edelson, Ph.D, Executive Director
Anthony Morgali, Producer, ARI Media
Denise Fulton, Administrative Director
Conducts research on the causes, diagnosis and treatment of autism. The institute also offers a quarterly newsletter that reviews worldwide research, referrals to health care professionals and clinics serving autistic people, advocacy, continuing education and more.

7674 Autism Services Center
929 4th Ave.
P.O. Box 507
Huntington, WV 25701-0507   304-525-8014
                                       Fax: 304-525-8026
                                  www.autismservicescenter.org
Ralph N Bentley, President
Jimmie Beirne, Ph.D, CEO
The Autism Services Center assists families and agencies to meet the needs of individuals with autism and other developmental disabilities by offering services such as technical assistance in designing treatment programs, a hotline providing informational packets to callers, supported employment, day programs, residential services and more.

7675 Autism Society of Minnesota
Autism Society of Minnesota
2380 Wycliff St.
Suite 102
St. Paul, MN 55114   651-647-1083
                                       Fax: 651-642-1230
                                           info@ausm.org
                                           www.ausm.org
Ellie Wilson, Executive Director
Dawn Brasch, Senior Director, Finance & Operations
Kelly Thomalla, Senior Director, Integration & Advancement
The Autism Society of Minnesota (AuSM) is a nonprofit membership organization dedicated to the education, advocacy, and support of individuals and families who have been affected by autism.

7676 Autism Treatment Center of America
2080 S Undermountain Rd
Sheffield, MA 01257-9643   413-229-2100
                                            877-766-7473
                                       Fax: 413-229-8931
                                 correspondence@option.org
                                  www.autismtreatmentcenter.org
Barry Neil Kaufman, Founder & CEO
Clyde Haberman, Senior Teacher & Director of Development
Blair Borgeson, Developmental Therapist
The Autism Treatment Center of America provides innovative training programs for parents and professionals caring for children challenged by Autism, Autism Spectrum Disorders, Pervasive Developmental Disorders (PDD) and other development difficulties. The center's Son-Rise Program teaches a comprehensive system of treatment and education designed to help families and caregivers enable their children to improve in all areas of learning.

7677 Autistic Self Advocacy Network (ASAN)
PO Box 66122
Washington, DC 20035   info@autisticadvocacy.org
                              autisticadvocacy.org
Julia Bascom, Executive Director
Zoe Gross, Director, Operations
Samantha Crane, Legal Directory & Director, Public Policy
Promotes a world in which equal access, rights and opportunities are available to autistic people, through advocacy and empowerment.

7678 Beck Institute for Cognitive Behavior Therapy
1 Belmont Ave
Suite 700
Bala Cynwyd, PA 19004   610-664-3020
                                       Fax: 610-709-5336
                                       info@beckinstitute.org
                                       www.beckinstitute.org
Aaron T Beck, Ph.D, President Emeritus
Judith S Beck, Ph.D, President
Lisa Pote, Executive Director
The Beck Institute for Cognitive Behavior Therapy serves as a training ground for cognitive therapists and cognitive behavior therapists. The institute provides online resources, training workshops and CBT therapy for the public and mental health professionals.

7679 Best Buddies
907-1243 Islington Ave
Toronto, ON, Canada M8X-1Y9   416-531-0003
                                            888-779-0061
                                       Fax: 416-531-0325
                                       info@bestbuddies.ca
                                           bestbuddies.ca
Daniel J Greenglass, Co-Chair
Sarah McCarthy, Program Coordinator
Kimberly Janohan, Program Support
Best Buddies offers programs for people with intellectual or developmental disabilities including those with Down syndrome, autism, cerebral palsy, traumatic brain injury and other undiagnosed disabilities. Programs include schooling, transition programs, sports, scholarships and more.

7680 Biologically Inspired Cognitive Architectures Society
4450 Rivanna River Way
Suite 3707
Fairfax, VA 22030-4441   703-910-3014
                                       Fax: 877-532-0197
                                       info@bicasociety.org
                                           bicasociety.org
Alexei V Samsonovich, President-Treasurer
Antonio Chella, Chair
Kamilla R Johannsdottir, Secretary
The Biologically Inspired Cognitive Architectures Society brings together researchers from disjointed fields and communities in order to combine their knowledge into forming a larger, unifying framework for the study of cognitive architectures.

7681 Brain Injury Alliance of Texas
9050 N Capital of Texas Hwy
Building 3, Suite 130
Austin, TX 78759   512-326-1212
                                            800-392-0040
                                       Fax: 512-478-3370
                                           www.texasbia.org
Kelly Ramsey, President
Greg Walton, Vice President
Mendi West, Secretary-Treasurer
The Brain Injury Alliance of Texas is a community of people with brain injuries, their families and the professionals that serve them. The alliance offers information, support groups, prevention strategies, educational opportunities, public policy advocacy, a resource library and more.

7682 Brain Injury Association of America (BIAA)
3057 Nutley St.
Suite 805
Fairfax, VA 22031-1931   703-761-0750
                                       Fax: 703-761-0755
                                           info@biausa.org
                                           www.biausa.org
Susan H. Connors, President & Chief Executive Officer
Shana De Caro, Chairwoman
Page Melton Ivie, Vice Chairwoman
The Brain Injury Association of America is a national organization serving and representing individuals, families and professionals who are touched by a traumatic brain injury (TBI). Its mission is to improve the quality of life for people affected by brain injury through the advancement of research, treatment, education and awareness.
1980

7683 Brain Injury Association of New York State
4 Pine W Plaza
Suite 402
Albany, NY 12205   518-459-7911
                                           800-444-6443
                                      Fax: 518-482-5285
                                      info@bianys.org
                                           bianys.org

Barry Dain, President
Eileen Reardon, Executive Director
Debbie Berenda-Chilandese, Director of Finance & Administration
The Brain Injury Association of New York State is a statewide non-profit membership organization that provides education, advocacy and community support services leading to improved outcomes for children and adults with brain injuries and their families. The association also offers chapters and support groups throughout the state, prevention programs, mentoring programs, speakers bureau and publications library.

7684 BroadFutures
National Youth Transitions Center
2013 H St, NW
5th Floor
Washington, DC 20006   202-521-4304
                                      info@broadfutures.org
                                           broadfutures.org

Bradley P Holmes, Chairman
Carolyn K Jeppsen, CEO & President
Diana Eisenstat, Secretary
BroadFutures offers transitional programs for youth with learning disabilities. The mission of the organization is to assit these youth in overcoming barriers to employment.

7685 Center Academy
6710 86th Ave. N
Pinellas Park, FL 33782   727-541-5716
                                      Fax: 727-544-8186
                                      infopp@centeracademy.com
                                           www.centeracademy.com

Mack R. Hicks, Founder & Chair
Andrew P. Hicks, Chief Executive Officer & Clinical Director
Eric V. Larson, President & Chief Operating Officer
Center Academy assists children with learning disabilities, difficulties in concentration and underdeveloped social skills. Programs offered include high impact learning, community involvement opportunities, ADHD schools, autism and asperger's schools, dyslexia treatment, special education schools and more.

7686 Cerebral Palsy Associations of New York State
Central Office & Metropolitan Services
330 W 34th St
15th Floor
New York, NY 10001-2488   212-947-5770
                                      information@cpofnys.org
                                           www.cpofnys.org

Stephen C Lipinski, Chairman
Susan Constantino, President & CEO
Michael A Alvaro, Executive Vice President
The Cerebral Palsy Associations of New York is a multi-service organization that provides services and programs for individuals with cerebral palsy and developmental disabilities, as well as resources for families.

7687 Child Neurology Society
1000 W County Rd E
Suite 290
Saint Paul, MN 55126   651-486-9447
                                      Fax: 651-486-9436
                                      nationaloffice@childneurologysociety.org
                                           www.childneurologysociety.org

Kenneth Mack, President
Roger Larson, Executive Director
Sue Hussman, Associate Director
The Child Neurology Society is designed for patiens, parents, and professionals alike, with the aim of promoting continued research, providing support, and offering informational resources and guidance on the subject of child neurology. Members include child neurologists and related medical professionals.

7688 Children and Adults with Attention-Deficit Hyperactivity Disorder
CHADD
4601 Presidents Dr
Suite 300
Lanham, MD 20706   301-306-7070
                                      Fax: 301-306-7090
                                      affiliate-services@chadd.org
                                           www.chadd.org

Michael MacKay, President
Leslie Kain, MBA, Executive Director
Robyn Maggio, MSW, Education & Training Coordinator
The Children and Adults with Attention-Deficit/Hyperactivity Disorder (CHADD) is a non-profit organization providing supports to people with ADHD. Some services offered include advocacy, education, employment, a resource directory, training programs, publications on research and more.

7689 Cognitive Neuroscience Society
267 Cousteau Place
Davis, CA 95618   916-850-0837
                                      cnsinfo@cogneurosociety.org
                                           www.cogneurosociety.org

Roberto Cabeza, Ph.D, Board Member
Marta Kutas, Ph.D, Board Member
Kate Tretheway, Executive Director
The Cognitive Neuroscience Society is committed to investigating the psychological, computational, and neuroscientific bases of cognition through research.

7690 Cognitive Science Society
108 E Dean Keeton
Stop A8000
Austin, TX 78712-1043   512-471-2030
                                      Fax: 512-471-3053
                                      cogsci@austin.utexas.edu
                                           www.cognitivesciencesociety.org

Susan Gelman, Chair
Terry Regier, Chair Elect
Anna Drummey, Executive Officer
The Cognitive Science Society brings together researchers from around the world who desire to understand the workings of the human mind. The society's mission is to promote the study of cognitive science and build connections between researchers in various areas of study (including Artificial Intelligence, Linguistics, Anthropology, Psychology, Neuroscience, Philosophy, and Education).

7691 Cognitive Science Student Association
University of California
Berkeley, CA   cssa.berkeley@gmail.com
                                           cssa.berkeley.edu

Timothy Guan, President
Harshali Wadge, Internal Vice President
Connor Brown, Outreach Coordinator
The Cognitive Science Student Association supports and enriches the academic life of anyone interested in the interdisciplinary field of cognitive science. Some programs offered by the association include guest lectures and information sessions, professor-student dinners, academic outreach program and California Cognitive Science Conference.

7692 Dementia Society of America
PO Box 600
Doylestown, PA 18901   800-336-3684
                                      knowdementia@dementiasociety.org
                                           www.dementiasociety.org

Kevin Jameson, President & Founder
The Dementia Society of America (DSA) is a nonprofit volunteer-run organization providing resources and information about dementia to individuals, corporations and organizations.

7693 Depression and Bipolar Support Alliance
55 E Jackson Blvd
Suite 490
Chicago, IL 60604
800-826-3632
Fax: 312-642-7243
dbsasocial@gmail.com
www.dbsalliance.org

William Gilmer, MD, Chair
Allen Doederlein, President
Cindy Specht, Executive Vice President

The Depression and Bipolar Support Alliance is a peer-directed national organization dedicated to offering supports to those living with depression or bipolar disorder. Some services they offer include peer support, education, advocacy and research.

7694 Epilepsy Foundation
8301 Professional Place E
Suite 200
Landover, MD 20785- 2353
800-332-1000
Fax: 301-459-1569
ContactUs@efa.org
www.epilepsy.com

Robert W Smith, Chair
Phillip M. Gattone, M.Ed, President & CEO
M. Vaneeda Bennett, Chief Development Officer

The Epilepsy Foundation is the national voluntary health agency dedicated to the welfare of people with epilepsy in the U.S. and their families. The organization works to ensure that people with seizures are able to participate in all life experiences; to improve how people with epilepsy are perceived, accepted and valued in society; and to promote research for a cure.

7695 FOCUS Center for Autism
126 Dowd Ave.
PO Box 452
Canton, CT 06019
860-693-8809
Fax: 860-693-0141
info@focuscenterforautism.org
www.focuscenterforautism.org

Patricia A. Cables, President
Timothy Grady, Secretary
Donna Swanson, Executive Director

FOCUS Center for Autism is a nonprofit center to help children and young adults with autism spectrum disorder, and other related disorders, achieve their full potential.

7696 Geneva Centre for Autism
112 Merton St.
Toronto, ON, Canada M4S-2Z8
416-322-7877
Fax: 416-322-5894
info@autism.net
www.autism.net

Abe Evreniadis, Chief Executive Officer
Kathy Shaw, Chief Financial Officer
Renita Paranjape, Senior Director, Programs & Services

The Geneva Centre for Autism's mission is to empower individuals with Autism Spectrum Disorder, and their families, to fully participate in their communities.

7697 International OCD Foundation
18 Tremont St
Suite 308
Boston, MA 02108
617-973-5801
Fax: 617-973-5803
info@iocdf.org
iocdf.org

Shannon A Shy, Esq, President
Jeff Szymanski, PhD, Executive Director
Pamela Layne, Director of Operations

The International OCD Foundation aims to provide resources for those living with OCD and their families. The foundation offers a research grant program, public education and a forum for professional networking.

7698 Lewy Body Dementia Association
912 Killian Hill Rd, SW
Lilburn, GA 30047
404-975-2322
Fax: 480-422-5434
lbda@lbda.org
www.lbda.org

Christina M Christie, President
Mike Koehler, CEO
Mark Wall, Vice President

The Lewy Body Dementia Association is a non-profit organization dedicated to raising awareness of the Lewy body dementias (LBD). The association offers services and information to people with LBD, their families and caregivers and works to promote research in the area.

7699 Life Development Institute
18001 N 79th Ave
Suite B-42
Glendale, AZ 85308
866-736-7811
Fax: 623-773-2788
info@life-development-inst.org
discoverldi.com

Robert Crawford, M.Ed, CEO
Veronica Lieb (Crawford), MA, President
Justin Coller, BS, Director of Operations

The Life Development Institute serves older adolescents and adults with learning disabilities, ADD and related disorders. The Institute's mission is to help program participants pursue responsible independent living, enhance academic/workplace literacy skills and facilitate employment or educational placements.

7700 Life Unlimited
Life Unlimited, Inc.
2135 Manor Way
Liberty, MO 64068
816-781-4332
www.lifeunlimitedinc.org

Erin Lankford, President
Scott Wingerson, Vice President
Jessie Smith, Secretary

Life Unlimited is a nonprofit working to provide support and services to individuals with developmental disabilities in the Kansas City Northland. Services include community living, day services, employment services, and recreation programs.

7701 Mental Health America (MHA)
500 Montgomery St.
Suite 820
Alexandria, VA 22314
703-684-7722
800-969-6642
Fax: 703-684-5968
info@mhanational.org
www.mhanational.org

Schroeder Stribling, President & Chief Executive Officer
Mary Giliberti, Chief Public Policy Officer
Jessica Kennedy, Chief of Staff & Chief Financial Officer

A nonprofit organization addressing issues related to mental health and mental illness. MHA works to improve the mental health of all Americans, especially individuals with mental disorders, through advocacy, education, research, and service.
Founded in 1909. 1909

7702 Multiple Sclerosis Association of America
375 Kings Hwy N
Cherry Hill, NJ 08034
800-532-7667
Fax: 856-661-9797
msaa@mymsaa.org
mymsaa.org

John McCorry, Chair
Gina Murdoch, President & CEO
Lauren Hooper, Northeast Regional Director

The Multiple Sclerosis Association of America is an organization dedicated to providing the most up-to-date resources for those affected by Multiple Sclerosis, including research, publications, assistive equipment, public education, and best practices and policy for professionals working with patients.

7703 NLP Comprehensive
PO Box 348
Indian Hills, CO 80454-0348   303-987-2224
                                      800-233-1657
                                 Fax: 303-987-2228
                                 learn@nlpco.com
                                 www.nlpco.com

Tom Dotz, President
Sharon DeBault, Director of Community Relations
Jamie Reaser, PhD, Director of Professional Relations
NLP Comprehensive provides a body of publications by Steve and Connirae Andreas) on the subject of NLP (Neuro-linguistic programming), as well as training.

7704 NLP University - Dynamic Learning Center
NLP University
PO Box 1112
Ben Lomond, CA 95005   831-336-3457
                         Fax: 503-738-9546
                         teresanlp@aol.com
                         www.nlpu.com

Robert B Dilts, Founder & Director of Training
Teresa Epstein, Coordinator
Deborah Bacon Dilts, Trainer
NLP (neuro-lingusitic programming) University seeks to create a context in which professionals of different backgrounds can develop fundamental and advanced NLP skills for applications relevant to their profession. The University provides guidance, training, certification, culture, and community support to those interested in exploring the global potential of Systemic NLP.

7705 National Alliance on Mental Illness (NAMI)
3803 N Fairfax Dr
Suite 100
Arlington, VA 22203   703-524-7600
                         800-950-6264
                         888-999-6264
                    Fax: 703-524-9094
                    info@nami.org
                    www.nami.org

Steve Pitman, J.D., President
Mary Giliberti, J.D., CEO
Cheri Villa, M.P.A, Chief Operating Officer
NAMI is a grassroots mental health organization working to provide people with mental health issues the technical assistance, tools and referrals to resources they need in order to manage the challenges they face.

7706 National Association for Developmental Disabilities (NADD)
12 Hurley Ave.
Kingston, NY 12401   845-331-4336
                         info@thenadd.org
                         thenadd.org

Jeanne M. Farr, CEO
Jeffrey Schmunk, Operations Manager
Michelle Jordan, Office Manager
NADD is a non-profit membership association established for professionals, care providers and families to promote understanding of and services for individuals who have developmental disabilities and mental health needs. The mission of NADD is to advance mental wellness for persons with developmental disabilities through the promotion of excellence in mental health care.

7707 National Association for Down Syndrome
1460 Renaissance Dr
Suite 102
Park Ridge, IL 60068   630-325-9112
                         info@nads.org
                         www.nads.org

Steve Connors, President
Diane Urhausen, Executive Director
Linda Smarto, Director, Programs and Advocacy
The National Association for Down Syndrome provides services and information to those with Down Syndrome and their families. The association's mission is to maintain a strong network of support systems within their own organization and with medical, educational and school service professionals who work with children and adults with Down Syndrome.

7708 National Association of Cognitive- Behavioral Therapists
102 Gilson Ave
Weirton, WV 26062   304-224-2534
                         800-253-0167
                         nacbt@nacbt.org
                         www.nacbt.org

Aldo R Pucci, Ph.D, President
The association's mission is to promote the teaching and practice of cognitive-behavioral psychotherapy and to support those professionals and students seeking to practice it. Some services offered by the association include educational videos, membership, CBT certification, workshops and more.

7709 National Association of Epilepsy Centers
600 Maryland Ave SW
Suite 835W
Washington, DC 20024   202-524-6767
                         888-525-6232
                    Fax: 202-484-1244
                    info@naec-epilepsy.org
                    www.naec-epilepsy.org

Nathan B Fountain, MD, President
Ellen Riker, MHA, Executive Director
Johanna Gray, MPA, Deputy Director
The National Association of Epilepsy Centers educates public and private policy makers and regulators about appropriate patient care standards, reimbursement and medical services policies. The association is designed to complement the efforts of existing scientific and charitable epilepsy organizations.

7710 National Ataxia Foundation
600 Hwy 169 S
Suite 1725
Minneapolis, MN 55426   763-553-0020
                         Fax: 763-553-0167
                         naf@ataxia.org
                         www.ataxia.org

William P Sweeney, President
Charlene Danielson, Treasurer
Joel Sutherland, Executive Director
The National Ataxia Foundation is a non-profit, membership-supported organization established to help improve the lives of persons affected by ataxia and their families through support, education, and research.

7711 National Autism Association
1 Park Ave
Suite 1
Portsmouth, RI 02871   401-293-5551
                         877-622-2884
                    Fax: 401-293-5342
                    naa@nationalautism.org
                    nationalautismassociation.org

Lori McIlwain, Board Chairperson
Wendy Fournier, President
Kelly Vanicek, Executive Director
The mission of the National Autism Association is to educate and empower families affected by autism and other neurological disorders, while advocating on behalf of those who cannot fight for their own rights. The association offers programs as well as educational resources.

7712 National Down Syndrome Congress
30 Mansell Ct
Suite 108
Roswell, GA 30076   770-604-9500
                         800-232-6372
                    Fax: 770-604-9898
                    info@ndsccenter.org
                    www.ndsccenter.org

Kishore Vellody, MD, President
David Tolleson, Executive Director
MaryKate Vandemark, Office Manager
The National Down Syndrome Congress provides information, advocacy and support concerning all aspects of life for individuals with Down syndrome. It is the purpose of the Congress to create a national climate in which all people will recognize and embrace the value and dignity of people with Down syndrome.

7713 **National Down Syndrome Society**
8 E 41st St
8th Floor
New York, NY 10017
212-460-9330
800-221-4602
Fax: 212-979-2873
info@ndss.org
www.ndss.org

Sara Weir, MS, President
Josh Hill, Executive Assistant
Ashley Helsing, Director of Government Relations
Non-profit organization dedicated to increasing public awareness about Down syndrome as well as engaging in research, education and advocacy. The organization distributes informative materials, encourages and supports the activities of local parent support groups, sponsors conferences and scientific symposiums and undertakes major advocacy efforts.

7714 **National Hydrocephalus Foundation**
12413 Centralia Rd
Lakewood, CA 90715-1653
562-924-6666
888-857-3434
Fax: 562-924-6666
www.nhfonline.org

Michael Fields, President & Treasurer
Debbi Fields, Executive Director
Sarah Dunn, Junior Director
The National Hydrocephalus Foundation assembles and disseminates information pertaining to hydrocephalus, its treatments and outcomes. The foundation also establishes and facilitates a communication network among affected families and individuals.

7715 **Oak-Leyden Developmental Services**
411 Chicago Ave
Oak Park, IL 60302
708-524-1050
Fax: 708-524-2469
info@oak-leyden.org
www.oak-leyden.org

Melissa Wyatt, President
Bertha Magana, Executive Director
Nancy Thomas, Director of Human Resources
Oak-Leyden Developmental Services works to help people with developmental disabilities meet life's challenges and reach their highest potential. Services offered by the organization include Early Intervention Program, Vocational Evaluation, Developmental Training Program, Supported Employment Program, Community Integrated Living Arrangements and Multi-disciplinary Clinic.

7716 **Ontario Federation for Cerebral Palsy**
104-1630 Lawrence Ave W
Toronto, ON, Canada M6L-1C5
416-244-9686
877-244-9686
Fax: 416-244-6543
info@ofcp.ca
www.ofcp.ca

Victor Gascon, President
Nilu Alizadeh, Supervisor
Cindy DeGraaff, Planning Services Manager
The Ontario Federation for Cerebral Palsy is dedicated to assisting individuals with cerebral palsy through research, financial resources, education, recreation programs, housing and life planning.

7717 **Society for Cognitive Rehabilitation**
668 Exton Commons
Exton, PA 19341
127-647-2369
www.societyforcognitiverehab.org

Kit Malia, President
Rita Carroll, Secretary
Pat Benfield, Treasurer
The Society for Cognitive Rehabilitation is a non-profit organization committed to the advancement of cognitive rehabilitation therapy across the globe.

7718 **St. John Valley Associates**
291 Newberry Dr
Suite 105
Madawaska, ME 04756
207-728-7197
800-339-9502
Fax: 207-728-3825

Robin Jackson-Eldridge, Program Director
A non-profit association with the mission of empowering adult citizens with intellectual disabilities. The association offers center-based community supports and residential supports to help members develop a sense of independence. *$75.00*

7719 **TEACCH Autism Program**
100 Renee Lynne Ct
Carrboro, NC 27510
919-966-2174
Fax: 919-966-4127
teacch@unc.edu
teacch.com

Laura G Klinger, Ph.D, Executive Director
Lauren Turner-Brown, Ph.D, Assistant Director
Rebecca Mabe, Assistant Director, Business & Operations
TEACCH Autism Program offers community-based services, training programs and research to help those with Autism Spectrum Disorder. Some programs offered by TEACCH include clinical evaluations, intervention, consultation and training, living and learning centers, supported employment and more.

7720 **The Arc of North Carolina**
343 E Six Forks Rd
Suite 320
Raleigh, NC 27609
919-782-4632
800-662-8706
Fax: 919-782-4634
info@arcnc.org
www.arcnc.org

John Nash, Executive Director
Melinda Plue, Director of Advocacy & Chapter Development
Nicole Kiefer, Housing Resources Coordinator
The Arc of North Carolina is committed to providing services for people with intellectual and developmental disabilities. Services include advocacy, housing, supported employment and other supports.

7721 **The Arc of the United States**
1825 K St NW
Suite 1200
Washington, DC 20006
202-534-3700
800-433-5255
Fax: 202-534-3731
info@thearc.org
www.thearc.org

Peter Berns, Chief Executive Officer
Ruben Rodriguez, Chief Operating Officer
Julie Ward, Senior Executive Officer, Public Policy
The Arc promotes and protects the rights of people with intellectual and developmental disabilities and actively supports their inclusion and participation in the community throughout their lifetimes. The Arc's clients include people with autism, Down syndrome, Fragile X syndrome, and various other developmental disabilities. Some services offered by The Arc include public policy advocacy, education and vocational services.

7722 **The Hemispherectomy Foundation**
8235 Lethbridge Rd
Millersville, MD 21108
410-987-5221
lynn@hemifoundation.org
hemifoundation.homestead.com

Kristi Hall, President, CEO & Co-Founder
Cris A Hall, Executive Director & Co-Founder
Jane Stefanik, Vice President & Chief Financial Officer
The Hemispherectomy Foundation is a non-profit organization dedicated to providing emotional, financial and educational support to individuals and their families who have undergone, or will undergo, a hemispherectomy or similar brain surgery.

7723 Tourette Association of America
42-40 Bell Blvd
Suite 205
Bayside, NY 11361 　　　　　718-224-2999
Fax: 718-279-9596
support@tourette.org
www.tourette.org
Amanda Talty, President & CEO
Tracey Costikyan-Alexander, VP, Resource Development & Chapter Services
Diana Felner, VP, Public Policy
Non-profit organization with the mission of researching and controlling the effects of Tourette syndrome. Some services they offer include seminars, conferences and support groups. The association publishes brochures, flyers, educational materials and papers on treatment and research.

7724 United Cerebral Palsy
1825 K St NW
Suite 600
Washington, DC 20006 　　　　202-776-0406
800-872-5827
Fax: 202-776-0414
info@ucp.org
ucp.org
Diane Wilush, Chair
Armando Contreras, President & CEO
Ellie Collinson, Chief Program Officer
United Cerebral Palsy educates, advocates, and provides support services to ensure a life without limits for people with cerebral palsy and other disabilities. Some services offered include networking, educational information, assistive technology information, research, public policy resources and more.

Camps

7725 Adventure Learning Center at Eagle Village
4507 170th Ave
Hersey, MI 49639-8785 　　　　231-832-2234
800-748-0061
Fax: 231-832-1468
alcinfo@eaglevillage.org
www.eaglevillage.org
Cathey Prudhomme, President/CEO
Jim McCain, Director of Support Services/CFO
Craig Weidner, Director of Advancement
Offers a variety of fun camp experiences with a low staff-to-camper ratio and exciting, challenging activities. This program accepts youth, ages 5-17, who are high risk or special needs - behavioral problems, emotionally unstable or Attention Deficit. The camping experience includes canoeing, hiking, swimming and high adventure activities. Half-week, one-week, and two-week sessions June-August. Coed.

7726 CNS Camp New Connections
Mclean Hospital Child/Adolescent Program
115 Mill St
Mailstop115
Belmont, MA 02478-1064 　　　　617-855-2000
800-333-0338
Fax: 617-855-2833
mcleaninfo@mclean.harvard.edu
www.mcleanhospital.org
Roya Ostovar PhD, Center Director
Scott L. Rauch, MD., President and Psychiatrist in Ch
Joseph Gold MD, Clinical Director
Four-week summer day camp for children ages 7-17 who have pervasive developmental disorders, Asperger's Syndrome, autism spectrum disorders and non-verbal learning disabilities. The camp is designed to help children develop social skills through fun activities including: communication games, swimming, field trips, drama, and arts and crafts. *$4500.00*

7727 Camp ASCCA
Alabama's Special Camp for Children and Adults
PO Box 21
5278 Camp Ascca Dr.
Jacksons Gap, AL 36861 　　　　256-825-9226
Fax: 256-269-0714
info@campascca.org
www.campascca.org
Matt Rickman, Camp Director
John Stephenson, Administrator
Jocelyn Jones, Secretary
Camp Evoked Potential is held one week out of the year for children aged 6-18 with epilepsy at Camp ASCCA. Fully funded by The Epilepsy Foundation, persons wishing to attend the camp must apply. The camp provides a barrier free setting situated on 230 acres of wooded land at Lake Martin. The camp is staffed with medical personnel trained to care for children with all types of disabilities and provides a variety of camp activities.
1976

7728 Camp Baker
Greater Richmond ARC
7600 Beach Rd
Chesterfield, VA 23838-6513 　　　804-748-4789
Fax: 804-796-6880
richmondarc.org
Robert L. Sommerville, Chair - Officer
Thomas G. Haskins, Vice Chair - Officer
Chriss Mumford, Secretary Officer
An organization created by families, for families that has grown to provide a continuum of programs and services for individuals with developmental disablties acroos the lifespan, helping each person achieve his or her potential and improving the quality of life for everyone in the community.

7729 Camp Buckskin
PO Box 389
Ely, MN 55731 　　　　763-432-9177
info@campbuckskin.com
www.campbuckskin.com
Tom Bauer, Camp Co-Director
Mary Bauer, Camp Co-Director
Camp is located in Ely, Minnesota. Buckskin helps children with underdeveloped social skills realize their potentials and abilities. Teaches a combination of traditional camp activities, academic activities, and social skills. Ages 6-18.

7730 Camp Candlelight
Epilepsy Foundation Arizona
941 S Park Lane
Tempe, AZ 85281 　　　　602-282-3515
800-332-1000
AZ@EFA.org
epilepsyaz.org/events/campcandlelight
Suzanne Matsumori, Executive Director
Min Skivington, Program Manager
Camp Candlelight provides children ages 8 to 17 a unique camp experience that mixes traditional summer camp with special sessions that teach campers about their seizures and gives them resources to manage the challenges that the seizures represent. Staff inclues a neurologist, several nurses, and a school psychologist, in addition to traditional camp staff who are given specialized training in responding appropriately to the needs of kids with epilepsy.

7731 Camp Civitan
Civitan Foundation
12635 N. 42nd Street
Phoenix, AZ 85032 　　　　602-953-2944
www.civitanfoundationaz.com
Dawn Trapp, Executive Director
Camp Civitan offers week long summer camp programs, and weekend programs throughout the year, to children with developmental disabilities. The camp is fully wheelchair accessible, is staffed by medical professionals and there is a 2:1 ratio of campers to staff. Camp Civitan offers campers the experience of traditional camp activities including, swimming, adaptive sports, fishing, music, arts and crafts, and talent shows.
1968

7732   Camp Horizons
127 Babcock Hill Rd
PO Box 323
South Windham, CT 06266- 323   860-456-1032
                                    Fax: 860-456-4721
                                    www.camphorizons.org
Adam Milne, Chairman
L. Sanford Rice, Treasurer
Kathleen McNAboe, VP
Bordering Lake Probus, the facilities at the camp are equipped to
accomodate a wide range of activities and programs for campers
with developmental disabilities, or other challenging emotional
and social needs. There is a 5:1 camper-counselor ratio with a
schedule of three programs in the morning and four in the
afternoon.

7733   Camp Huntington
56 Bruceville Rd.
High Falls, NY 12440-5100   845-687-7840
                                       855-707-2267
                                    Fax: 855-707-2267
                                    www.camphuntington.com
Daniel Falk, Executive Director
Dylan Sloan, Program Director
Margaret Short, Health Director
A co-ed residential summer camp specifically designed to focus
on adaptive and therapeutic recreation. Campers include those
with learning and developmental disabilities, ADD/HD, Autism
Spectrum Disorders, Asperger's, PDD, and other special needs.
Programs focus on recreation and social skills, independence,
and participation.

7734   Camp Krem
Camping Unlimited
102 Brook Lane
Boulder Creek, CA 95006   831-338-3210
                                 campkrem@campingunlimited.org
                                       campingunlimited.org
Christina Krem DiGirolamo, Camp Director
Leon Wong, Head of Camper Services
Kristen Carter, Virtual Program Coordinator
Camp Krem - Camping Unlimited offers year-round and summer
camping programs for children and adults with developmental
disabilities. With a variety of different programs and many facili-
ties on the campground such as a swimming pool, arts and crafts
building, amphitheater, music pavilion, and archery range, Camp
Krem provides its campers with recreation, education, and
adventure opportunities.

7735   Camp Nissokone
YMCA Camping Services
1401 Broadway
Suite A
Detroit, MI 48226-8929   313-267-5300
                                    www.ymcadetroit.org
Doug Grimm, Vice President Camping Services
David Marks, Director
A six week summer resident camp program for boys and girls
whose learning and behavior styles have made successful participation in the traditional camp program difficult. All camp activities have a special emphasis on building self-esteem and peer
relationships. Strong in waterfront, nature, campcrafts and a
special arts program.

7736   Camp Nuhop
1077 Township Rd. 2916
Perrysville, OH 44864   419-938-7151
                                    www.nuhop.org
Trevor Dunlap, Executive Director & CEO
Chris Clyde, Associate Director
Matt Poland, Director, Outdoor Education
A summer residential program for youth ages 6-18 with learning
disabilities, behavioral disorders, or other neuroatypical disor-
ders. Activities include outdoor education and team-building
workshops. The staff-to-camper ratio is 3:7 or 3:8.

7737   Camp Ramapo
Ramapo for Children
Rt. 52/Salisbury Turnpike
PO Box 266
Rhinebeck, NY 12572   845-876-8403
                                    Fax: 845-876-8414
                                 office@ramapoforchildren.org
                                 www.ramapoforchildren.org
Matthew McKnight, Camp Director
Lenora Sealey, Associate Camp Director
A residential summer camp for youth ages 6-16 with social, emo-
tional, or learning challenges.

7738   Camp ReCreation
9272 Madison Ave.
Orangeville, CA 95662   916-988-6835
                                 camprecreation@outlook.com
                                    www.camprecreation.org
Kathi Barber, Camp Director
Camp ReCreation offers residential summer camps and year
round programs for children, teens, and adults with developmental disabilities. The summer camp is held at Camp Ronald Mc-
Donald in Lassen National Forest. With a 1:1 staff to camper
ratio, Camp ReCreation offers wide variety of camp activities,
and campers wishing to participate must fill out a camper
application.
1983

7739   Camp Royall
250 Bill Ash Rd.
Moncure, NC 27559   919-542-1033
                                    Fax: 919-533-5324
                                 camproyall@autismsociety-nc.org
                                 www.autismsociety-nc.org/camp-royall
Sara Gage, Director
A week-long overnight and day camp for children and adults with
autism. Campers participate in traditional camp activities such as
swimming, boating, hiking, and arts and crafts. Counselor-to-camper ratio is 1:1 or 1:2, depending on the campers'
needs.

7740   Camp Ruggles
PO Box 353
Chepachet, RI 02814   401-567-8914
                                 campruggles@gmail.com
                                    www.campruggles.org
Jim Field, Executive Director
Ethan Roe, Assistant Director
Camp Ruggles is located in Glocester, RI and is a summer day
camp for children with emotional and behavioral disabilities. The
camp offers 240 hours of supervised therapeutic care for children
ages 6-12.

7741   Camp Sisol
Jewish Community Center of Greater Rochester/JCC
1200 Edgewood Ave.
Rochester, NY 14618   585-461-2000
                                    Fax: 585-461-0805
                                 bettertogether@jccrochester.org
                                    www.jccrochester.org
Josh Weinstein, Chief Executive Officer
Coed, ages 5-16. Camp Sisol accommodates children with special
needs.

7742   Camp World Light
Florida Baptist Convention
1230 Hendricks Ave
Jacksonville, FL 32207-8619   904-396-2351
                                       800-226-8584
                                    Fax: 904-396-6470
                                    www.campworldlight.com
Anne Wilson, Camp Director
Delicia Garland, Ministry Assistant to Director
Camp is located in Marianna, Florida. One-week sessions
June-July for girls with ADD. Ages 3-12. Activities include
arts/crafts, challenge/rope courses, clowning, community ser-
vice, dance, drama, drawing/painting, leadership development,
performing arts and sailing.

7743   Camp-A-Lot and Camp-A-Little
The Arc of San Diego
3030 Market Street
San Diego, CA 92102   619-685-1175
                                        Fax: 619-234-3759
                                        info@arc-sd.com
                                        www.arc-sd.com
Anthony J. DeSalis, President & Chief Executive Officer
Programs of The Arc of San Diego, Camp - A - Lot (ages 18 and
up) and Camp - A - Little (ages 5-17) offer recreational summer
camp opportunities for individuals with physical and developmental disabilities.

7744   Casowasco Camp, Conference and Retreat Center
158 Casowasco Dr
Moravia, NY 13118-3498   315-364-8756
                                        Fax: 315-364-7636
                                        info@casowasco.org
Mike Huber, Executive Director
Shelly Sherboneau, CRM Coordinating Registrar
Kevin Dunn, Casowasco Assistant Director
Camp is located in Moravia, New York. Summer sessions for chil-
dren with ADD. Coed, ages 6-18 and families.

7745   Center Academy at Pinellas Park
6710 86th Ave. N
Pinellas Park, FL 33782   727-541-5716
                                        Fax: 727-544-8186
                                        infopp@centeracademy.com
                                        www.centeracademy.com
Mack R. Hicks, Founder & Chair
Andrew P. Hicks, Chief Executive Officer & Clinical Director
Eric V. Larson, President & Chief Operating Officer
Specifically designed for the learning disabled child and other
children with difficulties in concentration, strategy, social skills,
impulsivity, distractibility and study strategies. Programs offered
include attention training, visual-motor remediation, socialization skills training, relaxation training, and more.

7746   Dallas Academy
950 Tiffany Way
Dallas, TX 75218   214-324-1481
                                        Fax: 214-327-8537
                                        www.dallas-academy.com
Elizabeth Murski, Head of School
Dallas Academy is a school for children with diagnosed learning
differences such as autism, ADD/ADHD, dyslexia, and more.
The academy offers a number of summer camps and programs.

7747   Eagle Hill School: Summer Program
242 Old Petersham Road
P.O. Box 116
Hardwick, MA 01037- 0116   413-477-6000
                                        Fax: 413-477-6837
                                        admission@ehs1.org
                                        www.ehs1.org
Peter J. Mc Donald, Headmaster
Marilyn Waller, President
Alden Bianchi, Vice President
For children ages 9-19 with specific learning (dis)abilities and/or
Attention Deficit Disorder, this summer program is designed to
remediate academic and social deficits while maintaining prog-
ress achieved during the school year. Electives and sports activi-
ties are combined with the academic courses to address the needs
of the whole person in a camp-like atmosphere.

7748   Englishton Park Academic Remediation
Englishton Park Presbyterian
P.O.Box 228
Lexington, IN 47138-228   812-889-2046
                                        ThomasLisaBarnett@etczone.com
                                        www.englishtonpark.org
Lisa Barnett, Director
Thomas Barnett, Co-Director
Camp is located in Lexington, Indiana. Two-week sessions for
children with ADD. Boys and girls, ages 7-12.

7749   Florida Sheriffs Caruth Camp
Florida Sheriffs Youth Ranches
2486 Cecil Webb Place
Boys Ranch, FL 32060   386-842-5501
                                        800-765-3797
                                        Fax: 386-842-2429
                                        fsyr@youthranches.org
                                        www.youthranches.org
Roger Bouchard, President
Bill Frye, Executive Vice President
Janet Bass, Vice President of Operations
Camp is located in Inglis, Florida. One-week sessions for chil-
dren with ADD. Coed, ages 10-15.

7750   Gow School Summer Programs
2491 Emery Rd.
South Wales, NY 14139   716-687-2004
                                        Fax: 716-687-2003
                                        summer@gow.org
                                        www.gow.org
Matthew Fisher, Director
Co-ed summer programs for students ages 8-16 with dyslexia or
similar learning disabilities. Offers a blend of morning academics, afternoon/evening traditional camp activities and weekend
overnights.

7751   Hill School of Fort Worth
4817 Odessa Ave.
Fort Worth, TX 76133   817-923-9482
                                        Fax: 817-923-4894
                                        hillschool@hillschool.org
                                        www.hillschool.org
Roxann Breyer, Head of School
Matt Errico, Dean, Student Success
Jimmy Cessna, Registrar
Provides an alternative learning environment for students with
learning differences. Hill School caters to individuals with disabilities by offering smaller class sizes and individualized learning programs. Offers an academic summer program during the
month of June.

7752   Indian Acres Camp for Boys
1712 Main St
Fryeburg, ME 04037-4327   207-935-2300
                                        Fax: 954-349-7812
                                        geoff@indianacres.com
                                        www.indianacres.com
Michael Burness, Assistant Director
Mary Beth 'Bert' Wiig, Head Counselor, Camp Forest Acre
Lisa Newman, Director
Camp is located in Fryeburg, Florida. Four and seven-week ses-
sions June-August for boys with ADD ages 7-16.

7753   Lab School of Washington
4759 Reservoir Rd NW
Washington, DC 20007-1921   200-965-6600
                                        www.labschool.org
Katherine Schantz, Head of School
Diana Meltzer, Associate Head of School
Laurelle Sheedy McCready, Associate Head of School for Fin
The Lab School six week summer session includes individualized
reading, spelling, writing, study skills and math programs. A
multisensory approach addresses the needs of bright learning disabled children. Related services such as speech/language therapy
and occupational therapy are integrated into the curriculum. Ele-
mentary/Intermediate; Junior High/High School.

7754   Lions Den Outdoor Learning Center
600 Kiwanis Dr
Eureka, MO 63025-2212   636-938-5245
                                        Fax: 636-938-5289
                                        www.wymancenter.org
David Hilliard, President
Theresa Mayberry, Executive VP
Kristine Ramsey, Sr. VP
Varied programs for developmentally disabled children, ages 6
and up, includes daily living, socialization and language skills.
Sports, tent camping, crafts, and nature study are also offered.
Sliding scale tuition for 2 weeks.

7755   Maplebrook School
5142 Route 22
Amenia, NY 12501   845-373-9511
                                     Fax: 845-373-7029
admissions@maplebrookschool.org
www.maplebrookschool.org
Donna Konkolics, Head of School
Roger Fazzone, President
Jennifer Scully, Assistant Head, Postsecondary Studies
A coeductional boarding school which offers a six week camp for
children with learning differences and ADD.

7756   Marvelwood Summer
Marvelwood School
476 Skiff Mountain Road
PO Box 3001
Kent, CT 06757-3001   860-927-0047
                                     Fax: 860-927-0021
www.marvelwood.org
Alfred C Brooks, President
Arthur F Goodearl, Jr, Head Of School
The emphasis in this summer program is on diagnosis and
remediation of individual reading, spelling, writing, mathemat-
ics and study problems. Offered to ages 12-16.

7757   New Horizons Summer Day Camp
YMCA of Orange County
13821 Newport Ave.
Suite 150
Tustin, CA 92780   714-508-7616
newhorizons@ymcaoc.org
www.ymcaoc.org/new-horizons
Jeff McBride, Chief Executive Officer
New Horizons is a program by the YMCA offering day camps for
adults with developmental disabilities. Outings in the community
are supervised and create an environment that fosters social interaction, skill building, and friendship.

7758   New Jersey YMHA/YWHA Camps Milford
21 Plymouth St
Fairfield, NJ 07004-1686   973-575-3333
                                           800-776-5657
                                     Fax: 973-575-4188
info@njycamps.org
www.njycamps.org
Leonard Robinson, President
Bruce Nussman, President
Camp is located in Milford, Pennsylvania. Summer sessions for
children with ADD. Coed, ages 6-17 and families.

7759   Oakland School & Camp
128 Oakland Farm Way
Troy, VA 22974   434-293-9059
                                     Fax: 434-296-8930
information@oaklandschool.net
www.oaklandschool.net
Carol Williams, Head of School
A highly individualized program that stresses improving reading
ability. Subjects taught are reading, English composition, math
and word analysis. Recreational activities include horseback riding, sports, swimming, tennis, crafts, archery and camping. For
girls and boys, ages 7-13. Students who attend the summer camp
often have a variety of learning disabilities, such as ADHD, dyslexia, visual/auditory processing disorders, and more.

7760   Outside In School Of Experiential Education, Inc.
PO Box 639
Greensburg, PA 15601   724-837-1518
                                     Fax: 724-837-0801
www.myoutsidein.org
Michael C. Henkel, Executive Director
Camp programs primarily focus on substance abuse, but some
services are available for special needs related to school/work.
Programs are for boys ages 13-18.

7761   Phelps School Academic Support Program
583 Sugartown Rd.
Malvern, PA 19355   610-644-1754
                                     Fax: 610-540-0156
admis@thephelpsschool.org
www.thephelpsschool.org
Charles A. McGeorge, Head of School
The Phelps School is a day and boarding school for grades 6-12.
They run an Academic Support Program for English, Reading,
Mathematics, and Study Skills for students who have diagnosed
learning differences.

7762   Quest Camp
907 San Ramon Valley Blvd.
Suite 202
Danville, CA 94526   925-743-2900
                                           800-313-9733
                                     Fax: 925-743-1937
www.questcamps.com
Robert B. Field, PhD., Founder & Executive Director
Debra Forrester-Field, MA, Administrative Director
Aprilyn Artz, MA, Clinical Director
Quest Camps are designed using the Quest Camp Therapeutic
System developed specifically to help and reduce a campers psy-
chological disability. With locations in San Francisco East Bay,
California, Huntington Beach, California, and Pittsburgh, Pennsylvania, camps have a 6:1 camper to staff ratio, with campers receiving sport instruction and participate in physical activity, arts,
and games.
1989

7763   Raven Rock Lutheran Camp
17912 Harbaugh Valley Road
P.O.Box 136
Sabillasville, MD 21780-136   410-303-2108
                                           800-321-5824
Brenda Minnich, Executive Director
Christ-centered program for youth and developmentally disabled
adults.

7764   Rimland Services for Autistic Citizens
1265 Hartrey Ave.
Evanston, IL 60202   847-328-4090
                                     Fax: 847-328-8364
                                     TTY: 847-328-4090
www.rimland.org
Lorraine Ganz, President
Barbara Cooper, Secretary
Services include residential living, community day services, and
health and wellness programs.

7765   Rolling Hills Country Day Camp
P.O.Box 172
Marlboro, NJ 07746   732-308-0405
                                     Fax: 732-780-4726
info@rollinghillsdaycamp.com
www.rollinghillsdaycamp.com
Billy Breitner, Director
Summer sessions for children with ADD. Coed, ages 3-12.

7766   SOAR Summer Adventures
226 SOAR Lane
PO Box 388
Balsam, NC 28707   828-456-3435
                                     Fax: 801-820-3050
admissions@soarnc.org
www.soarnc.org
John Willson, Executive Director
A nonprofit adventure program working with disadvantaged
youth diagnosed with learning disabilities in an outdoor, challenge-based environment. Focuses on esteem building and social
skills development through rock climbing, backpacking, whitewater rafting, mountaineering, sailing, snorkeling, and more. Offers two week, one month, and semester programs. Locations
include North Carolina, Florida, Wyoming, California, New
York, Belize, Costa Rica, and the Caribbean.

7767 Sherman Lake YMCA Outdoor Center
6225 N 39th St
Augusta, MI 49012-9722 269-731-3000
Fax: 269-731-3020
shermanlakeymca@ymcasl.org
www.shermanlakeymca.org

Luke Austenfeld, Executive Director
Jean Henderson, Business Manager
Lorrie Syverson, Director of Camping, Education &
Summer camping sessions for campers with ADD and spina bifida. Coed, ages 6-15 and families, seniors.

7768 Squirrel Hollow Summer Camp
The Bedford School
5665 Milam Rd.
Fairburn, GA 30213 770-774-8001
Fax: 770-774-8005
info@thebedfordschool.org
www.thebedfordschool.org

Betsy Box, Admissions Director
Jeff James, Head of School
Allison Day, Associate Head of School
A remedial summer program for children with academic needs held on the campus of The Bedford School in Fairburn, Georgia. It serves children ages 6-14.

7769 Summer@Carroll
Carroll School
25 Baker Bridge Rd.
Lincoln, MA 01773 781-259-8342
summeradmissions@carrollschool.org
www.carrollschool.org

Kristin Curry, Director
Donna Brown, Assistant Director
Summer@Carroll is a unique educational experience designed for children with language-based learning disabilities entering grades 1-9 in the Fall. Carroll's five-week, full-day program provides specialized reading support as well as writing and math classes. Classes are formed according to age and skill level, typically with eight or fewer students in a class.

7770 Summit Camp
55 W 38th St.
4th Floor
New York, NY 10018 570-253-4381
info@summitcamp.com
www.summitcamp.com

Shepherd Baum, Director
Leah Love, Assistant Director
Thea Mullis, Travel Director
The camp is located in Honesdale, Pennsylvania, and is for children ages 8-19 who have a variety of developmental, social, or learning challenges. In addition to traditional camp activities, Summit Camp has a strong focus on social skills development and interpersonal growth.

7771 Sunnyhill Adventures
6555 Sunlit Way
Dittmer, MO 63023 636-274-9044
sunnyhilladventures.org

Rob Darroch, Director
Summer camps and year-round programs are offered for youth and adults of all abilities.

7772 Talisman Summer Camp
64 Gap Creek Rd.
Zirconia, NC 28790 828-697-6313
info@talismancamps.com
www.talismancamps.com

Linda Tatsapaugh, Operations Director & Owner
Robiyn Mims, Admissions Director & Owner
Cory Greene, Camp Director
Talisman Summer Camp is located 40 minutes south of Asheville, North Carolina. Offers a program of hiking, rafting, climbing, and caving for young people with autism, ADHD and learning disabilities. Coed, ages 6-22.

7773 Timbertop Camp for Youth with Learning Disabilities
PO Box 423
Plover, WI 54467 715-869-6262
info@timbertopcamp.org
www.timbertopcamp.org

Pete Matthai, Camp Director
Timbertop Camp is a seven-day outdoor camp for children and youth with learning disabilities. Campers participate in traditional camp activities as well as activities that focus on enhancing cooperative abilities, interpersonal relationships, and self-esteem. The program includes nature exploration, canoeing, arts and crafts, archery, fishing, games, reading instruction, and campfires.

7774 Triangle Y Ranch YMCA
YMCA of Southern Arizona
PO Box 1111
Tucson, AZ 85702 520-623-5511
Fax: 520-624-1518
www.tucsonymca.org

Dane Woll, President and CEO
Kerry Dufour, V.P. Chief Development Officer
Cathy Scheirman, Chief Financial Officer
Summer camp programs for children and young adults ages 6-17. Camp offers horseback riding, sports, story telling, arts & crafts, swimming, archery and nature programs.

7775 Wendell Johnson Speech And Hearing Clinic
University Of Iowa
250 Hawkins Dr
Iowa City, IA 52242-1025 319-335-3500
Fax: 319-335-8851
dorothy-albright@uiowa.edu
www.uiowa.edu

Dorothy Albright, Department Administration
Lauren Eldridge, Undergraduate Academic Programs
Mary Jo Yotty, Graduate Programs
The clinic offers assessment and remediation for communication disorders in adults and children. The clinic also offers a Intensive Summer Residential Clinic for school age children needing intervention services because of speech, language, hearing and/or reading problems.

Books

7776 A Miracle to Believe In
Option Indigo Press
2080 S Undermountain Rd
Sheffield, MA 01257-9643 413-229-8727
800-714-2779
Fax: 413-229-8727

Barry Neil Kaufman, Author
A group of people from all walks of life come together and are transformed as they reach out, under the direction of the Kaufmans, to help a little boy the medical world had given up as hopeless. This heartwarming journey of loving a child back to life will not only inspire you, the reader, but presents a compelling new way to deal with life's traumas and difficulties.
379 pages
ISBN 0-449201-08-2

7777 ADD: Helping Your Child
Warner Books
1271 Avenue of the Americas
New York, NY 10020-1300 212-522-7200
Fax: 212-522-7989

Barbara Smalley, Author
Bruce Paonessa, Vice President
Elizabeth Nunuz, Manager
The definitive guide to helping children with AD/HD *$ 12.95*
224 pages Paperback
ISBN 0-446670-13-8

7778   ADHD Book of Lists: A Practical Guide for Helping Children and Teens with ADDs
Jossey-Bass
111 River St
Hoboken, NJ 7030-5773   201-748-6000
                                    Fax: 201-748-6008
                                      info@wiley.com
                                      www.wiley.com
Sandra F Rief, Author
Information about Attention Deficit/Hyperactivity Disorder including strategies, supports, and interventions that have been found to be the most effective. For teachers, parents, and counselors. *$29.95*
320 pages
ISBN 0-787965-91-X

7779   ADHD in the Schools: Assessment and Intervention Strategies
Guilford Press
72 Spring St
New York, NY 10012-4019   212-431-9800
                                         800-365-7006
                                    Fax: 212-966-6708
                                      info@guilford.com
                                      www.guilford.com
George J DuPaul, Author
Gary Stoner, Co-Author
This landmark volume emphasizes the need for a team effort among parents, community-based professionals, and educators. Provides practical information for educators that is based on empirical findings. Chapters focus on: how to identify and assess students who might have ADHD; the relationship between ADHD and learning disabilities; how to develop and implement classroom-based programs; communication strategies to assist physicians; and the need for community-based treatments. *$36.00*
269 pages Hardcover
ISBN 0-898622-45-X

7780   ADHD with Comorbid Disorders: Clinical Assessment and Management
Guilford Press
72 Spring St
New York, NY 10012-4019   212-431-9800
                                         800-365-7006
                                    Fax: 212-966-6708
                                      info@guilford.com
                                      www.guilford.com
Steven R Pliszka, MD, Author
Caryn Leigh Carlson, Co-Author
James M Swanson, Co-Author
$44.00
Cloth
ISBN 1-572304-78-2

7781   Adolescents with Down Syndrome: Toward a More Fulfilling Life
Brookes Publishing
P.O.Box 10624
Baltimore, MD 21285-624   410-337-9580
                                         800-638-3775
                                    Fax: 410-337-8539
                              custserv@brookespublishing.com
                                    www.brookespublishing.com
Maria Sustrova, Author
Lauren Smith, Western Region Sales Representat
Jeannine Blimline, Central Region Sales Representat
Written for health care professionals, psychologists, other developmental disabilities practitioners, educators, and parents, it covers biomedical concerns; behavioral, psychological, and psychiatric challenges; and education, employment, recreation, community, and legal concerns. *$35.95*
416 pages Paperback
ISBN 1-55766 -81-9

7782   Adult ADD: The Complete Handbook: Everything You Need to Know About How to Cope with ADD
Prima Publishing
P.O.Box 1260
Rocklin, CA 95677-1260   916-787-7000
                                         800-632-8676
                                    Fax: 916-787-7001
David B Sudderth, Author
In simple and friendly terms, the authors offer help to those leading frustrating lives. They provide coping mechanisms, both psychological and an up-to-date guide to the latest technology *$14.95*
272 pages
ISBN 0-761507-96-5

7783   All About Attention Deficit Disorders, Revised
Parent Magic
800 Roosevelt Rd
Glen Ellyn, IL 60137-5839   630-208-0031
                                         800-442-4453
                                    Fax: 630-208-7366
                                      www.parentmagic.com
Thomas Phelan, Owner
A psychologist and expert on ADD outlines the symptoms, diagnosis and treatment of this neurological disorder. *$12.95*
248 pages Paperback
ISBN 1-889140-11-2

7784   Assistive Technology for Individuals with Cognitive Impairments Handbook
Idaho Assistive Technology Project
University of Idaho
1187 Alturas Dr.
Moscow, ID 83843- 2268   208-885-3557
                                         800-432-8324
                                    Fax: 208-885-6102
                                      idahoat@uidaho.edu
                                      www.idahoat.org
Ron Seiler, Project Director
A handbook designed to provide resources and information on finding and acquiring assistive technology for individuals with cognitive impairments.

7785   Attention Deficit Disorder
Sage Publications
2455 Teller Road
Thousand Oaks, CA 91320   800-818-7243
                                    Fax: 800-583-2665
                                      info@sagepub.com
                                      www.sagepub.com
Sara Miller McCune, Founder, Publisher, Chairperson
Blaise R Simqu, President & CEO
A book providing helpful suggestions for both home and classroom management of students with attention deficit disorder.

7786   Attention Deficit Disorder and Learning Disabilities
Books on Special Children
P.O.Box 305
Congers, NY 10920-305   845-638-1236
                                    Fax: 845-638-0847
Barbara Ingersoll, Author
Introduces ADD and learning disabilities. This is an easy reading book. Gives definitions and discusses some effective and controverial medication, dietary, biofeedback, cognitive therapy, and many more issues. *$15.95*
246 pages Softcover
ISBN 0-385469-31-4

7787   Attention Deficit Disorder in Adults Workbook
Taylor Publishing Company
7211 Circle S. Road
Austin, TX 78745-5007   214-637-2800
                                         800-225-3687
                                    Fax: 214-819-8220
                                      Rings@balfour.com
                                      www.balfour.com
Don Percenti, CEO
Workbook for adults with ADD. *$17.99*
192 pages Paperback
ISBN 0-878338-50-0

7788 Attention Deficit Disorder: A Different Perception
Underwood Books
PO Box 1919
Nevada City, CA 95959-1919   800-788-3123
                              www.underwoodbooks.com

Thorn Hartmann, Author
Supports theory linking ADD to the genetic makeup of men and women who hunted for their food in prehistoric times. Also links second hand smoke to disruptive behavior. *$9.95*
180 pages Paperback
ISBN 0-887331-56-4

7789 Attention Deficit Disorders: Assessment & Teaching
Brooks/Cole Publishing Company
10650 Toebben Drive
Independence, KY 41051   859-525-2230
                              Fax: 859-282-5700
                              www.brookscole.com

Janet W Lerner, Author
A handy resource that offers teachers, school psychologists, councelors, social workers, administrators, and parents practical advice for working with children who have attention deficit disorders. *$18.95*
258 pages Paperback
ISBN 0-534250-44-0

7790 Attention-Deficit Hyperactivity Disorder: Symptoms and Suggestons for Treatment
Slosson Educational Publications Inc.
538 Buffalo Rd
East Aurora, NY 14052-280   716-652-0930
                              888-756-7766
                              Fax: 800-655-3840
                              slosson@slosson.com
                              www.slosson.com

Thomas W Phelan, Author
Steven Slosson, President
John Slosson, Vice President
An exhaustive review of current research and decades of experience as practicing school-based professionals, as well as being a parent of an ADHD child, have culminated in this brief, to-the-point, and yet informed ADHD package which has recieved tremendous reviews. Well-grounded answers and suggestions which would facillitate behavior, learning, social-emotional functioning, and other factors in preschool and adolesence are discussed. Answers most commonly asked questions about ADHD/ADD. *$60.00*
61 pages

7791 Attention-Deficit/Hyperactivity Disorder, What Every Parent Wants to Know
Brookes Publishing
P.O.Box 10624
Baltimore, MD 21285-0624   410-337-9580
                              800-638-3775
                              Fax: 410-337-8539
                              custserv@brookespublishing.com
                              www.brookespublishing.com

Lauren Rohe, Regional Sales Consultant
Jeff Stickler, Educational Sales Representative
Sam Schissler, Educational Sales Representative
New easy-to-understand, non-technical edition helps teachers and parents get accessible answers to their ADHD. *$21.95*
304 pages Paperback
ISBN 1-557663-98-X

7792 Augmenting Basic Communciation in Natural Contexts
Brookes Publishing
P.O.Box 10624
Baltimore, MD 21285-0624   410-337-9580
                              800-638-3775
                              Fax: 410-337-8539
                              custserv@brookespublishing.com
                              www.brookespublishing.com

Lauren Rohe, Regional Sales Consultant
Jeff Stickler, Educational Sales Representative
Sam Schissler, Educational Sales Representative

Here you will find the techniques needed to establish a basic communication system for people of all ages with cognitive disabilities or motor sensory impairments. *$41.95*
304 pages Paperback
ISBN 1-55766 -43-6

7793 Autism 24/7: A Family Guide to Learning at Home & in the Community
Autism Society of North Carolina Bookstore
505 Oberlin Rd
Suite 230
Raleigh, NC 27605-1345   919-743-0204
                              800-442-2762
                              Fax: 919-743-0208
                              info@autismsociety-nc.org
                              www.autismsociety-nc.org

David Lax, Manager
Martina Ballen, Chair
Beverly Moore, Vice Chair
Parents are encouraged to focus on skill sets and behaviors that most negatively affect family functioning, and replacing these behaviors with acceptable alternatives. *$19.95*

7794 Autism Handbook: Understanding & Treating Autism & Prevention Development
Oxford University Press
2001 Evans Rd
Cary, NC 27513-2010   919-677-0977
                              800-445-9714
                              Fax: 919-677-1303
                              custserv.us@oup.com
                              www.oup-usa.org

Thomas Carty, Senior Vice President
Simon Li, Regional Director
Adam Glazer, Director
$25.00
320 pages
ISBN 0-195076-67-2

7795 Autism and Learning
Taylor & Francis
7625 Empire Dr
Florence, KY 41042-2919   212-695-6599
                              800-634-7064
                              Fax: 212-563-2269
                              orders@taylorandfrancis.com
                              www.taylorandfrancis.com

Rita Jordan, Author
Stuart Powell, Co-Author
This book is about how a cognitive perception on the way in which individuals with autism think and learn may be applied to particular curriculum areas.
160 pages Paperback
ISBN 1-853464-21-X

7796 Autism in Adolescents and Adults
Springer Publishing
11 W 42nd St
Floor 15
New York, NY 10036-8002   212-431-4370
                              Fax: 212-460-1575
                              service-ny@springer.com
                              www.springerjournals.com

Eric Schopler, Editor
$63.00
456 pages
ISBN 0-306410-57-5

7797 Autism...Nature, Diagnosis and Treatment
Autism Society of North Carolina Bookstore
505 Oberlin Rd
Suite 230
Raleigh, NC 27605-1345   919-743-0204
                              800-442-2762
                              Fax: 919-743-0208
                              jchampion@autismsociety-nc.com
                              www.autismbookstore.com

David Lax, Manager
Covers perspectives, issues, neurobiological issues and new directions in diagnosis and treatment. *$49.00*

7798 Autism: Explaining the Enigma
Wiley Publishers
111 River St
Suite 2000
Hoboken, NJ 7030-5773   201-748-6000
                                    Fax: 201-748-6088
                                        info@wiley.com
                                        www.wiley.com

Uta Firth, Author
Explains the nature of autism. *$27.95*

7799 Autism: From Tragedy to Triumph
Branden Books
Po Box 812094
Wellesley, MA 02482   617-734-2045
                                    Fax: 781-790-1056
                                    www.brandenbooks.com

Carol Johnson, Author
Julia Crowder, Co-Author
A new book that deals with the Lovaas method and includes a foreward by Dr. Ivar Lovaas. The book is broken down into two parts — the long road to diagnosis and then treatment. *$12.95*

7800 Autism: Identification, Education and Treatment
Routledge (Taylor & Francis Group)
7625 Empire Dr
Florence, KY 41042-2919   212-695-6599
                                        800-634-7064
                                    Fax: 212-563-2269
                              orders@taylorandfrancis.com
                                        www.routledge.com

Dianne Zager, Editor
Jeffrey Lin, Director
Francis Chua, Manager
Chapters include medical treatments, early intervention and communication development in autism. *$36.00*
ISBN 0-805820-44-7

7801 Autism: The Facts
Oxford University Press
2001 Evans Rd
Cary, NC 27513-2010   919-677-0977
                                        800-445-9714
                                    Fax: 919-677-1303
                                   custserv.us@oup.com
                                        www.oup-usa.org

Simon Cohen, Author
Patrick Bolton, Co-Author
$22.50
128 pages
ISBN 0-192623-27-3

7802 Autistic Adults at Bittersweet Farms
Routledge (Taylor & Francis Group)
7625 Empire Dr
Florence, KY 41042-2919   212-695-6599
                                        800-634-7064
                                    Fax: 212-563-2269
                              orders@taylorandfrancis.com
                                        www.routledge.com

Norman Giddan PhD, Author
Jane Giddan MA, Co-Author
Jefferey Lin, Director
A touching view of an inspirational residential care program for autistic adolescents and adults. Also available in softcover. *$94.95*
Hardcover
ISBN 1-560240-42-3

7803 Be Quiet, Marina!
Star Bright Books
13 Landsdowne St
Cambridge, MA 02139   617-354-1300
                                    Fax: 617-354-1399
                              orders@starbrightbooks.com
                                    www.starbrightbooks.com

Kirsten Debear, Author

A noisy little girl with cerebral palsy and a quiet little girl with Down Syndrome learn to play together and eventually become best friends. *$16.95*
40 pages Hardcover
ISBN 1-887734-79-1

7804 Breakthroughs: How to Reach Students with Autism
Aquarius Health Care Media
30 Forest Road
PO Box 249
Millis, MA 02054   508-376-1244
                                    Fax: 508-376-1245
                                     aqvideos@tiac.net
                              www.aquariusproductions.com

Leslie Krussman, President/Producer
Joseph Wellington, Distribution Coordinator
Anne Baker, Billing & Accounting
A hands-on, how-to program for reaching students with autism, featuring Karen Sewell, Autism Society of America's teacher of the year. Here Sewell demonstrates the successful techniques she's developed over a 20-year career. A separate 250 page manual ($59) is also available which covers math, reading, fine motor, self help, social adaptive, vocational and self help skills as well as providing numerous plan reproducibles and an exhaustive listing of equipment and materials resources. Video. *$99.00*

7805 Bus Girl: Selected Poems
Brookline Books
8 Trumbull Rd
Suite B-001
Northampton, MA 01060   617-734-6772
                                        800-666-2665
                                    Fax: 617-734-3952
                                    brbooks@yahoo.com
                                  www.brooklinebooks.com

Gretchen Josephson, Author
Lula O Lubchenco, Editor
Poems written over several decades by a young woman with Down Syndrome. *$14.95*
144 pages Paperback
ISBN 1-57129-41-9

7806 Change Your Brain, Change Your Life: The Breakthrough Program for Conquering Depression
Three Rivers Press
3rd Floor
175 Broadway
New York, NY 10019   212-782-9000
                                    Fax: 212-940-7860
                                  www.randomhouse.com

Daniel G Amen MD, Author
Clinical neuroscientist and psychiatrist Amen uses nuclear brain imaging to diagnose and treat behavioral problems. He explains how the brain works, what happens when things go wrong, and how to optimize brain function. Five sections of the brain are discussed, and case studies clearly illustrate possible problems. *$15.00*
352 pages
ISBN 0-812929-98-5

7807 Child and Adolescent Therapy: Cognitive-Behavioral Procedures, Third Edition
Guilford Press
72 Spring Street
New York, NY 10012-4019   212-431-9800
                                        800-365-7006
                                    Fax: 212-966-6708
                                     info@guilford.com
                                       www.guilford.com

Chris Jennison, Publisher Emeritus, Education
Seymour Weingarten, Editor-in-Chief
Jody Falco, Managing Editor: Periodicals
Incorporating significant developments in treatment procedures, theory and clinical research, new chapters in this second edition examine the current status of empirically supported interventions and developmental issues specific to work with adolescents. *$45.00*
432 pages Cloth
ISBN 1-572305-56-8

**7808 Cognitive Behavioral Therapy for Adult Asperger
Syndrome**
Autism Society of North Carolina Bookstore
505 Oberlin Rd
Ste 230
Raleigh, NC 27605-1345

919-743-0204
800-442-2762
Fax: 919-743-0208
jchampion@autismsociety-nc.org
www.autismbookstore.com

David Lax, Manager
Text is prepared with case studies and examples from the author's
own experiences working as a cognitive-behavioral therapist
specializing in adults and adolescents with dual diagnosis, autism spectrum disorders, mood disorders, and anxiety disorders.

**7809 Communication Development in Children with Down
Syndrome**
Brookes Publishing
P.O.Box 10624
Baltimore, MD 21285-0624

410-337-9580
800-638-3775
Fax: 410-337-8539
custserv@brookespublishing.com
www.brookespublishing.com

Lauren Rohe, Regional Sales Consultant
Jeff Stickler, Educational Sales Representative
Sam Schissler, Educational Sales Representative
This book offers an extensive, detailed explanation of communication development in children with Down syndrome relative to
their advancing cognitive skills. It introduces a critical framework for assessing and treating hearing, speech, and language
problems and provides explicit intervention methods and tested
clinical protocols.
Paperback
ISBN 1-55766-50-5

**7810 Comprehensive Guide to ADD in Adults: Research,
Diagnosis & Treatment**
ADD Warehouse
300 NW 70th Ave
Suite 102
Plantation, FL 33317-2360

954-792-8100
800-233-9273
Fax: 954-792-8545
websales@addwarehouse.com
www.addwarehouse.com

Harvey C Parker, Owner
The first to provide broad coverage of the burgeoning field. Written for professionals who diagnose and treat adults with ADD, it
provides information from psychologists and physicians on the
most current research and treatment issues *$50.95*
426 pages
ISBN 0-876307-60-8

7811 Concentration Cockpit: Explaining Attention Deficits
Educators Publishing Service
P.O.Box 9031
Cambridge, MA 02139-9031

617-367-2700
800-225-5750
Fax: 617-547-0412
CustomerService.EPS@schoolspecialty.com
eps.schoolspecialty.com

Rick Holden, President
Melvin D Levine, Author
This eight-page pamphlet explains the administration of The
Concentration Cockpit, a newly revised poster that helps children
with attention deficits gain insight into their problems and moni-
tor their progress in grappling with these problems. *$64.50*
ISBN 0-838820-59-X

7812 Coping with ADD/ADHD
Rosen Publishing Group
29 E 21st St
New York, NY 10010-6209

212-420-1600
800-237-9932
Fax: 888-436-4643
www.rosenpublishing.com

Jaydene Morrison, Author

At least 3.5 million American youngsters suffer from attention
deficit disorder. This book defines the syndrome and provides
specific information about treatment and counseling. *$16.95*
ISBN 0-823920-70-4

7813 Count Us In
Exceptional Parent Library
P.O.Box 1807
Englewood Cliffs, NJ 7632-1207

201-947-6000
800-535-1910
Fax: 201-947-9376

Jason Kingsley, Author
Mitchell Levitz, Co-Author
Offers information on growing up with Downs Syndrome. *$9.95*

**7814 Culture and the Restructuring of Community Mental
Health**
Greenwood Publishing Group
130 Cremona Drive
Santa Barbara, CA 93117

805-968-1911
800-368-6868
Fax: 866-270-3856
CustomerService@abc-clio.com
www.greenwood.com

William A Vega, Author
John W Murphy, Co-Author
Michael Millman, Editor, American History
Examines treatment, organizational planning and research issues
and offers a critique of the theoretical and programmatic aspects
of providing mental health services to traditionally underserved
populations. $45.00-$52.95. *$95.00*
168 pages Hardcover
ISBN 0-313268-87-8

7815 Difficult Child
Bantam Books
1745 Broadway, 10th Floor
New York, NY 10019

212-782-9000
Fax: 212-302-7985
BBDPublicity@randomhouse.com
www.randomhouse.com/bantamdell

Stanley Turecki, Author
Leslie Tonner, Co-Author
The classic and definitive work on parenting hard-to-raise children with new sections on ADHD and the latest medications for
childhood disorders. *$15.95*
302 pages Paperback
ISBN 0-553380-36-2

7816 Disability Culture Perspective on Early Intervention
Through the Looking Glass
3075 Adeline Street
Suite 120
Berkeley, CA 94703-2212

510-848-1112
800-644-2666
Fax: 510-848-4445
TTY: 510-848-1005
TLG@lookingglass.org
www.lookingglass.org

Megan Kirshbaum PhD, Author
For parents with physical or cognitive disabilities and their families. Available in braille, large print or cassette. *$2.00*
12 pages

7817 Down Syndrome
Aquarius Health Care Media
30 Forest Road
PO Box 249
Millis, MA 02054-1066

508-376-1244
888-440-2963
Fax: 508-376-1245
www.aquariusproductions.com

Lesile Kussmann, Owner
This is an excellent video for families who have just had a baby
with Down Syndrome as well as professionals in the field of genetics and nursing. Through honest and open discussion, parents
of children with Down Syndrome express the feelings and concerns they had during the early years of their child's life. Preview
option available. *$150.00*
Video

7818 Driven to Distraction
Simon & Schuster/Touchstone Publishing
1230 Avenue of the Americas
Fl 11
New York, NY 10020- 1513
212-698-7000
Fax: 212-698-7009
www.simonsays.com

Edward M Hallowell, MD, Author
John J Ratey, MD, Co-Author
A practical book discussing adult as well as child attention deficit disorder (ADD). Non-technical, realistic and optimistic, it is an informative how-to manual for parents and consumers. *$23.00*

7819 Dyslexia over the Lifespan
Educators Publishing Service
PO Box 9031
Cambridge, MA 02139-9031
617-367-2700
800-225-5750
Fax: 617-547-0412
eps@schoolspecialty.com
www.epsbooks.com

Margaret B Rawston, Author
Discusses the educational and career development of 56 dyslexic boys from a private school that was one of the first to have a program to detect and treat developmental language disabilities. *$18.00*
224 pages
ISBN 0-838816-70-3

7820 Embracing the Monster: Overcoming the Challenges of Hidden Disabilities
Paul H Brookes Publishing Company
PO Box 10624
Baltimore, MD 21285-624
410-337-9580
800-638-3775
Fax: 410-337-8539
www.brookespublishing.com

Veronica Crawford M.A., Author
Larry B Silver, MD, Foreword/Commentary
The author shares her experience of living with LD, ADHD and bipolar disorder to give readers an awareness of the challenges of living with hidden disabilities and what can be done to help *$24.95*
272 pages paperback
ISBN 1-557665-22-2

7821 Encounters with Autistic States
Jason Aronson
400 Keystone Industrial Park
Dunmore, PA 18512-1507
800-782-0015
Fax: 201-840-7242

Theodore Mitrani, Author
This book explores and explands the work of the late Frances Tustin, which was devoted to the psychoanalytic understanding of the bewildering elemental world of the autistic child. *$50.00*
448 pages Hardcover
ISBN 0-765700-62-

7822 Families of Adults With Autism: Stories & Advice For the Next Generation
Autism Society of North Carolina Bookstore
505 Oberlin Road
Suite 230
Raleigh, NC 27605-1345
919-743-0204
800-442-2762
Fax: 919-743-0208
books@autismsociety-nc.org
www.autismbookstore.com

Tracey Sheriff, Chief Executive Officer
Paul Wendler, Chief Financial Officer
David Laxton, Director of Communications
This book's unique point of view is that of a parent who's been there and done that and is now willing to tell the reader what it was like. *$19.95*

7823 Family Therapy for ADHD: Treating Children, Adolescents and Adults
Guilford Press
72 Spring St
New York, NY 10012-4019
800-365-7006
www.guilford.com

Craig A Everett, Author
Sandra Volgy Everett, Co-Author
Presents an innovative approach to assesing and treating ADHD in the family context. *$29.00*
Paperback
ISBN 1-572304-38-3

7824 Fighting for Darla: Challenges for Family Care & Professional Responsibility
Teachers College Press
1234 Amsterdam Ave
New York, NY 10027-6602
212-678-3929
Fax: 212-678-4149
tcpress@tc.columbia.edu

Mary Lynch, Manager
Susan M Klein, Co-Author
Samuel Guskin, Co-Author
Follows the story of Darla, a pregnant adolescent with autism. *$18.95*
161 pages
ISBN 0-807733-56-3

7825 Fragile Success
Brookes Publishing
PO Box 10624
Baltimore, MD 21285-624
410-337-9580
800-638-3775
Fax: 410-337-8539
www.brookespublishing.com

Virginia Walker Sperry, Author
A book about the lives of autistic children, whom the author has followed from their early years at the Elizabeth Ives School in New Haven, CT, through to adulthood. *$27.50*
ISBN 1-557664-58-7

7826 Getting Our Heads Together
Thoms Rehabilitation Hospital
68 Sweeten Creek Rd
Asheville, NC 28803-2318
828-274-2400
Fax: 828-274-9452

Kathi Petersen, Director Planning/Communication
Edgardo Diez MD, Medical Director Brain Injury
Kathy Price, Director Admissions
A handbook for families of head injured patients - available in Spanish as well as English. *$4.00*
40 pages Paperback

7827 Getting a Grip on ADD: A Kid's Guide to Understanding & Coping with ADD
Educational Media Corporation
1443 Old York Rd
Warmister, PA 18794
763-781-0088
800-448-9041
Fax: 215-956-9041
www.educationalmedia.com

Kim Frank Ed.S., Author
Susan Smith-Rex Ed.D., Co-Author
Free catalog of resources.
64 pages Yearly

7828 Getting the Best for Your Child with Autism
Autism Society of North Carolina Bookstore
505 Oberlin Road
Suite 230
Raleigh, NC 27605-1345
919-743-0204
800-442-2762
Fax: 919-743-0208
books@autismsociety-nc.org
www.autismbookstore.com

Tracey Sheriff, Chief Executive Officer
Paul Wendler, Chief Financial Officer
David Laxton, Director of Communications
This treatment guide helps parents navigate the complex and overwhelming world of Autism. *$16.95*

7829 Group Activity for Adults with Brain Injury
Sage Publications
2455 Teller Road
Thousand Oaks, CA 91320   805-499-0721
                                 800-818-7243
                            Fax: 805-499-0871
                                 info@sagepub.com
                                 www.sagepub.com
Sara Miller McCune, Founder, Publisher, Executive Chairman
Blaise R Simqu, President & CEO
Tracey A. Ozmina, Executive Vice President & Chief Operating Officer
This manual addresses attention, memory, reasoning, and language skills in group settings. *$53.00*

7830 Guide to Successful Employment for Individuals with Autism
Brookes Publishing
P.O.Box 10624
Baltimore, MD 21285-0624   410-337-9580
                                 800-638-3775
                            Fax: 410-337-8539
                        custserv@brookespublishing.com
                             www.brookespublishing.com
Marcia Daltow Smith, Author
Ronald G Belcher, Co-Author
Patricia D Juhrs, Co-Author
Describing all aspects of job placement, this book details strategies for assessing workers, networking for job opportunities, and tailoring job supports to each individual. Also illustrates how to help individuals with autism become productive workers, and with detailed descriptions of specific jobs help provide ideas for employment. *$ 32.95*
336 pages Paperback
ISBN 1-55766 -71-5

7831 Handbook of Autism and Pervasive Developmental Disorders
Autism Society of North Carolina Bookstore
505 Oberlin Road
Suite 230
Raleigh, NC 27605-1345   919-743-0204
                                 800-442-2762
                            Fax: 919-743-0208
                        books@autismsociety-nc.org
                            www.autismbookstore.com
David Laxton, Director of Communications
Paul Wendler, Chief Financial Officer
Tracey Sheriff, Chief Executive Officer
A list of contributors address such topics as characteristics of autistic syndromes and interventions. *$125.00*

7832 Handbook of Career Planning for Students with Special Needs
Pro- Ed Publications
8700 Shoal Creek Boulevard
Austin, TX 78757-6897   512-451-3246
                                 800-897-3202
                            Fax: 512-451-8542
                        general@proedinc.com
                            www.proedinc.com
Donald D Hammill, Owner
Courtney King, Marketing Coordinator
Thomas F. Harrington, Editor
The practitioner's guide will show you how to help special needs adolescents and young adults overcome barriers to employment by identifying goals and problems, assessing interests and aptitudes, involving client families and developing communication skills. *$42.00*
358 pages

7833 Helping People with Autism Manage Their Behavior
Indiana Resource Center For Autism
2853 E 10th St
Bloomington, IN 47408-2696   812-855-6508
                            Fax: 812-855-9630
                        prattc@indiana.edu
                            www.iidc.indiana.edu
David Mank, Executive Director
Scott Bellini, Assistant Director

Covers the broad topic of helping people with autism manage their behavior. *$7.00*

7834 Helping Your Hyperactive: Attention Deficit Child
Crown Publishing Company (Random House)
1745 Broadway
New York, NY 10019-4305   212-782-9000
                                 800-632-8676
                            Fax: 212-572-6066
                        crownpublishing.com
John Taylor, Author
$19.95
ISBN 1-559584-23-8

7835 Hidden Child: The Linwood Method for Reaching the Autistic Child
Woodbine House
6510 Bells Mill Road
Bethesda, MD 20817-1636   301-897-3570
                                 800-843-7323
                            Fax: 301-897-5838
                        info@woodbinehouse.com
                            www.woodbinehouse.com
Irv Shapell, Owner
Sabine Oishi, Co-Author
Chronicle of the Linwood Children's Center's successful treatment program for autistic children. *$17.95*
286 pages Paperback
ISBN 0-933149-06-9

7836 How To Reach and Teach Children and Teens with Dyslexia
Jossey-Bass
111 River St
Hoboken, NJ 7030-5773   201-748-6000
                            Fax: 201-748-6008
                        info@wiley.com
                            www.wiley.com
Cynthia M Stowe, Author
This practical resource gives educators at all levels essential information, techniques, and tolls for understanding dyslexia and adapting teaching methods in all subject areas to meet the learning style, social, and emotional needs of students who have dyslexia. *$ 22.95*
340 pages
ISBN 0-130320-18-8

7837 Hyperactive Child, Adolescent, and Adult: ADD Through the Lifespan
Oxford University Press
198 Madison Ave
New York, NY 10016-4308   212-726-6000
                            www.us.oup.com/us
Paul H Wender, Author
Comprehensive general review. Update on previous research by the author, offering a basic text. Published by Ccnnecticut Association for Children & Adults with Learning Disabilities (CACLD). *$8.75*
162 pages
ISBN 0-195113-49-7

7838 Identifying and Treating Attention Deficit Hyperactivity Disorder
Learning Disabilities Association of America
461 Cochran Rd.
Suite 245
Pittsburgh, PA 15228   412-341-1515
                            Fax: 412-344-0224
                        info@ldaamerica.org
                            www.ldaamerica.org
Cindy Cipoletti, Executive Director
Aaron Goldstein, Director, Federal & State Engagement
Nina DelPrato, Administrative Manager
A resource guide for families and educators on the identification and treatment of Attention Deficit Hyperactivity Disorder (ADHD).

7839 In Search of Wings: A Journey Back from Traumatic Brain Injury
Lash & Associates Publishing/Training
100 Boardwalk Drive, Suite 150
Youngsville, NC 27596
919-556-0300
Fax: 919-556-0900
orders@lapublishing.com
www.lapublishing.com

Marilyn Lash, President
Bob Cluett, CEO
Bill Herrin, Director of Graphics & Design
The true story of one woman coping with traumatic brain injury after a car accident that affected her cognitive skills and memory *$14.95*
233 pages
ISBN 1-882332-00-8

7840 In Their Own Way
Alliance for Parental Involvement in Education
375 Hudson Street
New York, NY 10014
212-366-2000
Fax: 212-366-2933
ecommerce@us.penguingroup.com
http://us.penguingroup.com

Thomas Armstrong, Author
John Makinson, Chairman and Chief Executive
Coram Williams, CFO
For the parents whose children are not thriving in school, Armstrong offers insight into individual learning styles. *$11.95*

7841 Jumpin' Johnny Get Back to Work, A Child's Guide to ADHD/Hyperactivity
Ste 15-5
25 Van Zant St
Norwalk, CT 6855-1729
203-838-5010
Fax: 203-866-6108
CACLD@optonline.net
www.CACLD.org

Beryl Kaufman, Executive Director
Written primarily for elementary age youngsters with ADHD to help them understand their disability. Also valuable as an educational tool for parents, siblings, friends and classmates. Includes two pages on medication. *$12.50*
24 pages

7842 Keys to Parenting a Child with Attention Deficit Disorder
Barron's Educational Series
250 Wireless Blvd
Hauppauge, NY 11788-3924
631-434-3311
800-645-3476
Fax: 631-434-3723
barrons@barronseduc.com
barronseduc.com

Manuel H Barron, CEO
Francine McNamara MSW CSW, Co/Author
This book shows how to work with the child's school, effectively manage the child's behavior and act as the child's advocate. *$6.95*
160 pages Paperback
ISBN 0-812014-59-6

7843 Keys to Parenting a Child with Downs Syndrome
Barron's Educational Series
250 Wireless Blvd
Hauppauge, NY 11788-3924
631-434-3311
800-645-3476
Fax: 631-434-3723
barrons@barronseduc.com
barronseduc.com

Manuel H Barron, CEO
Lucy Guarino
Down Syndrome poses many challenges for children and their families. This book prepares parents and guardians to raise a child with Down Syndrome by discussing adjustment, advocacy, health and behavior, education and planning for greater independence. *$5.95*
160 pages Paperback
ISBN 0-812014-58-8

7844 Keys to Parenting the Child with Autism
Barron's Educational Series
250 Wireless Blvd
Hauppauge, NY 11788-3924
631-434-3311
800-645-3476
Fax: 631-434-3723
barrons@barronseduc.com
barronseduc.com

Manuel H Barron, CEO
Parents of children with autism will find a solid balance between home and practical information in this book. It explains what autism is and how it is diagnosed, then advises parents on how to adjust to their child and give the best care. *$6.95*
208 pages Paperback
ISBN 0-812016-79-3

7845 LD Child and the ADHD Child: Ways Parents & Professionals Can Help
1406 Plaza Dr
Winston Salem, NC 27103-1470
336-768-1374
800-222-9796
Fax: 336-768-9194
southern@blairpub.com
www.blairpub.com

Carolyn Sakowski, President
Susan H Stevens, Author
Book about learning disabilities available to parents. Stevens cuts through the jargon and complex theories which usually characterize books on the subject to present effective and practical techniques that parents can employ to help their child succeed at home and at school. New edition adds information about ADHD children. *$12.95*
201 pages Paperback
ISBN 0-895871-42-4

7846 Let Community Employment be the Goal for Individuals with Autism
Indiana Resource Center For Autism
2853 E 10th St
Bloomington, IN 47408-2601
812-855-9396
800-825-4733
Fax: 812-855-9630
prattc@indiana.edu
www.iidc.indiana.edu

David Mank, Executive Director
Scott Bellini, Assistant Director
A guide designed for people who are responsible for preparing individuals with autism to enter the work force. *$7.00*

7847 Making the Writing Process Work
Brookline Books
8 Trumbull Rd
Suite B-001
Northampton, MA 01060
617-734-6772
800-666-2665
Fax: 617-734-3952
brbooks@yahoo.com
www.brooklinebooks.com

Karen R Harris, Author
Steve Grahm, Co-Author
Making the Writing Process Work: Strategies for Composition and Self-Regulation is geared toward students who have difficulty organizing their thoughts and developing their writing. The specific strategies teach students how to approach, organize, and produce a final written product. *$24.95*
240 pages Paperback
ISBN 1-57129 -10-9

7848 Management of Autistic Behavior
Sage Publications
2455 Teller Road
Thousand Oaks, CA 91320
805-499-0721
800-818-7243
Fax: 800-583-2665
info@sagepub.com
www.sagepub.com

Sara Miller McCune, Founder, Publisher, Executive Chairman
Blaise R Simqu, President & CEO
Tracey A. Ozmina, Executive Vice President & Chief Operating Officer

This excellent reference is a comprehensive and practical book that tells what works best with specific problems. *$41.00*
450 pages

7849 Managing Attention Deficit Hyperactivity in Children: A Guide for Practitioners
John Wiley & Sons Inc
111 River St
Hoboken, NJ 07030-5774   201-748-6000
800-825-7550
Fax: 201-748-6088
info@wiley.com
www.wiley.com

Warren J Baker, President
Michael Goldstein, Co-Author
Matthe S Kissner, CEO
Offers information about human personality, structure and dynamics, assessment and adjustment. *$27.50*
214 pages Hardcover
ISBN 0-471121-58-9

7850 Neurobiology of Autism
Johns Hopkins University Press
2715 N Charles St
Baltimore, MD 21218-4363   410-516-6900
Fax: 410-516-6968
www.press.jhu.edu

William Brody, President
Thomas L Kemper, Co-Author
Margaret L Bauman, M.D., Co-Author
This book discusses recent advances in scientific research that point to a neurobiological basis for autism and examines the clinical implications of this research. *$28.00*
272 pages
ISBN 0-801880-47-5

7851 Out of the Fog: Treatment Options and Coping Strategies for ADD
Hyperion
1500 Broadway
3rd Floor
New York, NY 10036   212-563-6500
800-331-3761
Fax: 212-456-0176
www.hyperionbooks.com

Robert Miller, President
Suzanne Levert, Co-Author
Discusses the recent recognition of attention deficit disorder as a problem that is not outgrown in adolescence, and cogently summarizes the stumbling blocks this affliction creates in the pursuit of a career or attainment of a healthy family life *$14.95*
300 pages
ISBN 0-786880-87-2

7852 Overcoming Dyslexia
Vintage-Random House
3rd Fl
1745 Broadway
New York, NY 10019-4305   212-782-9000
Fax: 212-302-7985
www.randomhouse.com/vintage

Markus Dohle, CEO
Sally Shawitz, M.D., Author
Yale neuroscientist Shaywitz demystifies the roots of dyslexia (a neurologically based reading difficulty affecting one in five children) and offers parents and educators hope that children with reading problems can be helped. *$15.00*
432 pages
ISBN 0-679781-59-5

7853 Parent Survival Manual
Springer Publishing Company
11 W 42nd St
15th Floor
New York, NY 10036   212-431-4370
877-687-7476
Fax: 212-941-7842
cs@springerpub.com
www.springerpub.com

Ursula Springer, President
Ted Nardin, CEO
Edie Lambiase, CFO
A guide to crises resolution in autism and related developmental disorders. *$39.95*

7854 Parent's Guide to Down Syndrome: Toward a Brighter Future
Brookes Publishing
PO Box 10624
Baltimore, MD 21285-0624   410-337-9580
800-638-3775
Fax: 410-337-8539
custserv@brookespublishing.com
www.brookespublishing.com

Siegfried Pueschel MD PhD, Author
Highlights developmental stages and shows the advances that improve a child's quality of life. Includes discussions on easing the transition from home to school and choosing integration and curricular priorities, as well as guidelines for confronting adolescent and adult issues such as social and sexual needs and independent living and vocational options. *$21.95*
352 pages
ISBN 1-557664-52-8

7855 Parenting Attention Deficit Disordered Teens
CACLD
25 Van Zant Street
Norwalk, CT 06855-1729   203-838-5010
Fax: 203-866-6108
CACLD@optonline.net
cacld.org

Beryl Kaufman, Executive Director
Detailed outline of the various problems of adolescents with ADHD. Published by Connecticut Association for Children & Adults with Learning Disabilities (CACLD). *$3.25*
14 pages

7856 Parents Helping Parents: A Directory of Support Groups for ADD
Novartis Pharmaceuticals Division
59 State Route 10
East Hanover, NJ 7936-1005   862-778-7500
800-742-2422

Paulo Costa, CEO

7857 Please Don't Say Hello
Human Sciences Press
233 Spring St
New York, NY 10013-1522   212-229-2859
800-221-9369
Fax: 212-463-0742
isbndb.com

Charles Stenken, Author
Jaroslav Chobot, Author
Zirul Evany, Author
With the support and love of his family, and through them the neighborhood children, a nine-year-old autistic boy is able to emerge from his shell. *$10.95*
47 pages Paperback
ISBN 0-89885 -99-8

7858   Preventable Brain Damage
Springer Publishing Company
11 W 42nd St
15th Floor
New York, NY 10036   212-431-4370
                                      877-687-7476
                                Fax: 212-941-7842
                                cs@springerpub.com
                                www.springerpub.com
Donald L Templer, Author
Lawrence C Hartlage, Co-Author
Ursula Springer, President
Offers information on brain injuries from motor vehicle acci-
dents, contact sports and injuries of children. *$35.95*
256 pages

7859   Reading, Writing and Speech Problems in Children
International Dyslexia Association
40 York Rd.
4th Floor
Baltimore, MD 21204   410-296-0232
                                Fax: 410-321-5069
                                info@dyslexiaida.org
                                dyslexiaida.org
Samuel Torrey Orton, Author
This book provides reading, reading and speech execerises for
educating people with dyslexia. *$20.00*
259 pages
ISBN 0-89079-79-1

7860   Reality of Dyslexia
Brookline Books
8 Trumbull Rd
Suite B-001
Northampton, MA 01060   617-734-6772
                                      800-666-2665
                                Fax: 617-734-3952
                                brbooks@yahoo.com
                                www.brooklinebooks.com
John Osmond, Author
An informative and sensitive study of living with dyslexia which
affects one in 25. He introduces the reader to the subject by sharing the difficulties of his dyslexic son. He then uses the personal
accounts of other children and adult dyslexics, even entire dyslexic families, to illuminate the problems they encounter. *$14.95*
150 pages Paperback
ISBN 1-57129-17-6

**7861   Relationship Development Intervention with Young
Children**
Jessica Kingsley Publishers
400 Market St
Suite 400
Philadelphia, PA 19106   215-922-1161
                                Fax: 215-992-1417
                                orders@jkp.com
                                www.jkp.com
Steven E Gustein, Author
Rachelle Sheely, Co-Author
Social and emotional development activities for Asperger Syndrome, Autism, PDD and NLD. Comprehensive set of activities
emphasizes foundation skills for younger children between the
ages of two and eight. Covers skills such as social referencing,
regulating behvior, conversational reciprocity, and synchronized
actions. For use in therapeutic settings as well as schools and parents. *$22.95*
256 pages
ISBN 1-843107-14-7

7862   Rethinking Attention Deficit Disorder
Brookline Books
8 Trumbull Rd
Suite B-001
Northampton, MA 01060-4533   617-734-6772
                                      800-666-2665
                                Fax: 617-734-3952
                                brbooks@yahoo.com
                                www.brooklinebooks.com
Miriam Cherkes-Julkowski, Author

In contrast to the common focus on behavioral symptoms of attention disorders, this book emphasizes internal factors that make attention regulation difficult. In-depth discussions of social,
emotional, and academic consequences and appropriate interventions are provided. *$27.95*
250 pages Paperback
ISBN 1-571290-30-7

7863   Riddle of Autism: A Psychological Analysis
Jason Aronson
4501 Forbes Blvd
Suite 200
Lanham, MD 20706-4346   301-459-3366
                                      800-782-0015
                                Fax: 301-429-5746
                                www.rowmanlittlefield.com
Jason Aronson, Author
James Lyons, President/CEO
Stanley Plotnick, Chairman
Dr. Victor examines the myths that cloud an understanding of this
disorder and describes the meanings of its specific behavioral
symptoms. *$30.00*
356 pages Paperback
ISBN 1-568215-73-8

**7864   SCATBI: Scales Of Cognitive Ability for Traumatic
Brain Injury**
Sage Publications
2455 Teller Road
Thousand Oaks, CA 91320   805-499-0721
                                      800-818-7243
                                Fax: 805-499-0871
                                happiness@option.org
                                www.sagepub.com
Sara Miller McCune, Founder, Publisher, Executive Chairman
Blaise R Simqu, President & CEO
*Tracey A. Ozmina, Executive Vice President & Chief Operating
Officer*
Assesses cognitive and linguistic abilities of adolescent and adult
parents with head injuries. *$287.00*

7865   Sex Education: Issues for the Person with Autism
Indiana Resource Center For Autism
2853 E 10th St
Bloomington, IN 47408-2696   812-855-6508
                                      800-825-4733
                                Fax: 812-855-9630
                                iidc@indiana.edu
                                www.iidc.indiana.edu
David Mank, Executive Director
Scott Bellini, Assistant Director
Discusses issues of sexuality and provides methods of instruction
for people with autism. *$4.00*

7866   Son-Rise: The Miracle Continues
2080 S Undermountain Rd.
Sheffield, MA 01257   413-229-2100
                                      800-562-7171
                                correspondence@option.org
                                www.autismtreatmentcenter.org
Barry Neil Kaufman, Founder & CEO
Clyde Haberman, Senior Teacher & Director of Development
Blair Borgeson, Developmental Therapist
The center's Son-Rise Program teaches a comprehensive system
of treatment and education designed to help families and care-
givers enable their children to dramatically improve in all areas of
learning. *$12.95*
343 pages
ISBN 0-915811-53-7

7867   Soon Will Come the Light
Future Horizons Inc
721 W Abram St
Arlington, TX 76013-6995   817-277-0727
                                      800-479-0727
                                Fax: 817-277-2270
                                www.fhautism.com
Wayne Gilpin, Owner
Jennifer Gilpin, Vice President
Annette Vick, Manager

Offers new perspectives on the perplexing disability of autism. *$19.95*

7868 Successful Job Search Strategies for the Disabled: Understanding the ADA
Wiley Publishing
605 3rd Ave
New York, NY 10158-180   212-850-6000
                                     Fax: 212-850-6088
                                        www.wiley.com

Jeffrey G Allen, Author
Following a concise overview of the Americans with Disabilities Act (ADA), covers such topics as job identification, self-assessment, job leads, resumes, disability disclosure, interviewing, and accommodating specific disabilities. Includes dozen of relevant and instructive situation analyses, case examples, and answers to commonly asked questions. *$165.00*
229 pages

7869 Taking Charge of ADHD Complete Authoritative Guide for Parents
Guilford Press
72 Spring St
New York, NY 10012-4019   212-431-9800
                                          800-365-7006
                                     Fax: 212-966-6708
                                       info@guilford.com
                                        www.guilford.com

Russell A Barkley, Author
Revised and updated to incorporate the most current information on ADHD and its treatment. Provides parents with the knowledge, guidance and confidence they need to ensure that their child receives the best care possible. Also in cloth at $40.00 (ISBN# 1-57230-600-9 *$18.95*
331 pages Paperback
ISBN 1-572305-60-1

7870 Teaching Children with Autism: Strategies for Initiating Positive Interactions
Brookes Publishing
P.O.Box 10624
Baltimore, MD 21285-0624   410-337-9580
                                          800-638-3775
                                     Fax: 410-337-8539
                              custserv@brookespublishing.com
                                 www.brookespublishing.com

Robert L. Koegel, Author
Lynn Kern Koegel, Co-Author
Robert Miller, Sales Director
Offers strategies for initiating positive interactions and improving learning opportunities. This guide begins with an overview of characteristics and long-term strategies and proceeds through discussions that detail specific techniques for normalizing environments, reducing disruptive behavior, improving language and social skills, and enhancing generalization. *$39.95*
256 pages Paperback
ISBN 1-557661-80-4

7871 Teaching and Mainstreaming Autistic Children
Love Publishing Company
9101 E Kenyon Ave
Suite 2200
Denver, CO 80237-1854   303-221-7333
                                     Fax: 303-221-7444
                                     www.lovepublishing.com

Stan Love, Owner
Peter Knoblock, Author
Dr. Knoblock advocates a highly organized, structured environment for autistic children, with teachers and parents working together. His premise is that the learning and social needs of autistic children must be analyzed and a daily program designed with interventions that respond to this functional analysis of their behavior. *$24.95*
ISBN 0-89108 -11-9

7872 Techniques for Aphasia Rehab: (TARGET) Generating Effective Treatment
Speech Bin
1965 25th Ave
Vero Beach, FL 32960-3062   772-770-0007
                                          800-477-3324
                                     Fax: 772-770-0006
                                   store.schoolspecialty.com

Mary Jo Santo Pietro, Co-Author
Robert Goldfarb, Co-Author
TARGET is the kind of resource aphasia clinicians beg for. A practical resource that answers not only the what and how questions of treatment, but also the why. It describes dozens of treatment methods and gives you practical exercises and activities to implement each technique. It shows you how to treat all components of the disability, language disorder, overall impairment, communication problems, and the needs of the person with aphasia. *$45.00*
384 pages
ISBN 0-93785 -50-5

7873 Teenagers with ADD
Woodbine House
6510 Bells Mill Rd
Bethesda, MD 20817-1636   301-897-3570
                                          800-843-7323
                                     Fax: 301-897-5838
                                   info@woodbinehouse.com
                                     www.woodbinehouse.com

Irv Shapell, Owner
Chris A Ziegler Dendy, M.S., Author
This best selling guide to understanding and coping with teenagers with attention deficit disorder (ADD) provides complete coverage of the special issues and challenges faced by these teens. Based on current diagnostic criteria and the latest literature and research in the field, the book discusses diagnosis, medical treatment, family and school life, intervention, advocacy, legal rights, and options after high school. Parents find strategies for dealing with their teen's difficult behaviors. *$18.95*
370 pages Paperback
ISBN 0-933149-69-7

7874 Understanding Down Syndrome: An Introduction for Parents
Brookline Books
8 Trumbull Rd
Suite B-001
Northampton, MA 01060-4533   617-734-6772
                                          800-666-2665
                                     Fax: 617-734-3952
                                     brbooks@yahoo.com
                                   www.brooklinebooks.com

Cliff Cunningham, Author
Using positive and readable language, this book helps parents understand Down Syndrome. Medical details are explained in lay terms, and advice is given on working with professionals, obtaining services, and treatment techniques that help the child. Cunningham alerts families to potential problems, the prospects for the child in schooling and the passage to adulthood. Revised 1996. *$14.95*
Softcover
ISBN 1-57129 -09-5

7875 Valley News Dispatch
New York Families For Autistic Children
95-16 Pitkin Avenue
Ozone Park, NY 11417-2834   718-641-3441
                                     Fax: 718-641-2228

Cheryl L. Marsh, Chairperson
Robert Burt, Treasurer
Education, recreation and support services for families and children with developmental disabilities.

7876 Verbal Behavior Approach: How to Teach Children with Autism & Related Disorders
Autism Society of North Carolina Bookstore
505 Oberlin Road
Suite 230
Raleigh, NC 27605-1345
919-743-0204
800-442-2762
Fax: 919-743-0208
books@autismsociety-nc.org
www.autismbookstore.com
David Laxton, Director of Communications
Paul Wendler, Chief Financial Officer
Tracey Sheriff, Chief Executive Officer
Provides full descriptions of how to teach the verbal operants that make up expressive languate which include: manding, tacting, echoing and intraverbal skills. *$19.95*

7877 Without Reason: A Family Copes with two Generations of Autism
Books on Special Children
721 W Abram St
Arlington, TX 76013-6995
817-277-0727
800-489-0727
Fax: 817-277-2270
Wayne Tilton, President
The author discovers his son has autism. He delves into problems of the autistic person and explains reasons for their actions. *$20.95*
292 pages Hardcover

7878 Women with Attention Deficit Disorder: Embracing Disorganization at Home and Work
Underwood-Miller
708 Westover Dr
Lancaster, PA 17601-1242
Addresses the millions of withdrawn little girls and chronically overwhelmed women with ADD who go undiagnosed because they don't fit the stereotypical notion of people with ADD. *$11.95*
288 pages
ISBN 1-887424-05-9

7879 You Mean I'm Not Lazy, Stupid or Crazy?!: A Self-Help Book for Adults with ADD
Simon & Schuster
1230 Avenue Of The Americas
11th Floor
New York, NY 10020-1513
212-698-7000
Fax: 212-698-7099
www.simonsays.com
Kate Kelly, Author
Peggy Ramundo, Co-Author
Practical advice on controlling adult ADD, a straightforward guide explains how to get along in groups, become organized, improve memory, and pursue professional help. *$15.00*
464 pages
ISBN 0-684815-31-1

7880 You and Your ADD Child
Nelson Publications
1 Gateway Plz
Port Chester, NY 10573-4674
914-481-5490
Fax: 914-937-8950
Paul Warren MD, Author
Jody Capehart M.Ed., Co-Author
$12.99
252 pages Paperback
ISBN 0-785278-95-8

Journals

7881 Annals of Dyslexia
International Dyslexia Association
40 York Road
4th Floor
Baltimore, MD 21204
410-296-0232
Fax: 410-321-5069
info@dyslexiaida.org
dyslexiaida.org/annals-of-dyslexia
Denise Douce, Director, Publications & Resources
IDA is a clearinghouse of scientific data and practice-based information related to dyslexia. Provides community-based referrals and information fact sheets in response to thousands of emails, calls & letters. Our annual conference attracts thousands of outstanding researchers, clinicians, parents, teachers, psychologists, educational therapists and people with dyslexia.
Tri-annual

7882 Journal of Cognitive Rehabilitation
Neuroscience Publishers
6555 Carrollton Ave
Indianapolis, IN 46220-1664
317-257-9672
Fax: 317-257-9674
neuroscience.cnter.com
Odie L Bracy, Executive Director
Publication for therapists, family and patient, designed to provide information relevant to the rehabilitation of impairment resulting from brain injury. *$50.00*
36-48 pages Quarterly

Magazines

7883 AWARE
National Fibromyalgia Association
1000 Bristol Street North
Suite 17-247
Irvine, CA 92660
714-921-0150
Fax: 714-921-6920
www.fmaware.org
Lynne Matallana, President/Founder
Mark Dobrilovic, Board of Director
John Fry, PhD, Board of Director
Magazine published three times a year with membership only.

7884 Attention
Children & Adults with ADHD
8181 Professional Place
Suite 150
Landover, MD 20785- 2264
301-306-7070
800-233-4050
Fax: 301-306-7090
webmaster@chadd.org
www.chadd.org
Bryan Goodman, Director
A bi-monthly publication from CHADD. Free with membership.
Bi-monthly

Newsletters

7885 ADHD Report
Guilford Press
72 Spring St
New York, NY 10012-4019
212-431-9800
800-365-7006
Fax: 212-966-6708
info@guilford.com
www.guilford.com
Russell A Barkley PhD, Editor
Presents the most up-to-date information on the evaluation, diagnosis and management of ADHD in children, adolescents and

adults. This important newsletter is an invaluable resource for all professionals interested in ADHD. *$49.95*
16 pages BiMonthly
ISSN 1065-8025

7886 Arc Connection Newsletter
Arc of Tennessee
151 Athens Way
Suite 100
Nashville, TN 37228
615-248-5878
800-835-7077
Fax: 615-248-5879
info@thearctn.org
thearctn.org

John Lewis, President
John H. Shouse, VP,Planning & Rules committee Chair
Donna Lankford, Secretary
Quarterly publication from the ARC of Tennessee. *$ 10.00*
12 pages Quarterly

7887 Arc Light
Arc of Arizona
5610 S Central Ave
Phoenix, AZ 85040-3090
602-268-6101
800-252-9054
Fax: 602-268-7483
thearcaz@gmail.com

Cindy Waymire, Editor
For people with intellectual and developmental disabilities.
Quarterly

7888 Autism Research Review International
Autism Research Institute
4182 Adams Ave
San Diego, CA 92116-2599
619-281-7165
Fax: 619-563-6840
br@autismresearchinstitute.com
autism.com

Steve Edelson, Executive Director
The Autism Research Institute has pubished this quarterly newsletter, Autism Research Review International (ARRI), since 1987. The ARRI has received worldwide praise for it's thoroughness and objectivity in reporting the current developments in biomedical and educational research. The latest findings are gleaned from a computer search of the 25,000 scientific and medical articles published every week. *$18.00*
8 pages Quarterly

7889 BIATX Newsletter
Brain Injury Association of Texas
316 W 12th Street
Suite 405
Austin, TX 78701-1845
512-326-1212
800-392-0040
Fax: 512-478-3370
www.texasbia.org

Judith Abner, Director
Penny Phillips, President
Donna Kuhlmann, Chairman
A online quarterly e-newsletter, as well as news and updates on the Brain Injury Association of Texas.

7890 BIAWV Newsletter
Brain Injury Association of America
PO Box 574
Institute, WV 25112-0574
304-766-4892
800-356-6443
Fax: 304-766-4940
biawv@aol.com

Peggy Brown, Director
Mike Davis, President

7891 Best Buddies Times
Best Buddies Times
907-1243 Islington Ave
Toronto, ON, Canada
416-531-0003
888-779-0061
Fax: 416-531-0325
info@bestbuddies.ca
www.bestbuddies.ca

Steven Pinnock, Director
Emily Bolyea-Kyere, Regional Program Manager
Bi-annual newsletter.

7892 Chadder
Children & Adults with Attention Deficit Disorder
4601 Presidents Drive
Suite 300
Lanham, MD 20706
301-306-7070
Fax: 301-306-7090
www.chadd.org

Michael MacKay, President
Ruth Hughes, CEO
Susan Buningh, Executive Editor
Quarterly newsletter
Quarterly

7893 Cognitive Therapy Today
Beck Institute for Cognitive Therapy & Research
One Belmont Avenue
Ste 700
Bala Cynwyd, PA 19004-1610
610-664-3020
Fax: 610-709-5336
info@beckinstitute.org
www.beckinstitute.org

Judith S Beck, Director
Aaron T Beck, President
Cognitive Therapy TodayT features articles on a wide range of topics in CBT by leading clinicians from around the world. Articles have addressed evaluating psychotherapies; CBT and special populations, such as soldiers, the elderly, or diagnoses such as schizophrenia; conceptualizing emotions; cross-cultural issues and many other issues of interest to clinicians. You will also find information on workshops, speaking engagements by Beck Institute faculty and more.

7894 Down Syndrome News
National Down Syndrome Congress
30 Mansell Court
Suite 108
Roswell, GA 30076
770-604-9500
800-232-6372
Fax: 770-604-9898
info@ndsccenter.org
www.ndsccenter.org

Jim Faber, President
Marilyn Tolbert, 1st VP
Carole J. Guess, 2nd Vice President
Must become a member to receive the newsletter.

7895 Focus Times Newsletter
Focus Alternative Learning Center
126 Dowd Avenue
PO Box 452
Canton, CT 06019-0452
860-693-8809
Fax: 860-693-0141
info@focuscenterforautism.org
www.focus-alternative.org

Marcia Bok, President
Claudia Godburn, Secretary
Rita Barredo, Treasurer
Monthly online newsletter on autism.

7896 Imagine!
Imagine!
1400 Dixon Ave.
Lafayette, CO 80026-2790
303-665-7789
imaginecolorado.org

Rebecca Novinger, Executive Director
Jeff Tucker, Director of Human Resources
Jenna Corder, Director of Client Relations

For people of all ages with cognitive, developmental, physical & health related needs, so they may live lives of independence & quality in their homes and communities.
12-16 pages quarterly

7897 NAMI Advocate
National Alliance on Mental Illness
3803 N Fairfax Dr
Suite 100
Arlington, VA 22203-3080
703-524-7600
800-950-6264
Fax: 703-524-9094
www.nami.org

Suzanne Vogel-Scibilia, President
Our mission is to provide you with the technical assistance, tools and referrals to resources you need to build organizational capacity and achieve the goals of the NAMI Standards of Excellence.

7898 NLP News
NLP Comprehensive
PO.Box 348
Indian Hills, CO 80454-648
303-987-2224
800-233-1657
Fax: 303-987-2228
www.nlpco.com

Christian Miller, Editor
Tom Dotz, President
Tom Hoobyar, Director Of Planning
An online e-newsletter on Neuro-linguistic programming.

7899 Pure Facts
Feingold Association of the US
10955 Windjammer Dr. S
Indianapolis, IN 46256
631-369-9340
help@feingold.org
www.feingold.org

Deborah Lehner, Executive Director
Relationship between foods, food additives and behaviorial or learning challenges.

7900 REACH
TEACCH
100 Renee Lynn Ct
Carrboro, NC 27510
919-966-2174
Fax: 919-966-4127
teacch@unc.edu
www.teacch.com

Dr. Laura Klinger, Director
Walter Kelly, Business Officer
Rebecca Mabe, Assistant Director of Business
Free online newsletter.

7901 Rettsyndrome.org
4600 Devitt Dr
Cincinnati, OH 45246
513-874-3020
800-818-7388
Fax: 513-874-2520
admin@rettsyndrome.org
www.rettsyndrome.org

Peter White, Chair
Gordon Rich, Chief Operating Officer
Steven Kaminsky, Ph.D, Chief Science Officer
Rettsyndrome.org offers informational resources and programs for those affected by Rett syndrome as well as their families.

7902 Weekly Wisdom
Autism Treatment Center of America
2080 S Undermountain Rd
Sheffield, MA 01257-9643
413-229-2100
877-766-7473
Fax: 413-229-3202
www.son-rise.org

Barry Kausman, Owner
Weekly Wisdom is available through a free email subscription.

Audio/Visual

7903 ADD, Stepping Out of the Dark
Child Development Media
5632 Van Nuys Blvd
Suite 286
Van Nuys, CA 91401-4602
818-989-7221
800-405-8942
Fax: 818-989-7826

Margie Wagner, Owner
A powerful, effective video, ideal for health professionals, educators and parents providing a visual montage designed to promote an understanding and awareness of attention deficit disorder. Based on actual accounts of those who have ADD, including a neurologist, an office worker, and parents of children with ADD. The DVD allows the viewer to feel the frustration and lack of attention that ADD brings to many. *$52.95*
Video

7904 ADHD in Adults
Guilford Press
72 Spring St
New York, NY 10012-4019
212-431-9800
800-365-7006
Fax: 212-966-6708
info@guilford.com
www.guilford.com

Russell A Barkley, Editor
This program integrates information on ADHD with the actual experiences of four adults who suffer from the disorder. Representing a range of professions, from a lawyer to a mother working at home, each candidly discusses the impact of ADHD on his or her daily life. These interviews are augmented by comments from family members and other clinicians who treat adults with ADHD. *$99.00*
DVD 1906
ISBN 0-898629-86-1

7905 ADHD: What Can We Do?
Guilford Press
72 Spring St
New York, NY 10012-4019
212-431-9800
800-365-7006
Fax: 212-966-6708
info@guilford.com

Russell A Barkley, Editor
A video program that introduces teachers and parents to a variety of the most effective technologies for managing ADHD in the classroom, at home, and on family outings. *$99.00*
DVD 1906
ISBN 0-898629-72-1

7906 ADHD: What Do We Know?
Guilford Press
72 Spring St
New York, NY 10012-4019
212-431-9800
800-365-7006
Fax: 212-966-6708
info@guilford.com
www.guilford.com

Bob Matloff, President
Russell A Barkley, Editor
An introduction for teachers and special education practitioners, school psychologists and parents of ADHD children. Topics outlined in this video include the causes and prevalence of ADHD, ways children with ADHD behave, other conditions that may accompany ADHD and long-term prospects for children with ADHD. *$99.00*
DVD 1906
ISBN 0-898629-71-3

7907   Around the Clock: Parenting the Delayed AD HD Child
Guilford Press
72 Spring St
New York, NY 10012-4019
212-431-9800
800-365-7006
Fax: 212-966-6708
info@guilford.com

Joan F Goodman, Editor
Susan Hoban, Editor
This videotape provides both professionals and parents a helpful look at how the difficulties facing parents of ADHD children can be handled. Video. *$150.00*
VHS 1994
ISBN 0-898629-68-3

7908   Attention Deficit Disorder: Adults
Aquarius Health Care Media
30 Forest Road
Millis, MA 02054
508-376-1244
888-440-2963
Fax: 508-376-1245
www.aquariusproductions.com

Lesile Kussmann, President/Owner
Joseph Wellington, Distribution Coordinator
Anne Baker, Billing & Accounting
Adults with ADD talk about how the disorder that went undiagnosed for so many years has affected their choice of spouses and work, and what they have found to help them. Biofeedback, which is growing as a treatment, is explained and demonstrated by its founder, Dr. Joel Lubar. Medical treatments like antidepressants and stimulants are also discussed, along with behavioral changes that can help the person with ADD and his or her spouse and family. *$149.00*
Video

7909   Attention Deficit Disorder: Children
Aquarius Health Care Media
30 Forest Rd
PO Box 249
Millisrn, MA 02054-7159
508-376-1244
888-440-2963
Fax: 508-376-1245
www.aquariusproductions.com

Lesile Kussmann, President/Owner
Everyone has been impulsive or easily distracted for different periods of time, so these symptoms that are hallmarks of Attention Deficit Disorder (ADD) have also led to criticism that too many people are being diagnosed with this biochemical brain disorder. This program examines who is being diagnosed, and what treatments are working. An innovative private school specializing in alternative education is profiled, and tips on structuring the school and home environment are included. *$149.00*
Video

7910   Autism: A World Apart
Fanlight Productions C/O Icarus Films
32 Court Street
Brooklyn, NY 11201-1731
718-488-8900
800-876-1710
Fax: 718-488-8642
info@fanlight.com
www.fanlight.com

Ben Achtenberg, Owner
Nicole Johnson, Publicity Coordinator
Anthony Sweeney, Marketing Director
In this documentary, three families show us what the textbooks and studies cannot: what it's like to live with autism day after day; to raise and love children who may be withdrawn and violent and unable to make personal connections with their families. 29 minutes. *$195.00*
VHS/DVD 1988
ISBN 1-572950-39-0

7911   Autism: the Unfolding Mystery
Aquarius Health Care Media
30 Forest Road
PO Box 249
Millis, MA 02054
508-376-1244
Fax: 508-376-1245
www.aquariusproductions.com

Lesile Kussmann, Owner
Explore what it means to be autistic, how you can recognize the signs of autism in your child, and hear about new treatments and programs to help children learn to deal with the disorder. *$145.00*
DVD 1905

7912   Biology Concepts Through Discovery
Educational Activities Software
5600 W 83rd Street
Suite 300, 8200 Tower
Bloomington, MN 55437
800-447-5286
Fax: 239-225-9299
info@edmentum.com
http://www.ea-software.com

Vin Riera, President/CEO
Rob Rueckel, CFO
Dave Adams, Chief Academic Officer
These videos, available in English and Spanish versions, encourage learning by presenting interactive problem solving in an effective VISUAL/AUDITORY style. *$89.00*
Video

7913   Concentration Video
Learning disAbilities Resources
6 E Eagle Road
Havertown, PA 19083
610-446-6126
800-869-8336
Fax: 610-525-8337
rcooper-ldr@comcast.net

An instructional video which provides a perspective about attention problems, possible causes and solutions. *$19.95*
Video

7914   Educating Inattentive Children
ADD Warehouse
300 Northwest 70th Avenue
Suite 102
Plantation, FL 33317-2360
954-792-8100
800-233-9273
Fax: 954-792-8545
websales@addwarehouse.com
www.addwarehouse.com

Harvey C Parker, Owner
Ideal for in-service to regular and special educators concerning the problems inattentive, elementarty and secondary students experience. *$49.00*
Video

7915   Getting Started with Facilitated Communication
Facilitated Communication Institute, Syracuse Univ
230 Huntington Hal
Syracuse, NY 13244-1
315-443-4752
Fax: 315-443-2258
http://thefci.syr.edu

Annegret Schubert, Director
Describes in detail how to help individuals with autism and/or severe communication difficulties to get started with facilitated communication.
Video

7916   How to Cope with ADHD: Diagnosis, Treatment & Myths
Aquarius Health Care Media
30 Forest Road
PO Box 249
Millis, MA 02054
508-376-1244
Fax: 508-376-1245
www.aquariusproductions.com

Lesile Kussmann, President/Owner
Learn how ADHD is diagnosed, clear up some of the myths, explain the treatmens that are availiable, and give you tips on how you can help your child at home. *$145.00*
DVD 1905

7917 I Just Want My Little Boy Back
Autism Treatment Center Of America
2080 South Undermountain Road
Sheffield, MA 01257
413-229-2100
800-714-2779
happiness@option.org
www.option.org

Samahria Lyt Kaufman, Co-Founder and Co-Director
Dane Griffith, Director of Administrative Services
Bears Kaufman, Co-Founder and Co-Director
A great video for parents and professionals caring for children with special needs. Join one British family and their autistic son before, during and after their journey to America to attend The Son-Rise Program at The Autism Treatment Center of America. This informative, inspirational and deeply moving story not only captures the joy, tears, challenges and triumps of this amazing little boy and his family, but also serves as a powerful introduction to the attitude and principles of the program. *$25.00*

7918 It's Just Attention Disorder
Western Psychological Services
625 Alaska Avenue
Torrance, CA 90503-5124
424-201-8800
800-648-8857
Fax: 424-201-6950
customerservice@wpspublish.com
wpspublish.com

Gregg Gillmar, VP
This ground-breaking videotape takes the critical first steps in treating attention-deficit disorder: it enlists the inattentive or hyperactive child as an active participant in his or her treatment. *$99.50*
Video

7919 Understanding ADHD
Aquarius Health Care Videos
30 Forest Road
PO Box
Millis, MA 02054
508-376-1244
Fax: 508-376-1245
www.aquariusproductions.com

Leslie Kussmann, President/Owner
A look at some of the controversies surrounding Attention Deficit Hyperactivity Disorder. This video shows how the disorder is diagnosed and presents strategies for living with a child with the disorder. Diverse and candid opinions from teachers, social workers, a behavior specialist, a pediatrician and a parent with ADHD twins. Recommended for child development students, social workers, and caregivers. Preview option available. *$120.00*
Video

7920 Understanding Attention Deficit Disorder
CACLD
25 Van Zant Street
Norwalk, CT 6855-1713
203-838-5010
Fax: 203-866-6108
CACLD@optonline.net
www.CACLD.org

Beryl Kaufman, Executive Director
Helen Bosch, President
A video in an interview format for parents and professionals providing the history, symptoms, methods of diagnosis and three approaches used to ease the effects of attention deficit disorder. Published by Connecticut Association for Children & Adults with Learning Disabilities (CACLD). *$20.00*
45 Minutes VHS

7921 Understanding Autism
Fanlight Productions C/O Icarus Films
32 Court Street
Brooklyn, NY 11201
718-488-8900
800-876-1710
Fax: 718-488-8642
info@fanlight.com
www.fanlight.com

Ben Achtenberg, Owner
Susan Newman, Editor

Parents of children with autism discuss the nature and symptoms of this lifelong disability and outline a treatment program based on behavior modification principles. 19 minutes *$199.00*
VHS/DVD 1993
ISBN 1-572951-00-1

7922 We're Not Stupid
Media Projects Inc
5215 Homer St
Dallas, TX 75206-6623
214-826-3863
Fax: 214-826-3919
mail@mediaprojects.org
www.mediaprojects.org

Fonya Naomi Mondell, Producer
We're Not Stupid is an insightful and very personal video that gives a voice to people who are struggling with learning disabilities. It was made by filmmaker Fonya Naomi Mondell, who is also living with learning differences. The filmmaker camptures the personal stories of young people from all walks of life who discuss what it's like to live with Attention Deficit Disorder and Dyslexia. Their comments are open, honest and direct, and their determination to manage their condition shines through. *$125.00*
Video

7923 Why Won't My Child Pay Attention?
ADD Warehouse
300 Northwest 70th Avenue
Suite 102
Plantation, FL 33317-2360
954-792-8100
800-233-9273
Fax: 954-792-8545
www.addwarehouse.com

Sam Goldstein, Ph.D, Author
Michael Goldstein, M.D., Co-Author
Practical and reassuring videotape, noted child psychologist tells parents about two of the most common and complex problems of childhood: inattention and hyperactivity. *$49.50*
224 pages Hardcover 1992
ISBN 0-471530-77-8

Software

7924 Cogrehab
Life Science Associates
1 Fenimore Rd
Bayport, NY 11705-2115
631-472-2111
Fax: 631-472-8146

Joann Mandriota, President
Divided into six groups for diagnosis and treatment of attention, memory and perceptual disorders to be used by and under the guidance of a professional. $95.-$1,950

Support Groups

7925 Autism Society of America
4340 East-West Highway
Suite 350
Bethesda, MD 20814
301-657-0881
800-328-8476
Fax: 301-657-0869
info@autism-society.org
www.autism-society.org

Scott Badesch, President/CEO
Jennifer Repella, VP Programs
John Dabrowski, CFO
ASA is the largest and oldest grassroots organization within the autism community, with more than 200 chapters and over 20,000 members and supporters nationwide. ASA is the leading source of education, information and referral about autism and has been the leader in advocacy and legislative initiatives for more than three decades.

7926 National Autism Hotline
Autism Services Center
929 4th Ave
PO Box 507
Huntington, WV 25701-1408   304-525-8014
                                  Fax: 304-525-8026
                          www.autismservicescenter.org

Mike Grady, CEO
Jimmie Beirne, COO
Nathel Lewis, ASC Training Coordinator
Service agency for individuals with autism and developmental
disabilities, and their families. Assists families and agencies attempting to meet the needs of individuals with autism and other
developmental disabilities. Makes available technical assistance
in designing treatment programs and more. The hotline provides
informational packets to callers and assists via telephone when
possible.

7927 National Health Information Center
Office Of Disease Prevention And Health Promotion
P.O.Box 1133
Washington, DC 20013-1133   301-565-4167
                                       800-336-4797
                                       301-468-7394
                                   Fax: 301-984-4256
                               www.health.gov/nhic

Jessica Rowden, Sec Dept. Health Human Services
William Corr, J.D., Deputy Secretary
National health information center provides information referral
and support. NHIC links consumers and health professionals to
organizations that are best able to provide reliable health
information.

Dexterity

Associations

7928 American Amputee Foundation
1805 Wewoka Dr
North Little Rock, AR 72116   501-835-9290
Fax: 501-835-9292
www.americanamputee.org

Catherine J Walden, Executive Director

Serves primarily as a national information clearinghouse and referral center assisting amputees and their families. The foundation researches and gathers information including studies, product information, services, self-help publications and review articles written within the field.

7929 American Board for Certification in Orthotics, Prosthetics & Pedorthics
330 John Carlyle St
Suite 210
Alexandria, VA 22314   703-836-7114
Fax: 703-836-0838
info@abcop.org
www.abcop.org

Eric Ramcharran, CPO, President
Catherine Carter, Executive Director
Samlane Ketevong, Director, Certification Services

The American Board for Certification in Orthotics, Prosthetics and Pedorthics is the national certifying and accrediting body for the orthotic and prosthetic professions.

7930 American Physical Therapy Association
1111 N Fairfax St
Alexandria, VA 22314-1488   703-684-2782
800-999-2782
Fax: 703-684-7343
consumer@apta.org
www.apta.org

Sharon L. Dunn, President
Matthew Hyland, Vice President
Kip Schick, Secretary

The American Physical Therapy Association fosters advancements in physical therapy practice, research and education. The association offers courses, career counceling, advocacy, publications and more.

7931 American Stroke Association
7272 Greenville Ave
Dallas, TX 75231   888-478-7653
strokeconnection@heart.org
www.strokeassociation.org/STROKEORG

John Warner, Presiednt
James Postl, Chairman
Nancy Brown, Chief Executive Officer

The American Stroke Association offers educational materials, seminars, conferences and transportation for those effected by strokes as well as their families, caregivers and interested professionals.

7932 Charcot-Marie-Tooth Association
PO Box 105
Glenolden, PA 19036   610-499-9264
800-606-2682
Fax: 610-499-9267
info@cmtausa.org
www.cmtausa.org

Gilles Bouchard, Chairman
Amy J Gray, CEO
Kim Magee, Director of Finance

The Charcot-Marie-Tooth Association supports the development of new drugs to treat CMT, to improve the quality of life for people with CMT and to search for a cure. The association also offers a resource center, emotional support group, treatment options, genetic testing, medication and more.

7933 Dyspraxia Foundation USA
1012 Windsor Rd
Highland Park, IL 60035   847-780-3311
foundation@mail.dyspraxiausa.org
www.dyspraxiausa.org

Warren Fried, President & Founder
Theresa A Bidwell, Vice President

Dyspraxia Foundation USA is a non-profit organization centered on understanding, accepting and educating on issues connected to Developmental Dyspraxia.

7934 Epilepsy Foundation
8301 Professional Place E
Suite 200
Landover, MD 20785- 2353   800-332-1000
Fax: 301-459-1569
ContactUs@efa.org
www.epilepsy.com

Robert W Smith, Chair
Philip M Gattone, M.Ed, President & CEO
M. Vaneeda Bennett, Chief Development Officer

The Epilepsy Foundation is the national voluntary agency dedicated to the welfare of people with epilepsy in the U.S. and their families. The organization works to ensure that people with seizures are able to participate in all life experiences and to prevent, control and cure epilepsy through research, education, advocacy and services.

7935 International Parkinson and Movement Disorder Society
555 East Wells Street
Suite 1100
Milwaukee, WI 53202- 3823   414-276-2145
Fax: 414-276-3349
info@movementdisorders.org
www.movementdisorders.org

Christopher Goetz, MD, President
Susan Fox, PhD, Secretary
Victor Fung, MBBS, PhD, FRACP, Treasurer

A professional society of clinicians, scientists, and other healthcare professionals who are interested in Parkinson's disease, related neurodegenerative and neurodevelopmental disorders, hyperkinetic movement disorders, and abnormalities in muscle tone and motor control.

7936 Lewy Body Dementia Association
912 Killian Hill Road S.W.
Lilburn, GA 30047   404-975-2322
Fax: 480-422-5434
www.lbda.org

Mike Koehler, CEO
Shannon McCarty-Caplan, Vice President
Christina M. Christie, President

A nonprofit organization dedicated to raising awareness of the Lewy body dementias (LBD), supporting people with LBD, their families and caregivers and promoting scientific advances.

7937 Multilingual Children's Association
20 Woodside Ave
San Francisco, CA 94127   415-690-0026
Fax: 415-341-1137
www.multilingualchildren.org

The Multilingual Children's Association is focused on the day-to-day joys and challenges of raising bilingual and multilingual children.

7938 National Amputation Foundation
40 Church St
Malverne, NY 11565-1735   516-887-3600
516-887-3600
Fax: 516-887-3667
amps76@aol.com
www.nationalamputation.org

Paul Bernacchio, President
William Sturges, 1st Vice President
Al Pennacchia, 2nd Vice President

Information & resources for amputees. Scholarship programs for college students with major limb amputation. Free donated durable medical equipment open to anyone in need locally-as items need to be picked up.
Quarterly

7939 National Commission on Orthotic and Prosthetic Education
330 John Carlyle Street
Suite 200
Alexandria, VA 22314- 5760
703-836-7114
Fax: 703-836-0838
info@ncope.org
www.ncope.org
Robin C Seabrook, Executive Director
Jonathan D. Day, CPO
Dominique Mungo, Residency Program Manager
The mission of NCOPE is to be recognized authority for the development and accreditation of O&P education and residency standards leading to competent patient care in the changing healthcare environment. NCOPE develops, applies, and assures standards for orthotic and prosthetic education through accreditation and approval to promote exemplary patient care.

7940 National Institute of Neurological Disorders and Stroke
National Institutes of Health
PO Box 5801
Bethesda, MD 20824
800-352-9424
www.ninds.nih.gov
Nina Schor, Deputy Director
The mission of the National Institute of Neurological Disorders and Stroke is to reduce the burden of neurological disease by supporting neuroscience research, funding and conducting training and career development programs, and disseminating scientific information on neurological health.

7941 National Stroke Association
9707 E Easter Ln
Suite B
Centennial, CO 80112-3754
303-649-9299
800-787-6537
Fax: 303-649-1328
www.stroke.org
James Baranski, CEO
Sharon Jaunchowski, Executive VP
Teran Nash, Customer Relations
The only national health organization solely committed to stroke prevention, treatment, rehabilitation and community reintegration. Provides packaged training programs, on-site assistance, physician, patient and family education materials to acute and rehab hospitals. Develops workshops; operates the Stroke Information & Referral Center and produces professional publications such as Stroke: Clinical Updates and the Journal of Stroke and Cerebrovascular Diseases.

7942 World Chiropractic Alliance
2950 N Dobson Rd
Suite 3
Chandler, AZ 85224-1819
480-786-9235
800-347-1011
Fax: 480-732-9313
www.worldchiropracticalliance.org
Terry A Rondberg, Founder/CEO
Richard Barwell, President
Dedicated to protecting and strengthening chiropractic around the world. Serving as a watchdog and advocacy organization, we place our emphasis on education and political action.

Books

7943 Carpal Tunnel Syndrome
Arthritis Foundation
1330 W Peachtree St
Suite 100
Atlanta, GA 30309
404-872-7100
800-283-7800
Fax: 404-872-0457
help@arthritis.org
www.arthritis.org
John H Klippel, President/CEO
Daniel T. McGowan, Chairman Of The Board
Rowland W. Chang, Vice Chair
The Arthritis Foundation is committed to raising awareness and reducing the unacceptable impact of arthritis, a disease which must be taken as seriously as other chronic diseases because of its devastatng consequences.

7944 Don't Feel Sorry for Paul
Harper Collins Publishing
76 Ninth Ave
New York, NY 10011
800-843-2665
www.barnesandnoble.com
Bernard Wolf, Author
Ann Ledden, Vice President
Lorna Metzler, Manager
Paul is seven but was born with deformities of both hands and feet. Paul must wear a prosthesis on both feet so that he can walk. He has a third prosthesis for his right hand. The third prosthesis has a pair of hooks Paul uses as fingers.
94 pages Hardcover
ISBN 0-39731 -88-0

7945 Functional Restoration of Adults and Children with Upper Extremity Amputation
Demos Medical Publishing
11 West 42nd Street
15th Floor
New York, NY 10036-8804
212-683-0072
800-532-8663
Fax: 212-683-0118
www.demosmedpub.com
Robert Meier III, Author
Diane Atkins, OTR, Co-Author
Provides a comprehensive reference to the surgery, prosthetic fitting, and rehabilitation of individuals sustaining an arm amputation. Covers the recent advancements in prosthetics and rehabilitation. *$165.00*
384 pages
ISBN 1-888799-73-0

Magazines

7946 ABC Mark of Merit Newsletter
Amer Board for Cert in Otthotics & Prosthetics
330 John Carlyle St
Suite 210
Alexandria, VA 22314-5760
703-836-7114
Fax: 703-836-0838
info@abcop.org
www.abcop.org
Timothy E. Miller, CPO
Curt A. Bertram, President Elect
James H. Wynne, CPO
An online bi-monthly newsletter.

7947 Active Living Magazine
American Amputee Foundation
PO Box 94227
North Little Rock, AR 72190
501-835-9290
Fax: 501-835-9292
www.americanamputee.org
Catherine J Walden, Executive Director
A print magazine published four times a year.

7948 Stroke Connection Magazine
American Heart Association
7272 Greenville Ave
Dallas, TX 75231-5129
214-373-6300
888-478-7653
Fax: 214-706-5231
www.strokeassociation.org/STROKEORG/
John Caswell, Editor
Debra Lockwood, Chairman
Nancy Brown, CEO
Free magazine for stroke survivors and their family caregivers.

Newsletters

7949   Advocacy Pulse
American Stroke Association
7272 Greenville Ave
Dallas, TX 75231-5129   214-373-6300
                                         888-478-7653
                                    Fax: 214-706-5231
            www.strokeassociation.org/STROKEORG/
Ralph Sacco, President/Director
Debra Lockwood, Chairman
Nancy Brown, CEO

7950   NINDS Notes
Ntn'l Institute of Neurological Disorders & Stroke
P.O.Box 5801
Bethesda, MD 20284   301-496-5751
                                         800-352-9424
                                    Fax: 202-944-3295
                                         sbaa@sbaa.org

Caroline Lewis, Executive Officer
Story C. Landis, Director
Denise Dorsey, Chief Administrative Officer
A print newsletter published three times a year.

7951   Noteworthy Newsletter
Ntn'l Comm on Orthotic & Prosthetic Education
330 John Carlyle Street
Suite 200
Alexandria, VA 22314- 5760   703-836-7114
                                    Fax: 703-836-0838
                                         info@ncope.org
                                         www.ncope.org
Robin C Seabrook, Executive Director
Jonathan D. Day, CPO
Dominique Mungo, Residency Program Manager
The mission of NCOPE is to be recognized authority for the de-
velopment and accreditation of O&P education and residency
standards leading to competent patient care in the changing
healthcare environment. NCOPE develops, applies, and assures
standards for orthotic and prosthetic education through accreditation and approval to promote exemplary patient care.

7952   Stroke Smart Magazine
National Stroke Association
9707 E Easter Ln
Suite B
Centennial, CO 80112-3754   303-649-9299
                                         800-787-6537
                                    Fax: 303-649-1328
                                         www.stroke.org
James Baranski, CEO
Sharon Jaunchowski, Executive VP
Teran Nash, Customer Relations
The only national health organization solely committed to stroke
prevention, treatment, rehabilitation and community reintegra-
tion. Provides packaged training programs, on-site assistance,
physician, patient and family education materials to acute and
rehab hospitals. Develops workshops; operates the Stroke Information & Referral Center and produces professional publications
such as Stroke: Clinical Updates and the Journal of Stroke and
Cerebrovascular Diseases.

Hearing

Associations

7953 Alexander Graham Bell Association for the Deaf and Hard of Hearing
3417 Volta Pl. NW
Washington, DC 20007   202-337-5220
Fax: 202-337-8314
TTY: 202-337-5221
info@agbell.org
agbell.org

Emilio Alonso-Mendoza, Chief Executive Officer
Lisa Chutjian, Chief Development Officer
Gayla H. Guignard, Chief Strategy Officer
The Alexander Graham Bell Association for the Deaf and Hard of Hearing (AG Bell) is the world's oldest and largest membership organization promoting the use of spoken language by children and adults who are hearing impaired. Members include parents of children with hearing loss, adults who are deaf or hard of hearing, educators, audiologists, speech-language pathologists, physicians and other professionals in fields related to hearing loss and deafness.

7954 American Academy of Audiology (AAA)
11480 Commerce Park Dr.
Suite 220
Reston, VA 20191   703-790-8466
Fax: 703-790-8631
infoaud@audiology.org
www.audiology.org

Peter E. Gallagher, Executive Director
Kathryn Werner, Vice President, Public Affairs
Amy Miedema, Vice President, Communications & Membership
The American Academy of Audiology is the world's largest professional organization for audiologists. The Academy is dedicated to providing quality hearing care services through professional development, education, research, and increased public awareness of hearing and balance disorders.

7955 American Association of People with Disabilities (AAPD)
2013 H St. NW
5th Floor
Washington, DC 20006   202-521-4316
800-840-8844
communications@aapd.com
www.aapd.com

Maria Town, President & Chief Executive Officer
Jasmin Bailey, Manager, Business Operations
Christine Liao, Programs Director
Nonprofit cross-disability member organization dedicated to ensuring economic self-sufficiency and political empowerment for Americans with disabilities. AAPD works in coalition with other disability organizations for the full implementation and enforcement of disability nondiscrimination laws, particularly the Americans With Disabilities Act (ADA) of 1990 and the Rehabilitation Act of 1973.

7956 American Cochlear Implant Alliance
P.O. Box 103
McLEAN, VA 22101-103   703-534-6146
info@acialliance.org
www.acialliance.org

Craig A. Buchman, Chair
Teresa A. Zwolan, Vice Chair
Nancy M. Young, Secretary
A not-for-profit membership organization created with the purpose of eliminating barriers to cochlear implantation by sponsoring research, driving heightened awareness and advocating for improved access to cochlear implants for patients of all ages across the US.

7957 American Society for Deaf Children
PO Box 23
Woodbine, MD 21797   800-942-2732
info@deafchildren.org
deafchildren.org

Alisha Joslyn-Swob, President
Mark Drolsbaugh, Vice President
Rachel Berman, Secretary
The American Society for Deaf Children provides information for the caretakers of deaf children so children can have full communication access in their home, school and community. The society covers areas such as visual language, audiologists, healthcare providers, assistive technology and more.

7958 American Speech-Language-Hearing Association
2200 Research Blvd
Rockville, MD 20850-3289   301-296-5700
800-638-8255
actioncenter@asha.org
www.asha.org

Gail J. Richard, President
Elise Davis-Mcfaland, President-Elect
Margot L. Beckerman, Chair
Provides information for both the general public and physicians in an easy-to-access manner. The subjects of focus are speech, hearing and language disorders.

7959 American Tinnitus Association (ATA)
PO Box 424049
Washington, DC 20042-4049   800-634-8978
ata.org

Torryn Brazell, Chief Executive Officer
David Hadley, Chair
Gordon Mountford, Vice Chair
ATA is an organization dedicated to finding cures for tinnitus and hyperacusis. ATA's research program focuses on providing seed grants for new areas of tinnitus scientific exploration.

7960 Association of Adult Musicians with Hearing Loss
AAMHL, Inc.
P.O. Box 522
Rockville, MD 20848   301-838-0443
info@musicianswithhearingloss.org
www.musicianswithhearingloss.org

Wendy Cheng, President
Jennifer Castellano, Secretary
Janice Rosen, Treasurer
The Association of Adult Musicians with Hearing Loss creates a space for adult musicians with hearing loss to discuss the challenges they face in making and listening to music. The association also offers opportunities for public performance.

7961 Association of Late-Deafened Adults
8038 Macintosh Ln
Suite 2
Rockford, IL 61107-5336   815-332-1515
TTY: 815-332-1515
www.alda.org

Rick Brown, President
Cynthia Moynihan, Vice President
Matt Ferrara, Treasurer
The Association of Late-Deafened Adults supports the empowerment of late-deafened people by offering programs and information resources on a variety of topics: technology, disability laws, airline travel and more.

7962 Better Hearing Institute
1444 I St NW
Suite 700
Washington, DC 20005   202-449-1100
800-327-9355
Fax: 202-216-9646
www.betterhearing.org

Sergei Kochkin, Ph.D, Executive Director
The Better Hearing Institute is a non-profit corporation that educates the public about the neglected problem of hearing loss and what can be done about it. Its mission is to erase the stigma and end the embarassment that prevents millions of people from seeking help for hearing loss.

7963 Center for Hearing and Communication
50 Broadway
6th Floor
New York, NY 10004
917-305-7700
Fax: 917-305-7888
TTY: 917-305-7999
info@chchearing.org
chchearing.org

Laurie Hanin, Executive Director
Ellen Lafargue, Co-Director Speech & Hearing Services
Kshitija Sarpotdar, Director of Finance
The Center for Hearing and Communication provides hearing health services to people of all ages who have hearing loss. Some of its services include free hearing screenings, complete hearing evaluations, pediatric services and more.

7964 Communication Service for the Deaf
3520 Gateway Lane
Sioux Falls, SD 57106
866-642-6410
Fax: 605-362-2806
TTY: 866-273-3323
inquiry@c-s-d.org
www.c-s-d.org

Dr. Benjamin Soukup, Founder, Chairman & CEO
Christopher Soukup, President
Brad Hermes, CFO
CSD's mission is to create greater opportunities for Deaf and hard of hearing individuals to reach their full potential. Through global leadership and the development of innovative technologies, CSD provides tools conducive to a positive and fully integrated life.

7965 Conference of Educational Administrators of Schools and Programs for the Deaf
PO Box 116
Washington Grove, MD 20880
202-999-2204
TTY: 204-866-6248
ceasd@ceasd.org
www.ceasd.org

Barbara Raimondo, Executive Director
Dr. David Geeslin, President
Stacey Katz Shapiro, Secretary
CEASD provides an opportunity for professional educators to work together for the improvement of schools and educational programs for individuals who are deaf or hard of hearing. The organization brings together a rich composite of resources and reaches out to both enhance educational programs and influence educational policy makers.

7966 Council of American Instructors of the Deaf (CAID)
PO Box 377
Bedford, TX 76095-0377
817-354-8414
Fax: 817-354-8414
caid@swbell.net
www.caid.org

Keith Mousley, President
Helen Lovato, Office Manager
The CAID continues to follow the tradition begun in 1850 and recognizes the value of bringing fellow teaching professionals together to share experiences and ideas for the purpose of improving learning opportunities for deaf and hard of hearing children, adolescents and young adults.

7967 Deaf REACH
3521 12th St NE
Washington, DC 20017-2545
202-832-6681
Fax: 202-832-8454
deaf-reach.org

Sarah E. Brown, Executive Director
Annette Reichman, President
Jonathan Tomar, Vice-President
The psychosocial rehabilitation approach, ulitzed by all Deaf-REACH programs, provides the solid foundation to member's success. Participants are activly involved in establishing the format and level of highly individualized service delivery that they receive. The concept, which has achieved national acclaim, involves teaching members necessary life skills, thus minimizing the need for assistance from a service professional. This is part of what distinguishes the approach at Deaf-REACH.

7968 Deaf Women United
PO Box 61
South Barre, VT 5670
info@dwu.org
www.dwu.org

Alana Beal, President
Keri Darling, Vice President
Caroline Koo, Secretary
It is committed to continuing a community of support of Deaf women from all walks of life.

7969 Deafness Research Foundation
363 Seventh Avenue,
10th Floor
New York, NY 10001-3904
212-257-6140
866-454-3924
Fax: 212-257-6139
TTY: 888-435-6104
info@hearinghealthfoundation.org
www.drf.org

Shari Eberts, Chairman
Mark Angelo, President
Robert Boucai, Principal
Founded in 1958, the Deafness Research Foundation is the leading source of private funding for basic and clinical research in the hearing science. The DRF is committed to making lifelong hearing health a national priority by funding research and implementing education projects in both the government and private sectors.

7970 Dogs for the Deaf
10175 Wheeler Rd
Central Point, OR 97502-9360
541-826-9220
800-990-3647
Fax: 541-826-6696
TTY: 541-826-9220
info@dogsforthedeaf.org
dogsforthedeaf.org

Robin Dickson, CEO
Vaughan Maurice, General Manager
Janine Bol, Finance Director
Rescues dogs from shelters and professionally trains them for people with special needs such as: deafness, autism for children, seniors, stroke victims, cerebral palsy, etc.

7971 Ear Foundation
1817 Patterson St
Nashville, TN 37203-2110
615-329-7849
800-545-4327
Fax: 615-329-7935
www.earfoundation.org

Suzanne Wyatt, Executive Director
National, nonprofit organization committed to integrating the hearing and balance impaired into the mainstream of society through public awareness and medical education. Also administers The Meniere's Network, a national network of patient support groups providing people with the opportunity to share experiences and coping strategies.

7972 Georgiana Institute
736 Harmony Street
New Orleans, LA 70115
203-994-8215
georgianainstitute@snet.net
www.georgianainstitute.org

Annabel Stehli, President
The information source for Auditory Integration Training (AIT)/Digital Auditory Aerobics (DAA).

7973 HEAR Center
301 E Del Mar Blvd
Pasadena, CA 91101-2714
626-796-2016
Fax: 626-796-2320
info@hearcenter.org
hearcenter.org

Ellen Simon, Executive Director
Deborah Lorino, Office Manager
Berenice Castro, Accounting Supervisor
Auditory and verbal program designed to help hearing impaired children, infants and adults lead normal and productive lives. Seeks to develop auditory techniques to aid people who have communication problems due to deafness. Offers diagnostic

evaluations for speech and hearing. Individual auditory, verbal training and speech-language therapy.

7974 Hearing Education and Awareness for Rockers
1405 Lyon St
San Francisco, CA 94115-2914   415-409-3277
                                             Fax: 415-409-5683
                                             info@hearnet.com
                                             www.hearnet.com

Kathy Peck, Executive Director
Joseph Monatano, Chief of Audiology
Flash Gordon, Primary Care Physician
H.E.A.R.'s mission is the prevention of hearing loss and tinnitus among musicians and music fans (especially teens) through education awareness and grassroots outreach advocacy.

7975 Hearing Industries Association
1444 I Street, N.W.
Suite 700
Washington, DC 20005   202-449-1090
                                         Fax: 202-216-9646
                                         mjones@bostrom.com
                                         www.hearing.org
It provides a comprehensive source of information about hearing loss - how to prevent it, identify it, evaluate it, and treat it.

7976 Hearing Loss Association of America
7910 Woodmont Ave
Suite 1200
Bethesda, MD 20814   301-657-2248
                                         Fax: 301-913-9413
                                         inquiry@hearingloss.org
                                         www.hearingloss.org

Barbara Kelley, Executive Director
Lise Hamlin, Director of Public Policy
Carla Beyer-Smolin, National Chapter & Membership Coordinator
The mission of the Hearing Loss Association of America is to open the world of communication to people with hearing loss by offering information, education, resources, advocacy and training.

7977 Hearing, Speech and Deafness Center (HSDC)
1625 19th Ave.
Seattle, WA 98122   206-323-5770
                                              888-222-5036
                                         Fax: 206-328-6871
                                         TTY: 800-761-2821
                                         clinics@hsdc.org
                                         www.hsdc.org

Lindsay Klarman, Executive Director
Hearing, Speech & Deaf Center (HSDC) is a nonprofit for clients who are deaf, hard of hearing, or who face other communication barriers such as speech challenges. Their mission is to foster inclusive and accessible communities through communication, advocacy, and education.

7978 House Ear Institute
2100 W 3rd St
Los Angeles, CA 90057-1944   213-483-4431
                                              800-388-8612
                                         Fax: 213-484-8789
                                         TTY: 213-484-2642
                                         www.hei.org

James Boswell, CEO
John.W House, M.D, President
Daniel. M Graham, Executive Vice President Develop
Offers pediatric hearing tests, otologic and audiologic evaluation and treatment, rehabilitation, hearing aid dispensing, and cochlear implant services. Outreach programs focus on families with hearing impaired children.

7979 International Catholic Deaf Association
7202 Buchanan St
Landover Hills, MD 20784-2236   301-429-0697
                                         Fax: 301-429-0698
                                         homeoffice@icda-us.org
                                         icda-us.org

Jean Cox, President
Kate Slosar, Vice President
T.K Hill, Secretary

An organization of Catholic deaf people and hearing people in the church working with the deaf in the united states of America.

7980 International Hearing Dog
5901 E 89th Ave.
Henderson, CO 80640-8315   303-287-3277
                                         Fax: 303-287-3425
                                         info@hearingdog.org
                                         www.hearingdog.org

Valerie Foss-Brugger, President
Robert Cooley, Field Representative
Andrea Paul, Vetinary Technician
Trains and places Hearing dogs with deaf or hard-of-hearing persons, with or without multiple disabilities, nationwide, free of charge to the recipient.

7981 International Hearing Society
16880 Middlebelt Rd
Suite 4
Livonia, MI 48154   734-522-7200
                                         Fax: 734-522-0200
                                         interact@ihsinfo.org
                                         ihsinfo.org

Annette Cross, BC-HIS, President
Kathleen Mennillo, MBA, Executive Director
Fran Vincent, Director, Membership & Marketing
The International Hearing Society (IHS) represents hearing healthcare professionals worldwide. Members include professionals engaged in the practice of testing human hearing and selecting, fitting and dispensing hearing instruments. IHS offers accreditation programs, advocacy, education and training in support of these services.

7982 League for the Hard of Hearing
50 Broadway
6th Fl
New York, NY 10004-3810   917-305-7700
                                         TTY: 917-305-7999
                                         www.lhh.org

Laurie Hanin, Executive Director
Ellen Pfeffer Lafargue, Au.D, Director
Dorene Watkins, Coordinator
The Center for Hearing and Communication is a leading hearing center offering state-of-the-art hearing testing, hearing aid fitting, speech therapy and full range of services for people of all ages with hearing loss. Visit our offices in New York City and Florida for services that meet all of your hearing and communication needs.

7983 Lexington School for the Deaf: Center for the Deaf
30th Avenue and 75th St
Jackson Heights, NY 11370   718-350-3300
                                         Fax: 718-899-9846
                                         TTY: 718-350-3056
                                         generalinfo@lexnyc.org
                                         www.lexnyc.org

Regina Carroll PhD, CEO/Executive Director
Philip W. Bravin, President
Gregory Hlibok, Vice President
Offers a comprehensive range of services to deaf, hard of hearing and speech impaired persons from infancy to elderly through its affiliate agencies: The Center for Mental Health Services; The Lexington Hearing and Speech Center, Lexington Vocational Services, and the Lexington School for the Deaf. The Lexington Center also provides services through its research division which houses the only federally funded Rehabilitation Engineering Center.

7984 Michigan Association for Deaf and Hard of Hearing
5236 Dumond Court
Suite C
Lansing, MI 48917-6001   517-487-0066
                                              800-968-7327
                                         Fax: 517-487-0202
                                         www.madhh.org

Nancy Asher, Executive Director
Pat Walton, Office Manager
MADHH is a statewide collaboration agency dedicated to improving the lives of people who are deaf or hard of hearing through leadership in education, advocacy and services.

7985 Mississippi Speech-Language-Hearing Association
PO Box 22664
Jackson, MS 39225
800-664-6742
Fax: 601-510-7833
admin@mshausa.org
www.mshausa.org

Claudette Edwards, President
Ricki Garrett, Executive Director
The Mississippi Speech-Language-Hearing Association is the statewide organization supporting audiologists and speech-language pathologists in Mississippi by offering them resources, information, and professional development opportunities so they could better serve their clients.

7986 National Alliance of Black Interpreters
P.O. Box 90532
Washington, DC 20090-532
202-810-4451
www.naobidc.org
It provides professional training to promote excellence and empowerment in the profession of sign language interpretation.

7987 National Association of Hearing Officials
PO Box 4999
Midlothian, VA 23112-17
www.naho.org
Bonny M Fetch CALJ, President
The mission of the National Association of Hearing Officials is to improve the administrative hearing process and thereby benefit hearing officials, their employing agencies, and the individuals they serve through promoting professionalism and by providing traininf, continuing education, a national forum for discussion of issues, and leadership concerning administrative harings.

7988 National Association of Parents with Children in Special Education
3642 E Sunnydale Dr.
Chandler Heights, AZ 85142
800-754-4421
Fax: 800-424-0371
contact@napcse.org
www.napcse.org

George Giuliani, President
NAPCSE is a national membership organization dedicated to rendering all possible support and assistance to parents whose children receive special education services, both in and outside of school.

7989 National Association of Special Education Teachers
1250 Connecticut Ave., NW
Suite 200
Washington, DC 20036-2643
800-754-4421
Fax: 800-754-4421
contactus@naset.org
www.naset.org

Roger Pierangelo, Executive Director
George Giuliani, Executive Director
The National Association of Special Education Teachers (NASET) is a national membership organization dedicated to rendering all possible support and assistance to those preparing for or teaching in the field of special education. NASET was founded to promote the profession of special education teachers and to provide a national forum for their ideas.

7990 National Association of the Deaf
8630 Fenton Street
Suite 820
Silver Spring, MD 20910- 3819
301-587-1788
Fax: 301-587-1791
TTY: 301-587-1789
www.nad.org

Howard A. Rosenblum, CEO
Shane H. Feldman, COO
Marc P. Charmatz, Staff Attorney
Nation's largest organization safeguarding the accessability and civil rights of 28 million deaf and hard of hearing Americans in education, employment, health care, and telecommunications. Focuses on grassroots advocacy and empowerment, captioned media deafness-related information and publications, legal assistance, and policy development.

7991 National Black Association for Speech Language and Hearing
P.O. Box 779
Pennsville, NJ 08070
877-936-6235
Fax: 877-936-6235
nbaslh@nbaslh.org
www.nbaslh.org

Cathy Runnels, Interim
Kia N. Johnson, Parliamentarian
Martine Elie, Treasurer
The mission of the National Black Association of Speech-Language and Hearing is to maintain a viable mechanism through which the needs of black professionals, students and individuals with communication disorders can be met.

7992 National Black Deaf Advocates
PO Box 32
Frankfort, KY 40602
585-475-2411
800-421-1220
Fax: 585-475-6500
president@nbda.org
www.nbda.org

Benro Ogunyipe, President
Cory Parker, VP
Sharon.D White, Secretary
The Mission of the National Black Deaf Advocate is to promote the leadership development, economic and educational opportunities, social equality, and to safeguard the general health and welfare of Black deaf and hard of hearing people.

7993 National Catholic Office of the Deaf
7202 Buchanan St
Landover Hills, MD 20784-2299
301-577-1684
Fax: 301-577-1684
TTY: 301-577-4184
info@ncod.org
www.ncod.org

Consuelo Martinez Wild, Executive Director
Helps coordinate efforts of deaf or hard of hearing people who are involved in the ministry, acts as a resource center, assists bishops and pastors become available to the deaf and hard of hearing.

7994 National Cued Speech Association
1300 Pennsylvania Ave, NW
Suite 190-713
Washington, DC 20004
917-439-5126
800-459-3529
Fax: 866-269-9877
info@cuedspeech.org
www.cuedspeech.org

Anne Huffman, President
Sarina Roffe, Executive Director
Ben Lachman, Director of Development
Champions effective communication, language development and literacy through the use of cued speech.

7995 National Deaf Women's Bowling Association
9244 E Mansfield Ave
Denver, CO 80237-1915
303-771-9018
ndwbast@gmail.com

Gayle Willingham, President
Ali Martinez, VP
Holds world Deaf Bowling Torunament annually in July. Also holds Las Vegas Scratch Classic annually in October.

7996 National Hearing Conservation Association
3030 W 81st Ave
Westminster, CO 80031
303-224-9022
Fax: 303-458-0002
nhcaoffice@hearingconservation.org
www.hearingconservation.org

Jennifer Tufts, President
Beth Cooper, President Elect
Nancy Wojcik, Secretary/Treasurer
The mission of the NHCA is to prevent hearing loss due to noise and other environmental factors in all sectors of society.

7997 National Institute on Deafness and Other Communication Disorders
National Institutes of Health
31 Center Dr.
MSC 2320
Bethesda, MD 20892-2320   301-827-8183
            800-241-1044
          TTY: 800-241-1055
        nidcdinfo@nidcd.nih.gov
           www.nidcd.nih.gov

Debara L. Tucci, Director
Judith A. Cooper, Deputy Director
Timothy J. Wheeles, Executive Officer
The National Institute on Deafness and Other Communication Disorders supports and conducts research to help prevent, detect and diagnose disabilities that affect hearing, balance, taste, smell, voice, speech, and communication.
1988

7998 National Student Speech Language Hearing Association
2200 Research Blvd
Suite 450
Rockville, MD 20850-3289   301-296-5650
            800-498-2071
         Fax: 301-296-8580
        TTY: 301-296-5650
          nsslha@asha.org
           www.nsslha.org

Patricia A. Prelock, PhD, President
Elizabeth S. McCrea, President-Elect
Shelly S. Chabon, Immediate Past President
The American Speech-Language-Hearing Association is committed to ensuring that all people with speech, language, and hearing disorders receive services to help them communicate effectively.

7999 Registry of Interpreters for the Deaf
333 Commerce St
Alexandria, VA 22314-2801   703-838-0030
         Fax: 703-838-0454
         TTY: 7038380459
          ridinfo@rid.org
            rid.org

Brenda Walke Prudhomme, President
Kelly L. Flores, VP
Dawn Whitcher, Secretary
The Registry of Interpreters for the Deaf, Inc. (RID), a national membership organization, plays a leading role in advocating for excellence in the delivery of interpretation and transliteration services between people who use sign language and people who use spoken language. In collaboration with the Deaf community, RID supports our members and encourages the growth of the profession through the establishment of a national standard for qualified sign language interpreters and transliterators, o

8000 Sight & Hearing Association
1246 University Ave. W.,
Suite #226
St. Paul, MN 55104- 4125   651-645-2546
            800-992-0424
         Fax: 651-645-2742
        mail@sightandhearing.org
        www.sightandhearing.org

Kathy Webb, Executive Director
Karen Klevar, Screening Director
Bernice Burgy, Program Assistant
It is a nonprofit organization with a mission to enable lifetime learning by identifying preventable loss of vision and hearing in children.

8001 Spring Dell Center
6040 Radio Station Rd
La Plata, MD 20646-3368   301-934-4561
         Fax: 301-870-2439
        info@springdellcenter.org
        www.springdellcenter.org

Patsy Finch, President
Badgley CPA, Treasurer
Jean Hubbard, Secretary

Since 1967, Spring Dell center has been, bridging the gap to enhance the lives of developmentally disabled people. Spring Dell's goal is to empower people in every aspect of their lives through the implementation of two programs, employment/vocational services and residential services including transportation. Spring Dell offers transportation door-to-door for persons with developmental disabilities, including day care programs, supportive environment, residential and any other transportation.

8002 Starkey Hearing Foundation
P.O. Box 41514
Minneapolis, MN 55441   866-354-3254
        info@starkeyfoundation.org
       www.starkeyhearingfoundation.org

Richard S. Brown, President
Brady Forseth, Executive Director
Keith Becker, Senior Director of Operations
The Starkey Hearing Foundation works to assist those with hearing impairments by offering hearing aids and aftercare services.

8003 Telecommunications for the Deaf and Hard of Hearing
8630 Fenton St
Suite 121
Silver Spring, MD 20910-3803   301-563-9122
         Fax: 301-589-3797
        TTY: 301-589-3006
          tdiforaccess.org

Claude L Stout, Executive Director
James House, Director of Public Relations
John Skjeveland, Business Manager
Promoting equal access to telecommunications and media for people who are deaf, late-deafened, hard of hearing or deaf-blind through consumer education and involvement; technical assistance and consulting; applications of exisiting and emerging technologies; networking and collaboration; uniformity of standards; and national policy development and advocacy.

8004 The Davis Center
110 Wesley St.
PO Box 508
Manlius, NY 13104   862-251-4637
         Fax: 862-251-4642
       npdunn@thedaviscenter.com
       www.thedaviscenter.com

Dorinne S. Davis, Director
Offers sound-based therapies supporting positive change in learning, development, and wellness. All ages/all disabilities. Uses The Davis Model of Sound Intervention, an alternative approach.

8005 United States Deaf Ski & Snowboard Association
76 Kings Gate N
Rochester, NY 14617   585-286-2780
         info@usdssa.org
          usdssa.org

Anthony Di Giovani, Officer
It provides means for deaf people to get together to share their love for skiing and sponsor races for deaf skiers.

8006 Vestibular Disorders Association
5018 NE 15th Ave.
P.O. Box 13305
Portland, OR 97211   503-229-7705
         800-837-8428
        Fax: 503-229-8064
         info@vestibular.org
         www.vestibular.org

Sue Hickey, President
Cynthia Ryan, MBA, Executive Director
Kerrie Denner, Outreach Coordinator
The mission of the Vestibular Disorders Association is to serve people with vestibular disorders by providing access to information, offering a support network, and elevating awareness of the challenges associated with these disorders. They also aim to support and empower vestibular patients on their journey back to balance.

Camps

8007 ASD Summer Camp
Alabama Institute for Deaf & Blind
205 E South St
P.O. Box 698
Talladega, AL 35160

256-761-3214
Fax: 256-761-3278
TTY: 256-761-3215
wiggins.lavina@aidb.state.al.us
www.aidb.org

Paul Millard, Principal
The Alabama School for the Deaf Summer Enrichment Camp is designed especially for deaf and hard of hearing children ages 6-15. Recreation activities include swimming, skating, outdoor games, horseback riding, field trips, arts and craft. Tuition is free.

8008 Aspen Camp
4862 Snowmass Creek Rd.
Snowmass, CO 81654

970-315-0513
TTY: 970-315-0513
hi@aspencamp.org
www.aspencamp.org

Karen Immerson, Vice President
Eric Kaika, Treasurer
Open to the deaf community, including family members and friends as well as those who are deaf, deaf blind, hard of hearing, and late deafened, Camp Aspen provides year round programs for youth and adults.

8009 Camp Alexander Mack
Indiana Deaf Camps Foundation
P.O.Box 158
Milford, IN 46542

574-658-4831
www.campmack.org

Galen Jay, Interim Executive Director
Lauren Carrick, Director of Development/Facility Manager
Amber Barrett, Food Service
Our program is intentionally designed to provide campers with life changing experiences that lead to a formation of personal faith within a safe faith community.

8010 Camp Bishopswood
Diocese of Maine Episcopal
143 State St
Portland, ME 04101

207-772-1953
800-244-6062
Fax: 207-773-0095
mike@bishopswood.org
www.bishopswood.org

Laurie Kazilionis, President
Robert Johnston, VP
Jeff Mansir, Treasurer
Camp is located in Hope, Maine. One to seven-week sessions for hearing impaired children June-August. Coed, ages 7-16.

8011 Camp CaPella
PO Box 552
Holden, ME 04429

207-843-5104
www.campcapella.org

Deb Breindel, Director
Provides summer camp sessions for children with disabilities.

8012 Camp Chris Williams
Lions 11 B-2 and MADHH
5236 Dumond Court
Suite C
Lansing, MI 48917-6001

586-778-4188
Fax: 586-285-1842
TTY: 586-285-1842

Nancy Asher, Executive Director
An exciting summer camp experience for deaf and hard of hearing youth and their siblings ages 8-14.

8013 Camp Comeca & Retreat Center
United Methodist Church
75670 Road 417
Conzad, NE 69130

308-784-2808
www.campcomeca.com

Camp is located in Cozad, Nebraska. Summer sessions for campers with diabetes and hearing impairment. Coed, ages 6-19, families, seniors, single adults.

8014 Camp Emanuel
PO Box 752343
Dayton, OH 45475

937-477-5504
crawford@campemanuel.org
www.campemanuel.weebly.com

Brian Demarke, President
Stephanie Ackner, Vice President
Mary Foreman, Secretary
Camp Emanuel is a camp for hearing impaired and hearing youth. There are day sessions for children 5-14 and overnight resident sessions for children and teens 9-17. The camp aims to promote descision making, self-esteem, and acceptance by integrating non-hearing children with hearing children.

8015 Camp Grizzly
NorCal Services For Deaf & Hard Of Hearing
4044 N Freeway Blvd.
Sacramento, CA 95843

916-349-7500
Fax: 916-349-7578
TTY: 916-349-7500
campgrizzly@norcalcenter.org
www.campgrizzly.org

Molly Bowen, Program Leader
Cheryl Bella, Program Leader
A program of NorCal Services for Deaf & Hard of Hearing, Camp Grizzly is a coed camp for children aged 7-18 who have a hearing impairment. Camp Grizzly takes place at the Camp Lodestar campground facilities and offers sporting activities, performing and creative arts, hiking, swimming, playgrounds and campfires.

8016 Camp Isola Bella
410 Twin Lakes Rd.
Salisbury, CT 06079

860-824-5558
Fax: 860-824-4276
TTY: 860-596-0110
ibdirector@asd-1817.org
asd-1817.org/programs/camp-isola-bella

David Guardino, Director
A camp for hearing-impaired children ages 8-17. Qualified deaf and hearing staff members with experience in education, child care and counseling are employed at the camp.

8017 Camp Joy
3325 Swamp Creek Rd
Schwenksville, PA 19473-1518

610-754-6878
Fax: 610-754-7880
www.campjoy.com

Angus Murray, Camp Director
A special needs camp for kids and adults (ages 4-80+) with developmental disabilities such as autism, brain injury, neurological disorder, visual and/or hearing impairments, Angelman and Down syndromes, and other developmental disabilities.

8018 Camp Juliena
Georgia Center of the Deaf and Hard of Hearing
2296 Henderson Mill Rd.
Suite 115
Atlanta, GA 30345

404-381-8447
888-297-9461
Fax: 404-297-9465
info@gcdhh.org
www.gcdhh.org/camp-juliena

Jimmy Peterson, Executive Director
Andrea Alston, Coordinator, Community Outreach
A week-long residential summer camp for deaf or hard of hearing youth. Activities help campers develop leadership, team-building, social, and communication skills.

8019 Camp Mark Seven
Mark Seven Deaf Foundation
144 Mohawk Hotel Rd.
Old Forge, NY 13420

315-207-5706
TTY: 315-357-6089
registrar@campmark7.org
www.campmark7.org

Dave Staehle, Camp Director

A camp program for hard-of-hearing, deaf and hearing people. Coed, open to all ages. The camp is located on the Fourth Lake in the Adirondack Mountains.

8020 Camp Meadowood Springs
77650 Meadowood Rd.
Weston, OR 97886
541-276-2752
Fax: 541-276-7227
camp@meadowoodsprings.org
www.meadowoodsprings.org

Michelle Nelson, Camp Director
This camp is designed to help children with communication disorders and learning differences. A full range of activities in recreational and clinical areas is available.

8021 Camp Pacifica
California Lions Camp
1836 K Street
Merced, CA 95340-4818
559-373-0961
deafcamppacifica@gmail.com
camp-pacifica.org

Angelica Martinez, Camp Director
John Martinez, Assistant Director
Camp Pacifica provides a summer camp experience for children, boys and girls, aged 7-15 who have a hearing impairment. The camp is located in the foothills of Sierra on 52 acres of forested woodland. Activities include, but are not limited to, archery, canoeing, ropes course, swimming, horseback riding, and riflery. The camp costs $360, plus a registration fee.
1978

8022 Camp Ramah in the Poconos
2100 Arch St.
Philadelphia, PA 19103
215-885-8556
Fax: 215-885-8905
info@ramahpoconos.org
www.ramahpoconos.org

Rabbi Joel Seltzer, Executive Director
Rachel Dobbs Schwartz, Camp Director
Bruce I. Lipton, Director, Finance & Operations
Camp is located in Lakewood, Pennsylvania. Summer sessions for children with developmental and intellectual disabilities.

8023 Camp Shocco for the Deaf
216 North St. E
PO Box 602
Talladega, AL 35161
800-264-1225
Camp Shocco for the Deaf is a Christian Camp for children and teens with a hearing impairment, whose parents are deaf or are siblings of a person that are deaf. The camp runs for 1 week and offers a range of camp activities.

8024 Camp Taloali
15934 N Santiam Hwy. SE
PO Box 32
Stayton, OR 97383
503-400-6547
campadmin@taloali.org
www.taloali.org

Randall Smith, Camp Administrator
Summer sessions for children who are deaf, hard of hearing, or have a hearing impairment. Camp Taloali emphasizes communication, leadership, and social development.

8025 Camp Tekoa
United Methodist Camp Tekoa
PO Box 1793
Flat Rock, NC 28731-1793
828-692-6516
Fax: 828-697-3288
www.camptekoa.org

John Isley, Executive Director
Dave Bollen, Assistant Director
Karen Rohrer, Business Manager
Offers special needs camp programs for individuals with developmental disabilities.

8026 Cochlear Implant Camp
Listen Foundation
6950 E Belleview Ave.
Suite 203
Greenwood Village, CO 80111
303-781-9440
cochlearimplantcamp@gmail.com
www.listenfoundation.org/cicamp

Janette Cantwell, Camp Director
Held at the YMCA Rockies Estes Park Center, the camp offers a wide range of activities for children from 3-17 years old with cochlear implants. The camp is 4 days and 3 nights, held during the summer and also offers programs for parents and families. The cost is $800 for a family of four.

8027 Deaf Kid's Kamp
Sproul Ranch, Inc.
42263 50th Street West
Suite 610
Quartz Hill, CA 93536
661-675-3323
877-399-5449
www.deafkidskamp.com

Buffy Sproul, Executive Director
Our purpose is to meet the needs of deaf children outside of the classroom setting. These needs, as we have defined them, would include but are not limited to: social contact with peers; contact with the culture of the Deaf Community; educational and recreational programs not available in most school settings.

8028 Father Drumgoole Connelly Summer Camp
MIV: Mount Loretto
6581 Hylan Blvd
Staten Island, NY 10309-3830
718-317-2600
Fax: 718-317-2830
www.mountloretto.org

Stephen Rynn, Executive Director
Maryann Virga, Executive Assistant
Loretta Polanish, Executive Secretary
Summer sessions for children with epilepsy, hearing impairment and developmental disabilities. Coed, ages 5-13.

8029 Lions Camp Crescendo
1480 Pine Tavern Rd.
PO Box 607
Lebanon Junction, KY 40150
502-264-0120
wibblesb@aol.com
www.lccky.org

Billie J. Flannery, Administrator
Organization dedicated to enhancing quality of life for youths, including those with disabilities, through the delivery of a traditional camping experience.

8030 Lions Camp Kirby
1735 Narrows Hill Rd
Upper Black Eddy, PA 18972
610-982-5731

Alice Breon, Camp Director
Offers 2-week camps for deaf and hearing impaired children and their siblings in eastern Pennsylvania.

8031 Lions Camp Merrick
PO Box 56
Nanjemoy, MD 20662
301-870-5858
Fax: 301-246-9108
info@lionscampmerrick.org
www.lionscampmerrick.org

Heidi A. Fick, Executive Director
Donna Wadsworth, Office Administrator
This recreational camp for special needs children offers a complete waterfront program including swimming, canoeing and fishing for ages 6-16. Designed for children who are deaf, blind, or have type 1 diabetes. Also helps children to learn to deal with their special conditions.

8032 Lions Wilderness Camp for Deaf Children, Inc.
Lions Wilderness Camp Headquarters
PO Box 8
Roseville, CA 95661-9998
lionscampfordeaf@gmail.com
www.lionswildcamp.org

David Velasquez, Camp Program Director

Lions Wilderness Camp gives deaf children aged 7-15 an outdoor camp experience helping children to learn outdoor skills and enjoy nature.

8033 Sandcastle Day Camp
Children's Beach House
1800 Bay Ave
Lewes, DE 19958
302-645-9184
Fax: 302-645-9467
www.cbhinc.org

Martha P. Tschantz, President
Maryann Helms, Vice President
Linda M. Fischer, Secretary
Camp is located in Lewes, Delaware. Four-week sessions June-August for Delaware children with hearing impairment or speech/communication impairment. Coed, ages 6-12.

8034 Sertoma Camp Endeavor
Sertoma Camp Endeavor
P.O.Box 910
Dundee, FL 33838-0910
863-439-1300
Fax: 863-439-1300

Jeff Nunemaker, Executive Director
The intergration of deaf, hard of hearing and hearing youngsters is a unique characteristic of our camping program. Both hearing, deaf and hard of hearing children have the opportunity to learn about themselves and each other in an informal and empowering setting.

8035 Texas Lions Camp
PO Box 290247
Kerrville, TX 78029
830-896-8500
Fax: 830-896-3666
tlc@lionscamp.com
www.lionscamp.com

Stephen S. Mabry, President & CEO
Karen-Anne King, Vice President, Summer Camps
Milton Dare, Director, Development
Texas Lions Camp is a camp dedicated to serving children ages 7-16 in Texas with physical disabilities. While at camp, campers will participate in a variety of activities and be encouraged to become more independent and self-confident.

8036 YMCA Camp Fitch
12600 Abels Rd.
North Springfield, PA 16430
814-922-3219
877-863-4824
Fax: 814-922-7000
registrar@campfitchymca.org
campfitchymca.org

Tom Parker, Executive Director
Joe Wolnik, Summer Camp Director
Brandy Duda, Outdoor Education Director
Camp is located in North Springfield, Pennsylvania. Camp programs include sessions for children with diabetes or epilepsy.

8037 Youth Leadership Camp
National Association of the Deaf
8630 Fenton Street
Suite 820
Silver Spring, MD 20910
301-587-1788
Fax: 301-587-1791
www.nad.org

Christopher Wagnor, President
Melissa S. Draganac-Hawk, VP
Howard A. Rosenblum, CEO
Sponsored by the National Association of the Deaf, this camp emphasizes leadership training for deaf teenagers and young adults. In addition to many recreational activities and sports, there are academic offerings and camp projects.

Books

8038 A Basic Course in American Sign Language
TJ Publishers
2544 Tarpley Rd
Suite 108
Carrollton, TX 75006-2288
972-416-0800
800-999-1168
Fax: 972-416-0944
customerservice@tjpublishers.com
www.tjpublishers.com

Tom Humphries, Author
Carol Padden, Co-Author
Terrence J O'Rouke, Co-Author
The first three DVDs in this series are designed to illustrate and demonstrate each of the exercises and dialogues presented in A Basic Course in American Sign Language. Four Deaf teachers and three hearing students provide a variety of models for the exercises. *$35.95*
288 pages Spiral Bound
ISBN 0-932666-42-6

8039 A Basic Course in Manual Communication
National Association of the Deaf
8630 Fenton St.
Suite 820
Silver Spring, MD 20910
301-338-6380
Fax: 301-587-1791
TTY: 301-810-3182
www.nad.org

Terrence J. O'Rourke, Author
Teachers ASL grammar and vocabulary.

8040 A Basic Vocabulary: American Sign Languagefor Parents and Children
TJ Publishers
2544 Tarpley Rd
Suite 108
Carrollton, TX 75006-2288
972-416-0800
800-999-1168
Fax: 972-416-0944
customerservice@tjpublishers.com
www.tjpublishers.com

Terrence J O'Rouke, Author
Tanner Beach, Director
Carefully selected words and signs include those that children use every day. Alphabetically organized vocabulary incorporates developmental lists helpful to both deaf and hearing children and over 1000 clear sign language illustrations. *$9.95*
240 pages Softcover
ISBN 0-932666-00-0

8041 A Loss for Words
HarperCollins Publishers
10 E 53rd St
New York, NY 10022-5244
212-207-7901
800-242-7737
Fax: 212-702-2586
spsales@harpercollins.com
www.harpercollins.com

Lou Ann Walker, Author
From the time she was a toddler, Lou Ann Walker was the ears and voice for her deaf parents. Their family life was warm and loving, but outside the home, they faced a world that misunderstood and often rejected them. *$13.00*
224 pages Paperback 1987
ISBN 0-060914-25-4

8042 Access for All: Integrating Deaf, Hard of Hearing and Hearing Preschoolers
Gallaudet University Bookstore
800 Florida Avenue NorthEast
Washington, DC 20002-3600
202-651-5530
Fax: 202-651-5489
gupress@gallaudet.edu
http://www.gallaudet.edu

Stephanie Cawthon, Ph.D., Book Review Editor
Peter V. Paul, Ph.D., Editor, Literary Issues
Ye Wang, Ph.D., Senior Associate Editor

This exciting new 90 minute videotape and manual describes a model program for integrating deaf and hard of hearing children in early education.
169 pages Book & Video

8043 Advanced Sign Language Vocabulary: A Resource Text for Educators
Charles C. Thomas
2600 S First St
Springfield, IL 62704-4730
217-789-8980
800-258-8980
Fax: 217-789-9130
books@ccthomas.com
www.ccthomas.com

Michael P. Thomas, President
Elizabeth E Wolf, Co-Author
A resource text for educators, interpreters, parents and sign language instructors. *$53.95*
202 pages Spiral Paper
ISBN 0-398057-22-0

8044 American Sign Language Handshape Dictionary
Gallaudet University Press
800 Florida Ave NE
Washington, DC 20002-3600
773-568-1550
800-621-2736
Fax: 773-660-2235
TTY: 888-630-9347
gupress@gallaudet.edu
www.gupress.gallaudet.edu

Richard A Tennant, Author
Marianne Gluszak Brown, Co-Author
Valerie Nelson-Metlay, Illustrator
The new DVD shows how each sign is formed from beginning to end. Users can watch a sign at various speeds to learn precisely how to master it themselves. Together, the new edition of The American Sign Language Handshape Dictionary and its accompanying DVD presents students, sign language teachers, and deaf and hearing people alike with the perfect combination for enhancing communication skills in both ASL and English. *$45.00*
408 pages Hardcover
ISBN 1-563680-43-2

8045 American Sign Language Phrase Book
TJ Publishers
2544 Tarpley Rd
Suite 108
Carrollton, TX 75006-2288
972-416-0800
800-999-1168
Fax: 972-416-0944
customerservice@tjpublishers.com
www.tjpublishers.com

Lou Fant, Author
Terrence O'Rourke, Principal
Tanner Beach, Director
The author provides interesting, realistic and meaningful situations. Sign language is learned through novel remarks cleverly organized around everyday topics. *$18.95*
362 pages Softcover
ISBN 0-809235-00-5

8046 American Sign Language: A Look at Its History, Structure & Community
TJ Publishers
2544 Tarpley Rd
Suite 108
Carrollton, TX 75006-2288
972-416-0800
800-999-1168
Fax: 972-416-0944
customerservice@tjpublishers.com
www.tjpublishers.com

Charlotte Baker-Shenk, Author
Carol Padden, Co-Author
Terrence O'Rourke, Principal
Answers basic questions about American Sign Language. What is it? What is its history? Who uses it? What is the Deaf community? Why is ASL important? What are the building blocks of ASL?

What is the relationship between ASL and body language? What are examples of ASL -grammar? *$4.95*
22 pages Softcover
ISBN 0-93266 -01-9

8047 At Home Among Strangers
Gallaudet University Press
800 Florida Ave NE
Washington, DC 20002-3600
773-568-1550
800-621-2736
Fax: 773-660-2235
TTY: 888-630-9347
gupress@gallaudet.edu
www.gupress.gallaudet.edu

Jerome D Schein, Author
T. Alan Hurwitz, President
Paul Kelly, Vice President Adm And Finance
At Home Among Strangers presents an engrossing portrait of the Deaf community as a complex, nationwide social network that offers unique kinship to deaf people across the country. *$36.95*
264 pages Paperback
ISBN 1-563681-41-2

8048 BPPV: What You Need to Know
Vestibular Disorders Association
5018 NE 15th Ave
Portland, OR 97211-5331
503-229-7705
800-837-8428
Fax: 503-229-8064
veda@vestibular.org
www.vestibular.org

P J Haybach, Author
Lisa Haven, Executive Director
Jerry Underwood, Managing Director
The aim of this book is to present basic information about benign paroxysmal positional vertigo (BPPV) including what it is, causes, how it is diagnosed, various treatments currently in use, and strategies for coping with the symptoms associated with BPPV. *$29.95*
207 pages Hardcover
ISBN 0-963261-14-2

8049 Ben's Story: A Deaf Child's Right to Sign
Gallaudet University Bookstore
800 Florida Avenue NorthEast
Washington, DC 20002-3600
202-651-5530
Fax: 202-651-5489
gupress@gallaudet.edu
http://www.gallaudet.edu

Stephanie Cawthon, Ph.D., Book Review Editor
Peter V. Paul, Ph.D., Editor, Literary Issues
Ye Wang, Ph.D., Senior Associate Editor
This is a mother's story of how she responded to the diagnosis of her son's deafness and how she struggled to have her son educated using sign language.
267 pages Softcover
ISBN 0-930323-47-5

8050 Book of Name Signs: Naming in American Sign Language
DawnSign Press
6130 Nancy Ridge Dr
San Diego, CA 92121-3223
858-625-0600
800-549-5350
Fax: 858-625-2336
info@dawnsign.com
www.dawnsign.com

Joe Dannis, President
Sam Supalla, Author
To explain how a name sign is chosen in the Deaf community, professor and researcher Sam Supalla wrote this valuable resource book. Revealing fascinating insights about the origins of ASL name signs, Supalla shows how they serve the same function as given names used in the hearing community. He also details how the history of the name sign system dates back to the early years of deaf education in America. Included for reference is a list of more than 500 name signs available for selection. *$12.95*
120 pages Paperback 1992
ISBN 0-915035-30-4

8051 **Chelsea: The Story of a Signal Dog**
Gallaudet University Bookstore
800 Florida Ave NE
Washington, DC 20002-3600   202-651-5855
                                   866-204-0504
                                   Fax: 773-660-2235
                                   TTY: 202-651-5855
                                   gupress@gallaudet.edu
                                   www.clerccenter.gallaudet.edu
Paul Ogden, Author
T. Alan Hurwitz, President
Paul Kelly, Vice President Adm. And Finance
This is a story of a young deaf couple and their Belgian sheepdog,
who acts as their ears. It explains how these dogs are trained and
paired with their new owners.
169 pages

8052 **Children of a Lesser God**
Gallaudet University Bookstore
800 Florida Ave NE
Washington, DC 20002-3600   202-651-5855
                                   866-204-0504
                                   Fax: 773-660-2235
                                   TTY: 202-651-5855
                                   gupress@gallaudet.edu
                                   www.clerccenter.gallaudet.edu
Mark Medoff, Author
T. Alan Hurwitz, President
Paul Kelly, Vice President Adm. And Finance
The movie that won the hearts of thousands. This is a story of a
deaf woman who refuses to succumb to the hearing people's im-
age of what a deaf person should be.
91 pages Softcover
ISBN 0-822202-03-4

8053 **Choices in Deafness: A Parent's Guide to
Communication Options**
Woodbine House
6510 Bells Mill Rd
Bethesda, MD 20817-1636   301-897-3570
                                   800-843-7323
                                   Fax: 301-897-5838
                                   info@woodbinehouse.com
                                   www.woodbinehouse.com
Irv Shapell, Owner
Sue Schwartz, PhD., Editor
A useful aid in choosing the appropriate communication option
for a child with a hearing loss. Experts present the following communication options: Auditory-Verbal Approach, Bilin-
gual-Bicultural Approach, Cued Speech, Oral Approach, and
Total Communication. This new edition explains medical causes
of hearing loss, the diagnostic process, audiological assessment,
and cochlear implants. Children and parents also offer their personal experiences. *$24.95*
400 pages Paperback
ISBN 1-890627-73-7

8054 **Cochlear Implants for Kids**
Alexander Graham Bell Association
3417 Volta Pl NW
Washington, DC 20007-2737   202-337-5220
                                   Fax: 202-337-8314
                                   info@agbell.org
Warren Estabrooks MEd, Editor
Alexander T. Graham, Executive Director
Susan Boswell, Director of Communications and Marketing
Designed to educate readers about cochlear implants, including
surgery, the importance of rehabilitation and the significance of
parents' and professionals' roles. *$12.49*
404 pages Paperback
ISBN 0-882002-08-2

8055 **Cognition, Education and Deafness: Directions for
Research and Instruction**
Gallaudet University Press
800 Florida Ave NE
Washington, DC 20002-3600   773-568-1550
                                   800-621-2736
                                   Fax: 773-660-2235
                                   TTY: 888-630-9347
                                   gupress@gallaudet.edu
David S Martin, Editor
T. Alan Hurwitz, President
Paul Kelly, Vice President Adm. And Finance
This groundbreaking book integrates the work of 54 contributors
to the 1984 symposium on cognition, education, and deafness. It
focuses on cognition and deaf students' growth and development,
problem-solving strategies, thinking processes, language development, reading methodology, measurement of potential, and intervention programs. *$50.00*
248 pages Paperback
ISBN 1-563681-49-8

8056 **College and University Programs for Deaf and Hard of
Hearing Students**
Gallaudet & NTID
800 Florida Avenue NE
Gallaudet University
Washington, DC 20002   202-651-5000
                                   800-451-8834
                                   Fax: 202-651-5508
                                   www.lulu.com
S. Benaissa, & L. Dunning, Co-Authors
J. DeCaro, M. Karchmer, Co-Authors
J Hochgesang, Co-Author
Compiled by Gallaudet University and the National Technical In-
stitute for the Deaf, this publication is a guide to accessibility for
deaf and hard of hearing students in American colleges and uni-
versities. Available through LuLu Publishing. *$11.50*
240 pages Paperback
ISBN 9-998242-81-9

8057 **Come Sign with Us**
Gallaudet University Press
800 Florida Ave NE
Washington, DC 20002-3600   773-568-1550
                                   800-621-2736
                                   Fax: 773-660-2235
                                   TTY: 888-630-9347
                                   gupress@gallaudet.edu
                                   www.gupress.gallaudet.edu
Jan C Hafer, Author
Robert M Wilson, Co-Author
T. Alan Hurwitz, President
This fun guide for parents and educators on teaching hearing chil-
dren how to sign has been thoroughly revised with completely
new activities that provide contexts for practice. *$39.95*
160 pages Paperback
ISBN 1-563680-51-3

8058 **Comprehensive Reference Manual for Signers and
Interpreters**
Charles C. Thomas
2600 S First St
Springfield, IL 62704-4730   217-789-8980
                                   800-258-8980
                                   Fax: 217-789-9130
                                   books@ccthomas.com
                                   www.ccthomas.com
Michael P. Thomas, President
Cheryl M. Hoffman, Author
A classic in sign language literature since its introduction over
two decades ago, this updated and expanded sixth edition of
Comprehensive Reference Manual for Signers and Interpreters
contains almost seven thousand entries, including vocabulary
and idioms, with cross-references and sign descriptions. It is intended primarily for interpreters, but it can also be used effectively by signers who have at least a working knowledge of sign
language. *$59.95*
404 pages Spiral Paper 1909
ISBN 0-398078-58-4

8059   Comprehensive Signed English Dictionary
Gallaudet University Press
800 Florida Ave NE
Washington, DC 20002-3600   773-568-1550
                                          800-621-2736
                                     Fax: 773-660-2235
                                     TTY: 888-630-9347
                                     gupress@gallaudet.edu
                                     www.gupress.gallaudet.edu

Harry Bornstein, Editor
Karen L. Saulnier, Editor
Lillian B. Hamilton, Editor
The Comprehensive Signed English Dictionary is the premier
volume of the Signed English series. This complete dictionary
more than 3,100 signs, including signs reflecting lively, contemporary vocabulary. *$45.00*
464 pages Casebound
ISBN 0-913580-81-3

**8060   Conversational Sign Language II: An Intermediate
Advanced Manual**
Gallaudet University Press
800 Florida Ave NE
Washington, DC 20002-3600   773-568-1550
                                          800-621-2736
                                     Fax: 773-660-2235
                                     TTY: 888-630-9347
                                     gupress@gallaudet.edu
                                     www.gupress.gallaudet.edu

William J Madsen, Author
T. Alan Hurwitz, President
Paul Kelly, Vice President Adm. And Finance
This book presents English words and their American Sign Language (ASL) equivalents in 63 lessons. Part one covers 750
words and their signs. Part two deals with the interpretation of
220 English idioms (which have over 300 usages in ASL). Part
three presents over 300 ASL idioms and colloquialisms prevalent
in informal conversations. *$17.95*
236 pages Paperback
ISBN 0-913580-00-7

8061   Deaf Empowerment: Emergence, Struggle and Rhetoric
Gallaudet University Press
800 Florida Ave NE
Washington, DC 20002-3600   773-568-1550
                                          800-621-2736
                                     Fax: 773-660-2235
                                     TTY: 888-630-9347
                                     gupress@gallaudet.edu
                                     www.gupress.gallaudet.edu

Katherine A Jankowski, Author
T. Alan Hurwitz, President
Paul Kelly, Vice President Adm. And Finance
Employing the methodology successfully used to explore other
social movements in America, this meticulous study examines
the rhetorical foundation that motivated Deaf people to work for
social change during the past two centuries. *$49.95*
192 pages Hardcover
ISBN 1-563680-61-0

**8062   Deaf History Unveiled: Interpretations from the New
Scholarship**
Gallaudet University Press
800 Florida Ave NE
Washington, DC 20002-3600   773-568-1550
                                          800-621-2736
                                     Fax: 773-660-2235
                                     TTY: 888-630-9347
                                     gupress@gallaudet.edu
                                     www.gallaudet.edu

John Vickrey Van Cleve, Editor
T. Alan Hurwitz, President
Paul Kelly, Vice President Adm. And Finance
Deaf History Unveiled features 16 essays, including work by
Harlan Lane, Renate Fischer, Margret Winzer, William McCagg,
and other noted historians in this field. Readers will discover the
new themes driving Deaf history, including a telling comparison
of the similar experiences of Deaf people and African Americans,

both minorities with identifying characteristics that cannot be
hidden to thwart bias. *$ 36.95*
316 pages Paperback
ISBN 1-563680-87-4

8063   Deaf Like Me
Gallaudet University Press
800 Florida Ave NE
Washington, DC 20002-3600   773-568-1550
                                          800-621-2736
                                     Fax: 773-660-2235
                                     TTY: 888-630-9347
                                     gupress@gallaudet.edu
                                     www.gupress.gallaudet.edu

Thomas S Spradley, Author
James P Spradley, Co-Author
T. Alan Hurwitz, President
Deaf Like Me is the moving account of parents coming to terms
with their baby girl's profound deafness. The love, hope, and anxieties of all hearing parents of deaf children are expressed here
with power and simplicity. *$16.95*
292 pages Paperback
ISBN 0-930323-11-4

8064   Deaf Parents and Their Hearing Children
Through the Looking Glass
3075 Adeline Street
Suite 120
Berkeley, CA 94703   510-848-1112
                                          800-644-2666
                                     Fax: 510-848-4445
                                     tlg@lookingglass.org
                                     www.lookingglass.org

Maureen Block, J.D., President
Thomas Spalding, Treasurer
Alice Nemon, Secretary
The focus of this review article is on families with Deaf parents
and hearing children. We provide a brief description of the Deaf
community, their language, and culture; describe communication
patterns and parenting issues in Deaf-parented families, examine
the role of the hearing child in a Deaf family and how that experience affects their functioning in the hearing world; and discuss
important considerations and resources for families, educators,
and health care and service providers. *$2.00*
8 pages

8065   Deaf in America: Voices from a Culture
TJ Publishers
2544 Tarpley Rd
Suite 108
Carrollton, TX 75006-2288   972-416-0800
                                          800-999-1168
                                     Fax: 972-416-0944
                                     customerservice@tjpublishers.com
                                     www.tjpublishers.com

Carol Padden, Author
Tom Humphries, Co-Author
Terrence O'Rourke, Principal
Now available in paperback, this book opens deaf culture to outsiders, inviting readers to imagine and understand a world of silence. This book shares the joy and satisfaction many people have
with their lives and shows that deafness may not be the handicap
most hearing people think. *$15.95*
134 pages Softcover
ISBN 0-674194-24-1

8066   EASE Program: Emergency Access Self Evaluation
Telecommunications for the Deaf (TDI)
8630 Fenton St
Suite 604
Silver Spring, MD 20910-3822   301-589-3786
                                     Fax: 301-589-3797
                                     tdi-online.org

Claude L Stout, Executive Director
Gloria Carter, Executive Secretary
James House, Public Relations Director
A complete training, testing, maintenance and self evaluation
program that helps emergency service providers prepare for

emergency calls from TTY users and to comply with the American with Disabilities Act. *$35.00*
48 pages

8067   Encyclopedia of Deafness and Hearing Disorders
Powell's Books
1005 W Burnside St
Portland, OR 97209-3114   503-228-4651
                                           800-873-7323
                                           help@powells.com
                                           www.powells.com

Carol Turkington, Author
Michael Powell, Owner
Presents the most current information on deafness and hearing disorders in an authoritative A-to-Z compendium. *$7.50*
294 pages Hardcover
ISBN 0-816056-15-3

8068   Expressive and Receptive Fingerspelling for Hearing Adults
Gallaudet University Bookstore
800 Florida Ave NE
Washington, DC 20002-3600   202-651-5855
                                           866-204-0504
                                           Fax: 773-660-2235
                                           TTY: 202-651-5855
                                           gupress@gallaudet.edu
                                           www.clerccenter.gallaudet.edu

LaVera M Guillory, Author
T. Alan Hurwitz, President
Paul Kelly, Vice President Adm. And Finance
Here is a new and meaningful way for adults to increase their comfort with fingerspelling. The system is based on the principles of phonetics rather than letters of the English alphabet.
42 pages Softcover
ISBN 0-875110-55-X

8069   Eye-Centered: A Study of Spirituality of Deaf People
National Catholic Office for the Deaf
7202 Buchanan St
Hyattsville, MD 20784-2236   301-577-1684
                                           Fax: 301-577-1684
                                           info@ncod.org
                                           www.ncod.org

Bill Key, Author
Arvilla Rank, Executive Director
Deacon Patrick Graybill, Vice President
The findings of the five-year De Sales Project conducted by The National Catholic Office for the Deaf. *$16.70*
167 pages

8070   For Hearing People Only
Harris Communications
15155 Technology Dr
Eden Prairie, MN 55344   800-825-6758
                                           Fax: 952-906-1099
                                           TTY: 952-388-2152
                                           info@harriscomm.com
                                           www.harriscomm.com

Ray Harris, CEO
For Hearing People Only answers some of the most common questions hearing people ask about Deaf culture and how Deaf people communicate and live. *$72.00*
868 pages Paperback
ISBN 9-705876-00-7

8071   From Gesture to Language in Hearing and Deaf Children
Gallaudet University Press
800 Florida Ave NE
Washington, DC 20002-3600   773-568-1550
                                           800-621-2736
                                           Fax: 773-660-2235
                                           TTY: 888-630-9347
                                           gupress@gallaudet.edu
                                           www.gupress.gallaudet.edu

Virginia Volterra, Editor
Carol J. Erting, Editor

In 21 essays on communicative gesturing in the first two years of life, this vital collection demonstrates the importance of gesture in a child's transition to a linguistic system. *$45.95*
358 pages Paperback
ISBN 1-563680-78-5

8072   From Mime to Sign Package
TJ Publishers
2544 Tarpley Rd
Suite 108
Carrollton, TX 75006-2288   972-416-0800
                                           800-999-1168
                                           Fax: 972-416-0944
                                           customerservice@tjpublishers.com
                                           www.tjpublishers.com

Gilbert C Eastman, Author
Terrence O'Rourke, Principal
Tanner Beach, Director
More than 1,000 photographs illustrate how natural gestures, mime and facial expressions used every day can become the basis for learning sign language. *$27.95*
183 pages Softcover
ISBN 0-932666-34-5

8073   GA and SK Etiquette
Telecommunications for the Deaf
8630 Fenton Street
Suite 604
Silver Spring, MD 20910- 3822   301-589-3786
                                           Fax: 301-589-3797
                                           www.tdi-online.org

Claude L Stout, Executive Director
Keith Cagle, Co-Author
Roy Miller, President
Promoting equal access to telecommunications and media for people who are deaf, late-deafened, hard-of-hearing or deaf-blind through consumer education and involvement; technical assistance and consulting; applications of exisiting and emerging technologies; networking and collaboration; uniformity of standards; and national policy development and advocacy. *$11.95*
54 pages Paperback
ISBN 0-961462-17-5

8074   Gallaudet Survival Guide to Signing
Gallaudet University Press
800 Florida Ave NE
Washington, DC 20002-3600   773-568-1550
                                           800-621-2736
                                           Fax: 773-660-2235
                                           TTY: 888-630-9347
                                           gupress@gallaudet.edu
                                           www.gallaudet.edu

Jon Mitchiner, Manager
Leonard G. Lane, Author
Jan Skrobisz, Illustrator
Features 500 of the most frequently used signs with clear illustrations and descriptions for each one. *$9.95*
218 pages Paperback
ISBN 0-930323-67-X

8075   Goldilocks and the Three Bears: Told in Signed English
Gallaudet University Press
800 Florida Ave NE
Washington, DC 20002-3600   773-568-1550
                                           800-621-2736
                                           Fax: 773-660-2235
                                           TTY: 888-630-9347
                                           gupress@gallaudet.edu
                                           www.gupress.gallaudet.edu

Harry Bornstein, Author
Karen L Saulnier, Co-Author
T. Alan Hurwitz, President
Goldilocks and the Three Bears offers children ages 3 - 8 all of the fun their parents had when they first read about the little girl with the golden curls who turned the Bears' house upside down. *$21.95*
48 pages Hardcover
ISBN 1-563680-57-2

8076 **Hearing Impaired Children and Youth with Developmental Disabilities**
Gallaudet University Bookstore
800 Florida Ave NE
Washington, DC 20002-3600   202-651-5855
866-204-0504
Fax: 773-660-2235
TTY: 202-651-5855
gupress@gallaudet.edu

Evelyn Cherow, Editor
T. Alan Hurwitz, President
Paul Kelly, Vice President Adm. And Finance
The insights of 24 experts help clarify relationships between hearing impairment and developmental difficulties and propose interdisciplinary cooperation as an approach to the problems created. *$29.95*
394 pages Hardcover
ISBN 0-913580-97-X

8077 **Hollywood Speaks: Deafness and the Film Entertainment Industry**
University of Illinois Press
1325 S Oak St
MC-566
Champaign, IL 61820-6903   217-333-0950
Fax: 217-244-8082
uipress@uillinois.edu
www.press.uillinois.edu

Willis G. Regier, Director
John S. Schuchman, Author
Kathy O'Neill, Assistant To The Director
How deafness has been treated in movies and how it provides yet another window onto social history in addition to a fresh angle from which to view Hollywood. *$27.00*
200 pages Paperback 1999
ISBN 0-252068-50-8

8078 **I Have a Sister, My Sister is Deaf**
HarperCollins Publishers
10 E 53rd St
New York, NY 10022-5244   212-207-7901
800-242-7737
Fax: 212-702-2586
spsales@harpercollins.com
www.harpercollins.com

Jeanne Whitehouse Peterson, Author
Deborah Kogan Ray, Illustrator
Ann Ledden, Vice President
An emphatic, affirmative look at the relationship between siblings, as a young deaf child is affectionately described by her older sister. This Coretta Scott King Honor Award winner helps young children develop an understanding that deaf children share the same interests as hearing children. *$6.99*
32 pages Paperback 1984
ISBN 0-064430-59-6

8079 **Independence Without Sight or Sound**
AFB Press
2 Penn Plaza
Suite 1102
New York, NY 10121-2006   212-502-7600
800-232-5463
Fax: 888-545-8331
afbweb@afb.net
www.afb.org

Richard Obnen, Chairman Of The Board
Carl Augusto, President and CEO
Rick Bozeman, Chief Financial Officer
This practical guidebook covers the essential aspects of communicating and working with deaf-blind persons. Full of valuable information on subjects such as how to talk with deaf-blind people, adapt orientation and mobility techniques for deaf-blind travelers, and interact with deaf-blind individuals socially, this useful manual also contains a substantial resource section detailing sources of information and adapted equipment. *$39.95*
193 pages Paperback
ISBN 0-891282-46-4

8080 **Innovative Practices for Teaching Sign Language Interpreters**
Gallaudet University Press
800 Florida Ave NE
Washington, DC 20002-3600   773-568-1550
800-621-2736
Fax: 773-660-2235
TTY: 888-630-9347
gupress@gallaudet.edu
www.gupress.gallaudet.edu

Cynthia B Roy, Editor
Researchers now understand interpreting as an active process between two languages and cultures, with social interaction, sociolinguistics, and discourse analysis as more appropriate theoretical frameworks. Roy's penetrating new book acts upon these new insights by presenting six dynamic teaching practices to help interpreters achieve the highest level of skill. *$45.95*
200 pages Hardcover
ISBN 1-563680-88-2

8081 **Intermediate Conversational Sign Language**
Gallaudet University Press
800 Florida Ave NE
Washington, DC 20002-3600   773-568-1550
800-621-2736
Fax: 773-660-2235
TTY: 888-630-9347
gupress@gallaudet.edu
www.gupress.gallaudet.edu

Willard J Madsen, Author
This fully illustrated text offers a unique approach to using American Sign Language (ASL) and English in a bilingual setting. Each of the 25 lessons involve sign language conversation using colloquialisms that are prevalent in informal conversations. *$31.50*
400 pages Softcover
ISBN 0-913580-79-1

8082 **Interpretation: A Sociolinguistic Model**
Sign Media
4020 Blackburn Ln
Burtonsville, MD 20866-1167   301-421-0268
800-475-4756
Fax: 301-421-0270
info@signmedia.com
www.signmedia.com

Verden Ness, President
Dennis Cokely, Author
This text presents a sociolinguistically sensitive model of the interpretation process. The model applies to interpretation in any two languages although this one focuses on ASL and English. *$22.95*
199 pages
ISBN 0-932130-10-0

8083 **Interpreting: An Introduction**
Registry of Interpreters for the Deaf
333 Commerce St
Alexandria, VA 22314-2801   703-838-0030
Fax: 703-838-0454
TTY: 703-838-0459
ridinfo@rid.org
www.rid.org

Nancy J Frishberg, Author
Shane Feldman, Executive Director
Don Roose, Director
This text is written by a practicing interpreter and includes information on history, terminology, research, competence, setting and a comprehensive bibliography. *$24.95*
249 pages Softcover
ISBN 0-916883-07-8

8084 **Joy of Signing**
Gospel Publishing House
1445 N Boonville Ave
Springfield, MO 65802-1894   417-862-8000
800-641-4310
Fax: 417-862-5881
www.gospelpublishing.com

Lottie L Riekehof, Author

This manual on signing includes illustrations, information on sign origins, practice sentences, and step-by-step descriptions of hand positions and movements. *$23.99*
352 pages Hardcover
ISBN 0-882435-20-5

8085   Kid-Friendly Parenting with Deaf and Hard of Hearing Children
Gallaudet University Press
800 Florida Ave NE
Washington, DC 20002-3600   773-568-1550
                                          800-621-2736
                                     Fax: 773-660-2235
                                     TTY: 888-630-9347
                                 gupress@gallaudet.edu
                              www.gupress.gallaudet.edu
Daria Medwid, Author
Denise Chapman Weston, Co-Author
At each chapter's beginning, experts (some deaf, some hearing), including I. King Jordan, Jack Gannon, Merv Garretson, and others, offer their insights on the subject discussed. Designed for parents with various styles, Kid-Friendly Parenting is a complete, step-by-step guide and reference to raising a deaf or hard of hearing child. *$35.95*
320 pages Paperback
ISBN 1-563680-31-9

8086   Laurent Clerc: The Story of His Early Years
Gallaudet University Press
800 Florida Ave NE
Washington, DC 20002-3600   773-568-1550
                                          800-621-2736
                                     Fax: 773-660-2235
                                     TTY: 888-630-9347
                                 gupress@gallaudet.edu
                              www.gupress.gallaudet.edu
Cathryn Carroll, Author
T. Alan Hurwitz, President
Paul Kelly, Vice President Adm. And Finance
In his own voice, Clerc vividly relates the experiences that led to his later progressive teaching methods. Especially influential was his long stay at the Royal National Institute for the Deaf in Paris, where he encountered sharply distinct personalities - the saintly, inspiring deaf teacher Massieu, the vicious Dr. Itard and his heartless experiments on deaf boys, and the Father of the Deaf, Abbe Sicard, who could hardly sign. *$13.95*
208 pages Paperback
ISBN 0-930323-23-8

8087   Linguistics of American Sign Language: An Introduction
Gallaudet University Press
800 Florida Ave NE
Washington, DC 20002-3600   773-568-1550
                                          800-621-2736
                                     Fax: 773-660-2235
                                     TTY: 888-630-9347
                                 gupress@gallaudet.edu
                              www.gupress.gallaudet.edu
Clayton Valli, Author
Ceil Lucas, Co-Author
Kristin J Mulrooney, Co-Author
Completely reorganized to reflect the growing intricacy of the study of ASL linguistics, the 5th edition presents 26 units in seven parts. Part One: Introduction presents a revision of Defining Language and an entirely new unit, Defining Linguistics. Part Two: Phonology has been completely updated with new terminology and examples. *$75.00*
560 pages Hardcover
ISBN 1-563682-83-4

8088   Literacy & Your Deaf Child: What Every Parent Should Know
Gallaudet University Press
800 Florida Ave NE
Washington, DC 20002-3600   773-568-1550
                                          800-621-2736
                                     Fax: 773-660-2235
                                     TTY: 888-630-9347
                                 gupress@gallaudet.edu
                              www.gupress.gallaudet.edu
David A Stewart, Author
Bryan R Clarke, Co-Author
T. Alan Hurwitz, President
Literacy and Your Deaf Child begins by introducing some common concepts, among them the importance of parental involvement in a deaf child's education. It outlines how children acquire language and describes the auditory and visual links to literacy. *$24.95*
240 pages Paperback
ISBN 1-563681-36-6

8089   Mask of Benevolence: Disabling the Deaf Community, The
DawnSign Press
6130 Nancy Ridge Dr
San Diego, CA 92121-3223   858-625-0600
                                          800-549-5350
                                     Fax: 858-625-2336
                                   info@dawnsign.com
                                    www.dawnsign.com
Joe Dannis, President
Harlan Lane, Author
Dr. Harlan Lane does not view deafness as a handicap but rather a different state from hearing. Deaf people are a societal minority and should be treasured, not eradicated. *$12.95*
360 pages Paperback 1992
ISBN 1-581210-09-5

8090   Mother Father Deaf: Living Between Sound and Silence
Harvard University Press
79 Garden St
Cambridge, MA 02138-1423   617-495-2600
                                          800-405-1619
                                    Fax: 617- 49- 589
                             contact_hup@harvard.edu
                                 www.hup.harvard.edu
William Sisler, President
Paul Preston, Author
The book explores the intimate intersection of families like his own - families which embody the conflicts and resolutions of two often opposing world views, the Deaf and the Hearing. Although I have normal hearing, both of my parents are profoundly deaf. *$19.50*
278 pages Paperback
ISBN 0-674587-48-0

8091   My First Book of Sign
Gallaudet University Press
800 Florida Ave NE
Washington, DC 20002-3600   773-568-1550
                                          800-621-2736
                                     Fax: 773-660-2235
                                     TTY: 888-630-9347
                                 gupress@gallaudet.edu
                              www.gupress.gallaudet.edu
Pamela J Baker, Author
Patricia Bellan Gillen, Illustrator
T. Alan Hurwitz, President
Full-color book gives alphabetically grouped signs for 150 words most frequently used by young children. *$22.95*
80 pages Hardcover
ISBN 0-930323-20-3

8092 My Signing Book of Numbers
Gallaudet University Press
800 Florida Ave NE
Washington, DC 20002-3600

773-568-1550
800-621-2736
Fax: 773-660-2235
TTY: 888-630-9347
gupress@gallaudet.edu
www.gupress.gallaudet.edu

Patricia Bellan Gillen, Author
This full-color book helps children learn their numbers in sign language. Each two-page spread of this delightfully illustrated book has the appropriate number of things or creatures for the numbers 0 through 20. *$22.95*
56 pages Hardcover
ISBN 0-930323-37-8

8093 Nursery Rhymes from Mother Goose
Gallaudet University Press
800 Florida Ave NE
Washington, DC 20002-3600

773-568-1550
800-621-2736
Fax: 773-660-2235
TTY: 888-630-9347
gupress@gallaudet.edu
www.gupress.gallaudet.edu

Harry Bornstein, Author
Karen L Saulnier, Co-Author
Patricia Peters, Illustrator
Young readers, both hearing and deaf, will learn the special charm of rhyme while also discovering new vocabulary and new ways to experience English through signing. As they learn and memorize their favorite verses, children will also strengthen their language skills in a fun, entertaining way. *$21.95*
64 pages Hardcover
ISBN 0-930323-99-8

8094 Outsiders in a Hearing World: A Sociology of Deafness
Sage Publications
2455 Teller Rd
Thousand Oaks, CA 91320-2218

805-499-9774
800-818-7243
Fax: 805-499-0871
www.sagepub.com

Paul C Higgins, Author
An introduction to the social world of deaf people. The author gives a sociologists view of what it's like to be deaf. *$72.95*
208 pages Hardcover 1980
ISBN 0-803914-22-3

8095 Perigee Visual Dictionary of Signing
Harris Communications
15155 Technology Dr
Eden Prairie, MN 55344

800-825-6758
Fax: 952-906-1099
TTY: 952-388-2152
info@harriscomm.com
www.harriscomm.com

Ray Harris, CEO
An A-to-Z guide to American Sign Language vocabulary. *$15.28*
478 pages Softcover
ISBN 9-780399-51-9

8096 Phone of Our Own: The Deaf Insurrection Against Ma Bell
Gallaudet University Press
800 Florida Ave NE
Washington, DC 20002-3600

773-568-1550
800-621-2736
Fax: 773-660-2235
TTY: 888-630-9347
gupress@gallaudet.edu
www.gupress.gallaudet.edu

Harry G Lang, Author
T. Alan Hurwitz, President
Paul Kelly, Vice President Adm. And Finance
A recount of the history of the teletypewriter, from the three deaf engineers who developed the acoustic coupler that made mass communication on TTY's feasible, through the deaf community's twenty-year struggle against the government and AT&T to have TTY's produced and distributed. *$36.50*
256 pages Hardcover
ISBN 1-563680-90-4

8097 Place of Their Own: Creating the Deaf Community in America
Gallaudet University Press
800 Florida Ave NE
Washington, DC 20002-3600

773-568-1550
800-621-2736
Fax: 773-660-2235
TTY: 888-630-9347
gupress@gallaudet.edu
www.gallaudet.edu

John V Van Cleve, Author
Barry A Crouch, Co-Author
T. Alan Hurwitz, President
Traces development of American deaf society to show how deaf people developed a common language and sense of community. Views deafness as the distinguishing characteristic of a distinct culture. *$22.95*
224 pages Paperback
ISBN 0-930323-49-1

8098 PreReading Strategies
Gallaudet University Bookstore
800 Florida Ave NE
Washington, DC 20002-3600

202-651-5855
866-204-0504
Fax: 773-660-2235
TTY: 202-651-5855
gupress@gallaudet.edu

David R Schleper, Author
T. Alan Hurwitz, President
Paul Kelly, Vice President Adm. And Finance
Here is a wealth of good advice for preparing students to understand what they read, building comprehension and enjoyment. *$14.95*
65 pages

8099 Quad City Deaf & Hard of Hearing Youth Group: Tomorrow's Leaders for our Community
Independent Living Research Utilization ILRU
2323 S Shepherd Dr
Houston, TX 77019-7019

713-520-9058
Fax: 713-520-5785
ilru@ilru.org

Lex Frieden, Director
Rose Sheperd, Manager
IICIL staff see this program as a way to develop young leaders for themovement. Emphasis is given to providing oppportunities for members of the youth group to develop skills in planning and organizing activities.

8100 Religious Signing: A Comprehensive Guide for All Faiths
TJ Publishers
P.O. Box 702701
Dallas, TX 75370

972-416-0800
800-999-1168
Fax: 972-416-0944
TTY: 301-585-4440
TJPubinc@aol.com
www.tjpublishers.com

Elaine Costello, Author
Terrence O'Rourke, Principal
Tanner Beach, Director
Contains over 500 religious signs for all denominations and their meanings illustrated by clear upper torso illustrations that show movements of hand, body and face. Includes a section on signing favorite verses, prayers and blessings. *$18.95*
219 pages Softcover
ISBN 0-553342-44-4

8101 Seeing Voices
Vintage and Anchor Books
1745 Broadway
3rd Floor
New York, NY 10019   212-782-9000
                      Fax: 212-572-6066
           vintageanchor@randomhouse.com
                  www.randomhouse.com

Oliver Sacks, Author
Madeline McIntosh, President/Sales/Operations
Markus Dohle, Chairman/CEO
Well known for his exploration of how people respond to neurological impairments, Dr Sacks explores the world of the deaf and discovers how deaf people respond to their loss of hearing and how they develop language. A highly readable introduction to deaf people, deaf culture and American Sign Language. *$13.95*
240 pages Softcover 2000
ISBN 0-375704-07-8

8102 Sign Language Interpreting and Interpreter Education
Oxford University Press
2001 Evans Rd
Cary, NC 27513-2009   919-677-0977
                      800-445-9714
                 Fax: 919-677-1303
               custserv.us@oup.com
                     www.oup.com

Marc Marschark, Editor
Rico Peterson, Editor
Elizabeth A Winston, Editor
Provides a coherent picture of the field as a whole, including evaluation of the extent to which current practices are supported by validating research. The first comprehensive source, suitable as both a reference book and a textbook for interpreter training programs and a variety of courses on bilingual education, psycholinguistics and translation, and cross-linguistic studies. *$65.00*
328 pages Hardcover
ISBN 0-195176-94-4

8103 Signed English Starter, The
Gallaudet University Press
800 Florida Ave NE
Washington, DC 20002-3600   773-568-1550
                      800-621-2736
                 Fax: 773-660-2235
                 TTY: 888-630-9347
              gupress@gallaudet.edu
              www.gupress.gallaudet.edu

Harry Bornstein, Author
Karen L Saulnier, Co-Author
T. Alan Hurwitz, President
A first course in Signed English for adults and children, the book is fully illustrated (several figures per page), and it is organized in a way that leads to rewarding learning quite rapidly. The authors of this new and exciting text believe firmly that Signed English must be made as easy as possible if it is going to be as useful (and used) as it can and should be. The book explains the rationale for the Signed English system and the conventions used to teach it. *$18.50*
232 pages Paperback
ISBN 0-913580-82-1

8104 Signing Family: What Every Parent Should Know About Sign Communication, The
Gallaudet University Press
800 Florida Ave NE
Washington, DC 20002-3600   773-568-1550
                      800-621-2736
                 Fax: 773-660-2235
                 TTY: 888-630-9347
              gupress@gallaudet.edu
              www.gupress.gallaudet.edu

David A Stewart, Author
Barbara Luetke-Stahlman, Co-Author
T. Alan Hurwitz, President
This reader-friendly book shows parents how to create a set of goals around the communication needs of their deaf child. De-

scribes in even-handed terms the major signing options available, from American Sign Language to Signed English. *$29.95*
192 pages Paperback
ISBN 1-563680-69-6

8105 Signing for Reading Success
Gallaudet University Press
800 Florida Ave NE
Washington, DC 20002-3600   773-568-1550
                      800-621-2736
                 Fax: 773-660-2235
                 TTY: 888-630-9347
              gupress@gallaudet.edu
              www.gupress.gallaudet.edu

Jan C Hafer, Author
Robert M Wilson, Co-Author
T. Alan Hurwitz, President
This booklet provides summaries of four research students on the usefulness of signing for reading achievement. *$7.95*
24 pages Paperback
ISBN 0-930323-18-1

8106 Signing: How to Speak with Your Hands
TJ Publishers
2427 Bond Street
Suite 108
University Park, IL 60466- 2288   972-416-0800
                      800-999-1168
                 Fax: 972-416-0944
           customerservice@tjpublishers.com
                  www.tjpublishers.com

Elaine Costello, Author
Terrence O'Rourke, Principal
Tanner Beach, Director
Presents 1,200 basic signs with clear illustrations in logical topical groupings. Linguistic principles are described at the beginning of each chapter, giving insight into the rules which govern American Sign Language. *$19.95*
248 pages Softcover
ISBN 0-553375-39-3

8107 Signs Across America
Gallaudet University Press
800 Florida Ave NE
Washington, DC 20002-3600   773-568-1550
                      800-621-2736
                 Fax: 773-660-2235
                 TTY: 888-630-9347
              gupress@gaHaudet.edu
              www.gupress.gallaudet.edu

Edgar H Shroyer, Author
Susan P Shroyer, Co-Author
T. Alan Hurwitz, President
A look at regional variations in ASL. Signs for selected words collected from 25 different states. More than 1,200 signs illustrated in the text. *$28.95*
304 pages Paperback
ISBN 0-913580-96-1

8108 Signs for Me: Basic Sign Vocabulary for Children, Parents & Teachers
TJ Publishers
2427 Bond Street
Suite 108
University Park, IL 60466- 2288   972-416-0800
                      800-999-1168
                 Fax: 972-416-0944
                  www.tjpublishers.com

Ben Bahan, Author
Joe Dannis, Co-Author
Terrence O'Rourke, Principal
Sign language vocabulary for preschool and elementary school children introduces household items, animals, family members, actions, emotions, safety concerns and other concepts. *$14.95*
112 pages Softcover
ISBN 0-915035-27-8

8109 Signs for Sexuality: A Resource Manual
Planned Parenthood of Western Washington
2001 E Madison St
Seattle, WA 98122-2959   206-328-7715
                                  Fax: 206-328-6810
                              www.plannedparenthood.org
Marlyn Minken, Author
Laurie Rosen-Ritt, Co-Author
Cecile Richards, President
An important book for those who want to listen to and talk with other people about feelings, loving and caring. *$40.00*
122 pages Softcover

8110 Signs of the Times
Gallaudet University Press
800 Florida Ave NE
Washington, DC 20002-3600   773-568-1550
                                     800-621-2736
                                 Fax: 773-660-2235
                                 TTY: 888-630-9347
                                 gupress@gallaudet.edu
                              www.gupress.gallaudet.edu
Edgar H Shroyer, Author
Susan P Shroyer, Illustrator
T. Alan Hurwitz, President
An excellent beginner's contact signing book that fills the gap between sign language dictionaries and American Sign Language text. Designed for use as a classroom text. *$34.95*
448 pages Softcover
ISBN 0-913580-76-7

8111 Silent Garden, The
Gallaudet University Press
800 Florida Ave NE
Washington, DC 20002-3600   773-568-1550
                                     800-621-2736
                                 Fax: 773-660-2235
                                 TTY: 888-630-9347
                                 gupress@gallaudet.edu
                              www.gupress.gallaudet.edu
Paul W Ogden, Author
T. Alan Hurwitz, President
Paul Kelly, Vice President Adm. And Finance
The author explain the broad range of hearing loss types, from minor to profound. Parents also are advised about what type of school their child should attend and what kinds of professional help will be best for the entire family. The book describes all forms of communication, including choices in signing from American Sign Language to the various manual systems based upon English. Technological alternatives are presented also, including when and when not to consider cochler implants. *$34.95*
304 pages
ISBN 1-563680-58-0

8112 Sing Praise Hymnal for the Deaf
LifeWay Christian Resources
1 Lifeway Plz
MSN 146
Nashville, TN 37234-1001   615-251-2000
                                     800-458-2772
                                 Fax: 615-251-3899
                                   www.lifeway.com
Thom Rainer, President/CEO
Jerry Rhyne, CFO/ VP Finance And Buisness
Tim Vineyard, VP Technology And CIO
Designed to be used by interpreters to the deaf, sign-language students, and deaf members of the congregation, this special combined hymnal edition offers 234 of the most popular hymns. *$12.95*
Hardcover 2000
ISBN 0-767314-09-3

8113 TDI National Directory & Resource Guide: Blue Book
Telecommunications for the Deaf
8630 Fenton Street
Suite 604
Silver Spring, MD 20910- 3822   301-589-3786
                                 Fax: 301-589-3797
                                   www.tdi-online.org
Claude L Stout, Executive Director

Promoting Equal Access to Telecommunications and Media for People who are Deaf, Late-Deafened, Hard-of-Hearing or Deaf-Blind. *$ 20.00*
600 pages Annual

8114 Theoretical Issues in Sign Language Research
University of Chicago Press
1427 E 60th St
Chicago, IL 60637-2902   773-702-7700
                                 Fax: 773-702-9756
                              sales@press.uchicago.edu
                              www.press.uchicago.edu
Donald A Collins, President
Susan D Fischer, Author
Patricia Siple, Co-Author
These volumes are an outgrowth of a conference held at the University of Rochester in 1986, dealing with the four traditional core areas of phonology, morphology, syntax and semantics. *$29.95*
348 pages Paperback 1990
ISBN 0-226251-52-7

8115 We CAN Hear and Speak
Alexander Graham Bell Association
3417 Volta Pl. NW
Washington, DC 20007   202-337-5220
                                 Fax: 202-337-8314
                                 TTY: 202-337-5221
                                   info@agbell.org
                                     agbell.org
Carol Flexer Ph.D, Author
Catherine Richards MA, Co-Author
Written by parents for families of children who are deaf or hard of hearing, this work describes auditory-verbal terminology and approaches and contains personal narratives written by parents and their children who are deaf or hard of hearing. *$6.98*
184 pages Softcover

8116 Week the World Heard Gallaudet, The
Gallaudet University Press
800 Florida Ave NE
Washington, DC 20002-3600   202-651-5000
                                     800-621-2736
                                 Fax: 202-651-5508
                              gupress@gallaudet.edu
                              www.gupress.gallaudet.edu
Jack R Gannon, Author
T. Alan Hurwitz, President
Paul Kelly, Vice President Adm. And Finance
This day-to-day description of the events surrounding the Deaf President Now movement at Gallaudet University includes full color and black and white photographs and interviews with people involved in the events of that week. *$49.95*
176 pages Hardcover
ISBN 0-930323-54-8

8117 What is Auditory Processing?
Abilitations - Speech Bin
P.O.Box 922668
Norcross, GA 30010-2668   770-449-5700
                                     800-850-8602
                                 Fax: 770-510-7290
                                 info@speechbin.com
                                 www.speechbin.com
Susan Bell, Author
What is Auditory Processing? It is and information-packed 16-page booklet created to explain auditory processing and it's disorders and offers practical suggestions for coping with this problem. It describes the listening process and tells how to help children with auditory processing problems. It shows what families and teachers can do to help children who have trouble remembering and understanding what they hear and offers easy-to-use activities and practical suggestions. *$ 22.69*
16 pages Softcover

8118   You and Your Deaf Child: A Self-Help Guidefor Parents of Deaf and Hard of Hearing Children
Gallaudet University Press
800 Florida Ave NE
Washington, DC 20002-3600

773-568-1550
800-621-2736
Fax: 773-660-2235
TTY: 888-630-9347
gupress@gallaudet.edu
www.gupress.gallaudet.edu

John W Adams, Author
T. Alan Hurwitz, President
Paul Kelly, Vice President Adm. And Finance
Eleven chapters focus on such topics as feelings about hearing loss, the importance of communication in the family, and effective behavior management. Many chapters contain practice activities and questions to help parents retain skills taught in the chapter and check their grasp of the material. Four appendices provide references, general resources, and guidelines for evaluating educational programs. $29.95
224 pages Paperback
ISBN 1-563680-60-2

Journals

8119   ADARA
1022 7th St NE
Washington, DC 20002

301-293-8969
Fax: 301-293-9698
TTY: 301-293-8969
adaraorg@gmail.com
www.adara.org

John Gournaris, Ph.D, President
Kathy Schwabeland, MA, Vice President
Denise Thew Hackett, Ph.D, JADARA Editor
ADARA's mission is to improve service excellence for those who are deaf or hard of hearing. The ADARA Update is a quarterly newsletter published by the association, offering information on events, resources, legislation, employment opportunities and other matters related to the field. JADARA is another publication by them presenting research results, articles on deafness, social services, mental health and other areas of interest.

8120   American Journal of Audiology
American Speech-Language-Hearing Association
2200 Research Blvd
Rockville, MD 20850-3289

240-632-2081
800-638-8255
Fax: 301-296-8580
actioncenter@asha.org
www.asha.org

Gary Dunham, Editor-in-Chief
Bridget Murray Law, Managing Editor
Carol Polovoy, Assistant Managing Editor
Articles concern screening, assesment, and treatment techniques; prevention; professional issues; supervision; administration. Includes clinical forums, clinical reviews, letters to the editor, or research reports that emphasize clinical practice.
2 x year

8121   Hearing Professional
International Hearing Society
16880 Middlebelt Rd
Ste 4
Livonia, MI 48154-3374

734-522-7200
800-521-5247
Fax: 734-522-0200
akovach@ihsinfo.org
www.ihsinfo.org

Kathleen Mennillo, MBA, Executive Director
Provides authoritative technical and business information that will help hearing aid specialists serve the hearing impaired.
bi-monthly

8122   Journal of Speech, Language and Hearing Research
American Speech-Language-Hearing Association
2200 Research Blvd
Rockville, MD 20850-3289

301-296-5700
800-638-8255
Fax: 301-296-8580
actioncenter@asha.org
www.asha.org

Gary Dunham, Editor-in-Chief
Bridget Murray Law, Managing Editor
Carol Polovoy, Assistant Managing Editor
Pertains broadly to studies of the processess and disorders of hearing, language, and speech diagnosis and treatment of such disorders.

8123   Journal of the Academy of Rehabilitative Audiology
Academy of Rehabilitative Audiology
PO Box 2323
Albany, NY 12220-0323

ara@audrehab.org
www.audrehab.org

Anne D. Olsen, Editor
A peer-reviewed journal published annually.

8124   Literature Journal, The
Gallaudet University
800 Florida Ave NE
Washington, DC 20002-3695

202-651-5488
800-621-2736
Fax: 202-651-5508
Oluyinka.Fakunle@gallaudet.edu

Charles C Welsh-Charrier, Author
T. Alan Hurwitz, President
Paul Kelly, Vice President Adm. And Finance
This book includes extensive examples of student and teacher entries taken from actual journals of deaf high school students. $12.95
44 pages Spiral Bound

8125   Sign Language Studies
Gallaudet University Press
800 Florida Ave NE
Washington, DC 20002-3695

202-651-5488
800-621-2736
Fax: 202-651-5508
gupress@gallaudet.edu
www.gupress.gallaudet.edu

Ceil Lucas, Editor
T. Alan Hurwitz, President
Paul Kelly, Vice President Adm. And Finance
Presents a unique forum for revolutionary papers on signed languages and other related disciplines, including linguistics, anthropology, semiotics, and deaf studies, history, and literature. $55.00
Quarterly

8126   Volta Review
Alexander Graham Bell Association
3417 Volta Pl. NW
Washington, DC 20007

202-337-5220
Fax: 202-337-8314
TTY: 202-337-5221
vreditor@agbell.org
agbell.org

Emilio Alonso-Mendoza, Chief Executive Officer
Professionally refereed journal that publishes articles and research on education, rehabilitation and communicative development of people who have hearing impairments. Also includes subscription to Volta Voices, up-to-date magazine, bimonthly.
Biannual

Magazines

8127   Endeavor Magazine
American Society for Deaf Children
PO Box 23
Woodbine, MD 21797   800-942-2732
                                                info@deafchildren.org
                                                www.deafchildren.org
Tami Dominguez, Editor
ASDC's qurterly publication featuring committee reports, stories, and fun.
Quarterly

8128   Hearing Health Magazine
Deafness Research Foundation
363 Seventh Avenue
10th Floor
New York, NY 10001-3904   212-257-6140
                                                      866-454-3924
                                                 Fax: 212-257-6139
                                                        info@drf.org
                                                        www.drf.org
Andrea Boidman, Executive Director
Andrea Delbanco, Senior Editor
Yishane Lee, Editor
Serves as a source of quality information and provides the tools
and resources to help people seek treatment for and manage hearing loss. Each issue features relevant and timely information on
the latest research, articles written by leading authorities in the
field, news about the latest technology, and human interest stories
about those living with hearing loss.

8129   Hearing Life Magazine
Hearing Loss Association of America
7910 Woodmont Ave
Ste 1200
Bethesda, MD 20814-7022   301-657-2248
                                                 Fax: 301-913-9413
                                               inquiry@hearingloss.org
                                                  www.hearingloss.org
Barbara Kelley, Executive Director
Formerly known as Hearing Loss Magazine, this official publication of the Hearing Loss Association of America helps individuals with hearing loss live a better life.
Bi-Monthly

8130   Tinnitus Today
American Tinnitus Association
PO Box 424049
Washington, DC 20042-4049   800-634-8978
                                                   ringingears.ata.org
Joy Onozuka, Managing Editor
The magazine contains up-to-date medical and research news,
feature articles on urgent tinnitus issues, questions and answers,
self-help suggestions and letters to the editor from others with
tinnitus. *$35.00*
28 pages 3 x year

Newsletters

8131   ASHA Leader, The
American Speech-Language-Hearing Association
2200 Research Blvd
Rockville, MD 20850-3289   301-215-6710
                                                      800-638-8255
                                                 Fax: 301-296-8580
                                                      leader@asha.org
                                                        www.asha.org
Gary Dunham, Editor-in-Chief
Bridget Murray Law, Managing Editor
Carol Polovoy, Assistant Managing Editor
Association publication containing news, notices of events and
activities and information for members on issues facing the profession of audiology and speech-language pathology. *$80.00*
35 pages 2 x month

8132   American Annals of the Deaf
Gallaudet University Press
800 Florida Ave NE
Washington, DC 20002-3600   202-651-5000
                                                      800-621-2736
                                                 Fax: 202-651-2736
                                                       paul.3@osu.edu
                                            www.gupress.gallaudet.edu
Peter V. Paul, Editor, Literary Issues
T. Alan Hurwitz, President
Paul Kelly, Vice President Adm. And Finance
Quarterly publication from the Conference of Educational Administrators Serving the Deaf. *$55.00*
Quarterly

8133   Canine Listener
Dogs for the Deaf
10175 Wheeler Rd
Central Point, OR 97502   541-826-9220
                                                      800-990-3647
                                                      800-990-3647
                                                 Fax: 541-826-6696
                                                 TTY: 541-826-9220
                                             info@dogsforthedeaf.org
                                                  dogsforthedeaf.org
Marvin Rhodes, Chair
Susan Bahr, Vice Chair
Kelly Gonzales, Development Director
Provides information on Hearing Dogs, placements, dog training,
and other news about happenings at Dogs for the Deaf.
Quarterly

8134   Cochlear Implants In Children: Ethics and Choices
Gallaudet University Press
800 Florida Ave NE
Washington, DC 20002-3600   202-651-5000
                                                      800-621-2736
                                                 Fax: 202-651-5508
                                               gupress@gallaudet.edu
                                            www.gupress.gallaudet.edu
John B Christiansen, Author
Irene W Leigh, Co-Author
T. Alan Hurwitz, President
Designed to educate readers about cochlear implants, including
surgery, the importance of rehabilitation and the significance of
parents' and professionals' roles. *$55.00*
340 pages Casebound
ISBN 1-563681-16-1

8135   Communique
Michigan Association for Deaf Hard of Hearing
5236 Dumond Court
Suite C
Lansing, MI 48917-6001   517-487-0066
                                                      800-968-7327
                                                 Fax: 517-487-2586
Nancy Asher, Executive Director
Pat Walton, Office Manager
Provides leadership through advocacy and education. The association conducts leadership training for youth, information and referral services, interpreter referral, legislative advocacy, and a
variety of other services.
4-8 pages Bi-annually

8136   Connect - Commmunity News
Hearing, Speech & Deafness Center (HSDC)
1625 19th Ave.
Seattle, WA 98122   206-323-5770
                                                      888-222-5036
                                                 Fax: 206-328-6871
                                                 TTY: 800-761-2821
                                                     clinics@hsdc.org
                                                        www.hsdc.org
Lindsay Klarman, Executive Director
Connect is the quarterly eNews of the Hearing, Speech & Deafness Center. HSDC is is a nonprofit for clients who are deaf, hard
of hearing, or who face other communication barriers such as
speech challenges.
8 pages Annual

8137   Deaf Catholic
International Catholic Deaf Association
7202 Buchanan St
Landover Hills, MD 20784-2236   301-429-0697
                                        Fax: 301-429-0698
                                        homeoffice@icda-us.org
                                        www.icda-us.org
Jean Cox, President
Kate Slosar, Vice President
TK Hill, Treasurer
Newsletter reporting the news of the Archdiocese, Deaf
Apostolate and each of the Catholic Deaf Organizations. *$20.00*
16 pages Quarterly

8138   International Hearing Dog, Inc.
International Hearing Dog
5901 E 89th Ave.
Henderson, CO 80640-8315   303-287-3277
                                        Fax: 303-287-3425
                                        info@hearingdog.org
Valerie Foss-Brugger, Executive Director
Samuel Cheris, Chairman
Matt Bailey, Treasurer
International Hearing Dog, Inc. trains rescued shelter dogs for
people who are deaf or hard-of-hearing, with and without disabil-
ities, all at no cost to the recipient. Since 1979, 1300 dogs have
been placed throughout all 50 states and Canada.
4-8 pages Quarterly

8139   League Letter
Center for Hearing and Communication
50 Broadway
6th Floor
New York, NY 10004-3810   917-305-7700
                                        Fax: 917-305-7888
                                        TTY: 917-305-7999
                                        info@chchearing.org
                                        www.lhh.org
Laurie Hanin, Executive Director
Ellen Lafargue, Au.D., CCC, Director, Hearing Technology
Lois Kam Heymann, M.A., CCC, Director, Communication
Quarterly

8140   Listner
HEAR Center
301 E Del Mar Blvd
Pasadena, CA 91101-2714   626-796-2016
                                        Fax: 626-796-2320
                                        info@hearcenter.org
                                        www.hearcenter.org
Ellen Simon, Executive Director
Berenice Castro, Accounting Supervisro
Debbie Lorino, Office Manager
Chronicals current events, spotlights pediatric and adult clients
as well as community outreach events.
Semi-Quarterly

8141   NAD E-Zine
National Association of the Deaf
8630 Fenton Street
Suite 820
Silver Spring, MD 20910- 3819   301-587-1788
                                        Fax: 301-587-1791
                                        TTY: 301-587-1789
                                        www.nad.org
Bobbie Beth Scoggins, President
Christopher Wagner, Vice President
Includes up-to-the-minute information about the NAD, including
Board news, advocacy, outreach and community activities, as
well as NAD Conference and other information.

8142   NAHO News
National Association of Hearing Officials
PO Box 4999
Midlothian, VA 23112-17   701-328-3260
                                        www.naho.org
Joy Wezelman, Editor
Janice Deshais, Editor
National Association of Hearing Officials newsletter.

8143   On the Level
Vestibular Disorders Association
5018 NE 15th Ave
Portland, OR 97211-5331   503-229-7705
                                        800-837-8428
                                        Fax: 503-229-8064
                                        veda@vestibular.org
                                        www.vestibular.org
Lisa Haven PhD, Executive Director
Jerry Underwood, Director
Vincente Honrubia, Director
Contents of each issue include information about local support
groups, a calendar of conferences and training opportunities for
health professionals, a list of donors, and special items indexed
below. *$5.00*
12 pages Quarterly

8144   Pinnacle Newsletter
Academy of Rehabilitative Audiology
PO Box 26532
Minneapolis, MN 55426-532   952-920-0484
                                        Fax: 952-920-6098
                                        sherri.smith@va.gov
                                        www.audrehab.org
John Greer Clark, Editor
Diana Derry, Co-Editor
Sherri Smith, Ph.D.,, Content Editor
Academy of Rehabilitative Audiology newsletter.

8145   Soundings Newsletter
American Hearing Research Foundation
8 South Michigan Avenue
Suite 1205
Chicago, IL 60603- 4539   312-726-9670
                                        Fax: 312-726-9695
                                        www.american-hearing.org
Sharon Parmet, Executive Director
Promote, conduct and furnish financial assistance for medical research into the cause, prevention and cure of deafness, impaired
hearing and balance disorders; encourage the collaboration of
clinical and laboratory research; encourage and improve teaching
in the medical aspects of hearing problems; and disseminate the
most reliable scientific knowledge to physicians, hearing
professionals and the public.
Quarterly

8146   Spring Dell Center Newsletter
Spring Dell Center
6040 Radio Station Rd
La Plata, MD 20646-3368   301-934-4561
                                        Fax: 301-870-2439
                                        www.springdellcenter.org
Donna Retzlaff, Executive Director
Jody Loper, President
Brett Hamorsky, Vice President
Quarterly

8147   Vision Magazine
National Catholic Office of the Deaf
7202 Buchanan St
Hyattsville, MD 20784-2236   301-577-1684
                                        Fax: 301-577-1684
                                        info@ncod.org
                                        www.ncod.org
Arvilla Rank, Editor/Executive Director
Published as a pastoral service for the deaf and hard of hearing.
Provides information to members and others working in ministry.
$15.00
Quarterly

Audio/Visual

8148 Christmas Stories
Video Learning Library
15838 N 62nd St
Scottsdale, AZ 85254-1988

480-596-9970
800-383-8811
Fax: 480-596-9973
www.videolearning.com

Jim Spencer, Owner
Told by popular deaf story-tellers, the stories included are A Christmas Carol, Night Before Christmas, Story of the First Christmas Tree, Birth of Christ, The Great Walled City, and Little Match Girl. *$29.95*
Video/80 Mins 1986
ISBN 1-882257-02-2

8149 Fantastic Series Videotape Set
Gallaudet University Press
800 Florida Ave NE
Washington, DC 20002-3695

202-651-5488
800-621-2736
Fax: 202-651-5489
gupress@gallaudet.edu
www.gupress.gallaudet.edu

Rita Corey, Director
T. Alan Hurwitz, President
Paul Kelly, Vice President Adm. And Finance
These videotapes offer a blend of entertainment and information to both deaf and hearing children ages 6-10. A total of eight tapes in the series. *$254.00*
Video 8 VHS
ISBN 1-563680-12-2

8150 Fantastic: Colonial Times, Chocolate, and Cars
Gallaudet University Press
800 Florida Ave NE
Washington, DC 20002-3695

202-651-5488
800-621-2736
Fax: 202-651-5489
gupress@gallaudet.edu
www.gupress.gallaudet.edu

Rita Corey, Director
T. Alan Hurwitz, President
Paul Kelly, Vice President Adm. And Finance
Young viewers visit Colonial Williamsburg in Virginia to see various crafts. Other parts show chocolate being made, and films of old cars. *$39.95*
Video
ISBN 1-563680-06-8

8151 Fantastic: Dogs at Work and Play
Gallaudet University Press
800 Florida Ave NE
Washington, DC 20002-3695

202-651-5488
800-621-2736
Fax: 202-651-5489
gupress@gallaudet.edu
www.gupress.gallaudet.edu

Rita Corey, Director
T. Alan Hurwitz, President
Paul Kelly, Vice President Adm. And Finance
See how dogs are trained, including Fantastic's own hearing-ear dog, police dogs, plus puppies, and dogs in space? *$39.95*
Video
ISBN 1-563680-03-3

8152 Fantastic: Exciting People, Places and Things!
Gallaudet University Press
800 Florida Ave NE
Washington, DC 20002-3695

202-651-5488
800-621-2736
Fax: 202-651-5489
gupress@gallaudet.edu
www.gupress.gallaudet.edu

Rita Corey, Director
T. Alan Hurwitz, President
Paul Kelly, Vice President Adm. And Finance

Welcomes young viewers for a trip to a crayon factory, a jump rope tournament, and mime by actor Bernard Bragg. *$39.95*
Video
ISBN 1-563680-01-7

8153 Fantastic: From Post Offices to Dairy Goats
Gallaudet University Press
800 Florida Ave NE
Washington, DC 20002-3695

202-651-5488
800-621-2736
Fax: 202-651-5489
gupress@gallaudet.edu
www.gupress.gallaudet.edu

Rita Corey, Director
T. Alan Hurwitz, President
Paul Kelly, Vice President Adm. And Finance
In this video children follow the route of a letter from the mailbox through the post office to its final destination. Also, they visit dairy goats and other animals. *$39.95*
Video
ISBN 1-563680-05-X

8154 Fantastic: Imagination, Actors, and 'Deaf Way'
Gallaudet University Press
800 Florida Ave NE
Washington, DC 20002-3695

202-651-5488
800-621-2736
202-651-5508
Fax: 202-651-5489
gupress@gallaudet.edu
www.gupress.gallaudet.edu

Rita Corey, Director
T. Alan Hurwitz, President
Paul Kelly, Vice President Adm. And Finance
Deaf clowns, mimes, and actors display the wonders of imagination, along with performances at the international cultural celebration 'Deaf Way.' *$39.95*
Video
ISBN 1-563680-04-1

8155 Fantastic: Roller Coasters, Maps, and Ice Cream!
Gallaudet University Press
800 Florida Ave NE
Washington, DC 20002-3695

202-651-5488
800-621-2736
Fax: 202-651-5489
gupress@gallaudet.edu

Rita Corey, Director
T. Alan Hurwitz, President
Paul Kelly, Vice President Adm. And Finance
In this program Mike Montangino leads the way on rides at Kings Dominion, and also to see how maps are drawn, and how ice cream is made. *$39.95*
Video
ISBN 1-563680-07-6

8156 Fantastic: Skiing, Factories, and Race Hores
Gallaudet University Press
800 Florida Ave NE
Washington, DC 20002-3695

202-651-5488
800-621-2736
Fax: 202-651-5489
gupress@gallaudet.edu

Rita Corey, Director
T. Alan Hurwitz, President
Paul Kelly, Vice President Adm. And Finance
Snow Skiing starts this program, which continues in a factory where 'who-knows-what' is made. Also, young viewers learn about horse care, and also about the making of Oreos. *$39.95*
Video
ISBN 1-563680-08-4

8157 Fantastic: Wonderful Worlds of Sports and Travel
Gallaudet University Press
800 Florida Ave NE
Washington, DC 20002-3695
202-651-5488
800-621-2736
Fax: 202-651-5489
gupress@gallaudet.edu

Rita Corey, Director
T. Alan Hurwitz, President
Paul Kelly, Vice President Adm. And Finance
In this program, young viewers ride on a train, watch deaf athletes compete, and see actor Bernard Bragg perform 'The Lion and the Mouse.' *$39.95*
Video
ISBN 1-563680-02-5

8158 Fingerspelling: Expressive and Receptive Fluency
DawnSign Press
6130 Nancy Ridge Dr
San Diego, CA 92121-3223
858-625-0600
800-549-5350
Fax: 858-625-2336
info@dawnsign.com
www.dawnsign.com

Joe Dannis, President
Joyce Linden Groode, Fingerspelling Teacher
Improve your fingerspelling with this new video guide. A 24-page instructional booklet is included with fingerspelling practice suggestions. *$29.95*
120 Minutes
ISBN 1-581210-46-9

8159 Getting Better
Vestibular Disorders Association
5018 NE 15th Ave
Portland, OR 97211-5331
503-229-7705
800-837-8428
Fax: 503-229-8064
veda@vestibular.org
www.vestibular.org

Cynthia Ryan MBA, Executive Director
Tony Staser,, Development Director
Vicente Honrubia, Director
Interviews with physicians, physical therapists, psychologists, social workers, and patients on Managing Symptoms, Diagnosis & Treatment, and Cognitive/Psychological Impacts. *$24.95*
Video

8160 Helping the Family Understand
Vestibular Disorders Association
5018 NE 15th Ave
Portland, OR 97211-5331
503-229-7705
800-837-8428
Fax: 503-229-8064
veda@vestibular.org
www.vestibular.org

Cynthia Ryan MBA, Executive Director
Tony Staser,, Development Director
Vicente Honrubia, Director
Interviews with physicians, physical therapists, psychologists, social workers, and patients on Managing Symptoms, Diagnosis & Treatment and Cognitive/Psychological Impacts. *$24.95*
Video

8161 Managing Your Symptoms
Vestibular Disorders Association
5018 NE 15th Ave
Portland, OR 97211-5331
503-229-7705
800-837-8428
Fax: 503-229-8064
veda@vestibular.org
www.vestibular.org

Cynthia Ryan MBA, Executive Director
Tony Staser,, Development Director
Vicente Honrubia, Director
Interviews with physicians, physical therapists, psychologists, social workers, and patients. on Managing Symptoms, Diagnosis & Treatment, and Cognitive/Psychological Impacts. *$24.95*
Video

Sports

8162 American Hearing Impaired Hockey Association
4214 W. 77th Place
Chicago, IL 60652-1618
978-922-0955
Fax: 312-829-2098
kkmm2won@aol.com
www.ahiha.org

Stan Mikita, President
Cheryl Hager, General Manager
Helen Tovey, Registrar, USA Hockey Reg.
The American Hearing Impaired Hockey Association provides deaf and hard of hearing hockey players the opportunity to learn about and improve their hockey skills through our program. We offer these hockey players the opportunity to be coached by a coaching staff with college, national and international experience.

8163 USA Deaf Sports Federation
102 N Krohn Pl
PO Box 910338
Lexington, KY 40591-0338
605-367-5760
Fax: 605-782-8441
TTY: 605-367-5761

Jack C Lamberton, President
Mark Apodaca, VP Of Financial Affairs
William J Bowman, VP Of International Affairs
The USA Deaf Sports Federation's purpose was to foster and regulate uniform rules of competition and provide social outlets for deaf members and their friends; serve as a parent organization for regional sports organizations; conduct annual athletic competitions; and assist in the participation of U.S. teams in international competition.

Support Groups

8164 Dial-a-Hearing Screening Test
Occupational Hearing Services Inc.
300 S Chester Rd
Suite 301
Swarthmore, PA 19081-1800
610-544-7700
800-622-3277
Fax: 610-543-2802

George Biddle, President/Owner
James Biddle, Vice President
Phyllis Biddle, Treasurer
A national telephone resource providing information about hearing impairments and deafness. Dial-A-Hearing Screening Test: national test number for free telephone hearing test: 1-800-222-EARS, MON-FRI: 9:00 AM to 5:00 PM Eastern time.

Mobility

Associations

8165 Academy of Spinal Cord Injury Professionals
206 S. 6th St
Springfield, IL 62701   217-321-2488
Fax: 217-525-1271
www.academyscipro.org
Destiny Nance-Evans, Director Of Memebership Services
Kim Ruff, Director Of Education
An interdisciplinary organization dedicated to advancing the care of people with spinal cord injury/dysfunction, providing resources, research, and insights for SCI/D professionals.

**8166 Academy of Spinal Cord Injury Professionals:
Psychologists, Social Workers & Counselors**
Academy of Spinal Cord Injury Professionals
206 S. 6th St.
Springfield, IL 62701   217-321-2488
Fax: 217-525-1271
www.academyscipro.org/
Heather Russell, President, PSWC Section
Lisa Beck, President, Academy of Spinal Cord Injury Professionals
Toby Huston, Vice President
Organizes and operates for scientific and educational purposes to advance and improve the psychosocial care of persons with spinal cord impairment, develops and promotes education and research related to the psychosocial care of persons with spinal cord injury, recognizes psychologists and social workers whose careers are devoted to the problems of spinal cord impairment.

8167 Acid Maltase Deficiency Association
P.O. Box 700248
San Antonio, TX 78270-0248   210-494-6144
Fax: 210-490-7161
TiffanyLHouse@aol.com
www.amda-pompe.org
Tiffany House, President
The Acid Maltase Deficiency Association offers resource materials to help raise awareness and provide education and insight into Pompe disease (a.k.a. Acid Maltase Deficiency), a rare genetic disease derived from the family of Lysosomal Storage Disease. The association offers information for patients, their families, as well as medical professionals.

8168 American Academy of Osteopathy
The Pyramids
3500 DePauw Blvd.
Suite 1100
Indianapolis, IN 46268-1136   317-879-1881
Fax: 317-879-0563
info@academyofosteopathy.org
www.academyofosteopathy.org
Sherri Quarles, Interim Executive Director & Accountant
Michael P. Rowane, DO, MS, FAOO, President
The mission of the American Academy of Osteopathy is to teach, advocate, and research the science, art and philosophy of osteopathic medicine, emphasizing the integration of osteopathic principles, practice and manipulative treatment in patient care.

**8169 American Association of Neuromuscular &
Electrodiagnostic Medicine**
2621 Superior Drive NW
Rochester, MN 55901   507-288-0100
Fax: 507-288-1225
aanem@aanem.org
www.aanem.org
Shirlyn A. Adkins, JD, Executive Director
Scott Gerdes, Finance Director
Lori Nierman, Office Manager
The American Association of Neuromuscular & Electrodiagnostic Medicine (AANEM) is a nonprofit membership association dedicated to the advancement of neuromuscular (NM), musculoskeletal, and electrodiagnostic (EDX) medicine.

8170 American Back Society
St. Joseph's Professional Center
2647 E. 14th St.
Suite 401
Oakland, CA 94601   510-536-9929
Fax: 510-536-1812
www.chiroweb.com/hp/abs/index.html
Philip E. Greenman, D.O., FAAO, President
Alexander Hadjipavlou, MD, MSc, 1st Vice President
Stephen Esses, BSc, MD, 2nd Vice President
The American Back Society is a non-profit organization dedicated to providing an interdisciplinary educational forum for healthcare professionals committed to relieving pain and diminishing impairment in patients suffering from neck and back conditions through proper diagnosis and treatment.

8171 American Parkinson Disease Association
135 Parkinson Avenue
Staten Island, NY 10305   800-223-2732
Fax: 718-981-4399
apda@apdaparkinson.org
www.apdaparkinson.org
Leslie A. Chambers, President & CEO
Stephanie Paul, Vice President, Development and Marketing
Robin Kornhaber, MSW, Vice President, Programs and Services
APDA was founded in 1961 with the dual purpose to find the curefor Parkinson's disease, and to assist Americans living with Parkinson's disease live a quality life.

8172 American Spinal Injury Association
9702 Gayton Rd.
Suite 306
Richmond, VA 23238   877-274-2724
asia.office@asia-spinalinjury.org
www.asia-spinalinjury.org
Patty Duncan, Executive Director
Carolyn Moffatt, Association Manager
Kim Ruff, Administrative Assistant
Professional association for physicans and other health professionals working in all aspects of spinal cord injury.

8173 American Stroke Association
7272 Greenville Ave
Dallas, TX 75231   888-478-7653
strokeconnection@heart.org
www.strokeassociation.org/STROKEORG
John Warner, President
James Postl, Chairman
Nancy Brown, Chief Executive Officer
The American Stroke Association offers educational materials, seminars, conferences and transportation for those effected by strokes as well as their families, caregivers and interested professionals.

8174 Amytrophic Lateral Sclerosis Association
1275 K Street NW
Suite 250
Washington, DC 20005   202-407-8580
Fax: 202-464-8869
alsinfo@alsa-national.org
www.alsa.org
Barbara Newhouse, President/CEO
Calaneet Balas, Executive Vice President, Strategy
Gregory L. Mitchell, Executive Vice President, Finance & Administration
The ALS association is the only national not-for-profit health organization dedicated soley to lead the fight against ALS. The Association covers all the bases-research, patient and community services, public education, and advocacy-in providing help and hope to those facing the disease. The mission is to lead the fight to cure and treat ALS through global cutting edge research, and to empower people with Lou Gehrig's disease to live fuller lives & provide them with compassion, care and support.

8175 Arthritis Foundation
1355 Peachtree St NE
6th Floor
Atlanta, GA 30309   404-872-7100
                                          800-283-7800
                                          www.arthritis.org
Laurie Stewart, Secretary/Vice Chair
Rowland W. (Bing) Chang, Chair
Frank Longobardi, Treasurer
Offers information and referrals regarding educational materials
and programs, fund-raising, support groups, seminars and conferences, and aids Americans with arthritis in accessing optimal
care.

**8176 Association for Neurologically Impaired Brain Injured
Children**
61-35 220th St
Oakland Gardens, NY 11364   718-423-9550
                                          Fax: 718-423-9838
                                          jdebiase@anibic.org
                                          www.anibic.org
Vincent Tancredi, Chief Financial Officer
John F DeBiase, Executive Director
Rachel Plakstis, MSC Director
ANIBIc is a voluntary, multi-service organization that is dedi-
cated to serving individuals with severe learning disabilities,
neurological impairments and other developmental disabilities.
Services include: residential, vocational, family support services, recreation (children and adults), respite (adult), in home
support services, counseling and traumatic brain injury services
(adults).

8177 Capital Area Parkinsons Society
PO Box 27565
Austin, TX 78755-2565   512-371-3373
                                          www.capitalareaparkinsons.org
Tereasa Ford, President
Deborah Bryson, Vice President
Donna Hohm, Secretary
Founded in 1984, the Capital Area Parkinson's Society addresses
the needs for those impacted by Parkinson's disease in central
Texas. The organization offers a multitude of support groups, re-
sources, monthly meetings, exercise programs and a community
for people afflicted by Parkinson's and their care partners.

8178 Children's Hemiplegia & Stroke Association
4101 W. Green Oaks Blvd
Suite 305-149
Arlington, TX 76016   www.chasa.org
Nancy Atwood, Executive Director & Founder
Jana Smoot White, President
Patti Scrivano, Vice President
Founded in 1996, CHASA offers support and information to fam-
ilies of infants, children and young adults who have hemiplegia,
hemiparesis or hemiplegic cerebral palsy.

8179 Christopher & Dana Reeve Paralysis Resource Center
636 Morris Turnpike
Suite 3A
Short Hills, NJ 07078   973-467-8270
                                          800-225-0292
                                          InfoSpecialist@ChristopherReeve.org
                                          www.christopherreeve.org
John M Hughes, Chairman
John E McConnell, Vice Chairman
Peter Wilderotter, President & CEO
The Paralysis Resource Center's goal is to provide support and
information to those living with paralysis and their caregivers.
Some programs offered include financial grants, a family support
program, advocay programs, a lending library, rehabilitation cen-
ters, a veteran program and a resource guide about paralysis.

8180 Consortium of Multiple Sclerosis Centers
3 University Plaza Dr.
Suite 116
Hackensack, NJ 07601   201-487-1050
                                          Fax: 862-772-7275
                                          www.mscare.org
June Halper, Chief Executive Officer
Gary Cutter, PhD, President
Lisa Skutnik, Chief Operating Officer

CMSC provides leadership in clinical research and education; develops vehicles to share information and knowledge among members; disseminates information to the health care community and
to persons affected by Multiple Sclerosis; and develops and implements mechanisms to influence health care delivery.

8181 Cure SMA
Cure SMA
925 Busse Rd
Elk Grove Village, IL 60007   800-886-1762
                                          info@curesma.org
                                          www.curesma.org
Jill Jarecki, Chief Scientific Officer
Kenneth Hobby, President
Richard Rubenstein, Chair
Cure SMA is the largest international organization dedicated
solely to eradicating spinal muscular atrophy (SMA) by promot-
ing and supporting research, helping families cope with SMA
through informational programs and support, and educating the
public and professional community about SMA.

8182 Dystonia Advocacy Network
One East Wacker Drive
Suite 2810
Chicago, IL 60601   dystonia-advocacy.org
Established in 2007, The Dystonia Advocacy Network (DAN) is
an organization of dystonia-affected individuals and organiza-
tions united in speaking on legislative and public policy issues
which impact the dystonia community.

8183 Epilepsy Foundation
8301 Professional Place E
Suite 200
Landover, MD 20785- 2353   800-332-1000
                                          Fax: 301-459-1569
                                          ContactUs@efa.org
                                          www.epilepsy.com
Robert W Smith, Chair
Phillip M. Gattone, M.Ed, Preisdent & CEO
M. Vaneeda Bennett, Chief Development Officer
The organization works to ensure that people with epilepsy are
able to participate in all life experiences; to improve how people
with epilepsy are perceived and treated in society; and to promote
research for a cure.

8184 Friends of Disabled Adults and Children
4900 Lewis Rd
Stone Mountain, GA 30083   770-491-9014
                                          866-977-1204
                                          www.fodac.org
Chris Brand, President
Pam Holley, Director of Administration
Betty Felder, DME Office Manager
FODAC's mission is to provide durable medical equipment
(DME) at lost cost to the disabled and their families, and to en-
hance the quality of life for individuals with disabilities or
illnesses.

**8185 Head Injury Rehabilitation And Referral Service, Inc.
(HIRRS)**
11 Taft Court
Suite 100
Rockville, MD 20850   301-309-2228
                                         Fax: 301-309-2278
                                         tbi@headinjuryrehab.org
                                         www.headinjuryrehab.org
Maggie Hunter, Director of Admissions and Quality Assurance
Robert Cousland, Director of Rehabilitation
Ricardo Hunter, President
Head Injury Rehabilitation and Referral Services, Inc. (HIRRS)
is a private not-for-profit agency that provides comprehensive
brain injury support including long-term living, daily programs,
vocational supports and services to individuals that live in the
community. The agency is located in Rockville, MD, but serves
the DC Metropolitan area.

8186 International Parkinson and Movement Disorder Society
555 East Wells St.
Suite 1100
Milwaukee, WI 53202-3823   414-276-2145
                          Fax: 414-276-3349
                     info@movementdisorders.org
                     www.movementdisorders.org
Christopher Goetz, MD, President
Susan Fox, PhD, Secretary
Victor Fung, MBBS, PhD, FRACP, Treasurer
The International Parkinson and Movement Disorder Society
(MDS) is a professional society of clinicians, scientists, and other
healthcare professionals who are interested in Parkinson's dis-
ease, related neurodegenerative and neurodevelopmental disor-
ders, hyperkinetic movement disorders, and abnormalities in
muscle tone and motor control.

8187 Lewy Body Dementia Association
912 Killian Hill Road S.W.
Lilburn, GA 30047   404-975-2322
                          Fax: 480-422-5434
                               www.lbda.org
Christina M. Christie, President
Shannon McCarty-Caplan, Vice President
Mike Koehler, CEO
The Lewy Body Dementia Association (LBDA) is a nonprofit or-
ganization dedicated to raising awareness of the Lewy body
dementias (LBD), supporting people affected by LBD, and pro-
moting scientific advances.

8188 Mobility International USA
132 E Broadway
Suite 343
Eugene, OR 97401   541-343-1284
                          Fax: 541-343-6812
                          TTY: 541-343-1284
                     clearinghouse@miusa.org
                               www.miusa.org
Susan Sygall, Chief Executive Officer
Cindy Lewis, Director, Programs
A US based national nonprofit organization dedicated to empowering people with disabilities around the world through leadership development, training and international exchange to ensure
inclusion of people with disabilities in international exchange
and development programs. The National Clearinghouse on Disability & Exchange, a joint project managed by MIUSA, provides
free information and referrals.

8189 Multiple Sclerosis Association of America
375 Kings Hwy N
Cherry Hill, NJ 08034   800-532-7667
                          Fax: 856-661-9797
                          msaa@mymsaa.org
                               mymsaa.org/
John McCorry, Chair
Monica Derbes Gibson, Vice Chair
Steve Bruneau, Treasurer
MSAA is a national non-profit organization dedicated to enrich-
ing the quality of life for evryone affected by Multiple Sclerosis
through vital services and support.

8190 Multiple Sclerosis Foundation
6520 N. Andrews Ave
Fort Lauderdale, FL 33309-2132   954-776-6805
                               800-225-6495
                          Fax: 954-938-8708
                          admin@msfocus.org
                               www.msfocus.org
Jules Kuperberg, Executive Director
Alan Segaloff, Co- Executive Director
Kasey Minnis, Director, Operations & Communications
A national, nonprofit organization that provides free support ser-
vices and public education for persons with Multiple Sclerosis,
newsletters, toll-free phone support, information, referrals, home
care, assitive technology, and support groups.

8191 NBIA Disorders Association
2082 Monaco Ct.
El Cajon, CA 92019-4235   619-588-2315
                          Fax: 619-588-4093
                          info@NBIAdisorders.org
                          www.nbiadisorders.org
Patricia Wood, President
Coleen Lukoff, Development Director
Melissa Woods, Social Media Director
NBIA provides support to families, educates the public and accel-
erates research with collaborators from around the world.

8192 National Association for Continence
P.O. Box 1019
Charleston, SC 29402   800-252-3337
                          sgregg@nafc.org
                               www.nafc.org
Katherine F. Jeter, EdD, Founder
Steven G. Gregg, PhD, Executive Director
Donna Deng, Chairperson
NAFC's mission is to educate the public about the causes, diagnosis, categories, treatment options and management alternatives
for incontinence, voiding dysfunction and related pelvic floor
disorders; to network with other organizations and agencies; to
elevate the visibility and priority given to these areas; and to advocate on behalf of consumers who suffer from such symptoms as
a result of disease or other illness.

8193 National Center for Health, Physical Activity and Disability
4000 Ridgeway Dr.
Birmingham, AL 35209   800-900-8086
                          Fax: 205-313-7475
                          email@nchpad.org
                               www.nchpad.org
James Rimmer, Principal Investigator
Angela Grant, Business Manager
Jeff Underwood, Program Director
NCHPAD promotes health for people with disability through in-
creased participation in all types of physical and social activities.
These include fitness and aquatic activities, recreational and
sports programs, adaptive equipment usage, and more.
1999

8194 National Coalition for Assistive and Rehab Technology
54 Towhee Court
East Amhurst, NY 14051   716-839-9728
                          Fax: 716-839-9624
                          info@ncart.us
                               www.ncart.us
Don Clayback, Executive Director
Doug Westerdahl, President
Greg Packer, Vice President
The coalition's mission is to ensure proper and appropriate access
to complex rehab and assistive technologies.

8195 National Council on Independent Living (NCIL)
P.O. Box 31260
Washington, DC 20006   202-207-0334
                               844-778-7961
                          Fax: 202-207-0341
                          TTY: 202-207-0340
                          ncil@ncil.org
                               www.ncil.org
Darrell Llynn Jones, Interim Executive Director
Jenny Sichel, Director, Operations
Denise Law, Coordinator, Member Services
A national cross-disability grassroots organization, NCIL ad-
vances independent living and the rights of people with disabili-
ties through consumer-driven advocacy.

8196 National Fibromyalgia Association
3857 Birch St.
Suite 312
Newport Beach, CA 92660   nfa@fmaware.org
                               www.fmaware.org
Lynne Matallana, President/Founder
National Fibromyalgia Association's mission is to develop and
execute programs dedicated to improving the quality of life for
people with fibromyalgia.

8197 National Mobility Equipment Dealers Association
3327 West Bearss Ave
Tampa, FL 33618   813-264-2697
                                         866-948-8341
                                    Fax: 813-962-8970
                                      info@nmeda.org
                                      www.nmeda.com

Chad Blake, President
Richard May, Vice President
Bill Koeblitz, Secretary
The National Mobility Equipment Dealers Association
(NMEDA) is a non-profit trade association dedicated creating
and expanding oppotunities of safe transportation for people with
disabilities in vehicles modified to fit their specific needs.

8198 National Spasmodic Dysphonia Association
300 Park Blvd.
Suite 335
Itasca, IL 60143   800-795-6732
                                    Fax: 630-250-4505
                                   nsda@dysphonia.org
                                    www.dysphonia.org

Charlie Reavis, President
Marcia Sterling, Treasurer
Kimberly Kuman, Executive Director
The National Spasmodic Dysphonia Association (NSDA) is a
not-for-profit organization dedicated to advancing medical research into the causes of and treatments for SD, promoting physician and public awareness of the disorder, and providing support
to those affected by SD through symposiums, support groups, and
on-line resources.

8199 National Spasmodic Torticollis Association
9920 Talbert Ave
Fountain Valley, CA 92708   714-378-9837
                                         800-487-8385
                                   NSTAmail@aol.com
                                    www.torticollis.org

Ken Price, President/Treasurer
Diane Truong, Vice President
Janelle Lazzo, Secretary
The mission of the National Spasmodic Torticollis Association is
to support the needs and well being of individuals affected by
Spasmodic Torticollis; to promote awareness and education; and
to advance research for more treatments and a cure.

8200 Paralyzed Veterans of America
801 18th St. NW
Washington, DC 20006-3517   800-424-8200
                                   TTY: 800-795-4327
                                         info@pva.org
                                         www.pva.org

Charles Brown, National President
Marcus Murray, National Secretary
Carl Blake, Executive Director
A national organization serving veterans and individuals with
spinal cord injury/disorder (SCI/D), as well as their family mem-
bers and caregivers.

8201 Parkinson's Disease Research Society
Northwestern Medicine Central DuPage Hospital
25 N. Winfield Rd
4 North Tower
Winfield, IL 60190   630-933-4384
                                    Fax: 630-933-3077
                                   parkinsonsprogress.org

Carol A. Santi, President
Alex Katz, Vice President
Mitchell King, Treasurer
The PDRS mandate is to mount a concerted effort to intensify the
research, both in the basic science laboratory as well as with clini-
cal trials, to advance the diagnosis, treatment and prevention of
Parkinson's disease.

8202 Simon Foundation for Continence
P.O. Box 815
Wilmette, IL 60091   847-864-3913
                                         800-237-4666
                                    Fax: 847-864-9758
                             webmaster@simonfoundation.org
                                www.simonfoundation.org

Cheryl B. Gartley, Founder/President
Elizabeth A. LaGro, Vice President, Communications & Education
Services
Twila Yednock, Director of Special Events
The Simon Foundation is known throughout the world for its innovative educational projects and tireless efforts on behalf of
people with loss of bladder and bowel control. The mission of the
foundation is to remove the stigma surrounding incontinence and
to provide help for people with incontinence, their families, and
the healthcare professionals who provide care for people with
incontinence.

8203 Society for Progressive Supranuclear Palsy
30 E. Padonia Road,
Suite 201
Timonium, MD 21093   800-457-4777
                                    Fax: 410-785-7009
                                      info@curepsp.org
                                         www.psp.org

Janet Edmunson, Med, Chair
Dan Johnson, Vice-Chair
George S. Jankiewicz, CPA, CFP,, Treasurer
Members of the Board of Directors of CurePSP accept the major
responsibility of implementing the mission of the Foundation for
PSP | CBD and Related Brain Diseases. Board members are ac-
tively involved in continually defining and redefining the mission and participating in strategic planning to review purposes,
programs, priorities, funding needs, and levels of achievement.

8204 United Spinal Association
120-34 Queens Blvd
Ste 320
Kew Gardens, NY 11415   718-803-3782
                                    Fax: 718-803-0414
                                    www.unitedspinal.org
United Spinal Association is dedicated to enhancing the quality
of life of all people living with spinal cord injuries and disorders,
including veterans, and providing support and information to
loved ones, care providers and professionals.

8205 Vermont Back Research Center
1 S Prospect St
Burlington, VT 05405   802-656-3131
                                    Fax: 802-660-9243
                                       learn@uvm.edu
                                        www.uvm.edu
Conducts research aimed at reducing back-related disability following injury or acute pain episodes. Current research includes
studies of posture, seating, vibration, materials handling, and exercise. The Center develops and tests assistive devices, and promotes employment of people with back disorders and rapid return
to work after injury. The staff provides a variety of information
services, including bibliographic searches and fact finding.

8206 World Chiropractic Alliance
2683 Via De La Valle
Suite G 629
Del Mar, CA 92014   480-786-9235
                                         866-789-8073
                                    Fax: 480-732-9313
                             www.worldchiropracticalliance.org

Linda Bevel, Manager
Terry A Rondberg DC, Founder/CEO
The World Chiropractic Alliance was founded in 1989 as a
non-profit organization dedicated to protecting and strengthening chiropractic around the world. Since its inception, the WCA
has played an important role in the global chiropractic community. In 1998, it was granted status as a Non-Governmental Organization (NGO) associated with the United Nations Department
of Public Information.

Camps

8207 Camp Esperanza
Southern California Chapter
West 6th Street
Suite 1250
Los Angeles, CA 90017   323-954-5760
                                     800-954-2873
                                Fax: 213-954-5790
                                jziegler@arthritis.org
                                     www.arthritis.org

Jennifer Ziegler, Camp Director
Lindsey Gonzales, Regional Director, Human Resources
Manuel Loya, Chief Executive Officer
A one-week camp in August that allows children with arthritis to participate in such activities as horseback riding, swimming, etc. in a fun-filled environment.

8208 Easterseals Camp Stand by Me
Easterseals Washington
17809 S Vaughn Rd. NW
PO Box 289
Vaughn, WA 98394   253-884-2722
                        campadmin@wa.easterseals.com
                        www.easterseals.com/washington
Cathy Bisaillon, President & CEO
Angela Cox, Camp Director
Camp Stand By Me provides a safe, barrier-free environment for children and adults with any disability to experience all aspects of camp without limitations. Respite weekends offered throughout the year. Activities include campfires, fishing, swimming, sports, archery, and more.

8209 Hillcroft Services
501 W Air Park Dr.
Muncie, IN 47303   765-284-4166
                                     www.hillcroft.org

Debbie Bennett, President & CEO
Abby Halstead, Chief Financial Officer
Jessica Hammett, Chief Operations Officer
Offers a summer camp program for children with autism spectrum disorders.

8210 Illinois Wheelchair Sport Camps
University of Illinois
1207 S Oak St.
Champaign, IL 61820   217-333-1970
                                Fax: 217-244-0014
                                sportscamp@illinois.edu
                        www.disability.illinois.edu/camps
Wheelchair sport programs including track, basketball, and individual skills camps. Hosted at the University of Illinois.

8211 Rising Treetops at Oakhurst
111 Monmouth Rd.
Oakhurst, NJ 07755   732-531-0215
                                Fax: 732-531-0292
                                info@risingtreetops.org
                                www.risingtreetops.org
Robert Pacenza, Executive Director
Charles Sutherland, Camp Director
Lori Schenck, Assistant Director, Services
A summer and day camp for adults and children with special needs, including autism and physical and intellectual disabilities. Campers experience traditional camp activities while gaining skills for greater independence.

8212 Twin Lakes Camp
1451 E Twin Lakes Rd
Hillsboro, IN 47949-8004   765-798-4000
                                outdoors@twinlakescamp.com
                                www.twinlakescamp.com
Jon Beight, Executive Director
Duane Bush, Guest Service
Dan Daily, Program Director
Provides a summer camp program for special needs children and young adults. Campers suffer from a wide range of maladies including crippling accidents, Spina Bifida, epilepsy, Cerebral Palsy, Muscular Dystrophy, Quadriplegia, Paraplegia, and other disabling diseases. Campers range in age from 8 to 27.

8213 YMCA Camp Fitch
12600 Abels Rd.
North Springfield, PA 16430   814-922-3219
                                     877-863-4824
                                Fax: 814-922-7000
                                registrar@campfitchymca.org
                                     campfitchymca.org
Tom Parker, Executive Director
Joe Wolnik, Summer Camp Director
Brandy Duda, Outdoor Education Director
Camp is located in North Springfield, Pennsylvania. Camp programs include sessions for children with diabetes or epilepsy.

Books

8214 Adapted Physical Education and Sport
Human Kinetics, Inc.
1607 N Market Street
Champaign, IL 61820-2220   217-351-5076
                                     800-747-4457
                                Fax: 217-351-1549
                                     info@hkusa.com
                                     www.naspem.org

Joseph P Winnick EdD, Author
Scott Kimberly, Owner
Rainer Martens, President/Treasurer
Designed as a resource for both present and future physical education leaders, this book is an exceptional book for teaching exceptional children. It emphasizes the physical education of young people with disabilities. *$68.00*
592 pages Hardcover
ISBN 0-736052-16-X

8215 Arthritis Bible
Inner Traditions - Bear & Company
PO Box 388
Rochester, VT 05767-0388   802-767-3174
                                     800-246-8648
                                Fax: 802-767-3726
                        customerservice@innertraditions.com
                                     www.innertraditions.com
Craig Weatherby, Author
Leonid Gordin MD, Co-Author
A comprehensive guide to the alternative therapies and conventional treatments for Arthritic diseases including Osteoarthritis, Rheumatoid Arthritis, Gout, Fibromyalgia and more. *$16.95*
272 pages Paperback 1999
ISBN 0-892818-25-5

8216 Arthritis Helpbook: A Tested Self Management Program for Coping with Arthritis
Da Capo Press
44 Farnsworth Street,
Boston, MA 02210   617-252-5200
                                Fax: 617-252-5265
                                     www.dacapopress.com
Kate Lorig, Author
James Fries, Co-Author
The Arthritis Helpbook is the world's leading guide to coping with joint pain, and has been used by more than 600,000 readers over its twenty years in print. It succeeds because of its tested advice, its hundreds of useful hints, and its emphasis on self-management-helping people with arthritis and fibromyalgia to achieve their own health goals. *$18.95*
Paperback
ISBN 0-738210-38-2

8217 Arthritis Sourcebook
McGraw-Hill Professional
7500 Chavenelle Rd
Dubuque, IA 52002-9655   563-584-6000
                                     877-833-5524
                                Fax: 614-759-3749
                                     www.mhprofessional.com
Earl J Brewer Jr MD, Author
Kathy Cochran Angel, Co-Author

A comprehensive guide to the latest information on treatments, medications, and alternative therapies for arthritis. *$ 16.95*
272 pages Paperback
ISBN 0-737303-81-6

8218   Arthritis, What Exercises Work: Breakthrough Relief for the Rest of Your Life
MacMillan - St. Martin's Press
175 5th Ave
New York, NY 10010-7703   646-307-5151
                                        Fax: 212-420-9314
                                press.inquiries@macmillanusa.com
                                        www.us.macmillan.com
Dava Sorbel, Author
Arthur C Klein, Co-Author
What is the most powerful arthritis treatment ever developed to help restore you to a healthy, pain-free, and vigorous life—for the rest of your life? It's exercise. Here are the right exercised for your kind of arthritis, pain-level, age, occupation, and hobbies. *$14.99*
200 pages Paperback 1995
ISBN 0-312130-25-2

8219   Arthritis: A Take Care of Yourself Health Guide
Da Capo Press
44 Farnsworth Street,
Boston, MA 02210   617-252-5200
                                        Fax: 617-252-5265
                                        www.dacapopress.com
James F Fries, Author
Donald M Vickery, Co-Author
In this updated book the author draws on new research to recommend exercises and new pain medications for both arthritis and fibromyalgia. *$18.95*
Paperback 1909
ISBN 0-738202-25-8

8220   Disability and Sport
Human Kinetics, Inc.
1607 N Market Street
Champaign, IL 61820-2220   217-351-5076
                                          800-747-4457
                                        Fax: 217-351-1549
                                        info@hkusa.com
                                        www.naspem.org
Karen P DePauw, Author
Susan J Gavron, Co-Author
Scott Kimberley, Owner
Provides a comprehensive and practical look at the past, present, and future of disability sport. Topics covered are inclusive of youth through adult participation with in-depth coverage of the essential issues involving athletes with disabilities. This new edition has updated references and new chapter-opening outlines that assist with individual study and class discussions. *$48.00*
408 pages Hardcover
ISBN 0-736046-38-0

8221   Fitness Programming for Physical Disabilities
Human Kinetics, Inc.
1607 N Market Street
Champaign, IL 61820-2220   217-351-5076
                                          800-747-4457
                                        Fax: 217-351-1549
                                        info@hkusa.com
                                        www.naspem.org
Patricia D Miller, Editor
Scott Kimberley, Owner
Rainer Martens, President/Treasurer
A book offering information for developing and conducting exercise programs for groups that included people with physical disabilities. A dozen authorities in exercise science and adapted exercise programming explain how to effectively and safely modify existing programs for individuals with physical disabilities. *$42.00*
232 pages Paperback
ISBN 0-873224-34-5

8222   Freedom from Arthritis Through Nutrition
Tree of Life Publications
PO Box 126
Joshua Tree, CA 92252-0126   760-366-2937
                                        Fax: 760-366-2937
                                        www.treelifebooks.com
Philip J Welsh DDS ND, Author
Bianca Leonardo ND, Co-Author
Reveals the results of 60 years of research on arthritis by noted nutritionist, Dr. Philip J. Welsh, D.D.S. N.D. Here you will find simple, natural, inexpensive, tested ways of coping with the various forms of arthritis, using only nutrition and other natural methods. There are no drugs or gadgets in this program. *$24.95*
255 pages Softcover

8223   Functional Electrical Stimulation for Ambulation by Paraplegics
Krieger Publishing Company
1725 Krieger Drive
PO Box 9542
Malabar, FL 32950   321-724-9542
                                          800-724-0025
                                        Fax: 321-951-3671
                                        info@krieger-publishing.com
                                        www.krieger-publishing.com
Daniel Graupe, Author
Kate H Kohn, Co-Author
FES is employed to enable spinal cord injury patients who are complete paraplegics to stand and ambulate without bracing. The text covers 12 years of amulation experience. *$49.50*
210 pages Paperback 1994
ISBN 0-894648-45-4

8224   Guide to Managing Your Arthritis
Arthritis Foundation
1330 W. Peachtree St
Suite 100
Atlanta, GA 30309   404-872-7100
                                          800-283-7800
                                        Fax: 404-237-8153
                                        AFOrders@pbd.com
                                        www.arthritis.org
Mary Anne Dunkin, Author
John Klippel, President/CEO
Cecile Perich, Chairman
Expert reviewers answer questions about basic arthritis facts, treatments, research, surgery and more. Also, specific information about six common conditions: rheumatoid arthritis, osteoarthritis, osteoporosis, fibromyalgia, lupus and gout. *$9.95*
193 pages Paperback
ISBN 0-912423-28-5

8225   How to Deal with Back Pain and Rheumatoid Joint Pain: A Preventive and Self Treatment Manua
Global Health Solutions
2146 Kings Garden Way
Falls Church, VA 22043-2593   703-848-2333
                                          800-759-3999
                                        Fax: 703-848-0028
                                        information@watercure.com
                                        www.watercure.com
Fereydoon Batmanghelidj, Author
Xiaopo Batmanjhelidj, President
Kristin Swan, Administrator
The physiology of pain production and its direct relationship to chronic regional dehydration of some joint spaces is explained: Special movements that would create vacuum in the disc spaces and draw water and the displaced discs into the vertebral joints are demonstrated. *$14.95*
100 pages Paperback
ISBN 0-962994-20-0

8226   **Inclusive Games**
Human Kinetics
1607 N Market Street
PO Box 5076
Champaign, IL 61825- 5076   217-351-5076
800-747-4457
Fax: 217-351-1549
info@hkusa.com
www.humankinetics.com

Susan L Kasser, Author
Scott Kimberley, Owner
Rainer Martens, President/Treasurer
Features more than 50 games, helpful illustrations, and hundreds of game variations. The book shows how to adapt games so that children of every ability level can practice, play and improve their movement skills together. The game finder makes it easy to locate an appropriate game according to its name, approximate grade level, difficulty within the grade level, skills required/developed, and number of players. *$17.95*
120 pages Paperback
ISBN 0-873226-39-9

8227   **Inside The Halo and Beyond: The Anatomy of a Recovery**
WW Norton & Company
500 5th Ave
New York, NY 10110-2   212-354-5500
Fax: 212-869-0856
www.wwnorton.com

Maxine Kumin, Author
W Drake McFeely, Chairman/President
Stephen King, VP Finance/CFO
A skilled horsewoman and lifelong athlete, poet Kumin was 73 when a riding accident left her with two broken vertebrae in her neck. Kumin survived in the face of overwhelming odds that she would be paralyzed for the rest of her life. Miraculously, however, she was walking again within weeks of the accident; now, though one hand and an arm remain partially immobilized, her life has largely resumed its normal course. Here is the journal of her first nine months of recovery. *$ 13.95*
192 pages Softcover
ISBN 0-393049-00-0

8228   **Life on Wheels: For the Active Wheelchair User**
Patient-Centered Guides
1005 Gravenstein Highway North
Sebastopol, CA 95472   707-827-7000
Fax: 707-829-0104
support@oreilly.com
www.oreilly.com

Gary Karp, Author
For 1.5 million Americans, life includes a wheelchair for mobility. Life on Wheels is for people who want to take charge of their life experience. Author Gary Karp describes medical issues (paralysis, circulation, rehab, cure research); day-to-day living (exercise, skin, bowel and bladder, sexuality, home access, maintaining a wheelchair); and social issues (self-image, adjustment, friends, family, cultural attitudes, activism). *$24.00*
565 pages Paperback 1999
ISBN 1-565922-53-0

8229   **Paralysis Resource Guide**
Christopher and Dana Reeve Paralysis Resource Ctr
636 Morris Turnpike
Suite 3A
Short Hills, NJ 07078   973-467-8270
800-539-7309
Fax: 973-912-9433
information@christopherreeve.org
www.paralysis.org

John M. Hughes, Chairman
John E. McConnell, Vice Chair
Matthew Reeve, Vice Chair
A comprehensive information tool for people affected by paralysis and for those who care for them. English or Spanish.
336 pages

8230   **Primer on the Rheumatic Diseases**
Arthritis Foundation
1330 W. Peachtree St
Suite 100
Atlanta, GA 30309-2111   404-872-7100
800-933-7023
Fax: 404-237-8153
AFOrders@pbd.com
www.arthritis.org

Rob Shaw, President
Patience White M.D., Editor
John H. Klippel, Editor
The leading professional book about arthritis and related diseases, the Primer is published by Springer and the Arthritis Foundation. *$79.95*
724 pages Softcover
ISBN 0-387356-64-8

8231   **Sport Science Review: Adapted Physical Activity**
Human Kinetics
1607 N Market Street
Champaign, IL 61820-2220   217-351-5076
800-747-4457
Fax: 217-351-1549
info@hkusa.com
www.naspem.org

Rainer Martens, President/Treasurer
Scott Kimberley, Owner
Jill Wikgren, COO
This issue of Sport Science Review examines the newly emerging academic discipline of adapted physical activity. Researchers from diverse academic backgrounds and parts of the world review the issues and controversies surrounding inclusion in physical education and sport. *$15.00*
96 pages Paperback
ISBN -073602-07-9

8232   **Still Me**
Random House
1745 Broadway
3rd Floor
New York, NY 10019-4305   212-782-9000
Fax: 212-572-6066
vintageanchor@randomhouse.com
www.randomhouse.com

Christopher Reeve, Author
Markus Dohle, Chairman/CEO
Madeline McIntosh, President
The man who was Superman begins with his debilitating riding accident, then weaves back and forth between past and present, creating a thorough biography of Reeve's life. *$7.99*
336 pages Paperback 1999
ISBN 0-345432-41-4

8233   **When Your Student Has Arthritis**
Arthritis Foundation
2970 Peachtree Rd NW
PO Box 932915, Ste 200
Atlanta, GA 31193-2915   404-237-8771
800-933-7023
Fax: 404-237-8153
aforders@arthritis.org
www.afstore.org

Rob Shaw, President
An overview of arthritis, including juvenile rhuematoid arthritis and treatment. Also includes a school activities checklist for students, education rights, and how teachers can help.
28 pages

8234   **Yoga for Fibromyalgia: Move, Breathe, and Relax to Improve Your Quality of Life**
Mobility Limited
PO Box 838
Morro Bay, CA 93443-0838   805-772-3560
800-366-6038
Fax: 805-772-4717
shsh@mobilityltd.com
www.mobilityltd.com

Shoosh Lettick Crotzer, Director

The first book devoted exclusively to managing the symptoms of fibromyalgia; the comprehensive program of 26 illustrated poses, breathing techniques, and guided visualization and relaxation sessions can be practiced regardless of age or experience. The Living with Fibromyalgia section discusses lifestyle concerns. *$14.95*
128 pages 1908

Journals

8235   Topics in Spinal Cord Injury Rehabilitation
American Spinal Injury Association
9702 Gayton Rd.
Suite 306
Richmond, VA 23238   877-274-2724
asia.office@asia-spinalinjury.org
www.asia-spinalinjury.org
Patty Duncan, Executive Director
Carolyn Moffatt, Association Manager
Kim Ruff, Administrative Assistant
Clinical, peer-reviewed information for physiatrists, PTs, OTs, rehabilitation nurses, psychologists, neurologists, orthopedists, and others.

Magazines

8236   Arthritis Today
Arthritis Foundation
1330 W. Peachtree St.
Suite 100
Atlanta, GA 30309   404-872-7100
800-933-7023
Fax: 404-237-8153
info.ga@arthritis.org
www.arthritis.org
Dan McGowan, Chairman
Rowland W. Chang, Vice Chair
Ann M. Palmer, President and CEO
Magazine for patients, physicians, public authorities and others with an interest in the field of arthritis. (Price noted paid for yearly subscription) *$12.95*
Bi-Monthly

8237   Fibromyalgia AWARE Magazine
National Fibromyalgia Association
2121 S Towne Centre Pl
suite 30
Orange, CA 92865-6124   714-921-0150
Fax: 714-921-6920
fmaware.org
Lynne Matallana, Editor In Chief
Malina Anderson, CFO
Eroll Landy, Treasurer
Addresses the needs and concerns of people affected by fibromyalgia and overlapping conditions. *$35.00*
3 times a year

8238   New Mobility
Leonard Media Group
120-34 Queens Blvd.
Suite 330
Kew Gardens, NY 11415   800-404-2898
www.newmobility.com
Jean Dobbs, Publisher & Editorial Director
Josie Byzek, Executive Editor
Ian Ruder, Editor
The full-service, full-color lifestyle magazine for the disability community. The award-winning magazine is contemporary, witty and candid. Produced by professional journalists and visual artists, the magazine's voice is uncompromising and unsentimental, yet practical, knowing and friendly. The magazine covers issues that matter to readers: medical news, and cure research; jobs, benefits and civil rights; sports, recreation and travel; product news, technology and innovation. *$27.95*
Monthly

8239   PALAESTRA: Forum of Sport, Physical Education and Recreation for Those with Disabilities
Challenge Publications Limited
1807 N. Federal Drive
Urbana, IL 61801   217-359-5940
800-327-5557
Fax: 217-359-5975
www.palaestra.com
David P Beaver EdD, Fonding Editor
Martin.E Block, Editor-in-Chief
Julian U. Stein, Associate Editor
The most comprehensive resource on sport, physical education and recreation for individuals with disabilities, their parents and professionals in the field of adapted physical activity. Published in cooperation with US Paralympics and AAHPERD's Adapted Physical Activity Council. Informative yet entertaining and delivers valuable insights for consumers, families and professionals in the field. Published quarterly.

8240   PN/Paraplegia News
PVA Publications
2111 E Highland Ave
Suite 180
Phoenix, AZ 85016-4702   602-224-0500
888-888-2201
Fax: 602-224-0507
www.pn-magazine.com
Richard Hoover, Editor
Ann Santos, Assistant Editor
Packed with timely information on spinal-cord-injury research, new products, legislation that impacts people with disabilities, accessible travel, computer options, car/van adaptations, news for veterans, housing, employment, health care and all issues affecting wheelers and caregivers around the world.

8241   Spirit Magazine
Special Olympics International
1133 19th St NW
Washington, DC 20036-3604   202-628-3630
Fax: 202-824-0200
info@specialolympics.org
www.specialolympics.org
Kathy Smallwood, Editor
Timothy P Shriver PhD, Chariman/CEO
J Brady Lum, President/COO
This magazine reflects the power of Special Olympics to build bridges between people with and without intellectual disabilities and spark personal insight, compassion and gratitude for life.
Quarterly

8242   Strides Magazine
North American Riding for the Handicapped Assoc
7475 Dakin Street
Suite 600
Denver, CO 80221-6920   303-452-1212
800-369-7433
Fax: 303-252-4610
Carol Nickell, CEO
Sheila Dietrich, Executive Director
William Scebbi, CEO
This engaging magazine is a non-technical, yet accurate journal that focuses on the work of NARHA. Rider profiles, how-to articles, editorials and instructional columns seek to educate a general readership of the diverse aspects of equine facilitated therapy and activities. Each seasonal issue carries a theme.
Quarterly

8243   Stroke Connection Magazine
American Stroke Association
7272 Greenville Ave
Dallas, TX 75231-5129   214-373-6300
888-478-7653
Fax: 214-706-1191
www.strokeassociation.org
Ralph Sacco, President/Director
Nancy Brown, CEO
Debra Lockwood, Chairman
From in-depth information on conditions such as aphasia, central pain, high blood pressure and depression, to tips for daily living from healthcare professionals and other stroke survivors. Stroke

Connection keeps you abreast of how to cope, how to reduce your risk of stroke and how to make the most of each day.
6 issues

Newsletters

8244   **A World Awaits You**
Mobility International USA
132 E Broadway
Suite 343
Eugene, OR 97401

541-343-1284
Fax: 541-343-6812
TTY: 541-343-1284
clearinghouse@miusa.org
www.miusa.org/away

Susan Sygall, Chief Executive Officer
Cindy Lewis, Director, Programs
Includes interviews with people with disabilities who have participated in a wide range of international exchange programs.
Annually

8245   **ABS Newsletter**
American Back Society
2648 International Blvd
Suite 502
Oakland, CA 94601-1547

510-536-9929
Fax: 510-536-1812
info@americanbacksoc.org
www.americanbacksoc.org

Scott Haldeman, President
Aubrey Swartz MD, Executive Director
Keeps subscribers current with timely topics on the diagnosis and treatment of a wide spectrum of painful and disabling conditions of the spine.

8246   **Arthritis Foundation Great West Region**
Arthritis Foundation
115 N.E. 100th St
Suite 350
Seattle, WA 98125

206-547-2707
888-391-9389
Fax: 206-547-2805
tzuehl@arthritis.org
www.arthritis.org

Scott Weaver, CEO
Kelsey Birnbaum, Vice President, Development
Deborah Genge, Vice President, Development
Offers regional updates, information on activities and events, resources and medical research for members.
Newsletter

8247   **Arthritis Update**
Arthritis Foundation
1330 W. Peachtree St.
Suite 100
Atlanta, GA 30309

404-872-7100
info.uny@arthritis.org
www.arthritis.org

Dan McGowan, Chairman
Rowland W. Chang, Vice Chair
Ann M. Palmer, President and CEO
Offers chapter updates, information on activities and events, resources and medical research for members.
Newsletter

8248   **CurePSP Magazine**
Society for Progressive Supranuclear Palsy
2648 International Blvd
Suite 502
Hunt Valley, MD 21031-1002

410-785-7004
800-457-4777
Fax: 410-785-7009
info@curepsp.org
www.psp.org

Richard Gordon Dyne DMin, President
Janet Edmunson, Chair
Dan Johnson, Vice Chair
Informs readers of findings in the area of PSP.

8249   **EpilepsyUSA Magazine**
Epilepsy Foundation of America
8301 Professional Pl
Landover, MD 20785-2237

301-459-3700
Fax: 301-577-2684
www.epilepsyfoundation.org

Brien J Smith Md, Chair
Mark E Nini, Senior Vice Chair
Richard P Denness, President/CEO
The Epilepsy Foundation's award-winning magazine, epilepsyUSA, is published online four times a year. The magazine is one of the only publications of its kind devoted entirely to news and up-to-the-minute information about epilepsy.

8250   **Exchange**
ALS Association
27001 Agoura Rd
Suite 250
Agoura Hills, CA 91301-5105

818-340-0182
800-782-4747
Fax: 818-880-9006
www.alsa.org

Gary A Leo, CEO
Morton Charlestein, Chairman
Andrew Soffel, Chairman
Covers a broad range of subjects including stories about the lives of ALS patients, special events, research and public policy in the ALS community.
4-6 times/year

8251   **Fibromyalgia Online**
National Fibromyalgia Association
2121 S Towne Centre Pl
suite 300
Ornage, CA 92865-6124

714-921-0150
Fax: 714-921-6920
www.fmaware.org

Lynne Matallana, President/Editor In Chief
Malina Anderson, CFO
Eroll Landy, Treasurer
An educational resource for patients and healthcare professionals that brings the latest news on fibrmyalgia and overlapping conditions.
Monthly

8252   **Focus**
Arthritis Foundation
1330 W. Peachtree St.
Suite 100
Atlanta, GA 30309

404-872-7100
info.coh@arthritis.org
www.arthritis.org

Dan McGowan, Chairman
Rowland W. Chang, Vice Chair
Ann M. Palmer, President and CEO
Offers chapter updates, information on activities and events, resources and medical research for members.
Newsletter

8253   **Joint Efforts**
Arthritis Foundation
1330 W. Peachtree St.
Suite 100
Atlanta, GA 30309

404-872-7100
800-464-6240
Fax: 415-356-1240
info.nca@arthritis.org
www.arthritis.org

Dan McGowan, Chairman
Rowland W. Chang, Vice Chair
Ann M. Palmer, President and CEO
Offers chapter updates, information on activities and events, resources and medical research for members.
Newsletter

8254 **MIUSA's Global Impact Newsletter**
Mobility International USA
132 E Broadway
Suite 343
Eugene, OR 97401   541-343-1284
                                              Fax: 541-343-6812
                                              TTY: 541-343-1284
                                         clearinghouse@miusa.org
                                                  www.miusa.org

Susan Sygall, Chief Executive Officer
Cindy Lewis, Director, Programs
Each issue features photos, alumni updates, highlights from recent activities, and new publications.
Quarterly

8255 **Motivator**
Multiple Sclerosis Association of America
706 Haddonfield Rd
Cherry Hill, NJ 8002-2652   856-488-4500
                                                   800-532-7667
                                              Fax: 856-661-9797
                                             jmasino@mymsaa.org
                                            www.msassociation.org

Andrea L GriesS, Editor
Susan W Courtney, Sr Writer & Creative Director
Amanda Bednar, Contributing Writer
MSAA's 48-plus page magazine highlights and explains many vital issues of importance to our readers affected by MS. These include cover and feature stories about a variety of topics such as depression, assistive technology, the role of pets and service animals, parents with MS, and clinical trials, to name a few.
48 pages Quarterly

8256 **New York Arthritis Reporter**
New York Chapter of the Arthritis Foundation
122 East 42nd Street
New York, NY 10168-1898   212-984-8700
                                              Fax: 212-878-5960
                                            info.ny@arthritis.org
                                                 www.arthritis.org

Phyllis Geraghty, Editor
Ross Alfieri, President
Daniel T. McGowan, Chair
Provides public access to current arthritis information and resources on important health issues.
Quarterly

8257 **SCI Psychosocial Process**
American Assoc of Spinal Cord Injury Psych/Soc Wor
75-20 Astoria Blvd
East Elmhurst, NY 11370   718-803-3782
                                                   800-404-2898
                                              Fax: 718-803-0414
                                            info@unitedspinal.org
                                              www.unitedspinal.org

David C. Cooper, Chairman
Patrick W. Maher, Vice Chairman
Joseph Gaskins, President and CEO
The purpose of this e journal is disseminating information of value to psychologists, social workers and other psychological caring for spinal cord injured persons.
2 time a year

8258 **SCILIFE**
National Spinal Cord Injury Association
75-20 Astoria Blvd
East Elmhurst, NY 11370   718-803-3782
                                                   800-404-2898
                                              Fax: 718-803-0414
                                             info@spinalcord.org
                                              www.unitedspinal.org

David C. Cooper, Chairman
Patrick W. Maher, Vice Chairman
Joseph Gaskins, President and CEO
Filled with issue-driven articles, and news of interest to the SCI community and the larger disability community.
Bi-monthly

Audio/Visual

8259 **A Wheelchair for Petronilia**
Fanlight Productions C/O Icarus Films
32 Court St.
21st Floor
Brooklyn, NY 11201-1731   718-488-8900
                                                   800-876-1710
                                              Fax: 718-488-8642
                                               info@fanlight.com
                                                 www.fanlight.com

Bob Gliner, Director
Jonathan Miller, President
Meredith Miller, Sales Manager
Profiles a program, organized and run by Guatemalans with disabilities, which trains them to manufacture and repair cheap, sturdy wheelchairs designed for conditions in developing countries. 28 Minutes.
VHS/DVD
ISBN 1-572953-98-5

8260 **Beyond the Barriers**
Aquarius Health Care Videos
30 Forest Road
PO Box 249
Millis, MA 02054   508-376-1244
                                                   888-440-2963
                                              Fax: 508-376-1245

Mark Wellman, Director
Leslie Kussmann, President/Producer
For too many years, paraplegics, amputees, quadraplegics and the blind have felt trapped by their disabilities. No more! Mark Wellman and other disabled adventurers, rock climb the desert towers of Utah, sail in British Columbia, body-board the big waves of Pipeline and Waimea Bay, scuba dive with sea lions in Mexico and hand glide the California coast. This film delivers the simple message: Don't give up, and never give in. If you can't ever lose, then you can't ever win. Preview option.
Video/47 Mins

8261 **Breathing Lessons: The Life and Work of Mark O'Brien**
Fanlight Productions C/O Icarus Films
32 Court St.
21st Floor
Brooklyn, NY 11201-1731   718-488-8900
                                                   800-876-1710
                                              Fax: 718-488-8642
                                               info@fanlight.com
                                                 www.fanlight.com

Jessica Yu, Director
Jonathan Miller, President
Meredith Miller, Sales Manager
Breathing Lessons breaks down barriers to understanding by presenting an honest and intimate portrait of a complex, intelligent, beautiful and interesting person, who happens to be disabled.
$225.00
Video/35 Mins 1996
ISBN 1-572958-41-3

8262 **Complete Armchair Fitness**
CC-M Productions
7755 16th St NW
Washington, DC 20012-1460   202-882-7432
                                                   800-453-6280
                                              Fax: 202-882-7432
                                             www.armchairfitness.com

Robert Mason, Manager
Armchair Fitness video series. 4 DVDs: Armchair Fitness Aerobic, Armchair Fitness Gentle, Armchair Fitness Strength and Armchair Fitness Yoga. *$120.00*
Video

8263 How Come You Walk Funny?
Fanlight Productions C/O Icarus Films
32 Court St.
21st Floor
Brooklyn, NY 11201-1731   718-488-8900
                                 800-876-1710
                             Fax: 718-488-8642
                             info@fanlight.com
                             www.fanlight.com

Tina Hahn, Director
Jonathan Miller, President
Meredith Miller, Sales Manager
Profiles a unique experiment in reverse integration: a school where non disabled kids attend a kindergarten designed for children with physical disabilities. The kids and families tackle their differences and discover common ground through finding a way that all can play. *$ 179.00*
Video/47 Mins 2004
ISBN 1-572958-84-7

8264 Key Changes: A Portrait of Lisa Thorson
Fanlight Productions C/O Icarus Films
32 Court St.
21st Floor
Brooklyn, NY 11201-1731   718-488-8900
                                 800-876-1710
                             Fax: 718-488-8642
                             info@fanlight.com
                             www.fanlight.com

Cindy Marshall, Director
Jonathan Miller, President
Meredith Miller, Sales Manager
A documentary profiling Lisa Thorson, a gifted vocalist who uses a wheelchair. Ms. Thorson defines herself as a performer first, a person with a disability second, and this thoughtful portrait respects that distinction. Her work as a jazz singer is at the heart of the film, reflecting her philosophy that the biggest contribution that she can make to the struggle for the rights of people with disabilities is doing her art the best way she can. *$149.00*
Video/28 Mins 1993
ISBN 1-572959-30-4

8265 Wheelchair Bowling
American Wheelchair Bowling Association
PO Box 69
Clover, VA 24534-69   434-454-2269
                             Fax: 434-454-6276
                             garyryan210@gmail.com
                             www.awba.org

Dick Schaaf, Author
Dave Roberts, Executive Secretary Treasurer
In addition to providing historical background, it includes principles of the game from keeping score through ball drilling for the wheelchair bowler. Through profiles of wheelchair bowlers, the text covers ball delivery, spare making techniques and special equipment that can be used. *$9.95*
96 pages

8266 Yoga for Arthritis
Mobility Limited
601 Morro Bay Blvd
Suite E
Morro Bay, CA 93442-2000   805-772-3560
                                 800-366-6038
                             Fax: 805-772-4717
                             shsh@mobilityltd.com
                             www.mobilityltd.com

Shoosh Crotzer, Owner/Executive Director
A yoga-based program with five separate segments, which includes breathing and relaxation techniques, stretching and strengthening routines, and aerobic exercises. This 52-minute program can also be performed seated. Available on DVD or VHS; DVD includes Spanish version. *$19.95*
Video

8267 Yoga for MS and Related Conditions
Mobility Limited
601 Morro Bay Blvd
Suite E
Morro Bay, CA 93442-2000   805-772-3560
                                 800-366-6038
                             Fax: 805-772-4717
                             shsh@mobilityltd.com
                             www.mobilityltd.com

Shoosh Crotzer, Owner/Executive Director
A yoga-based program. Shows assisted versions of each exercise for those who require it; is available with an optional Instructional Guidebook with illustrations, alternative positions, and hints. This 48-minute program can also be performed seated. Available on DVD or VHS; DVD includes Spanish version. *$19.95*
Video

Sports

8268 Access to Sailing
423 E Shoreline Village Drive
Long Beach, CA 90802   562-901-9999
                             www.accesstosailing.org

Duncan Milne, Founder/Executive Director
Cliff Larson, Director
Gaile Oslapas, Assistant Director
Provides therapeutic rehabilitation to disabled and disadvantaged children and adults, through interactive sailing outings.

8269 Achilles Track Club
42 West 38th Street
Suite 400
New York, NY 10018-6241   212-354-0300
                             Fax: 212-354-3978

Richard Traum PhD, President/Founder
Mary Bryant, Vice President
Kathleen Bateman, Director
Organization whose goal is to guide disabled athletes into the able-bodied community.

8270 Adaptive Sports Center
PO Box 1639
Crested Butte, CO 81224-1639   970-349-2296
                                 866-349-2296
                             Fax: 970-349-2077
                             info@adaptivesports.org
                             www.adaptivesports.org

Christopher Hensley, Executive Director
Chris Read, CTRS Program Director
Ella Fahrlander, Development Director
Year round adaptive, adventure recreation program located at the base of Crested Butte Mountain Resort, Crested Butte,CO. The Adaptive Sports Centers provides adaptive downhill and cross country ski lessons, ski rentals and snowboarding lessons in the winter. Offers a variety of wilderness based programs in the summer including multi-day trips into the back country, extensive cycling programs, canoeing, and white water rafting.

8271 American Wheelchair Bowling Association
PO Box 69
Clover, VA 24534-69   434-454-2269
                             Fax: 434-454-6276
                             garyryan210@gmail.com
                             www.awba.org

Joseph L. Fox, Chairman
Wayne Webber, Vice Chairperson
Paul Kenney, Treasurer
A non-profit organization, composed of wheelchair bowlers, dedicated to encouraging, developing, and regulating wheelchair bowling and wheelchair bowling leagues.

8272   Chesapeake Region Accessible Boating
177 Defense Hwy.
Suite 9
Annapolis, MD 21401   410-266-5722
                                       info@crabsailing.org
                                       crabsailing.org

Brad La Tour, President
Paul Bollinger, Executive Director
Sarah Winchester, Operations Manager
Chesapeake Region Accessible Boating (CRAB) provides opportunities for the disabled and their friends to sail the Chesapeake Bay. Programs include group sails for organizations representing special guests, sailing clinics and camps, SailFree Sundays for families, and regattas for those who wish to race.

8273   Disabled Sports Program Center
Disabled Sports USA Far West
PO Box 9780
Truckee, CA 96162-7780   530-581-4161
                                       Fax: 530-581-3127

Doug Pringle, President
Marilyn Cummings,, Office Manager
Haakon Lang-Ree, Manager
Founded in 1967, Disabled Sports USA Far West is dedicated to innovative programs that provide an environment with positive therapeutic and psychological outcomes. Individuals are empowered to reach their full potential. Our programs allow individuals of all abilities to discover their own strengths and interests.

8274   Disabled Sports USA
451 Hungerford Dr
Suite 100
Rockville, MD 20850-5102   301-217-0960
                                       Fax: 301-217-0968
                                       www.disabledsportsusa.org

Kirk Bauer, Executive Director
Kathy Chandler, Executive Director
Kathy Celo, Operations
Provides year-round sports and recreation opportunities for people with physical disabilities, veterans and non-veterans alike, such as sanctioned regional and national events in alpine and Nordic skiing, cycling, shooting swimming, table tennis, track and field, volleyball, and weightlifting. The organization handles physical disabilities which restrict mobility, including amputations paraplegia, quadriplegia, cerebral palsy, head injury, mulitple sclerosis, muscular dystrophy, and more.

8275   Disabled Watersports Program
Mission Bay Aquatic Center
1001 Santa Clara Pl
San Diego, CA 92109   858-488-1000
                                       Fax: 858-488-9625
                                       mbac@sdsu.edu
                                       www.missionbayaquaticcenter.com

Kevin Starw, Director
Kevin Waldick, Asst. director
Eric Fehrs, Maintenance Director
Devoted to providing accessible water sports and recreational opportunities for individuals with disabilities. Specially designed equipment makes water skiing, wake boarding, keelboat sailing, windsurfing, rowing, surfing, and kayaking possible for people with varying levels of mobility and ability.

8276   Galvin Health and Fitness Center
Rehabilitation Institute of Chicago
345 East Suuperior St.
Chicago, IL 60611   312-238-1000
                                       800-354-7342
                                       800-354-REHA
                                       Fax: 312-238-5017
                                       sports@ric.org
                                       http://www.ric.org

Jude Reyes, Chair
Mike P. Kransy, Vice Chair
Thomas Reynolds III, Vice Chair
The RIC Sports and Fitness Program offers people with physical disabilities an on-site fitness center, specialized exercise classes and services, and adult and junior competitive and recreational sports opportunities, including the recreational/social Caring for Kids program for youth ages 7-17. Most programs are provided free of charge or for a nominal fee.

8277   Guide to Wheelchair Sports and Recreation
Paralyzed Veterans of America
801 18th St. NW
Washington, DC 20006-3517   800-424-8200
                                       TTY: 800-795-4327
                                       info@pva.org
                                       www.pva.org

Charles Brown, National President
Marcus Murray, National Secretary
Carl Blake, Executive Director
This guide lists descriptions of adaptive sports and recreation, activity and equipment directories, and additional resources for people with disabilities.
28 pages Booklet

8278   Handicapped Scuba Association International
Handicapped Scuba Association
1104 El Prado
San Clemente, CA 92672-4637   949-498-4540
                                       Fax: 949-498-6128
                                       www.hsascuba.com

Jim Gatacre, President
Patricia Derk, Vice President
A nonprofit volunteer organization dedicated to improving the physical and social well being of those with special needs through the exhilarating sport of scuba diving. An educational program for able bodied scuba instructors to learn to teach and certify people with special needs. Accessible travel opportunities.

8279   Lakeshore Foundation
4000 Ridgeway Dr
Birmingham, AL 35209-5563   205-313-7400
                                       Fax: 205-313-7475
                                       information@lakeshore.org
                                       www.lakeshore.org

Jeff Underwood, President & CEO
Beth Curry, Chief Program Officer
Jen Remick, Director, Communications & Membership
Promotes independence for persons with physically disabling conditions and provides opportunities to pursue active, healthy lifestyles.

8280   National Disability Sports Alliance
25 W Independence Way
Kingston, RI 02881-1124   401-792-7130
                                       Fax: 401-792-7132
                                       http://nationaldisabilitysportsalliance.webs.
Jerry McCole, Executive Director
Serves to present disabled athletes with the opportunity to perform in many different sports. Participants range from the beginning athlete to the elite, international caliber athlete.

8281   National Skeet Shooting Association
5931 Roft Rd
San Antonio, TX 78253-9261   210-688-3371
                                       800-877-5338
                                       Fax: 210-688-3014
                                       nsca@nssa-nsca.com
                                       www.mynssa.com

Michael Hampton, Jr., Executive Director
Royce Graff, NSSA Director
Amber Schwarz, NSC Assistant Director
Offers information on sporting clay targets for the disabled hunter.

8282   National Sports Center for the Disabled
33 Parsenn Rd
PO Box 1290
Winter Park, CO 80482   970-726-1518
                                       Fax: 970-726-4112
                                       volunteer@nscd.org
                                       nscd.org

Kim Easton, President & CEO
Diane Eustace, Marketing Director
Beth Fox, Outreach & Education Director
The center's mission is to provide quality outdoor sports and therapeutic recreation programs that positively impact the lives of people with physical, cognitive, emotional, or behavioral challenges. Winter programming includes alpine skiing, snowboarding, ski racing, show shoeing, and cross-country ski-

ing. Summer sports include rafting, sailing, kayaking, camping, hiking, horseback riding, fishing, and rock climbing.
6-8 pages Quarterly

8283 National Wheelchair Poolplayers Association
90 Flemons Dr
Somerville, AL 35670 256-778-0449
Fax: 703-817-1215
www.nwpainc.org

Jeffrey Dolezal, President
Bob Calderon, Secretary
Ken Force, Editor
Works together with other groups, organizations, and tournaments to update rules to include wheelchair players.

8284 Ontario Cerebral Palsy Sports Association
P.O. Box 60082
Ottawa, ON, Canada K1T-0K9 613-723-1806
866-286-2772
Fax: 613-723-6742

Amanda Fader, Executive Director
Don Sinclair, President
Lorette Dupuis, Vice President
Organization that provides, promotes and coordinates competitive opportunities as well as encourages individual excellence through sport for athletes within the cerebral palsy family. To that end, OCPSA recruits, develops and supports athletes, coaches and volunteers.

8285 Professional Association of Therapeutic Horsemanship International (PATH Intl.)
PO Box 33150
Denver, CO 80233 303-452-1212
800-369-7433
Fax: 303-252-4610
pathintl@pathintl.org
www.pathintl.org

Kathy Alm, Chief Executive Officer
Carrie Garnett, Director, Membership & Operations
Kaye Marks, Director, Marketing & Communications
A national nonprofit equestrian organization dedicated to serving individuals with disabilities by giving disabled individuals the opportunity to ride horses. Establishes safety standards, provides continuing education, and offers networking opportunities for both its individuals and center members. Produces educational materials including fact sheets, brochures, booklets, audio-visual tapes, a directory, and PATH Intl. magazine Strides.

8286 Special Olympics
1133 19th St NW
Washington, DC 20036-3604 202-393-1251
Fax: 202-715-1146
info@specialolympics.org
www.specialolympics.org

Timothy P Shriver PhD, Chariman/CEO
J Brady Lum, President/COO
Stephen M Carter, Lead Director/CEO/Vice Chair
A year-round worldwide program that promotes physical fitness, sports training and athletic competition for children and adults with intellectual disabilities.

8287 Special Olympics International
1133 19th St NW
Washington, DC 20036-3604 202-393-1251
Fax: 202-715-1146
info@specialolympics.org
www.specialolympics.org

Timothy P Shriver PhD, Chariman/CEO
J Brady Lum, President/COO
Stephen M Carter, Lead Director/CEO/Vice Chair
Provides year-round training and athletic competition in a variety of well-coached, Olympic-type sparts for persons with developmental disabilities. Offers opportunities to develop physical fitness, prepare for entry into school and community sports programs. Athletes express courage, experience joy and participate in gifts, skills and friendship with their families and other Special Olympics athletes. Local information can be provided by regional offices.

8288 US Paralympics
United States Olympic Committee
1 Olympic Plaza
Colorado Springs, CO 80909 719-866-2030
888-222-2313
Fax: 719-866-2029
www.teamusa.org/us-paralympics

Scott Blackmun, CEO
Alan Ashley, Chief of Sport Performance
Lisa Baird, Chief Marketing Officer
A division of the US Olympic Committee focused on enhancing programs, funding and opportunities for persons with physical disabilities to participate in Paralympic sports.

8289 United Foundation for Disabled Archers
20 NE 9th Ave. Glenwood,
PO Box 251
Glenwood, MN 56334- 251 320-634-3660
info@uffdaclub.com
www.uffdaclub.com

Daniel James Hendricks, President
Russ Kalk, Vice President
Debbie Kalk, Treasurer
It is the mission of the United Foundation for Disabled Archers to promote and provide a means to practice all forms of archery for any physically challenged person.

8290 Wheelchair Sports, USA
PO Box 5266
Kendall Park, NJ 08824-5266 732-266-2634
Fax: 732-355-6500

Kelly Behlmann, Owner
Gregg Baumgraten, Chairperson
Denise Hutchins, Vice-Chairperson
Initiates, stimulates and promotes the growth and development of wheelchair sports.

Support Groups

8291 Information Hotline
Arthritis Foundation, Southeast Region Inc
1330 W. Peachtree St.
Suite 100
Atlanta, GA 30309 404-872-7100
800-933-7023
Fax: 404-237-8153
info.ga@arthritis.org
www.arthritis.org

Dan McGowan, Chairman
Rowland W. Chang, Vice Chair
Ann M. Palmer, President and CEO
The mission of the Arthritis Foundation is to improve lives through leadership in the prevention, control and cure of arthritis and related diseases.

8292 Kids on the Block Programs
9385 Gerwig Lane
Suite C
Maryland, MD 21157-2893 410-290-9095
800-368-5437
Fax: 410-290-9358
www.kotb.com

Aric Darroe, President
Jane Thuman, Vice President
Christina Grogan, Marketing Manager
Features life-size puppets in educational programs that enlighten children and adults on the issues of disability awareness, medical and educational differences, and social concerns.

General Disorders

Associations

8293   AIDS United
1424 K Street, N.W.
Ste 200
Washington, DC 20005-1511   202-408-4848
888-234-2437
Fax: 202-408-1818
info@aidsunited.org
www.aidsunited.org
Jesse Milan Jr., JD, Interim President & CEO
Matthew J. Kessler, Vice President, Operations
Cody Barnett, Commuications Coordinator
AIDS United advocates for people living with or affected by
HIV/AIDS and the organizations that serve them. AIDS United's
mission is to end the AIDS epidemic in the United States through
strategic grantmaking, capacity building, policy/advocacy, technical assistance and formative research.

**8294   American Academy for Cerebral Palsy and
Developmental Medicine**
555 East Wells
Suite 1100
Milwaukee, WI 53202   414-918-3014
Fax: 414-276-2146
info@aacpdm.org
www.aacpdm.org
Tamara Wagester, Executive Director
Erin Trimmer, Senior Meetings Manager
Heather Schrader, Membership & Administrative Manager
Professional health academy offering multidisciplinary scien-
tific education and promoting excellence in research and services
in the area of cerebral palsy and other childhood-onset
disabilities.

8295   American Academy of Allergy, Asthma & Immunology
555 E Wells St.
Ste 1100
Milwaukee, WI 53202-3823   414-272-6071
Fax: 414-272-6070
info@aaaai.org
www.aaaai.org
Thomas A. Fleisher, M.D.; FAAAAI, President
An association of medical professionals and specialists that
places focus on research and treatment for allergic and immunologic diseases, as well as improved patient care.

**8296   American Academy of Otolaryngology - Head and Neck
Surgery**
1650 Diagonal Rd
Alexandria, VA 22314-2857   703-836-4444
Fax: 703-683-5100
TTY: 703-519-1585
www.entnet.org
James c. Denneny III, M.D., Executive Vice President & CEO
Sujana S. Chandrasekhar, M.D., President
Carol R. Bradford, Director, Academic
The American Academy of Otolaryngology-Head and Neck Sur-
gery (AAO-HNS) is an organization representing specialists who
treat the ear, nose, throat, and related structures of the head and
neck.

**8297   American Academy of Physical Medicine and
Rehabilitation**
9700 W Bryn Mawr Ave
Ste 200
Rosemont, IL 60018-5701   847-737-6000
877-227-6799
Fax: 847-737-6001
info@aapmr.org
www.aapmr.org
*Thomas E. Stautzenbach, Executive Director & Chief Executive Of-
ficer*
Gregory M. Worsowicz, President
Darryl L. Kaelin, Vice President

This national medical specialty society represents more than
6,500 physical medicine and rehabilitation physicians, whose patients include people with physical disabilities and chronic, disabling illnesses. The academy's mission is to maximize quality of
life, minimize the incidence and prevalence of impairments and
disability, promote societal health and enhance the understanding and development of the specialty. The organization offers
information, referrals, and patient materials.

8298   American Association for Respiratory Care
9425 N. MacArthur Blvd.
Ste 100
Irving, TX 75063-4706   972-243-2272
Fax: 972-484-2720
info@aarc.org
www.aarc.org
Tom Kallstrom, Executive Director
Steve Bowden, IT, General Inquiries
AARC's mission is to advance the science, technology, ethics and
art of respiratory care through research and education for its
members and to teach the general public about pulmonary health
and disease prevention.

**8299   American Association of Cardiovascular and Pulmonary
Rehabilitation**
330 N. Wabash Avenue
Suite 2200
Chicago, IL 60611   312-321-5146
Fax: 312-673-6924
aacvpr@aacvpr.org
www.aacvpr.org
Adam T. deJong, President
Megan Cohen, Executive Director
Jessica Eustice, Director Of Corporate Relations
The mission of American Association of Cardiovascular and Pul-
monary Rehabilitation is to reduce morbidity, mortality, and dis-
ability from cardiovascular and pulmonary diseases through
education, prevention, rehabilitation, research, and aggressive
disease management.

8300   American Brain Tumor Association
8550 W. Bryn Mawr Ave
Ste 550
Chicago, IL 60631-4106   773-577-8750
800-886-2282
Fax: 773-577-8738
info@abta.org
www.abta.org
Elizabeth Wilson, President & CEO
Martha Carlos, Chief Communications Officer
Kerri Mink, Chief Operating Officer
A non-profit organization founded in 1973 dedicated to the elimi-
nation of brain tumors through research and patient education
services.

8301   American Diabetes Association
2451 Crystal Dr.
Suite 900
Arlington, VA 22202   800-342-2383
askada@diabetes.org
www.diabetes.org
Tracey D. Brown, Chief Executive Officer
Charlotte Carter, Chief Financial Officer
Charles Henderson, Chief Development Officer
Funds diabetes research, information and advocacy. The mission
of the Association is to prevent and cure diabetes and to improve
the lives of all people affected by diabetes.

8302   American Group Psychotherapy Association
25 E. 21st St.
6th Floor
New York, NY 10010-6207   212-477-2677
877-668-2472
Fax: 212-979-6627
info@agpa.org
www.agpa.org
Marsha S. Block, Chief Executive Officer
Eleanor F. Counselman, EdD; CGP, President
Nina Brown, Secretary
AGPA serves as the national voice specific to the interests of
group psychotherapy. Its 4,100 members and 31 affiliate societies

provide a wealth of professional, educational and social support for group psychotherapists in the United States and around the world.

8303 American Head and Neck Society
11300 W. Olympic Blvd
Ste 600
Los Angeles, CA 90064-1663 310-437-0559
Fax: 310-437-0585
www.ahns.info

Dennis Kraus, MD, President
Jonathan Irish, MD, Vice President
Brian B. Burkey, MD; MEd, Secretary

AHNS is a professional organization, formed in 1998 to promote research and education in head and neck oncology. The AHNS offers clinical practice guidelines, details of events, grants, and patient information. It aims to promote and advance the knowledge of prevention, diagnosis, treatment, and rehabilitation of neoplasms and other diseases of the head and neck.

8304 American Lung Association
55 W. Wacker Dr.
Ste 1150
Chicago, IL 60601 312-781-1100
800-548-8252
Fax: 202-452-1085
info@lung.org
www.lung.org

Harold P. Wimmer, President & CEO
Sue Swan, National Chief Development Officer
Sally Draper, National Vice President, Development

The ALA is an organization dedicated to combating tobacco use, eliminating lung diseases, and improving air quality through research, education, and advocacy. The association provides knowledge beneficial to patients, patients' families, and medical professionals and specialists.

8305 American SIDS Institute
528 Raven Way
Naples, FL 34110 239-431-5425
Fax: 239-431-5536
prevent@sids.org
www.sids.org

Marc Peterzell, JD, Chairman
Betty McEntire, PhD, Executive Director & CEO
Nicole Dobson, MD, Board Member

American SIDS Institute is a national nonprofit health care organization that is dedicated to the prevention of sudden infant death and the promotion of infant health through an aggressive, comprehensive nationwide program of research, clinical services, education and family support.

8306 American Sexual Health Association
P.O. Box 13827
Research Triangle Park, NC 27709-3827 919-361-8400
Fax: 919-361-8425
info@ashasexualhealth.org

Lynn Barclay, President & CEO
Deborah Arrindell, Vice President, Health Policy

The American Sexual Health Association is a trusted source of information on sexual health, relationships, and measures to prevent adverse sexual health

8307 American Society of Pediatric Hematology/Oncology
8735 West Higgins Rd.
Ste. 300
Chicago, IL 60631 847-375-4716
Fax: 847-375-6483
info@aspho.org
www.aspho.org

Sally Weir, Executive Director
Steve Biddle, Education Consultant
Jackie Holcomb, Education Manager

ASPHO is multidisciplinary organization dedicated to promoting optimal care of children and adolescents with blood disorders and cancer by advancing research, education, treatment and professional practice.

8308 American Thoracic Society
25 Broadway
18th Floor
New York, NY 10004-2755 212-315-8600
Fax: 212-315-6498
atsinfo@thoracic.org
www.thoracic.org

Steve Crane, Executive Director
Nicola Black, Associate Director, Governance Activities
Jennifer A. Ian, Director, Member Services & Chapter Relations

The American Thoracic Society is dedicated to research, public health education, and patient care in relation to pulmonary disease, critical illness, and sleep disorders.

8309 Aplastic Anemia and MDS International Foundation
100 Park Ave
Ste 108
Rockville, MD 20850 301-279-7202
800-747-2820
Fax: 301-279-7205
help@aamds.org
www.aamds.org

John Huber, Executive Director
Angie Onofre, Director of Patient Programs and Services
Leigh Clark, Patient Educator

This organization, formerly known as Aplastic Anemia Foundation of America, provides a resource directory for patient assistance, produces educational material and supports research into AA and MDS.

8310 Arizona Hemophilia Association
826 North 5th Ave
Phoenix, AZ 85003 602-955-3947
info@hemophiliaz.org
www.arizonahemophilia.org

Cindy Komar, Chief Executive Officer
Chelsea Bolyard, Program Director
Yleana Highes, Director, Client Services

The Arizona Hemophilia Association (AHA) is a volunteer based nonprofit organization working to support, educate, and advocate for families affected by bleeding disorders in Arizona.

8311 CPATH Cerebral Palsy Awareness Transition Hope
5501A Balcones
Suite 160
Austin, TX 78731 866-742-7284
info@cpathtexas.com
www.cpathtexas.com

Victoria Polega, President
Marielle Deckard, Secretary
Jamie Eppele, Director, Devleopment

CPATH is a non-profit organization whose mission is to provide resources, support, and financial assistance to families and individuals living with cerebral palsy.

8312 Canadian Cancer Society
55 St. Clair Avenue W.
Ste 300
Toronto, ON, Canada M4V- 2Y7 416-961-7223
888-939-3333
Fax: 416-961-4189
TTY: 866-786-3934
ccs@cancer.ca
www.cancer.ca

Anne V,zina, Interim President & CEO
Martin Kabat, Chief Executive Officer
Lesley Ring, Vice President, Development & Marketing

A national community-based organization of volunteers whose mission is the eradication of cancer and the enhancement of the quality of life for people living with cancer.

8313 Canadian Diabetes Association
1400-522 University Ave
Toronto, ON, Canada M5G-2R5 416-363-3373
800-226-8464
Fax: 416-408-7015
info@diabetes.ca
www.diabetes.ca

Doug Macnamara, President & CEO
Paul Kilbertus, Senior Director, Strategic Communications

The mission of the Canadian Diabetes Association is to promote the health of Canadians through diabetes research, education, service and advocacy.

8314 Canadian Lung Association
1750 Courtwood Cres.
Ottawa, ON, Canada K2C-2B5
613-569-6411
888-566-5864
Fax: 613-569-8860
info@lung.ca
www.lung.ca

Terry Dean, President & CEO
The Canadian Lung Association is a non-profit and volunteer-based health charity, dedicated to improving lung health in the Canadian community through research, education, prevention and advocacy.

8315 Childhood Cancer Canada Foundation
21 St. Clair Ave E
Ste 801
Toronto, ON, Canada M4T-1L9
416-489-6440
800-363-1062
Fax: 416-489-9812
info@childhoodcancer.ca
www.childhoodcancer.ca

Clare Davenport, President & CEO
Natasha Bowes, Senior Manager, Fund Development
Patricia Zareba, Fund Development Manager
A national, volunteer governed, charitable organization dedicated to improving the quality of life for children with cancer. The foundation raises funds to assist with cancer research undertakings across Canada.

8316 Childhood Leukemia Foundation
807 Mantoloking Rd
Brick, NJ 08723
732-920-8860
888-253-7109
www.clf4kids.org

Barbara Haramis, Executive Director & Founder
Barb Estelle, Chief Operating Officer
Kim Wetmore, Director, Development
The CLF is a national, non-profit organization providing education, information, support, and advocacy for patients of cancer and their families. the foundation works closely with health professionals, social workers, and specialists to offer a variety of programs that aim to enrich the lives of children living with cancer.

8317 Emphysema Foundation for Our Right to Survive
PO Box 20241
Kansas City, MO 64119-0241
866-363-2673
www.emphysema.net

Linda Watson, President
Debbie Snodell, Secretary
EFFORTS is a non-profit organization that takes an active role in promoting research for more effective treatments and perhaps a cure for emphysema and related lung diseases. It also works to further education about the disease and provides a support mailing list for members.

8318 Environmental Health Center: Dallas
8345 Walnut Hill Lane
Ste 220
Dallas, TX 75231-4205
214-368-4132
Fax: 214-691-8432
contact@ehcd.com
www.ehcd.com

William J Rea, Director
Chris Rea, Business Manager
Yaqin Pan, M.D., Research Physician
Clinic providing patient care in the areas of Immunotherapy, Nutrition, Physical Therapy, Chemical Depuration, Energy Balancing, Electromagnetic Sensitivity Testing, Psychological Support Services, Family Practice Medicine and Internal Medicine. Provides services for individuals whose diseases are caused by environmental factors.

8319 Epilepsy Foundation of Alabama
3929 Airport Blvd
Suite 3-310
Mobile, AL 36609-2235
251-341-0170
800-626-1582

Donna Dodson, Executive Director
Paige Norris, Outreach & Program Director
David Toenes, Director, Client Services
The Epilepsy Foundation of Alabama provides health service programs and public education on behalf of people with seizures and epilepsy. Some of their services include emergency medication assistance, information referral, training, employer education, and camping trips.

8320 Eunice Kennedy Shriver National Institute of Child Health and Human Development (NICHD)
National Institutes of Health (NIH)
31 Center Dr.
Bldg 31, Rm 2A32
Bethesda, MD 20892-2425
301-496-5097
800-370-2943
Fax: 866-760-5947
TTY: 888-320-6942
nichdinformationresourcecenter@mail.nih.gov
www.nichd.nih.gov

Diana W. Bianchi, Director
The Eunice Kennedy Shriver National Institute of Child Health and Human Development, part of the federal National Institutes of Health, conducts and supports basic, translational, and clinical research in the biomedical, behavioral, and social sciences related to child and maternal health, in medical rehabilitation, and in the reproductive sciences.

8321 Fragile X Family
Fanlight Productions
c/o Icarus Films
32 Court Street, 21st Floor
Brooklyn, NY 11201
718-488-8900
800-876-1710
Fax: 718-488-8642
info@fanlight.com
www.fanlight.com

Ben Achtenberg, Founder, Owner
Eric Kutner, Producer
Fragile X Family takes viewers inside the lives of a developmentally disabled family who are affected by Fragile X Syndrome, an inherited chromosomal disorder. *$149.00*
VHS/VIDEO
ISBN 1-572954-14-0

8322 Herpes Resource Center
American Social Health Association
P.O. Box 13827
Research Triangle Park, NC 27709-3827
919-361-8400
800-227-8922
Fax: 919-361-8425
customerservice@ashastd.org
www.ashastd.org/stdsstis/herpes/

Lynn Barclay, President & CEO
The Herpes Resource Center (HRC) focuses on increasing education, public awareness, and support to anyone concerned about herpes.

8323 IKUS Life Enrichment Services
O-1859 Lake Michigan Dr. NW
Grand Rapids, MI 49534
616-677-5251
Fax: 616-677-2955
info@ikuslife.org
www.ikuslife.org

Scott Blakeney, Executive Director
Amy DeMott, Director, Programs & Services
Nikki Outhier, Director, Development
IKUS Life Enrichment Services helps individuals with disabilities learn new skills and experience greater freedom by providing support, recreation and educational services. IKUS also provides respite services to caregivers and families.

8324 International Academy of Biological Dentistry and Medicine
19122 Camellia Bend Circle
Suite 101
Spring, TX 77379   281-651-1745
                                            Fax: 281-651-1745
                                            drdawn@drdawn.net
                                            www.iabdm.org

Dr. Dawn Ewing, Executive Director
The IABDM promotes non-toxic diagnostic and therapeutic approaches in dentistry and hosts seminars on biological diagnosis and therapy.

8325 International Academy of Oral Medicine & Toxicology
8297 ChampionsGate Blvd
Ste 193
ChampionsGate, FL 33896-8387   863-420-6373
                                            Fax: 863-419-8136
                                            info@iaomt.org
                                            www.iaomt.org

Mark Wisniewski, President
Tammy DeGregorio, Executive Vice President
Kym Smith, Executive Director
A non-profit organization dedicated to funding solid peer-reviewed scientific research in the area of toxic substances used in dentistry as well as providing continuing education and carefully reviewed procedures, protocols, and methodologies to reduce the risk for patients and professionals.

8326 International Association for Cancer Victors & Friends
P.O. Box 745
Lakeport, CA 95453   408-834-5300
                                            Fax: 408-264-9659
                                            www.cancervictors.net
The Cancer Victors and Friends, also known as The International Association of Cancer Victors and Friends, or IACVF, is dedicated to disseminating information about alternative and complimentary methods for treating cancer and other diseases. It encompasses hundreds of clinics and practitioners as well as multiple avenues for information, including the website, printed information, chapter meetings, guest speakers, promotional videos, books, and conventions.
a.k.a. Cancer Victors & Friends

8327 International Association of Hygienic Physicians
4620 Euclid Blvd
Youngstown, OH 44512-1633   330-788-0526
                                            Fax: 330-788-0093
                                            www.iahp.net

Alec Burton, Co-Founder
Mark A. Huberman, Secretary/Treasurer
The International Association of Hygienic Physicians (IAHP) is a professional association for licensed, primary care physicians (Medical Doctors, Osteopaths, Chiropractors, and Naturopaths) who specialize in Therapeutic Fasting Supervision as an integral part of Hygienic Care.

8328 International Medical and Dental Hypnotherapy Association
8852 SR 3001
RR 2
Laceyville, PA 18623-9417   570-869-1021
                                            800-553-6886
                                            Fax: 570-869-1249
                                            www.hypnosisalliance.com/imdha
Linda Otto, Executive Director
Robert Otto, President & CEO
Christie Boecker, Membership Services Coordinator
The association provides and encourages education programs to further, the knowledge, understanding, and application of hypnosis in complementary healthcare; encourages research and scientific publication in the field of hypnosis; and advocates for further recognition and acceptance of hypnosis as an important tool in healthcare and focus for scientific research.

8329 International Myeloma Foundation
12650 Riverside Dr
Ste 206
North Hollywood, CA 91607- 3421   818-487-7455
                                            800-452-2873
                                            Fax: 818-487-7454
                                            theimf@myeloma.org
                                            www.myeloma.org

David Girard, Executive Director
Susie Novis, President
Diane Moran, Senior Vice President, Strategic Planning
The IMF serves myeloma patients, family members, and the medical community, offering a wide range of programs in the areas of Research, Education, Support, and Advocacy.

8330 International Ventilator Users Network (IVUN)
50 Crestwood Executive Ctr.
Suite 440
St. Louis, MO 63126-1916   314-534-0475
                                            Fax: 314-534-5070
                                            info@ventusers.org
                                            www.ventnews.org

Mark Mallinger, President & Chairperson
Frederick M. Maynard, Vice President
Marny K. Eulberg, Secretary
To enhance the lives and independence of individuals using ventilators by promoting education, networking and advocacy. IVUN is an affiliate of Post-Polio Health International.

8331 Leukemia & Lymphoma Society
3 International Dr
Ste 200
Rye Brook, NY 10573   914-949-5213
                                            800-955-4572
                                            Fax: 914-949-6691
                                            supportservices@lls.org
                                            www.lls.org

Louis DeGennaro, President & CEO
Piper Medcalf, Executive Director
Nancy Hallberg, Chief Marketing Officer
The Leukemia and Lymphoma Society is the world's largest voluntary health organization dedicated to funding blood cancer research, education and patient services. The society offers information and support for patients of various blood cancer types, including leukemia, lymphoma, Hodgkin's disease and myeloma. It also offers services and resources to help improve the quality of life of patients and their families.

8332 Little People of America
250 El Camino Real
Ste 218
Tustin, CA 92780   714-368-3689
                                            888-572-2001
                                            Fax: 714-368-3367
                                            info@lpaonline.org
                                            www.lpaonline.org

Joanna Campbell, Executive Director
Gary Arnold, President
April Brazier, Senior Vice President
Little People of America is a national non-profit organization that provides support and information to people of short stature and their families. Short stature is generally caused by one of the more than 200 medical conditions known as dwarfism. LPA offers information on employment, education, disability rights, adoption, medical issues, clothing, adaptive products, and the many stages of parenting a short-statured child - from birth to adult.

8333 Lowe Syndrome Association
P.O. Box 417
Chicago Ridge, IL 60415   216-630-7723
                                            www.lowesyndrome.org

Lisa Waldbaum, President
Jane Gallery, Treasurer
Tiffany Johnson, Director, Medical & Scientific Affairs
The organization aims to foster communication, provide education, and support research into Lowe Syndrome.

8334 Lymphoma Canada
Formerly The Lymphoma Foundation Canada
6860 Century Ave
Ste 202
Mississauga, ON, Canada L5N-2W5   905-858-5967
                                         866-659-5556
                                         info@lymphoma.ca
                                         www.lymphoma.ca
Robin Markowitz, Chief Executive Officer
Lorna Warwick, National Director, Education & Services
Charlene Ragin, Marketing & Communications
Lymphoma Canada provides, at no cost and in both official languages: electronic and print materials on the Hodgkin lymphoma, non-Hodgkin lymphoma and CLL, peer and caregiver support groups, educational forums and advocacy on behalf of patients. Lymphoma Canada also funds Canadian research.

8335 Merrimack Hall Performing Arts Center
3320 Triana Blvd SW.
Huntsville, AL 35805   256-534-6455
                             info@merrimackhall.com
                             www.merrimackhall.com
Merrimack Hall Performing Arts Center is a nonprofit organization offering an array of programs including camps, classes, and social events, for children and adults with special needs. More than 500 individuals with special needs participate in Merrimack Hall's Happy Programs which are designed to provide participants with visual and performing arts education, as well as cultural activities.

8336 Myositis Association
1940 Duke St.
Suite 200
Alexandria, VA 22314   800-821-7356
                             tma@myositis.org
                             www.myositis.org
Bob Goldberg, Executive Director
Theresa Reynolds Curry, Communications Manager
Aisha Morrow, Operations Manager
The aim of TMA's programs and services is to provide information, support, advocacy and research for those concerned about myositis, as well as serving those affected by these diseases. Support groups offer members the chance to share and discuss their concerns with people in similar situations.

8337 National Association for Children of Alcoholics
10920 Connecticut Ave
Ste 100
Kensington, MD 20895-3007   301-468-0985
                                   888-554-2627
                                   Fax: 301-468-0987
                                   nacoa@nacoa.org
                                   www.nacoa.org
Sis Wenger, President & CEO
Steve Hornberger, Program Director
National non-profit membership and affiliate organization working on behalf of children of alcohol and drug dependent parents to help eliminate the adverse impact of drug use on children through public awareness, policy, advocacy, education, and support.

8338 National Association for Home Care & Hospice
228 7th St SE
Washington, DC 20003-4306   202-547-7424
                                   Fax: 202-547-3540
                                   webmaster@nahc.org
                                   www.nahc.org
Val J. Halamandris, President
Lucy Andrews, Vice Chair
Karen Marshall Thompson, Secretary
This is a non-profit trade association representing various home care, hospice and health aid organizations. With services aimed at assiting the chronically ill and disabled, the NAHC offers information on how to choose a home care provider and a zip code driven locator for home care and hospice.

8339 National Association for Medical Direction of Respiratory Care
8618 Westwood Center Dr
Ste 210
Vienna, VA 22182-2273   703-752-4359
                               Fax: 703-752-4360
                               www.namdrc.org
Phillip Porte, Executive Director
Vickie Parshall, Director, Member Services
Karen Lui, RN, Associate Executive Director
NAMDRC's primary mission is to improve access to quality care for patients with respiratory disease by removing regulatory and legislative barriers to appropriate treatment.

8340 National Association for Proton Therapy
1155 15th St NW
Ste 500
Washington, DC 20005   202-495-3133
                              Fax: 202-530-0659
                              info@proton-therapy.org
                              www.proton-therapy.org
Leonard Arzt, Executive Director
The National Association for Proton Therapy (NAPT) is registered as an independent, non-profit, public benefit corporation providing education and awareness for the public, professional and governmental communities. It promotes the therapeutic benefits of proton therapy for cancer treatment in the U.S. and abroad.

8341 National Association of Anorexia Nervosa and Associated Disorders
750 E Diehl Road
Ste 127
Naperville, IL 60563   630-577-1333
                              Fax: 847-433-4632
                              anadhelp@anad.org
                              www.anad.org
Laura Zinger, Executive Director
Deb Prinz, Director, Community Relations
A non-profit organization that seeks to alleviate the problems of eating disorders, especially anorexia nervosa and bulimia nervosa, by promoting eating disorder awareness, prevention and recovery through supporting, educating, and connecting individuals, families and professionals.

8342 National Association of Chronic Disease Diseases
325 Swanton Way
Decatur, GA 30030   770-458-7400
                           Fax: 770-458-7401
                           jrobitscher@chronicdisease.org
                           www.chronicdisease.org
John W. Robitscher, Chief Executive Officer
Namvar Zohoori, President
John Patton, Director, Communications
A national public health association founded in 1988 to link the chronic disease program directors of each state and U.S. territory to provide a national forum for chronic disease prevention and control efforts. NACDD aims to mobilize national efforts to reduce chronic diseases and the associated risk factors.

8343 National Association to Advance Fat Acceptance
P.O. Box 4662
Foster City, CA 94404-0662   916-558-6880
                                    Fax: 916-558-6881
                                    www.naafaonline.com
Founded in 1969, the National Association to Advance Fat Acceptance (NAAFA) is a non-profit, all volunteer, civil rights organization dedicated to protecting the rights and improving the quality of life for fat people. NAAFA works to eliminate discrimination based on body size and provide fat people with the tools for self-empowerment through advocacy, public education, and support.

8344 National Cancer Institute
9609 Medical Center Dr.
Rockville, MD 20850   800-422-6237
                                               TTY: 800-332-8615
                                                   nciinfo@nih.gov
                                                    www.cancer.gov

Norman E. Sharpless, Director
Douglas R. Lowy, Principal Deputy Director
James Doroshow, Deputy Director, Clinical & Translational
Research
The National Cancer Institute conducts and supports research,
training, health information dissemination, and programs related
to cancer, cancer rehabilitation, and the care of cancer patients.
1975

8345 National Diabetes Information Clearinghouse
NI of Diabetes and Digestive and Kidney Diseases
31 Center Dr.
Bethesda, MD 20892   800-860-8747
                                               TTY: 866-569-1162
                                             healthinfo@niddk.nih.gov
                                            www.diabetes.niddk.nih.gov

Griffin P. Rodgers, Director
Gregory G. Germino, Deputy Director
Camille Hoover, Executive Officer
An information and referral service of the National Institute of
Diabetes and Digestive and Kidney Diseases, one of the National
Institutes of Health. The clearinghouse responds to written inquiries, develops and distributes publications about diabetes, and
provides referrals to diabetes organizations, including support
groups. The NDIC maintains a database of patient and professional education materials, from which literature searches are
generated.

8346 National Digestive Diseases Information Clearinghouse
NI of Diabetes and Digestive and Kidney Diseases
31 Center Dr.
Bethesda, MD 20892   800-860-8747
                                               TTY: 866-569-1162
                                             healthinfo@niddk.nih.gov
                                            www.digestive.niddk.nih.gov

Griffin P. Rodgers, Director
Gregory G. Germino, Deputy Director
Camille Hoover, Executive Officer
Information and referral service of the National Institute of Diabetes and Digestive and Kidney Diseases. A central information
resource on the prevention and management of digestive diseases, the clearinghouse responds to written inquiries, develops
and distributes publications about digestive diseases, provides
referrals to digestive disease organizations and support groups,
and maintains a database of patient and professional education
materials from which literature searches are generated.

8347 National Fibromyalgia Association
3857 Birch St.
Suite 312
Newport Beach, CA 92660   nfa@fmaware.org
                                                    www.fmaware.org

Lynne Matallana, Founder
National Fibromyalgia Association's mission is to develop and
execute programs dedicated to improving the quality of life for
people with fibromyalgia.

8348 National Hemophilia Foundation
7 Penn Plaza
Suite 1204
New York, NY 10001   212-328-3700
                                                      888-463-6643
                                                 Fax: 212-328-3777
                                                 info@hemophilia.org
                                                  www.hemophilia.org

Leonard Valentino, President & CEO
Dawn Rotellini, Chief Operating Officer
Kevin Mills, Chief Scientific Officer
The National Hemophilia Foundation is dedicated to finding
better treatments and cures for bleeding and clotting disorders
and to preventing the complications of these disorders through
education, advocacy and research. Established in 1948, the National Hemophilia Foundation has chapters throughout the
country.

8349 National Kidney and Urologic Diseases Information Clearinghouse
NI of Diabetes and Digestive and Kidney Diseases
31 Center Dr.
Bethesda, MD 20892   800-860-8747
                                               TTY: 866-569-1162
                                             healthinfo@niddk.nih.gov
                                            www.kidney.niddk.nih.gov

Griffin P. Rodgers, Director
Gregory G. Germino, Deputy Director
Camille Hoover, Executive Officer
NKUDIC was established in 1987 to increase knowledge and understanding about diseases of the kidneys and urologic system
among people with these conditions and their families, health
care professionals, and the general public.

8350 National Organization for Albinism and Hypopigmentation
P.O. Box 959
East Hampstead, NH 03826-0959   603-887-2310
                                                      800-473-2310
                                                 Fax: 800-648-2310
                                                    info@albinism.org
                                                    www.albinism.org

Michael McGowan, Executive Director
Diana McCown, Vice-chair
Kris Baker, Secretary
Organization offering information and support to people with al-
binism, their families and the prodessionals who work with them.

8351 National Organization for Rare Disorders
55 Kenosia Ave
Danbury, CT 06810   203-744-0100
                                                 Fax: 203-263-9938
                                              orphan@rarediseases.org
                                                    rarediseases.org

Marshall Summar, MD, Chairman
Peter Saltonstall, President & CEO
Pamela Gavin, Chief Operating Officer
The National Organization for Rare Disorders (NORD) is an organization serving individuals with rare diseases and the organizations that serve them. NORD offers educational programs,
advocacy, research and patient services.

8352 National Organization on Fetal Alcohol Syndrome
1200 Eton Ct NW
3rd Fl
Washington, DC 20007-3239   202-785-4585
                                                      800-666-6327
                                                 Fax: 202-466-6456
                                                information@nofas.org
                                                      www.nofas.org

Tom Donaldson, President
Kathleen Tavenner Mitchell, Vice President
Andy Kachor, Communications Director
Dedicated to eliminating birth defects caused by alcohol con-
sumption during pregnancy and improving the qualtiy of life for
those individuals and families affected.

8353 Post-Polio Health International
50 Crestwood Executive Ctr.
Suite 440
St. Louis, MO 63126   314-534-0475
                                                 Fax: 314-534-5070
                                                   info@post-polio.org
                                                    www.post-polio.org

Mark Mallinger, President
Frederick M. Maynard, Vice President
Brian M. Tiburzi, Executive Director
To enhance the lives and independence of polio survivors, home
ventilator users, their caregivers and families, and health profes-
sionals through education, networking, and advocacy.

8354 **Prader-Willi Syndrome Association USA**
8588 Potter Park Dr
Ste 500
Sarasota, FL 34238   941-312-0400
                                    800-926-4797
                              Fax: 941-312-0142
                                   www.pwsausa.org
Ken Smith, Executive Director
Jack Hannings, Development Director
Donny Moore, Development & Communications Specialist
National, nonprofit public charity that works for the benefit of individuals with Prader-Willi syndrome and their families. Dedicated to serving individuals affected by Prader-Willi syndrome (PWS) their families, and interested professionals, providing information, education, and support services to its members.

8355 **Simonton Cancer Center**
P.O. Box 6607
Malibu, CA 90264-6607   818-879-7904
                                    800-459-3424
                              Fax: 310-457-0421
                   simontoncancercenter@msn.com
                              www.simontoncenter.com
Dr. O. Carl Simonton, Founder
Edward Gilbert, MD, Medical Director
Karen Smith Simonton, Executive / Program Director
The Simonton Cancer Center is a non-profit organization dedicated to improving the health and lives of cancer patients and their families through psycho-social oncology.

8356 **Special Care Dentistry Association**
330 N. Wabash Avenue
Ste 2000
Chicago, IL 60611-4245   312-527-6764
                              Fax: 312-673-6663
                                   scda@scdaonline.org
                                   www.scdaonline.org
Kristin Dee, Executive Director
Miriam Robbins, President
Jeffrey Hicks, President-Elect
The Special Care Dentistry Association serves as a resource to all oral health care professionals who serve or are interested in serving patients with special needs through education and networking to increase access to oral healthcare for patients with special needs.

8357 **Spina Bifida Association**
1600 Wilson Blvd
Ste 800
Arlington, VA 22209   202-944-3285
                                    800-621-3141
                              Fax: 202-944-3295
                                   sbaa@sbaa.org
                        www.spinabifidaassociation.org
Sara Struwe, President & CEO
Lee Towns, National Director, Communications & Outreach
Elizabeth Merck, National Director, Development
Non-profit organization whose mission is to promote the prevention of spina bifida and to enhance the lives of all affected. Addresses the specific needs of the spina bifida community and serves as the national representative of almost 60 chapters. Services include Toll free 800 information and referral service, as well as legislative updates.

8358 **Spina Bifida and Hydrocephalus Association of Canada**
167 Lombard Ave
Suite 472
Winnipeg, MB R3B 0T6,   204-925-3650
                                    800-565-9488
                              Fax: 204-925-3654
                                   info@sbhac.ca
                                   www.sbhac.ca
Susana Scott, President
Linda Randall, Vice President
Bonnie Hidlebaugh, National Manager, Communications & Development Coordinator
The Spina Bifida and Hydrocephalus Association of Canada has been working on behalf of people with spina bifida and/or hydrocephalus and their families.

8359 **Sunburst Projects**
Sunburst Projects United States Headquarters
2143 Hurley Way
Suite 240
Sacramento, CA 95825   916-440-0889
                              Fax: 916-440-1208
                        admin@sunburstprojects.org
                              www.sunburstprojects.org
Jacob Bradley-Rowe, Executive Director
Sunburst Projects is a international organization that works to keep families together by providing services and support for youth who are infected or affected by HIV/AIDS.

8360 **Taking Control of Your Diabetes (TCOYD)**
990 Highland Dr
Suite 312
Solana Beach, CA 92075   858-755-5683
                                    800-998-2693
                              Fax: 858-755-6854
                                   info@tcoyd.org
                                   www.tcoyd.org
Steven Edelman, MD, Founder & Director
Sandra Bourdette, Co-Founder & Executive Director Emeritus
Jennifer Braidwood, Director of Marketing & Special Projects
Taking Control of Your Diabetes works to educate and motivate people with diabetes to take a more active role in managing their condition. The organization also offers continuing education programs for medical professionals caring for people with diabetes.

8361 **United Brachial Plexus Network, Inc.**
32 William Rd
Reading, MA 01867   781-315-6161
                                   ubpn@ubpn.org
                                   www.ubpn.org
Richard Looby, President
Dan Aldrich, Co- Vice President & Traumatic BPI Group
The United Brachial Plexus Network, Inc. provides education, information, and assistance for those affected by Brachial Plexus Palsy by offering information, contacts, resources, parent matching, and assistance developing chapters or support groups throughout the United States and the world.

8362 **World Service Office of Overeaters Anonymous**
6075 Zenith Crt NE
Rio Rancho, NM 87144-6424   505-891-2664
                              Fax: 505-891-4320
                                   info@oa.org
                                   www.oa.org
Sarah Armstrong, Managing Director
OA aims to provide physical, emotional, and practical support for those seeking to improve their dietary habits. OA encourages members to develop a food plan with a health care professional and a sponsor.

Camps

8363 **ADA Camp GranADA**
American Diabetes Association
55 E Monroe St.
Suite 3420
Chicago, IL 60603   312-346-1805
                              illinoiscamps@diabetes.org
                                   www.diabetes.org
Camp GranADA is an American Diabetes Association resident camp located in Monticello, Illinois at the 4H Memorial Campground. For children with diabetes, ages 8-16.

8364 **ADA Camp Needlepoint**
American Diabetes Association
375 Bishops Way
Brookfield, WI 53005   414-778-5500
                              campsupport@diabetes.org
                                   www.diabetes.org
Becky Barnett, Camp Director
Camp Needlepoint is a summer camp for children who have type 1 diabetes. Coed, ages 8-16. The camp takes place at the YMCA Camp St. Croix in Hudson, Wisconsin.

8365   ADA Teen Adventure Camp
American Diabetes Association
55 E Monroe St.
Suite 3420
Chicago, IL 60603   312-346-1805
                    illinoiscamps@diabetes.org
                         www.diabetes.org
Paula Williams, Contact
Camping for teenagers with diabetes. Coed, ages 14 to 17. Camp dates are early in August. Located at the YMCA Camp Duncan in Ingleside, Illinois.

8366   ADA Triangle D Camp
American Diabetes Association
55 E Monroe St.
Suite 3420
Chicago, IL 60603   312-346-1805
                    illinoiscamps@diabetes.org
                         www.diabetes.org
Triangle D Camp is a resident camp program located at the YMCA Camp Duncan in Ingleside, Illinois. Activities include swimming, row boating, canoeing, camp games, sports, and diabetes education. For children ages 9-13 with diabetes.

8367   Adam's Camp
56 Inverness Drive East
Suite 250
Englewood, CO 80112   .   303-563-8290
                    contact@adamscamp.org
                    www.adamscampcolorado.org
Brian Conly, Executive Director
Paige Heydon, Director, Finance & Development
Adam's Camp is a nonprofit organization, with multiple locations across the United States, providing therapeutic programs and recreational camps for children, and the families of children with special needs and developmental delays.

8368   Adventure Day Camp
3480 Commission Ct
Lake Ridge, VA 22192   703-491-1444
                    office@princewilliamacademy.com
                    www.princewilliamacademy.com
Dr. Samia Harris, Founder & Executive Director
Rebecca Nykwest, Communications Director
Lindsay Chickering, Office Manager
Camping for children with asthma/respiratory ailments and cancer. Coed, ages 2-13.

8369   Agassiz Village
238 Bedford St
Suite B
Lexington, MA 02420-3477   781-860-0200
                         Fax: 781-860-0352
                         www.agassizvillage.org
Cliff Simmonds, Executive Director
Thomas Semeta, Camp Director
Warren Soar, Facility Director
Agassiz Village offers a variety of activities for all campers, boys and girls, younger camper and teens, and programs for physically challenged children and teens. By participating in daily activities, campers build a cooperative and positive community of different races, ages, ethnic and cultural backgrounds while enhancing confidence and individuality. Camp is located in Poland, Maine. For ages 8-17.

8370   Arizona Camp Sunrise
American Cancer Society
PO Box 27872
Tempe, AZ 85285   602-952-7550
                                 800-865-1582
                         Fax: 602-404-1118
                         www.azcampsunrise.org
Barbara Nicholas, Director
Leigh Ansley, Manager
Melissa Lee, Camp Director
Provides one-week summer camping sessions to children aged 8-16 who have had, or currently have, cancer. The classes range from sports and outdoor games to dance and drama, arts, crafts, and cooking. Other activities planned for the campers include horseback riding, a trip to a lake, a dance, and learning to make friendship bracelets.

8371   Bearskin Meadow Camp
Diabetic Youth Families
5167 Clayton Rd
Suite F
Concord, CA 94521   925-680-4994
                         Fax: 925-680-4863
                             info@dyf.org
                             www.dyf.org
Davey Warner, Executive Director
Kaylor Glassman, Director, Programs
Marissa Clarke-Howard, Director, Development & Communications
Bearskin Meadow Camp, is a camp program offered by the Diabetes Youth Families organization to children (7-13), teens (14-17), and families who are affected by type 1 diabetes. The camp has traditional camp activities as well as educational opportunities for campers.

8372   Becket Chimney Corners YMCA Camps and Outdoor Center
748 Hamilton Rd
Becket, MA 01223   413-623-8991
                         Fax: 413-623-5890
                         cburke@bccymca.org
                         www.bccymca.org
Drew Lipsher, Chair
David Smith, Vice Chair
Christine Kalakay, Chief Financial Officer
Half-week and one-week sessions for campers with asthma/respiratory ailments. Coed, ages 3 and up, families, seniors, single adults.

8373   Breckenridge Outdoor Education Center
PO Box 697
Breckenridge, CO 80424   970-453-6422
                                 800-383-2632
                         Fax: 970-453-4676
                             boec@boec.org
                             www.boec.org
Sonya Norris, Executive Director
Karen Skruch, Finance Director
Jeff Inouye, Ski Program Director
Breckenridge Outdoor Education Center (BOEC) provides year round educational outdoor experiences to individuals with physical and intellectual disabilities. Some programs BOEC offer include, Adaptive Ski and Ride School, Wilderness Programs and adaptive programs for individuals with brain injuries, multiple sclerosis, and Parkinson's Disease.
1976

8374   Bright Horizons Summer Camp
Sickle Cell Disease Association of Illinois
8100 S. Western Avenue
Chicago, IL 60620   773-526-5016
                                 866-798-1097
                         Fax: 773-526-5012
                sicklecelldisease-illinois@scdai.org
Darryl H. Armstrong, Chair
TaLana Hughes, Executive Director
Anquineice Brown, Outreach Coordinator
Camping for children with blood disorders, ages 7-13. The joys of learning include instruction in first aid, swimming and water safety, boating, horseback riding and bowling plus arts and crafts. In addition, there is a traditional menu of camp pleasures, like hayrides, cookouts, nature hikes and sing-a-longs.

8375   Camp ASCCA
Alabama Easter Seal Society
PO Box 21
5278 Camp Ascca Dr.
Jacksons Gap, AL 36861   256-825-9226
                         Fax: 256-269-0714
                         info@campascca.org
                         www.campascca.org
Matt Rickman, Camp Director
John Stephenson, Administrator
Jocelyn Jones, Secretary
Camp ASCCA is for children and adults with disabilities or health impairements. Camp ASCCA strives to help these individuals

achieve equality, independence and dignity in a safe environment.
1976

8376   Camp Aldersgate
2000 Aldersgate Road
Little Rock, AR 72205   501-225-1444
                                          Fax: 501-225-2019
                                      hello@campaldersgate.net
                                      www.campaldersgate.net
Sonya S. Murphy, Chief Executive Officer
Shelley Myers, Chief Operating Officer & Chief Financial Officer
Brooke Wilson, Director, Communications
Camp Aldersgate is a nonprofit organization, offering summer,
weekend camps, and year-round social service programs to children, teens and adults with special needs. The camp promotes outdoor recreation and socialization in a completely accessible
environment.

8377   Camp Alpine
Alpine Alternatives
2518 E. Tudor Road
Ste 105
Anchorage, AK 99507-1105   907-561-6655
                                              800-361-4174
                                          Fax: 907-563-9232
                                    alpinealternatives@arctic.net
                             www.alpinealternatives.org/programs.html
Margaret Webber, Executive Director
LaVerne Lee, Day Outings Director & Camp Alpine Director
Offers programs aimed at helping disabled youth expand their horizons, master new skills, make new friends, and increase motor
coordination. Most importantly, participants experience growth
in self-confidence and independence that affects all aspects of an
individual's life. Camp services are open to all, regardless of type
of disability or age. Activities include canoeing, hiking, swimming, outdoor games, sports, nature identification and much
more.

8378   Camp Anuenue
250 Williams St. NW
Atlanta, GA 30303   808-595-7500
                                              888-227-2345
                                          Fax: 808-595-7502
                                             www.cancer.org
Pamela K. Meyerhoffer, Chair
Robert E. Youle, Vice Chairman
Douglas K. Kelsey, Board Scientific Officer
(1 week) June, children with or recovered from cancer.

8379   Camp Beausite NW
PO Box 1227
Port Hadlock, WA 98339   360-732-7222
                                           campbeausitenw.org
Raina Baker, Executive Director
The camp is located in Chimacum, Washington. Campers range
from 7-65 in age and includes those with developmental disabilities, cerebral palsy, autism, Down syndrome, and other physical
or mental disabilities. The camp offers five week-long overnight
summer camp sessions for adults and children.

8380   Camp Beyond The Scars
Burn Institute
8825 Aero Drive
Suite 200
San Diego, CA 92123-2269   858-541-2277
                                          Fax: 858-541-7179
                                      ccoppenrath@burninstitute.org
                             www.burninstitute.org/camp-beyond-the-scar s
Susan Day, Executive Director
Tessa Haviland, Director, Marketing & Events
Benjamin Hemmings, Director, Operations
Camp Beyond the Scars, is a weeklong sleepaway summer camp
for children aged 8-17 who have survived a burn injury. Staffed
by adult burn survivors, healthcare professionals, and off-duty
firefighters, the camp provides an inclusive environment for burn
survivors to participate in activities including, swimming, basketball, volleyball, archery, golf, and arts and crafts. The camp is
free of charge, and is hosted at a camp facility in Romano,
California.
1987

8381   Camp Boggy Creek
30500 Brantley Branch Rd.
Eustis, FL 32736   352-483-4200
                                              866-462-6449
                                          Fax: 352-483-0589
                                      info@campboggycreek.org
                                          www.boggycreek.org
June Clark, President & CEO
Lisa Hicks, Chief Development Officer
David Mann, Camp Director
Year-round sessions for children with a variety of chronic or
life-threatening illnesses including cancer, hemophilia, epilepsy,
heart defects, HIV, spina bifida and respiratory ailments. Coed,
ages 7-16.

8382   Camp Bon Coeur
300 Ridge Rd.
Suite K
Lafayette, LA 70506   337-233-8437
                                          Fax: 337-233-4160
                                        info@heartcamp.com
                                          www.heartcamp.com
Susannah Craig, Executive Director
Chelsea Doyle, Summer Program Coordinator
Jessica Becnel, Family Support Group Coordinator
A week-long summer camp program for children ages 7-16 with
heart defects. Activities include canoeing, swimming, archery,
art, sports, and teambuilding and personal development
activities.

8383   Camp Breathe Easy
American Lung Association
2452 Spring Rd. SE
Smyrna, GA 30080
Camp Breathe Easy is a summer camp for children ages 6-13 with
asthma. Campers learn asthma self-management techniques and
coping strategies as well as participate in activities such as swimming, fishing, canoeing, sports, and arts and crafts. The camp is
operated by the Georgia Chapter of the American Lung Association and held at Camp Twin Lakes in Rutledge, GA.

8384   Camp Can Do
Administrative Office
3 Unami Trail
Chalfont, PA 18914   717-273-6525
                                         campcandoforever.org
Tom Prader, Director, Patient Camp
Stephanie Cole, Director, Patient Camp
Caitlyn McLarnon, Director, Sibling Camp
Camp Can Do is for children ages 8-17 who have been diagnosed
with cancer in the last five years. The camp also offers a session
for siblings of children with cancer.

8385   Camp Carefree
American Diabetes Association
Lions Camp Pride
154 Camp Pride Way
New Durham, NH 03855   campsupport@diabetes.org
                                          www.diabetes.org
Phyllis Woestemeyer, Director
Camp Carefree is a American Diabetes Association summer camp
for children with diabetes. The camp is located at Lions Camp
Pride in New Durham, New Hampshire.

8386   Camp Catch-a-Rainbow
American Cancer Society
250 Williams St. NW
Atlanta, GA 30303   808-595-7500
                                              888-227-2345
                                          Fax: 808-595-7502
                                             www.cancer.org
Pamela K. Meyerhoffer, Chair
Robert E. Youle, Vice Chairman
Douglas K. Kelsey, Board Scientific Officer
Camp Catch-a-Rainbow's programs are available completely
free to any child in MI or IN who has or has had cancer, between
the ages of 4 and 20, with their doctor's approval. Family Camp is
reserved for those campers who have attended camp during that
year's summer sessions and their families. Day, week, adult retreat, and family camp are available options.

8387 Camp Cheerful
Achievement Centers For Children
15000 Cheerful Lane
Strongsville, OH 44136-5420   440-238-6200
                                      Fax: 440-238-1858
                            www.achievementcenters.org
Sally Farwell, President & CEO
Scott Peplin, Executive Vice President & CFO
Deborah Osgood, Vice President, Development & Marketing
Camp Cheerful provides a number of day and overnight camping
options for children and adults who have disabilities. The camp
hosts traditional camp activities as well as year-round therapeutic
horseback riding sessions and an accessible high ropes challenge
course during the summer. The focus of activities is to increase
the quality of life while encouraging confidence and
independence.

8388 Camp Christmas Seal
American Lung Association of Oregon
102 W McDowell Rd
Phoenix, AZ 85003-1213   602-258-7505
                                      Fax: 202-452-1805
                                     info@lungoregon.org
                                     www.lungoregon.org
Kathryn A. Forbes, Chairman
John F. Emanuel, Vice Chair
Harold Wimmer, President/CEO
Camp is located in Sisterhood, Oregon. Sessions for children
with asthma/respiratory ailments. Coed, ages 8-15.

8389 Camp Classen YMCA
YMCA of Greater Oklahoma City
10840 Main Camp Rd
Davis, OK 73030   580-369-2272
                                      Fax: 580-369-2284
                                     www.itsmycamp.org
Ford C. Price, Chair
Tricia Everest, Vice Chairman
Mike Grady, President & CEO
Camp is located in Davis, Oklahoma. Sessions for children and
adults with diabetes. Coed, ages 8-17, families, seniors and sin-
gle adults.

8390 Camp Conrad Chinnock
Diabetes Camping And Educational Services, Inc.
2400 E. Katella Ave.
Suite 800
Anaheim, CA 92806   844-744-2267
                                      Fax: 909-752-5354
                                  info@diabetescamping.org
                                  www.diabetescamping.org
Rocky Wilson, Executive Director
Ryan Martz, Development & Program Director
Dale Lissy, Camp Manager
Camp Conrad Chinnock offers year round recreational, social,
and educational opportunities for children and families with type
1 diabetes.

8391 Camp Courage North
True Friends
37569 Courage North Dr.
Lake George, MN 56458   952-852-0101
                                     800-450-8376
                                      Fax: 952-852-0123
                                     info@truefriends.org
                                     www.truefriends.org
John Leblanc, President & CEO
Conor McGrath, Senior Director, Camp & Operations
Jon Salmon, Director, Programs
Camp Courage North provides summer camp sessions for indi-
viduals with disabilities.

8392 Camp Discovery - Illinois
American Diabetes Association
55 E Monroe St.
Suite 3420
Chicago, IL 60603   312-346-1805
                                  illinoiscamps@diabetes.org
                                     www.diabetes.org

Camp Discovery is a day camp program for children ages 4-9 with
diabetes. The camp is held at HealthTrack Sports and Wellness in
Glen Ellyn, Illinois.

8393 Camp Discovery Kansas
American Diabetes Association
608 W Douglas Ave.
Wichita, KS 67203   316-684-6091
                                  campsupport@diabetes.org
                                     www.diabetes.org
Camp is located at Rock Springs 4-H Center in Junction City. For
children and teens ages 8-16 with diabetes.

8394 Camp Echoing Hills
36272 County Rd. 79
Warsaw, OH 43844   740-327-2311
                                     www.ehvi.org
Lauren Unger, Camp Administrator
Summer camp for children and adults with physical, intellectual
and developmental disabilities.

8395 Camp Eden Wood
True Friends
6350 Indian Chief Rd.
Eden Prairie, MN 55346   952-852-0101
                                     800-450-8376
                                      Fax: 952-852-0123
                                     info@truefriends.org
                                     www.truefriends.org
John Leblanc, President & CEO
Conor McGrath, Senior Director, Camp & Operations
Jon Salmon, Director, Programs
Offers resident camp programs for children, teenagers and adults
with developmental, physical or multiple disabilities. Fishing,
creative arts, golf, sports and other activities are available. Respite care weekend camps year round for children, teenagers and
adults. Guided vacations for teens and adults with developmental
disabilities or other unique needs.

8396 Camp Floyd Rogers
PO Box 541058
Omaha, NE 68154   402-885-9022
                                director@campfloydrogers.com
                                  www.campfloydrogers.com
Dylan Helberg, Camp Director
Carrie Busing, Operations Director
A camp for diabetic children. Coed, ages 8-18. Campers enjoy ac-
tivities, participate in special events, engage in evening pro-
grams, and they meet other children their own age with diabetes.

8397 Camp Glengarra
Girl Scouts - Foothills Council
33 Jewett Pl
Utica, NY 13501-4715   315-733-1909
                                      Fax: 315-733-1909
Natalie Brown, Executive Director
Karen Lubecki, Director
Camp Glengarra is located on 500+ acres of fields and forests,
about eight miles west of Camden. This Girl Scout Camp hosts a
myriad of programs throughout the year as well as summer day
and resident camp. Summer sessions for girls 5-17 with ADD or
asthma/respiratory ailments.

8398 Camp Glyndon
American Diabetes Association
800 Wyman Park Dr
Suite 110
Baltimore, MD 21211-2837   410-265-0075
                                     800-342-2383
                                      Fax: 410-235-4048
                                     askada@diabetes.org
                              www.childrenwithdiabetes.com
Heather Magoon, Director
Camp is located in Nanjemoy, Maryland. One and two-week ses-
sions July-August for children with diabetes and their families.
Coed, ages 8-16.

8399   Camp H.U.G.
Arizona Hemophilia Association
826 North 5th Ave
Phoenix, AZ 85003   602-955-3947
                                    info@arizonahemophilia.org
                        www.arizonahemophilia.org/camp-programs
Leigh Goldstein, Executive Director
Vickie Parra, Programs & Conferences Manager
Jessica Jackson, Finance Manager
Camp H.U.G (Hemophilia Uniting Generations) is a weekend
camp program of the Arizona Hemophilia Association. The camp
is for families who have a member with hemophilia, WWD,
and/or other bleeding disorders.

8400   Camp Harkness
The Arc Eastern Connecticut
125 Sachem St.
Norwich, CT 06360   860-889-4435
                                            Fax: 860-889-4662
                                            info@thearcect.org
                                thearcect.org/camp-harkness
Kathleen Stauffer, Chief Executive Officer
A week-long summer camp program for individuals with intellec-
tual and developmental disabilities. The camp is held at Camp
Harkness in Waterford, CT.

8401   Camp Heartland
One Heartland
26001 Heinz Rd.
Willow River, MN 55795   888-216-2028
                                    helpkids@oneheartland.org
                                        www.oneheartland.org
Patrick Kindler, Executive Director
Katie Donlin, Operations Manager
Kadien Bartels-Merkel, Program Director
A program of One Heartland, a nonprofit organization working to
provide camping programs for children with serious illnesses or
experiencing social isolation, Camp Heartland is a weeklong
summer camp for children, ages 7-15, who are infected or af-
fected by HIV/AIDS. The camp is held in Willow River,
Minnesota.

8402   Camp Hertko Hollow
4200 University Ave.
Suite 320
Des Moines, IA 50266   515-471-8523
                                                   855-502-8500
                                            Fax: 515-288-2531
                                        www.camphertkohollow.com
Jessica Thornton, Executive Director
Deb Holwegner, Camp Director
Camp Hertko Hollow is an educational and recreational summer
camp program for children and teens ages 6-17 with diabetes.
Campers participate in traditional camp activities and learn about
living with diabetes.

8403   Camp Hickory Hill
PO Box 1942
Columbia, MO 65205   573-445-9146
                                    camphickoryhill@gmail.com
                                        www.camphickoryhill.com
Jessica Bernhardt, Camp Director
Educates diabetic children concerning diabetes and its care. In
addition to daily educational sessions on some aspects of diabe-
tes, campers participate in swimming, sailing, arts and crafts and
overnight camping. Coed, ages 7-17.

8404   Camp Ho Mita Koda
14040 Auburn Rd.
Newbury, OH 44065   440-739-4095
                                    info@camphomitakoda.org
                                        www.camphomitakoda.org
Ian Roberts, Executive Director
Eric Brown, Camp Director
Camp Ho Mita Koda is a summer camp for children with type 1 diabetes. The camp aims to provide outdoor activities while also educating and building life skills for children with diabetes. Offers
overnight camp, family camp, specialty camp, and leadership
development programs.

8405   Camp Hodia
Idaho Diabetes Youth Programs, Inc.
5439 W Kendall St.
Boise, ID 83706   208-891-1023
                                            info@hodia.org
                                            www.hodia.org
Lisa Gier, Executive Director
Morgan Coenen, Director, Programs
Ciera Miller, Director, Marketing
Offers a variety of educational camp programs for children and
teens with type 1 diabetes.

8406   Camp Hollywood HEART
One Heartland
26001 Heinz Rd.
Willow River, MN 55795   888-216-2028
                                            Fax: 612-824-6303
                                    helpkids@oneheartland.org
                                        www.oneheartland.org
Patrick Kindler, Executive Director
Katie Donlin, Operations Manager
Kadien Bartels-Merkel, Program Director
A program of One Heartland, a nonprofit organization working to
provide camping programs for children with serious illnesses or
experiencing social isolation. Camp Hollywood HEART is a
weeklong summer camp for youths, ages 15-20, who are infected
or affected by HIV/AIDS. The camp is held in Malibu, California
and is partnership camp between One Heartland and Hollywood
Heart.

8407   Camp Honor
Arizona Hemophilia Association
826 North 5th Ave
Phoenix, AZ 85003   602-955-3947
                                    info@arizonahemophilia.org
                        www.arizonahemophilia.org/camp-programs
Leigh Goldstein, Executive Director
Vickie Parra, Programs & Conferences Manager
Jessica Jackson, Finance Manager
Camp Honor offers a week long summer camp to children affected by an inherited bleeding disorders. The cost of the camp is
$35 for a single camper and $50 dollars for a family (2 or more
campers). Camp Honor offers children the chance to partcipate in
outdoor activities and educational opportunities. In order to attend the camp there is an application process.

8408   Camp Independence
National Kidney Foundation
30 East 33rd Street
New York, NY 10016   770-452-1539
                                                   800-622-9010
                                            Fax: 212-689-9261
                                            info@kidney.org
                                            www.kidneyga.org
Gregory W. Scott, Chair
Beth Piraino, President
Bruce Skyer, CEO
Camp Independence is Georgia's a overnight, week-long summer
camp providing essential medical care, treatment & fun for kids
with kidney disease and transplants. Camp Independence recognizes that campers are normal children but have special needs
providing these children with opportunities for development &
individual growth, peer support & normal life experiences. Activities include swimming, arts & crafts, fishing and
horsebackriding, in addition to archery, games and sports, and
ceramics.

8409   Camp Jened
United Cerebral Palsy Association New York
P.O.Box 483
Rock Hill, NY 12775-483   845-434-2220
                                            Fax: 845-434-2253
Michael Branam, Executive Director
Camp is located in Rock Hill, New York. Sessions for adults with
severe developmental and physical disabilities. Coed, ages
18-99.

786

8410   Camp John Warvel
American Diabetes Association
8604 Allisonville Rd.
Suite 140
Indianapolis, IN 46250   317-352-9226
                                       campsupport@diabetes.org
                                               www.diabetes.org
A camp program for children and teens ages 7-17 with diabetes.
The camp is held at Camp Crosley in North Webster, Indiana.

8411   Camp Joslin
The Barton Center for Diabetes Education, Inc.
30 Ennis Rd.
PO Box 356
North Oxford, MA 01537-0356   508-987-2056
                                          Fax: 508-987-2002
                                            info@bartoncenter.org
                                             www.bartoncenter.org
Lynn Butler-Dinunno, Executive Director
Jenna Dufresne, Director, Health Services
Sarah Balko, Director, Camps & Programs
Camp for boys ages 6-16 with diabetes. This program offers active summer sports and activities, supplemented by medical treatment and diabetes education.

8412   Camp Joy
3325 Swamp Creek Rd
Schwenksville, PA 19473-1518   610-754-6878
                                          Fax: 610-754-7880
                                               www.campjoy.com
Robert G Griffith, President
A special needs camp for kids and adults (ages 4-80+) with developmental disabilities such as autism, brain injury, neurological disorder, visual and/or hearing impairments, Angelman and Down syndromes, and other developmental disabilities.

8413   Camp Ko-Man-She
Diabetes Dayton
2555 S Dixie Dr.
Suite 112
Dayton, OH 45409   937-220-6611
                                          Fax: 937-224-0240
                                        admin@diabetesdayton.org
                                      www.diabetesdaytoncamp.com
Susan McGovern, Executive Director
Camp Ko-Man-She is located in Bellefontaine, Ohio, and is held annually for children with diabetes. The camp's goal is for children to socialize with other children who also have diabetes and to have fun outdoors in a medically supervised setting. Co-ed, ages 8-17.

8414   Camp Kweebec
157 Game Farm Rd.
Schwenksville, PA 19473   610-667-2123
                                          Fax: 610-667-6376
                                              info@kweebec.com
                                               www.kweebec.com
Les Weiser, Owner/Director
Maddy Weiser, Owner/Director
Rachel Weiser, Associate Director, Director of
Camp is located in Schwenksville, Pennsylvania. Sessions for children and adults with diabetes. Coed, ages 6-16, families, seniors and single adults.

8415   Camp L-Kee-Ta
940 Golden Valley Drive
Bettendorf, IA 52722   319-752-3639
                                               800-798-0833
                                          Fax: 319-753-1410
                                                www.gseiwi.org
Teresa Colgan, Chair
Jill Dashner, 1st Vice chiar
Anna Gibney, Development Manager
Camp is located in Danville, Iowa. Half-week and one-week sessions June-August for children with asthma/respiratory ailments. Girls, ages 7-18 and families.

8416   Camp Latgawa
Oregon-Idaho Conference Center
13250 S Fork Little Butte Creek Rd
Eagle Point, OR 97524- 5593   541-826-9699
                                        camplatgawa@hotmail.com
                                           latgawa.gocamping.org/
Eva LaBonty, Director
Camp Latgawa provides year round hospitality for groups up to 90 people. The bunk/dormitory style facilities are heated and have restrooms and showers either in the cabin or nearby.

8417   Camp Libbey
Maumee Valley Girl Scout Center
2244 Collingwood Blvd
Toledo, OH 43620-1147   419-243-8216
                                               800-860-4516
                                          Fax: 419-245-5357
                                    www.girlscoutsofwesternohio.org
Jody Wainscott, Chair
Ellen Iobst, 1st Vice Chair
Susan Gantz Matz, 2nd Vice Chair
Camp for girls 7-18 with asthma/respiratory ailments, diabetes, epilepsy and muscular dystrophy is located in Defiance, Ohio.

8418   Camp MITIOG
Share, Inc
7615 N. Platte Purchase Drive
Kansas City, MO 64118   816-221-4450
                                               877-221-4450
                                          Fax: 816-221-1420
                                         midlands@midlandsmc.org
                                             www.midlandsmc.org
Mike Hale, President/Financial Officer
Pam Mathena, Adm. Assistant to MMC Financial Officer
Donna Fletcher, Congregational Consultant
Camp is located in Excelsior Springs, Missouri. One-week summer sessions for children with spina bifida. Coed, ages 6-16.

8419   Camp Magruder
17450 Old Pacific Hwy.
Rockaway Beach, OR 97136   503-355-2310
                                          Fax: 503-355-8701
                                          troy@campmagruder.org
                                            www.campmagruder.org
Troy Taylor, Camp Director
Hope Montgomery, Program Director
Rik Gutzke, Facilities Manager
Camp is located in Rockaway Beach, Oregon. Sessions for teens and adults with developmental disabilities through Camp Hope.

8420   Camp Nejeda
Camp Nejeda Foundation
910 Saddlebrook Road
P.O. Box 156
Stillwater, NJ 07875   973-383-2611
                                          Fax: 973-383-9891
                                            info@campnejeda.org
Ernest Post, MD, Secretary
Scott Ross, President
Bill Vierbuchen, Executive Director
For children with diabetes, ages 7-15. Provides an active and safe camping experience which enables the children to learn about and understand diabetes. Activities include boating, swimming, fishing, archery, as well as camping skills.

8421   Camp Not-A-Wheeze
2689 E Michelle Way
Gilbert, AZ 85234   602-336-6575
                                          Fax: 602-336-6576
                                       info@campnotawheeze.org
                                           campnotawheeze.org
Alan Crawford, Camp Director
Week-long summer camp for children aged 7-14 with moderate to severe asthma living in Arizona. Campers attending Camp Not-A- Wheeze, participate in a wide range of activities such as, horseback riding, hiking, canoeing, and fishing as well as an asthma education class. Those wishing to attend must fill out and send in a camper application.

8422 **Camp Okizu**
Okizu Foundation
83 Hamilton Dr.
Suite 200
Novato, CA 94949-5755
415-382-9083
Fax: 415-382-8384
info@okizu.org
www.okizu.org

Suzie Randall, Executive Director
Heather Ferrier, Director, Family Services
Sarah Uldricks, Director, Marketing & Special Events
Camp Okizu offers a variety of medically supervised, residential camp programs for families who have a child diagnosed with cancer. Programs are offered throughout the year free of charge.

8423 **Camp Paivika**
PO Box 3367
Crestline, CA 92325
909-338-1102
Fax: 909-338-2502
camppaivika@abilityfirst.org
www.abilityfirst.org/camp-paivika

Kelly Kunsek, Camp Director
Lauren Wilson, Program Director
Tina Ronning-Fraynd, Coordinator, Camper Services
As a program of AbilityFirst, Camp Paivika offers overnight summer programs for children, teens and adults with developmental and physical disabilities. The camp is completely accessible and the staff is trained to provide any assistance or personal care a camper needs. Located in San Bernardino National Forest, Camp Paivika provides a traditional summer camp experience in a safe and fun environment.
1947

8424 **Camp Pelican**
PO Box 10235
New Orleans, LA 70181
888-617-1118
Fax: 866-295-3803
camppelican@gmail.com
www.camppelican.org

A week-long overnight summer camp for children with pulmonary disorders, including severe asthma and cystic fibrosis, living in the state of Louisiana.

8425 **Camp Rainbow**
Phoenix Childrens Hospital
1919 E Thomas Rd
Phoenix, AZ 85016
602-933-1000
888-908-5437
camprainbow@phoenixchildrens.com
www.phoenixchildrens.org

Emilie Jarboe, Camp Director
Camp Rainbow is for children aged 7-17 who have or had cancer or a chronic blood disorder. The camp is offered for one week during the summer, held at camp Friendly Pines in Prescott, Arizona. Campers must be patients of Phoenix Children's Hospital's Center for Cancer and Blood Disorders, with the camp offering participants the opportunity to experience traditional camp activities including but not limited to, horseback riding, canoeing, fishing, swimming, and archery.

8426 **Camp Reach for the Sky**
The Seany Foundation
3530 Camino del Rio N
Suite 101
San Diego, CA 92108
858-551-0922
www.theseanyfoundation.org

Amy Robins, Co-Founder, The Seany Foundation
Paula Lutzky, Chief Financial Officer
Emily Brody, Director, Marketing & Media
Previously run by the American Cancer Society, Camp Reach for the Sky (CR4TS) is now run by The Seany Foundation and provides an opportunity for children with cancer and their siblings to attend a free summer camp. Camp Reach for the Sky offers a multiple programs, including a Resident Oncology Camp, a Sibling Camp and Day Camps.

8427 **Camp Ronald McDonald at Eagle Lake**
2555 49th Street
Sacramento, CA 95817
916-734-4230
Fax: 916-734-4238
info@rmhcnc.org
www.campronald.org

Catherine Ithurburn, Chief Executive Officer
Pip Pipkins, Camp Manager
Camp Ronald McDonald at Eagle Lake collaborates with other nonprofit organizations to provide week long summer camp opportunities for children with special medical needs, financial hardship and/or emotional, developmental or physical disabilities. The camp is fully accessible.

8428 **Camp Ronald McDonald for Good Times**
4560 Fountain Avenue
Los Angeles, CA 90029
323-666-6400
Fax: 626-744-9969
www.campronaldmcdonald.org

Erica Mangham, Executive Director
Brian Crater, Associate Executive Director
Chad Edwards, Program Director
Free year-round residential camping for children with cancer and their families.

8429 **Camp Sawtooth**
Oregon-Idaho Conference Center
P.O.Box 68
Fairfield, ID 83327-68
800-593-7539
sawtooth@gocamping.org
www.gocamping.org

David Hargreaves, Director
Camp located 35 miles north of fairfield, centrally located for all of southern Idaho.

8430 **Camp Seale Harris**
Southeastern Diabetes Education Services
500 Chase Park S.
Ste 104
Birmingham, AL 35244
205-402-0415
Fax: 205-402-0416
info@campsealeharris.org
www.campsealeharris.org

Rhonda McDavid, Executive Director
John Latimer, Director, Camp & Community Programs
Shelby Harrison, Manager, Communications & Events
Offering overnight, family, day and community program camps, Camp Seale Harris is a nonprofit organization that offers residential camps for children and teens with diabetes. With multiple programs in Alabama, the volunteer camp counselors are trained adults living with diabetes, to better help the camp attendees gain independence in learning to manage their diabetes. Camp programs run all year round.
1949

8431 **Camp Setebaid**
Setebaid Services, Inc.
PO Box 196
Winfield, PA 17889-0196
570-524-9090
Fax: 570-523-0769
info@setebaidservices.org
www.setebaidservices.org

Mark Moyer, Executive Director
Camping sessions for children with diabetes. The camp also hosts a family day for children with diabetes and their families.

8432 **Camp Smile-A-Mile**
Smile-A-Mile Place
1600 2nd Ave. S.
Birmingham, AL 35233
205-323-8427
Fax: 205-323-6220
info@campsam.org
www.campsam.org

Bruce Hooper, Executive Director
Kellie Reece, Chief Operating Officer
Katie Langley, Special Events Director
Camp Smile-A-Mile offers 7 different educational camp opportunities for children and their families who have been affected by childhood cancer in Alabama. The programs run all year long, in a variety of formats.

8433 **Camp Sunburst**
Sunburst Projects United States Headquarters
2143 Hurley Way
Suite 240
Sacramento, CA 95825 916-440-0889
Fax: 916-440-1208
admin@sunburstprojects.org
www.sunburstprojects.org
Jacob Bradley-Rowe, Executive Director
Camp Sunburst is a youth oriented leadership camp that promotes and creates an environment to help youth learn self confidence to change negative social patterns and break cycles of HIV/AIDS infections. Activities campers will participate in include, boating, swimming, art, dance, and sports.

8434 **Camp Sunrise**
Johns Hopkins Hospital
600 North Wolfe Street
CMSC 800
Baltimore, MD 21287-5904 410-955-5311

Sherryce Robinson, Mission Delivery Manager
Kira Elring, Regional Mission Director
Gloria Jetter, Regional Executive Director
Week long summer camp in White Hall, MD., for children ages 6-18 who have been diagnosed with or have survived cancer. Camp sunrise also has a 'day camp' program available for children ages 4-5. Camp activities include sports & games, swimming, arts & crafts, and nature hikes.

8435 **Camp Sunshine Dreams**
PO Box 28232
Fresno, CA 93729-8232 stephanie@campsunshinedreams.org
www.campsunshinedreams.com
Stephanie Scharbach, Contact
Pam Aiello, Contact
Camp Sunshine Dreams provides a summer camp experience to children aged 8-15 with cancer and their siblings.

8436 **Camp Sweeney**
PO Box 918
Gainesville, TX 76241 940-665-2011
Fax: 940-665-9467
info@campsweeney.org
www.campsweeney.org
Ernie Fernandez, Camp Director
Bob Cannon, Program Director
Billie Hood, Business Manager
Camp Sweeney teaches self-care and self-reliance to children ages 5-18 with type 1 diabetes. Campers participate in activities such as swimming, fishing, horseback riding and arts and crafts while learning how to self manage their diabetes.

8437 **Camp Tall Turf**
816 Madison SE
Grand Rapids, MI 49507 616-452-7906
Fax: 616-452-7907
info@tallturf.org
www.tallturf.org
Eric Brown, Chair
Ed Van Poolen, Vice Chair
Miriam DeJong, Director of Programs
Camp is located in Walkerville, Michigan. Summer camping sessions for youth with asthma/respiratory ailments and ADD. Coed, ages 8-16.

8438 **Camp Taylor**
Camp Taylor, Inc.
8224 West Grayson Rd.
Modesto, CA 95358-9094 209-545-3853
camp@kidsheartcamp.org
www.kidsheartcamp.org
Kimberlie Gamino, Founder & Executive Director
With several programs, Camp Taylor provides youth, teens, and the families of children with heart disease the opportunity to go to a free medically supervised summer sleepaway camp. Campers are able to enjoy activities such as, swimming, snorkeling, horseback riding, rock-wall, skits, archery, and heart education.
Founded in 2002. 2002

8439 **Camp Vacamas**
256 Macopin Rd
West Milford, NJ 07480 973-838-0942
877-428-8222
www.vacamas.org
Felix A. Urrutia, Executive Director
Kristin Short, Camp Director
Karen Wendolowski, Executive Secretary
Disadvantaged children with asthma or sickle cell anemia, ages 8-16, are offered special programs in canoeing, backpacking, camping, music and leadership training. Sliding scale tuition. Year round programs for youth at risk groups. Conference center facility open for group rentals.

8440 **Camp Waziyatah**
530 Mill Hill Rd
Waterford, ME 04088-4011 207-583-2267
Fax: 509-357-2267
info@wazi.com
wazi.com
Gregg Parker, Owner/Director
Mitch Parker, Owner/Director
Camp is located in Waterford, Massachusetts. Three, four and seven-week sessions June-August for campers with cancer and diabetes. Coed, ages 8-15 and families, single adults.

8441 **Camp WheezeAway**
YMCA Camp Chandler
880 South Lawrence Street
Mongtomery, AL 36104 334-229-4362
jikner@ymcamontgomery.org
ymcamontgomery.org/camp/wheezeaway
Jennifer Ikner, Contact
For children ages 8-12 with moderate to severe asthma, Camp WheezeAway offers week long summer camp programs that foster confidence building skills. The camp is free and managed by medical professionals. Those with children wishing to attend must apply to the camp and complete a selection process.

8442 **Camp del Corazon**
11615 Hesby St
North Hollywood, CA 91601-3620 818-754-0312
Fax: 818-754-0377
info@campdelcorazon.org
www.campdelcorazon.org
Kevin Shannon, President & Medical Director
Chrissie Endler, Executive Director
Kristina Caberto Wallace, Director of Development & Operations
Camp del Corazon, is a nonprofit corporation offering a no cost summer camp and other programs to children aged 7-17 living with heart disease. Campers or their guardians must fill out a camp application, with acceptance into the camp dependant upon a nurse review of the parent and cardiology portions of the application.
1995

8443 **Camps for Children & Teens with Diabetes**
Diabetes Society
1165 Lincoln Ave
Suite 300
San Jose, CA 95125-3052 408-287-3785
800-989-1165
Fax: 408-287-2701
info@diabetessociety.org
Sharon Ogbor, Executive Director
Thomas Smith, Director
Since 1974, sponsors up to 20 day camps, family camps and resident camps for children 4 through 17. These camps provide an opportunity for children with diabetes to go to camp, meet other children and gain a better understanding of their diabetes. The total experience can help campers develop more confidence in their abilities to control their diabetes effectively while enjoying the traditional camp experience. Camps are located throughout CA and parts of Nevada.

8444 **Cedar Ridge Camp**
4120 Old Routt Road
Louisville, KY 40299 502-267-5848
Fax: 502-267-0116
info@cedarridgecamp.com
www.cedarridgecamp.com
Andrew Hartmans, Executive Director
Half-week, one and two-week sessions for children with diabetes, developmental disabilities and muscular dystrophy. Coed, ages 6-17.

8445 **Children's Hospital Burn Camps Program**
13123 E 16th Ave.
PO Box 580
Aurora, CO 80045 720-777-8295
Fax: 720-777-7270
learnmore@noordinarycamps.org
www.noordinarycamps.org
Trudy Boulter, Camp Director
Tim Schuetz, Outreach Coordinator
The Children's Hospital Colorado Burn Camps Program provides rehabilitation and reintegration opportunities for children, teens, adults, and families who have been affected by burn injuries. The Camps Program has partnerships with 7 hospitals across the United States and offers year round programs.

8446 **Clara Barton Camp**
The Barton Center for Diabetes Education, Inc.
30 Ennis Rd.
PO Box 356
North Oxford, MA 01537-0356 508-987-2056
Fax: 508-987-2002
info@bartoncenter.org
www.bartoncenter.org
Lynn Butler-Dinunno, Executive Director
Jenna Dufresne, Director, Health Services
Sarah Balko, Director, Camps & Programs
Camp for girls ages 6-16 with diabetes. Campers participate in traditional camp activities and receive diabetes education. Activities include swimming, boating, sports, dance, music and arts and crafts.

8447 **Diabetes Camp**
Tanager Place
1614 W Mount Vernon Rd.
Mount Vernon, IA 52314 319-363-0681
Fax: 319-365-6411
campmail@tanagerplace.org
www.camptanager.org
Donald Pirrie, Camp Director
Provides recreational activities for children and teens with diabetes. The camp has on-site 24-hour physician and nursing staff. Ages 6-17.

8448 **Dr. Moises Simpser VACC Camp**
Nicklaus Children's Hospital
3200 SW 62nd Ave.
Suite 203
Miami, FL 33155-4076 305-662-8222
Fax: 786-268-1765
bela.florentin@mch.com
www.vacccamp.com
Bela Florentin, Camp Coordinator
Tania Diaz, Camp Clinical Coordinator
VACC Camp is a week-long overnight camp program for ventilation-assisted children and their families. The program includes sailing, swimming, field trips to local attractions, campsite entertainment, structured games, free play, and more. Parents have formal and informal opportunities to network among themselves.

8449 **Dream Street**
Dream Street Foundation
324 S. Beverly Dr.
Suite 500
Beverly Hills, CA 90212 424-333-1371
Fax: 310-388-0302
www.dreamstreetfoundation.org
Patty Grubman, Founder
Run by The Dream Street Foundation, Dream Street Camps provide camping programs for children (aged 4-14) and young adults (18-24) with chronic and life threatening illnesses. The kids pro-

gram runs in California, with the young adults program running in Arizona. The programs are free of charge, and campers can participate in different activities such as, swimming, arts and crafts, sports, horseback riding, and archery.

8450 **EDI Camp**
Wyman Center
600 Kiwanis Dr
St. Louis, MO 63025-2212 636-938-5245
Fax: 636-938-5289
www.wymancenter.org
David Hilliard, President
Theresa Mayberry, Senior Vice President
Youngsters with diabetes learn how to care for themselves while participating in a wide variety of outdoor activities and trips. The camp, managed and financed by the American Diabetes Association Greater St. Louis Affiliate, offers camperships to children from the Greater St. Louis area, ages 7-16, but nonresidents may also apply.

8451 **Easterseals Camp ASCCA**
PO Box 21
5278 Camp Ascca Dr.
Jacksons Gap, AL 36861 256-825-9226
Fax: 256-269-0714
info@campascca.org
www.campascca.org
Matt Rickman, Camp Director
John Stephenson, Administrator
Jocelyn Jones, Secretary
Easterseals Camp ASCCA is Alabama's Special Camp for Children and Adults, offering therapeutic recreation for children and adults with both physical and intellectual disabilities. The camp is located on 260 acres of barrier free woodland on Lake Martin and campers experience a wide variety of educational and recreational activities, including but not limited to: horseback riding, fishing, tubing, swimming, environmental education, arts, canoeing, and zip-lining. 1 week camp fees are $750.00.
1976

8452 **FCYD Camp Utada**
Foundation for Children and Youth with Diabetes
1995 W 9000 S
West Jordan, UT 84088 801-566-6913
www.fcydcamputada.org
Dave Okubo, MD, Co-Founder & Trustee
Elizabeth Elmer, Co-Founder & Trustee
Nathan Gedge, Co-Founder & Trustee
Camping for children with diabetes. Coed, ages 1-18 and families.

8453 **Father Drumgoole Connelly Summer Camp**
MIV Mount Loretto
6581 Hylan Blvd
Staten Island, NY 10309-3830 718-317-2600
Fax: 718-317-2830
www.mountloretto.org
Stephen Rynn, Executive Director
Maryann Virga, Executive Assistant
Loretta Polanish, Executive Secretary
Summer sessions for children with epilepsy, hearing impairment and developmental disabilities. Coed, ages 5-13.

8454 **Florida Diabetes Camp**
Florida Camp for Children & Youth with Diabetes
PO Box 14136
Gainesville, FL 32604-2136 352-334-1321
Fax: 352-334-1326
www.floridadiabetescamp.org
Gary Cornwell, Executive Director
Chris Stakely, Assistant Director
Janet Silverstein, Medical Director
Camp is located in Florida. Offers weekend and summer camps for children with type 1 diabetes.

8455 Friends Academy Summer Camps
Duck Pond Rd
Locust Valley, NY 11560   516-393-4207
                              Fax: 516-465-1720
                              camp@fa.org
                              www.fasummercamp.org
Rich Mack, Camp Director
Summer sessions for children with diabetes. Coed, ages 3-14, families.

8456 God's Camp
Episcopal Church of Hawaii
68-729 Farrington Hwy
Waialua, HI 96791-9314   808-637-6241
                              808-637-5505
                              Fax: 808-637-5505
                              www.campmokuleia.org
Debbie Alemeda, Manager
Episcopal Church tent camping, 5 nights, July. Church groups, family reunions, weddings, other organizations.

8457 Growing Together Diabetes Camp
ETMC
1000 S. Beckham
Tyler, TX 75701   903-597-0351
                       800-232-8318
                       info@etmc.org
                       www.etmc.org
Marty Wiggins, Development Director
Vicki Jowell, Director
Elmer G. Ellis, President
A summer camp for youths ages 6 to 15 with Type 1 or Type 2 diabetes.

8458 Happiness Is Camping
62 Sunset Lake Rd.
Hardwick, NJ 07825   908-362-6733
                          Fax: 908-362-5197
                          rich@happinessiscamping.org
                          www.happinessiscamping.org
Laura San Miguel, President
Julie McMahon, Secretary
Beth Fuchs, Treasurer
Happiness Is Camping is a camp for children with cancer and their siblings, ages 6-16.

8459 Happy Camp
Merrimack Hall Performing Arts Center
3320 Triana Blvd SW.
Huntsville, AL 35805   256-534-6455
                            info@merrimackhall.com
                            www.merrimackhall.com/happy-headquarters
For ages 3-12, Happy Camp is Merrimack Hall's annual half-day performing arts camp for children with special needs. Open to children with a wide range of physical or intellectual disabilities at any art level, activities include: music, theater, dance, and visual art. Happy Camp has a 1:1 staff-to-camper ratio. Camp time is from 9am - 12pm every day of the week.

8460 Hemophilia Camp
Tanager Place
1614 W Mount Vernon Rd.
Mount Vernon, IA 52314   319-363-0681
                              Fax: 319-365-6411
                              campmail@tanagerplace.org
                              www.camptanager.org
Donald Pirrie, Camp Director
A six-day camp for children with hemophilia and other bleeding disorders. The camp has onsite 24-hour physician and nursing staff.

8461 Kiwanis Camp Wyman
Wyman Center
600 Kiwanis Dr
Eureka, MO 63025-2212   636-938-5245
                             Fax: 636-938-5289
                             www.wymancenter.org
Keat Wilkins, Chairman
Dave Hilliard, President/CEO
Tom Etzkorn, VP, Executive Resource Officer

Summer sessions for youth with diabetes. Coed, ages 8-16, run in conjunction with the American Diabetes Association. Call for program description.

8462 Kota Camp
Junior League Of Little Rock
401 South Scott Street
Little Rock, AR 72201   501-375-5557
                             info@jllr.org
                             www.jllr.org/community/kota-camp/
Maradyth McKenzie, President
Tabitha McNulty, President Elect
Jenna Martin, Treasurer
Kota Camp is offered to children aged 6-16 with disabilities or medical conditions. Kota derived from a word used by the Quapaw Native American Tribe indigenous to Arkansas, means friend, and reflects the goals of the camp. Children with a disability bring a sibling or friend without a disability, to create a environment of inclusion, participate in camp activities, and promote an understanding of those with special needs. The camp is held at Camp Aldersgate in Little Rock.

8463 Lions Camp Tatiyee
5283 W White Mountain Blvd
Lakeside, AZ 85929   480-380-4254
                          pam@camptatiyee.org
                          camptatiyee.org
Richard Page, President
Lions Camp Tatiyee is the only organization in Arizona providing a week long summer camp for individuals with special needs. There is no cost for the camp and all of the programs are adaptable. Some activities that campers can participate in are, go-karting, fishing, art, games, cooking, rock wall, swimming, dances and campfires.

8464 Makemie Woods Camp
Presbytery of Eastern Virginia
P.O.Box 39
Barhamsville, VA 23011   757-566-1496
                              800-566-1496
                              Fax: 757-566-8803
Mike Burcher, Director
Sherri Egerton, Program Director
Karen Broughman, Office Manager
Residential Christian camp that tailors each group and individual goals. Counselors serve as teachers, friends and activity leaders. For children 8-18 with diabetes.

8465 Makemie Woods Camp/Conference Retreat
Presbytery of Eastern Virginia
P.O.Box 39
Barhamsville, VA 23011   757-566-1496
                              800-566-1496
                              Fax: 757-566-8803
Mike Burcher, Director
Sherri Egerton, Program Director
Karen Broughman, Office Manager
Counselors serve as teachers, friends and activity leaders. The individual is important within the small group. No camper is lost in the crowd, but is an integral partner in the group process. Residential Christian Camp and conference center. Summer camp for children 8-18 and special camp for children with diabetes.

8466 Marist Brothers Mid-Hudson Valley Camp
PO Box 197
Esopus, NY 12429   845-384-6620
                        info@maristbrotherscenter.org
Amy Reinwald-Earle, Camp Director, Special Children
Brother Owen Ormsby, Executive Director
Scott Kuhner, Director of Operations
The camp provides week-long summer sessions for children who have a variety of special needs/illnesses, such as cancer, HIV, deaf or mental disabilities. Each session is specific to the special need/illness.

8467 MedCamps of Louisiana
102 Thomas Rd.
Suite 615
West Monroe, LA 71291   318-329-8405
                               Fax: 318-329-8407
                               info@medcamps.com
                               www.medcamps.com
Caleb Seney, Executive Director
Kacie Hobson, Camp Director
Offers camp programs for children with chronic illnesses and physical or developmental disabilities.

8468 Mountaineer Spina Bifida Camp
534 New Goff Mountain Rd.
Charleston, WV 25313   info@drewsday.org
                               www.drewsday.org
Suzie Humphreys, Contact
A summer camp for individuals with spina bifida. Campers can participate in activities such as swimming, wheelchair hockey, baseball, and more.

8469 Muscular Dystrophy Association Free Camp
222 S. Riverside Plaza
Suite 1500
Chicago, IL 60606   907-276-2131
                               800-572-1717
                               Fax: 907-276-0946
                               www.mdausa.org
R. Rodney Howell, MD, Chairman
Steven M. Derks, President/CEO
Julie Faber, EVP/CFO
MDA Camp provides a wide range of activities for those who have limited mobility or are in wheelchairs. The camp offers may outdoor sporting activities, art's & crafts and talent shows.

8470 NeSoDak
Lutherans Outdoors in South Dakota
2001 S Summit Ave.
Sioux Falls, SD 57197   605-947-4440
                               800-888-1464
                               nesodak@losd.org
                               www.losd.org/nesodak
Vicki Foss, Director
Located in Waubay, South Dakota, NeSoDak provides camp programs for a range of ages. Hosts Camp Gilbert, a summer camp program for children with diabetes.

8471 Open Hearts Camp
The Edward J. Madden Open Hearts Camp
250 Monument Valley Rd.
Great Barrington, MA 01230   413-528-2229
                               hearts@openheartscamp.org
                               www.openheartscamp.org
David Zaleon, Executive Director
Camp program for children who have had and are fully recovered from open heart surgery or a heart transplant. Four two-week sessions by age group. Small camp - around 15 campers per session.

8472 Phantom Lake YMCA Camp
S110W30240 YMCA Camp Rd.
Mukwonago, WI 53149   262-363-4386
                               office@phantomlakeymca.org
                               www.phantomlakeymca.org
Karin Mulrooney, Chair
Sara Hacker, Secretary
Bill Canfield, Treasurer
Phantom Lake Camp offers day and residential camping sessions for children ages 3-17. All programs are open to individuals with disabilities.

8473 Rapahope Children's Retreat Foundation
205 Lambert Ave.
Suite A
Mobile, AL 36604   251-476-9880
                               info@rapahope.org
                               www.rapahope.org
Melissa McNichol, Executive Director
Roz Dorsett, Assistant Director
Rapahope is an organization that offers a one week long summer camp for children who have, or who have had cancer. For children ages 7-17, the camp offers a wide range of summer camp activi-

ties, including but not limited to, swimming, kayaking, horseback riding, and arts. The camp is offered at no cost to campers or their families.

8474 Roundup River Ranch
8333 Colorado River Rd.
Gypsum, CO 81637   970-524-2267
                               Fax: 888-524-2477
                               info@roundupriverranch.org
                               www.roundupriverranch.org
Ruth B. Johnson, President & Chief Executive Officer
Sterling Nell Leija, Director of Operations
Kendra Perkins, Camp Director
Roundup River Ranch provides traditional camp experiences for children and their families with chronic and serious illnesses. The Ranch is located in Gypsum, Colorado, with all programs offered free of charge.

8475 STIX Diabetes Programs
PO Box 8308
Spokane, WA 99203   509-484-1366
                              Fax: 509-955-1329
                              stix@stixdiabetes.org
                              www.stixdiabetes.org
Tonya Kobluk, Director, Administration & Camps
Cindy Schneider, Director, Community Outreach
Jill Strom, Director, Development
STIX Diabetes Programs is a non-profit organization providing camp experiences for children and teens with diabetes. STIX offers a three-day non-residential day camp for children ages 6-8; a week-long residential camp for youth ages 9-16; and an excursion-based Adventure Camp for teens ages 16-19.

8476 Shady Oaks Camp
16300 Parker Rd.
Homer Glen, IL 60491   708-301-0816
                              Fax: 708-301-5091
                              soc16300@sbcglobal.net
                              www.shadyoakscamp.org
Scott Steele, Executive Director
Katie Clark, Camp Director
Gary Schaid, Assistant Director
Shady Oaks Camp provides summer camp programs for children and adults with cerebral palsy and similar disabilities.

8477 Sherman Lake YMCA Summer Camp
Sherman Lake YMCA Outdoor Center
6225 N 39th St
Augusta, MI 49012   269-731-3000
                              Fax: 269-731-3020
                              shermanlakeymca@ymcasl.org
                              www.shermanlakeymca.org
Luke Austenfeld, Executive Director
Jean Henderson, Business Manager
Lorrie Syverson, Director, Camping, Education & Retreat Services
Summer camping sessions for campers with ADD and spina bifida. Coed, ages 6-15 and families, seniors.

8478 Strength for the Journey
Oregon-Idaho Conference Center
1505 SW 18th Ave
Portland, OR 97201-2524   503-226-7931
                              800-593-7539
                              suttlelake@gocamping.org
                              www.gocamping.org
Jane Petke, Suttle Lake Camp Director
Geneva Cook, Camping Registrar
Camp is located near Sisters, Oregon at Suttle Lake Camp. Strength for the Journey is a program for adults living with HIV/AIDS.

8479 Summer Camp for Children with Muscular Dystrophy
Muscular Dystrophy Association - USA
222 S. Riverside Plaza
Suite 1500
Chicago, IL 60606
520-529-2000
800-572-1717
Fax: 520-529-5300
mda@mdausa.org
www.mdausa.org

R. Rodney Howell, MD, Chairman
Steven M. Derks, President/CEO
Pete Morgan, EVP/COO
Offers a wide range of activities such as adaptive sports, swimming, fishing, archery, scavenger hunts, dances & talent shows, art's & crafts, karaoke, and campfires.

8480 Suttle Lake Camp
29551 Suttle Lake Rd.
Sisters, OR 97759
541-595-6663
suttlelake@gocamping.org
suttlelake.gocamping.org

Daniel Petke, Co-Director
Jane Petke, Co-Director
Offers a variety of camp programs, including sessions for individuals with HIV/AIDS.

8481 TSA CT Kid's Summer Event
Tourette Syndrome Association of Connecticut (TSA)
c/o Massachusetts Chapter
39 Godfrey Street
Taunton, MA 02780
617-277-7589
www.tsact.org

Tom Meehan, Chairman
Peter Tavolacci, Vice-Chairman
Paul Nazario, Treasurer
TSA of Connecticut sponsors summer events for children with TS/Tourette Syndrome activities of which include minature golf in addition to an Annual Conference. The kids' program at this annual conference provides children who have TS a unique opportunity to meet other children like them who also struggle with TS. Entertainment includes puppeteers, magicians, learning karate from the experts, getting face paintings and more.
uniqu pages

8482 Texas Lions Camp
PO Box 290247
Kerrville, TX 78029
830-896-8500
Fax: 830-896-3666
tlc@lionscamp.com
www.lionscamp.com

Stephen S. Mabry, President & CEO
Karen-Anne King, Vice President, Summer Camps
Milton Dare, Director, Development
Texas Lions Camp is a camp dedicated to serving children ages 7-16 in Texas with physical disabilities. While at camp, campers will participate in a variety of activities and be encouraged to become more independent and self-confident.

8483 The Hole in the Wall Gang Camp
565 Ashford Center Rd.
Ashford, CT 06278
860-429-3444
info@holeinthewallgang.org
www.holeinthewallgang.org

James H. Canton, Chief Executive Officer
Padraig Barry, Chief Strategy Officer
Kevin Magee, Chief Financial Officer
The Hole in the Wall Gang Camp offers summer and weekend camp experiences for children and the siblings of children with serious illnesses. Located in Ashford, Connecticut, campers are able to participate in traditional camp activities in a medically safe environment.

8484 Twin Lakes Camp
1451 E Twin Lakes Rd
Hillsboro, IN 47949-8004
765-798-4000
outdoors@twinlakescamp.com
www.twinlakescamp.com

Jon Beight, Executive Director
Dan Daily, Program Director
Duane Bush, Guest Service

Provides a summer camp program for special needs children and young adults. Campers suffer from a wide range of maladies including crippling accidents, Spina Bifida, epilepsy, Cerebral Palsy, Muscular Dystrophy, Quadriplegia, Paraplegia, and other disabling diseases. Campers range in age from 8 to 27.

8485 Wisconsin Lions Camp
Wisconsin Lions Foundation
3834 County Rd. A
Rosholt, WI 54473
715-677-4969
877-463-6953
Fax: 715-677-4527
info@wisconsinlionscamp.com
www.wisconsinlionscamp.com

Evett Hartvig, Executive Director
Andrea Yenter, Camp Director
Phillip Potter, Assistant Camp Director
Provides camp programs for youth and adults in Wisconsin with disabilities, including autism, intellectual disabilities, diabetes, epilepsy, visual impairments, and hearing impairments. ACA accredited, located in central Wisconsin, near Stevens Point.

8486 Y Camp
YMCA of Greater Des Moines
1192 166th Drive
Boone, IA 50036
515-432-7558
Fax: 515-432-5414
ycamp@dmymca.org
www.y-camp.org

David Sherry, Executive Director
Mike Havlik, Program Director- Environmental
Alex Kretzinger, Program Director- Summer Camp
Camp is located in Boone, Iowa. Year-round one and two-week sessions for boys and girls with cancer, diabetes, asthma, cystic fibrosis, hearing impaired and other disabilities. Coed, ages 6-16 and families.

8487 YMCA Camp Fitch
12600 Abels Rd.
North Springfield, PA 16430
814-922-3219
877-863-4824
Fax: 814-922-7000
registrar@campfitchymca.org
campfitchymca.org

Tom Parker, Executive Director
Joe Wolnik, Summer Camp Director
Brandy Duda, Outdoor Education Director
Camp is located in North Springfield, Pennsylvania. Camp programs include sessions for children with diabetes or epilepsy.

8488 YMCA Camp Ihduhapi
Minneapolis YMCA Camping Services
15200 Hanson Blvd.
Andover, MN 55304
763-230-9622
info@campihduhapi.org
campihduhapi.org

Kerry Pioske, Camp Executive
Josh Cobb, Overnight Camp Director
Devin Hanson, Day Camp Director
Camp is located in Loretto, Minnesota. Summer sessions for campers with asthma/respiratory ailments and epilepsy. Coed, ages 7-16.

8489 YMCA Camp Kitaki
Lincoln YMCA
570 Fallbrook Blvd.
Suite 210
Lincoln, NE 68521
402-434-9200
Fax: 402-434-9208
info@ymcalincoln.org
www.ymcalincoln.org

Barb Bettin, President/CEO
J.P. Lauterbach, COO
Misty Muff, Chief Administrative Officer
Camp is located in Louisville, Nebraska. Summer sessions for children with cystic fibrosis. Coed, ages 7-17 and families.

8490   YMCA Camp Shady Brook
YMCA of the Pikes Peak Region (PPYMCA)
316 N. Tejon Street
Colorado Springs, CO 80903   719-329-7227
                              Fax: 719-272-7026
                              campinfo@ppymca.org
                              www.campshadybrook.org

Sonny Adkins, Executive Director
Laura Petersen, Program Director
Patrick Casey, Facility Director
Camp is located in Sedalia, Colorado. One-week sessions for campers with HIV. Boys and girls 7-16. Also families, seniors and single adults.

8491   YMCA Camp jewell
YMCA of Greater Hartford
6 Prock Hill Road
P.O. Box 8
Colebrook, CT 06021   860-379-2782
                              888-412-2267
                              Fax: 860-379-8715
                              camp.jewell@ghymca.org
                              www.ghymca.org

Eric Tucker, Executive Director
Camp is located in Colebrook, Connecticut. Two-week sessions for children with cancer. Coed, ages 8-16. Also families.

8492   YMCA Camp of Maine
305 Winthrop Center Rd
P.O. Box 446
Winthrop, ME 04364   207-395-4200
                              Fax: 207-395-7230
                              info@maineycamp.org
                              www.maineycamp.org

Tom Christensen, CVO
Rebecca Henry, Vice CVO
Marty Allen, Treasurer
Activities include arts and crafts, nature study, hiking, and overnight camping, dancing, and singing. Summer session dates run from June through August; for ages 8-16.

8493   YMCA Outdoor Center Campbell Gard
4803 Augspurger Road
Hamilton, OH 45011   513-867-0600
                              Fax: 513-867-0127
                              camp@gmvymca.org
                              www.ccgymca.org

Pete Fasano, Executive Director
Katie Depew, Summer Program Director
Tom Andrews, Facilities and Properties Manager
Camp is located in Hamilton, Ohio. Camping sessions for children and young adults with developmental disabilities. Runs overnight and day sessions for ages 7-22 and families.

Books

8494   A Woman's Guide to Living with HIV Infection
Johns Hopkins University Press
2715 N Charles St
Baltimore, MD 21218-4363   410-516-6900
                              800-548-1784
                              Fax: 410-516-6998
                              jwehmueller@press.jhu.edu
                              www.press.jhu.edu

Rebecca A Clark M.D., PhD, Author
Robert T Maupin Jr. M.D. FACOG, Co-Author
Jill Hayes Hammer PhD, Co-Author
A resource for women with HIV that discusses coping with the diagnosis, finding a physician, recognizing symptoms, and preventing complications. Explains the latest treatment options and advice on coping with gynecologic infections. *$18.00*
328 pages Hardback

8495   ABC of Asthma, Allergies & Lupus
Global Health Solutions
2146 Kings Garden Way
PO Box 3189
Falls Church, VA 22043-2593   703-848-2333
                              800-759-3999
                              Fax: 703-848-0028
                              information@watercure.com
                              www.watercure.com

Fereydoon Batmanghelidj MD, Author
Xiaopo Batmanghelidj, President
Kristin Swan, Administrator
This book introduces new approaches in preventing and treating asthma, allergies and lupus without toxic chemicals. It also offers new insight on how to prevent and treat children's asthma. *$ 17.00*
240 pages
ISBN 0-962994-26-x

8496   AIDS Sourcebook
Omnigraphics
615 Griswold Street
Suite 520
Detroit, MI 48226   610-461-3548
                              800-234-1340
                              Fax: 800-875-1340
                              contact@omnigraphics.com
                              www.omnigraphics.com

Peter Ruffner, Co-Founder
Fred Ruffner, Co-Founder
Basic consumer health information about the Human Immunodeficiency Virus (HIV) and Acquired Immunodeficiency Syndrome (AIDS), including facts about its origins, stages, types, transmission, risk factors, and prevention, and featuring details about diagnostic testing, antiretroviral treatments, and co-occurring infections. *$ 85.00*
600 pages 5th Edition 1911
ISBN 0-780811-47-8

8497   AIDS and Other Manifestations of HIV Infection
Elsevier Inc
30 Corporate Dr
Suite 400
Burlington, MA 01803-4252   781-313-4700
                              800-545-2522
                              Fax: 800-568-5136
                              usbkinfo@elsevier.com
                              www.elsevier.com

Gary Wormser MD, Editor
A comprehensive overview of the biological properties of this etiologic viral agent, its clinicopathological manifestations, the epidemiology of its infection, and present and future therapeutic options. *$249.95*
1000 pages 2004
ISBN 0-127640-51-7

8498   AIDS in the Twenty-First Century: Disease and Globalization
Palgrav Macmillan
175 5th Ave
New York, NY 10010-7703   888-330-8477
                              Fax: 800-672-2054
                              onlinesupportusa@palgrave.com
                              www.palgrave-usa.com

Gabriella Georgiades, Editor
Alan Whiteside, Author
Tony Barnett, Co-Author
The authors — exprets in the field for over 15 years — argue that it is vital to not only look at AIDS in terms of prevention and treatment, but to also consider consequences which affect households, communities, companies, governments, and countries. This is a major contribution toward understanding the global public health crisis, as well as the relationship between poverty, inequality, and infectious diseases. *$32.00*
464 pages
ISBN 1-403997-68-5

8499   Adult Leukemia: A Comprehensive Guide for Patients and Families
O'Reilly Media Inc
1005 Gravenstein Hwy N
Sebastopol, CA 95472-2811
707-827-7000
800-998-9938
Fax: 707-829-0104
order@oreilly.com
www.oreilly.com

Linda Lamb, Editor
Barb Lackritz, Author
For the tens of thousands of Americans with adult leukemia, Adult Leukemia: A Comprehensive Guide for Patients and Families addresses diagnosis, medical tests, finding a good oncologist, treatments, side effects, getting emotional and other support, resources for further study, and much more. The book includes real-life stories from those who have battled leukemia themselves. *$29.95*
536 pages Paperback
ISBN 0-596500-01-7

8500   Advanced Breast Cancer: A Guide to Living with Metastic Disease
O'Reilly Media Inc
1005 Gravenstein Hwy N
Sebastopol, CA 95472-2811
707-827-7000
800-998-9938
Fax: 707-829-0104
order@oreilly.com
www.oreilly.com

Linda Lamb, Editor
Musa Mayer, Author
This is the only book on breast cancer that deals honestly with the realities of living with metastic disease, yet offers hope and comfort. All aspects of facing the disease are covered, including: coping with the shock of recurrence, seeking information and making treatment decisions, communicating effectively with medical personnel finding support, and handling disease progression and end-of-life issues. A comprehensive guide, it also provides updated resources and treatment developments. *$24.95*
532 pages Paperback 1998
ISBN 1-565925-22-X

8501   Allergies Sourcebook
Omnigraphics
615 Griswold Street
Suite 520
Detroit, MI 48226
610-461-3548
800-234-1340
Fax: 800-875-1340
contact@omnigraphics.com
www.omnigraphics.com

Peter Ruffner, Co-Founder
Fred Ruffner, Co-Founder
Basic comsumer health information about the immune system and allergic disorders, including rhinitis (hay fever), sinusitis, conjunctivitis, asthma, atopic dermatitis, and anaphylaxis, and allergy triggers such as pollen, mold, dust mites, animal dander, chemicals, foods and additives, and medications; along with facts about allergy diagnosis and treatment, tips on avoiding triggers and preventing symptoms, a glossary of related terms, and directories of resources for additional help and info. *$95.00*
608 pages 4th Edition 1911

8502   Allergies and Asthma: What Every Parent Needs to Know (2nd Edition)
American Academy of Pediatrics
345 Park Blvd.
Itasca, IL 60143
800-433-9016
Fax: 847-434-8000
mcc@aap.org
www.aap.org

Mark Del Monte, Chief Executive Officer & Executive Vice President
Christine Bork, Chief Development Officer & Sr. Vice President, Development
Roberta Bosak, Chief Administrative Officer & Sr. Vice President, HR

Consumer resource for parents who need answers and information about their children's allergies and asthma. Covers advice on identifying allergies and asthma, preventing attacks, minimizing triggers, understanding medications, explaining allergies to young children, and helping children manage symptoms. *$14.95*
174 pages Paperback; eBook available 1910
ISBN 1-581104-45-6

8503   Alternative Approach to Allergies
Harper Collins Publishers
10 E 53rd St
New York, NY 10022-5244
212-207-7901
800-242-7737
Fax: 212-702-2586
spsales@harpercollins.com
www.harpercollins.com

Theron G Randolph M.D., Author
Ralph W Moss PhD, Co-Author
Here is the book that revolutionized the way allergies and other common illnesses were diagnosed and treated.
ISBN 0-060916-93-1

8504   Alzheimer Disease Sourcebook
Omnigraphics
615 Griswold Street
Suite 520
Detroit, MI 48226
610-461-3548
800-234-1340
Fax: 800-875-1340
contact@omnigraphics.com
www.omnigraphics.com

Peter Ruffner, Co-Founder
Fred Ruffner, Co-Founder
Alzheimer Disease Sourcebook, Fifth Edition provides updated information about causes, symptoms, and stages of AD and other forms of dementia, including mild cognitive impairment, corticobasal degeneration, dementia with Lewy bodies, frontotemporal dementia, Huntington disease, Parkinson disease, and dementia caused by infections. *$95.00*
600 pages 1911
ISBN 0-780811-50-8

8505   Alzheimer Disease Sourcebook, 4th Edition
Omnigraphics
615 Griswold Street
Suite 520
Detroit, MI 48226
610-461-3548
800-234-1340
Fax: 800-875-1340
contact@omnigraphics.com
www.omnigraphics.com

Peter Ruffner, Co-Founder
Fred Ruffner, Co-Founder
Basic consumer health information about alzheimer disease, other dementias, and related disorders, including multi-infarct dementia, dementia with lewy bodies, frontotemporal dementia (pick disease), Wernicke-Korsakoff syndrome (alcohol-related dementia), AIDS dementia complex, Huntington disease, Creutzfeldt-Jacob disease, and delirium. *$84.00*
603 pages
ISBN 0-780810-01-3

8506   Amyotrophic Lateral Sclerosis: A Guide for Patients and Families
Demos Medical Publishing
11 West 42nd Street
15th Floor
New York, NY 10036
212-683-0072
800-532-8663
Fax: 212-683-0118
support@demosmedical.com
www.demosmedpub.com

Richard Winters, Executive Editor
Beth Kaufman Barry, Publisher
Noreen Henson, Executive Director of Demos Heal
This comprehensive guide covers every aspect of the management of ALS. Beginning with discussions of its clinical features of the disease, diagnosis, and an overview of symptom management, major sections deal with medical and rehabilitative management, living with ALS, managing advanced disease and

end-of-life issues, and reources that can provide support and assistance. *$29.95*
470 pages 2001
ISBN 1-888799-28-5

8507   Arthritis Sourcebook.
Omnigraphics
615 Griswold Street
Suite 520
Detroit, MI 48226

610-461-3548
800-234-1340
Fax: 800-875-1340
contact@omnigraphics.com
www.omnigraphics.com

Peter Ruffner, Co-Founder
Fred Ruffner, Co-Founder
Basic consumer health information about osteoarthritis, rheumatoid arthritis, other rheumatic disorders, infectious forms of arthritis, and diseases with symptoms linked to arthritis, and facts
about diagnosis, pain management, and surgical therapies.
$84.00
567 pages 2nd Edition
ISBN 0-780806-67-2

8508   Asthma Sourcebook.
Omnigraphics
615 Griswold Street
Suite 520
Detroit, MI 48226

610-461-3548
800-234-1340
Fax: 800-875-1340
contact@omnigraphics.com
www.omnigraphics.com

Peter Ruffner, Co-Founder
Fred Ruffner, Co-Founder
Provides information about asthma, including symptoms, reme-
dies and research updates. *$84.00*
581 pages 2nd Edition
ISBN 0-780808-66-9

**8509   Asthma and Allergy Answers: A Patient Education
Library**
Asthma and Allergy Foundation of America
8201 Corporate Dr
Suite 1000
Landover, MD 20785

202-466-7643
800-727-8462
Fax: 202-466-8940
info@aafa.org
www.aafa.org

Amy Patterson, Senior Director of Administration & Governance
Jacqui Vok, Director of Programs and Services
William McLin, M.Ed., President/CEO
This resource contains 50 reproducible fact sheets for patients on
a variety of popular asthma and allergy topics. Information is
written in a patient-friendly question and answer format and
packaged in a durable binder for easy storage and use. *$50.00*

8510   Back & Neck Sourcebook.
Omnigraphics
615 Griswold Street
Suite 520
Detroit, MI 48226

610-461-3548
800-234-1340
Fax: 800-875-1340
contact@omnigraphics.com
www.omnigraphics.com

Peter Ruffner, Co-Founder
Fred Ruffner, Co-Founder
Basic consumer health information about back and neck pain, spinal cord injuries, and related disorders, such as degenerative disk
disease, osteoarthritis, scoliosis, sciatica, spina bifida, and spinal
stenosis, and featuring facts about maintaining spinal health,
self-care, rehabilitative care, chiropractic care, spinal surgeries,
and complementary therapies. *$84.00*
607 pages 2nd Edition
ISBN 0-780807-38-9

8511   Being Close
National Jewish Health
1400 Jackson St
Denver, CO 80206-2761

303-398-1002
877-225-5654
Fax: 303-398-1125
allstetterw@njc.org
www.nationaljewish.org

Michael Salem M.D., President/CEO
William Allstetter, Director Media/External Relation
A booklet offering information to patients suffering from a respiratory disorder such as emphysema, asthma or tuberculosis, that
discusses sexual problems and feelings.

**8512   Bittersweet Chances: A Personal Journey o f Living and
Learning in the Face of Illness**
PublishAmerica
PO Box 151
Frederick, MD 21705-151

301-695-1707
Fax: 301-631-9073
support@publishamerica.com
www.publishamerica.com

Dana Selenke Broehl, Author
Recounts Doug and Dana Broehl's journey of growth through the
darkness of cystic fibrosis and the renewed hope of a double lung
transplant. *$24.95*
189 pages Softcover
ISBN 1-413713-24-6

8513   Blood and Circulatory Disorders Sourcebook
Omnigraphics
615 Griswold Street
Suite 520
Detroit, MI 48226

610-461-3548
800-234-1340
Fax: 800-875-1340
contact@omnigraphics.com
www.omnigraphics.com

Peter Ruffner, Co-Founder
Fred Ruffner, Co-Founder
Blood and Circulatory Disorders Sourcebook, Third Edition offers facts about blood function and composition, the maintenance
of a healthy circulatory system, and the types of concerns that
arise when processes go awry. It discusses the diagnosis and treatment of many common blood cell disorders, bleeding disorders,
and circulatory disorders, including anemia, hemochromatosis,
leukemia, lymphoma, hemophilia, hypercoagulation,
thrombophilia, atherosclerosis, blood pressure irregularities,
coronary *$84.00*
634 pages 2nd Edition
ISBN 0-780807-46-4

**8514   Blooming Where You're Planted: Stories From The
Heart**
Meeting Life's Challenges
9042 Aspen Grove Lane
Madison, WI 53717-2700

608-824-0402
Fax: 608-824-0403
help@MeetingLifesChallenges.com
www.makinglifeeasier.com

Shelley Peterman Schwatz, Editor
Author Shelley Peterman Schwarz takes you on her journey of
self-discovery and change following her diagnosis of multiple
sclerosis in 1979. Her personal stories are warm and humorous,
and insightful. This 138-page book will motivate and inspire you
to rise above life's challenges and live life to its fullest. *$12.95*
138 pages 1998
ISBN 0-891854-01-1

**8515   Brain Allergies: The Psychonutrient and Magnetic
Connections**
McGraw-Hill

William Philpott PhD, Author
Dwight Keating PhD, Author
Linus Pauling PhD, Author
A complete overview of the concept of brain allergies - the theory
that exposure to certain foods and other substances triggers men-

tal disorders in people so predisposed, and that such disturbances can be cured by eliminating these substances. *$16.95*
ISBN 0-658003-98-1

8516 Brain Disorders Sourcebook
Omnigraphics
615 Griswold Street
Suite 520
Detroit, MI 48226
610-461-3548
800-234-1340
Fax: 800-875-1340
contact@omnigraphics.com
www.omnigraphics.com

Peter Ruffner, Co-Founder
Fred Ruffner, Co-Founder
Brain Disorders Sourcebook, Third Edition provides readers with updated information about brain function, neurological emergencies such as a brain attack (stroke) or seizure, and symptoms of brain disorders. It describes the diagnosis, treatment, and rehabilitation therapies for genetic and congenital brain disorders, brain infections, brain tumors, seizures, traumatic brain injuries, and degenerative neurological disorders such as Alzheimer disease and other dementias, Parkinson disease, and am *$84.00*
600 pages 2nd Edition
ISBN 0-780807-44-0

8517 Breast Cancer Sourcebook
Omnigraphics
615 Griswold Street
Suite 520
Detroit, MI 48226
610-461-3548
800-234-1340
Fax: 800-875-1340
contact@omnigraphics.com
www.omnigraphics.com

Peter Ruffner, Co-Founder
Fred Ruffner, Co-Founder
Breast Cancer Sourcebook, Fourth Edition, provides updated information about breast cancer and its causes, risk factors, diagnosis, and treatment. Readers will learn about the types of breast cancer, including ductal carcinoma in situ, lobular carcinoma in situ, invasive carcinoma, and inflammatory breast cancer, as well as common breast cancer treatment complications, such as pain, fatigue, lymphedema, hair loss, and sexuality and fertility issues. Information on preventive therapies, nutrition *$84.00*
600 pages 3rd Edition
ISBN 0-780810-30-3

8518 Breathe Free
Lotus Press
P.O. Box 325
Twin Lakes, WI 53181
262-889-8561
800-824-6396
Fax: 262-889-8591
lotuspress@lotuspress.com
www.lotuspress.com

Daniel Gagnon, Author
Amanda Morningstar, Author
An expose on respiratory diseases and their natural treatment. Learn how you can heal and/or manage common colds/flu, earaches/asthma, allergies/hay fever, pleurisy/pneumonia, coughs/sore throats, bronchitis/emphysema, AIDS and ARC related respiration infection. Covers information you wish your doctor would share with you such as what is happening to your body. *$14.95*
179 pages
ISBN 9-780914-95-5

8519 Cancer Sourcebook
Omnigraphics
615 Griswold Street
Suite 520
Detroit, MI 48226
610-461-3548
800-234-1340
Fax: 800-875-1340
contact@omnigraphics.com
www.omnigraphics.com

Peter Ruffner, Co-Founder
Fred Ruffner, Co-Founder

Cancer Sourcebook, Sixth Edition provides updated information about common types of cancer affecting the central nervous system, endocrine system, lungs, digestive and urinary tracts, blood cells, immune system, skin, bones, and other body systems. It explains how people can reduce their risk of cancer by addressing issues related to cancer risk and taking advantage of screening exams. *$84.00*
1105 pages 5th Edition
ISBN 0-780809-47-5

8520 Cancer Sourcebook for Women
Omnigraphics
615 Griswold Street
Suite 520
Detroit, MI 48226
610-461-3548
800-234-1340
Fax: 800-875-1340
contact@omnigraphics.com
www.omnigraphics.com

Peter Ruffner, Co-Founder
Fred Ruffner, Co-Founder
Cancer Sourcebook for Women, Fourth Edition offers updated information about gynecologic cancers and other cancers of special concern to women, including breast cancer, cancers of the female reproductive organs, and cancers responsible for the highest number of deaths in women. It explains cancer risks-including lifestyle factors, inherited genetic abnormalities, and hormonal medications-and methods used to diagnose and treat cancer. *$84.00*
687 pages 5th Edition
ISBN 0-780808-67-6

8521 Cardiovascular Diseases and Disorders Sourcebook, 3rd Edition
Omnigraphics
615 Griswold Street
Suite 520
Detroit, MI 48226
610-461-3548
800-234-1340
Fax: 800-875-1340
contact@omnigraphics.com
www.omnigraphics.com

Peter Ruffner, Co-Founder
Fred Ruffner, Co-Founder
Cardiovascular Diseases and Disorders Sourcebook, Third Edition, provides information about the symptoms, diagnosis, and treatment heart diseases and vascular disorders. It includes demographic and statistical data, an overview of the cardiovascular system, a discussion of risk factors and prevention techniques, a look at cardiovascular concerns specific to women, and a report on current research initiatives. *$84.00*
687 pages Hard cover
ISBN 0-780807-39-6

8522 Childhood Cancer Survivors: A Practical Guide to Your Future
O'Reilly Media Inc
1005 Gravenstein Hwy N
Sebastopol, CA 95472-2811
707-827-7000
800-998-9938
Fax: 707-829-0104
order@oreilly.com
www.oreilly.com

Linda Lamb, Editor
Nancy Keene, Author
Wendy Hobbie, Co-Author
More than 250,000 people have survived childhood cancer - a cause for celebration. Authors Keene, Hobbie, and Ruccione chart the territory of long-term survivorship: relationships; overcoming employment or insurance discrimination; maximizing health; follow-up schedules; medical late effects. The stories of over sixty survivors - their challenges and triumphs - are told. Includes medical history record-keeper. *$27.95*
464 pages Paperback 1906
ISBN 0-596528-51-5

8523   Childhood Cancer: A Parent's Guide to Solid Tumor Cancers
O'Reilly Media Inc
1005 Gravenstein Highway North
Sebastopol, CA 95472

707-827-7000
800-889-8969
Fax: 707-829-0104
order@oreilly.com
www.oreilly.com

Childhood Cancer: A Parent's Guide to Solid Tumor Cancers features a wealth of resources for parents of children with solid tumor cancers, plus many stories of veteran parents. Parents will encounter medical facts simply explained, practical advice to ease their daily lives, and tools to be strong advocates for their child. Includes a passport to record patient's medical history. *$29.95*
560 pages Paperback
ISBN 0-596500-14-9

8524   Childhood Diseases and Disorders Sourcebook, 2nd Edition
Omnigraphics
615 Griswold Street
Suite 520
Detroit, MI 48226

610-461-3548
800-234-1340
Fax: 800-875-1340
contact@omnigraphics.com
www.omnigraphics.com

Peter Ruffner, Co-Founder
Fred Ruffner, Co-Founder
Basic consumer health information about medical problems often encountered in pre-adolescent children, including respiratory tract ailments, ear infections, sore throats, disorders of the skin and scalp, digestive and genitourinary diseases, infectious diseases, inflammatory disorders, chronic physical and developmental disorders, allergies, and more. *$84.00*
600 pages Hard cover
ISBN 0-780810-31-0

8525   Childhood Leukemia: A Guide for Families, Friends & Caregivers
O'Reilly Media Inc
1005 Gravenstein Hwy N
Sebastopol, CA 95472-2811

707-827-7000
800-998-9938
Fax: 707-829-0104
order@oreilly.com
www.oreilly.com

Linda Lamb, Editor
Nancy Keene, Author
The second edition of this comprehensive guide offers detailed and precise medical information for parents that includes day-to-day practical advice on how to cope with procedures, hospitalization, family and friends, school, and social, emotional, and financial issues. It features a wealth of tools for prents and contains significant updates on treatments and procedures. *$29.95*
528 pages 4th Edition 1910 •
ISBN 0-596500-15-7

8526   Children with Cerebral Palsy: A Parents' Guide
Woodbine House
6510 Bells Mill Road
Bethesda, MD 20817-1636

301-897-3570
800-843-7323
Fax: 301-897-5838
info@woodbinehouse.com
www.woodbinehouse.com

Irvin Shapell, Owner
Beth Binns, Special Marketing Manager
Sarah Glenner, Office Receptionist;
A classic primer for parents that provides a complete spetrum of information and compassionate advice about cerebral palsy and its effect on their child's development and education. *$18.95*
481 pages
ISBN 0-933149-82-4

8527   Chronic Fatigue Syndrome: Your Natural Gu ide to Healing with Diet, Herbs and Other Methods
Random House Publishing
1745 Broadway
3rd Floor
New York, NY 10019-4305

212-782-9000
Fax: 212-572-6066
ecustomerservice@randomhouse.com
www.randomhouse.com

Susanna Porter, Editor
Michael T Murray N.D.
Explains specific measures sufferers can take to improve stamina, mental energy, and physical abilities. *$15.00*
208 pages
ISBN 1-559584-90-6

8528   Coffee in the Cereal: The First Year with Multiple Sclerosis
Pathfinder Publishing

520-647-0158
800-977-2282
bill@pathfinderpublishing.com
www.pathfinderpublishing.com

Moorhead recounts the experience of her first year with multiple sclerosis with a vitality unique in the often gloomy world of personal medical histories. *$14.95*
96 pages
ISBN 0-934793-07-7

8529   Colon & Rectal Cancer: A Comprehensive Guide for Patients & Families
O'Reilly Media Inc
1005 Gravenstein Hwy N
Sebastopol, CA 95472-2811

707-827-7000
800-998-9938
Fax: 707-829-0104
order@oreilly.com
www.oreilly.com

Linda Lamb, Editor
Lorraine Johnston, Author
The fourth most common cancer, colon and rectal cancer is diagnosed in 130,000 new cases in the United States each year. Patients and families need uo-to-date and in-depth information to participate wisely in treatment decisions (e.g., knowing what sexual and fertility issues to discuss with the doctor before surgery). This book covers coping with tests and treatment side effects, caring for ostomies, finding supportt, and other practical issues. *$24.95*
544 pages Paperback 1999
ISBN 1-565926-33-1

8530   Colon Health: Key to a Vibrant Life
Norwalk Press
P.O.Box 190526
Boise, ID 83719-526

928-445-5567
Fax: 928-445-5567

Norman Walker MD, Editor
Includes complete glossary of terms and index of referrals.

8531   Complementary Alternative Medicine and Multiple Sclerosis
Demos Medical Publishing
11 West 42nd Street
15th Floor
New York, NY 10036

212-683-0072
800-532-8663
Fax: 212-683-0118
support@demosmedical.com
www.demosmedpub.com

Richard Winters, Executive Editor
Beth Kaufman Barry, Publisher
Noreen Henson, Executive Director of Demos Heal
Offers reliable information on the relevance, safety, and effectiveness of various alternative therapies that are not typically considered in discussions of MS management, yet are in widespread use. *$24.95*
304 pages
ISBN 1-932603-54-9

8532 **Conquering the Darkness: One Story of Recovering from a Brain Injury**
Paragon House
1925 Oakcrest Avenue
Suite 7
Saint Paul, MN 55113-2619
651-644-3087
800-447-3709
Fax: 651-644-0997
info@paragonhouse.com
www.paragonhouse.com

Rosemary Yokoi, Publicity Director
Gordon Anderson, Executive Director
Deborah Quinn, Author
The course of recovery from a brain injury by a woman who lived through it. *$15.95*
276 pages 1998
ISBN 1-557787-63-8

8533 **Coping with Cerebral Palsy**
Rosen Publishing
29 East 21st Street
New York, NY 10010
800-237-9932
Fax: 888-436-4643
www.rosenpublishing.com

Laura Anne Gilman, Author
This second edition book provides parents of children and adults with cerebral palsy the answers to more than 300 questions that have been carefully researched. It represents 40 years of experience by the author and is presented in a highly readable, jargon-free manner. *$31.95*
ISBN 0-823931-50-1

8534 **Curing MS: How Science is Solving the Mysteries of Multiple Sclerosis**
Random House Publishing
1745 Broadway
3rd Floor
New York, NY 10019-4305
212-782-9000
Fax: 212-572-6066
www.randomhouse.com

Howard L Weiner M.D., Author
Founder-director of the Multiple Sclerosis Center at Mass General Hospital discusses what ends up as a deconstruction of the last 30 years of his own and general MS research and of experience in treating patients with the puzzling disorder. Weiner summarizes what is currently known about treatments and the potential for a cure. *$14.95*
352 pages 1905
ISBN 0-307236-04-8

8535 **Cystic Fibrosis: A Guide for Patient and Family**
Lippincott Williams & Wilkins
16522 Hunters Green Parkway
PO Box 1620
Hagerstown, MD 21741-1620
301-223-2300
800-638-3030
Fax: 301-223-2400
orders@lww.com
www.lww.com

David M Orenstein MD, Author
Text is designed specifically for patients with cystic fibrosis and their families. Explains the disease process, outlines the fundamentals of diagnosing and screening, and addresses the challenges of treatment for those living with CF. Includes new material on carrier testing, infection control, and more. *$51.50*
448 pages 3rd Edition
ISBN 0-781741-52-1

8536 **Diabetes Sourcebook.**
Omnigraphics
615 Griswold Street
Suite 520
Detroit, MI 48226
610-461-3548
800-234-1340
Fax: 800-875-1340
contact@omnigraphics.com
www.omnigraphics.com

Peter Ruffner, Co-Founder
Fred Ruffner, Co-Founder

Diabetes Sourcebook, Fourth Edition contains updated information for people seeking to understand the risk factors, complications, and management of diabetes. It discusses medical interventions, including the use of insulin and oral diabetes medications, self-monitoring of blood glucose, and complementary and alternative therapies. *$84.00*
627 pages 4th Edition
ISBN 0-780810-05-1

8537 **Digestive Diseases & Disorders Sourcebook**
Omnigraphics
615 Griswold Street
Suite 520
Detroit, MI 48226
610-461-3548
800-234-1340
Fax: 800-875-1340
contact@omnigraphics.com
www.omnigraphics.com

Peter Ruffner, Co-Founder
Fred Ruffner, Co-Founder
Digestive Diseases and Disorders Sourcebook provides basic information for the layperson about common disorders of the upper and lower digestive tract. It also includes information about medications and recommendations for maintaining a healthy digestive tract in addition to a glossary of important terms and a directory of digestive diseases organizations are also provided. *$84.00*
323 pages Hard cover
ISBN 0-780803-27-5

8538 **Duchenne Muscular Dystrophy**
Oxford University Press
198 Madison Ave
New York, NY 10016-4308
212-726-6000
800-445-9714
Fax: 919-677-1303
custserv.us@oup.com

William Lamsback, Editor
Alan Emery, Author
Francesco Muntoni, Co-Author
Identification of the genetic defect responsible for Duchenne Muscular Dystrophy and isolation of the protein dystrophin have led to the development of new theories for the disease's pathogenesis. This title incorporates these advances from the field of molecular biology, and describes the resultant opportunities for screening, prenatal diagnosis, genetic counselling and management. *$135.00*
282 pages 3rd Edition 2003
ISBN 0-198515-31-6

8539 **Ear, Nose, and Throat Disorders Sourcebook**
Omnigraphics
615 Griswold Street
Suite 520
Detroit, MI 48226
610-461-3548
800-234-1340
Fax: 800-875-1340
contact@omnigraphics.com
www.omnigraphics.com

Peter Ruffner, Co-Founder
Fred Ruffner, Co-Founder
Ear, Nose and Throat Disorders Sourcebook, Second Edition, provides consumers with updated health information on the most common disorders of the ear, nose, and throat. The book also includes descriptions of current diagnostic tests, discussion of common surgical procedures, including cosmetic surgery on the nose and ears, a glossary of related medical terms, and a directory of sources for further help and information. *$84.00*
631 pages 2nd Edition
ISBN 0-780808-72-0

8540   Eating Disorders Sourcebook.
Omnigraphics
615 Griswold Street
Suite 520
Detroit, MI 48226
610-461-3548
800-234-1340
Fax: 800-875-1340
contact@omnigraphics.com
www.omnigraphics.com

Peter Ruffner, Co-Founder
Fred Ruffner, Co-Founder
Provides general imformation, causes and treatments of eating disorders. *$84.00*
557 pages 2nd Edition
ISBN 0-780809-48-2

8541   Educational Issues Among Children with Spina Bifida
Spina Bifida Association of America
1600 Wilson Boulevard
Suite 800
Arlington, VA 22209
202-944-3285
800-621-3141
Fax: 202-944-3295
sbaa@sbaa.org
www.sbaa.org

Ana Ximenes, Chair
Sara Struwe, President & CEO
Mark Bohay, National Web Initiatives & Development Manager
Children with spina bifida/ hydrocephalus often show unique learning strengths and weaknesses that affect their schoolwork. Parents and schools need to work together to help the young people meet their physical, social, emotional, and academic goals.

8542   Epilepsy, 199 Answers: A Doctor Responds to His Patients' Questions
Demos Medical Publishing
11 West 42nd Street
15th Floor
New York, NY 10036
212-683-0072
800-532-8663
Fax: 212-683-0118
support@demosmedical.com
www.demosmedpub.com

Richard Winters, Executive Editor
Beth Kaufman Barry, Publisher
Noreen Henson, Executive Director of Demos Heal
An epilepsy specialist answers questions about the causes, diagnosis, and treatments, and how to live and work with this brain disorder. Includes an epilepsy history timeline, patient health record form, resources, and a glossary. *$19.95*
180 pages
ISBN 1-932603-35-2

8543   Epilepsy: Patient and Family Guide
Demos Medical Publishing
11 West 42nd Street
15th Floor
New York, NY 10036
212-683-0072
800-532-8663
Fax: 212-683-0118
support@demosmedical.com
www.demosmedpub.com

Richard Winters, Executive Editor
Beth Kaufman Barry, Publisher
Noreen Henson, Executive Director of Demos Heal
A guide for adults with epilepsy and for parents of children with the disorder explains the nature and diversity of seizures, the risks and benefits of the various antiepileptic drugs, and medical and surgical therapies. *$16.95*
408 pages
ISBN 1-932603-41-7

8544   Ethnic Diseases Sourcebook
Omnigraphics
615 Griswold Street
Suite 520
Detroit, MI 48226
610-461-3548
800-234-1340
Fax: 800-875-1340
contact@omnigraphics.com
www.omnigraphics.com

Peter Ruffner, Co-Founder
Fred Ruffner, Co-Founder
Ethnic Diseases Sourcebook provides health information about genetic and chronic diseases that affect ethnic and racial minorities in the United States. Information about mental health services, women's health, and tips for improving health are also included, along with a glossary and a list of resources for additional help and informatio methods, treatment options, and current research initiatives. *$84.00*
648 pages Hard cover
ISBN 0-780803-36-7

8545   From Where I Sit: Making My Way with Cerebral Palsy
Scholastic
557 Broadway
New York, NY 10012-3962
124-484-2800
Fax: 212-343-6934
www.scholastic.com

Dick Robinson, Chairman & CEO
Maureen O'Connell, Executive Vice President, Chief
Kyle Good, Senior Vice President, Corporate
An autobiographical account of a young woman explores how it feels to live with cerebral palsy while struggling to have a full life despite the challenges facing her every day. *$13.00*
136 pages
ISBN 0-590395-84-X

8546   Genetics and Spina Bifida
Spina Bifida Association of America
1600 Wilson Boulevard
Suite 800
Arlington, VA 22209
202-944-3285
800-621-3141
Fax: 202-944-3295
sbaa@sbaa.org
www.sbaa.org

Ana Ximenes, Chair
Sara Struwe, President & CEO
Mark Bohay, National Web Initiatives & Development Manager
Spina bifida is a birth defect involving incomplete formation of the spine.

8547   Growing Up with Epilepsy: A Pratical Guide for Parents
Demos Medical Publishing
11 West 42nd Street
15th Floor
New York, NY 10036
212-683-0072
800-532-8663
Fax: 212-683-0118
support@demosmedical.com
www.demosmedpub.com

Richard Winters, Executive Editor
Beth Kaufman Barry, Publisher
Noreen Henson, Executive Director of Demos Heal
Developed to help parents with the uniques challenges that this disorder presents *$19.95*
168 pages
ISBN 1-888799-74-9

8548   Guide to Living with HIV Infection: Developed at the Johns Hopkins AIDS Clinic
Johns Hopkins Universty Press
2715 N Charles St
Baltimore, MD 21218-4363
410-516-6900
800-548-1784
Fax: 410-516-6998
webmaster@jhupress.jhu.edu
www.press.jhu.edu

William Brody, President
John G Bartlett, M.D., Author
Ann K Finkbeiner, Co-Author

A handbook and reference for people living with HIV infection and their families, friends, and caregivers. *$19.95*
408 pages 6th Edition
ISBN 0-801884-85-6

8549 Handbook of Chronic Fatigue Syndrome
John Wiley & Sons
1 Wiley Dr.
Somerset, NJ 08875-1272
732-469-4400
800-225-5945
Fax: 732-302-2300
onlinelibrary.wiley.com

Leonard A. Jason, Editor
Discusses diagnosis and treatment as well as the history, phenomenology, symptomatology, assessment, and pediatric and community issues. Introduces phase-based therapy and nutritional approaches. *$ 110.00*
794 pages 2003
ISBN 0-471415-12-1

8550 Handbook of Epilepsy
Lippincott, Williams & Wilkins
Philadelphia, PA 19106-3713
215-521-8300
800-777-2295
Fax: 301-824-7390

J Lippincott, CEO
Pocket-sized reference provides concise, up-to-date, clinically oriented reviews of each of the major areas of diagnosis and management of epilepsy. *$42.95*
272 pages
ISBN 0-781743-52-4

8551 Healthy Breathing
National Jewish Health
1400 Jackson St
Denver, CO 80206-2761
303-270-2708
877-225-5654
Fax: 303-398-1125
physicianline@njhealth.org
www.nationaljewish.org

Richard A. Schierburg, Chair
Robin Chotin, Vice Chair
Don Silversmith, Vice Chair
Offers patients with lung or respiratory disorders information on exercise and healthy breathing.

8552 Heart of the Mind
New World Library
14 Pamaron Way
Novato, CA 94949
415-884-2100
800-972-6657
Fax: 415-884-2199
ami@newworldlibrary.com
www.newworldlibrary.com
Provides common NLP problems and several new techniques.
208 pages
ISBN 1-577311-56-6

8553 Hepatitis Sourcebook
Omnigraphics
615 Griswold Street
Suite 520
Detroit, MI 48226
610-461-3548
800-234-1340
Fax: 800-875-1340
contact@omnigraphics.com
www.omnigraphics.com

Peter Ruffner, Co-Founder
Fred Ruffner, Co-Founder
Hepatitis Sourcebook provides basic consumer health information about hepatitis A, hepatitis B, hepatitis C, and other types of hepatitis, including autoimmune hepatitis, alcoholic hepatitis, nonalcoholic steatohepatitis, and toxin-induced hepatitis. It gives the facts about risk factors, prevention, transmission, screening and diagnostic methods, treatment options, and current research initiatives. *$84.00*
570 pages Hard cover
ISBN 0-780807-49-5

8554 Hip Function & Ambulation
Spina Bifida Association of America
1600 Wilson Boulevard
Suite 800
Arlington, VA 22209
202-944-3285
800-621-3141
Fax: 202-944-3295
sbaa@sbaa.org
www.sbaa.org

Ana Ximenes, Chair
Sara Struwe, President & CEO
Mark Bohay, National Web Initiatives & Development Manager
The ability to walk is important in our society, despite recent advances in wheelchair design and wheelchair accessibility. It also is a desire of children with spina bifida.

8555 Hydrocephalus: A Guide for Patients, Families & Friends
O'Reilly Media Inc
1005 Gravenstein Hwy N
Sebastopol, CA 95472-2811
707-827-7000
800-998-9938
Fax: 707-829-0104
order@oreilly.com
www.oreilly.com

Linda Lamb, Editor
Chuck Toporek, Author
Kellie Robinson, Author
Hydrocephalus is a life-threatening condition often referred to as, water on the brain, that is treated by surgical placement of a shunt system. Hydrocephalus: A Guide for Patients, Families and Friends educates families so they can select a skilled neurosurgeon, understand treatments, participate in care, know what symptoms need attention, discover where to turn for support, keep records needed for follow-up treatments, and make wise lifestyle choices. *$19.95*
379 pages Paperback 1999
ISBN 1-565924-10-X

8556 Hypertension Sourcebook
Omnigraphics
615 Griswold Street
Suite 520
Detroit, MI 48226
610-461-3548
800-234-1340
Fax: 800-875-1340
contact@omnigraphics.com
www.omnigraphics.com

Peter Ruffner, Co-Founder
Fred Ruffner, Co-Founder
This Sourcebook describes the known causes and risk factors associated with essential (or primary) hypertension, secondary hypertension, prehypertension, and other hypertensive disorders. The book also provides information about blood pressure management strategies, including dietary changes, weight loss, exercise, and medications. *$ 84.00*
588 pages Hard cover
ISBN 0-780806-74-0

8557 Immune System Disorders Sourcebook.
Omnigraphics
615 Griswold Street
Suite 520
Detroit, MI 48226
610-461-3548
800-234-1340
Fax: 800-875-1340
contact@omnigraphics.com
www.omnigraphics.com

Peter Ruffner, Co-Founder
Fred Ruffner, Co-Founder
Immune System Disorders Sourcebook provides information about inherited, acquired, and autoimmune diseases including primary immune deficiency, acquired immunodeficiency syndrome (AIDS), lupus, multiple sclerosis, type one diabetes, rheumatoid arthritis, and Graves' disease. Tips for coping with an immune disorder, caregiving, and treatments are presented along with a glossary and directory of additional resourcesories of additional resources. *$84.00*
643 pages 2nd Edition
ISBN 0-780807-48-8

8558 Informed Touch; A Clinician's Guide To The Evaluation Of Myofascial Disorders
Inner Traditions/Bear And Company
One Park Street
PO Box 388
Rochester, VT 05767-0388   802-767-3174
                                          800-246-8648
                                     Fax: 802-767-3726
                     customerservice@innertraditions.com
                              www.innertraditions.com

Rob Meadows, VP Sales/Marketing
Jessica Arsenault, Sales Associate
Donna Finando, LAc, LMT, Author
A Clinician's guide to the evaluation and treatment of myofascial disorders. *$30.00*
224 pages
ISBN 0-892817-40-5

8559 Injured Mind, Shattered Dreams: Brian's Survival from a Severe Head Injury
Brookline Books
8 Trumbull Rd,
Northampton, MA 01060-4533   413-584-0184
                                          800-666-2665
                                     Fax: 413-584-6184
                              brbooks@yahoo.com
                            www.brooklinebooks.com
Brian, headed for normal adulthood, crashes his car and suffers a severe head injury. This book speaks to the issues in his recovery and the victory a family can achieve through caring advocacy and faith. *$17.95*
Paperback
ISBN 0-91479 -95-6

8560 Interdisciplinary Clinical Assessment of Young Children with Developmental Disabilities
Brookes Publishing
P.O.Box 10624
Baltimore, MD 21285-0624   410-337-9580
                                          800-638-3775
                                     Fax: 410-337-8539
                         custserv@brookespublishing.com
                            www.brookespublishing.com

Paul H. Brookes, Chairman
Jeffrey D. Brookes, President
Melissa A. Behm, Executive Vice President
Offers insight from veteran team members on interdisciplinary team assessments. Professionals organizing a team as well as students preparing for practice will find advice on how practitioners gather information, approach assessment, make decisions, and face the challenges of their individual fields. Includes case studies and appendix of photocopiable questionnaires for clinicians and parents. *$44.95*
796 pages Hardcover
ISBN 1-557664-50-1

8561 Introduction to Spina Bifida
Spina Bifida Association of America
1600 Wilson Boulevard
Suite 800
Arlington, VA 22209   202-944-3285
                                          800-621-3141
                                     Fax: 202-944-3295
                                   sbaa@sbaa.org
                                      www.sbaa.org

Ana Ximenes, Chair
Sara Struwe, President & CEO
Mark Bohay, National Web Initiatives & Development Manager
An aid for parents, family and nonmedical people who care for a child with spina bifida. *$7.00*

8562 It's All in Your Head: The Link Between Mercury Amalgams and Illness
Avery Publishing Group
299 W. Houston Street
New York, NY 10014   212-859-1100
                                     Fax: 212-859-1150
                              info@programexchange.com
Dr. Higgins's critique of the use of mercury, a toxic element and environmental hazard, in dentistry. For those suffering mercury

poisoning, the book examines a number of conventional and alternative treatments.
208 pages

8563 Joslin Guide to Diabetes: A Program for Managing Your Treatment
Joslin Diabetes Center
1 Joslin Pl
Boston, MA 02215-5306   617-732-2400
                                     Fax: 617-732-2452
                                      www.joslin.org

Richard S Beaser, M.D., Author
Amy Campbell,Ms, RD, CDE, Co-Author
Ralph M. James, Chairperson of the Board
Discusses the causes of diabetes, the role of diet and exercise, meal planning and complications. Also provide information on drawing blood, mixing and injecting insulin, special challenges, living with diabetes. *$16.95*
352 pages Revised Edition

8564 Journey to Well: Learning to Live After Spinal Cord Injury
Altarfire Publishing
1835 Oak Terrace
Newcastle, CA 95658
Margie Williams, Author
The author's close-up view of what life is like during and after such an incident, including her experience with institutional medicine and insurance companies (for better and for worse), and her determined - and ultimately successful - effort to rehabilitate herself and reconstruct her life. *$15.95*
251 pages
ISBN 0-965555-82-8

8565 Ketogenic Diet: A Treatment for Children and Others with Epilepsy
Demos Medical Publishing
11 West 42nd Street
15th Floor
New York, NY 10036   212-683-0072
                                          800-532-8663
                                     Fax: 212-683-0118
                           support@demosmedical.com
                              www.demosmedpub.com

Richard Winters, Executive Editor
Beth Kaufman Barry, Publisher
Noreen Henson, Executive Director of Demos Heal
Patient education reference on the use of the ketogenic diet to conrol epilepsy in children. *$24.95*
328 pages Paperback
ISBN 1-932603-18-2

8566 Latex Allergy in Spina Bifida Patients
Spina Bifida Association of America
1600 Wilson Boulevard
Suite 800
Arlington, VA 22209   202-944-3285
                                          800-621-3141
                                     Fax: 202-944-3295
                                   sbaa@sbaa.org
                                      www.sbaa.org

Ana Ximenes, Chair
Sara Struwe, President & CEO
Mark Bohay, National Web Initiatives & Development Manager
The Spina Bifida Association (SBA) serves adults and children who live with the challenges of Spina Bifida.

8567 Learning Among Children with Spina Bifida
Spina Bifida Association of America
1600 Wilson Boulevard
Suite 800
Arlington, VA 22209   202-944-3285
                                          800-621-3141
                                     Fax: 202-944-3295
                                   sbaa@sbaa.org
                                      www.sbaa.org

Ana Ximenes, Chair
Sara Struwe, President & CEO
Mark Bohay, National Web Initiatives & Development Manager

The Spina Bifida Association (SBA) serves adults and children who live with the challenges of Spina Bifida.

8568 Let's Talk About Having Asthma
Rosen Publishing
29 E 21st St
New York, NY 10010-6209

212-420-1600
800-237-9932
Fax: 888-436-4643
www.rosenpublishing.com

Marianna Johnstone, Co-Author
Elizabeth Weitzman, Co-Author
Kelly Chambers, Marketing Assistant
Many kids suffer from asthma, which can overtake them suddenly, causing them terror as they struggle for breath. This book talks about the causes and treatments for asthma, as well as precautions sufferers should take. *$21.95*
ISBN 0-823950-32-8

8569 Leukemia Sourcebook
Omnigraphics
615 Griswold Street
Suite 520
Detroit, MI 48226

610-461-3548
800-234-1340
Fax: 800-875-1340
contact@omnigraphics.com
www.omnigraphics.com

Peter Ruffner, Co-Founder
Fred Ruffner, Co-Founder
This Sourcebook provides health information about adult and childhood leukemias focusing on the diagnosis and treatments for leukemia, including chemotherapy, radiation, drug therapy, and transplantation of peripheral blood stem cells or marrow. Also included are tips for nutrition, pain and fatigue control, recognizing possible long-term and late effects of leukemia treatment, along with a glossary and directories of additional resources. *$84.00*
564 pages Hard cover
ISBN 0-780806-27-6

8570 Life After Trauma: A Workbook for Healing
Guilford Press
72 Spring St
New York, NY 10012-4019

212-431-9800
800-365-7006
Fax: 212-966-6708
info@guilford.com
www.guilford.com

Denaour Rosenbloom, Author
Mary Beth Williams, Co-Author
Barbar E Watkins, Co-Author
A self-help book on how to deal with trauma. *$19.95*
300 pages Paperback 1910
ISBN 1-606236-08-6

8571 Life Line
National Hydrocephalus Foundation
12413 Centralia St
Lakewood, CA 90715-1653

562-402-3523
888-857-3434
888-260-1789
Fax: 562-924-6666

Debbi Fields, Executive Director
Michael Fields, President/Treasurer
Jaynie Dunn, Secretary
National Hydrocephalus Foundation quarterly newsletter. *$35.00*
12 pages Quarterly

8572 Lipomas & Lipomyelomeningocele
Spina Bifida Association of America
1600 Wilson Boulevard
Suite 800
Arlington, VA 22209

202-944-3285
800-621-3141
Fax: 202-944-3295
sbaa@sbaa.org
www.sbaa.org

Ana Ximenes, Chair
Sara Struwe, President & CEO
Mark Bohay, National Web Initiatives & Development Manager
The Spina Bifida Association (SBA) serves adults and children who live with the challenges of Spina Bifida.

8573 Liver Disorders Sourcebook
Omnigraphics
615 Griswold Street
Suite 520
Detroit, MI 48226

610-461-3548
800-234-1340
Fax: 800-875-1340
contact@omnigraphics.com
www.omnigraphics.com

Peter Ruffner, Co-Founder
Fred Ruffner, Co-Founder
Liver Disorders Sourcebook contains basic consumer health information about the liver, how it works, and how to keep it healthy through diet, vaccination, and other preventive care measures. Readers will learn about the symptoms and treatment options for such diseases as hepatitis, primary biliary cirrhosis, Wilson's disease, hemochromatosis, liver failure, cancer of the liver, and disorders related to drugs and other toxins. *$84.00*
580 pages Hard cover
ISBN 0-780803-83-1

8574 Living Beyond Multiple Sclerosis: A Woman's Guide
Hunter House
PO Box 2914
Alameda, CA 94501-914

510-865-5282
800-266-5592
Fax: 510-865-4295
www.hunterhouse.com

Judith Lynn Nichols, Author
Lily Jung, Foreword
This collection of e-mail conversations provides anecdotal and personal information contributed by women with multiple sclerosis. *$14.95*
256 pages
ISBN 0-897932-93-6

8575 Living Well with Asthma
Guilford Press
72 Spring St
New York, NY 10012-4019

212-431-9800
800-365-7006
Fax: 212-966-6708
info@guilford.com
www.guilford.com

Cynthia L Divino, Author
Michael R Freedman, Co-Author
Samuel J Rosenberg, Co-Author
Meeting the needs of a growing clinical population, this reader-friendly, practical book offers a lifeline to asthma patients attempting to understand and cope with the psychological ramifications of their illness and its treatment. *$15.95*
213 pages Paperback
ISBN 1-572300-51-4

8576 Living Well with Chronic Fatigue Syndrome and Fibromyalgia
Harper Collins Publishers
10 E 53rd St
New York, NY 10022-5244

212-207-7901
800-242-7737
Fax: 212-702-2586
spsales@harpercollins.com
www.harpercollins.com

Mary J Shomon, Author

From the author of Living Well With Hypothyroidism, a comprehensive guide to the diagnosis and treatment of chronic fatigue syndrome and fibromyalgia—vital help for the millions of people suffering from pain, fatigue, and sleep problems. *$14.95*
416 pages 2004
ISBN 0-060521-25-2

8577   Living Well with HIV and AIDS
Bull Publishing
PO Box 1377
Boulder, CO 80306-1377
303-545-6350
800-676-2855
Fax: 303-545-6354
www.bullpub.com

David Sobel, MPH, Author
Virginia Gonzalez MPH, Co-Author
Daina Laurent MPH, Co-Author
New drugs and drug combinations have turned HIV/AIDS into a long-term illness rather than a death sentence. Practical advice on mental adjustments and physical vigilance is outlined. *$18.95*
245 pages 3rd Edition
ISBN 0-923521-52-6

8578   Living With Spinal Cord Injury Series
Fanlight Productions C/O Icarus Films
32 Court St.
21st Floor
Brooklyn, NY 11201
718-488-8900
800-876-1710
Fax: 718-488-8642
info@fanlight.com
www.fanlight.com

Barry Corbet, Producer
Jonathan Miller, President
Meredith Miller, Sales Manager
The producer, himself injured in a helicopter crash, brings a unique perspective to this classic three-part series on coming to terms with spinal cord injury. These films offer enduring proof that a tough break doesn't have to mean a ruined life. *$210.00*
VHS 1973

8579   Living with Brain Injury: A Guide for Families
Delmar Cengage Learning
PO Box 6904
Florence, KY 41022-6904
800-354-9706
Fax: 800-487-8488

Richard C Senelick MD, Author
Karla Dougherty, Co-Author
A consumer text to aid people living with brain-injured survivors, includes facts on neuroplasticity, experimental rehabilitation research, and the process of rehabilitation itself. *$19.95*
225 pages Softcover 2001
ISBN 1-891525-09-3

8580   Living with Spina Bifida: A Guide for Families and Professionals
University of North Carolina at Chapel Hill
116 S Boundary St
Chapel Hill, NC 27514-3808
919-966-3561
800-848-6224
Fax: 919-962-2704
uncpress@unc.edu
www.uncpress.unc.edu
Adrian Sandler MD, Author
A handbook that addresses patients' biopsychosocial and developmental needs from birth through adolescence and into adulthood. Sandler's holistic approach encourages families to focus more on the child and less on the disability while providing abundant information about this condition. *$20.95*
296 pages 2004
ISBN 0-807855-47-8

8581   Lung Cancer: Making Sense of Diagnosis, Treatment, and Options
O'Reilly Media Inc
1005 Gravenstein Hwy N
Sebastopol, CA 95472-2811
707-827-7000
800-998-9938
Fax: 707-829-0104
order@oreilly.com
www.oreilly.com

Linda Lamb, Editor
Lorraine Johnston, Author
Straightforward language and the words of patients and their families are the hallmarks of this book on the number one cancer killer in the US. Written by a widely respected author and patient advocate, Lung Cancer: Making Sense of Diagnosis, Treatment, & Options has been meticulously reviewed by top medical experts and physicians. Readers will find medical facts simply explained, advice to ease their daily life, and tools to be strong advocates for themselves or a family member. *$ 27.95*
530 pages Paperback 2001
ISBN 0-596500-02-5

8582   Lung Disorders Sourcebook
Omnigraphics
615 Griswold Street
Suite 520
Detroit, MI 48226
610-461-3548
800-234-1340
Fax: 800-875-1340
contact@omnigraphics.com
www.omnigraphics.com

Peter Ruffner, Co-Founder
Fred Ruffner, Co-Founder
Lung Disorders Sourcebook offers information about specific types of lung disorders, including diagnosis, treatment, and prevention issues. The book offers advice for preventing some types lung disorder that are acquired by asbestos, radon, and other environmental exposures. *$84.00*
657 pages Hard cover
ISBN 0-780803-39-8

8583   Lupus: Alternative Therapies That Work
Inner Traditions
PO Box 388
Rochester
VT, 05 0388-802-
800-246-8648
802-767-3726
TTY: customerserv
info@innertraditions.com
www.innertraditions.com

Sharon Moore, Author
A comprehensive guise to noninvasive, nontoxic therapies for lupus - written by a lupus survivor. *$14.95*
256 pages 2000
ISBN 0-892818-89-1

8584   MAGIC Touch
MAGIC Foundation for Children's Growth
6645 North Ave
Oak Park, IL 60302-1057
708-383-0808
800-362-4423
Fax: 708-383-0899
mary@magicfoundation.org
www.magicfoundation.org

Mary Andrews, CEO
Dianne Kremidas, Executive Director
Pam Pentaris, Office Manager
Provides support and education regarding growth disorders in children and related adult disorders, including adult GHD. Dedicated to helping children whose physical growth is affected be a medical problem by assisting families of afflicted children through local support groups, public education/awareness, newsletters, specialty divisions and programs for the children.
36-40 pages Quarterly

8585 Management of Autistic Behavior
Sage Publications
2455 Teller Road
Thousand Oaks, CA 91320   805-499-0721
                                  800-818-7243
                            Fax: 805-499-0871
                             info@sagepub.com
                             www.sagepub.com
Sara Miller McCune, Founder, Publisher, Executive Chairman
Blaise R Simqu, President & CEO
Tracey A. Ozmina, Executive Vice President & Chief Operating Officer
Comprehensive and practical book that tells what works best with specific problems. *$51.00*
450 pages Paperback
ISBN 0-890791-96-1

8586 Management of Genetic Syndromes
John Wiley & Sons
111 River St
Hoboken, NJ 07030-5774   201-748-6000
                                  201-748-6088
                             info@wiley.com
Suzanne B Cassidy, Editor
Judith E Allanson, Editor
Edited by two of the field's most highly esteemed experts, this landmark volume provides: A precise reference of the physical manifestations of common genetic syndromes, clearly written for professionals and families, Extensive updates, particularly in sections on diagnostic criteria and diagnostic testing, pathogenesis, and management, A tried-and-tested, user-friendly format, with each chapter including information on incidence, etiology and pathogenesis, diagnostic criteria and testing, and d *$204.95*
720 pages 3rd Edition
ISBN 0-470191-41-5

8587 Managing Post Polio: A Guide to Living Well with Post Polio
ABI Professional Publications
PO Box 149
St Petersburg, FL 33731-149   727-556-0950
                                       800-551-7776
                                 Fax: 727-556-2560
                                 www.abipropub.com
Lauro S Halstead MD, Editor
Edited by Lauro S. Halstead, M.D., Managing Post-Polio, 2nd Edition, provides a comprehensive overview dealing with the medical, psychological, vocational, and many other challenges of living with post-polio syndrome. With contributions from over 15 healthcare professionals, the majority of whom are polio survivors themselves, Managing Post-Polio distills and summarizes the wealth of information presented from over the past 20 plus years.
256 pages
ISBN 1-886236-17-8

8588 Meniere's Disease
Vestibular Disorders Association
5018 NE 15th Avenue
Portland, OR 97211   800-837-8428
                       Fax: 503-229-8064
                        info@vestibular.org
                        www.vestibular.org
P. Ashley Wackym, Chair
Cynthia Ryan MBA, Executive Director
Tony Staser, Development Director
VEDA's website contains a wealth of information on the symptoms, diagnosis and treatment of various types of vestibular disorders. *$5.00*

8589 Menopause without Medicine
Hunter House
PO Box 2914
Alameda, CA 94501-914   510-865-5282
                                  800-266-5592
                            Fax: 510-865-4295
                            www.hunterhouse.com
Linda Ojeda PhD, Author

Menopause Without Medicine provides complete information on the symptoms of menopause - hot flashes, fatigue, sexual changes, depression and osteoporosis - and how to alleviate them. *$18.95*
304 pages 5th Edition
ISBN 0-897934-05-3

8590 Movement Disorders Sourcebook
Omnigraphics
615 Griswold Street
Suite 520
Detroit, MI 48226   610-461-3548
                             800-234-1340
                        Fax: 800-875-1340
                        contact@omnigraphics.com
                        www.omnigraphics.com
Peter Ruffner, Co-Founder
Fred Ruffner, Co-Founder
This Sourcebook provides health information about neurological movement disorders, their symptoms, causes, diagnostic tests, and treatments. Readers will learn about Essential Tremor, Parkinson's Disease, Dystonia, and many other early-onset and adult-onset movement disorders. Information about mobility and assistive technology aids is included, along with a glossary and a listing of additional resources. *$84.00*
600 pages Hard cover
ISBN 0-780810-34-1

8591 Multiple Sclerosis and Having a Baby
Inner Traditions
PO Box 388
Rochester, VT 05767-0388   802-767-3174
                                     800-246-8648
                               Fax: 802-767-3726
                        customerservice@innertraditions.com
                               www.innertraditions.com
Judy Graham, Author
Everything you need to know about conception, pregnancy and parenthood. *$12.95*
160 pages 2001
ISBN 0-892817-88-7

8592 Multiple Sclerosis: 300 Tips for Making Life Easier
Demos Medical Publishing
11 West 42nd Street
15th Floor
New York, NY 10036   212-683-0072
                             800-532-8663
                        Fax: 212-683-0118
                        support@demosmedical.com
                        www.demosmedpub.com
Richard Winters, Executive Editor
Beth Kaufman Barry, Publisher
Noreen Henson, Executive Director of Demos Heal
This latest book in the Making Life Easier series features tip, techniques and shortcuts for conserving time and energy so you can do more of the things you want to do. These tips should help increase the number of good days you have while encouraging you to develop your own techniques for making life easier. *$16.95*
128 pages
ISBN 1-932603-21-2

8593 Multiple Sclerosis: A Guide for Families
Demos Medical Publishing
11 West 42nd Street
15th Floor
New York, NY 10036   212-683-0072
                             800-532-8663
                        Fax: 212-683-0118
                        support@demosmedical.com
                        www.demosmedpub.com
Richard Winters, Executive Editor
Beth Kaufman Barry, Publisher
Noreen Henson, Executive Director of Demos Heal
Guide for living and coping with multiple sclerosis. *$24.95*
256 pages
ISBN 1-932603-10-7

8594 Multiple Sclerosis: A Guide for the Newly Diagnosed
Demos Medical Publishing
11 West 42nd Street
15th Floor
New York, NY 10036

212-683-0072
800-532-8663
Fax: 212-683-0118
support@demosmedical.com
www.demosmedpub.com

Richard Winters, Executive Editor
Beth Kaufman Barry, Publisher
Noreen Henson, Executive Director of Demos Heal
A must-have title for anyone who has recently been diagnosed with MS and a good idea for family members and friends. *$19.95*
256 pages
ISBN 1-932603-27-1

8595 Multiple Sclerosis: The Guide to Treatment and Management
Demos Medical Publishing
11 West 42nd Street
15th Floor
New York, NY 10036

212-683-0072
800-532-8663
Fax: 212-683-0118
support@demosmedical.com
www.demosmedpub.com

Richard Winters, Executive Editor
Beth Kaufman Barry, Publisher
Noreen Henson, Executive Director of Demos Heal
A current guide to modern therapies. *$24.95*
216 pages
ISBN 1-932603-15-4

8596 Muscular Dystrophies
Oxford University Press
198 Madison Avenue
New York, NY 10016

212-726-6000
800-445-9714
Fax: 919-677-1303
custserv.us@oup.com
www.oup.com

Alan E.H. Emery, Author
Describes the opportunities for management of more than 30 types of MD through respiratory care, physiotherapy and surgical correction of contractures, and examines the potential for effective treatment utilizing the new techniques of gene and cell therapy *$165.00*
330 pages
ISBN 0-192632-91-4

8597 Muscular Dystrophy in Children: A Guide for Families
Demos Medical Publishing
11 West 42nd Street
15th Floor
New York, NY 10036

212-683-0072
800-532-8663
Fax: 212-683-0118
support@demosmedical.com

Richard Winters, Executive Editor
Beth Kaufman Barry, Publisher
Noreen Henson, Executive Director of Demos Heal
Defines the available medical options at every stage of the disease and offers guidance even when it may seem that little or nothing can be done. Includes a glossary and suggestions for furhter reading. *$19.95*
144 pages Paperback
ISBN 1-888799-33-1

8598 Muscular Dystrophy: The Facts
Oxford University Press
198 Madison Avenue
New York, NY 10016

212-726-6000
800-445-9714
Fax: 919-677-1303
custserv.us@oup.com
www.oup.com

Peter Harper, Author

A good first book for individuals and families faced with the likelihood or reality of a muscular dystrophy diagnosis. *$22.50*
178 pages
ISBN 0-192632-17-5

8599 My House is Killing Me! The Home Guide for Families with Allergies and Asthma
Johns Hopkins University Press
2175 N Charles St
Baltimore, MD 21218-4363

410-516-6900
800-548-1784
Fax: 410-516-6968
webmaster@jhupress.jhu.edu
www.press.jhu.edu

Jeffrey C May, Author
Jonathan M Samet, M.D., Foreword
Kathleen Keane, Director
Chemical consultant May describes where and how the various parts of a residence can cause temporary or chronic illness for those with allergies or other sensitivities. *$20.95*
352 pages
ISBN 0-801867-30-9

8600 Neuropsychiatry of Epilepsy
Cambridge University Press
100 Brookhill Dr
West Nyack, NY 10994

845-353-7500
845-353-4141
www.cambridge.org

Michael R Trimble, Editor
Bettina Schmitz, Editor
Covers the practical implications of ongoing research, and offers a diagnostic and management perspective. Topics include cognitive aspects, nonepileptic attacks, and clinical aspects. For professionals treating epileptic patients. *$104.00*
232 pages 2nd Edition 1911
ISBN 0-521154-69-7

8601 Nick Joins In
Spina Bifida Association of America
1600 Wilson Boulevard
Suite 800
Arlington, VA 22209

202-944-3285
800-621-3141
Fax: 202-944-3295
sbaa@sbaa.org
www.sbaa.org

Ana Ximenes, Chair
Sara Struwe, President & CEO
Mark Bohay, National Web Initiatives & Development Manager
When Nick, who is in a wheelchair, enters a regular classroom for the first time, he realizes that he has much to contribute. *$17.00*

8602 No More Allergies
Random House
1745 Broadway
3rd Floor
New York, NY 10019-4305

212-782-9000
Fax: 212-572-6066
www.randomhouse.com

Markus Dohle, CEO
Gary Null PhD, Author
Null redefines a health problem that afflicts 40 million Americans: More than mere hay fever, contemporary allergic reactions include chronic fatigue syndrome, Alzheimer's disease, and even HIV infection. These conditions, he explains, occur when our immune systems break down. This ground-breaking book now prescribes effective solutions. *$23.00*
464 pages 1992
ISBN 0-679743-10-1

8603 No Time for Jello: One Family's Experience
Brookline Books
8 Trumbull Rd,
Northampton, MA 01060-4533

413-584-0184
800-666-2665
Fax: 413-584-6184
brbooks@yahoo.com
www.brooklinebooks.com

One family's story of their attempts to remediate and cure the effects of a cerebral palsied condition the oldest son was born with. The Bratts traveled traditional routes, through distinguished medical centers in Boston, and nontraditional routes in a search for treatments that would help their son. *$17.95*

Softcover
ISBN 0-91479 -56-5

8604 Nocturnal Asthma
National Jewish Health
1400 Jackson Street
Denver, CO 80206
303-270-2708
877-225-5654
Fax: 303-398-1125
allstetterw@njc.org
nationaljewish.org

Rich Schierburg, Chair
Robin Chotin, Vice Chair
Michael Salem, M.D., President and CEO
Offers information to patients about how to understand and manage asthma at night.

8605 Obesity
Spina Bifida Association of America
1600 Wilson Boulevard
Suite 800
Arlington, VA 22209
202-944-3285
800-621-3141
Fax: 202-944-3295
sbaa@sbaa.org
www.sbaa.org

Ana Ximenes, Chair
Sara Struwe, President & CEO
Mark Bohay, National Web Initiatives & Development Manager
The Spina Bifida Association (SBA) serves adults and children who live with the challenges of Spina Bifida. *$8.00*

8606 Obesity Sourcebook
Omnigraphics
615 Griswold Street
Suite 520
Detroit, MI 48226
610-461-3548
800-234-1340
Fax: 800-875-1340
contact@omnigraphics.com
www.omnigraphics.com

Peter Ruffner, Co-Founder
Fred Ruffner, Co-Founder
Discusses diseases and other problems associated with obesity. *$78.00*
376 pages
ISBN 0-780803-33-6

8607 Occulta
Spina Bifida Association of America
1600 Wilson Boulevard
Suite 800
Arlington, VA 22209
202-944-3285
800-621-3141
Fax: 202-944-3295
sbaa@sbaa.org
www.sbaa.org

Ana Ximenes, Chair
Sara Struwe, President & CEO
Mark Bohay, National Web Initiatives & Development Manager
The Spina Bifida Association (SBA) serves adults and children who live with the challenges of Spina Bifida. *$8.00*

8608 Official Patient's Sourcebook on Bell's Palsy
Icon Group International
9606 Tierra Grande Street
Suite 205
San Diego, CA 92126
Fax: 858-635-9414
orders@icongroupbooks.com
www.icongroupbooks.com
Provides patients with guidance on where and how to look for information covering virtually all topics related to bell's palsy (also Antoni's Palsy; facial nerve palsy; facial palsy; facial paralysis; idiopathic facial palsy; idiopathic facial paralysis), from the essentials to the most advanced areas of research. *$24.95*
ISBN 0-597835-20-9

8609 Official Patient's Sourcebook on Cystic Fibrosis
Icon Group International
9606 Tierra Grande Street
Suite 205
San Diego, CA 92126
Fax: 858-635-9414
orders@icongroupbooks.com
icongroupbooks.com
For parents who have decided to make education and research an integral part of the treatment process. Although it also gives information useful to doctors, caregivers and other health professionals, it tells paretns where and how to look for information covering virtually all topics related to cystic fibrosis (also fbrocystic disease of pancreas; mucosis; mucoviscidosis; pancreatic fibrosis), from the essentials to the most advanced areas of research. *$28.95*
356 pages
ISBN 0-597831-46-7

8610 Official Patient's Sourcebook on Muscular Dystrophy
Icon Group International
9606 Tierra Grande Street
Suite 205
San Diego, CA 92126
Fax: 858-635-9414
orders@icongroupbooks.com
icongroupbooks.com
Created for patients who have decided to make education and research an integral part of the treatment process. Although it also gives information useful to doctors, caregivers and other health professionals, it tells patients where and how to look for information covering virtually all topics related to muscular dystrophy. *$24.95*
268 pages
ISBN 0-597832-10-2

8611 Official Patient's Sourcebook on Osteoporosis
Icon Group International
9606 Tierra Grande Street
Suite 205
San Diego, CA 92126
Fax: 858-635-9414
orders@icongroupbooks.com
icongroupbooks.com
Provides patients with guidance on where and how to look for information covering virtually all topics related to bell's palsy (also Antoni's Palsy; Facial Nerve Palsy; Facial palsy; Facial Paralysis; Idiopathic Facial Palsy; Idiopathic facial paralysis), from the essentials to the most advanced areas of research. *$34.95*
ISBN 0-597833-04-4

8612 Official Patient's Sourcebook on Post-Polio Syndrome: A Revised and Updated Directory
Icon Group International
9606 Tierra Grande Street
Suite 205
San Diego, CA 92126
Fax: 858-635-9414
orders@icongroupbooks.com
icongroupbooks.com
A sourcebook created for patients who have decided to make education and Internet-based research an integral part of the treatment process. Although it gives information useful to doctors, caregivers and other health professionals, it also tells patients where and how to look for information covering virtually all topics related to post-polio syndrome, from the essentials to the most advanced areas of research. *$28.95*
124 pages
ISBN 0-597835-31-4

8613 Official Patient's Sourcebook on Primary Pulmonary Hypertension
Icon Group International
9606 Tierra Grande Street
Suite 205
San Diego, CA 92126
Fax: 858-635-9414
orders@icongroupbooks.com
icongroupbooks.com
Provides patients with guidance on where and how to look for information covering virtually all topics related to primary pulmonary hypertension (also familial primary pulmonary hypertension; idiopathic pulmonary hypertension; primary obliterative pulmonary vascular disease; primary pulmonary vas-

cular disease; and pulmonary hypertension), from the essentials to the most advanced areas of research. *$24.95*
ISBN 0-597831-54-8

8614 Official Patient's Sourcebook on Pulmonary Fibrosis
Icon Group International
9606 Tierra Grande Street
Suite 205
San Diego, CA 92126   Fax: 858-635-9414
                           orders@icongroupbooks.com
                           icongroupbooks.com
Provides patients with guidance on where and how to look for information covering virtually all topics related to idiopathic pulmonary fibrosis (also alveolocapillary block; cryptogenic fibrosing alveolitis; diffuse fibrosing alveolitis; fibrosing alveolitis; Hamman-Rich syndrome; and idiopathic diffuse interstitial pulmonary fibrosis), from the essentials to the most advanced areas of research. *$24.95*
ISBN 0-597831-65-3

8615 Official Patient's Sourcebook on Scoliosis
Icon Group International
9606 Tierra Grande Street
Suite 205
San Diego, CA 92126   Fax: 858-635-9414
                           orders@icongroupbooks.com
                           icongroupbooks.com
Provides patients with guidance on where and how to look for information covering virtually all topics related to scoliosis (also Idiopathic scoliosis; Kyphoscoliosis; Paralytic scoliosis; Sciatic scoliosis), from the essentials to the most advanced areas of research. *$28.95*
ISBN 0-597829-90-X

8616 Official Patient's Sourcebook on Sickle Cell Anemia
Icon Group International
9606 Tierra Grande Street
Suite 205
San Diego, CA 92126   Fax: 858-635-9414
                           orders@icongroupbooks.com
                           icongroupbooks.com
Provides patients with guidance on where and how to look for information covering virtually all topics related to sickle cell anemia (also Hb S disease; Hemoglobin S disease; Hemoglobin SS disease; sickle cell disease; sickle cell trait), from the essentials to the most advanced areas of research. *$28.95*
ISBN 0-597831-57-2

8617 Official Patient's Sourcebook on Ulcerative Colitis
Icon Group International
9606 Tierra Grande Street
Suite 205
San Diego, CA 92126   Fax: 858-635-9414
                           orders@icongroupbooks.com
                           icongroupbooks.com
Provides patients with guidance on where and how to look for information covering virtually all topics related to ulcerative colitis (also Chronic Non-Specific Ulcerative Colitis; Colitis Gravis; Idiopathic Non-Specific Ulcerative Colitis; Idiopathic proctocolitis; Inflammatory bowel disease (IBD); Nonspecific ulcerative colitis), from the essentials to the most advanced areas of research. *$34.95*
ISBN 0-597834-09-1

8618 One Day at a Time: Children Living with Leukemia
Gareth Stevens Publishing
111 East 14th Street
Suite #349
New York, NY 10003   800-542-2595
                           Fax: 877-542-2596
                           customerservice@gspub.com
                           www.garethstevens.com
Focus on Hanna, two years old, and 3 year old Frederick. Both diagnosed with Leukemia and follows them as they are treated for their illness. Includes such daily routines as eating breakfast, washing and playing. *$16.95*
56 pages Hardcover
ISBN 1-55532 -13-6

8619 Options: Revolutionary Ideas in the War on Cancer
People Against Cancer
P.O.Box 10
604 East Street
Otho, IA 50569   515-972-4444
                                 800-662-2623
                           Fax: 515-972-4415
                           info@PeopleAgainstCancer.org
                           www.peopleagainstcancer.com
Frank D. Wiewel, Executive Director/Founder
Publication of People Against Cancer, a nonprofit, grassroots public benefit organization dedicated to 'New Directions in the War on Cancer.' We help people to find the best cancer treatment. We are a democratic organization of people with cancer, their loved ones and citizens working together to protect and enhance medical freedom of choice.

8620 Osteoporosis Sourcebook
Omnigraphics
615 Griswold Street
Suite 520
Detroit, MI 48226   610-461-3548
                                 800-234-1340
                           Fax: 800-875-1340
                           contact@omnigraphics.com
                           www.omnigraphics.com
Peter Ruffner, Co-Founder
Fred Ruffner, Co-Founder
Discusses causes, risk factors, treatments and traditional and non-traditional pain management issues concerning osteoporosis. *$ 84.00*
568 pages Hard cover
ISBN 0-780802-39-1

8621 Parent's Guide to Allergies and Asthma
Allergy & Asthma Network Mothers of Asthmatics
Ste 150
PO Box 7474
Fairfax Station, VA 22039-7474   703-323-9170
                                 800-756-5525
                           Fax: 703-323-9173
                           custsvc@parent-institute.com
                           www.parent-institute.com
John H Wherry, Ed.D, President
A up-to-date, easy-to-read resource offering essential information on asthma and allergies.

8622 Partial Seizure Disorders: A Guide for Patients and Families
O'Reilly Media Inc
1005 Gravenstein Hwy N
Sebastopol, CA 95472-2811   707-827-7000
                                 800-998-9938
                           Fax: 707-829-0104
                           order@oreilly.com
                           www.oreilly.com
Linda Lamb, Editor
Mitzi Waltz, Author
Partial Seizure Disorders helps patients and families get an accurate diagnosis of this condition, understand medications and their side effects, and learn coping skills and other adjuncts to medication. It walks readers through developmental and school issues for young children; adult issues such as employment and driving; working with an existing health plan; and getting further help through advocacy and support organizations, articles, and online resources. *$19.95*
288 pages Paperback
ISBN 0-596500-03-3

8623 Penitent, with Roses: An HIV+ Mother Reflects
University Press of New England
1 Court St
Ste 250
Lebanon, NH 03766-1358   603-448-1533
                                 800-421-1561
                           Fax: 603-448-7006
                           www.upne.com
Paula W Peterson, Author
Peterson, a married, middle-class, Jewish mother, was diagnosed with full-blown AIDS four years into her marriage and 11 months

after her son was born. In seven poignant autobiographical essays and a collection of letters to her uninfected, four-year-old son, the author maintains an upbeat tone and describes her unsuccessful attempts to find the source of her infection (her husband tested negative), her relationships with her doctors, and her work as an HIV activist. *$ 26.95*
256 pages 2001
ISBN 1-584651-28-4

8624 Plan Ahead: Do What You Can
Spina Bifida Association of America
1600 Wilson Boulevard
Suite 800
Arlington, VA 22209
　　　　　　　　　　　　202-944-3285
　　　　　　　　　　　　800-621-3141
　　　　　　　　　　Fax: 202-944-3295
　　　　　　　　　　　　sbaa@sbaa.org
　　　　　　　　　　　　www.sbaa.org

Ana Ximenes, Chair
Sara Struwe, President & CEO
Mark Bohay, National Web Initiatives & Development Manager
Folic aciid information for women at risk for recurrence. *$15.00*

8625 Post-Polio Syndrome: A Guide for Polio Survivors and Their Families
Yale University Press
PO Box 209040
New Haven, CT 6520-9040
　　　　　　　　　　　　203-432-0960
　　　　　　　　　　　　203-432-0948
　　　　　　language.yalepress@yale.edu

Julie K Silver M.D., Author
Laro S Halstead, M.D., Foreword
A guide for polio survivors, their families, and their health care providers offers expert advice on all aspects of post-polio syndrome. Based on the author's experience treating post-polio patients, Silver discusses issues of critical importance, including how to find the best medical care, deal with symptoms, sustain mobility, manage pain, approach insurance issues, and arrange a safe living environment. *$ 19.50*
304 pages 2002
ISBN 0-300088-08-3

8626 Prader-Willi Syndrome: Development and Manifestations
Cambridge University Press
32 Avenue of the Americas
New York, NY 10013-2473
　　　　　　　　　　　　212-924-3900
　　　　　　　　　　　　212-691-3239
　　　　　　　　　　　　www.cambridge.org

Joyce Whittington, Author
Tony Holland, Co-Author
Seeks to identify and provide the latest findings about how best to manage the complex medical, nutritional, psychological, educational, social and therapeutic needs of people with PWS. *$130.00*
230 pages 2004
ISBN 0-521840-29-3

8627 Preventing Secondary Conditions Associated with Spina Bifida or Cerebral Palsy
Spina Bifida Association of America
1600 Wilson Boulevard
Suite 800
Arlington, VA 22209
　　　　　　　　　　　　202-944-3285
　　　　　　　　　　　　800-621-3141
　　　　　　　　　　Fax: 202-944-3295
　　　　　　　　　　　　sbaa@sbaa.org
　　　　　　　　　　　　www.sbaa.org

Ana Ximenes, Chair
Sara Struwe, President & CEO
Mark Bohay, National Web Initiatives & Development Manager
This report is for health professionals, parents and teachers. *$3.00*

8628 Prostate and Urological Disorders Sourcebook
Omnigraphics
615 Griswold Street
Suite 520
Detroit, MI 48226
　　　　　　　　　　　　610-461-3548
　　　　　　　　　　　　800-234-1340
　　　　　　　　　　Fax: 800-875-1340
　　　　　　　　contact@omnigraphics.com
　　　　　　　　　www.omnigraphics.com

Peter Ruffner, Co-Founder
Fred Ruffner, Co-Founder
Prostate and Urological Disorders Sourcebook provides information about prostate cancer and other prostate problems, such as prostatitis and benign prostatic hyperplasia. A glossary of andrological terms and a directory of resources for additional help and information are also included. *$84.00*
604 pages Hard cover
ISBN 0-780807-97-6

8629 Protecting Against Latex Allergy
Spina Bifida Association of America
1600 Wilson Boulevard
Suite 800
Arlington, VA 22209
　　　　　　　　　　　　202-944-3285
　　　　　　　　　　　　800-621-3141
　　　　　　　　　　Fax: 202-944-3295
　　　　　　　　　　　　sbaa@sbaa.org
　　　　　　　　　　　　www.sbaa.org

Ana Ximenes, Chair
Sara Struwe, President & CEO
Mark Bohay, National Web Initiatives & Development Manager
Because awareness and proper action may help prevent an allergic reation, learning about latex allergy is especially important for parents, health care workers and anyone who is exposed to latex regulary. *$20.00*

8630 Questions and Answers: The ADA and Personswith HIV/AIDS
US Department of Justice
950 Pennsylvania Ave. NW
Washington, DC 20530
　　　　　　　　　　　　202-307-0663
　　　　　　　　　　　　800-514-0301
　　　　　　　　　　Fax: 202-307-1197
　　　　　　　　　　TTY: 800-514-0383
　　　　　　　　　　　　www.ada.gov

Rebecca B. Bond, Chief
Anne Raish, Principal Deputy Chief
Christina Galindo-Walsh, Deputy Chief
A 16-page publication explaining the requirements for employers, businesses and nonprofit agencies that serve the public, and state and local governments to avoid discriminating against persons with HIV/AIDS.

8631 Raynaud's Phenomenon
Arthritis Foundation
1330 W. Peachtree Street
Suite 100
Atlanta, GA 30309
　　　　　　　　　　　　404-872-7100
　　　　　　　　　　　　800-283-7800
　　　　　　　　　　Fax: 404-872-0457
　　　　　　　　　　　　arthritis.org

Daniel T. McGowan, Chair
Michael V. Ortman, Vice Chair
Ann M. Palmer, CEO/President
The Arthritis Foundation is the largest national nonprofit organization that supports the more than 100 types of arthritis and related conditions. Founded in 1948, with headquarters in Atlanta, the Arthritis Foundation has multiple service points located throughout the country.

8632 Reaching the Autistic Child: A Parent Training Program
Brookline Books
8 Trumbull Rd,
Northampton, MA 01060-4533
　　　　　　　　　　　　413-584-0184
　　　　　　　　　　　　800-666-2665
　　　　　　　　　　Fax: 413-584-6184
　　　　　　　　　　brbooks@yahoo.com

Detailed case studies of social and behavioral change in autistic children and their families show parents how to implement the principles for improved socialization and behavior. *$15.95*
Softcover
ISBN 1-571290-56-7

8633 Respiratory Disorders Sourcebook
Omnigraphics
615 Griswold Street
Suite 520
Detroit, MI 48226
610-461-3548
800-234-1340
Fax: 800-875-1340
contact@omnigraphics.com
www.omnigraphics.com

Peter Ruffner, Co-Founder
Fred Ruffner, Co-Founder
Respiratory Disorders Sourcebook provides up-to-date information about infectious, inflammatory, occupational, and other types of respiratory disorders. Tips for managing chronic respiratory diseases and suggestions for ways to promote lung health are presented, and the book concludes with a glossary of related terms and a list of additional resources. *$84.00*
638 pages Hard cover
ISBN 0-780810-07-5

8634 SPINabilities: A Young Person's Guide to Spina Bifida
Spina Bifida Association of America
1600 Wilson Boulevard
Suite 800
Arlington, VA 22209
202-944-3285
800-621-3141
Fax: 202-944-3295
sbaa@sbaa.org
www.sbaa.org

Ana Ximenes, Chair
Sara Struwe, President & CEO
Mark Bohay, National Web Initiatives & Development Manager
A cool and practical book for young adults becoming independent. *$22.30*

8635 Seizures and Epilepsy in Childhood: A Guide
John Hopkins University Press
2715 N Charles St
Baltimore, MD 21218-4363
410-516-6900
800-548-1784
Fax: 410-516-6998
webmaster@jhupress.jhu.edu
www.press.jhu.edu

Kathleen Keane, Director
Eileen P G Vining MD, Co-Author
Diana J Pillas, Co-Author
The award-winning Seizures and Epilepsy in Childhood is the standard resource for parents in need of comprehensive medical information about their child with epilepsy. *$54.00*
432 pages 3rd Edition
ISBN 0-801870-51-4

8636 Sexuality and the Person with Spina Bifida
Spina Bifida Association of America
1600 Wilson Boulevard
Suite 800
Arlington, VA 22209
202-944-3285
800-621-3141
Fax: 202-944-3295
sbaa@sbaa.org
www.sbaa.org

Ana Ximenes, Chair
Sara Struwe, President & CEO
Mark Bohay, National Web Initiatives & Development Manager
Dr Sloan foucuses on sexual development, sexual activity and other important issues. *$11.00*

8637 Sinus Survival: A Self-help Guide
Penguin Group
375 Hudson St
New York, NY 10014-3658
212-366-2372
Fax: 212-366-2933
insidesales@penguingroup.com
us.penguingroup.com

Robert S Ivker, Author

Self-help manual for sufferers of bronchitis, sinusitis, allergies, and colds. *$15.95*
336 pages Paperback 2000
ISBN 1-101798-02-6

8638 Social Development and the Person with Spina Bifida
Spina Bifida Association of America
1600 Wilson Boulevard
Suite 800
Arlington, VA 22209
202-944-3285
800-621-3141
Fax: 202-944-3295
sbaa@sbaa.org
www.sbaa.org

Ana Ximenes, Chair
Sara Struwe, President & CEO
Mark Bohay, National Web Initiatives & Development Manager
Examines how spina bifida and hydrocephalus may influence development and learning social skills.

8639 Solving the Puzzle of Chronic Fatigue
Essential Science Publishing
1216 S 1580 W
Ste A
Orem, UT 84058-4906
801-224-6228
800-336-6308
Fax: 801-224-6229
info@essentialscience.net
www.essentialsciencepublishing.com

Michael Rosenbaum, Author
Murray Susser, Co-Author
Although primarily a book about CFS, this comprehensive study also provides a detailed overview of candidiasis, including its causes and best approaches for treatment. *$14.95*
190 pages
ISBN 0-943685-11-7

8640 Son Rise: The Miracle Continues
New World Library
14 Pamaron Way
Novato, CA 94949
415-884-2100
800-972-6657
Fax: 415-884-2199
ami@newworldlibrary.com
www.newworldlibrary.com

Barry Neil Kaufman, Author
Documents Raun Kaufman's astonishing development from a lifeless, autistic child into a highly verbal, lovable youngster with no traces of his former condition. Details Raun's extraordinary progress from the age of four into young adulthood, also shares moving accounts of five families that successfully used the Son-Rise Program to reach their own special children. *$14.96*
372 pages
ISBN 0-915811-53-7

8641 Steps to Independence: Teaching Everyday Skills to Children with Special Needs
Spina Bifida Association of America
1600 Wilson Boulevard
Suite 800
Arlington, VA 22209
202-944-3285
800-621-3141
Fax: 202-944-3295
sbaa@sbaa.org
www.sbaa.org

Ana Ximenes, Chair
Sara Struwe, President & CEO
Mark Bohay, National Web Initiatives & Development Manager
A guide to help parents teach life skills to their disabled child. *$34.25*

8642 Stroke Sourcebook
Omnigraphics
615 Griswold Street
Suite 520
Detroit, MI 48226   610-461-3548
                                            800-234-1340
                                       Fax: 800-875-1340
                                   contact@omnigraphics.com
                                       www.omnigraphics.com

Peter Ruffner, Co-Founder
Fred Ruffner, Co-Founder
Basic Consumer Health Information about Stroke, Including Ischemic, Hemorrhagic, and Mini Strokes, as Well as Risk Factors, Prevention Guidelines, Diagnostic Tests, Medications and Surgical Treatments, and Complications of Stroke.

8643 Stroke Sourcebook, 2nd Edition
Omnigraphics
615 Griswold Street
Suite 520
Detroit, MI 48226   610-461-3548
                                            800-234-1340
                                       Fax: 800-875-1340
                                   contact@omnigraphics.com
                                       www.omnigraphics.com

Peter Ruffner, Co-Founder
Fred Ruffner, Co-Founder
Stroke Sourcebook, Second Edition provides updated information about stroke, its causes, risk factors, diagnosis, acute and long-term treatment, and recent innovations in poststroke care. Information on rehabilitation therapies, prevention strategies, and tips on caring for a stroke survivor is also included, along with a glossary of related terms and a directory of organizations that offer additional information to stroke survivors and their families. *$84.00*
626 pages Hard cover
ISBN 0-780810-35-8

8645 Succeeding With Interventions For Asperger Syndrome Adolescents
Autsim Society of North Carolina Bookstore
505 Oberlin Road
Suite 230
Raleigh, NC 27605-1345   919-743-0204
                                            800-442-2762
                                       Fax: 919-743-0208
                                  books@autismsociety-nc.org
                                     www.autismbookstore.com

Tracey Sheriff, Chief Executive Officer
David Laxton, Director of Communications
Paul Wendler, Chief Financial Officer
This book includes a very useful outline of all the therapy sessions, which can be used as a template by a practitioner for creating their own interaction therapy intervention for adolescents.

8646 Symptomatic Chiari Malformation
Spina Bifida Association of America
1600 Wilson Boulevard
Suite 800
Arlington, VA 22209   202-944-3285
                                            800-621-3141
                                       Fax: 202-944-3295
                                            sbaa@sbaa.org
                                            www.sbaa.org

Ana Ximenes, Chair
Sara Struwe, President & CEO
Mark Bohay, National Web Initiatives & Development Manager
The Spina Bifida Association (SBA) serves adults and children who live with the challenges of Spina Bifida.

8647 Taking Charge
Spina Bifida Association of America
1600 Wilson Boulevard
Suite 800
Arlington, VA 22209   202-944-3285
                                            800-621-3141
                                       Fax: 202-944-3295
                                            sbaa@sbaa.org

Ana Ximenes, Chair
Sara Struwe, President & CEO
Mark Bohay, National Web Initiatives & Development Manager
Teenagers talk about life and physical disabilities. *$7.95*

8648 Ten Things I Learned from Bill Porter
New World Library
14 Pamaron Way
Novato, CA 94949   415-884-2100
                                            800-972-6657
                                       Fax: 415-884-2199
                                  ami@newworldlibrary.com
                                     www.newworldlibrary.com

Shelly Ackerman, Author
Bill Porter worked for the Watkins Corp, selling household products door-to-door in one of Portland's worst neighborhoods. Afflicted with cerebral palsy and burdened with continual pain, Porter was determined not to live on government disability and went on to become Watkin's top-grossing salesman in Portland, the Northwest, and the US. This book was written by the woman who worked as Porter's typist and driver and later became his friend and cospeaker. *$20.00*
192 pages
ISBN 1-577312-03-1

8649 Thyroid Disorders Sourcebook
Omnigraphics
615 Griswold Street
Suite 520
Detroit, MI 48226   610-461-3548
                                            800-234-1340
                                       Fax: 800-875-1340
                                   contact@omnigraphics.com
                                       www.omnigraphics.com

Peter Ruffner, Co-Founder
Fred Ruffner, Co-Founder
Thyroid Disorders Sourcebook provides essential information about thyroid and parathyroid function, diseases, and treatments. Also presented are symptoms, risk factors, diagnosis, treatments, thyroid effects on the body, and the impact of environmental conditions on the thyroid. *$84.00*
573 pages Hard cover
ISBN 0-780807-45-7

8650 Tourette Syndrome: The Facts
Oxford University Press
198 Madison Avenue
New York, NY 10016   212-726-6000
                                            800-445-9714
                                       Fax: 919-677-1303
                                      custserv.us@oup.com
                                            www.oup.com

Mary Robertson, Co-Editor
Andrea Cavanna, Co-Editor
Johnathan Keats, Author
The causes of the syndrome, how it is diagnosed, and the ways in which it can be treated. *$35.00*
122 pages
ISBN 0-198523-98-X

8651 Tourette's Syndrome: Finding Answers and Getting Help
O'Reilly Media Inc
1005 Gravenstein Hwy N
Sebastopol, CA 95472-2811   707-827-7019
                                            800-889-8969
                                       Fax: 707-824-8268
                                        order@oreilly.com
                                            www.oreilly.com

Tourette's Syndrome is a neurological disorder usually diagnosed in childhood and characterized by tics, physical jerks, and involuntary vocalizations. Tourette's can be a devastating disability. The good news is that it's very treatable. Tourette's Syn-

drome helps you secure a diagnosis, understand medical interventions, get healthcare coverage, and manage Tourette's in family life, school, community, and workplace. *$24.95*
416 pages Paperback
ISBN 0-596500-07-6

8652 Tourette's Syndrome: Tics, Obsessions, Compulsions: Developmental Psychopathology
John Wiley & Sons
111 River Street
Hoboken, NJ 07030-5774 201-748-6000
Fax: 201-748-6088
www.wiley.com

Peter Booth Wiley, Chairman
Stephen M. Smith, President & CEO
John Kitzmacher, EVP, CFO
Contains 21 contributions compromising the work of researchers associated with the Yale Child Study Center, which has been at the forefront of research on Tourette's syndrome and associated disorders. *$85.00*
600 pages
ISBN 0-471113-75-1

8653 Treating Epilepsy Naturally: A Guide to Alternative and Adjunct Therapies
McGraw-Hill Company
P.O.Box 182605
Columbus, OH 43218 800-338-3987
Fax: 609-308-4480
customer.service@mheducation.com
www.mcgraw-hill.com

David Levin, President and CEO
Patrick Milano, Chief Administrative Officer & CFO
Stephen Laster, Chief Digital Officer
Offers alternative treatments to replace and to complement traditional therapies and sound advice to find the right health practitioner. *$15.95*
288 pages
ISBN 0-658013-79-3

8654 Understanding Asthma
National Jewish Health
1400 Jackson Street
Denver, CO 80206 303-270-2708
877-225-5654
Fax: 303-398-1125
allstetterw@njc.org
nationaljewish.org

Rich Schierburg, Chair
Robin Chotin, Vice Chair
Michael Salem, M.D., President and CEO
Offers a brief introduction to asthma and then goes into the physiology of asthma, the triggers of asthma, and diagnosis and monitoring of asthma.
27 pages

8655 Understanding Asthma: The Blueprint for Breathing
Allergy & Asthma Network Mothers of Asthmatics
8229 Boone Boulevard
Suite 260
Vienna, VA 22182 800-878-4403
Fax: 703-288-5271
www.aanma.org

Michael Amato, Chair
Tonya Winders, President & CEO
Brenda Silvia-Torma, Project Manager
A layman's guide to asthma facts based on a presentation from the first national asthma patient conference.

8656 Understanding Cystic Fibrosis
University Press of Mississippi
3825 Ridgewood Road
Jackson, MS 39211-6492 601-432-6205
800-737-7788
Fax: 601-432-6217
press@ihl.state.ms.us
www.upress.state.ms.us

Leila W. Salisbury, Director
Craig Gill, Assistant Director/Editor-in-Chief
Anne Stascavage, Managing Editor

A reference for CF patients and their families. *$14.00*
128 pages
ISBN 0-878059-67-9

8657 Understanding Multiple Sclerosis
University Press of Mississippi
3825 Ridgewood Road
Jackson, MS 39211-6492 601-432-6205
800-737-7788
Fax: 601-432-6217
press@ihl.state.ms.us
www.upress.state.ms.us

Melissa Stauffer, Author
Craig Gill, Assistant Director/Editor-in-Chief
Anne Stascavage, Managing Editor
Two psychologists discuss their roles with a member who has multiple sclerosis. Includes chapters on adolescents with multiple sclerosis, employment, and research. *$14.00*
136 pages
ISBN 1-578068-03-7

8658 Urologic Care of the Child with Spina Bifida
Spina Bifida Association of America
1600 Wilson Boulevard
Suite 800
Arlington, VA 22209 202-944-3285
800-621-3141
Fax: 202-944-3295
sbaa@sbaa.org

Ana Ximenes, Chair
Sara Struwe, President & CEO
Mark Bohay, National Web Initiatives & Development Manager
The Spina Bifida Association (SBA) serves adults and children who live with the challenges of Spina Bifida.

8659 Usher Syndrome
NI on Deafness & Other Communication Disorders
31 Center Dr.
MSC 2320
Bethesda, MD 20892-2320 301-827-8183
800-241-1044
TTY: 800-241-1055
nidcdinfo@nidcd.nih.gov
www.nidcd.nih.gov

Debara L. Tucci, Director
Judith A. Cooper, Deputy Director
Timothy J. Wheeles, Executive Officer
Explains what is Usher Syndrome, who is affected by Usher syndrome, what causes Usher syndrome, how is Usher syndrome treated, and what research is being conducted on Usher syndrome.

8660 What Everyone Needs to Know About Asthma
Allergy & Asthma Network Mothers of Asthmatics
8229 Boone Boulevard
Suite 260
Vienna, VA 22182 800-878-4403
Fax: 703-288-5271
www.aanma.org

Michael Amato, Chair
Tonya Winders, President & CEO
Brenda Silvia-Torma, Project Manager
Offers information and facts on gaining control of asthma, asthma triggers and monitoring asthma disorders.

8661 When the Road Turns: Inspirational Stories About People with MS
Health Communications
3201 SouthWest 15th Street
Deerfield Beach, FL 33442 954-360-0909
800-441-5569
Fax: 954-360-0034

An inspiring collection of stories written by people living with multiple sclerosis. *$10.36*
300 pages
ISBN 1-558749-07-1

8662 **Young Person's Guide to Spina Bifida**
Spina Bifida Association of America
1600 Wilson Boulevard
Suite 800
Arlington, VA 22209

202-944-3285
800-621-3141
Fax: 202-944-3295
sbaa@sbaa.org

Ana Ximenes, Chair
Sara Struwe, President & CEO
Mark Bohay, National Web Initiatives & Development Manager
Gives practical tips and suggestions for becoming independent and managing your health. *$19.00*

8663 **Your Child and Asthma**
National Jewish Health
1400 Jackson Street
Denver, CO 80206

303-270-2708
877-225-5654
Fax: 303-398-1125
allstetterw@njc.org
nationaljewish.org

Rich Schierburg, Chair
Robin Chotin, Vice Chair
Michael Salem, M.D., President and CEO
A booklet offering information to parents and family about their child with asthma. Offers information on diagnosis, treatments, triggers and family concerns.

8664 **Your Cleft Affected Child**
Hunter House Inc. Publisher
PO Box 2914
Alameda, CA 94501-914

510-865-5282
800-266-5592
Fax: 510-865-4295
www.hunterhouse.com

Carrie T Gruman Trinker, Author
The book also provides in-depth information, guidance, and support on a wide variety of relevant topics, from feeding to surgery to helping a child cope until his/her cleft has been fully corrected. *$ 16.95*
288 pages Paperback
ISBN 0-897931-85-4

8665 **Your Guide to Bowel Cancer**
Oxford University Press
2001 Evans Road
Cary, NC 27513

919-677-0977
800-445-9714
Fax: 919-677-1303
www.us.oup.com

Offers information and public awareness on the disease of bowel cancer. *$18.95*
ISBN 0-340927-46-1

Journals

8666 **AIDS: The Official Journal of the International AIDS Society**
Lippincott Williams & Wilkins
2 Commerce Square
2001 Market St.
Philadelphia, PA 19103

215-521-8300
Fax: 215-521-8902
customerservice@lww.com
lww.com

JA Levy, Co Editor
B. Autran, Co Editor
R. A Coutinho, Co Editor
The latest groundbreaking research on HIV and AIDS. *$ 433.00*
18 per year

8667 **American Journal of Orthopsychiatry**
American Psychological Association
750 1st Street NorthEast
Washington, DC 20002-4242

202-336-5500
800-374-2721
Fax: 202-336-5502
TTY: 202-336-6123
www.apa.org

Nadine J. Kaslow, President
Norman B. Anderson, PhD, CEO & EVP
Bonnie Markham, Treasurer
Mental health issues from multidisciplinary and interprofessionals perspectives: clinical, research and expository approaches. *$45.00*
160 pages Quarterly

8668 **Annals of Otology, Rhinology and Laryngology**
Annals Publishing Company
4507 Laclede Ave
Saint Louis, MO 63108-2103

314-367-4987
Fax: 314-367-4988
www.annals.com

Ken Cooper, President
Richard J. Smith, Editor
Monica L. Bergers, Editor's Assistant
Original, peer-reviewed articles in the fields of otolaryngology - head and neck medicine and surgery, broncho-esophagology, audiology, speech, pathology, allery, and maxillofacial surgery. Official journal of the American Laryngological Association/American Broncho-Esophagological Association. *$170.00*
112 pages Monthly

8669 **Archives of Neurology**
American Medical Association
P.O.Box 10946
Chicago, IL 60654

312-670-7827
800-262-2350
Fax: 312-464-4184
subscriptions@jamanetwork.com
jamanetwork.com

Margaret Vanner, Manager
Mission is to publish scientific information primarily important to those physicians caring for people with neurologic disorders, but also for those interested in the structure and function of the normal and diseased nervous system. *$235.00*
198 pages Monthly

8670 **Cleft Palate-Craniofacial Journal**
American Cleft Palate-Craniofacial Association
2455 Teller Rd.
Thousand Oaks, CA 91320

800-818-7243
Fax: 800-583-2665
journal@acpa-cpf.org
www.cpcjournal.org

Jack C. Yu, Editor
A peer-reviewed, interdisciplinary, international journal dedicated to current research on etiology, prevention, diagnosis, and treatment in all areas pertaining to craniofacial anomalies. Publishes 10 issues a year.

8671 **Developmental Medicine & Childhood Neurology**
American Academy for Cerebral Palsy/Dev. Medicine
555 East Wells
Suite 1100
Milwaukee, WI 53202

414-918-3014
Fax: 414-276-2146
info@aacpdm.org
www.aacpdm.org

Tamara Wagester, Executive Director
Clinical research into the wide range of neurological conditions and disabilities that affect children.

8672 Journal of Head Trauma Rehabilitation
Lippincott, Williams & Wilkins
P.O.Box 1620
Hagerstown, MD 21740   301-223-2300
                                                  800-638-3030
                                             Fax: 301-223-2400
                                              orders@lww.com
                                                  www.lww.com
John D Corrigan PhD, ABPP, Editor
Scholarly journal designed to provide information on clinical
management and rehabilitation of the head-injured for the prac-
ticing professional. Published bimonthly. *$113.96*

Magazines

8673 Coping with Cancer Magazine
Media America
P.O.Box 682268
Franklin, TN 37068-2268   615-790-2400
                                             Fax: 615-794-0179
                                                copingmag.com
Provides knowledge, hope and inspiration, its readers include
cancer patients (survivors) and their families, caregivers,
healthcare teams and support group leaders. *$19.95*
53 pages 6 x year

8674 CurePSP Magazine
Society for Progressive Supranuclear Palsy
Suite 201
30 E. Padonia Road
Timonium, MD 21093   410-785-7004
                                                  800-457-4777
                                             Fax: 410-785-7009
                                              info@curepsp.org
                                                  www.psp.org
John T. Burhoe, Chair
Everett R. Cook, Vice Chair
Richard Gordon Zyne, President-CEO
Quarterly newsletter. The society's mission is to promote and
fund research into finding the cause and cure for progressive
supranuclear palsy (PSP). Provides information, support and ad-
vocacy to persons diagnosed with PSP, their families and care-
givers. Educates physicians and allied health professionals on
PSP and how to improve patient care.

8675 EpilepsyUSA
Epilepsy Foundation
8301 Professional Place
Landover, MD 20785-2353   301-459-3700
                                                  800-332-1000
                                             Fax: 301-459-1569
                                              ContactUs@efa.org
                                         epilepsyfoundation.org
Warren Lammert, Chair
Phil Gattone, President and CEO
May J. Liang, Secretary
Magazine reporting on issues of interest to people with epilepsy
and their families. *$15.00*
22 pages Bi-Monthly

8676 MSFOCUS Magazine
Multiple Sclerosis Foundation
6520 North Andrews Avenue
Fort Lauderdale, FL 33309-2130   954-776-6805
                                                  888-673-6287
                                             Fax: 954-351-0630
                                             support@msfocus.org
                                                 www.msfocus.org
Jules Kuperberg, Executive Director
Alan Segaloff, Executive Director
Natalie Blake, Program Services Director
Contemporary national, nonprofit organization that provides free
support services and public education for persons with Multiple
Sclerosis, newsletters, toll-free phone support, information, re-
ferrals, home care, assistive technology and support groups.
48 pages Quarterly

8677 Orthotics and Prosthetics Almanac
American Orthotic & Prosthetics Association
330 John Carlyle Street
Suite 200
Alexandria, VA 22314   571-431-0876
                                             Fax: 571-431-0899
                                              info@aopanet.org
                                                  www.aopanet.org
Anita L. Lampear, President
Charles H. Dankmeyer, Vice President
Thomas F. Fise, JD, Executive Director
Features articles covering current professional, patient care, gov-
ernment, business and National Office activities affecting the
orthotics and prosthetics profession and industry. *$40.00*
80 pages Monthly
ISSN 1061-46 1

8678 PDF News
Parkinson's Disease Foundation
1359 Broadway
Suite 1509
New York, NY 10018   212-923-4700
                                                  800-457-6676
                                             Fax: 212-923-4778
                                              info@pdf.org
                                                  www.pdf.org
Howard D. Morgan, Chair
Woodruff Atwell, Ph.D., Vice Chair
Stephen Ackerman, Treasurer
8-12 pages Quarterly

8679 POZ Magazine
212 W 35th St
New York, NY 10001   212-242-2163
                                                  800-973-2376
                                             Fax: 212-675-8505
                                              website@poz.com
                                                  poz.com
A health magazine written for individuals who are HIV+, their
friends and families. POZ provides the latest treatment information, investigative journalism and survivor profiles.

8680 SCI Life
National Spinal Cord Injury Association
11300 Rockville Pike
Suite 803
Rockville, MD 20852   301-468-3902
                                             Fax: 301-468-3904
                                              info@ilcreations.com
                                                  ilcreations.com
SCI/LIFE is dedicated to the presentation of news concerning
people with spinal cord injuries caused by trauma or disease.
Quarterly/Free

8681 Spine
Lippincott, Williams & Wilkins
530 Walnut St
Philadelphia, PA 19106-3603   215-521-8300
                                             Fax: 215-521-8411
                                          customerservice@lww.com
James N Weinstein DO MSc, Editor
Publishes original papers on theoretical issues and research con-
cerning the spine and spinal cord injuries. *$9.00*
26 Issues Year

Newsletters

8682 ACPOC News
Assoc of Children's Prosthetic-Orthotic Clinics
6300 N River Rd
Suite 727
Rosemont, IL 60018-4226   847-698-1637
                                             Fax: 847-823-0536
                                              acpoc@aaos.org
                                                  www.acpoc.org
David B. Rotter,CPO, President
Jorge A. Fabregas, Vice President
Hank White,PT,PhD, Secretary-Treasurer

Quarterly publication from the Association of Children's Pros-
thetic/Orthotic Clinics. Included with membership.
40 pages Quarterly

8683   AID Bulletin
Project AID Resource Center
P.O. Box 5190
Kent, OH 44242-0001   330-672-3000
                                        Fax: 330-672-4724
                                            info@kent.edu
                                            www.kent.edu/

Beverly Warren, President
Todd A. Diacon, Provost & SVP
Gregg S. Floyd, Sr. Vice President
Has the latest news on upcoming conferences, literature, developments in programs and/or services for disabled persons who
are substance abusers. Offers articles on their experiences, ideas
and questions of others in this field which includes providers and
consumers. *$7.50*

8684   AIDS Alert
AHC Media LLC
PO Box 550669
Atlanta, GA 30355   404-262-5436
                                             800-688-2421
                                        Fax: 404-262-5560
                                            www.ahcpub.com/
Joy Daughtery Dickinson, Senior Managing Editor
Source of AIDS news and advice for health care professionals.
Covers up-to-the-minute developments and guidance on the en-
tire spectrum of AIDS challenges, including treatment, educa-
tion, precautions, screening, diagnosis and policy. *$499.00*
Monthly

8685   Adaptive Tracks
Adaptive Sports Center
P.O.Box 1639
Crested Butte, CO 81224   970-349-2296
                                             866-349-2296
                                        Fax: 970-349-2077
                                        info@adaptivesports.org
                                        www.adaptivesports.org
Christopher Hensley, Executive Director
Chris Read, CTRS, Program Director
Ella Fahrlander, Development Director
The Adaptive Sports Center (ASC) of Crested Butte, Colorado is
a non-profit organization that provides year-round recreation activities for people with disabilities and their families. The ASC
provides adaptive snowboarding downhill skiing, cross country
skiing as well as backcountry trips. Summer activities include a
variety of wilderness-based programs, multi-day trips into the
back country, extensive cycling programs, canoeing, and white
water rafting.
6 pages Quarterly

8686   Arthritis Self-Management
Rapaport Publishing, Inc.
150 W 22nd St
Ste 800
New York, NY 10011-2421   212-989-0200
                                        Fax: 212-989-4786
                                    ASMcustserv@cdsfulfillment.com
                                    www.arthritisselfmanagement.com
Richard A Rapaport, President
Maryanne Schott Turner, Director of Manufacturing
Richard Boland, Art Director
Arthritis Self-Management publishes practical 'how-to' informa-
tion for the growing number of people with arthritis who want to
know more about managing their condition. We focus on the
day-to-day and long-term aspects of arthritis in a positive and upbeat style, giving our subscribers up-to-date news, facts, and advice to help them make informed decisions about their health.
$9.97
BiMonthly

8687   Breaking Ground
Tennessee Council on Developmental Disabilities
404 James Robertson Pkwy
Suite 130
Nashville, TN 37243- 0228   615-532-6615
                                        Fax: 615-532-6964
                                        TTY: 615-741-4562
                                            tnddc@tn.gov
                                            www.tn.gov/cdd
Stephanie Brewer cook, Chair
Roger D. Gibbens,, Vice Chair
Wanda Willis, Executive Director
Newsletter
20 pages 6 x Year

8688   Breaking New Ground News Note
Purdue University
225 West University Street
West Lafayette, IN 47907   765-494-4600
                                             800-825-4264
                                        Fax: 765-496-1356
                                        engineering.purdue.edu/
Paul Jones, Project Manager
Bill Field, Project Director
Denise Heath, Project Asst.
News, practical ideas and success stories of and for farmers and
other agricultural workers with physical disabilities.
2 pages Quarterly

8689   Diabetes Self-Management
Rapaport Publishing, Inc.
150 W 22nd St
Ste 800
New York, NY 10011-2421   212-989-0200
                                        Fax: 212-989-4786
                                    www.diabetesselfmanagement.com
Richard A Rapaport, President
Maryanne Schott Turner, Director of Manufacturing
Richard Boland, Art Director
Publishes practical how-to information, focusing on the
day-to-day and long-term aspects of diabetes in a positive and up-
beat style. Gives subscribers up-to-date news, facts and advice to
help them maintain their wellness and make informed decisions
regarding their health. *$9.97*
BiMonthly

8690   Directions
Families of Spinal Muscular Dystrophy
925 Busse Road
Elk Grove Village, IL 60007   847-367-7620
                                             800-886-1762
                                        Fax: 847-367-7623
                                            info@fsma.org
                                            www.fsma.org
Richard Rubenstein, Chair
Kenneth Hobby, President
Sue Kovach, Director of Finance
$35.00
60-70 pages Quarterly

8691   IAL News
International Association of Laryngectomees
925B Peachtree Street NE
Suite 316
Atlanta, GA 30309   866-425-3678
                                            www.larynxlink.com
Wade Hampton, President
Susan Reeves, Administrative Manager
Jodi Knott, Director, Voice Institute
Focuses on rehabilitation and well-being of persons who have
had laryngectomy surgery.

8692 Informer
Simon Foundation
P.O. Box 815
Wilmette, IL 60091   847-864-3913
                                              800-237-4666
                                         Fax: 847-864-9758
                                   info@simonfoundation.org
                                        simonfoundation.org
Cheryle Gartley, President and Founder
Elizabeth T. LaGro, VP, Communications & Education
Twila Yednock, Director of Special Events
Publishes items of interest to people with bladder or bowel incon-
tinence, including medical articles, helpful devices, publications
and a pen pal list. Quarterly newsletter.
Quarterly

8693 Moisture Seekers
Sjogren's Syndrome Foundation
6707 Democracy Boulevard
Suite 325
Bethesda, MD 20817   301-530-4420
                                              800-475-6473
                                         Fax: 301-530-4415
                                          tms@sjogrens.org
                                           www.sjogrens.org
Kenneth Economou, Chair
Steven Taylor, CEO
Sheriese DeFruscio, VP of Development
Newsletter of the organization for lay people and professionals
interested in Sjogren's Syndrome. Contains medical news, cur-
rent research, and essential tips for daily living. *$25.00*
15-16 pages Monthly

8694 Momentum
National Multiple Sclerosis Society
Ste 6
421 New Karner Rd
Albany, NY 12205-3838   518-464-0850
                                              800-344-4867
                                         Fax: 518-464-1232
                                            nyr@nmss.org
                                     www.nationalmssociety.org
Eli Rubenstein, Chair
Cynthia Zagieboylo, President & CEO
Sherri Giger, EVP, Marketing
News and information on research progress, medical treatments,
patient services, therapeutic claims and activities.

8695 Options
People Against Cancer
P.O. Box 10
604 East Street
Otho, IA 50569   515-972-4444
                                              800-662-2623
                                         Fax: 515-972-4415
                                 info@PeopleAgainstCancer.org
                                   www.peopleagainstcancer.com
Frank D. Wiewel, Executive Director/Founder
Publication of People Against Cancer, a nonprofit, grassroots
public benefit organization dedicated to 'New Directions in the
War on Cancer.' We help people to find the best cancer treatment.
We are a democratic organization of people with cancer, their
loved ones and citizens working together to protect and enhance
medical freedom of choice.
8 pages Quarterly

8696 PDF Newsletter
Parkinson's Disease Foundation
1359 Broadway
Suite 1509
New York, NY 10018   212-923-4700
                                              800-457-6676
                                         Fax: 212-923-4778
                                              info@pdf.org
                                              www.pdf.org
Howard D. Morgan, Chair
Woodruff Atwell, Ph.D., Vice Chair
Stephen Ackerman, Treasurer

The Parkinson's Disease Foundation (PDF) is a leading national
presence in Parkinson's disease research, education and public
advocacy.
12-16 pages Quarterly

8697 Parkinson Report
National Parkinson Foundation
200 SE 1st Street
Suite 800
Miami, FL 33131   800-473-4636
                                          www.parkinson.org
John L. Lehr, President & CEO
Leilani Pearl, SVP & Chief Communications Officer
Articles, reports and news on Parkinson's disease and the activi-
ties of the National Parkinson Foundation.
32 pages Quarterly

8698 Post-Polio Health
Post-Polio Health International
50 Crestwood Executive Ctr.
Suite 440
St. Louis, MO 63126   314-534-0475
                                         Fax: 314-534-5070
                                      editor@post-polio.org
                                          www.post-polio.org
Brian M. Tiburzi, Editor
Post-Polio Health supports Post-Polio Health International's ed-
ucational, research, and advocacy efforts. Offers information
about relevant events. Published in February, May, August and
November.
12 pages Quarterly

8699 Prader-Willi Alliance of New York Newsletter
244 5th Avenue
Suite D-110
New York, NY 10001   800-442-1655
                                    alliance@prader-willi.org
                                        www.prader-willi.org
Rachel Johnson, Executive Director
The Prader-Willi Foundation is a national, nonprofit public char-
ity that works for the benefit of individuals with Prader-Willi syn-
drome and their families. *$20.00*
Quarterly

8700 Quality Care Newsletter
National Association for Continence
P.O. Box 1019
Charleston, SC 29402-1019   843-352-2559
                                              800-BLA-DER
                                         Fax: 843-352-2563
                                     memberservices@nafc.org
                                              www.nafc.org
Donna Deng, Chairman
Nancy Hicks, Vice Chaiperson
Steven Gregg, Executive Director
Newsletter from NAFC. By donating $25 and becomming a Qual-
ity Care donor, you may receive our quarterly newsletter. *$25.00*
14-16 pages Quarterly

**8701 Rasmussen's Syndrome and Hemispherectomy Support
Network Newsletter**
55 Kenosia Avenue
Danbury, CT 06810   203-744-0100
                                         Fax: 203-798-2291
                           http://www.rarediseases.org/rare-disease-info
Ronald J. Bartek, Chair
Sheldon M. Schuster, Vice Chair
Peter L. Saltonstall, President & CEO
National, not-for-profit organization dedicated to providing in-
formation and support to individuals affected by Rasmussen's
Syndrome and hemispherectomy. Publishes a periodic newsletter
and disseminates reprints of medical journal articles concerning
Rasmussen's Syndrome and its treatments. Maintains a support
network that provides encouragement and information to individ-
uals affected by Rasmussen's Syndrome and their families.

8702 SCI Psychosocial Process
Amer Assn of Spinal Cord Injury Psych & Soc Wks
75-20 Astoria Blvd
East Elmhurst, NY 11370   718-803-3782
                                       800-404-2898
                                  Fax: 718-803-0414
                           info@unitedspinal.org
                           http://www.unitedspinal.org/

David C. Cooper, Chairman
Patrick W. Maher, Vice Chairman
Joseph Gaskins, President and CEO
Quarterly newsletter.

8703 Special Care in Dentistry
Blackwell Publishing
350 Main St
Malden, MA 02148   781-388-0200
                                  Fax: 781-388-8210
                          www.blackwellpublishing.com

Peter Booth Wiley, Chairman
Stephen M. Smith, President & CEO
John Kitzmacher, EVP, CFO
$125.00
48 pages BiMonthly

8704 TSA Newsletter
Tourette Syndrome Association
42-40 Bell Boulevard
Bayside, NY 11361   718-224-2999
                                       800-237-0717
                                  Fax: 718-279-9596
                                   ts@tsa-usa.org
                                   www.tsa-usa.org

Stephen M. McCall, President
National non-profit membership organization whose mission is
to identify the cause of, find the cure for, and control the effects of
this disorder. A growing number of local chapters nationwide
provide educational materials, seminars, conferences and support groups for over 35,000 members.
Quarterly

8705 Teens & Asthma
American Lung Association
530 7th St SE
Washington, DC 20003   202-546-5864
                                  Fax: 202-546-5607
                                    www.epa.gov/

Rolando E Bates Jr, CEO
Tips from other teens with asthma to help those having it get on
with the serious business of having fun with the rest of their lives.
Online/Free

8706 Tethering Cord
Spina Bifida Association of America
PO Box 5801
Bethesda, MD 20824   800-352-9424
                                    www.ninds.nih.gov
Nina Schor, Deputy Director
Tethered spinal cord syndrome is a neurological disorder caused
by tissue attachments that limit the movement of the spinal cord
within the spinal column. Attachments may occur congenitally at
the base of the spinal cord (conus medullaris) or they may de-
velop near the site of an injury to the spinal cord.

8707 Tourette Syndrome Association Children's Newsletter
42-40 Bell Boulevard
Bayside, NY 11361   718-224-2999
                                       800-237-0717
                                  Fax: 718-279-9596
                                   ts@tsa-usa.org
                                   tsa-usa.org

Stephen M. McCall, President
National, nonprofit membership organization. Mission is to identify the cause of, find the cure for, and control the effects of this
disorder. A growing number of local chapters nationwide provide
educational materials, seminars, conferences and support groups
for over 35,000 members.

8708 Ventilator-Assisted Living
International Ventilator Users Network
50 Crestwood Executive Ctr.
Suite 440
St. Louis, MO 63126-1916   314-534-0475
                                  Fax: 314-534-5070
                                  info@ventusers.org
                                   www.ventnews.org

Brian M. Tiburzi, Editor
Articles for home mechanical ventilator users, health profession-
als and industry professionals.
Bi-monthly

8709 Voice of the Diabetic
NFB Diabetes Action Network
200 E. Wells St.
at Jernigan Place
Baltimore, MD 21230   410-659-9314
                                  Fax: 410-685-5653
                                      nfb@nfb.org
                                      www.nfb.org

Newsletter containing personal stories and practical guidelines
by blind diabetics and medical professionals, medical news, resource column and a recipe corner.

Sports

8710 National Sports Center for the Disabled
33 Parsenn Rd
PO Box 1290
Winter Park, CO 80482   970-726-1518
                                  Fax: 970-726-4112
                                   volunteer@nscd.org
                                       nscd.org

Kim Easton, President & CEO
Diane Eustace, Marketing Director
Beth Fox, Outreach & Education Director
Organization providing year-round recreation for children and
adults with disabilities. Winter programming includes alpine skiing, snowboarding, ski racing, show shoeing, and cross-country
skiing. Summer sports include rafting, sailing, kayaking, camping, hiking, horseback riding, fishing, and rock climbing.

**8711 Rehabilitation Institute of Chicago's Virginia
Wadsworth Sports Program**
345 East Suuperior St.
Chicago, IL 60611   312-238-1000
                                       800-354-7342
                                       800-354-REHA
                                  Fax: 312-238-5017
                                     sports@ric.org
                                       www.ric.org

Jude Reyes, Chair
mike P. Kransy, Vice Chair
Thomas Reynolds III, Vice Chair
RIC's Center for Health and Fitness is a full service fitness center
for individuals with disablilties and the administrative offices for
RIC's Wirtz Sports Program. Eighteen different sport and recreation programs are offered free of charge. The facility is adjacent
to RIC's main building and also is the location of a branch of The
National Center for Physical Activity and Disability (NCPAD), a
joint project operated by the University of Illinois-Chigcago.

8712 Special Hockey International (SHI)
93 Bell Farm Rd.
Suite 120B
Barrie, ON, Canada L4M-5G1   specialhockeyinternational.org
Mike Dwyer, President
Bill Weishuhn, Treasurer
The organization has teams throughout North America and Eu-
rope, attracting over 70 teams to its annual tournament.

Support Groups

8713 AAN's Toll-Free Hotline
Allergy and Asthma Network Mothers of Asthmatics
8229 Boone Boulevard
Suite 260
Vienna, VA 22182
800-878-4403
Fax: 703-288-5271
www.aanma.org

Michael Amato, Chair
Tonya Winders, President & CEO
Brenda Silvia-Torma, Project Manager
Offers answers to questions regarding allergies and asthma, provides referrals and support to assist the patient and his or her family.

8714 Breaking New Ground Resource Center
Purdue University
225 S University St
West Lafayette, IN 47907
765-494-5088
800-825-4264
Fax: 765-496-1356
bng@ecn.purdue.edu
engineering.purdue.edu/

Bill Field, Project Director
Paul Jones, Project Manager
Steve Swain, Rural Rehab Specialist
A resource center devoted to helping farmers and ranchers with physical disabilities. Resource materials and a free newsletter are available to anyone.

8715 Clearinghouse on Disability Information: Office Special Education & Rehabilitative Service
U S Department of Education
400 Maryland Ave SW
Washington, DC 20202-1
202-245-7549
800-872-5327
Fax: 202-245-7614
www.ed.gov

Arne Duncan, Secretary Of Education
Tony Miller, Deputy Secretary
Martha Kanter, Under Secretary
Provides information to people with disabilities or anyone requesting information, by doing research and providing documents in response to inquiries. The information provided includes areas of federal funding for disability-related programs. Information provided may be useful to disabled individuals and their families, schools and universities, teacher's and/or school administrators, and organizations who have persons with disabilities as clients.

8716 Compassionate Friends, The
P.O.Box 3696
Oak Brook, IL 60522
630-990-0010
877-969-0010
Fax: 630-990-0246
nationaloffice@compassionatefriends.org
compassionatefriends.org

Patrick O'Donnell, President
Georgia Cockerham, Vice President
Lisa Corrao, COO
Peer support for bereaved parents, grandparents and siblings, offering over 600 chapters in the United States. The organization also offers a quarterly magazine, We Need Not Walk Alone, and TCF resources of brochures, DVDs, and memorial wristbands for the bereaved parent, grandparent and sibling.

8717 Cornerstone Services
777 Joyce Rd.
Joliet, IL 60436
815-741-7600
877-444-0304
Fax: 815-723-1177
cornerstoneservices.org

Ben Stortz, President & Chief Executive Officer
Kim Hudgens, Vice President & Chief Operating Officer
Ken Mihelich, Vice President & Chief Financial Officer
Cornerstone Services provides progressive, comprehensive services for people with disabilities, promoting choice, dignity and the opportunity to live and work in the community. Established in 1969, the agency provides developmental, vocational, residential and behavior health services.
1969

8718 Disability Network
Ste 54
3600 S Dort Hwy
Flint, MI 48507
810-742-1800
Fax: 810-742-2400
TTY: 810-742-7647
tdn@disnetwork.org
www.disnetwork.org

Bruce Chargo, Chairman
Diane Brown, Treasurer/ Vice Chairman
Mike Zelley, President & CEO
The Disability Network's mission is to realize consumer empowerment, self determination, full inclusion and participation of all people in the communities through independent living philosophy and the unequivocal implementation of the Americans with Disabilities Act

8719 Disability and Health: National Center for Birth Defects and Developmental Disabilities
Centers for Disease Control and Prevention
1600 Clifton Road
Atlanta, GA 30333
404-498-3012
800-232-4636
800-CDC-INFO
Fax: 404-498-3060
cdcinfo@cdc.gov
www.cdc.gov/ncbddd/dh

Dr. Tom Frieden, Director
Sherri A. Berger, COO
Carmen Villar, Chief of Staff
Located within the new CDC, National Center for Birth Defects and Developmental Disabilities, the Disability and Health section, operates a ralatively small program that primarily supports: data collection on the prevalence of people with disabilities & their health status and risk factors for poor health and well-being; research on measures of disability, functioning and health; health promotion intervention studies; and dissemination of health information.

8720 Easterseals
141 W Jackson Blvd.
Suite 1400A
Chicago, IL 60604
312-726-6200
800-221-6827
Fax: 312-726-1494
info@easterseals.com
www.easterseals.com

Kendra E. Davenport, President & CEO
Glenda Oakley, Chief Financial Officer
Marcy Traxler, Senior Vice President, Network Advancement
Easterseals provides services, education, outreach and advocacy for people with disabilities, veterans, senior citizens and their families. Programs include early intervention, workforce development, adult day care, adult services, mental health services, and more.

8721 Epilepsy Foundation
8301 Professional Place E
Suite 200
Landover, MD 20785- 2353
800-332-1000
Fax: 301-459-1569
ContactUs@efa.org
www.epilepsy.com

Robert W Smith, Chair
Philip M Gattone, M.Ed, President & CEO
M. Vaneeda Bennett, Chief Development Officer
Offers information, referrals and support groups for those diagnosed with epilepsy.

8722 Family Support Project for the Developmentally Disabled
3424 Kossuth Ave
Bronx, NY 10467-2410
718-519-5000
Fax: 718-519-4902
www.nyc.gov/html/hhc/ncbh/home.html

William Walsh, Vice President
Sheldon McLeod, COO

8723   Head Injury Hotline
Brain Injury Resource Center
P.O.Box 84151
Seattle, WA 98124-5451   206-621-8558
                                     Fax: 206-329-0912
                                   brain@headinjury.com
                                   www.headinjury.com

Hugh R. MacMahon, Neurology
Constance Miller, Founder
Paul M. Kuroiwa, Performance management consultant
Disseminates head injury information and provides referrals to
facilitate adjustment to life following head injury. Organizes
seminars for professionals, head injury survivors, and their
families.

**8724   International Braille and Technology Center for the
Blind**
National Federation of the Blind
200 E. Wells St.
at Jernigan Place
Baltimore, MD 21230   410-659-9314
                                     Fax: 410-685-5653
                                          nfb@nfb.org
                                   nfb.org/programs-services

John Berggren, Executive Director, Operations
World's largest and most complete evaluation and demonstration
center of all assistive technology used by the blind from around
the world. Includes all braille, synthetic speech, print-to-speech
scanning, internet and portable devices and programs. Available
for tours by appointment to blind persons, employers, technology
manufacturers, teachers, parents and those working in the
assistive technology field.

8725   Lung Line Information Service
National Jewish Health
1400 Jackson Street
Denver, CO 80206   877-225-5654
                                          877-225-5654
                                     Fax: 303-398-1125
                                      allstetterw@njc.org
                                      nationaljewish.org

Rich Schierburg, Chair
Robin Chotin, Vice Chair
Michael Salem, M.D., President & CEO
A free information service answering questions, sending literature and giving advice to patients with immunologic or respiratory illnesses. The Line is an educational service and not a
substitute for medical care. Diagnosis or suggested treatment will
not be provided for a caller's specific condition.

8726   NCI's Contact Center
National Cancer Institute
9609 Medical Center Dr.
Rockville, MD 20850   800-422-6237
                                     TTY: 800-332-8615
                                        nciinfo@nih.gov
                                        www.cancer.gov

Norman E. Sharpless, Director
Douglas R. Lowy, Principal Deputy Director
*James Doroshow, Deputy Director, Clinical & Translational
Research*
The NCI Contact Center provides accurate, up-to-date information on cancer to patients and their families, health professionals
and the general public. The Contact Center can provide specific
information in understandable language about particular types of
cancer, as well as information on second opinions and the
availability of clinical trials.

8727   National AIDS Hotline
Centers for Disease Control and Prevention
1600 Clifton Road
Atlanta, GA 30333   404-639-3311
                                          800-232-4636
                                          800-CDC-INFO
                                     Fax: 404-498-3060
                                          www.cdc.gov

Dr. Tom Frieden, Director
Sherri A. Berger, COO
Carmen Villar, Chief of Staff

Offers free confidential information and publications on HIV infection and AIDS.

8728   PPAL Support Groups
Parent Professional Advocacy League
77 Rumford Ave.
Waltham, MA 02453   866-815-8122
                                     Fax: 617-542-7832
                                         info@ppal.net
                                         www.ppal.net

Lisa Lambert, Executive Director
Meri Viano, Associate Director
Joel Khattar, Program Manager
The Parent Professional Advocacy League (PPAL) provides fam-
ily support services and support groups for parents and families
of children with emotional, behavioral, and mental health needs.

8729   PXE International
Ste 404
4301 Connecticut Ave NW
Washington, DC 20008- 2369   202-362-9599
                                     Fax: 202-966-8553
                                          info@pxe.org
                                          www.pxe.org

Patrick F. Terry, President
Sharon Terry, CEO
Terry M. Dermaid, Executive Director
Provides support for individuals and families affected by
psukdoxanthoma elasticum (PXE), and resources for healthcare
professionals. PXE causes select elastic tissue to mineralize, and
effects the skin, eyes, cardiovascular, and GI systems.

8730   Parent Assistance Network
Good Samaritan Hospital
10 E. 31st Street
Kearney, NE 68847   308-865-7100
                                          800-235-9905
                                     Fax: 308-865-2924
                                sheilameyer@catholichealth.net

Randy DeFreece, President
Kent Barney, Chairman
Mary Henning, Vice Chairman
Provides information and emotional support to all parents and es-
pecially to parents of children with disabilities in the central Ne-
braska area. Ongoing activities include parent support group
meetings, parent-to-parent networking and referrals and Respite
Care provider trainings.

8731   Post-Polio Support Group
Adventist Hinsdale Hospital
120 N Oak St
Hinsdale, IL 60521-3829   630-856-9000
                                     Fax: 630-856-6000
                                   www.keepingyouwell.com

David Crane, President
Information and support for polio patients and their families;
meets the fourth Wednesday of each month.

8732   Prevent Child Abuse America
288 South Wabash Avenue
10th floor
Chicago, IL 60604   312-663-3520
                                          800-244-5373
                                          800-CHI-DREN
                                     Fax: 312-939-8962
                               mailbox@preventchildabuse.org
                                   preventchildabuse.org

Fred M. Riley, Chair
David Rudd, Vice Chair
James Hmurovich, President & CEO
Through public education, community partnerships and support
services, PCAMW helps everyone play a role in prevention. We
share information on prevention stategies and effective parenting
at community forums and events and advocate for polices and services that keep children safe. We operate PhoneFriend, a telephone support line for children at home without adult supervision
and conduct personal safety workshops in schools, camps and
libraries.

8733 Son-Rise Program
2080 S Undermountain Rd.
Sheffield, MA 01257-9643   413-229-2100
                                           877-766-7473
                                       Fax: 413-229-8931
                              www.autismtreatmentcenter.org

Barry Neil Kaufman, Founder & CEO
Clyde Haberman, Senior Teacher & Director of Development
Blair Borgeson, Developmental Therapist

The center's Son-Rise Program teaches a comprehensive system
of treatment and education designed to help families and caregivers enable their children to dramatically improve in all areas of
learning.

8734 Special Children
1306 Wabash Ave
Belleville, IL 62220-3370   618-234-6876
                                       Fax: 618-234-6150
                                       specialchildren.net

Kathleen Cullen, Administrator

A nonprofit agency serving children with developmental disabilities ages birth to 6 years

8735 Support Works
1607 Dilworth Rd W
Charlotte, NC 28203-5213   704-331-9500
                                       www.supportworks.org

Joel Fisher, Manager

SupportWorks helps people find and form support groups. An 8
page publication Power Tools, clearly walks new group leaders
through steps of putting together a healthy self-help group.
SupportWorks also has a telephone conference program which allows people with similar diseases or other nonprofit issues to
meet by phone conference for free or at very low cost.

8736 Toll-Free Information Line
Asthma and Allergy Foundation of America
8201 Corporate Drive
Suite 1000
Landover, MD 20785   202-466-7643
                                           800-727-8462
                                        800-7 A-THMA
                                       Fax: 202-466-8940
                                           info@aafa.org
                                               aafa.org

Lynn Hanessian, Chair
Yolanda Miller, SVP & COO
Lynda Mitchell, VP, Food Allergies

The Asthma and Allergy Foundation of America (AAFA) provides practical information, community based services and support through a national network of chapters and support groups.
AAFA develops health education, organizes state and national
advocacy efforts and funds research to find better treatments and
cures.

8737 Visiting Nurse Association of America
2121 Crystal Drive
Suite 750
Arlington, VA 22202   571-527-1520
                                           888-866-8773
                                       Fax: 571-527-1527
                                       webadmin@vnaa.org
                                               vnaa.org

Mary B. DeVeau, Chair
Linnea Windel, Vice Chair
Tracey Moorhead, President & CEO

The VNAA is the official national association for not-for-profit,
community based home health organizations known as the Visiting Nurse Associations (VNA's). They created the profession of
home health care more then 100 years ag. They have a united mission to bring compassionate, high-quality and cost-effective
home care to individuals in their communities.

Speech & Language

Books

8644 Stuttering
NI on Deafness & Other Communication Disorders
31 Center Dr.
MSC 2320
Bethesda, MD 20892-2320
301-827-8183
800-241-1044
TTY: 800-241-1055
nidcdinfo@nidcd.nih.gov
www.nidcd.nih.gov

Debara L. Tucci, Director
Judith A. Cooper, Deputy Director
Timothy J. Wheeles, Executive Officer
Describes how speech is produced, treatments for stuttering and research supported by the federal government.

Associations

8738 Academic Language Therapy Association
14070 Proton Rd.
Suite 100
Dallas, TX 75244
972-233-9107
Fax: 972-490-4219
office@altaread.org
www.altaread.org

Janna Curry-Dobbs, President
Jo Ann Handy, VP Membership
Susan Louchen, VP Public Relations
The Academic Language Therapy Associationr (ALTA) is a non-profit national professional organization with the purpose of establishing, maintaining, and promoting standards of education, practice and professional conduct for Certified Academic Language Therapists. Academic Language Therapy is an educational, structured, comprehensive, phonetic, multisensory approach for the remediation of dyslexia and/or written-language disorders.
1986

8739 American Speech-Language-Hearing Association
2200 Research Blvd.
Rockville, MD 20850-3289
301-296-5700
800-638-8255
actioncenter@asha.org
www.asha.org

Gail J. Richard, President
Elise Davis-Mcfaland, President-Elect
Margot L. Beckerman, Chair
The American Speech-Language Association is the professional, scientific, and credentialing association for members and affiliates who are speech-language pathologists, audiologists, and speech, language, and hearing scientists in the United States and internationally. ASHA provides information for the public, professionals, students, and the research community related to hearing, balance, speech, language and swallowing disorders.

8740 Aphasia Hope Foundation
P.O. Box 79701
Houston, TX 77279
855-764-4673
jstradinger@comcast.net
www.aphasiahope.org

Sandy Caudell, Program Director
Judi Stradinger, Executive Director
Aphasia Hope Foundation is a nonprofit foundation whose mission is to promote research into the prevention and cure of aphasia and to ensure that all survivors of aphasia and their caregivers are aware of and have access to the best possible tratments.

8741 Association of Language Companies
9707 Key West Ave.
Suite 100
Rockville, MD 20850
240-404-6511
Fax: 301-990-9771
info@alcus.org
www.alcus.org

Christopher Carter, President
Rick Antezana, Vice President
Lenani P. Craig, Treasurer
The Association of Language Companies (ALC) is a national trade association representing businesses that provide translation, interpretation, localization, and language training services.

8742 Autism Research Institute
4182 Adams Ave.
San Diego, CA 92116-2599
866-366-3361
www.autism.com

Stephen Edelson, Executive Director
Rebecca McKenney, Office Manager
Christopher Flynn, Treasurer
Conducts research on the causes, diagnosis, and treatment of autism and publishes a quarterly newsletter that reviews worldwide research. Literature on causes and treatment available. Refers patients and families to health care professionals and clinics.

8743 Autism Services Center
929 4th Ave.
P.O. Box 507
Huntington, WV 25701-0507
304-525-8014
Fax: 304-525-8026
www.autismservicescenter.org

Jimmie Beirne, Chief Executive Officer
Jodi Fields, Director
Barbara Bragg, Director
Provides developmental disabilities services with a specialty in autism. Services include case management, residential, personal care, assessments and evaluations, supported employment, independent living and family support.

8744 Autism Treatment Center of America
2080 S Undermountain Rd.
Sheffield, MA 01257-9643
413-229-2100
877-766-7473
Fax: 413-229-8931
correspondence@option.org
www.autismtreatmentcenter.org

Barry Neil Kaufman, Founder & CEO
Clyde Haberman, Senior Teacher & Director of Development
Blair Borgeson, Developmental Therapist
The Autism Treatment Center of America provides innovative training programs for parents and professionals caring for children challenged by Autism, Autism Spectrum Disorders, Pervasive Developmental Disorders (PDD) and other development difficulties. The center's Son-Rise Program teaches a comprehensive system of treatment and education designed to help families and caregivers enable their children to dramatically improve in all areas of learning.

8745 Carl and Ruth Shapiro Family National Center for Accessible Media
WGBH Educational Foundation
1 Guest St.
Boston, MA 02135-2016
617-300-3400
Fax: 617-300-1035
TTY: 617-300-2489
ncam@wgbh.org
ncam.wgbh.org

Donna Danielewski, Director
Geoff Freed, Director of technology projects and Web media standards
Madeleine Rothberg, Senior Subject Matter Expert
The Carl and Ruth Shapiro Family National Center for Accessible Media (NCAM) is a research and development facility dedicated to addressing barriers to media and emerging technologies for people with disabilities in their homes, schools, workplaces, and communities.

Speech & Language / Associations

8746 Childhood Apraxia of Speech Association
416 Lincoln Ave.
2nd Fl.
Pittsburgh, PA 15209   412-343-7102
                             www.apraxia-kids.org
Mary Sturm, President
Michele R. Atkins, Executive Director
Joshua Zellers, Treasurer
The Childhood Apraxia of Speech Association is a nonprofit publicly funded charity whose mission is to strengthen the support systems in the lives of children with apraxia so that each child is afforded their best opportunity to develop speech and communication.

8747 Deafness and Communicative Disorders Branch of Rehab Services Administration Office
Special Education and Rehab Services
400 Maryland Ave., SW
Washington, DC 20202   800-872-5327
                             www.ed.gov
Kimberly Richey, Secretary Of Education
Promotes improved rehabilitation services for deaf and hard of hearing people and individuals with speech or language impairments. Provides technical assistance to public and private agencies and individuals.

8748 Dysphagia Research Society
2800 West Higgins Rd.
Suite 440
Hoffman Estates, IL 60169   888-775-7361
                             Fax: 847-885-8393
                             info@dysphagiaresearch.org
                             www.dysphagiaresearch.org
Gary H. McCullough, President
Sudarshan R. Jadcherla, President Elect
Susan Langmore, Secretary/Treasurer
The Dysphagia Research Society is a nonprofit organization with the purpose of enhancing and encouraging research pertinent to normal and disordered swallowing, to promote the dissemination of knowledge related to normal and disordered swallowing, and to provide a multidisciplinary forum for presentation of research into normal and disordered swallowing.

8749 Hearing, Speech and Deafness Center (HSDC)
Hearing, Speech & Deafness Center (HSDC)
1625 19th Ave.
Seattle, WA 98122   206-323-5770
                             888-222-5036
                             Fax: 206-328-6871
                             TTY: 800-761-2821
                             clinics@hsdc.org
                             www.hsdc.org
Lindsay Klarman, Executive Director
Hearing, Speech & Deaf Center (HSDC) is a nonprofit for clients who are deaf, hard of hearing, or who face other communication barriers such as speech challenges. Their mission is to foster inclusive and accessible communities through communication, advocacy, and education.

8750 International Cluttering Association
705 Tilbury Court
Sun City Center, FL 33573   elanouette@tampabay.rr.com
                             associations.missouristate.edu/ica
Charley Adams, Ph.D., Chair
Susanne Cook, Chair Elect
Katarzyna Wesierska, Secretary
They work to increase awareness of the communication disorder of cluttering worldwide among speech-language therapists/logopedists, healthcare professionals, people with cluttering, and the public.

8751 International Fluency Association
Northern Illinois University
Dept. of Communicative Disorders
DeKalb, IL 60115-2899   www.theifa.org
Elaine Kelman, President
Nan Bernstein Ratner, President Elect
Shelly Jo Kraft, Treasurer
The International Fluency Association is a not-for-profit, international, interdisciplinary organization devoted to the understanding and management of fluency disorders, and to the improvement in the quality of life for persons with fluency disorders.

8752 Lindamood-Bell Home Learning Process
CA   805-541-3836
                             800-233-1819
                             www.lindamoodbell.com
Nanci Bell, Founder/Director
Patricia C. Lindamood, Founder/Director
Lindamood-Bell Learning Process is dedicated to enhancing human learning. Lindamood-Belll programs teach children and adults to read, spell, comprehend, and express language.
1986

8753 Myositis Association
1940 Duke St.
Suite 200
Alexandria, VA 22314   800-821-7356
                             tma@myositis.org
                             www.myositis.org
Bob Goldberg, Executive Director
Linda Kobert, Communications Director
Aisha Morrow, Operations Manager
The aim of TMA's programs and services is to provide information, support, advocacy and research for those concerned about myositis, as well as serving those affected by these diseases. Support groups offer members the chance to share and discuss their concerns with people in similar situations.

8754 National Aphasia Association
P.O. Box 87
Scarsdale, NY 10583   800-922-4622
                             naa@aphasia.org
                             www.aphasia.org
Darlene S. Williamson, President
Daniel Martin, Vice President Strategic Planning
Barbara Kessler, Vice President Community Outreach & Education
The National Aphasia Association (NAA) is a nonprofit organization that promotes public education, research, rehabilitation and support services to assist people with aphasia and their families.

8755 National Association of Special Education Teachers
1250 Connecticut Ave., NW
Suite 200
Washington, DC 20036-2643   800-754-4421
                             Fax: 800-754-4421
                             contactus@naset.org
                             www.naset.org
Roger Pierangelo, Executive Director
George Giuliani, Executive Director
The National Association of Special Education Teachers (NASET) is a national membership organization dedicated to rendering all possible support and assistance to those preparing for or teaching in the field of special education. NASET was founded to promote the profession of special education teachers and to provide a national forum for their ideas.

8756 National Black Association for Speech-Language and Hearing
P.O. Box 779
Pennsville, NJ 08070   877-936-6235
                             Fax: 877-936-6235
                             nbaslh@nbaslh.org
                             www.nbaslh.org
Cathy Runnels, Interim Chair
Kia N. Johnson, Parliamentarian
Martine Elie, Treasurer
The mission of the National Black Association of Speech-Language and Hearing is to maintain a viable mechanism through which the needs of black professionals, students and individuals with communication disorders can be met.

8757 National Cued Speech Association
1300 Pennsylvania Ave, NW
Suite 190-713
Washington, DC 20004   917-439-5126
                                          800-459-3529
                                    Fax: 866-269-9877
                                    info@cuedspeech.org
                                    www.cuedspeech.org
Anne Huffman, President
Sarina Roffe, Executive Director
Ben Lachman, Director of Development
The association champions effective communication, language development and literacy through the use of cued speech. Families are informed about Cued Speech along with other communication options.

8758 National Fragile X Foundation
2100 M St., NW
Suite 170, P.O. Box 302
Washington, DC 20037-1233   800-688-8765
                                          www.fragilex.org
Tony Ferlenda, Chief Executive Officer
Linda Sorensen, Chief Operating Officer
Jayne Dixon Weber, Director of Education & Support Services
Unites the fragile X community to enrich lives through educational and emotional support, promote public and professional awareness and advance research toward improvemed treatments and cure for fragile X syndrome.

8759 National Spasmodic Dysphonia Association
300 Park Blvd.
Suite 335
Itasca, IL 60143   800-795-6732
                                    Fax: 630-250-4505
                                    NSDA@dysphonia.org
                                    www.dysphonia.org
Charlie Reavis, President
Marcia Sterling, Treasurer
Kimberly Kuman, Executive Director
The National Spasmodic Dysphonia Association (NSDA) is a not-for-profit organization dedicated to advancing medical research into the causes of and treatments for SD, promoting physician and public awareness of the disorder, and providing support to those affected by SD through symposiums, support groups, and on-line resources.

8760 National Stuttering Association
119 W. 40th St.
14th Fl.
New York, NY 10018   212-944-4050
                                          800-937-8888
                                    Fax: 212-944-8244
                                    info@westutter.org
                                    www.westutter.org
Gerald Maguire, Chairman
Evan Sherman, Vice Chairman
Bob Wellington, Treasurer
A nonprofit organization dedicated to bringing hope, dignity, support, education, and empowerment to children and adults who stutter and their families, and the professionals who serve them.

8761 National Tourette Syndrome Association
42-40 Bell Blvd.
Suite 205
Bayside, NY 11361   888-4TO-URET
                                          www.tsa-usa.org
John Miller, President & CEO
Diana Felner, VP Public Policy
Sonji Mason-Vidal, VP Finance & Administration
The Tourette Association is dedicated to making life better for all people affected by Tourette and Tic Disorders.

8762 Providence Speech and Hearing Center
1301 Providence Ave.
Orange, CA 92868-3892   714-923-1521
                                          855-901-7742
                                    Fax: 714-639-2593
                                    pshc@pshc.org
                                    www.pshc.org
Bruce May, President
Kevin Timone, Vice President - Fund Development
Randy Free, Vice President - Finance
Mission is to provide the highest quality services available in the identification, diagnosis, treatment and prevention of speech, language and hearing disorders for persons of all ages.

8763 Scottish Rite Center for Childhood Language Disorders
1733 16th St., NW
Washington, DC 20009-3103   202-323-3579
                                    Fax: 202-464-0487
                                    council@scottishrite.org
                                    www.scottishrite.org
Bill Sizemore, Executive Director
Offers speech-language evaluations and treatment, hearing screening and consultations to children ages birth through adolescence. Bilingual services are also available.

8764 Stern Center for Language and Learning
183 Talcott Rd.
Suite 101
Williston, VT 05495-9209   802-878-2332
                                    learning@sterncenter.org
                                    www.sterncenter.org
Blanche Podhajski, President
Michael Shapiro, Chief Operating Officer
Moneer Greenbaum, Director of Development
The Stern Center is a nonprofit learning center dedicated to helping children and adults reach their full potential. Stern Center professionals evaluate and teach all kinds of learners, including those with learning disabilities such as dyslexia or attention deficit disorders.

8765 Stuttering Foundation of America
1805 Moriah Woods Blvd.
Suite 3
Memphis, TN 38117   901-761-0343
                                          800-992-9392
                                    Fax: 901-761-0484
                                    info@stutteringhelp.org
                                    www.stutteringhelp.org
Jane Fraser, President
Dennis Drayna, Director
Joseph R. G. Fulcher, Director
Provides resources, services, and support to those who stutter and their families, as well as support for research into the causes of stuttering.

8766 Texas Speech-Language-Hearing Association
2025 M St., NW
Suite 800
Washington, DC 20036-2342   855-330-8742
                                          888-729-8742
                                    Fax: 512-463-9468
                                    staff@txsha.org
                                    www.txsha.org
Judy Rudebusch Rich, President
Erin Bellue, VP of Educational & Scientific Affairs
Shannon Butkus, VP of Social & Governmental Policy
Mission is to encourage and promote the role of the speech-language pathologist and audiologist as a professional in the delivery of clinical services to persons with communications disorders. Encourages basic scientific study of processes of individual human communication with reference to speech, hearing and language.

8767 The Cherab Foundation
2301 NE Savannah Rd
Suite 1771
Jensen Beach, FL 34957   772-335-5135
                                    help@cherab.org
                                    cherabfoundation.org
Lisa Geng, Founder & President
Jolie Abreu, Vice President

The Cherab Foundation is a world-wide nonprofit organization working to improve the communication skills and education of all children with speech and language delays and disorders. The Cherab Foundation is committed to assisting with the development of new therapeutic approaches, preventions, and cures to neurologically-based speech disorders.

8768   The Davis Center
110 Wesley St.
PO Box 508
Manlius, NY 13104

862-251-4637
Fax: 862-251-4642
npdunn@thedaviscenter.com
www.thedaviscenter.com

Dorinne S. Davis, Director
Offers sound-based therapies supporting positive change in learning, development, and wellness. All ages/all disabilities. Uses The Davis Model of Sound Intervention, an alternative approach.

8769   Wendell Johnson Speech And Hearing Clinic
University Of Iowa
Iowa City, IA 52242-1025

319-335-8736
Fax: 319-335-8851
TTY: 319-335-8736
speech-path-aud@uiowa.edu
clas.uiowa.edu/comsci/clinical-services

Ann Fennell, Clinical Coordinator
The clinic offers assessment and remediation for communication disorders in adults and children. The clinic also offers a Intensive Summer Residential Clinic for school age children needing intervention services because of speech, language, hearing and/or reading problems.

Camps

8770   CNS Camp New Connections
Mclean Hospital Child/Adolescent Program
Mailstop115
115 Mill Street
Belmont, MA 02478

617-855-2000
800-333-0338
Fax: 617-855-2833
mcleaninfo@partners.org
mcleanhospital.org

Scott L. Rauch, MD, President & Chief Psychiatrist
Blaise Aguirre, Clinical Staff
Alan Barry, Clinical Staff
Four-week summer day camp for children ages 7-17 who have pervasive developmental disorders, Asperger's Syndrome, autism spectrum disorders and non-verbal learning disabilities. The camp is designed to help children develop social skills through fun activities including: communication games, swimming, field trips, drama, and arts and crafts. *$4500.00*

8771   Camp Meadowood Springs
77650 Meadowood Rd.
Weston, OR 97886

541-276-2752
Fax: 541-276-7227
camp@meadowoodsprings.org
www.meadowoodsprings.org

Michelle Nelson, Camp Director
This camp is designed to help children with communication disorders and learning differences. A full range of activities in recreational and clinical areas is available.

8772   Camp Royall
250 Bill Ash Rd.
Moncure, NC 27559

919-542-1033
Fax: 919-533-5324
camproyall@autismsociety-nc.org
www.autismsociety-nc.org/camp-royall

Sara Gage, Director
A week-long overnight and day camp for children and adults with autism. Campers participate in traditional camp activities such as swimming, boating, hiking, and arts and crafts. Counselor-to-camper ratio is 1:1 or 1:2, depending on the campers' needs.

8773   Camp Sisol
Jewish Community Center of Greater Rochester/JCC
1200 Edgewood Ave.
Rochester, NY 14618

585-461-2000
Fax: 585-461-0805
bettertogether@jccrochester.org
www.jccrochester.org

Josh Weinstein, Chief Executive Officer
Coed, ages 5-16. Camp Sisol accommodates children with special needs.

8774   Childrens Beach House
100 West 10th Street
Suite 411
Wilmington, DE 19801-1674

302-655-4288
Fax: 302-655-4216
www.cbhinc.org

Martha P. Tschantz, President
Mary Helms, Vice President
Richard T Garrett, Executive Director
Camp is located in Lewes, Delaware. Four-week sessions June-August for Delaware children with hearing impairment or speech/communication impairment. Coed, ages 6-12.

8775   New Horizons Summer Day Camp
YMCA of Orange County
13821 Newport Ave.
Suite 150
Tustin, CA 92780

714-508-7616
newhorizons@ymcaoc.org
www.ymcaoc.org/new-horizons

Jeff McBride, Chief Executive Officer
New Horizons is a program by the YMCA offering day camps for adults with developmental disabilities. Outings in the community are supervised and create an environment that fosters social interaction, skill building, and friendship.

8776   Sequanota Lutheran Conference Center and Camp
PO Box 245
Jennerstown, PA 15547

814-629-6627
contact@sequanota.com
www.sequanota.com

Rev. Nathan Pile, Executive Director
Angie Pile, Director, Business Management
Ann Ferry, Director, Hospitality
Runs Camp Bethesda, a summer camp for adults with developmental and intellectual disabilities. For ages 18 and up.

8777   Talisman Summer Camp
64 Gap Creek Rd.
Zirconia, NC 28790

828-697-6313
info@talismancamps.com
www.talismancamps.com

Linda Tatsapaugh, Operations Director & Owner
Robyn Mims, Admissions Director & Owner
Cory Greene, Camp Director
Talisman Summer Camp is located 40 minutes south of Asheville, North Carolina. Offers a program of hiking, rafting, climbing, and caving for young people with autism, ADHD and learning disabilities. Coed, ages 6-22.

8778   Wendell Johnson Speech & Hearing Clinic
University Of Iowa
250 Hawkins Dr
Iowa City, IA 52242-1025

319-335-8736
Fax: 319-335-8851
kathy-miller@uiowa.edu
www.uiowa.edu

Chuck Wieland, President
Hans Hoerschelman, Vice President
Josh Smith, Budget Officer
The clinic offers assessment and remediation for communication disorders in adults and children. The clinic also offers a Intensive Summer Residential Clinic for school age children needing intervention services because of speech, language, hearing and/or reading problems.

8779 YMCA Camp Fitch
12600 Abels Rd.
North Springfield, PA 16430   814-922-3219
                                 877-863-4824
                            Fax: 814-922-7000
                      registrar@campfitchymca.org
                              campfitchymca.org

Tom Parker, Executive Director
Joe Wolnik, Summer Camp Director
Brandy Duda, Outdoor Education Director
Camp is located in North Springfield, Pennsylvania. Camp programs include sessions for children with diabetes or epilepsy.

Books

8780 Autism 24/7: A Family Guide to Learning at Home & in the Community
Autism Society of North Carolina Bookstore
Ste 230
505 Oberlin Rd
Raleigh, NC 27605-1345   919-743-0204
                            800-442-2762
                       Fax: 919-743-0208
                 jchampion@autismsociety-nc.org
                 http://www.autismsociety-nc.org/

Sharon Jeffries-Jones, Chair
Elizabeth Phillippi, Vice Chair
Tracey Sheriff, Chief Executive Officer
Parents are encouraged to focus on skill sets and behaviors that most negatively affect family functioning, and replacing these behaviors with acceptable alternatives. *$19.95*

8781 Autism Handbook: Understanding & Treating Autism & Prevention Development
Oxford University Press
2001 Evans Road
Cary, NC 27513   919-677-0977
                            800-445-9714
                       Fax: 919-677-1303
                  http://www.oup.com/us/

Oxford University Press USA is the US branch of Oxford University Press in Oxford, England (OUP UK), which is a department of Oxford University and is the oldest and largest continuously operating university press in the world. *$25.00*
320 pages
ISBN 0-195076-67-2

8782 Autism and Learning
Taylor & Francis
37-41 Mortimer St
London, UK W1T 3   http://www.informatandm.com
Stuart Powell, Author
Rita Jordan, Editor
This book is about how a cognitive perception on the way in which individuals with autism think and learn may be applied to particular curriculum areas.
160 pages Paperback
ISBN 1-853464-21-X

8783 Autism in Adolescents and Adults
Springer Publishing
233 Spring St
New York, NY 10013   877-283-3229
                        ainy@aveda.com
                   http://aveda.edu/new-york

Eric Schopler, Editor
Gary B. Mesibov, Editor
This book is a great history lesson in the development of understanding about autism spectrum disorders, and is a testament to how far research and services in the field have come. This book contains lots of information about what general thinking and services used to be like, in an era when still little was understood about these disorders. *$ 63.00*
456 pages
ISBN 0-306410-57-5

8784 Autism...Nature, Diagnosis and Treatment
Autism Society of North Carolina Bookstore
Ste 230
505 Oberlin Rd
Raleigh, NC 27605-1345   919-743-0204
                            800-442-2762
                       Fax: 919-743-0208
                 http://www.autismsociety-nc.org/

Sharon Jeffries-Jones, Chair
Elizabeth Phillippi, Vice.Chair
Paul Wendler, Chief Financial Officer
Covers perspectives, issues, neurobiological issues and new directions in diagnosis and treatment. *$49.00*

8785 Autism: Explaining the Enigma
Wiley Publishers
111 River Street
Hoboken, NJ 07030-5774   201-748-6000
                       Fax: 201-748-6088
                       http://as.wiley.com

Peter Booth Wiley, Chairman
Stephen M. Smith, President & CEO
John Kitzmacher, EVP, CFO
Explains the nature of autism. *$27.95*

8786 Autism: From Tragedy to Triumph
Branden Publishing Company
17 Station St
Brookline, MA 2445-7995   617-730-5757
                 http://www.yogainthevillage.com
Karen Wenc, Teaching Staff
Veronica Wolff, Teaching Staff
Annie Hoffman, Teaching Staff
A new book that deals with the Lovaas method and includes a foreward by Dr. Ivar Lovaas. The book is broken down into two parts — the long road to diagnosis and then treatment. *$12.95*

8787 Autism: Identification, Education and Treatment
Routledge (Taylor & Francis Group)
270 Madison Ave
New York, NY 10016-601   212-576-1411
            http://books.google.co.in/books/about/Autism.
Dianne Zager, Editor
Chapters include medical treatments, early intervention and communication development in autism. *$36.00*
ISBN 0-805820-44-7

8788 Autism: The Facts
Oxford University Press
2001 Evans Road
Cary, NC 27513   919-677-0977
                            800-445-9714
                       Fax: 919-677-1303
         http://www.oup.com/us/corporate/contact/?view
Simon Baron-Cohen, Co-Author
Patrick Bolton, Co-Author
$22.50
128 pages
ISBN 0-192623-27-3

8789 Autistic Adults at Bittersweet Farms
Routledge (Taylor & Francis Group)
12660 Archbold-Whitehouse Rd.
Whitehouse, OH 43571   419-875-6986
                 http://www.bittersweetfarms.org/
Robert St. Clair, President
Matt Anderson, VP
Jan Toczynski, Secretary
A touching view of an inspirational residential care program for autistic adolescents and adults. Also available in softcover. *$94.95*
Hardcover
ISBN 1-560240-42-3

Speech & Language / Books

8790 Beyond Baby Talk: From Sounds to Sentences, a Parent's Guide to Language Development
Prima Publishing
P.O.Box 1260
Rocklin, CA 95677-1260   916-787-7000
                                800-632-8676
                                Fax: 916-787-7001
Fernando Bueno, Editor in Chief
Julie Asbury, Managing Editor
Christopher Buffa, Sr. Editor
The authors discuss the best ways to help your child develop the all-important skill of communication and to recognize the signs of language development problems. *$15.95*
224 pages
ISBN 0-761526-47-1

8791 Breaking the Speech Barrier: Language Develpment Through Augmented Means
Brookes Publishing
P.O.Box 10624
Baltimore, MD 21285-0624   410-337-9580
                                800-638-3775
                                Fax: 410-337-8539
                                custserv@brookespublishing.com
                                readplaylearn.com
Paul Brookes, Owner
This resource describes the creation of the System for Augmenting Language (SAL) for school-age youth with developmental disabilities and offers important insights into the language development of children who are not learning to communicate typically. *$39.95*
224 pages Paperback
ISBN 1-557663-90-0

8792 Breakthroughs: How to Reach Students with Autism
Aquarius Health Care Media
Ste 230
505 Oberlin Rd
Raleigh, NC 27605-1345   919-743-0204
                                800-442-2762
                                Fax: 919-743-0208
                                jchampion@autismsociety-nc.org
                                www.autismtreatmentcenter.org
Sharon Jeffries-Jones, Chair
Elizabeth Phillippi, Vice Chair
Tracey Sheriff, CEO
A hands-on, how-to program for reaching students with autism, featuring Karen Sewell, Autism Society of America's teacher of the year. Here Sewell demonstrates the successful techniques she's developed over a 20-year career. A separate 250 page manual ($59) is also available which covers math, reading, fine motor, self help, social adaptive, vocational and self help skills as well as providing numerous plan reproducibles and an exhaustive listing of equipment and materials resources. Video. *$99.00*

8793 Childhood Speech, Language & Listening Problems
Wiley Publishing
605 3rd Ave
New York, NY 10158-180   212-850-6000
                                Fax: 212-850-6088
                                http://books.google.co.in/books/about/Childho
Patricia McAleer Hamaguchi
Language pathologist Hamaguchi employs her 15 years of experience to show parents how to recognize the most common speech, language, and listening problems. *$16.95*
224 pages Paperback
ISBN 0-471387-53-3

8794 Cognitive Behavioral Therapy for Adult Asperger Syndrome
Autism Society of North Carolina Bookstore
Ste 230
505 Oberlin Rd
Raleigh, NC 27605-1345   919-743-0204
                                800-442-2762
                                Fax: 919-743-0208
                                jchampion@autismsociety-nc.org
                                http://www.autismsociety-nc.org
Sharon Jeffries-Jones, Chair
Elizabeth Phillippi, Vice Chair
Tracey Sheriff, CEO
Text is prepared with case studies and examples from the author's own experiences working as a cognitive-behavioral therapist specializing in adults and adolescents with dual diagnosis, autism spectrum disorders, mood disorders, and anxiety disorders.

8795 Communication Development and Disorders in African American Children
Brookes Publishing
P.O.Box 10624
Baltimore, MD 21285-0624   410-337-9580
                                800-638-3775
                                Fax: 410-337-8539
                                custserv@brookespublishing.com
Paul Brooks, Owner
Research, Assessment, and Intervention. This text presents research on communication disorders and language development in African American children. Also addresses multicultural aspects of service delivery and intervention and discusses issues in assessing, diagnosing, and treating communication disorders. *$39.00*
400 pages Paperback
ISBN 1-55766 -53-3

8796 Communication Development in Children with Down Syndrome
Brookes Publishing
P.O.Box 10624
Baltimore, MD 21285-0624   410-337-9580
                                800-638-3775
                                Fax: 410-337-8539
                                custserv@brookespublishing.com
Paul Brooks, Owner
This book offers an extensive, detailed explanation of communication development in children with Down syndrome relative to their advancing cognitive skills. It introduces a critical framework for assessing and treating hearing, speech, and language problems and provides explicit intervention methods and tested clinical protocols.
Paperback
ISBN 1-55766 -50-5

8797 Coping for Kids Who Stutter
Speech Bin
P.O.Box 1579
Appleton, WI 54912   419-589-1425
                                888-388-3224
                                Fax: 888-388-6344
                                info@speechbin.com
                                www.speechbin.com
James R. Henderson, Chairman
Joseph M. Yorio, President & CEO
Rick Holden, EVP, Educators Publishing Service
Informative book for children and adults about stuttering and how to manage it. *$15.95*
32 pages
ISBN 0-93785 -43-2

8798 Disorders of Motor Speech: Assessment, Treatment, and Clinical Characterization
Brookes Publishing
P.O.Box 10624
Baltimore, MD 21285-0624   410-337-9580
                                800-638-3775
                                Fax: 410-337-8539
                                custserv@brookespublishing.com
Paul Brooks, Owner

826

This book provides a probing examination of normal, dysarthric, and apraxic speech. Great for speech-language pathologists, neurologists, physical or occupational therapists, and physiatrists. *$47.00*
400 pages Hardcover
ISBN 1-55766 -23-1

8799 **Employment for Individuals with Asperger Syndrome or Non-Verbal Learning Disability**
Jessica Kingsley Publishers
400 Market Street
Suite 400
Philadelphia, PA 19106-2513　　　　　215-922-1161
　　　　　　　　　　　　　　　　866-416-1078
　　　　　　　　　　　　　　　Fax: 215-922-1474
　　　　　　　　　　　　　　　orders@jkp.com
　　　　　　　　　　　　　　　www.jkp.com
Laurie Schlesinger, Vp Of Sales & Marketing
Yvona Fast, Author
Most people with Non-Verbal Learning Disorder (NLD) or Asperger Syndrome (AS) are underemployed. This book sets out to change this. With practical and technical advice on everything from job hunting to interview techniques, from 'fitting in' in the workplace to whether or not to disclose a diagnosis, this book guides people with NLD or AS successfully through the employment mine field. There is also information for employers, agencies and careers counsellors on AS and NLD as 'invisible' disabili *$22.95*
272 pages
ISBN 1-843107-66-X

8800 **Encounters with Autistic States**
Jason Aronson
400 Keystone Industrial Park
Dunmore, PA 18512-1507　　　　　800-782-0015
This book explores and explands the work of the late Frances Tustin, which was devoted to the psychoanalytic understanding of the bewildering elemental world of the autistic child. *$50.00*
448 pages Hardcover
ISBN 0-765700-62-

8801 **Kitten Who Couldn't Purr**
William Morrow & Company
1350 Avenue of the Americas
New York, NY 10019-4702　　　　　212-261-6500
　　　　　　　　　　　　　　　Fax: 212-261-6925
　　　　http://www.goodreads.com/book/show/2319648.Th
Otis Chandler, CEO & Co-Founder
Eve Titus, Author
Jonathan the kitten doesn't know how to purr to say thank you, so he sets off to find someone to teach him. *$12.95*
32 pages

8802 **Language Disabilities in Children and Adolescents**
McGraw-Hill School Publishing
PO Box 182605
Columbus, OH 43218　　　　　800-338-3987
　　　　　　　　　　　　　　　Fax: 609-308-4480
　　　　　　　　　customer.service@mheducation.com
　　　　　　　　　　　　　　　mcgraw-hill.com
David Levin, President and CEO
Patrick Milano, Chief Administrative Officer & CFO
Stephen Laster, Chief Digital Officer
A comprehensive review of research in language disabilities.

8803 **Late Talker: What to Do If Your Child Isn't Talking Yet**
St Martin's Griffin
175 5th Ave
New York, NY 10010-7703　　　　　646-307-5151
　　　　　　　　　　　　　　　888-330-8477
　　　　　　　　　　　　　　　Fax: 212-674-6132
　　　　　　　　　customerservice@mpsvirginia.com
Marilyn C Agin, Author
This handbook offers advice on ways to identify the warning signs of a speech disorder, information on how to get the right kind of evaluations and therapy, ways to obtain appropriate services through the school system and health insurance, at-home activities that parents can do with their child to stimulate speech, benefits of nutritional supplementation, and advice from experi-

enced parents who've been there on what to expect and what you can do to be your child's best advocate. *$13.95*
256 pages Paperback
ISBN 0-312309-24-4

8804 **Let Community Employment be the Goal for Individuals with Autism**
Indiana Resource Center For Autism
1905 North Range Road
Bloomington, IN 47408-9801　　　　　812-855-6508
　　　　　　　　　　　　　　　800-825-4733
　　　　　　　　　　　　　　　Fax: 812-855-9630
　　　　　　　　　　　　　　　iidc@indiana.edu
　　　　　　　　　　　　　　　www.iidc.indiana.edu/irca
Cathy Pratt, Director
Catherine Davies, Educational Consultant
Pamela Anderson, Outreach/Resource Specialist
A guide designed for people who are responsible for preparing individuals with autism to enter the work force. *$7.00*

8805 **Lollipop Lunch**
Speech Bin-Abilitations
P.O.Box 1579
Appleton, WI 54912-1579　　　　　419-589-1425
　　　　　　　　　　　　　　　888-388-3224
　　　　　　　　　　　　　　　Fax: 888-388-6344
　　　　　　　　　　　　　　　info@speechbin.com
　　　　　　　　　　　　　　　www.speechbin.com
James R. Henderson, Chairman
Joseph M. Yorio, President & CEO
Rick Holden, EVP, Educators Publishing Service
Cleverly illustrated stories and activities for phonological and language development. *$19.95*
128 pages
ISBN 0-937857-54-8

8806 **Management of Autistic Behavior**
Sage Publications
2455 Teller Road
Thousand Oaks, CA 91320　　　　　805-499-0721
　　　　　　　　　　　　　　　800-818-7243
　　　　　　　　　　　　　　　Fax: 805-499-0871
　　　　　　　　　　　　　　　info@sagepub.com
　　　　　　　　　　　　　　　www.sagepub.com
Sara Miller McCune, Founder, Publisher, Chairperson
Blaise R Simqu, President & CEO
Tracey A. Ozmina, Executive Vice President & Chief Operating Officer
This excellent reference is a comprehensive and practical book that tells what works best with specific problems. *$41.00*
450 pages

8807 **Motor Speech Disorders**
WB Saunders Company
14 Main Street
Southampton, NY 11968-2822　　　　　631-283-5050
　　　　　　　　　　　　　　　800-523-1649
　　　　　　　　　　　　　　　Fax: 631-283-2290
　　　　　　　　　　　　　　　info@saunders.com
　　　　　　　　　　　　　　　www.wbsaunders.com
Joseph R Duffy PhD, Author
Professional text on rehabilitation techniques for motor speech disorders. *$74.00*
592 pages
ISBN 0-323024-52-5

8808 **Neurobiology of Autism**
Johns Hopkins University Press
National Library of Medicine
Building 38A
Bethesda, MD 20894　　　　　410-516-6900
　　　　　　　　　　　　　　　888-346-3656
　　　　　　　　　　　　　　　888-FIN- NLM
　　　　　　　　　　　　　　　Fax: 410-516-6998
　　　　　　　　　　　　　　　info@ncbi.nlm.nih.gov
　　　　http://www.ncbi.nlm.nih.gov/pubmed/17919129
Pardo CA, Co-Author
Ebarhat CG, Co-Author

This book discusses recent advances in scientific research that point to a neurobiological basis for autism and examines the clinical implications of this research. *$28.00*
272 pages
ISBN 0-801880-47-5

8809 Nonverbal Learning Disabilities at Home: A Parent's Guide
Jessica Kingsley Publishers
400 Market Street
Suite 400
Philadelphia, PA 19106   215-922-1161
                                 866-416-1078
                            Fax: 215-922-1474
                            hello.usa@jkp.com
                                  www.jkp.com

Jessica Kingsley, Chairman & Managing Director
Jemima Kingsley, Director
Octavia Kingsley, Production Director
Explores the variety of daily life problems children with NLD may face, and provides practical strategies for parents to help them cope and grow, from preschool age through their challenging adolescent years. *$19.95*
272 pages Paperback
ISBN 1-853029-40-0

8810 Parent Survival Manual
Springer Publishing Company
11 West 42nd Street
8th Floor
New York, NY 10036   212-355-1501
                            Fax: 212-355-7370
                    christieseducation@christies.edu
                    http://www.christieseducation.com

Craig Lickliter, Manager
A guide to crises resolution in autism and related developmental disorders. *$39.95*

8811 Perspectives: Whole Language Folio
Gallaudet University Bookstore
PO Box 35009
Charlotte, NC 28235-5009   202-651-5750
                                 800-995-0550
                            Fax: 202-651-5744
                         www.cpcc.edu/disabilities

Edwin A. Dalrymple, Chairman
Judith N. Allison, Vice Chair
Tony Zeiss, President
The 19 articles in this collection offer practical help to teachers seeking to emphasize whole language strategies in their classroom. *$9.95*
64 pages

8812 Please Don't Say Hello
Human Sciences Press
233 Spring St
New York, NY 10013   877-283-3229
                            ainy@aveda.com
                            aveda.edu/new-york

Phyllis Terri Gold, Author
With the support and love of his family, and through them the neighborhood children, a nine-year-old autistic boy is able to emerge from his shell. *$10.95*
47 pages Paperback
ISBN 0-89885 -99-8

8813 Promoting Communication in Infants and Young Children: 500 Ways to Succeed
Speech Bin-Abilitations
P.O.Box 1579
Appleton, WI 54912-1579   419-589-1425
                                 888-388-3224
                            Fax: 888-388-6344
                            info@speechbin.com
                                www.speechbin.com

James R. Henderson, Chairman
Joseph M. Yorio, President & CEO
Rick Holden, EVP, Educators Publishing Service
This practical reference for parents, caregivers and professional service providers how to promote communication development in infants and young children. Gives down-to-earth information and activities to help your youngest children succeed. It provides step-by-step suggestions for stimulationg children's speech and language skills. Paperback. *$14.95*
ISBN 0-937857-72-6

8814 Reading, Writing and Speech Problems in Children
International Dyslexia Association
40 York Rd.
4th Floor
Baltimore, MD 21204   410-296-0232
                            Fax: 410-321-5069
                            info@dyslexiaida.org
                                 dyslexiaida.org

Samuel Torrey Orton, Author
This book provides reading, reading and speech execerises for educating people with dyslexia. *$20.00*
259 pages
ISBN 0-89079 -79-1

8815 Relationship Development Intervention with Young Children
Taylor & Francis Group
73 Collier St.
London, N1 9BE   44- 0 -0 78
                            Fax: 44- 0 -0 78
                            hello.usa@jkp.com
                    http://www.jkp.com/jkp/distributors.php

Jessica Kingsley, Chairman
Jemima Kingsley, Director
Octavia Kingsley, Production Director
Social and emotional development activities for Asperger Syndrome, Autism, PDD and NLD. Comprehensive set of activities emphasizes foundation skills for younger children between the ages of two and eight. Covers skills such as social referencing, regulating behvior, conversational reciprocity, and synchronized actions. For use in therapeutic settings as well as schools and parents. *$22.95*
256 pages
ISBN 1-843107-14-7

8816 Riddle of Autism: A Psychological Analysis
Jason Aronson
Ste 200
4501 Forbes Blvd
Lanham, MD 20706   301-459-3366
                                 800-462-6420
                            Fax: 301-429-5746
                            customercare@nbnbooks.com
                                http://www.nbnbooks.com

Jason Brockwell, Sales Staff
Michael Sullivan, Sales
Mark Cozy, Sales Staff
Dr. Victor examines the myths that cloud an understanding of this disorder and describes the meanings of its specific behavioral symptoms. *$30.00*
356 pages Paperback
ISBN 1-568215-73-8

8817 Self-Therapy for the Stutterer
Stuttering Foundation of America
1805 Moriah Woods Blvd.
Suite 3
Memphis, TN 38117   901-761-0343
                                 800-992-9392
                            Fax: 901-761-0484
                                www.stutterhelp.org

Jane Fraser, President
Jean Gruss, Journalist
Robert M. Kurtz, Chairman & CEO
A guide to help adults who stutter overcome the problem on their own. *$3.00*
191 pages Paperback
ISBN 0-933388-32-2

8818 Sex Education: Issues for the Person with Autism
Indiana Resource Center For Autism
1905 North Range Road
Bloomington, IN 47408-9801   812-855-6508
                                              800-825-4733
                                         Fax: 812-855-9630
                                     www.iidc.indiana.edu/irca

Cathy Pratt, Director
Catherine Davies, Educational Consultant
Pamela Anderson, Outreach/Resource Specialist
Discusses issues of sexuality and provides methods of instruction
for people with autism. *$4.00*

8819 Son-Rise: The Miracle Continues
2080 South Undermountain Road
Sheffield, MA 01257   413-229-2100
                                              800-714-2779
                                         sonrise@option.org
                                             www.option.org
Samahria Lyt Kaufman, Co-Founder and Co-Director
Dane Griffith, Director of Administrative Services
Bears Kaufman, Co-Founder and Co-Director
Part One is the astonishing record of Raun Kaufman's development from an autistic child into a loving, brilliant youngster who
shows no traces of his former condition. Part Two follows Raun's
development after the age of four, teaching the limitless possibilities of the Son-Rise Program. Part Three shares moving accounts
of five other ordinary families who became extraordinary when
they used the Son-Rise Program to reach their own unreachable
children. *$12.95*
343 pages
ISBN 0-915811-53-7

8820 Sound Connections for the Adolescent
Speech Bin
P.O.Box 1579
Appleton, WI 54912-1579   419-589-1425
                                              888-388-3224
                                         Fax: 888-388-6344
                                         info@speechbin.com
                                          www.speechbin.com
James R. Henderson, Chairman
Joseph M. Yorio, President & CEO
Rick Holden, EVP, Educators Publishing Service
A resource to help older elementary and secondary students un-
derstand their sound systems an how it functions. It targets skills
critical for academic achievement: phonological awareness, pho-
nemic relationships, phonemic processing, listening and memory
and teaches linguistic rules they need to succeed. *$19.95*
Paperback

8821 Talkable Tales
Speech Bin-Abilitations
P.O.Box 1579
Appleton, WI 54912-1579   419-589-1425
                                              888-388-3224
                                         Fax: 888-388-6344
                                          www.speechbin.com
James R. Henderson, Chairman
Joseph M. Yorio, President & CEO
Rick Holden, EVP, Educators Publishing Service
Read-a-rebus stories and pictures targeting most consonant pho-
nemes for K-5 children. *$25.95*
128 pages
ISBN 0-93783-44-0

**8822 Teaching Children with Autism: Strategies for Initiating
Positive Interactions**
Brookes Publishing
P.O.Box 10624
Baltimore, MD 21285-0624   410-337-9585
                                              888-337-8808
                                         Fax: 410-337-8539
                                  custserv@healthpropress.com
                                   http://www.healthpropress.com
Melissa A. Behm, President
Mary Magnus, Director
Strategies for initiating positive interactions and improving learn-
ing opportunities. This guide begins with an overview of charac-
teristics and long-term strategies and proceeds through

discussions that detail specific techniques for normalizing environments, reducing disruptive behavior, improving language and
social skills, and enhancing generalization. *$32.95*
256 pages Paperback
ISBN 1-55766 -80-4

8823 Teaching and Mainstreaming Autistic Children
Love Publishing Company
9101 East Kenyon Avenue
Suite 2200
Denver, CO 80237   303-221-7333
                                         Fax: 303-221-7444
                                   http://www.lovepublishing.com/
Peter Knoblock, Author
Dr. Knoblock advocates a highly organized, structured environment for autistic children, with teachers and parents working together. His premise is that the learning and social needs of autistic
children must be analyzed and a daily program designed with interventions that respond to this functional analysis of their behavior. *$24.95*
ISBN 0-89108 -11-9

**8824 Techniques for Aphasia Rehab: (TARGET) Generating
Effective Treatment**
Speech Bin
P.O.Box 1579
Appleton, WI 54912-1579   419-589-1425
                                              888-388-3224
                                         Fax: 888-388-6344
                                          www.speechbin.com
James R. Henderson, Chairman
Joseph M. Yorio, President & CEO
Rick Holden, EVP, Educators Publishing Service
Practical treatment manual for use by aphasia clinicians. *$45.00*
384 pages
ISBN 0-93785 -50-5

**8825 Understanding & Controlling Stuttering: A
Comprehensive New Approach Based on the Valsa Hyp**
National Stuttering Association
119 West 40th Street
14th Floor
New York, NY 10018   212-944-4050
                                              800-937-8888
                                         Fax: 212-944-8244
                                         info@westutter.org
                                          www.nsastutter.org
Kenny Koroll, Chair
Tammy Flores, Executive Director
Stephanie Coopen, Family Programs Administrator
Demonstrates how physical and psychological factors may inter-
act to stimulate and perpetuate stuttering through a Valsalva-Stut-
tering cycle. *$25.00*
176 pages
ISBN 7-929773-01-3

**8826 Verbal Behavior Approach: How to Teach Children with
Autism & Related Disorders**
Autism Society of North Carolina Bookstore
Ste 230
505 Oberlin Rd
Raleigh, NC 27605-1345   919-743-0204
                                              800-442-2762
                                         Fax: 919-743-0208
                                   http://www.autismsociety-nc.org
Sharon Jeffries-Jones, Chair
Elizabeth Phillippi, Vice Chair
Tracey Sheriff, CEO
Provides full descriptions of how to teach the verbal operants that
make up expressive languate which include: manding, tacting,
echoing and intraverbal skills. *$19.95*

8827   **Without Reason: A Family Copes with two Generations of Autism**
Books on Special Children
721 W Abram St
Arlington, TX 76013-6995   817-277-0727
                                          800-489-0727
                                          Fax: 817-277-2270
                                          http://www.fhautism.com/
R. Wayne Gilpin, President
Jennifer Gilpin Yacio, Vice President and Editorial Director
David Reasor, CPA and Administrative Director
The author discovers his son has autism. He delves into problems of the autistic person and explains reasons for their actions. *$20.95*
292 pages Hardcover

Journals

8828   **American Journal of Speech-Language Pathology**
American Speech-Language-Hearing Association
2200 Research Boulevard
Rockville, MD 20850-3289   301-296-5700
                                          800-638-8255
                                          Fax: 301-296-8580
                                          nsslha@asha.org
                                          www.asha.org
Elizabeth S. McCrea, PhD, CCC-SLP, President
Barbara K. Cone, PhD, CCC-A, Vice President for Academic Affairs in Audiology
Carolyn W. Higdon, EdD, CCC-SLP, Vice President for Finance
This is a quarterly journal of clinical practice for speech-language pathologists and language researchers. This journal will be online only beginning January 2010.

8829   **Journal of Speech, Language and Hearing Research**
American Speech-Language-Hearing Association
2200 Research Boulevard
Rockville, MD 20850-3289   301-296-5700
                                          800-638-8255
                                          Fax: 301-296-8580
                                          nsslha@asha.org
                                          www.asha.org
Elizabeth S. McCrea, PhD, CCC-SLP, President
Barbara K. Cone, PhD, CCC-A, Vice President for Academic Affairs in Audiology
Carolyn W. Higdon, EdD, CCC-SLP, Vice President for Finance
This bimonthly journal contains basic, as well as applied research in normal and disordered communication processes. It will be available online only beginning January 2010.

8830   **Language, Speech, and Hearing Services in Schools**
International Fluency Association
Northern Illinois University
Dept. of Communicative Disorders
DeKalb, IL 60115-2899   www.theifa.org
David Shapiro, President
Norimune Kawat, Secretary
Rachel Everard, Treasurer
This is a quarterly journal focusing on research appropriate to speech-language pathologists and audiologists in schools. The journal will only be available online beginning in January 2010.

Magazines

8831   **Communication Outlook**
Artificial Language Laboratory
220 Trowbridge Road
East Lansing, MI 48824   517-353-8332
                                          Fax: 517-353-4766
                                          artling@msu.edu
                                          www.msu.edu
Lou Anna K. Simon, President
Satish Udpa, EVP for Administrative Services
Bill Beekman, VP & Secretary
Communication Outlook (CO) is an international quarterly magazine, which focuses on the techniques and technology of augmentative and alternative communication. CO provides information on technological developments for persons experiencing communication handicaps due to neurological, sensory or neuromuscular conditions. *$18.00*
32 pages Quarterly

Newsletters

8832   **Access Academics & Research**
American Speech-Language-Hearing Association
2200 Research Boulevard
Rockville, MD 20850-3289   301-296-5700
                                          800-638-8255
                                          Fax: 301-296-8580
                                          nsslha@asha.org
                                          www.asha.org
Elizabeth S. McCrea, PhD, CCC-SLP, President
Barbara K. Cone, PhD, CCC-A, Vice President for Academic Affairs in Audiology
Carolyn W. Higdon, EdD, CCC-SLP, Vice President for Finance
Dedicated to the specific needs of academic and clinical faculty, PhD students and researchers. The e-newsletter was developed as part of the Focused Initiative on the PhD Shortage in Higher Education.

8833   **Access Audiology**
American Speech-Language-Hearing Association
2200 Research Boulevard
Rockville, MD 20850-3289   301-296-5700
                                          800-638-8255
                                          Fax: 301-296-8580
                                          nsslha@asha.org
                                          www.asha.org
Elizabeth S. McCrea, PhD, CCC-SLP, President
Barbara K. Cone, PhD, CCC-A, Vice President for Academic Affairs in Audiology
Carolyn W. Higdon, EdD, CCC-SLP, Vice President for Finance
Dedicated to the specific needs of all professionals interested in hearing, balance, and the field of audiology. Each issue spotlights a specific topic of interest and relevance to audiologists.

8834   **Access SLP Health Care**
American Speech-Language-Hearing Association
2200 Research Boulevard
Rockville, MD 20850-3289   301-296-5700
                                          800-638-8255
                                          Fax: 301-296-8580
                                          nsslha@asha.org
                                          www.asha.org
Elizabeth S. McCrea, PhD, CCC-SLP, President
Barbara K. Cone, PhD, CCC-A, Vice President for Academic Affairs in Audiology
Carolyn W. Higdon, EdD, CCC-SLP, Vice President for Finance
An e-newsletter dedicated to the specific needs of speech-language pathologists in healthcare settings. Each issue of Access SLP Health Care features recent legislative activity impacting SLPs and provides information on clinical issues, continuing education opportunities, and ASHA web-based resources.

8835   **Access Schools**
American Speech-Language-Hearing Association
2200 Research Boulevard
Rockville, MD 20850-3289   301-296-5700
                                          800-638-8255
                                          Fax: 301-296-8580
                                          nsslha@asha.org
                                          www.asha.org
Elizabeth S. McCrea, PhD, CCC-SLP, President
Barbara K. Cone, PhD, CCC-A, Vice President for Academic Affairs in Audiology
Carolyn W. Higdon, EdD, CCC-SLP, Vice President for Finance
Dedicated to the specific needs of school-based speech-language pathologists. Each Access Schools e-newsletter features recent legislative activity impacting school SLPs and provides information on clinical issues, continuing education opportunities, and ASHA web-based resources.

8836   Autism Research Review International
Autism Research Institute
4182 Adams Avenue
San Diego, CA 92116-2599   619-281-7165
                                      866-366-3361
                                  Fax: 619-563-6840
                                        autism.com

Stephen Edelson, Executive Director
Jane Johnson, Managing Director
Valerie Paradiz, Director
Provides clearly written summaries of articles selected from computer searches. *$18.00*
8 pages Quarterly

8837   Communicologist
Texas Speech-Language-Hearing Association
Ste 200
918 Congress Ave
Austin, TX 78701-2342   512-494-1128
                                      888-729-8742
                                  Fax: 512-494-1129

Judith Keller, President
Larry Higdon, Director
Melanie McDonald, President Elect
A forum for distributing current information relevant to the practices of speech-language pathology and audiology across the state. Provides TSHA membership with the latest news from the Executive Board and Task Forces, as well as information about regional associations, distinguished service providers, the TSHA Annual Convention, and committee honors and nominations. Also contains advertisements of interest to the field.

8838   Connect
Hearing, Speech & Deafness Center (HSDC)
1625 19th Ave.
Seattle, WA 98122   206-323-5770
                                      888-222-5036
                                  Fax: 206-328-6871
                                  TTY: 800-761-2821
                                    clinics@hsdc.org
                                        www.hsdc.org

Lindsay Klarman, Executive Director
A newsletter that addresses concerns of those affected by speech and language disorders. HSDC is a nonprofit for clients who are deaf, hard of hearing, or who face other communication barriers such as speech challenges.
8 pages Quarterly

8839   NSSLHA Now
Ntn'l Student Speech Language Hearing Association
2200 Research Boulevard
Rockville, MD 20850-3289   301-296-5700
                                      800-638-8255
                                  Fax: 301-296-8580
                                    nsslha@asha.org
                                        www.asha.org

Elizabeth S. McCrea, PhD, CCC-SLP, President
Barbara K. Cone, PhD, CCC-A, Vice President for Academic Affairs in Audiology
Carolyn W. Higdon, EdD, CCC-SLP, Vice President for Finance
Published three times per year.

8840   On Cue
National Cued Speech Association
1300 Pennsylvania Avenue, NW
Suite 190-713
Washington, DC 20004   301-915-8009
                                      800-459-3529
                                    www.cuedspeech.org

Shannon Howell, President
Penny Hakim, 1st Vice President
John Brubaker, VP Fundraising
Published several times a year and mailed to members of the Association.

8841   Stuttering & Your Child: Help For Parents
Stuttering Foundation of America
18005 Moriah Woods Blvd
PO Box 11749, Suite 3
Memphis, TN 38111-0749   901-761-0343
                                      800-992-9392
                                  Fax: 901-761-0484
                                  info@stutteringhelp.org
                                  www.StutteringHelp.org

Jane Fraser, President
Dennis Drayna, Director
Joseph R. G. Fulcher, Director
The Stuttering Foundation provides resources, services and support to those who stutter and their families, as well as support research into the cause of stuttering. The Stuttering Foundation provides a referral list of speech-language pathologists and referrals to other information including research on stuttering, intensive workshops and camps. *$10.00*

8842   Stuttering Foundation Newsletter
Stuttering Foundation of America
P.O.Box 11749
Memphis, TN 38111-0749   901-761-0343
                                      800-992-9392
                                  Fax: 901-761-0484
                                  info@stutteringhelp.org
                                  www.stutteringhelp.org

Jane Fraser, President
Jean Gruss, Journalist
Robert M. Kurtz, Chairman & CEO

8843   Voice
Providence Speech and Hearing Association
1301 Providence Avenue
Orange, CA 92868   714-923-1521
                                      855-901-7742
                                  Fax: 714-744-3841
                                      pshc@pshc.org
                                        www.pshc.org

Lewis Jaffe, President
Bret Rathwick, Vice President - Finance
Casey Immel, Treasurer
People of all ages with speech and hearing problems by providing specialized products and services.

Audio/Visual

8844   Autism: A World Apart
Fanlight Productions
c/o Icarus Films
32 Court Street, 21st Floor
Brooklyn, NY 11201   718-488-8900
                                      800-876-1710
                                  Fax: 718-488-8642
                                    info@fanlight.com
                                      www.fanlight.com

Ben Achtenberg, Owner, Founder
Nicole Johnson, Publicity Coordinator
Anthony Sweeney, Marketing Director
In this documentary, three families show us what the textbooks and studies cannot: what it's like to live with autism day after day; to raise and love children who may be withdrawn and violent and unable to make personal connections with their families. 29 minutes.
VHS/DVD
ISBN 1-572950-39-0

8845   Autism: the Unfolding Mystery
Aquarius Health Care Media
18 N Main St
Sherborn, MA 1770-1066   508-650-1616

Lesile Kussmann, Owner
Explore what it means to be autistic, how you can recognize the signs of autism in your child, and hear about new treatments and programs to help children learn to deal with the disorder. *$145.00*
DVD

8846 **Getting Started with Facilitated Communication**
Facilitated Communication Institute, Syracuse Univ
370 Huntington Hall
Syracuse, NY 13244-1   315-443-9657
                                             Fax: 315-443-9218

Annegret Schubert, Producer
Describes in detail how to help individuals with autism and/or severe communication difficulties to get started with facilitated communication.
Video

8847 **I Just Want My Little Boy Back**
Autism Treatment Center Of America
2080 South Undermountain Road
Sheffield, MA 01257   413-229-2100
                                                 800-714-2779
                                          happiness@option.org
                                          http://www.option.org
Samahria Lyt Kaufman, Co-Founder and Co-Director
Dane Griffith, Director of Administrative Services
Bears Kaufman, Co-Founder and Co-Director
A great video for parents and professionals caring for children with special needs. Join one British family and their autistic son before, during and after their journey to America to attend The Son-Rise Program at The Autism Treatment Center of America. This informative, inspirational and deeply moving story not only captures the joy, tears, challenges and triumps of this amazing little boy and his family, but also serves as a powerful introduction to the attitude and principles of the program. *$25.00*

8848 **Understanding Autism**
Fanlight Productions
c/o Icarus Films
32 Court Street, 21st Floor
Brooklyn, NY 11201   718-488-8900
                                                 800-876-1710
                                            Fax: 718-488-8642
                                             info@fanlight.com
                                              www.fanlight.com
Ben Achtenberg, Owner, Founder
Nicole Johnson, Publicity Coordinator
Anthony Sweeney, Marketing Director
Parents of children with autism discuss the nature and symptoms of this lifelong disability and outline a treatment program based on behavior modification principles. 19 minutes
VHS/DVD
ISBN 1-572951-00-1

Support Groups

8849 **Autism Society of America**
4340 East West Highway
Suite 350
Bethesda, MD 20814-3067   301-657-0881
                                                 800-328-8476
                                            Fax: 301-657-0869
                                          www.autism-society.org
Mary Beth Collins, Director of Programs
Tonia Ferguson, Senior Director of Content
Scott Badesch, President/Chief Executive Officer
ASA is the largest and oldest grassroots organization within the autism community, with a nationwide network of chapters and over 20,000 members and supporters nationwide. ASA is the leading source of education, information and referral about autism and has been the leader in advocacy and legislative initiatives for more than four decades.

8850 **Friends: National Association of Young People who Stutter**
38 S Oyster Bay Rd
Syosset, NY 11791-5033   866-866-8335
                                             lcaggiano@aol.com
                                          www.friendswhostutter.org
Lee Caggiano, President
A national organization created to provide a network of love and support for children and teenagers who stutter, their families, and the professionals who work with them.

8851 **National Health Information Center**
US Department of Health
P.O.Box 1133
Washington, DC 20013-1133   301-565-4167
                                                 800-336-4797
                                                 301-468-7394
                                            Fax: 301-984-4256
                                          healthypeople@hhs.gov
                                          http://www.healthypeople.gov
Jonathan Fielding, Chair
Shirika Kumanyika, Vice Chair
A health information referral service that puts health professionals and consumers who have health questions in touch with those organizations that are best able to provide answers.

8852 **Speech Pathways**
410 Meadow Creek Drive
Suite 206
Westminster, MD 21158   410-374-0555
                                                 800-961-2724
                                            Fax: 410-374-8620
                                    kim.bell@speechpathways.net
                                              speechpathways.net
Kimberly A. Bell, Owner
Karie Hadley, Therapist
Erica Hamilton, Therapist
We realize that parent and family support is critical to a child's success, in therapy as well as in life. We offer support at local and regional levels along with traditional speech and language services, and a wide variety of specialized pediatric programs. Our support groups/services are open to the larger community as well as to our clients.

8853 **The Cherab Foundation**
2301 NE Savannah Rd
Suite 1771
Jensen Beach, FL 34957   772-335-5135
                                               help@cherab.org
                                             cherabfoundation.org
Lisa Geng, Founder & President
Jolie Abreu, Vice President
The Cherab Foundation is a world-wide nonprofit organization working to improve the communication skills and education of all children with speech and language delays and disorders.

Visual

Associations

8854 American Academy of Ophthalmology
655 Beach St
San Francisco, CA 94109   415-561-8540
866-561-8558
Fax: 415-561-8575
customer_service@aao.org
aao.org

Cynthia Ann Bradford, MD, President
David W Parke II, MD, CEO
Maria M Aaron, MD, Secretary for Annual Meeting
The American Academy of Ophthalmology is an association of
doctors who provide comprehensive eye care, including medical,
surgical and optical care. The academy is dedicated to advancing
the profession of ophthalmology through programs, public
education, courses and advocacy.

8855 American Action Fund for Blind Children and Adults
1800 Johnston St.
Baltimore, MD 21230-4914   410-659-9315
actionfund@actionfund.org
www.actionfund.org

Barbara Loos, President
Ramona Walhof, Vice President
Sandra Halverson, Second Vice President/Medical Transcriptionist
A service agency which specializes in providing to blind people
help which is not readily available to them from government programs or other existing service systems. The services are planned
especially to meet the needs of blind children, the elderly blind,
and the deaf-blind.

8856 American Council of Blind Lions
148 Vernon Ave.
Louisville, KY 40206   502-897-1472
carla40206@gmail.com
www.acb.org/affiliate-ACBL

Carla Ruschival, President
The American Council of Blind Lions (ACBL) works to educate
members of local Lions Clubs about the needs and concerns of
blind or visually impaired people. The ACBL is open to members
from across the United States and encourages blind persons to
join their local clubs and participate in civic projects.

8857 American Council of the Blind
1703 N Beauregard St
Suite 420
Alexandria, VA 22311   202-467-5081
800-424-8666
Fax: 703-465-5085
info@acb.org
www.acb.org

Eric Bridges, Executive Director
Tony Stephens, Director, Advocacy & Governmental Affairs
The American Council of the Blind (ACB) is an association working to increase the independence, security, and opportunity for all
blind or visually impaired individuals. The Council primarily focuses on developing and maintaining policies to implement the
services needed for the blind or visually impaired.

8858 American Council of the Blind Radio Amateurs
19821 Vineyard Ln.
Saratoga, CA 95070   408-257-1034
acbra@acb.org
www.acbhams.org

John Glass, President
A special interest affiliate of the American Council of the Blind,
the American Council of the Blind Radio Amateurs (ACBRA)
promotes the interest of FCC licensed amaetur radio operators.
The ACBRA is made up of legally blind and fully sighted radio
amateurs.

8859 American Foundation for the Blind
2 Penn Plaza
Suite 1102
New York, NY 10121   800-232-5463
www.afb.org

Kirk Adams, President & CEO
Darren M. Davis, Executive Administrator Executive Office
The American Foundation for the Blind (AFB) is a national non-
profit that is dedicated to removing barriers, creating solutions,
and expanding possibilities for the blind and visually impaired.
The AFB is focused on spreading access to technology, elevating
the quality of information and tools for professional who serve
people with vision loss, and the promotion of independent living
for those with vision loss.

8860 American Optometric Association
243 N Lindbergh Blvd
Floor 1
St. Louis, MO 63141-7881   800-365-2219
www.aoa.org

Christopher J. Quinn, O.D, President
Barbara L. Horn, O.D, Vice President
William T. Reynolds, O.D, Secretary-Treasurer
The American Optometric Association (AOA) advocates for improving the quality and availability of eye and vision care. The
AOA represents more than 44,000 doctors of optometry,
optometric professionals, and optometry students and works to
set professional standards, lobby government and organizations
on behalf of the profession, and provide research and education
leadership.

8861 American Printing House for the Blind
American Printing House for the Blind, Inc.
1839 Frankfort Ave.
Louisville, KY 40206-0085   502-895-2405
800-223-1839
Fax: 502-899-2284
info@aph.org
www.aph.org

The American Printing House for the Blind (APH) is the world's
largest nonprofit organization creating educational and independent living products for blind and visually impaired individuals. APH promotes independence through the manufacturing of
specialized materials and products for blind persons. The APH is
the official supplier of educational materials in the United States
below a college level.

8862 Associated Services for the Blind and Visually Impaired
919 Walnut Street
Philadelphia, PA 19107-5237   215-627-0600
Fax: 215-922-0692
asbinfo@asb.org
www.asb.org

Karla S. McCaney, President & CEO
Beth Deering, Chief Program Officer
Sylvia Purnell, Director of Learning & Development
Associated Services for the Blind and Visually Impaired (ASB),
is a private, nonprofit organization working to provide services,
education, training, and resources to promote self-esteem, independence, and self determination in people who are blind or visually impaired. In addition, ASB advocates for the rights of blind
and visually impaired persons through community actions and
public education.

**8863 Association for Education & Rehabilitationof the Blind
& Visually Impaired**
5680 King Centre Dr.
Suite 600
Alexandria, VA 22315   703-671-4500
Fax: 703-671-6391
aer@aerbvi.org
www.aerbvi.org

Neva Fairchild, President
Sergio Oliva, Secretary
Jennifer Wheeler, Treasurer
The Association for Education and Rehabilitation of the Blind
and Visually Impaired (AER) is an international, nonprofit membership organization that supports professionals who provide education and rehabilitation services to people with visual
impairments. The AER provides professional development and

growth opportunities for its members and advocates to maintain specialized blind services.

8864 Association for Macular Diseases
The Association for Macular Diseases, Inc.
210 E 64th St
New York, NY 10065   212-605-3719
                                    association@retinal-research.org
                                                    macula.org

Bernard Landou, President
The Association for Macular Diseases provides support and assistance to individuals with macular disease, their caregivers, and professional community.

8865 Association for Research in Vision and Ophthalmology
1801 Rockville Pike
Suite 400
Rockville, MD 20852-5622   240-221-2900
                                            Fax: 240-221-0370
                                                   arvo@arvo.org
                                                    www.arvo.org

The Association for Research in Vision and Ophthalmology (ARVO) advances research and understanding of the visual system and the preventing, treating, and curing visual disorders. ARVO is an international organization of 12,000 researches from 75 countries performing both clinical and basic research.

8866 Association for Vision Rehabilitation and Employment
174 Court St
Binghamton, NY 13901   607-724-2428
                                            Fax: 607-771-8045
                                              avreinfo@avreus.org
                                                  www.avreus.org

Ken Fernald, President & CEO
Jenn Small, Chief Operating Officer
Anthony Saccento, Chief Financial Officer
The Association for Vision Rehabilitation and Employment, Inc. (AVRE) is a private, nonprofit organization providing rehabilitation and employment services for people who are blind or visually impaired in the Twin Tiers of New York and Pennsylvania. Services include Low Vision, Early Intervention, Orientation and Mobility, Vision Rehabilitation Therapy, and employment preparation and placement.

8867 Association of Blind Citizens
PO Box 246
Holbrook, MA 02343   781-961-1023
                                            Fax: 781-961-0004
                                       president@blindcitizens.org
                                              www.blindcitizens.org
The Association of Blind Citizens (ABC) is a membership organization advocating for, and advancing opportunities in education, employment, cultural, and recreational activities for blind and visually impaired persons.

8868 Blind Children's Center
4120 Marathon St
Los Angeles, CA 90029-3584   323-664-2153
                                     info@blindchildrenscenter.org
                                     www.blindchildrenscenter.org
Sarah E. Orth, Chief Executive Officer
Fernanda Armenta-Schmitt, Director, Education & Family Services
A nonprofit organization working to foster the development and education of children from birth to the 2nd grade who are blind or visually impaired. The Blind Children's Center serves about 100 children a year through a variety of family centered programs including the infant, preschool, and elementary.

8869 Blind Information Technology Specialists
8761 E Placita Bolivar
Tucson, AZ 85715-5650   520-232-2100
                                                  www.bits-acb.org
Tom L. Jones, President
Earlene Hughes, Vice President
David Tanner, Secretary
The Blind Information Technology Specialists (BITS) is a nonprofit organization fostering the career development of computer professionals, promoting the use of computer technology and improved information access for people who are blind or visually impaired.

8870 Blinded Veterans Association
1001 King St.
Suite 300
Alexandria, VA 22314   800-669-7079
                                                     bva@bva.org
                                                     www.bva.org
Thomas Zampieri, National President
Joseph D. McNeil, Sr., National Vice President
Donald D. Overton, Jr., Executive Director
The Blinded Veterans Association locates blinded veterans who need assistance, guides them through the rehabilitation process and acts as advocates for them before Congress and the Department of Veterans Affairs in securing the benefits they have earned through their service to the nation. The association also promotes access to technology, practical use of the latest research as well as offering programs for blinded veterans.

8871 Braille Institute of America
741 N Vermont Ave.
Los Angeles, CA 90029-3594   323-663-1111
                                                   800-272-4553
                                            Fax: 323-663-0867
                                           la@brailleinstitute.org
                                           www.brailleinstitute.org
Peter A. Mindnich, President
Gloria Coulston, Vice President, Program Delivery
Nancy N. Neibrugge, Vice President, Program Content
The Braille Institute is a nonprofit organization providing assistance to blind and visually impaired individuals. The institute offers a variety of free programs, classes, and services at 5 regional centers in Southern California.

8872 California State Library Braille and Talking Book Library
PO Box 942837
Sacramento, CA 94237-0001   916-654-0640
                                                   800-952-5666
                                              btbl@library.ca.gov
                                                  www.btbl.ca.gov
A division of the California State Library, the Braille and Talking Book Library (BTBL) is a free service offering braille and audiobook to readers in Northern California who cannot read due to a visual or physical disability. The BTBL is an affiliate of the National Service for the Blind and Physically Handicapped.

8873 Canine Helpers for the Handicapped
Canine Helpers for the Handicapped, Inc.
5699 Ridge Rd.
Lockport, NY 14094   716-433-4035
                                                 chhdogs@aol.com
A nonprofit organization dedicated to training dogs in order to assist people with disabilities and promote independence.

8874 Caption Center
Media Access Group at WGBH
One Guest St.
Boston, MA 02135   617-300-3600
                                            Fax: 617-300-1020
                                                  access@wgbh.org
Pat McDonald, Director
The Caption Center was the world's first captioning agency providing access to television for viewers who are visually impaired and/or hard of hearing. The Center develops new solutions and uses closed captioning and descriptive video to promote access to technology.

8875 Central Association for the Blind & Visually Impaired
507 Kent St.
Utica, NY 13501   315-797-2233
                                                   877-719-9996
                                                    www.cabvi.org
Edward P. Welsh, Chair
Kenneth C. Thayer, Vice Chair
Richard Evans, Treasurer
It assists people who are blind or visually impaired to achieve their highest levels of independence.

8876 Chicago Lighthouse for People who are Blind and Visually Impaired
1850 W Roosevelt Rd
Chicago, IL 60608-1298
312-666-1331
Fax: 312-243-8539
TTY: 312-666-8874
www.chicagolighthouse.org
Bruce R. Hague, Chairman
Sandra C. Forsythe, Vice Chairman
Janet P. Szlyk, President
A non profit agency committed to providing the highest quality educational, clinical, vocational, and rehabilitation services for children, youth and adults who are blind or visually impaired, including deaf blind and multi disabled. Also respects personal dignity and partners with individuals to enhance independent living and self sufficiency. This agency is a leader, innovator and advocate for people who are blind or visually impaired, enhancing the quality of life for all individuals.

8877 Clovernook Center for the Blind and Visually Impaired
7000 Hamilton Ave
Cincinnati, OH 45231-5240
513-522-3860
888-234-7156
Fax: 513-728-3946
TTY: 513-522-3860
contact@clovernook.org
www.clovernook.org
Alfred J. Tuchfarber, Chair
Wilbert F. Schwartz, Vice Chair
Mark Jackson, Treasurer
Mission is to promote independence and foster the highest quality of life for people with visual impairments, including those with additional disabilities. We provide comprehensive program services including training and support for independent living, orientation and mobility instruction, vocational training, job placement, counseling, recreation, and youth services. Meaningful employment opportunities are also provided to individuals who are blind or visually impaired.

8878 Clovernook Printing House, The Clovernook Center for the Blind and Visually Impaired
7000 Hamilton Ave
Cincinnati, OH 45231-5240
513-522-3860
888-234-7156
Fax: 513-728-3946
contact@clovernook.org
www.clovernook.org
Alfred J. Tuchfarber, Chair
Wilbert F. Schwartz, Vice Chair
Mark Jackson, Treasurer
Clovernook also offers Braille Transcription Services including: Literary Books, Literary Magazines, Religious Materials, Instructional Manuals, ADA Conformance Materials, Literary Textbook Materials, Menus, Braille Alphabet Cards, and Forms. In addition, our Business Operations provide meaningful employment opportunities for individuals who are blind or visually impaired, while at the same time manufacturing high-quality products for customers across the country. $145.00
591 pages
ISBN 1-930956-48-7

8879 College of Optometrists in Vision Development
215 W Garfield Rd
Ste 200
Aurora, OH 44202-7884
330-995-0718
888-268-3770
Fax: 330-995-0719
info@covd.org
www.covd.org
David A. Damari, President
Kara Heying, Vice President
Christine Allison, Secretary-Treasurer
The College of Optometrists in Vision Development (COVD) is an international membership association of eye care professionals including optometrists, optometry students, and vision therapists. Members of COVD provide developmental vision care, vision therapy and vision rehabilitation services for children and adults.

8880 College of Syntonic Optometry
2052 W Morales Dr.
Pueblo West, CO 81007
719-547-8177
877-559-0541
Fax: 719-547-3750
Syntonics@q.com
www.collegeofsyntonicoptometry.com
Hans Lessmann, O.D, FCOVD, President
Robert Fox, O.D, FCOVD, FCSO, Vice President
Larry Wallace, O.D, Ph.D, Education Director
The College of Syntonic Optometry is an international organization dedicated to furthering Phototherapy in the treatment of the visual system. Members of the college include optometrists, and health care professionals.

8881 Columbia Lighthouse for the Blind
1825 K St. NW
Suite 1103
Washington, DC 20006
202-454-6400
Fax: 202-955-6401
info@clb.org
www.clb.org
Tony Cancelosi, President & CEO
Jocelyn Hunter, Senior Director, Communications
Toya Horten, Director, Administrative Operations
Columbia Lighthouse for the Blind (CLB) helps blind and visually impaired individuals in Washington, DC. CLB's services include training and consultation in assistive technology, employment skills, career placement, low vision care, and counseling and rehabilitation services.

8882 DeafBlind Division of the National Federation of the Blind
200 E. Wells St.
at Jernigan Place
Baltimore, MD 21230
410-659-9314
Fax: 410-685-5653
nfb@nfb.org
www.nfb.org
Alice Eaddy, Division President
The nation's largest and most influential membership organization of blind persons, with a two-fold purpose: to help blind persons achieve self-confidence and self respect and to act as a vehicle for collective self-expression by the blind. The NFB improves blind people's lives through advocacy, education, research, technology, and programs encouraging independence and self-confidence. It is the leading force in the blindness field today and is the voice of the nations blind.

8883 Desert Blind & Handicapped Association
Desert Blind and Handicapped Association, Inc.
777 E Tahquitz Canyon Way
Suite 200
Palm Springs, CA 92262
760-969-5025
info@desertblind.org
Thomas Samulski, Executive Director
George Holliday, Treasurer
The Desert Blind & Handicapped Association provides free transportation for individuals who are blind or have a disability.

8884 Eye Bank Association of America
1101 17th St NW
Suite 400
Washington, DC 20036
202-775-4999
Fax: 202-429-6036
www.restoresight.org
Kevin P. Corcoran, CAE, President & CEO
Bernie Dellario, Director, Finance
Stacey Gardner, Director, Education
The Eye Bank Association of America (EBAA) is a nonprofit organization advocating the restoration of sight by advancing donation, transplantation, and research. The EBAA is the oldest transplant association in the United States.

8885 Fidelco Guide Dog Foundation
103 Vision Way
Bloomfield, CT 06002   860-243-5200
                                   Fax: 860-769-0567
                                   admissions@fidelco.org
                                   www.fidelco.org

Karen C. Tripp, Chair
G. Kenneth Bernhard, Esq., Vice Chair
Gregg Barratt, Chief of Staff
The Fidelco Guide Dog Foundation creates increased freedom
and independence for men and women who are blind by providing
them with guide dogs.

8886 Fight for Sight
381 Park Ave S
Suite 809
New York, NY 10016   212-679-6060
                                   Fax: 212-679-4466
                                   Arthur@fightforsight.org
                                   www.fightforsight.org

Arthur Makar, Executive Director
Janice Benson, Associate Director
Fight for Sight is a nonprofit charity working to support eye and
vision research through the providing of funds to scientists starting their careers.

8887 Foundation Fighting Blindness
7168 Columbia Gateway Dr.
Suite 100
Columbia, MD 21046   410-423-0600
                                   800-683-5555
                                   TTY: 410363713951
                                   info@FightBlindness.org
                                   www.blindness.org

William T. Schmidt, Chief Executive Officer
Valerie Navy-Daniels, Chief Development Officer
Stephen M. Rose, PhD, Chief Research Officer
The Foundation Fighting Blindness (FFB) works to promote research in order to prevent, treat and restore vision. FFB is currently the world's leading private funder of retinal disease
research, funding over 100 research grants and 150 researchers.

8888 Guide Dogs for the Blind
PO Box 151200
San Rafael, CA 94915   800-295-4050
                                   information@guidedogs.com
                                   www.guidedogs.com

Christine Benninger, Chief Executive Officer & President
Cathy Martin, Chief Financial Officer & Treasurer
Brent Ruppel, Vice President, Community Operations
Guide Dogs for the Blind empowers lives by creating exceptional
partnerships between people, dogs, and communities. All of their
services provided free of charge of charge to their clients, including personalized training and extensive post-graduation support,
plus financial assistance for veterinary care, if needed.

8889 Guiding Eyes for the Blind
611 Granite Springs Rd
Yorktown Heights, NY 10598-3499   914-245-4024
                                   800-942-0149
                                   Fax: 914-245-1609
                                   info@guidingeyes.org
                                   www.guidingeyes.org

Thomas Panek, President & Chief Executive Officer
Guiding Eyes for the Blind is a nonprofit organization providing
guide dogs for individuals who are blind or visually impaired.

8890 Horizons for the Blind
125 Erick St.
A103
Crystal Lake, IL 60014   815-444-8800
                                   800-318-2000
                                   Fax: 815-444-8830
                                   mail@horizons-blind.org
                                   www.horizons-blind.org

Camille Caffarelli, Executive Director
Jeff T. Thorsen, First Vice President & Treasurer
Keith Myers, Second Vice President
Horizons for the Blind is a nonprofit organization working to im-
prove the quality of life for people who are blind or visually im-

paired by increasing access to consumer products, services, culture, arts, education, and recreation.

8891 Independent Visually Impaired Entrepreneurs
                                   818-238-9321
                                   abazyn@bazyncommunications.com
                                   www.ivie-acb.org

Ardis Bazyn, President
The Independent Visually Impaired Entrepreneurs (IVIE) is a national organization for visually impaired business owners. The
IVIE offers an annual convention, planning a program of interest
for business owners.

8892 Institute for Families
1300 N Vermont Ave.
Suite 1004
Los Angeles, CA 90027   323-361-4649
                                   Fax: 323-665-7869
                                   info@instituteforfamilies.org
                                   instituteforfamilies.org

Gary Huffaker, Chairperson
Institute for Families is a nonprofit organization providing support and information for families of children with vision loss. The
Institute provides guidance through a resource and referral network; referring families to organizations specializing in meeting
the needs of children with specific vision loss problems.

8893 International Association of Audio Information Services
                                   800-280-5325
                                   iaaismember@gmail.com
                                   www.iaais.org

Marjorie Moore, President
Maryfrances Evans, Vice-President
The International Association of Audio Information Services
(IAAIS) is a membership organization that works to turn text into
speech and providing information through broadcast, telephone
or internet. IAAIS connects and supports organizations that deliver equal access information for people with disabilities
worldwide.

8894 Jewish Braille Institute International
JBI International
110 E 30th St
New York, NY 10016-7393   212-889-2525
                                   800-433-1531
                                   Fax: 212-689-3692
                                   admin@jbilibrary.org
                                   www.jbilibrary.org

Dr. Ellen Isler, President & Cheif Executive Officer
Israel A. Taub, Vice President & Cheif Financil Officer
The Jewish Braille Institute (JBI) International is a nonprofit organization working to meet the Jewish and general cultural needs
of the blind and visually impaired.

8895 Keystone Blind Association
3056 East State St.
Hermitage, PA 16148   724-347-5501
                                   Fax: 724-347-2204
                                   info@keystoneblind.org
                                   www.keystoneblind.org

Jonathan Fister, President/ CEO
Karen Anderson, Board Member
Sam Bellich, Board Member
The Keystone Blind Association works to education, and employ
individuals with vision loss. Headquartered in Hermitage, the As-
sociation has offices in Meadville and New Castle, Pennsylvania.

8896 Lighthouse Guild
250 West 64th Street
New York, NY 10023   800-284-4422
                                   www.lighthouseguild.org

Calvin W. Roberts, President & CEO
James M. Dubin, Chairman
Lawrence E. Goldschmidt, Vice Chairman & Treasurer
Lighthouse Guild is a not-for-profit vision & healthcare organization, addressing the needs of people who are blind or visually
impaired, including those with multiple disabilities or chronic
medical conditions.

8897   Lions Clubs International
300 W 22nd St
Oak Brook, IL 60523-8842   630-571-5466
                                        Fax: 630-571-8890
                                        TTY: 630-571-6533
                                        lions@lionsclubs.org
                                        www.lionsclubs.org
Benedict Ancar, Director
Jui-Tai Chang, Director
Jaime Garcia Cepeda, Director
Our 46,000 clubs and 1.35 million members make us the world's largest service club organization. We're also one of the most effective. Our members do whatever is needed to help their local communities. Everywhere we work, we make friends. With children who need eyeglasses, with seniors who don't have enough to eat and with people we may never meet.

8898   Macular Degeneration Foundation
PO Box 531313
Henderson, NV 89053-1313   702-450-2908
                                        888-633-3937
                                        liz@eyesight.org
                                        www.eyesight.org
Liz Trauernicht, President/Director of Communications
Julie Zavala, VP/Asst Director of Operations
David Seftel, M.D., MBA, Executive Vice President/Director of Research Development
The Macular Degeneration Foundation is dedicated to those who have and will develop macular degeneration. We offer this growing community the latest information, news, hope and encouragement.

8899   National Alliance of Blind Students NABS Liaison
American Council of the Blind
1155 15th St NW
Ste 1004
Washington, DC 20005-2706   202-467-5081
                                        800-424-8666
                                        Fax: 202-467-5085
                                        info@acb.org
                                        www.acb.org
Jill Gaus, President
Lynn Jansen, Vice President
Debby Lieberman, Secretary
A student affiliate of the American Council of the Blind which is a national organization of blind and visually impaired high school and college students who believe that every blind and visually impaired student has the right to an equal and accessible education. Also encourages blind and visually impaired students to challenge their limits and reach their potential.

8900   National Association for Parents of Children with Visual Impairments (NAPVI)
PO Box 317
Watertown, MA 02471-317   617-972-7441
                                        800-562-6265
                                        Fax: 617-972-7444
                                        spedex.com@gmail.com
                                        www.spedex.com
Susan LaVenture, Executive Director
Julie Urban, President
Venetia Hayden, Vice President
A non profit organization of, by and for parents committed to providing support to the parents of children who have visual impairments. Also a national organization that enables parents to find information and resources for their children who are blind or visually impaired including those with additional disabilities. NAPVI also provides leadership, support, and training to assist parents in helping children reach their potential.

8901   National Association for Visually Handicapped (NAVH)
111 E 59th S
Fl 6
New York, NY 10022-1202   212-889-3141
                                        800-829-0500
                                        Fax: 212-821-9707
                                        TTY: 212-821-9713
                                        info@lighthouse.org
                                        www.lighthouse.org
Alan R. Morse, President & CEO
Lawrence E. Goldschmidt, Deputy Chair & Secretary
Himanshu R. Shah, CFO
NAVH is unique in the services it offers to the hard of seeing™ worldwide and is the only non-profit organization solely dedicated to providing assistance to this population. NAVH runs senior support groups, provides individual consultations, informational materials, training in the use of visual aids, and numerous other tools to ensure that the visually impaired can remain independent and lead fulfilling lives.

8902   National Association of Blind Educators
National Federation of the Blind
200 E. Wells St.
at Jernigan Place
Baltimore, MD 21230   410-659-9314
                                        Fax: 410-685-5653
                                        nfb@nfb.org
                                        www.nfb.org
Cayte Mendez, Division President
Membership organization of blind teachers, professors and instructors in all levels of education. Provides support and information regarding professional responsibilities, classroom techniques, national testing methods and career obstacles. Publishes The Blind Educator, national magazine specifically for blind educators.

8903   National Association of Blind Lawyers
National Federation of the Blind
200 E. Wells St.
at Jernigan Place
Baltimore, MD 21230   410-659-9314
                                        Fax: 410-685-5653
                                        nfb@nfb.org
                                        www.nfb.org
Scott LaBarre, President
Membership organization of blind attorneys, law students, judges and others in the law field. Provides support and information regarding employment, techniques used by the blind, advocacy, laws affecting the blind, current information about the American Bar Association and other issues for blind lawyers.

8904   National Association of Blind Merchants (NABM)
National Federation of the Blind
7450 Chapman Hwy.
Suite 319
Knoxville, TN 37920   888-687-6226
                                        president@merchants-nfb.org
                                        blindmerchants.org
Nicky Gacos, President
Harold Wilson, First Vice President
Ed Birmingham, Second Vice President
Serving as an advocacy and support group, NABM is a membership organization of blind persons employed in self-employment work or the Randolph-Sheppard Vending Program. The organization provides information on issues affecting blind merchants, including rehabilitation, social security, and tax.

8905   National Association of Blind Rehabilitation Professionals
National Federation of the Blind
200 E. Wells St.
at Jernigan Place
Baltimore, MD 21230   410-659-9314
                                        Fax: 410-685-5653
                                        nfb@nfb.org
                                        www.nfb.org
Amy Porterfield, Division President
Membership organization.

8906 **National Association of Blind Students**
National Federation of the Blind
200 E. Wells St.
at Jernigan Place
Baltimore, MD 21230
410-659-9314
Fax: 410-685-5653
nfb@nfb.org
www.nfb.org

Trisha Kulkarni, Division President
For over 30 years this national organization of blind students has provided support, information, and encouragement to blind college and university students. NABS leads the way in offering resources in issues such as national testing, accessible textbooks and materials, overcoming negative attitudes about blindness from school personnel, developing new techniques of accomplishing laboratory or field assignments, and many other college experiences.

8907 **National Association of Blind Teachers**
American Council of the Blind
1155 15th St NW
Ste 1004
Washington, DC 20005-2706
202-467-5081
800-424-8666
Fax: 202-467-5085
johnbuckley25@hotmail.com
www.blindteachers.net

Jill Gaus, President
Lynn Jansen, Vice President
Debby Lieberman, Secretary
Works to advance the teaching profession for blind and visually impaired people, protects the interest of teachers, presents discussions and solutions for special problems encountered by blind teachers and publishes a directory of blind teachers in the US.

8908 **National Association of Blind Veterans**
PO Box 784957
Winter Garden, FL 34778
321-948-1466
president@nabv.org
www.nabv.org

Dwight Sayer, President
Gene Huggins, 1st Vice President
Larry Ball, 2nd Vice President
A nationwide organization of blind and visually impaired veterans striving to serve fellow veterans who have lost their sight in the service of country or have lost their sight after serving country.

8909 **National Association of Guide Dog Users**
National Federation of the Blind
1003 Papaya Dr
Tampa, FL 33619-4629
813-626-2789
800-558-8261
888-624-3841
president@nagdu.org
www.nagdu.org

Marion Gwizdala, President
Provides information and support for guide dog users and works to secure high standards in guide dog training. Addresses issues of discrimination of guide dog users and offers public education about guide dog use. Biennial newsletter available: Harness Up!

8910 **National Association to Promote the Use of Braille**
National Federation of the Blind
39481 Gallaudet Dr
Apt 127
Fremont, CA 94538
510-248-0100
877-558-6524
Fax: 818-344-7930
mwillows@sbcglobal.net
www.nfbcal.org

Nadine Jacobson, President
Robert Jaquiss, Vice President
Linda Mentink, Second Vice President
Dedicated to securing improved Braille instruction, increasing the number of braille materials available to the blind and providing information of braille in securing independence, education and employment for the blind.

8911 **National Beep Baseball Association**
1501 41st NW
Apt G1
Rochester, MN 55901
866-400-4551
www.nbba.org

Stephen A. Guerra, Secretary
It facilitates and provides the adaptive version of America's favorite pastime for the blind, low vision and legally blind.

8912 **National Braille Association**
95 Allens Creek Rd
Bldg 1 Ste 202
Rochester, NY 14618- 3252
585-427-8260
Fax: 585-427-0263
nbaoffice@nationalbraille.org
www.nationalbraille.org

David Shaffar, Executive Director
Jan Carroll, President
Whitney Gregory-Williams, Vice President
The only national organization dedicated to the professional development of individuals who prepare and produce braille materials.

8913 **National Braille Press**
88 Saint Stephen St
Boston, MA 02115-4312
617-266-6160
888-965-8965
888-965-8965
Fax: 617-437-0456
contact@nbp.org
www.nbp.org

Brian A. Mac Donald, President
Kimberley Ballard, Vice President
Tony Grima, Vice President of Braille Publications
The guiding purposes of National Braille Press are to promote the literacy of blind children through braille, and to provide access to information that empowers blind people to actively engage in work, family, and commuity affairs.

8914 **National Center for Vision and Child Development**
Lighthouse Guild
250 West 64th Street
New York, NY 10023
800-284-4422
www.lighthouseguild.org

Calvin W. Roberts, President & CEO
James M. Dubin, Chairman
Lawrence E. Goldschmidt, Vice Chairman & Treasurer
The worldwide leader in helping people of all ages who are blind or partially sighted overcome the challenges of vision loss.

8915 **National Diabetes Action Network for the Blind**
National Federation of the Blind
200 E. Wells St.
at Jernigan Place
Baltimore, MD 21230
410-659-9314
Fax: 410-685-5653
bernienfb75@gmail.com
www.nfb.org

Debbie Wunder, Division President
Leading support and information organization of persons losing vision due to diabetes. Provides personal contact and resource information with other blind diabetics about non-visual techniques of independently managing diabetes, monitoring glucose levels, measuring insulin and other matters concerning diabetes. Publishes Voice of the Diabetic, the leading publication about diabetes and blindness.

8916 **National Eye Institute**
National Institutes of Health
31 Center Dr.
MSC 2510
Bethesda, MD 20892-2510
301-496-5248
2020@nei.nih.gov
www.nei.nih.gov

Michael F. Chiang, Director
Santa Tumminia, Deputy Director
Melanie Reagan, Acting Executive Officer
To conduct and support research for blinding eye diseases, visual disorders, mechanisms of visual function, and the preservation of sight.

8917 **National Federation of the Blind**
200 E. Wells St.
at Jernigan Place
Baltimore, MD 21230
410-659-9314
Fax: 410-685-5653
nfb@nfb.org
www.nfb.org

Mark A. Riccobono, President
John Berggren, Executive Director, Operations
Anil Lewis, Executive Director, Blindness Initiatives
The National Federation of the Blind (NFB) works to help blind
people achieve self-confidence, self-respect and self-determination and to achieve complete integration into society on a basis of
equality. The Federation provides public educations, information
and referral services, scholarships, literature and publications,
adaptive equipment, advocacy services, legal services,
employment assistance and more.

8918 **National Industries for the Blind**
1310 Braddock Pl
Alexandria, VA 22314-1691
703-310-0500
Fax: 703-998-8268
info@nib.org
www.nib.org

Gary J. Krump, Chairperson
Ronald Tascarella, Vice Chairperson
A nonprofit organization that represents over 100 associated industries serving people who are blind in thirty-six states. These
agencies serve people who are blind or visually impaired and help
them to reach their full potential. Services include job and family
counseling, job skills training, instruction in Braille and other
communication skills, children's programs and more.

8919 **National Library Service for the Blind and Physically
Handicapped (NLS)**
1291 Taylor St NW
Washington, DC 20011
202-707-5100
800-424-8567
Fax: 202-707-0712
nls@loc.gov
www.loc.gov/nls

Administers a national library service that provides Braille and
recorded books and magazines on free loan to anyone who cannot
read standard print because of visual or physical disabilities.
Annual

8920 **National Organization of Parents of Blind Children**
National Federation of the Blind
200 E. Wells St.
at Jernigan Place
Baltimore, MD 21230
410-659-9314
Fax: 410-685-5653
nfb@nfb.org
www.nfb.org

Carlton Walker, Division President
Support information and advocacy organization of parents of
blind or visually impaired children. Addresses issues ranging
from help to parents of a newborn blind infant, mobility and
braille instruction, education, social and community participation, development of self-confidence and other vital factors
involved in growth of a blind child.

8921 **New Eyes for the Needy**
549 Millburn Avenue
PO Box 332
Short Hills, NJ 07078-332
973-376-4903
Fax: 973-376-3807
neweyesfortheneedy@verizon.net
www.neweyesfortheneedy.org

Susan Dyckman, Executive Director
Marianne Muench Busby, Vice President
Barbara Daney, Treasurer
New Eyes provides new prescription glasses for poor children
and adults in the U.S. through a voucher system.

8922 **Prevent Blindness America**
211 W Wacker Drive
Suite 1700
Chicago, IL 60606
312-363-6001
800-331-2020
Fax: 312-363-6052
info@preventblindness.org
www.preventblindness.org

James E. Anderson, Chair
Kira Baldanado, Director
Arzu Bilazer, Creative Director
The nation's leading volunteer eye health and safety organization
dedicated to fighting blindness and saving sight. Also touches the
lives of millions of people each year through public and professional education, advocacy, certified vision screening training,
community and patient service programs and research.

8923 **Seeing Eye, The**
10 Washington Valley Rd
PO Box 375
Morristown, NJ 07963-0375
973-539-4425
Fax: 973-539-0922
info@seeingeye.org
www.seeingeye.org

Peggy Gibbon,, Director of Canine Development
James A Kutsch Jr, President/CEO
Dolores Holle, VMD,, Director of Canine Medicine & Surgery
An organization that concentrates on its mission to enhance the
independence, dignity, and self confidence of blind people
through the use of seeing eye dogs. The Seeing Eye will be an organization that concentrates on its mission to enhance the independence, dignity, and self confidence of blind people through
the use of Seeing Eye dogs, and on improving its ability to fulfill
this mission. We will maintain and nuture the spirit of our founders and adhere to the highest standards of respect

8924 **Society for the Blind**
1238 S St.
Sacramento, CA 95811
916-452-8271
Fax: 916-492-2483
info@societyfortheblind.org
societyfortheblind.org

Shari Roeseler, Executive Director
Shane Snyder, Director of Programs
Serving 26 counties in Northern California, Society for the Blind
is a full service, nonprofit, agency providing services and programs for people who are blind or have low vision. services include the Low Vision Clinic, Braille Classes, computer training,
support groups, living skills instruction, mobility training, and
the Products for Independence Store.

8925 **United States Association of Blind Athletes**
1 Olympic Plaza
Colorado Springs, CO 80909-3508
719-866-3224
Fax: 719-866-3400
mlucas@usaba.org
www.usaba.org

Mark A. Lucas, Executive Director
Ryan Ortiz, Assistant Executive Director
John Potts, Goalball High Performance Director
USABA is a Colorado-based 501(c) (3) organization that provides life-enriching sports opportunities for every individual
with a visual impairment. A member of the U.S. Olympic Committee, USABA provides athletic opportunities in various sports
including, but not limited to track and field, nordic and alpine skiing, biathlon, judo, wrestling, swimming, tandem cycling,
powerlifting and goalball (a team sport for the blind and visually
impaired).

8926 **United States Blind Golfers Association**
125 Gilberts Hill Rd
Lehighton, PA 18235
615-679-9629
info@usblindgolf.com
www.usblindgolf.com

Jim Baker, President
Diane Wilson, Vice President
Tony Schiros, Board Member
It encourages and enhances opportunities of blind and visually
impaired golfers to compete in golf.

8927 United States Braille Chess Association
1881 N. Nash St.
Unit 702
Arlington, VA 22209 516-223-8685
www.americanblindchess.org
LA Pietrolungo, President
Alan Dicey, Vice President
Jay Leventhal, Secretary
It is dedicated to encourage and assist in the promotion and advancement of correspondence and over-the board chess among chess enthusiasts who are blind or visually impaired.

8928 Vermont Association for the Blind and Visually Impaired
60 Kimball Ave
South Burlington, VT 05403 802-863-1358
800-639-5861
Fax: 802-863-1481
general@vabvi.org
www.vabvi.org
James Mooney, President
Thomas Chase, Vice President
Debbie Balserus, Secretary
The Vermont Association for the Blind and Visually Impaired (VABVI), a non-profit organization founded in 1926, is the only private agency to offer free training, services and support to visually impaired Vermonters. Each year we serve hundreds of children from birth to age 22 and adults age 55 and over.

8929 Vision Forward Association
912 N. Hawley Road
Milwaukee, WI 53213 414-615-0100
855-878-6056
Fax: 414-256-8748
www.vision-forward.org
Terri Davis, Executive Director
Jacci Borchardt, Program Director
Jacque Cline, Human Resources Director
Its mission is to empower, educate, and enhance the lives of individuals impacted by vision loss through all of life's transitions.

8930 Vision World Wide
Apt 302
5707 Brockton Dr
Indianapolis, IN 46220-5481 317-254-1332
800-431-1739
Fax: 317-251-6588
www.visionww.org
Patricia L Prince, President
A non profit organization dedicated to improving the lives of the vision impaired through direct interaction and indirectly through the caregiving community. Also serve both the totally blind and those with various degrees and forms of vision loss.

8931 Visions Center on Blindness (VCB)
111 Summit Park Rd.
Spring Valley, NY 10977 845-354-3003
888-245-8333
info@visionsvcb.org
www.visionsvcb.org
Nancy D. Miller, Executive Director & CEO
Natalia S. Young, Chief Operating Officer
Carlos Cabrera, Chief Financial Officer
VISIONS VCB is a 35-acre year round residential rehabilitation and training center in Rockland County, New York. VCB offers comprehensive overnight training and vision rehabilitation facilities.

8932 Visually Impaired Veterans of America
American Council of the Blind
1155 15th St NW
Ste 1004
Washington, DC 20005-2706 202-467-5081
800-424-8666
Fax: 202-467-5085
www.acb.org
Jill Gaus, President
Lynn Jansen, Vice President
Debby Lieberman, Secretary
Maintain, promote and foster the well bring and rehabilitation of all visually Impaired Veterans of the Armed Forces of the United States of America who are eligible to receive from the Veterans

Administration; develops and encourages the practice of high standards of personal professional conduct among Visually Impaired Veterans; maintain, promote, and foster public confidence and awareness In Visually Impaired Veterans.

8933 Washington Ear
12061 Tech Rd.
Silver Spring, MD 20904 301-681-6636
Fax: 301-625-1986
information@washear.org
www.washear.org
Terry Pacheco, President
Amir Rahimi, Secretary
John F. Anderschat, Treasurer
A nonprofit organization providing reading and information services for blind, visually impaired and physically disabled people who cannot effectively read print, see plays, watch television programs and films, or view museum exhibits. Ear free services strive to substitute hearing for seeing, improving the lives of people with limited or no vision by enabling them to be well-informed, fully productive members of their families, their communities and the working world.

Camps

8934 Camp Barakel
P.O.Box 159
Fairview, MI 48621-0159 989-848-2279
Fax: 989-848-2280
info@campbarakel.org
www.campbarakel.org
Paul Gardner, Camp Director
Hannah Gardner, Music Coordinator
Jon Ford, Head Lifeguard
Five-day Christian camp experience in mid-August for campers ages 18-55 who are physically disabled, visually impaired, upper trainable mentally impaired or educable mentally impaired, bus transportation provided from locations in Lansing, Flint and Bay City, Michigan.

8935 Camp Bloomfield
Wayfinder Family Services
5300 Angeles Vista Blvd.
Los Angeles, CA 90043 323-295-4555
Fax: 323-296-0424
JLucas@WayfinderFamily.org
www.wayfinderfamily.org
Miki Jordan, Chief Executive Officer
Jay Allen, President & Chief Operating Officer
Fernando Almodovar, Chief Financial Officer
Camp Bloomfield is a summer camp with week long sessions for children and youth who are blind, visually impaired or multi-disabled. The 45 acre campground offers campers a variety of activities, specifically designed to meet the needs of the children, with campers attending at no cost.

8936 Camp Challenge
8914 US Highway 50 East
Bedford, IN 47421 812-834-5159
info@gocampchallenge.com
www.gocampchallenge.com
One and two-week sessions for campers with developmental and or physical disabilities, hearing impairment and the blind/visually impaired. Ages 6-99 and families.

8937 Camp Lawroweld
288 West Side Rd.
Weld, ME 04285 207-585-2984
bchase@nnec.org
www.camplawroweld.org
Trevor Schlisner, Director
Camp is located in Weld, Maine. Offers various camp sessions, including a week-long camp for individuals who are blind or visually impaired.

8938   Camp Lighthouse
Columbia Lighthouse for the Blind
1825 K St. NW
Suite 1103
Washington, DC 20006   202-454-6400
                                     Fax: 202-955-6401
                                         info@clb.org
                                         www.clb.org

Tony Cancelosi, President & CEO
Jocelyn Hunter, Senior Director, Communications
Toya Horten, Director, Administrative Operations
Camp Lighthouse is a one week day camp program for children ages 6-12 with visual impairments. Activities include games, recreation, arts and crafts, field trips, and braille activities.

8939   Camp Lou Henry Hoover
Girl Scouts of Washington Rock Council
201 East Grove Street
Westfield, NJ 07090   908-518-4400
                                     Fax: 908-232-4508
                                      girlscouts@gshnj.org
                                         www.gshnj.org

Samantha Basek, Field Executive
Susan Brooks, CEO
Camp is located in Middleville, New Jersey. Sessions for girls who are blind/visually impaired, ages 7-18.

8940   Camp Merrick
PO Box 56
Nanjemoy, MD 20662   301-870-5858
                                     Fax: 301-246-9108
                                   info@lionscampmerrick.org
                                     www.lionscampmerrick.org

Heidi A. Fick, Executive Director
Donna Wadsworth, Office Administrator
Programs offered April-January for children who are blind/visually impaired, hearing impaired or diabetic. Coed, ages 6-16.

8941   Camp Winnekeag
257 Ashby Road
Ashburnham, MA 01430   978-827-4455
                                     Fax: 978-827-4551
                                 sneconference@sneconline.org
                                     www.campwinnekeag.com

Frank Tochterman, Religious Leader
Camp is located in Ashburnham, Massachusetts. Camping sessions for blind/visually impaired children. Coed, ages 8-16.

8942   Enchanted Hills Camp for the Blind
Lighthouse for the Blind
1155 Market St.
10th Floor
San Francisco, CA 94103   415-431-1481
                                     Fax: 415-863-7568
                                    info@lighthouse-sf.org
                                     www.lighthouse-sf.org

W. Brandon Cox, Chief Operating Officer
Michelle Knapik, Chief Financial Officer
Enchanted Hills Camp for the Blind is located on 311 acres of land on Mt. Veeder, offering programs for children, teens, adults, deaf-blind, seniors, and families of the blind. The camp gives campers the experience of traditional summer camp but is adapted to meet the needs of the campers.

8943   Highbrook Lodge
Cleveland Sight Center
1909 E 101st St.
Cleveland, OH 44106   216-791-8118
                                     Fax: 216-791-1101
                                     TTY: 216-791-8119
                              info@clevelandsightcenter.org
                                 www.clevelandsightcenter.org

Larry Benders, President & CEO
Kevin Krencisz, Chief Financial & Administrative Officer
Jassen Tawil, Director, Business Development & Customer Success
Camp is located in Chardon, Ohio. Summer sessions for children, adults and families who are blind or have low vision. Sessions inclide a wide range of outdoor camp activities. Camp activities focus on gaining independent skills, mobility, orientation and self-confidence in an accessible and traditional camp setting.

8944   Indian Creek Camp
Kentucky Tennessee Conference
150 Cabin Circle Drive
Liberty, TN 37095   615-548-4411
                                     Fax: 615-548-4029
                                     www.indiancreekcamp.com

Ken Wetmore, Director
Marty Sutton, Asst. Director
Toni Stephens, Program Director
Camp is located in Liberty, Tennessee. Summer sessions for children and adults who are blind/visually impaired. Coed, ages 7-17, families and seniors.

8945   Kamp A-Komp-Plish
9035 Ironsides Rd
Nanjemoy, MD 20662-3432   301-870-3226
                                         301-934-3590
                                     Fax: 301-870-2620
                                   recreation@melwood.org

Jonathan Rondeau, Chief Program Officer
Bekah Carmichael, Director
Doria Fleisher, Associate Director
Camp is located in Nanjemoy, Maryland. Half-week, one-week and two-week sessions for blind/visually impaired children and those with developmental disabilities and mobility limitation. Coed, ages 8-16.

8946   Kamp Kaleo
46872 Willow Springs Rd.
Burwell, NE 68823   308-346-5083
                                    kampkaleo@gmail.com
                                      www.kampkaleo.com

David Butz, Camp Administrator
Offers an overnight summer camp for individuals with developmental disabilities. In addition to regular camp activities, there is a strong focus on religious education.

8947   National Camps for Blind Children
Christian Record Services
5900 S 58th St.
Suite M
Lincoln, NE 68516   402-488-0981
                                     Fax: 402-488-7582
                                    info@christianrecord.org
                                      www.christianrecord.org

Diane Thurber, President
Lonnie Kreiter, Vice President, Finance
Christian Record Services runs National Camps for Blind Children, summer camps for individuals who are considered legally blind.

8948   Texas Lions Camp
PO Box 290247
Kerrville, TX 78029   830-896-8500
                                     Fax: 830-896-3666
                                      tlc@lionscamp.com
                                       www.lionscamp.com

Stephen S. Mabry, President & CEO
Karen-Anne King, Vice President, Summer Camps
Milton Dare, Director, Development
Texas Lions Camp is a camp dedicated to serving children ages 7-16 in Texas with physical disabilities. While at camp, campers will participate in a variety of activities and be encouraged to become more independent and self-confident.

8949   VISIONS Vacation Camp for the Blind (VCB)
VISIONS Center on Blindness
111 Summit Park Rd.
Spring Valley, NY 10977   845-354-3003
                                         888-245-8333
                                      info@visionsvcb.org
                                       www.visionsvcb.org

Krystal Findley-Jones, Director
A nonprofit agency that promotes the independence of people of all ages who are blind or visually impaired. Camp offers Braille classes, computers with large print and voice output, support groups, discussions, cooking classes, personal and home management training, and large print and Braille books.

8950 Wendell Johnson Speech And Hearing Clinic
University Of Iowa
250 Hawkins Dr
Iowa City, IA 52242-1025   319-335-8736
                                       Fax: 319-335-8851
                                  kathy-miller@uiowa.edu
                                             www.uiowa.edu
Chuck Wieland, President
Hans Hoerschelman, Vice President
Josh Smith, Budget Officer
The clinic offers assessment and intervention for communication disorders in adults and children as well as an audiology clinic. The clinic also offers several summer programs for children with hearing, speech, language, autism and/or reading disorders, including a summer residential program for teens who stutter.

8951 YMCA Camp Chingachgook on Lake George
Capital District YMCA
1872 Pilot Knob Rd.
Kattskill Bay, NY 12844   518-656-9462
                                       Fax: 518-656-9362
                               chingachgook@cdymca.org
                                  www.lakegeorgecamp.org
Jine Andreozzi, Executive Director
Mike Obermayer, Director, Summer Program
Carol Lewis, Office Manager
Offers sailing programs for people with disabilities.

Books

8952 A Christian Approach to Overcoming Disability: A Doctor's Story
Routledge (Taylor & Francis Group)
711 Third Ave.
New York, NY 10017   212-216-7800
                                       Fax: 212-564-7854
                             orders@taylorandfrancis.com
                                         www.routledge.com
Dr. Elaine Leong Eng, M.D.
A personal account of Dr. Elaine Leong Eng and her career move from obstetrician/gynecologist to full-time mom, as she faces the diagnosis of impending visual impairment. Dr. Eng offers personal experience and faith-based, psychological techniques for coping with disability.
142 pages Hardcover

8953 AFB Directory of Services for Blind and Visually Impaired Persons in the US and Canada
American Foundation for the Blind/AFB Press
2 Penn Plaza
Suite 1102
New York, NY 10121   212-502-7600
                                             800-232-5463
                                       Fax: 888-545-8331
                                         afbinfo@afb.net
                                               www.afb.org
Carl Augusto, President & Chief Executive Officer
Rick Bozeman, Finance Director, Chief Financial Officer
Kelly Bleach, Chief Administrative Officer
Comprehensive print resource containing more that 2,500 local, state, regional, and national services throughout the US and Canada for persons who are blind or visually impaired. *$79.95*
624 pages Paperback/onlin
ISBN 0-891288-05-3

8954 About Children's Eyes
National Association for Visually Handicapped
111 East 59th Street
New York, NY 10022-1202   212-821-9384
                                             800-829-0500
                                       Fax: 212-821-9707
                                      info@lighthouse.org
                                         lighthouse.org/navh
Mark G. Ackermann, President / CEO
How to identify the child with a visual problem. LightHouse acquired NAVH.

8955 About Children's Vision: A Guide for Parents
National Association for Visually Handicapped
111 East 59th Street
New York, NY 10022-1202   212-821-9384
                                             800-829-0500
                                       Fax: 212-821-9707
                                      info@lighthouse.org
                                         lighthouse.org/navh
Mark G. Ackermann, President / CEO
Offers a better understanding of the normal and possible abnormal development of a child's eyesight. LightHouse acquired NAVH. *$.50*

8956 Access to Art: A Museum Directory for Blind and Visually Impaired People
American Foundation for the Blind/AFB Press
2 Penn Plaza
Suite 1102
New York, NY 10121   212-502-7600
                                             800-232-5463
                                       Fax: 888-545-8331
                                         afbinfo@afb.net
                                               www.afb.org
Carl R. Augusto, President & Chief Executive Officer
Rick Bozeman, Finance Director, Chief Financial Officer
Kelly Bleach, Chief Administrative Officer
Details the access facilities of over 300 museums, galleries and exhibits in the United States. Also included are organizations offering art-related resources such as, art classes, competitions and traveling exhibits. *$19.95*
144 pages Large Print
ISBN 0-891281-56-8

8957 African Americans in the Profession of Blindness Services
Mississippi State University
P.O.Box 6189
Mississippi State, MS 39762   662-325-2001
                                       Fax: 662-325-8989
                                       TTY: 662-325-2694
                                  nrtc@colled.msstate.edu
                                         www.blind.msstate.edu
Jacqui Bybee, Research Associate II
Douglas Bedsaul, Research and Training Coordinator
Anne Carter, Research and Training Coordinator
This study investigated the level of participation by African Americans in vocational rehab. (VR) services to persons who are visually impaired. Using surveys and interviews with all state VR directors, national census data and national RSA data, it was found nationally that African Americans are substantially under-represented in the service provider ranks, yet over-represented as clients. *$20.00*
61 pages Paperback

8958 Age-Related Macular Degeneration
National Association for Visually Handicapped
111 East 59th Street
New York, NY 10022-1202   212-821-9384
                                             800-829-0500
                                       Fax: 212-821-9707
                                      info@lighthouse.org
                                         lighthouse.org/navh
Mark G. Ackermann, President / CEO
A large booklet offering information and up-to-date research on Macular Degeneration. Also available in Russian. Revised in 2007. LightHouse acquired NAVH. *$5.00*

8959 American Anals of the Deaf Reference
800 Florida Ave NE
Washington, DC 20002-3600   202-651-5530
                                       Fax: 202-651-5489
                                     gupress@gallaudet.edu
                                  gupress.gallaudet.edu/annals
Stephanie Cawthon, Ph.D., Book Review Editor
Peter V. Paul, Ph.D., Editor, Literary Issues
Ye Wang, Ph.D., Senior Associate Editor
The controlled scope of GUPress operations allows the continuance of a highly focused commitment to individual titles that has contributed significantly to its 20 years of leadership in publishing on Deaf issues. Gallaudet University Press brings unmatched

experience and knowledge to the marketplace for books on and for the Deaf community, its advocates, and scholars invested in the study of deaf society.

8960   Americans with Disabilities Act Guide for Places of Lodging: Serving Guests Who Are Blind
US Department of Justice
950 Pennsylvania Ave. NW
Washington, DC 20530   202-307-0663
                                              800-514-0301
                                         Fax: 202-307-1197
                                         TTY: 800-514-0383
                                              www.ada.gov

Rebecca B. Bond, Chief
Anne Raish, Principal Deputy Chief
Christina Galindo-Walsh, Deputy Chief
A 12-page publication explaining what hotels, motels, and other places of transient lodging can do to accommodate guests who are blind or have low vision.

8961   Art and Science of Teaching Orientation and Mobility to Persons with Visual Impairments
American Foundation for the Blind/AFB Press
2 Penn Plaza
Suite 1102
New York, NY 10121   212-502-7600
                                              800-232-5463
                                         Fax: 888-545-8331
                                              afbinfo@afb.net
                                              www.afb.org

Carl R. Augusto, President & Chief Executive Officer
Rick Bozeman, Finance Director, Chief Financial Officer
Kelly Bleach, Chief Administrative Officer
Comprehensive decription of the techniques of teaching orientation and mobility, presented along with considerations and strategies for sensitive and effective teaching. Hardcover. Paperback also available. *$48.00*
200 pages
ISBN 0-891282-45-9

8962   Awareness Training
Landmark Media
3450 Slade Run Drive
Falls Church, VA 22042   703-241-2030
                                              800-342-4336
                                         Fax: 703-536-9540
                                         info@landmarkmedia.com

Michael Hartogs, President
Peter Hartogs, VP New Business & Development
Richard Hartogs, VP Acquisitions
Covers disabilities of various types — vision, hearing, speech disorders, loss of limbs, loss of mobility, or mental/emotional limitations and how to integrate such individuals into various business and educational settings. It is a 4-part series designed to identify and enable others to interact effectively with those suffering such disabilities. *$495.00*
Set of 4

8963   Babycare Assistive Technology
Through the Looking Glass
3075 Adeline Street
Suite 120
Berkeley, CA 94703   510-848-1112
                                              800-644-2666
                                         Fax: 510-848-4445
                                              tlg@lookingglass.org
                                              www.lookingglass.org

Maureen Block, J.D., President
Thomas Spalding, Treasurer
Alice Nemon, Secretary
Available in braille, large print or cassette. Provides an overview of the baby care assistive technology work at Through The Looking Glass including a discussion of TLG's intervention model, the impact of babycare equipment and guidelines for equipment development. *$2.00*
8 pages

8964   Babycare Assistive Technology for Parents with Physical Disabilties
Through the Looking Glass
3075 Adeline Street
Suite 120
Berkeley, CA 94703   510-848-1112
                                              800-644-2666
                                         Fax: 510-848-4445
                                              tlg@lookingglass.org
                                              www.lookingglass.org

Maureen Block, J.D., President
Thomas Spalding, Treasurer
Alice Nemon, Secretary
Examines the provision of babycare equipment through the lens of ithe infant/parent relationship, the lens of the family system, and through the lens of culture. Availiable in braille, large print or cassette. *$2.00*
7 pages

8965   Basic Course in American Sign Language
TJ Publishers
P.O. Box 702701
Dallas, TX 75370   972-416-0800
                                              800-999-1168
                                         Fax: 972-416-0944
                                         TTY: 301-585-4440
                                              TJPubinc@aol.com
                                              www.tjpublishers.com/

Tom Humphries, Author
Carol Padden, Co-Author
Terrance J O'Rourke, Co-Author
Accompanying videotapes and textbooks include voice translations. Hearing students can analyze sound for initial instruction, or opt to turn off the sound to sharpen visual acuity. Package includes the Basic Course in American Sign Language text, Student Study Guide, the original four 1-hour videotapes plus the ABCASI Vocabulary videotape. *$139.95*
280 pages

8966   Behavioral Vision Approaches for Persons with Physical Disabilities
Optometric Extension Program Foundation
7754 Braegger Road
Three Lakes, WI 54562   714-250-0176
                                              Info@depf.org
                                              www.depf.org

Kristin R. Jungbluth, President
Eric J. Lindberg, VP
Barbara Kuntz, Secretary
A discussion of the behavioral vision/neuro-motor approach to providing directions for prescriptive and therapeutic services for the visually handicapped child or adult. *$49.50*
197 pages

8967   Belonging
Dial Books
375 Hudson St
New York, NY 10014-3657   212-366-2000
                                         Fax: 212-414-3394
                                              www.penguin.com/

Deborah Kent, Author
Meg attended special schools for the blind until she was ready for high school. She decided that she wanted to go to a regular high school. She and her mother practiced her walks to school and studied the layout of the building prior to school starting, but Meg was unprepared for the trip when there were 1,500 students. She adjusted quickly to the crowds and the pace of the new school.
200 pages Hardcover
ISBN 0-80370 -30-1

8968   Berthold Lowenfeld on Blindness and Blind People
American Foundation for the Blind/AFB Press
2 Penn Plaza
Suite 1102
New York, NY 10121   212-502-7600
                                                  800-232-5463
                                            Fax: 888-545-8331
                                               afbinfo@afb.net
                                                   www.afb.org
Carl R. Augusto, President & Chief Executive Officer
Rick Bozeman, Finance Director, Chief Financial Officer
Kelly Bleach, Chief Administrative Officer
These writings of the pioneering educator, author and advocate
range over a forty-year period include various ground-breaking
papers for the blind educator, a remembrance of Helen Keller
and other essays on education, sociology and history. *$21.95*
254 pages Paperback
ISBN 0-891281-01-0

8969   Blind and Vision-Impaired Individuals
Mainstream
Ste 830
3 Bethesda Metro Ctr
Bethesda, MD 20814-6301   301-961-9299
                                                  800-247-1380
                                            Fax: 301-654-6714
Charles Moster
Mainstreaming blind individuals into the workplace. *$ 2.50*
12 pages

**8970   Blindness and Early Childhood Development Second
Edition**
American Foundation for the Blind/AFB Press
2 Penn Plaza
Suite 1102
New York, NY 10121   212-502-7600
                                                  800-232-5463
                                            Fax: 888-545-8331
                                               afbinfo@afb.net
                                                       afb.org
Carl R. Augusto, President & Chief Executive Officer
Rick Bozeman, Finance Director, Chief Financial Officer
Kelly Bleach, Chief Administrative Officer
A review of current knowledge on motor and locomotor develop-
ment, perceptual development, language and cognitive pro-
cesses, and social, emotional and personality development.
Paperback. *$34.95*
384 pages
ISBN 0-891281-23-8

**8971   Blindness: What it is, What it Does and How to Live with
it**
American Foundation for the Blind/AFB Press
2 Penn Plaza
Suite 1102
New York, NY 10121   212-502-7600
                                                  800-232-5463
                                            Fax: 888-545-8331
                                               afbinfo@afb.net
                                                   www.afb.org
Carl R. Augusto, President & Chief Executive Officer
Rick Bozeman, Finance Director, Chief Financial Officer
Kelly Bleach, Chief Administrative Officer
A classic work on how blindness affects self-perception and so-
cial interaction and what can be done to restore basic skills, mo-
bility, daily living and an appreciation of life's pleasures. *$15.95*
396 pages Paperback
ISBN 0-891282-05-

8972   Books are Fun for Everyone
Nat'l Lib Svc/Blind And Physically Handicapped
1291 Taylor Street North West
Washington, DC 20011   202-707-5100
                                            Fax: 202-707-0712
                                            TTY: 202-707-0744
                                                   nls@loc.gov
                                               www.loc.gov/nls
Karen Keninger, Director

8973   Books for Blind & Physically Handicapped Individuals
Nat'l Lib Svc/Blind And Physically Handicapped
1291 Taylor Street North West
Washington, DC 20011   202-707-5100
                                            Fax: 202-707-0712
                                            TTY: 202-707-0744
                                                   nls@loc.gov
                                               www.loc.gov/nls
Karen Keninger, Director
A free national library program of braille and recorded materials
for blind and physically handicapped persons.

8974   Books for Blind and Physically Handicapped Individuals
Nat'l Lib Svc/Blind And Physically Handicapped
1291 Taylor Street North West
Washington, DC 20011   202-707-5100
                                            Fax: 202-707-0712
                                            TTY: 202-707-0744
                                                   nls@loc.gov
                                               www.loc.gov/nls
Karen Keninger, Director
A free national library program of braille and recorded materials
for blind and physically handicapped persons is administered by
the National Library Service for the Blind and Physically Handicapped Library of Congress.
Annual

8975   Braille Book Bank, Music Catalog
National Braille Association
95 Allens Creek Road
Building 1, Suite 202
Rochester, NY 14618   585-427-8260
                                            Fax: 585-427-0263
                                      nbaoffice@nationalbraille.org
                                          www.nationalbraille.org
Jan Carroll, President
Cindi Laurent, Vice President
David Shaffer, Executive Director
Offers hundreds of musical titles in print form, braille and on cas-
sette.
62 pages

8976   Braille: An Extraordinary Volunteer Opportunity
Nat'l Lib Svc/Blind And Physically Handicapped
1291 Taylor Street North West
Washington, DC 20011   202-707-5100
                                            Fax: 202-707-0712
                                            TTY: 202-707-0744
                                                   nls@loc.gov
                                               www.loc.gov/nls
Karen Keninger, Director

8977   Burns Braille Transcription Dictionary
American Foundation for the Blind/AFB Press
2 Penn Plaza
Suite 1102
New York, NY 10121   212-502-7600
                                                  800-232-5463
                                            Fax: 888-545-8331
                                               afbinfo@afb.net
                                                       afb.org
Carl R. Augusto, President & Chief Executive Officer
Rick Bozeman, Finance Director, Chief Financial Officer
Kelly Bleach, Chief Administrative Officer
A handy, portable guide that is a quick reference for anyone who
needs to check print-to-braille and braille-to-print meanings and
symbols. Paperback. *$21.95*
96 pages 96 pages
ISBN 0-891282-32-7

8978 Can't Your Child See? A Guide for Parents of Visually Impaired Children
Sage Publications
2455 Teller Road
Thousand Oaks, CA 91320 805-499-0721
800-818-7243
Fax: 805-499-0871
info@sagepub.com
www.sagepub.com
Sara Miller McCune, Founder, Publisher, Executive Chairman
Blaise R Simqu, President & CEO
Tracey A. Ozmina, Executive Vice President & Chief Operating Officer
This second edition offers parents optimistic, practical guidelines for helping visually impaired children reach their full potential. *$26.00*
279 pages Paperback

8979 Career Perspectives: Interviews with Blindand Visually Impaired Professionals
American Foundation for the Blind/AFB Press
2 Penn Plaza
Suite 1102
New York, NY 10121 212-502-7600
800-232-5463
Fax: 888-545-8331
afbinfo@afb.net
afb.org
Carl R. Augusto, President & Chief Executive Officer
Rick Bozeman, Finance Director, Chief Financial Officer
Kelly Bleach, Chief Administrative Officer
Profiles of 20 successful archivers who describe in their own words what it takes to pursue and attain professional success in a sighted world. Available in large print, cassette and braille. *$19.95*
96 pages
ISBN 0-891281-70-2

8980 Careers in Blindness Rehabilitation Services
Mississippi State University
P.O.Box 6189
Mississippi State, MS 39762 662-325-2001
Fax: 662-325-8989
TTY: 662-325-2694
nrtc@colled.msstate.edu
www.blind.msstate.edu
Jacqui Bybee, Research Associate II
Douglas Bedsaul, Research and Training Coordinator
Anne Carter, Research and Training Coordinator
In a follow-up study in a series examining the substantial under-representation of African Americans as professionals in blindness services, researchers questioned college students about their knowledge, opinions and interests in blindness services. *$15.00*
54 pages Paperback

8981 Cataracts
National Association for Visually Handicapped
111 East 59th Street
New York, NY 10022-1202 212-821-9384
800-829-0500
Fax: 212-821-9707
info@lighthouse.org
lighthouse.org/navh
Mark G. Ackermann, President / CEO
A booklet offering information about Cataracts, diagnosis and treatment of this common condition. LightHouse acquired NAVH. *$ 4.00*

8982 Characteristics, Services, & Outcomes of Rehab. Consumers who are Blind/Visually Impaired
Mississippi State University
P.O.Box 6189
Mississippi State, MS 39762 662-325-2001
Fax: 662-325-8989
TTY: 662-325-2694
nrtc@colled.msstate.edu
www.blind.msstate.edu
Jacqui Bybee, Research Associate II
Douglas Bedsaul, Research and Training Coordinator
Anne Carter, Research and Training Coordinator
Issues regarding the efficacy of separate state agencies providing specialized vocational rehabilitation (VR) services to consumers who are blind have generated spirited discussions within the rehabilitation community throughout the history of the state-federal program. In this monograph, RRTC researches report results of their investigation of services provided to blind consumers in separate and general (combined) rehabilitation agencies. *$20.00*
45 pages Paperback

8983 Childhood Glaucoma: A Reference Guide for Families
NAPVI
1 North Lexington Avenue
White Plains, NY 10601 617-972-7441
800-562-6265
Fax: 617-972-7444
napvi@guildhealth.org
www.napvi.org
Julie Urban, President
Venetia Hayden, Vice President
Susan LaVenture, Executive Director
A vaulable tutorial and resource covering all aspects from genetics through diagnosis, sibling relationships and more.
36 pages

8984 Children with Visual Impairments: A Guide For Parents
American Foundation for the Blind/AFB Press
105 East 22nd Street
New York, NY 10010 212-949-4800
childrensaidsociety.org
William D. Weisberg, Ph.D., President & CEO
Drema Brown, VP of Education
Katherine Eckstein, Chief of Staff
Written by parents and professional, this book presents a comprehensive overview of the issues that are crucial to the healthy development of children with mild to severe visual impaiments. It also offers insight from parents about coping with the emotional aspects of raising a child with special needs. *$16.95*
416 pages
ISBN 0-933149-36-0

8985 Classification of Impaired Vision
National Association for Visually Handicapped
111 East 59th Street
New York, NY 10022-1202 212-821-9384
800-829-0500
Fax: 212-821-9707
info@lighthouse.org
lighthouse.org/navh
Mark G. Ackermann, President / CEO
Designed to provide a foundation for a better understanding of teaching reading, writing, and listning skills to students with visual impairments from preschool age through adult levels. LightHouse acquired NAVH. *$57.95*
322 pages
ISBN 0-398066-93-2

8986 Communication Skills for Visually Impaired Learners
Charles C. Thomas
2600 S First St
Springfield, IL 62704-4730 217-789-8980
800-258-8980
Fax: 217-789-9130
books@ccthomas.com
www.ccthomas.com
Michael P. Thomas, President
Randall Harley, Author
Mila Truan, Author

This book has been designed to provide a foundation for a better understanding of teaching reading, writing, and listening skills to students with visual impairments from preschool age through adult levels. The plan of the book incorporates the latest research findings with the practical experiences learned in the classroom. *$57.95*
322 pages Paperback
ISBN 0-398066-93-2

8987 Comprehensive Examination of Barriers to Employment Among Persons who are Blind or Impaire
Mississippi State University
P.O.Box 6189
Mississippi State, MS 39762

662-325-2001
Fax: 662-325-8989
TTY: 662-325-2694
nrtc@colled.msstate.edu
www.blind.msstate.edu

Jacqui Bybee, Research Associate II
Douglas Bedsaul, Research and Training Coordinator
Anne Carter, Research and Training Coordinator
A multi-phase research project designed to: identify barriers to employment; identify and develop innovative successful strategies to overcome these barriers; develop methods for others to utilize these strategies; disseminate this information to rehabilitation providers; replicate the use of selected strategies in other settings. *$20.00*
90 pages Paperback

8988 Contrasting Characteristics of Blind and Visually Impaired Clients
Mississippi State University
P.O.Box 6189
Mississippi State, MS 39762

662-325-2001
Fax: 662-325-8989
TTY: 662-325-2694
nrtc@colled.msstate.edu
www.blind.msstate.edu

Jacqui Bybee, Research Associate II
Douglas Bedsaul, Research and Training Coordinator
Anne Carter, Research and Training Coordinator
This report examines cases in the National Blindness and Low Vision Employment Database to identify and profile environmental and personal characteristics of clients who are blind or visually impaired and who were achieving successful and unsuccessful retention of competitive jobs. A total of 787 cases were analyzed. *$15.00*
44 pages Paperback

8989 Dancing Cheek to Cheek
Blind Children's Center
4120 Marathon Street
Los Angeles, CA 90029-3584

323-664-2153
info@blindchildrenscenter.org
www.blindchildrenscenter.org

Laura Meyers, Co-Author
Pamela Lansky, Co-Author
Beginning social, play and language interactions. *$ 10.00*
23 pages

8990 Development of Social Skills by Blind and Visually Impaired Students
American Foundation for the Blind/AFB Press
2 Penn Plaza
Suite 1102
New York, NY 10121

212-502-7600
800-232-5463
Fax: 888-545-8331
afbinfo@afb.net
www.afb.org

Carl R. Augusto, President & Chief Executive Officer
Rick Bozeman, Finance Director, Chief Financial Officer
Kelly Bleach, Chief Administrative Officer
Offers an examination of the social interactions of blind and visually impaired children in mainstreamed settings and the community that highlights the need to teach social interaction skills to children and provide them with support. Paperback. *$45.95*
232 pages
ISBN 0-891282-17-4

8991 Diabetic Retinopathy
National Association for Visually Handicapped
111 East 59th Street
New York, NY 10022-1202

212-821-9384
800-829-0500
Fax: 212-821-9707
info@lighthouse.org
lighthouse.org/navh

Mark G. Ackermann, President / CEO
A booklet offering information about Diabetic Retinopathy. LightHouse acquired NAVH.

8992 Diversity and Visual Impairment: The Influence of Race, Gender, Religion and Ethnicity
American Foundation for the Blind
2 Penn Plaza
Suite 1102
New York, NY 10121

212-502-7600
800-232-5463
Fax: 888-545-8331
afbinfo@afb.net
www.afb.org

Carl R. Augusto, President & Chief Executive Officer
Rick Bozeman, Finance Director, Chief Financial Officer
Kelly Bleach, Chief Administrative Officer
Cultural, social, ethnic, gender, and religious issues can influence the way an individual perceives and copes with a visual impairment. *$45.95*
480 pages
ISBN 0-891283-83-8

8993 Do You Remember the Color Blue: The Questions Children Ask About Blindness
Viking Books
375 Hudson Street
New York, NY 10014-3657

212-366-2000
Fax: 212-366-2933
ecommerce@us.penguingroup.com
www.us.penguingroup.com

John Makinson, Chairman & CEO
The author answers thirteen thought-provoking questions that children have asked her over the years about being blind.
78 pages
ISBN 0-670880-43-4

8994 Don't Lose Sight of Glaucoma
National Eye Institute
2020 Vision Place
Building 31 Room 6a32
Bethesda, MD 20892-3655

301-496-5248
800-869-2020
Fax: 301-402-1065
2020@nei.nih.gov
www.nei.nih.gov

Provides information about glaucoma for people at higher risk, answers questions about causes and symptoms, and discusses diagnosis and types of treatment.

8995 Early Focus: Working with Young Children Who Are Blind or Visually Impaired & Their Families
American Foundation for the Blind/AFB Press
2 Penn Plaza
Suite 1102
New York, NY 10121

212-502-7600
800-232-5463
Fax: 888-545-8331
afbinfo@afb.net
www.afb.org

Carl R. Augusto, President & Chief Executive Officer
Rick Bozeman, Finance Director, Chief Financial Officer
Kelly Bleach, Chief Administrative Officer
Describes early intervention techniques used with blind and visually impaired children and stresses the benefits of family involvement and transdisciplinary teamwork. Paperback. *$32.95*
176 pages
ISBN 0-891282-15-7

8996 Encyclopedia of Blindness and Vision Impairment Second Edition
Facts on File
132 West 31st Street
17th Floor
New York, NY 10001
800-322-8755
Fax: 800-678-3633
CustServ@InfobaseLearning.com
www.factsonfile.com

Jill Sardenga, Author
Susan Shelly, Co-Author
Alan Shelly MD, Co-Author
Designed to provide both laymen and professionals with concise, practical information on the second most common disability in the U.S. *$65.00*
340 pages Hardcover
ISBN 0-816042-80-2

8997 Equals in Partnership: Basic Rights for Families of Children with Blindness
NAPVI
1 North Lexington Avenue
White Plains, NY 10601
617-972-7441
800-562-6265
Fax: 617-972-7444
napvi@guildhealth.org
www.napvi.org

Julie Urban, President
Venetia Hayden, Vice President
Susan LaVenture, Executive Director
A comprehensive compilation of educational advocacy materials to help parents better understand the special needs of their children with visual impairments and to assist them in accessing appropriate services for their children.

8998 Eye Research News
Research to Prevent Blindness
645 Madison Avenue
Floor 21
New York, NY 10022-1010
212-752-4333
800-621-0026
Fax: 212-688-6231
www.rpbusa.org

Diane S. Swift, Chair
Brian F. Hofland, PhD, President
David H. Brenner, VP & Secretary
Yearly publication from Research to Prevent Blindness. Free.
4 pages Yearly

8999 Eye and Your Vision
National Association for Visually Handicapped
111 East 59th Street
New York, NY 10022-1202
212-821-9384
800-829-0500
Fax: 212-821-9707
info@lighthouse.org
lighthouse.org/navh

Mark G. Ackermann, President / CEO
A large booklet offering information, with illustrations, on the eye. Includes information on protection of eyesight, how the eye works and vision disorders. Available in Russian and Spanish also. LightHouse acquired NAVH. *$5.00*

9000 Eye-Q Test
National Association for Visually Handicapped
111 East 59th Street
New York, NY 10022-1202
212-821-9384
800-829-0500
Fax: 212-821-9707
info@lighthouse.org
lighthouse.org/navh

Mark G. Ackermann, President / CEO
Five questions and answers to assist in knowing more about vision. Also available in Spanish and Russian. LightHouse acquired NAVH.

9001 Family Context and Disability Culture Reframing: Through the Looking Glass
Through the Looking Glass
3075 Adeline Street
Suite 120
Berkeley, CA 94703
510-848-1112
800-644-2666
Fax: 510-848-4445
tlg@lookingglass.org
www.lookingglass.org

Maureen Block, J.D., President
Thomas Spalding, Treasurer
Alice Nemon, Secretary
This article provides an overview of the issues and guiding perspectives underlying 'Through the Lookinglass' eighteen years of work with families. Available in braille, large print or cassette. *$2.00*
5 pages

9002 Family Guide to Vision Care (FG1)
American Optometric Association
243 North Lindbergh Boulevard
Floor 1
Saint Louis, MO 63141-7881
800-365-2219
aoa.org

David A. Cockrell, OD, President
Andrea P. Thau, OD, Vice President
Barry Barresi, Executive Director
Offers information on the early developmental years of your vision, finding a family optometrist and how to take care of your eyesight through the learning years, the working years and the mature years.

9003 Family Guide: Growth & Development of the Partially Seeing Child
National Association for Visually Handicapped
111 East 59th Street
New York, NY 10022-1202
212-821-9384
800-829-0500
Fax: 212-821-9707
info@lighthouse.org
lighthouse.org/navh

Mark G. Ackermann, President / CEO
Offers information for parents and guidelines in raising a partially seeing child. LightHouse acquired NAVH. *$.60*

9004 Fathers: A Common Ground
Blind Children's Center
4120 Marathon Street
Los Angeles, CA 90029-3584
323-664-2153
info@blindchildrenscenter.org
www.blindchildrenscenter.org

Paula Schmitt, Co-Author
Fernanda Armenta-Schmitt, Co-Author
Exploring the concerns and roles of fathers of children with visual impairments. *$10.00*
50 pages

9005 Fighting Blindness News
Foundation Fighting Blindness
7168 Columbia Gateway Drive
Suite 100
Columbia, MD 21046
410-423-0600
800-683-5555
Fax: 410-363-2393
TTY: 800-683-5551
info@FightBlindness.org
www.blindness.org

Offers information on medical updates, donor programs, assistive devices, resources and clinical trial information for persons with visual impairments, blindness and retinal degenerative diseases.
2x Year

9006 **First Steps**
Blind Children's Center
4120 Marathon Street
Los Angeles, CA 90029-3584   323-664-2153
                                    info@blindchildrenscenter.org
                                    www.blindchildrenscenter.org

Tanni L. Anthony, Co-Author
Fernanda Armenta-Schmitt, Co-Author

A handbook for teaching young children who are visually impaired. Designed to assist students, professionals and parents working with children who are visually impaired. Visit our website for many publications addressing training very young children who are blind or visually impaired. *$35.00*
203 pages

9007 **Foundations of Orientation and Mobility**
American Foundation for the Blind/AFB Press
2 Penn Plaza
Suite 1102
New York, NY 10121   212-502-7600
                            800-232-5463
                            Fax: 888-545-8331
                            afbinfo@afb.net
                            www.afb.org

Carl R. Augusto, President & Chief Executive Officer
Rick Bozeman, Finance Director, Chief Financial Officer
Kelly Bleach, Chief Administrative Officer

This text has been updated and revised and includes current research from a variety of disciplines, an international perspective, and expanded contents on low vision, aging, multiple disabilities, accessibility, program design and adaptive technology from more that 30 eminent subject experts. *$79.95*
775 pages
ISBN 0-891289-46-3

9008 **Foundations of Rehabilitation Counseling with Persons Who Are Blind or Visually Impaired**
American Foundation for the Blind/AFB Press
2 Penn Plaza
Suite 1102
New York, NY 10121   212-502-7600
                            800-232-5463
                            Fax: 888-545-8331
                            afbinfo@afb.net
                            www.afb.org

Carl R. Augusto, President & Chief Executive Officer
Rick Bozeman, Finance Director, Chief Financial Officer
Kelly Bleach, Chief Administrative Officer

Rehabilitation professionals have long recognized that the needs of people who are blind or visually impaired are unique and requie a special knowledge and expertise to provide and corrdinate rehabilitation services. *$59.95*
477 pages
ISBN 0-891289-45-3

9009 **General Facts and Figures on Blindness**
Prevent Blindness America
211 West Wacker Drive
Suite 1700
Chicago, IL 60606   800-331-2020
                           info@preventblindness.org
                           www.preventblindness.org

Paul G. Howes, Chairman
Hugh R. Parry, President & CEO,Prevent Blindness America
Jerome Desserich, Vice President & Chief Financial Officer

9010 **Get a Wiggle On**
American Alliance for Health, Phys. Ed. & Dance
1900 Association Drive
Reston, VA 20191-1598   703-476-3400
                               800-213-7193
                               Fax: 703-476-9527
                               aahperd.org

Dolly D. Lambdin, President
E. Paul Roetert, CEO
Marybell Avery, Director

Gives teachers and parents practical suggestions for helping blind and visually impaired infants grow and learn like other children. *$5.00*
80 pages
ISBN 0-88314 -77-2

9011 **Gift of Sight**
RP Foundation Fighting Blindness
1401 W Mount Royal Ave
Baltimore, MD 21217-4245   410-225-9409
                                  800-683-5555
                                  Fax: 410-225-3936

A pamphlet offering information on the Retina Donor Program, which studies diseased, human retinal tissue in their search for a cure of retinal degenerative diseases.

9012 **Glaucoma**
Glaucoma Research Foundation
251 Post Street
Suite 600
San Francisco, CA 94108   415-986-3162
                                 800-826-6693
                                 Fax: 415-986-3763
                                 question@glaucoma.org
                                 glaucoma.org

Andrew L. Iwach, MD, Chair
Robert L. Stamper, MD, Vice Chair
Thomas M. Brunner, President and CEO

Offers information on what glaucoma is, the causes, treatments, types of glaucoma, eye exams and prevention.

9013 **Glaucoma: The Sneak Thief of Sight**
National Association for Visually Handicapped
Fl 6
22 W 21st St
New York, NY 10010-6943   212-242-4438
                                 800-3 C-NCOS
                                 Fax: 631-736-0371
                                 customerservice@cancos.com
                                 cancos.com

Denise Green, Owner

A pamphlet describing the disease, treatment and medications. Also available in Russian and Spanish. Revised in 1999. *$3.50*

9014 **Guidelines and Games for Teaching Efficient Braille Reading**
American Foundation for the Blind/AFB Press
2 Penn Plaza
Suite 1102
New York, NY 10121   212-502-7600
                            800-232-5463
                            Fax: 888-545-8331
                            afbinfo@afb.net
                            www.afb.org

Carl R. Augusto, President & Chief Executive Officer
Rick Bozeman, Finance Director, Chief Financial Officer
Kelly Bleach, Chief Administrative Officer

Based on research in the areas of rapid reading and precision teaching, these guidelines represent a unique adaptation of a general reading program to the needs of braille readers. Paperback. *$24.95*
116 pages Paperback
ISBN 0-891281-05-4

9015 **Guidelines for Comprehensive Low Vision Care**
National Association for Visually Handicapped
111 East 59th Street
New York, NY 10022-1202   212-821-9384
                                 800-829-0500
                                 Fax: 212-821-9707
                                 info@lighthouse.org
                                 lighthouse.org/navh

Mark G. Ackermann, President / CEO

A description of the proper method to conduct a low vision evaluation.LightHouse acquired NAVH. *$.50*

9016 **Handbook for Itinerant and Resource Teachers of Blind Students**
National Federation of the Blind
200 East Wells St
Baltimore, MD 21230-4914   410-659-9314
                                  nfb@iamdigex.net
Doris Willoughby, Author
Sharon L Monthei, Co-Author
The Handbook provides help to teachers, school administrators or other school personnel that have experience with blind or visually impaired students. The Handbook devotes 45 pages to Braille and how to teach Braille for parents and teachers. There are other chapters offering information on the law, physical education, fitting in socially, testing and evaluation, home economics, daily living skills and more. *$23.00*
533 pages Softcover
ISBN 0-962412-20-1

9017 **Handbook of Information for Members of the Achromatopsia Network**
P.O.Box 214
Berkeley, CA 94701-214   510-540-4700
                                Fax: 510-540-4767
                                www.achromat.org

9018 **Health Care Professionals Who Are Blind or Visually Impaired**
American Foundation for the Blind
2 Penn Plaza
Suite 1102
New York, NY 10121   212-502-7600
                            800-232-5463
                            Fax: 888-545-8331
                            afbinfo@afb.net
                            afb.org
Carl R. Augusto, President & Chief Executive Officer
Rick Bozeman, Finance Director, Chief Financial Officer
Kelly Bleach, Chief Administrative Officer
This resource is essential reading for older students and young adults who are blind or visually impaired, their families, and the professionals who work with them. *$21.95*
160 pages
ISBN 0-891283-88-9

9019 **Heart to Heart**
Blind Children's Center
4120 Marathon Street
Los Angeles, CA 90029-3584   323-664-2153
                            info@blindchildrenscenter.org
                            www.blindchildrenscenter.org
Nancy Chernus-Mansfield, Co-Author
Dori Hayashi, Co-Author
Parents of children who are blind and partially sighted talk about their feelings. *$10.00*
12 pages

9020 **Heartbreak of Being A Little Bit Blind**
National Association for Visually Handicapped
111 East 59th Street
New York, NY 10022-1202   212-821-9384
                            800-829-0500
                            Fax: 212-821-9707
                            info@lighthouse.org
                            lighthouse.org/navh
Mark G. Ackermann, President / CEO
Summary of what it means to have impaired vision; includes illustrations. LightHouse acquired NAVH.

9021 **Helen Keller National Center Newsletter**
141 Middle Neck Road
Sands Point, NY 11050   516-944-8900
                            800-225-0411
                            Fax: 516-944-7302
                            hkncinfo@hknc.org
                            www.hknc.org
Joseph McNulty, Executive Director
The center provides evaluation and training in vocational skills, adaptive technology and computer skills, orientation and mobility, independent living, communication, speech-language skills, creative arts, fitness and leisure activities.

9022 **Helping the Visually Impaired Child with Developmental Problems**
Teachers College Press
1234 Amsterdam Avenue
New York, NY 10027   212-678-3929
                            800-575-6566
                            Fax: 212-678-4149
                            tcpress@tc.columbia.edu
                            www.teacherscollegepress.com
Mary Lynch, Manager
Brian Ellerbeck, Executive Acquisitions Editor
Marie Ellen Larcada, Senior Acquisitions Editor
This book aims to explore the human consequences of severe visual problems combined with other handicaps. The application of child development research to educational interventions, the need for educational and rehabilitative services that serve the human and the special needs of children and their families and the promise of technology in helping to expand communicative possibilities are also discussed. *$18.95*
216 pages Paperback
ISBN 0-807729-02-7

9023 **History and Use of Braille**
American Council of the Blind
2200 Wilson Boulevard
Suite 650
Arlington, VA 22201-3354   202-467-5081
                            800-424-8666
                            Fax: 703-465-5085
                            info@acb.org
                            acb.org
Kim Charlson, President
Jeff Thom, 1st Vice President
Melanie Brunson, Executive Director
A system of touch reading and writing for blind persons in which raised dots represent the letters of the alphabet.

9024 **How to Thrive, Not Just Survive**
American Foundation for the Blind/AFB Press
2 Penn Plaza
Suite 1102
New York, NY 10121   212-502-7600
                            800-232-5463
                            Fax: 888-545-8331
                            afbinfo@afb.net
                            www.afb.org
Carl R. Augusto, President & Chief Executive Officer
Rick Bozeman, Finance Director, Chief Financial Officer
Kelly Bleach, Chief Administrative Officer
Practical, hands-on guide for parents, teachers, and everyone involved in helping children develop the skills necessary for socialization, orientations and mobility, and leisure and recreational activities. Some of the subjects covered are eating, dressing, personal hygiene, self-esteem and etiquette. *$24.95*
104 pages Paperback
ISBN 0-89128 -48-7

9025 **Hub**
SPOKES Unlimited
1006 Main Street
Klamath Fals, OR 97601   541-883-7547
                            Fax: 541-885-2469
                            spokesunlimited.org
Wendy Howard, Executive Director
Celeste Wolf, Clerical Support Specialist II
Newsletter on rehabilitation, peer counseling, blindness, visual impairments, information and referral.

9026 **If Blindness Comes**
National Federation of the Blind
200 E. Wells St.
at Jernigan Place
Baltimore, MD 21230   410-659-9314
                            Fax: 410-685-5653
                            nfb@nfb.org
                            www.nfb.org
Kenneth Jerrigan, Editor
An introduction to issues relating to vision loss and provides a positive, supportive philosophy about blindness. It is a general information book which includes answers to many common ques-

tions about blindness, information about services and programs for the blind and resource listings. Contact the Materials Center.

9027 If Blindness Strikes Don't Strike Out
2600 South 1st Street
Springfield, IL 62704

217-789-8980
800-258-8980
Fax: 217-789-9130
books@ccthomas.com
www.ccthomas.com

Bob Stork, Owner

9028 Imagining the Possibilities: Creative Approaches to Orientation and Mobility Instructio
American Foundation for the Blind
2 Penn Plaza
Suite 1102
New York, NY 10121

212-502-7600
800-232-5463
Fax: 888-545-8331
afbinfo@afb.net
afb.org

Carl R. Augusto, President & Chief Executive Officer
Rick Bozeman, Finance Director, Chief Financial Officer
Kelly Bleach, Chief Administrative Officer
Innovative and varied approaches to O&M techniques and teaching and dynamic suggestions on how to analyze learning styles are just some of the important topics included. *$49.95*
378 pages
ISBN 0-891283-82-X

9029 Increasing Literacy Levels: Final Report
Mississippi State University
P.O.Box 6189
Mississippi State, MS 39762

662-325-2001
Fax: 662-325-8989
TTY: 662-325-2694
nrtc@colled.msstate.edu
www.blind.msstate.edu

Jacqui Bybee, Research Associate II
Douglas Bedsaul, Research and Training Coordinator
Anne Carter, Research and Training Coordinator
This study is composed of three research projects to identify and analyze the appropriate use of and instruction in Braille, optical devices and other technologies as they relate to literacy and employment of individuals who are blind or visually impaired. *$20.00*
148 pages Paperback

9030 Information on Glaucoma
Glaucoma Research Foundation
251 Post Street
Suite 600
San Francisco, CA 94108

415-986-3162
800-826-6693
Fax: 415-986-3763
question@glaucoma.org
www.glaucoma.org

Andrew L. Iwach, MD, Chair
Robert L. Stamper, MD, Vice Chair
Thomas M. Brunner, President and CEO

9031 Intervention Practices in the Retention of Competitive Employment
Mississippi State University
P.O.Box 6189
Mississippi State, MS 39762

662-325-2001
Fax: 662-325-8989
TTY: 662-325-2694
nrtc@colled.msstate.edu
www.blind.msstate.edu

Jacqui Bybee, Research Associate II
Douglas Bedsaul, Research and Training Coordinator
Anne Carter, Research and Training Coordinator
This study investigated the methods by which an individual can retain competitive employment after the onset of a significant vision loss. Interviews were conducted with 89 rehabilitation counselors across the US Strategies that contribute to successful job retention were identified as well as best rehabilitation practices in job retention. *$15.00*
60 pages Paperback

9032 Know Your Eye
American Council of the Blind
2200 Wilson Boulevard
Suite 650
Arlington, VA 22201-3354

202-467-5081
800-424-8666
Fax: 703-465-5085
info@acb.org
acb.org

Kim Charlson, President
Jeff Thom, 1st Vice President
Melanie Brunson, Executive Director

9033 Large Print Loan Library
National Association for Visually Handicapped
111 East 59th Street
New York, NY 10022-1202

212-821-9384
800-829-0500
Fax: 212-821-9707
info@lighthouse.org
lighthouse.org/navh

Mark G. Ackermann, President / CEO
A huge large print catalog of all the publications, fiction and non-fiction, cassette tapes, books-on-tape and videos available for the visually impaired from the loan library of the National Association for the Visually Handicapped. LightHouse acquired NAVH.

9034 Large Print Loan Library Catalog
National Association for Visually Handicapped
111 East 59th Street
New York, NY 10022-1202

212-821-9384
800-829-0500
Fax: 212-821-9707
info@lighthouse.org
lighthouse.org/navh

Mark G. Ackermann, President / CEO
Listing of over 7,000 commercially published and NAVH large print books available through NAVH on a loan basis. Includes a limited selection of titles available for purchase. LightHouse acquired NAVH.

9035 Large Print Recipies for a Healthy Life
123601 Wilshire
Los Angeles, CA 90025

310-826-8280
800-481-EYES
Fax: 310-458-8179

Judith Caditz PhD, Author
$21.95
283 pages
ISBN 0-962236-82-9

9036 Learning to Play
Blind Children's Center
4120 Marathon Street
Los Angeles, CA 90029-3584

323-664-2153
info@blindchildrenscenter.org
www.blindchildrenscenter.org

Susan L. Recchia, Co-Author
Presenting play activities to the pre-school child who is visually impaired. *$10.00*
12 pages

9037 Let's Eat
Blind Children's Center
4120 Marathon Street
Los Angeles, CA 90029-3584

323-664-2153
info@blindchildrenscenter.org
www.blindchildrenscenter.org

Jill Brody, Co-Author
Lynne Webber, Co-Author
Feeding a child with visual impairment. *$10.00*
28 pages

9038 Library Services for the Blind
South Carolina State University
300 College Street NorthEast
P.O. Box 7491
Orangeburg, SC 29117

803-536-7045
Fax: 803-536-8902
reference@scsu.edu
library.scsu.edu

Adrienne C. Webber, Dean, Library/Information Services
Ramona S. Evans, Administrative Specialist
Ruth A. Hodges, Reference & Information Specialist
News and information on developments in library services for
readers who are blind and physically disabled.

9039 Lifestyles of Employed Legally Blind People
Mississippi State University
P.O. Box 6189
Mississippi State, MS 39762

662-325-2001
Fax: 662-325-8989
TTY: 662-325-2694
nrtc@colled.msstate.edu
www.blind.msstate.edu

Jacqui Bybee, Research Associate II
Douglas Bedsaul, Research and Training Coordinator
Anne Carter, Research and Training Coordinator
Results from a telephone survey show that visually impaired respondents are involved in a wide variety of activities with little
restrictions on their range of activities. Sighted respondents
tended to spend more time in child care, obtaining goods and services, attending to self-care activities and engaging in social activities, while visually impaired respondents spent more time in
education and passive activities. This report is a study of expenditures and time use. *$ 10.00*
193 pages Paperback

9040 Lion
Lion's Clubs International
300 West 22nd Street
Oak Brook, IL 60523-8842

630-571-5466
Fax: 630-571-8890
TTY: 630-571-6533
www.lionsclubs.org/

Joseph Preston, International President
Jitsuhiro Yamada, 1st Vice President
Robert E. Corlew, 2nd Vice President
Publication for the blind.

9041 Living with Achromatopsia
P.O. Box 214
Berkeley, CA 94701-214

510-540-4700
Fax: 510-540-4767
www.achromat.org

Frances Futterman, Author
Consists entirely of comments from persons who know firsthand
about living with achromatopsia.

**9042 Low Vision Questions and Answers: Definitions, Devices,
Services**
American Foundation for the Blind/AFB Press
2 Penn Plaza
Suite 1102
New York, NY 10121

212-502-7600
800-232-5463
Fax: 888-545-8331
afbinfo@afb.net
afb.org

Carl R. Augusto, President & Chief Executive Officer
Rick Bozeman, Chief Financial Officer
Kelly Bleach, Chief Administrative Officer
What does low vision mean? What do low vision services cost?
What diseases cause low vision? Answers to these and other ques-
tions are presented in a comprehensive format with accompany-
ing photographs. $50.00/pack of 25.
21 pages Pamphlet
ISBN 0-891281-96-7

9043 Low Vision: Reflections of the Past, Issues for the Future
American Foundation for the Blind/AFB Press
2 Penn Plaza
Suite 1102
New York, NY 10121

212-502-7600
800-232-5463
Fax: 888-545-8331
afbinfo@afb.net
www.afb.org

Carl R. Augusto, President & Chief Executive Officer
Rick Bozeman, Chief Financial Officer
Kelly Bleach, Chief Administrative Officer
Background papers and a strategies section are used to identify
the shifting needs of visually impaired persons and the resources
that may be needed to address them. Paperback. *$34.95*
Paperback
ISBN 0-891282-18-1

9044 Mainstreaming and the American Dream
American Foundation for the Blind/AFB Press
2 Penn Plaza
Suite 1102
New York, NY 10121

212-502-7600
800-232-5463
Fax: 888-545-8331
afbinfo@afb.net
www.afb.org

Carl R. Augusto, President & Chief Executive Officer
Rick Bozeman, Chief Financial Officer
Kelly Bleach, Chief Administrative Officer
Based on in-depth interviews with parents and professionals, this
research monograph presents information on the needs and aspirations of parents of blind and visually impaired children. Paperback. *$34.95*
256 pages Paperback
ISBN 0-891281-91-7

9045 Mainstreaming the Visually Impaired Child
NAPVI
1 North Lexington Avenue
White Plains, NY 10601

617-972-7441
800-562-6265
Fax: 617-972-7444
napvi@guildhealth.org
www.napvi.org

Julie Urban, President
Venetia Hayden, Vice President
Susan LaVenture, Executive Director
A unique, informative guide for teachers and educational profes-
sionals that work with the visually impaired. *$10.00*
121 pages Paper

9046 Making Life More Livable
American Foundation for the Blind
2 Penn Plaza
Suite 1102
New York, NY 10121

212-502-7600
800-232-5463
Fax: 888-545-8331
afbinfo@afb.net
www.afb.org

Carl R. Augusto, President & Chief Executive Officer
Rick Bozeman, Chief Financial Officer
Kelly Bleach, Chief Administrative Officer
Shows how simple adaptations in the home and environment can
make a big difference in the lives of blind and visually impaired
older persons. The suggestions offered are numerous and specific, ranging from how to mark food cans for greater visibility to
how to get out of the shower safley. Large print. *$24.95*
128 pages
ISBN 0-891283-87-0

9047 Meeting the Needs of People with Vision Loss: Multidisciplinary Perspective
Resources for Rehabilitation
22 Bonad Road
Winchester, MA 01890
781-368-9080
Fax: 781-368-9096
orders@rfr.org
www.rfr.org

Susan L Greenblatt, Editor

Written by rehabilitation professionals, physicians, and a sociologist, this book discusses how to provide appropriate information and how to serve special populations. Chapters on the role of the family, diabetes and vision loss, special needs of children and adolescents, adults with hearing and vision loss. *$29.95*
ISBN 0-929718-07-0

9048 Model Program Operation Manual: Business Enterprise Program Supervisors
Mississippi State University
P.O. Box 6189
Mississippi State, MS 39762
662-325-2001
Fax: 662-325-8989
TTY: 662-325-2694
nrtc@colled.msstate.edu
www.blind.msstate.edu

Jacqui Bybee, Research Associate II
Douglas Bedsaul, Research and Training Coordinator
Anne Carter, Research and Training Coordinator

This monograph serves as a Model Program Operation Manual for Business Enterprise Program Supervisors who administer Randolph-Sheppard vending facilities under the Randolph-Sheppard Act. A wide variety of topics are covered including the role of the State Committee of Blind Venders, the role and responsibilities of the Vending Facility Operator, model qualification, for potential Facility Managers, guidelines for location of vending facilities and policies for closing vending facilities. *$20.00*
199 pages Paperback

9049 More Alike Than Different: Blind and Visually Impaired Children
American Foundation for the Blind/AFB Press
2 Penn Plaza
Suite 1102
New York, NY 10121
212-502-7600
800-232-5463
Fax: 888-545-8331
www.afb.org

Carl R. Augusto, President & Chief Executive Officer
Rick Bozeman, Chief Financial Officer
Kelly Bleach, Chief Administrative Officer

Offers photographs of blind and visually impaired children around the world learning to read and write, travel independently and performing basic living skills. Covers the most recent technological advances and demonstrates the universality of educational needs and goals. Paperback. $100.00/pack of 25.
ISBN 0-891281-69-0

9050 Mothers with Visual Impairments who are Raising Young Children
American Foundation for the Blind/AFB Press
2 Penn Plaza
Suite 1102
New York, NY 10121
212-502-7600
800-232-5463
Fax: 888-545-8331
afbinfo@afb.net
www.afb.org

Carl R. Augusto, President & Chief Executive Officer
Rick Bozeman, Chief Financial Officer
Kelly Bleach, Chief Administrative Officer

Available in braille, large print or cassette. *$2.00*
16 pages

9051 Move With Me
Blind Children's Center
4120 Marathon Street
Los Angeles, CA 90029-3584
323-664-2153
info@blindchildrenscenter.org
www.blindchildrenscenter.org

Doris Hug, Co-Author
Nancy Chernus-Mansfield, Co-Author

A parent's guide to movement development for babies who are visually impaired. *$10.00*
12 pages

9052 National Eye Institute
National Institute of Health
31 Center Dr.
MSC 2510
Bethesda, MD 20892-2510
301-496-5248
2020@nei.nih.gov
www.nei.nih.gov

Michael F. Chiang, Director
Santa Tuminia, Deputy Director
Melanie Reagan, Acting Executive Officer

To conduct and support research for blinding eye diseases, visual disorders, mechanisms of visual function, and the preservation of sight.

9053 Orientation and Mobility Primer for Families and Young Children
American Foundation for the Blind/AFB Press
2 Penn Plaza
Suite 1102
New York, NY 10121
212-502-7600
800-232-5463
Fax: 888-545-8331
afbinfo@afb.net
www.afb.org

Carl R. Augusto, President & Chief Executive Officer
Rick Bozeman, Chief Financial Officer
Kelly Bleach, Chief Administrative Officer

Practical information for helping a child learn about his or her environment right from the start. Covers sensory training, concept development and orientation skills. Paperback. *$14.95*
48 pages
ISBN 0-891281-57-6

9054 Out of the Corner of My Eye: Living with Vision Loss in Later Life
American Foundation for the Blind/AFB Press
2 Penn Plaza
Suite 1102
New York, NY 10121
212-502-7600
800-232-5463
Fax: 888-545-8331
www.afb.org

Carl R. Augusto, President & Chief Executive Officer
Rick Bozeman, Chief Financial Officer
Kelly Bleach, Chief Administrative Officer

A personal account of students' vision loss and subsequent adjustment that is full of practical advice and cheerful encouragement, told by an 87 year old retired college teacher who has maintained her independence and zest for life. Available in paperback or on audio cassette. *$23.95*
120 pages
ISBN 0-891281-82-1

9055 Out of the Corner of My Eye: Living with Macular Degeneration
American Foundation for the Blind/AFB Press
2 Penn Plaza
Suite 1102
New York, NY 10121
212-502-7600
800-232-5463
Fax: 888-545-8331
afbinfo@afb.net
www.afb.org

Carl R. Augusto, President & Chief Executive Officer
Rick Bozeman, Chief Financial Officer
Kelly Bleach, Chief Administrative Officer

A personal account of students' vision loss and subsequent adjustment that is full of practical advice and cheerful encourage-

ment, told by an 87 year old retired college teacher who has maintained her independence and zest for life. *$29.95*
168 pages Paperback
ISBN 0-891238-31-2

9056   Pain Erasure: the Bonnie Prudden Way
Ballantine Books
1540 Broadway
New York, NY 10036-4039   212-751-2600
                                         Fax: 212-572-4949
Bonnie Prudden, Author
Revolutionary breakthrough in pain relief involves trigger points-tender areas where muscles have been damaged from falls, childhood ailments, poor posture, and the stresses of daily life.

9057   Patient's Guide to Visual Aids and Illumination
National Association for Visually Handicapped
111 East 59th Street
New York, NY 10022-1202   212-821-9384
                                              800-829-0500
                                         Fax: 212-821-9707
                                         info@lighthouse.org
                                         lighthouse.org/navh
Mark G. Ackermann, President / CEO
A reference booklet offering information on aids for the visually impaired. LightHouse acquired NAVH. *$.75*

9058   Pediatric Visual Diagnosis Fact Sheets
Blind Children's Center
4120 Marathon Street
Los Angeles, CA 90029-3584   323-664-2153
                                         info@blindchildrenscenter.org
                                         blindchildrenscenter.org
Sarah E. Orth, CEO
Collection of fact sheets addressing commonly encountered eye conditions, diagnostic tests and materials. *$10.00*
10 pages

9059   Perkins Activity and Resource Guide: A Handbook for Teachers
Perkins School for the Blind
175 North Beacon Street
Watertown, MA 02472   617-924-3434
                                         Fax: 617-972-7363
                                         info@perkins.org
                                         www.perkins.org
Frederic M. Clifford, Chair of the Board
Philip L. Ladd, Vice Chair of the Board
Leslie Nordon, Secretary
This is a comprehensive, two volume guide with over 1,000 pages of activities, resources and instructional strategies for teachers and parents of students with visual and multiple disabilities. *$80.00*

9060   Personal Reader Update
Personal Reader Department
9 Centennial Dr
Peabody, MA 01960-7906   978-977-2000
                                              800-343-0311
                                         Fax: 978-977-2409
Offers information on new services, assistive devices and technology for the blind.

9061   Preschool Learning Activities for the Visually Impaired Child
NAPVI
1 North Lexington Avenue
White Plains, NY 10601   617-972-7441
                                              800-562-6265
                                         Fax: 617-972-7444
                                         napvi@guildhealth.org
                                         www.napvi.org
Julie Urban, President
Venetia Hayden, Vice President
Susan LaVenture, Executive Director
This guide for parents offers games and activities to keep visually impaired children active during the preschool years. *$8.00*
91 pages Paperback

9062   Reaching, Crawling, Walking... Let's Get Moving
Blind Children's Center
4120 Marathon Street
Los Angeles, CA 90029-3584   323-664-2153
                                         info@blindchildrenscenter.org
                                         www.blindchildrenscenter.org
Susan S. Simmons, Co-Author
Sharon O'Mara Maida, Co-Author
Orientation and mobility for preschool children who are visually imapired. *$10.00*
24 pages

9063   Reading Is for Everyone
Nat'l Lib Svc/Blind And Physically Handicapped
1291 Taylor Street North West
Washington, DC 20011   202-707-5100
                                         Fax: 202-707-0712
                                         TTY: 202-707-0744
                                         nls@loc.gov
                                         www.loc.gov/nls
Karen Keninger, Director

9064   Reading with Low Vision
Nat'l Lib Svc/Blind And Physically Handicapped
1291 Taylor Street North West
Washington, DC 20011   202-707-5100
                                         Fax: 202-707-0712
                                         TTY: 202-707-0744
                                         nls@loc.gov
                                         www.loc.gov/nls
Karen Keninger, Director

9065   Recording for the Blind & Dyslexic
20 Roszel Road
Princeton, NJ 08540   800-221-4792
                                         Fax: 609-987-8116
                                         Custserv@LearningAlly.org
                                         www.learningally.org/
Brad Grob, Chairman
Harold J. Logan, Vice Chairman
Andrew Friedman, President & CEO
Provides recorded and computerized textbooks, library services and other educational resources to people who cannot effectively read standard print because of visual impairment, dyslexia or other physical disability. RFB&D is now Learning Ally.

9066   Reference and Information Services From NLS
Nat'l Lib Svc/Blind And Physically Handicapped
1291 Taylor Street North West
Washington, DC 20011   202-707-5100
                                         Fax: 202-707-0712
                                         TTY: 202-707-0744
                                         nls@loc.gov
                                         www.loc.gov/nls
Karen Keninger, Director

9067   Resource List for Persons with Low Vision
American Council of the Blind
2200 Wilson Boulevard
Suite 650
Arlington, VA 22201-3354   202-467-5081
                                              800-424-8666
                                         Fax: 703-465-5085
                                         info@acb.org
                                         acb.org
Kim Charlson, President
Jeff Thom, 1st Vice President
Melanie Brunson, Executive Director

9068   Rose-Colored Glasses
Human Sciences Press
233 Spring St
New York, NY 10013-1522   212-229-2859
                                              800-221-9369
                                         Fax: 212-463-0742
After a vacation, Deborah was excited about going back to school. Renewing old friendships, she met a classmate who seemed stuck up. Deborah learned that Melanie was in a recent accident resulting in impaired vision. She did not wish to wear her glasses, which were rose-colored and very funny looking. With Deborah's help, Miss Davis, the teacher showed a blurry film and

then had Melanie speak about her impaired vision. When Melanie began to participate in the class they accepted her. *$16.95*
30 pages Hardcover
ISBN 0-87705 -08-8

9069   See A Bone
Facts on File
132 West 31st Street
14th Floor
New York, NY 10001   212-967-8800
                                       800-683-5433
                                    Fax: 212-760-0862
                               info@northernleasing.com
                                    northernleasing.com

Mark Donnell, President
$65.00
352 pages
ISBN 0-816042-80-2

9070   See What I Feel
Britannica Film Company
345 4th Street
San Francisco, CA 94107   415-928-8466
                                    Fax: 415-928-5027

Dave Bekowich, Owner
A blind child tells her friends about her trip to the zoo. Each experience was explained as a blind child would experience it. A teacher's guide comes with this video.
Film

9071   Selecting a Program
Blind Children's Center
4120 Marathon Street
Los Angeles, CA 90029-3584   323-664-2153
                         info@blindchildrenscenter.org
                          www.blindchildrenscenter.org
Deborah Chen, Co-Author
Mary Ellen McCann, Co-Author
A free guide for parents of infants and preschoolers with visual impairments.
28 pages

9072   Show Me How: A Manual for Parents of Preschool Blind Children
American Foundation for the Blind/AFB Press
2 Penn Plaza
Suite 1102
New York, NY 10121   212-502-7600
                                       800-232-5463
                                    Fax: 888-545-8331
                                       afbinfo@afb.net
                                          www.afb.org

Carl R. Augusto, President & Chief Executive Officer
Rick Bozeman, Chief Financial Officer
Kelly Bleach, Chief Administrative Officer
A practical guide for parents, teachers and others who help preschool children attain age-related goals. Covers issues on playing precautions, appropriate toys and facilitating relationships with playmates. Paperback. *$12.95*
56 pages
ISBN 0-891281-13-4

9073   Sign of the Times
Fanlight Productions
c/o Icarus Films
32 Court Street, 21st Floor
Brooklyn, NY 11201   718-488-8900
                                       800-876-1710
                                    Fax: 718-488-8642
                                     info@fanlight.com
                                      www.fanlight.com

Ben Achtenberg, Owner, Founder
Profiles a public school in the heart of Los Angeles - an American microcosm where over 300 languages are spoken, and where cultures and races collide. Fairfax High, publicized as the site of gang activity and murder, has long been a focus for bad press. But something very right is going on in this school. A Sign of the Times offers a positive example of how the American dream and American education are still alive

9074   Special Technologies Alternative Resources
210 McMorran Boulevard
Port Huron, MI 48060   810-987-7323
                                      877-987-READ
                                   star@sccl.lib.mi.us

Arnold H. Larson, Chairman
Kathleen J. Wheelihan, Vice Chairman
Arlene M. Marcetti, Board Member
Addresses the needs of a very unique diverse group of people by offering a full range of library services for people who cannot read standard print. Provides reading material in specialized formats that permit individuals with disabilities to have access to the written word, delivering to customer's mailboxes free of charge. Talking Book Machines, recorded books and magazines, descriptive videos, large print editions and braille books and magazines.

9075   Standing on My Own Two Feet
Blind Children's Center
4120 Marathon Street
Los Angeles, CA 90029-3584   323-664-2153
                         info@blindchildrenscenter.org
                          www.blindchildrenscenter.org
Lorie Lynn LaPrelle, Author
A guide to constructing mobility devices for children who are visually impaired. *$10.00*
38 pages

9076   Starting Points
Blind Children's Center
4120 Marathon Street
Los Angeles, CA 90029-3584   323-664-2153
                         info@blindchildrenscenter.org
                          www.blindchildrenscenter.org
Deborah Chen, Co-Author
Jamie Dote-Kwan, Co-Author
Basic information for the classroom teacher of 3 to 8 year olds whose multiple disabilities include visual impairment. *$35.00*
157 pages
ISBN 0-891280-61-8

9077   Step-By-Step Guide to Personal Management for Blind Persons
American Foundation for the Blind/AFB Press
2 Penn Plaza
Suite 1102
New York, NY 10121   212-502-7600
                                       800-232-5463
                                    Fax: 888-545-8331
                                       afbinfo@afb.net
                                          www.afb.org

Carl R. Augusto, President & Chief Executive Officer
Rick Bozeman, Chief Financial Officer
Kelly Bleach, Chief Administrative Officer
A manual of techniques in the areas of hygiene, grooming, clothing, shopping and child care. *$19.95*
136 pages Spiralbound
ISBN 0-891280-61-8

9078   Student Teaching Guide for Blind and Visually Impaired College Students
American Foundation for the Blind/AFB Press
2 Penn Plaza
Suite 1102
New York, NY 10121   212-502-7600
                                       800-232-5463
                                    Fax: 888-545-8331
                                       afbinfo@afb.net
                                          www.afb.org

Carl R. Augusto, President & Chief Executive Officer
Rick Bozeman, Chief Financial Officer
Kelly Bleach, Chief Administrative Officer
A comprehensive resource designed to enable the student to enter the classroom of a university or college with confidence. Large print. *$14.95*
52 pages
ISBN 0-891281-42-8

9079 Survey of Direct Labor Workers Who Are Blind & Employed by NIB
Mississippi State University
P.O.Box 6189
Mississippi State, MS 39762
662-325-2001
Fax: 662-325-8989
TTY: 662-325-2694
nrtc@colled.msstate.edu
www.blind.msstate.edu

Jacqui Bybee, Research Associate II
Douglas Bedsaul, Research and Training Coordinator
Anne Carter, Research and Training Coordinator
This report is a follow-up to surveys by National Industries for the Blind in 1983 and 1987 and summarizes the results of a national survey of approximately 500 legally blind direct labor workers. *$10.00*
101 pages Paperback

9080 Talk to Me
Blind Children's Center
4120 Marathon Street
Los Angeles, CA 90029-3584
323-664-2153
info@blindchildrenscenter.org
www.blindchildrenscenter.org

Nancy Chernus-Mansfield, Co-Author
Linda Kekelis, Co-Author
A language guide for parents of children who are visually impaired. *$10.00*
11 pages

9081 Talk to Me II
Blind Children's Center
4120 Marathon Street
Los Angeles, CA 90029-3584
323-664-2153
Fax: 323-665-3828
info@blindchildrenscenter.org
www.blindchildrenscenter.org

Nancy Chernus-Mansfield, Co-Author
Linda Kekelis, Co-Author
A sequel to Talk to Me *$10.00*
15 pages

9082 Talking Books & Reading Disabilities
Nat'l Lib Svc/Blind And Physically Handicapped
1291 Taylor Street North West
Washington, DC 20011
202-707-5100
Fax: 202-707-0712
TTY: 202-707-0744
nls@loc.gov
www.loc.gov/nls

Karen Keninger, Director

9083 Talking Books for People with Physical Disabilities
Nat'l Lib Svc/Blind And Physically Handicapped
1291 Taylor Street North West
Washington, DC 20011
202-707-5100
Fax: 202-707-0712
TTY: 202-707-0744
nls@loc.gov
www.loc.gov/nls

Karen Keninger, Director

9084 Teaching Orientation and Mobility in the Schools: An Instructor's Companion
American Foundation for the Blind
2 Penn Plaza
Suite 1102
New York, NY 10121
212-502-7600
800-232-5463
Fax: 888-545-8331
afbinfo@afb.net
www.afb.org

Carl R. Augusto, President & Chief Executive Officer
Rick Bozeman, Chief Financial Officer
Kelly Bleach, Chief Administrative Officer
This book, with its useful forms, checklists, and tips, will help O&M instructors and teachers of visually impaired students master the arts of planning schedules, organizing equipment and work routines, working with school personnel and educational team members, and effectively providing instruction to children with diverse needs. *$ 45.95*
176 pages
ISBN 0-891283-91-1

9085 Teaching Visually Impaired Children
Charles C. Thomas
2600 S First St
Springfield, IL 62704-4730
217-789-8980
800-258-8980
Fax: 217-789-9130
books@ccthomas.com
www.ccthomas.com

Michael P. Thomas, President
A comprehensive resource for the classroom teacher who is working with a visually impaired child for the first time, as well as a systematic overview of education for the specialist in visual disabilities. It approaches instructional challenges with clear explanations and practical suggestions, and it addresses common concerns of teachers in a reassuring and positive manner. Also available in cloth. *$49.95*
352 pages Paper 2004
ISBN 0-398074-77-7

9086 Textbook Catalog
National Braille Association
95 Allens Creek Road
Building 1, Suite 202
Rochester, NY 14618
585-427-8260
Fax: 585-427-0263
nbaoffice@nationalbraille.org
www.nationalbraille.org

Jan Carroll, President
Cindi Laurent, Vice President
David Shaffer, Executive Director
Lists hundreds of scholarly, college and professional textbooks offered in large print, braille or on cassette for visually impaired readers.
80 pages

9087 Three Rivers News
Carnegie Library of Pitts. Library for the Blind
4724 Baum Boulevard
Pittsburgh, PA 15213
412-687-2440
800-242-0586
Fax: 412-687-2442

Kathleen Kappel, Executive Director
Loans recorded books/magazines and playback equipment, large print books and described videos to western PA residents unable to use standard printed materials due to a visual, physical, or physically-based reading disability.
12 pages Quarterly

9088 To Love this Life: Quotations by Helen Keller
American Foundation for the Blind/AFB Press
2 Penn Plaza
Suite 1102
New York, NY 10121
212-502-7600
800-232-5463
Fax: 888-545-8331
www.afb.org

Carl R. Augusto, President & Chief Executive Officer
Rick Bozeman, Chief Financial Officer
Kelly Bleach, Chief Administrative Officer
Inspirational work that offers the penetrating observations of Helen Keller, the beloved deaf-blind champion of the rights of people with disabilities. Also available on cassette at $21.95 (ISBN# 0-89128-348-X) *$21.95*
144 pages Hardcover
ISBN 0-891283-47-1

9089 **Touch the Baby: Blind & Visually Impaired Children As Patients**
American Foundation for the Blind/AFB Press
2 Penn Plaza
Suite 1102
New York, NY 10121
212-502-7600
800-232-5463
Fax: 888-545-8331
afbinfo@afb.net
www.afb.org

Carl R. Augusto, President & Chief Executive Officer
Rick Bozeman, Chief Financial Officer
Kelly Bleach, Chief Administrative Officer
A how-to manual for health care professionals working in hospitals, clinics and doctors' offices. Teaches the special communication and touch-related techniques needed to prevent blind and visually impaired patients from withdrawing from the healthcare workers and the outside world. $25.00/pack of 25.
13 pages
ISBN 0-891281-97-5

9090 **Transition Activity Calendar for Students with Visual Impairments**
Mississippi State University
P.O.Box 6189
Mississippi State, MS 39762
662-325-2001
Fax: 662-325-8989
TTY: 662-325-2694
nrtc@colled.msstate.edu
www.blind.msstate.edu

Jacqui Bybee, Research Associate II
Douglas Bedsaul, Research and Training Coordinator
Anne Carter, Research and Training Coordinator
The Transition Activity Calendar guides the student with a visual disability through the maze of college preparation. Beginning in junior high school, clearly written steps are listed for each grade level. Students planning to enter college after high school graduation can check-off their accomplishments each step of the way. The calendar helps students focus on their goals while providing reminders of tasks yet to be completed. It can be used in a self-directed manner or in a group format. *$4.25*
16 pages Paperback

9091 **Transition to College for Students with Visual Impairments: Report**
Mississippi State University
P.O.Box 6189
Mississippi State, MS 39762
662-325-2001
Fax: 662-325-8989
TTY: 662-325-2694
nrtc@colled.msstate.edu
www.blind.msstate.edu

Jacqui Bybee, Research Associate II
Douglas Bedsaul, Research and Training Coordinator
Anne Carter, Research and Training Coordinator
A report offering results from telephone interviews of college students with visual impairments and mail surveys of college officials which examines the transition experience of successful college students. General domains in the study include demographics, educational history, computers, specialized and adaptive equipment, resources, college preparation, problems adjusting to college and O&M skills. A literature review covers preparing for college, task timelines,and classroom, labs and tests. *$20.00*
151 pages Paperback

9092 **Unseen Minority: A Social History of Blindness in the United States**
American Foundation for the Blind/AFB Press
2 Penn Plaza
Suite 1102
New York, NY 10121
212-502-7600
800-232-5463
Fax: 888-545-8331
abfinfo@abf.org
www.afb.org

Carl R. Augusto, President & Chief Executive Officer
Rick Bozeman, Chief Financial Officer
Kelly Bleach, Chief Administrative Officer

A lively narrative, with anecdotes, that recounts how the blind overcame discrimination to gain full participation in the social, educational, economic and legislative spheres. Hardcover. *$59.95*
573 pages Paperback
ISBN 0-891288-96-1

9093 **Vision Enhancement**
UN Printing
122
1790 E 54th St
Indianapolis, IN 46220-3454
317-254-1332
800-431-1739
Fax: 317-251-6588
www.visionww.org

Patricia L Price, Managing Editor
Designed to encourage and support individuals with vision loss, family members, and caregivers. *$25.00*
72-78 pages Quarterly

9094 **Visual Impairment: An Overview**
American Foundation for the Blind/AFB Press
2 Penn Plaza
Suite 1102
New York, NY 10121
212-502-7600
800-232-5463
Fax: 888-545-8331
afbinfo@afb.net
www.afb.org

Carl R. Augusto, President & Chief Executive Officer
Rick Bozeman, Chief Financial Officer
Kelly Bleach, Chief Administrative Officer
An overall look at the most common forms of vision loss and their impact on the individual. Includes drawings as well as photographs that stimulate how people with vision loss see. Paperback. *$19.95*
56 pages
ISBN 0-891281-74-0

9095 **Visual Impairments And Learning**
Sage Publications
2455 Teller Road
Thousand Oaks, CA 91320
805-499-0721
800-818-7243
Fax: 805-499-0871
info@sagepub.com
www.sagepub.com

Sara Miller McCune, Founder, Publisher, Executive Chairman
Blaise R Simqu, President & CEO
Tracey A. Ozmina, Executive Vice President & Chief Operating Officer
The major focus of this new, third edition is to present a new way of thinking about individuals with visual impairment so that they are viewed as participating members of a seeing world despite their reduced visual functioning. *$40.00*
213 pages
ISBN 0-890798-68-3

9096 **Walking Alone and Marching Together**
National Federation of the Blind
200 E. Wells St.
at Jernigan Place
Baltimore, MD 21230
410-659-9314
Fax: 410-685-5653
nfb@nfb.org
www.nfb.org

Floyd Matson, Author
The history of the organized blind movement, this book spans more than 50 years of civil rights, social issues, attitudes and experiences of the blind. Published in 1990, it has been read by thousands of blind and sighted persons and is used in colleges, libraries and programs across the country as an important tool in understanding blindness and it's impact on both personal lives and the society at large.

9097 **What Do You Do When You See a Blind Person- and What Don't You Do?**
American Foundation for the Blind/AFB Press
2 Penn Plaza
Suite 1102
New York, NY 10121   212-502-7600
                                            800-232-5463
                                       Fax: 888-545-8331
                                         afbinfo@afb.net
                                                 afb.org

Carl R. Augusto, President & Chief Executive Officer
Rick Bozeman, Chief Financial Officer
Kelly Bleach, Chief Administrative Officer
Examples of real-life situations that teach sighted persons how to interact effectively with blind persons. Topics covered include how to help someone across the street, how not to distract a guide dog and how to take leave of a blind person. *$25.00*
8 pages
ISBN 0-891281-95-5

9098 **What Museum Guides Need to Know: Access for the Blind and Visually Impaired**
American Foundation for the Blind/AFB Press
2 Penn Plaza
Suite 1102
New York, NY 10121   212-502-7600
                                            800-232-5463
                                       Fax: 888-545-8331
                                         afbinfo@afb.net
                                             www.afb.org

Carl R. Augusto, President & Chief Executive Officer
Rick Bozeman, Chief Financial Officer
Kelly Bleach, Chief Administrative Officer
Explains how blind and visually impaired museum-goers experience art and offers pointers on greeting people, asking if help is needed and teaching about a specific work of art. Contains information on access laws, resources, training guides and guidelines for preparing large print, cassette and braille materials. *$14.95*
64 pages Paperback
ISBN 0-891281-58-4

9099 **Work Sight**
Lighthouse Guild
250 West 64th Street
New York, NY 10023   800-284-4422
                                  www.lighthouseguild.org

Calvin W. Roberts, President & CEO
James M. Dubin, Chairman
Lawrence E. Goldschmidt, Vice Chairman & Treasurer
Intended for employers and employees who have concerns about vision loss and job performance. *$25.00*

9100 **World Through Their Eyes**
Lighthouse Guild
250 West 64th Street
New York, NY 10023   800-284-4422
                                  www.lighthouseguild.org

Calvin W. Roberts, President & CEO
James M. Dubin, Chairman
Lawrence E. Goldschmidt, Vice Chairman & Treasurer
Intended to help nursing home staff understand how residents with impaired vision perceive the world. Concrete suggestions help staff provide better care to visually impaired residents. *$25.00*

9101 **You Seem Like a Regular Kid to Me**
American Foundation for the Blind/AFB Press
2 Penn Plaza
Suite 1102
New York, NY 10121   212-502-7600
                                            800-232-5463
                                       Fax: 888-545-8331
                                         afbinfo@afb.net
                                             www.afb.org

Carl R. Augusto, President & Chief Executive Officer
Rick Bozeman, Chief Financial Officer
Kelly Bleach, Chief Administrative Officer
An interview with Jane, a blind child, tells other children what it's like to be blind. Jane explains how she gets around, takes care of herself, does her school work, spends her leisure time and even pays for things when she can't see money.
16 pages
ISBN 0-891289-21-6

Journals

9102 **Journal of Visual Impairment and Blindness**
Sheridan Press,
450 Fame Ave
Hanover, PA 17331-1585   717-632-3535
                                             800-352-2210
                                        Fax: 717-633-8929
                                  www.sheridanreprints.com

Sharon Shively, Editor
Published in braille, regular print and on ASC II disk and cassette, this journal contains a wide variety of subjects including rehabilitation, psychology, education, legislation, medicine, technology, employment, sensory aids and childhood development as they relate to visual impairments. $130 annual individual subscription, $180 annual institutional subscription.
64 pages Monthly
ISSN 0145-48 x

Magazines

9103 **Braille Forum**
American Council of the Blind
2200 Wilson Boulevard
Suite 650
Arlington, VA 22201-3354   202-467-5081
                                             800-424-8666
                                        Fax: 703-465-5085
                                             info@acb.org
                                             www.acb.org

Kim Charlson, President
Jeff Thom, 1st Vice President
Melanie Brunson, Executive Director
Offered in print, braille, cassette, IBM computer disk and e-mail. $25 per format per year for companies and non-US residents.
48 pages Magazine

9104 **Braille Montior**
National Federation of the Blind
200 E. Wells St.
at Jernigan Place
Baltimore, MD 21230   410-659-9314
                                        Fax: 410-685-5653
                                     nfbpublications@nfb.org
                                             www.nfb.org

Gary Wunder, Editor
The Braille Monitor is the leading publication of the National Federation of the Blind. It covers the events and activities of the NFB and addresses the many issues and concerns of the blind. *$40.00*
11 times a year

9105 **Dialogue Magazine**
Blindskills Inc.
P.O. Box 5181
Salem, OR 97304-0181   503-581-4224
                                             800-860-4224
                                        Fax: 503-581-0178
                                     info@blindskills.com
                                     www.blindskills.com

Marja Byers, Executive Director
B.T. Kimbrough, Editor
Publishes quarterly magazine in braille, large-type, cassette and email of news items, technology and articles of special interest to visually impaired youth and adults. Annual subscription cost $35 for braille, large print or cassette, $20 for email. *$35.00*
Quarterly

9106 **Future Reflections**
Deaf-Blind Division of the Ntn'l Fed of the Blind
200 E. Wells St.
at Jernigan Place
Baltimore, MD 21230

Fax: 410-659-9314
Fax: 410-685-5653
nfbpublications@nfb.org
www.nfb.org

Deborah Kent Stein, Editor
A magazine for parents and teachers of blind children.

9107 **Guide Magazine**
The Seeing Eye
P.O.Box 375
10 Washington Valley Road
Morristown, NJ 7963

973-539-4425
Fax: 973-539-0922
info@seeingeye.org
seeingeye.org

James A. Kutsch, Jr., Ph.D., President & CEO
Robert Pudlak, CFO & Director of Administration & Finance
Glenn Cianci, Director of Facilities Management
The Guide offers stories of inspiration from our graduates and
news of the latest program developments.

9108 **JBI Voice**
Jewish Braille Institute of America
110 Est 30th Street
New York, NY 10016

212-889-2525
800-433-1531
Fax: 212-689-3692
admin@jbilibrary.org
www.jbilibrary.org

Judy E. Tenney, Chairman
Thomas G. Kahn, Viec Chairman
Dr. Ellen Isler, President and CEO
Monthly recorded magazine emphasizing Jewish current events
and culture.

9109 **Jewish Braille Review**
Jewish Braille Institute of America
110 Est 30th Street
New York, NY 10016

212-889-2525
800-433-1531
Fax: 212-689-3692
admin@jbilibrary.org
www.jbilibrary.org

Judy E. Tenney, Chairman
Thomas G. Kahn, Viec Chairman
Dr. Ellen Isler, President and CEO
The JBI seeks the integration of Jews who are blind, visually impaired and reading disabled into the Jewish community and society in general. More than 20,000 men, women and children in 50
countries receive a broad variety of JBI services.

9110 **Musical Mainstream**
Nat'l Lib Svc/Blind And Physically Handicapped
1291 Taylor Street North West
Washington, DC 20011

202-707-5100
Fax: 202-707-0712
TTY: 202-707-0744
nls@loc.gov
www.loc.gov/nls

Karen Keninger, Director
Articles selected from print music magazines.
Quarterly

9111 **Opportunity**
National Industries for the Blind
1310 Braddock Place
Alexandria, VA 22314-1691

703-310-0500
Fax: 703-998-8268
services@nib.org
www.nib.org

The Honorabl Krump, Esq., Chairman
Louis J. Jablonski, Jr., Vice Chairman
Kevin A. Lynch, President and Chief Executive Officer
Offers information and articles on the newest technology, equip-
ment, services and programs for blind and visually impaired
persons.
Quarterly

9112 **Providing Services for People with Vision Loss:**
Multidisciplinary Perspective
Resources for Rehabilitation
22 Bonad Road
Winchester, MA 01890-1302

781-368-9080
Fax: 781-368-9096
orders@rfr.org
www.rfr.org

Susan L Greenblatt, Editor
A collection of articles by ophthalmologists and rehabilitation
professionals, including chapters on operating a low vision service, starting self-help programs, mental health services, aids and
techniques that help people with vision loss. *$19.95*
136 pages
ISBN 0-929718-02-0

Newsletters

9113 **AFB News**
American Foundation for the Blind/AFB Press
2 Penn Plaza
Suite 1102
New York, NY 10121

212-502-7600
800-232-5463
Fax: 888-545-8331
afbinfo@afb.net
www.afb.org

Carl R. Augusto, President & Chief Executive Officer
Rick Bozeman, Chief Financial Officer
Kelly Bleach, Chief Administrative Officer
National newsletter for general readership about blindness and
visual impairments featuring people, programs, services and
activities.
12 pages Quarterly

9114 **ASB Visions Newsletter**
ASB
919 Walnut Street
Philadelphia, PA 19107-5237

215-627-0600
Fax: 215-922-0692
asbinfo@asb.org
www.asb.org

Karla S. McCaney, President & CEO
Beth Deering, Chief Program Officer
Sylvia Purnell, Director of Learning & Development
Newsletter associated services for the blind and visually im-
paired.

9115 **Adaptive Services Division**
District of Columbia Public Library
901G St NW,
Rm 215
Washington, DC 20001-4531

202-727-2142
Fax: 202-727-0322
TTY: 202-559-5368
lbph.dcpl@dc.gov
www.dclibrary.org

Venetia Demson, Chief, Adaptive Services
DC Regional Library for the blind, deaf and physically handicapped. Provides adaptive technology and training programs.
8 pages Quarterly

9116 **Alumni News**
Guide Dogs for the Blind
P.O.Box 151200
San Rafael, CA 94915-1200

415-499-4000
800-295-4050
Fax: 415-499-4035
guidedogs.com

Bob Burke, Chairman
Stuart Odell, Vice Chairman
Chris Benninger, President and CEO
Restricted to graduates only.

9117 Annual Report/Newsletter
National Accreditation Council for Agencies/Blind
Rm 1004
15 E 40th St
New York, NY 10016-401   212-683-5068
                                      Fax: 212-683-4475
Ruth Westman, Executive Director
Provides standards and a program of accreditation for schools
and organizations which serve children and adults who are blind
or vision impaired.

9118 Association for Macular Diseases Newsletter
210 East 64th Street
New York, NY 10065   212-605-3719
                                      Fax: 212-605-3795
                           association@retinal-research.org
                                              macula.org
Bernard Landou, President
Mary Fern Breheny, Board Member
Patricia Dahl, Board Member
Not-for-profit organization promotes education and research in
this scarcely explored field. Acts as a nationwide support group
for individuals and their families endeavoring to adjust to the restrictions and changes brought about by macular disease. Offers
hotline, educational materials, quarterly newsletter, support
groups, referrals and seminars for persons and families affected
by macular disease.

9119 Awareness
NAPVI
1 North Lexington Avenue
White Plains, NY 10601   617-972-7441
                                           800-562-6265
                                      Fax: 617-972-7444
                              napvi@guildhealth.org
                                        www.napvi.org
Julie Urban, President
Venetia Hayden, Vice President
Susan LaVenture, Executive Director
Newsletter offering regional news, sports and activities, confer-
ences, camps, legislative updates, book reviews, audio reviews,
professional question and answer column and more for the visu-
ally impaired and their families.
Quarterly

9120 BTBL News
Braille and Talking Book Library
P.O. Box 942837
Sacramento, CA 94237-0001   916-654-0261
                                           800-952-5666
                                      Fax: 916-654-1119
                                   btbl@library.ca.gov
                                        www.btbl.ca.gov
Janet Coles, Editor
Christopher Berger, Senior Librarian
Olena Bilyk, Web Developer
BTBL News, the quarterly newsletter of the California Braille
and Talking Book Library, features articles on topics of interest to
library customers, including information about new services, ex-
isting services, events, staff and more.

9121 Canes and Trails
Guide Dogs for the Blind
P.O.Box 151200
San Rafael, CA 94915-1200   415-499-4000
                                           800-295-4050
                                      Fax: 415-499-4035
                                          guidedogs.com
Bob Burke, Chairman
Stuart Odell, Vice Chairman
Chris Benninger, President and CEO
A quarterly newsletter for orientation and mobility specialists, re-
habilitation professionals, teachers, and service providers in the
field of blindness and visual impairment.

9122 Community Connection
Guide Dogs for the Blind
P.O.Box 151200
San Rafael, CA 94915-1200   415-499-4000
                                           800-295-4050
                                      Fax: 415-499-4035
                                          guidedogs.com
Bob Burke, Chairman
Stuart Odell, Vice Chairman
Chris Benninger, President and CEO
A newsletter produced for our volunteers and other friends of
Guide Dogs.

9123 DVH Quarterly
University of Arkansas at Little Rock
2801 S University Ave
Little Rock, AR 72204-1000   501-569-3000
Bob Brasher, Editor
Mary Boaz, Manager
Offers information on upcoming events, conferences and work-
shops on and for visual disabilities. Book reviews, information
on the newest resources and technology, educational programs,
want ads and more.
Quarterly

9124 Deaf-Blind Perspective
National Consortium on Deaf-Blindness
345 North Monmouth Avenue
Monmouth, OR 97361   503-838-8391
                                           800-438-9376
                                      Fax: 503-838-8150
                                      TTY: 800-854-7013
Ingrid Amerson, Child Development Center
Lyn Ayer, Center on Deaf & Blindness
Robert Ayres, Evaluation and Research
A free publication with articles, essays, and announcements
about topics related to people who are deaf-blind. Published two
times a year (Spring and Fall) by the Teaching Research Institute
of Western Oregon University, its purpose is to provide information and serve as a forum for discussion and sharing ideas.

9125 Fidelco
Fidelco Guide Dog Foundation
103 Vision Way
Bloomfield, CT 06002   860-243-5200
                                      Fax: 860-769-0567
                                       info@fidelco.org
                                            fidelco.org
Karen C. Tripp, Chairman
G. Kenneth Bernhard, Vice Chairman
Eliot D. Matheson, CEO
A newsletter published by Fidelco Guide Dog Foundation.

9126 Focus
Visually Impaired Center
1422 W Court St
Flint, MI 48503-5008   810-767-4014
                                      Fax: 810-767-0020
Charles Tommasulo, Executive Director
Newsletter offering information for the visually impaired person
in the forms of legislative and law updates, ADA information,
support groups, hotlines, and articles on the newest technology in
the field.
Quarterly

9127 Gleams Newsletter
Glaucoma Research Foundation
2345 Yale Street
2nd Floor
Palo Alto, CA 94306   650-328-3388
                                           800-826-6693
                                      Fax: 415-986-3763
                                   info@glaucoma.org
Tom Brunner, CEO
Offers updated medical & research information on glaucoma. Included are glaucoma treatant and coping tips, legsilative information, professional articles and book reviews.
6 pages Quarterly

9128   Guide Dog News
Guide Dogs for the Blind
P.O.Box 151200
San Rafael, CA 94915-1200   415-499-4000
                                             800-295-4050
                                         Fax: 415-499-4035
                                             guidedogs.com
Bob Burke, Chairman
Stuart Odell, Vice Chairman
Chris Benninger, President and CEO
Read about changes to our teaching techniques, our new Adult
Learning Program, vet tips, and find news about our graduates.

9129   Guideway
Guide Dog Foundation for the Blind
371 East Jericho Turnpike
Smithtown, NY 11787-2976   631-930-9000
                                             800-548-4337
                                         Fax: 631-930-9009
                                             info@guidedog.org
                                             www.guidedog.org
James C. Bingham, Chairman
Alphonce J. Brown, Jr., Vice Chairman
Wells B. Jones, CEO
Offers updates and information on the foundation's activities and
guide dog programs. In print form but is also available on
cassette.
Monthly

9130   Guild Briefs
Catholic Guild for The Blind
65 East Wacker Place
Suite 1010
Chicago, IL 60601   312-236-8569
                                         Fax: 312-236-8128
                                             www.guildfortheblind.org
Brett Christenson, President
Laura Rounce, Vice President
David Tabak, Executive Director
Monthly publication for individuals who are blind or visually im-
paired. It contains articles on topics such as service programs,
scholarships, education, seniors, research, and government.
12 pages monthly

9131   IAAIS Report
Int'l Association of Audio Information Services
3920 Willshire Dr
Lawrence, KS 66049-3673   412-434-6023
                                             800-280-5325
                                             www.iaais.org
Stuart Holland, President
Marjorie Williams, 1st Vice President
Linda Hynson, Secretary
Newsletter for persons interested in radio reading services. *$7.00*
Quarterly

9132   Insight
Eye Bank Association of America
Ste 1010
1015 18th Street NorthWest
Washington, DC 20036   202-775-4999
                                         Fax: 202-429-6036
                                             info@restoresight.org
                                             www.restoresight.org
Colleen Bayus, Communications Manager
An electronic newsletter.

9133   LampLighter
Columbia Lighthouse for the Blind
1825 K St. NW
Suite 1103
Washington, DC 20006   202-454-6400
                                         Fax: 202-955-6401
                                             info@clb.org
                                             www.clb.org
Tony Cancelosi, President & CEO
Jocelyn Hunter, Senior Director, Communications
Toya Horten, Director, Administrative Operations
Columbia Lighthouse for the Blind's monthly newsletter. Pro-
vides information on community news and events.

9134   Library Users of America Newsletter
American Council of the Blind
2200 Wilson Boulevard
Suite 650
Arlington, VA 22201-3354   202-467-5081
                                             800-424-8666
                                         Fax: 703-465-5085
                                             info@acb.org
                                             www.acb.org
Kim Charlson, President
Jeff Thom, 1st Vice President
Melanie Brunson, Executive Director
Published twice yearly, the newsletter contains much information
about library services of particular interest to blind and visually
impaired patrons, and is available in the following formats:
Braille, audiocassette, large print and e-mail.

9135   Light the Way
Blind Children's Center
4120 Marathon Street
Los Angeles, CA 90029-3584   323-664-2153
                                             info@blindchildrenscenter.org
                                             blindchildrenscenter.org
Sarah E. Orth, CEO
Newsletter of the Blind Childrens Center, a family-centered
agency which serves young children with visual impairments.
The center-based and home-based services help the children to
acquire skills and build their independence. The center utilizes its
expertise and experience to serve families and professionals
worldwide through support services, education and research.

9136   Lighthouse Publication
Chicago Lighthouse
1850 West Roosevelt Road
Chicago, IL 60608-1298   312-666-1331
                                         Fax: 312-243-8539
                                         TTY: 312-666-8874
                                             publications@chicagolighthouse.org
                                             www.thechicagolighthouse.org
Janet P. Szlyk, Ph.D., President & Chief Executive Officer
Mary Lynne Januszewski, Executive Vice President/CFO
Melanie M. Hennessy, SVP

9137   Lights On
Fight for Sight
Ste 809
391 Park Ave S
New York, NY 10016-8806   212-679-6060
                                         Fax: 212-679-4466
Mary Prudden, Executive Director
A newsletter published by Fight for Sight.

9138   Listen Up
Recording for the Blind & Dyslexic
20 Roszel Rd
Princeton, NJ 8540-6206   609-452-0606
                                             866-732-3585
                                         Fax: 609-520-7990
                                             www.learningally.org
John Kelly, CEO
RFB&D's bi-monthly electronic newsletter for members.

9139   Long Cane News
American Foundation for the Blind/AFB Press
2 Penn Plaza
Suite 1102
New York, NY 10121   212-502-7600
                                             800-232-5463
                                         Fax: 888-545-8331
                                             afbinfo@afb.net
                                             www.afb.org
Carl R. Augusto, President & Chief Executive Officer
Rick Bozeman, Chief Financial Officer
Kelly Bleach, Chief Administrative Officer
SemiAnnual

9140 **Magnifier**
Macular Degeneration Foundation
P.O.Box 531313
Henderson, NV 89053
702-450-2908
888-633-3937
liz@eyesight.org
www.eyesight.org

Liz Trauernicht, President & Director of Communications
Julie Zavala, VP & Asst. Director of Operations
David Seftel, EVP & Dircetor, R & D
The Magnifier is the distributed without charge via email and by regular mail to those without access to the Internet. It features breaking news, clinical trails, clarifies recent reports in the media, announces new Internet resources and informs the public of important additions to the web site.

9141 **NAVH Update**
National Association of Visually Handicapped
111 East 59th Street
New York, NY 10022-1202
212-821-9384
800-829-0500
Fax: 212-821-9707
info@lighthouse.org
lighthouse.org/navh

Mark G. Ackermann, President / CEO
A newsletter published by the National Association of Visually Impaired. LightHouse acquired NAVH.

9142 **NBA Bulletin**
National Braille Association
95 Allens Creek Road
Building 1, Suite 202
Rochester, NY 14618
585-427-8260
Fax: 585-427-0263
nbaoffice@nationalbraille.org
www.nationalbraille.org

Jan Carroll, President
Cindi Laurent, Vice President
David Shaffer, Executive Director
Published quarterly and included int he price of the regular and student NBA membership.

9143 **NLS News**
Nat'l Lib Svc/Blind And Physically Handicapped
1291 Taylor Street North West
Washington, DC 20011
202-707-5100
Fax: 202-707-0712
TTY: 202-707-0744
nls@loc.gov
www.loc.gov/nls

Karen Keninger, Director
Newsletter on current program developments.
Quarterly

9144 **NLS Newsletter**
Nat'l Lib Svc/Blind And Physically Handicapped
1291 Taylor Street North West
Washington, DC 20011
202-707-5100
Fax: 202-707-0712
TTY: 202-707-0744
nls@loc.gov
www.loc.gov/nls

Karen Keninger, Director
Newsletter on the service's volunteer activities.
Quarterly

9145 **PBA News**
Prevent Blindness America
211 West Wacker Drive
Suite 1700
Chicago, IL 60606
800-331-2020
info@preventblindness.org
www.preventblindness.org

Paul G. Howes, Chairman
Hugh R. Parry, President & CEO,Prevent Blindness America
Jerome Desserich, Vice President & Chief Financial Officer
Newsletter is filled with the information you need to protect your eyes, preserve your sight, and educate yourself about your own eye condition or that of a family member. Publication offered three times yearly.
3 times yearly

9146 **Planned Giving Department of Guide Dogs for the Blind**
Guide Dogs for the Blind
P.O.Box 151200
San Rafael, CA 94915-1200
415-499-4000
800-295-4050
Fax: 415-499-4035
guidedogs.com

Bob Burke, Chairman
Stuart Odell, Vice Chairman
Chris Benninger, President and CEO
A newsletter published by Guide Dogs for the Blind.

9147 **Playback**
Recording for the Blind & Dyslexic
20 Roszel Road
Princeton, NJ 08540
800-221-4792
Fax: 609-987-8116
Custserv@LearningAlly.org
www.learningally.org/

Brad Grob, Chairman
Harold J. Logan, Vice Chairman
Andrew Friedman, President & CEO
A publication dedicated to our unit's family of members, volunteers, supporters and staff. RFB&D is now Learning Ally.
3x Year

9148 **Quarterly Update**
National Association for Visually Handicapped
111 East 59th Street
New York, NY 10022-1202
212-821-9384
800-829-0500
Fax: 212-821-9707
info@lighthouse.org
lighthouse.org/navh

Mark G. Ackermann, President / CEO
Quarterly newsletter offering information on new products for the visually impaired, advances in medical treatments, new books available in the NAVH large print loan library and any new/updated booklets. Free. LightHouse acquired NAVH.

9149 **RP Messenger**
Texas Association of Retinitis Pigmentosa
P.O.Box 8388
Corpus Christi, TX 78468-8388
361-852-8515
Fax: 361-852-8515
tarp@homebiz101.com

Dorothy Steifel, Executive Director
A bi-annual newsletter offering information on Retinitis Pigmentosa. *$15.00*
BiAnnual

9150 **SCENE**
Braille Institute
527 North Dale Avenue
Anaheim, CA 92801
714-821-5000
800-272-4553
Fax: 714-527-7621
oc@brailleinstitute.org
brailleinstitute.org

Lester M. Sussman, Chairman
Peter A. Mindnich, President
Jon K. Hayashida, OD, FAAO, Vice President, Programs & Services
Offers information on the organization, question and answer column, articles on the newest technology and more for visually impaired persons.

9151 **STAR**
Special Technologies Alternative Resources
210 McMorran Boulevard
Port Huron, MI 48060
810-987-7323
877-987-READ
star@sccl.lib.mi.us
www.sccl.lib.mi.us

Arnold H. Larson, Chairman
Kathleen J. Wheelihan, Vice Chairman
Arlene M. Marcetti, Board Member
A newsletter published by Special Technologies Alternative Resources.

9152 Seeing Eye Guide
The Seeing Eye
P.O.Box 375
10 Washington Valley Road
Morristown, NJ 07963   973-539-4425
                                    Fax: 973-539-0922
                                    info@seeingeye.org
                                          seeingeye.org

James A. Kutsch, Jr., Ph.D., President & CEO
Randall Ivens, Director of Human Resources
Robert Pudlak, CFO & Director of Adninistration & Finance
A quarterly publication from Seeing Eye.
Quarterly

9153 Shared Visions
Vista Center for the Blind & Visually Impaired
413 Laurel St
Santa Cruz, CA 95060-4904   831-458-9766
                                        800-705-2970
                                    Fax: 831-426-6233
                                information@vistacenter.org
Pam Brandin, Executive Director
A quarterly publication for Blind and Visually Impaired individu-
als from Vista Center for the Blind and Visually Impaired.

9154 Sharing Solutions: A Newsletter for Support Groups
Lighthouse Guild
250 West 64th Street
New York, NY 10023   800-284-4422
                                    www.lighthouseguild.org
Calvin W. Roberts, President & CEO
James M. Dubin, Chairman
Lawrence E. Goldschmidt, Vice Chairman & Treasurer
A newsletter for members and leaders of support groups for older
adults with impaired vision. The letter provides a forum for sup-
port groups members to network and share information, printed
in a very large type format.

9155 Sightings Newsletter
Schepens Eye Research Institute
20 Staniford Street
Boston, MA 02114   617-912-0100
                                    Fax: 617-912-0110
                                  www.schepens.harvard.edu
Michael Gilmore, Director
Mary E. Leach, Director of Public Affairs
Frances Ng, Director of Human Resources
Publication of prominent center for research on eye, vision, and
blinding diseases; dedicated to research that improves the understanding, management, and prevention of eye diseases and visual
deficiencies; fosters collaboration among its faculty members;
trains young scientists and clinicians from around the world; promotes communication with scientists in allied fields; leader in the
worldwide dispersion of basic scientific knowledge of vision.

9156 Smith Kettlewell Rehabilitation Engineering Research Center
2318 Fillmore Street
San Francisco, CA 94115   415-345-2000
                                    Fax: 415-345-8455
                                        rerc@ski.org
                                             ski.org
John Brabyn, Ph.D., CEO/Executive Director
Ruth S. Poole, COO
Arthur Jampolsky, Director
Reports on technology and devices for persons with visual im-
pairments.

9157 Student Advocate
National Alliance of Blind Students NABS Liaison
Ste 1004
1155 15th St NW
Washington, DC 20005-2706   202-467-5081
                                        800-424-8666
                                    Fax: 202-467-5085
                                    www.blindstudents.org
Melanie Brunson, Executive Director
A newsletter created by members of NABS and for any interested
parties.

9158 TBC Focus
Chicago Public Library Talking Books Center
400 South State Street
Chicago, IL 60605   312-747-4300
                                        800-757-4654
                                    Fax: 312-747-1609
                                      www.chipublib.org
Linda Johnson Rice, President
Christopher Valenti, VP
Christina Benitez, Secretary
Published quarterly by the Chicago Public Library Talking Book
Center. Free of charge.
4 pages Quarterly

9159 Talking Books Topics
Nat'l Lib Svc/Blind And Physically Handicapped
1291 Taylor Street North West
Washington, DC 20011   202-707-5100
                                    Fax: 202-707-0712
                                    TTY: 202-707-0744
                                          nls@loc.gov
                                       www.loc.gov/nls
Karen Keninger, Director
New recorded books and program news
Bi-monthly

9160 Upstate Update
New York State Talking Book & Braille Library
222 Madison Avenue
Albany, NY 12230-1   518-474-5935
                                        800-342-3688
                                    Fax: 514-474-5786
                                    TTY: 518-474-7121
                                  nyslweb@mail.nysed.gov
                                      www.nysl.nysed.gov
*Bernard A. Margolis, State Librarian & Asst. Commissioner for Li-
braries*
Loretta Ebert, Research Library Director
Liza Duncan, Technical Services & Systmes
Books on audio cassette, cassette players, braille books, summer
reading programs, braille writer, magnifiers, closed-circuit T.V.,
large-print photocopier, cassette books and magazines, children's books on cassette, reference materials on blindness and
other handicaps.
4 pages Quarterly

9161 Visual Aids and Informational Material
National Association for Visually Handicapped
111 East 59th Street
New York, NY 10022-1202   212-821-9384
                                        800-829-0500
                                    Fax: 212-821-9707
                                      info@lighthouse.org
                                      lighthouse.org/navh
Mark G. Ackermann, President / CEO
A complete listing of the visual aids NAVH carries such as magnifiers, talking clocks, large print playing cards, etc. LightHouse
acquired NAVH. *$2.50*
65 pages

9162 Voice
Vermont Assn for the Blind & Visually Impaired
60 Kimball Avenue
South Burlington, VT 05403   802-863-1358
                                        800-639-5861
                                    Fax: 802-863-1481
                                     General@vabvi.org
                                             vabvi.org
Thomas Chase, President
Stephen Pouliot, Executive Director
Kathleen Quinlan, Director of Operations
The Voice is a newsletter published by Vermont Association for
the Blind and Visually Impaired.

9163 Voice of Vision
GW Micro
725 Airport North Office Park
Fort Wayne, IN 46825   260-489-3671
                                    Fax: 260-489-2608
                                      www.gwmicro.com
Dan Weirich, Owner

Offers product reviews, product announcements, tips for making systems or applications more accessible, or explanations of concepts of interest to any computer user or would-be computer user. This association newsletter is available in braille, in large print, on audio cassette and on 3.5 or 5.25 IBM format diskette.
Quarterly

Audio/Visual

9164 Aging and Vision: Declarations of Independence
American Foundation for the Blind/AFB Press
2 Penn Plaza
Suite 1102
New York, NY 10121   212-502-7600
                                      800-232-5463
                                 Fax: 888-545-8331
                                    afbinfo@afb.net
                                       www.afb.org

Carl R. Augusto, President & Chief Executive Officer
Rick Bozeman, Chief Financial Officer
Kelly Bleach, Chief Administrative Officer
A very personal look at five older people who have successfully coped with visual impairment and continue to lead active, satisfying lives. Their stories are not only inspirational, but also provide practical, down-to-earth suggestions for adapting to vision loss later in life. 18 minute video tape. Also available in PAL, $52.95, 0-89128-276-9. *$42.95*
VHS
ISBN 0-891282-20-3

9165 Blindness, A Family Matter
American Foundation for the Blind/AFB Press
2 Penn Plaza
Suite 1102
New York, NY 10121   212-502-7600
                                      800-232-5463
                                 Fax: 888-545-8331
                                    afbinfo@afb.net
                                       www.afb.org

Carl R. Augusto, President & Chief Executive Officer
Rick Bozeman, Chief Financial Officer
Kelly Bleach, Chief Administrative Officer
A frank exploration of the effects of an individual's visual impairment on other members of the family and how those family members can play a positive role in the rehabilitation process. Features interviews with three families whose 'success stories' provide advice and encouragement, as well as interviews with newly blinded adults currently involved in a rehabilitation program. 23 minute video tape. Also available in PAL, $49.95, 0-89128-271-8. *$43.95*
VHS
ISBN 0-891282-22-X

9166 Building Blocks: Foundations for Learning for Young Blind and Visually Impaired Children
American Foundation for the Blind/AFB Press
2 Penn Plaza
Suite 1102
New York, NY 10121   212-502-7600
                                      800-232-5463
                                 Fax: 888-545-8331
                                    afbinfo@afb.net
                                       www.afb.org

Carl R. Augusto, President & Chief Executive Officer
Rick Bozeman, Chief Financial Officer
Kelly Bleach, Chief Administrative Officer
Presents the essential components of a successful early intervnetion program, including collaboration with family members, positive relationships between parents and professionals, public education, and attention to important programming components such as space exploration, braille readiness, orientation and mobility, play, cooking and music. Includes interviews with parents. Available in English or Spanish. 10 minute video tape. Also available in PAL, $33.95, 0-89128-268-8. *$26.95*
VHS
ISBN 0-891282-14-9

9167 Choice Magazine Listening
85 Channel Drive
Port Washington, NY 11050   516-883-8280
                                      888-724-6423
                                      888-724-6423
                                 Fax: 516-944-5849
                                  choicemag@aol.com
                          www.choicemagazinelistening.org

Pamela Loeser, Editor in Chief
Ann Schlegel-Kyrkostas, Associate Editor
David Graham Pade, Associate Editor
A free audio anthology is available bi-monthly to visually impaired/physically disabled or dislexic persons nationwide. Playable on the special free 4-track cassette playback equipment which is provided by the Library of Congress through the National Library Service. Each issue features eight hours of unabridged magazine articles, short stories, poetry and media selections from over 100 sources. College level and older. Bimonthly distribution.
Bi-Monthly

9168 Heart to Heart
Blind Children's Center
4120 Marathon St
Los Angeles, CA 90029-3584   323-664-2153
                          info@blindchildrenscenter.org
                          www.blindchildrenscenter.org

Nancy Chernus-Mansfield, Co-Author
Dori Hayashi, Co-Author
Parents of blind and partially sighted children talk about their feelings. *$35.00*
VHS/DVD

9169 Juggler
Beacon Press
24 Farnsworth Street
Boston, MA 02210   617-742-2110
                                 Fax: 617-723-3097
                                       beacon.org

Helene Atwan, Executive Director
Andre was the young son of a wealthy, early Quebec fur trader. Because he was almost totally blind, he was overly protected by his family, and his movement outside his home was very limited.
Film

9170 Let's Eat Video
Blind Children's Center
4120 Marathon Street
Los Angeles, CA 90029-3584   323-664-2153
                          info@blindchildrenscenter.org
                             blindchildrenscenter.org

Jill Brody, Co-Author
Lynne Webber, Co-Author
Babies and toddlers with visual impairments lack one major avenue of exploration, and this significantly infulences their awareness, perceptions, and anticipation of the food which is presented to them. *$35.00*
VHS/DVD

9171 Look Out for Annie
Lighthouse Guild
250 West 64th Street
New York, NY 10023   800-284-4422
                               www.lighthouseguild.org

Calvin W. Roberts, President & CEO
James M. Dubin, Chairman
Lawrence E. Goldschmidt, Vice Chairman & Treasurer
Depicts an older woman coping with her vision loss. It focuses on the emotional issues surrounding vision loss and conveys the idea that both the person with the vision disorder and their family and friends will need to make adjustments. *$25.00*
Video

9172 Not Without Sight
American Foundation for the Blind/AFB Press
PO Box 1020
Sewickley, PA 15143-920   412-741-1142
                                        800-232-3044
                                     Fax: 412-741-0609
                                          www.afb.org
Carl R Augusto, President/CEO
Tracy Charlovich, Css
This video describes the major types of visual impairment and
their causes and effects on vision, while camera simulations ap-
proximate what people with each impairment actually see. Also
demonstrates how people with low vision make the best use of the
vision they have. 20 minute video tape, $49.95. *$42.95*
VHS 17 min
ISBN 0-891282-27-3

9173 Out of Left Field
American Foundation for the Blind/AFB Press
2 Penn Plaza
Suite 1102
New York, NY 10121   212-502-7600
                                        800-232-5463
                                     Fax: 888-545-8331
                                       afbinfo@afb.net
                                            afb.org
Carl R. Augusto, President & Chief Executive Officer
Rick Bozeman, Chief Financial Officer
Kelly Bleach, Chief Administrative Officer
Illustrates how youngsters who are blind or visually impaired in-
tegrated with their sighted peers in a variety of recreational and
athletic activities. 17 minute video tape. Also available in PAL,
$33.95, 0-89128-270-X. *$29.95*
VHS 17 minutes
ISBN 0-891282-28-0

9174 See What I'm Saying
Fanlight Productions
c/o Icarus Films
32 Court Street, 21st Floor
Brooklyn, NY 11201   718-488-8900
                                        800-876-1710
                                     Fax: 718-488-8642
                                       info@fanlight.com
                                         www.fanlight.com
Ben Achtenberg, Founder, Owner
The documentary follows Patricia, who is deaf and from a Span-
ish-speaking family, through her first year at the Kendall Demonstration Elementary School of Gallaudet University.
VHS/DVD

9175 See for Yourself
Lighthouse Guild
250 West 64th Street
New York, NY 10023   800-284-4422
                                     www.lighthouseguild.org
Calvin W. Roberts, President & CEO
James M. Dubin, Chairman
Lawrence E. Goldschmidt, Vice Chairman & Treasurer
This video features older adults with impaired vision who have
been helped by vision rehabilitation. *$50.00*

9176 Shape Up 'n Sign
Harris Communications
15155 Technology Dr
Eden Prairie, MN 55344-2273   952-906-1180
                                        800-825-6758
                                     Fax: 952-906-1099
                                       info@harriscomm.com
Robert Harris, Owner
An aerobic exercise tape introducing the basic sign language for
deaf and hearing children ages six to ten. *$29.95*
30 Minutes DVD

9177 Sight by Touch
Landmark Media
3450 Slade Run Drive
Falls Church, VA 22042   703-241-2030
                                        800-342-4336
                                     Fax: 703-536-9540
                                   info@landmarkmedia.com
Michael Hartogs, President
Peter Hartogs, VP New Business & Development
Beverly Weisenberg, Sales Rep
This video features the life and importance of Louis Braille. Vi-
sion-impaired performers and teachers demonstrate how Braille
has benefitted their lives, and how improvements are constantly
being made. *$195.00*
Video

9178 Taping for the Blind
3935 Essex Lane
Houston, TX 77027   713-622-2767
                                     Fax: 713-622-2772
                                          www.afb.org
Carl R. Augusto, President & Chief Executive Officer
Rick Bozeman, Chief Financial Officer
Robin Vogel, VP, Resource Development
An independent non profit educational organization funded by
corporations, listeners and individuals, with a mission to turn
sight into sound, enriching the lives of individuals with visual,
physical and learning disabilities. Founded in 1967 to read materials not availiable through other sources onto standard audio cassettes in our custom recording division. In 1978, Houston Taping
fFor The Blind signed on the air. Reading several dozen popular
magazines and best selling books on the air.

9179 We Can Do it Together!
American Foundation for the Blind/AFB Press
2 Penn Plaza
Suite 1102
New York, NY 10121   212-502-7600
                                        800-232-5463
                                     Fax: 888-545-8331
                                       afbinfo@afb.net
                                            afb.org
Carl R. Augusto, President & Chief Executive Officer
Rick Bozeman, Chief Financial Officer
Kelly Bleach, Chief Administrative Officer
This video illustrates a transdisciplinary team orientation and
mobility program for students with severe visual and multiple im-
pairments, covering both adapted communication systems used
to teach mobility skills and basic indoor mobility in the school.
For mobility instructors, administrators, teachers of the visually
and severely handicapped, occupational, physical and speech
therapists and parents. Discussion guide included. 10 minute
video tape. Also available in PAL, $33.95, 0-89128-267-X.
$26.95
VHS
ISBN 0-891282-13-0

Sports

9180 American Blind Bowling Association
1209 Somerset Road
Raleigh, NC 27610   919-755-0700
                                        www.abba1951.org
Thomas Lester, President
A.J. Inglesby, 1st Vice President
James Benton, 2nd Vice President
Promotes blind bowling throughout the US and Canada by sanc-
tioning blind bowling leagues and conducting a National Tourna-
ment. Current membership exceeds 2,000 people in the United
States and Canada.

9181 Basketball: Beeping Foam
Maxi Aids
42 Executive Blvd.
Farmingdale, NY 11735-4710   631-752-0521
800-522-6294
Fax: 631-752-0689
TTY: 631-752-0738
sales@maxiaids.com
www.maxiaids.com

Elliot Zaretsky, Founder, President & CEO
This sound-making basketball enables the visually impaired to play basketball and other games. *$36.95*

9182 Blind Outdoor Leisure Development
P.O.Box 6639
Snowmass Village, CO 81615   970-923-0578
Fax: 970-923-7338
challengeaspen.org

Jimmy Yeager, President
Jack Kennedy, VP
Grayson Stover, Secretary
Outdoor recreation for the blind. Winter program of skiing with guides plus numerous summer programs for the visually impaired.

9183 Challenge Golf
otivation Media
1245 Milwaukee Ave
Glenview, IL 60025-2400   847-827-9057
Fax: 847-297-6829

Dorothy Bauer, Coordinator
A plain-language video, Challenge Golf is packed with information for beginners or veterans. Peter Longo covers 5 handicaps (one-arm, one-leg, in a seated position, blind, and arthritis) clearly and concisely, on how to play golf with a physical disability. In color, complete with special effects, graphs and real handicapped golfers at play. *$38.95*
Home Edition

9184 US Association of Blind Athletes
1 Olympic Plaza
Colorado Springs, CO 80909   719-630-0422
Fax: 719-630-0616
www.usaba.org

Mark A. Lucas, MS, Executive Director
Ryan Ortiz, Assistant Executive Director
John Potts, Goalball High Performance director
Provides athletic opportunities and training in competitive sports for visually impaired and blind individuals throughout the US Competitions indlcude local, regional and national events, internation events, and the Winter and Summer Paralympic Games.

9185 United States Blind Golf Association
3094 Shamrock St N
Tallahassee, FL 32309-2735   520-648-1088
info@usblindgolf.com
www.blindgolf.com

Dick Pomo, President
Provides blind and vision impaired gold tournaments to members.

Support Groups

9186 Braille Institute Orange County Center
527 North Dale Avenue
Anaheim, CA 92801   714-821-5000
800-272-4553
Fax: 714-527-7621
oc@brailleinstitute.org
brailleinstitute.org

Lester M. Sussman, Chairman
Peter A. Mindnich, President
Jon K. Hayashida, OD, FAAO, Vice President, Programs & Services
Offers services, publications, information and programs free of charge to blind and visually impaired persons of all ages.

9187 Consumer and Patient Information Hotline
Prevent Blindness America
211 West Wacker Drive
Suite 1700
Chicago, IL 60606   800-331-2020
info@preventblindness.org
www.preventblindness.org/

Paul G. Howes, Chairman
Hugh R. Parry, President & CEO,Prevent Blindness America
Jerome Desserich, Vice President & Chief Financial Officer
A toll-free line offering free information on a broad range of vision, eye health and safety topics including sports eye safety, diabetic retinopathy, glaucoma, cataracts, children's eye disorders and more.

9188 Department of Ophthalmology Information Line
Eye & Ear Infirmary
1855 W Taylor St
Chicago, IL 60612-7242   312-996-6590
Fax: 312-996-7770
eyeweb@uic.edu
www.uic.edu

Jospeh White, President
Offers eye clinic and physician referrals to persons suffering from vision disorders as well as offers emergency information.

9189 Lighthouse International Information and Resource Service
111 East 59th Street
New York, NY 10022-1202   212-821-9384
800-829-0500
Fax: 212-821-9707
info@lighthouse.org
lighthouse.org

Mark G. Ackermann, President / CEO
Provides information about eye diseases, low vision, age-related vision loss, adaptive technology, optical devices, large print and braille publishers, helps people find low vision services, vision rehabilitation services, and support groups across the U.S.; offers large selection of consumer products.

9190 National Association for Parents of Children with Visual Impairments (NAPVI)
1 North Lexington Avenue
White Plains, NY 10601   617-972-7441
800-562-6265
Fax: 617-972-7444
napvi@guildhealth.org
www.napvi.org

Julie Urban, President
Venetia Hayden, Vice President
Susan LaVenture, Executive Director
In 1979, a group of parents responding to their own needs founded NAPVI, the National Association for Parents of the Visually Impaired, Inc. Never before was there a self-help organization specific to the needs of families of children with visual impairments. Since that time, NAPVI has grown and helped families across the US and in other countries.

9191 VUE: Vision Use in Employment
Carroll Center for the Blind
770 Centre Street
Newton, MA 02458-2597   617-969-6200
800-852-3131
Fax: 617-969-6204
www.carroll.org

Joseph Abely, President
Brian Charlson, Director of Technology
Diane M. Newark, Chief Development Officer
Provides engineering solutions plus training to help people keep jobs despite their vision loss.

9192   **Washington Connection**
American Council of the Blind
1703 N. Beauregard St
Ste 420
Alexandria, VA 22311   202-467-5081
                                                   800-424-8666
                                             Fax: 703-465-5085
                                                   info@acb.org
                                                   www.acb.org/wc

Kim Charlson, President
Jeff Thom, 1st Vice President
Eric Bridges, Executive Director
Coverage of issues affecting blind people via legislative information, participates in law-making, legislative training seminars and networking of support resources across the US.

2020 Annual Disability Statistics Compendium

List of Tables

Table 1.1 Resident Population – States: 2017 to 2020

Geography	2017	2018	2019	2020 [1]
U.S.	320,842,721	327,167,439	328,239,523	329,504,815
AL	4,796,532	4,887,871	4,903,185	4,922,663
AK	716,592	737,438	731,545	725,368
AZ	6,908,516	7,171,646	7,278,717	7,439,168
AR	2,949,813	3,013,825	3,017,804	3,020,858
CA	39,052,156	39,557,045	39,512,223	39,273,649
CO	5,516,225	5,695,564	5,758,736	5,801,720
CT	3,537,144	3,572,665	3,565,287	3,561,894
DE	947,351	967,171	973,764	986,302
DC	684,065	702,455	705,749	708,536
FL	20,683,330	21,299,325	21,477,737	21,777,656
GA	10,246,239	10,519,475	10,617,423	10,735,354
HI	1,370,850	1,420,491	1,415,872	1,408,226
ID	1,696,598	1,754,208	1,787,065	1,845,631
IL	12,625,584	12,741,080	12,671,821	12,559,183
IN	6,568,754	6,691,878	6,732,219	6,755,447
IA	3,103,193	3,156,145	3,155,070	3,167,157
KS	2,856,162	2,911,510	2,913,314	2,917,100
KY	4,372,996	4,468,402	4,467,673	4,477,027
LA	4,580,488	4,659,978	4,648,794	4,636,548
ME	1,322,156	1,338,404	1,344,212	1,333,280
MD	6,786,014	6,042,718	6,045,680	6,039,168
MA	6,006,403	6,902,197	6,892,503	6,893,349
MI	9,853,848	9,995,915	9,986,857	10,005,488
MN	5,520,151	5,611,179	5,639,632	5,637,415
MS	2,922,300	2,986,530	2,976,149	2,949,108
MO	5,959,960	6,126,452	6,137,428	6,160,572
MT	1,036,512	1,062,305	1,068,778	1,070,633
NE	1,892,212	1,929,268	1,934,408	1,910,229
NV	2,961,838	3,034,392	3,080,156	3,159,862
NH	1,325,207	1,356,410	1,359,711	1,369,826
NJ	8,903,054	8,908,520	8,882,190	8,866,369
NM	2,054,508	2,095,428	2,096,829	2,103,947
NY	19,608,509	19,542,209	19,453,561	19,342,277
NC	10,071,642	10,383,620	10,488,084	10,634,814
ND	738,859	760,077	762,062	762,179
OH	11,485,462	11,689,442	11,689,100	11,696,589
OK	3,851,546	3,943,079	3,956,971	4,004,290
OR	4,103,141	4,190,713	4,217,737	4,235,391
PA	12,602,223	12,807,060	12,801,989	12,808,018
RI	1,044,426	1,057,315	1,059,361	1,064,254
SC	4,933,516	5,084,127	5,148,714	5,215,144
SD	852,604	882,235	884,659	904,399
TN	6,614,699	6,770,010	6,829,174	6,909,363
TX	27,844,511	28,701,845	28,995,881	29,354,409
UT	3,076,547	3,161,105	3,205,958	3,264,928
VT	617,936	626,299	623,989	624,318
VA	8,257,571	8,517,685	8,535,519	8,565,201
WA	7,301,382	7,535,591	7,614,893	7,697,393
WV	1,787,062	1,805,832	1,792,147	1,790,562
WI	5,725,670	5,813,568	5,822,434	5,838,186
WY	568,664	577,737	578,759	574,367

Citation: Paul, S., Rafal, M., & Houtenville, A. (2021). Annual Disability Statistics Compendium: 2021 (Table 1.1). Durham, NH: University of New Hampshire, Institute on Disability. Note: Authors' calculations using the U.S. Census Bureau, American Community Survey, Public Use Microdata Sample, 2017-2020, which is subject to sampling variation.
[1] The U.S. Census Bureau recommends to exercise caution when comparing 2020 estimates from the American Community Survey with prior years. See introduction for more details.

Table 1.2 State Resident Population – Projections: 2015 to 2030

State	2015	2020	2025	2030
U.S.	322,365,787	335,804,546	349,439,199	363,584,435
AL	4,663,111	4,728,915	4,800,092	4,874,243
AK	732,544	774,421	820,881	867,674
AZ	7,495,238	8,456,448	9,531,537	10,712,397
AR	2,968,913	3,060,219	3,151,005	3,240,208
CA	40,123,232	42,206,743	44,305,177	46,444,861
CO	5,049,493	5,278,867	5,522,803	5,792,357
CT	3,635,414	3,675,650	3,691,016	3,688,630
DE	927,400	963,209	990,694	1,012,658
DC	506,323	480,540	455,108	433,414
FL	21,204,132	23,406,525	25,912,458	28,685,769
GA	10,230,578	10,843,753	11,438,622	12,017,838
HI	1,385,952	1,412,373	1,438,720	1,466,046
ID	1,630,045	1,741,333	1,852,627	1,969,624
IL	13,097,218	13,236,720	13,340,507	13,432,892
IN	6,517,631	6,627,008	6,721,322	6,810,108
IA	3,026,380	3,020,496	2,993,222	2,955,172
KS	2,852,690	2,890,566	2,919,002	2,940,084
KY	4,351,188	4,424,431	4,489,662	4,554,998
LA	4,673,721	4,719,160	4,762,398	4,802,633
ME	1,388,878	1,408,665	1,414,402	1,411,097
MD	6,208,392	6,497,626	6,762,732	7,022,251
MA	6,758,580	6,855,546	6,938,636	7,012,009
MI	10,599,122	10,695,993	10,713,730	10,694,172
MN	5,668,211	5,900,769	6,108,787	6,306,130
MS	3,014,409	3,044,812	3,069,420	3,092,410
MO	6,069,556	6,199,882	6,315,366	6,430,173
MT	999,489	1,022,735	1,037,387	1,044,898
NE	1,788,508	1,802,678	1,812,787	1,820,247
NV	3,058,190	3,452,283	3,863,298	4,282,102
NH	1,456,679	1,524,751	1,586,348	1,646,471
NJ	9,255,769	9,461,635	9,636,644	9,802,440
NM	2,041,539	2,084,341	2,106,584	2,099,708
NY	19,546,699	19,576,920	19,540,179	19,477,429
NC	10,010,770	10,709,289	11,449,153	12,227,739
ND	635,133	630,112	620,777	606,566
OH	11,635,446	11,644,058	11,605,738	11,550,528
OK	3,661,694	3,735,690	3,820,994	3,913,251
OR	4,012,924	4,260,393	4,536,418	4,833,918
PA	12,710,938	12,787,354	12,801,945	12,768,184
RI	1,139,543	1,154,230	1,157,855	1,152,941
SC	4,642,137	4,822,577	4,989,550	5,148,569
SD	796,954	801,939	801,845	800,462
TN	6,502,017	6,780,670	7,073,125	7,380,634
TX	26,585,801	28,634,896	30,865,134	33,317,744
UT	2,783,040	2,990,094	3,225,680	3,485,367
VT	673,169	690,686	703,288	711,867
VA	8,466,864	8,917,395	9,364,304	9,825,019
WA	6,950,610	7,432,136	7,996,400	8,624,801
WV	1,822,758	1,801,112	1,766,435	1,719,959
WI	5,882,760	6,004,954	6,088,374	6,150,764
WY	528,005	530,948	529,031	522,979

Citation: Paul, S., Rafal, M., & Houtenville, A. (2021). Annual Disability Statistics Compendium: 2021 (Table 1.2). Durham, NH: University of New Hampshire, Institute on Disability. Note: Sourced from the U.S. Census Bureau, 2005, Interim State Population Projections, Table 6, which is subject to sampling variation.

Table 1.3 Civilians Living in the Community for the United States and States, by Disability Status: 2020

State	Total	Disability [1] Count	%	No Disability Count	%
U.S.	328,293,917	44,061,818	13.4	284,232,099	86.6
AL	4,908,912	828,999	16.9	4,079,913	83.1
AK	703,146	85,876	12.2	617,270	87.8
AZ	7,420,020	1,028,797	13.9	6,391,223	86.1
AR	3,014,116	578,536	19.2	2,435,580	80.8
CA	39,123,202	4,409,276	11.3	34,713,926	88.7
CO	5,764,939	644,775	11.2	5,120,164	88.8
CT	3,555,183	435,857	12.3	3,119,326	87.7
DE	982,331	145,696	14.8	836,635	85.2
DC	706,629	74,492	10.5	632,137	89.5
FL	21,695,068	3,085,765	14.2	18,609,303	85.8
GA	10,671,030	1,440,292	13.5	9,230,738	86.5
HI	1,365,210	164,933	12.1	1,200,277	87.9
ID	1,841,020	266,684	14.5	1,574,336	85.5
IL	12,541,886	1,530,941	12.2	11,010,945	87.8
IN	6,753,016	985,158	14.6	5,767,858	85.4
IA	3,164,622	412,569	13.0	2,752,053	87.0
KS	2,898,795	408,313	14.1	2,490,482	85.9
KY	4,462,819	820,799	18.4	3,642,020	81.6
LA	4,615,615	761,512	16.5	3,854,103	83.5
ME	1,332,120	218,850	16.4	1,113,270	83.6
MD	6,005,118	694,317	11.6	5,310,801	88.4
MA	6,887,330	858,405	12.5	6,028,925	87.5
MI	10,001,947	1,468,729	14.7	8,533,218	85.3
MN	5,634,769	650,592	11.5	4,984,177	88.5
MS	2,934,741	523,114	17.8	2,411,627	82.2
MO	6,143,005	901,112	14.7	5,241,893	85.3
MT	1,066,483	158,996	14.9	907,487	85.1
NE	1,905,612	218,665	11.5	1,686,947	88.5
NV	3,145,192	422,943	13.4	2,722,249	86.6
NH	1,367,525	183,112	13.4	1,184,413	86.6
NJ	8,852,661	999,280	11.3	7,853,381	88.7
NM	2,090,104	357,004	17.1	1,733,100	82.9
NY	19,324,301	2,370,697	12.3	16,953,604	87.7
NC	10,533,083	1,487,892	14.1	9,045,191	85.9
ND	756,157	83,908	11.1	672,249	88.9
OH	11,687,765	1,752,373	15.0	9,935,392	85.0
OK	3,985,175	711,189	17.8	3,273,986	82.2
OR	4,232,126	637,697	15.1	3,594,429	84.9
PA	12,799,353	1,856,929	14.5	10,942,424	85.5
RI	1,059,413	158,237	14.9	901,176	85.1
SC	5,179,851	789,480	15.2	4,390,371	84.8
SD	901,635	108,967	12.1	792,668	87.9
TN	6,891,933	1,110,307	16.1	5,781,626	83.9
TX	29,247,594	3,573,362	12.2	25,674,232	87.8
UT	3,258,478	342,360	10.5	2,916,118	89.5
VT	623,385	84,485	13.6	538,900	86.4
VA	8,430,315	1,061,601	12.6	7,368,714	87.4
WA	7,635,653	1,035,051	13.6	6,600,602	86.4
WV	1,787,384	349,832	19.6	1,437,552	80.4
WI	5,834,849	704,481	12.1	5,130,368	87.9
WY	571,301	78,581	13.8	492,720	86.2

Citation: Paul, S., Rafal, M., & Houtenville, A. (2021). Annual Disability Statistics Compendium: 2021 (Table 1.3). Durham, NH: University of New Hampshire, Institute on Disability. Note: Authors' calculations using the U.S. Census Bureau American Community Survey, Public Use Microdata Sample with Experimental Weights, 2020, which is subject to sampling variation.
[1] The U.S. Census uses a series of six questions to identify persons with vision, hearing, cognitive, ambulatory, self-care, and independent living disabilities. The cognitive, ambulatory, self-care, and independent living related questions are not asked of individuals less than five years old and the independent living related question is not asked of individuals less than 15 years old. See glossary for more information.

Table 1.4 Civilians Living in the Community for the United States and States – Hearing Disability: 2020

State	Total	Disability	Hearing [1] Count	Hearing [1] % Total	Hearing [1] % Disability
U.S.	328,293,917	44,061,818	11,926,360	3.6	27.1
AL	4,908,912	828,999	220,753	4.5	26.6
AK	703,146	85,876	32,646	4.6	38.0
AZ	7,420,020	1,828,797	311,570	4.2	30.3
AR	3,014,116	578,536	147,166	4.9	25.4
CA	39,123,202	4,409,276	1,146,710	2.9	26.0
CO	5,764,939	644,775	209,961	3.6	32.6
CT	3,555,183	435,857	112,099	3.2	25.7
DE	982,331	145,696	31,986	3.3	22.0
DC	706,629	74,492	10,935	1.5	14.7
FL	21,695,068	3,085,765	824,531	3.8	26.7
GA	10,671,030	1,440,292	353,073	3.3	24.5
HI	1,365,210	164,933	49,850	3.7	30.2
ID	1,841,020	266,684	83,534	4.5	31.3
IL	12,541,886	1,530,941	401,173	3.2	26.2
IN	6,753,016	985,158	274,955	4.1	27.9
IA	3,164,622	412,569	127,400	4.0	30.9
KS	2,898,795	408,313	124,183	4.3	30.4
KY	4,462,819	820,799	213,786	4.8	26.0
LA	4,615,615	761,512	185,499	4.0	24.4
ME	1,332,120	218,850	66,153	5.0	30.2
MD	6,005,118	694,317	166,905	2.8	24.0
MA	6,887,330	858,405	221,054	3.2	25.8
MI	10,001,947	1,468,729	385,228	3.9	26.2
MN	5,634,769	650,592	200,985	3.6	30.9
MS	2,934,741	523,114	129,243	4.4	24.7
MO	6,143,005	901,112	256,565	4.2	28.5
MT	1,066,483	158,996	57,364	5.4	36.1
NE	1,905,612	218,665	74,595	3.9	34.1
NV	3,145,192	422,943	127,104	4.0	30.1
NH	1,367,525	183,112	58,127	4.3	31.7
NJ	8,852,661	999,280	245,532	2.8	24.6
NM	2,090,104	357,004	109,889	5.3	30.8
NY	19,324,301	2,370,697	540,207	2.8	22.8
NC	10,533,083	1,487,892	402,210	3.8	27.0
ND	756,157	83,908	28,918	3.8	34.5
OH	11,687,765	1,752,373	460,012	3.9	26.3
OK	3,985,175	711,189	228,019	5.7	32.1
OR	4,232,126	637,697	190,384	4.5	29.9
PA	12,799,353	1,856,929	489,122	3.8	26.3
RI	1,059,413	158,237	43,033	4.1	27.2
SC	5,179,851	789,480	219,772	4.2	27.8
SD	901,635	108,967	32,642	3.6	30.0
TN	6,891,933	1,110,307	308,734	4.5	27.8
TX	29,247,594	3,573,362	956,480	3.3	26.8
UT	3,258,478	342,360	97,290	3.0	28.4
VT	623,385	84,485	28,117	4.5	33.3
VA	8,430,315	1,061,601	298,942	3.5	28.2
WA	7,635,653	1,035,051	301,416	3.9	29.1
WV	1,787,384	349,832	106,735	6.0	30.5
WI	5,834,849	704,481	205,742	3.5	29.2
WY	571,301	78,581	28,031	4.9	35.7

Citation: Paul, S., Rafal, M., & Houtenville, A. (2021). Annual Disability Statistics Compendium: 2021 (Table 1.4). Durham, NH: University of New Hampshire, Institute on Disability. Note: Authors' calculations using the U.S. Census Bureau American Community Survey, Public Use Microdata Sample with Experimental Weights, 2020, which is subject to sampling variation.
[1] The hearing disability question asks people of all ages, "Is this person deaf or does he/she have serious difficulty hearing?" See glossary for more information.

Table 1.5 Civilians Living in the Community for the United States and States – Vision Disability: 2020

State	Total	Disability	Vision [1] Count	Vision [1] % Total	Vision [1] % Disability
U.S.	328,293,917	44,061,818	8,032,555	2.4	18.2
AL	4,908,912	828,999	151,483	3.1	18.3
AK	703,146	85,876	17,125	2.4	19.9
AZ	7,420,020	1,028,797	199,050	2.7	19.3
AR	3,014,116	578,536	113,939	3.8	19.7
CA	39,123,202	4,409,276	815,164	2.1	18.5
CO	5,764,939	644,775	117,504	2.0	18.2
CT	3,555,183	435,857	72,627	2.0	16.7
DE	982,331	145,696	21,474	2.2	14.7
DC	706,629	74,492	13,357	1.9	17.9
FL	21,695,068	3,085,765	579,706	2.7	18.8
GA	10,671,030	1,440,292	267,049	2.5	18.5
HI	1,365,210	164,933	28,030	2.1	17.0
ID	1,841,020	266,684	43,005	2.3	16.1
IL	12,541,886	1,530,941	273,621	2.2	17.9
IN	6,753,016	985,158	166,421	2.5	16.9
IA	3,164,622	412,569	60,573	1.9	14.7
KS	2,898,795	408,313	72,271	2.5	17.7
KY	4,462,819	820,799	160,559	3.6	19.6
LA	4,615,615	761,512	176,501	3.8	23.2
ME	1,332,120	218,850	29,672	2.2	13.6
MD	6,005,118	694,317	110,879	1.8	16.0
MA	6,887,330	858,405	127,524	1.9	14.9
MI	10,001,947	1,468,729	226,334	2.3	15.4
MN	5,634,769	650,592	86,472	1.5	13.3
MS	2,934,741	523,114	112,774	3.8	21.6
MO	6,143,005	901,112	159,576	2.6	17.7
MT	1,066,483	158,996	27,902	2.6	17.5
NE	1,905,612	218,665	35,606	1.9	16.3
NV	3,145,192	422,943	80,566	2.6	19.0
NH	1,367,525	183,112	28,959	2.1	15.8
NJ	8,852,661	999,280	188,166	2.1	18.8
NM	2,090,104	357,004	81,008	3.9	22.7
NY	19,324,301	2,370,697	400,048	2.1	16.9
NC	10,533,083	1,487,892	277,591	2.6	18.7
ND	756,157	83,908	14,001	1.9	16.7
OH	11,687,765	1,752,373	288,995	2.5	16.5
OK	3,985,175	711,189	149,202	3.7	21.0
OR	4,232,126	637,697	100,770	2.4	15.8
PA	12,799,353	1,856,929	308,195	2.4	16.6
RI	1,059,413	158,237	24,913	2.4	15.7
SC	5,179,851	789,480	165,258	3.2	20.9
SD	901,635	108,967	17,136	1.9	15.7
TN	6,891,933	1,110,307	233,660	3.4	21.0
TX	29,247,594	3,573,362	762,228	2.6	21.3
UT	3,258,478	342,360	61,382	1.9	17.9
VT	623,385	84,485	12,485	2.0	14.8
VA	8,430,315	1,061,601	195,034	2.3	18.4
WA	7,635,653	1,035,051	184,918	2.4	17.9
WV	1,787,384	349,832	65,028	3.6	18.6
WI	5,834,849	704,481	113,580	1.9	16.1
WY	571,301	78,581	13,234	2.3	16.8

Citation: Paul, S., Rafal, M., & Houtenville, A. (2021). Annual Disability Statistics Compendium: 2021 (Table 1.5). Durham, NH: University of New Hampshire, Institute on Disability. Note: Authors' calculations using the U.S. Census Bureau American Community Survey, Public Use Microdata Sample with Experimental Weights, 2020, which is subject to sampling variation.
[1] The vision disability question asks people of all ages, "Is this person blind or does he/she have serious difficulty seeing even when wearing glasses?" See glossary for more information.

Table 1.6 Civilians Living in the Community for the United States and States – Cognitive Disability: 2020

State	Total	Disability Count	Cognitive [1] Count	Cognitive [1] % Total	Cognitive [1] % Disability
U.S.	328,293,917	44,061,818	17,472,328	5.3	39.7
AL	4,908,912	828,999	332,659	6.8	40.1
AK	703,146	85,876	30,476	4.3	35.5
AZ	7,420,020	1,028,797	381,966	5.1	37.1
AR	3,014,116	578,536	235,288	7.8	40.7
CA	39,123,202	4,409,276	1,712,586	4.4	38.8
CO	5,764,939	644,775	262,993	4.6	40.8
CT	3,555,183	435,857	181,946	5.1	41.7
DE	982,331	145,696	59,440	6.1	40.8
DC	706,629	74,492	37,545	5.3	50.4
FL	21,695,068	3,085,765	1,189,899	5.5	38.6
GA	10,671,030	1,440,292	602,424	5.6	41.8
HI	1,365,210	164,933	66,432	4.9	40.3
ID	1,841,020	266,684	103,197	5.6	38.7
IL	12,541,886	1,530,941	594,723	4.7	38.8
IN	6,753,016	985,158	410,825	6.1	41.7
IA	3,164,622	412,569	158,449	5.0	38.4
KS	2,898,795	408,313	167,373	5.8	41.0
KY	4,462,819	820,799	329,349	7.4	40.1
LA	4,615,615	761,512	307,858	6.7	40.4
ME	1,332,120	218,850	98,865	7.4	45.2
MD	6,005,118	694,317	274,188	4.6	39.5
MA	6,887,330	858,405	381,434	5.5	44.4
MI	10,001,947	1,468,729	605,393	6.1	41.2
MN	5,634,769	650,592	280,348	5.0	43.1
MS	2,934,741	523,114	207,001	7.1	39.6
MO	6,143,005	901,112	352,778	5.7	39.1
MT	1,066,483	158,996	59,084	5.5	37.2
NE	1,905,612	218,665	78,418	4.1	35.9
NV	3,145,192	422,943	145,288	4.6	34.4
NH	1,367,525	183,112	74,488	5.4	40.7
NJ	8,852,661	999,280	370,585	4.2	37.1
NM	2,090,104	357,004	137,904	6.6	38.6
NY	19,324,301	2,370,697	945,681	4.9	39.9
NC	10,533,083	1,487,892	591,176	5.6	39.7
ND	756,157	83,908	32,609	4.3	38.9
OH	11,687,765	1,752,373	704,666	6.0	40.2
OK	3,985,175	711,189	268,792	6.7	37.8
OR	4,232,126	637,697	273,021	6.5	42.8
PA	12,799,353	1,856,929	752,904	5.9	40.5
RI	1,059,413	158,237	68,828	6.5	43.5
SC	5,179,851	789,480	287,649	5.6	36.4
SD	901,635	108,967	36,263	4.0	33.3
TN	6,891,933	1,110,307	433,984	6.3	39.1
TX	29,247,594	3,573,362	1,398,229	4.8	39.1
UT	3,258,478	342,360	145,785	4.5	42.6
VT	623,385	84,485	37,463	6.0	44.3
VA	8,430,315	1,061,601	414,962	4.9	39.1
WA	7,635,653	1,035,051	428,414	5.6	41.4
WV	1,787,384	349,832	133,387	7.5	38.1
WI	5,834,849	704,481	262,593	4.5	37.3
WY	571,301	78,581	24,720	4.3	31.5

Citation: Paul, S., Rafal, M., & Houtenville, A. (2021). Annual Disability Statistics Compendium: 2021 (Table 1.6). Durham, NH: University of New Hampshire, Institute on Disability. Note: Authors' calculations using the U.S. Census Bureau American Community Survey, Public Use Microdata Sample with Experimental Weights, 2020, which is subject to sampling variation.
[1] The cognitive disability question asks people 5 years and older "Because of a physical, mental, or emotional condition, does this person have serious difficulty concentrating, remembering, or making decisions?" See glossary for more information.

Table 1.7 Civilians Living in the Community for the United States and States – Ambulatory Disability: 2020

State	Total	Disability	Ambulatory [1] Count	% Total	% Disability
U.S.	328,293,917	44,061,818	21,779,183	6.6	49.4
AL	4,908,912	828,999	431,880	8.8	52.1
AK	703,146	85,876	33,954	4.8	39.5
AZ	7,420,020	1,028,797	496,304	6.7	48.2
AR	3,014,116	578,536	315,908	10.5	54.6
CA	39,123,202	4,409,276	2,189,487	5.6	49.7
CO	5,764,939	644,775	275,548	4.8	42.7
CT	3,555,183	435,857	211,634	6.0	48.6
DE	982,331	145,696	73,705	7.5	50.6
DC	706,629	74,492	35,641	5.0	47.8
FL	21,695,068	3,085,765	1,573,331	7.3	51.0
GA	10,671,030	1,440,292	717,521	6.7	49.8
HI	1,365,210	164,933	83,464	6.1	50.6
ID	1,841,020	266,684	125,525	6.8	47.1
IL	12,541,886	1,530,941	765,685	6.1	50.0
IN	6,753,016	985,158	483,538	7.2	49.1
IA	3,164,622	412,569	187,005	5.9	45.3
KS	2,898,795	408,313	194,694	6.7	47.7
KY	4,462,819	820,799	419,237	9.4	51.1
LA	4,615,615	761,512	386,483	8.4	50.8
ME	1,332,120	218,850	97,164	7.3	44.4
MD	6,005,118	694,317	347,058	5.8	50.0
MA	6,887,330	858,405	399,187	5.8	46.5
MI	10,001,947	1,468,729	725,063	7.2	49.4
MN	5,634,769	650,592	288,674	5.1	44.4
MS	2,934,741	523,114	285,221	9.7	54.5
MO	6,143,005	901,112	452,385	7.4	50.2
MT	1,066,483	158,996	70,707	6.6	44.5
NE	1,905,612	218,665	103,043	5.4	47.1
NV	3,145,192	422,943	217,033	6.9	51.3
NH	1,367,525	183,112	84,440	6.2	46.1
NJ	8,852,661	999,280	509,600	5.8	51.0
NM	2,090,104	357,004	176,199	8.4	49.4
NY	19,324,301	2,370,697	1,256,967	6.5	53.0
NC	10,533,083	1,487,892	757,204	7.2	50.9
ND	756,157	83,908	35,040	4.6	41.8
OH	11,687,765	1,752,373	864,433	7.4	49.3
OK	3,985,175	711,189	355,425	8.9	50.0
OR	4,232,126	637,697	286,807	6.8	45.0
PA	12,799,353	1,856,929	922,666	7.2	49.7
RI	1,059,413	158,237	72,218	6.8	45.6
SC	5,179,851	789,480	393,126	7.6	49.8
SD	901,635	108,967	50,389	5.6	46.2
TN	6,891,933	1,110,307	578,314	8.4	52.1
TX	29,247,594	3,573,362	1,733,569	5.9	48.5
UT	3,258,478	342,360	130,852	4.0	38.2
VT	623,385	84,485	36,707	5.9	43.4
VA	8,430,315	1,061,601	514,963	6.1	48.5
WA	7,635,653	1,035,051	468,255	6.1	45.2
WV	1,787,384	349,832	186,523	10.4	53.3
WI	5,834,849	704,481	344,251	5.9	48.9
WY	571,301	78,581	35,156	6.2	44.7

Citation: Paul, S., Rafal, M., & Houtenville, A. (2021). Annual Disability Statistics Compendium: 2021 (Table 1.7). Durham, NH: University of New Hampshire, Institute on Disability. Note: Authors' calculations using the U.S. Census Bureau American Community Survey, Public Use Microdata Sample with Experimental Weights, 2020, which is subject to sampling variation.
[1] The ambulatory disability question asks people 5 years old or older, "Does this person have serious difficulty walking or climbing stairs?" See glossary for more information.

875

Table 1.8 Civilians Living in the Community for the United States and States – Self-Care Disability: 2020

State	Total	Disability Count	Self-Care [1] Count	Self-Care [1] % Total	Self-Care [1] % Disability
U.S.	328,293,917	44,061,818	8,916,136	2.7	20.2
AL	4,908,912	828,999	157,901	3.2	19.0
AK	703,146	85,876	14,700	2.1	17.1
AZ	7,420,020	1,028,797	173,693	2.3	16.9
AR	3,014,116	578,536	113,560	3.8	19.6
CA	39,123,202	4,409,276	1,023,667	2.6	23.2
CO	5,764,939	644,775	104,946	1.8	16.3
CT	3,555,183	435,857	101,218	2.8	23.2
DE	982,331	145,696	27,585	2.8	18.9
DC	706,629	74,492	17,375	2.5	23.3
FL	21,695,068	3,085,765	594,272	2.7	19.3
GA	10,671,030	1,440,292	274,533	2.6	19.1
HI	1,365,210	164,933	35,120	2.6	21.3
ID	1,841,020	266,684	46,467	2.5	17.4
IL	12,541,886	1,530,941	323,243	2.6	21.1
IN	6,753,016	985,158	194,747	2.9	19.8
IA	3,164,622	412,569	82,235	2.6	19.9
KS	2,898,795	408,313	73,058	2.5	17.9
KY	4,462,819	820,799	159,039	3.6	19.4
LA	4,615,615	761,512	161,720	3.5	21.2
ME	1,332,120	218,850	38,551	2.9	17.6
MD	6,005,118	694,317	139,583	2.3	20.1
MA	6,887,330	858,405	185,966	2.7	21.7
MI	10,001,947	1,468,729	298,319	3.0	20.3
MN	5,634,769	650,592	141,241	2.5	21.7
MS	2,934,741	523,114	106,859	3.6	20.4
MO	6,143,005	901,112	189,833	3.1	21.1
MT	1,066,483	158,996	25,811	2.4	16.2
NE	1,905,612	218,665	39,766	2.1	18.2
NV	3,145,192	422,943	80,697	2.6	19.1
NH	1,367,525	183,112	37,918	2.8	20.7
NJ	8,852,661	999,280	226,571	2.6	22.7
NM	2,090,104	357,004	66,628	3.2	18.7
NY	19,324,301	2,370,697	557,025	2.9	23.5
NC	10,533,083	1,487,892	294,990	2.8	19.8
ND	756,157	83,908	15,044	2.0	17.9
OH	11,687,765	1,752,373	343,234	2.9	19.6
OK	3,985,175	711,189	126,095	3.2	17.7
OR	4,232,126	637,697	129,316	3.1	20.3
PA	12,799,353	1,856,929	382,485	3.0	20.6
RI	1,059,413	158,237	33,276	3.1	21.0
SC	5,179,851	789,480	153,432	3.0	19.4
SD	901,635	108,967	21,845	2.4	20.0
TN	6,891,933	1,110,307	210,263	3.1	18.9
TX	29,247,594	3,573,362	687,821	2.4	19.2
UT	3,258,478	342,360	51,436	1.6	15.0
VT	623,385	84,485	15,787	2.5	18.7
VA	8,430,315	1,061,601	212,003	2.5	20.0
WA	7,635,653	1,035,051	194,200	2.5	18.8
WV	1,787,384	349,832	69,286	3.9	19.8
WI	5,834,849	704,481	149,620	2.6	21.2
WY	571,301	78,581	12,156	2.1	15.5

Citation: Paul, S., Rafal, M., & Houtenville, A. (2021). Annual Disability Statistics Compendium: 2021 (Table 1.8). Durham, NH: University of New Hampshire, Institute on Disability. Note: Authors' calculations using the U.S. Census Bureau American Community Survey, Public Use Microdata Sample with Experimental Weights, 2020, which is subject to sampling variation.
[1] The self-care disability question asks people 5 years old or older, "Does this person have difficulty dressing or bathing?" See glossary for more information.

Table 1.9 Civilians Living in the Community for the United States and States – Independent Living Disability: 2020

State	Total	Disability	Independent Living [1] Count	% Total	% Disability
U.S.	328,293,917	44,061,818	16,356,212	5.0	37.1
AL	4,908,912	828,999	299,401	6.1	36.1
AK	703,146	85,876	25,111	3.6	29.2
AZ	7,420,020	1,028,797	356,287	4.8	34.6
AR	3,014,116	578,536	204,897	6.8	35.4
CA	39,123,202	4,409,276	1,816,893	4.6	41.2
CO	5,764,939	644,775	221,283	3.8	34.3
CT	3,555,183	435,857	177,196	5.0	40.7
DE	982,331	145,696	48,980	5.0	33.6
DC	706,629	74,492	29,914	4.2	40.2
FL	21,695,068	3,085,765	1,117,016	5.1	36.2
GA	10,671,030	1,440,292	508,218	4.8	35.3
HI	1,365,210	164,933	74,107	5.4	44.9
ID	1,841,020	266,684	85,433	4.6	32.0
IL	12,541,886	1,530,941	604,018	4.8	39.5
IN	6,753,016	985,158	357,588	5.3	36.3
IA	3,164,622	412,569	142,808	4.5	34.6
KS	2,898,795	408,313	142,645	4.9	34.9
KY	4,462,819	820,799	299,296	6.7	36.5
LA	4,615,615	761,512	265,335	5.7	34.8
ME	1,332,120	218,850	72,708	5.5	33.2
MD	6,005,118	694,317	260,343	4.3	37.5
MA	6,887,330	858,405	336,748	4.9	39.2
MI	10,001,947	1,468,729	564,667	5.6	38.4
MN	5,634,769	650,592	248,077	4.4	38.1
MS	2,934,741	523,114	194,715	6.6	37.2
MO	6,143,005	901,112	329,938	5.4	36.6
MT	1,066,483	158,996	52,956	5.0	33.3
NE	1,905,612	218,665	76,082	4.0	34.8
NV	3,145,192	422,943	143,238	4.6	33.9
NH	1,367,525	183,112	69,984	5.1	38.2
NJ	8,852,661	999,280	399,678	4.5	40.0
NM	2,090,104	357,004	121,521	5.8	34.0
NY	19,324,301	2,370,697	1,005,562	5.2	42.4
NC	10,533,083	1,487,892	527,954	5.0	35.5
ND	756,157	83,908	27,280	3.6	32.5
OH	11,687,765	1,752,373	638,349	5.5	36.4
OK	3,985,175	711,189	240,795	6.0	33.9
OR	4,232,126	637,697	233,745	5.5	36.7
PA	12,799,353	1,856,929	718,130	5.6	38.7
RI	1,059,413	158,237	62,375	5.9	39.4
SC	5,179,851	789,480	275,842	5.3	34.9
SD	901,635	108,967	36,936	4.1	33.9
TN	6,891,933	1,110,307	396,596	5.8	35.7
TX	29,247,594	3,573,362	1,230,934	4.2	34.4
UT	3,258,478	342,360	114,102	3.5	33.3
VT	623,385	84,485	28,381	4.6	33.6
VA	8,430,315	1,061,601	391,127	4.6	36.8
WA	7,635,653	1,035,051	368,541	4.8	35.6
WV	1,787,384	349,832	127,766	7.1	36.5
WI	5,834,849	704,481	262,731	4.5	37.3
WY	571,301	78,581	21,985	3.8	28.0

Citation: Paul, S., Rafal, M., & Houtenville, A. (2021). Annual Disability Statistics Compendium: 2021 (Table 1.9). Durham, NH: University of New Hampshire, Institute on Disability. Note: Authors' calculations using the U.S. Census Bureau American Community Survey, Public Use Microdata Sample with Experimental Weights, 2020, which is subject to sampling variation.
[1] The independent living disability question asks people 15 years old or older, "Because of a physical, mental, or emotional condition, does this person have difficulty doing errands alone such as visiting a doctor's office or shopping?" See glossary for more information.

877

Table 3.1 Employment — Civilians with Disabilities Ages 18-64 Years Living in the Community for the United States and States: 2020

State	Total	Employed Count	% [1]	State	Total	Employed Count	% [1]
U.S.	21,523,050	7,975,590	37.0	MO	452,325	165,594	36.6
AL	434,220	134,813	31.0	MT	73,328	30,570	41.6
AK	40,730	15,943	39.1	NE	98,096	47,190	48.1
AZ	488,802	185,961	38.0	NV	208,600	75,984	36.4
AR	297,304	90,963	30.5	NH	87,215	38,586	44.2
CA	2,064,229	754,024	36.5	NJ	451,856	184,429	40.8
CO	338,603	140,975	41.6	NM	180,015	55,210	30.6
CT	198,105	75,629	38.1	NY	1,092,557	369,415	33.8
DE	69,127	29,882	43.2	NC	745,123	247,881	33.2
DC	46,410	13,990	30.1	ND	37,939	19,783	52.1
FL	1,345,230	473,940	35.2	OH	874,248	322,005	36.8
GA	757,956	273,580	36.0	OK	373,359	141,445	37.8
HI	67,460	30,070	44.5	OR	315,368	115,612	36.6
ID	130,917	55,265	42.2	PA	883,490	319,732	36.1
IL	716,876	280,534	39.1	RI	78,954	31,881	40.3
IN	514,248	200,603	39.0	SC	380,650	131,970	34.6
IA	197,212	88,714	44.9	SD	49,716	23,178	46.6
KS	206,067	90,996	44.1	TN	557,495	187,386	33.6
KY	447,045	144,725	32.3	TX	1,809,900	735,016	40.6
LA	395,171	131,928	33.3	UT	187,415	89,131	47.5
ME	109,097	37,563	34.4	VT	43,494	13,600	31.2
MD	335,712	135,066	40.2	VA	511,784	206,152	40.2
MA	413,228	157,271	38.0	WA	529,586	205,993	38.8
MI	759,317	255,465	33.6	WV	176,780	48,905	27.6
MN	307,760	132,435	43.0	WI	335,325	145,765	43.4
MS	269,622	77,077	28.5	WY	37,984	15,765	41.5

Citation: Paul, S., Rafal, M., & Houtenville, A. (2021). Annual Disability Statistics Compendium: 2021 (Table 3.1). Durham, NH: University of New Hampshire, Institute on Disability. Note: Authors' calculations using the U.S. Census Bureau American Community Survey, Public Use Microdata Sample with Experimental Weights, 2020, which is subject to sampling variation.
[1] The percentage of people employed with disabilities.

Table 3.2 Employment – Civilians without Disabilities Ages 18-64 Years Living in the Community for the United States and States: 2020

State	Total	Employed Count	% [1]	State	Total	Employed Count	% [1]
U.S.	178,475,229	133,949,072	75.0	MO	3,226,772	2,509,999	77.7
AL	2,516,017	1,829,058	72.6	MT	553,646	431,340	77.9
AK	395,524	284,271	71.8	NE	1,026,166	837,282	81.5
AZ	3,900,699	2,858,690	73.2	NV	1,710,089	1,234,255	72.1
AR	1,478,506	1,089,012	73.6	NH	762,360	607,616	79.7
CA	22,364,711	16,186,174	72.3	NJ	4,969,902	3,746,983	75.3
CO	3,307,379	2,594,672	78.4	NM	1,058,682	739,019	69.8
CT	1,988,949	1,531,669	77.0	NY	10,863,050	7,878,359	72.5
DE	510,792	384,148	75.2	NC	5,662,705	4,230,313	74.7
DC	443,787	335,428	75.5	ND	406,661	337,439	82.9
FL	11,459,108	8,551,983	74.6	OH	6,148,772	4,705,417	76.5
GA	5,823,262	4,277,124	73.4	OK	2,005,129	1,492,061	74.4
HI	727,711	551,080	75.7	OR	2,271,151	1,722,123	75.8
ID	941,857	730,164	77.5	PA	6,840,367	5,206,072	76.1
IL	6,984,533	5,310,745	76.0	RI	584,159	445,139	76.2
IN	3,574,075	2,757,682	77.1	SC	2,701,777	1,991,650	73.7
IA	1,674,271	1,358,117	81.1	SD	470,935	387,308	82.2
KS	1,508,097	1,209,026	80.1	TN	3,651,972	2,748,163	75.2
KY	2,244,032	1,677,545	74.7	TX	16,151,018	11,931,351	73.8
LA	2,378,364	1,655,184	69.5	UT	1,757,473	1,393,824	79.3
ME	689,847	549,307	79.6	VT	336,815	266,731	79.1
MD	3,346,635	2,601,681	77.7	VA	4,666,601	3,594,038	77.0
MA	3,943,738	3,049,824	77.3	WA	4,208,860	3,212,277	76.3
MI	5,307,054	3,936,053	74.1	WV	878,406	620,238	70.6
MN	3,084,851	2,526,218	81.8	WI	3,191,886	2,562,566	80.2
MS	1,477,260	1,044,734	70.7	WY	298,816	237,920	79.6

Citation: Paul, S., Rafal, M., & Houtenville, A. (2021). Annual Disability Statistics Compendium: 2021 (Table 3.2). Durham, NH: University of New Hampshire, Institute on Disability. Note: Authors' calculations using the U.S. Census Bureau American Community Survey, Public Use Microdata Sample with Experimental Weights, 2020, which is subject to sampling variation.
[1] The percentage of people employed without disabilities.

Table 3.3 Employment – Civilians with Hearing Disabilities Ages 18–64 Years Living in the Community for the United States and States: 2020

State	Total	Employed Count	Employed % [1]
U.S.	3,892,160	2,041,592	52.4
AL	78,335	40,258	51.3
AK	10,938	5,751	52.5
AZ	94,116	49,896	53.0
AR	54,745	25,177	45.9
CA	354,809	177,668	50.0
CO	73,967	40,715	55.0
CT	32,611	17,518	53.7
DE	9,494	5,626	59.2
DC	5,564	1,835	32.9
FL	219,303	112,200	51.1
GA	120,130	64,996	54.1
HI	13,013	8,184	62.8
ID	27,364	16,555	60.4
IL	130,344	68,989	52.9
IN	98,230	56,090	57.1
IA	41,213	26,001	63.0
KS	42,717	22,649	53.0
KY	80,821	35,567	44.0
LA	63,721	31,896	50.0
ME	23,824	12,390	52.0
MD	49,298	28,166	57.1
MA	72,827	38,406	52.7
MI	124,812	64,447	51.6
MN	63,589	38,318	60.2
MS	45,163	17,398	38.5
MO	83,736	43,003	51.3
MT	15,522	8,805	56.7
NE	23,572	15,849	67.2
NV	47,397	22,670	47.8
NH	17,803	11,346	63.7
NJ	74,168	42,421	57.1
NM	36,469	14,841	40.6
NY	157,252	75,887	48.2
NC	132,998	66,992	50.3
ND	10,289	7,658	74.4
OH	153,063	75,533	49.3
OK	88,825	47,046	52.9
OR	62,064	29,805	48.0
PA	140,841	73,632	52.2
RI	16,031	8,716	54.3
SC	68,861	35,132	51.0
SD	10,248	5,841	56.9
TN	109,927	51,366	46.7
TX	359,165	201,081	55.9
UT	35,381	22,875	64.6
VT	10,337	5,431	52.5
VA	97,911	54,788	55.9
WA	102,759	57,531	55.9
WV	36,541	14,362	39.3
WI	61,018	37,337	61.1
WY	9,034	4,948	54.7

Citation: Paul, S., Rafal, M., & Houtenville, A. (2021). Annual Disability Statistics Compendium: 2021 (Table 3.3). Durham, NH: University of New Hampshire, Institute on Disability. Note: Authors' calculations using the U.S. Census Bureau American Community Survey, Public Use Microdata Sample with Experimental Weights, 2020, which is subject to sampling variation.
[1] The percentage of people employed with hearing disabilities.

Table 3.4 Employment – Civilians with Vision Disabilities Ages 18–64 Years Living in the Community for the United States and States: 2020

State	Total	Employed Count	% [1]
U.S.	4,001,765	1,823,152	45.5
AL	77,960	28,425	36.4
AK	8,519	3,582	42.0
AZ	93,680	46,328	49.4
AR	54,374	21,712	39.9
CA	399,073	184,676	46.2
CO	64,421	33,492	51.9
CT	34,562	16,755	48.4
DE	9,941	6,608	66.4
DC	7,272	2,798	38.4
FL	256,657	121,230	47.2
GA	148,627	67,244	45.2
HI	12,668	7,289	57.5
ID	22,722	9,316	40.9
IL	130,572	65,983	50.5
IN	87,596	40,909	46.7
IA	28,725	15,992	55.6
KS	37,620	19,785	52.5
KY	91,077	35,610	39.0
LA	94,157	40,737	43.2
ME	13,744	5,462	39.7
MD	53,577	25,172	46.9
MA	62,098	26,632	42.8
MI	113,933	49,000	43.0
MN	41,257	20,691	50.1
MS	60,798	22,356	36.7
MO	80,522	36,604	45.4
MT	12,229	6,188	50.6
NE	16,481	10,460	63.4
NV	43,016	17,675	41.0
NH	13,324	10,051	75.4
NJ	92,214	51,771	56.1
NM	38,719	15,774	40.7
NY	186,845	85,920	45.9
NC	139,827	55,212	39.4
ND	5,197	3,057	58.8
OH	142,230	64,117	45.0
OK	79,447	31,997	40.2
OR	50,231	21,191	42.1
PA	145,494	64,715	44.4
RI	11,258	4,435	39.3
SC	81,307	34,422	42.3
SD	6,161	3,463	56.2
TN	123,565	47,625	38.5
TX	401,256	185,800	46.3
UT	35,265	19,524	55.3
VT	7,200	2,399	33.3
VA	96,694	42,813	44.2
WA	95,070	44,650	46.9
WV	31,827	12,373	38.8
WI	53,424	28,676	53.6
WY	7,332	4,456	60.7

Citation: Paul, S., Rafal, M., & Houtenville, A. (2021). Annual Disability Statistics Compendium: 2021 (Table 3.4). Durham, NH: University of New Hampshire, Institute on Disability. Note: Authors' calculations using the U.S. Census Bureau American Community Survey, Public Use Microdata Sample with Experimental Weights, 2020, which is subject to sampling variation.
[1] The percentage of people employed with vision disabilities.

Table 3.5 Employment – Civilians with Cognitive Disabilities Ages 18–64 Years Living in the Community for the United States and States: 2020

State	Total	Employed Count	% [1]
U.S.	9,849,570	2,875,776	29.1
AL	192,265	45,699	23.7
AK	15,956	3,553	22.2
AZ	219,667	60,201	27.4
AR	130,636	26,019	19.9
CA	919,852	253,169	27.5
CO	161,903	55,950	34.5
CT	96,654	29,432	30.4
DE	32,117	10,970	34.1
DC	27,694	8,165	29.4
FL	605,236	167,633	27.6
GA	357,918	99,007	27.6
HI	29,038	8,212	28.2
ID	63,533	21,225	33.4
IL	326,990	97,937	29.9
IN	237,153	75,243	31.7
IA	91,886	34,557	37.6
KS	93,165	37,007	39.7
KY	203,496	51,802	25.4
LA	179,537	41,513	23.1
ME	60,211	15,983	26.5
MD	154,837	50,890	32.8
MA	220,624	70,617	32.0
MI	360,622	96,806	26.8
MN	164,045	62,403	38.0
MS	114,184	25,474	22.3
MO	205,196	59,746	29.1
MT	34,068	11,461	33.6
NE	44,371	15,473	34.8
NV	84,260	26,144	31.0
NH	41,169	14,427	35.0
NJ	196,560	61,397	31.2
NM	83,607	19,094	22.8
NY	495,885	137,256	27.6
NC	328,710	83,170	25.3
ND	17,453	7,159	41.0
OH	408,289	127,689	31.2
OK	162,084	45,491	28.0
OR	161,926	48,786	30.1
PA	428,476	122,586	28.6
RI	41,006	13,238	32.2
SC	159,580	40,239	25.2
SD	20,531	8,812	42.9
TN	245,767	67,826	27.5
TX	781,028	244,409	31.2
UT	92,752	37,224	40.1
VT	25,317	5,855	23.1
VA	225,121	72,699	32.2
WA	262,226	77,661	29.6
WV	76,493	16,092	21.0
WI	152,783	57,240	37.4
WY	15,693	5,135	32.7

Citation: Paul, S., Rafal, M., & Houtenville, A. (2021). Annual Disability Statistics Compendium: 2021 (Table 3.5). Durham, NH: University of New Hampshire, Institute on Disability. Note: Authors' calculations using the U.S. Census Bureau American Community Survey, Public Use Microdata Sample with Experimental Weights, 2020, which is subject to sampling variation.
[1] The percentage of people employed with cognitive disabilities.

Table 3.6 Employment – Civilians with Ambulatory Disabilities Ages 18-64 Years Living in the Community for the United States and States: 2020

State	Total	Employed Count	Employed % [1]	State	Total	Employed Count	Employed % [1]
U.S.	9,304,426	2,231,962	23.9	MO	212,648	46,989	22.0
AL	213,213	39,986	18.7	MT	28,431	7,451	26.2
AK	12,711	3,350	26.3	NE	37,649	10,060	26.7
AZ	204,359	49,039	23.9	NV	92,749	20,748	22.3
AR	148,090	31,866	21.5	NH	33,390	9,695	29.0
CA	847,093	217,626	25.6	NJ	184,855	50,049	27.0
CO	121,355	26,713	22.0	NM	81,991	16,886	20.5
CT	79,555	19,290	24.2	NY	489,832	109,354	22.3
DE	32,060	10,439	32.5	NC	346,149	76,820	22.1
DC	16,644	2,690	16.1	ND	11,098	4,478	40.3
FL	595,899	147,844	24.8	OH	378,809	85,814	22.6
GA	351,607	85,486	24.3	OK	162,722	40,273	24.7
HI	24,776	6,774	27.3	OR	121,827	27,746	22.7
ID	53,708	15,943	29.6	PA	388,037	93,690	24.1
IL	295,296	74,732	25.3	RI	30,960	8,714	28.1
IN	234,283	58,568	24.9	SC	172,933	32,575	18.8
IA	73,801	21,337	28.9	SD	19,149	5,964	31.1
KS	87,144	25,750	29.5	TN	262,920	54,386	20.6
KY	213,037	40,999	19.2	TX	776,387	204,994	26.4
LA	181,128	40,390	22.2	UT	62,541	18,309	29.2
ME	43,985	8,968	20.3	VT	14,936	3,446	23.0
MD	145,071	42,664	29.4	VA	219,233	59,366	27.0
MA	151,922	37,303	24.5	WA	205,776	49,998	24.2
MI	335,762	71,725	21.3	WV	88,775	13,906	15.6
MN	117,141	31,911	27.2	WI	148,136	38,765	26.1
MS	137,470	26,259	19.1	WY	15,383	3,834	24.9

Citation: Paul, S., Rafal, M., & Houtenville, A. (2021). Annual Disability Statistics Compendium: 2021 (Table 3.6). Durham, NH: University of New Hampshire, Institute on Disability. Note: Authors' calculations using the U.S. Census Bureau American Community Survey, Public Use Microdata Sample with Experimental Weights, 2020, which is subject to sampling variation.
[1] The percentage of people employed with ambulatory disabilities.

Table 3.7 Employment – Civilians with Self-Care Disabilities Ages 18–64 Years Living in the Community for the United States and States: 2020

State	Total	Employed Count	Employed % [1]
U.S.	3,533,797	497,108	14.0
AL	71,247	8,335	11.6
AK	5,669	1,195	21.0
AZ	71,184	10,028	14.0
AR	48,855	5,131	10.5
CA	352,197	44,417	12.6
CO	44,897	7,051	15.7
CT	31,576	3,460	10.9
DE	9,891	1,735	17.5
DC	5,859	906	15.4
FL	215,745	37,594	17.4
GA	128,478	16,330	12.7
HI	10,892	1,605	14.7
ID	19,329	1,791	9.2
IL	118,986	18,554	15.5
IN	78,669	11,065	14.0
IA	30,786	7,203	23.3
KS	30,334	5,223	17.2
KY	77,294	9,618	12.4
LA	71,344	8,772	12.2
ME	16,227	1,518	9.3
MD	50,532	7,186	14.2
MA	61,919	10,504	16.9
MI	130,807	14,328	10.9
MN	57,626	9,323	16.1
MS	45,214	6,142	13.5
MO	85,185	11,176	13.1
MT	11,211	1,803	16.0
NE	15,501	2,481	16.0
NV	33,200	7,238	21.8
NH	11,115	2,189	19.6
NJ	80,649	15,630	19.3
NM	31,483	4,863	15.4
NY	190,755	25,600	13.4
NC	125,254	18,211	14.5
ND	3,969	725	18.2
OH	133,012	19,828	14.9
OK	53,858	6,974	12.9
OR	56,499	5,038	8.9
PA	144,718	20,573	14.2
RI	14,966	2,335	15.6
SC	67,946	6,581	9.6
SD	6,928	1,889	27.2
TN	90,385	9,410	10.4
TX	291,484	37,806	12.9
UT	25,987	4,979	19.1
VT	6,741	917	13.6
VA	81,771	14,785	18.0
WA	85,577	12,830	14.9
WV	29,763	2,852	9.5
WI	64,507	10,248	15.8
WY	5,776	1,133	19.6

Citation: Paul, S., Rafal, M., & Houtenville, A. (2021). Annual Disability Statistics Compendium: 2021 (Table 3.7). Durham, NH: University of New Hampshire, Institute on Disability. Note: Authors' calculations using the U.S. Census Bureau American Community Survey, Public Use Microdata Sample with Experimental Weights, 2020, which is subject to sampling variation.
[1] The percentage of people employed with self-care disabilities.

Table 3.8 Employment – Civilians with Independent Living Disabilities Ages 18–64 Years Living in the Community for the United States and States: 2020

State	Total	Employed Count	% [1]	State	Total	Employed Count	% [1]
U.S.	7,794,788	1,381,112	17.7	MO	166,104	30,514	18.3
AL	152,411	19,737	12.9	MT	28,151	6,065	21.5
AK	11,540	1,253	10.8	NE	33,094	7,153	21.6
AZ	178,940	30,415	16.9	NV	70,376	12,259	17.4
AR	102,900	8,135	7.9	NH	31,660	7,869	24.8
CA	767,722	125,885	16.3	NJ	166,623	36,105	21.6
CO	121,349	22,814	18.8	NM	63,135	11,050	17.5
CT	73,481	13,785	18.7	NY	417,950	63,812	15.2
DE	24,374	4,673	19.1	NC	255,714	35,263	13.7
DC	17,642	2,839	16.0	ND	11,788	2,607	22.1
FL	481,715	80,682	16.7	OH	309,899	60,043	19.3
GA	273,196	47,004	17.2	OK	125,016	26,179	20.9
HI	27,610	5,774	20.9	OR	120,654	21,206	17.5
ID	44,129	8,583	19.4	PA	333,211	58,876	17.6
IL	273,766	53,291	19.4	RI	29,370	5,919	20.1
IN	193,052	35,124	18.1	SC	133,245	19,466	14.6
IA	67,441	17,252	25.5	SD	15,021	3,661	24.3
KS	71,787	15,793	21.9	TN	192,586	25,207	13.0
KY	164,651	27,943	16.9	TX	612,312	114,496	18.6
LA	138,097	18,370	13.3	UT	65,604	18,307	27.9
ME	41,049	7,323	17.8	VT	14,964	2,878	19.2
MD	119,116	20,344	17.0	VA	182,451	38,829	21.2
MA	153,812	33,616	21.8	WA	194,469	40,588	20.8
MI	293,708	47,301	16.1	WV	63,758	7,986	12.5
MN	122,655	30,991	25.2	WI	129,745	31,579	24.3
MS	100,802	11,311	11.2	WY	10,943	2,957	27.0

Citation: Paul, S.; Rafal, M.; & Houtenville, A. (2021). Annual Disability Statistics Compendium: 2021 (Table 3.8). Durham, NH: University of New Hampshire, Institute on Disability. Note: Authors' calculations using the U.S. Census Bureau American Community Survey, Public Use Microdata Sample with Experimental Weights, 2020, which is subject to sampling variation.
[1] The percentage of people employed with independent living disabilities.

Table 3.9 Employment Gap – Civilians Ages 18–64 Years Living in the Community for the United States and States, by Disability Status: 2020

State	Disability [1]	No Disability [2]	Gap (% pts) [3]
U.S.	37.0	75.0	37.9
AL	31.0	72.6	41.5
AK	39.1	71.8	32.6
AZ	38.0	73.2	35.1
AR	30.5	73.6	43.0
CA	36.5	72.3	35.7
CO	41.6	78.4	36.7
CT	38.1	77.0	38.8
DE	43.2	75.2	31.9
DC	30.1	75.5	45.3
FL	35.2	74.6	39.3
GA	36.0	73.4	37.3
HI	44.5	75.7	31.1
ID	42.2	77.5	35.2
IL	39.1	76.0	36.8
IN	39.0	77.1	38.0
IA	44.9	81.1	36.1
KS	44.1	80.1	35.9
KY	32.3	74.7	42.3
LA	33.3	69.5	36.1
ME	34.4	79.6	45.1
MD	40.2	77.7	37.4
MA	38.0	77.3	39.2
MI	33.6	74.1	40.4
MN	43.0	81.8	38.7
MS	28.5	70.7	42.1
MO	36.6	77.7	41.0
MT	41.6	77.9	36.2
NE	48.1	81.5	33.3
NV	36.4	72.1	35.6
NH	44.2	79.7	35.4
NJ	40.8	75.3	34.4
NM	30.6	69.8	39.1
NY	33.8	72.5	38.6
NC	33.2	74.7	41.4
ND	52.1	82.9	30.7
OH	36.8	76.5	39.6
OK	37.8	74.4	36.5
OR	36.6	75.8	39.1
PA	36.1	76.1	39.9
RI	40.3	76.2	35.8
SC	34.6	73.7	39.0
SD	46.6	82.2	35.5
TN	33.6	75.2	41.5
TX	40.6	73.8	33.1
UT	47.5	79.3	31.7
VT	31.2	79.1	47.8
VA	40.2	77.0	36.7
WA	38.8	76.3	37.4
WV	27.6	70.6	42.9
WI	43.4	80.2	36.7
WY	41.5	79.6	38.0

Citation: Paul, S., Rafal, M., & Houtenville, A. (2021). Annual Disability Statistics Compendium: 2021 (Table 3.9). Durham, NH: University of New Hampshire, Institute on Disability. Note: Authors' calculations using the U.S. Census Bureau American Community Survey, Public Use Microdata Sample with Experimental Weights, 2020, which is subject to sampling variation.

[1] The percentage of people employed with disabilities.
[2] The percentage of people employed without disabilities.
[3] The difference in percentage points of people employed with and without disabilities.

Aging

ADHD: What Can We Do?, 7905
ARC Of Southeast Los Angeles-Southeast
  Industries, 6375
Activities in Action, 7454
Administration on Aging, 3215
Advocacy Centre for the Elderly (ACE), 592
Aging & Vision News, 7587
Aging Brain, 2201
Aging Life Care Association, 7336
Aging News Alert, 7588
Aging Services of Michigan, 7337
Aging Services of South Carolina, 7338
Aging Services of Washington, 7339
Aging and Disability Services, 3755, 7340
Aging and Disability Services Division, 3529
Aging and Disability: Crossing Network Lines,
  2202
Aging and Family Therapy: Practitioner
  Perspectives on Golden Pond, 7457
Aging and Rehabilitation II: The State of the
  Practice, 2203
Aging and Vision: Declarations of Independence,
  9164
Aging in America, 7341
Aging in Stride, 7458
Aging in the Designed Environment, 7459
Aging with a Disability, 7460
Alabama Department of Senior Services, 3252
Alabama VA Benefits Regional Office -
  Montgomery, 5472
Alaska Commission on Aging, 3263
Albany County Department for Aging and Albany
  Social Services, 3573
Albany VA Medical Center: Samuel S Stratton,
  5605
Aleda E Lutz VA Medical Center, 5566
Alexandria VA Medical Center, 5549
Alliance for Aging Research, 7343
Alliance for Retired Americans, 7344
Alvin C York VA Medical Center, 5662
Amarillo VA Healthcare System, 5667
American Aging Association, 7345
American Association of Retired Persons, 7347
American Geriatrics Society, 7349
American Planning Association, 7350
American Society on Aging, 7353
American Wheelchair Bowling Association, 8271
Amyotrophic Lateral Sclerosis: A Guide for
  Patients and Families, 8506
Area Agency on Aging of Southwest Arkansas,
  7607
Area Agency on Aging: Region One, 7608
Arizona Division of Aging and Adult Services,
  3275
Arkansas Division of Aging & Adult Services,
  3284
Asheville VA Medical Center, 5621
Association for Gerontology in Higher Education,
  7358
Association for International Practical Training,
  2603
Association of Jewish Aging Services, 7359
Association on Aging with Developmental
  Disabilities, 7360
Atlanta Regional Office, 5519
Atlanta VA Medical Center, 5520
Attention Getter, 1557
Attention Teens, 1558
Augusta VA Medical Center, 5521
Baltimore Regional Office, 5554
Baltimore VA Medical Center, 5555
Bath VA Medical Center, 5607
Battle Creek VA Medical Center, 5567
Bay Pines VA Medical Center, 5513
Biloxi/Gulfport VA Medical Center, 5577
Blindness, A Family Matter, 9165
Boise Regional Office, 5527
Boise VA Medical Center, 5528
Boston VA Regional Office, 5560
Bronx VA Medical Center, 5608
Brooklyn Campus of the VA NY Harbor
  Healthcare System, 5609

Buffalo Regional Office - Department of Veterans
  Affairs, 5610
Building Blocks: Foundations for Learning for
  Young Blind and Visually Impaired Children,
  9166
Butler VA Medical Center, 5643
CARF International, 648, 1916, 7363
California Department of Aging, 3292
Cambia Health Foundation, 649, 3059
Can America Afford to Grow Old?, 4512
Canandiagua VA Medical Center, 5611
Caring for Those You Love: A Guide to
  Compassionate Care for the Aged, 7462
Carl T Hayden VA Medical Center, 5479
Carl Vinson VA Medical Center, 5522
Castle Point Campus of the VA Hudson Valley
  Healthcare System, 5612
Center for Disability and Elder Law, Inc., 4487
Center for Positive Aging, 7367
Change Your Brain, Change Your Life: The
  Breakthrough Program for Conquering
  Depression, 7806
Cheyenne VA Medical Center, 5699
Children of Aging Parents, 7368
Chillicothe VA Medical Center, 5629
Cincinnati VA Medical Center, 5630
Clement J Zablocki VA Medical Center, 5694
Cleveland Regional Office, 5631
Coatesville VA Medical Center, 5644
Colmery-O'Neil VA Medical Center, 5542
Colorado Association of Homes and Services for
  the Aging, 7369
Colorado Department of Aging & Adult Services,
  3307
Colorado Springs Independence Center, 3906
Colorado/Wyoming VA Medical Center, 5499
Columbia Foundation, 2846
Columbia Regional Office, 5657
Communication Skills for Working with Elders,
  2256
Complementary Alternative Medicine and Multiple
  Sclerosis, 8531
Connecticut Commission on Aging, 3316
Coping and Caring: Living with Alzheimer's
  Disease, 7464
Court-Related Needs of the Elderly and Persons
  with Disabilities, 4519
CurePSP Magazine, 8674
DSHS/Aging & Adult Disability Services
  Administration, 3764
Dayton VA Medical Center, 5632
DeafBlind Division of the National Federation of
  the Blind, 8882
Delaware Department of Health and Social
  Services, 3323
Delaware VA Regional Office, 5506
Denver VA Medical Center, 5500
Des Moines VA Medical Center, 5537
Des Moines VA Regional Office, 5538
District of Columbia Office on Aging, 3332
Duchenne Muscular Dystrophy, 8538
Durham VA Medical Center, 5623
Dwight D Eisenhower VA Medical Center, 5543
East Orange Campus of the VA New Jersey
  Healthcare System, 5600
Edith Nourse Rogers Memorial Veterans Hospital,
  5561
Edward Hines Jr Hospital, 5529
Ehrman Medical Library, 4793
El Paso VA Healthcare Center, 5669
Elder Abuse and Mistreatment, 7465
Elder Visions Newsletter, 7593
ElderLawAnswers.com, 4529
Elgin Training Center, 6661
Employment for Individuals with Asperger
  Syndrome or Non-Verbal Learning Disability,
  8799
Enabling News, 7594
Erie VA Medical Center, 5645
Eugene J Towbin Healthcare Center, 5482
Explore Your Options, 7466
Facilitating Self-Care Practices in the Elderly,
  2307
Falling in Old Age, 7467

Family Intervention Guide to Mental Illness, 7468
Family-Guided Activity-Based Intervention for
  Toddlers & Infants, 5257
Fanlight Productions, 24
Fargo VA Medical Center, 5627
Fayetteville VA Medical Center, 5483, 5624
Films & Videos on Aging and Sensory Change,
  5260
Florida Adult Services, 3347
Fort Howard VA Medical Center, 5556
Foundations of Orientation and Mobility, 9007
Gainesville Division, North Florida/South Georgia
  Veterans Healthcare System, 5514
Georgia Department of Aging, 3362
The Gerontological Society of America, 7450
Gerontology: Abstracts in Social Gerontology,
  7486
Getting Better, 8159
Golf Xpress, 448
Grand Island VA Medical System, 5588
Grand Junction VA Medical Center, 5501
Hampton VA Medical Center, 5680
Handbook of Assistive Devices for the
  Handicapped Elderly, 7469
Handbook on Ethnicity, Aging and Mental Health,
  7470
Harry S Truman Memorial Veterans' Hospital,
  5579
Hartford Regional Office, 5502
Hawaii Executive Office on Aging, 3378
Health Care of the Aged: Needs, Policies, and
  Services, 7471
Health Promotion and Disease Prevention in
  Clinical Practice, 7472
Healthy Aging Association, 7377
Helping the Family Understand, 8160
Honolulu VBA Regional Office, 5525
Houston Regional Office, 5670
Hunter Holmes McGuire VA Medical Center, 5681
Huntington Regional Office, 5689
Huntington VA Medical Center, 5690
Idaho Commission on Aging, 3383
Illinois Department on Aging, 3399
Independence Economic Development, 4497
Independent Living Office, 5031
Independent Living Resources, 4341
Indiana Association for Home and Hospice Care
  (IAHHC), 721
Indianapolis Regional Office, 5533
Innovations, 7596
Institute on Aging, 7610
Insurance Solutions: Plan Well, Live Better, 5034
Interstitial Cystitis Association, 5353
Iowa City VA Medical Center, 5539
Iowa Department on Aging, 3415
Iron Mountain VA Medical Center, 5568
Jack C. Montgomery VA Medical Center, 5634
Jackson Regional Office, 5578
James A Haley VA Medical Center, 5515
James E Van Zandt VA Medical Center, 5646
Jerry L Pettis Memorial VA Medical Center, 5486
John D Dingell VA Medical Center, 5569
John J Pershing VA Medical Center, 5580
John L McClellan Memorial Hospital, 5484
Jonathan M Wainwright Memorial VA Medical
  Center, 5685
Justice in Aging, 7384
Kansas City VA Medical Center, 5581
Kansas Department on Aging, 3424
Kansas VA Regional Office, 5544
Kentucky Office of Aging Services, 3429
Knoxville VA Medical Center, 5540
Laurel Grove Hospital: Rehab Care Unit, 6082
LeadingAge, 7387
LeadingAge Arizona, 7388
LeadingAge California, 7389
LeadingAge Connecticut, 7390
LeadingAge Gulf States, 7391
LeadingAge Illinois, 7392
LeadingAge Indiana, 7393
LeadingAge Iowa, 7394
LeadingAge Kentucky, 7395
LeadingAge Maine & New Hampshire, 7396
LeadingAge Massachusetts, 7397

VA Pittsburgh Healthcare System, Highland Drive Division, 5653
VA Pittsburgh Healthcare System, University Drive Division, 5652
VA Puget Sound Health Care System, 5688
VA Salt Lake City Healthcare System, 5677
VA San Diego Healthcare System, 5497
VA Sierra Nevada Healthcare System, 5594
VA Southern Nevada Healthcare System, 5595
VA Western NY Healthcare System, Batavia, 5619
VA Western NY Healthcare System, Buffalo, 5620
Vermont Department of Aging, 3747
Vermont Department of Disabilities, Aging and Independent Living, 3749
Vermont Division of Disability & Aging Services, 3753
Vermont VA Regional Office Center, 5678
Veteran Benefits Administration - Anchorage Regional Office, 5478
Visiting Nurse Association of America, 8737
Visually Impaired Seniors as Senior Companions: A Reference Guide, 7483
WG Hefner VA Medical Center - Salisbury, 5625
Waco Regional Office, 5674
Washington County Disability, Aging and Veteran Services, 3650
Washington DC VA Medical Center, 5512
We Can Do it Together!, 9179
West Palm Beach VA Medical Center, 5518
West Texas VA Healthcare System, 5675
West Virginia Department of Aging, 3780
Wilkes-Barre VA Medical Center, 5654
William Jennings Bryan Dorn VA Medical Center, 5659
William S Middleton Memorial VA Hospital Center, 5696
Wilmington VA Medical Center, 5507
Winston-Salem Regional Office, 5626
Wisconsin Bureau of Aging, 3790
Wisconsin VA Regional Office, 5697
Work, Health and Income Among the Elderly, 7484
Wyoming Department of Aging, 3798
Wyoming/Colorado VA Regional Office, 5701
Yoga for Fibromyalgia: Move, Breathe, and Relax to Improve Your Quality of Life, 8234
Young Person's Guide to Spina Bifida, 8662

AIDS

AHF Federation, 584
AIDS Alert, 8684
AIDS Healthcare Foundation, 585, 2645
AIDS Sourcebook, 8496
AIDS United, 8293
AIDS Vancouver, 586
AIDS and Other Manifestations of HIV Infection, 8497
AIDS in the Twenty-First Century: Disease and Globalization, 8498
AIDS: The Official Journal of the International AIDS Society, 8666
Access & Information Network, 589
Camp Heartland, 1061, 8401
Camp Hollywood HEART, 862, 8406
Camp Starlight, 1212
Camp Sunburst, 877, 8433
Caremark Healthcare Services, 6646
Children with Disabilities, 5129
CrescentCare Legal Services, 4490
FC Search, 3193
Glaser Progress Foundation, 3163
Guide to Living with HIV Infection: Developed at the Johns Hopkins AIDS Clinic, 8548
HEAL: Health Education AIDS Liaison, 1937
HIV Infection and Developmental Disabilities, 2319
Harborview Medical Center, Low Vision Aid Clinic, 7021
Health Resources & Services Administration: State Bureau of Health, 3449
Health Resources and Services Administration (HRSA), 3224
Legal Action Center, 4500

Legal Counsel for Health Jusice, 4501
Legislative Network for Nurses, 4546
Levi Strauss Foundation, 2684
Living Well with Chronic Fatigue Syndrome and Fibromyalgia, 8576
Living Well with HIV and AIDS, 8577
A Loving Spoonful, 582
Miami VA Medical Center, 5516
Michigan Association for Deaf, and Hard of Hearing, 3468
Michigan Protection & Advocacy Service, 3481
National AIDS Hotline, 8727
Penitent, with Roses: An HIV+ Mother Reflects, 8623
Questions and Answers: The ADA and Personswith HIV/AIDS, 8630
Ryan White HIV/AIDS Program, 793
Sight by Touch, 9177
Strength for the Journey, 1220, 8478
Sunburst Projects, 8359
Suttle Lake Camp, 1221, 8480
Vinfen Corporation, 6811
Visiting Nurse Association of North Shore, 6812
WORLD, 816

Alternative Therapies

The ACNM Foundation, Inc., 2859
Academy for Guided Imagery, 2565
Academy of Integrative Health & Medicine (AIHM), 588
Accreditation Commission for Acupuncture & Oriental Medicine, 590
Accreditation Commission for Midwifery Education (ACME), 591
American Academy of Medical Acupuncture, 597
American Academy of Osteopathy, 8168
American Acupuncture Council, 601
American Association of Acupuncture and Oriental Medicine (AAAOM), 602
American Association of Neuromuscular & Electrodiagnostic Medicine, 8169
American College of Advancement in Medicine (ACAM), 612
American College of Nurse Midwives (ACNM), 613
American Herb Association Newsletter, 4945
American Migraine Foundation, 1912, 2927
American Sexual Health Association, 8306
American Society for the Alexander Technique (AmSAT), 624
American Society of Clinical Hypnosis (ASCH), 625
Aromatherapy Book: Applications and Inhalations, 4952
Aromatherapy for Common Ailments, 4953
Association for Applied Psychophysiology and Biofeedback (AAPB), 632
Ayurvedic Institute, 2570
Bach Flower Therapy: Theory and Practice, 4958
Bastyr Center for Natural Health, 641
Beliefs, Values, and Principles of Self Advocacy, 4960
Brain Allergies: The Psychonutrient and Magnetic Connections, 8515
Center for Mind-Body Medicine, 657
Chinese Herbal Medicine, 4978
Chronic Fatigue Syndrome: Your Natural Gu ide to Healing with Diet, Herbs and Other Methods, 8527
Colon Health: Key to a Vibrant Life, 8530
Council of Colleges of Acupuncture & Oriental Medicine, 669
Creating Wholeness: Self-Healing Workbook Using Dynamic Relaxation, Images and Thoughts, 4986
Curing MS: How Science is Solving the Mysteries of Multiple Sclerosis, 8534
The Davis Center, 804, 8004, 8768
Designing and Using Assistive Technology: The Human Perspective, 2270
Disabled Athlete Sports Association (DASA), 681
Divided Legacy: A History of the Schism in Medical Thought, The Bacteriological Era, 2285

Dr. Ida Rolf Institute (DIRI), 688
Environmental Health Center: Dallas, 8318
Esalen Institute, 694
Everybody's Guide to Homeopathic Medicines, 5005
Feldenkrais Guild of North America (FGNA), 702
Flying Manes Therapeutic Riding, Inc., 703
Handbook of Chronic Fatigue Syndrome, 8549
Healing Herbs, 5019
Health Action, 713
Heart of the Mind, 8552
Herb Research Foundation, 5349
Homeopathic Educational Services, 717
Imagery in Healing Shamanism and Modern Medicine, 5027
Informed Touch; A Clinician's Guide To The Evaluation Of Myofascial Disorders, 8558
International Association of Hygienic Physicians, 8327
International Association of Yoga Therapists (IAYT), 724
International Childbirth Education Association, 1940
International Clinic of Biological Regeneration (ICBR), 727
It's All in Your Head: The Link Between Mercury Amalgams and Illness, 8562
JoanBorysenko.Com, 5354
Journal of Midwifery & Women's Health (JMWH), 2120
Living Beyond Multiple Sclerosis: A Woman's Guide, 8574
Living an Idea: Empowerment and the Evolution of an Alternative School, 1855
Long Beach Department of Health and Human Services, 3300
Los Angeles County Department of Health Services, 3301
Lupus: Alternative Therapies That Work, 8583
National Association for Holistic Aromatherapy (NAHA), 747
National Association to Advance Fat Acceptance, 8343
National Center for Homeopathy, 1950
National Certification Commission for Acupuncture and Oriental Medicine, 760
National Guild of Hypnotists (NGH), 765
National Headache Foundation, 2808
National University of Natural Medicine (NUNM), 770
Nothing is Impossible: Reflections on a New Life, 5069
Nutritional Desk Reference, 5070
Nutritional Influences on Illness:, 5071
Optometric Extension Program Foundation, 2857
Our Own Road, 5283
Pacific Institute of Aromatherapy, 778
Pain Erasure, 5151
Pain Erasure: the Bonnie Prudden Way, 9056
Professional Association of Therapeutic Horsemanship International (PATH Intl.), 788, 8285
Small Wonder, 1887
Solving the Puzzle of Chronic Fatigue, 8639
Structural Integration: The Journal of the Rolf Institute, 2142
Therapeutic Touch International Association (TTIA), 808
Tourette's Syndrome: Tics, Obsessions, Compulsions: Developmental Psychopathology, 8652
United States Trager Association, 811
Upledger Institute International (UII), 813
Weiner's Herbal, 5115

Amputation

American Amputee Foundation, 7928
Amputee Coalition, 628
Baylor Institute for Rehabilitation, 6982
Botsford Center For Rehabilitation & Health Improvement-Redford, 6815
Breaking New Ground Resource Center, 8714
Camp No Limits California, 865

Amythrophic Lateral Sclerosis

Art & Music Therapies

Arthritis

Asthma

Attention Deficit Disorder

Autism

Behavioral Disorders

Birth Defects

Blind/Deaf

Brain Injuries

Cancer

Cerebral Palsy

Chiropractics

Chronic Disabilities

Cleft Palate

Cognitive Disorders

Cystic Fibrosis

Dementia

Dental Issues

Depression

Developmental Disabilities

Change, Inc., 660
Cheyenne Village, 5777
Children's Beach House, 928
Civitan Foundation, 2641
Clausen House, 6406
Clay Tree Society, 665
Clearbrook, 5841
Colton-Redlands-Yucaipa Regional Occupational Program (CRY-ROP), 5750
Communication Development and Disorders in African American Children, 8795
Communitas Supportive Care Society, 667
Community Employment Services, 5751
Community Gatepath, 6407
Comprehensive Rehabilitation Center of Naples Community Hospital, 6559
Connecticut Office of Protection and Advocacy for Persons with Disabilities, 3319
CranstonArc, 3091
DOCS: Developmental Observation Checklist System, 2512
Datahr Rehabilitation Institute, 6527
Desert Haven Enterprises, 5753
Developmental Disabilities Resource Center (DDRC), 5779
Developmental Disabilities in Infancy and Childhood, 5133
Developmental Disabilities: A Handbook for Interdisciplinary Practice, 2277
Developmental Services Center, 2514
Devereux Advanced Behavioral Health - Florida, 6563
Devereux Advanced Behavioral Health Colorado, 6510
Devereux Advanced Behavioral Health Florida - Titusville Campus, 6562
Devereux Threshold Center for Autism, 6566
Dictionary of Developmental Disabilities Terminology, 4991, 5134
Directory for Exceptional Children, 1968
Directory of Members, 4992
Donaldsville Area Arc, 6751
Dynamic Dimensions, 5781
Dyspraxia Foundation USA, 7933
Eastern Colorado Services for the Developmentally Disabled (ECSDD), 5782
Easterseals, 690, 8720
Easterseals Gilchrist Marchman Child Development Center, 6657
Elwyn, 691
Elwyn Delaware, 4626, 6544
FYI, 2152
Family Support Project for the Developmentally Disabled, 8722
Family-Centered Service Coordination: A Manual for Parents, 5141
Federal Laws of the Mentally Handicapped: Laws, Legislative Histories and Admin. Documents, 4533
Fellow Insider, 2154
Field Notes, 2155
Foundation Industries, 6754
Fragile X Family, 8321
Frank Olean Center, 3093
Gateway Center of Monterey County, 6428
Gateway Industries: Castroville, 6429
Glenkirk, 5844
Goodwill Life Skills Development Program, 5809
Goodwill's Community Employment Services, 5811
Goodwill's JobWorks, 5813
The Guided Tour, Inc., 5454
Handbook of Developmental Education, 2324
Happiness Bag, 992
Hartford Foundation for Public Giving, 2726
HealthSouth Sports Medicine & Rehabilitation Center, 6113
Hockanum Greenhouse, 6531
Illinois Life Span Program, 5845
Inclusion, 2111
Independence, 7595
Information Services for People with Developmental Disabilities, 5032
Innabah Camps, 1245

Institute for Basic Research in Developmental Disabilities, 4797
Intellectual and Developmental Disabilities (IDD), 2112
James L. Maher Center, 3095
Jersey Cape, 5963
Joseph P Kennedy Jr Foundation, 2743
Kamp Kaleo, 1090, 8946
Katy Isaacson Elaine Gordon Lodge, 1148
Keep the Promise: Managed Care and People with Disabilities, 5042
Kennedy Job Training Center, 5847
Kent County Arc, 2890
Knox County Board of Developmental Disabilities, 5848
Lambs Farm, 5850
Lambton County Developmental Services (LCDS), 735
Legacy, 7597
Life Unlimited, 7700
Life-Span Approach to Nursing Care for Individuals with Developmental Disabilities, 2367
Lifelong Leisure Skills and Lifestyles for Persons with Developmental Disabilities, 5046
Lions Den Outdoor Learning Center, 7754
LoSeCa Foundation, 740
Lutherdale Bible Camp, 1344
MAGIC Foundation for Children's Growth, 2803
MAGIC Touch, 8584
Mainstay Life Services Summer Program, 1246
Match-Sort-Assemble Pictures, 1863
Match-Sort-Assemble SCHEMATICS, 1864
Member Update, 2165
Minnesota Governor's Council on Developmental Disabilities, 3492
Missouri Division Of Developmental Disabilities, 3505
Montgomery County Arc, 3112
Mosholu Day Camp, 1152
Music Therapy for the Developmentally Disabled, 40
NACDD Annual Conference, 1749
Napa Valley PSI Inc., 5760
National Association for Developmental Disabilities (NADD), 7706
National Association of Councils on Developmental Disabilities (NACDD), 750
National Association of State Directors of Developmental Disabilities Services (NASDDDS), 752
National Theatre Workshop of the Handicapped (NTWH), 51
Nevada Governor's Council on Developmental Disabilities, 5944
New Directions For People With Disabilities, 5450
New Directions for People with Disabilities, 2619
New Hampshire Bureau of Developmental Services, 3542
New Hampshire Developmental Disabilities Council, 3546
New Horizons Summer Day Camp, 896, 7757, 8775
Nuvisions For Disabled Artists, Inc., 56
Oak-Leyden Developmental Services, 7715
Parallels in Time, 5075
Parents and Friends, Inc, 5762
Pioneer Center for Human Services, 6678
Porterville Sheltered Workshop, 5765
President's Committee on People with Intellectual Disabilities, 3240
Prime Time, Inc., 1336
Primrose Center, 5817
Professional Fit Clothing, 1379
Project Independence, 5766
Quest, Inc., 5819, 6599
Quest, Inc. - Tampa Area, 5820, 6600
Raven Rock Lutheran Camp, 7763
Rehabilitation Opportunities, 6779
Relaxation Techniques for People with Special Needs, 5291
Rhode Island Arc, 3096
Richmond Research Training Center (RRTC), 6043
Sebasticook Farms-Great Bay Foundation, 6770

Sequanota Lutheran Conference Center and Camp, 1249, 8776
Sexuality and the Developmentally Handicapped, 5157
Shore Training Center, 5854
Sibpage, 2175
SleepSafe Beds, 165
Social Vocational Services, 5769
Special Services Summer Day Camp, 1154
Spring Dell Center, 8001
St. Francis Camp On The Lake, 1053
St. John Valley Associates, 7718
St. Paul Abilities Network, 798
Steps to Independence: Teaching Everyday Skills to Children with Special Needs, 8641
Summit Camp, 1155, 7770
Sundial Special Vacations, 5453
TERI, 5106
Teacher Education Division (TED), 1956
Tennessee Council on Developmental Disabilities, 3698
Thumb Industries, 6831
Torah Alliance of Families of Kids with Disabilities, 5617
Toyei Industries, 6362
Trips Inc., 5455
United Foundation for Disabled Archers, 8289
Unity Language System, 198
Unyeway, 5773
VBS Special Education Teaching Guide, 2481
Ventures Travel, 5456
Waban Projects, 817
Warren Achievement Center, 6700
Wisconsin Badger Camp, 1347
YAI: National Institute for People with Disabilities, 821
YMCA Outdoor Center Campbell Gard, 1200, 8493
Young Children with Special Needs: A Developmentally Appropriate Approach, 2563

Diabetes

ADA Annual Scientific Sessions, 1722
ADA Camp 180, 1119
ADA Camp Aspire, 1122
ADA Camp GranADA, 963, 8363
ADA Camp Needlepoint, 8364
ADA Teen Adventure Camp, 964, 8365
ADA Triangle D Camp, 965, 8366
American Diabetes Association, 8301
The Barton Center, 1037
The Barton Center Camp Joslin, 1038
The Barton Center Clara Barton Camp, 1039
The Barton Center Danvers Day Camp, 1040
The Barton Center Family Camp, 1041
The Barton Center Worcester Day Camp, 1042
Bearskin Meadow Camp, 856, 8371
Camp AZDA, 842
Camp Adam Fisher, 1258
Camp Buck, 1092
Camp Carefree, 1098, 1161, 8385
Camp Carolina Trails, 1162
Camp Classen YMCA, 8389
Camp Comeca & Retreat Center, 8013
Camp Conrad Chinnock, 860, 8390
Camp Daypoint, 1339
Camp Discovery - Illinois, 8392
Camp Discovery Kansas, 1001, 8393
Camp Endres, 1203
Camp Floyd Rogers, 1086, 8396
Camp Freedom, 1231
Camp Gilbert, 1264
Camp Glyndon, 8398
Camp Hamwi, 1177
Camp Hertko Hollow, 998, 8402
Camp Hickory Hill, 1074, 8403
Camp Ho Mita Koda, 1179, 8404
Camp Hodia, 959, 8405
Camp Hope, 1350
Camp ICANDO, 1310
Camp John Warvel, 985, 8410
Camp Jordan, 1324
Camp Joslin, 8411

Camp Ko-Man-She, 1181, 8413
Camp Korelitz, 1182
Camp Kudzu, 951
Camp Kweebec, 8414
Camp Libbey, 8417
Camp Lo-Be-Gon, 1204
Camp Midicha, 1048
Camp Needlepoint, 1342
Camp Nejeda, 1110, 8420
Camp New Horizons North, 1289
Camp New Horizons South, 1290
Camp NoLoHi, 1292
Camp Planet D, 1002
Camp Sandcastle, 1295
Camp Seale Harris, 825, 8430
Camp Setebaid, 1238, 8431
Camp Sioux, 1171
Camp Sugar Falls, 1275
Camp Sweeney, 1298, 8436
Camp Sweet Betes, 1004
Camp Tiponi, 1188
Camp Waziyatah, 8440
Camps for Children & Teens with Diabetes, 1326, 8443
Canadian Diabetes Association, 8313
Cedar Ridge Camp, 8444
Center for the Partially Sighted, 6400
Clara Barton Camp, 8446
Coast to Coast Home Medical, 243
Comprehensive Rehabilitation Center at Lee Memorial Hospital, 6558
Diabetes Camp, 8447
Diabetes Network of East Hawaii, 3370
Diabetes Self-Management, 8689
Diabetes Sourcebook., 8536
EDI Camp, 8450
FCYD Camp Utada, 1314, 8452
Florida Diabetes Camp, 939, 8454
Friends Academy Summer Camps, 8455
Gales Creek Diabetes Camp, 1217
Growing Together Diabetes Camp, 8457
Immune System Disorders Sourcebook., 8557
JDRF, 732
Joslin Guide to Diabetes: A Program for Managing Your Treatment, 8563
Kids Rock The World Day Camp, 1315
Kiwanis Camp Wyman, 8461
Kluge Children's Rehabilitation Center, 6308
Makemie Woods Camp, 8464
Makemie Woods Camp/Conference Retreat, 8465
Meeting the Needs of People with Vision Loss: Multidisciplinary Perspective, 9047
National Diabetes Action Network for the Blind, 8915
National Institute of Diabetes and Digestive and Kidney Diseases, 3230
NeSoDak, 1265, 8470
No More Allergies, 8602
The Rainbow Club, 926
Raleigh Rehabilitation and Healthcare Center, 7178
Resources for People with Disabilities and Chronic Conditions, 5094
STIX Diabetes Programs, 1337, 8475
Taking Control of Your Diabetes (TCOYD), 8360
Vermont Overnight Camp, 1320
Voice of the Diabetic, 8709
Y Camp, 8486

Diet & Nutrition

Feingold Association of the US, 701
Genova Diagnostics, 706, 4810
National Association of Anorexia Nervosa and Associated Disorders, 8341
Pure Facts, 7899

Down Syndrome

Adolescents with Down Syndrome: Toward a More Fulfilling Life, 7781
Biomedical Concerns in Persons with Down's Syndrome, 2228
Bobby Dodd Institute (BDI), 6617

Bus Girl: Selected Poems, 7805
Camp Oginali, 1273
Clockworks, 5249
Communication Development in Children with Down Syndrome, 7809, 8796
Down Syndrome, 7817
Down Syndrome Camp, 1069
Down Syndrome News, 7894
Down Syndrome Society of Rhode Island, 3092
Early Communication Skills for Children with Down Syndrome, 2287
Keys to Parenting a Child with Downs Syndrome, 7843
National Association for Down Syndrome, 7707
National Down Syndrome Congress, 7712
National Down Syndrome Society, 7713
Parent's Guide to Down Syndrome: Toward a Brighter Future, 7854
Teaching Children with Down Syndrome about Their Bodies, Boundaries, and Sexuality, 5182
Teaching Reading to Children with Down Syndrome: A Guide for Parents and Teachers, 2456
Understanding Down Syndrome: An Introduction for Parents, 7874

Dyslexia

Annals of Dyslexia, 7881
Annual Conference on Dyslexia and Related Learning Disabilities, 1734
Assets School, 5828
Dyslexia Training Program, 1826
Dyslexia over the Lifespan, 7819
Gow School Summer Programs, 1146, 7750
How To Reach and Teach Children and Teens with Dyslexia, 7836
Individualized Keyboarding, 1841
Instrumental Music for Dyslexics: A Teaching Handbook, 31
International Dyslexia Association, 1941
International Dyslexia Association of DC, 3335
International Dyslexia Association: Arizona Branch, 3279
International Dyslexia Association: Austin Branch, 3710
International Dyslexia Association: Central California Branch, 3299
International Dyslexia Association: Central Ohio Branch, 3623
International Dyslexia Association: Florida Branch, 3352
International Dyslexia Association: Georgia Branch, 3366
International Dyslexia Association: Hawaii Branch, 3380
International Dyslexia Association: Illinois Branch, 3400
International Dyslexia Association: Indiana Branch, 3407
International Dyslexia Association: Iowa Branch, 3409
International Dyslexia Association: Kansas/Missouri Branch, 3420
International Dyslexia Association: Louisiana Branch, 3497
International Dyslexia Association: Maryland Branch, 3450
International Dyslexia Association: New Jersey Branch, 3553
International Dyslexia Association: North Carolina Branch, 3605
International Dyslexia Association: Oregon Branch, 3642
International Dyslexia Association: Pennsylvania Branch, 3652
International Dyslexia Association: Rocky Mountain Branch, 3313
International Dyslexia Association: Tennessee Branch, 3694
International Dyslexia Association: Upper Midwest Branch, 3485
International Dyslexia Association: Virginia Branch, 3756

International Dyslexia Association: Washington State Branch, 3766
International Dyslexia Association: Wisconsin Branch, 3786
Learning Disabilities Sourcebook, 3rd Ed., 35
Let's Write Right: Teacher's Edition, 2365
Louisiana Center for Dyslexia and Related Learning Disorders, 3434
Many Faces of Dyslexia, 1861
Mozart Effect: Tapping the Power of Music to Heal the Body, Strengthen the Mind, 37
Multisensory Teaching of Basic Language Skills: Theory and Practice, 2379
Music and Dyslexia: A Positive Approach, 43
Overcoming Dyslexia, 7852
Overcoming Dyslexia in Children, Adolescents and Adults, 2383
Pre-Reading Screening Procedures, 2540
Reading, Writing and Speech Problems in Children, 7859, 8814
Reality of Dyslexia, 7860
Recording for the Blind & Dyslexic, 9065
Sandhills School, 2587
Southwest Branch of the International Dyslexia Association, 3571
Stern Center for Language and Learning, 8764
TESTS, 2443
Teaching of Reading: A Continuum from Kindergarten through College, The, 2553
To Teach a Dyslexic, 1901
We're Not Stupid, 7922

Education & Counseling

ACA Annual Conference, 1721
ADA National Network, 583
ATIA Conference, 1728
Adapting Early Childhood Curricula for Children with Special Needs (9th Edition), 2195
Advocates for Children of New York (AFC), 593
Alaska Department of Education: Special Education, 2016
American Counseling Association (ACA), 614, 1984
American Disabled for Attendant Programs Today (ADAPT), 616, 7348
American Journal of Occupational Therapy (AJOT), 2085
American Journal of Public Health (AJPH), 5203
American Occupational Therapy Association (AOTA), 620
American Public Health Association, 7351
American Public Health Association (APHA), 622
American Red Cross, 623
Applied Rehabilitation Counseling (Springer Series on Rehabilitation), 2209
Assistive Technology Industry Association (ATIA), 631
Brookline Books, 1987
Building the Healing Partnership: Parents, Professionals and Children with Chronic Illnesses, 2232
Burton Blatt Institute (BBI), 647
Camp Independence, 949, 8408
Cape Organization for Rights of the Disabled (CORD), 4132
Case Management Society of America (CMSA), 653
Center for Inclusive Design and Innovation, 656, 1918
Center for Workplace Compliance, 4488
Chicago Lawyers' Committee for Civil Rights Under Law, 4489
Childhood Disablity and Family Systems(Routledge Library Editions) (Volume 5), 2242
Children's Specialized Hospital Medical Library - Parent Resource Center, 4784
Choices: A Guide to Sex Counseling with Physically Disabled Adults, 2245
Coalition for Health Funding, 666
Council of Parent Attorneys and Advocates (COPAA), 670
Counseling & Values, 2097

Religious Signing: A Comprehensive Guide for All Faiths, 8100
Room Valet Visual-Tactile Alerting System, 432
See What I'm Saying, 9174
Seeing Voices, 8101
Sertoma Camp Endeavor, 942, 8034
Shape Up 'n Sign, 9176
Show Me How: A Manual for Parents of Preschool Blind Children, 9072
Sign Language Interpreting and Interpreter Education, 8102
Sign Language Studies, 8125
Sign of the Times, 9073
Signaling Wake-Up Devices, 434
Signed English Schoolbook, 2428
Signed English Starter, The, 8103
Signing Family: What Every Parent Should Know About Sign Communication, The, 8104
Signing Naturally Curriculum, 1886
Signing for Reading Success, 8105
Signing: How to Speak with Your Hands, 8106
Signs Across America, 8107
Signs for Me: Basic Sign Vocabulary for Children, Parents & Teachers, 8108
Signs for Sexuality: A Resource Manual, 8109
Signs of the Times, 8110
Silent Garden, The, 8111
Sing Praise Hymnal for the Deaf, 8112
Smoke Detector with Strobe, 435
Sonic Alert, 191
Sonic Alert Alarm Clock with Bed Shaker, 166
Sound & Fury, 5297
Soundings Newsletter, 8145
Speech Adjust-A-Tone Basic, 192
Speech and the Hearing-Impaired Child, 2434
Starkey Hearing Foundation, 272, 8002
Store @ HDSC Product Catalog, 395
Strobe Light Signalers, 438
TDI National Directory & Resource Guide: Blue Book, 8113
TTYs: Telephone Device for the Deaf, 194
Telecommunications for the Deaf and Hard of Hearing, 8003
Test of Early Reading Ability Deaf or Hard of Hearing, 2555
Texas School of the Deaf, 2076
Theoretical Issues in Sign Language Research, 8114
There's a Hearing Impaired Child in My Class, 2473
Thinklabs One Stethoscope, 256
To Love this Life: Quotations by Helen Keller, 9088
Toward Effective Public School Program for Deaf Students, 2474
USA Deaf Sports Federation, 8163
Ultratec, 273
Usher Syndrome, 8659
Vestibular Disorders Association, 8006
Vision Magazine, 8147
Volta Review, 8126
We CAN Hear and Speak, 8115
Week the World Heard Gallaudet, The, 8116
Weitbrecht Communications, Inc. (WCI), 397
What is Auditory Processing?, 8117
You and Your Deaf Child: A Self-Help Guidefor Parents of Deaf and Hard of Hearing Children, 8118
Youth Leadership Camp, 8037
iLuv SmartShaker 2, 167

Hemophilia

Arizona Hemophilia Association, 8310
Bright Horizons Summer Camp, 8374
Camp Ailihpomeh, 1279
Camp Brave Eagle, 984
Camp H.U.G., 846, 8399
Camp High Hopes, 1131
Camp Honor, 847, 8407
Camp Hot-to-Clot, 1232
Camp Klotty Pine, 1341
Camp Little Oak, 1134
Hemophilia Camp, 8460

National Hemophilia Foundation, 2996, 8348

Herbal Medicine

American Botanical Council (ABC), 609
American Herbalists Guild (AHG), 618
HerbalEGram, 2160
HerbalGram, 2108

Human Interaction Disabilities

Camp Akeela, 1226
Camp Buckskin, 1056, 7729
Camp Connect, 1099
Eagle Hill School: Summer Program, 1033, 7747
Taking Part: Introducing Social Skills to Young Children, 2552

Immune Deficiencies

IDF National Conference, 1747
Immune Deficiency Foundation, 720, 2853
POZ Magazine, 8679
YMCA Camp Shady Brook, 8490

Incontinence

Duraline Medical Products Inc., 246
Informer, 8692
Kleinert's, 380
MOMS Catalog, 384
National Association for Continence, 8192
Quality Care Newsletter, 8700
Simon Foundation for Continence, 8202
Specialty Care Shoppe, 1387

Language Disorders

Academic Language Therapy Association, 8738
American Speech-Language-Hearing Association, 7958, 8739
Association of Language Companies, 8741
Beyond Baby Talk: From Sounds to Sentences, a Parent's Guide to Language Development, 8790
International Fluency Association, 8751
Language Arts: Detecting Special Needs, 2356
Language Disabilities in Children and Adolescents, 8802
Language and Communication Disorders in Children, 2358
Lindamood-Bell Home Learning Process, 8752
OWLS: Oral and Written Language Scales LC/OE & WE, 2531
PAT-3: Photo Articulation Test, 2532
Peabody Early Experiences Kit (PEEK), 2533
Peabody Language Development Kits (PLDK), 2535
Perspectives: Whole Language Folio, 8811
Preventing Academic Failure - Teachers Handbook, 2399
RULES: Revised, 2543
Receptive-Expressive Emergent-REEL-2 Language Test, 2nd Edition, 2544
Teaching Language-Disabled Children: A Communication/Games Intervention, 2452
Teaching Reading to Disabled and Handicapped Learners, 2457
Test of Language Development: Primary, 2556
Test of Phonological Awareness, 2559
Woodcock Reading Mastery Tests, 2562

Learning Disabilities

AEPS Child Progress Record: For Children Ages Three to Six, 1798
AEPS Child Progress Report: For Children Ages Birth to Three, 2489
AEPS Curriculum for Birth to Three Years, 2191
AEPS Curriculum for Three to Six Years, 1799
AEPS Data Recording Forms: For Children Ages Birth to Three, 2490

AEPS Data Recording Forms: For Children Ages Three to Six, 1800
AEPS Family Interest Survey, 1801
AEPS Family Report: For Children Ages Birth to Three, 4933
AEPS Measurement for Birth to Three Years, 2491
AEPS Measurement for Three to Six Years, 2492
AIR: Assessment of Interpersonal Relations, 2493
AVKO Educational Research Foundation, 1909
Academic Therapy Publications, 1982
Activity-Based Approach to Early Intervention, 2nd Edition, 2193
Adaptive Education Strategies Building on Diversity, 2197
Adaptive Mainstreaming: A Primer for Teachers and Principals, 3rd Edition, 2495
Advanced Language Tool Kit, 1803
Ages & Stages Questionnaires, 2496
All Kinds of Minds, 1804
Alphabetic Phonics Curriculum, 2204
Alternative Educational Delivery Systems, 2205
American College Testing Program, 2497
American School Counselor Association, 1913
Arkansas Department of Special Education, 2017
Assessing Students with Special Needs, 2498
Assessment Log & Developmental Progress Charts for the CCPSN, 2213, 2499
Assessment of Learners with Special Needs, 2500
Assessment: The Special Educator's Role, 2219
Assistive Technology, 174
Association of Educational Therapists (AET), 635
Association on Higher Education & Disability (AHEAD), 640, 1915
BOSC: Directory of Facilities for People with Learning Disabilities, 1961
Beacon Therapeutic Diagnostic and Treatment Center, 6643
Beginning Reasoning and Reading, 1811
Behind Special Education, 2227
Benchmark Measures, 2501
BroadFutures, 7684
Buy!, 1813
CAI, Career Assessment Inventories for the Learning Disabled, 2233
CEC Catalog, 2088
CEC Pioneers Division (CEC-PD), 1917
CREVT: Comprehensive Receptive and Expressive Vocabulary Test, 2503
Camp Nuhop, 1183, 7736
Camp Starfish, 1032
Carolina Curriculum for Infants and Toddlers with Special Needs (3rd Edition), 2235
Carolina Curriculum for Preschoolers with Special Needs, 2236
Catalyst, 2091
Center Academy, 7685
Center Academy at Pinellas Park, 935, 7745
Charis Hills Camp, 1300
Chemists with Disabilities Committee - American Chemical Society, 5225
Children's Understanding of Disability, 4886
Christian Approach to Overcoming Disability: A Doctor's Story, 4979
Clovernook Printing House, The Clovernook Center for the Blind and Visually Impaired, 8878
Cognitive Approaches to Learning Disabilities, 2250
College Internship Program at the Berkshire Center, 6792
Colorado Department of Education: Special Education Service Unit, 2019
Communicating with Parents of Exceptional Children, 2254
Complete Handbook of Children's Reading Disorders: You Can Prevent or Correct LDs, 2258
Complete Learning Disabilities Resource Guide, 1963
Complete Resource Guide for Pediatric Disorders, 1965
Complete Resource Guide for People with Chronic Illness, 1966
Computer Access/Computer Learning, 2259

Lowe's Syndrome

Lung Disorders

Massage Therapy

Mental Disabilities

Multiple Disabilities

TLC Speech-Language/Occupational TherapyCamps, 2551, 5909, 6781
Take a Chance, 5416
TalkTrac Wearable Communicator, 195
Talkable Tales, 8821
Understanding & Controlling Stuttering: A Comprehensive New Approach Based on the Valsa Hyp, 8825
Voice Amplified Handsets, 199
Wendell Johnson Speech & Hearing Clinic, 8778

Spina Bifida

Agassiz Village, 8369
Camp MITIOG, 1075, 8418
Educational Issues Among Children with Spina Bifida, 8541
Genetics and Spina Bifida, 8546
In the Middle, 5269
Introduction to Spina Bifida, 8561
Latex Allergy in Spina Bifida Patients, 8566
Learning Among Children with Spina Bifida, 8567
Lipomas & Lipomyelomeningocele, 8572
Mountaineer Spina Bifida Camp, 1338, 8468
Obesity, 8605
Occulta, 8607
Plan Ahead: Do What You Can, 8624
SPINabilities: A Young Person's Guide to Spina Bifida, 8634
Sexuality and the Person with Spina Bifida, 8636
Sherman Lake YMCA Summer Camp, 8477
Social Development and the Person with Spina Bifida, 8638
Spina Bifida Association, 8357
Spina Bifida Program of Children's National Medical Center, 6553
Spina Bifida and Hydrocephalus Association of Canada, 8358
Symptomatic Chiari Malformation, 8646
Taking Charge, 8647
Urologic Care of the Child with Spina Bifida, 8658

Spinal Cord Injuries

ASIA Annual Scientific Meeting, 1727
Academy of Spinal Cord Injury Professionals, 8165
Academy of Spinal Cord Injury Professionals: Psychologists, Social Workers & Counselors, 8166
American Spinal Injury Association, 8172
Camp PossAbility, 988
Christopher & Dana Reeve Foundation, 4785
Christopher & Dana Reeve Paralysis Resource Center, 8179
Cure SMA, 8181
Directions, 8690
Functional Electrical Stimulation for Ambulation by Paraplegics, 8223
Guide to Wheelchair Sports and Recreation, 8277
Head Injury Rehabilitation And Referral Service, Inc. (HIRRS), 8185
Journey to Well: Learning to Live After Spinal Cord Injury, 8564
Living With Spinal Cord Injury Series, 8578
National Coalition for Assistive and Rehab Technology, 8194
National Fibromyalgia Association, 8196, 8347
NeuroControl Corporation, 5371
PVA Adaptive Sports, 5510
PVA Summit & Expo, 1755
Paralysis Resource Guide, 8229
Paralyzed Veterans of America, 5432, 8200
SCI Life, 8680
SCI Psychosocial Process, 8702
Shirley Ryan AbilityLab, 794
Southeastern Paralyzed Veterans of America, 5523
Spinal Cord Dysfunction, 2436
Spine, 8681
Sports 'N Spokes Magazine, 5420
Tethering Cord, 8706
Topics in Spinal Cord Injury Rehabilitation, 8235
United Spinal Association, 8204

VA North Texas Health Veterans Affairs Care System: Dallas VA Medical Center, 5673

Stroke

American Stroke Association, 7931, 8173
Children's Hemiplegia & Stroke Association, 8178
National Stroke Association, 7941
Stroke Sourcebook, 2nd Edition, 8643

Theater & Dance Therapies

American Dance Therapy Association (ADTA), 4
Disability and Social Performance: Using Drama to Achieve Successful Acts, 22
National Association for Drama Therapy, 48
National Theatre of the Deaf, 52
Non-Traditional Casting Project, 55
Phoenix Dance, 5286

Tinnitus

American Tinnitus Association (ATA), 627, 7959
Tinnitus Today, 8130

Tourette Syndrome

TSA CT Kid's Summer Event, 8481
TSA Newsletter, 8704
Tourette Association of America, 7723
Tourette Association of America National Education Conference, 1761
Tourette Syndrome Association Children's Newsletter, 8707
Twitch and Shout, 5302

Visual Impairments

AAO Annual Meeting, 1720
AER Annual International Conference, 1723
AFB Center on Vision Loss, 2946
AFB Directory of Services for Blind and Visually Impaired Persons in the US and Canada, 8953
AFB News, 9113
AFB Press, 1981
About Children's Eyes, 8954
About Children's Vision: A Guide for Parents, 8955
Access to Art: A Museum Directory for Blind and Visually Impaired People, 8956
Adaptek Systems, 170
Adaptive Services Division, 9115
Adjustable Folding Support Cane for the Blind, 491
African Americans in the Profession of Blindness Services, 8957
Age-Related Macular Degeneration, 8958
Ai Squared, 5316
All Terrain Cane, 492
American Academy of Ophthalmology, 8854
American Anals of the Deaf Reference, 8959
American Blind Bowling Association, 9180
American Council of Blind Lions, 8856
American Council of the Blind, 3, 8857
American Council of the Blind Radio Amateurs, 8858
American Foundation for the Blind, 2951, 8859
American Optometric Association, 8860
American Printing House for the Blind, 8861
Americans with Disabilities Act Guide for Places of Lodging: Serving Guests Who Are Blind, 8960
Amerock Corporation, 2784
Annual Report/Newsletter, 9117
Arizona Rehabilitation State Services for the Blind and Visually Impaired, 3276
Arkenstone: The Benetech Initiative, 1401
Art and Science of Teaching Orientation and Mobility to Persons with Visual Impairments, 8961
Assemblies of God Center for the Blind, 4770
Associated Services for the Blind and Visually Impaired, 4828, 8862

Association for Education & Rehabilitationof the Blind & Visually Impaired, 8863
Association for Macular Diseases, 8864
Association for Macular Diseases Newsletter, 9118
Association for Research in Vision and Ophthalmology, 8865
Association for Vision Rehabilitation and Employment, 8866
Association of Blind Citizens, 8867
Awareness, 9119
Babycare Assistive Technology, 8963
Babycare Assistive Technology for Parents with Physical Disabilties, 8964
Backgammon Set: Deluxe, 5393
Basketball: Beeping Foam, 9181
Beam, 7650
Berthold Lowenfeld on Blindness and Blind People, 8968
Beyond Sight, Inc., 494
Big Button Talking Calculator with Function Replay, 495
Big and Bold Low Vision Timer, 276
Blind Babies Foundation, 2653
Blind Children's Center, 8868
Blind Children's Center Annual Meeting, 1738
Blind Children's Fund, 2879
Blind Information Technology Specialists, 8869
Blind Outdoor Leisure Development, 9182
Blind and Vision-Impaired Individuals, 8969
Blinded Veterans Association, 8870
Blinded Veterans Association National Convention, 1739
Blindness, 5242
Blindness and Early Childhood Development Second Edition, 8970
Blindness: What it is, What it Does and How to Live with it, 8971
Board Games: Peg Solitaire, 5394
Board Games: Snakes and Ladders, 5395
Bold Line Paper, 481
Books are Fun for Everyone, 8972
Books for Blind and Physically Handicapped Individuals, 8974
Braille Calendar, 482
Braille Documents, 5244
Braille Elevator Plates, 496
Braille Forum, 9103
Braille Institute Orange County Center, 9186
Braille Institute of America, 8871
Braille Notebook, 483
Braille Paper, 1435
Braille Playing Cards, 5396
Braille Timer, 279
Braille Touch-Time Watches, 497
Braille: An Extraordinary Volunteer Opportunity, 8976
Braille: Bingo Cards, Boards and Call Numbers, 5397
Braille: Greeting Cards, 484
Braille: Rook Cards, 5398
Brailon Plastic Sheets, 1436
Bureau Of Exceptional Education And Student Services, 3343
Burns Braille Transcription Dictionary, 8977
California Department of Education: Special Education Division, 2018
California State Library Braille and Talking Book Library, 4602, 8872
Camp Barakel, 8934
Camp Bloomfield, 858, 8935
Camp Can-Do, 1285
Camp Challenge, 1010, 8936
Camp Dogwood, 1163
Camp Inter-Actions, 1100
Camp Lawroweld, 1016, 8937
Camp Lighthouse, 929, 8938
Camp Lou Henry Hoover, 8939
Camp Mauchatea, 1253
Camp Webber, 840
Camp Winnekeag, 8941
Can't Your Child See? A Guide for Parents of Visually Impaired Children, 8978
Can-Do Products Catalog, 141
Canine Helpers for the Handicapped, 652, 8873

Women

Camp Lighthouse, 929
Center for Mind-Body Medicine, 657
Children's National Medical Center, 664
Chronicle Guide to Grants, 3188
Coalition for Health Funding, 666
Department of Medicine and Surgery Veterans Administration, 5465
Department of Veterans Affairs Regional Office - Vocational Rehab Division, 5466
Department of Veterans Benefits, 5467
Disability Rights International (DRI), 678
Disabled American Veterans, 5509
District of Columbia Center for Independen t Living, 3930
District of Columbia Department of Employment Services, 5799
District of Columbia Public Library: Services for the Deaf Community, 4627
District of Columbia Regional Library for the Blind and Physically Handicapped, 4628
Eugene and Agnes E Meyer Foundation, 2738
Eye Bank Association of America Annual Meeting, 1746
Federal Benefits for Veterans and Dependents, 5469
Federal Student Aid Information Center, 2739
GEICO Philanthropic Foundation, 2740
Georgetown University Center for Child and Human Development, 4629
Goodwill of Greater Washington, 5800
Guide Service of Washington, 5449
HEATH Resource Center at the National Youth Transitions Center, 709
Habilitation Benefits Coalition, 710
Institute for Educational Leadership (IEL), 722
Jacob and Charlotte Lehrman Foundation, 2741
Joseph P Kennedy Jr Foundation, 2743
Kiplinger Foundation, 2744
Laurent Clerc National Deaf Education Cent er, 736
Montgomery County Arc, 3112
Morris and Gwendolyn Cafritz Foundation, 2745
NACDD Annual Conference, 1749
National Association of City and County he alth Officials, 749
National Association of Councils on Develo pmental Disabilities (NACDD), 750
National Certification Commission for Acup uncture and Oriental Medicine, 760
National Council on Independent Living (NCIL), 762, 3931
National Disability Rights Network (NDRN), 763
National Health Council, 766
National Institute on Disability, Independ ent Living, and Rehabilitation Research (NIDILRR), 767, 4630
National Women's Health Network (NWHN), 772
PVA Adaptive Sports, 5510
PVA Summit & Expo, 1755
Paddy Rossbach Youth Camp, 930
Palladium, 5801
Partnership to Improve Patient Care, 782
Paul and Annetta Himmelfarb Foundation, 2746
Primary Care Collaborative, 787
Public Welfare Foundation, 2747
RESNA Annual Conference, 1758
Rehabilitation Research and Development Center, 5491
Rehabilitation Services Administration, 5802
Sister Cities International, 2623
Student Guide, 3214
TASH, 801
The District of Columbia Office of Human Rights (OHR), 5803
US Department of Veterans Affairs National Headquarters, 5470
VA Medical Center, Washington DC, 5511
Washington DC VA Medical Center, 5512

Florida

Abilities of Florida: An Affiliate of Service Source, 5804
Able Trust, 2748

Able Trust, The, 5805
Adult Day Training, 3933
Alpha One: Bangar, 4116
American Academy of Pain Medicine (AAPM), 598
American Academy of Pain Medicine Foundati on, 599, 2749
American Disabled Golfers Association (ADGA), 615
Arc of Florida, 2750
Bank of America Client Foundation, 2751
Barron Collier Jr Foundation, 2752
Bay Pines VA Medical Center, 5513
Birth Defect Research for Children (BDRC), 643
Brevard County Talking Books Library, 4631
Broward County Talking Book Library, 4632
CIL of Central Florida, 3934
Camiccia-Arnautou Charitable Foundation, 2753
Camp Amigo, 931
Camp Boggy Creek, 932
Camp No Limits Florida, 933
Camp Thunderbird, 934
Caring and Sharing Center for Independent Living, 3935
Caring and Sharing Center: Pasco County, 3936
Center Academy at Pinellas Park, 935
Center for Independent Living in Central Florida, 3937
Center for Independent Living of Broward, 3938
Center for Independent Living of Florida Keys, 3939
Center for Independent Living of N Florida, 3940
Center for Independent Living of NW Florid a, 3941
Center for Independent Living of North Central Florida, 3942
Center for Independent Living of North Cen tral Florida, 3943
Center for Independent Living of S Florida, 3944
Center for Independent Living of SW Florida, 3945
Centers of Excellence Leadership Conferenc e, 1741
Chatlos Foundation, 2754
Coalition for Independent Living Options: Okeechobee, 3946
Coalition for Independent Living Options: Fort Pierce, 3947
Coalition for Independent Living Options, 3948
Coalition for Independent Living Options: Stuart, 3949
Dade County Talking Book Library, 4633
Dialysis at Sea Cruises, 5445
Disability Matters, 1745
Disability Rights Florida, 677
Dr. Moises Simpser VACC Camp, 936
Dream Oaks Camp, 937
Easterseals Camp Challenge, 938
Edyth Bush Charitable Foundation, 2755
Enable America Inc., 693
FPL Group Foundation, 2756
Federal Grants & Contracts Weekly, 3194
Florida Diabetes Camp, 939
Florida Division of Blind Services, 4634, 5806
Florida Division of Vocational Rehabilitation, 5807
Florida Fair Employment Practice Agency, 5808
Florida Instructional Materials Center for the Visually Impaired (FIMC-VI), 4635
Foundation & Corporate Grants Alert, 3201
Gainesville Division, North Florida/South Georgia Veterans Healthcare System, 5514
Goodwill Life Skills Development Program, 5809
Goodwill Temporary Staffing, 5810
Goodwill's Community Employment Services, 5811
Goodwill's Job Connection Center, 5812
Goodwill's JobWorks, 5813
Hand Camp, 940
Hillsborough County Talking Book Library Tampa-Hillsborough County Public Library, 4636
Jacksonville Public Library: Talking Books /Special Needs, 4637

James A Haley VA Medical Center, 5515
Jefferson Lee Ford III Memorial Foundation, 2757
Jessie Ball duPont Fund, 2758
Kris' Camp, 941
Lakeland Adult Day Training, 3951
Lee County Library System: Talking Books Library, 4638
Lighthouse Central Florida, 3952, 5814
Lost Tree Village Charitable Foundation, 2759
Louis de la Parte Florida Mental Health Institute Research Library, 4639
Miami Foundation, The, 2760
Miami VA Medical Center, 5516
Miami-Dade County Disability Services and Independent Living (DSAIL), 3953
Mount Sinai Medical Center, 2761
National Parkinson Foundation, 2762
Norwegian Cruise Line, 5451
Ocala Adult Day Training, 3954
One-Stop Service Center, 5815
Orange County Library System: Audio-Visual Department, 4640
Palm Beach Habilitation Center, 5816
Pearlman Biomedical Research Institute, 4641
Pinellas Park Adult Day Training, 3955
Pinellas Talking Book Library for the Blind and Physically Handicapped, 4642
Primrose Center, 5817
Project SEARCH, 5818
Publix Super Markets Charities, 2763
Quest, Inc., 5819
Quest, Inc. - Tampa Area, 5820
SCCIL at Titusville, 3956
Seagull Industries for the Disabled, 5822
Self Reliance, 3957
Sertoma Camp Endeavor, 942
Space Coast Center for Independent Living, 3958
St. Petersburg Regional Office, 5517
Suncoast Center for Independent Living, Inc., 3959
Talking Book Service: Mantatee County Central Library, 4643
Talking Books Library for the Blind and Physically Handicapped, 4644
Talking Books/Homebound Services, 4645
The Cherab Foundation, 803, 2764
University of Miami: Bascom Palmer Eye Institute, 4646
University of Miami: Mailman Center for Child Development, 4647
Upledger Institute International (UII), 813
West Florida Regional Library, 4648
West Palm Beach VA Medical Center, 5518
Young Onset Parkinson Conference, 1762
disAbility Solutions for Independent Livin g, 3960

Georgia

Aerie Experiences, 943
Arc Of Georgia, 2765
Arms Wide Open, 3961
Athens Talking Book Center-Athens-Clarke County Regional Library, 4649
Atlanta Regional Office, 5519
Atlanta VA Medical Center, 5520
Augusta Talking Book Center, 4650
Augusta VA Medical Center, 5521
Bain, Inc. Center For Independent Living, 3962
Bainbridge Subregional Library for the Blind & Physically Handicapped, 4651
Camp Breathe Easy, 944
Camp Caglewood, 945
Camp Dream, 946
Camp Hawkins, 948
Camp Independence, 949
Camp Juliena, 950
Camp Kudzu, 951
Camp Twin Lakes, 953
Camp Twin Lakes: Rutledge, 954
Camp Twin Lakes: Will-A-Way, 955
Carl Vinson VA Medical Center, 5522
Center for Inclusive Design and Innovation, 656
Columbus Subregional Library For The Blind And Physically Handicapped, 4652

Hawaii

Idaho

Illinois

Peoria Area Community Foundation, 2811
Polk Brothers Foundation, 2812
Progress Center for Independent Living, 4015
Progress Center for Independent Living: Bl ue
 Island, 4016
Regional Access & Mobilization Project, 4017
Regional Access & Mobilization Project: Be
 lvidere, 4018
Regional Access & Mobilization Project: De Kalb,
 4019
Regional Access & Mobilization Project: Fr eeport,
 4020
Retirement Research Foundation, 2813
Rimland Services for Autistic Citizens, 978
Ronald McDonald House Charities (RMHC), 792
Rotary Youth Exchange, 2621
Sears-Roebuck Foundation, 2814
Sertoma Centre, 5853
Shady Oaks Camp, 979
Shirley Ryan AbilityLab, 794
Shore Training Center, 5854
Siragusa Foundation, 2815
Skokie Accessible Library Services, 4679
Soyland Access to Independent Living (SAIL),
 4021
Soyland Access to Independent Living: Char
 leston, 4022
Soyland Access to Independent Living: Shel
 byville, 4023
Soyland Access to Independent Living: Sull ivan,
 4024
Springfield Center for Independent Living, 4025
Square D Foundation, 2816
Stone-Hayes Center for Independent Living, 4026
The Workshop, 5855
Thresholds, 809, 5856
Timber Pointe Outdoor Center, 980
University of Illinois at Chicago: Lions of Illinois
 Eye Research Institute, 4680
VA Illiana Health Care System, 5532
Vocational Rehabilitation Services, 5743, 5857
Voices of Vision Talking Book Center at DuPage
 Library System, 4681
WP and HB White Foundation, 2817
Washington County Vocational Workshop, 5858
Washington Square Health Foundation, 2818
West Central Illinois Center for Independent
 Living, 4027
West Central Illinois Center for Independe nt
 Living: Macomb, 4028
Wheat Ridge Ministries, 2819
Will Grundy Center for Independent Living, 4029

Indiana

ADEC Resources for Independence, 5859
Allen County Public Library, 4682
American Camp Association (ACA), 610
Anderson Woods, 981
Arc Northwest Indiana, 5860
Arc of Indiana, 2820
Assistive Technology Training and Informat ion
 Center (ATTIC), 4030
Association of Independent Camps, 636
BI-County Services, 5861
Ball Brothers Foundation, 2821
Bartholomew County Public Library, 4683
CHAMP Camp, 982
Camp About Face, 983
Camp Brave Eagle, 984
Camp John Warvel, 985
Camp Little Red Door, 986
Camp Millhouse, 987
Camp PossAbility, 988
Camp Red Cedar, 990
Camp Riley, 991
Carey Services, 5862
Community Foundation of Boone County, 2822
DAMAR Services, 4031
Elkhart Public Library for the Blind and Physically
 Handicapped, 4684
Evansville Association for the Blind, 5863
Everybody Counts Center for Independent Living,
 4032

Feingold Association of the US, 701
Four Rivers Resource Services, 4033, 5864
Future Choices Independent Living Center, 4034
Gateway Services/JCARC, 5865
Goodwill of Central & Southern Indiana, 5866
Happiness Bag, 992
Hillcroft Services, 993
Hoosier Burn Camp, 994
Independent Living Center of Eastern Indiana
 (ILCEIN), 4035
Indiana Association for Home and Hospice Care
 (IAHHC), 721
Indiana Civil Rights Commission, 5867
Indiana Deaf Camp, 995
Indiana Disability Employment Initiative, 5868
Indiana Resource Center for Autism, 4685
Indiana University: Multipurpose Arthritis Center,
 4686
Indianapolis Regional Office, 5533
Indianapolis Resource Center for Independe nt
 Living, 4036
John W Anderson Foundation, 2823
Lake County Public Library Talking Books
 Service, 4687
League for the Blind and Disabled, 4037
Martin Luther Homes of Indiana, 4038
New Hope Services, 5869
New Horizons Rehabilitation, 5870
Noble of Indiana, 5871
Paladin, 5872
Putnam County Comprehensive Services, 5873
Richard L Roudebush VA Medical Center, 5534
Ruben Center for Independent Living, 4039
SILC, Indiana Council on Independent Livin g
 (ICOIL), 4040
Southern Indiana Center for Independent Living,
 4041
Southern Indiana Resource Solutions, 5874
Special Services Division: Indiana State Library,
 4688
St. Joseph Hospital Rehabilitation Center, 4689
Sycamore Rehabilitation Services, 5875
Talking Books Service Evansville Vanderburgh
 County Public Library, 4690
VA North Indiana Health Care System: Fort
 Wayne Campus, 5535
VA Northern Indiana Health Care System: Marion
 Campus, 5536
Wabash Independent Living Center & Learning
 Center (WILL), 4042

Iowa

Access, Inc., 5876
Arc of Iowa, 2824
Black Hawk Center for Independent Living, 4043
Camp Albrecht Acres, 996
Camp Courageous of Iowa, 997
Camp Hertko Hollow, 998
Camp Sunnyside, 999
Camp Tanager, 1000
Central Iowa Center for Independent Living, 4044
Des Moines VA Medical Center, 5537
Des Moines VA Regional Office, 5538
Evert Conner Rights & Resources CIL, 4045
Hall-Perrine Foundation, 2825
Hope Haven, 4046
Iowa Career Connection, 5877
Iowa City VA Medical Center, 5539
Iowa Civil Rights Commission, 5878
Iowa Department for the Blind Library, 4691
Iowa Economic Development Authority, 5879
Iowa Registry for Congenital and Inherited
 Disorders, 4692
Iowa Valley Community College, 5880
Iowa Vocational Rehabilitation Services, 5881
Knoxville VA Medical Center, 5540
League of Human Dignity, Center for Indepe ndent
 Living, 4047
Library Commission for the Blind, 4693
Mid-Iowa Health Foundation, 2826
New Focus, 5882
Principal Financial Group Foundation, 2827
Siouxland Community Foundation, 2828

South Central Iowa Center for Independent Living,
 4049
Universal Pediatrics, 812
VA Central Iowa Health Care System, 5541
Youth MOVE National, 822

Kansas

Advocates for Better Living For Everyone
 (A.B.L.E.), 4051
Arc of Kansas, 2829
Association for Applied Psychophysiology and
 Biofeedback (AAPB), 632
Camp Discovery Kansas, 1001
Camp Planet D, 1002
Camp Quality Kansas, 1003
Camp Sweet Betes, 1004
Center for Independent Living SW Kansas: L
 iberal, 4052
Center for Independent Living Southwest Kansas,
 4053
Center for Independent Living Southwest Ka nsas:
 Dodge City, 4054
Center for the Improvement of Human
 Functioning, 4694
Central Kansas Library Systems Headquarter s
 (CSLS), 4695
Coalition for Independence, 4055
Colmery-O'Neil VA Medical Center, 5542
Cowley County Developmental Services, 4056
Dwight D Eisenhower VA Medical Center, 5543
Hutchinson Community Foundation, 2830
Independence, 4057
Independent Connection, 4058
Independent Connection: Abilene, 4059
Independent Connection: Beloit, 4060
Independent Connection: Concordia, 4061
Independent Living Resource Center, 3876, 4062
Kansas Human Rights Commission, 5883
Kansas Services for the Blind & Visually
 Impaired, 4063
Kansas VA Regional Office, 5544
Kansas Vocational Rehabilitation Agency, 5884
LINK: Colby, 4064
Living Independently in Northwest Kansas: Hays,
 4065
Manhattan Public Library, 4696
Northwest Kansas Library System Talking Books,
 4697
Prairie IL Resource Center, 4066
Prairie Independent Living Resource Center, 4067
Resource Center for Independent Living: Emporia,
 4070
Resource Center for Independent Living: Ar kansas
 City, 4071
Resource Center for Independent Living: Bu
 rlington, 4072
Resource Center for Independent Living: Co
 ffeyville, 4073
Resource Center for Independent Living: El
 Dorado, 4074
Resource Center for Independent Living: Ft Scott,
 4075
Resource Center for Independent Living: Ot tawa,
 4076
Resource Center for Independent Living: Ov erland
 Park, 4077
Resource Center for Independent Living: To peka,
 4078
Richard W Higgins Charitable Foundation, 2831
Robert J Dole VA Medical Center, 5545
South Central Kansas Library System, 4698
Southeast Kansas Independent Living (SKIL),
 4079
Southeast Kansas Independent Living:
 Independence, 4080
Southeast Kansas Independent Living: Chanu te,
 4081
Southeast Kansas Independent Living: Colum bus,
 4082
Southeast Kansas Independent Living: Fredo nia,
 4083
Southeast Kansas Independent Living: Hays, 4084

Southeast Kansas Independent Living: Pitts burg, 4085
Southeast Kansas Independent Living: Sedan, 4086
Southeast Kansas Independent Living: Yates Center, 4087
State Library of Kansas, 4699
Three Rivers Independent Living Center, 4088
Three Rivers Independent Living Center: Clay, 4089
Three Rivers Independent Living Center: Ma nhattan, 4090
Three Rivers Independent Living Center: Se neca, 4091
Three Rivers Independent Living Center: To peka, 4092
Topeka & Shawnee County Public Library Talking Books Service, 4700
Topeka Independent Living Resource Center, 4093
Whole Person: Nortonville, 4094
Whole Person: Nortonville, The, 4095
Whole Person: Prairie Village, 4096
Whole Person: Prairie Village, The, 4097
Whole Person: Tonganoxie, 4098
Wichita Public Library/Talking Book Service, 4701
Wichita Public Library/Talking Book Servic e, 4702

Kentucky

Arc of Kentucky, 2832
Camp Quality Kentuckiana, 989, 1005
Center for Accessible Living, 4099
Center for Accessible Living: Murray, 4100
Center for Independent Living: Kentucky Department for the Blind, 4101
Children's Alliance, 662
Disability Coalition of Northern Kentucky, 4102
Disability Resource Initiative, 4103
Disabled American Veterans Headquarters, 5468
EnTech: Enabling Technologies of Kentuckiana, 4703
Independence Place, 4104
Kentucky Commission on Human Rights, 5885
Kentucky Office for the Blind, 5886
Kentucky Talking Book Library - Kentucky Dept. for Libraries and Archives, 4704
Kentucky Vocational Rehabilitation Agency, 5887
Kids Cancer Alliance, 1006
Lexington VA Medical Center, 5546
Lions Camp Crescendo, 1007
Louisville Free Public Library, 4705
Louisville VA Medical Center, 5547
Louisville VA Regional Office, 5548
Pathfinders for Independent Living, 4105
Pioneer Vocational/Industrial Services, 5888
SILC Department of Vocational Rehabilitation, 4106
The Center for Courageous Kids, 1008

Louisiana

Alexandria VA Medical Center, 5549
Arc of Louisiana, 2833
Baton Rouge Area Foundation, 2834
Blind Services, 5889
COEA The Arc of East Ascension, 5890
Camp Bon Coeur, 1009
Camp Challenge, 1010
Camp Pelican, 1011
Camp Quality Louisiana, 1012
Central Louisiana State Hospital Medical and Professional Library, 4706
Community Foundation of Shreveport-Bossier, 2835
Disability Rights Louisiana, 679
Louisiana Lions Camp, 1013
Louisiana Rehabilitation Services, 5891
Louisiana State Library, 4707
Louisiana State University Genetics Sectio n of Pediatrics, 4708
MedCamps of Louisiana, 1014
New Horizons: Central Louisiana, 4107

New Horizons: Northeast Louisiana, 4108
New Horizons: Northwest Louisiana, 4109
New Orleans VA Medical Center, 5550
Resources for Independent Living: Baton Rouge, 4110
Resources for Independent Living: Metairie, 4111
Shreveport VA Medical Center, 5551
Southwest Louisiana Independence Center: L ake Charles, 4112
Southwest Louisians Independence Center: Lafayette, 4113
State Library of Louisiana: Services for the Blind and Physically Handicapped, 4709
The Arc Westbank, 5892
Vocational Rehabilitation Program, 5893
Volunteers of America of Greater New Orlea ns, 4114
W Troy Cole Independent Living Specialist, 4115

Maine

Alpha One: South Portland, 4117
BCR Foundation, 2836
Bangor Public Library, 4710
Bangor Veteran Center: Veterans Outreach Center, 5894
Camp CaPella, 1015
Camp Lawroweld, 1016
Camp No Limits Maine, 1017
Camp Sunshine, 854, 952, 1018, 1018
Camp sNOw Maine, 1019
Cary Library, 4711
Creative Work Systems, 5895
Division for the Blind and Visually Impair ed, 5896
High School Students Guide to Study, Travel, and Adventure Abroad, 2609
Lewiston Public Library, 4712
Maine Commission on Disability & Employmen t, 5897
Maine Department of Labor, 5898
Maine Human Rights Commission, 5899
Maine State Library, 4713
Maine VA Regional Office, 5552
Motivational Services, 4118
No Limits Foundation, 2837
Northeast Occupational Exchange, 5900
Pine Tree Camp, 1020
Portland Public Library, 4715
Shalom House, 4119
Togus VA Medical Center, 5553
UNUM Charitable Foundation, 2838
Waban Projects, 817
Waterville Public Library, 4716
Women to Women Healthcare, 818

Maryland

AAIDD Annual Meeting, 1719
APSE National Conference, 1725
ASHA Convention, 1726
Accreditation Commission for Midwifery Education (ACME), 591
American Association on Health and Disabil ity (AAHD), 604
American Association on Intellectual and Developmental Disabilities (AAIDD), 605
American College of Nurse Midwives (ACNM), 613
American Health Assistance Foundation, 2839
American Occupational Therapy Association (AOTA), 620
American Occupational Therapy Foundation, 2840
American Society of Clinical Hypnosis (ASCH), 625
Anxiety and Depression Association of Amer ica (ADAA), 629
Arc of Maryland, 2841
Ardmore Developmental Center, 5901
Association for International Practical Training, 2603
Association of People Supporting Employmen t First (APSE), 638

Association of University Centers on Disabilities (AUCD), 639
Baltimore Community Foundation, 2842
Baltimore Regional Office, 5554
Baltimore VA Medical Center, 5555
Broadmead, 4120
CASA Inc., 4262
CQL Accreditation, 1740
Camp Great Rock, 1021
Camp Littlefoot, 1022
Camp No Limits Maryland, 1023
Camp SunSibs, 1024
Camp Sunrise, 1025
Candlelighters Childhood Cancer Foundation, 2843
Change, Inc., 660
Children's Fresh Air Society Fund, 2844
Clark-Winchcole Foundation, 2845
Columbia Foundation, 2846
Community Health Funding Report, 3190
Corporate Giving Program, 2847
Council of Parent Attorneys and Advocates (COPAA), 670
Council of State Administrators of Vocational Rehabilitation (CSAVR), 671
Cystic Fibrosis Foundation, 2848
Deaf Camps, Inc., 1026
Department of Physical Medicine & Rehabilitation at Sinai Hospital, 672
Disability Funding News, 3192
Eastern Shore Center for Independent Living, 4121
Easterseals Camp Fairlee, 1027
Family Run Executive Director Leadership Association (FREDLA), 696
Fort Howard VA Medical Center, 5556
Foundation Fighting Blindness, 2849
Freedom Center, 4122
George Wasserman Family Foundation, 2850
Giant Food Foundation, 2851
Goodwill Industries International, 707
Grand Lodge of the International Association of Machinists and Aerospace Workers, 708
Harry and Jeanette Weinberg Foundation, 2852
Housing Unlimited, 4123
Humanity & Inclusion (HI), 719
IDF National Conference, 1747
Immune Deficiency Foundation, 720, 2853
Independence Now, 4124
Independence Now: The Center for Independent Living, 4125
Johns Hopkins University Dana Center for Preventive Ophthalmology, 4717
Johns Hopkins University: Asthma and Allergy Center, 4718
Kennedy Krieger Institute, 2854
League at Camp Greentop, 1028
Lions Camp Merrick, 1029
Making Choices for Independent Living, 4126
Maryland Commission on Civil Rights (FEPA), 5902
Maryland Department of Disabilities, 5903
Maryland State Department of Education, 5905
Maryland State Library for the Blind and Physically Handicapped, 4719
Maryland Veterans Centers, 5557
Melwood, 5906
Montgomery County Department of Public Libraries/Special Needs Library, 4720
NFB Career Mentoring, 5907
National 4-H Council, 2618
National Epilepsy Library (NEL), 4721
National Federation of Families for Children's Mental Health (NFFCMH), 764
National Federation of the Blind, 2856
National Federation of the Blind Jernigan Institute, 4722
National Institute on Aging, 4723
National Rehabilitation Information Center (NARIC), 4724
Office of Fair Practices, 5908
Optometric Extension Program Foundation, 2857
Perry Point VA Medical Center, 5558
Red Notebook, 4725
Resources for Independence, 4127

RespectAbility, 791
Ryan White HIV/AIDS Program, 793
Sjogren's Syndrome Foundation, 2858
Social Security Library, 4726
Society for Post-Acute and Long-Term Care
    Medicine (AMDA), 795
Southern Maryland Center for LIFE, 4128
TLC Speech-Language/Occupational Therapy
    Camps, 5909
The ACNM Foundation, Inc., 2859
Trace Research and Development Center, 4727
United States Trager Association, 811
VA Maryland Health Care System, 5559
Warren Grant Magnuson Clinical Center, 4728
Youth for Understanding International Exchange,
    2630

Massachusetts

Abbot and Dorothy H Stevens Foundation, 2860
Adlib, 4129
Arc of Cape Cod, 4130
Arc of Massachusetts, The, 2861
Arc of Northern Bristol County, 2862
Boston Center for Independent Living, 4131
Boston Foundation, 2863
Boston Globe Foundation, 2864
Boston University Arthritis Center, 4729
Boston University Center for Human Genetics,
    4730
Boston University Robert Dawson Evans
    Memorial Dept. of Clinical Research, 4731
Boston VA Regional Office, 5560
Braille and Talking Book Library, Perkins School
    for the Blind, 4732
Brigham and Women's Hospital: Asthma and
    Allergic Disease Research Center, 4733
Brigham and Women's Hospital: Robert B
    Brigham Multipurpose Arthritis Center, 4734
Bushrod H Campbell and Ada F Hall Charity
    Fund, 2865
Camp Howe, 1030
Camp Jabberwocky, 1031
Camp Starfish, 1032
Cape Organization for Rights of the Disabled
    (CORD), 4132
Caption Center, 4735
Center for Interdisciplinary Research on
    Immunologic Diseases, 4736
Center for Living & Working: Fitchburg, 4133
Center for Living & Working: Framingham, 4134
Center for Living & Working: Worcester, 4135
Clipper Ship Foundation, 2866
Community Foundation of Western
    Massachusetts, 2867
Developmental Evaluation and Adjustment Fa
    cilities, 4136
Eagle Hill School: Summer Program, 1033
Edith Nourse Rogers Memorial Veterans Hospital,
    5561
Executive Office of Labor & Workforce Deve
    lopment, 5910
Family Voices, 697
Federation for Children with Special Needs, 700
Feldenkrais Guild of North America (FGNA), 702
Frank R and Elizabeth Simoni Foundation, 2868
Friendly Ice Cream Corp Contributions Prog ram,
    2869
Gateway Arts Center: Studio, Craft Store &
    Gallery, 5911
Greater Worcester Community Foundation, 2870
Harvard University Howe Laboratory of
    Ophthalmology, 4737
Hyams Foundation, 2871
Independence Associates, 4137
Independent Living Center of Stavros: Gree nfield,
    4138
Independent Living Center of Stavros: Spri ngfield,
    4139
Independent Living Center of the North Sho re &
    Cape Ann, 4140
Kamp for Kids at Camp Togowauk, 1034
Labouré College Library, 4738
Learning Disabilities Worldwide, 739

Life-Skills, Inc., 5912
Massachusetts Commission Against Discrimin
    ation (FEPA), 5913
Massachusetts Commission for the Blind, 5914
Massachusetts Governor's Commission on
    Employment of People with Disabilities, 5915
Massachusetts Rehabilitation Commission, 4739,
    5916
MetroWest Center for Independent Living, 4141
Multi-Cultural Independent Living Center of
    Boston, 4142
New England Regional Genetics Group, 4714
Northampton VA Medical Center, 5562
Northeast Independent Living Program, 4143
Open Hearts Camp, 1035
Parent Professional Advocacy League (PPAL), 779
Raytheon Company Contributions Program, 2872
Renaissance Clubhouse, 4144
Scandinavian Exchange, 2622
Schepens Eye Research Institute, 4740
Southeast Center for Independent Living, 4145
Student Independent Living Experience
    Massachusetts Hospital School, 4146
Summer@Carroll, 1036
TJX Foundation, 2873
Talking Book Library at Worcester Public Library,
    4741
The Barton Center, 1037
The Barton Center Camp Joslin, 1038
The Barton Center Clara Barton Camp, 1039
The Barton Center Danvers Day Camp, 1040
The Barton Center Family Camp, 1041
The Barton Center Worcester Day Camp, 1042
The Beveridge Family Foundation, Inc., 2874
The Bridge Center, 1043
The Rainbow Club, 926
VA Boston Healthcare System: Brockton Division,
    5563
VA Boston Healthcare System: Jamaica Plain
    Campus, 5564
VA Boston Healthcare System: West Roxbury
    Division, 5565
Vermont Overnight Camp, 1320
Viability, 814, 5917
Work Inc., 5918
Youth as Self Advocates (YASA), 823

Michigan

Aleda E Lutz VA Medical Center, 5566
Alternating Hemiplegia of Childhood Foundation,
    2648
Ann Arbor Area Community Foundation, 2876
Ann Arbor Center for Independent Living, 4147
Arc Michigan, 4148
Arc of Michigan, 2877
Arc/Muskegon, 4149
Artificial Language Laboratory, 4742
Bad Axe: Blue Water Center for Independent
    Living, 4150
Battle Creek VA Medical Center, 5567
Bay Area Coalition for Independent Living, 4151
Berrien Community Foundation, 2878
Blind Children's Fund, 2879
Burger School for the Autistic, 4743
Camp Barefoot, 1044
Camp Catch-A-Rainbow, 1045
Camp Chris Williams, 1046
Camp Grace Bentley, 1047
Camp Midicha, 1048
Camp Quality North Michigan, 1049
Camp Quality South Michigan, 1050
Capital Area Center for Independent Living, 4152
Caro: Blue Water Center for Independent Li ving,
    4153
Center for Independent Living of Mid-Michigan,
    4154
Chi Medical Library, 4744
Community Connections of Southwest Michigan,
    4155
Community Foundation of Monroe County, 2880
Cowan Slavin Foundation, 2881
Cristo Rey Handicappers Program, 4156
Daimler Chrysler, 2882

Department of Health & Human Services, 5919
Detroit Center for Independent Living, 4157
Disability Advocates of Kent County, 4158
Disability Connection, 4159
Disability Network Southwest Michigan, 4160
Disability Network of Mid-Michigan, 4161
Disability Network of Oakland & Macomb, 4162
Disability Network/Lakeshore, 4163
Division on Deaf, DeafBlind & Hard of Hear ing,
    5920
Echo Grove Camp, 1051
Frank & Mollie S VanDervoort Memorial Foun
    dation, 2883
Fremont Area Community Foundation, 2884
Glaucoma Laser Trial, 4745
Grand Rapids Foundation, 2885
Grand Traverse Area Community Living
    Management Corporation, 4164
Grand Traverse Area Library for the Blind and
    Physically Handicapped, 4746
Granger Foundation, 2886
Great Lakes/Macomb Rehabilitation Group, 4165
Harvey Randall Wickes Foundation, 2887
Havirmill Foundation, 2888
Hope Network Neuro Rehabilitation, 718
Indian Trails Camp, 1052
Iron Mountain VA Medical Center, 5568
JARC, 4166
John D Dingell VA Medical Center, 5569
Kelly Services Foundation, 2889
Kent County Arc, 2890
Kent District Library for the Blind and Physically
    Handicapped, 4747
Kresge Foundation, 2891
Lanting Foundation, 2892
Lapeer: Blue Water Center for Independent
    Living, 4167
Livingston Center for Independent Living, 4168
Macomb Library for the Blind & Physically
    Handicapped, 4748
Michigan Braille and Talking Book Library, 4749
Michigan Commission for the Blind: Independent
    Living Rehabilitation Program, 4169
Michigan Commission for the Blind: Detroit, 4170
Michigan Department of Civil Rights, 5921
Michigan Library for the Blind and Physically
    Handicapped, 4750
Michigan Rehabilitation Services, 5922
Michigan VA Regional Office, 5570
Michigan Workforce Development Agency, 5923
Michigan's Assistive Technology Resource, 4751
Mideastern Michigan Library Co-op, 4752
Monroe Center for Independent Living, 4171
Muskegon Area District Library for the Bli nd and
    Physically Handicapped, 4753
Northland Library Cooperative, 4754
Oakland County Library for the Visually &
    Physically Impaired, 4755
Port Huron: Blue Water Center for Independ ent
    Living, 4172
Rollin M Gerstacker Foundation, 2893
Sandusky: Blue Water Center for Independen t
    Living, 4173
Southeastern Michigan Commission for the Blind,
    4174
Spartan Stuttering Laboratory, 797
St. Clair County Library Special Technologies
    Alternative Resources (S.T.A.R.), 4756
St. Francis Camp On The Lake, 1053
Steelcase Foundation, 2894
Straits Area Services, Inc. (SAS), 5924
Student Disability Services (SDS), 800
Superior Alliance for Independent Living (SAIL),
    4175
The Creative Mobility Group, LLC, 5462
Trail's Edge Camp, 1054
University of Michigan: Orthopaedic Research
    Laboratories, 4757
Upper Peninsula Library for the Blind, 4758
VA Ann Arbor Healthcare System, 5571
Vet Center Readjustment Counseling Service, 5572
Washtenaw County Library for the Blind &
    Physically Handicapped, 4759

Wayne County Regional Library for the Blind, 4760
Wayne State University: CS Mott Center for Human Genetics and Development, 4761
disAbility Connections, 4176

Minnesota

Access North Center for Independent Living of Northeastern MN, 4177
Accessible Space, Inc., 4178
Accreditation Commission for Acupuncture & Oriental Medicine, 590
Advocates for Developmental Disabilities, 594
Arc of Minnesota, 2895
AuSM Summer Camp, 1055
Burnett Foundation, 2896
Camp Buckskin, 1056
Camp Confidence, 1057
Camp Courage North, 1059
Camp Eden Wood, 1060
Camp Heartland, 1061
Camp Hollywood HEART, 862
Camp Knutson, 1062
Camp Odayin, 1063
Camp Odayin Family Camp, 1064
Camp Odayin Residential Camp, 1065
Camp Odayin Summer Camp, 1066
Camp Odayin Winter Camp, 1067
Century College, 4762
Closing the Gap's Annual Conference, 1742
Communication Center/Minnesota State Services for the Blind, 4763
Courage Center, 4179
Cristo Vive International: Minnesota Camp, 1068
Deluxe Corporation Foundation, 2897
Down Syndrome Camp, 1069
Duluth Public Library, 4764
Freedom Resource Center for Independent Living: Fergus Falls, 4180
General Mills Foundation, 2898
Hugh J Andersen Foundation, 2899
Independent Life Styles, 4406
James R Thorpe Foundation, 2900
Jay and Rose Phillips Family Foundation, 2901
Jewish Vocational Service of Jewish Family and Children's Services, 5925
Metropolitan Center for Independent Living, 4181
Minneapolis Foundation, 2902
Minneapolis VA Medical Center, 5573
Minnesota Association of Centers for Independent Living, 4182
Minnesota Department of Employment & Economic Development: State Services for the Blind, 5926
Minnesota Department of Employment and Economic Development: Vocational Rehab Services, 5927
Minnesota Department of Human Rights (FEPA), 5928
Minnesota Library for the Blind and Physically Handicapped, 4765
Miracle-Ear Children's Foundation, 2855
OPTIONS, 4183
Options Interstate Resource Center for Independent Living, 4184
Ordean Foundation, 2903
Otto Bremer Foundation, 2904
PACER Center (Parent Advocacy Coalition for Educational Rights), 776
Perry River Home Care, 4185
Rochester Area Foundation, 2905
SMILES, 4186
SMILES: Mankato, 4187
Southeastern Minnesota Center for Independent Living: Red Wing, 4188
Southeastern Minnesota Center for Independent Living: Rochester, 4189
Special U, 4766
St. Cloud VA Medical Center, 5574
St. Paul Regional Office, 5575
True Friends, 1070
University of Minnesota at Crookston, 2625
Ventures Travel, 5456

Vinland Center Lake Independence, 4191
Wilderness Inquiry, 5457

Mississippi

AbilityWorks, 5929
Alpha Home Royal Maid Association for the Blind, 4192
Arc of Mississippi, 2906
Biloxi/Gulfport VA Medical Center, 5577
Blind and Physically Handicapped Library Services, 4767
Gulf Coast Independent Living Center, 4193
Jackson Regional Office, 5578
LIFE of Mississippi, 4195
LIFE of Mississippi: Biloxi, 4196
LIFE of Mississippi: Greenwood, 4197
LIFE of Mississippi: Hattiesburg, 4198
LIFE of Mississippi: McComb, 4199
LIFE of Mississippi: Meridian, 4200
LIFE of Mississippi: Oxford, 4201
LIFE of Mississippi: Tupelo, 4202
Mississippi Department of Rehabilitation Services, 5930
Mississippi Employment Security Commission, 5931
Mississippi Library Commission, 4768
Mississippi Library Commission\Talking Book and Braille Services, 4769
National Research and Training Center on Blindness and Low Vision, 5932

Missouri

Access II Independent Living Center, 4203
Allen P & Josephine B Green Foundation, 2907
American Academy of Environmental Medicine (AAEM), 596
American Academy of Environmental Medicine Annual Conference, 1732
Anheuser-Busch, 2908
Arc of the US Missouri Chapter, 2909
Assemblies of God Center for the Blind, 4770
Bootheel Area Independent Living Services, 4204
Camp Barnabas, 1072
Camp Encourage, 1073
Camp Hickory Hill, 1074
Camp MITIOG, 1075
Camp No Limits Missouri, 1076
Camp Quality Central Missouri, 1077
Camp Quality Greater Kansas City, 1078
Camp Quality Northwest Missouri, 1079
Camp Quality Ozarks, 1080
Church of the Nazarene, 4771
Coalition for Independence: Missouri Branch Office, 4205
Delta Center for Independent Living, 4206
Disability Resource Association, 4207
Disabled Athlete Sports Association (DASA), 681
Easterseals Midwest, 4208
Greater Kansas City Community Foundation & Affiliated Trusts, 2910
Greater St Louis Community Foundation, 2911
H&R Block Foundation, 2912
Harry S Truman Memorial Veterans' Hospital, 5579
Independent Living Center of Southeast Missouri, 4209
International Clinic of Biological Regeneration (ICBR), 727
International Ventilator Users Network (IVUN), 730
James S McDonnell Foundation, 2913
John J Pershing VA Medical Center, 5580
Judevine Center for Autism, 4772
Kansas City VA Medical Center, 5581
Lutheran Blind Mission, 4773
Lutheran Charities Foundation of St Louis, 2914
Midland Empire Resources for Independent Living (MERIL), 4210
Missouri Commission on Human Rights, 5933
Missouri Governor's Council on Disability, 5934
Missouri Vocational Rehabilitation Agency, 5935

National Car Rental System, 5460
Northeast Independent Living Services, 4211
On My Own, 4212
Ozark Independent Living, 4213
Paraquad, 4214
People to People International, 2620
Places for People, 4215
Post-Polio Health International, 785
RA Bloch Cancer Foundation, 2915
RAIL, 4216
SEMO Alliance for Disability Independence, 4217
Southwest Center for Independent Living (S CIL), 4219
Southwestern Center for Independent Living, 4190
St. Louis Regional Office, 5582
St. Louis VA Medical Center, 5583
Sunnyhill Adventures, 1081
Sunnyhill, Inc., 4220
Tri-County Center for Independent Living, 4221
University of Missouri: Columbia Arthritis Center, 4774
Veteran's Voices Writing Project, 5471
Victor E Speas Foundation, 2916
Vocational Rehabilitation Services for the Blind, 5936
West Central Independent Living Solutions, 4222
Whole Person, The, 4223
Whole Person: Kansas City, 4224
Wolfner Talking Book & Braille Library, 4775
Wonderland Camp, 1082

Montana

American College of Advancement in Medicine (ACAM), 612
Big Sky Kids Cancer Camps, 1083
Camp Mak-A-Dream, 1084
Charles Campbell Childrens Camp, 1085
Disability Employment & Transitions, 5937
Living Independently for Today and Tomorrow w, 4225
MonTECH, 4776
Montana Human Rights Bureau (FEPA), 5938
Montana Independent Living Project, Inc., 4226
Montana State Library-Talking Book Library, 4777
Montana VA Regional Office, 5584
North Central Independent Living Services, 4227
Summit Independent Living Center: Kalipsell, 4228
Summit Independent Living Center: Hamilton, 4229
Summit Independent Living Center: Missoula, 4230
Summit Independent Living Center: Ronan, 4231
V A Montana Healthcare System, 5585
VA Montana Healthcare System, 5586
Vet Center, 5576, 5587

Nebraska

Arc of Nebraska, 2917
Camp Floyd Rogers, 1086
Camp Kindle, 863, 1087
Camp Quality Heartland, 1088
Center for Independent Living of Central Nebraska, 4232
Cooper Foundation, 2918
Easterseals Nebraska Camp, 1089
Grand Island VA Medical System, 5588
Kamp Kaleo, 1090
League of Human Dignity: Lincoln, 4233
League of Human Dignity: Norfolk, 4234
League of Human Dignity: Omaha, 4235
Lincoln Regional Office, 5589
Lincoln VA Medical Center, 5590
Mosaic, 2919
Mosaic Of De, 3929
Mosaic of Axtell Bethpage Village, 4236
Mosaic of Beatrice, 4237
Mosaic: Pontiac, 4010
Mosaic: York, 4238
National Camps for Blind Children, 1091

North Carolina

Valley Association for Independent Living:
Harlingen, 4420
Waco Regional Office, 5674
West Texas VA Healthcare System, 5675
William Stamps Farish Fund, 3146
World Federation for Mental Health, 819

Utah

Action X-Treme Camp, 1307
Active Re-Entry, 4421
Active Re-Entry: Vernal, 4422
Camp Giddy-Up, 1308
Camp Hobe, 1309
Camp ICANDO, 1310
Camp Kostopulos, 1311
Camp Nah-Nah-Mah, 1312
Central Utah Independent Living Center, 4423
Discovery Camp, 1313
FCYD Camp Utada, 1314
Kids Rock The World Day Camp, 1315
Marriner S Eccles Foundation, 3148
National Care Planning Council, 754
OPTIONS for Independence, 4424
OPTIONS for Independence: Brigham Satellit e,
4425
Overnight Camps, 1316
Pathfinders Camp, 1317
Questar Corporation Contributions Program, 3149
Red Rock Center for Independence, 4426
Utah Assistive Technology Program (UTAP) Utah
State University, 4428
Utah Department of Human Services: Division of
Services for People with Disabilities, 6031
Utah Division of Veterans Affairs, 5676
Utah Employment Services, 6032
Utah Governor's Committee on Employment for
People with Disabilities (GCEPD), 6033
Utah Independent Living Center, 4429
Utah Independent Living Center: Minersville,
4430
Utah Independent Living Center: Tooele, 4431
Utah State Library Division: Program for the Blind
and Disabled, 4848
Utah State Office for Rehabilitation (USOR), 6034
Utah State Office of Rehabilitation: Vocational
Rehabilitation, 6035
Utah State Office of Rehabilitation: Service s for the
Blind and Visually Impaired, 6036
VA Salt Lake City Healthcare System, 5677
Veterans Support Center (VSC), 6037

Vermont

Camp Thorpe, 1318
National Center for PTSD, 4849
Silver Towers Camp, 1319
Vermont Assistive Technology Program, 4432
Vermont Center for Independent Living: Ben
nington, 4433
Vermont Center for Independent Living: Chi
ttenden, 4434
Vermont Center for Independent Living: Mon
tpelier, 4435
Vermont Community Foundation, 3150
Vermont Department of Disabilities, Aging and
Independent Living (DAIL), 6038
Vermont Department of Labor, 6039
Vermont Department of Libraries - Special
Services Unit, 4850
Vermont Department of Libraries -Special
Services Unit, 4851
Vermont Division of Vocational Rehabilitat ion,
6040
Vermont VA Regional Office Center, 5678
Vermont Veterans Centers, 5679

Virginia

ACA Annual Conference, 1721
ADA Annual Scientific Sessions, 1722
AER Annual International Conference, 1723
ASIA Annual Scientific Meeting, 1727

Access Independence, 4436
Access Services, 4852
Alexandria Library Talking Book Service, 4853
American Academy of Audiology (AAA), 595
American Academy of Audiology Conference,
1731
American Chiropractic Association (ACA), 611
American Counseling Association (ACA), 614
American National Bank and Trust Company, 2783
Appalachian Independence Center, 4437
Arc of Virginia, 3151
Arlington County Department of Libraries, 4854
Beacon Tree Foundation, 642, 3152
Blinded Veterans Association National
Convention, 1739
Blue Ridge Independent Living Center, 4438
Blue Ridge Independent Living Center:
Christianburg, 4439
Blue Ridge Independent Living Center: Low
Moor, 4440
Braille Circulating Library for the Blind, 4855
Brain Injury Association of America (BIAA), 646
Camp Dickenson, 1321
Camp Easterseals UCP, 1322
Camp Foundation, 3153
Camp Holiday Trails, 1323
Camp Jordan, 1324
Camp Loud And Clear, 1325
Campagna Center, 6041
Camps for Children & Teens with Diabetes, 1326
Central Rappahannock Regional Library, 4856
Civitan Acres, 1327
Clinch Independent Living Services, 4441
Community Foundation of Richmond & Central
Virginia, 3154
Council for Exceptional Children (CEC), 668, 4857
Council for Exceptional Children Annual
Convention and Expo, 1744
Didlake, 6042
Disability Funders Network (DFN), 674
Disability Resource Center, 3950, 4442
Disability:IN, 680
ENDependence Center of Northern Virginia, 4443
Equal Access Center for Independence, 4444
From the State Capitals: Public Health, 3205
Hampton VA Medical Center, 5680
Hunter Holmes McGuire VA Medical Center, 5681
Independence Empowerment Center, 4445
Independence Resource Center, 4446
Independent Living Center Network: Department
of the Visually Handicapped, 4447
International Chiropractors Association (ICA), 726
International Student Exchange Programs (I SEP),
2612
James Branch Cabell Library, 4858
John Randolph Foundation, 3155
Junction Center for Independent Living, 4448
Junction Center for Independent Living: Du ffield,
4449
Loudoun County Adaptive Recreation Camps,
1328
Lynchburg Area Center for Independent Living,
4450
March of Dimes, 742
Mental Health America (MHA), 744
NEXT Conference & Exposition, 1752
National Association of State Directors of
Developmental Disabilities Services
(NASDDDS), 752
National Council on the Aging Conference, 1754
National Rehabilitation Association (NRA), 769
National Right to Work Legal Defense
Foundation, 3156
National Vaccine Information Center (NVIC), 771
Newport News Public Library System, 4859
Norfolk Foundation, 3157
Northern Virginia Resource Center for Deaf and
Hard of Hearing Persons, 4860
Oakland School & Camp, 1329
Peidmont Independent Living Center, 4451
Peninsula Center for Independent Living, 4452
Piedmont Independent Living Center, 4453
Resources for Independent Living, 3891, 4454
Richmond Research Training Center (RRTC), 6043

Roanoke City Public Library System, 4861
Roanoke Regional Office, 5682
Robey W Estes Family Foundation, 3158
Salem VA Medical Center, 5683
ServiceSource Disability Resource Center, 6044
SourceAmerica, 6045
Staunton Public Library Talking Book Center,
4862
University of Virginia Health System General
Clinical Research Group, 4863
Valley Associates for Independent Living (VAIL),
4455
Valley Associates for Independent Living:
Lexington, 4456
Virginia Autism Resource Center, 4864
Virginia Beach Foundation, 3159
Virginia Beach Public Library Special Services
Library, 4865
Virginia Chapter of the Arthtitis Foundation, 4866
Virginia Department for the Blind and Vision
Impaired (DBVI), 6046
Virginia Department of Veterans Services, 5684
Virginia State Library for the Visually and
Physically Handicapped, 4867
Volunteers of America (VOA), 815
Woodrow Wilson Rehabilitation Center Training
Program, 4457

Washington

ADA National Network, 583
Alliance for People with Disabilities: Sea ttle, 4458
Alliance of People with Disabilities: Redmond,
4459
Arc of Washington State, 3160
Bastyr Center for Natural Health, 641
Ben B Cheney Foundation, 3161
Business Enterprise Program (BEP), 5734, 6047
Camp Beausite NW, 1330
Camp Goodtimes, 1331
Camp Killoqua, 1332
Camp Korey, 1333
Camp Sealth, 1334
Community Foundation of North Central
Washington, 3162
Community Services for the Blind and Parti ally
Sighted Store: Sight Connection, 4460
Department of Services for the Blind (DSB), 6048
Department of Social & Health Services: Division
of Vocational Rehabilitation, 6049
Department of Social & Health Services:
Developmental Disabilities Administration
(DDA), 6050
DisAbility Resource Connection: Everett, 4461
Easterseals Camp Stand by Me, 1335
Glaser Progress Foundation, 3163
Greater Tacoma Community Foundation, 3164
Inland Northwest Community Foundation, 3165
Jonathan M Wainwright Memorial VA Medical
Center, 5685
Kitsap Community Resources, 4462
Medina Foundation, 3166
Meridian Valley Clinical Laboratory, 4868
Norcliffe Foundation, 3167
Ophthalmic Research Laboratory Eye
Institute/First Hill Campus, 4869
Prime Time, Inc., 1336
SL Start Washington, 6051
STIX Diabetes Programs, 1337
Seattle Regional Office, 5686
Spokane Center for Independent Living, 4463
Spokane VA Medical Center, 5687
Stewardship Foundation, 3168
Tacoma Area Coalition of Individuals with
Disabilities, 4464
VA Puget Sound Health Care System, 5688
Washington Talking Book and Braille Library,
4870
Western Washington University, 2627
Weyerhaeuser Company Foundation, 3169
Wheelchair Getaways, 5463

West Virginia

925

Appalachian Center for Independent Living, 4465
Appalachian Center for Independent Living: Spencer, 4466
Arc Of West Virginia, The, 3170
Bernard McDonough Foundation, 3171
Cabell County Public Library/Talking Book Department/Subregional Library for the Blind, 4871
Division of Rehabilitation Services: Staff Library, 4872
High Technology Foundation, 715, 3172
Huntington Regional Office, 5689
Huntington VA Medical Center, 5690
Job Accommodation Network (JAN), 733
Kanawha County Public Library, 4873
Louis A Johnson VA Medical Center, 5691
Martinsburg VA Medical Center, 5692
Mountain State Center for Independent Living, 4467
Mountain State Center for Independent Living, 4468
Mountaineer Spina Bifida Camp, 1338
Northern West Virginia Center for Independent Living, 4469
Ohio County Public Library Services for the Blind and Physically Handicapped, 4874
Talking Book Department, Parkersburg and Wood County Public Library, 4875
US Department Veterans Affairs Beckley Vet Center, 5693
West Virginia Autism Training Center, 4876
West Virginia Division of Rehabilitation Services (DRS), 6052
West Virginia Library Commission, 4877
West Virginia School for the Blind Library, 4878
WorkForce West Virginia, 6053

Wisconsin

AACRC Annual Conference, 1717
Able Trek Tours, 5439
American Academy for Cerebral Palsy and Developmental Medicine Annual Conference, 1730

Arc of Dunn County, 3173
Arc of Eau Claire, 3174
Arc of Fox Cities, 3175
Arc of Racine County, 3176
Arc of Wisconsin Disability Association, 3177
Arc-Dane County, 3178
Association of Children's Residential Centers (ACRC), 634
Association of Educational Therapists (AET), 635
Brown County Library, 4879
Camp Daypoint, 1339
Camp Kee-B-Waw, 1340
Camp Klotty Pine, 1341
Camp Needlepoint, 1342
Center for Independent Living of Western Wisconsin, 4470
Clement J Zablocki VA Medical Center, 5694
Department of Workforce Development: Vocational Rehabilitation, 6054
Easter Seal Camp Wawbeek, 1343
Eye Institute of the Medical College of Wisconsin and Froedtert Clinic, 4880
Faye McBeath Foundation, 3179
Helen Bader Foundation, 3180
Independence First, 4471
Independence First: West Bend, 4472
Inspiration Ministries, 4473
Johnson Controls Foundation, 3181
Lutherdale Bible Camp, 1344
Lynde and Harry Bradley Foundation, 3182
Mid-State Independent Living Consultants: Wausau, 4474
Mid-state Independent Living Consultants: Stevens Point, 4475
Milwaukee Foundation, 3183
North Country Independent Living, 4476
North Country Independent Living: Ashland, 4477
Northwestern Mutual Life Foundation, 3184
Options for Independent Living, 4478
Options for Independent Living: Fox Valley, 4479
Phantom Lake YMCA Camp, 1345
SB Waterman & E Blade Charitable Foundation, 3186
Society's Assets: Elkhorn, 4480
Society's Assets: Kenosha, 4481

Society's Assets: Racine, 4482
Timbertop Camp for Youth with Learning Disabilities, 1346
Tomah VA Medical Center, 5695
William S Middleton Memorial VA Hospital Center, 5696
Wisconsin Badger Camp, 1347
Wisconsin Elks/Easterseals Respite Camp, 1348
Wisconsin Lions Camp, 1349
Wisconsin Regional Library for the Blind & Physically Handicapped, 4881
Wisconsin VA Regional Office, 5697

Wyoming

Arc of Natrona County, 3187
Camp Hope, 1350
Casper Vet Center, 5698
Cheyenne VA Medical Center, 5699
Department of Workforce Services: Vocational Rehabilitation, 6055
Eagle View Ranch, 1351
RENEW: Gillette, 4483
RENEW: Rehabilitation Enterprises of North Eastern Wyoming, 4484
Rehabilitation Enterprises of North Eastern Wyoming: Newcastle, 4485
Sheridan VA Medical Center, 5700
Wyoming Department of Workforce Services: Unemployment Insurance Division, 6056
Wyoming Services for Independent Living, 4486
Wyoming Services for the Visually Impaired, 4882
Wyoming State Rehabilitation Council (SRC), 6057
Wyoming's New Options in Technology (WYNOT) - University of Wyoming, 4883

Amplified Phones, 172
Amplified Portable Phone, 173
Amplify Life, 1093
Amputee Coalition, 628, 930, 5223
Amtrak, 5425
Amyotrophic Lateral Sclerosis: A Guide for
    Patients and Families, 8506
Amytrophic Lateral Sclerosis Association, 8174
Anaheim Veterans Center, 6380
Analog Switch Pad, 1400
Andalusia Health Services, 2632
Anderson Woods, 981
Andrew Heiskell Braille and Talking Book Library,
    4790
Angel River Health and Rehabilitation, 7105
Anglo California Travel Service, 5442
Anheuser-Busch, 2908
Anixter Center, 5839
Ann Arbor Area Community Foundation, 2876
Ann Arbor Center for Independent Living, 4147
Annals of Dyslexia, 7881
Annals of Otology, Rhinology and Laryngolo gy,
    8668
Annals Publishing Company, 8668
Annandale Village, 6615
Anne and Henry Zarrow Foundation, 3056
Annual Conference on Dyslexia and Related
    Learning Disabilities, 1734
Annual Report Sarkeys Foundation, 4949
Annual Report/Newsletter, 9117
Annual TASH Conference, 1735
Antecedent Control: Innovative Approaches to
    Behavioral Support, 2207
Anthesis, 5747
Anthony Brothers Manufacturing, 5391
Anthracite Region Center for Independent Living,
    4347
Antioch College, 2601
Anxiety and Depression Association of Amer ica
    (ADAA), 629, 7668
Anxiety-Free Kids: An Interactive Guide for
    Parents and Children, 2208
APA Access, 2144
Aphasia Hope Foundation, 8740
Aplastic Anemia and MDS International
    Foundation, 8309
Appalachian Center for Independent Living, 4465
Appalachian Center for Independent Living:
    Spencer, 4466
Appalachian Independence Center, 4437
Applied Kinesiology: Muscle Response in
    Diagnosis, Therapy and Preventive Medicine,
    4950
Applied Rehabilitation Counseling (Springe r
    Series on Rehabilitation), 2209
Approaching Equality, 4510
Apria Healthcare, 360, 6524
Apria Healthcare Group, Inc., 360, 6524
APSE, 1725
APSE National Conference, 1725
Aqua Massage International, 240
Aquarius Health Care Media, 5239, 7804, 7817,
    7908, 7909, 7911, 7916, 8792, 8845
Aquarius Health Care Videos, 5007, 5170, 5275,
    5276, 5277, 5279, 5282, 5283, 5292, 5295,
    5297, 5301, 5303, 7919, 8260
Aquatic Access, 332
A AR P Fulfillment, 4540
Arbors at Canton Subacute And Rehabilitation
    Center, 7182
Arbors at Dayton, 7183
Arbors at Marietta, 7184
Arbors at Milford, 7185
Arbors at New Castle, 7066
Arbors at Sylvania, 7186
Arbors at Toledo Subacute and Rehab Centre, 7187
Arbors East Subacute and Rehabilitation Center,
    7181
The Arc, 1736
The Arc - Iberville, 6763
The Arc Caddo-Bossier, 6764
Arc Connection Newsletter, 4951, 7886
The Arc Eastern Connecticut, 919, 8400
ARC Fresno-Kelso Activity Center, 6371
ARC Gateway, 3341

The Arc Gloucester, 5975, 1112
Arc Light, 7887
The Arc Los Angeles and Orange Counties, 5771
Arc Massachusetts, 4944
Arc Michigan, 4148
Arc National Convention, The, 1736
Arc Northwest Indiana, 5860
Arc Of Alabama, The, 2633
Arc of Alaska, 2635
The Arc of Allen County, 2065
The Arc of Anchorage, 2635
Arc of Anderson County, 3101
Arc of Arizona, 7887
The Arc of Arizona, 2638
Arc of Arkansas, 2643
Arc of Bergen and Passaic Counties, 5954
Arc of Blackstone, 4372
Arc of Blackstone Valley, 3088
Arc of California, 2649
The Arc of Camden County, 5971
Arc of Cape Cod, 4130
Arc of Central Alabama, 5704
Arc of Colorado, 2712
Arc of Connecticut, 2720
Arc of Davidson County, 3102
Arc of Delaware, 2733, 3327
Arc of Dunn County, 3173
Arc of Eau Claire, 3174
Arc of Florida, 2750
Arc of Fox Cities, 3175
Arc Of Georgia, 2765
Arc of Hamilton County, 3103
Arc of Hawaii, 2776
ARC of Hunterdon County, The, 5948
Arc of Illinois, 2785
The Arc of Illinois, 5845
Arc of Indiana, 2820
Arc of Iowa, 2824
Arc of Kansas, 2829
Arc of Kentucky, 2832
Arc of Louisiana, 2833
Arc of Maryland, 2841
Arc of Massachusetts, The, 2861
ARC of Mercer County, 5949
Arc Of Meriden-Wallingford, Inc., 6525
Arc of Michigan, 2877
Arc of Minnesota, 2895
Arc of Mississippi, 2906
ARC of Monmouth, 5950
Arc of Natrona County, 3187
Arc of Nebraska, 2917
Arc of New Jersey, 2928
The Arc of New Jersey, 2060
Arc of New Mexico, 2942
Arc of North Carolina, 3018
The Arc of North Carolina, 7720
Arc of North Dakota, 3027
Arc of Northern Bristol County, 2862
Arc of Northern Rhode Island, 3089
Arc of Ohio, 3031
Arc of Oregon, 3058
Arc of Pennsylvania, 3064
Arc of Racine County, 3176
The Arc of San Diego, 887, 7743
ARC Of San Diego-ARROW Center, 6372
ARC Of San Diego-Rex Industries, The, 6373
ARC Of San Diego-South Bay, 6374
Arc of South Carolina, 3098
ARC Of Southeast Los Angeles-Southeast
    Industries, 6375
Arc of Tennessee, 3104, 4951, 7886
Arc of Texas, The, 3116
Arc of the District of Columbia, 2737, 4934
The Arc of the East Bay, 6498
The Arc of the United States, 5380, 7721
Arc of the US Missouri Chapter, 2909
Arc of Utah, 3147
Arc of Virginia, 3151
Arc of Washington County, 3105
Arc of Washington State, 3160
Arc Of West Virginia, The, 3170
Arc of Williamson County, 3106
Arc of Wisconsin Disability Association, 3177
The Arc San Francisco, 5752
Arc South County Chapter, 3087

The Arc Tampa Bay, 6610
The Arc Westbank, 5892
ARC's Government Report, 4934
Arc-Dane County, 3178
Arc-Diversified, 3107
Arc/Muskegon, 4149
ARC: VC Community Connections West, 6376
ARC: VC Ventura, 6377
ARCA - Dakota County Technical College, 4935
ARCA Newsletter, 4935
Arcadia Foundation, 3065
Arcadia University, 2605
Architect Magazine, 1781
Archives of Neurology, 8669
Arctic Access, 3812
Arden Rehabilitation And Healthcare Center, 7017
Arden Rehabilitation and Healthcare Center, 7232
Ardence, 6213
Ardmore Developmental Center, 5901
Area Access, 300, 300
Area Agency on Aging of Southwest Arkansas,
    7607
Area Agency on Aging: Region One, 7608
Area Cooperative Educational Services (ACES),
    5788
Arena Stage, 6, 7623
Argentum, 7355
ARISE, 4269
ARISE: Oneida, 4270
ARISE: Oswego, 4271
ARISE: Pulaski, 4272
Arista Surgical Supply Company, 509
Arista Surgical Supply Company/AliMed, 156,
    518, 519, 564
Arizona State Department of Health Services, 2184
Arizona Autism Resources, 2638
Arizona Braille and Talking Book Library, 4585
Arizona Bridge to Independent Living, 3821, 4967
Arizona Bridge to Independent Living: Phoenix,
    3822
Arizona Bridge to Independent Living: Mesa, 3823
Arizona Camp Sunrise, 8370
Arizona Camp Sunrise & Sidekicks, 841
Arizona Center for Disability Law, 3280
Arizona Center for the Blind and Visually
    Impaired, 6342
Arizona Center on Aging, 7356
Arizona Civil Rights Division, 5736
Arizona Community Foundation, 2639
Arizona Department of Economic Security, 3273,
    5734, 5735
Arizona Department of Health Services, 3274,
    2185, 2309
Arizona Developmental Disabilities Plannin g
    Council (ADDPC), 5732
Arizona Division of Aging and Adult Services,
    3275
Arizona Hemophilia Association, 8310, 846, 847,
    8399, 8407
Arizona Industries for the Blind, 6343
Arizona Instructional Resource Center for Students
    who are Blind or Visually Impaired, The, 2640
Arizona Rehabilitation State Services for the Blind
    and Visually Impaired, 3276
Arizona State Library, 4585
Arjo Inc, 204, 205, 334, 337, 338
ArjoHuntleigh, 134, 134, 146, 152
Arkansas Assistive Technology Projects, 3283
Arkansas Department of Special Education, 2017
Arkansas Department of Workforce Services, 5740
Arkansas Division of Aging & Adult Services,
    3284
Arkansas Division of Developmental Disabilities
    Services, 3285
Arkansas Division of Services for the Blind, 3286
Arkansas Division of Services for the Blind, 5743
Arkansas Governor's Developmental Disabili ties
    Council, 3287
Arkansas Independent Living Council, 3829
Arkansas Lighthouse for the Blind, 6364
Arkansas Regional Library for the Blind and
    Physically Handicapped, 4593
Arkansas Rehabilitation Services (ARS), 5741
Arkansas School for the Blind, 4594
Arkenstone: The Benetech Initiative, 1401

C

I

M

National Association of Blind Merchants (NABM), 748, 8904
National Association of Blind Rehabilitati on Professionals, 8905
National Association of Blind Students, 8906
National Association of Blind Teachers, 8907
National Association of Blind Veterans, 8908
National Association of Chronic Disease Di seases, 8342
National Association of City and County he alth Officials, 749
National Association of Cognitive- Behavioral Therapists, 7708
National Association of Colleges and Employers, 1947
National Association of Councils on Develo pmental Disabilities (NACDD), 750
National Association of Counties, 7420
National Association of Disability Represe ntatives (NADR), 751
National Association of Disability Representatives, 1750
National Association of Epilepsy Centers, 7709
National Association of Guide Dog Users, 8909
National Association of Hearing Officials, 7987, 8142
National Association of Nutrition and Aging Services Programs (NANASP), 7421
National Association of Parents with Child ren in Special Education, 1948, 7988
National Association of School Psychologists, 2003
National Association of School Psychologists, 2205, 2244, 2362, 2542
National Association of Special Education Teachers, 7989, 8755
National Association of State Directors of Developmental Disabilities Services (NASDDDS), 752
National Association of State Directors of Special Education, 1949
National Association of State Units on Aging, 7598
National Association of States United for Aging and Disabilities, 7422
National Association of the Deaf, 7990, 4543, 4557, 8037, 8039, 8141
National Association of Visually Handicapped, 9141
National Association to Advance Fat Acceptance, 8343
National Association to Promote the Use of Braille, 8910
National Ataxia Foundation, 7710
National Autism Association, 7711
National Autism Hotline, 7926
National Autism Resources, 1870
National Beep Baseball Association, 8911
National Birth Defect Registry, 5364
National Black Association for Speech Language and Hearing, 7991
National Black Association for Speech-Lang uage and Hearing, 8756
National Black Deaf Advocates, 7992
National Braille Association, 4801, 8912, 8975, 9086, 9142
National Braille Press, 8913
National Brain Tumor Foundation - National Brain Tumor Society, 5365
National Bullying Prevention Center Newsle tter, 2166
National Business & Disability Council, 5366, 5985
National Business & Disability Council (NBDC), 753
National Camps for Blind Children, 1091, 8947
National Cancer Institute, 3225, 8344, 8726
National Car Rental System, 5460
National Care Planning Council, 754
National Catholic Office for the Deaf, 8069
National Catholic Office of the Deaf, 7993, 8147
National Center for College Students with Disabilities (NCCSD), 755
National Center for Education in Maternal and Child Health (NCEMCH), 756

National Center for Health, Physical Activ ity and Disability, 757, 8193
National Center for Homeopathy, 1950
National Center for Learning Disabilities, 2004
National Center for PTSD, 4849
National Center for Vision and Child Development, 8914
National Center on Birth Defects and Developmental Disabilities, 4658
National Center on Caregiving at Family Caregiver Alliance (FCA), 2690
National Center on Deaf-Blindness (NCDB), 758, 7633
National Center on Disability and Journalism (NCDJ), 759
National Center on Elder Abuse, 7423
National Cerebral Palsy of American, 3730
National Certification Commission for Acup uncture and Oriental Medicine, 760
National Clearinghouse on Abuse in Later Life, 7424
National Clearinghouse on Family Support and Children's Mental Health, 2027
National Clearinghouse on Postsecondary Education, 1999
National Coalition for Assistive and Rehab Technology, 8194
National Coalition of Federal Aviation Employees with Disabilities, 3226
National Collaborative Workforce on Disability (NCWD/Youth), 761
National Commission on Orthotic and Prosth etic Education, 7939
The National Committee to Preserve Social Security, 7572
National Committee to Preserve Social Security & Medicare, 7425
National Conference on Building Codes and Standards, 1770
National Consortium on Deaf-Blindness, 7651, 9124
National Council for Aging Care, 7426
National Council of Architectural Registration Boards (NCARB), 1771
National Council on Aging, 7427, 7364, 7365, 7433, 7497, 7537, 7596, 7599, 7605
National Council on Disability, 3227, 4570, 5063
National Council on Independent Living (NCIL), 762, 3931, 8195
National Council on Multifamily Housing Industry, 1789
National Council on Rehabilitation Education (NCRE), 1951
National Council on the Aging, 7486
National Council on the Aging Conference, 1754
National Cued Speech Association, 7994, 8757, 8840
National Deaf Women's Bowling Association, 7995
National Diabetes Action Network for the Blind, 8915
National Diabetes Information Clearinghouse, 8345
National Digestive Diseases Information Clearinghouse, 8346
National Directory of Corporate Giving, 3212
National Disability Rights Network (NDRN), 763
National Disability Sports Alliance, 8280
National Down Syndrome Congress, 7712, 7894
National Down Syndrome Society, 7713
National Education Association of the United States, 1952
National Endowment for the Arts Office, 1784
National Endowment for the Arts: Office for AccessAbility, 49
National Epilepsy Library (NEL), 4721
National Eye Institute, 3228, 8916, 9052, 8994
National Eye Research Foundation, 2806
National Eye Research Foundation (NERF), 4676
National Falls Prevention Resource Center, 7428
National Family Association for Deaf-Blind, 7634, 7656
National Federation of Families for Children's Mental Health (NFFCMH), 764

National Federation of the Blind, 2856, 7635, 8917, 748, 5907, 7644, 8724, 8902, 8903, 8904, 8905, 8906, 8909, 8910, 8915, 8920, 9016, 9026, 9096, 9104
National Federation of the Blind Jernigan Institute, 4722
National Fibromyalgia Association, 8196, 8347, 7883, 8237, 8251
National Foundation for Ectodermal Dysplasias, 2807
National Foundation for Facial Reconstruction, 2995
National Foundation of Wheelchair Tennis, 2691
National Fragile X Foundation, 8758
National Gerontological Nursing Association, 7429
National Guild of Hypnotists (NGH), 765
National Headache Foundation, 2808
National Headquarters, 6959
National Health Council, 766
National Health Information Center, 7927, 8851
National Health Law Program (NHeLP), 4502
National Hearing Conservation Association, 7996
National Hemophilia Foundation, 2996, 8348
National Hemophilia Foundation - Western PA, 1232
National Hispanic Council on Aging, 7430
National Hookup, 5065
National Hospice & Palliative Care Organization (NHPCO), 7431
National Human Genome Research Institute, 2043
National Hydrocephalus Foundation, 7714, 8571
National Indian Council on Aging, 7593
National Indian Council on Aging, Inc., 7432
National Industries for the Blind, 8918, 9111
National Institue Health, 4728
National Institute of Arthritis and Muscul oskeletal and Skin Diseases, 3229
National Institute of Building Sciences, 1772, 1792, 1796
National Institute of Diabetes and Digesti ve and Kidney Diseases, 3230
National Institute of Environmental Health Sciences, 2052
National Institute of General Medical Scie nces, 2044
National Institute of Health, 9052
National Institute of Mental Health, 3231
National Institute of Neurological Disorders and Stroke, 3232, 7940
National Institute of Senior Centers, 7433
National Institute on Aging, 3233, 4723, 7434
National Institute on Deafness and Other Communication Disorders, 3234, 7997
National Institute on Disability, Independ ent Living, and Rehabilitation Research (NIDILRR), 767, 3235, 4630
National Institutes of Health, 7435, 2043, 3228, 3229, 3230, 3231, 3232, 3234, 7940, 7997, 8916
National Institutes of Health (NIH), 8320
National Jewish Health, 8511, 8551, 8604, 8654, 8663, 8725
National Jewish Medical & Research Center, 4617
National Kidney and Urologic Diseases Information Clearinghouse, 8349
National Kidney Foundation, 8408
National Lekotek Center, 4677, 5409
National Library of Medicine, 1462
National Library Office, 4820
National Library Service, 5330
National Library Service for the Blind and Physic, 7558
National Library Service for the Blind and Physically Handicapped (NLS), 50, 8919
National Library Service in Washington, 4821
National Mobility Equipment Dealers Associ ation, 8197
National Multiple Sclerosis Society, 7538, 8694
National Older Worker Career Center, 7436
National Organization for Albinism and Hypopigmentation, 8350
National Organization for Rare Disorders, 8351
National Organization of Parents of Blind Children, 8920
National Organization on Disability (NOD), 768, 5367

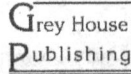

2022 Title List

Visit www.GreyHouse.com for Product Information, Table of Contents, and Sample Pages.

Opinions Throughout History

Opinions Throughout History: Church & State
Opinions Throughout History: The Death Penalty
Opinions Throughout History: Diseases & Epidemics
Opinions Throughout History: Drug Use & Abuse
Opinions Throughout History: The Environment
Opinions Throughout History: Free Speech & Censorship
Opinions Throughout History: Gender: Roles & Rights
Opinions Throughout History: Globalization
Opinions Throughout History: Guns in America
Opinions Throughout History: Immigration
Opinions Throughout History: Law Enforcement in America
Opinions Throughout History: National Security vs. Civil & Privacy Rights
Opinions Throughout History: Presidential Authority
Opinions Throughout History: Robotics & Artificial Intelligence
Opinions Throughout History: Social Media Issues
Opinions Throughout History: Voters' Rights
Opinions Throughout History: War & the Military
Opinions Throughout History: Workers Rights & Wages

This is Who We Were

This is Who We Were: Colonial America (1492-1775)
This is Who We Were: 1880-1899
This is Who We Were: In the 1900s
This is Who We Were: In the 1910s
This is Who We Were: In the 1920s
This is Who We Were: A Companion to the 1940 Census
This is Who We Were: In the 1940s (1940-1949)
This is Who We Were: In the 1950s
This is Who We Were: In the 1960s
This is Who We Were: In the 1970s
This is Who We Were: In the 1980s
This is Who We Were: In the 1990s
This is Who We Were: In the 2000s
This is Who We Were: In the 2010s

Working Americans

Working Americans—Vol. 1: The Working Class
Working Americans—Vol. 2: The Middle Class
Working Americans—Vol. 3: The Upper Class
Working Americans—Vol. 4: Children
Working Americans—Vol. 5: At War
Working Americans—Vol. 6: Working Women
Working Americans—Vol. 7: Social Movements
Working Americans—Vol. 8: Immigrants
Working Americans—Vol. 9: Revolutionary War to the Civil War
Working Americans—Vol. 10: Sports & Recreation
Working Americans—Vol. 11: Inventors & Entrepreneurs
Working Americans—Vol. 12: Our History through Music
Working Americans—Vol. 13: Education & Educators
Working Americans—Vol. 14: African Americans
Working Americans—Vol. 15: Politics & Politicians
Working Americans—Vol. 16: Farming & Ranching
Working Americans—Vol. 17: Teens in America
Working Americans—Vol. 18: Health Care Workers

Grey House Health & Wellness Guides

The Autism Spectrum Handbook & Resource Guide
Autoimmune Disorders Handbook & Resource Guide
Cardiovascular Disease Handbook & Resource Guide
Dementia Handbook & Resource Guide
Diabetes Handbook & Resource Guide
Nutrition, Obesity & Eating Disorders Handbook & Resource Guide

Consumer Health

Complete Mental Health Resource Guide
Complete Resource Guide for Pediatric Disorders
Complete Resource Guide for People with Chronic Illness
Complete Resource Guide for People with Disabilities
Older Americans Information Resource
Parenting: Styles & Strategies

Education

Complete Learning Disabilities Resource Guide
Educators Resource Guide
The Comparative Guide to Elem. & Secondary Schools
Special Education: A Reference Book for Policy & Curriculum Development

General Reference

American Environmental Leaders
Constitutional Amendments
Encyclopedia of African-American Writing
Encyclopedia of Invasions & Conquests
Encyclopedia of Prisoners of War & Internment
Encyclopedia of the Continental Congresses
Encyclopedia of the United States Cabinet
Encyclopedia of War Journalism
The Environmental Debate
Financial Literacy Starter Kit
From Suffrage to the Senate
The Gun Debate: Gun Rights & Gun Control in the U.S.
Historical Warrior Peoples & Modern Fighting Groups
Human Rights and the United States
Political Corruption in America
Privacy Rights in the Digital Age
The Religious Right and American Politics
Speakers of the House of Representatives, 1789-2021
US Land & Natural Resources Policy
The Value of a Dollar 1600-1865 Colonial to Civil War
The Value of a Dollar 1860-2019

Business Information

Business Information Resources
The Complete Broadcasting Industry Guide: Television, Radio, Cable & Streaming
Directory of Mail Order Catalogs
Environmental Resource Handbook
Food & Beverage Market Place
The Grey House Guide to Homeland Security Resources
The Grey House Performing Arts Industry Guide
Guide to Healthcare Group Purchasing Organizations
Guide to U.S. HMOs and PPOs
Guide to Venture Capital & Private Equity Firms
Hudson's Washington News Media Contacts Guide
New York State Directory
Sports Market Place

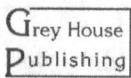

2022 Title List

Visit www.GreyHouse.com for Product Information, Table of Contents, and Sample Pages.

Statistics & Demographics

America's Top-Rated Cities
America's Top-Rated Smaller Cities
The Comparative Guide to American Suburbs
Profiles of America
Profiles of California
Profiles of Florida
Profiles of Illinois
Profiles of Indiana
Profiles of Massachusetts
Profiles of Michigan
Profiles of New Jersey
Profiles of New York
Profiles of North Carolina & South Carolina
Profiles of Ohio
Profiles of Pennsylvania
Profiles of Texas
Profiles of Virginia
Profiles of Wisconsin

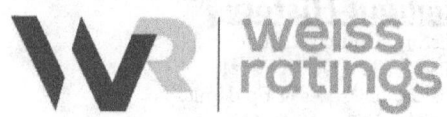

Weiss Financial Ratings

Financial Literacy Basics
Financial Literacy: How to Become an Investor
Financial Literacy: Planning for the Future
Weiss Ratings Consumer Guides
Weiss Ratings Guide to Banks
Weiss Ratings Guide to Credit Unions
Weiss Ratings Guide to Health Insurers
Weiss Ratings Guide to Life & Annuity Insurers
Weiss Ratings Guide to Property & Casualty Insurers
Weiss Ratings Investment Research Guide to Bond & Money Market
   Mutual Funds
Weiss Ratings Investment Research Guide to Exchange-Traded Funds
Weiss Ratings Investment Research Guide to Stock Mutual Funds
Weiss Ratings Investment Research Guide to Stocks

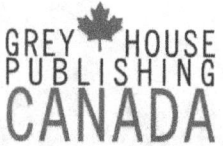

Canadian Resources

Associations Canada
Canadian Almanac & Directory
Canadian Environmental Resource Guide
Canadian Parliamentary Guide
Canadian Venture Capital & Private Equity Firms
Canadian Who's Who
Cannabis Canada
Careers & Employment Canada
Financial Post: Directory of Directors
Financial Services Canada
FP Bonds: Corporate
FP Bonds: Government
FP Equities: Preferreds & Derivatives
FP Survey: Industrials
FP Survey: Mines & Energy
FP Survey: Predecessor & Defunct
Health Guide Canada
Libraries Canada

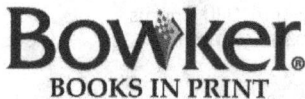

Books in Print Series

American Book Publishing Record® Annual
American Book Publishing Record® Monthly
Books In Print®
Books In Print® Supplement
Books Out Loud™
Bowker's Complete Video Directory™
Children's Books In Print®
El-Hi Textbooks & Serials In Print®
Forthcoming Books®
Law Books & Serials In Print™
Medical & Health Care Books In Print™
Publishers, Distributors & Wholesalers of the US™
Subject Guide to Books In Print®
Subject Guide to Children's Books In Print®

SALEM PRESS
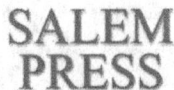

2022 Title List
Visit www.SalemPress.com for Product Information, Table of Contents, and Sample Pages.

LITERATURE

Critical Insights: Authors

Louisa May Alcott
Sherman Alexie
Isabel Allende
Maya Angelou
Isaac Asimov
Margaret Atwood
Jane Austen
James Baldwin
Saul Bellow
Roberto Bolano
Ray Bradbury
The Brontë Sisters
Gwendolyn Brooks
Albert Camus
Raymond Carver
Willa Cather
Geoffrey Chaucer
John Cheever
Joseph Conrad
Charles Dickens
Emily Dickinson
Frederick Douglass
T. S. Eliot
George Eliot
Harlan Ellison
Louise Erdrich
William Faulkner
F. Scott Fitzgerald
Gustave Flaubert
Horton Foote
Benjamin Franklin
Robert Frost
Neil Gaiman
Gabriel Garcia Marquez
Thomas Hardy
Nathaniel Hawthorne
Robert A. Heinlein
Lillian Hellman
Ernest Hemingway
Langston Hughes
Zora Neale Hurston
Henry James
Thomas Jefferson
James Joyce
Jamaica Kincaid
Stephen King
Martin Luther King, Jr.
Barbara Kingsolver
Abraham Lincoln
Mario Vargas Llosa
Jack London
James McBride
Cormac McCarthy
Herman Melville
Arthur Miller
Toni Morrison
Alice Munro
Tim O'Brien
Flannery O'Connor
Eugene O'Neill
George Orwell
Sylvia Plath
Edgar Allan Poe

Philip Roth
Salman Rushdie
J.D. Salinger
Mary Shelley
John Steinbeck
Amy Tan
Leo Tolstoy
Mark Twain
John Updike
Kurt Vonnegut
Alice Walker
David Foster Wallace
Edith Wharton
Walt Whitman
Oscar Wilde
Tennessee Williams
Virginia Woolf
Richard Wright
Malcolm X

Critical Insights: Works

Absalom, Absalom!
Adventures of Huckleberry Finn
Adventures of Tom Sawyer
Aeneid
All Quiet on the Western Front
Animal Farm
Anna Karenina
The Awakening
The Bell Jar
Beloved
Billy Budd, Sailor
The Book Thief
Brave New World
The Canterbury Tales
Catch-22
The Catcher in the Rye
The Color Purple
The Crucible
Death of a Salesman
The Diary of a Young Girl
Dracula
Fahrenheit 451
The Grapes of Wrath
Great Expectations
The Great Gatsby
Hamlet
The Handmaid's Tale
Harry Potter Series
Heart of Darkness
The Hobbit
The House on Mango Street
How the Garcia Girls Lost Their Accents
The Hunger Games Trilogy
I Know Why the Caged Bird Sings
In Cold Blood
The Inferno
Invisible Man
Jane Eyre
The Joy Luck Club
Julius Caesar
King Lear
The Kite Runner
Life of Pi
Little Women

Lolita
Lord of the Flies
The Lord of the Rings
Macbeth
The Metamorphosis
Midnight's Children
A Midsummer Night's Dream
Moby-Dick
Mrs. Dalloway
Nineteen Eighty-Four
The Odyssey
Of Mice and Men
The Old Man and the Sea
On the Road
One Flew Over the Cuckoo's Nest
One Hundred Years of Solitude
Othello
The Outsiders
Paradise Lost
The Pearl
The Poetry of Baudelaire
The Poetry of Edgar Allan Poe
A Portrait of the Artist as a Young Man
Pride and Prejudice
The Red Badge of Courage
Romeo and Juliet
The Scarlet Letter
Short Fiction of Flannery O'Connor
Slaughterhouse-Five
The Sound and the Fury
A Streetcar Named Desire
The Sun Also Rises
A Tale of Two Cities
The Tales of Edgar Allan Poe
Their Eyes Were Watching God
Things Fall Apart
To Kill a Mockingbird
War and Peace
The Woman Warrior

Critical Insights: Themes

The American Comic Book
American Creative Non-Fiction
The American Dream
American Multicultural Identity
American Road Literature
American Short Story
American Sports Fiction
The American Thriller
American Writers in Exile
Censored & Banned Literature
Civil Rights Literature, Past & Present
Coming of Age
Conspiracies
Contemporary Canadian Fiction
Contemporary Immigrant Short Fiction
Contemporary Latin American Fiction
Contemporary Speculative Fiction
Crime and Detective Fiction
Crisis of Faith
Cultural Encounters
Dystopia
Family
The Fantastic
Feminism

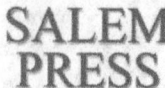
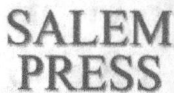
2022 Title List

Visit www.SalemPress.com for Product Information, Table of Contents, and Sample Pages.

Flash Fiction
Gender, Sex and Sexuality
Good & Evil
The Graphic Novel
Greed
Harlem Renaissance
The Hero's Quest
Historical Fiction
Holocaust Literature
The Immigrant Experience
Inequality
LGBTQ Literature
Literature in Times of Crisis
Literature of Protest
Love
Magical Realism
Midwestern Literature
Modern Japanese Literature
Nature & the Environment
Paranoia, Fear & Alienation
Patriotism
Political Fiction
Postcolonial Literature
Pulp Fiction of the '20s and '30s
Rebellion
Russia's Golden Age
Satire
The Slave Narrative
Social Justice and American Literature
Southern Gothic Literature
Southwestern Literature
Survival
Technology & Humanity
Truth & Lies
Violence in Literature
Virginia Woolf & 20th Century Women Writers
War

Critical Insights: Film
Bonnie & Clyde
Casablanca
Alfred Hitchcock
Stanley Kubrick

Critical Approaches to Literature
Critical Approaches to Literature: Feminist
Critical Approaches to Literature: Moral
Critical Approaches to Literature: Multicultural
Critical Approaches to Literature: Psychological

Critical Surveys of Literature
Critical Survey of American Literature
Critical Survey of Drama
Critical Survey of Graphic Novels: Heroes & Superheroes
Critical Survey of Graphic Novels: History, Theme, and Technique
Critical Survey of Graphic Novels: Independents & Underground Classics
Critical Survey of Graphic Novels: Manga
Critical Survey of Long Fiction
Critical Survey of Mystery and Detective Fiction
Critical Survey of Mythology & Folklore: Gods & Goddesses
Critical Survey of Mythology & Folklore: Heroes and Heroines
Critical Survey of Mythology & Folklore: Love, Sexuality, and Desire
Critical Survey of Mythology & Folklore: World Mythology
Critical Survey of Poetry
Critical Survey of Poetry: Contemporary Poets
Critical Survey of Science Fiction & Fantasy Literature
Critical Survey of Shakespeare's Plays
Critical Survey of Shakespeare's Sonnets
Critical Survey of Short Fiction
Critical Survey of World Literature
Critical Survey of Young Adult Literature

Cyclopedia of Literary Characters & Places
Cyclopedia of Literary Characters
Cyclopedia of Literary Places

Introduction to Literary Context
American Poetry of the 20th Century
American Post-Modernist Novels
American Short Fiction
English Literature
Plays
World Literature

Magill's Literary Annual
Magill's Literary Annual, 2022
Magill's Literary Annual, 2021
Magill's Literary Annual, 2020
Magill's Literary Annual (Backlist Issues 2019-1977)

Masterplots
Masterplots, Fourth Edition
Masterplots, 2010-2018 Supplement

Notable Writers
Notable African American Writers
Notable American Women Writers
Notable Mystery & Detective Fiction Writers
Notable Writers of the American West & the Native American Experience
Novels into Film: Adaptations & Interpretation
Recommended Reading: 600 Classics Reviewed

Grey House Publishing | Salem Press | H.W. Wilson | 4919 Route, 22 PO Box 56, Amenia NY 12501-0056

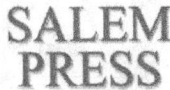
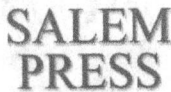
2022 Title List

Visit www.SalemPress.com for Product Information, Table of Contents, and Sample Pages.

HISTORY
The Decades

The 1910s in America
The Twenties in America
The Thirties in America
The Forties in America
The Fifties in America
The Sixties in America
The Seventies in America
The Eighties in America
The Nineties in America
The 2000s in America
The 2010s in America

Defining Documents in American History

Defining Documents: The 1900s
Defining Documents: The 1910s
Defining Documents: The 1920s
Defining Documents: The 1930s
Defining Documents: The 1950s
Defining Documents: The 1960s
Defining Documents: The 1970s
Defining Documents: The 1980s
Defining Documents: American Citizenship
Defining Documents: The American Economy
Defining Documents: The American Revolution
Defining Documents: The American West
Defining Documents: Business Ethics
Defining Documents: Capital Punishment
Defining Documents: Civil Rights
Defining Documents: Civil War
Defining Documents: The Constitution
Defining Documents: The Cold War
Defining Documents: Dissent & Protest
Defining Documents: Domestic Terrorism
Defining Documents: Drug Policy
Defining Documents: The Emergence of Modern America
Defining Documents: Environment & Conservation
Defining Documents: Espionage & Intrigue
Defining Documents: Exploration and Colonial America
Defining Documents: The First Amendment
Defining Documents: The Free Press
Defining Documents: The Great Depression
Defining Documents: The Great Migration
Defining Documents: The Gun Debate
Defining Documents: Immigration & Immigrant Communities
Defining Documents: The Legacy of 9/11
Defining Documents: LGBTQ+
Defining Documents: Manifest Destiny and the New Nation
Defining Documents: Native Americans
Defining Documents: Political Campaigns, Candidates & Discourse
Defining Documents: Postwar 1940s
Defining Documents: Prison Reform
Defining Documents: Secrets, Leaks & Scandals
Defining Documents: Slavery
Defining Documents: Supreme Court Decisions
Defining Documents: Reconstruction Era
Defining Documents: The Vietnam War
Defining Documents: U.S. Involvement in the Middle East
Defining Documents: World War I
Defining Documents: World War II

Defining Documents in World History

Defining Documents: The 17th Century
Defining Documents: The 18th Century
Defining Documents: The 19th Century
Defining Documents: The 20th Century (1900-1950)
Defining Documents: The Ancient World
Defining Documents: Asia
Defining Documents: Genocide & the Holocaust
Defining Documents: Nationalism & Populism
Defining Documents: Pandemics, Plagues & Public Health
Defining Documents: Renaissance & Early Modern Era
Defining Documents: The Middle Ages
Defining Documents: The Middle East
Defining Documents: Women's Rights

Great Events from History

Great Events from History: The Ancient World
Great Events from History: The Middle Ages
Great Events from History: The Renaissance & Early Modern Era
Great Events from History: The 17th Century
Great Events from History: The 18th Century
Great Events from History: The 19th Century
Great Events from History: The 20th Century, 1901-1940
Great Events from History: The 20th Century, 1941-1970
Great Events from History: The 20th Century, 1971-2000
Great Events from History: Modern Scandals
Great Events from History: African American History
Great Events from History: The 21st Century, 2000-2016
Great Events from History: LGBTQ Events
Great Events from History: Human Rights
Great Events from History: Women's History

Great Lives from History

Computer Technology Innovators
Fashion Innovators
Great Athletes
Great Athletes of the Twenty-First Century
Great Lives from History: African Americans
Great Lives from History: American Heroes
Great Lives from History: American Women
Great Lives from History: Asian and Pacific Islander Americans
Great Lives from History: Inventors & Inventions
Great Lives from History: Jewish Americans
Great Lives from History: Latinos
Great Lives from History: Scientists and Science
Great Lives from History: The 17th Century
Great Lives from History: The 18th Century
Great Lives from History: The 19th Century
Great Lives from History: The 20th Century
Great Lives from History: The 21st Century, 2000-2017
Great Lives from History: The Ancient World
Great Lives from History: The Incredibly Wealthy
Great Lives from History: The Middle Ages
Great Lives from History: The Renaissance & Early Modern Era
Human Rights Innovators
Internet Innovators
Music Innovators
Musicians and Composers of the 20th Century
World Political Innovators

Grey House Publishing | Salem Press | H.W. Wilson | 4919 Route, 22 PO Box 56, Amenia NY 12501-0056

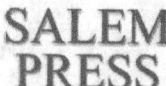
2022 Title List

Visit www.SalemPress.com for Product Information, Table of Contents, and Sample Pages.

History & Government
American First Ladies
American Presidents
The 50 States
The Ancient World: Extraordinary People in Extraordinary Societies
The Bill of Rights
The Criminal Justice System
The U.S. Supreme Court

SOCIAL SCIENCES
Civil Rights Movements: Past & Present
Countries, Peoples and Cultures
Countries: Their Wars & Conflicts: A World Survey
Education Today: Issues, Policies & Practices
Encyclopedia of American Immigration
Ethics: Questions & Morality of Human Actions
Issues in U.S. Immigration
Principles of Sociology: Group Relationships & Behavior
Principles of Sociology: Personal Relationships & Behavior
Principles of Sociology: Societal Issues & Behavior
Racial & Ethnic Relations in America
World Geography

HEALTH
Addictions, Substance Abuse & Alcoholism
Adolescent Health & Wellness
Aging
Cancer
Community & Family Health Issues
Integrative, Alternative & Complementary Medicine
Genetics and Inherited Conditions
Infectious Diseases and Conditions
Magill's Medical Guide
Nutrition
Parenting: Styles & Strategies
Psychology & Behavioral Health
Women's Health

Principles of Health
Principles of Health: Allergies & Immune Disorders
Principles of Health: Anxiety & Stress
Principles of Health: Depression
Principles of Health: Diabetes
Principles of Health: Nursing
Principles of Health: Obesity
Principles of Health: Pain Management
Principles of Health: Prescription Drug Abuse

SCIENCE
Ancient Creatures
Applied Science
Applied Science: Engineering & Mathematics
Applied Science: Science & Medicine
Applied Science: Technology
Biomes and Ecosystems
Earth Science: Earth Materials and Resources
Earth Science: Earth's Surface and History
Earth Science: Earth's Weather, Water and Atmosphere
Earth Science: Physics and Chemistry of the Earth
Encyclopedia of Climate Change
Encyclopedia of Energy
Encyclopedia of Environmental Issues
Encyclopedia of Global Resources
Encyclopedia of Mathematics and Society
Forensic Science
Notable Natural Disasters
The Solar System
USA in Space

Principles of Science
Principles of Anatomy
Principles of Astronomy
Principles of Behavioral Science
Principles of Biology
Principles of Biotechnology
Principles of Botany
Principles of Chemistry
Principles of Climatology
Principles of Computer-aided Design
Principles of Information Technology
Principles of Computer Science
Principles of Ecology
Principles of Energy
Principles of Fire Science
Principles of Geology
Principles of Marine Science
Principles of Mathematics
Principles of Microbiology
Principles of Modern Agriculture
Principles of Pharmacology
Principles of Physical Science
Principles of Physics
Principles of Programming & Coding
Principles of Robotics & Artificial Intelligence
Principles of Scientific Research
Principles of Sports Medicine & Kinesiology
Principles of Sustainability
Principles of Zoology

SALEM PRESS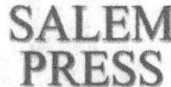

2022 Title List

SALEM PRESS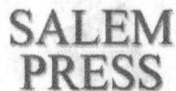

Visit www.SalemPress.com for Product Information, Table of Contents, and Sample Pages.

CAREERS

- Careers: Paths to Entrepreneurship
- Careers in Artificial Intelligence
- Careers in the Arts: Fine, Performing & Visual
- Careers in the Automotive Industry
- Careers in Biology
- Careers in Building Construction
- Careers in Business
- Careers in Chemistry
- Careers in Communications & Media
- Careers in Education & Training
- Careers in Engineering
- Careers in Environment & Conservation
- Careers in Financial Services
- Careers in Forensic Science
- Careers in Gaming
- Careers in Green Energy
- Careers in Healthcare
- Careers in Hospitality & Tourism
- Careers in Human Services
- Careers in Information Technology
- Careers in Law, Criminal Justice & Emergency Services
- Careers in the Music Industry
- Careers in Manufacturing & Production
- Careers in Nursing
- Careers in Physics
- Careers in Protective Services
- Careers in Psychology & Behavioral Health
- Careers in Public Administration
- Careers in Sales, Insurance & Real Estate
- Careers in Science & Engineering
- Careers in Social Media
- Careers in Sports & Fitness
- Careers in Sports Medicine & Training
- Careers in Technical Services & Equipment Repair
- Careers in Transportation
- Careers in Writing & Editing
- Careers Outdoors
- Careers Overseas
- Careers Working with Infants & Children
- Careers Working with Animals

BUSINESS

- Principles of Business: Accounting
- Principles of Business: Economics
- Principles of Business: Entrepreneurship
- Principles of Business: Finance
- Principles of Business: Globalization
- Principles of Business: Leadership
- Principles of Business: Management
- Principles of Business: Marketing

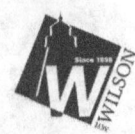

2022 Title List

Visit www.HWWilsonInPrint.com for Product Information, Table of Contents, and Sample Pages.

Core Collections

Children's Core Collection
Fiction Core Collection
Graphic Novels Core Collection
Middle & Junior High School Core
Public Library Core Collection: Nonfiction
Senior High Core Collection
Young Adult Fiction Core Collection

The Reference Shelf

Affordable Housing
Aging in America
Alternative Facts, Post-Truth and the Information War
The American Dream
Artificial Intelligence
The Business of Food
Campaign Trends & Election Law
College Sports
Democracy Evolving
The Digital Age
Embracing New Paradigms in Education
Food Insecurity & Hunger in the United States
Future of U.S. Economic Relations: Mexico, Cuba, & Venezuela
Global Climate Change
Guns in America
Hate Crimes
Immigration
Income Inequality
Internet Abuses & Privacy Rights
Internet Law
LGBTQ in the 21st Century
Marijuana Reform
Mental Health Awareness
National Debate Topic 2014/2015: The Ocean
National Debate Topic 2015/2016: Surveillance
National Debate Topic 2016/2017: US/China Relations
National Debate Topic 2017/2018: Education Reform
National Debate Topic 2018/2019: Immigration
National Debate Topic 2019/2021: Arms Sales
National Debate Topic 2020/2021: Criminal Justice Reform
National Debate Topic 2021/2022: Water Resources
National Debate Topic 2022/2023
New Frontiers in Space
Policing in 2020
Pollution
Prescription Drug Abuse
Propaganda and Misinformation
Racial Tension in a Postracial Age
Reality Television
Representative American Speeches, Annual Editions
Rethinking Work
Revisiting Gender
The South China Sea Conflict
Sports in America
The Supreme Court
The Transformation of American Cities
The Two Koreas
UFOs
Vaccinations
Voters' Rights
Whistleblowers

Current Biography

Current Biography Cumulative Index 1946-2021
Current Biography Monthly Magazine
Current Biography Yearbook

Readers' Guide to Periodical Literature

Abridged Readers' Guide to Periodical Literature
Readers' Guide to Periodical Literature

Indexes

Index to Legal Periodicals & Books
Short Story Index
Book Review Digest

Sears List

Sears List of Subject Headings
Sears: Lista de Encabezamientos de Materia

History

American Game Changers: Invention, Innovation & Transformation
American Reformers
Speeches of the American Presidents

Facts About Series

Facts About the 20th Century
Facts About American Immigration
Facts About China
Facts About the Presidents
Facts About the World's Languages

Nobel Prize Winners

Nobel Prize Winners: 1901-1986
Nobel Prize Winners: 1987-1991
Nobel Prize Winners: 1992-1996
Nobel Prize Winners: 1997-2001
Nobel Prize Winners: 2002-2018

Famous First Facts

Famous First Facts
Famous First Facts About American Politics
Famous First Facts About Sports
Famous First Facts About the Environment
Famous First Facts: International Edition

American Book of Days

The American Book of Days
The International Book of Days